Contemporary Surgical Management of Fractures and Complications

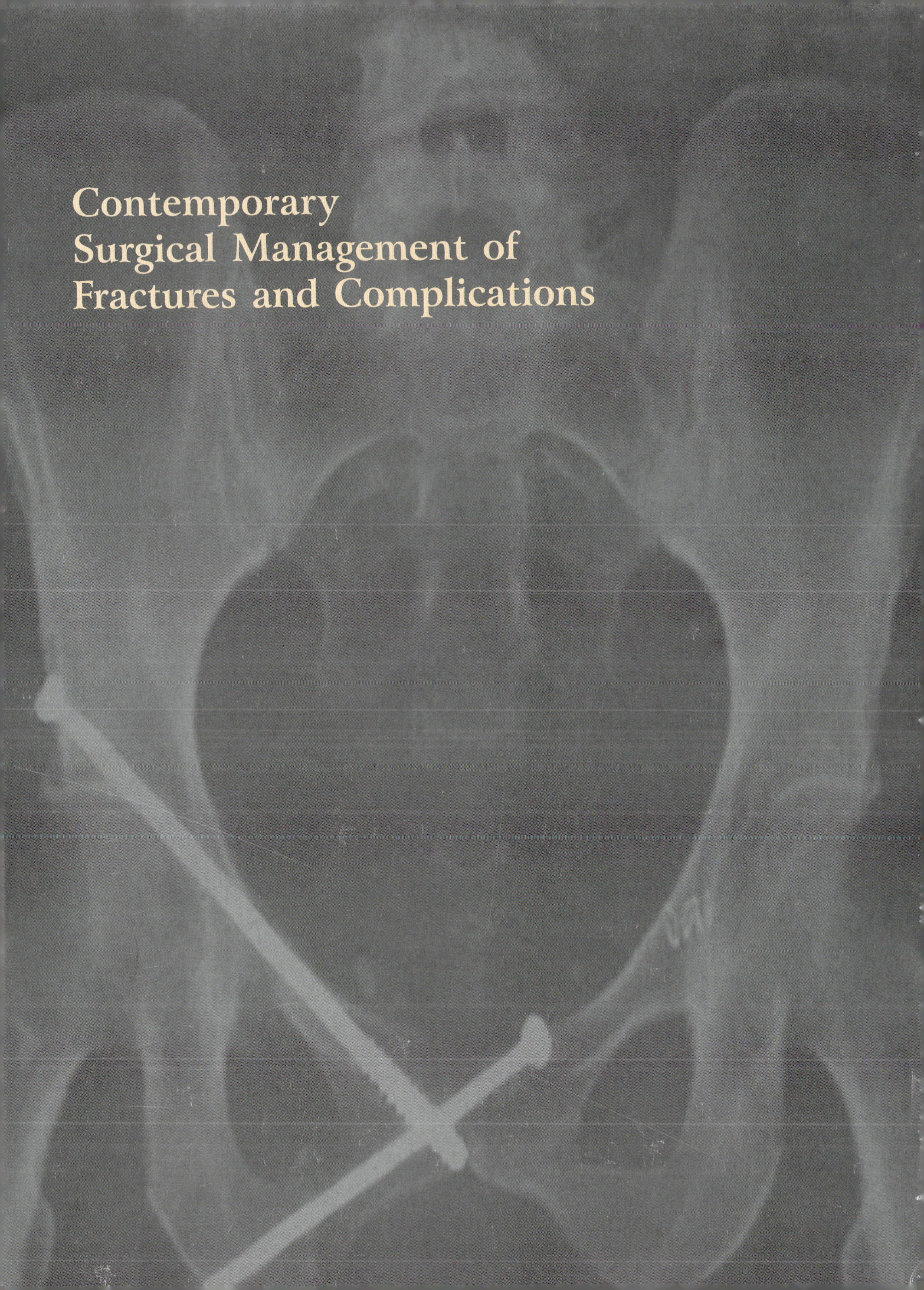

Volume 1: Upper Extremity and Spine

Contemporary Surgical Management of Fractures and Complications

Editors

ASIF ILYAS MD
Program Director of Hand and Upper Extremity Surgery Fellowship
Rothman Institute
Associate Professor of Orthopaedic Surgery
Thomas Jefferson University
Philadelphia, Pennsylvania, USA

SAQIB REHMAN MD
Director of Orthopaedic Trauma
Temple University Hospital
Associate Professor of Orthopaedic Surgery
Temple University
Philadelphia, Pennsylvania, USA

Foreword

JESSE B JUPITER MD

JAYPEE BROTHERS MEDICAL PUBLISHERS (P) LTD

New Delhi • Panama City • London • Philadelphia (USA)

Jaypee Brothers Medical Publishers (P) Ltd

Headquarters

Jaypee Brothers Medical Publishers (P) Ltd
4838/24, Ansari Road, Daryaganj
New Delhi 110 002, India
Phone: +91-11-43574357
Fax: +91-11-43574314
Email: jaypee@jaypeebrothers.com

Overseas Offices

JP Medical Ltd
83 Victoria Street, London
SW1H 0HW (UK)
Phone: +44-2031708910
Fax: +02-03-0086180
Email: info@jpmedpub.com

Jaypee-Highlights Medical Publishers Inc
City of Knowledge, Bld 237, Clayton
Panama City, Panama
Phone: +507-301-0496
Fax: +507-301-0499
Email: cservice@jphmedical.com

Jaypee Brothers Medical Publishers (P) Ltd
17/1-B Babar Road, Block-B, Shaymali
Mohammadpur, Dhaka-1207
Bangladesh
Mobile: +08801912003485
Email: jaypeedhaka@gmail.com

Jaypee Brothers Medical Publishers (P) Ltd
Shorakhute, Kathmandu
Nepal
Phone: +00977-9841528578
Email: jaypee.nepal@gmail.com

Website: www.jaypeebrothers.com
Website: www.jaypeedigital.com

Inquiries for bulk sales may be solicited at: jaypee@jaypeebrothers.com

Contemporary Surgical Management of Fractures and Complications

First Edition : **2013**

ISBN: 978-93-5025-964-1

Printed at: Ajanta Offset & Packagings Ltd., New Delhi

Dedicated to

My wife Erum and my children Dean, Amber and Sammy
for their inspiration to excel and their patience
with my ever-growing commitments.
My parents Qazi and Sajda Ilyas for their
commitment to my education and perfect guidance
through my personal and professional development.
And lastly, to my fellows and residents for continually challenging me
to better myself as a clinician and educator.

Asif Ilyas

The residents and fellows whom I have had the privilege to work with;
My mentors Drs William DeLong and Christopher Born as well as
the many other surgeons whom I have learned so much from;
My brother Asim, my wife Saadia, and
my children, Omar, Laila and Sofia for their support;
Omar, in particular, for reminding me that there is far more to life than work.
Most importantly, to my parents, Khalid and Sabeeha Rehman,
for being true role models and paving the way to help me achieve
my goals and aspirations.

Saqib Rehman

Contributors

Jamal Ahmad MD
Assistant Professor of
Orthopaedic Surgery
Thomas Jefferson University Hospital
Rothman Institute
Philadelphia, Pennsylvania, USA

Andrea Bauer MD
Orthopaedic Surgery Fellow
Massachusetts General Hospital
Boston, Massachusetts, USA

Stephen Becher MD
Orthopaedic Surgery Resident
Atlanta Medical Center
Atlanta, Georgia, USA

Pedro Beredjiklian MD
Chief, Hand Surgery Service
Rothman Institute
Associate Professor of
Orthopaedic Surgery
Thomas Jefferson University
Philadelphia, PA, USA

Christopher Born MD
Chief of Orthopaedic Trauma and
Director of the Weiss
Laboratory for
Orthopaedic Trauma Research
Rhode Island Hospital
Intrepid Heroes Professor of
Orthopaedic Surgery
The Apert Medical School of
Brown University
Providence, Rhode Island, USA

Wendy Bruinsma MD
Orthopaedic Surgery Fellow
Massachusetts General Hospital
Boston, Massachusetts, USA

Neal Chen MD
Assistant Professor of
Orthopaedic Surgery
Thomas Jefferson University
Philadelphia Hand Center
Philadelphia, Pennsylvania, USA

Peter Cole MD
Chief of Orthopaedic Surgery
Regions Hospital
Professor of Orthopaedic Surgery
University of Minnesota
St Paul, Minnesota, USA

Katharine Criner MD
Orthopaedic Surgery Resident
Temple University
Philadelphia, Pennsylvania, USA

William DeLong MD
Chief of Orthopaedic Surgery
St Luke's Health Network
Professor of Orthopaedic Surgery
Anatomy and Cell Biology
Temple University
Philadelphia, Pennsylvania, USA

River Elliott MD
Plastic Surgery Resident
University of the Pennsylvania
Philadelphia, Pennsylvania, USA

Christina Endress MD
Orthopaedic Surgery Resident
University of the Pennsylvania
Philadelphia, Pennsylvania, USA

Ryan Ficco MD
Orthopaedic Surgery Resident
University of Miami
Miami, Florida, USA

Abtin Foroohar MD
Orthopaedic Surgery Fellow
University of the Pennsylvania
Philadelphia, Pennsylvania, USA

John Fowler MD
Orthopaedic Surgery Resident
Temple University
Philadelphia, Pennsylvania, USA

Matthew Frank MD
Orthopaedic Surgery Resident
New Jersey Medical School
Newark, New Jersey, USA

Elie Ghanem MD
Orthopaedic Surgery Resident
Thomas Jefferson University
Philadelphia, Pennsylvania, USA

Melissa Gorman MD
Assistant Professor of
Orthopaedic Surgery
Louisiana State University
Health Science Center
New Orleans, Louisiana, USA

Steven Gross MD
Orthopaedic Surgery Resident
NYU-Hospital for Joint Diseases
New York, New York, USA

Christopher Haydel MD
Orthopaedic Trauma Fellow
Temple University Hospital
Philadelphia, Pennsylvania, USA

David Helfet MD
Director of Orthopaedic Trauma
Hospital for Special Surgery
Professor of Orthopaedic Surgery
Weill Medical College of Cornell
University
New York, New York, USA

Zhiyong Hou MD
Orthopaedic Research Fellow
Geisinger Medical Center
Danville, Pennsylvania, USA

Asif Ilyas MD
Program Director of Hand and Upper Extremity Surgery Fellowship
Rothman Institute
Associate Professor of Orthopaedic Surgery
Thomas Jefferson University
Philadelphia, Pennsylvania, USA

Kaan Irgit MD
Orthopaedic Research Fellow
Geisinger Medical Center
Danville, Pennsylvania, USA

Roman Isaac MD
Orthopaedic Surgery Resident
Thomas Jefferson University
Philadelphia, Pennsylvania, USA

Andrew Jawa MD
Assistant Professor of Orthopaedic Surgery
Boston University
Boston, Massachusetts, USA

Jesse Jupiter MD
Hansjorg Wyss/AO Professor of Orthopaedic Surgery
Harvard Medical School
Massachusetts General Hospital
Boston, Massachusetts, USA

Rishi Kanna MS
Consultant Spine Surgeon
Ganga Hospital
Coimbatore, Tamil Nadu, India

Stephen Kayiaros MD
Orthopaedic Trauma Fellow
Rhode Island Hospital
Providence, Rhode Island, USA

Emily Keener DO
Orthopaedic Surgery Resident
University of Medicine and Dentistry of New Jersey
Stratford, New Jersey, USA

Sanjit Konda MD
Orthopaedic Surgery Resident
NYU-Hospital for Joint Diseases
New York, USA

Stephen Kottmeier MD
Chief of Orthopaedic Trauma and Associate Chairman
Associate Professor of Orthopaedic Surgery
Stony Brook University Hospital
Stony Brook, New York, USA

Peter Krause MD
Director of Orthopaedic Trauma
Louisiana State University Public Hospital
Associate Professor of Orthopaedic Surgery and Residency Director
Louisiana State University Health Science Center
New Orleans, Louisiana, USA

Paul Lafferty MD
Assistant Professor of Orthopaedic Surgery
University of Minnesota
St Paul, Minnesota, USA

Charles Leinberry MD
Associate Professor of Orthopaedic Surgery
Thomas Jefferson University
Philadelphia, Pennsylvania, USA

Frank Liporace MD
Associate Professor of Orthopaedic Surgery
New Jersey Medical School
Newark, New Jersey, USA

Dean Lorich MD
Associate Director of Orthopaedic Trauma
Hospital for Special Surgery
Assistant Professor of Orthopaedic Surgery
Weill Medical College of Cornell University, New York, USA

Neil MacIntyre MD
Director of Orthopaedic Trauma
New Hannover Regional Medical Center
Wilmington, North Carolina, USA

Megan Manthe MD
Orthopaedic Surgery Resident
University of Florida, Shands
Jacksonville, Florida, USA

Jonas Matzon MD
Assistant Professor of Orthopaedic Surgery
Thomas Jefferson University
Philadelphia, Pennsylvania, USA

Matthew Mellon MD
Director of Orthopaedic Trauma
Total Orthopaedics and Sports Medicine
Massapequa, New York, USA

Matthew Mendez-Zfass MD
Orthopaedic Surgery Resident
University of Miami
Miami, Florida, USA

Chaitanya Mudgal MD
Interim Chief and Program Director of Orthopaedic Hand Service
Massachusetts General Hospital
Assistant Professor of Orthopaedic Surgery
Harvard Medical School
Boston, Massachusetts, USA

Valentin Neuhaus MD
Orthopaedic Surgery Research Fellow
Massachusetts General Hospital
Boston, Massachusetts, USA

Meredith Osterman MD
Orthopaedic Surgery Resident
Thomas Jefferson University
Philadelphia, Pennsylvania, USA

Frank Peters MD
Orthopaedic Surgery Fellow
Massachusetts General Hospital
Boston, Massachusetts, USA

Samuel Popinchalk MD
Orthopaedic Surgery Resident
Temple University
Philadelphia, Pennsylvania, USA

S Rajasekaran PhD
Chairman of Orthopaedic and
Spine Surgery, Ganga Hospital
Adjunct Professor of
Orthopaedic Surgery
Tamil Nadu Medical University
Coimbatore, Tamil Nadu, India

Saqib Rehman MD
Director of Orthopaedic Trauma
Temple University Hospital
Associate Professor of
Orthopaedic Surgery
Temple University
Philadelphia, Pennsylvania, USA

J Spence Reid MD
Chief, Division of Orthopaedic Trauma
Milton S Hershey Medical Center
Professor of Orthopaedic Surgery
Penn State University College of
Medicine
Hershey, Pennsylvania, USA

Michael Rivlin MD
Orthopaedic Surgery Resident
Thomas Jefferson University
Philadelphia, Pennsylvania, USA

ML Chip Routt Jr MD
Professor of Orthopaedic Surgery
University of Washington
Harborview Medical Center
Seattle, Washington, USA

Ajoy Prasad Shetty MS
Consultant Spine Surgeon
Ganga Hospital
Coimbatore, Tamil Nadu, India

Wade Smith MD
Professor of Orthopaedic Surgery
University of Colorado
Mountain Orthopaedic Trauma
Surgeons
Englewood, Colorado, USA

Dean Sotereanos MD
Professor of Orthopaedic Surgery
Drexel University College of Medicine
Allegheny General Hospital
Pittsburgh, Pennsylvania, USA

Brandon Steen MD
Orthopaedic Surgery Resident
Boston University
Boston, Massachusetts, USA

David Steinberg MD
Program Director of Hand
Upper Extremity and Microsurgery
Associate Professor of
Orthopaedic Surgery
University of the Pennsylvania
Philadelphia, Pennsylvania, USA

Michael Suk MD JD MPH FACS
Chairman, Department of
Orthopaedic Surgery
Geisinger Health System
Danville, Pennsylvania, USA

Nirmal Tejwani MD
Associate Director and Chief of
Orthopaedic Service
Bellevue Hospital
Professor of Orthopaedic Surgery
New York University Langone
Medical Center, New York, USA

Joseph Thoder MD
Chairman, Department of
Orthopaedic Surgery
Professor of Orthopaedic Surgery
Temple University
Philadelphia, Pennsylvania, USA

Richard Tosti MD
Orthopaedic Surgery Resident
Temple University
Philadelphia, Pennsylvania, USA

Uzoma Ukomadu MD
Orthopaedic Surgery Resident
Thomas Jefferson University
Philadelphia, Pennsylvania, USA

Aaron Venouziou MD
Orthopaedic Surgery Fellow
Allegheny General Hospital
Pittsburgh, Pennsylvania, USA

Fernando Vilella-Hernandez MD
Assistant Professor of
Orthopaedic Surgery
University of Miami
Jackson Memorial Hospital
Miami, Florida, USA

Barton Wax MD
Orthopaedic Surgery Resident
Louisiana State University Health
Science Center
New Orleans, Louisiana, USA

David Wellman MD
Instructor of Orthopaedic Surgery
Weill Medical College of Cornell
University, Hospital for Special
Surgery, New York, USA

Bruce Ziran MD
Director of Orthopaedic Trauma
Atlanta Medical Center
Atlanta, Georgia, USA

Foreword

It is a pleasure and honor to be asked by Dr Ilyas and Dr Rehman to write a foreword to their new fracture textbook. This is not just because I have had the true joy of seeing the growth in the academic career of Dr Ilyas since completing our Hand and Upper Limb Fellowship but also because that this is a text whose purpose is clearly defined and well achieved.

This is a twenty-first century text focusing less on historical highlights, background principles, and alternative treatments to internal fixation that formed the basis of what was considered standard formats for fracture texts in the past. Rather, the editors have decided to create a text that the practicing surgeon can have at his/her fingertips when faced with a clinical fracture problem. Accordingly, the reader will find a consistent format in each chapter emphasizing the surgical approaches, techniques of specific fracture fixation, as well as practical tips and "pitfalls". Complications and their management are to be found in each chapter. The chapters are well illustrated sprinkled throughout with excellent clinical examples.

What I found to be strength of this text is the list of contributing authors. While located throughout are the "usual suspects", the vast majority of contributors represent the "rising stars" of the next generation of thought leaders and fracture surgeons.

We are in the era of instant information, which will now be found in a variety of modalities from multiple websites, web-based how-to videos, industry educational sites or easy access journals. So too will the surgeon treating fractures find ready access to specific questions and techniques in *Contemporary Surgical Management of Fractures and Complications*.

Jesse B Jupiter MD
Hansjorg Wyss/AO Professor of Orthopaedic Surgery
Harvard Medical School
Massachusetts General Hospital
Boston, Massachusetts, USA

Preface

"The surgeon who has not had a complication has not done enough surgery."

We have all heard this quote at some point in our training or practice. Complications in fracture management are unfortunately a common occurrence. There are many reasons for the association of fractures with complications.

Patients can present at unpredictable times of the day, requiring urgent surgery by a surgeon who may be inexperienced in the necessary fracture management. Fracture surgery frequently utilizes bacteria-harboring implants which are placed in damaged soft tissue beds potentially inviting infections. Also, modern fracture management has witnessed a significant growth of new implants and biologics which are often quickly applied before their indications are well defined. Furthermore, there still exist significant deficits in our understanding of fracture healing. Why some fractures heal while others do not continue to elude us. And sometimes, the problem lies with the patient and subsequent lack of compliance with the prescribed postoperative regimen.

There are many outstanding textbooks which go to great lengths to describe proper techniques of fracture management. Nevertheless, complications will happen and correcting them can represent a significant challenge. Despite all the excellent references available to orthopaedic surgeons, it became apparent to us that there are few modern texts that actually focus on the management of complications at length. When we came together to discuss our aspirations and goals of this book, this deficit in our literature quickly came to the forefront.

What we have therefore set out to do was to present a concise, practical text for the orthopaedic surgeon who manages fractures on a regular or occasional basis. The goals of this book are to clearly describe the indications for surgery, provide appropriate surgical techniques, present tips for achieving good results, and offer an extensive case-based discussion on how to manage select complications. Whereas many other texts have given a more exhaustive review of the historical literature as well as basic principles of fracture management (including nonoperative management), we have chosen to go directly to the surgical management of fractures and their complications. Of course, this is not to downplay the importance of the basic principles of nonoperative fracture care or to imply all fractures be treated operatively. As such, this text should not be viewed as a comprehensive textbook of fracture management, but rather a practical and thorough text for the orthopaedic surgeon managing a fracture operatively and/or its complication.

This textbook contains several highlights. We have included focused "pearls and pitfalls" sections to allow the author to share important practical points on various surgical techniques with the reader. To this end, we have also tried to make generous use of figures and images to help illustrate the key concepts in each chapter. The section on "Author's preferred management of select complications" is what we feel is the most unique and important part of this textbook. Here we have included actual cases with complications such as nonunions, malunions and infections managed by the chapter contributors.

We sincerely hope that this textbook will be a useful addition to your library and that you will use it for years to come. Incurring a fracture is a significant event for a patient. Experiencing a subsequent complication from fracture management can further compromise a patient's outcome. As orthopaedic surgeons, it is our job not only to avoid these complications, but also to know how to effectively navigate through them when they occur. If this book helps you in this effort, then we have succeeded in our mission.

SAQIB REHMAN
ASIF ILYAS

Acknowledgments

First and foremost, this book would clearly not be possible without the generous contributions by an outstanding group of surgeons who authored the chapters. To these authors, we are sincerely grateful and appreciative of their efforts and for sharing their expertise with our readers. We have clearly learned much from them in the process of editing this text.

What would we be without our mentors who helped us start and mold our careers, showing us how to properly manage fractures, and most importantly, reminding us to "do the right thing" for our patients?

Although we consider ourselves educators, we have been fortunate to be surrounded by exemplary colleagues, residents and fellows who educate us on a daily basis through our exchanges, collaborations and daily clinical care. For this, and for their support with this project, we thank them.

We would also like to thank the wonderful people at Jaypee Brothers Medical Publishers (P) Ltd, New Delhi, India for their support throughout this process and particularly for letting us see our vision come to fruition.

Finally, it goes without saying that a project like this could not happen without the support of our wives and families. We sincerely thank them for their patience, understanding and encouragement throughout this process.

Contents

Volume 1: Upper Extremity and Spine

Asif Ilyas

1. **Phalangeal Fractures** 1
   Jonas Matzon, Elie Ghanem, Pedro Beredjiklian
2. **Metacarpal Fractures and Carpometacarpal Fracture-Dislocations** 30
   Charles Leinberry, Uzoma Ukomadu, Asif Ilyas
3. **Carpal Fractures and Perilunate Dislocations** 53
   Valentin Neuhaus, Andrea Bauer, Chaitanya Mudgal
4. **Scaphoid Fractures** 94
   Aaron Venouziou, Dean Sotereanos
5. **Distal Radius Fractures** 128
   Wendy Bruinsma, Frank Peters, Jesse Jupiter
6. **Forearm Fractures** 167
   Abtin Foroohar, River Elliott, Christina Endress, David Steinberg
7. **Olecranon Fractures** 192
   Brandon Steen, Andrew Jawa
8. **Radial Head Fractures and Terrible Triad Injuries** 223
   John Fowler, Joseph Thoder
9. **Distal Humerus Fractures** 249
   Asif Ilyas, Saqib Rehman
10. **Humeral Shaft Fractures** 276
    Richard Tosti, Asif Ilyas
11. **Proximal Humerus Fractures** 302
    David Wellman, Dean Lorich, David Helfet
12. **Glenoid and Scapula Fractures** 334
    Samuel Popinchalk, Neil MacIntyre
13. **Clavicle Fractures** 358
    Roman Isaac, Meredith Osterman, Michael Rivlin, Neal Chen
14. **Cervical Spine Fractures and Dislocations** 378
    S Rajasekaran, Rishi Kanna, Ajoy Prasad Shetty
15. **Thoracic and Lumbar Spine Fractures and Dislocations** 447
    S Rajasekaran, Rishi Kanna, Ajoy Prasad Shetty

Volume 2: Pelvis and Lower Extremity

Saqib Rehman

16. **Pelvic Ring and Sacral Injuries** 495
Stephen Kottmeier, ML Chip Routt Jr

17. **Acetabulum Fractures** 552
Bruce Ziran, Stephen Becher

18. **Femoral Head Fractures and Hip Dislocations** 581
Kaan Irgit, Zhiyong Hou, Wade Smith

19. **Femoral Neck Fractures** 611
Christopher Haydel, Saqib Rehman

20. **Intertrochanteric Femur Fractures** 654
Stephen Kayiaros, Christopher Born

21. **Subtrochanteric Femur Fractures** 672
Paul Lafferty, Emily Keener, Peter Cole

22. **Femoral Shaft Fractures** 708
Matthew Mendez-Zfass, Ryan Ficco, Fernando Vilella-Hernandez

23. **Distal Femur Fractures** 737
Matthew Mellon, William DeLong, Saqib Rehman

24. **Patellar Fractures** 766
Peter Krause, Melissa Gorman, Barton Wax

25. **Proximal Tibia Fractures** 785
J Spence Reid

26. **Tibial Shaft Fractures** 845
Saqib Rehman, Katharine Criner

27. **Distal Tibia Fractures** 894
Michael Suk, Megan Manthe, Saqib Rehman

28. **Ankle Fractures and Syndesmotic Injuries** 926
Nirmal Tejwani, Sanjit Konda, Steven Gross

29. **Hindfoot Fractures** 953
Frank Liporace, Matthew Frank

30. **Midfoot and Forefoot Fractures** 983
Jamal Ahmad

Index *I-i-xx*

Chapter 1

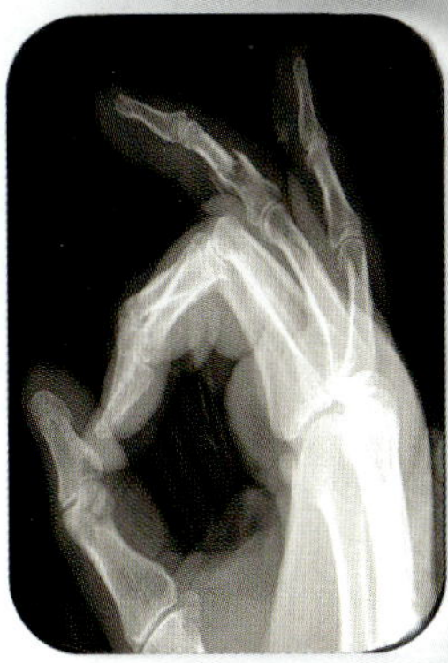

Phalangeal Fractures

Jonas Matzon, Elie Ghanem, Pedro Beredjiklian

Chapter Outline

Introduction
Diagnosis
Classification
Surgical Indications
- Closed Reduction Percutaneous Pinning
- Open Reduction and Internal Fixation
- External Fixation

Surgical Anatomy, Positioning and Approaches
- Applied Anatomy
- Positioning
- Approaches

Surgical Techniques
- Technique 1: Proximal Phalangeal Base Fracture
- Technique 2: Phalangeal Diaphyseal Fractures
- Technique 3: Condylar Fracture
- Technique 4: Middle Phalanx Base Fractures/PIP/Fracture-Dislocations
- Technique 5: Distal Phalanx Fractures

Outcomes
Complications
- Malunion
- Stiffness

Authors' Preferred Management of Select Complications
- Case 1: Malunion
- Case 2: Stiffness

Summary

Introduction

Fractures of the phalanges account for approximately 20% of all hand fractures in the United States and are nearly twice as common as metacarpal fractures peaking in the third decade for men and second decade for women.[1] The two most common mechanisms of injury are accidental fall and direct blow to the extremity.[1] Most phalangeal fractures occur in the proximal phalanx, followed by the distal phalanx and then the middle phalanx.[2] Although phalangeal fractures are common injuries, they can be frequently missed or underestimated, potentially leading to significant impairment of function.[3]

Treatment of phalangeal fractures is based on the presentation of the fracture, degree of displacement and difficulty in maintaining fracture reduction. However, the management of phalangeal fractures is heavily influenced by its intimate relationship with surrounding tendons, vulnerability to malalignment and the propensity toward swelling and stiffness. Subsequently, the cornerstone of treatment is restoration of normal alignment, minimizing swelling and rapid mobilization.

A wide array of treatment options exists for phalangeal fractures. Despite the abundance of treatment options for hand fractures, the literature remains unclear regarding which treatments are superior because there are currently very limited well-performed comparative prospective studies providing high levels of evidence.[4] Randomized controlled trials are difficult to perform because of the variation in fracture patterns and the many associated variables that are thought to affect treatment and outcome. Nonetheless, knowledge of the complex digital anatomy, fracture patterns, rehabilitation protocols and postoperative complications helps the surgeon to tailor treatment accordingly.

Diagnosis

A thorough physical examination of the entire hand and all the fingers should be performed for suspected phalangeal fractures. This starts with observation of the hand, focusing on the soft tissues and the resting posture of the fingers. Inspection should note signs of swelling, ecchymosis, wounds and finger alignment. A normal resting cascade should exist with all fingers pointing toward the scaphoid tubercle. Loss of digital length and normal knuckle contour may indicate fracture shortening or angulation. Next, all bones in the hand should be palpated to check for areas of tenderness and crepitation. The rotational alignment of the digits should be assessed and compared to the contralateral side during active finger flexion and extension. In flexion, all fingers should point toward the scaphoid tubercle and no scissoring or overlap should exist (Figs 1.1A to E).[5] Malalignment and malrotation of the finger is most evident with finger flexion. If active flexion is not possible, passive manipulation or wrist tenodesis can be performed to assess finger alignment. In extension, subtle rotational deformity can be detected by comparing orientation of the nail plates. Active flexion and extension of all interphalangeal (IP) and metacarpophalangeal (MP) joints should be verified to ensure intact flexor digitorum superficialis (FDS), flexor digitorum profundus (FDP), central slip and terminal tendon function. Finally, joint stability should be confirmed by assessing for collateral ligament sufficiency.

Most phalangeal fractures can be readily diagnosed with standard radiographs including posteroanterior (PA), lateral (LAT) and oblique (OBL) views (Figs 1.2A and B).[12] Focusing the radiographs on the effected phalanges rather than the hand in general can improve the diagnostic quality of the radiographs. The extent of angulation and displacement can often be the best assessed on true PA and lateral radiographs. Oblique radiographs frequently create an illusion of more angulation than truly exists.[13] Special traction views can be helpful in visualization of intra-articular fractures.

Although radiographs are typically adequate for the diagnosis of the majority of phalangeal fractures, fine-cut CT scans with high spatial and contrast resolution may be useful imaging technique for certain complex intra-articular fractures.[11,13] In certain centers, ultrasound has also been used to evaluate bony injuries in many areas of the body.[15,16] Tayal et al. performed a prospective observational study of adult patients with injuries of the hand using high-resolution ultrasound imaging and showed excellent sensitivity (90%) and specificity (98%) in the diagnosis of hand fractures compared to radiography and clinical examination.[16]

PHALANGEAL FRACTURES DIAGNOSIS: Pearls and Pitfalls

- Subtle fractures can cause a rotational deformity. Check for rotational alignment with active and passive finger flexion and extension and compare it to the contralateral extremity
- Standard PA and lateral views will readily identify a fracture and associated displacement and angulation. Oblique views can often exaggerate fracture angulation
- Traction radiographs are helpful in evaluating intra-articular fractures

Classification

Phalangeal fractures can be classified using the AO system. The AO classification can be cumbersome and difficult to apply clinically but is very useful in research. Phalangeal fractures are more commonly classified with descriptive characteristics. Relevant terms include the fracture location (head, neck, shaft or base), the fracture pattern (transverse, oblique, spiral or comminuted), the fracture deformity (translation, angulation or rotation) and the extent of soft-tissue and/or bone contamination (open or closed).

Transverse fractures are typically the result of a direct blow to the dorsum of the digit and, depending on the magnitude of the impact, variable degrees of comminution.[18] A combination of bending and axial compression will produce a comminuted fracture with an associated

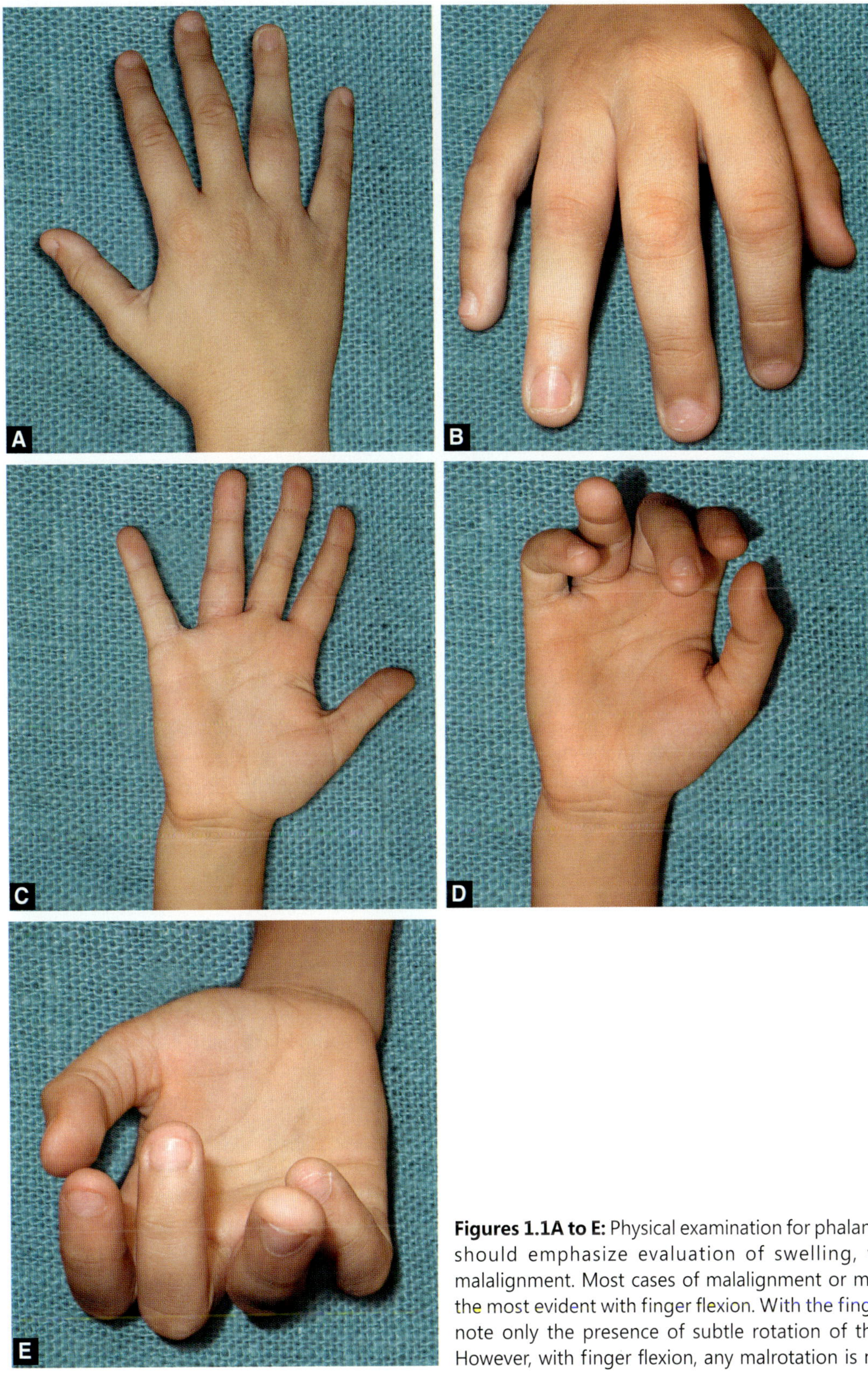

Figures 1.1A to E: Physical examination for phalangeal fractures should emphasize evaluation of swelling, wounds and malalignment. Most cases of malalignment or malrotation are the most evident with finger flexion. With the fingers extended, note only the presence of subtle rotation of the nail plates. However, with finger flexion, any malrotation is maximized.

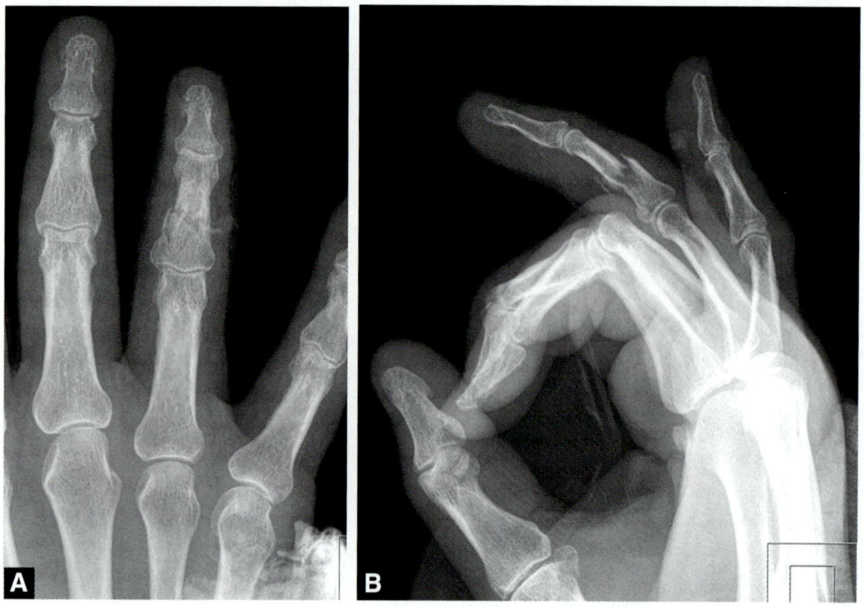

Figures 1.2A and B: The diagnosis of a phalangeal fracture can readily be made with posteroanterior and lateral views. To improve the diagnostic quality of the radiographs, the image intensifier should focus on the finger in question and not the hand in general.

butterfly fragment. A twisting injury will cause a spiral fracture with the fracture line oriented 45° to the shaft of the bone.[5] A combination of torque and axial load will produce a short oblique fracture with variable comminution.

Proximal phalangeal fractures usually angulate with an apex volar deformity.[5] The proximal fragment is flexed by the interossei insertions onto the proximal phalangeal base, and the distal fragment is pulled into hyperextension by the central slip.[20] Middle phalangeal fractures are less predictable with regard to angulation given that the extensor and flexor tendons and their accompanying forces cross the middle phalanx. Fractures proximal to the FDS insertion usually have an apex dorsal angulation secondary to the pull of the central slip, while fractures distal to the FDS insertion usually have an apex volar angulation secondary to the pull of the FDS. Distal phalangeal fractures are usually comminuted tuft or diaphyseal fractures secondary to a crush injury.[9] Because both the extensor and flexor tendons insert on the distal phalangeal base, these fractures do not usually demonstrate severe displacement.

Surgical Indications

The primary factors that determine management of phalangeal fractures are displacement, reducibility and stability. In general, nondisplaced fractures are treated with splinting and early motion. Fractures that are reducible and stable can similarly be treated with splinting and early motion. In contrast, extra-articular fractures that are reducible but unstable or displaced intra-articular fractures are best treated with operative reduction and fixation. Whenever possible, closed reduction and pinning should be utilized. However, fractures that are irreducible using closed techniques may require open reduction and internal fixation. Furthermore, fractures with open wounds, significant bone loss, tendon laceration and/or neurovascular injury are also indicated for surgical management.

Closed Reduction Percutaneous Pinning

Closed reduction percutaneous pinning (CRPP) is the preferred technique for the majority of unstable and/or reducible extra-articular phalangeal fractures (Fig. 1.3A). While Kirchner (K) wires do not compress the fracture, they can effectively hold a fracture until union. Since phalangeal fractures are intimately associated with tendons that are prone to adhesions, the advantage of percutaneous K-wire fixation is the avoidance of open soft tissue dissection and subsequent tendon adhesions. The disadvantages of this technique include its often unrecognized technical difficulty, its inability to achieve interfragmentary compression, the potential to tether soft tissues and the inability to institute early motion.[23]

Open Reduction and Internal Fixation

Open reduction and internal fixation (ORIF) is best indicated for intra-articular fractures, irreducible extra-articular fractures, or when rigid fixation is necessary. The advantage of ORIF is the ability to achieve anatomic reduction and institute early motion. However, the disadvantage of ORIF is the predilection toward tendon adhesions and joint fibrosis from soft tissue dissection, secondary swelling and hardware irritation.[17] Open reduction and internal fixation can be performed with interfragmentary screw fixation or plate fixation (Figs 1.3B and C).

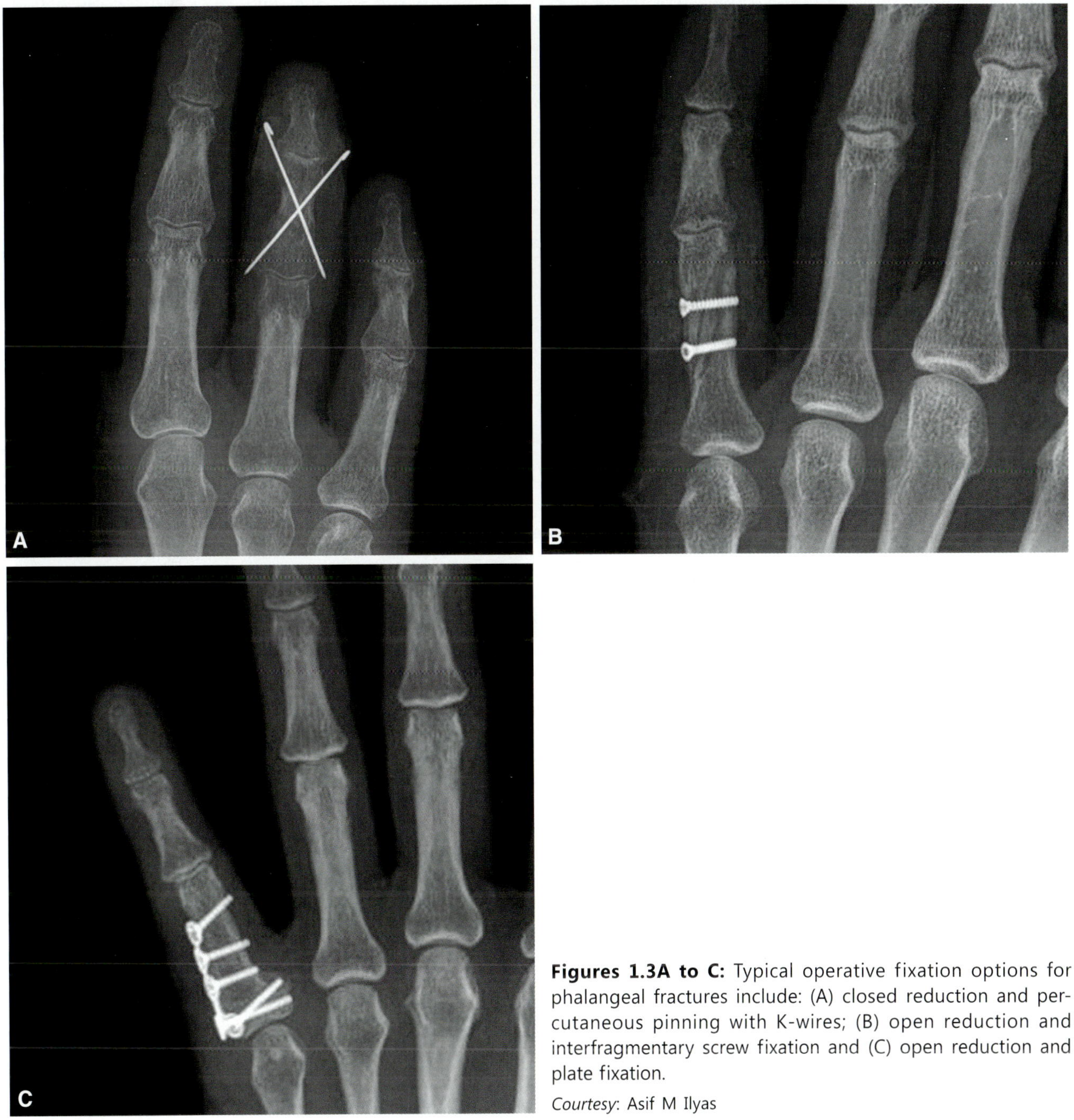

Figures 1.3A to C: Typical operative fixation options for phalangeal fractures include: (A) closed reduction and percutaneous pinning with K-wires; (B) open reduction and interfragmentary screw fixation and (C) open reduction and plate fixation.

Courtesy: Asif M Ilyas

External Fixation

External fixators can be used to treat a variety of hand fractures. While its advantages include minimal or no exposure of the fracture site and adequate stability, they have no compelling advantage over K-wires in the treatment of simple closed fractures of the phalanx.[19] Conversely, external fixators may be useful in bridging comminuted intra-articular fractures, or for temporary fixation of severe open fractures with bone loss and/or soft tissue loss.

PHALANGEAL FRACTURES SURGICAL INDICATIONS: Pearls and Pitfalls

- Most finger fractures can be treated nonoperatively. However, displaced and unstable fractures require operative fixation. We recommend utilizing closed reduction and percutaneous pinning whenever possible
- Pinning can provide near anatomic reduction while minimizing soft tissue manipulation, swelling and avoiding late hardware irritation
- Open reduction and internal fixation can provide stable anatomic reduction and early motion at the expense of possible tendon adhesions and joint stiffness
- External fixation is the best indicated in the management of complex hand injuries with extensive soft tissue injury, bone loss and/or contamination

Surgical Anatomy, Positioning and Approaches

Applied Anatomy

The phalanges have an intimate association with the surrounding extensor and flexor tendons. Although the extensor tendons to each of the fingers are well-defined units over the metacarpals, once they approach the phalanges they become much more complex (Fig. 1.4). At the MP joint the extensor tendon results in a sagittal band that acts as a sling around the MP joint attaching to the volar plate. The sagittal bands also centralize the extensor digitorum communis tendon and aid in MP extension. Distal to the MP joint, the intrinsics (lumbricals and interosseous muscles) join to create the lateral bands that insert into the dorsal extensor mechanism and concomitantly cover the entire lateral border of the proximal phalanx shaft. Dorsally, the transverse fibers of the interossei create the transverse retinacular ligament which acts as a sling over the proximal phalanx to aid in MP flexion. At the proximal interphalangeal (PIP) joint the common extensor tendon trifurcates into two lateral bands and a central slip. The central slip inserts at the base of the middle phalanx to extend the PIP joint. The lateral bands coalesce with the lateral slips from the intrinsics (interossei and lumbricals) to form the conjoined lateral bands. The two conjoined lateral bands coalesce into the terminal tendon, which

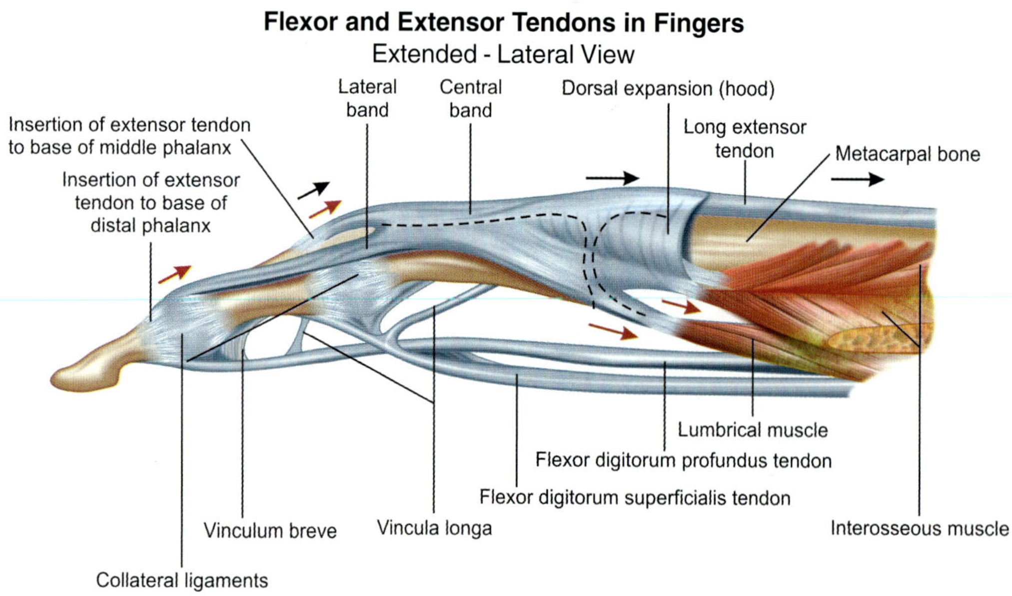

Figure 1.4: The phalanges are intimately associated with the extensor tendons (which reside dorsally and laterally) and the flexor tendons (which reside volarly). The extensor mechanism inserts at each joint to facilitate finger extension: the sagittal band forms a sling around the metacarpophalangeal joint, the central slip inserts at the base of the middle phalanx at the proximal interphalangeal joint, and the terminal slip inserts at the base of the distal phalanx at the distal interphalangeal joint.
Note: Black arrows indicate pull of long extensor tendon; red arrows indicate pull of interosseous and lumbrical muscles.

inserts at the base of the distal phalanx to extend the distal interphalangeal (DIP) joint. The triangular ligament prevents the conjoined lateral bands from volar subluxation while the transverse retinacular ligament prevents dorsal subluxation.

In comparison to the extensor system, the flexor system is more straightforward. Both the FDS and FDP travel together in the fibro-osseous sheath providing flexion of the PIP joint and the DIP joint, respectively. At the level of the proximal phalanx, FDS splits into two at Camper's chiasm inserting into either side of base of the middle phalanx while the FDP inserts into the base of the distal phalanx. The fibro-osseous sheath that the flexor tendons traverse through is composed of fibrous pulleys that provide structural stability and maintain the tendons close to the phalanges. There are five annular pulleys and three cruciate pulleys.

The neurovascular bundle lies on both the radial and ulnar sides of the flexor tendon sheath. In the fingers, the digital nerve lies volar and medial to the digital artery. Dorsal branches of the nerves give sensation to the dorsal aspect of the fingers distal to the PIP joint. At the DIP joint, the digital nerve trifurcates.

The IP joints are complex, uniaxial hinge joints. Stability is provided by both the articular conformity and the supporting soft tissue structures.[6] These soft tissue structures include the capsule, the collateral ligaments, the extensor tendon dorsally, the flexor tendon sheath and the volar plate.

Positioning

Positioning is universal for most hand surgical cases. The patient is placed supine on a well-padded operating room table with the affected upper extremity on a hand table. A nonsterile pneumatic tourniquet is placed on the proximal arm of the affected extremity.

Approaches

Surgical exposure of the phalanges involves careful navigation of the surrounding tendons and neurovascular structures. Choice of surgical approach depends on location, fracture pattern and choice of fixation. Regardless of surgical approach, manipulation of the tendon should be minimized to avoid secondary adhesions, tendon insertions should be protected to avoid disparities in motion, and swelling minimized to avoid joint fibrosis. Furthermore, incisions should be placed carefully to avoid soft tissue contractures and wound complications (Figs 1.5A and B).

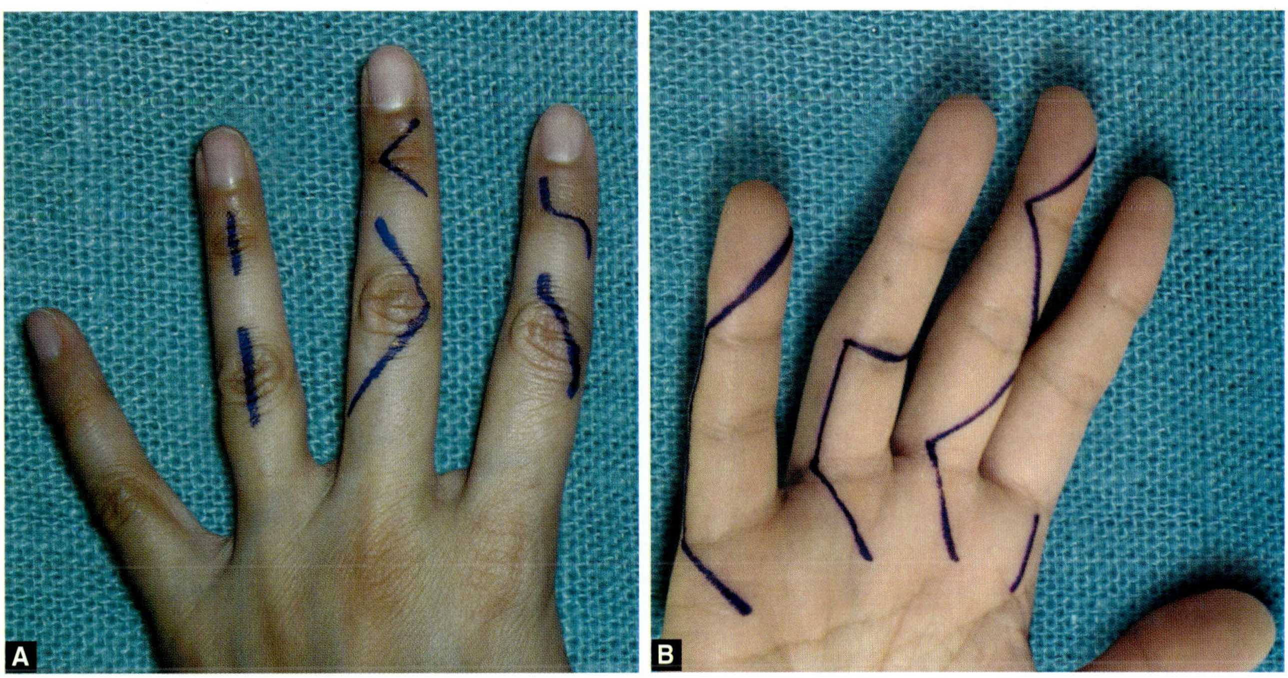

Figures 1.5A and B: Incisions should be placed carefully to avoid soft tissue contractures and wound complications. (A) Dorsally, incisions can be placed either longitudinally or obliquely across the extension crease. (B) Volarly, incisions should be placed away from the flexion creases utilizing a midaxial or Bruner techniques.

Courtesy: Asif M Ilyas

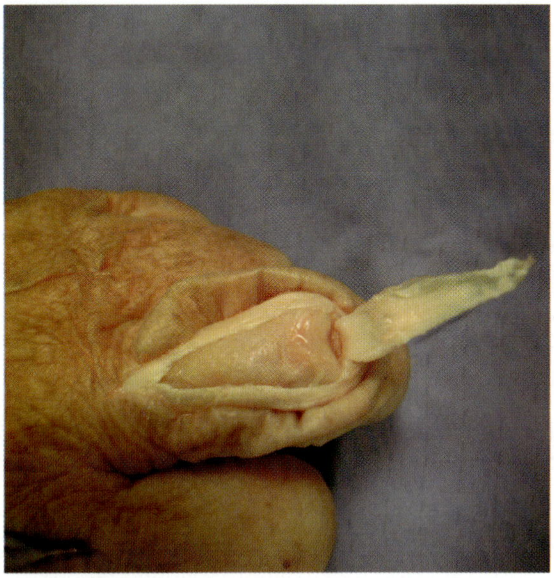

Figure 1.6: Dorsal exposure of the proximal phalanx may be performed with a longitudinal incision or through a distally based central slip (Chamay) flap.

Courtesy: Asif M Ilyas

Dorsal Approach

The dorsal approach provides excellent exposure to the shaft and base of the proximal phalanx. An incision is placed over the dorsal aspect of the finger and then a large skin flap is developed and retracted thereby exposing the dorsal extensor mechanism. At the proximal phalangeal level, the extensor mechanism can be either split longitudinally or elevated with a dorsally based central slip (Chamay) flap (Fig. 1.6).[7] Throughout the approach, violation of the central slip at the insertion of the base of the middle phalanx is avoided. For distal exposure of the proximal phalanx the Chamay approach provides the greatest exposure while protecting the central slip. At the middle phalanx level, the extensor mechanism is the best split longitudinally. However, exposure is significantly limited by both the central slip insertion proximally and terminal slip insertion distally. The middle phalanx is best approached through the midaxial approach.

Midaxial Approach

The midaxial approach offers better exposure of the medial or lateral aspect of the bone for plate application while minimizing trauma to the extensor apparatus[9] (Figs 1.7A to C). The decreased manipulation of the extensor mechanism with the midaxial exposure can therefore potentially reduce postoperative adhesions and contracture of the extensor apparatus.[10] At the level of the proximal phalanx, the lateral bands need to be either retracted dorsally or incised and reflected. Alternatively, a unilateral Littler intrinsic resection of the lateral band and oblique fibers may be performed to allow access to the proximal phalanx while reducing the risks of adhesion formation and stiffness.[9] Preservation of the contralateral lateral band retains important extensor power to the PIP joint and prevents deformity. At the level of the middle phalanx, midaxial exposure provides direct access to the lateral cortex without tendon interference.

Volar Approach

For some fracture patterns, it is necessary to obtain volar exposure. This occurs most commonly with PIP fracture-dislocations, especially when performing a hemi-hamate reconstruction. A Bruner incision is placed centered over the PIP flexion crease. The skin flap is carefully elevated taking care to protect the neurovascular bundles. The flexor sheath is carefully open between A2 and A4 using a transverse incision taking care not to injure the flexor tendons. The flexor tendons are retracted revealing the volar plate overlying the PIP joint. If necessary, the joint can be "shotgunned" to expose both articular surfaces (Fig. 1.8).

Surgical Techniques

Technique 1: Proximal Phalangeal Base Fracture

The surgical approach for proximal phalangeal base fractures is first determined by whether the fracture is intra- or extra-articular. Fractures not involving the joint can be treated using CRPP (Figs 1.9A to C). Alternatively, fractures that are intra-articular or not amenable to closed reduction can be treated with ORIF (Figs 1.10A to C).

Closed reduction is performed using longitudinal traction. The MP joint is then concomitantly flexed and the finger is derotated to restore normal rotation and cascade. After adequate reduction is verified on fluoroscopy, a 0.035 K-wire or 0.045 K-wire is passed percutaneously around each side of the metacarpal head with the MP joint flexed until the wire contacts the base of the proximal phalanx. The K-wires are advanced convergently. In order to maximize stability of the construct, the wires should not cross at the fracture site and preferably should

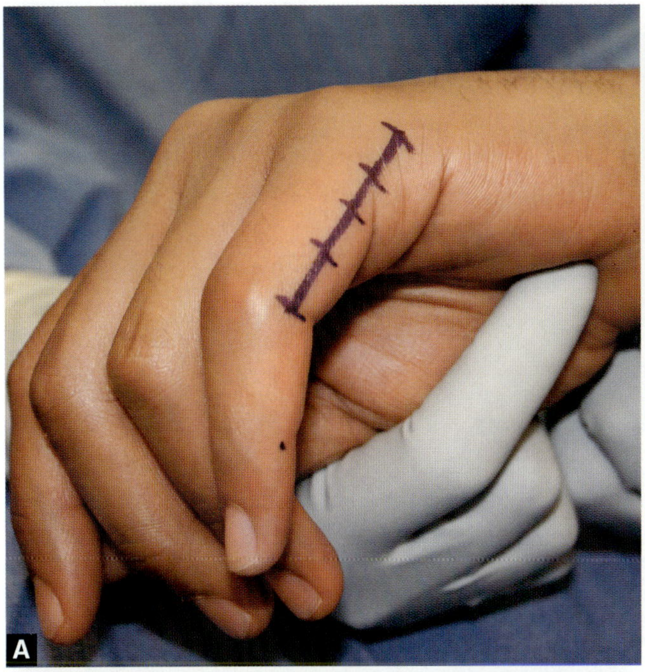

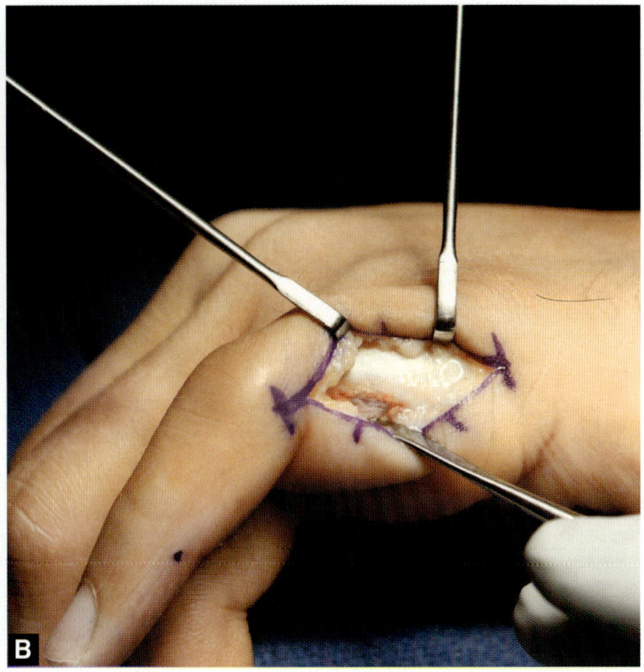

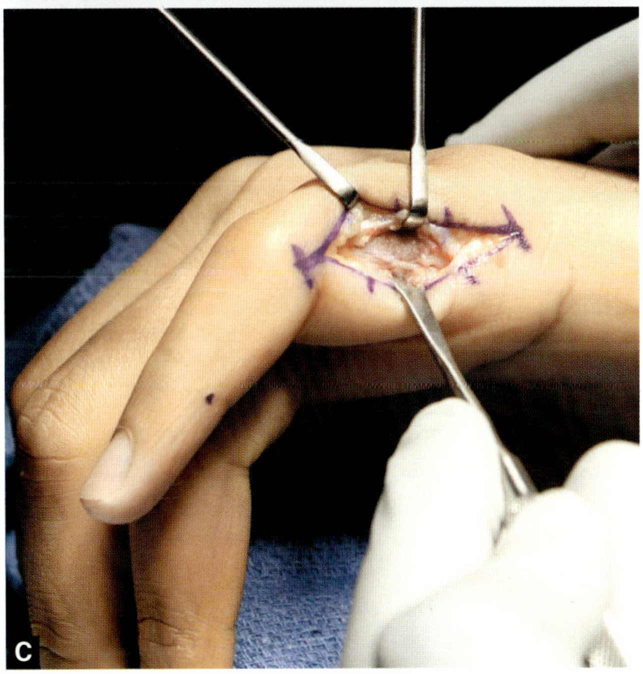

Figures 1.7A to C: Midaxial exposure of the proximal phalanx begins with (A) a lateral-based incision; (B) the lateral bands will be immediately encountered covering the lateral surface of the proximal phalanx. Exposure of the lateral cortex can be performed with; (C) dorsal retraction of the lateral band. Volar dissection should be avoided to prevent inadvertent injury to the digital neurovascular structures or the flexor tendons.

Courtesy: Asif M Ilyas

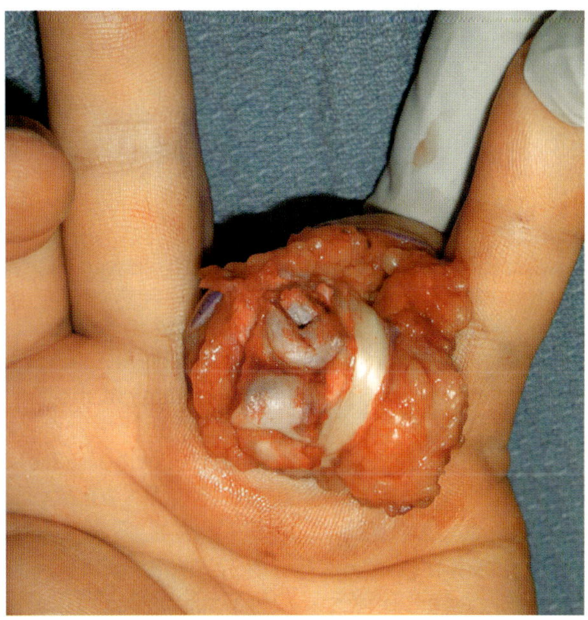

Figure 1.8: The "shotgun" exposure of the proximal interphalangeal joint is a volar exposure developed by opening the flexor tendon sheath between the A2 and A4 pulley and taking down the volar plate to expose the proximal interphalangeal joint. The joint is hyperextended 180° thereby exposing both articular surfaces.

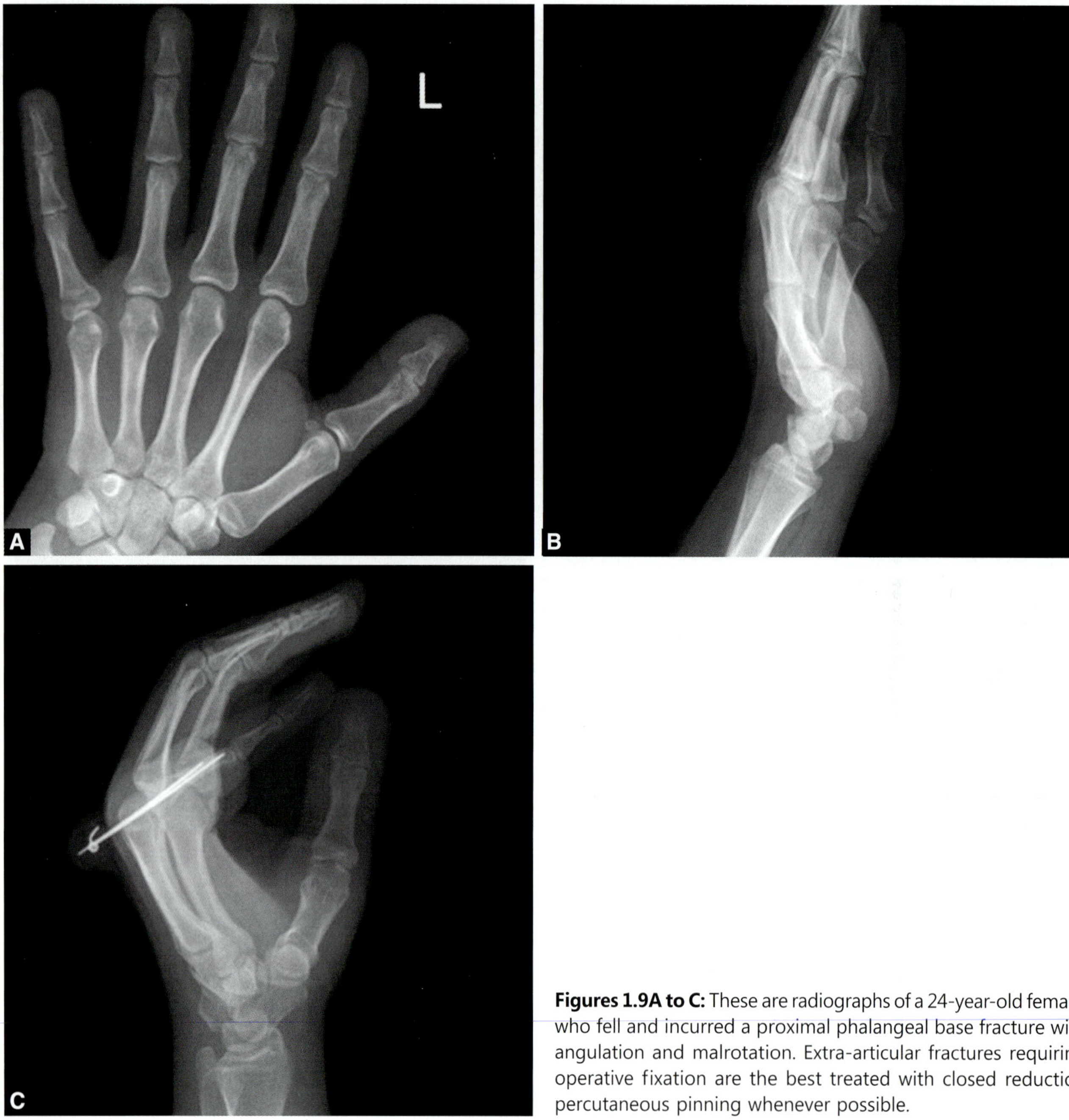

Figures 1.9A to C: These are radiographs of a 24-year-old female, who fell and incurred a proximal phalangeal base fracture with angulation and malrotation. Extra-articular fractures requiring operative fixation are the best treated with closed reduction percutaneous pinning whenever possible.

achieve bicortical purchase (Figs 1.10A to C). Fluoroscopy is used to confirm reduction of the fracture and position of the wires. The K-wires are bent and then cut short. A splint is applied in an intrinsic plus fashion (the MP joint is flexed and the PIP and DIP joints extended). Postoperatively, early PIP joint motion can be initiated to minimize stiffness. The K-wires can be removed by 3–4 weeks.

In cases requiring ORIF, the proximal phalanx may be approached either dorsally or midaxially (Figs 1.11A and B). Following fracture reduction, fixation can be achieved with 1.5 mm or 2.0 mm plate and screws. Restoration of fracture reduction and finger alignment is paramount and must be confirmed following ORIF. In addition, diligence should be paid to reduce prominence of the hardware and length of the screws in order to minimize soft tissue adhesions. Similarly, great care is taken to repair the extensor mechanism during closure. A splint is applied in an intrinsic plus fashion (the MP joint is flexed and the PIP and DIP

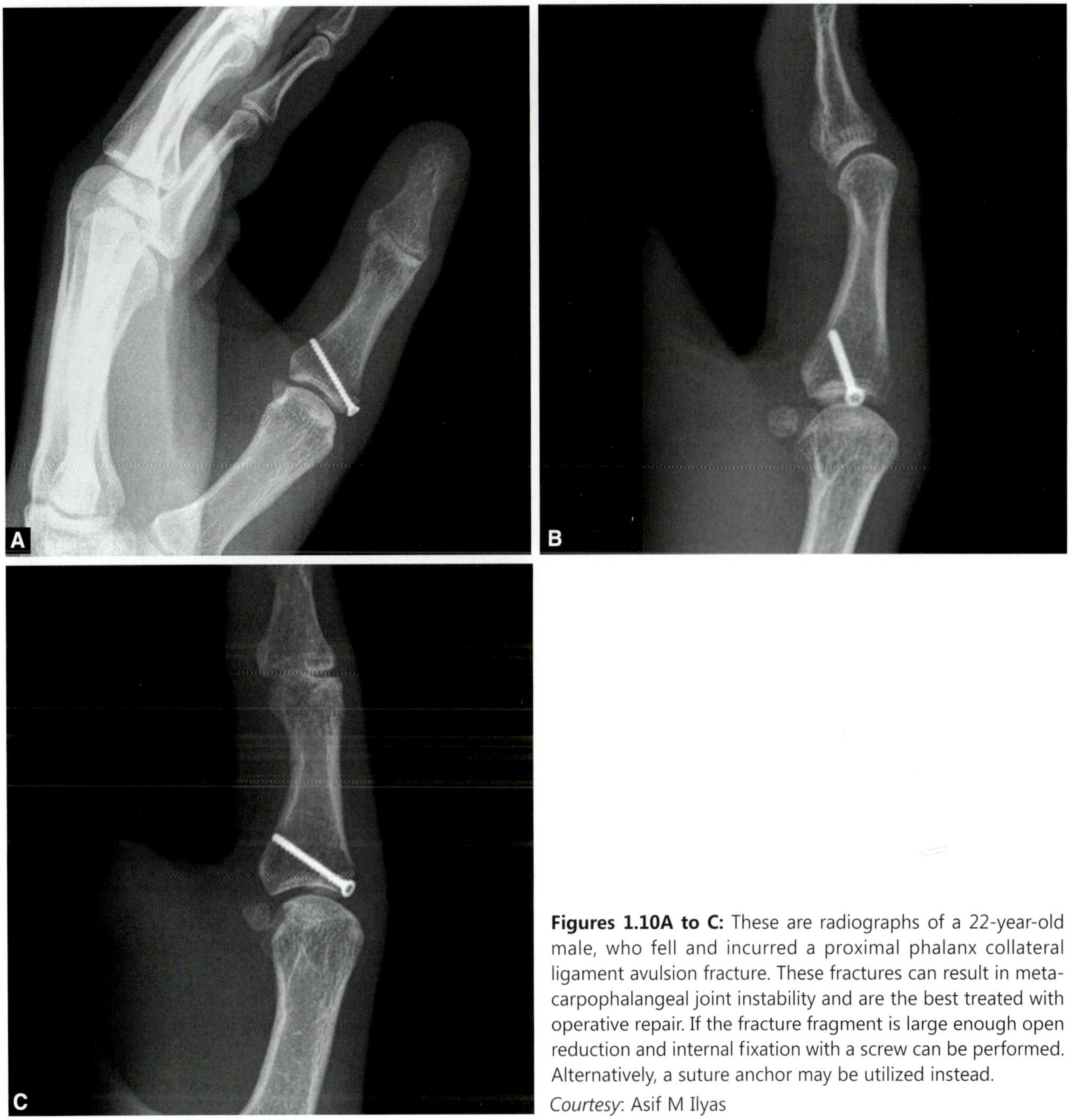

Figures 1.10A to C: These are radiographs of a 22-year-old male, who fell and incurred a proximal phalanx collateral ligament avulsion fracture. These fractures can result in metacarpophalangeal joint instability and are the best treated with operative repair. If the fracture fragment is large enough open reduction and internal fixation with a screw can be performed. Alternatively, a suture anchor may be utilized instead.
Courtesy: Asif M Ilyas

joints extended). Postoperatively, early motion and aggressive anti-edema measures are instituted.

Technique 2: Phalangeal Diaphyseal Fractures

Phalangeal diaphyseal fractures are susceptible to shortening, rotation and angulation. Operative treatment options include CRPP or ORIF. Closed reduction percutaneous pinning is best indicated for extra-articular fractures amenable to closed reduction (Figs 1.12A to F). Typically, multiple 0.035 K-wires or 0.045 K-wires are required. Before and after K-wire fixation it is imperative to confirm restoration of normal finger alignment. Fluoroscopy is also used to confirm reduction of the fracture

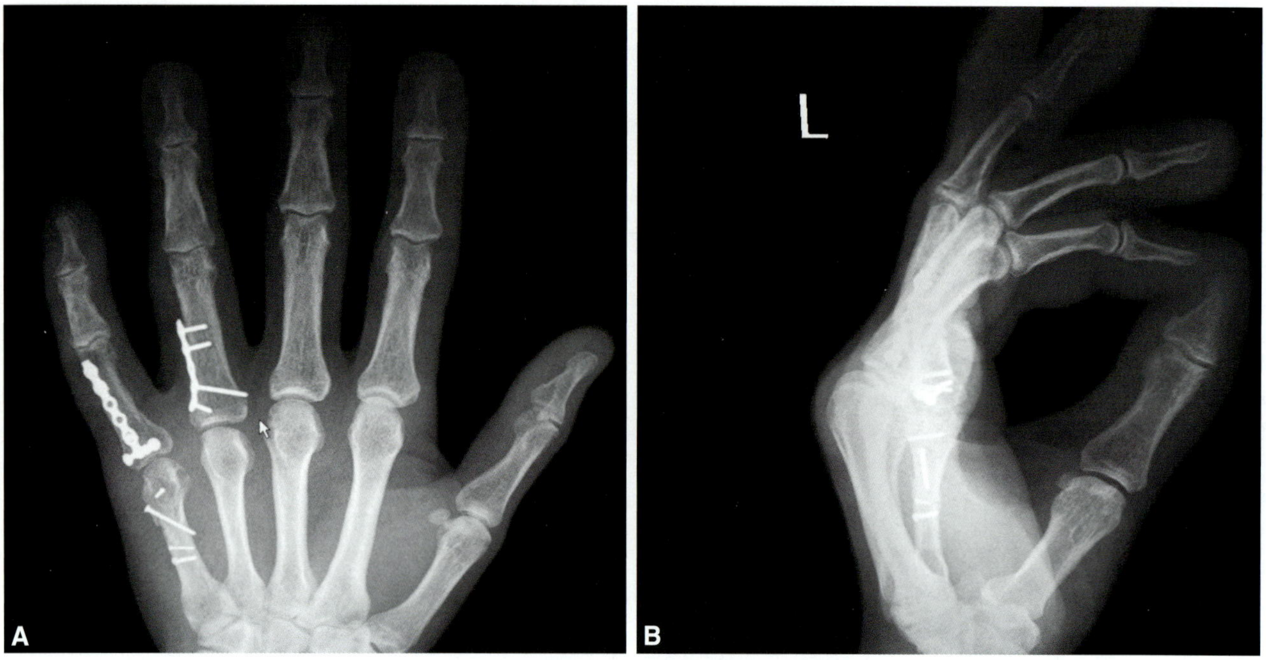

Figures 1.11A and B: Intra-articular fractures or multiple phalangeal fractures may be treated with open reduction and internal fixation through either a midaxial or dorsal approach.

and position of the wires. A splint is applied in an intrinsic plus fashion (the MP joint is flexed and the PIP and DIP joints extended). Postoperatively, early PIP joint motion can be initiated to minimize stiffness. The K-wires can be removed by 3–4 weeks.

Open reduction and internal fixation is the best indicated for fractures not amenable to closed reduction, intra-articular fractures and cases with multiple phalangeal fractures or rotationally unstable fractures (Figs 1.13A to D). Proximal phalanx fractures can be approached through either a dorsal or midaxial approach but middle phalanx fractures are the best approached midaxially. Open reduction and internal fixation can be performed utilizing either 1.5 mm or 2.0 mm plate and screws. For oblique or spiral fractures, the authors recommend ORIF using interfragmentary compression screws. For transverse fractures, they recommend plate and screw fixation. Before and after fixation it is imperative to confirm restoration of normal finger alignment. Fluoroscopy is also used to confirm reduction of the fracture and position of the hardware. Upon closure, the extensor mechanism is carefully repaired. A splint is applied in an intrinsic plus fashion (the MP joint is flexed and the PIP and DIP joints extended). Postoperatively, early motion and aggressive anti-edema measures are instituted.

Beyond tendon adhesions and joint stiffness, the most common problem following proximal phalanx ORIF is an extensor lag at the PIP joint, which can also develop into a fixed flexion contracture.[24] Prevention of this deformity relies on diligent extensor mechanism repair, emphasizing PIP joint extension at rest and early tendon gliding.[25]

PROXIMAL PHALANGEAL BASE FRACTURE AND PHALANGEAL DIAPHYSEAL FRACTURES: Pearls and Pitfalls

- Before and after fixation it is imperative to confirm restoration of normal finger alignment
- In order to avoid postoperative MP joint contracture and PIP extensor lag following CRPP, the fingers should be splinted in an intrinsic plus fashion
- In order to avoid an extensor lag of the PIP joint following ORIF, diligent extensor mechanism repair should be performed followed by early tendon gliding and PIP joint extension at rest
- In order to maximize finger motion and recovery, early motion and aggressive anti-edema modalities should be instituted as early as possible

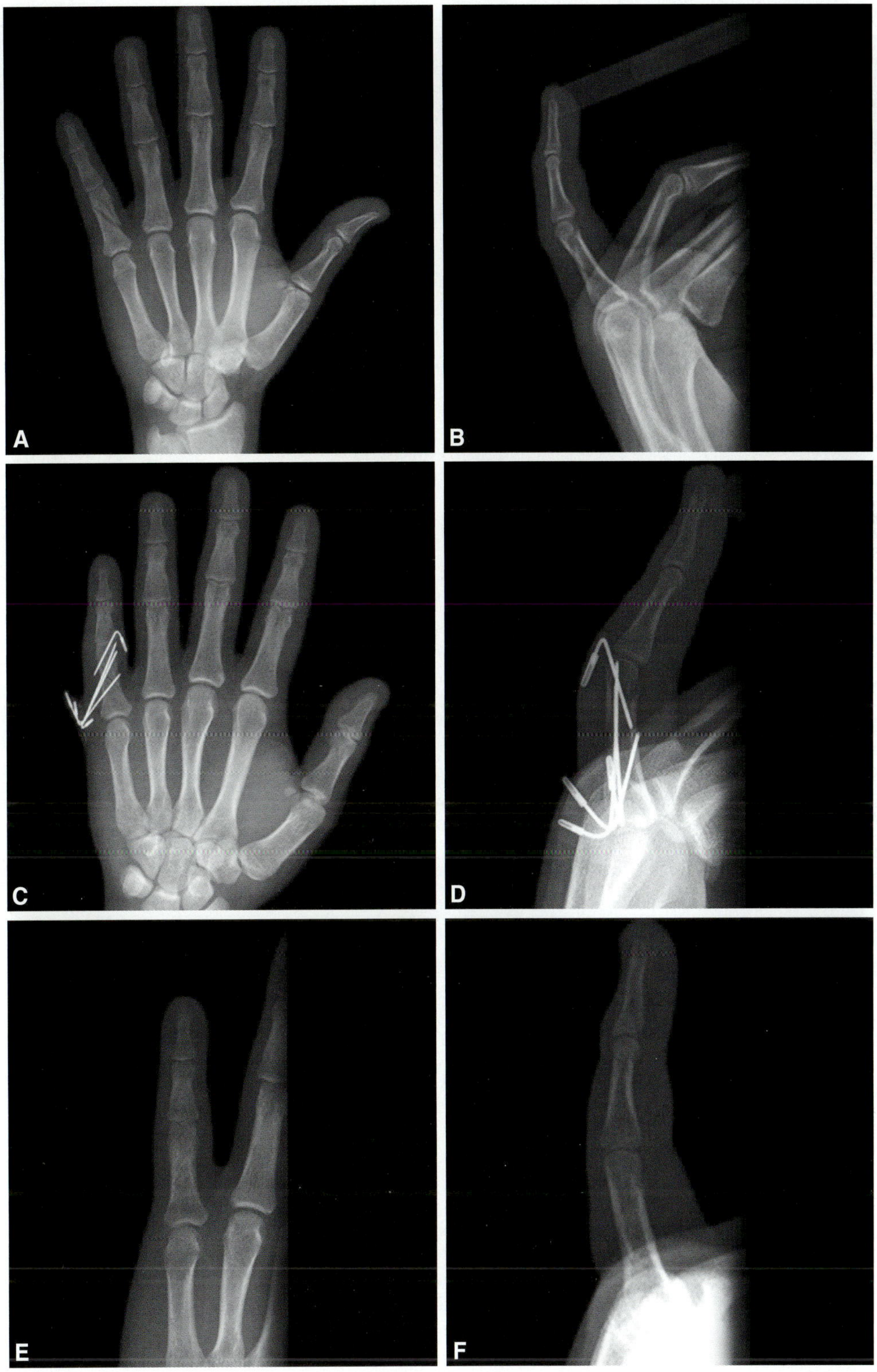

Figures 1.12A to F: These are radiographs of a 35-year-old female who fell and incurred a (A and B) diaphyseal fracture of the small finger proximal phalanx with malrotation; (C and D) the fracture was amenable to closed reduction and was treated with multiple 0.035 K-wires placed perpendicular to the fracture site. The K-wires were removed at 6 weeks postoperatively; (E and F) note the healed fracture in normal alignment at 3 months postoperatively.

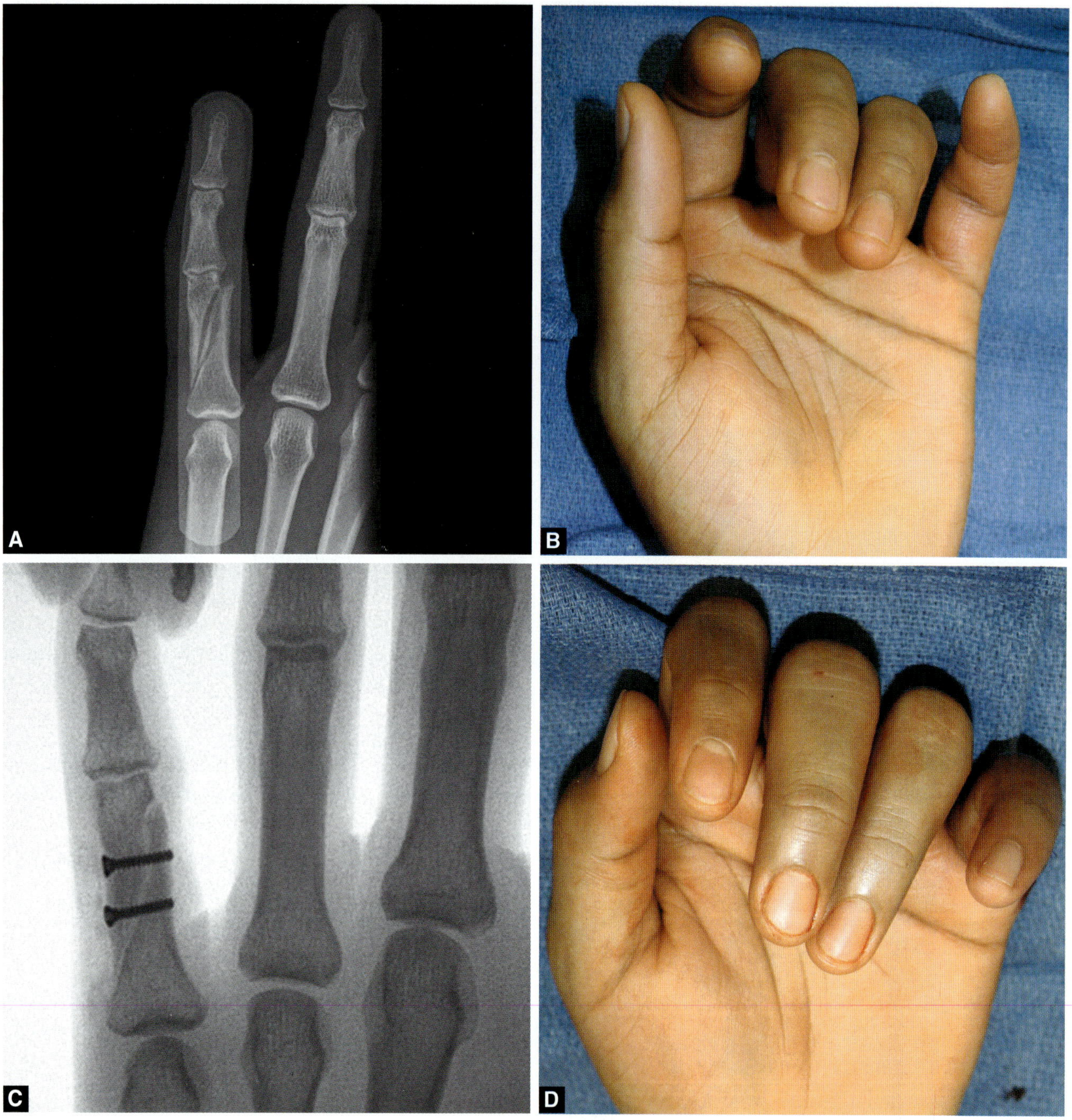

Figures 1.13A to D: This is a 32-year-old male who forcefully jammed his small finger and incurred a (A) long spiral diaphyseal proximal phalanx fracture with malrotation; (B) Preoperative examination identified malrotation of the finger. The fracture was deemed malrotated and unstable and was treated with (C) ORIF utilizing 2.0 mm interfragmentary compression screws; (D) Note restoration of normal finger alignment and rotation postoperatively.

Courtesy: Asif M Ilyas

Technique 3: Condylar Fracture

The two condyles at the head of the proximal or middle phalanx provide bony stability to the PIP and DIP joints, respectively (Fig. 1.14). Condylar fractures of the phalangeal head are typically the result of axial loading and lateral deviation. London described three fracture configurations with proximal phalanx condylar fractures: type I is a stable, undisplaced unicondylar fracture; type II is an unstable, displaced unicondylar fracture and type III is a comminuted bicondylar fracture.[26] Surgery is usually indicated, if there is any displacement, angulation or comminution. Surgical options include CRPP versus ORIF. In order to maximize articular reduction and achieve stable fixation that can facilitate early motion, the authors recommend ORIF through a midaxial approach. If the fracture is unicondylar, it can readily be repaired with 1.5 mm or 2.0 mm screws placed parallel to the joint surface. If the fracture in bicondylar, a 90° blade plate or a locking plate is utilized.

Technique 4: Middle Phalanx Base Fractures/PIP/Fracture-Dislocations

Middle phalanx base fractures represent a spectrum of difficult fractures that can be extra-articular but are the most commonly intra-articular. In the most cases, when the volar articular surface of the middle phalanx fractures, the PIP joint dislocates dorsally due to tension from the finger extensors on their distal attachment and shorten due to the FDS insertion volarly. Fractures involving less than one-third of the middle phalangeal surface with a well-reduced PIP joint is typically stable and can be treated non-surgically with a dorsal extension block splint and early motion. However, fractures with greater involvement of the articular surface or any displacement or instability of the PIP joint warrants surgical intervention. Surgical treatment options include: closed reduction and dorsal extension block pinning, dynamic external fixation, ORIF, hemi-hamate reconstruction, volar plate arthroplasty, implant arthroplasty or arthrodesis.

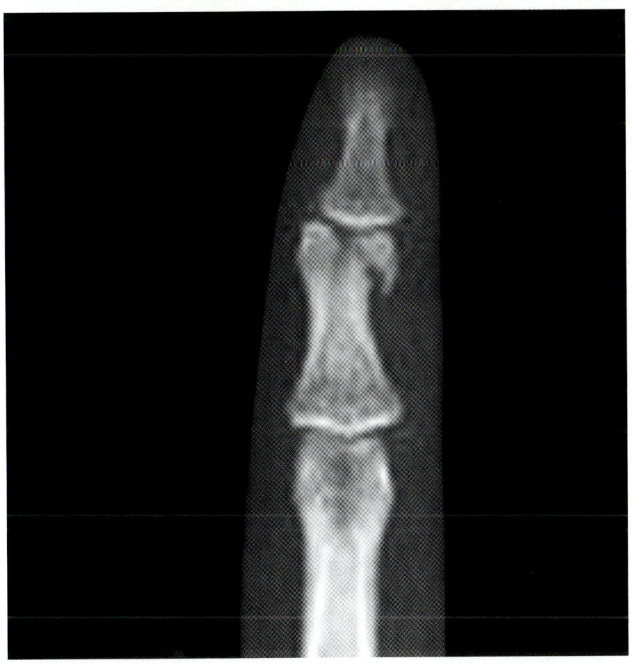

Figure 1.14: A condylar fracture of the middle phalanx is by definition intra-articular and can result in incongruency and potential angulation.

Dorsal Extension Block Pinning

Dorsal extension block pinning is effective in the management of intra-articuar middle phalanx base fractures when the PIP joint is amenable to closed reduction with gentle PIP flexion (Figs 1.15A to C). It is a straightforward technique and consists of directing a 0.035 K-wire or 0.045 K-wire retrograde through the head of a proximal phalanx fracture with the PIP joint flexed. Following pin placement concentric reduction of the PIP joint must be confirmed. Postoperatively, full active and passive finger motion is encouraged. The pin is removed by 3–4 weeks. Although a simple technique, tethering of the extensor mechanism by the pin can potentially lead to a PIP joint flexion contracture and stiffness. Furthermore, the presence of a transcutaneous intra-articular pins can potentially become infected and cause a septic arthritis of the PIP joint.[5] Most clinical series report mild residual flexion contractures at the PIP joint while recovering 80-90° of flexion.[41]

Dynamic External Fixation

Dynamic external fixation allows for indirect fracture reduction of the PIP joint fracture-dislocation using ligamentotaxis while maintaining PIP joint motion (Fig. 1.16).[32] Although potentially cumbersome and technically demanding, dynamic external fixation is inexpensive and affords early motion. The technique is performed with three 0.045 K-wires and dental rubber bands. All three K-wires are placed parallel to each other but perpendicular to the long axis of the digit. The first K-wire is placed through the head of the proximal phalanx in line with the rotational center of the joint. The second K-wire is placed at the distal aspect of the middle phalanx.

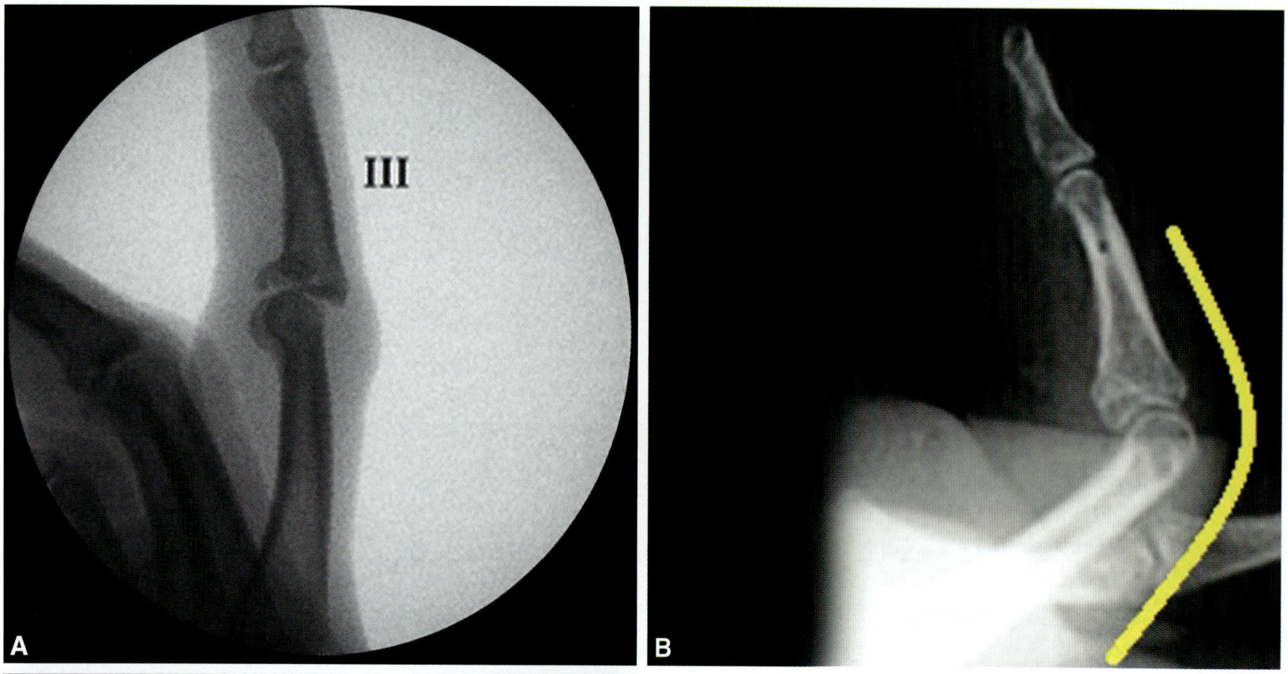

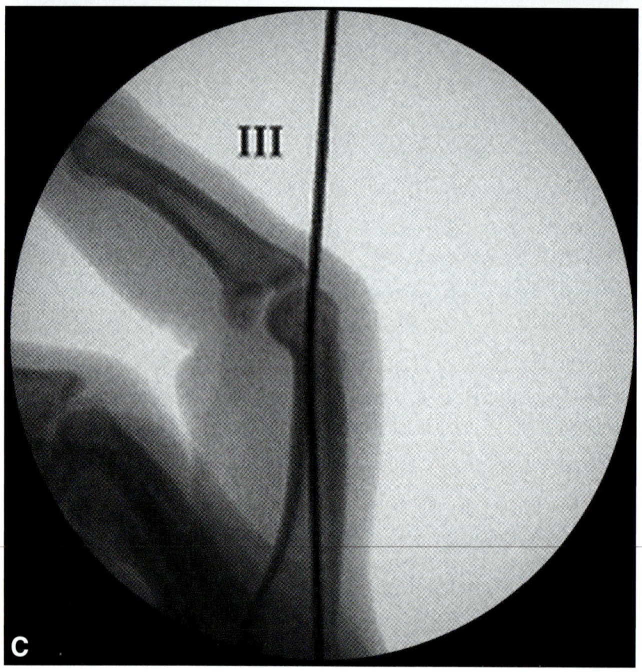

Figures 1.15A to C: Middle phalanx base fractures involving less than one-third of the middle phalangeal surface with a well-reduced proximal interphalangeal joint is typically stable and can be treated nonsurgically with a dorsal extension block splint and early motion. Alternatively, extension block pinning may be indicated in cases with a displaced proximal interphalangeal fracture-dislocation that is amenable to closed reduction can be treated with a pin placed across the proximal phalanx thereby reducing the proximal interphalangeal joint in flexion.

The third K-wire is placed in the proximal aspect of the middle phalanx. All wires are bent and angled upward. The first K-wire is then rotated under the second K-wire and over the third K-wire thereby providing a dorsal directed force at the middle phalanx base. The second K-wires are wrapped around the traversing first K-wire. Hooks are created at the end of the first and third K-wires, and dental rubber bands are applied to provide ligamentotaxis to distract and reduce the PIP joint. Additional bands are applied until a concentric reduction of the PIP joint is achieved. Once reduced active PIP joint flexion is encouraged.

Open Reduction Internal Fixation

Open reduction internal fixation is performed through a volar exposure to the PIP joint through a Bruner incision

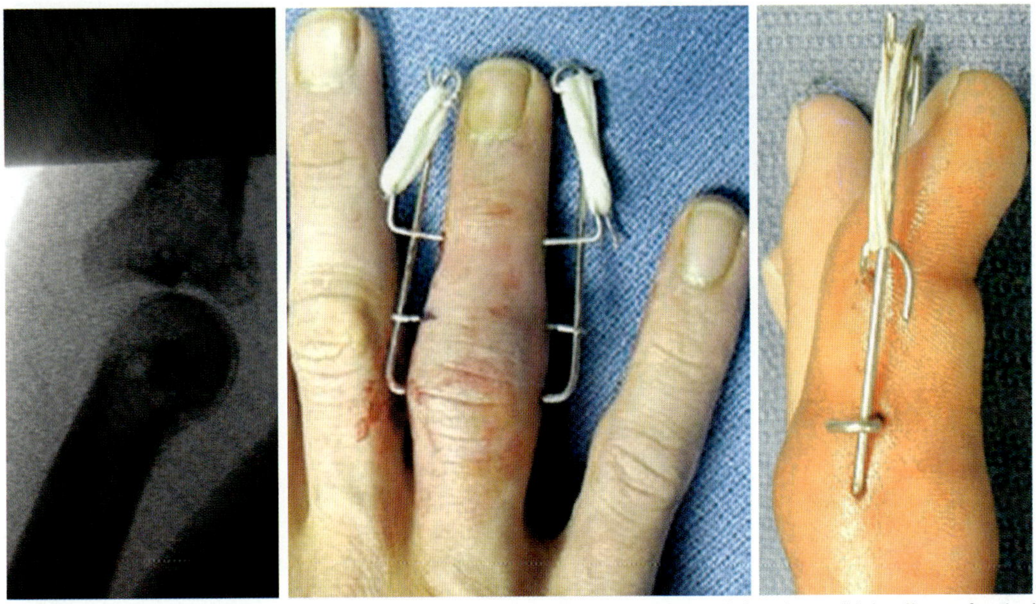

Figure 1.16: Middle phalanx base fractures can be treated with dynamic external fixation which allows for indirect fracture reduction of the proximal interphalangeal joint fracture-dislocation using ligamentotaxis while maintaining proximal interphalangeal joint motion. Three K-wires are placed. The first is placed through the rotational center of the head of the proximal phalanx. The second K-wire is placed in the proximal aspect of the middle phalanx and acts as the fulcrum. The third K-wire is placed in the distal aspect of the middle phalanx. Dental rubber bands are then applied between the first and third K-wires thereby distracting the proximal interphalangeal joint.

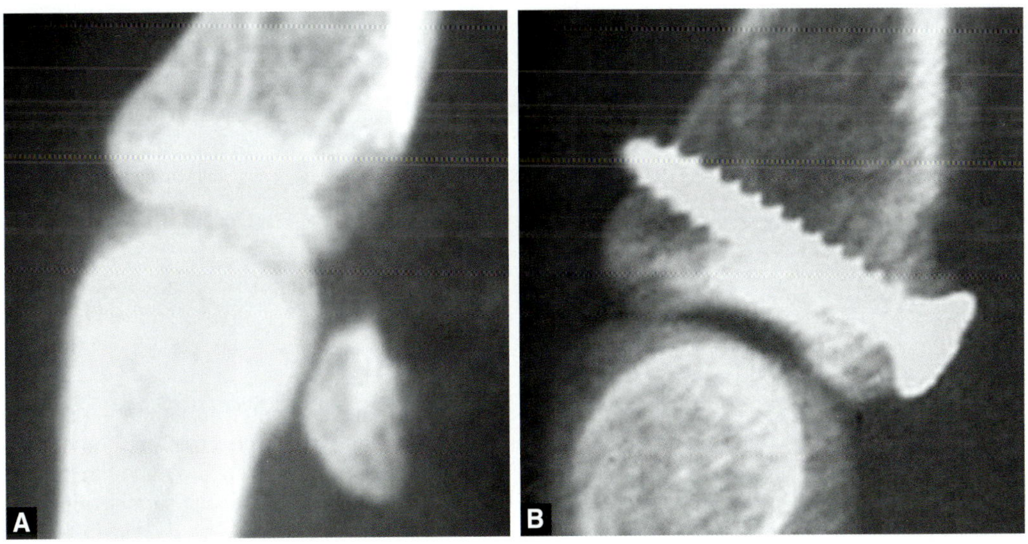

Figures 1.17A and B: Open reduction and internal fixation is performed through a standard volar approach. The flexor tendon sheath is opened between the A2 and A4 pulleys and the tendons are retracted. The volar plate is not taken down as the volar articular fragment will be attached to it. The fracture site is developed, debrided and the fracture is directly reduced and repaired with two to three 1.0 mm or 1.3 mm screws. Take care not to place the screws too proud volarly as they will irritate the extensor tendons. Also, avoid over-tightening as it may comminute the small volar articular fragment.

centered over the PIP flexion crease (Figs 1.17A and B). The PIP joint is exposed by carefully opening the flexor sheath between the A2 and A4 pulley at the PIP joint. The flexor tendons are retracted and the volar plate is opened transversely exposing the PIP joints. The collateral ligaments are carefully protected. The fracture is directly reduced and repaired with 1.3 mm or 1.5 mm screws placed in a volar to dorsal direction. Following fracture fixation concentric reduction of the PIP joint must be confirmed.

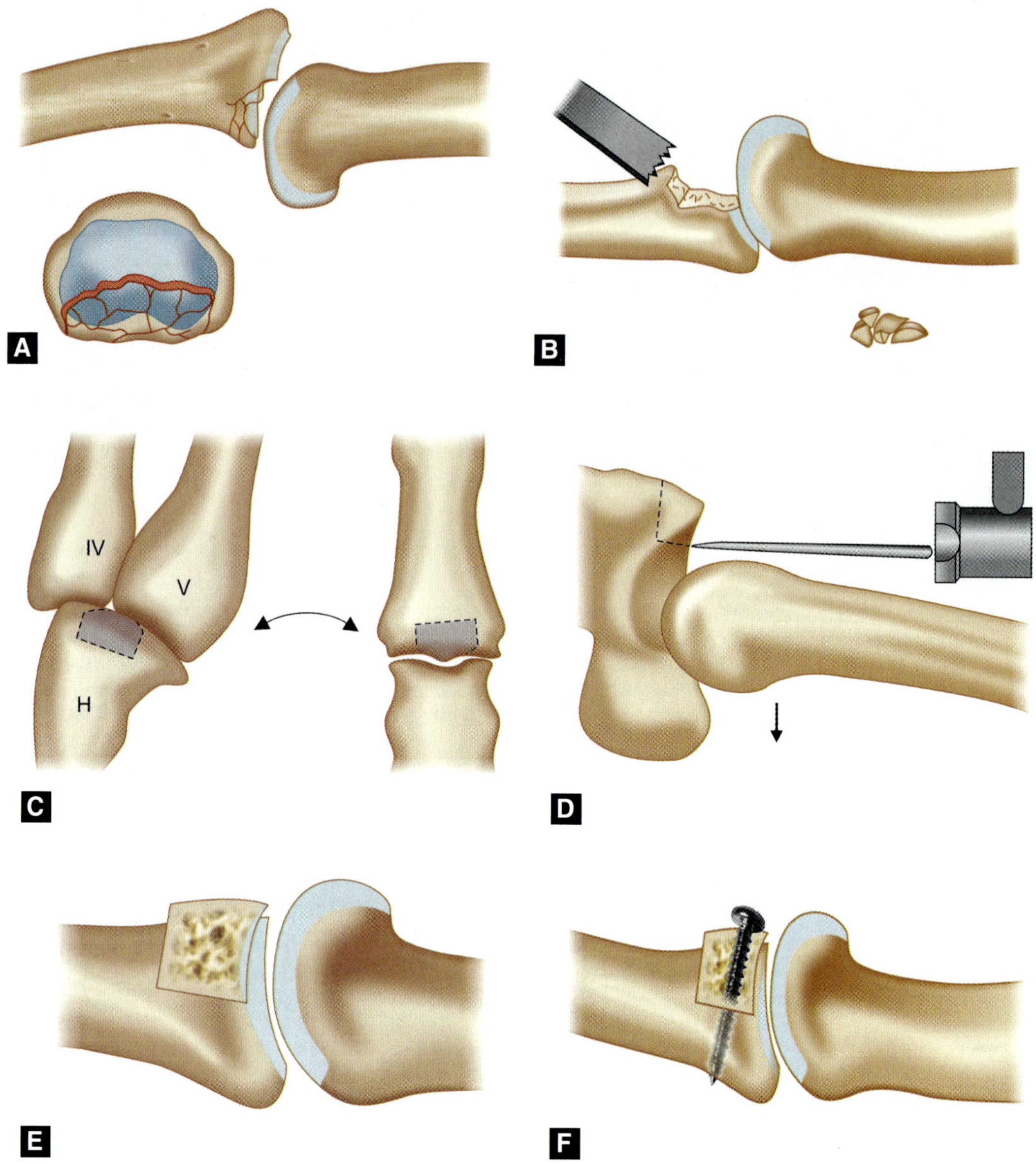

Figures 1.18A to F: Hemi-hamate reconstructions are indicated in cases with a proximal interphalangeal joint fracture-dislocation where the volar articular fragment is small, comminuted and/or not amenable to open reduction and internal fixation. (A) The fracture site is exposed volarly and the finger is shotgunned; (B) The comminution is debrided away and the defect is formed into a 'box' using a rongeur or saw; (C) The osteoarticular autograft is harvested from the distal articular surface of the hamate between the fourth and fifth metacarpal bases. Be precise in its measurement and take more rather than less; (D) With volar pressure on the metacarpal bases, use an osteotome or small oscillating saw to harvest the graft; (E) Place the bone graft in the defect and contour it as needed until a congruent joint is achieved. Make sure the graft is adequately large to provide complete volar articular coverage. (F) Fix the fragment with one to three 1.0 mm or 1.3 mm screws. Take care not to place the screws too proud volarly as they will irritate the extensor tendons.

Hemi-hamate Reconstruction

Hemi-hamate reconstruction is an osteochondral autograft used to reconstruct an unrepairable middle phalanx base fracture using a size-matched osteochondral hamate graft (Figs 1.18A to F). This technique is best indicated where 50% or more of the proximal articular surface has been lost. Furthermore, by restoring both articular congruity and osseous stability osteochondral autografting theoretically allows for more immediate rehabilitation with potentially early motion, less stiffness and possibly less post-traumatic arthritis.[30] It can be used acutely for the treatment of comminuted, unstable PIP dorsal lip fracture-dislocations but is also suitable as a salvage procedure for patients, who have redislocated after other surgical procedures.[35] Although this procedure replaces the disrupted articular surface at the base of the middle phalanx and recreates joint congruity, the long-term viability of this transplanted cartilage remains unknown. The technique involves a volar exposure to the PIP joint through a Bruner incision centered over the PIP flexion crease. The PIP joint is exposed by carefully opening the flexor sheath between the A2 and A4 pulley at the PIP joint. The flexor tendons are retracted and the PIP joint is exposed by debriding the volar plate and fracture comminution.[28] The collateral ligaments, however, are maintained and protected. The PIP joint is then hyper-extended. The hamate graft is obtained via a dorsal capsulotomy of the carpometacarpal joints of the ring and small fingers. The graft should be slightly larger than the measured defect to allow further contouring to the exact size and shape. The graft should be contoured to recreate the cup-like shape of the articular base of the middle phalanx. Depending on the size of the bone, two or three 1.3 mm or 1.5 mm screws are placed in a volar to dorsal direction to secure the graft to the base of the middle phalanx. Following fixation concentric reduction of the PIP joint is confirmed. Postoperatively, a dorsal extension block splint is applied with the PIP joint in 30° of flexion and full active flexion is allowed.

Arthroplasty

Multiple salvage treatment options exist for middle phalanx base PIP joint fracture-dislocations including volar plate arthroplasty, implant arthroplasty and arthrodesis. Volar plate arthroplasty is indicated for primary or secondary repair of a PIP fracture-dislocation. We typically recommend considering a volar plate arthroplasty for a secondary or reconstruction of a failed PIP fracture-dislocation repair or hemi-hamate reconstruction (Fig. 1.19). In addition, in cases with failed fixation or delayed diagnosis with a chronically dislocated PIP joint fracture-dislocation, implant arthroplasty or arthrodesis can also be considered (Figs 1.20A and B).

Eaton et al. in 1980 described volar plate arthroplasty to address the comminuted fragments at the volar base of the middle phalanx that were not amenable to ORIF.[33] The technique involves a standard volar approach to the PIP joint through a Bruner's incision. The PIP joint is exposed by opening the flexor pulley system between the A2 and A4 pulleys. The volar plate is released along its lateral borders from the collaterals and carefully raised off the middle phalanx base and retracted proximally. The collaterals are removed in its entirety. A shallow trough is created in the volar base of the middle phalanx at the junction with the articular surface. The PIP joint is reduced with gentle volar translation and PIP joint flexion, and a K-wire is placed across the reduced PIP joint in 10-20° of flexion. The volar plate is advanced into the defect and repaired with suture anchors or pull out wires. The K-wire is removed at 3–4 weeks.

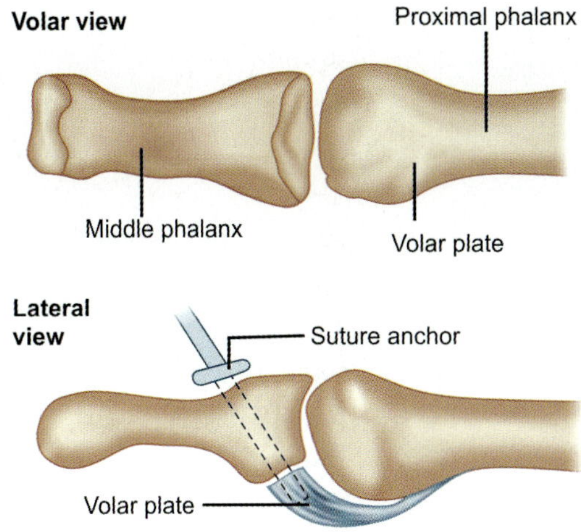

Figure 1.19: Volar plate arthroplasty depicted with repair using a pull out sutures. Alternatively, the volar plate may be repaired with a suture anchor placed in the middle phalanx base.

CONDYLAR FRACTURE AND MIDDLE PHALANX BASE FRACTURES: Pearls and Pitfalls

- Whenever possible, closed reduction with mild flexion and extension block splinting or pinning should be considered to minimize surgical exposure and potential secondary complications
- ORIF of PIP joint fracture-dislocations is predicated upon an adequately sized volar articular fragment with relatively little comminution
- Hemi-hamate reconstruction is effective in treating PIP joint fracture-dislocations but requires careful contouring and fixation of the graft into the volar articular defect

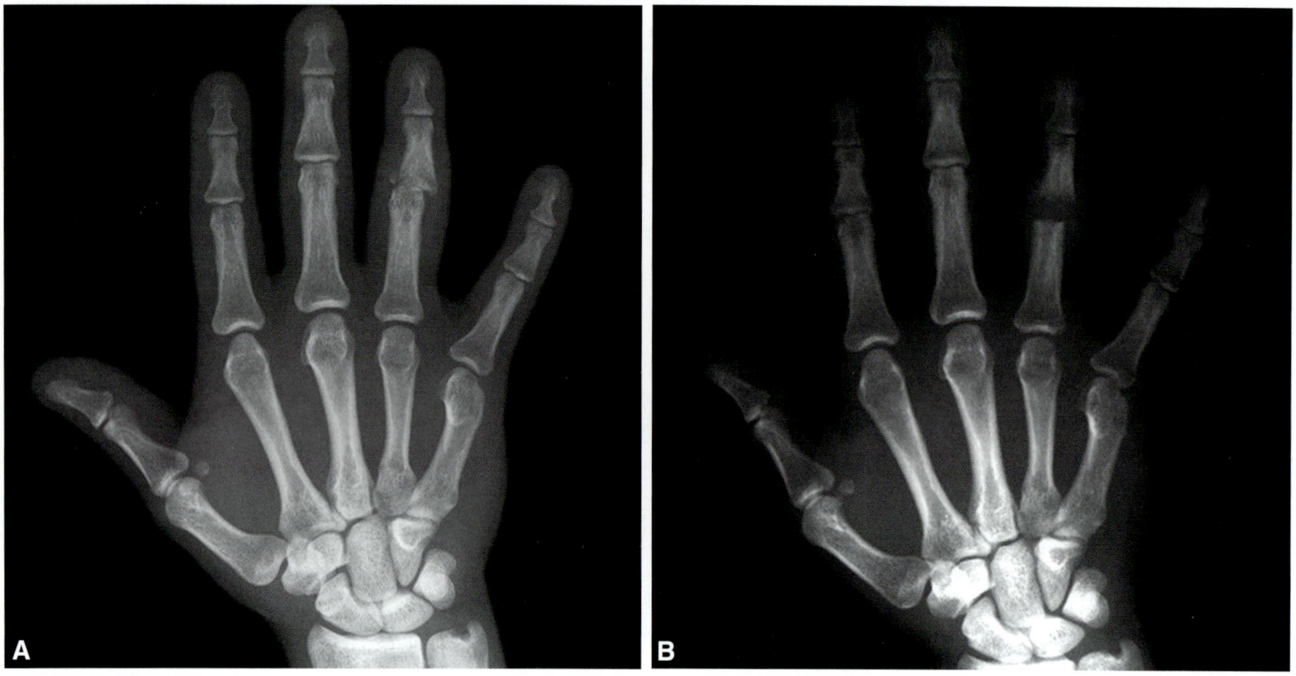

Figures 1.20A and B: These are radiographs of a 42-year-old female, who fell three months previously and presented with persistent ring finger pain, swelling and decreased range of motion. Radiographs demonstrated a chronic proximal interphalangeal joint fracture-dislocation with fixed dorsal dislocation of the middle phalanx and loss of the volar articular fragment. The patient was treated with a silicone implant proximal interphalangeal joint arthroplasty.
Courtesy: Asif M Ilyas

- Dynamic external fixation requires careful K-wire placement in order to establish the appropriate fulcrum and axis for ligamentotaxis across the PIP joint
- Volar plate arthroplasty is the best indicated for salvage cases and often results in some residual dorsal translation of the PIP joint
- Regardless of surgical treatment technique, concentric reduction of the PIP joint must be confirmed prior to exiting the case

Technique 5: Distal Phalanx Fractures

Distal phalanx fractures can consist of tuft fractures, shaft fractures or avulsion fractures of its base. Tuft fractures are typically minimally displaced unless associated with a concomitant soft tissue injury, and can typically be treated non-operatively with protective splinting and early motion. Similarly, distal phalanx shaft fractures can usually be treated non-operatively unless grossly malaligned and/or associated with a nail bed injury requiring operative repair. In these cases, percutaneous pinning with a 0.035 K-wire or 0.045 K-wire placed down the axis of the distal phalanx will provide reliable reduction to the fracture site and stability to the nail bed repair. The K-wire can be placed in the distal phalanx alone; however, the authors would recommend advancing the K-wire across the DIP joint into the middle phalanx to provide additional stability to the fracture site and any associated soft tissue repairs. Symptomatic DIP stiffness is uncommon following trans-articular pinning of the DIP joint.

Articular fractures at the base of the distal phalanx fractures typically are a product of an extensor or flexor tendon avulsion fracture resulting in "Mallet" fractures or "Jersey" finger fractures, respectively.

Jersey Finger Fracture Repair

This fracture is named after a common sports injury in which one player grabs the shirt of an opponent who pulls away suddenly causing the FDP tendon to avulse of the volar base of the distal phalanx with a fragment of bone. Clinically, it manifests as an extended DIP joint with inability to actively flex the joint. In small avulsion fractures, the bone can be debrided and the tendon repaired in standard fashion. However, when the fracture represents at least 30% of the articular surface of the distal phalanx then fracture repair is indicated. We recommend repairing the fracture through a volar approach utilizing a Bruner incision centered over the DIP joint. The fracture is mobilized and its FDP tendon insertion protected. If adequate fragment size is available the fracture can be repaired directly with 1.3 mm or 1.5 mm screws in a volar to dorsal direction with care being taken not to violate the germinal matrix on the dorsal surface of the distal phalanx shaft. Alternatively, a pull-out suture can be run through the tendon and fracture fragment and out through the dorsal cortex and repaired over a padded button on the nail.[38] A congruent DIP joint reduction must be confirmed prior to exiting the case. Postoperatively, a dorsal blocking splint in slight flexion at the DIP joint is applied and rehabilitation is started per flexor tendon repair protocol.

Mallet Fracture Repair

Avulsion fractures of the terminal slip of the extensor tendon off the dorsal distal phalanx base typically occurs when the extended digit sustains an axial loading or a forceful flexion.[5] Most cases can be treated with extension splinting of the DIP joint for 4–6 weeks. However, when more than 30% of the articular surface is involved, there is secondary subluxation of the DIP joint surgical repair is indicated, or if the injury presents in a delayed fashion surgical repair is indicated. Surgical treatment options include DIP joint pinning, tension band wiring,[39] extension block pinning[40] and compression pinning.[41] The authors recommend extension block pinning as it is an effective and straightforward technique that has provided reliable outcomes (Figs 1.21 A to C).[40] The technique first involves placing a dorsal blocking wire proximal to the avulsion fracture into the middle phalanx head, with the DIP joint flexed, thereby locking the avulsion fracture in a distal position. Next, a second K-wire is placed through the distal phalanx in a transarticular fashion across the DIP joint with it fully extended resulting in secondary reduction of the fracture site. In chronic cases, a small incision at the level of the fracture site is placed and both fracture ends are freshened up with a curette prior to reduction to enhance healing. Concentric reduction of the DIP joint and the fracture site must be confirmed prior to exiting the case. A protective splint for the DIP joint is fashioned leaving the PIP joint free. The pins are removed by 4-6 weeks.

Outcomes

Horton et al. performed a prospective randomized analysis of K-wire versus lag screw fixation for oblique phalangeal fractures and found no significant difference in the functional recovery rates or in the pain scores for the two groups, similar rates of malunion and no differences in range of motion (ROM) or grip strength.[8] However, the K-wire group had a higher rate of complications including pin site and wound infection and finger stiffness postulated due to tethering of the extensor mechanism.

Extension block pinning is simple to apply and allows the PIP joint to be placed in a lesser degree of flexion while preventing subluxation. Clinical series have been limited by small patient numbers but document the recovery of active PIP joint arc of motion averaging 85° after treatment.[31]

Ellis et al. evaluated their experience in treating unstable, dorsal, intra-articular, fracture-dislocations of the PIP joint with a dynamic external fixator. Fourteen patients were treated consecutively with eight available for final follow-up at an average of 26 months. Average PIP motion was 1–89° with a grip strength that was 92% relative to the contralateral hand. All patients had a concentric reduction, but five of eight patients had a slight step-off deformity or arthritis present.[29]

Calfee et al. described their experience with hemi-hamate reconstructions performed on 33 patients with unstable, comminuted PIP fracture-dislocations involving at least 50% of the volar middle phalangeal surface that was not amenable to ORIF.[36] Although, radiographic evaluation demonstrated loss of joint space in 43% of patients, the radiographic changes did not correlate with poorer outcomes. Restoration of PIP motion and disability of arm, shoulder and hand scores were similar between acute and chronic reconstructions.

Dionysian and Eaton described their long-term experience with volar plate arthroplasty used to manage both acute and chronic PIP joint fracture-dislocations. Seventeen patients were available for review at an average follow-up of 11 years. There were no complaints of pain at rest, although four showed signs of joint space narrowing and degeneration. Those cases performed

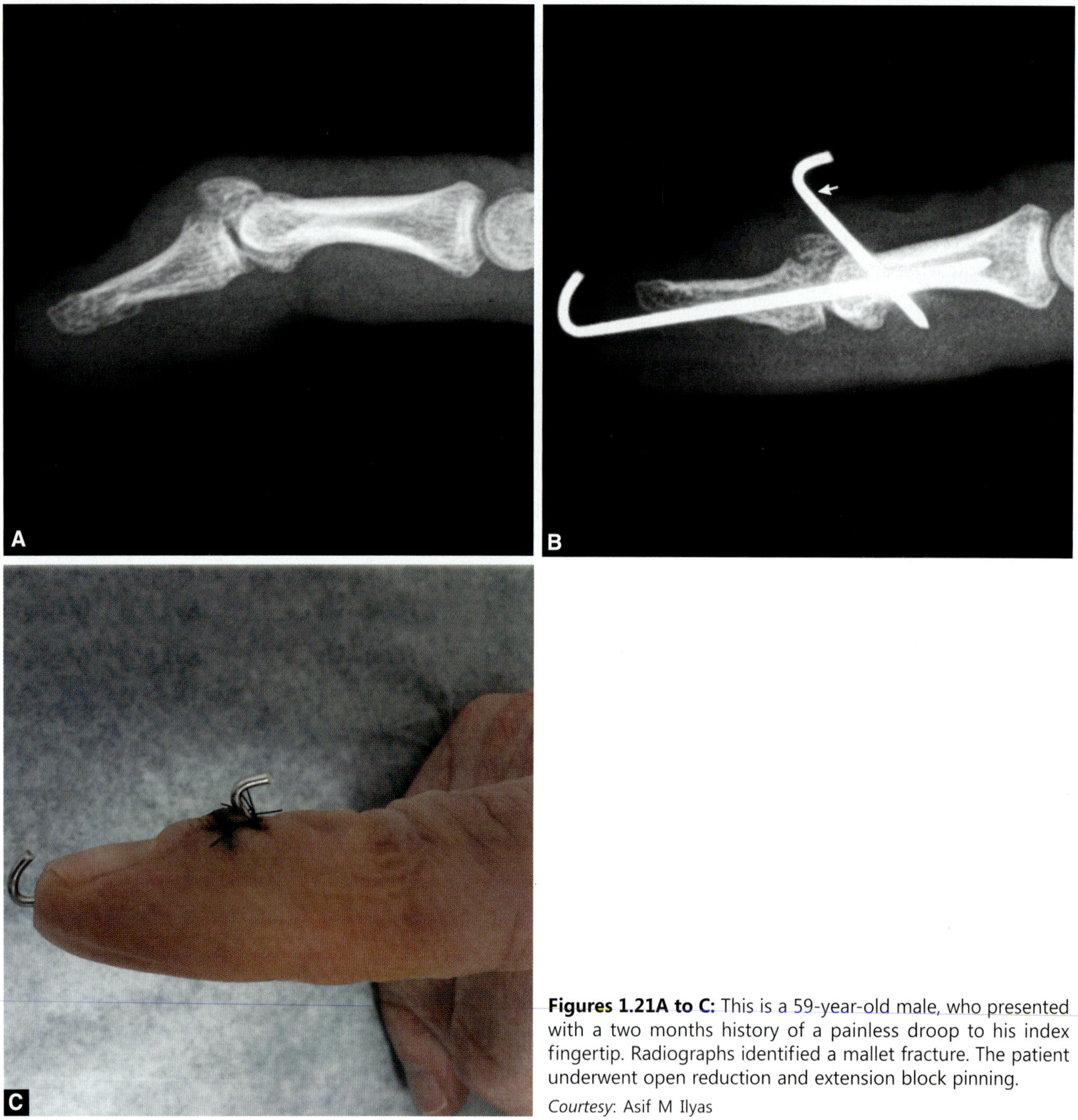

Figures 1.21A to C: This is a 59-year-old male, who presented with a two months history of a painless droop to his index fingertip. Radiographs identified a mallet fracture. The patient underwent open reduction and extension block pinning.
Courtesy: Asif M Ilyas

within four weeks from the time of injury achieved an average total arc of active motion of 85° versus 61° among those cases performed after four weeks (average, 20 weeks) from the time of injury.

Lubahn compared surgical and nonsurgical treatment of mallet injuries and concluded surgical treatment provided cosmetically and functionally better results than did closed treatment.[42] Complications in this series included skin breakdown, infection and secondary displacement. In contrast, Wehbe et al. reported 33% complication rate associated with surgical treatment of mallet injuries as opposed to a 9% rate with nonsurgical treatment, and therefore recommended nonsurgical treatment of the majority of mallet fractures.[43]

Complications

It has become a principle that stable fixation of phalangeal fractures enables early initiation of motion and maximizes the chance for a successful result.[22] Previous biomechanical studies in a phalangeal fracture model have revealed that plate fixation provides stability equal to or greater than that with K-wire and interosseous wiring.[44] Hence, plate fixation may offer substantial advantages because of its ability to control the anatomic alignment of fractures and allow early joint mobilization. Some investigators, however, have shown that a stable construct is but one of many determinants of outcome.[45] The severity of the fracture (comminution and articular involvement), soft tissue damage, poor reduction, poor fixation, surgical trauma and inadequate postoperative management are the main factors adversely affecting functional outcome.[46]

A disadvantage of plate fixation of phalanges is that they are bulky and may interfere with the excursion of the tendon apparatus. Some have suggested that this problem may outweigh the advantage of a stable plate fixation and that closed methods frequently offer a worthwhile alternative.[5] In recent years, technical advancements have been made with the use of mini-fragment plates, as well as the introduction of titanium plates with improved design and lower profile that interfere less with tendon gliding.[47] Despite the advances in plate profile, design and instrumentation, plate fixation of phalangeal fractures can be fraught with complications and unsatisfactory results.[24] For assessing the complications, the classification of Page and Stern is frequently used.[24] This defines any significant functional deficit or complication, such as ROM less than 180°, complex regional pain syndrome, infections and additional surgery including tenolysis.

Studies of plate fixation of phalangeal fractures have reported mixed results.[10,48] Kurzen et al. retrospectively reviewed 54 consecutive patients with 64 phalangeal fractures treated by open reduction and plate fixation (condylar plates, low profile included low profile titanium straight plates and T plates).[49] There was no difference if a dorsal tendon-splitting approach or a midaxial approach (28% stiffness with a midaxial approach vs 37% stiffness with dorsal approach) was used. Fifteen patients claimed persistent pain in the affected finger or the hand in general (27%). Page et al. encountered major complications in 36% of phalanx fractures, especially with open fractures, despite stable fixation and early mobilization.[24] Stiffness was the most frequent complication. The total combined complication rate for periarticular and intra-articular fractures was significantly higher than that for extra-articular diaphyseal fractures. Similarly, Page and Stern showed that the complication rate for periarticular fractures was higher than that for diaphyseal fractures.[24] Comminuted periarticular fractures of the phalangeal bones are difficult to manage in terms of restoration of finger movement.[50] Omokawa et al. prospectively evaluated clinical results for ORIF of unstable metaphyseal phalangeal fractures using a mini-titanium plate.[51] Statistical analysis revealed that patient age, intra-articular involvement and associated soft tissue injury significantly affected the range of finger motion at one year follow-up.

Malunion

Proximal phalangeal fracture malunion with volar angulation deformity may result in bone shortening, pseudoclaw deformity and a decrease in ROM of the joints of the finger, especially when the angle of deformity is greater than 25-30°.[52] For each millimeter of shortening in the proximal phalanx, the PIP joint should experience 12° of extensor lag. Angulation produces similar effects with 16° of apex palmar angulation producing 10° of extensor lag, 27° of angulation producing 24° of lag, and 46° of angulation producing 66° of lag.[53]

Treatment for malunited fractures of the middle phalangeal base varies from waiting until pain prompts arthrodesis or joint replacement[54] to osteochondral arthroplasty.[55] Correction of these angular deformities has previously been achieved by either a closing wedge or an opening wedge osteotomy at the fracture site.[56] However, these procedures do not restore the length of the bone to its initial prefracture length. Open reduction with osteotomy and K-wire internal fixation with or without bone graft has been reported in the literature.[34] To view the entire malunited base of the middle phalanx, the authors propose the hyperextension volar approach used by Eaton and Malerich to perform arthroplasties (the shotgun approach) combined with a thorough manipulation of the malunited fragments to restore the joint congruency and avoid residual dorsal subluxation.[33] According to Ishida et al. restoring the volar buttress by osteotomy and elevation of the volar lip is important for a better outcome, but they found that elevation of central depressed fragments was not feasible in comminuted, chronic cases.[34]

del Pinal et al. presented their results in the treatment of late presenting impaction fractures of the base of the middle phalanx treated by osteotomy with full exposure of the articular surface to restore the normal anatomy.[57] The restoration of the cup-shape contour of the middle phalangeal base was accomplished by osteotomy and mobilization of small osteochondral fragments. Rigid fixation was performed by cerclage wire, screws or a combination of these. Favorable results have been achieved in this challenging scenario in the short and middle-term in nine of ten patients. Previous surgery and moderate to severe wearing of the cartilage of the proximal phalanx head negatively affected the results.

Stiffness

Apart from malunion or nonunion, the chief concern associated with a proximal phalanx fracture is loss of motion in the PIP joint. Stiffness is defined as total ROM arc (MCP, PIP, DIP) less than 180°.[24] Ip et al. reported that 29% of finger fractures in their prospective study were associated with flexor or extensor tendon adhesions.[58] The causes of restricted finger motion after extra-articular phalangeal fractures include flexor tendon adhesion, extensor tendon adhesion, joint contracture, skin contracture, malunion of the phalanges or a combination of these factors.[59] Flexor tendon adhesion tends to occur with fractures of the proximal and middle phalanges[37] and are associated with fracture malalignment or displacement,[37] volar angulation,[12] crush injury[37] and prolonged immobilization.[59]

Enhanced understanding of the biology of fracture healing, better decision-making in initial fracture management, technical advances in implant design, improved surgical skills with respect to gliding structures and early controlled mobilization have contributed to reducing the incidence of complications.[9] Phalangeal fractures respond more unfavorably to immobilization than metacarpal fractures, with a predicted 84% return of motion compared to 96% return in metacarpal fractures.[60] If immobilization is continued longer than four weeks, the motion return drops to 66%. When plate fixation is required in the proximal phalanx, the lateral approach is preferred both to minimize extensor tendon interference and for improved biomechanical stability.[44] It has even been suggested to resect the lateral band and intrinsic tendon on the side of the surgical approach to minimize subsequent hardware interference.[9]

The adhesions that develop and lead to limitation of ROM are widespread and not only adjacent to the fracture site.[21] The location and density of the adhesions are variable and unrelated to the fracture type, the immobilization period or the interval between fracture and tenolysis. Yamazaki et al. performed flexor tenolysis on 12 fingers after phalangeal fractures treated either conservatively or with OIRF.[61] The authors posted satisfactory results regardless of fracture type (comminuted or transverse), time to mobilization following the fracture or the interval from fracture to tenolysis in patients with reasonable preoperative mobility of the finger. Only the preoperative total passive motion of the digit affected the total active motion achieved by tenolysis.

Authors' Preferred Management of Select Complications

Case 1: Malunion

A 51-year-old-female incurred a small finger fracture that was treated non-operatively. They presented six months after her injury for persistent finger malalignment and decreased grip strength (Figs 1.22A to F). Examination identified a healed fracture of the small finger proximal phalanx with overlapping of her small finger over the ring finger. She was diagnosed with a rotational malunion of the small finger proximal phalanx malunion. The patient was offered a corrective osteotomy.

Malunions are common with phalangeal fractures and can result in either an angular or rotational deformity. Minimal fracture malalignment can result in significant malunion. Treatment is based upon identifying the site of deformity and its subsequent correction. Rotational deformity is corrected with a transverse osteotomy perpendicular to the axis of rotation. In contrast, angular deformity requires an opening or closing wedge osteotomy. A closing wedge osteotomy is technically easier and heals more reliably; however, it risks shortening the moment arm of the extensor mechanism that can lead to an extensor lag.

Technique

A regional block is applied and the patient is sedated. To minimize tendon manipulation a midaxial incision is utilized. The lateral band of the extensor tendon is identified and retracted dorsally. The site of the malunion is typically

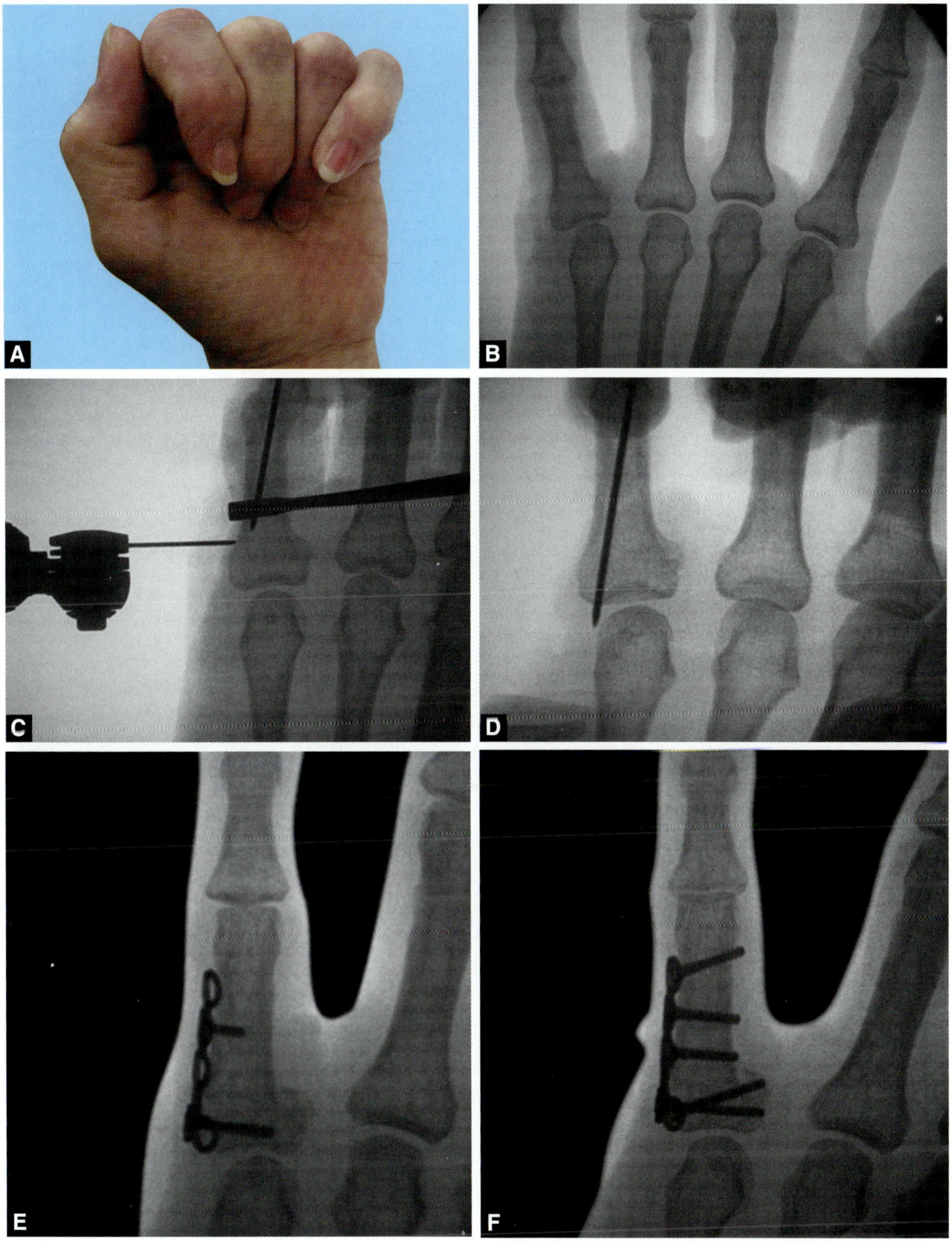

Figures 1.22A to F: This is a 51-year-old female, who presented with a small finger proximal phalanx malunion resulting in a rotational deformity of the finger. The patient underwent an osteotomy at the base of the proximal phalanx perpendicular to the longitudinal axis of the phalanx. The finger was derotated and pinned in a reduced position. A locking plate was applied that was initially fixed in standard compression utilizing non-locking screws above and below the osteotomy site followed by the placement of locking screws.

Courtesy: Asif M Ilyas

selected as the site of correction. A transverse osteotomy is placed perpendicular to the longitudinal axis of the phalanx. The finger is derotated and provisionally pinned in place. A 2.0 mm plate is applied laterally and fixed in compression. A minimum of two if not three screws are placed above and below the osteotomy site. The surgeons prefer to utilize locking screws, if possible to increase the stiffness of the construct after the osteotomy site is compressed. Prior to ending the case, normal rotation of the finger must be confirmed. Closure is performed in standard fashion. Rehabilitation is initiated utilizing standard ORIF protocol.

Case 2: Stiffness

A 42-year-old right-hand dominant male, who presented following a fall. His main complaint was pain and deformity over the MP joint of his dominant small finger. On evaluation, he was found to have an obvious rotational deformity of the small finger. Radiographs revealed the presence of an unstable and displaced small finger proximal phalangeal base fracture (Figs 1.23A to D). Surgical repair was recommended and ORIF was performed through a dorsal tendon splitting approach to the proximal phalanx using locking mini

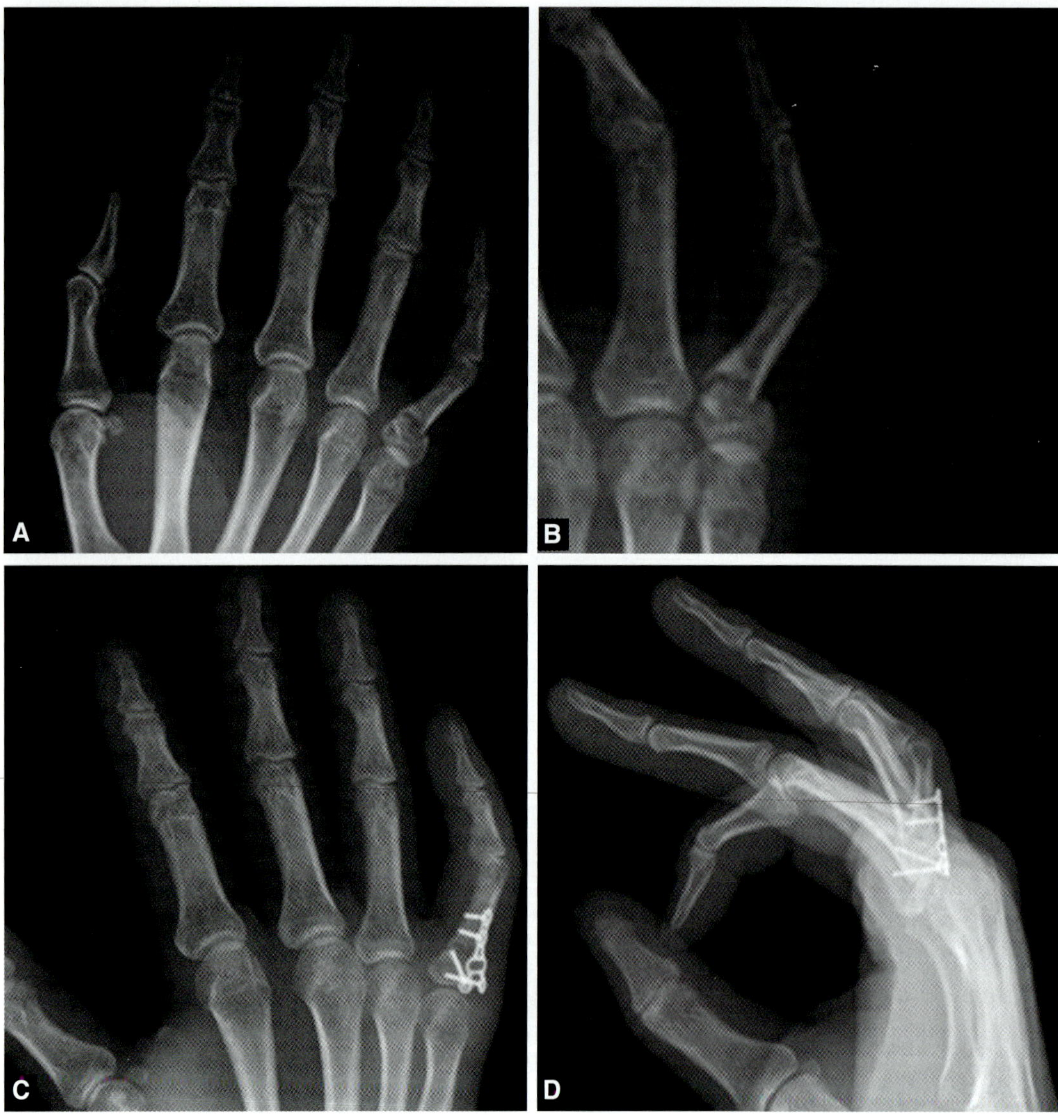

Figures 1.23A to D: This is a 42-year-old male, who presented with a small finger proximal phalanx fracture that was treated with open reduction and internal fixation. The patient developed persistent stiffness and subsequently, underwent removal of hardware, tenolysis and metacarpophalangeal joint capsulotomy.

plate and screws. The patient had an uneventful post-operative course including immobilization for two weeks followed by supervised therapy and the use of a protective ulnar gutter intrinsic plus splint. However, the patient experienced extensive swelling and stiffness despite diligent therapy, and by four months post-operatively the patient's arc of active MP joint motion was 20–30° and active PIP joint motion was 30–60°.

Joint stiffness is common following finger fracture fixation due to a combination of factors including tendon adhesions, joint contractures and skin contractures. Early management of stiffness is aimed at prevention. Modalities to prevent stiffness include early motion, tendon gliding and aggressive anti-edema measures. However, assuming the fracture is well-healed, surgical management for stiffness can be entertained three months or more after surgery and after therapy is no longer of benefit. The authors recommend removal of hardware, joint releases and tendon tenolysis.

Technique

A regional block is applied and the patient is sedated. The authors recommend utilizing the same incision used previously. The tendon is carefully split and the hardware removed. Typically, the extensor tendon will be quite adherent to the bone. Dissection using a freer or a tenolysis blade is used to elevate the tendon from the bone. Care must be taken not to injure the central slip distally. Tenolysis is completed once passive flexion of the finger results in independent motion between the bone and the tendon. Lastly, a joint release can be performed. The joints typically involved are either the MP or PIP joints. A contracted joint is confirmed by the presence of equal motion despite passive or active joint manipulation. In this case, the MP joint was contracted. The longitudinal extensor tendon split is extended proximally. The dorsal capsule is elevated from the extensor mechanism. A transverse dorsal capsulotomy is performed. The collateral ligaments are next approached and are sectioned slowly in a stepwise fashion until full passive MP joint flexion is achieved. Prior to closure, the patient is awakened and asked to actively range the finger to confirm adequate releases have been performed. Once satisfied, the wounds are closed and soft compression dressings are applied. Therapy is initiated within 48 hours after surgery with instructions to proceed with aggressive range of motion, tendon gliding and anti-edema modalities.

Summary

Phalangeal fractures are an extremely complex and diverse group of injuries. The treatment of each fracture is dependent on many variables, including location, stability and reducibility and associated soft tissue injuries. When managing these fractures, it is important to consider the overall functional goals. Surgeons have to balance the advantages and disadvantages of various surgical techniques to best treat individual patients.

References

1. Chung KC, Spilson SV. The frequency and epidemiology of hand and forearm fractures in the United States. J Hand Surg Am. 2001;26(5):908-15.
2. van Onselen EB, Karim RB, Hage JJ, et al. Prevalence and distribution of hand fractures. J Hand Surg Br. 2003;28(5): 491-5.
3. Perron AD, Brady WJ, Keats TE, et al. Orthopedic pitfalls in the emergency department: closed tendon injuries of the hand. Am J Emerg Med. 2001;19(1):76-80.
4. Henry MH. Fractures of the proximal phalanx and metacarpals in the hand: preferred methods of stabilization. J Am Acad Orthop Surg. 2008;16(10):586-95.
5. Kozin SH, Thoder JJ, Lieberman G. Operative treatment of metacarpal and phalangeal shaft fractures. J Am Acad Orthop Surg. 2000;8(2):111-21.
6. Bailie DS, Benson LS, Marymont JV. Proximal interphalangeal joint injuries of the hand. Part I: anatomy and diagnosis. Am J Orthop (Belle Mead NJ). 1996;25(7):474-7.
7. Chamay A. A distally-based dorsal and triangular tendinous flap for direct access to the proximal interphalangeal joint. Ann Chir Main. 1988;7(2):179-83.
8. Horton TC, Hatton M, Davis TR. A prospective randomized controlled study of fixation of long oblique and spiral shaft fractures of the proximal phalanx: closed reduction and percutaneous Kirschner wiring versus open reduction and lag screw fixation. J Hand Surg Br. 2003;28(1):5-9.
9. Freeland AE, Sud V, Lindley SG. Unilateral intrinsic resection of the lateral band and oblique fibers of the metacarpophalangeal joint for proximal phalangeal fracture. Tech Hand Up Extrem Surg. 2001;5(2):85-90.
10. Dabezies EJ, Schutte JP. Fixation of metacarpal and phalangeal fractures with miniature plates and screws. J Hand Surg Am. 1986;11(2):283-8.
11. Faccioli N, Foti G, Barillari M, et al. Finger fractures imaging: accuracy of cone-beam computed tomography and

multislice computed tomography. Skeletal Radiol. 2010; 39(11): 1087-95.

12. Coonrad RW, Pohlman MH. Impacted fractures in the proximal portion of the proximal phalanx of the finger. J Bone Joint Surg Am. 1969;51(7):1291-6.
13. Schreibman KL, Freeland A, Gilula LA, et al. Imaging of the hand and wrist. Orthop Clin North Am. 1997;28(4):537-82.
14. Lazar RD, Waters PM, Jaramillo D. The use of ultrasonography in the diagnosis of occult fracture of the radial neck. A case report. J Bone Joint Surg Am. 1998; 80(9):1361-4.
15. Marshburn TH, Legome E, Sargsyan A, et al. Goal-directed ultrasound in the detection of long-bone fractures. J Trauma. 2004;57(2):329-32.
16. Tayal VS, Antoniazzi J, Pariyadath M, et al. Prospective use of ultrasound imaging to detect bony hand injuries in adults. J Ultrasound Med. 2007;26(9):1143-8.
17. Stern PJ. Management of fractures of the hand over the last 25 years. J Hand Surg Am. 2000;25(5):817-23.
18. Tencer AF, Johnson KD, Kyle RF, et al. Biomechanics of fractures and fracture fixation. Instr Course Lect. 1993;42:19-55.
19. Freeland AE. External fixation for skeletal stabilization of severe open fractures of the hand. Clin Orthop Relat Res. 1987;(214):93-100.
20. Black DM, Mann RJ, Constine RM, et al. The stability of internal fixation in the proximal phalanx. J Hand Surg Am. 1986;11(5):672-7.
21. Green DP, Anderson JR. Closed reduction and percutaneous pin fixation of fractured phalanges. J Bone Joint Surg Am. 1973;55(8):1651-4.
22. Hastings H. Unstable metacarpal and phalangeal fracture treatment with screws and plates. Clin Orthop Relat Res. 1987;(214):37-52.
23. Barton NJ. Fractures of the hand. J Bone Joint Surg Br. 1984;66(2):159-67.
24. Page SM, Stern PJ. Complications and range of motion following plate fixation of metacarpal and phalangeal fractures. J Hand Surg Am. 1998;23(5):827-32.
25. Hardy MA. Principles of metacarpal and phalangeal fracture management: a review of rehabilitation concepts. J Orthop Sports Phys Ther. 2004;34(12):781-99.
26. London PS. Sprains and fractures involving the interphalangeal joints. Hand. 1971;3(2):155-8.
27. Glickel SZ, Barron OA. Proximal interphalangeal joint fracture dislocations. Hand Clin. 2000;16(3):333-44.
28. Williams RM, Kiefhaber TR, Sommerkamp TG, et al. Treatment of unstable dorsal proximal interphalangeal fracture/dislocations using a hemi-hamate autograft. J Hand Surg Am. 2003;28(5):856-65.
29. Ellis SJ, Cheng R, Prokopis P, et al. Treatment of proximal interphalangeal dorsal fracture-dislocation injuries with dynamic external fixation: a pins and rubber band system. J Hand Surg Am. 2007;32(8):1242-50.
30. Dionysian E, Eaton RG. The long-term outcome of volar plate arthroplasty of the proximal interphalangeal joint. J Hand Surg Am. 2000;25(3):429-37.
31. Twyman RS, David HG. The doorstop procedure. A technique for treating unstable fracture dislocations of the proximal interphalangeal joint. J Hand Surg Br. 1993; 18(6):714-5.
32. Ruland RT, Hogan CJ, Cannon DL, et al. Use of dynamic distraction external fixation for unstable fracture-dislocations of the proximal interphalangeal joint. J Hand Surg Am. 2008;33(1):19-25.
33. Eaton RG, Malerich MM. Volar plate arthroplasty of the proximal interphalangeal joint: a review of ten years' experience. J Hand Surg Am. 1980;5(3):260-8.
34. Ishida O, Ikuta Y. Results of treatment of chronic dorsal fracture-dislocations of the proximal interphalangeal joints of the fingers. J Hand Surg Br. 1998;23(6):798-801.
35. Capo JT, Hastings H, Choung E, et al. Hemicondylar hamate replacement arthroplasty for proximal interphalangeal joint fracture dislocations: an assessment of graft suitability. J Hand Surg Am. 2008;33(5):733-9.
36. Calfee RP, Kiefhaber TR, Sommerkamp TG, et al. Hemi-hamate arthroplasty provides functional reconstruction of acute and chronic proximal interphalangeal fracture-dislocations. J Hand Surg Am. 2009;34(7):1232-41.
37. Agee J. Treatment principles for proximal and middle phalangeal fractures. Orthop Clin North Am. 1992; 23(1): 35-40.
38. Cannon NM. Rehabilitation approaches for distal and middle phalanx fractures of the hand. J Hand Ther. 2003; 16(2):105-16.
39. Bischoff R, Buechler U, De RR, et al. Clinical results of tension band fixation of avulsion fractures of the hand. J Hand Surg Am. 1994;19(6):1019-26.
40. Ishiguro T, Itoh Y, Yabe Y, et al. Extension block with Kirschner wire for fracture dislocation of the distal inter-phalangeal joint. Tech Hand Up Extrem Surg. 1997;1(2):95-102.
41. Yamanaka K, Sasaki T. Treatment of mallet fractures using compression fixation pins. J Hand Surg Br. 1999;24(3):358-60.
42. Lubahn JD. Mallet finger fractures: a comparison of open and closed technique. J Hand Surg Am. 1989;14(2 Pt 2):394-6.
43. Wehbe MA, Schneider LH. Mallet fractures. J Bone Joint Surg Am. 1984;66(5):658-69.
44. Lu WW, Furumachi K, Ip WY, et al. Fixation for comminuted phalangeal fractures. A biomechanical study of five methods. J Hand Surg Br. 1996;21(6):765-7.

45. Duncan RW, Freeland AE, Jabaley ME, et al. Open hand fractures: an analysis of the recovery of active motion and of complications. J Hand Surg Am. 1993;18(3):387-94.
46. Pun WK, Chow SP, So YC, et al. Unstable phalangeal fractures: treatment by A.O. screw and plate fixation. J Hand Surg Am. 1991;16(1):113-7.
47. Lins RE, Myers BS, Spinner RJ, et al. A comparative mechanical analysis of plate fixation in a proximal phalangeal fracture model. J Hand Surg Am. 1996;21(6):1059-64.
48. Stern PJ, Wieser MJ, Reilly DG. Complications of plate fixation in the hand skeleton. Clin Orthop Relat Res. 1987;(214):59-65.
49. Kurzen P, Fusetti C, Bonaccio M, et al. Complications after plate fixation of phalangeal fractures. J Trauma. 2006; 60(4): 841-3.
50. Tan V, Beredjiklian PK, Weiland AJ. Intra-articular fractures of the hand: treatment by open reduction and internal fixation. J Orthop Trauma. 2005;19(8):518-23.
51. Omokawa S, Fujitani R, Dohi Y, et al. Prospective outcomes of comminuted periarticular metacarpal and phalangeal fractures treated using a titanium plate system. J Hand Surg Am. 2008;33(6):857-63.
52. Lee SG, Jupiter JB. Phalangeal and metacarpal fractures of the hand. Hand Clin. 2000;16(3):323-32, vii.
53. Vahey JW, Wegner DA, Hastings H. Effect of proximal phalangeal fracture deformity on extensor tendon function. J Hand Surg Am. 1998;23(4):673-81.
54. Peimer CA. Silicone rubber implant arthroplasty of MP joint in rheumatoid arthritis. J Hand Surg Am. 1987;12(1):154.
55. Ishida O, Ikuta Y, Kuroki H. Ipsilateral osteochondral grafting for finger joint repair. J Hand Surg Am. 1994;19(3):372-7.
56. Seitz WH, Jr, Froimson AI. Management of malunited fractures of the metacarpal and phalangeal shafts. Hand Clin. 1988;4(3):529-36.
57. Del PF, Garcia-Bernal FJ, Delgado J, et al. Results of osteotomy, open reduction, and internal fixation for late-presenting malunited intra-articular fractures of the base of the middle phalanx. J Hand Surg Am. 2005;30(5):1039.e1-14.
58. Ip WY, Ng KH, Chow SP. A prospective study of 924 digital fractures of the hand. Injury. 1996;27(4):279-85.
59. Schneider LH. Tenolysis and capsulectomy after hand fractures. Clin Orthop Relat Res. 1996;(327):72-8.
60. Shehadi SI. External fixation of metacarpal and phalangeal fractures. J Hand Surg Am. 1991;16(3):544-50.
61. Yamazaki H, Kato H, Uchiyama S, et al. Results of tenolysis for flexor tendon adhesion after phalangeal fracture. J Hand Surg Eur Vol. 2008;33(5):557-60.

Chapter 2

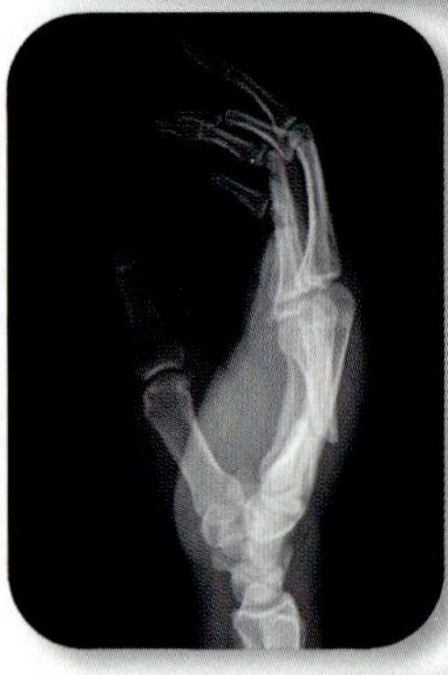

Metacarpal Fractures and Carpometacarpal Fracture-Dislocations

Charles Leinberry, Uzoma Ukomadu, Asif Ilyas

Chapter Outline

Introduction
Diagnosis
Classification
Surgical Indications
- Metacarpal Fractures
- Basal Thumb Metacarpal Fractures

Surgical Anatomy, Positioning and Approaches
- Surgical Anatomy
- Patient Positioning
- Surgical Approaches

Surgical Techniques
- Technique 1: Metacarpal Head Fractures: Screw Fixation
- Technique 2: Metacarpal Neck, Shaft or Base Fractures: Closed Reduction and Pinning
- Technique 3: Metacarpal Neck Fractures: Plate and Screw Fixation
- Technique 4: Metacarpal Shaft and Base Fractures: Plate and Screw Fixation
- Technique 5: Thumb Metacarpal Base Intra-articular 'Bennett' Fractures: Closed Reduction and Pinning
- Technique 6: Thumb Metacarpal Base Intra-articular 'Bennett' Fractures: Plate and Screw Fixation

Outcomes
Complications
Authors' Preferred Management of Select Complications
- Case 1: Finger Stiffness
- Case 2: Tendon Rupture

Summary

Introduction

Metacarpal fractures are among the most common fractures of the hand. The incidence is approximately 1.5 million injuries per year and is thought to represent up to 40% of all hand fractures.[1] Common etiologies include force imparted by an axial load or by direct trauma to the hand as is manifested by punching injuries or breaking a fall with one's hands. The far majority of metacarpal fractures are isolated fractures, most commonly involving the fifth metacarpal neck, but fractures of other metacarpals are also very common (Fig. 2.1).

Thumb metacarpal fractures account for nearly a quarter of all metacarpal fractures and represent the second most frequently injured metacarpal after the small finger. Fractures of the distal portion of the thumb metacarpal are rare, in fact the vast majority (> 80%) of fractures of the thumb metacarpal take place in the proximal metadiaphyseal region.[1] These fractures are usually caused by axially directed forces to the base of the thumb.

Fracture-dislocations at the carpometacarpal (CMC) joint are also commonly seen with hand trauma. These

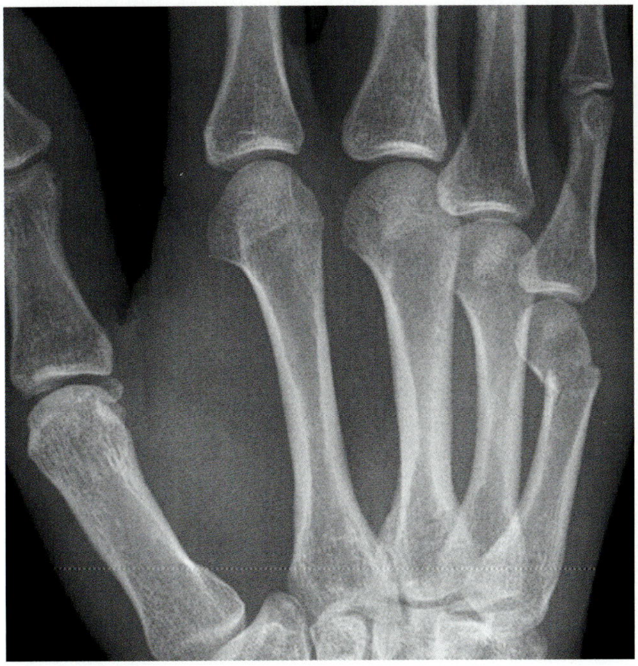

Figure 2.1: Isolated fifth metacarpal neck fracture.

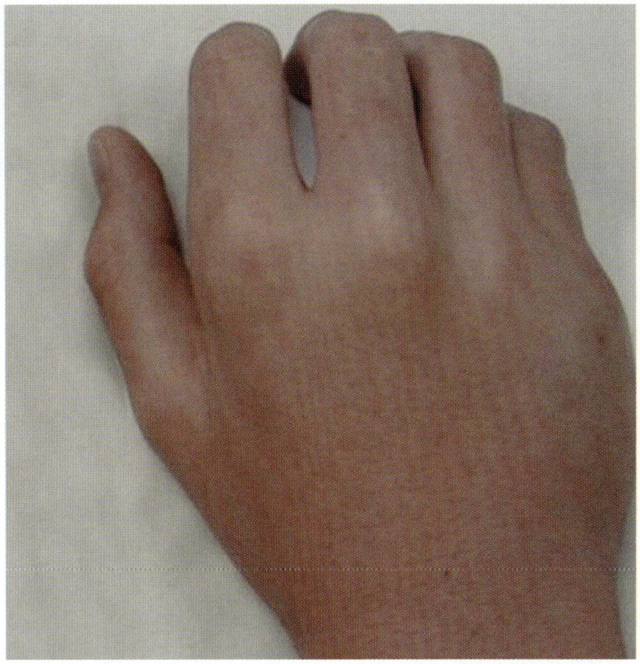

Figure 2.2: Inspection of the hand during the physical examination identifies ecchymosis and blunting or decreased prominence of the fifth metacarpal head, consistent with the fifth metacarpal neck fracture.

injuries typically result from a high axial load applied to the metacarpal head in a full fist position resulting in load transmission to the metacarpal base and CMC joint.

Diagnosis

A thorough history should be taken eliciting the mechanism of injury and history of previous fractures in the hand. The physical examination should begin with inspection focusing on swelling, bruising, ecchymosis, wounds or lacerations. Metacarpal neck fractures are commonly associated with open wounds and blunting of the corresponding metacarpal head (Fig. 2.2). In particular, open wounds around the metacarpophalangeal (MP) joints may represent an open fracture.

Furthermore, rotation and alignment of the fingers are assessed. Finger alignment may appear normal on extension, but upon flexion, malrotation may become evident (Fig. 2.3). If the patient is unable to actively flex the fingers, gentle passive flexion can be performed to identify the rotation of the fingers. In flexion, all fingertips should point to the distal pole of the scaphoid.

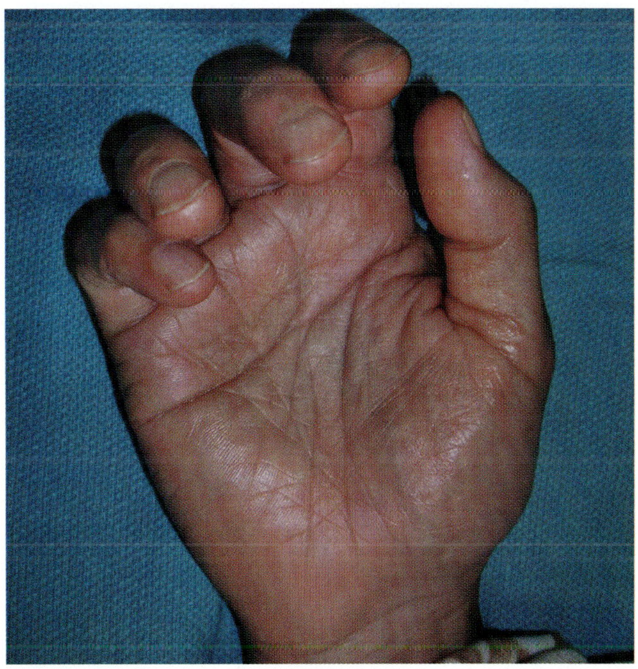

Figure 2.3: Note the external rotation of the ring finger with the fingers held in passive flexion. The patient had incurred an isolated ring finger metacarpal fracture.

Imaging studies are critical and can readily provide the diagnosis. The standard three-view radiographs should be performed including posteroanterior (PA), lateral and

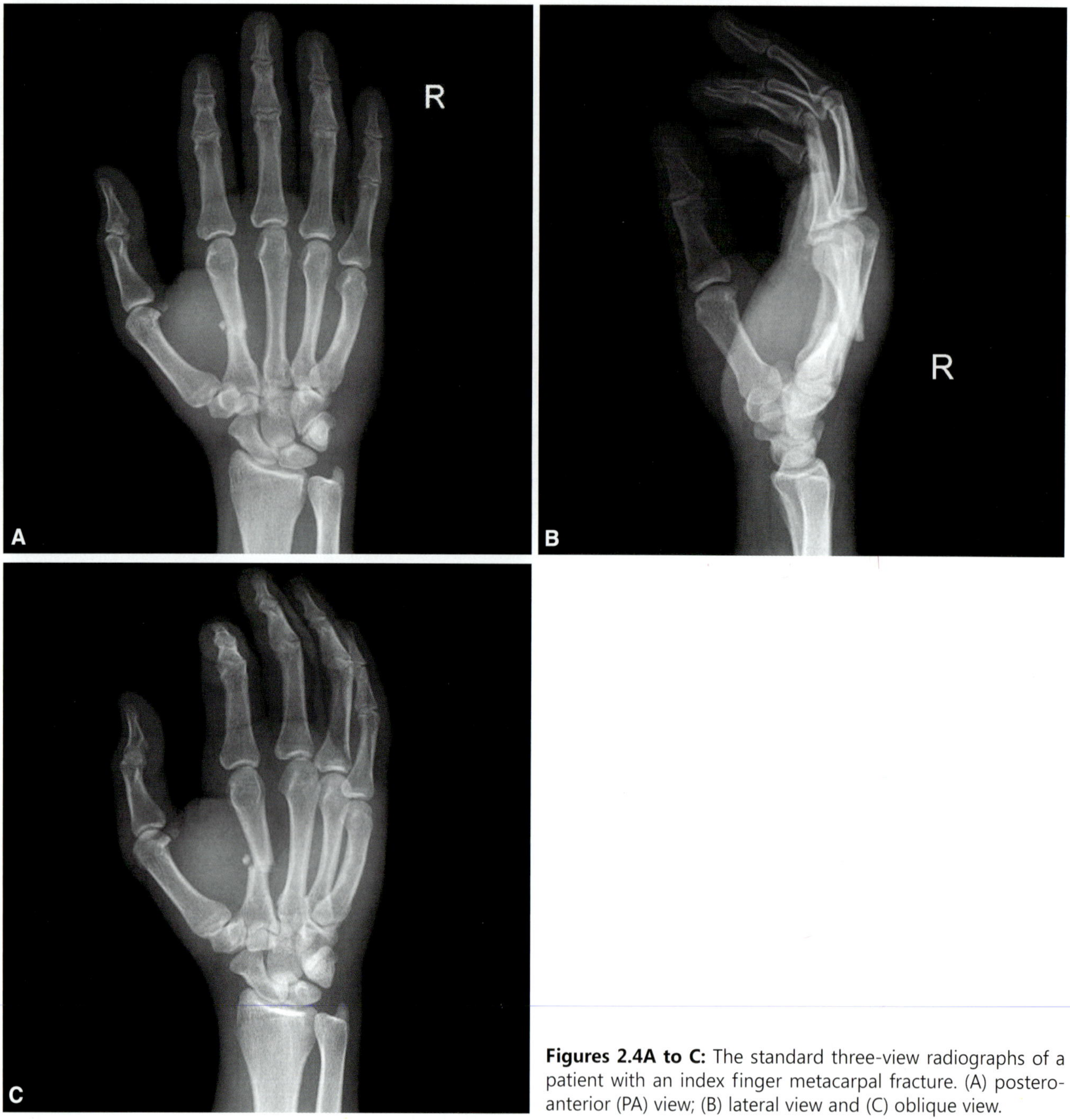

Figures 2.4A to C: The standard three-view radiographs of a patient with an index finger metacarpal fracture. (A) postero-anterior (PA) view; (B) lateral view and (C) oblique view.

oblique views (Figs 2.4A to C). Fractures are typically evident on radiographs, but occasionally, minimally displaced fractures may be subtle and only be evident on a single view. In addition, depending on the clinical suspicion, certain special views can be obtained. These views include the Brewerton view, which requires the MP joint to be flexed at 65° with the dorsum of the fingers lying flat on the X-ray plate and the tube angled 15° ulnar to radial. Computed tomography (CT) scanning can also be used and is best indicated for assessing intra-articular fractures such as of the metacarpal head or CMC joints (Figs 2.5A and B).

The standard maxim of performing a thorough physical examination as previously discussed is also applicable while evaluating the thumb metacarpal fracture. However, given

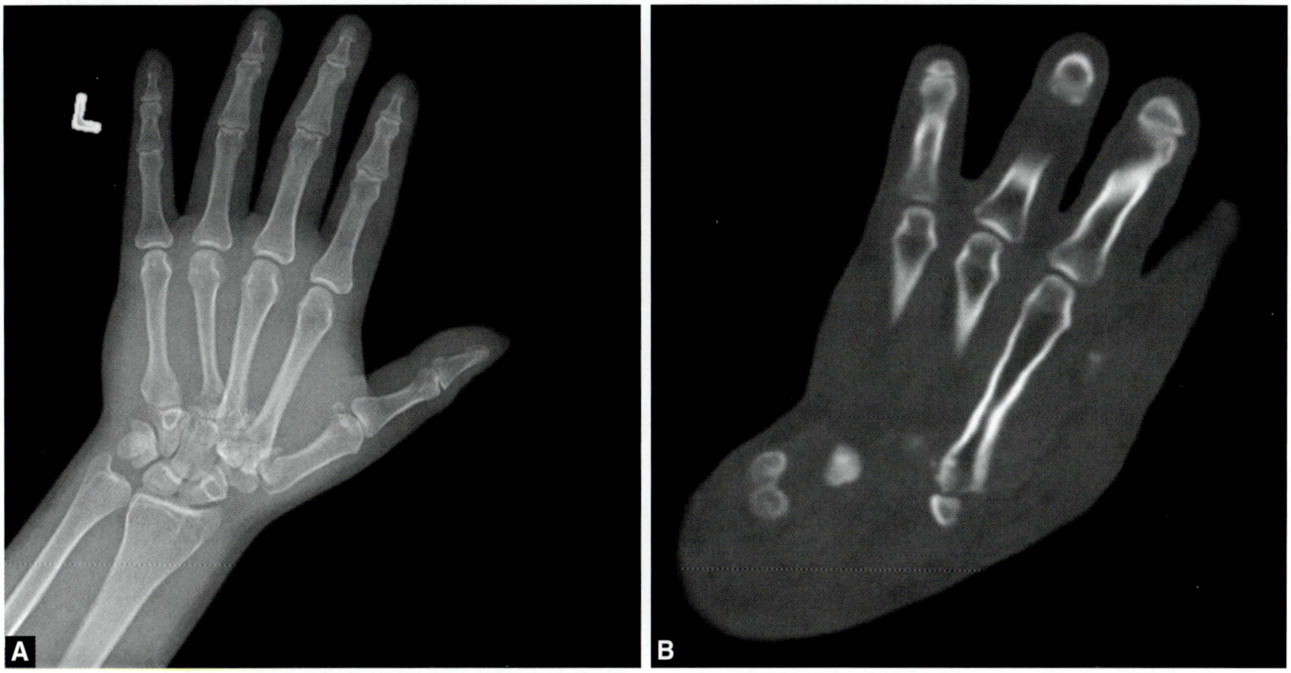

Figures 2.5A and B: A patient, who incurred a high-energy injury to the hand. Note the index metacarpal fracture-dislocation on (A) X-ray and (B) CT scan.

the oblique nature of the thumb metacarpal relative to the rest of the hand, proper imaging becomes even more critical. Here, true orthogonal views of the thumb (as opposed to the hand) require different positioning in order to fully appreciate the fracture anatomy. The true anteroposterior (AP) view is obtained by having the forearm pronated with the dorsum of the thumb lying on the X-ray cassette. A true lateral view is obtained by pronating the hand on the X-ray cassette and angling the X-ray source 10° from the vertical going from distal to proximal.

METACARPAL FRACTURES AND CARPOMETACARPAL FRACTURE-DISLOCATIONS DIAGNOSIS: Pearls and Pitfalls

- Scrutinize the hand for swelling, ecchymosis and open wounds. In particular, open wounds around the MP joint may indicate an open fracture
- Assessment of finger rotation is critical and is best assessed with active finger flexion, with comparison to the contralateral side. If active motion is not tolerated, attempt gentle passive flexion or passive wrist tenodesis. All fingers should point to the scaphoid with flexion
- Fractures are readily identified with the standard three radiographic views; however subtle injuries may only be identified on a single view. Advanced imaging such as CT scanning can be utilized but are best reserved for articular injuries

Classification

The classification of metacarpal fractures relies less on a standardized schema than it does on the location that guides general fracture description. As such metacarpal fracture classification is usually descriptive taking into account the following fracture qualities: location, pattern, morphology, displacement and skin integrity (Table 2.1). The classification parameters can further be divided into displaced versus nondisplaced fractures, stable versus unstable fractures, and reducible versus irreducible fractures.

Table 2.1: Classification of metacarpal fracture

Location	Base, shaft, neck, head
Pattern	Transverse, oblique, spiral
Morphology	Comminuted, segmented, wedge
Displacement	Angulation, shortening, translation, rotation
Skin Integrity	Open, closed

Basal thumb metacarpal fractures are classified into one of four types: (1) epibasal; (2) Bennett's; (3) Rolando's and (4) comminuted (Figs 2.6A to D). Thumb epibasal fractures are extra-articular fractures that occur in the proximal portion of the thumb metacarpal in a transverse or oblique pattern. Bennett's and Rolando fractures represent the two most common variations of intra-articular basal thumb metacarpal fractures (Figs 2.7A and B).

Bennett's fractures are two-part intra-articular fractures of the thumb metacarpal base. This fracture type consists of a volar-ulnar fragment called the Bennett's fragment, which is held in place by the anterior oblique ligament. The remainder of the metacarpal is pulled into a radial, dorsally subluxed, and shortened position by the pull of the abductor pollicis longus (APL) tendon.

Rolando's fractures of the thumb are classically described as three-part fractures that have a T- or Y-shaped configuration. However, the term is commonly used to describe all comminuted basal thumb metacarpal fractures. In addition to the fracture fragments found in the Bennett's fracture, the Rolando's fracture pattern also typically has an APL tendon avulsion fracture.

Fracture-dislocations at the CMC joint are usually classified and named by the involved metacarpal and direction of the CMC dislocation. Most commonly encountered is an isolated dislocation of the small metacarpal at the CMC joint. Often, a portion of the carpus

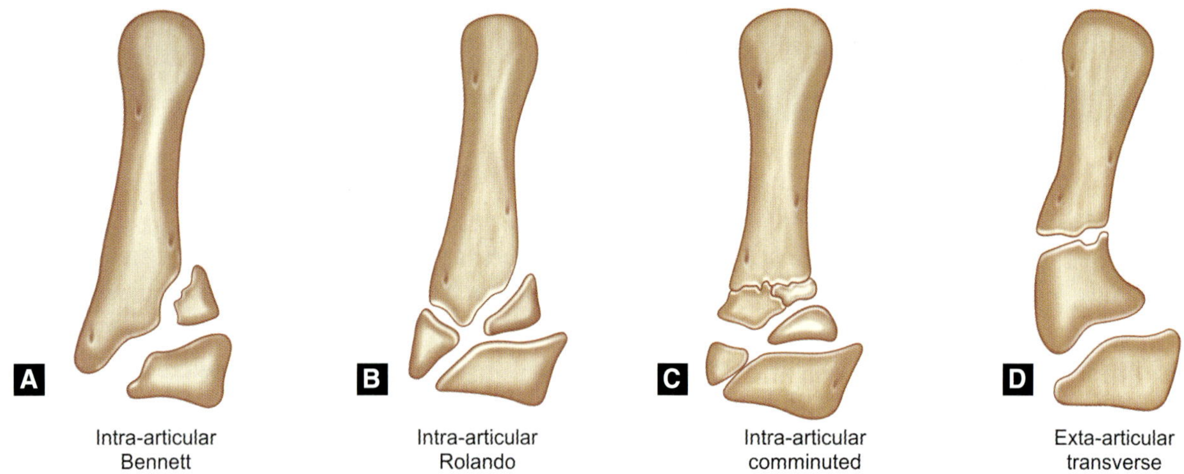

Figures 2.6A to D: Basal thumb metacarpal fractures are classified into one of the four types: (A) Bennett's; (B) Rolando's; (C) comminuted and (D) epibasal or extra-articular.

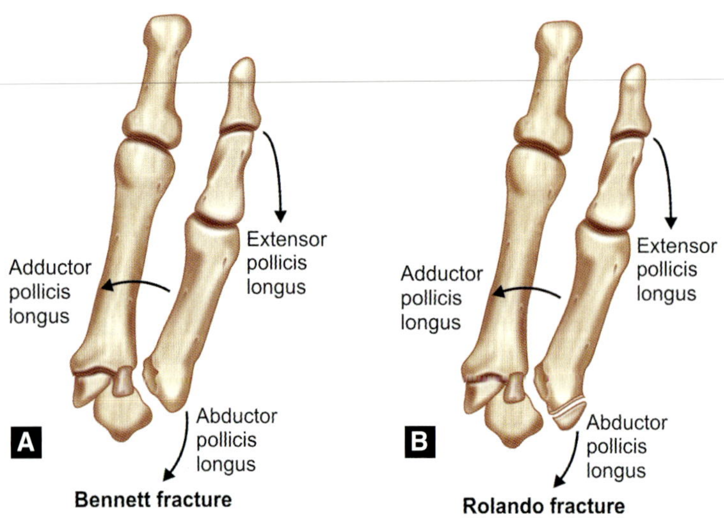

Figures 2.7A and B: Intra-articular basal thumb metacarpal fractures represent a continuity of injuries that are the product of deforming forces created by the abductor pollicis longus, extensor pollicis longus, and adductor pollicis longus tendons.

is also fractured in this injury pattern (e.g. fracture of the dorsal aspect of the hamate with dislocation of the ring or small metacarpals). Beyond recognizing the location of the fracture and the direction of the dislocation, the most important descriptive term is whether the injury is stable or not.

Surgical Indications

The surgical indications of metacarpal fractures are variable and are best divided by the location: head, neck, shaft or base. Surgical indications for basal thumb metacarpal fractures and CMC fractures are based upon fracture pattern and the extent of displacement.

Metacarpal Fractures

Surgical indications of metacarpal head fractures include more than 1 mm of displacement and/or any impediment to MP joint motion. Furthermore, "fight bite" fractures represent open fractures and warrant surgical intervention in the form of irrigation, debridement and fracture fixation.

Metacarpal neck fractures most commonly involve the fifth metacarpal and in the far majority of cases they can be treated nonoperatively. As malrotation is uncommon with metacarpal neck fractures, the primary indication is fracture angulation. Apex dorsal angulation greater than the following can be considered for surgical fixation:

- 15° for the index finger metacarpal neck fracture
- 25° for the middle finger metacarpal neck fracture
- 35° for the ring finger metacarpal neck fracture
- 45° for the small finger metacarpal neck fracture

Greater angulation is well-tolerated among the ulnar digits. In contrast, angulation is poorly tolerated in the index and middle finger metacarpals due to compromise of grip strength, volar prominence of the metacarpal head within the clenched fist, dorsal soft tissue compromise and extensor tendon entrapment. Treatment options include closed versus open reduction and pinning, intramedullary fixation, open reduction internal fixation with interfragmentary compression screws or with plate and screws.

Surgical indications for metacarpal shaft fracture depend on a number of variables including rotation, angulation, shortening, instability and multiplicity. Because of the strong intermetacarpal ligaments proximally and distally, instability and deformity are greater with the border index and small finger metacarpals and less with the middle and ring finger metacarpals. Surgical indications include:

- Any significant malrotation of the finger, either internal or external
- Angulation of greater than 10° for the index and middle, 20° for the ring and 30° for the small finger metacarpal shaft
- Shortening of greater than 3 mm
- Extensive comminution, particularly in the border metacarpals
- Multiple metacarpal fractures

Treatment options include closed versus open reduction and pinning, intramedullary fixation, open reduction internal fixation with interfragmentary compression screws or with plate and screws.

Surgical indications for metacarpal base fractures are similar to shaft fractures. However, base fractures are susceptible to the deforming forces of tendon insertions. The index and middle finger metacarpals are often displaced dorsally and shortened by the extensor carpi radialis longus (ECRL) and extensor carpi radialis brevis (ECRB) tendons, respectively. The small finger metacarpals may be displaced by the extensor carpi ulnaris (ECU) tendon insertion. Treatment options include closed versus open reduction and pinning, and open reduction internal fixation with plate and screws.

Basal Thumb Metacarpal Fractures

Surgical indications for extra-articular basal thumb metacarpal fractures are dependent on fracture angulation, displacement and instability. Although fracture deformity is better tolerated in the thumb ray, maintaining a reduction with closed treatment is often difficult to maintain. The distal fragment is susceptible to a number of deforming forces, including flexion and adduction caused by the flexor pollicis brevis (FPB) and adductor pollicis, and shortening caused by the extensor pollicis longus (EPL) and extensor pollicis brevis (EPB). Surgical indications include:

- Any significant malrotation, most commonly excessive pronation
- Angulation greater than 30° on the coronal plane
- Extensive comminution with shortening greater than 3 mm

Intra-articular basal thumb metacarpal fractures, including the Bennett's, Rolando's and comminuted types are all best treated operatively in order to counter the deforming forces, restore normal length to the thumb ray and reduce the trapeziometacarpal joint. Treatment options include closed versus open reduction and pinning and open reduction internal fixation with plate and screws. However, due to the often small nature of the articular fragments, indirect fracture reduction and distraction pinning or external fixation can also be utilized for intra-articular basal thumb metacarpal fractures.

Surgical Anatomy, Positioning and Approaches

Surgical Anatomy

The metacarpals have the shape of a traditional long bone, with prominent articular surfaces proximally and distally, a metaphyseal region consisting of the neck and base, and a middle diaphyseal region consisting of the shaft with strong cortical bone and a true intramedullary canal. The metacarpals are protected by a thick soft tissue envelope. Dorsally, the metacarpals are nearly subcutaneous and are covered only by their periosteum and the extensor tendons. As such, surgical exposure is routinely performed dorsally. The metacarpal head is spherical and bows volarly. It articulates with the base of the proximal phalanx and forms a multiaxial condyloid joint. The collateral ligaments provide varus-valgus restraint to the proximal phalanx and, along with the volar plate, also prevent its volar subluxation. Furthermore, the vascular supply to the distal metacarpal follows the collateral ligaments and enters at their sites of origin. Both proximally and distally, strong transverse intermetacarpal ligaments join one metacarpal to the other.

The metacarpals are naturally bowed apex dorsally. They form the arch of the hand and can be broken down into two general segments (Fig. 2.8). First is the rigid central pillar section which is provided by the index and middle finger metacarpals. Second is the mobile section consisting of the ring and small finger metacarpals. Metacarpal fractures tend to fall into an apex dorsal angulation due to the tension placed on the dorsal side and the deforming forces caused by intrinsic and lumbrical muscles. Therefore,

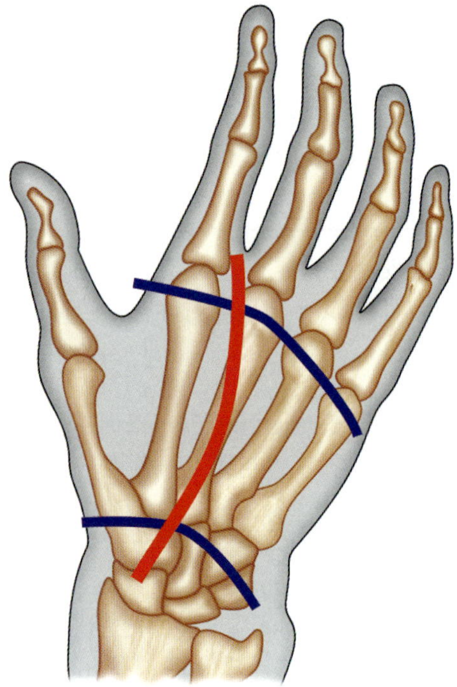

Figure 2.8: The hand consists of two arches formed by the metacarpals: a longitudinal arch (red line) and a transverse arch (blue lines).

since the index and long metacarpals provide the rigid pillar, very little, if any displacement or angulation should be accepted, usually less than 10° is tolerated assuming no rotational deformity. In contrast, given that the ring and small finger metacarpals are more mobile, up to 20–30° can be accepted with shaft fractures, but again with no rotational deformity.

Similar principles are espoused with the metacarpal neck fractures of the index, middle and ring finger metacarpals. However, much more controversy exists with fractures of the small finger metacarpal neck. Literature reviews have shown no true consensus to support a specific acceptable angulation, although typically less than 30–40° is most often considered to be acceptable for nonoperative treatment.[2] However, other studies have shown that more angulation, even up to 65° can be tolerated.[3] Moreover, Hunter and Cowen suggested that if the patient can extend the finger without an extensor lag, treat the small finger metacarpal neck fracture closed regardless of angulation.[3] Although, a clinical data to define acceptable small finger metacarpal neck fracture angulation is not available, cadaveric biomechanical studies have identified compromise of flexor tendon excursion, intrinsic strength and extension lag with fracture angulation greater than 30°.[4,5]

The base of the thumb metacarpal articulates with the trapezium in a double saddle joint that allows axial rotation as well as motion in both the flexion/extension and the abduction/adduction planes. The stability of this universal joint is derived from the complex of surrounding ligaments. The volar oblique ligament is an important joint stabilizer, in addition to the dorsoradial ligament (DRL) and superficial anterior oblique ligaments (SAOL). In intra-articular basal thumb metacarpal fractures, the Bennett's fragment is held and maintained reduced by the volar oblique ligament. The remainder of the metacarpal base is displaced dorsally and radially by APL (Figs 2.7A and B).

Patient Positioning

The patient is positioned supine with the hand on a radiolucent hand table. Since surgical approaches are typically performed dorsally with the wrist pronated, the surgeon is typically seated on the side next to the patient's head and the assistant sits in the patient's axilla. A pneumatic tourniquet is routinely used. A large, rolled-up towel is used to aid extension or flexion of the wrist. A fluoroscopic image intensifier is required.

Surgical Approaches

The metacarpal head and neck are approached dorsally through a longitudinal incision placed midline or centered over the intermetacarpal space, but proximal to the web space (Figs 2.9A and B). Blunt dissection is performed through the soft tissues while protecting branches of cutaneous nerves and vessels. The juncturae tendinae are identified, incised if necessary and tagged for later repair. Not repairing the juncturae can result in an extensor lag postoperatively. The sagittal band, which is confluent with the extensor tendon and envelopes the metacarpal head, is identified and the proximal portion is incised, thereby exposing the MP joint capsule and metacarpal neck. If necessary, the entire sagittal band may be incised longitudinally but diligent repair is necessary to avoid subluxation of the extensor tendon postoperatively. Alternatively, the extensor tendon may be split longitudinally, thereby exposing the MP joint capsule. To expose the metacarpal head, the joint capsule is capsulotomized longitudinally along its dorsal surface and elevated. The collateral ligaments and its vascular perforators are not violated in order to avoid MP joint instability or compromised perfusion to the distal metacarpal.

The metacarpal shaft and base are approached dorsally through a longitudinal incision (Figs 2.10A and B).

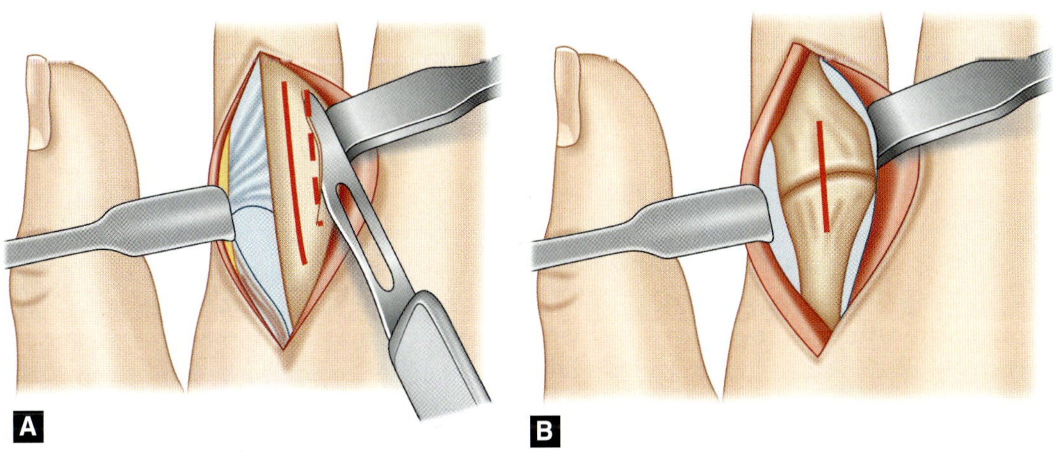

Figures 2.9A and B: Extensor mechanism including the extensor tendon and sagittal band envelopes the metacarpal head. The head may be exposed by either longitudinally incising the sagittal band or longitudinally splitting the extensor tendon. Sagittal band incision provides an excellent exposure to the metacarpal head and neck but requires diligent repair to avoid late tendon subluxation. Once the MP joint capsule is exposed, a dorsal longitudinal capsulotomy is performed and the joint capsule is elevated. Care must be exercised not to inadvertently compromise the collateral ligaments.

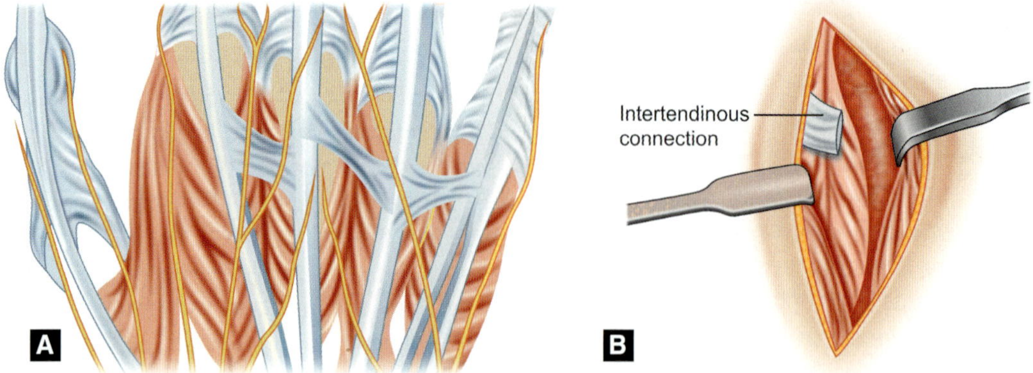

Figures 2.10A and B: The extensor tendons lie directly over the metacarpals dorsally. In order to expose the metacarpals, carefully retract the extensor tendons and incise the intertendinous connections (juncturae tendinae), if necessary, but tag them for later repair. Expose the dorsal surface of the metacarpal subperiosteally by sharply incising the dorsal periosteum and simultaneously retracting the periosteum and interossei musculature together away from the bone.

Blunt dissection is performed through soft tissues while protecting branches of cutaneous nerves and vessels. The extensor tendons are identified and retracted. The juncturae tendinae are identified, incised if necessary and tagged for later repair. The periosteum directly over the metacarpal shaft is identified and sharply incised longitudinally. The metacarpal is exposed subperiosteally and the interossei are reflected away. The periosteal layer is preserved for later repair over the hardware. Avoid exposing the metacarpal circumferentially. During metacarpal base exposure, avoid injuring the stout intermetacarpal ligaments. Basal thumb metacarpal fractures may be approached either volar-radial (Wagner approach) or dorsal-radial. The authors recommend the Wagner approach as it facilitates avoidance of the radial sensory nerve branches, provides excellent exposure to the radial and dorsal border of the thumb metacarpal and provides greater access to the Bennett's fragment (Fig. 2.11). The skin incision is placed along the base of the thumb at the junction of the glabrous and nonglabrous skin. Branches of the radial sensory nerve are identified and protected. The interval between the thenar musculature and APL tendon is developed, and the thumb metacarpal base is exposed subperiosteally. If necessary, the CMC joint may be entered with a longitudinal capsulotomy, thereby exposing the articular base of the thumb metacarpal.

Surgical Techniques

Technique 1: Metacarpal Head Fractures: Screw Fixation

Metacarpal head fractures typically represent impacted articular fractures requiring disimpaction and reduction. These fractures are best approached dorsally through either an extensor mechanism splitting approach or longitudinally splitting the sagittal band. The MP capsule will typically be hemorrhagic. The capsule is split exposing the articular surface. The joint should be irrigated and the fracture line carefully debrided of any soft tissue. The fracture is directly reduced either with the help of a dental pick, freer elevator or small "joystick" K-wires. Once the fracture is reduced, it is provisionally pinned with 0.028 or 0.035 K-wires. Our preference is to pin the fracture with the guidewires utilized for headless screws, assuming the fracture is large enough and amenable to a headless screw. Alternatively, definitive fixation may be achieved with 1.5 mm or 2.0 mm screws. Bicortical screw fixation is difficult as the metacarpal head is covered with articular cartilage along 270° of its surface in the sagittal plane. Screw fixation must, therefore, be unicortical or utilize headless compression screws. Alternatively, screws may be placed to exit along the nonarticular radial or ulnar border of the metacarpal head. Diligence must be paid to avoid prominence of the screw head on the articular surface.

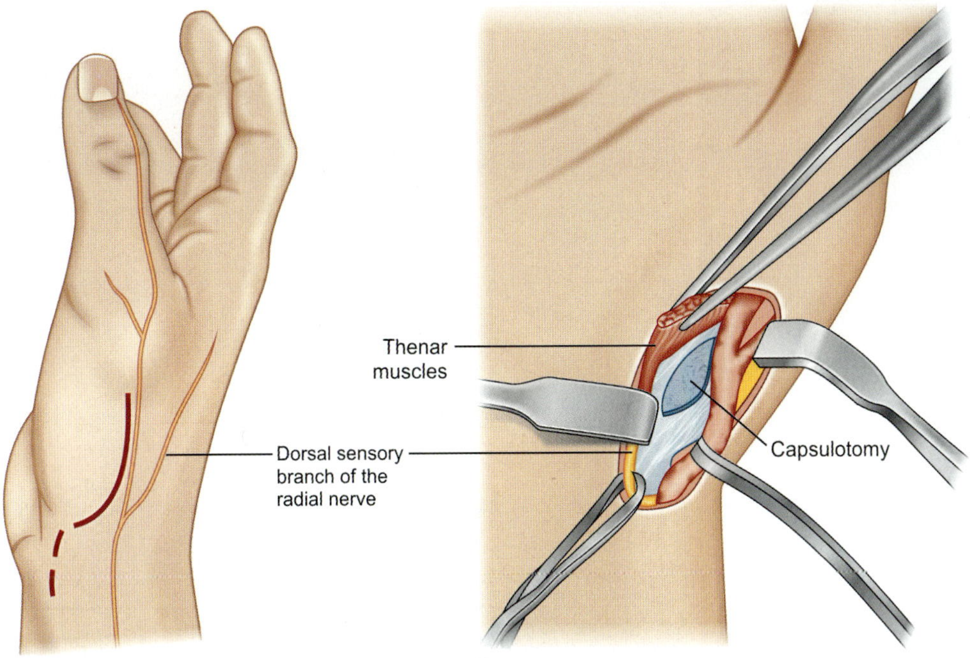

Figure 2.11: The Wagner approach provides an excellent exposure to the base of the thumb metacarpal and shaft. After placing the skin incision at the junction of the glabrous and nonglabrous skin, radial sensory nerve branches should be readily visible and must be diligently protected. The interval between the thenar musculature and APL tendon is developed, thereby exposing the CMC joint and radial border of the thumb metacarpal shaft. If necessary, a longitudinal capsulotomy may be performed to expose the articular surface of the thumb metacarpal base.

Alternatively, intramedullary screw fixation of subcapital metacarpal head or distal neck fractures may be achieved with a long headless compression screw (Figs 2.12A to C). The technique involves achieving closed or limited open reduction of the fracture. With the MP joint flexed, a percutaneous incision is placed over the metacarpal head. The extensor mechanism is split longitudinally. The guidewire for the headless compression screw is placed across the reduced fracture into the intramedullary canal and confirmed under image intensification. Once satisfied with the reduction, the head and distal shaft are opened with the cannulated drill, and a screw is placed over the guidewire. The screw is placed across the guidewire and seated just below the articular surface of the metacarpal head. The screw length should be approximately the length from the metacarpal head to the isthmus of the medullary canal.

Fracture reduction is confirmed directly as well as fluoroscopically. Passive manipulation of the joint should yield smooth motion unencumbered by the hardware and with good stability of the fracture site. Postoperatively, the patient is briefly immobilized in an intrinsic plus splint and early protected motion is initiated.

METACARPAL HEAD FRACTURES (SCREW FIXATION): Pearls and Pitfalls

- Articular fractures are often impacted and require disimpaction for optimal reduction
- The metacarpal head is covered with articular cartilage along 270° of its surface; therefore, to avoid hardware impingement, screws should be placed unicortically and countersunk. Alternatively, headless compression screws can be utilized
- Following fixation, passive manipulation of the joint should yield smooth motion unencumbered by the hardware and with good stability of the fracture site

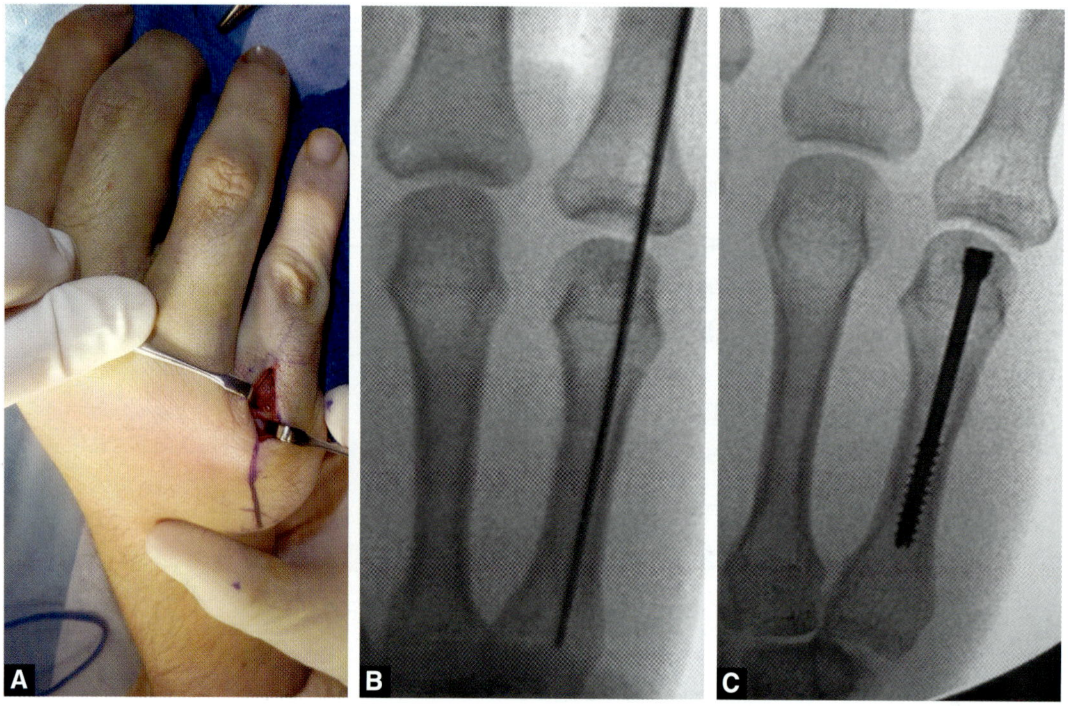

Figures 2.12A to C: In a 20-year-old male who incurred a displaced metacarpal neck fracture. (A) an incision was placed directly over the metacarpal head and the extensor mechanism was split; (B) with the fracture reduced, a guidewire was placed in a retrograde fashion and (C) a headless compression screw was placed over the guidewire. The length of the screw must be adequate enough to countersink the screw head while allowing for the screw threads to cross the isthmus of the metacarpal shaft.
Courtesy: Chaitanya Mudgal

Technique 2: Metacarpal Neck, Shaft or Base Fractures: Closed Reduction and Pinning

A number of closed or limited open reduction and pinning techniques are available for metacarpal neck, shaft or base fractures (Figs 2.13A to F). All techniques are acceptable but are predicated upon acceptable closed reduction. When applied appropriately, each technique can yield excellent results. Common closed reduction and pinning techniques include:

- Cross pinning
- Crucifix pinning
- Transverse pinning
- Bouquet pinning
- Intramedullary pinning
- Transarticular pinning

Our preferred technique for closed reduction and pinning of metacarpal neck or shaft fractures is either cross pinning or crucifix pinning. Metacarpal neck fractures are readily reduced by maximally flexing the MP joint followed by placing a dorsally directed axial load across the flexed proximal interphalangeal (PIP) joint and the proximal phalanx. Simultaneously, normal rotation of the fractured finger is restored by matching it to the other flexed fingers. Metacarpal shaft fractures are closed reduced in a similar fashion, except that in addition to the dorsally directed axial load across the flexed MP joint, a volarly directed counterforce is also applied across the fracture site.

Cross pinning the fracture is best achieved with 0.035 or 0.045 K-wires placed distal to the fracture site either at the collateral recess of the metacarpal head or at the flare of the metacarpal neck and is then advanced in a retrograde fashion. In order to maximize rotational control, the pins should be placed bicortical and not cross at the fracture site. The pins can be bent and cut short outside the skin, or cut below the skin to facilitate early motion.

Crucifix pinning is achieved by placing two pins across the distal fragment (Figs 2.14A and B). First, with the fracture reduced as described above, a 0.062 K-wire is

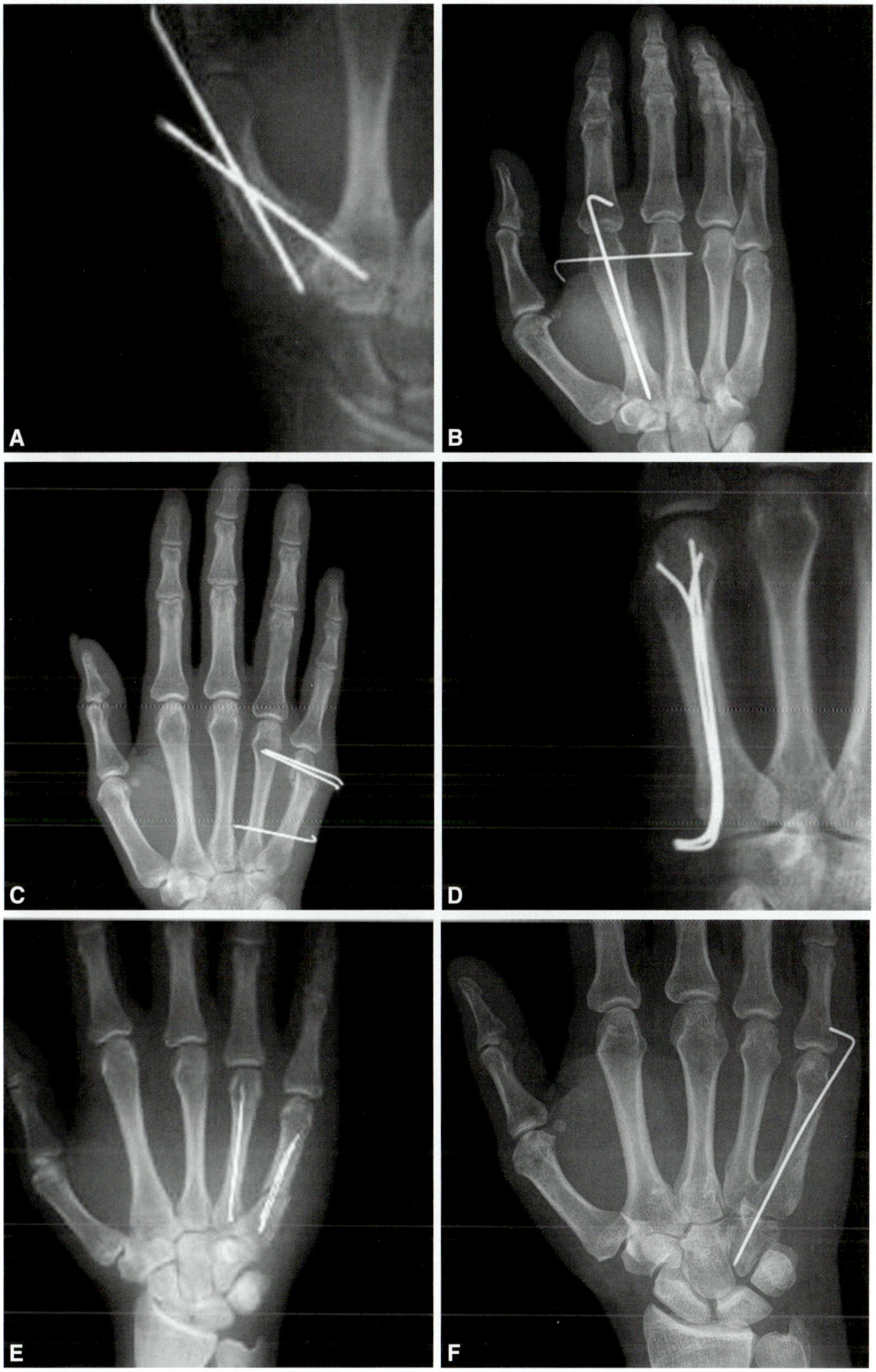

Figures 2.13A to F: Closed reduction and pinning techniques available for metacarpal neck, shaft or base fractures. (A) Cross pinning; (B) Crucifix pinning; (C) Transverse pinning; (D) Bouqet pinning; (E) Intramedullary nailing; (F) Transarticular pinning.

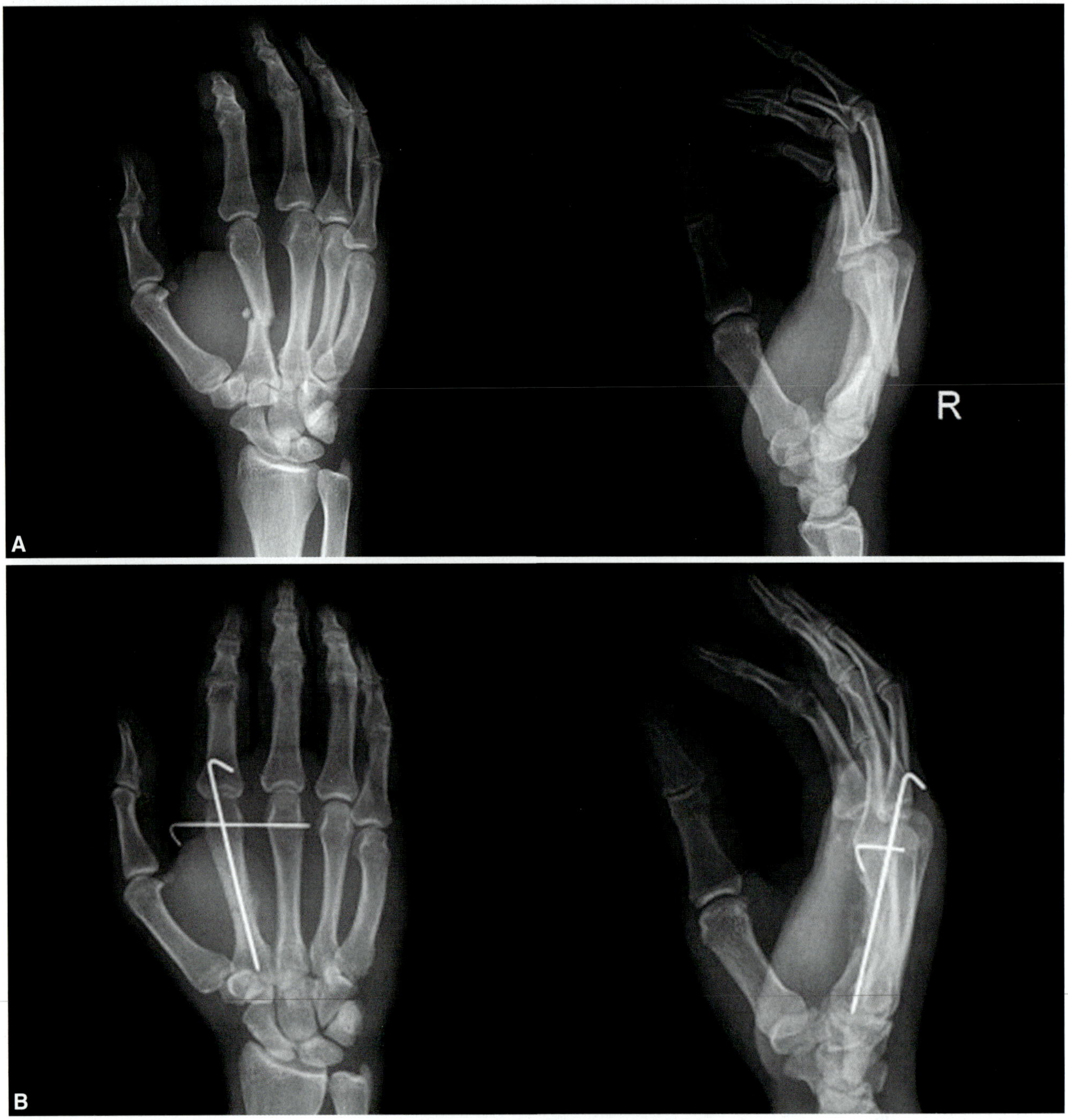

Figures 2.14A and B: Radiographs of an 18-year-old male (A) who incurred an index metacarpal fracture during an altercation that underwent crucifix pinning; (B) A 0.062 K-wire was placed percutaneously through the index metacarpal head down the intramedullary canal to reduce the fracture while a second 0.045 K-wire was placed transversely across the index metacarpal head and then into the long metacarpal's head to lock in normal rotation.

directed percutaneously across the reduced metacarpal head in a retrograde fashion. Second, with normal rotation of the metacarpal head confirmed, a 0.45 K-wire is directed laterally into the border metacarpal head and advanced bicortically into the next metacarpal head.

Intramedullary pinning may be performed freehand with standard 0.062 or 0.045 K-wires in either a retrograde or antegrade fashion. Alternatively, prefabricated intramedullary nails are available for fixation of metacarpal shaft fractures in an antegrade fashion (Figs 2.15A and B).

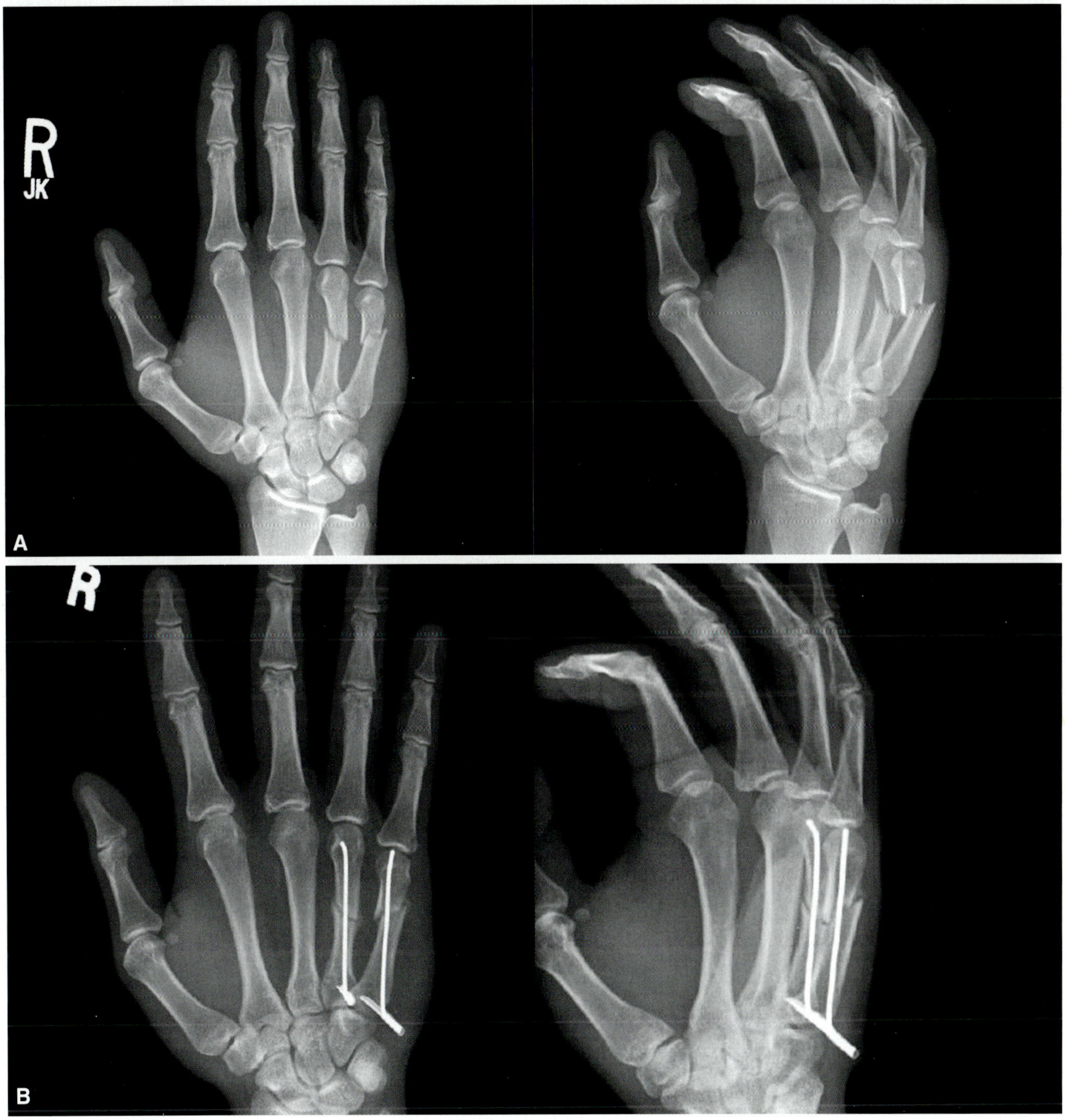

Figures 2.15A and B: Radiographs of a 22-year-old male (A) who incurred multiple metacarpal shaft fractures. (B) He underwent antegrade intramedullary pinning using prefabricated intramedullary nails.

Courtesy: Jorge Orbay

Our preferred technique for metacarpal base fractures or CMC fracture-dislocations is transarticular pinning. The fracture and/or dislocation should readily reduce with axial traction of the injured finger and volarly directed force across the fracture-dislocation site. Once reduced, a 0.062 or 0.045 K-wire is placed across the fracture-dislocation site in a retrograde fashion. The K-wire should be advanced across the CMC joint into the bones of the distal carpal row.

METACARPAL NECK, SHAFT OR BASE FRACTURES (CLOSED REDUCTION AND PINNING): Pearls and Pitfalls

- A number of percutaneous pinning techniques are available that can be successful in the management assuming adequate closed reduction has been achieved
- The normal shape of the metacarpals consists of a gentle bow with the apex dorsal. Overcorrection or overstraightening of metacarpals can result in decreased finger flexion. Rotation of fingers and restoration of composite grip should be assessed regularly during fixation of metacarpal fractures

Technique 3: Metacarpal Neck Fractures: Plate and Screw Fixation

Metacarpal neck fractures typically result from an axial compression and bending moment resulting in fracture and angulation at the metacarpal neck. Comminution is uncommon with isolated metacarpal neck fractures. The far majority of metacarpal neck fractures requiring operative reduction are amenable to closed reduction and pinning. However, plate and screw fixation for metacarpal neck fractures are indicated with fractures not amenable to closed reduction and pinning. These fractures are best approached dorsally. Exposure is facilitated by incising the juncturae tendinae, retracting the extensor tendons and exposing the metacarpal neck subperiosteally. If necessary, the sagittal band may be incised partly or entirely to expose the metacarpal distally. Distal exposure of the fracture site may be limited by the MP joint capsule, and it may be arthrotomized to increase exposure. Direct fracture reduction and interfragmentary screw fixation may be performed, if adequate length and obliquity of the fracture is available. More commonly, plate fixation with 1.5 or 2.0 mm screws facilitates consistent reduction of the fracture (Figs 2.16A to C). A minimum of two screws proximally into the shaft and two screws distally into the metacarpal head and neck is recommended. Distal bicortical fixation will be limited by articular cartilage on the volar side. Subsequently, stable fixation may be achieved by placing the distal screws obliquely into different planes or by utilizing a locking plate with unicortical locked screws.

Fracture reduction is confirmed directly as well as fluoroscopically. In particular, restoration of the normal gentle flexion of the metacarpal neck and normal rotation of the finger is directly confirmed with passive manipulation of the MP joint and tenodesis of the hand. Hardware prominence is also assessed. A plate applied too distally or screws placed too long on the volar side can obstruct MP joint motion. Postoperatively, the patient is briefly immobilized in an intrinsic plus splint and early protected motion is initiated.

METACARPAL NECK FRACTURES (PLATE AND SCREW FIXATION): Pearls and Pitfalls

- Majority of metacarpal neck fractures are amenable to closed reduction and pinning. However, in situations with fracture comminution or multiple metacarpal neck fractures, plate fixation may be utilized
- Because the metacarpal head is covered by articular cartilage along 270° of its surface, locking plates are well-indicated to be used to provide periarticular unicortical locking screw fixation of the head
- A dorsal plate applied too distally can result in extensor tendon irritation and/or obstruction to MP joint motion
- Rotation of the fingers and restoration of composite grip should be assessed regularly during fixation of metacarpal fractures

Technique 4: Metacarpal Shaft and Base Fractures: Plate and Screw Fixation

Plate and screw fixation of metacarpal shaft fractures may include interfragmentary compression (lag screw) fixation, compression plate fixation or bridge/locking plate fixation. Typically 2.0 mm screws are utilized for metacarpal fixation. Lag screw fixation is indicated for fractures with long spiral fractures without comminution. Compression plate

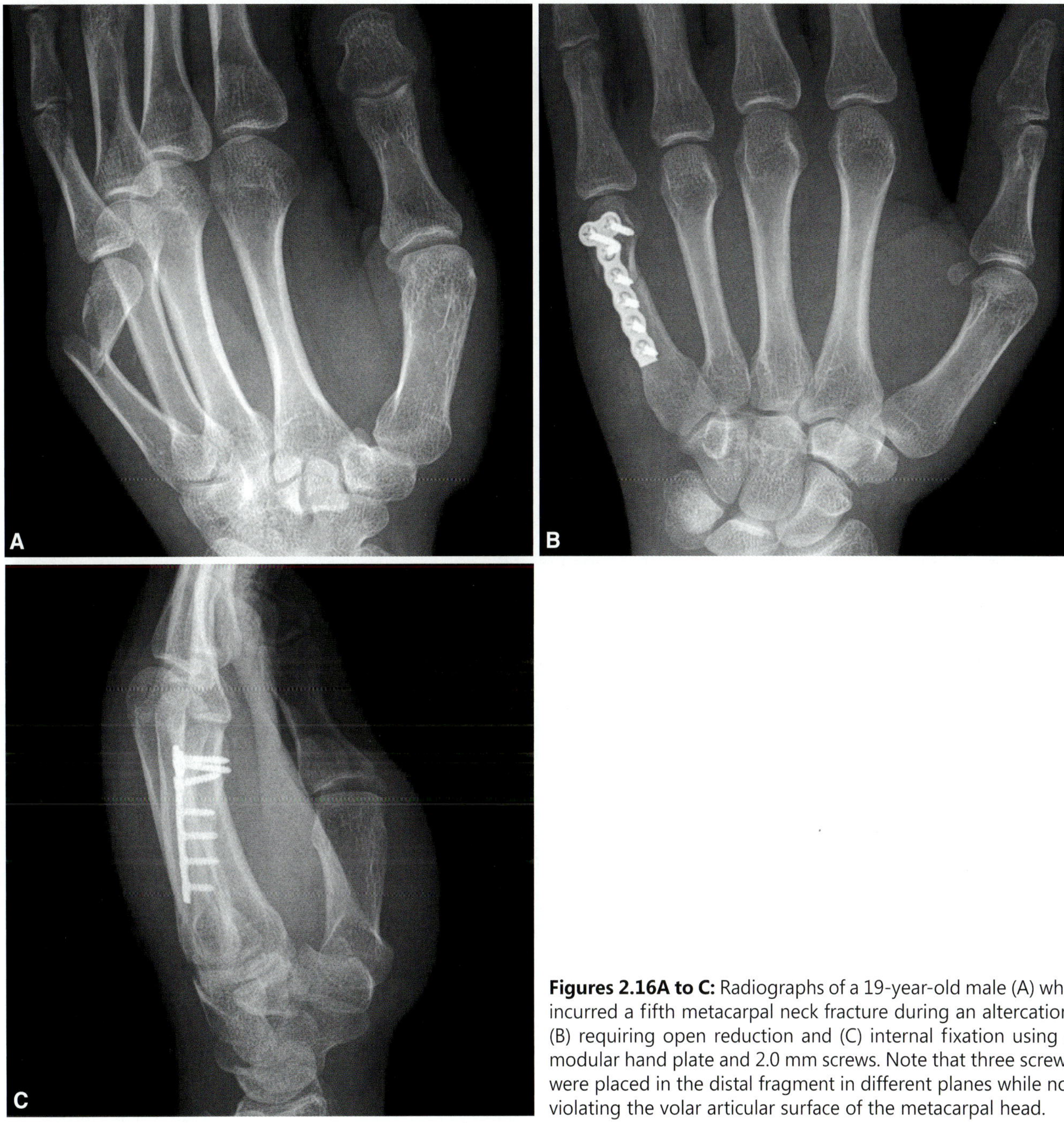

Figures 2.16A to C: Radiographs of a 19-year-old male (A) who incurred a fifth metacarpal neck fracture during an altercation; (B) requiring open reduction and (C) internal fixation using a modular hand plate and 2.0 mm screws. Note that three screws were placed in the distal fragment in different planes while not violating the volar articular surface of the metacarpal head.

fixation is best indicated for noncomminuted transverse or short oblique fractures. Bridge plating or locking plate fixation is best indicated for fractures associated with extensive comminution.

Dorsal exposure is utilized with subperiosteal dissection of the metacarpal. Intervening juncturae tendinae are incised and tagged for later repair. The fracture site is exposed, irrigated and debrided of interposing soft tissues. The fracture site is reduced, and normal length and rotation is restored.

In cases with long spiral oblique fractures, lag screw fixation achieves excellent compression and absolute stability of the fracture. The fracture is first reduced and held with either a fracture tenaculum or 0.035 K-wires. Using standard AO interfragmentary compression technique, the larger proximal drill hole is placed followed by the smaller distal drill hole. The length is measured and the proximal drill hole countersunk. The screw is placed with care not to fracture or shear across the fracture site. Typically, two to three screws are placed perpendicular to the fracture plane. Screws must be separated by a distance equal to or greater than twice the diameter of the screw. If necessary, a neutralization plate may be applied across the fracture site to offset the torsional forces on the metacarpal shaft and lag screws (Figs 2.17A and B).

In cases with transverse of short oblique fractures without comminution, compression plating is indicated. The fracture is first reduced and held with either a fracture tenaculum or 0.035 K-wires. A plate is selected that will provide at least two and preferably three screws proximal and distal to the fracture site. A slight convex bend is applied to the plate in order to maximize compression on the volar cortex with fixation. The plate is applied to the dorsal cortex and standard AO compression technique is utilized (Figs 2.18A and B). The first screw is placed in neutral mode or in the center of the screw hole in the hole closest to the fracture site. The second screw is placed in the closest hole opposite to the fracture site offset in compression mode or in the distal aspect of the hole. The remaining screws may then all be placed neutral, or the compression technique may be repeated. During compression plating, the fracture site must be closely scrutinized to avoid secondary loss of reduction.

In cases with extensive comminution, compression plating is not indicated and instead bridge plating should be utilized. If available, in this setting the authors would recommend utilizing a modular hand locking plate with two to three locking screws placed bicortically proximal and distal to the fracture site.

Fracture reduction is confirmed directly as well as fluoroscopically. In particular, restoration of the normal bow of the metacarpal shaft is confirmed on multiple fluoroscopic views. Also, normal rotation of the finger is directly confirmed with passive manipulation of the MP joint and tenodesis of the hand. Postoperatively, the patient is briefly immobilized in an intrinsic plus splint and early protected motion is initiated.

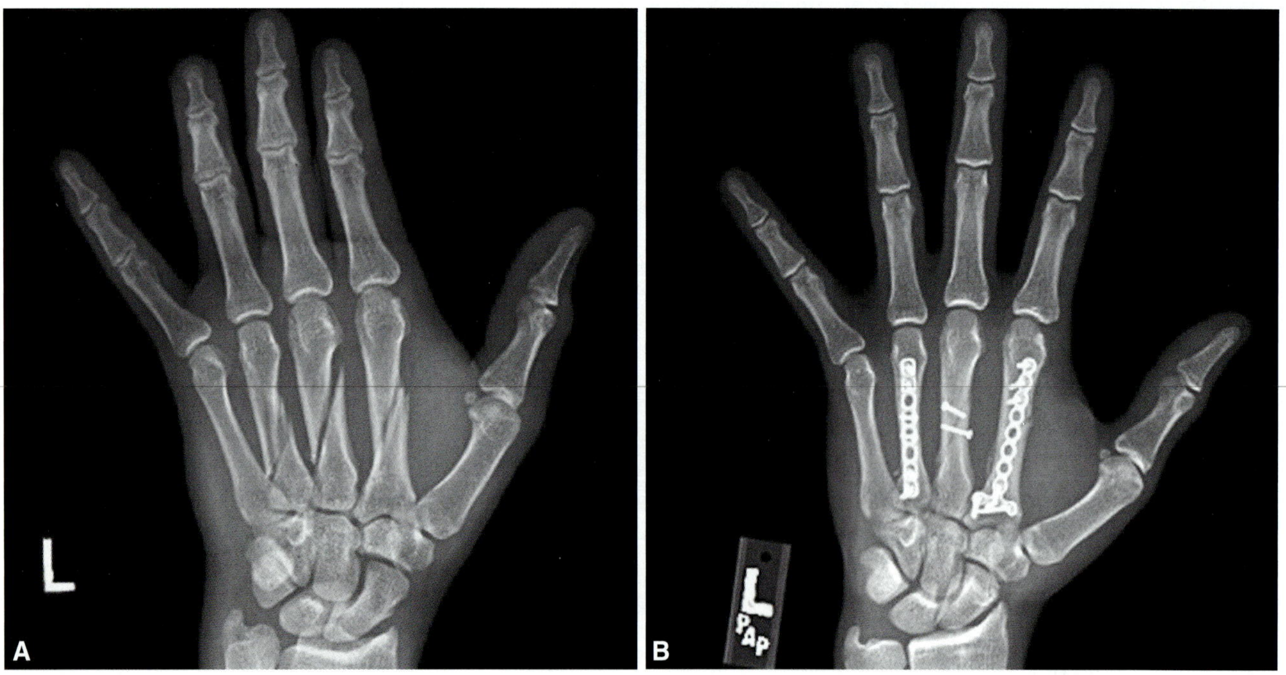

Figures 2.17A and B: Radiographs of a 25-year-old male, involved in a high speed motor vehicle accident (MVA), who injured his left hand (A) resulting in a long spiral fracture and comminution of the ring metacarpal, spiral fracture of the long metacarpal and comminuted fracture of the index metacarpal; (B) The ring metacarpal was treated with lag screw fixation followed by neutralization plating. The long metacarpal was treated with lag screw fixation alone and the index metacarpal fracture was treated with bridge plating.

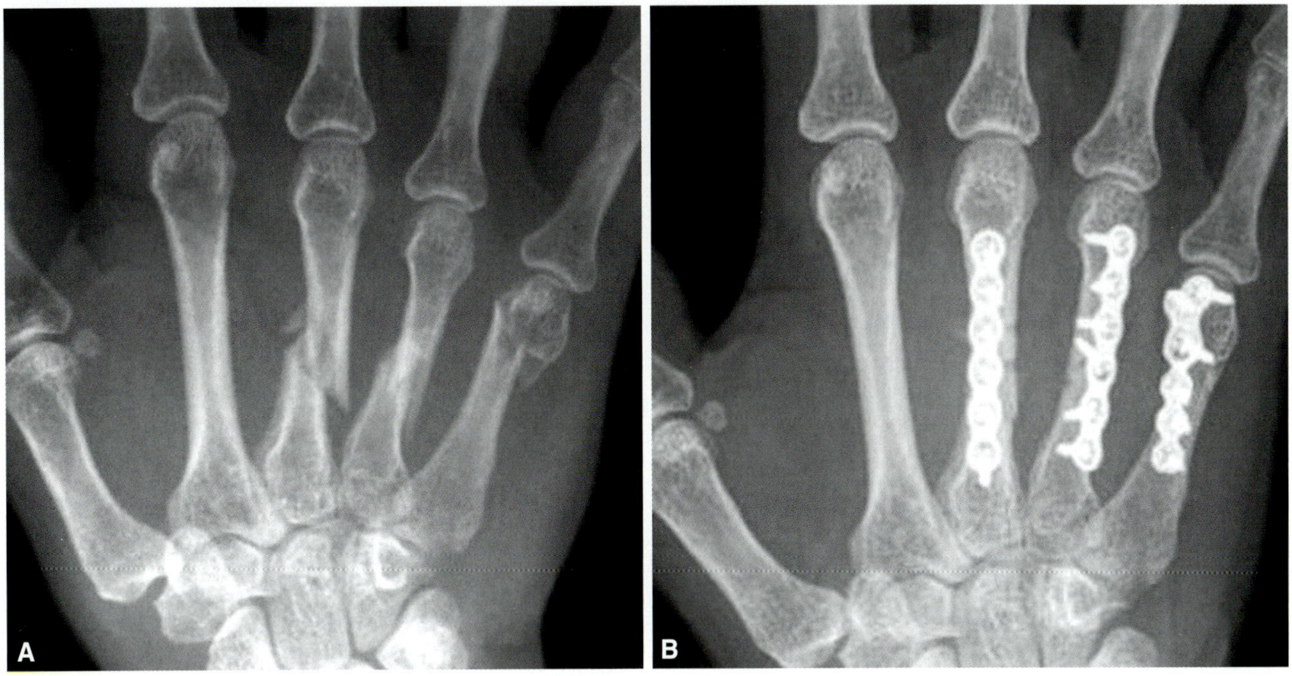

Figures 2.18A and B: Radiographs of a 52-year-old female involved in a motor vehicle accident (A) who incurred multiple metacarpal fractures; (B) In order to restore the length and rotation, the patient underwent plate fixation through a dorsal approach followed by early motion.

For fractures involving the base of the metacarpal, if adequate distal bone is not available for fixation, the plate can be temporarily placed across the CMC joint with proximal screw fixation into the distal carpal row. Limited motion occurs across the index and middle CMC joints; however, increasing motion occurs across the ring and small CMC joints. As such, plating across these joints can result in fatigue failure of the hardware and the authors would recommend routine removal of the hardware once the fracture is radiographically healed.

METACARPAL SHAFT AND BASE FRACTURES (PLATE AND SCREW FIXATION): Pearls and Pitfalls

- Lag screw or interfragmentary compression, fixation is best indicated for spiral fractures without comminution. A neutralization plate may be applied in addition to neutralize the torsional forces
- Compression plate fixation is best indicated for transverse or short oblique fractures
- Bridge plate fixation is best indicated for highly comminuted fractures
- Careful elevation and closure of the periosteal layer over the plate can minimize extensor tendon irritation
- The normal shape of the metacarpals consists of a gentle bow with the apex dorsal. Overcorrection or overstraightening of the metacarpal can result in decreased finger flexion. Rotation of the fingers and restoration of composite grip should be assessed regularly during fixation of metacarpal fractures

Technique 5: Thumb Metacarpal Base Intra-articular "Bennett" Fractures: Closed Reduction and Pinning

Closed reduction of intra-articular thumb metacarpal base "Bennett" fractures typically results in a fracture-subluxation of the first CMC joint. The volar-beak or "Bennett" fragment remains congruent while the remainder of the thumb metacarpal subluxes proximally. Successful closed reduction requires counteracting the deforming forces of the APL, EPL and adductor pollicis longus which cause shortening, extension and adduction of the thumb metacarpal respectively. The thumb metacarpal is axially distracted and extended while concomitantly applying

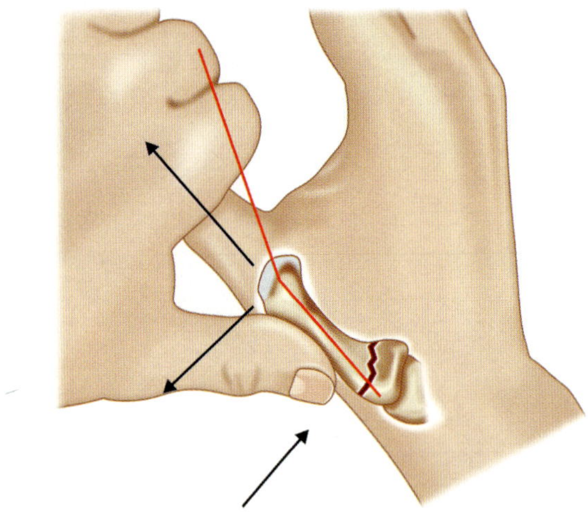

Figure 2.19: Successful closed reduction of Bennett's fractures require counteracting the deforming forces caused by the abductor pollicis longus (APL), extensor pollicis longus (EPL) and adductor pollicis longus. The thumb metacarpal is axially distracted and extended while concomitantly applying midline pressure at its base to reduce the intra-articular fracture.

midline pressure at its base (Fig. 2.19). With the fracture reduced, a 0.045 K-wire is directed across the base of the fracture into the reduced Bennett's fragment. This initial K-wire may also be advanced further into the index metacarpal base. A second, and possibly third, 0.45 K-wire is also placed across the fracture to reinforce fracture fixation (Figs 2.20A to D). Alternatively, with the fracture reduced, a 0.062 K-wire is directed retrograde from the distal shaft of the thumb metacarpal, across its base and into the trapezium. It is advantageous to have this initial K-wire positioned in the thumb metacarpal shaft so that the wire needs only to be advanced retrograde once the fracture is reduced. A second, 0.062 K-wire is placed transversely across the thumb metacarpal shaft into the index metacarpal resulting in indirect reduction of the Bennett's fragment. If desired, one or two 0.45 K-wires may then be advanced across the base of the thumb metacarpal, thereby achieving direct reduction of the Bennett's fragment.

THUMB METACARPAL BASE INTRA-ARTICULAR "BENNETT" FRACTURES (CLOSED REDUCTION AND PINNING): Pearls and Pitfalls

- One or two K-wires should be placed to reduce the Bennett's fracture. Careful fluoroscopic evaluation is warranted to confirm fracture fixation as the Bennett's fragment sits ulnar and volar relative to the thumb metacarpal base
- Successful closed reduction requires sustained neutralization of the deforming forces on the thumb metacarpal base. This can be achieved by placing a neutralizing pin across the trapeziometacarpal base or from the thumb metacarpal shaft into the index metacarpal shaft

Technique 6: Thumb Metacarpal Base Intra-articular "Bennett" Fractures: Plate and Screw Fixation

For open reduction, exposure of the thumb metacarpal base and Bennett's fragment is best achieved through the volar-radial (Wagner) approach. The interval between the thenar musculature and the APL tendon is developed, and the thumb metacarpal base is exposed subperiosteally. If necessary, the CMC joint may be entered with a longitudinal capsulotomy, thereby exposing the articular base of the thumb metacarpal. The fracture is reduced under direct visualization, provisionally reduced with a fracture tenaculum and fixed with 0.035 or 0.028 K-wires. If the Bennett's fragment is too small for screws, these K-wires can be cut short and left for definitive fixation. Preferably, one or two 1.5 or 2.0 mm screws are placed to reduce the fracture (Figs 2.21A and B). Alternatively, fracture reduction may be facilitated with plate fixation. Locking plate fixation is particularly appropriate with comminuted intra-articular thumb metacarpal base fractures, such as in the case of Rolando's fractures.

THUMB METACARPAL BASE INTRA-ARTICULAR "BENNETT" FRACTURES (PLATE AND SCREW FIXATION): Pearls and Pitfalls

- Careful fluoroscopic evaluation is warranted to confirm fracture fixation as the Bennett's fragment may be small and sits ulnar and volar relative to the thumb metacarpal base
- In cases of intra-articular comminution, a locking plate may be applied or alternatively, the fracture may be indirectly reduced and held with an external fixator. The external fixator half pins should be placed in the trapezium and thumb metacarpal shaft while holding the fracture out to length

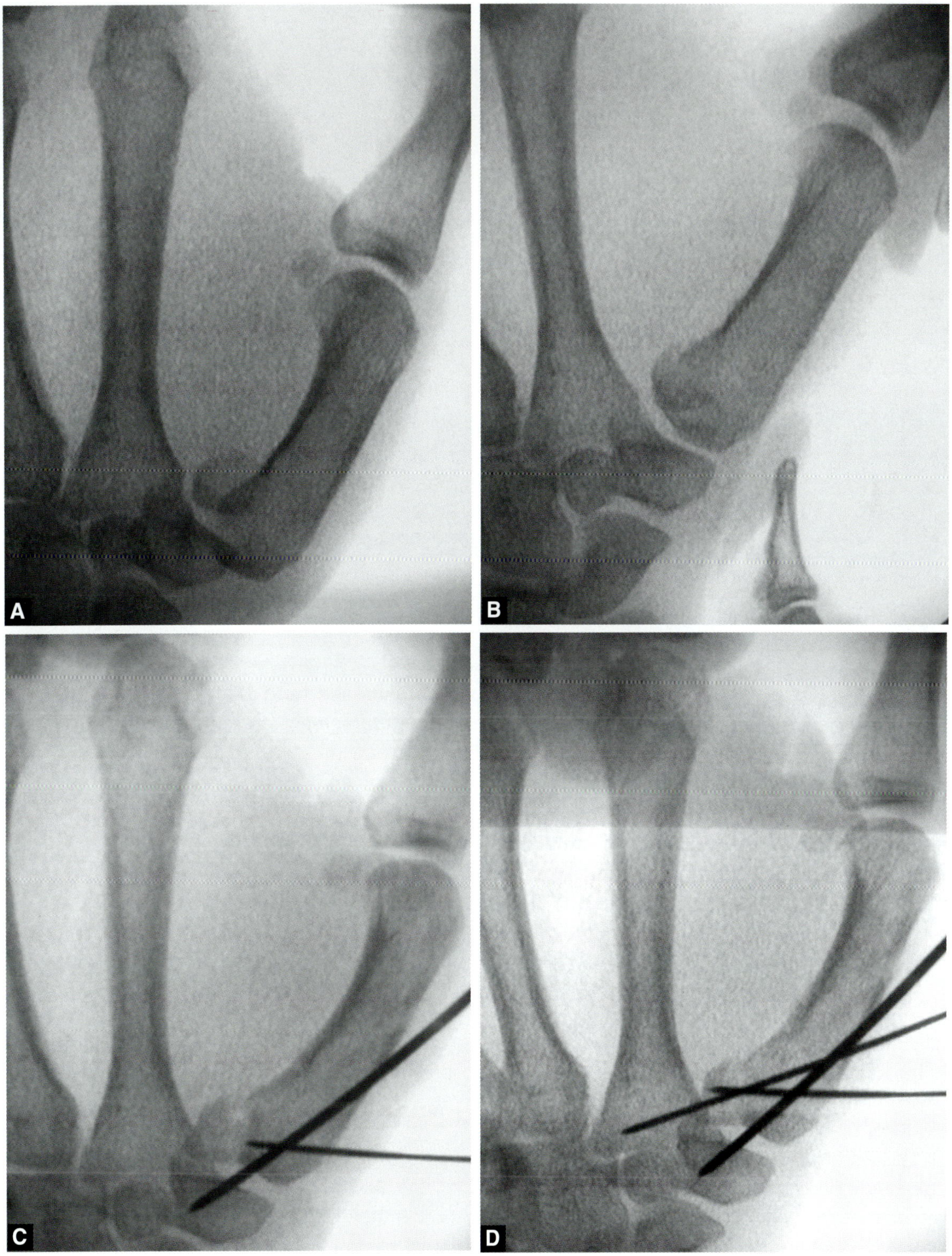

Figures 2.20A to D: Radiographs of a 43-year-old male who involved in a work accident resulting in (A and B) a displaced Bennett's fracture (C) with the fracture reduced, a 0.045 K-wire was directed across the base of the fracture into the reduced Bennett's fragment and advanced into the index metacarpal; (D) Two additional K-wires were placed to reinforce fixation including a transarticular K-wire across the thumb carpometacarpal (CMC) joint.

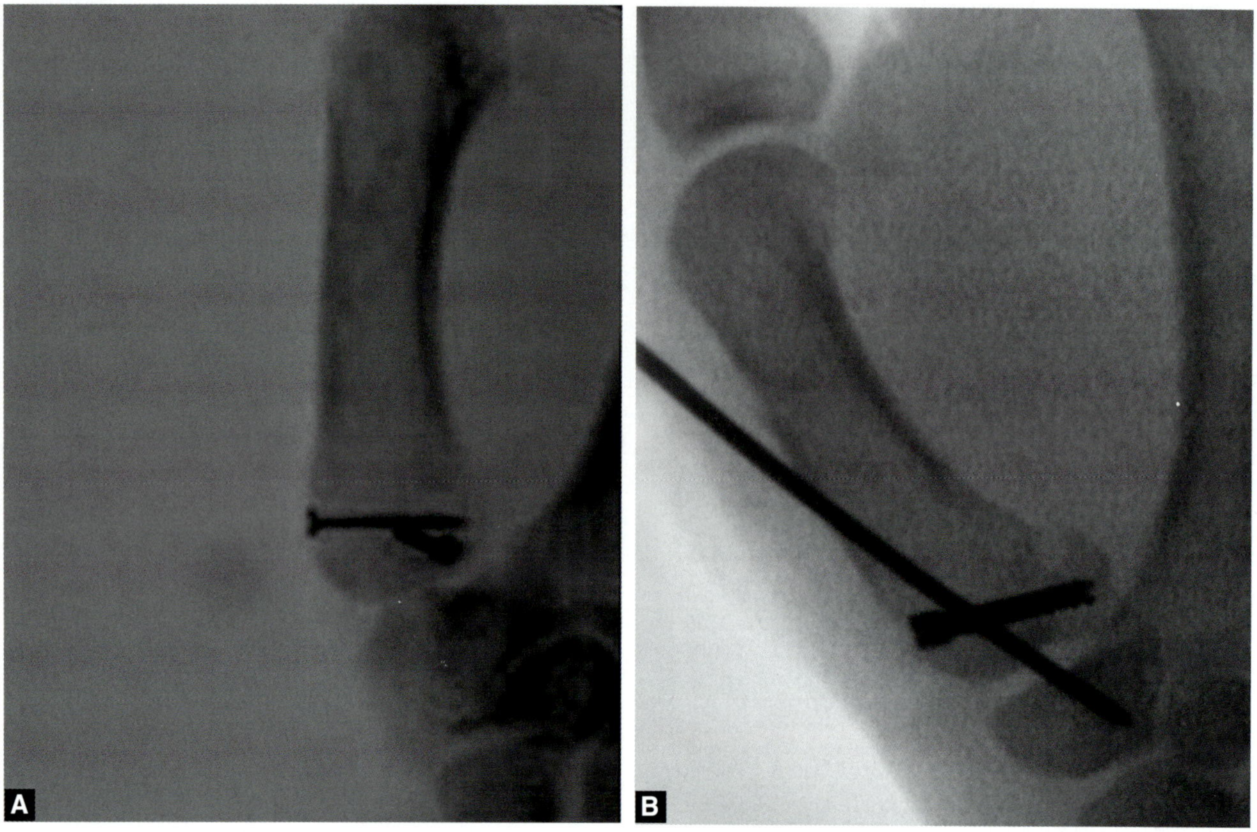

Figures 2.21A and B: Screw fixation of Bennett's fracture may be (A) achieved with headed or headless screws; (B) Fixation may be reinforced with a transarticular pin across the thumb carpometacarpal (CMC) joint.

Outcomes

Outcomes following operative fixation of metacarpal fractures have been consistently good. Bannasch et al. reported the results of 365 patients with open and closed metacarpal and phalangeal fractures that were treated with plate and screw fixation constructs.[6] No significant difference was found in terms of infection or union rates on comparing the open and closed groups of fractures. Ozer et al. reported the results of 52 patients with closed, displaced and extra-articular metacarpal fractures treated operatively using intramedullary or plate and screw fixation.[7] No significant differences were found between the techniques with regard to the disabilities of the arm, shoulder and hand (DASH) score, total active motion of the digit or radiographic evidence of healing. Furthermore, intramedullary fixation was not found to shorten operative times. Lutz et al. reported the results of 32 patients with a two-part Bennett's fractures treated by closed reduction and pinning or open reduction and lag screw fixation.[8] No significant difference was seen in the pain levels, pinch/grip strength, CMC joint range of motion or radiographic evidence of post-traumatic arthritis. The closed reduction group did, however, show a higher incidence of adduction deformity of the thumb metacarpal. Klasen described the results of 11 patients with CMC fracture-dislocations treated with open reduction and internal fixation using either screws or a bridging plate for combined fourth and fifth CMC fracture-dislocations.[9] The average follow-up was 6.6 years and at long-term follow-up 9 of the 11 patients treated operatively were found to have had full recovery of their hand function with no complaints.

Complications

Complications associated with metacarpal fracture fixation include stiffness, tendon injury, malunion and nonunion.

Stiffness of the MP joint is common following metacarpal fixation, particularly those involving metacarpal head and neck fractures. The combination of joint injury, swelling, immobilization and the insult of dorsal surgical intervention predisposes the MP joint to contracture or arthrofibrosis. The most effective management of MP joint stiffness is prevention. Stiffness may be avoided with rigid fixation, early motion and aggressive antiedema modalities. Stiffness may also result from extensor tendon adhesions, also known as extrinsic tightness of the hand. Management of extensor tendon adhesions is best done by prevention. Adhesions can be prevented by avoiding longitudinal incisions directly over the extensor tendons, early motion and antiedema modalities.

Extensor tendon injury can occur acutely or chronically. Acute or early tendon injury is uncommon and can occur from direct tendon injury caused by the fracture or during surgical exposure. Chronic or late tendon injury is more common and occurs from attritional injury from either the fracture callous or prominent hardware.

Nonunion following metacarpal fixation is uncommon; however, malunion is common and typically manifests as residual malrotation of the finger. During metacarpal fracture fixation, it is imperative to confirm restoration of normal rotation of the fingers before, during and after fixation. This is best achieved with active flexion, if possible, or passive tenodesis and finger flexion. Typically, finger malrotation is most evident during finger flexion.

Authors' Preferred Management of Select Complications

Case 1: Finger Stiffness

A 32-year-old male police officer was involved in an altercation, and incurred a displaced and rotated ring metacarpal fracture which was treated with open dorsal compression plate fixation (Fig. 2.22). Early range of motion exercises was initiated under the supervision of a therapist. However, despite 3 months of therapy, the patient lacked both active and passive flexion of the ring finger MP joint, thereby limiting flexion and compromising grip strength. Furthermore, the patient also demonstrated a mild extensor lag at the MP joint that was passively correctable.

MP joint stiffness is common following metacarpal fractures. If diligent therapy is unable to restore functional flexion of the joint, surgical intervention in the form of a joint release may be entertained. Furthermore, the authors recommend routine removal of the hardware, assuming the fracture is healed. In this case, there is not only MP joint stiffness manifested by limited flexion but also an extensor tendon adhesion resulting in an extensor lag.

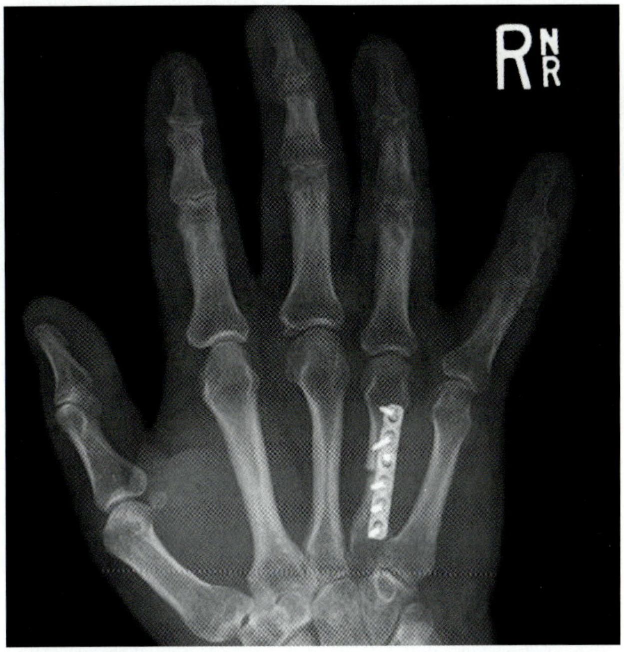

Figure 2.22: Radiograph of a 32-year-old male who underwent open dorsal compression plate fixation of a displaced and rotated ring metacarpal fracture. Postoperatively, the patient developed metacarpophalangeal (MP) joint stiffness and extensor tendon adhesions requiring surgical release.

Technique

The prior dorsal incision is utilized and the hardware is removed. The dorsal surface of the metacarpal is gently debrided to minimize cortical irregularity and the periosteum is then tightly closed. Attention is then turned to the MP joint. The extensor hood is identified overlying the MP joint. It is mobilized and retracted distally. Often the hood is adherent to the joint capsule and requires sharp dissection to separate. With the dorsal surface of the MP joint exposed, a transverse dorsal capsulotomy is performed. The joint is then passively manipulated to restore MP flexion. If additional range of motion is necessary, the collateral ligaments may be taken down carefully by releasing each side in a sequential limited step-wise manner. Finally, the extensor tendon is tenolysed by aggressively separating it from the surrounding tissue and overlying skin to maximize excursion. Postoperatively, aggressive range of motion is initiated with the help of a therapist beginning on postoperative day one.

Case 2: Tendon Rupture

A 19-year-old male incurred an epibasal thumb metacarpal fracture that underwent open dorsal plate

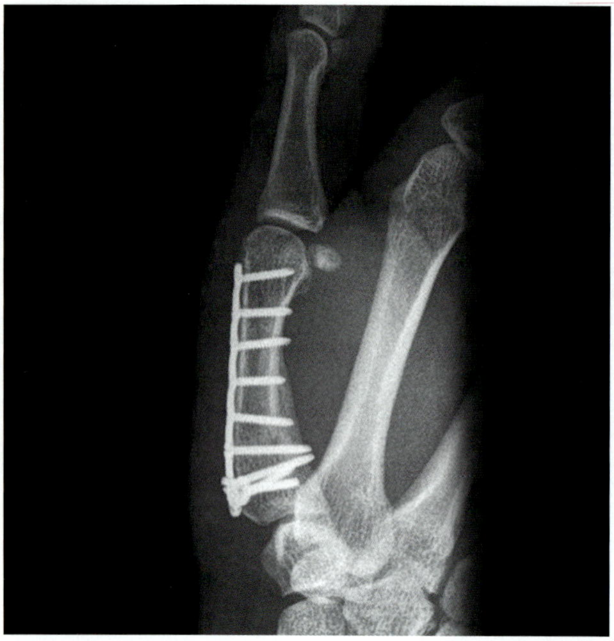

Figure 2.23: Radiographs of a 19-year-old male who underwent an open dorsal plate fixation of an epibasal thumb metacarpal fracture that resulted in a late attritional rupture of the extensor pollicic longus (EPL) tendon.

fixation (Fig. 2.23). He had an uneventful postoperative course. Approximately, 3 years following surgery, the patient returned with the sudden and painless inability to extend the interphalangeal (IP) joint of the thumb and weakness in extension of the MP joint.

Late extensor tendon rupture commonly occurs from chronic attrition of the tendon over the dorsally placed hardware. Surgical options include direct repair, tendon transfer, tenodesis or tendon grafting. Typically direct repair is not a viable option due to loss of integrity of the two tendon edges. Rupture of the extensor tendons over the finger metacarpals is readily treated with tenodesis to the neighboring extensor tendon. In case of EPL tendon rupture of the thumb, transfer of the extensor indicis propius (EIP) is best indicated.

Technique

The EIP is harvested at the level of the MP joint extensor hood. The EIP is differentiated from the extensor digitorum communis tendon to the index finger by its ulnar position at the hood. A second incision is placed approximately where the EPL tendon rupture is anticipated. The subcutaneous tissue under the skin bridge is bluntly dissected to access the EIP tendon and then the tendon is brought through the second incision. The EPL tendon is also identified. Using a standard tendon-weave technique, the EIP tendon is repaired to the EPL tendon. The transfer is tensioned so that the IP joint is in full extension and the MP joint is in only slight flexion. Postoperatively, the thumb is splinted in full extension and held for approximately 4 weeks, followed by tendon transfer rehabilitation under the supervision of a therapist.

Summary

Metacarpal fractures are one of the most common injuries that occur to our hands. Many of these fractures can be treated nonoperatively. When operative intervention is indicated, a wide array of surgical options is available. The goals of surgical intervention are accurate fracture reduction and early mobilization. Outcomes have indicated good results following surgical management. Complications are common and consist of joint stiffness, tendon injuries and malunion. The best management of these complications is prevention.

References

1. Diao E. Metacarpal fixation. Hand Clin. 1997;13(4):557-71.
2. Beredjiklian PK. Small finger metacarpal neck fractures. J Hand Surg Am. 2009;34(8):1524-6.
3. Hunter JM, Cowen NJ. Fifth metacarpal fractures in a compensation clinic population. A report on one hundred and thirty-three cases. J Bone Joint Surg Am. 1970;52(6): 1159-65.
4. Ali A, Hamman J, Mass DP. The biomechanical effects of angulated boxer's fractures. J Hand Surg Am. 1999;24(4): 835-44.
5. Birndorf MS, Daley R, Greenwald DP. Metacarpal fracture angulation decreases flexor mechanical efficiency in human hands. Plast Reconstr Surg. 1997;99(4):1079-83.
6. Bannsash H, Heermann AK, Iblher N, et al. Ten years stable internal fixation of metacarpal and phalangeal hand fractures-risk factors and outcome analysis show no increase of complications in the treatment of open compared with closed fractures. J Trauma. 2010;68(3):624-8.
7. Ozer K, Gillani S, Williams A, et al. Comparison of intramedullary nailing versus plate-screw fixation of extraarticular metacarpal fractures. J Hand Surg Am. 2008; 33(10):1724-31.
8. Lutz M, Sailer R, Zimmermann R, et al. Closed reduction transarticular Kirschner wire fixation versus open reduction internal fixation in the treatment of Bennett's fracture-dislocation. J Hand Surg Br. 2003;28(2):142-7.
9. Schortinghuis J, Klasen HJ. Open reduction and internal fixation of combined fourth and fifth carpometacarpal (fracture) dislocations. J Trauma. 1997;42(6):1052-5.

Chapter 3

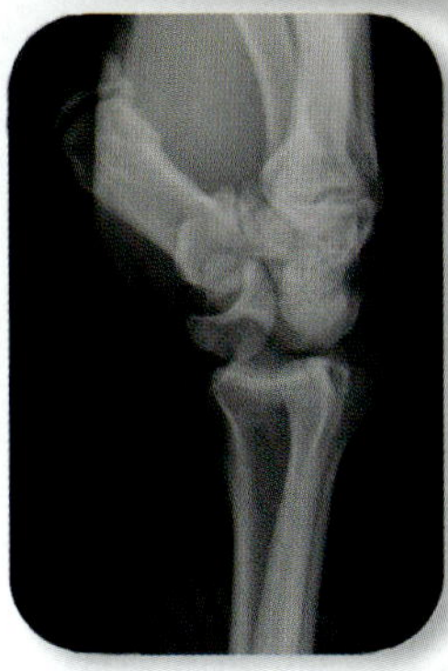

Carpal Fractures and Perilunate Dislocations

Valentin Neuhaus, Andrea Bauer, Chaitanya Mudgal

Chapter Outline

Introduction
Diagnosis
Classification
- Scaphoid Fractures
- Triquetral Fractures
- Trapezial Fractures
- Lunate Fractures
- Capitate Fractures
- Hamate Fractures
- Other Carpal Fractures

Surgical Indications
- Scaphoid Fractures
- Fractures of Other Carpal Bones
- Carpal Dislocations
- Radiocarpal Dislocations
- Axial Dislocations
- Transverse Dislocations

Surgical Anatomy, Positioning and Approaches
- Relevant Surgical and Applied Anatomy

Surgical Techniques
- Technique 1: Open Reduction and Internal Fixation (ORIF) of Scaphoid Fractures
- Technique 2: ORIF of Other Carpal Bone Fractures
- Technique 3: ORIF of Perilunate Dislocations

Outcomes
- Scaphoid Fractures
- Perilunate Dislocations

Complications
- Scaphoid Fractures
- Fractures of Other Carpal Bones
- Carpal Dislocations–Carpal Instability

Authors' Preferred Management of Select Complications
- Case 1: Chronic Scapholunate Dissociation Treated with Reduction and Association of the Scaphoid and Lunate Screw Repair
- Case 2: Failed Perilunate Dislocation Repair Salvaged with a Total Wrist Fusion
- Case 3: Lunate Avascular Necrosis Treated with a Proximal Row Carpectomy

Summary
- Fractures
- Dislocations

Introduction

Injuries to the carpal bones and ligaments can have a considerable impact on a patient's wrist function and quality of life. Normal motion of the hand is dependant upon the smooth articulation of the intricately aligned carpal bones and intercarpal ligaments. The radiocarpal and intercarpal articulations allow flexion, extension, as well as radial and ulnar deviation. Together these allow synchronized multidirectional movement which could be easily disturbed with osseous or ligamentous injuries. Therefore, prompt diagnosis and appropriate treatment of carpal injuries are paramount.

Fractures and dislocations of the carpal bones are rare. The scaphoid is the most commonly affected bone, accounting for up to 80% of carpal injuries. Around 2.5% of all wrist fractures are scaphoid fractures.[1] The incidence is about 1.5 fractures per 100,000 person a year,[1] rising up to 120 in at-risk populations such as soldiers.[2] The second most commonly injured carpal bone is the triquetrum comprising 5–20% of all carpal fractures. All other carpal bones are usually involved in less than 2% of all carpal fractures.[3] Pure dislocations are uncommon. Perilunate fracture-dislocations are more common than perilunate dislocations.[4] The transscaphoid perilunate fracture dislocation is encountered most often and is seen in more than 60% of wrist fracture-dislocations.

The mechanism of injury for the various carpal fractures and dislocations can range from a fall onto the outstretched hand to a motor vehicle collision. The history, clinical presentation and location of swelling and tenderness can guide the treating physician to the injury. Plain films must be obtained on all patients with suspected carpal injuries (Fig. 3.1), but the complex anatomy can often be difficult to interpret on radiographs alone. Therefore, if adequate suspicion exists then advanced imaging [such as, computed tomography (CT) or magnetic resonance imaging (MRI)] can be employed (Fig. 3.2).

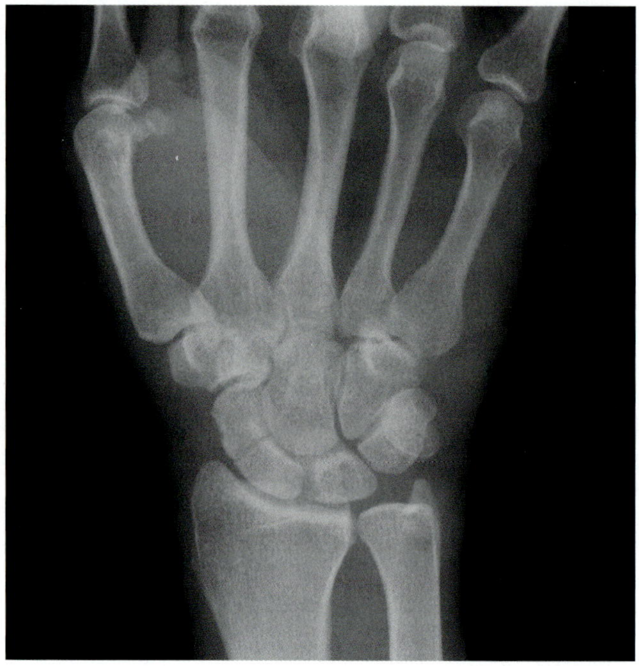

Figure 3.1: Standard posteroanterior radiograph identifying a fracture through the waist of the scaphoid.

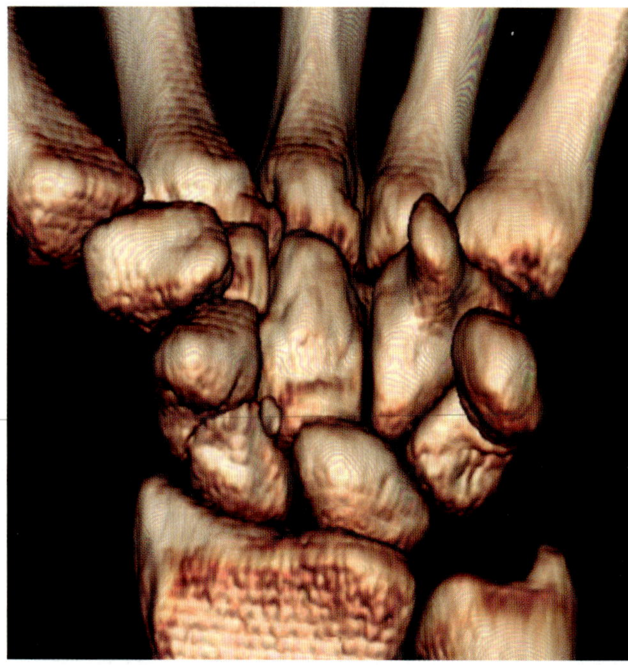

Figure 3.2: 3D reconstruction of the hand, showing eight carpal bones in two rows. The proximal row, also considered as the "intercalated segment" consisting of the scaphoid (with a waist fracture), the lunate and the triquetrum. The pisiform lies palmar-adjacent to the proximal row. The distal row consists of the trapezium, the trapezoid, the capitate and the hamate with the prominent hook.

Diagnosis

Accurate diagnosis begins with a thorough history. Several carpal injuries have characteristic injury mechanisms. For example, a fall onto an outstretched hand is a typical etiology for a scaphoid fracture. Whereas, hamate hook fractures are characteristically caused by club-sports such as golf. Patients typically present with pain and loss of function. A thorough history begins with the mechanism of injury and current symptoms, as well as information about the dominant limb and occupation. Past medical history is also relevant in the evaluation of carpal injuries. While issues specific to the hand, such as a pre-existing carpal tunnel syndrome or prior trauma to the wrist, may be important, medical issues unrelated to the hand, such as smoking and diabetes mellitus, are also critical to ascertain as they can play a major role in recovery and can ultimately affect outcome.

A physical examination begins with an inspection of both hands. Deformities, swelling, ecchymosis, lacerations and redness are noted. Palpation of the bony landmarks of the hand and wrist, including the distal radius, distal ulna, triangular fibrocartilage complex (TFCC), volar scaphoid tubercle, dorsal triquetrum, and the anatomic snuffbox can be performed, depending on the location of the patient's pain and swelling. To assess perfusion, we palpate the radial and ulnar pulses at the wrist, as well as the temperature and capillary refill of each digit. If in doubt, a Doppler examination may be performed. Any patient who is likely to go on to surgery should have an Allen's test documented as well. A full neurologic examination of the radial, median and ulnar nerves is also performed. Sensation to light touch can be unreliable, especially in the setting of trauma. We prefer to test pain sensation with a needle, as well as static 2-point discrimination. In motor testing, it is important to distinguish motion limited by pain from true neurologic dysfunction. Finally, some provocative testing may be warranted. These include Durkan and Phalen tests for median nerve compression. Grind and axial load tests of the thumb can be provocative of a scaphoid or trapezium fracture. A positive triquetrolunate and scapholunate ballottement tests may indicate a ligamentous injury.

Radiologic assessment begins with plain radiographs of the affected hand. A posteroanterior (PA) and lateral view of the wrist must be included and an oblique view is prudent as it often reveals details of subtle carpal fractures. On the PA view, Gilula's lines (Figs 3.3A to D) are examined for any discontinuities, and the lunate should appear trapezoidal.[5] Diastasis of the scaphoid and lunate, also known as the "Terry Thomas" sign can indicate scapholunate dissociation. A "cortical ring" sign caused by excessive scaphoid flexion, can also indicate scapholunate dissociation (Fig. 3.4). On the lateral view, the radius, lunate, capitate and the third metacarpal must be collinear with the wrist in the neutral position. Absence of the lunate in this line on the lateral view, as well as a triangular shaped lunate on the PA view, indicates a perilunate dislocation (Figs 3.5A and B).

Specialized views can then be added depending upon the area of interest. The "scaphoid view" is a PA view of the wrist in ulnar deviation. The surgeon should beware of a PA view taken in radial deviation, as the scaphoid flexes as the wrist deviates radially and therefore appears shorter, which can be misinterpreted as a fracture. The semipronated view can help to examine the radial side of the carpus, whereas the semisupinated view helps to clarify the bony structures at the ulnar side of the wrist. A PA view of a clenched fist is the most sensitive for identifying a scapholunate dissociation. Additional views in radial and ulnar deviation may help to detect carpal instabilities. In addition, radiographs of the uninjured wrist may be helpful for comparison. This is especially the case in children or in patients with suspected carpal instability where a normal anatomic variant may mimic an injury.

Particular mention must be made of the radiographic diagnosis of scaphoid fractures. This is an area of some controversy as the overall sensitivity and specificity of plain radiographs is only about 75%,[6] and the consequences of a missed scaphoid fracture can be significant. In addition, there is a lack of strong interobserver agreement in interpreting radiographs.[7] In cases where a scaphoid fracture is suspected but not visible on injury films, the surgeon has several options. Traditionally, bone scans were utilized but may be negative in the first 48 hours. Computed tomography and MRI are comparable in the diagnosis of an occult scaphoid fracture.[8] Both are subject to false-positive and false-negative results and are overall better at excluding occult fractures than they are at confirming them (sensitivity as low as 67%, specificity 89–96%).[8] We favor placing patients with a suspected scaphoid fracture in a thumb spica cast and repeating the clinical examination and radiographs in 10–14 days. This is similar to other authors who recommend immobilizing the wrist for 2 weeks because most of the occult fractures are visible after 2 weeks.[9] However, it has also been reported that up to 80% of these patients have no fracture and are unnecessarily immobilized and followed up.[9]

Advanced imaging, such as CT and MRI scanning, is often useful in the diagnosis and management of carpal injuries. In the acute setting, CT scanning can more clearly delineate fracture patterns and displacement,[6] as well as revealing occult fractures. We also routinely use CT scans in the management of scaphoid fractures to confirm union following both operative and nonoperative treatment.

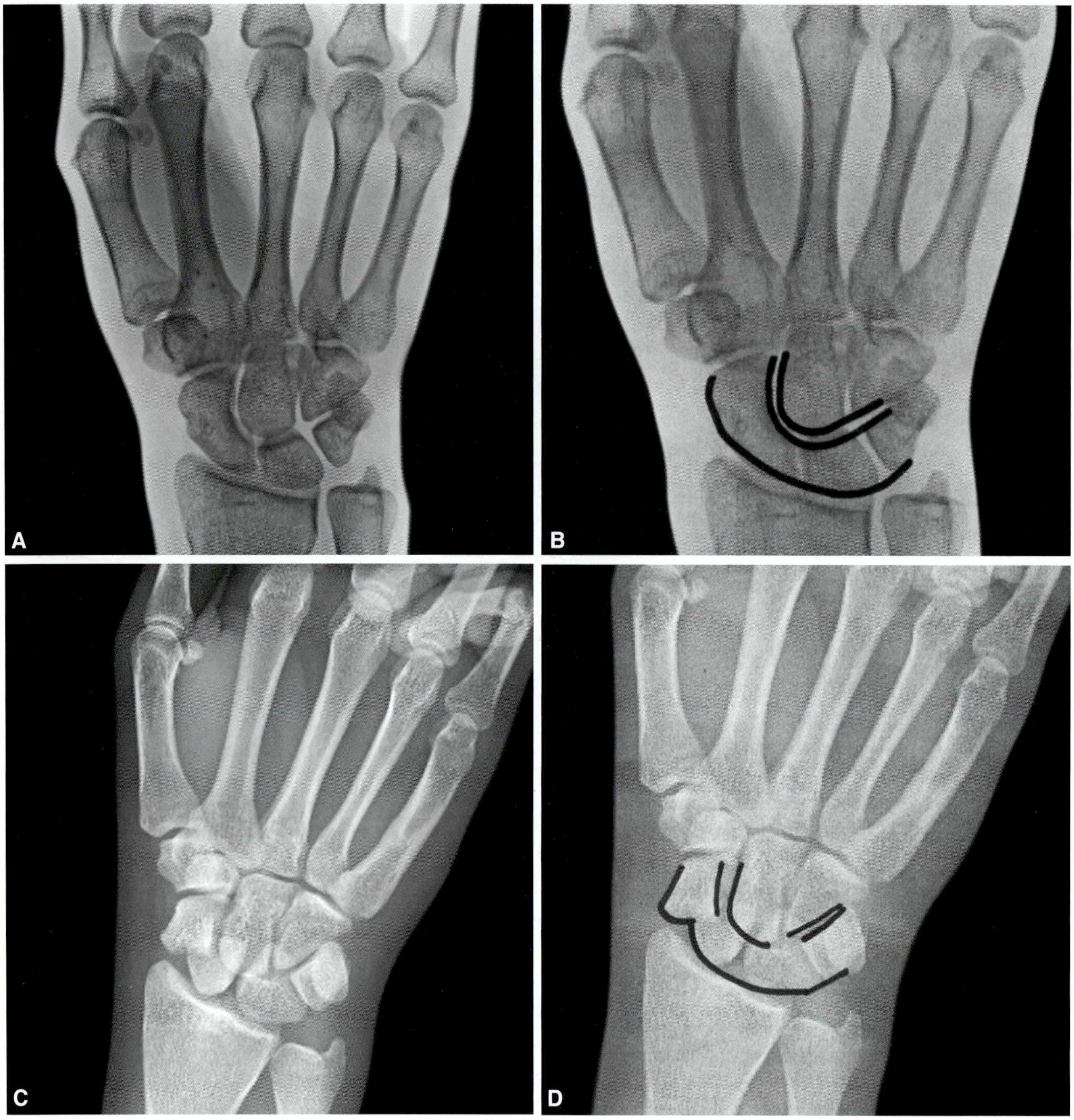

Figures 3.3A to D: The lines of Gilula on a posteroanterior view of the wrist help to detect fractures and instabilities: (A and B) Note the normal radiograph of the wrist and the subsequent lines of Gilula; (C and D) Now, note a trans-scaphoid perilunate dislocation with disruption of the lines of Gilula.

Alternatively, MRI scanning can also provide details on the osseous anatomy and also aide in identifying associated injuries, such as vascularity (Fig. 3.6) or intercarpal ligament tears. Magnetic resonance imaging has demonstrated a sensitivity of 89% and specificity of 89% in assessing scapholunate and lunotriquetral ligament tears, but microperforations within these ligaments can result in false-positive results.[10]

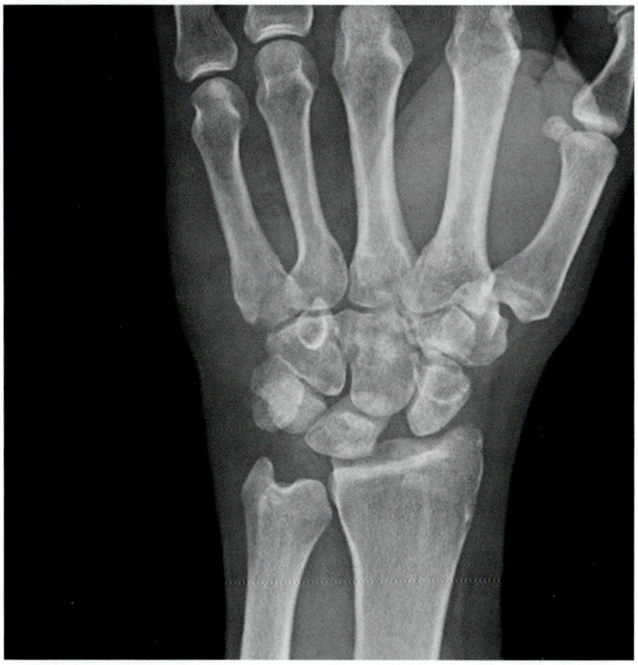

Figure 3.4: Scapholunate dissociation represents compromise of the scapholunate ligament resulting in a rotatory subluxation of the scaphoid showing a gap of more than 4 mm (also known as a Terry Thomas sign) between the scaphoid and lunate on this posteroanterior view as well as a "ring sign" of the distal pole of the scaphoid caused by abnormally increased flexion of the scaphoid.

CARPAL FRACTURES AND PERILUNATE DISLOCATIONS DIAGNOSIS: Pearls and Pitfalls

- Key physical exam findings to diagnose scaphoid fractures are tenderness in the "anatomic snuffbox", tenderness at the volar scaphoid tubercle and pain with axial compression of the thumb
- Every patient with a history of trauma to the wrist and wrist pain should have plain radiographs, at least PA and lateral views in neutral position. On the PA view, the three lines of Gilula must be continuous, and the lunate should be trapezoidal in shape. On the lateral view, the third metacarpal should be in colinear with the capitate, lunate and radius
- CT is useful in the diagnosis of an occult scaphoid fracture and to assess interval healing
- MRI is helpful in assessing occult scaphoid fractures, scaphoid vascularity and associated intercarpal ligament injuries

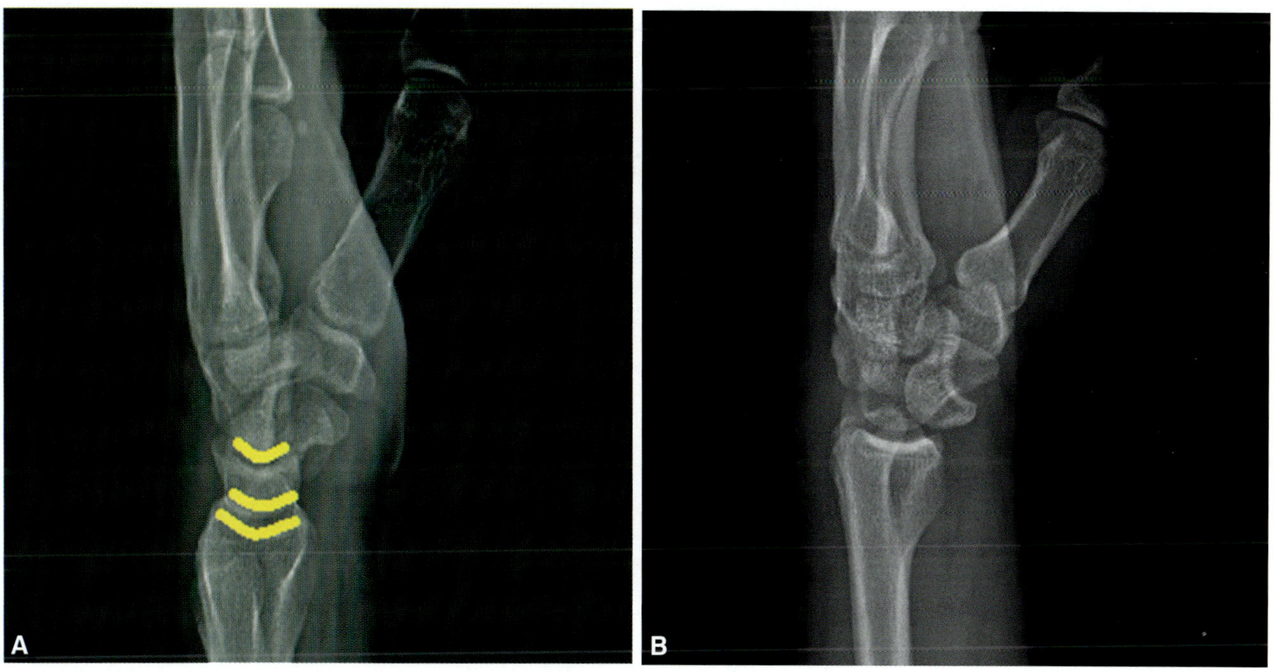

Figures 3.5A and B: Perilunate dislocations are best identified on the lateral view. (A) On a normal lateral view, the third metacarpal, capitate, lunate and radius should be all aligned; (B) However, in the case of a perilunate dislocation the lunate dislocates volarly (also known as a spilled tea cup sign) disrupting the normal alignment.

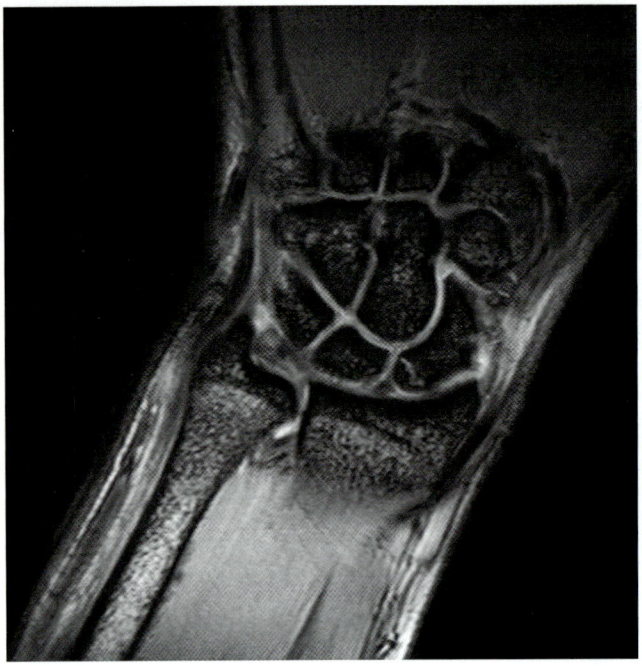

Figure 3.6: MRI of the wrist showing a vascularized proximal scaphoid pole fracture as signified by no signal change of either pole of the scaphoid across the fracture.

Classification

Classification schemes can be useful tools for communication and research, as well as to guide treatment and predict outcomes. Every carpal injury can simply be classified in descriptive terms:

- Which bone(s) is/are affected?
- Is the fracture line simple or comminuted?
- Are the fracture fragments displaced?
- Is there any dislocation?
- Is the fracture open or closed?

There is a considerable discrepancy in intra and interobserver reliability in fracture classifications. One reason is the difficulty in interpretating X-rays of the carpal bones. It is important to distinguish between simple and comminuted fractures. Comminution is defined as existence of 3 or more fragments. Cooney defined "displacement" in scaphoid fractures as presence of a gap between the fragments greater than 1 mm in any direction, scapholunate angulation greater than 45° or lunocapitate angle greater than 15° on lateral radiographs.[11] An offset of 1 mm in any carpal fracture is generally considered to represent a displaced fracture.

All carpal fractures and dislocations can be classified according to the AO/OTA format. This system is comprehensive but the numbering system can be cumbersome for general use. We find it the most useful for research purposes. For clinical purposes, we will highlight the Herbert[12] and Russe[13] classifications which are also commonly used.

Scaphoid Fractures

Herbert described the following classification of scaphoid fractures (Fig. 3.7) based on the radiographic appearance on plain X-rays:[12]

- Type A: Acute stable fractures
  - Type A1: Fractures of the tubercle
  - Type A2: Undisplaced crack fracture of the waist
- Type B: Acute unstable fractures
  - Type B1: Oblique fracture of distal third
  - Type B2: Displaced or mobile fractures of the waist
  - Type B3: Proximal pole fractures

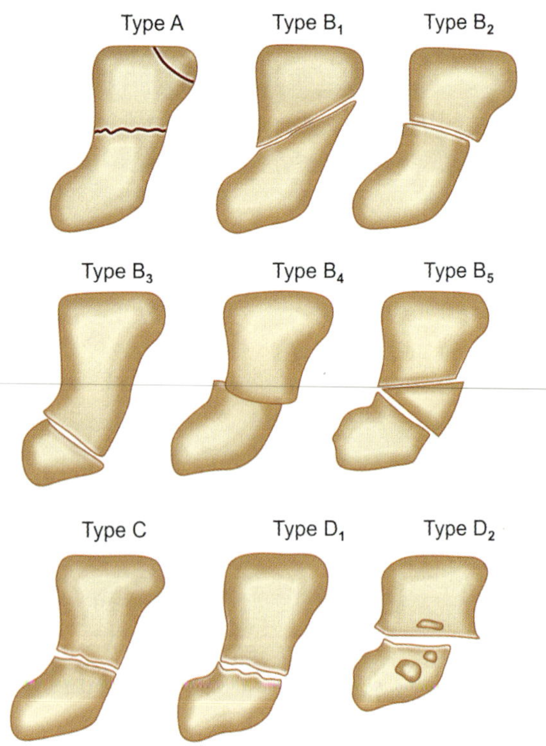

Figure 3.7: Herbert's classification of scaphoid fractures.

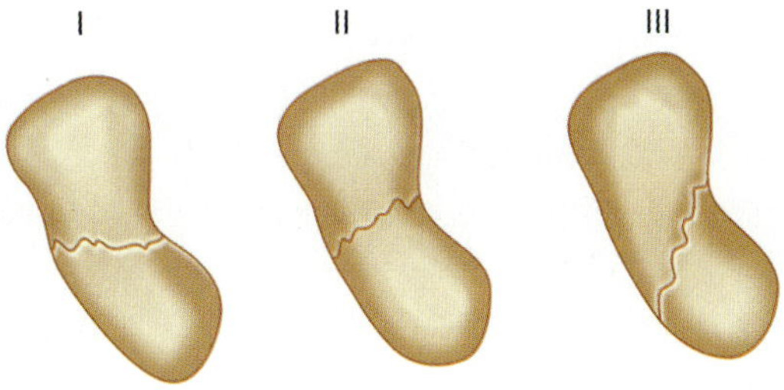

Figure 3.8: Russe's classification of scaphoid fractures.

- Type B4: Fracture dislocation of carpus
- Type B5: Comminuted fractures

- Type C: Delayed union
- Type D: Established nonunion
  - Type D1: Fibrous
  - Type D2: Sclerotic nonunion (pseudarthrosis)

This classification system is useful as it distinguishes between stable and unstable fractures, as well as acute fractures versus nonunions. However, it is based on the interpretation of plain radiographs and as such the intra- and interobserver reliability is low. Alternatively, the Russe's classification[13] distinguishes three types of scaphoid fractures based on the relationship of the fracture line to the long axis of the scaphoid (Fig. 3.8). Type 1 is a horizontal oblique fracture, Type 2 is a transverse fracture, and Type 3 is a vertical oblique fracture.

It is important to note that scaphoid fractures are commonly associated with other carpal fractures or a perilunate dislocation. Furthermore, concomitant intercarpal ligament injuries, such as rupture of the scapholunate ligament, have also been described in association with scaphoid fractures,[10] but the overall incidence of these ligamentous injuries is unknown. None of the above classifications take these ligamentous injuries into account.

Triquetral Fractures

Triquetral fractures are the second most commonly fractured carpal bone. These are classified simply as either avulsion fractures or body fractures. Ninety percent of all fractures of the triquetrum are bony avulsion of the dorsal radiotriquetral and intercarpal ligaments (Fig. 3.9). These occur due to forced hyperflexion or impact fractures of the ulnar styloid during hyperextension.[14] Fractures of the triquetral body are much less common and generally occur from falls on the outstretched hand (Figs 3.10A and B).

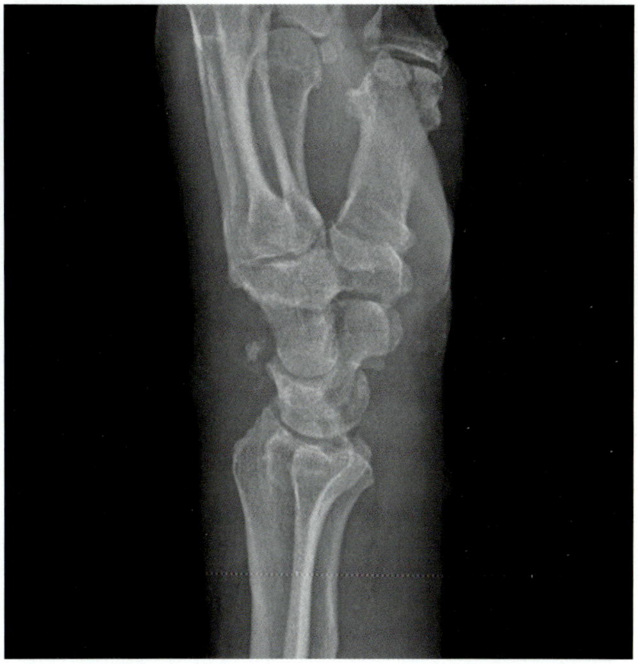

Figure 3.9: Triquetral avulsion fractures are best seen on lateral views.

Avulsion fractures are the best identified on the lateral view while body fractures are the best visualized on the PA view.

Trapezial Fractures

Trapezial fractures are the third most common carpal fracture, representing only 3–4% of all carpal fractures. They are divided into palmar ridge fractures and vertical fractures through the body. Due to force transmission, they can often be accompanied by fractures of the first metacarpal.

Lunate Fractures

Greater than 80% of the lunate surface is covered with cartilage. Within the lunate, only two small areas of blood supply are described on the palmar and dorsal surface. Teisen and Hjarbaek classified fractures of the lunate (Fig. 3.11) into five groups based on its vascular anatomy:[3]

- Group I: Fracture of the volar pole possibly affecting nutrient vessel
- Group II: Chip fracture not in the areas of nutrient vessels
- Group III: Fracture of the dorsal pole possibly affecting nutrient vessel

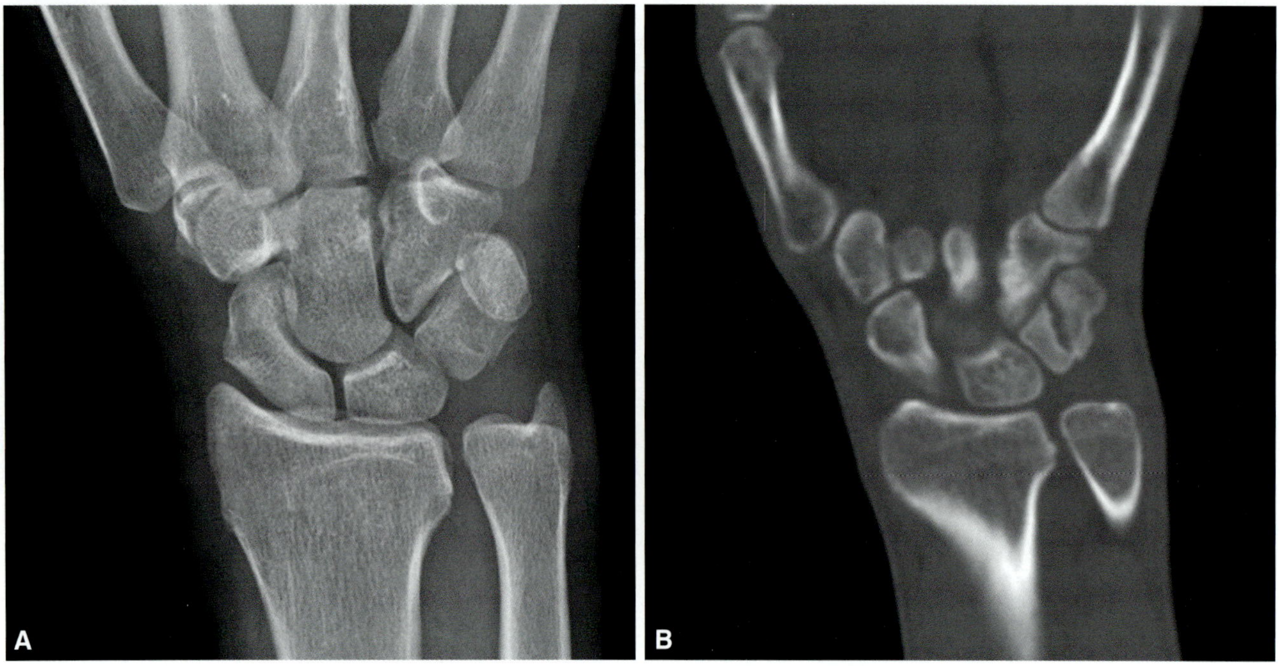

Figures 3.10A and B: Triquetral body fracture demonstrated on a (A) posteroanterior radiograph and on the corresponding; (B) CT scan.

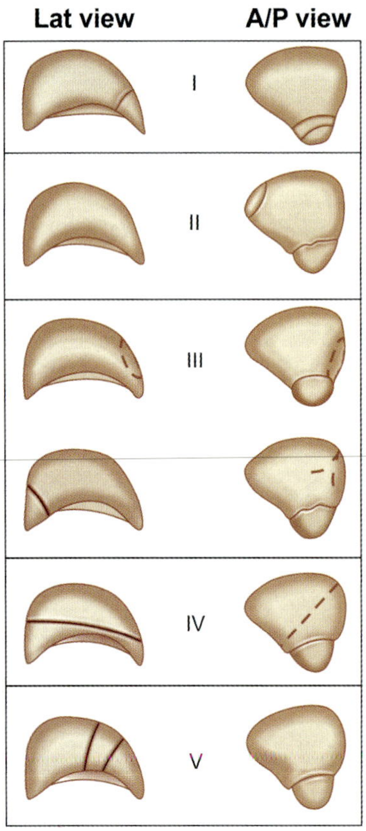

Figure 3.11: Teisen and Hjarbaek's classification of lunate fractures.

- Group IV: Sagittal fracture through the body
- Group V: Transverse fracture through the waist of the bone

Capitate Fractures

Fractures of the capitate may occur as a single injury but occurs more commonly in combination with other injuries. When combined with a scaphoid fracture, this is known as scaphocapitate fracture syndrome,[15] or alternatively as, a "greater arc" perilunate injury.

Hamate Fractures

Hamate fractures are classified as type I if the hook is involved and type 2 if the body is affected.[16] Type 1 is more common. Type 2 can be further divided into sagittal and coronal plane fractures. Coronal fractures of the hamate are often associated with carpometacarpal dislocations.

Other Carpal Fractures

Pisiform fractures are not specifically classified. Trapezoid fractures are very rare and are generally part of a more complex injury such as, a fracture-dislocation of the index finger.

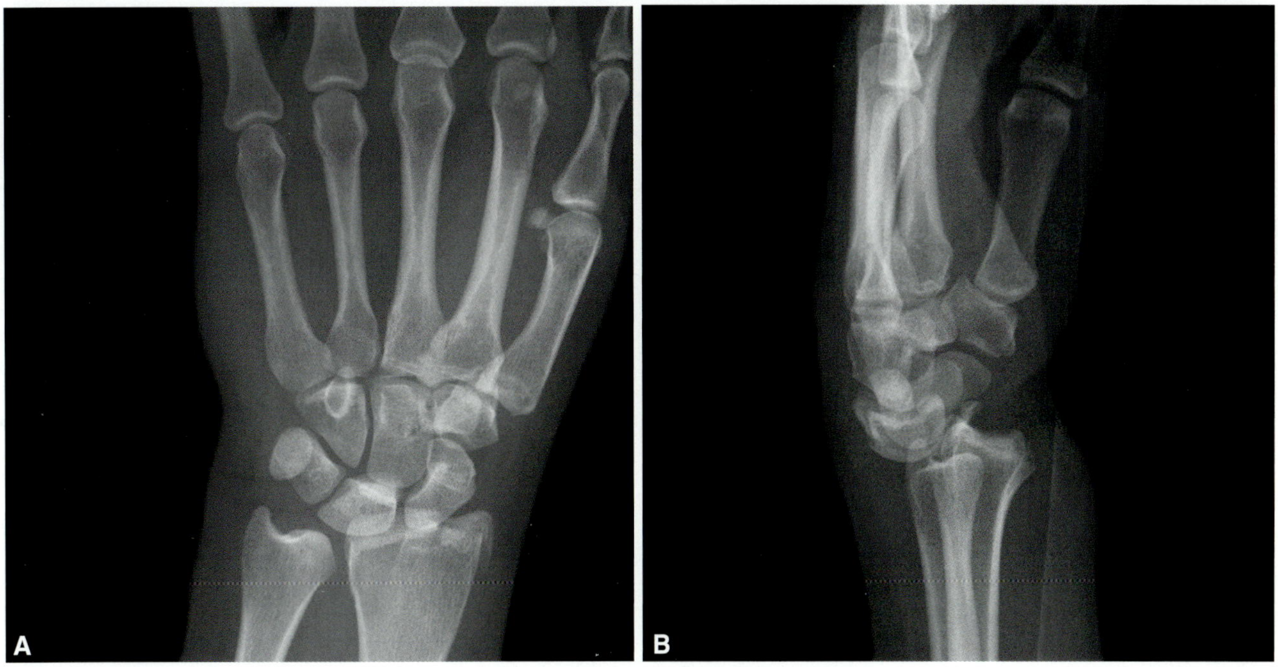

Figures 3.12A and B: Dorsally directed radiocarpal dislocation with an avulsion fracture of the radial styloid.
Courtesy: Asif M Ilyas

Carpal Dislocations

Because the proximal carpal row is more mobile than the distal row, the proximal row is at higher risk for dislocations. Still, carpal dislocations are uncommon. They usually result from high-energy hyperextension trauma to the wrist with ulnar deviation and intercarpal supination.[17] Due to the high-energy mechanisms, concomitant injuries must be ruled out. There are four patterns of carpal dislocations:

- Radiocarpal dislocations are uncommon. They are primarily a soft tissue injury but are usually associated with a bony avulsion of the radiocarpal ligaments of the distal radius (Figs 3.12A and B). They represent a ligamentous injury but are often misinterpreted as a dorsal Barton's distal radius fractures.[18]
- Axial dislocations are longitudinal separations of the finger rays.
- Isolated carpal bone dislocation, mostly described in rare case reports. Every single carpal bone can potentially dislocate.
- Transverse dislocations are the most common and include lunate and perilunate dislocations.[19]

Lunate dislocation is a dislocation of only the lunate, while the rest of the carpus remains aligned with the radius. This is in contrast to perilunate dislocations in which the lunate remains aligned with the radius but not with the carpus (Figs 3.13A and B). Most authors mention that perilunate dislocation precedes lunate dislocation,[17] that is, lunate and perilunate dislocations are different stages of the same injury progression. These dislocations may be purely ligamentous (also called lesser arc injuries) or associated with fractures of the radial styloid, scaphoid, capitate and/or triquetrum (also called greater arc injuries) (Figs 3.14A and B). Perilunate dislocations are 2–3 times more common than lunate dislocations, and the most commonly encountered perilunate injury is the transscaphoid fracture-dislocation.

According to Mayfield,[17] the stages of progressive perilunate instability may be classified as follows (Figs 3.15A and B):

- Stage I: The scapholunate interosseous ligament is disrupted, and the ligaments between scaphoid and radius are attenuated or torn. Scapholunate instability results and radiographs demonstrate a scapholunate diastasis.

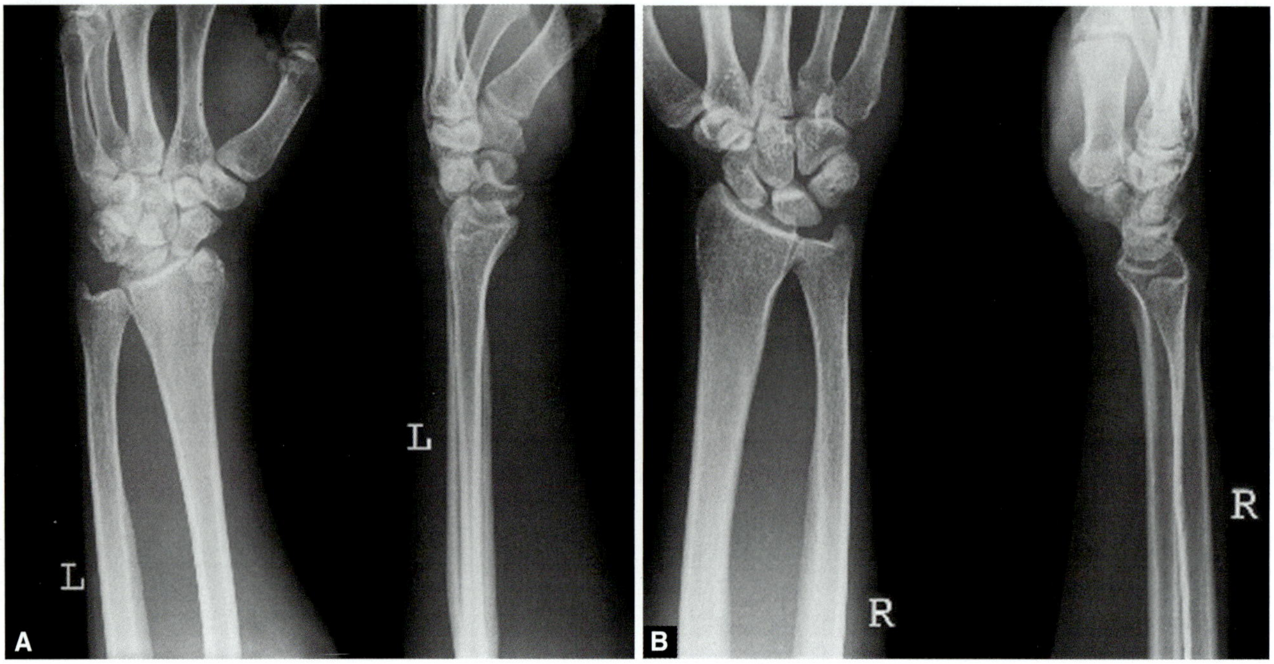

Figures 3.13A and B: In perilunate dislocation of the left wrist in this figure, the lunate remains aligned with the radius but not the carpus compared to the unaffected contralateral right side.
Source: Hans-Peter Simmen

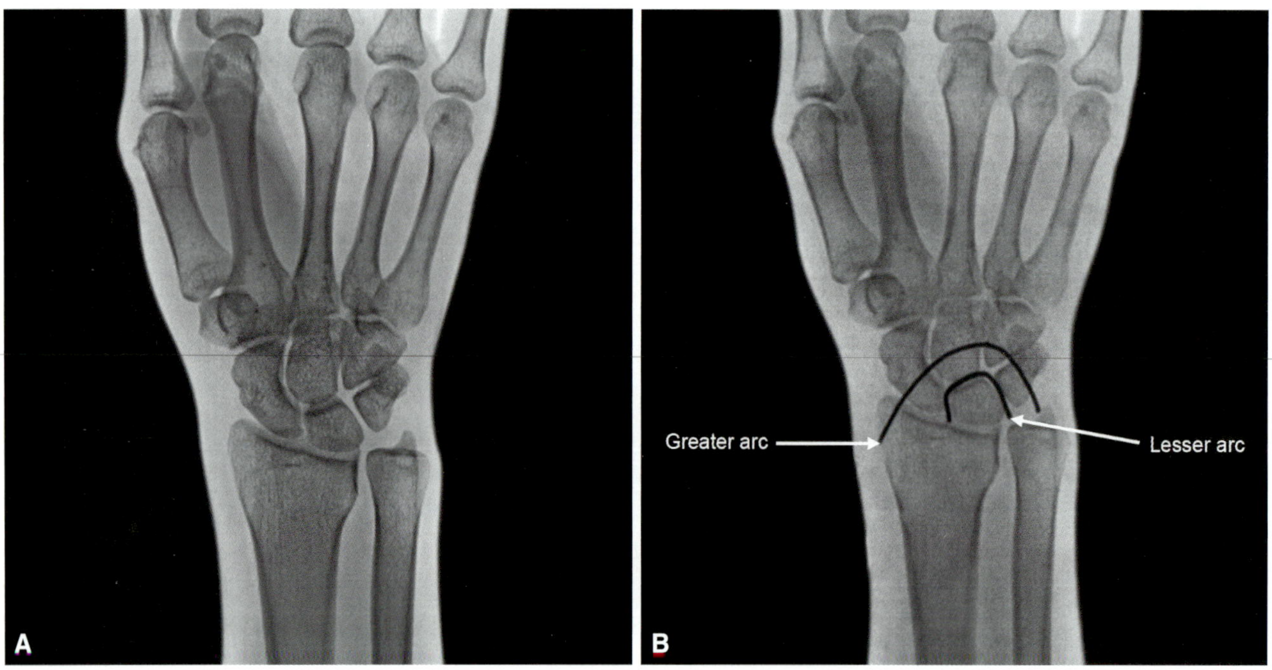

Figures 3.14A and B: Perilunate dislocations follow either a lesser arc or greater arc injury patterns depending on the path of injury and subsequent injury. A lesser arc injury consists of a strict ligamentous perilunate dislocation without a fracture. A greater arc injury consists of a perilunate dislocation with associated fractures of the radial styloid, scaphoid, capitate or triquetrum.

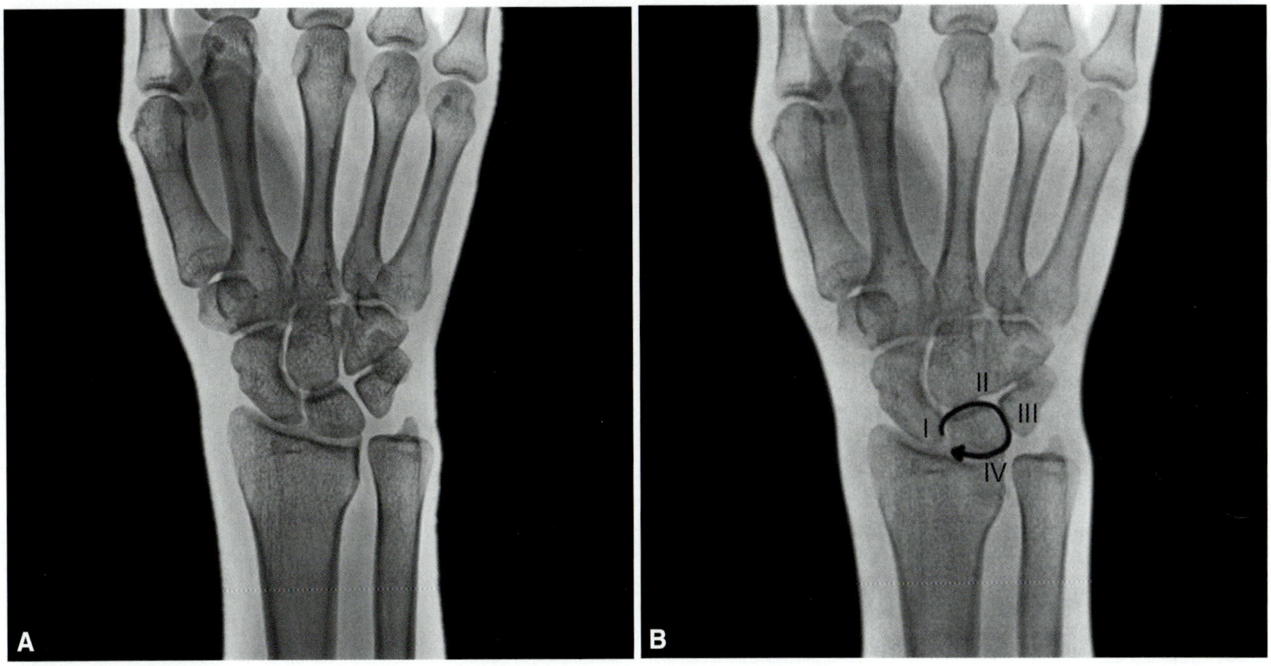

Figures 3.15A and B: Perilunate dislocations follow a circular path centered around the lunate. According to Mayfield, four dislocation stages are encountered: Stage I: scapholunate ligament injury; Stage II: midcarpal joint; Stage III: lunotriquetral ligament injury (carpus dislocates dorsally) and Stage IV: lunate dislocates volarly.

- Stage II: With progressive force the capitate is peeled away from the lunate as the radiocapitate ligaments are torn resulting in proximal migration of the capitate ensues.
- Stage III: The lunotriquetral interosseous ligament ruptures resulting in a dorsal perilunate dislocation. The lunate typically remains articulating with the radius
- Stage IV: The lunate freely rotates downward and dislocates into the carpal tunnel. The lateral radiographic view shows a palmarly dislocated lunate.

As the carpus dislocates progressively, it appears that the most common direction of force transmission is from radial to ulnar. Reverse injuries, i.e. from ulnar to radial have also been described but appear to be very uncommon. Once the carpus dislocates, there is dorsal displacement of the capitate on the lunate. This is accompanied by the inevitable muscle spasm that accompanies the most severe musculoskeletal injuries, displacing the capitate onto the dorsal aspect of the lunate. As the deforming force expends itself, the injury now starts to recoil back to its "anatomic" location. In doing so, the capitate has no place to fall back into and can actually impact the lunate with sufficient violence in effect displacing it volarly. This then leads to the lunate dislocation, thus completing the final stage of progressive perilunate instability.

Surgical Indications

Scaphoid Fractures

Nondisplaced, Herbert type A or minimally displaced (< 1 mm) scaphoid fractures can be treated non-operatively[12,20] (Figs 3.16A to D). Depending on the location and classification of the fracture a cast is applied for anywhere from 6–12 weeks. Distal pole fractures can be immobilized for a lesser period while waist fractures can require longer immobilization. Different types of casts are used, including above and below elbow, and with or without the thumb included. There is yet no clear evidence which cast should be used, but the authors prefer a short arm thumb spica cast. After consolidation and pain-free motion, occupational therapy can be started. The authors generally obtain a CT scan at 8–10 weeks to confirm healing.

In selected patients, nondisplaced and minimally-displaced waist fractures can be treated operatively with

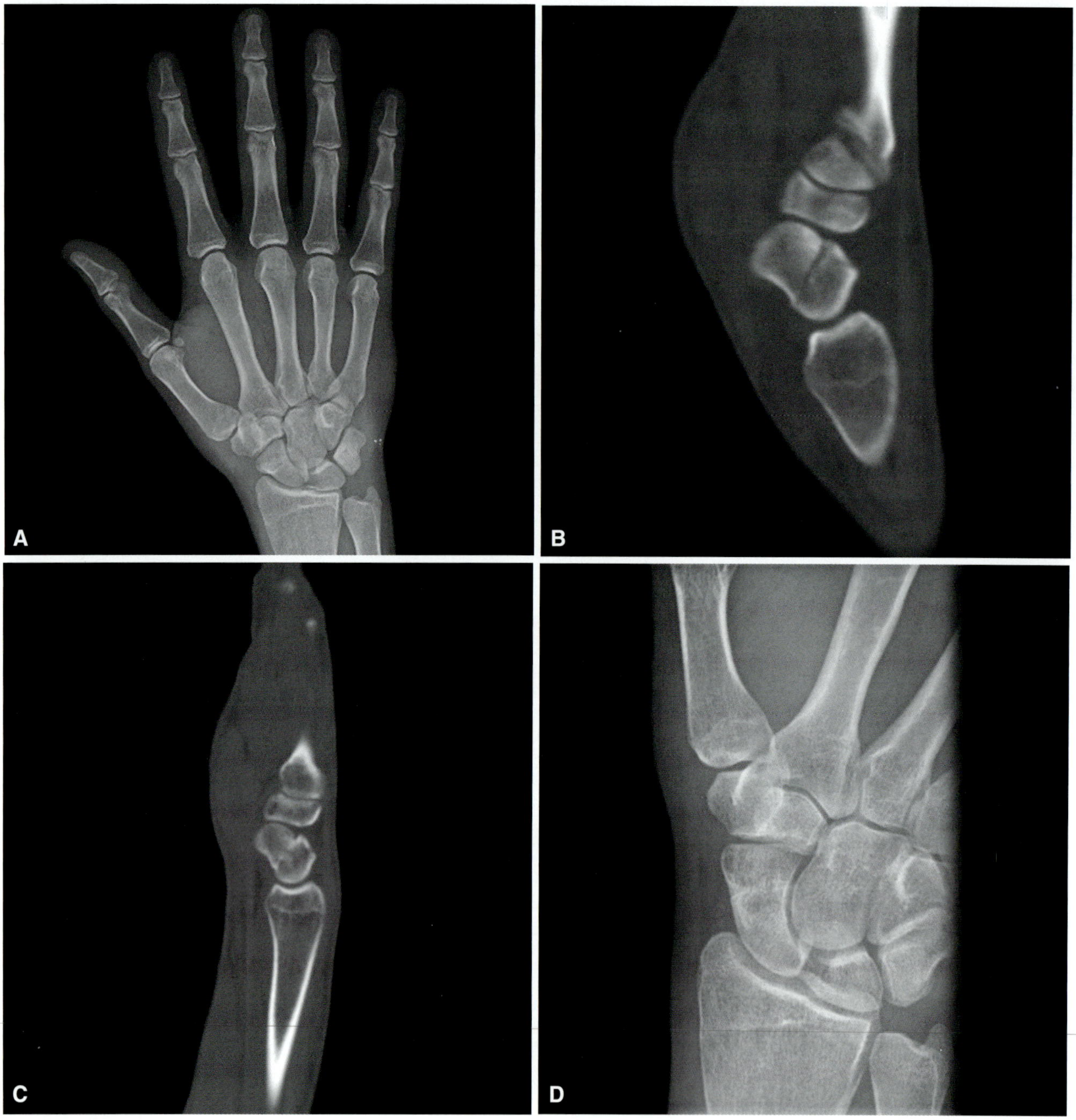

Figures 3.16A to D: This is a 26-year-old male patient who incurred a (A) nondisplaced scaphoid fracture treated nonoperatively with a short arm thumb spica cast for 12 weeks. Also shown are the (B) initial CT-scan; (C) CT-scan at 6 months follow-up and a (D) follow-up radiograph after 1 year demonstrating a healed scaphoid fracture.

minimally invasive techniques (Figs 3.17A to C). The benefit of this is a shorter duration of cast immobilization, with a shorter recovery, while risking an increased rate of complications[21] (Figs 3.18A to C). In a prospective study, Schädel-Höpfner[22] showed that operative treatment primarily facilitates earlier return to previous activity level, better functional status, less pain and higher patient satisfaction. However, a significant increase in the

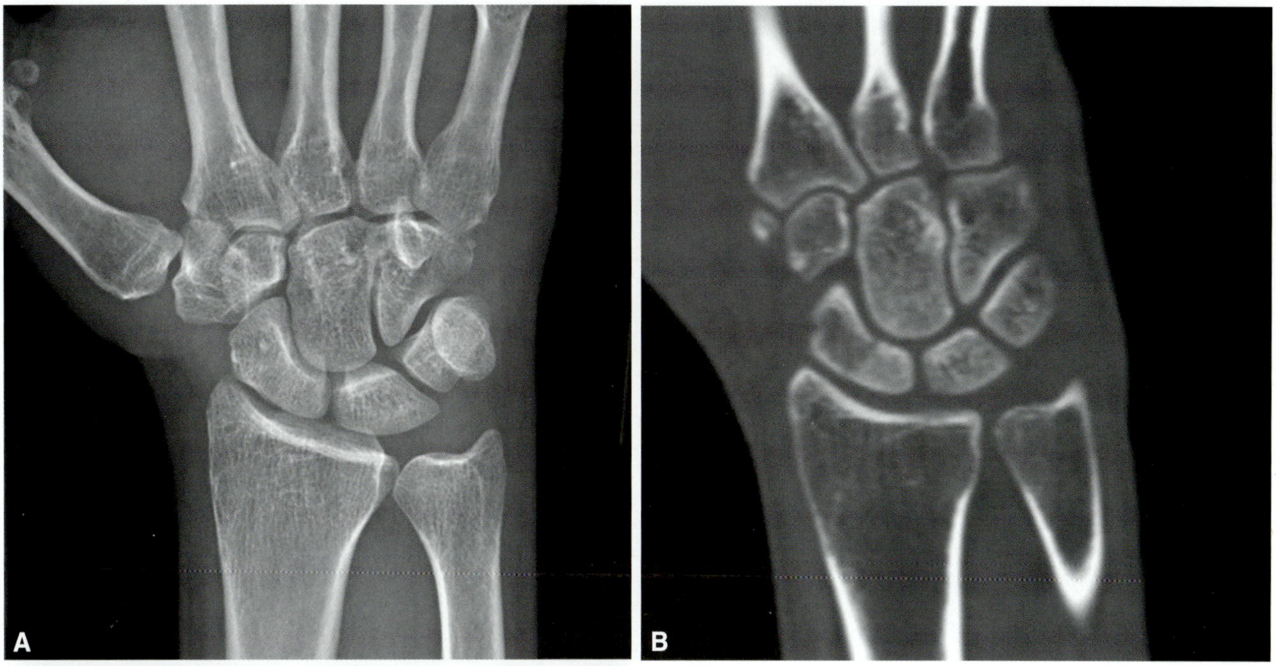

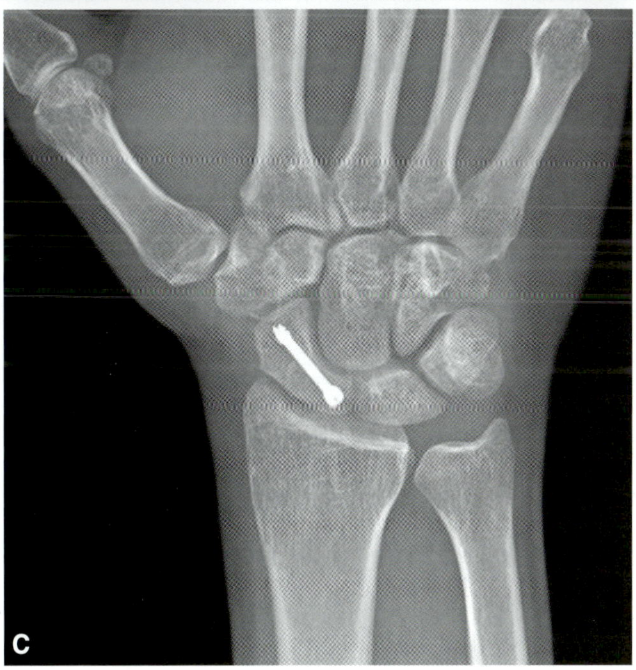

Figures 3.17A to C: This is a 42-year-old male patient who presented with pain in the anatomic snuff box following a fall on the outstretched hand with (A) negative radiographs. However, (B) CT scanning identified a nondisplaced scaphoid fracture. The patient's occupational demands did not allow for prolonged immobilization and therefore; (C) internal fixation with a cannulated compression screw was offered through a dorsal approach. Healing was uneventful.

prevalence of osteoarthritis in the scaphotrapezial joint in patients treated operatively was noted in a long-term follow-up study.[20] Both dorsal and volar percutaneous placement of interfragmentary compression screws have been described.[23,24] The authors prefer the dorsal percutaneous approach as it affords consistently reproducible central screw placement.

Operative treatment is indicated for all displaced or unstable (Herbert Type B), scaphoid fractures.[12] As increasing displacement is related to increasing risk of avascular necrosis and nonunion, early open reduction, or closed reduction, if feasible and internal fixation is the authors' treatment of choice for displaced fractures. Depending on the localization of the fracture, the amount

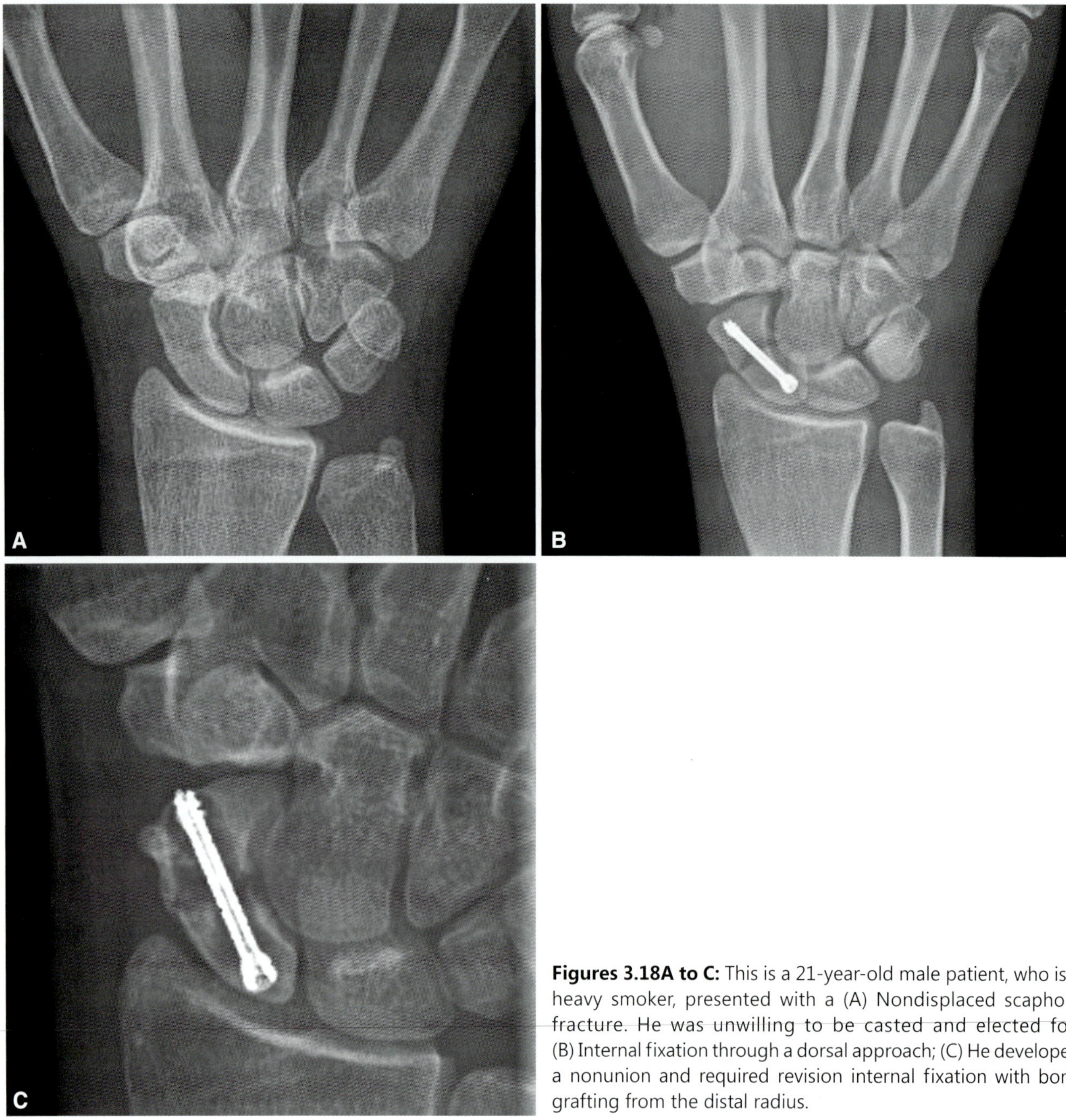

Figures 3.18A to C: This is a 21-year-old male patient, who is a heavy smoker, presented with a (A) Nondisplaced scaphoid fracture. He was unwilling to be casted and elected for; (B) Internal fixation through a dorsal approach; (C) He developed a nonunion and required revision internal fixation with bone grafting from the distal radius.

of displacement and the surgeon's preference of a dorsal or palmar approach is used. If closed reduction is successful, a percutaneous technique can be applied. The fragments can be fixed with a headless compression screw, a cannulated screw or Kirschner wires. We find closed manipulation to be extremely challenging in displaced fractures and prefer open reduction in these fractures. We also find Kirschner wires to provide inadequate stability and can potentially distract a fracture and as such mention it here only for historical value.

Fractures of the proximal pole and late-presenting scaphoid fractures should be considered for surgical treatment regardless of initial displacement.[23,25] A dorsal percutaneous approach may be chosen in most of these cases. Scaphoid fractures with concomitant severe soft-tissue injury, open wounds, associated carpal ligament injuries or concomitant fractures of the distal radius are often treated operatively regardless of initial displacement.[25] The exception to this generality is the minimally-displaced scaphoid fracture which presents in combination with a minimally-displaced distal radius fracture. If both are amenable to nonoperative treatment, they may together be treated nonoperatively as well.[26]

Overview

Nondisplaced fractures:

- Cast immobilization, duration dependent on fracture location
- Consider percutaneous fixation in active patients or those unable to be casted
- Consider open reduction and fixation of proximal pole or delayed diagnosed fractures

Displaced fractures:

Closed reduction if possible, otherwise open reduction and internal fixation

Fractures of Other Carpal Bones

As a rule of thumb, the authors recommend treating nondisplaced carpal fractures with cast immobilization for 4–6 weeks. Displaced fractures (> 1 mm) can be treated operatively to minimize risks of nonunion and osteoarthritis. A closed reduction and internal fixation may be tried. However, if adequate reduction is not achieved open reduction will be required. Kirschner wires are used in smaller fragments, whereas screws (mini-fragment, cannulated or headless compression screws) are preferred in larger fragments.

Bony avulsions of the triquetrum are typically treated nonoperatively.[14] A forearm-based splint or cast is typically applied for 4–6 weeks. Displaced fractures (> 1 mm) of the triquetral body should be treated operatively, especially if they are intra-articular. Most fractures of the trapezium, lunate and capitate may be treated nonoperatively. A short-arm cast is usually applied for 4–6 weeks. In cases of joint incongruity (> 1 mm), the authors recommend open reduction and internal fixation. In scaphocapitate syndrome, open reduction is required to derotate the capitates.[15] Most pisiform fractures are due to a direct trauma and are typically nondisplaced.[27] They can be treated with a removable splint. Although rare, pisiform nonunions are the best treated with excision.[27]

A type 1 hamate fracture or a hook of hamate fracture, may be treated nonoperatively with a short-arm cast.[14] As nonunion of the hook is common,[28] some authors recommend immobilizing the fingers to reduce the risk of nonunion. Late-presenting hook of hamate fractures can also be treated initially with a trial of casting, but are even more likely to go on to nonunion. Some surgeons treat every fracture of the hook of hamate with internal fixation (Kirschner wires or screws depending on the size of the fragment) fearing a painful nonunion of the hook. However, the "salvage" option remains excision for painful nonunions, generally leaving no gross functional impairment of the affected hand.[28] We prefer to treat all hook of hamate fractures nonoperatively at first, and treat symptomatic nonunions with hook excision. Type 2 fractures, especially coronal fractures, are often associated with subluxation or dislocation of the fourth and fifth carpometacarpal joints.[14] These fracture patterns are unstable and require surgical treatment. If closed reduction can be obtained, percutaneous fixation can be used. Otherwise, they are treated with open reduction and internal fixation. Any isolated hamate body fractures which are displaced (> 1 mm), also warrant open reduction and internal fixation.

Carpal Dislocations

Carpal dislocations are generally managed on an urgent basis. Any neurovascular compromise necessitates urgent closed reduction. Patients who have persistent neurologic symptoms after closed reduction or those who present late with neurovascular compromise may require an urgent open reduction and/or decompression. As these injuries are generally unstable injuries, operative repair usually follows.

Radiocarpal Dislocations

These injuries are unstable and typically warrant operative treatment. Nonoperative treatment can be cautiously employed where there is a concentric reduction in a compliant patient available for close follow-up. Otherwise, treatment of choice in purely ligamentous dislocation is open repair of the volar extrinsic ligamentous structures and temporary fixation with Kirschner wires or external fixation of the radiocarpal joint. Radiocarpal fracture-dislocations treatment consists of repair of the avulsion fractures of the distal radius, as well as open repair of the volar extrinsic ligaments of the wrist.

Axial Dislocations

These are rare injuries which are usually high-energy open fracture-dislocations and therefore, warrant open reduction and internal fixation.

Transverse Dislocations

Most perilunate dislocations are unstable or irreducible and therefore warrant operative management.[29,30] In selected cases (such as, severely ill patients), closed reduction and immobilization may be considered. But open ligament repair and internal fixation (Kirschner wires or screws between the scaphoid-lunate and lunate-triquetrum) generally leads to improved outcomes.[29,31] (Figs 3.19A to D). The authors prefer a combined dorsal and palmar approach which will be detailed in later sections. They recommend performing a concomitant carpal tunnel release at the time of surgery regardless of

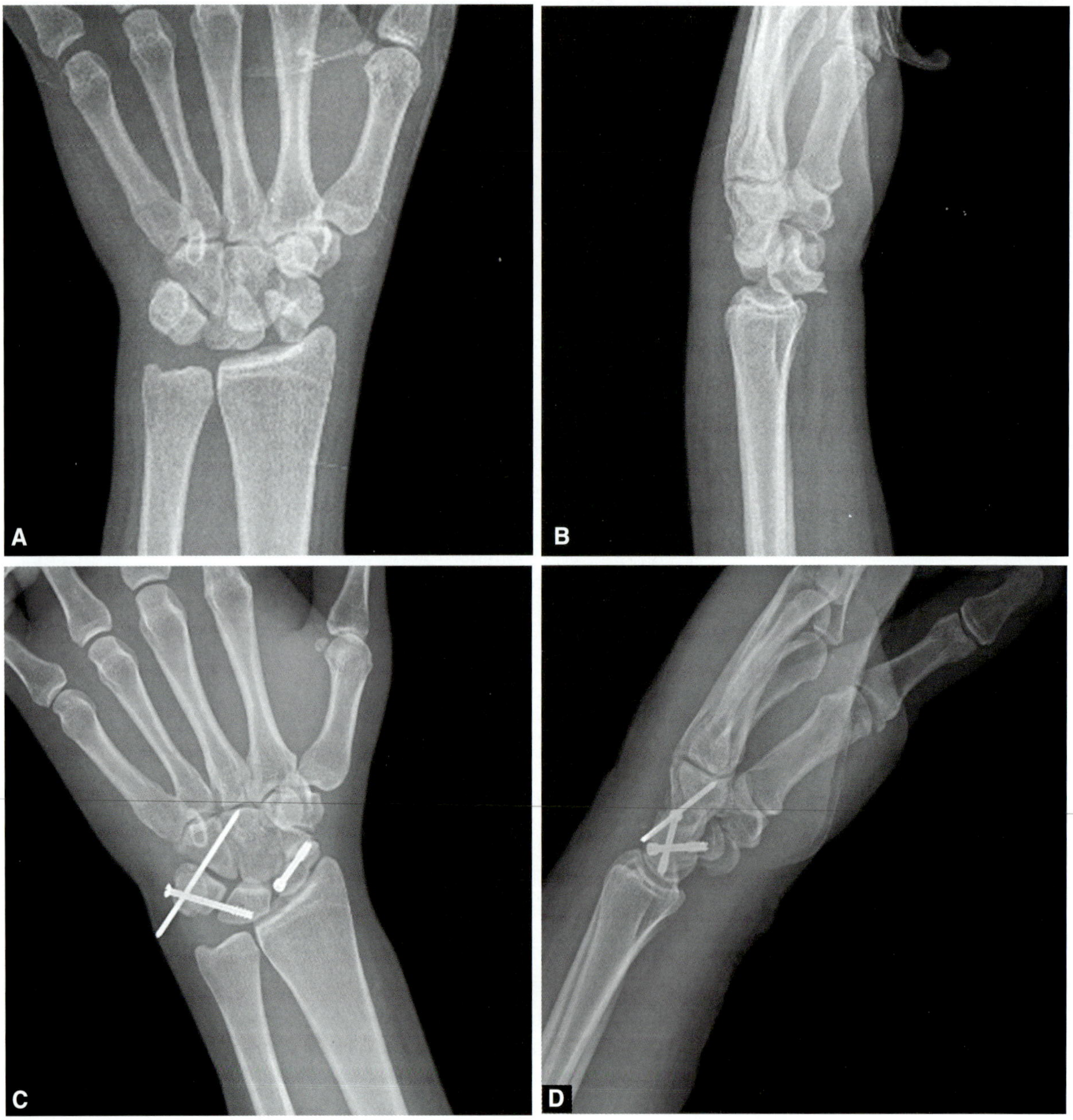

Figures 3.19A to D: This is a 40-year-old female who fell from a height sustaining a (A and B) trans-scaphoid perilunate dislocation; (C and D) a combined extensile volar approach with carpal tunnel release and lunate reduction followed by a dorsal approach with internal fixation of the scaphoid fracture and reduction with pinning of normal carpal alignment.

preoperative neurologic symptoms because there is nearly always a considerable amount of postoperative and post-traumatic swelling. The advantage of a palmar approach consists of repair of the important volar capsular ligaments, good access to the carpal tunnel and direct reduction of the lunate. The dorsal approach facilitates excellent exposure and direct reduction of the carpal bones. A cast or an external fixator is usually applied for 4–6 weeks. In special circumstances, the carpus may be spanned by an internal fixator, which usually consists of a plate fixed to the radius and third metacarpal. Not only does this allow excellent wound care in open injuries but also facilitates early, uncomplicated soft tissue coverage of wounds if needed. The disadvantage of this approach is the need for a second operative procedure to remove the plate 10–12 weeks after the index procedure.[32]

CARPAL FRACTURES AND PERILUNATE DISLOCATIONS SURGICAL INDICATIONS: Pearls and Pitfalls

- Cast immobilization is effective for nondisplaced and minimally displaced (< 1 mm) scaphoid fractures
- Surgical indications for scaphoid fractures include:
  - Displaced fractures
  - Proximal pole fractures
  - Delayed diagnosis/delayed healing
  - Any fracture in patients unable to be immobilized in a cast
- Neurovascular compromise is common with carpal dislocations and requires prompt reduction and decompression
- Radiocarpal and perilunate dislocations warrant open reduction and ligament repair to restore adequate stability

Surgical Anatomy, Positioning and Approaches

Relevant Surgical and Applied Anatomy

Surface Anatomy

Knowledge of the surface anatomy of the hand and wrist is important for the physical exam, as well as percutaneous and mini-open procedures. It must be remembered that carpal fractures are often high-energy injuries with significant soft tissue injury and disruption of the normal anatomic relationships.

On the volar surface, the scaphoid tubercle can be easily palpated just distal to the distal wrist crease, in line with the radial aspect of the long finger. It is also the first bony prominence palpable at the end of the flexor carpi radialis tendon at the level of the distal wrist crease. On the ulnar side of the palm, at the level of the distal wrist crease is the pisiform. If the examiner places the volar pad of their thumb on the pisiform and presses the thumb tip into the palm distally and radially, the hook of the hamate is felt as a deep resistance in the palm. In most circumstances, the hook of the hamate is 2 cm distal and 2 cm radial to the center of the pisiform. The tendons of the flexor carpi radialis (FCR) and palmaris longus (PL), when present can usually be palpated in the distal aspect of the volar forearm. In cases of severe swelling, the scaphoid tubercle can be used as a guide to the location of the FCR tendon, as it can be palpated immediately distal to the FCR tendon at the wrist. The pulse of the radial artery can be felt just radial to the FCR tendon.

On the dorsal surface, the waist of the scaphoid can be palpated in the anatomic snuffbox in line with the thumb ray between the tendons of the extensor pollicis brevis and extensor pollicis longus (EPL). Just proximal and radial to this is the radial styloid, which is generally easily palpable but can become obscured by swelling after trauma. Just ulnar to the scaphoid and distal to Lister's tubercle is a soft spot at the radiocarpal joint between the scaphoid and lunate. The lunate can be felt just ulnar to this soft spot, and ulnar to the lunate lies the dorsal aspect of the triquetrum.

Bones and Ligaments

The eight carpal bones are conventionally divided into a proximal and a distal row. The proximal row consists of (from radial to ulnar) the scaphoid (S), lunate (L), triquetrum (T) and pisiform (P). The distal row consists of the trapezium (T1), trapezoid (T2), capitate (C) and hamate (H) (Fig. 3.20). The relationships of the carpal bones (along with the distal radius and ulna) are maintained by the complex array of radiocarpal and intercarpal ligaments. These ligaments can be divided into palmar and dorsal radiocarpal ligaments, ulnocarpal ligaments, palmar and dorsal midcarpal ligaments and proximal and distal interosseous ligaments.[33]

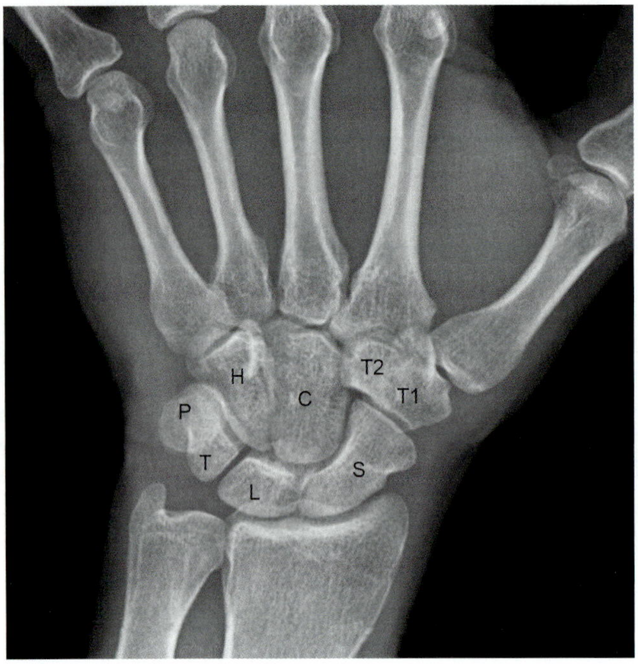

Figure 3.20: The carpal anatomy of the wrist: the scaphoid (S), lunate (L), triquetrum (T) and pisiform (P). The distal row consists of the trapezium (T1), trapezoid (T2), capitate (C) and hamate (H).

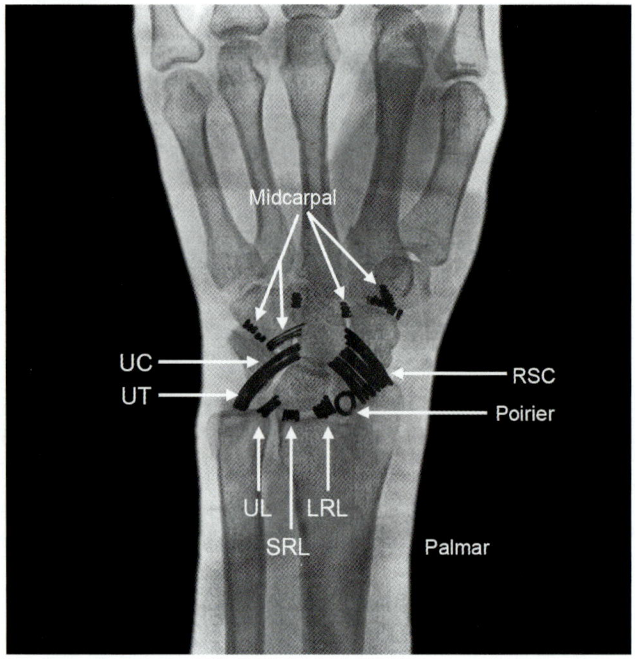

Figure 3.21: The palmar wrist ligaments: the radioscaphocapitate (RSC), radioscapholunate (ligament of Testut), long radiolunate (LRL), short radiolunate (SRL) and the ulnocarpal ligaments.

The volar radiocarpal ligaments (from radial to ulnar) are the radioscaphocapitate (RSC), radioscapholunate (ligament of Testut), long radiolunate (LRL) and short radiolunate (SRL) (Fig. 3.21). The space of Poirier is the defect in the volar ligaments through which the lunate dislocates palmarly in a perilunate dislocation. This space is created by the weak point between the RSC and the LRL ligaments. The radioscapholunate ligament (ligament of Testut) is the least like a true ligament and rather serves as a conduit for neurovascular structures.

The ulnocarpal ligaments are a continuation of the ligaments on the palmar side of the wrist, and wrap around the ulnar aspect of the wrist. These are the ulnolunate, ulnotriquetral and ulnocapitate ligaments. There is a single dorsal radiocarpal ligament with attachments to the distal radius, lunate and triquetrum (Fig. 3.22).

There are four volar midcarpal ligaments (scapho-trapezium-trapezoid, scaphocapitate, triquetrocapitate, triquetrohamate and palmar scaphotriquetral) and two dorsal midcarpal ligaments (dorsal intercarpal ligament and dorsal scaphotriquetral ligament). The palmar

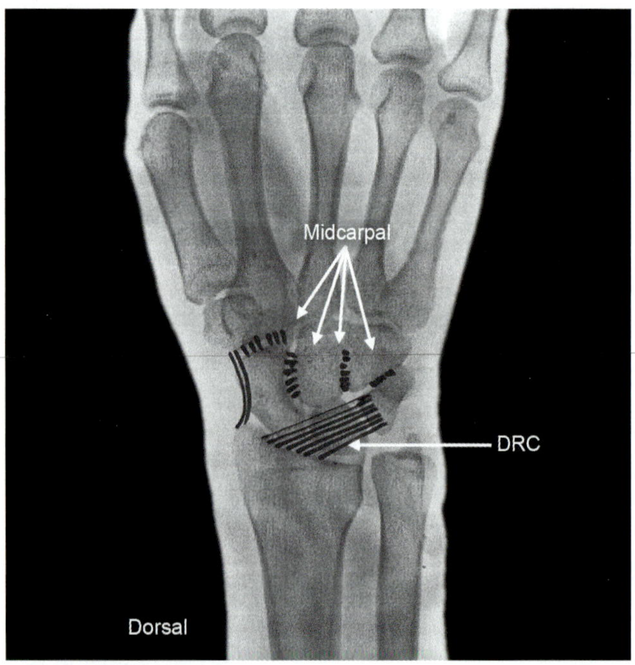

Figure 3.22: The dorsal wrist ligaments consist primarily of one single dorsal radiocarpal ligament (DRC), with attachments to the distal radius, lunate and triquetrum.

midcarpal ligaments are generally discrete intra-articular ligaments connecting two bones (or three in the case of the scaphotrapezium-trapezoid ligament), whereas the two dorsal midcarpal ligaments are broad capsular ligaments spanning several bones.

Individual carpal bones are connected via interosseous ligaments. In the proximal row, these are the scapholunate and lunotriquetral interosseous ligaments. In the distal row, there are the trapeziotrapezoid, trapeziocapitate and capitohamate interosseous ligaments.

Tendons

The tendons of the dorsal wrist are divided into six dorsal compartments. From radial to ulnar, they are: first (abductor pollicis longus and extensor pollicis brevis), second (extensor carpi radialis longus and brevis), third (EPL), fourth (extensor digitorum communis (four tendons) and extensor indicis), fifth (extensor digiti minimi) and sixth (extensor carpi ulnaris). The third compartment turns a corner around Lister's tubercle of the distal radius, increasing the mechanical advantage of the EPL.

Volarly, the flexor carpi radialis tendon is an important landmark, just ulnar to the radial artery. The flexor carpi ulnaris (FCU) tendon lies ulnar to the ulnar nerve and artery, and inserts onto the pisiform. The tendons of the flexor pollicis longus, flexor digitorum superficialis and profundus lie within the carpal tunnel at this level. These tendons are visualized during carpal tunnel release which is often done in combination with the exposure and repair of carpal injuries.

Nerves

In approaching carpal fractures either percutaneously or open, the course of the radial, median and ulnar nerves must be appreciated. The radial nerve at this level has already split into its terminal branches—the radial sensory nerve and the posterior interosseous nerve (PIN). The radial sensory nerve emerges from beneath the brachioradialis approximately 9 cm proximal to the radial styloid. It then arborizes, usually into 2–3 distinct branches before dividing further to provide sensation to the dorsoradial hand.[34] The terminal branch of the PIN lies in the floor of the fourth dorsal compartment. At this point, the PIN provides only sensation to the wrist joint, and many surgeons elect to perform a PI neurectomy at the time of any surgery on the dorsal wrist to mitigate possible wrist pain.

The median nerve gives off the palmar cutaneous branch toward its radial aspect in the volar forearm, anywhere from 0–5 cm proximal to the wrist crease. This branch then continues along the radial aspect of the PL tendon sheath to provide sensation to the palm. The median nerve properly enters the wrist via the carpal tunnel. The nerve will then give off the recurrent motor branch (to the thenar muscles), followed by the common digital nerves. The motor branch usually takes off from the radial aspect of the median nerve just after exiting the carpal tunnel (so called extraligamentous), or while in the carpal tunnel (subligamentous). However, other anatomical variations have also been described, so any surgery in this area must be done carefully under direct visualization.

The ulnar nerve runs along the radial aspect of the FCU tendon in the wrist, giving off the dorsal ulnar sensory branch about 7 cm proximal to the wrist crease. The remainder of the nerve then enters the hand via Guyon's canal. The anatomy of the ulnar nerve in this area is divided into three zones. Zone I describes the most proximal portion of Guyon's canal before the nerve branches into its superficial and deep components. The nerve then branches nearly vertically with the motor branch lying deep in Guyon's canal (Zone II) with the superficial branch just volar to it (Zone III). The deep branch then continues between the abductor digiti minimi and flexor digiti minimi brevis to supply the deep intrinsic muscles of the hand. The superficial branch innervates the palmaris brevis, as well as providing sensory branches to the ring and small fingers.

Vessels

The courses of the radial and ulnar arteries are important to understand in the management of carpal injuries. The radial artery courses through the volar forearm between the tendons of the brachioradialis and the FCR. It gives off two branches in the distal forearm; the superficial palmar branch (contribution to the superficial arch) and the palmar carpal branch (can usually be seen at the distal aspect of the pronator quadratus), as well as two branches at the wrist—the dorsal carpal branch and first dorsal metacarpal artery (can be seen during dorsal thumb base surgery). The artery then continues as the deep palmar branch, which passes dorsal to the base of the thumb in the anatomic snuff-box, before returning to the volar hand through the first webspace between the first dorsal interosseous and adductor pollicis muscles. Once there, it gives off branches to the thumb (princeps pollicis) and index finger (radialis indices) before terminating as the deep palmar arch.

The ulnar artery gives off carpal branches at the wrist which anastamose with similar branches of the radial artery. It then passes into the hand via Guyon's canal where it runs just radial to the ulnar nerve. Immediately, distal to the pisiform, the artery divides into deep and superficial palmar branches. The deep branch provides a minor contribution to the deep arch, while the superficial branch is the major contributor to the superficial arch.

Special mention of the vascular supply to the scaphoid is warranted. Because the proximal portion of the scaphoid is nearly all articular surface, the primary blood supply is retrograde via the distal portion of the scaphoid. Penetrating vessels to the distal scaphoid are branches of the radial artery, predominantly from the dorsal carpal branch mentioned earlier.

Positioning

We perform all of these procedures with the patient supine and the involved limb extended on a hand table and under tourniquet control applied to the upper arm. For dorsal approaches, a rolled towel is placed under the hand to allow wrist flexion which will generally improve visualization. For volar approaches, a lead hand may be helpful. Whenever possible, we prefer regional anesthesia (either an axillary or infraclavicular block). This allows decreased intraoperative use of narcotics while providing excellent postoperative pain relief.

Surgical Approaches

Nearly all of these fractures can be approached through two "workhorse" incisions about the wrist; the modified volar distal Henry approach and the midline dorsal approach. Both are described below along with others used for specific fractures.

The modified distal Henry approach follows the line of the FCR tendon in the distal forearm. When using this approach for a scaphoid fracture, we continue the incision at a 45° angle across the wrist crease, angling in line with the thumb ray. The skin and subcutaneous tissue are incised to the FCR sheath proximally and to the thenar musculature distally. The FCR sheath is then opened along its radial edge so as to avoid the palmar cutaneous branch of the median nerve. The tendon is retracted ulnarly and the floor of the sheath is incised along its radial edge as well to enter the space of Parona. The thenar musculature is split in line with the distal portion of the incision. The volar radiocarpal ligaments and capsule are then identified in the base of the wound and incised sharply in line with the skin incision. The surgeon may choose to tag them for later repair. The scaphoid is exposed. The capsule can then be elevated radially and ulnarly to expose the entire scaphoid, as well as the trapezium. Towards the distal pole of the scaphoid, it is essential to make a capsular incision in the scaphotrapezial joint. Furthermore, in order to achieve a central position for screw placement through the distal pole of the scaphoid, it is important to excise the volar lip of the trapezium and elevate the distal pole of the scaphoid to access the central portion of the distal pole.

The dorsal midline approach to the wrist begins with a midline incision, just ulnar to Lister's tubercle in line with the third metacarpal. Thick skin flaps are developed ulnarly and radially to expose the entire extensor retinaculum (Figs 3.23A and B). It is important to maintain the thickness of the flaps so that the dorsal cutaneous nerves will remain undisturbed in the flaps. The third dorsal compartment is identified (flexing and extending the thumb interphalangeal joint can help) and opened lengthwise. The EPL is brought out of the compartment. The second and fourth compartments are then elevated subperiosteally to reveal the dorsal wrist capsule. The capsule is then incised longitudinally in line with the midline skin incision (Fig. 3.24). Care is taken to avoid injury to the cartilage of the carpal bones or the scapholunate interosseous ligament. Again it is important to remember that anatomical relationships are likely to be altered in the setting of trauma.

The pisiform and hook of the hamate are volar structures that reside ulnar that are the best approached with the FCU approach. The incision runs along the FCU tendon in the distal forearm turning obliquely across the wrist in a radial direction in line between the hamate and the pisiform. The FCU sheath is opened along its radial edge, and the volar carpal ligament is divided in line with the skin incision to enter Guyon's canal. The ulnar artery

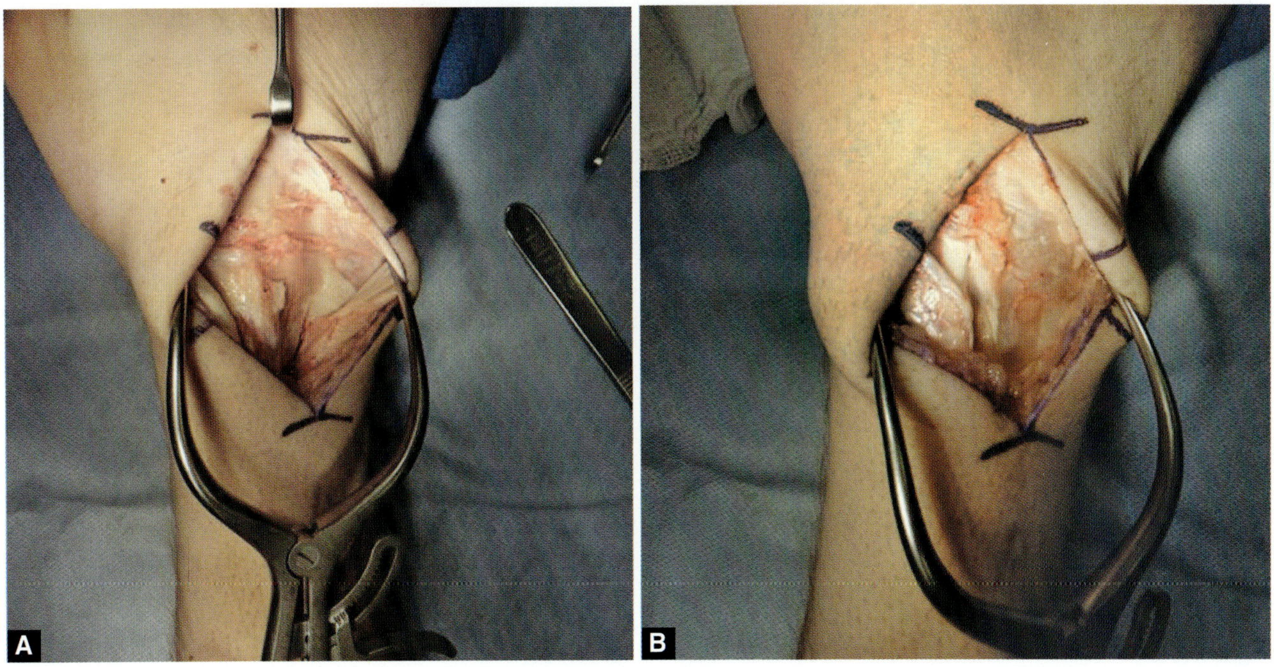

Figures 3.23A and B: The dorsal exposure of the wrist begins with splitting the interval between the tendons of the second and fourth dorsal compartments. Next, the (A) third dorsal compartment is approached and (B) opened to release the extensor pollicis longus which is retracted radially. The result is complete exposure of the dorsal capsule of the wrist.

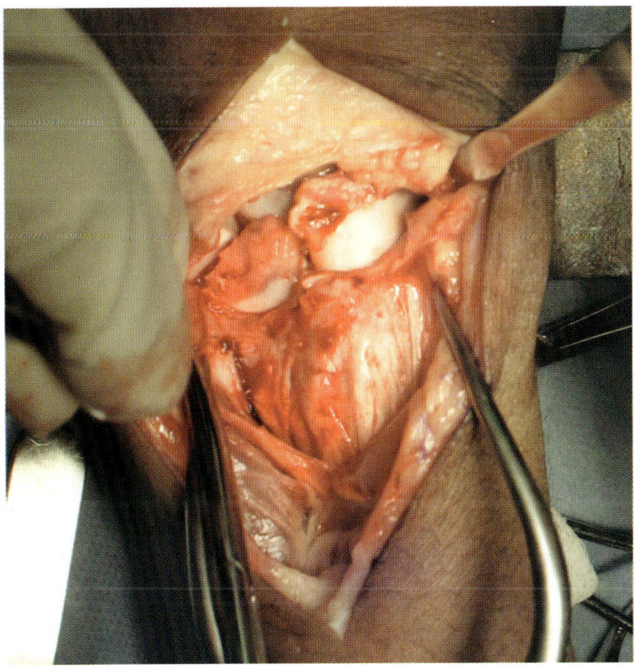

Figure 3.24: A dorsal view of the wrist in the case of a perilunate dislocation. Note rupture of the scapholunate ligament and displacement of the scaphoid and lunate.

and nerve can then be identified from proximal to distal. At the level of the pisiform, the ulnar nerve can be seen dividing into a superficial sensory and deep motor branch. Once identified, the nerve and artery can be gently retracted away from the area of interest (either the hamate hook or the pisiform). In situations where a carpal tunnel release is performed, at the same time, an extended approach is utilized. Distally, the approach lies in the proximal palm along a line which is collinear with the third webspace and then proximally lies ulnar to the median nerve and flexor tendons. This allows access to the ulnar corner of the distal radius and volar carpal ligaments, as well as the carpal tunnel. Through this same approach, the hook of the hamate can also be accessed easily.

The pisotriquetral joint can also be approached through a midlateral incision on the ulnar aspect of the hand. If this incision is used to excise the pisiform, care must be taken to stay completely subperiosteal on the pisiform as the ulnar artery and nerve are vulnerable at the radial aspect of the pisotriquetral joint.

Surgical Techniques

Technique 1: Open Reduction and Internal Fixation (ORIF) of Scaphoid Fractures

Acute scaphoid fractures can be treated via one of the three approaches: percutaneous volar, open volar or mini-open dorsal approach, all of which will be described below. Prior to any of these surgical procedures, a CT scan is obtained which we use to confirm the orientation of the fracture line, the displacement and the size of the scaphoid. Fixation is generally obtained with a 3.0 mm cannulated compression screw but occasionally a 2.4 mm screw is required.

Percutaneous Volar Scaphoid Fixation

We prefer a percutaneous volar technique for nondisplaced fractures of the scaphoid waist (Figs 3.25A to F). The patient is positioned supine with a hand table, as described previously. We begin with fluoroscopy to confirm the location of the fracture. Next, the volar scaphoid tubercle is palpated and marked. This can also be confirmed on fluoroscopy, if it is not readily apparent. We make a small incision direction over the tubercle just large enough to accommodate a drill guide. Blunt dissection is used to reach the bone. The incision should be large enough to allow the volar lip of the trapezium to be rongeured if necessary, so as to permit satisfactory placement of the guidewire and screw.

The guidewire is placed freehand on the tubercle and the entry point and trajectory are confirmed with fluoroscopy. The trajectory of the guidewire is generally in line with the thumb ray, aiming approximately 45° both dorsally and ulnarly. We then pass the guidewire into the superficial cortex of the distal fragment. The position of the entry point and the trajectory are again confirmed. If the positioning of the wire is incorrect, the wire can either be withdrawn and repositioned or left in place as a guide for appropriate placement of a second wire. Once the entry point and trajectory are acceptable, the guidewire is advanced into the proximal pole fragment and seated in the subchondral bone. The position of the guidewire is confirmed under fluoroscopy. We generally obtain AP and lateral views, as well as an ulnar-deviation anteroposterior view, semipronated and semisupinated oblique views. Live fluoroscopy is used between these views if there is any doubt about the positioning.

Once we are satisfied with the guidewire placement, a measuring device is used to determine the length of the guidewire, and we generally choose a screw about 4 mm shorter than the measured length. The cannulated drill is then inserted over the guidewire. We start the drill running prior to seating it on the bone to ensure that it is exactly in line with the guidewire. We then drill across the fracture site into the proximal fragment. If there is doubt about the length that has been drilled, fluoroscopy can be used. The drill is withdrawn carefully. In the event that the guidewire is removed with the drill, a second wire is placed freehand and confirmed on fluoroscopy. The screw is then inserted over the guidewire and compressed. The guidewire is removed and final fluoroscopic images are obtained.

Open Volar Scaphoid Fixation

An open volar approach is our preferred exposure for displaced fractures of the scaphoid waist. The patient is positioned supine with a hand table. The wrist is extended over a bump. An incision is placed obliquely across the volar wrist crease in line with the FCR tendon. The tendon is retracted ulnarly thereby exposing the distal pole of the scaphoid. The displaced scaphoid fracture at this point is usually readily apparent from fracture hematoma. To expose the waist of the fracture, the capsuloligamentous complex and the volar radiocarpal ligaments crossing at the waist is split longitudinally and tagged for later repair. The fracture site is irrigated and the fracture edges debrided of any interposed tissue. To facilitate reduction of the scaphoid fragments, we recommend placing 0.045 inch Kirschner wires into both fragments to use as joysticks. A freer elevator is placed at the proximal pole of the scaphoid so that it is visible. While the assistant holds the fracture fragments reduced, as well as the freer to visualize the proximal pole, the surgeon places the guidewire into the distal pole aiming for the freer, and driving it across into the proximal fragment. The positioning of the guidewire is confirmed with fluoroscopy with multiple views as discussed above, before continuing with measuring, drilling and placement of the compression screw. We ensure that the screw is advanced just below the subchondral bone of the scaphoid before removing the guidewire. Final fluoroscopic images are obtained. The wound is irrigated thoroughly. The capsuloligamentous

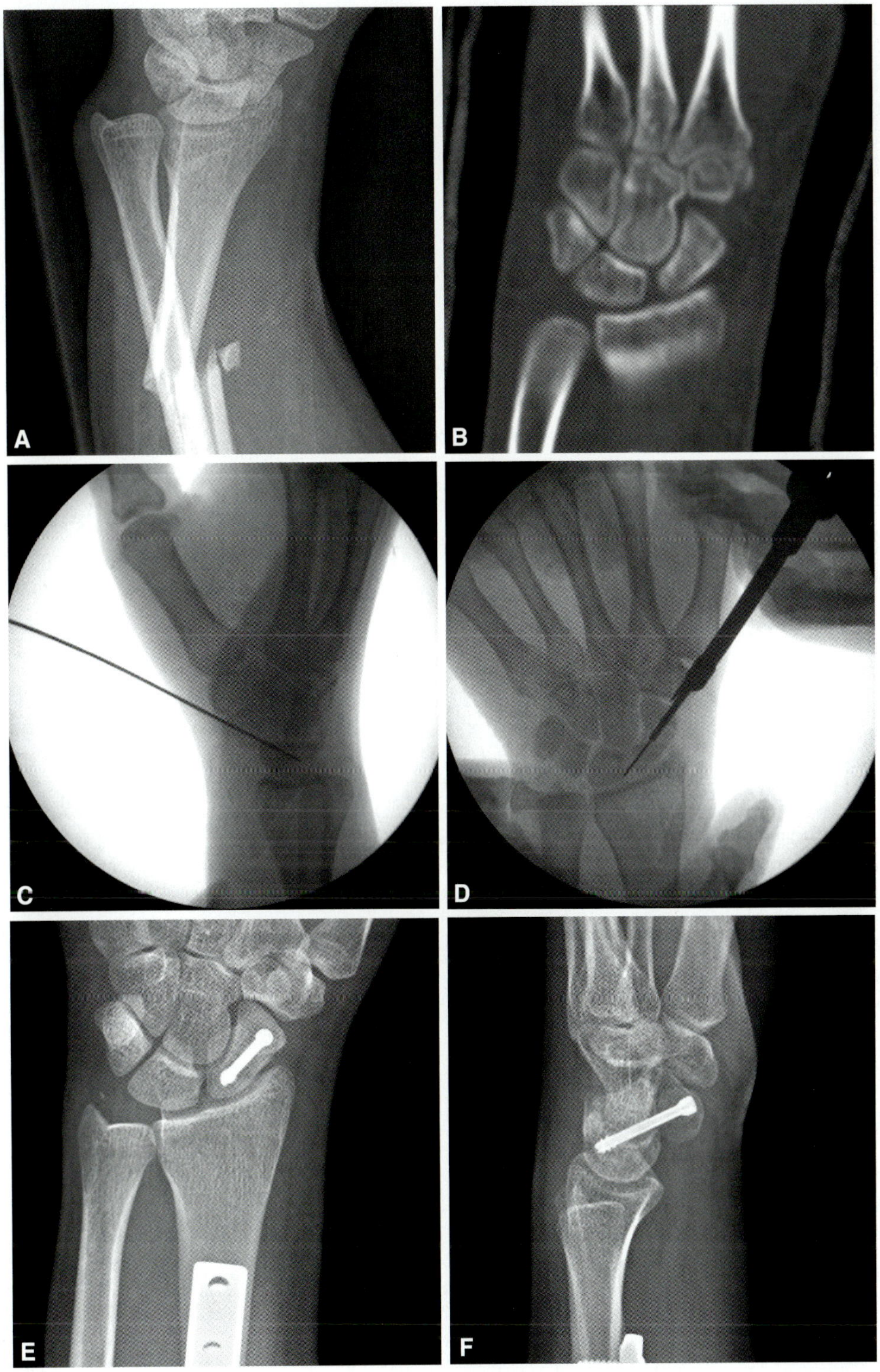

Figures 3.25A to F: A 23-year-old female fell (A) incurring a Galeazzi fracture that underwent operative fixation. Persistent wrist pain led to the identification of an (B) occult scaphoid fracture ultimately diagnosed by CT; (C and D) The scaphoid was fixed through a percutaneous volar approach. Orthogonal views are necessary to confirm appropriate placement of the guidewire into the central axis of the scaphoid. We recommend placing a screw 4 mm shorter than the measured length of the scaphoid to avoid inadvertent screw prominence; (E and F) Final radiographs confirm good reduction of the fracture and appropriate placement of the headless compression screw.

envelope is reapproximated with interrupted sutures. The skin is then closed with interrupted nylon sutures.

Mini-Open Dorsal Scaphoid Fixation

We use a mini-open dorsal approach for fractures of the proximal pole (Fig. 3.26). The same positioning is used except the wrist is pronated and volar-flexed over a bump. Fluoroscopy is used to determine the appropriate starting point at the proximal pole. A small longitudinal incision is made directly over this area, typically correlating to just distal to Lister's tubercle. The subcutaneous tissue is dissected bluntly to protect the sensory nerves, and the distal extent of the extensor retinaculum is identified. The EPL tendon is identified and retracted and the dorsal capsule is incised in the interval between the second and fourth extensor compartments. While opening the capsule, caution must be exercised to avoid causing iatrogenic injury to the scapholunate interosseous ligament.

Once satisfied the proximal pole is reduced, a guidewire is placed directly on the proximal pole at the junction of the proximal pole with the scapholunate ligament aiming down the axis of the thumb ray. Flexion of the wrist is vital at this stage as it allows the guidewire to enter the proximal pole at its central tip rather than its dorsal edge. Once the guidewire is advanced into the near fragment, multiple C-arm views are obtained to check both the starting point and trajectory. If the starting point is still not volar enough, the incision can be extended proximally to allow creation of a trough in the dorsal aspect of the distal radius. Once the guidewire position is confirmed, it is advanced to the subchondral bone of the distal scaphoid. The screw length is measured, and again we usually choose a screw 4 mm shorter than the measured length. The guidewire is overdrilled in the same manner as noted above, and we place the screw over the guidewire taking care to advance it below the surface of the cartilage before withdrawing the guidewire.

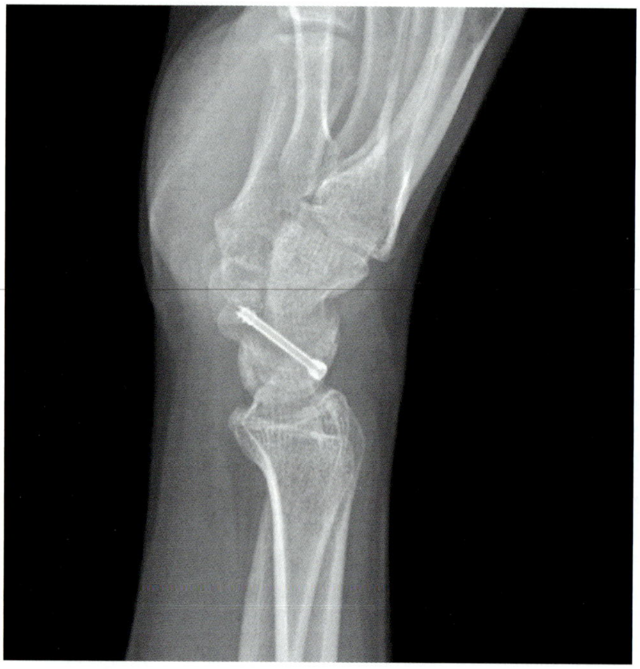

Figure 3.26: Mini-open dorsal approach and fixation of the scaphoid.

The wound is irrigated and closed.

Postoperative Management

Regardless of approach and fixation, all patients are placed into a well-padded short arm thumb spica splint at the conclusion of the procedure. We routinely see patients in follow-up within 1–2 weeks postoperatively. Patients with proximal pole fractures and those undergoing a formal volar open reduction are generally immobilized for an additional 4 weeks postoperatively, while those patients undergoing percutaneous fixation (either volar or dorsal) for waist fractures are converted to a removable splint and a rehabilitation program is commenced. A postoperative CT scan can be obtained at 6 weeks after surgery to assess union. After confirmation of evidence of union, a strengthening program is commenced and all splinting is discontinued. Contact sport is usually allowed after 12 weeks.

ORIF OF SCAPHOID FRACTURES: Pearls and Pitfalls

- Most scaphoid fractures can be treated through a percutaneous or mini-open approach
- The key to success is the starting point and positioning of the guidewire. Take your time. The guidewire must be positioned along the central axis of the scaphoid. The volar percutaneous approach can be improved by rongeuring the trapezium overlying the distal pole of the scaphoid
- Live fluoroscopy is very useful and the fluoroscope should be positioned to facilitate easy access throughout the case
- Avoid distraction at the fracture site; stable fixation and compression leads to union.

Technique 2: ORIF of Other Carpal Bone Fractures

Isolated and combined carpal fractures are generally approached through an extensile dorsal approach. The dorsal capsule can be opened widely to expose the entire carpus. Generally, we prefer to secure relationships between carpal bones with 0.045 inch or 0.062 inch Kirschner wires, which are left out of the skin. Coronal shear fractures of individual carpal bones can be reduced by hand under direct visualization and fixed with 1.5 mm or 2.0 mm headed screws if possible or with headless screws as needed. We do not lag these screws due to the already tenuous fixation of these small screws. Horizontal body fractures are fixed with headless cannulated compression screws. Flexion of the wrist over a bump may be necessary to expose the starting point for the screw guidewire in the carpal bone of interest. All of these require confirmation on fluoroscopy to ensure adequate reduction.

ORIF OF OTHER CARPAL BONE FRACTURES: Pearls and Pitfalls

- The carpal bones and fragments can be very small. Use hardware commensurate to the size of the fragment
- Exposure is often facilitated by flexing the wrist over a bump after adequate capsular elevation

Technique 3: ORIF of Perilunate Dislocations

In general, perilunate injuries cannot be treated through closed or percutaneous approaches. We recommend approaching both greater arc and lesser arc injuries through a combined dorsal and volar approach (Figs 3.27A and B). We will use fixation of a trans-scaphoid, transradial perilunate fracture-dislocation as a model for this approach (Figs 3.28A to G).

We routinely begin with a carpal tunnel release via an extensile volar approach. As the approach is extended

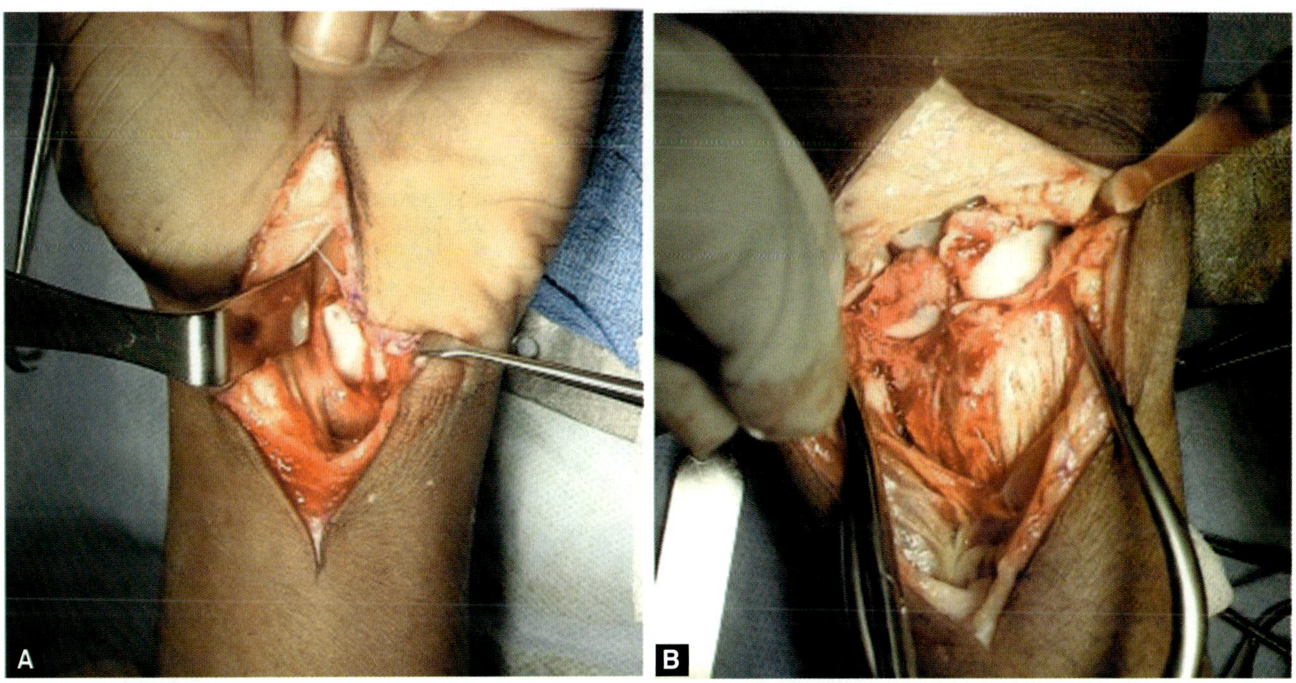

Figures 3.27A and B: Perilunate dislocations are approached through a combined volar and dorsal approach in order to maximize exposure and facilitate accurate reduction of the carpus as well as to provide access to repair the capsuloligamentous and interosseous ligament injuries.

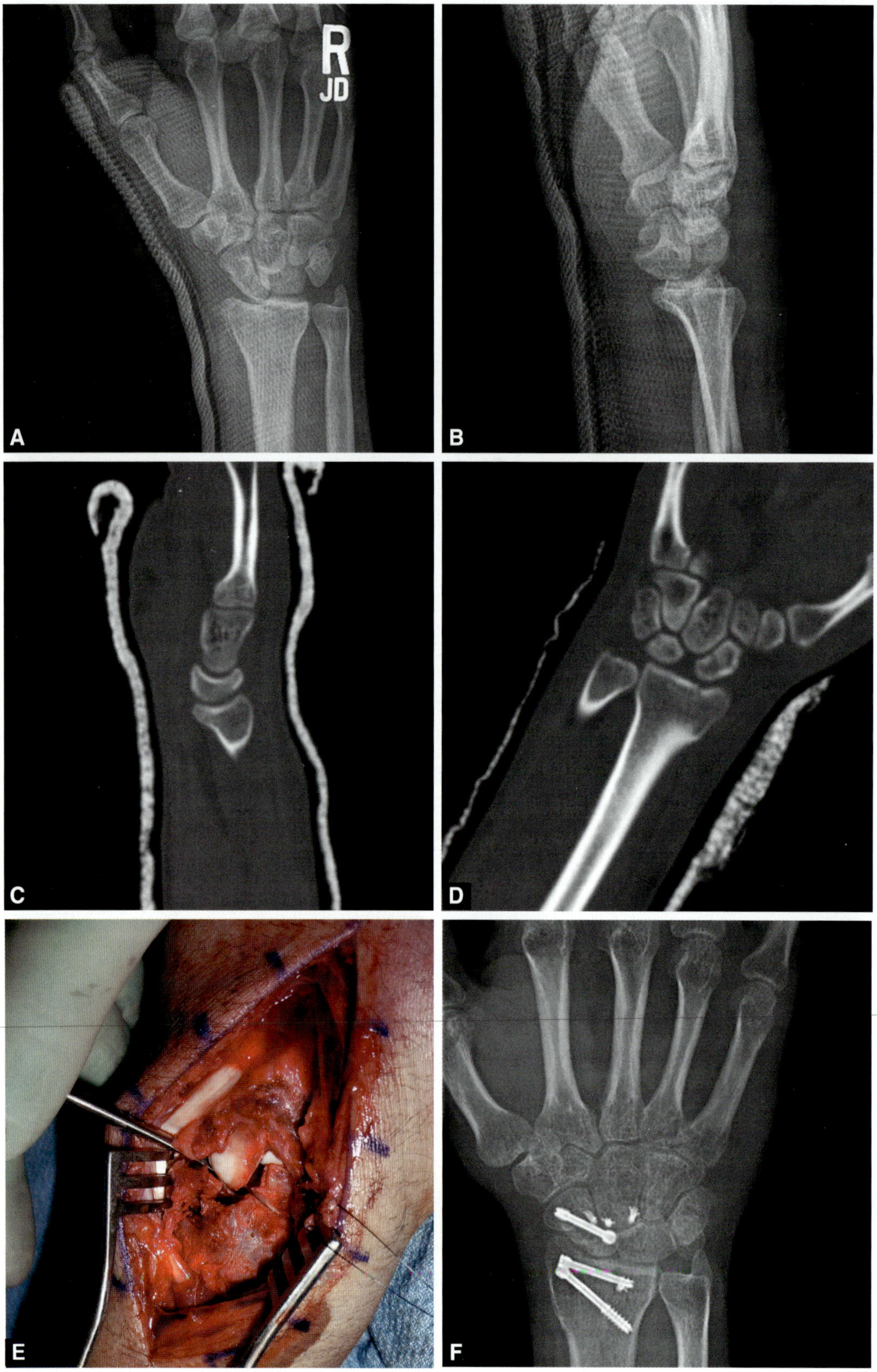

Figures 3.28A to F

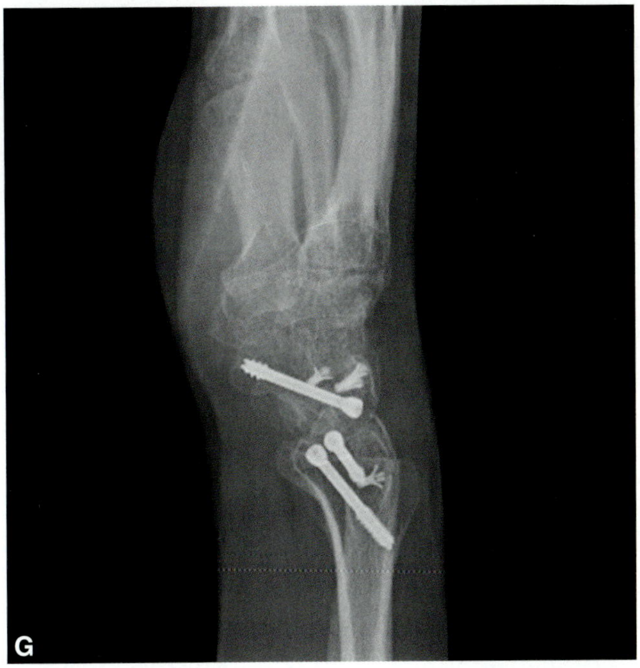

Figures 3.28A to G: A 26-year-old male fell from a height and presented with a (A and B) transscaphoid dorsal perilunate dislocation with a concomitant distal radius fracture and median nerve paresthesias; (C) A closed reduction was performed; (D) The post-reduction CT also showed a scapholunate diastasis, a scaphoid fracture and a distal radial styloid fracture; (E) Intra-operative dorsal exposure confirms both fracture of the scaphoid through its waist, as well as complete disruption of the scapholunate interosseous ligament. Furthermore fracture of the radial styloid and a metaphysal die-punch lesion is also identified in the distal radius. The repair followed the following steps: (1) repair of all fractures, (2) resotration and pinning of the normal carpal relationships, (3) repair of the scapholunate interosseous ligament, and (4) repair of the capsuloligamentous structures volarly and dorsally; (F and G) Posteroanterior and lateral radiographs taken at 6 months follow-up demonstrates all fractures to have healed with well-maintained carpal relationships.

proximally across the wrist with an oblique incision, an interval is developed between the finger flexor tendons and the ulnar neurovascular bundle. This allows excellent access to the volar capsular rent and for its subsequent repair. It must be remembered that the volar structure seen after retracting the flexor tendons is not the ligamentous rent but merely the capsular tear. It is only after debriding the edges of this, can the true ligamentous injury be appreciated. If the lunate is still dislocated volarly through the rent, it is reduced dorsally back into the carpus. Sutures are placed in this rent with braided nonabsorbable material and are left untied at this time. These will be tied later after all the manipulation required for bony reduction and stabilization is completed.

We then make an extensile dorsal approach to the wrist. There is often a capsular tear already, and if not, an inverted T-shaped incision is made in the capsule which in the most circumstances is quite friable. During this exposure, the dorsal ridge blood supply to the scaphoid is protected.

Once the carpus is adequately exposed, we begin with fixation of the scaphoid. This is done with a cannulated headless compression screw. We then proceed with ORIF of the radial styloid fracture which can be done via the same dorsal incision or through an additional small radial styloid incision. Care is taken to protect branches of the radial sensory nerve. These radial styloid fractures can generally be fixed with cannulated screws. Alternatively, a radial styloid plate may be applied.

After all fractures are fixed, we address the carpal instability. We prefer a "diamond configuration" of 0.045 inch or 0.062 inch Kirschner wires to secure the carpal relationships. We begin with reduction of the scapholunate interval. This can be done by using Kirschner wires as joysticks in the scaphoid and lunate or by pinning the lunate reduced to the radius, then bringing the scaphoid into alignment with the lunate. Once reduction is attained, a Kirschner wire is passed from the proximal scaphoid into the lunate under X-ray guidance. A second Kirschner wire is then placed from the distal scaphoid into the capitate for added fixation. It is imperative during this step to restore the normal scapholunate relationship including elimination of any scapholunate diastasis and restoration of the normal scapholunate angle of approximately 35–60° on the lateral view.

Usually, the lunotriquetral ligament is ruptured as well. Once the scapholunate reduction is complete, the lunotriquetral relationship should be re-established. A Kirschner wire is placed from the triquetrum into the lunate, followed by a second wire from the triquetrum into the hamate. This completes the diamond configuration. If portions of the scapholunate or lunotriquetral ligament are intact, they can then be reattached to their appropriate attachment points using mini suture anchors. Again, fluoroscopic confirmation of restoration of all carpal relationships is essential at this time.

Upon closure, the dorsal capsular repair is accomplished as best as possible. The EPL is exteriorized and the extensor retinaculum is closed deep to it. Attention is now turned back to the volar wound and the sutures placed in the volar capsular rent are now tied off. The wounds are irrigated and closed as usual and a thumb spica splint is placed.

Postoperatively, all patients are placed into a well-padded short arm thumb spica splint at the conclusion of the procedure. We routinely see patients in follow-up within 1–2 weeks postoperatively, at which point the postoperative splint is changed to a short-arm thumb spica cast. The patient will be immobilized for 8–12 weeks to allow sufficient time for the osseous and soft tissue injuries to heal. Unfortunately, early mobilization may compromise the carpal realignment. Preoperatively, it is imperative to emphasize the fact that prolonged immobilization is necessary and there is a high predilection towards post-traumatic stiffness and arthrosis.

ORIF OF PERILUNATE DISLOCATIONS: Pearls and Pitfalls

- An extensile volar approach allows concomitant decompression of the carpal tunnel and repair of the volar ligaments. Furthermore, if the lunate is incarcerated volarly, the extensile volar approach facilitates direct reduction of the lunate back into the radiocarpal joint
- An extensile dorsal approach allows assessment and direct restoration of the normal carpal relationships
- The order of repair should be: (1) fracture repair, (2) reduction and pinning of the carpal relationships, (3) interosseous ligament repair, if applicable and lastly, (4) capsuloligamentous repair
- The restoration of the normal anatomy of the scaphoid and lunate is critical

Outcomes

Injuries to the carpal bones and ligaments are often severe injuries which can lead to a wrist that is forever changed. Patients may develop long-term disability related to the original trauma, such as pain and post-traumatic osteoarthritis. Dislocations are especially prone to an unsatisfactory outcome with many patients having residual stiffness, weakness and eventual radiographic arthrosis. Prolonged cast immobilization may lead to poor outcomes as well. Patients treated in a cast can experience stiffness, muscular atrophy and disuse osteopenia. For scaphoid fractures in particular, a slower return to work and higher rate of nonunion have been reported.[35]

Scaphoid Fractures

Return to work is variable following scaphoid fractures. Among nonoperatively treated scaphoid fractures, 50% have returned to normal work by 3 months. This is in contrast to 80% treated operatively.[22] Furthermore, grip strength, range of motion and overall patient satisfaction is typically higher in the operative group. However, there are no differences in the two groups after 6 months. In the long-term follow-up, up to 20% of patients with healed fractures may complain of persistent pain, which some surgeons believe is related to damage to the cartilage at the time of injury.

The determination of union is difficult to establish, and the timing threshold for the diagnosis of nonunion is unclear. Time to union in nondisplaced fractures is shorter than in displaced scaphoid fractures treated with open reduction and internal fixation.[36] Those undergoing percutaneous screw fixation showed a quicker time to union (9 weeks) than those treated with a cast (14 weeks).[37] In displaced scaphoid fractures treated with ORIF, time to union usually varies between 3–5 months.[36]

Nondisplaced fractures of the scaphoid treated in a cast heal uneventfully in up to 95% of patients, whereas nondisplaced fractures treated operatively have union rates approaching 100%.[35] In our institution, we confirm union with a CT scan at 6–8 weeks post-treatment and follow this with a second CT scan at 3 months, if necessary. Risk factors for scaphoid fracture nonunion (Fig. 3.29) include fracture displacement, smoking[36] and

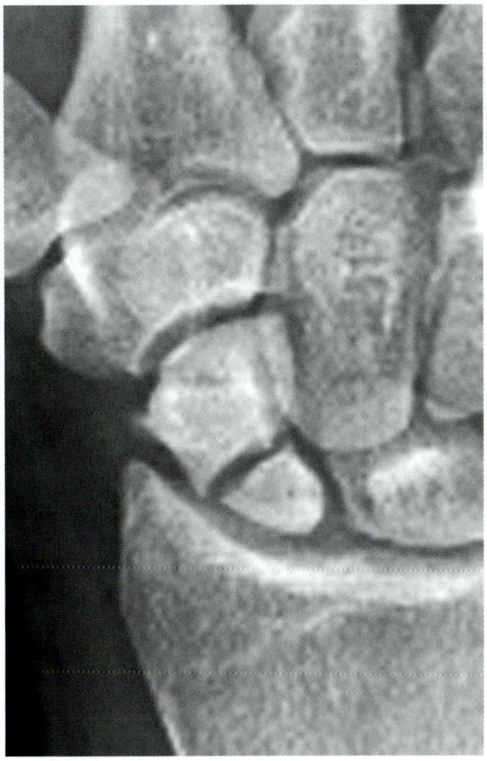

Figure 3.29: Radiographs demonstrating nonunion of the scaphoid. Note the displacement of the two poles of the scaphoid and cortication and spurring of the fracture site.

delay in diagnosis and/or treatment. More proximal fractures are also at higher risk for nonunion, with only 60% of proximal pole fractures healing uneventfully. This is believed to be related to the retrograde blood supply of the proximal scaphoid.

Perilunate Dislocations

These injuries are difficult to treat and large cohort outcome studies are lacking. Perilunate and trans-scaphoid perilunate fracture-dislocations seem to show a similar clinical and radiological outcome.[38] More than 50% of patients having a perilunate (fracture) dislocation had a fair or poor outcome according to Mayo wrist score.[38] They also demonstrated a predilection towards developing advanced midcarpal arthrosis within an average of approximately 4 years of follow-up.[39] After a mean follow-up of 4 years, more than 20% already had already undergone a salvage procedure.

Complications

Scaphoid Fractures

Delayed Union

More than 90% of scaphoid fractures treated non-operatively are healed after 3 months.[22] Those that do not are termed "delayed unions", and another 60% of these will heal without specific treatment or prolonged immobilization. Those fractures that do not heal after 6–12 months of treatment are generally termed non-unions.

Nonunion of the Scaphoid

Patients treated operatively or nonoperatively that have continued complaint of local pain after 4 months with demonstrated nonunion on CT scan are generally offered surgical intervention. There are a wide variety of techniques for addressing scaphoid nonunion. The treatment of the classic scaphoid waist fracture nonunion in patients without arthritic changes is debridement of the nonunion and bone grafting from the distal radius or the iliac crest (Figs 3.30A to C). The use of inlay bone graft was first described by Matti. Russe modified the technique by altering the approach from dorsal to volar; he reported union rate up to 90%.[13] These early surgical procedures for scaphoid nonunion generally did not include internal fixation. Occasionally, internal fixation with Kirschner wires was used in cases of movement at the graft site. This concept changed with Herbert who introduced the compression screw.[12] It is now generally agreed that the combination of compression and cancellous bone grafting is ideal for the treatment of scaphoid nonunion.

We first assess patients with scaphoid nonunions clinically, as well as with plain X-rays, CT scan and MRI. Often, plain X-rays of the contralateral wrist are helpful as well. CT scan helps define the nonunion site and alignment of the scaphoid. The MRI will identify whether the scaphoid, and in particular the proximal pole are vascularized. To help decide which surgical technique to use for each patient, we use the following algorithm:

- Where is the nonunion?
  - Waist-generally approached volarly
  - Proximal pole-generally approached dorsally

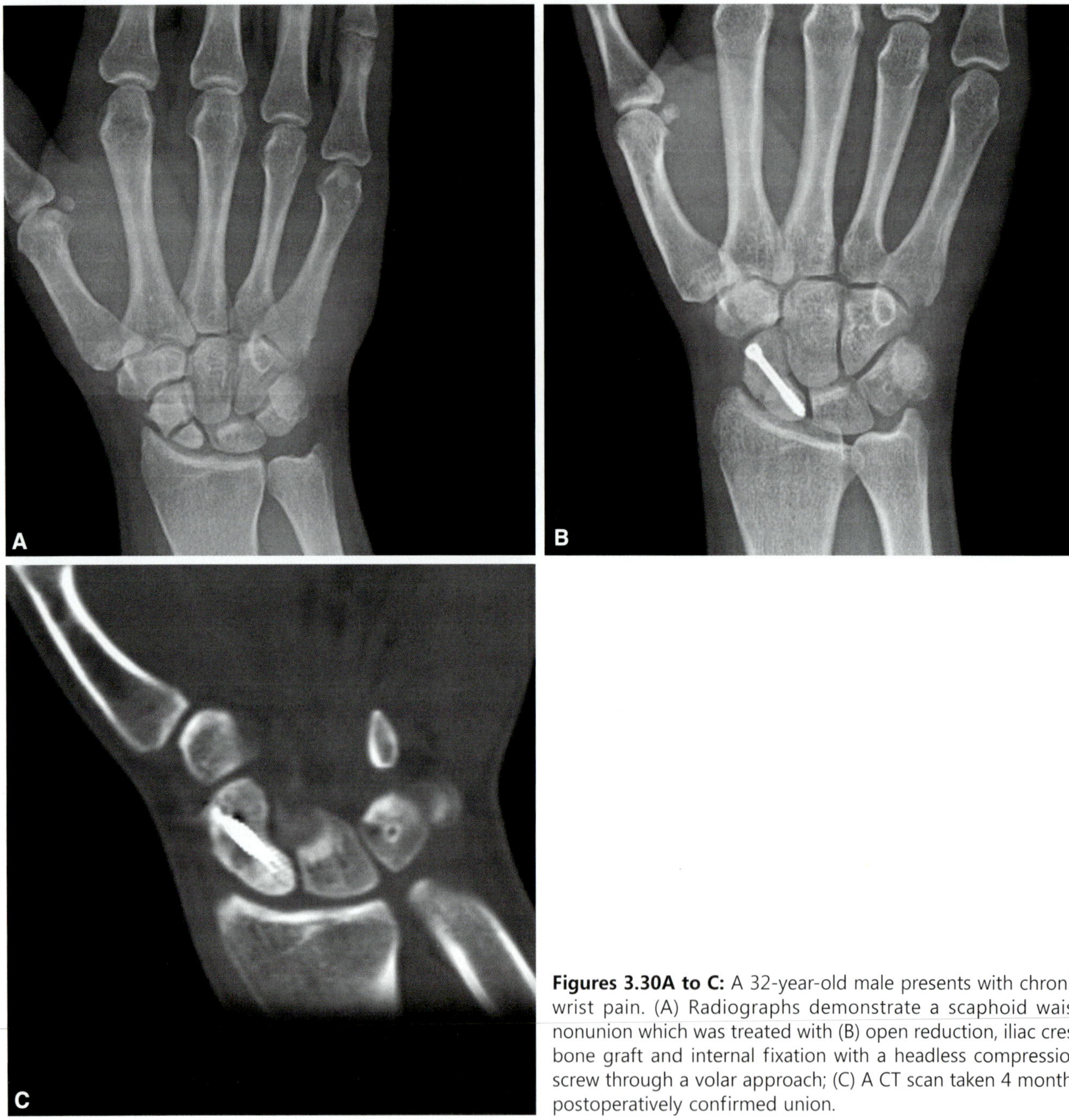

Figures 3.30A to C: A 32-year-old male presents with chronic wrist pain. (A) Radiographs demonstrate a scaphoid waist nonunion which was treated with (B) open reduction, iliac crest bone graft and internal fixation with a headless compression screw through a volar approach; (C) A CT scan taken 4 months postoperatively confirmed union.

- Is there cavitation at the nonunion site?
  - If so, bone graft is necessary.
- Is there a humpback deformity?
  - If so, structural bone graft is necessary.
- Is the proximal pole avascular?
  - If so, vascularized bone graft is necessary.

For scaphoid nonunions that have failed a surgical attempt at repair, salvage procedures include excision of the scaphoid with four bone fusion, proximal row carpectomy (PRC) or a complete wrist arthrodesis.

Malunion

Malunion of the scaphoid can lead to a "humpback deformity" with resultant dorsal intercalated segment instability (DISI) deformity and possible progression to osteoarthrits. An intrascaphoid angle of more than 35–45° may lead to unfavorable results. However, the treatment of scaphoid malunion is controversial. Given the difficulties with scaphoid alignment and healing, we currently do not recommend osteotomy for scaphoid malunion.

Osteoarthritis

Scaphoid nonunion advanced collapse (SNAC) wrist is a well-known complication following scaphoid nonunion. The progression of changes begins with cystic resorptive changes in the scaphoid, followed by radioscaphoid arthritis and finally generalized arthritis of the wrist[40] (Figs 3.31A and B). There is usually sparing of the lunate facet. The most commonly associated risk factors for development of a SNAC wrist are displacement and instability of the fracture. The patients complain of pain, swelling and stiffness. Depending on the site of nonunion and the amount of osteoarthritis, surgical treatment includes a PRC, 4-bone arthrodesis (Figs 3.32A to D), or complete wrist arthrodesis as the final procedure.[41] There are different techniques described, using Kirschner wires, screws or circular plates. Proximal row carpectomy seems more favorable for patients who require less grip strength at work.[42] With PRC an active range of motion of at least 50% of the unaffected side can be achieved and more than 75% of patients are pain free during resting conditions. We always perform a PIN denervation during any salvage procedure on the wrist.

Undisplaced, healed scaphoid fractures may also lead to osteoarthritis, although generally not to the extent of a SNAC wrist. Recent literature has also demonstrated a propensity toward osteoarthritis in nondisplaced scaphoid fractures treated operatively.[20] This commonly tends to affect the scaphotrapezial articulation and is thought to be related to the insertion of a retrograde screw. Further study is needed in this area to determine whether surgery is a risk for the development of osteoarthritis.

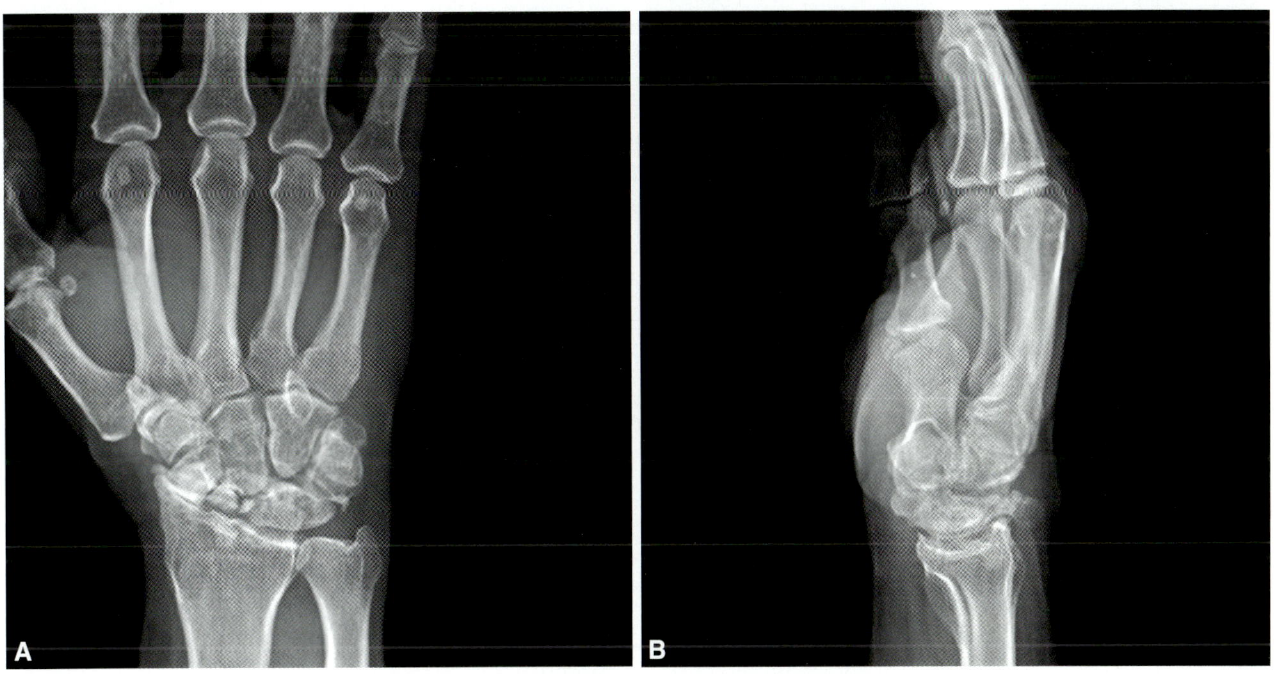

Figures 3.31A and B: A 59-year-old male with a long-standing history of pain in the wrist showing a scaphoid, nonunion advanced collapse.

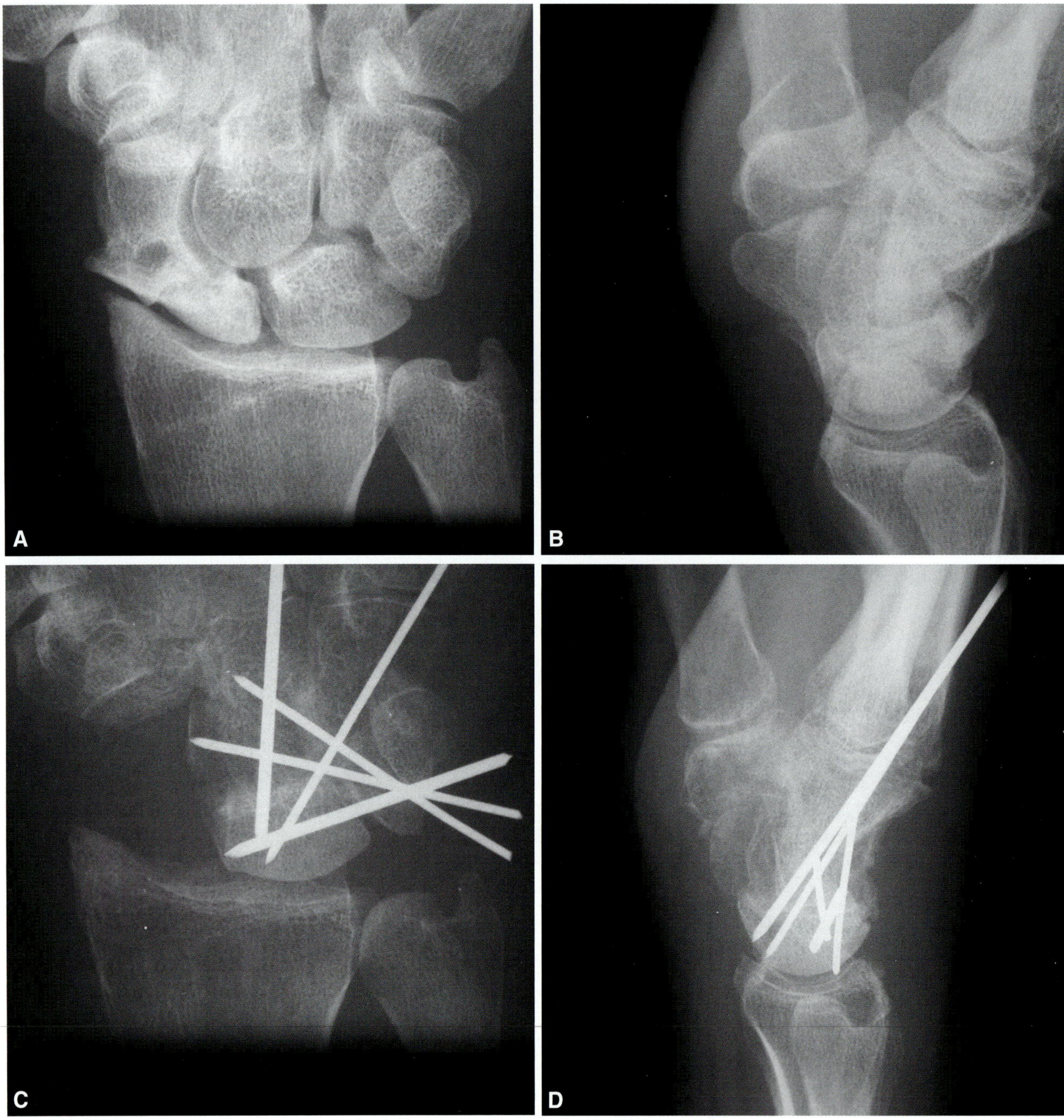

Figures 3.32A to D: A 30-year-old male was diagnosed with a (A and B) scaphoid-nonunion advanced collapse; (C and D) He was treated with a scaphoid excision and 4-bone arthrodesis with bone graft and Kirschner wire fixation.

Fractures of Other Carpal Bones

Hook of hamate fractures commonly progress to nonunion.[28] This is thought to occur due to its poor blood supply, commonly delayed presentation, and difficulty in immobilization that can result in persistent motion and subsequently poor healing at the fracture site. We prefer to treat symptomatic nonunions with excision of the fragment.

The retrograde blood supply of the capitate predisposes fractures of the capitate to nonunion and avascular necrosis.

When this occurs, we recommend debridement of the nonunion, bone grafting and internal fixation.

Very rarely, bony avulsion fractures of the triquetrum or the trapezium can progress to symptomatic nonunion and warrant further treatment, such as excision of the displaced fragment. Painful nonunions of pisiform fractures are also generally treated with excision.

Carpal Dislocations—Carpal Instability

The relationships of the carpal bones are dependent on the ligaments and trauma which affect either the bones themselves or their relationships via the ligaments may lead to instability. Carpal instability can occur either statically or dynamically.

Carpal instability can be divided broadly into dissociative (CID) and nondissociative (CIND) types.[43] CID is perhaps easier to understand as it encompasses instabilities caused by disruption of the proximal row carpal bones. These injuries include scapholunate and lunotriquetral ligament tears. CIND encompasses other carpal instabilities in which the bones of the proximal row remain aligned. These injuries include radiocarpal dislocations and carpal instability. A perilunate injury is usually a combination of CID and CIND.

Probably the most common carpal instability is from rupture of the scapholunate ligament. In case of a rupture of the scapholunate ligament, the scaphoid tends to flex palmar under axial pressure whereas the lunate tends to extend due to its shape. The lunate is often referred to as the "intercalated segment" of the proximal row because it is the link between the scaphoid and triquetrum. Extension of the lunate in a scapholunate ligament injury is therefore also known as DISI because the lunate is pointed dorsally. Similarly in case of a displaced scaphoid fracture the distal pole tends to flex while the proximal pole extends. Due to the intact scapholunate ligament, the lunate follows the proximal pole into extension, again resulting in DISI. In the lateral radiograph the scapholunate angle is usually greater than 60°.

Following rupture of the lunotriquetral ligament, the triquetrum remains in extension whereas the lunate is flexed. In the lateral radiograph, we can see the lunate palmar flexed, which is known as volar intercalated segment instability (VISI). In VISI, the scapholunate angle is less than 30°.

CT and MRI may help to establish the diagnosis. The gold standard in imaging diagnostics is a true lateral X-ray and the direct visualization during arthroscopy. Evidence-based medicine is lacking in the treatment of carpal instability. In the following section, we will describe one method of treatment for chronic scapholunate ligament rupture.

Authors' Preferred Management of Select Complications

Case 1: Chronic Scapholunate Dissociation Treated with Reduction and Association of the Scaphoid and Lunate Screw Repair

A 51-year-old man presents with a multiple year history of left wrist (Figs 3.33A to F). A specific antecedent trauma could not be recalled. His main complaint was of wrist pain that was worse with activities and heavy lifting. On physical exam, he had tenderness over the dorsal aspect of his left wrist. His range of motion of the left wrist was limited to 60° of flexion and 45° of extension, with pain throughout the arc of motion. Radiographs demonstrated widening of the scapholunate interval. An MRI was obtained which was consistent with a chronic scapholunate ligament tear (Figs 3.33C and D).

Treatment options for chronic scapholunate dissociation include:

- Open reduction with pinning and ligament repair/reconstruction
- Reduction and association of the scaphoid and lunate (RASL) fixation
- Salvage procedures, such as a proximal row carpectomy, scaphoid excision with 4-corner fusion or a total wrist fusion

To help decide which surgical technique to use for each patient, we use the following algorithm:

- Scapholunate dissociation without arthritic changes:
  - Open reduction and ligament repair/reconstruction with pinning
  - Open reduction and RASL screw fixation
- Scapholunate dissociation with arthritic changes limited to the radioscaphoid joint:
  - Proximal row carpectomy
- Scapholunate dissociation with arthritic changes extending into the midcarpal joint:
  - Scaphoid excision with 4-corner fusion

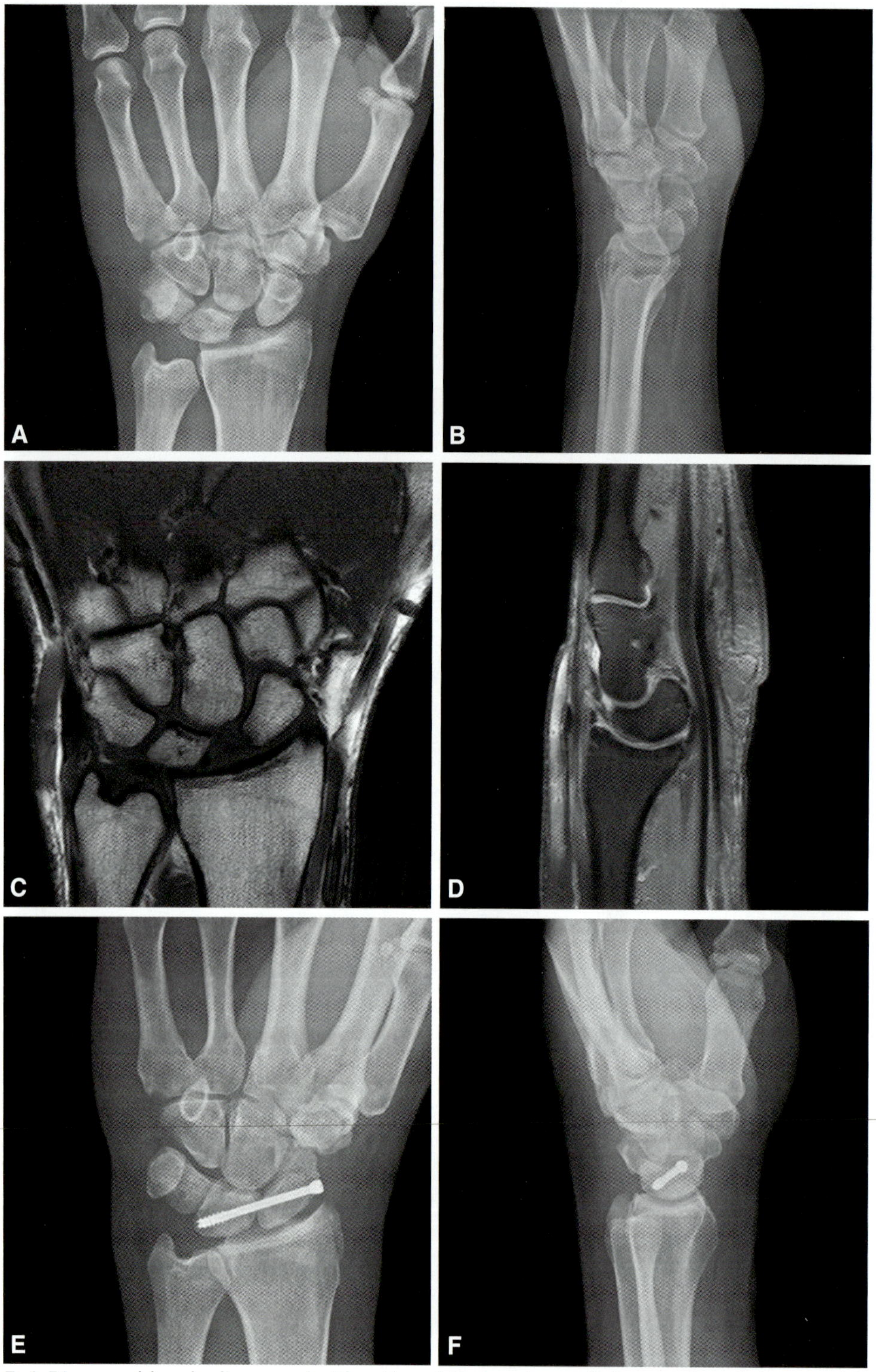

Figures 3.33A to F: A 51-year-old male diagnosed with a (A and B) chronic scapholunate dissociation on plain radiographs and (C and D) MRI. Note the DISI orientation on lateral images; (E) The patient underwent an open reduction through a midline dorsal approach; (F) Capsulotomy was performed with a proximally-based dorsal capsular flap in case a salvage may be necessary in the form of an interposition and proximal row carpectomy. The ligamentous surfaces of the scaphoid and lunate are decorticated to bleeding bone. The scapholunate relationship is restored and then fixed with a headless compression (RASL) screw placed over a guidewire directed across the scapholunate axis just distal to the radial styloid. This RASL screw should be placed just proud to aide in later removal; (E and F) Normal scapholunate relationship should be confirmed on anteroposterior and lateral views.

- Scapholunate dissociation with pancarpal arthritic changes:
  - Total wrist fusion: Total wrist arthroplasty

Technique

A midline dorsal approach to the wrist is utilized. A midline dorsal capsulotomy is performed. The scapholunate ligament is examined for potential re-approximation. The carpal relationships are examined. The scaphoid will typically be flexed and the lunate extended. First it is determined whether the scaphoid and lunate are mobile and reducible. If they are not reducible RASL screw fixation is aborted and a salvage procedure is undertaken.[44]

To perform the RASL, a 0.062 inch Kirschner wire is passed into the lunate taking into account its dorsiflexion and a similar 0.062 inch Kirschner wire is passed into scaphoid taking into account its volar flexion. After these wires are passed, the adjoining ligamentous surfaces of the scaphoid and lunate are decorticated. Using the Kirschner wires as joysticks the scapholunate relationship is restored. The reduction can temporarily be maintained with a fracture tenaculum. Once the scaphlunate relationship is re-established, a small incision is placed just distal to the radial styloid. This provides access to the radial aspect of the scaphoid for placement of the RASL headless compression screw across the scaphoid into the lunate. The screw head should be left slightly proud to facilitate later removal if needed. Radiographs are obtained to demonstrate restoration of the scapholunate angle laterally as well the scapholunate relationship on the AP view.

A layered closure of the tissues is performed with the EPL left exteriorized. Postoperatively, the patient is placed in a short-arm splint and later transitioned into a cast. The total duration of immobilization is 6 weeks.

Case 2: Failed Perilunate Dislocation Repair Salvaged with a Total Wrist Fusion

A 41-year-old male was involved in a high speed motor vehicle accident. (Figs 3.34A to F) Evaluation in the emergency room identified a severely swollen and tender wrist. Radiographs demonstrated a displaced perilunate dislocation. The patient was taken urgently to the operating room for a combined volar and dorsal open reduction and pinning of the carpus, suture anchor repair of the scapholunate ligament and carpal tunnel release. The patient was immobilized for 12 weeks in a thumb spica cast. The cast and pins were removed and the patient was begun on progressive range of motion and strengthening. At 12 months postoperatively, the patient presented with persistent pain and radiographs that identified scapholunate advanced collapse with pancarpal arthrosis.

Perilunate dislocations have a high predilection for developing post-traumatic arthritis. The risk increases with missed or delayed diagnosis. (Figs 3.35A to F) However, post-traumatic arthritis is common even with expeditious diagnosis and treatment. The most common pattern of post-traumatic arthritis following a perilunate dislocation is scapholunate advanced collapse. Treatment options include:

- Revision open reduction with pinning and ligament repair/reconstruction
- Proximal row carpectomy
- Scaphoid excision with 4-corner fusion
- Total wrist fusion

To help decide which surgical technique to use for each patient, we use the following algorithm:

- Recurrent perilunate dislocation or instability
  - Revision open reduction and ligament repair/reconstruction with pinning
- Scapholunate dissociation without arthritic changes:
  - Open reduction and ligament repair/reconstruction with pinning
  - Open reduction and RASL screw fixation
- Scapholunate dissociation with arthritic changes limited to the radioscaphoid joint:
  - Proximal row carpectomy
- Scapholunate dissociation with arthritic changes extending into the midcarpal joint:
  - Scaphoid excision with 4-corner fusion
- Scapholunate dissociation with pancarpal arthritic changes:
  - Total wrist fusion

Technique

When arthritic symptoms are already present, a number of salvage options are available and the patient must be

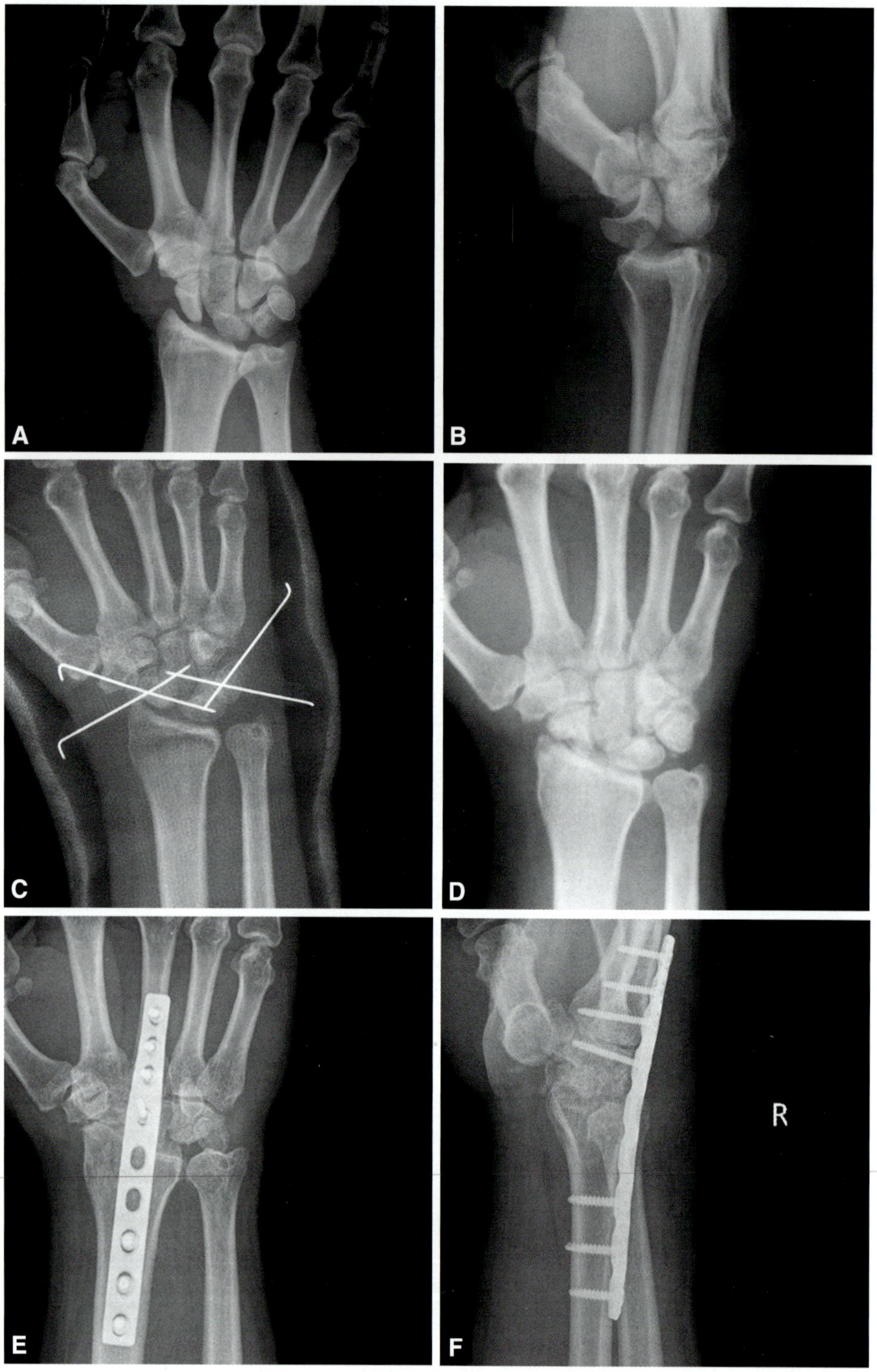

Figures 3.34A to F: A 41-year-old male laborer was involved in a motor vehicle accident and incurred a (A and B) perilunate dislocation. He underwent open reduction, pinning of the carpus in a diamond configuration and suture anchor repair of the scapholunate ligament. Postoperatively, he was immobilized in a short arm thumb spica; (C) Radiographs taken at 12 weeks prior to cast and pin removal identified mild interval scapholunate dissociation; (D) Radiographs taken 12 months postoperatively identified scapholunate advanced collapse with pancarpal arthritis. Patient also was complaining of persistent pain, weakness and difficulties with activities of daily living; (E and F) In order to control his pain and maximize his grip strength the patient underwent a total wrist fusion.

Courtesy: Asif M Ilyas

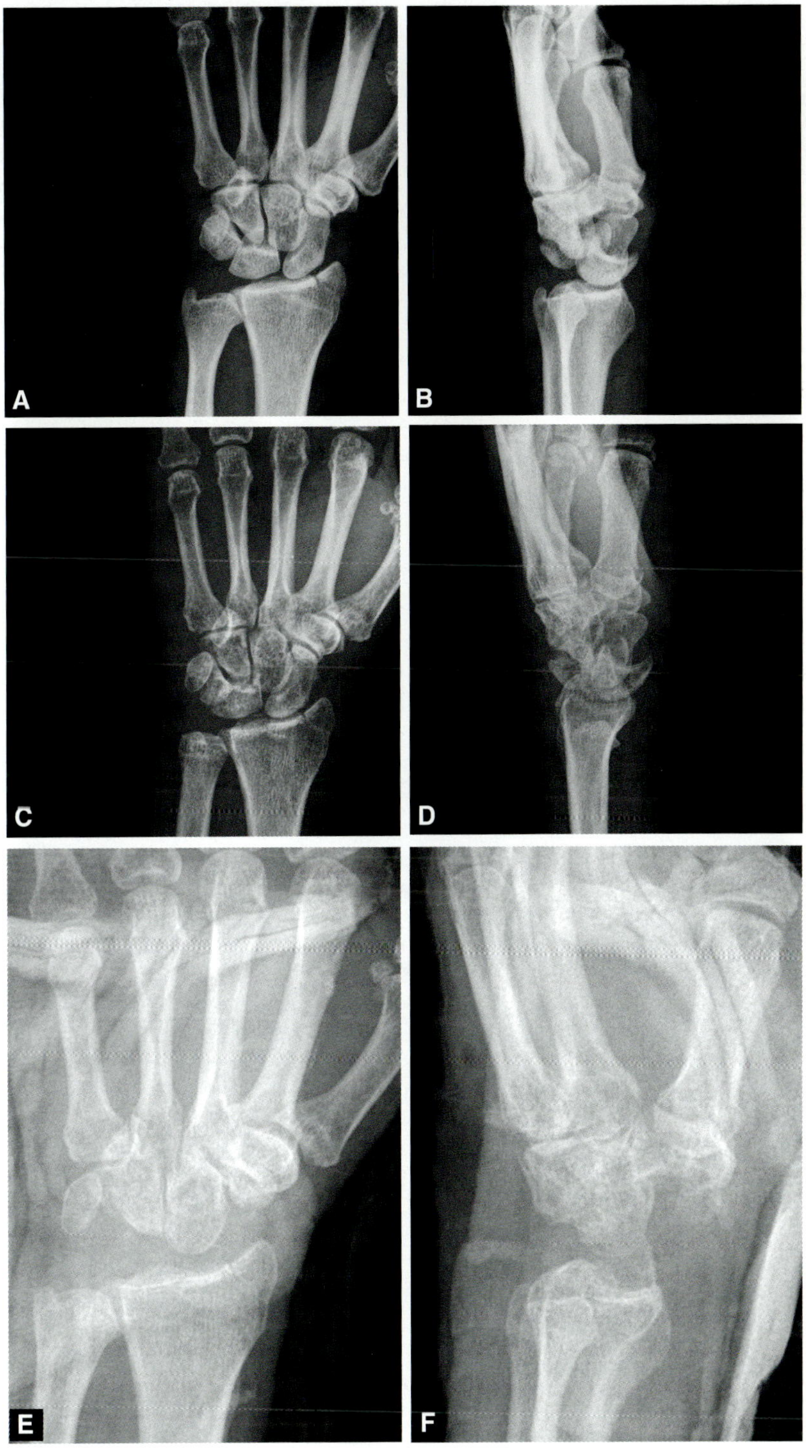

Figures 3.35A to F: A 51-year-old male fell from a height and presented to the emergency department with complaints of wrist pain and swelling. (A and B) Radiographs were taken that were interpreted as a minimally displaced distal radius fracture. A perilunate dislocation evident on the lateral view was missed. A splint was applied and the patient was ordered to follow-up as an outpatient. The patient ultimately returned to the emergency department with persistent wrist pain 3 months later; (C and D) Repeat radiographs demonstrated a healed radial styloid fracture but a persistent perilunate dislocation that was initially not diagnosed. The patient was taken to the operating room for an attempted open reduction. However, intraoperatively extensive chonrdrolysis of the lunate and scaphoid was identified and the wrist was salvaged to (E and F) a proximal row carpectomy. *Courtesy*: Asif M Ilyas

consented for a variety of procedures that will ultimately be dependent upon the actual status of the articular cartilage of the wrist joint assessed intraoperatively. The prior midline dorsal approach to the wrist is utilized. As this is a revision procedure, the EPL tendon must be carefully identified, dissected free and retracted. A standard dorsal capsulotomy is made. The articular surfaces of the radiocarpal and midcarpal joints are carefully examined. If pancarpal arthrosis is present then a total wrist fusion is indicated.

If not previously done, a PIN neurectomy is performed to minimize postoperative dorsal wrist joint pain. To minimize the number of joints that must fuse following a total wrist fusion, a PRC is performed. The proximal carpal bones also provide a source of bone graft. The articular surfaces of the distal radius and the base of the trapezoid, capitate and hamate is debrided down to bleeding cancellous bone. This may be performed with a rongeur or a high speed burr. Care must be taken to avoid injury to the TFCC and the distal radioulnar joint. Next, Lister's tubercle is taken down and through its base a curette is introduced to harvest bone graft from the distal radius. Finally, the wrist is reduced, compressed and aligned in slight wrist extension and ulnar deviation. A precontoured wrist fusion plate is applied and fixed using dynamic compression plating technique. The plate is centered in line with the axis of the distal radius and the third metacarpal. Once fixed, the fusion site is packed with the harvested bone graft. Postoperatively, the patient is immobilized in a splint or cast for 6–12 weeks until the union across the wrist fusion site is confirmed.

Case 3: Lunate Avascular Necrosis Treated with a Proximal Row Carpectomy

A 42-year-old female office worker fell while riding a bike and incurred a minimally displaced lunate body fracture. (Figs 3.36A to F) The patient was treated nonoperatively with a cast. After 8 weeks of cast immobilization radiographs demonstrated fracture union and the patient was begun on progressive motion and strengthening. The patient returned 6 months later with persistent wrist pain. Radiographs at that time demonstrated avascular necrosis of the lunate with collapse.

Avascular necrosis is the most common following fracture of the scaphoid; however, all of the carpal bones are at risk for avascular necrosis following trauma. In the case of the lunate, avascular necrosis is a well described phenomenon and is referred to as Kienbock's disease.[45] The etiology of Kienbock's disease is poorly understood but generally encompasses chronic processes that ultimately result in compromise of the lunate's perfusion. However, in this case, the history of a fracture readily explains the development of avascular necrosis. Treatment options include:

- Radial shortening
- Revascularization
- Proximal row carpectomy
- Total wrist fusion

To help decide which surgical technique to use for each patient, we use the following algorithm:

- Lunate shape maintained without arthritic changes
  - Radial shortening (with negative ulnar variance)
  - Revascularization
- Lunate collapse without arthritic changes
  - Proximal row carpectomy
- Lunate collapse with arthritic changes
  - Total wrist fusion

Technique

A midline dorsal approach to the wrist is utilized. The EPL tendon is identified and the third compartment is opened. The second and fourth extensor compartments are elevated subperiostally. A PIN neurectomy is performed. The dorsal capsulotomy is performed utilizing a proximally maintained "trap door" capsular flap which will be used later as an interposition flap to maximize longevity of the new articulation.[46] The scaphoid and triquetrum are excised first followed by the lunate last. The radial styloid tip is excised. Care must be taken to avoid injury to the volar radiocarpal ligaments in order to avoid late radiocarpal instability. Furthermore, great care must be taken to avoid injury to the distal radius lunate fossa and base of the capitate articular surfaces. However, if pre-existing arthritis is identified then salvage to a wrist fusion must be entertained.

Once the carpectomy has been performed the dorsal capsular flap is interposed over the lunate fossa and repaired to the volar capsule. The interval between the second and fourth compartments is repaired and the EPL is left exteriorized. The capitate is allowed to reduce

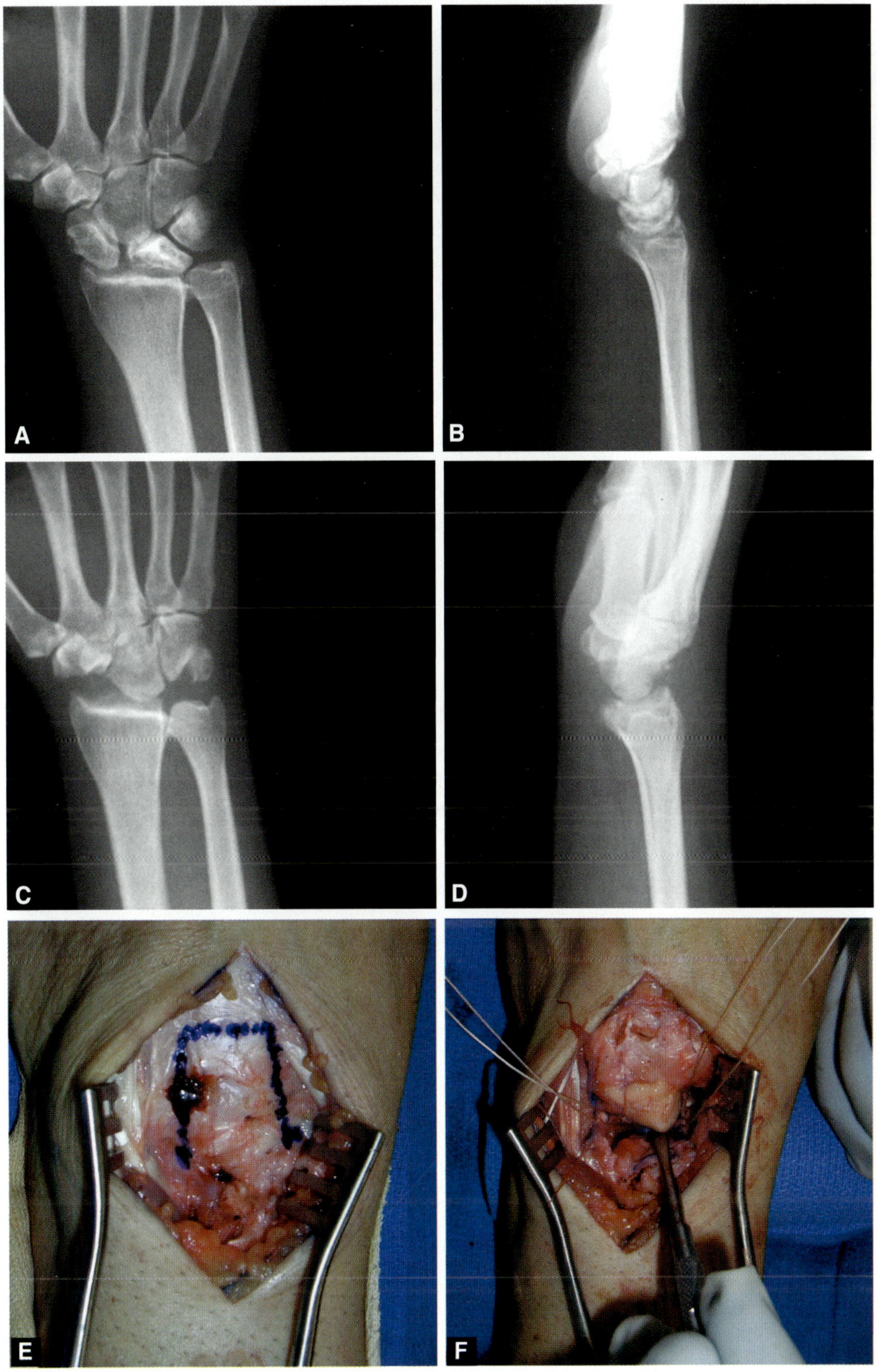

Figures 3.36A to F: A 42-year-old female had incurred a lunate fracture treated nonoperatively in a cast for 8 weeks. The patient presented 6 months later with persistent wrist pain. (A and B) Radiographs demonstrated avascular necrosis of the lunate. Patient was offered a (C and D) proximal row carpectomy with a (E and F) proximally based dorsal capsular interposition flap that was interposed between the base of capitates and lunate fossa.

Courtesy: Asif M Ilyas

proximally. The wounds are closed and a splint is applied for comfort. Early motion and strengthening is initiated.

Summary

Carpal fractures and perilunate dislocations are rare. The scaphoid is the most commonly affected bone being involved in up to 80% patients. The trans-scaphoid perilunate fracture dislocation is the most commonly encountered dislocation. The incidence of scaphoid fractures is about 1.5 fractures per 100,000 people a year. The mechanism is usually one of hyperextension. Clinical examination may guide further diagnostic assessment. An X-ray of the wrist, at least two views should be taken of every patient presenting with a trauma to the wrist and complaining of pain. Special attention must be paid to Gilula's lines, the Terry Thomas sign and the triangular shape of the lunate on a PA radiograph in case of dislocation. In unclear cases or in cases with fractures, a CT or MRI can add important information about the degree of displacement, the extent of injury and any other injuries to the carpus.

Fractures

We recommend treating undisplaced fractures with cast immobilization for 4–6 weeks. In case of scaphoid fractures the duration is longer, for up to 10–12 weeks. Patients with a very active lifestyle or those unwilling for cast treatment who have a nondisplaced scaphoid fracture can be suitable candidates for percutaneous fixation. Displaced articular fractures (> 1 mm) should be treated operatively to minimize risks of nonunion and osteoarthritis. A closed reduction and internal fixation may be tried. If adequate reduction fails, open reduction is mandatory. Kirschner wires are used in smaller fragments whereas screws (mini-fragment or headless compression screws) are preferred in bigger fragments. The amount of union is best assessed with CT. In case of painful nonunion we recommend open reduction, bone grafting and internal fixation.

Dislocations

These are emergency situations and an expeditious gentle closed reduction is mandatory. Open reduction and internal fixation is recommended as a definitive treatment to restore and maintain carpal relationships. The long-term aim is to prevent progression to chronic instability due to failed ligamentous healing or fracture nonunion.

References

1. Van Tassel DC, Owens BD, Wolf JM. Incidence estimates and demographics of scaphoid fracture in the US population. J Hand Surg Am. 2010;35(8):1242-5.
2. Wolf JM, Dawson L, Mountcastle SB, et al. The incidence of scaphoid fracture in a military population. Injury. 2009; 40(12):1316-9.
3. Teisen H, Hjarbaek J. Classification of fresh fractures of the lunate. J Hand Surg Br. 1988;13(4):458-62.
4. Herzberg G, Comtet JJ, Linscheid RL, et al. Perilunate dislocations and fracture-dislocations: a multicenter study. J Hand Surg Am. 1993;18(5):768-79.
5. Gilula LA. Carpal injuries: analytic approach and case exercises. AJR Am J Roentgenol. 1979;133(3):503-17.
6. Lozano-Calderon S, Blazar P, Zurakowski D, et al. Diagnosis of scaphoid fracture displacement with radiography and computed tomography. J Bone Joint Surg Am. 2006; 88(12):2695-703.
7. Bernard SA, Murray PM, Heckman MG. Validity of conventional radiography in determining scaphoid waist fracture displacement. J Orthop Trauma. 2010;24(7): 448-51.
8. Mallee W, Doornberg JN, Ring D, et al. Comparison of CT and MRI for diagnosis of suspected scaphoid fractures. J Bone Joint Surg Am. 2011;93(1):20-8.
9. Pillai A, Jain M. Management of clinical fractures of the scaphoid: results of an audit and literature review. Eur J Emerg Med. 2005;12(2):47-51.
10. Magee T. Comparison of 3-T MRI and arthroscopy of intrinsic wrist ligament and TFCC tears. AJR Am J Roentgenol. 2009;192(1):80-5.
11. Cooney WP, Dobyns JH, Linscheid RL. Fractures of the scaphoid: a rational approach to management. Clin Orthop Relat Res. 1980;(149):90-7.
12. Herbert TJ, Fisher WE. Management of the fractured scaphoid using a new bone screw. J Bone Joint Surg Br. 1984;66(1):114-23.
13. Russe O. Fracture of the carpal navicular. Diagnosis, non-operative treatment, and operative treatment. J Bone Joint Surg Am. 1960;42-A:759-68.
14. Papp S. Carpal bone fractures. Orthop Clin North Am. 2007;38(2):251-60.
15. Mudgal C, Lovell M. Scapho-capitate syndrome: distant fragment migration. Acta Orthop Belg. 1995;61(1):62-5.

16. Hirano K, Inoue G. Classification and treatment of hamate fractures. Hand Surg. 2005;10(2-3):151-7.
17. Mayfield JK, Johnson RP, Kilcoyne RK. Carpal dislocations: pathomechanics and progressive perilunar instability. J Hand Surg Am. 1980;5(3):226-41.
18. Ilyas AM, Mudgal CS. Radiocarpal fracture-dislocations. J Am Acad Orthop Surg. 2008;16(11):647-55.
19. Graham TJ. The inferior arc injury: an addition to the family of complex carpal fracture-dislocation patterns. Am J Orthop (Belle Mead NJ). 2003;32(9 Suppl):10-9.
20. Vinnars B, Pietreanu M, Bodestedt A, et al. Nonoperative compared with operative treatment of acute scaphoid fractures. a randomized clinical trial. J Bone Joint Surg Am. 2008;90(6):1176-85.
21. Buijze GA, Doornberg JN, Ham JS, et al. Surgical compared with conservative treatment for acute nondisplaced or minimally displaced scaphoid fractures: a systematic review and meta-analysis of randomized controlled trials. J Bone Joint Surg Am. 2010;92(6):1534-44.
22. Schadel-Hopfner M, Marent-Huber M, Gazyakan E, et al. Acute non-displaced fractures of the scaphoid: earlier return to activities after operative treatment. A controlled multicenter cohort study. Arch Orthop Trauma Surg. 2010; 130(9):1117-27.
23. Haisman JM, Rohde RS, Weiland AJ. Acute fractures of the scaphoid. J Bone Joint Surg Am. 2006;88(12):2750-8.
24. Jeon IH, Micic ID, Oh CW, et al. Percutaneous screw fixation for scaphoid fracture: a comparison between the dorsal and the volar approaches. J Hand Surg Am. 2009;34(2): 228-36.e1.
25. Ring D, Jupiter JB, Herndon JH. Acute fractures of the scaphoid. J Am Acad Orthop Surg. 2000;8(4):225-31.
26. Rutgers M, Mudgal CS, Shin R. Combined fractures of the distal radius and scaphoid. J Hand Surg Eur Vol. 2008; 33(4):478-83.
27. Lacey JD, Hodge JC. Pisiform and hamulus fractures: easily missed wrist fractures diagnosed on a reverse oblique radiograph. J Emerg Med. 1998;16(3):445-52.
28. Scheufler O, Andresen R, Radmer S, et al. Hook of hamate fractures: critical evaluation of different therapeutic procedures. Plast Reconstr Surg. 2005;115(2):488-97.
29. Weil WM, Slade JF, 3rd, Trumble TE. Open and arthroscopic treatment of perilunate injuries. Clin Orthop Relat Res. 2006;445:120-32.
30. Green DP, O'Brien ET. Classification and management of carpal dislocations. Clin Orthop Relat Res. 1980;(149):55-72.
31. Kremer T, Wendt M, Riedel K, et al. Open reduction for perilunate injuries—clinical outcome and patient satisfaction. J Hand Surg Am. 2010;35(10):1599-606.
32. Nourissat G, Mudgal CS, Ring D. Bridge plating of the wrist for temporary stabilization of concomitant radiocarpal, intercarpal, and carpometacarpal injuries: a report of two cases. J Orthop Trauma. 2008;22(5):368-71.
33. Berger RA. The ligaments of the wrist. A current overview of anatomy with considerations of their potential functions. Hand Clin. 1997;13(1):63-82.
34. Abrams RA, Ziets RJ, Lieber RL, et al. Anatomy of the radial nerve motor branches in the forearm. J Hand Surg Am. 1997;22(2):232-7.
35. Dias JJ, Wildin CJ, Bhowal B, et al. Should acute scaphoid fractures be fixed? A randomized controlled trial. J Bone Joint Surg Am. 2005;87(10):2160-8.
36. Trumble TE, Gilbert M, Murray LW, et al. Displaced scaphoid fractures treated with open reduction and internal fixation with a cannulated screw. J Bone Joint Surg Am. 2000; 82(5):633-41.
37. McQueen MM, Gelbke MK, Wakefield A, et al. Percutaneous screw fixation versus conservative treatment for fractures of the waist of the scaphoid: a prospective randomised study. J Bone Joint Surg Br. 2008;90(1):66-71.
38. Forli A, Courvoisier A, Wimsey S, et al. Perilunate dislocations and transscaphoid perilunate fracture-dislocations: a retrospective study with minimum ten-year follow-up. J Hand Surg Am. 2010;35(1):62-8.
39. Souer JS, Rutgers M, Andermahr J, et al. Perilunate fracture-dislocations of the wrist: comparison of temporary screw versus K-wire fixation. J Hand Surg Am. 2007;32(3): 318-25.
40. Mack GR, Bosse MJ, Gelberman RH, et al. The natural history of scaphoid non-union. J Bone Joint Surg Am. 1984; 66(4):504-9.
41. Strauch RJ. Scapholunate advanced collapse and scaphoid nonunion advanced collapse arthritis-update on evaluation and treatment. J Hand Surg Am. 2011;36(4):729-35.
42. Dacho AK, Baumeister S, Germann G, et al. Comparison of proximal row carpectomy and midcarpal arthrodesis for the treatment of scaphoid nonunion advanced collapse (SNAC-wrist) and scapholunate advanced collapse (SLAC-wrist) in stage II. J Plast Reconstr Aesthet Surg. 2008; 61(10):1210-8.
43. Larsen CF, Amadio PC, Gilula LA, et al. Analysis of carpal instability: I. Description of the scheme. J Hand Surg Am. 1995;20(5):757-64.
44. Rosenwasser MP, Miyasajsa KC, Strauch RJ. The RASL procedure: reduction and association of the scaphoid and lunate using the Herbert screw. Tech Hand Up Extrem Surg. 1997;1(4):263-72.
45. Divelbiss B, Baratz ME. Kienbock Disease. J Am As Surg Hand. 2001;1(1):61-72.
46. Ilyas AM. Proximal row carpectomy with a dorsal capsule interposition flap. Tech Hand Up Extrem Surg. 2010;14(3): 136-40.

Chapter 4

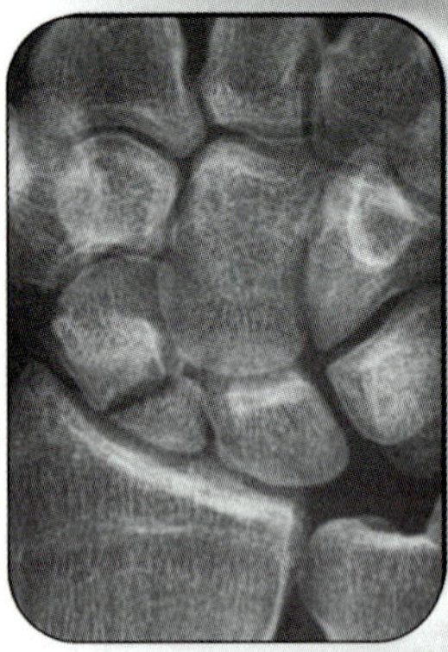

Scaphoid Fractures

Aaron Venouziou, Dean Sotereanos

Chapter Outline

Introduction
Diagnosis
Classification
Surgical Indications
- Nonoperative Treatment
- Operative Treatment
- Implants

Surgical Anatomy, Positioning and Approaches
- Applied Anatomy
- Positioning
- Approaches

Surgical Techniques
- Technique 1: Volar ORIF of Scaphoid Fractures
- Technique 2: Dorsal ORIF of Scaphoid Fractures
- Technique 3: Volar Percutaneous Fixation of Scaphoid Fractures
- Technique 4: Dorsal Percutaneous Fixation of Scaphoid Fractures

Outcomes
Complications
- Nonunions
- Avascular Necrosis
- Arthritis

Authors' Preferred Management of Select Complications
- Case 1: Proximal Pole Scaphoid Fracture Nonunion with Avascular Necrosis
- Case 2: Scaphoid Nonunion without Avascular Necrosis
- Case 3: Scaphoid Nonunion Advanced Collapse Wrist: Four Corner Fusion with Scaphoid Excision

Summary

Introduction

Fractures of the scaphoid are common injuries, representing 60–70% of carpal fractures. They are frequently the result of a fall on the outstretched hand. Scaphoid fractures may appear in any age group from the young to the elderly but are most common in adolescents and young adult males. These injuries are rarely seen in children because the distal radial physis usually fails first. Similarly, scaphoid fractures are uncommon in the elderly as the distal radial metaphysis also fails first. Scaphoid fractures are often misdiagnosed as sprained wrists.

The proper and timely diagnosis of these fractures is a key for successful treatment. Once diagnosed, the fracture can be managed by closed, open or percutaneous methods. It has been a standard practice to treat majority of scaphoid fractures with immobilization in a short-arm cast and it continues to be the most common method of treatment. The problem with this approach is that the treatment is often prolonged for many months and the outcome is unpredictable, particularly with unstable fractures. Internal fixation has an advantage of providing compression and a rigid construct with higher rates of union and earlier return to sports and activities. However, an open approach risks stripping of critical blood supply to the scaphoid and also disruption of important carpal ligaments, such as the radioscaphocapitate ligament (RSCL). Percutaneous techniques have been developed, providing the benefits of open reduction internal fixation (ORIF) with a smaller incision, preservation of the carpal ligaments and blood supply.

The most frequent complications of scaphoid fractures reported in the literature include delayed union, malunion and nonunion, avascular necrosis (AVN), stiffness, residual pain and wound problems. Nonunion is the most common complication after scaphoid fracture treatment, particularly with unstable fractures. If left untreated, patients may develop pain, instability and eventually carpal collapse that can lead to intercarpal or radiocarpal arthritis. Thus, scaphoid nonunions are typically treated operatively to avoid arthritic changes.[1]

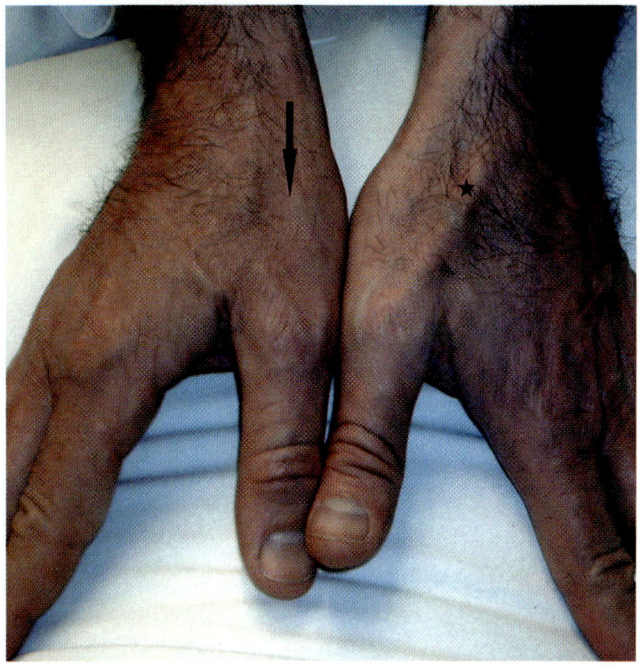

Figure 4.1: Typical edema seen in the anatomical snuffbox in a patient with a scaphoid injury of his right hand (arrow). The extensor pollicis longus (EPL) is not visible in the right hand in contrast with the uninjured side (asterisk).

Diagnosis

Early diagnosis and treatment of scaphoid fractures is critical for a satisfactory outcome. The diagnostic criteria of a scaphoid fracture include an appropriate history, clinical suspicion and objective documentation (radiographs or other imaging modality) of the fracture.

Scaphoid fractures usually result from a fall on the extended wrist. There may be a history of participation in contact sports, a fall or an accident. Physical examination findings are typically subtle on inspection. Most patients will demonstrate tenderness over the anatomical snuff box or over the distal scaphoid tubercle, pain with longitudinal compression of the thumb, and possibly edema over the anatomical snuff box (Fig. 4.1), limited range of motion with pain at the extremes of motion, especially with flexion and radial deviation. Reduced grip strength may also be noted. The overall sensitivity of the clinical examination has been reported as high as 100%, although specificity approaches only 74%.[2]

Plain radiographs remain the standard initial imaging technique of suspected acute scaphoid fractures. The American College of Radiology (ACR) has recommended four views for a suspected scaphoid fracture. These include a posteroanterior (PA), lateral, semipronated oblique and PA with ulnar deviation (Figs 4.2A to D). Scaphoid fractures are not identified on initial plain radiographs in 16% of cases and can take up to 1–2 weeks to become evident on plain films.[3] Several variables that will direct treatment must be scrutinized from the radiographs, including the site of the fracture (distal pole, waist or proximal pole), extent of displacement, presence of comminution and disruption of intercarpal relationships.

Typically, patients with clinical findings suspicious for scaphoid fracture but negative initial radiographs are treated with 2 weeks of cast immobilization followed by repeated examination and radiographic studies. Although this remains an accepted treatment option, it may result in unnecessary immobilization. If initial X-rays are negative and there is a strong suspicion of scaphoid fracture, a

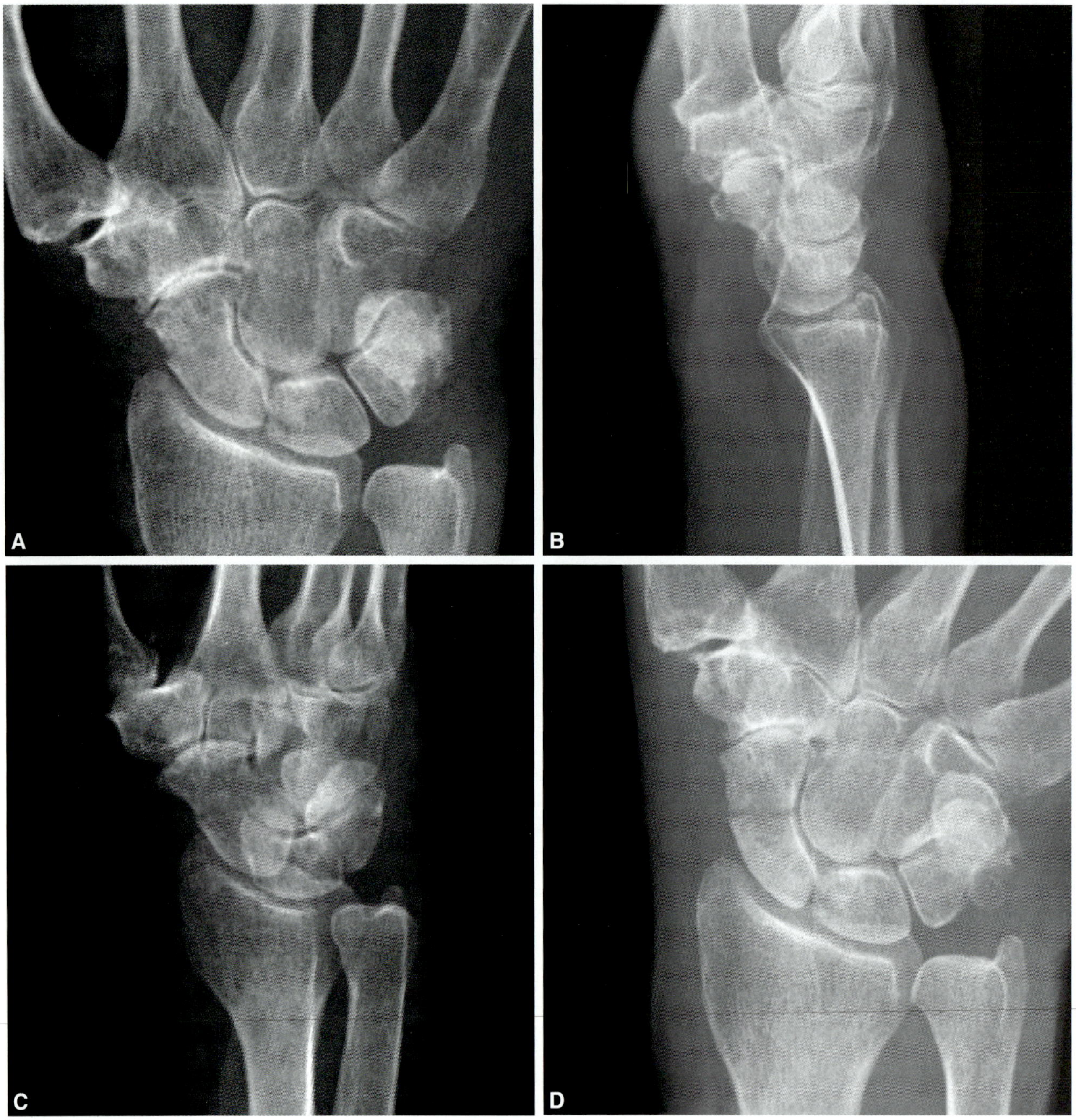

Figures 4.2A to D: Standard scaphoid radiographic series includes 4 views. Note how the standard (A) posteroanterior (PA) and (B) lateral view of the wrist do not demonstrate an obvious scaphoid fracture. However, (C) the semipronated oblique and (D) the PA with ulnar deviation (or scaphoid view) clearly demonstrates a nondisplaced scaphoid waist fracture. The fracture is stable because there is no displacement or comminution.

magnetic resonance imaging (MRI) scan is recommended. Magnetic resonance imaging has been reported to have excellent sensitivity (100%) and specificity (95–100%) for assessment of acute fractures.[4] Magnetic resonance imaging features suggestive of fracture include the presence of a fracture line, displayed by decreased signal intensity on T1 images and increased signal intensity around the fracture line on T2 images from surrounding

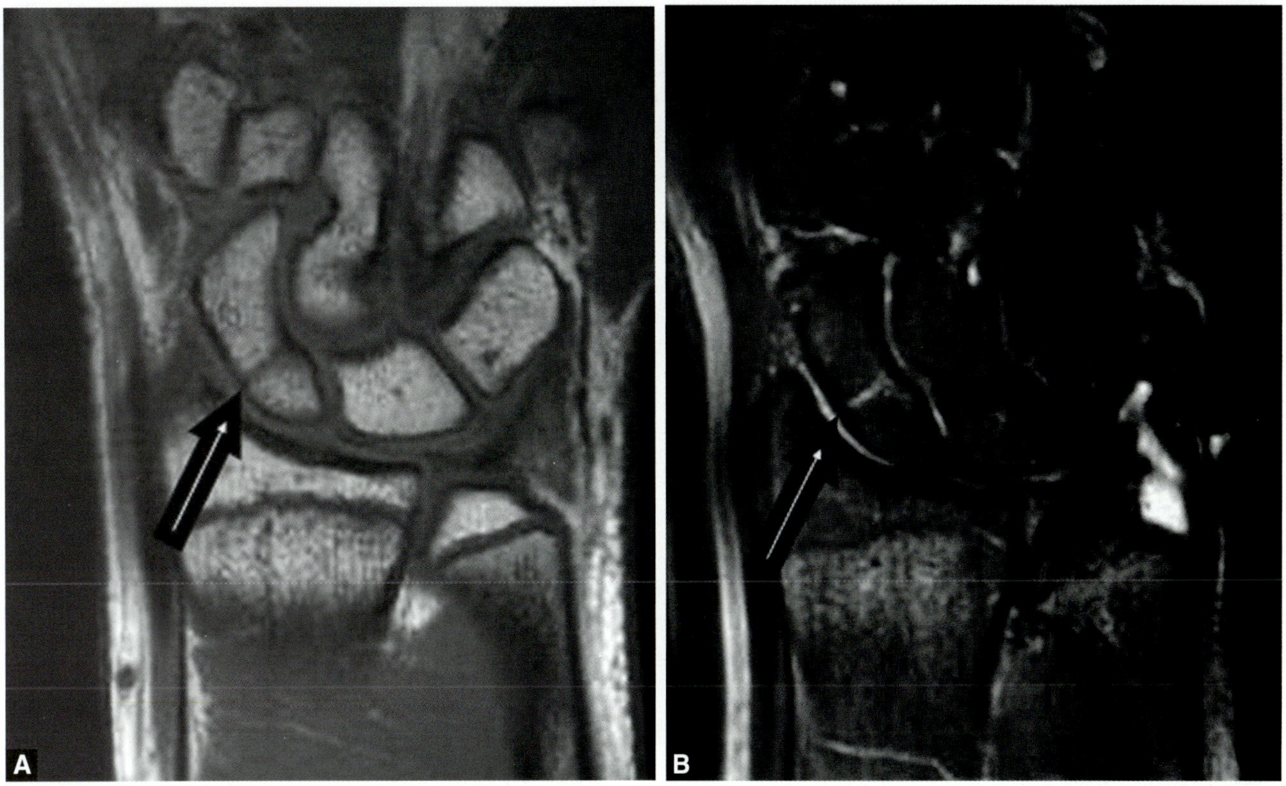

Figures 4.3A and B: Magnetic resonance imaging scans of a scaphoid waist fracture. (A) The T1-weighted image reveals a nondisplaced fracture through the waist of scaphoid (arrow); (B) The T2-weighted image with fat suppression shows edema in the region of the fracture (arrow).

edema (Figs 4.3A and B). Magnetic resonance imaging with gadolinium enhancement has also an important role in diagnosing scaphoid AVN.[4] Alternatively, a technetium bone scan has also been shown to be 100% sensitive in identifying acute fractures. However, a bone scan demonstrates a low specificity. Moreover, unlike an MRI, it may not be positive within first few days following injury.

Computerized tomography scan is useful in assessing fracture displacement and angulation. Moreover, it is the study of choice in determining fracture union or evaluation of suspected nonunions.

SCAPHOID FRACTURES DIAGNOSIS:
Pearls and Pitfalls

- Anatomic snuffbox tenderness and scaphoid tubercle tenderness are sensitive but not specific in diagnosing a scaphoid fracture
- In patients with a suspected scaphoid fracture, but negative radiographs, diagnosis is best made with an MRI or repeat radiographic evaluation after 2 weeks of immobilization
- CT scanning is recommended in the evaluation of scaphoid displacement, fracture union, and nonunion
- MRI with gadolinium is recommended for the evaluation of scaphoid AVN

Classification

Scaphoid fractures have been classified by fracture plane, location and stability. Fractures are localized within the proximal, middle (waist) or distal third of the bone. Most scaphoid fractures occur at the waist (70%), followed by the proximal pole (20%) and then the distal pole (10%). Herbert's classification system is the most commonly used, as it identifies the fractures that need operative fixation, either due to inherent instability or delayed union/ nonunion (Table 4.1). Fractures are divided into four types: (1) Type A, stable acute fractures; (2) Type B, unstable acute

Table 4.1: Herbert and Fisher's classification of scaphoid fractures

Acute Fractures-Stable	A1	Tubercle fracture
	A2	Incomplete waist fracture
Acute Fractures-Unstable	B1	Complete waist fracture
	B2	Complete transverse waist fracture
	B3	Proximal pole fracture
	B4	Trans-scaphoid perilunate dislocation
Delayed Union	C	Delayed union
Nonunion	D1	Fibrous union
	D2	Pseudoarthrosis

fractures; (3) Type C, delayed unions; and (4) Type D, established nonunions (Table 4.1).[5]

Surgical Indications

The ultimate goal of scaphoid fracture treatment is to obtain and maintain anatomical alignment while preserving vascularity until complete fracture union has occurred. Thus, the treatment of acute scaphoid fractures depends primarily on the location and stability of the fracture. Generally, the management of scaphoid fractures can be divided into three main categories: (1) nonoperative treatment with cast immobilization, (2) percutaneous fixation and (3) ORIF.

Nonoperative Treatment

Nonoperative treatment is usually indicated for distal pole fractures. These are typically avulsion or impaction fractures of the scaphoid tuberosity. As they are are well vascularized, they are routinely treated for 4–6 weeks in a short-arm thumb spica splint. Incomplete and non-displaced stable scaphoid waist fractures traditionally have been treated in a short- or long-arm cast. Many investigators have shown that union rates of greater than 90% can be achieved with prompt recognition and continuous immobilization.

Operative Treatment

Percutaneous fixation is best indicated for nondisplaced scaphoid fractures in patients who desire immediate return to activities. Acute unstable scaphoid fractures are a relative indication for percutaneous fixation. With unstable fractures, percutaneous fixation must be performed with the fracture reduced and aligned. When this cannot be achieved closed, open reduction is indicated. As with the open fixation, the volar approach is favored for waist fractures and the dorsal approach for proximal pole fractures.

Table 4.2: Criteria for displacement and instability of scaphoid fractures

- Displacement greater than 1 mm
- Lateral intrascaphoid angle greater than 35°
- Bone loss or comminution
- Perilunate fracture-dislocation
- Dorsal intercalated segmental instability (DISI) deformity
- Proximal pole fractures

Open reduction internal fixation is the treatment of choice for unstable or displaced scaphoid fractures. It has the advantage of facilitating anatomical reduction, rigid fixation and early motion. The criteria for displacement and instability includes displacement greater than 1 mm, lateral intrascaphoid angle greater than 35°, the presence of bone loss or comminution, scaphoid fractures associated with perilunate dislocation, presence of dorsal intercalated segmental instability (DISI) alignment, and proximal pole fractures (Table 4.2).[6] Other indications for ORIF are concomitant fractures of the distal radius and a delayed presentation/diagnosis of the scaphoid fracture. The surgical approach depends on the location of the fracture. The dorsal approach is preferred for the fixation of a proximal pole fracture; whereas fractures of the waist and distal third of the scaphoid are best approached through a volar approach.

Implants

Headless compression screws have undoubtedly become the primary option for fixing scaphoid fractures. In the early 1980s, Herbert developed a special screw system, which became the gold standard for the treatment of scaphoid fractures.[5] This headless double-thread screw permits fixation in both fragments. The pitch difference between the two threads also provides interfragmentary compression. The next major development in headless screw design was cannulation. This modification simplified the accurate placement of the screw within the scaphoid bone by using a thin guidewire placed under fluoroscopic control. Currently, several manufacturers have developed cannulated headless compression screws, either partially or fully threaded. Few clinical comparative studies between those screws exist, and the selection of the implant is a matter of surgeon preference. Besides the headless cannulated screw set, instrumentation to consider having on hand during the case includes a small power drive drill, Kirschner (K) wires and a mini C-arm. Alternatively, K-wires and headed partially threaded screws can also be used. Wires provide variable stability and also risk fracture distraction and are noted only for historical value. Headed screws can provide good fracture compression but risk articular injury.

Surgical Anatomy, Positioning and Approaches

Applied Anatomy

The word "scaphoid" is derived from the Greek word "skaphee", meaning "skiff" or "boat". The complex three-dimensional shape of the scaphoid hinders fracture diagnosis, the degree of displacement between fragments and the accuracy of screw or wire placement.

The scaphoid is the largest and most radial bone in the proximal row. It has five articulating surfaces and is almost entirely covered by cartilage, limiting ligamentous attachment and vascular supply. The scaphoid contacts the radius, lunate, capitate, trapezium and trapezoid, and serves as a mechanical link between the proximal and distal carpal rows. It is divided into the proximal pole, the waist and the distal pole with tubercle (Fig. 4.4A). The proximal surface is biconvex and articulates with the radius. A large concave sulcus opposite the radial articular facet acts as a socket for the radial aspect of nearly spherical capitate head (Fig. 4.4B). The distal pole is flexed with respect to the proximal pole and has separate articular surfaces for the trapezium and trapezoid distally.

There are multiple ligamentous attachments to the scaphoid (Fig. 4.5). The scapholunate interosseous ligament (SLIL) is a stout ligament connecting the scaphoid to the lunate and inserts into the proximal pole. The SLIL is C-shaped and attaches exclusively along the dorsal, proximal and volar margins of the articulating surfaces.

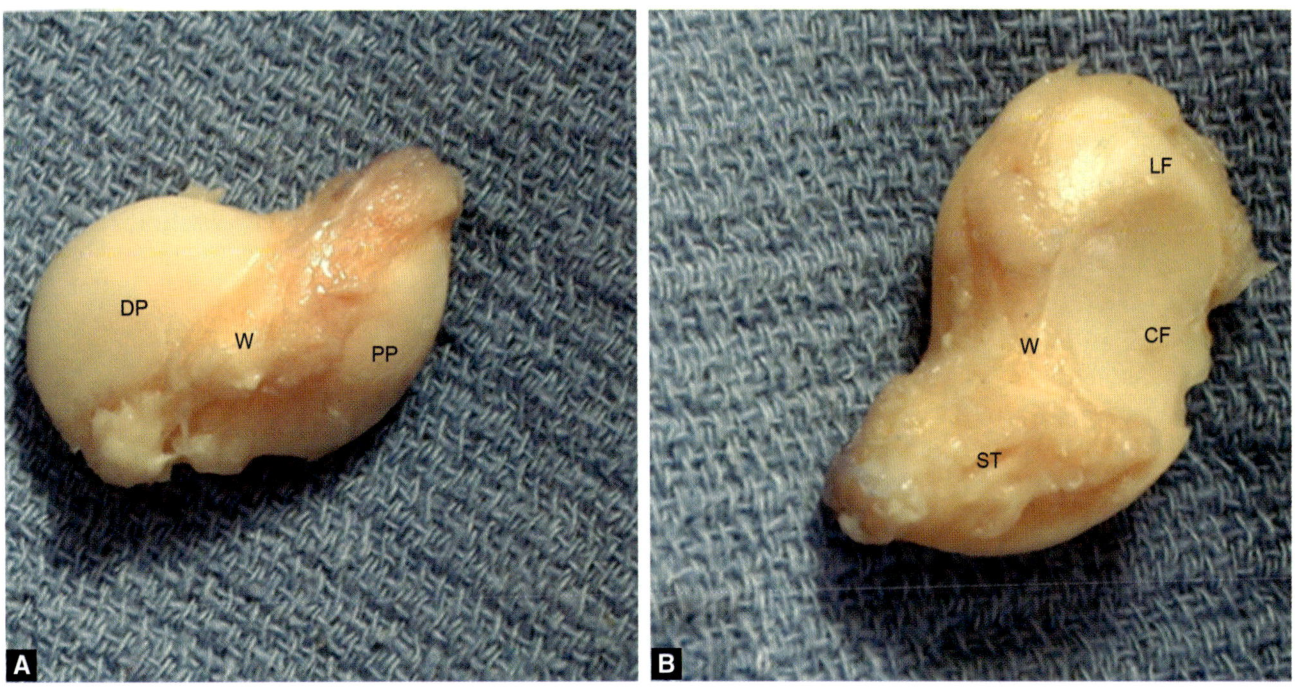

Figures 4.4A and B: An anatomical specimen of the scaphoid. (A) Dorsal surface (PP: Proximal pole, W: Waist, DP: Distal pole); (B) Volar surfaces (LF: Lunate facet, CF: Capitate facet, ST: Scaphoid tubercle). Note the complex shape and the fact that the scaphoid is almost entirely covered by articular cartilage.

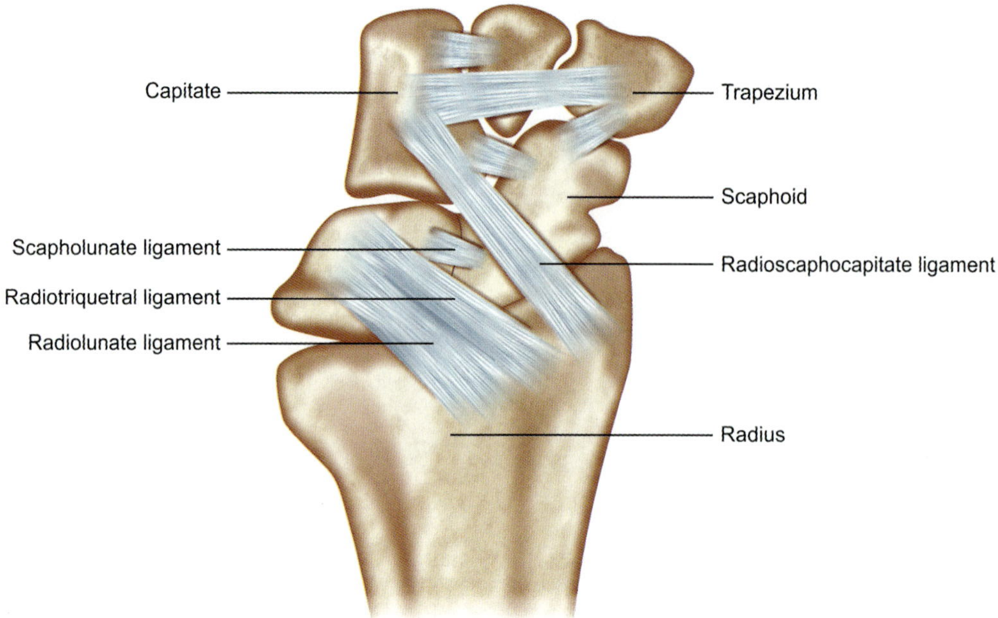

Figure 4.5: The volar radiocarpal ligaments. Note how the radioscaphocapitate ligament (RSCL) crosses the waist of the scaphoid.

The dorsal part serves as primary restraint to dorsal-volar translation. The palmar component has important contributions to rotational stability of the scapholunate joint. The RSCL originates from radial styloid, lies in volar concavity of the scaphoid waist, and proceeds ulnarly toward capitate, acting as a fulcrum around which the scaphoid rotates. The scaphocapitate ligament (SCL) originates from the volar distal scaphoid at the border between the trapezoid facet and the capitate facet. It inserts into the volar waist of the capitate distal to the RSCL. This ligament, along with the scaphotrapezial ligament, functions as a primary restraint of the distal pole. The dorsal surface is the attachment site for the dorsal intercarpal (DIC) ligament and radial collateral ligaments. The DIC ligament is a weak capsular ligament that functions as a stabilizer of the wrist and a dorsal hammock restraint for the proximal pole of the capitate.[7]

The scaphoid receives its blood supply through ligamentous attachments. Gelberman has shown that blood supply to the scaphoid is derived from tributaries of the radial artery. Dorsal branches supply 70–80% of the blood flow to the scaphoid, whereas volar perforators supply the remaining 20–30%. Palmar branches enter through the distal third of the bone, whereas dorsal branches enter through the middle third. The proximal scaphoid is supplied by retrograde blood flow from these vessels. Therefore, injuries to the proximal third of the scaphoid are at a high risk of AVN.[8]

The ability of the intercarpal and radiocarpal ligaments to stabilize the intercalated proximal carpal row is dependent on the integrity of scaphoid. An unstable scaphoid fracture allows dorsal rotation of the lunate as its ligamentous attachments to the triquetrum become predominant. The proximal pole of the scaphoid rotates with lunate while the distal pole remains flexed by virtue of its attachments to trapezium and trapezoid. The result is apex dorsal (and radial) angulation through the fracture of the scaphoid, so-called humpback deformity (Fig. 4.6). This deformity produces an alteration of carpal kinematics even if the fracture heals, which may lead to carpal collapse and arthritic changes.

Positioning

The patient is positioned supine with the hand on a radiolucent hand table. For a volar approach, whether open or closed, the surgeon should be seated with dominant hand at outer end of the table. For a dorsal approach, this position is reversed. A pneumatic tourniquet is routinely used. A large, rolled-up towel is used to aid

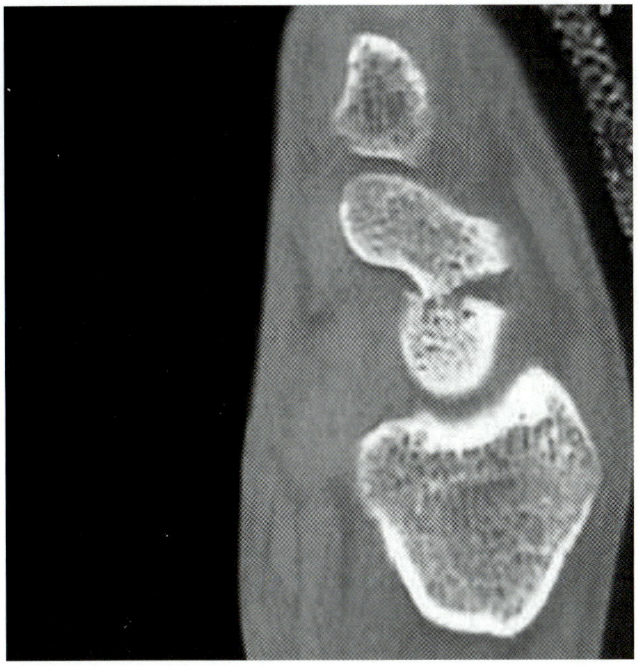

Figure 4.6: Computerized tomography scan demonstrating humpback deformity of scaphoid nonunion.

extension or flexion of the wrist. A fluoroscopic image intensifier is mandatory to perform the operation. We prefer to use the mini C-arm to minimize the radiation exposure.

Approaches

The volar approach to the scaphoid provides excellent visualization and access while minimizing risk to its blood supply. This approach is indicated for unstable scaphoid fractures at the middle or distal third, and for scaphoid waist nonunions, especially in the presence of a humpback deformity. In case of a humpback deformity, this approach provides excellent exposure for reduction of the scaphoid angulation with bone grafts, and for fixation with cannulated compression screws. This approach is contraindicated for proximal pole fractures. Structures at risk with this approach are the radial artery and palmar cutaneous branch of the median nerve.

The dorsal approach is indicated for proximal pole fractures. This approach may also be used for transscaphoid perilunate dislocations and for scaphoid nonunions, when a vascularized bone graft (VBG) from the distal radius is needed. The dorsal exposure has benefits of sparing the volar ligaments of the wrist. However, the exposure may place perfusion of the scaphoid at risk if taken too far distally.

Surgical Techniques

Technique 1: Volar ORIF of Scaphoid Fractures

Volar ORIF of scaphoid fractures are best indicated for displaced scaphoid fractures (Figs 4.7A to G and 4.8A to C).

Surgical Technique

A 3–4 cm, hockey-stick incision is centered over the scaphoid tuberosity (Fig. 4.7A). The distal part of the incision is gently curved toward the base of the thumb metacarpal, and the proximal part is carried over the flexor carpi radialis (FCR) tendon for about 3 cm. The FCR sheath is divided sharply and a blunt self-retaining retractor is placed into the wound (Fig. 4.7B). The dissection is continued between the FCR tendon, which is retracted ulnarly, and the radial artery, which is retracted radially. The floor of the FCR tendon sheath is sharply incised exposing the volar joint capsule (Fig. 4.7C). The palmar branch of the radial artery is typically ligated as it enters the palm just proximal to scaphoid tuberosity. The capsule is incised longitudinally in line with the skin incision with care to avoid damaging the articular cartilage of the scaphoid (Fig. 4.7D). Proximally, there is a thickening of the capsule which corresponds to the RSCL and long radiolunate ligament. These ligaments must be preserved for later repair. Distally, the capsule is divided up to the scaphotrapezial joint. The self-retaining retractor is placed deeper along the incised capsule providing direct visualization of the scaphoid (Figs 4.7E and F).

The scaphoid is irrigated to remove the hematoma. Any intervening synovium trapped within the fracture site is removed. Next, anatomical fracture reduction is performed to correct any step-offs and rotational or angular deformities. The wrist is positioned in extension over a bump of towels. Kirschner wires may be placed into the proximal and distal fragments and used as joysticks to assist with fracture reduction. Provisional fixation can be secured with a 0.045 inch K-wire that is placed out of the way for definitive fixation with a cannulated screw. The provisional K-wire maintains the reduction and serves as an antirotational wire. Sometimes, to place the screw in the center of the scaphoid along the long axis, it is necessary to remove a small portion of the trapezium (Fig. 4.7G). A guidewire is then placed from the scaphoid tubercle and is aimed toward the apex of the proximal pole (Figs 4.8A to C). The central position of the wire is confirmed with fluoroscopy. The cannulated drill is then used to drill over the guidewire, and an appropriately measured compression screw is placed making sure that the screw is buried deep to the articular surface. The screw length should be typically 2–4 mm shorter than the measured length to allow for compression and subchondral placement. The fracture site must be visualized as the screw is placed to confirm that the reduction is not lost during this process. The position and length of the screw are verified with fluoroscopy, and once that is confirmed to be satisfactory, the initial provisional K-wire may be removed (Figs 4.8B and C). At this time, the

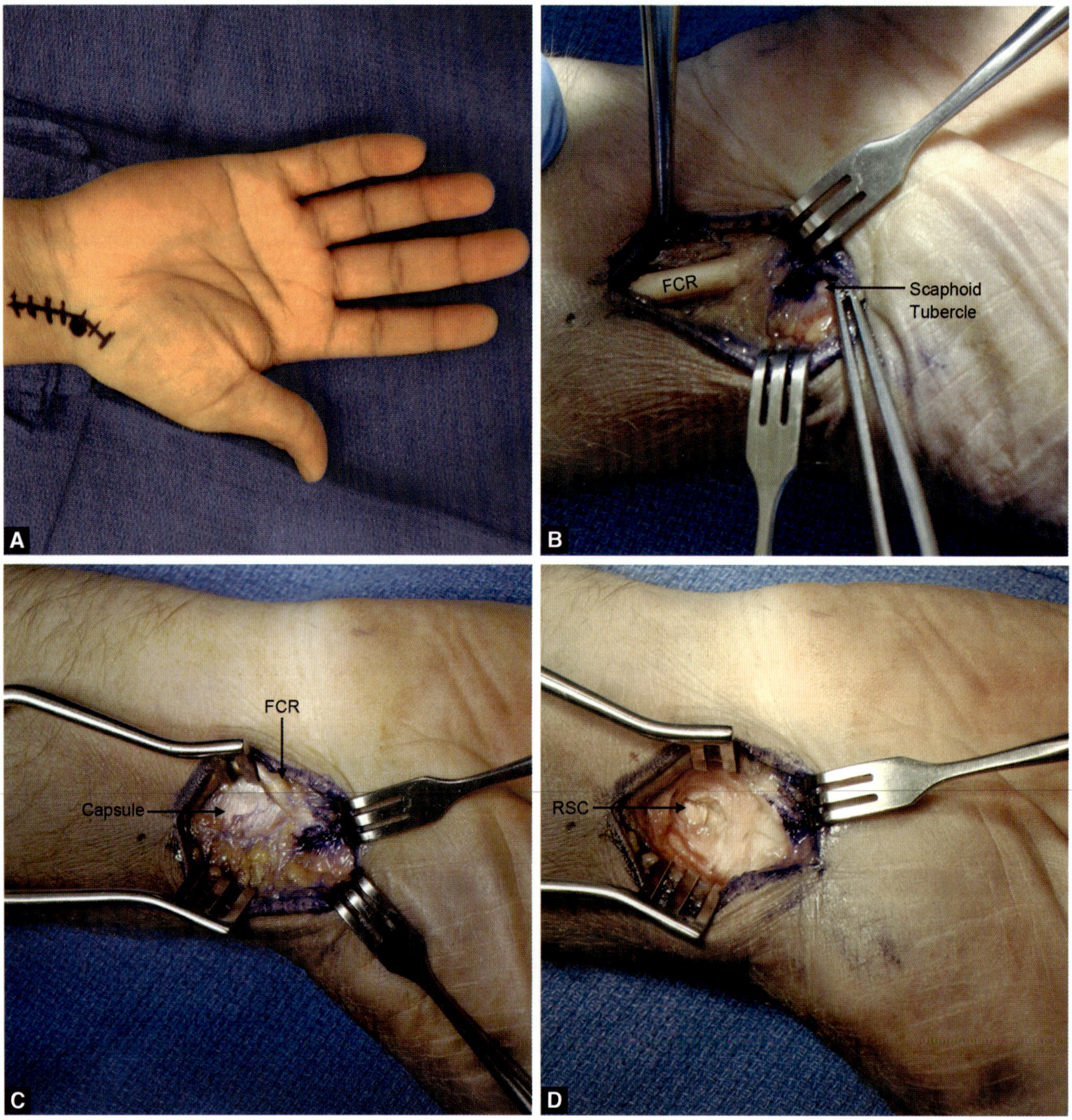

Figures 4.7A to D

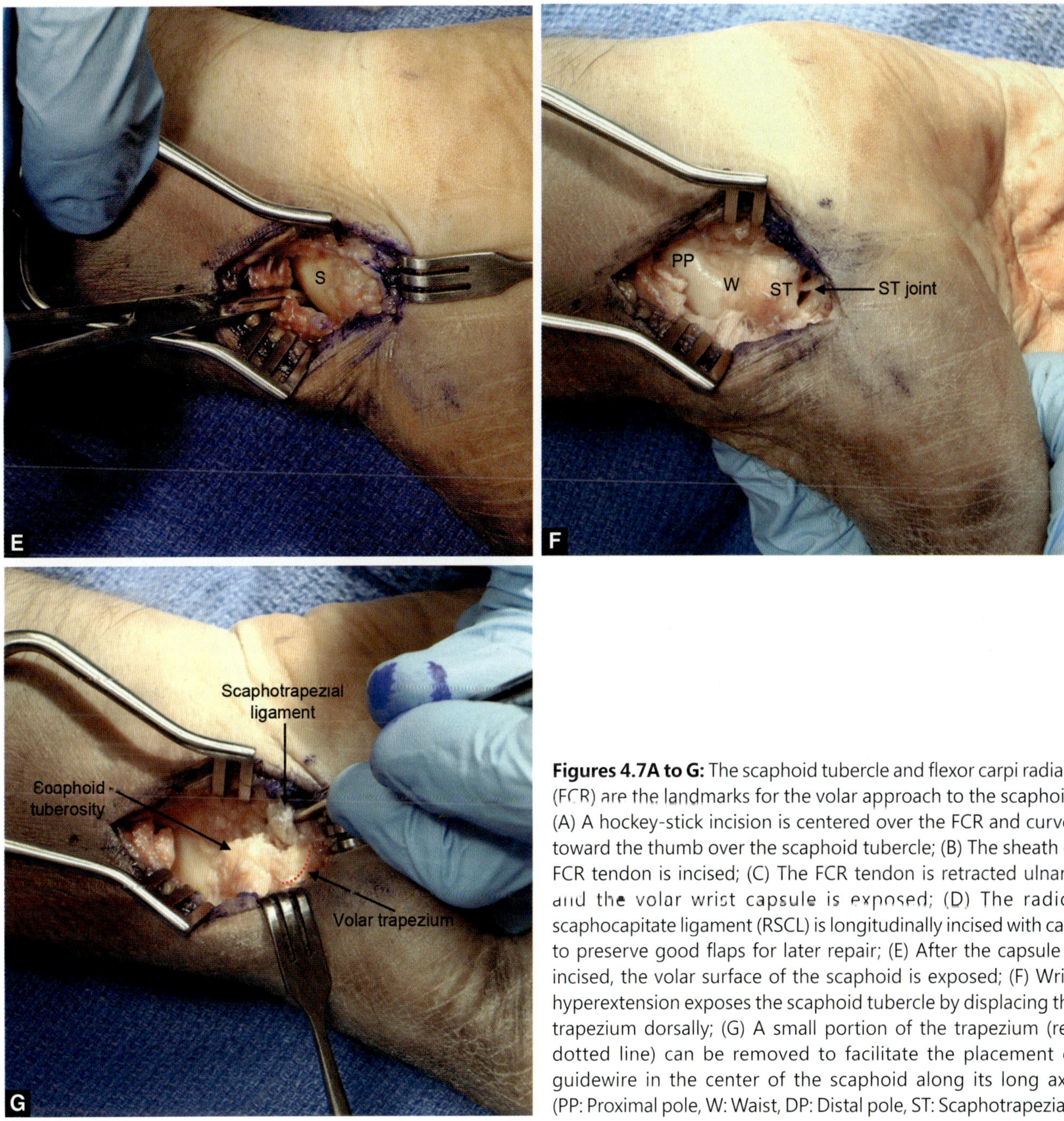

Figures 4.7A to G: The scaphoid tubercle and flexor carpi radialis (FCR) are the landmarks for the volar approach to the scaphoid. (A) A hockey-stick incision is centered over the FCR and curves toward the thumb over the scaphoid tubercle; (B) The sheath of FCR tendon is incised; (C) The FCR tendon is retracted ulnarly and the volar wrist capsule is exposed; (D) The radio-scaphocapitate ligament (RSCL) is longitudinally incised with care to preserve good flaps for later repair; (E) After the capsule is incised, the volar surface of the scaphoid is exposed; (F) Wrist hyperextension exposes the scaphoid tubercle by displacing the trapezium dorsally; (G) A small portion of the trapezium (red dotted line) can be removed to facilitate the placement of guidewire in the center of the scaphoid along its long axis (PP: Proximal pole, W: Waist, DP: Distal pole, ST: Scaphotrapezial).

tourniquet is released and meticulous hemostasis is achieved. The wound is copiously irrigated and the capsule is closed with interrupted 3-0 absorbable sutures. The skin is closed with interrupted nylon sutures in a horizontal mattress fashion. A thumb spica splint is applied.

Postoperatively, a thumb spica splint is applied for the first 2 weeks until suture removal. Once sutures are removed, the patient is encouraged to work on active digit and wrist motion. Patients are allowed to return to work light duty, with a removable orthoplast thumb spica splint. Heavy manual work or contact sports are not allowed for at least 6 weeks or until evidence of radiographic fracture union. Radiographs are typically obtained at 6 and 12 weeks postoperatively.

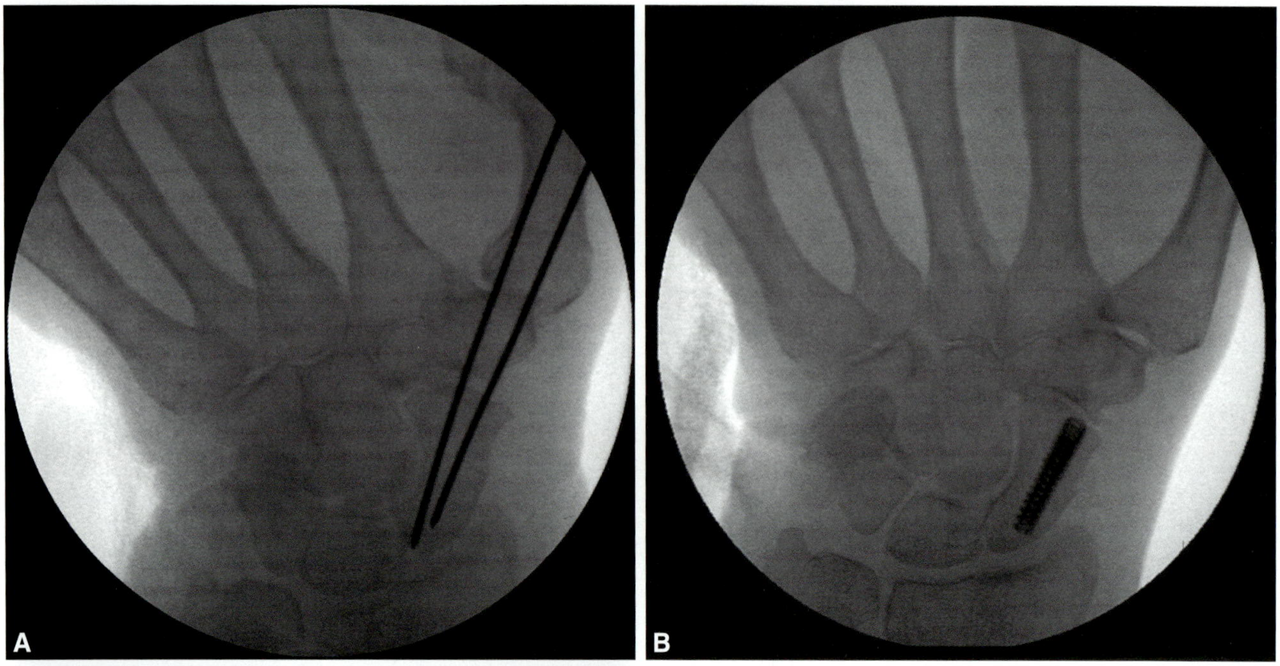

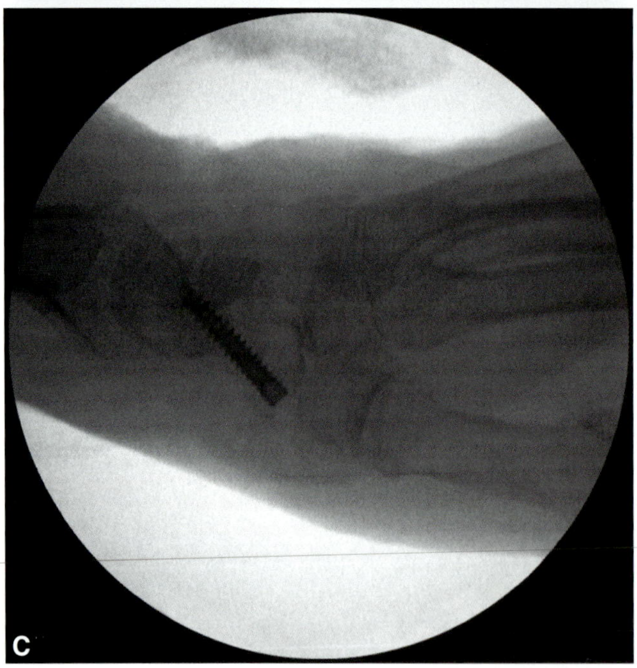

Figures 4.8A to C: Volar fixation of the scaphoid begins with reduction and Kirschner (K) wire fixation. (A) Two K-wires are placed in the scaphoid. The first K-wire is used for provisional fixation and to provide antirotational control. The second pin is placed along the center axis of the scaphoid and serves as a guidewire. The final position and length of the screw on (B) anteroposterior (AP) and (C) lateral views are verified with fluoroscopy.

VOLAR ORIF OF SCAPHOID FRACTURES: Pearls and Pitfalls

- The FCR tendon is the landmark to the volar aspect of the scaphoid
- Extend the approach distal enough to identify the scaphotrapezial joint and remove volar portion of the trapezium to achieve central placement of the guidewire
- Always use an antirotational wire to prevent rotational displacement of the fracture
- Select a 4 mm shorter cannulated screw than the measured guidewire length to adequately bury the screw below the articular surface
- Anatomical closure of the volar capsule is essential to prevent carpal instability

Technique 2: Dorsal ORIF of Scaphoid Fractures

Dorsal ORIF of scaphoid fractures are best indicated for proximal pole fractures or scaphoid nonunions requiring VBG placement (Figs 4.9A to E and 4.10).

Surgical Technique

A standard 3 cm longitudinal incision is made over the dorsum of the wrist centered just distal and ulnar to the Lister's tubercle (Fig. 4.9A). Superficial dissection is performed with care to protect the branches of the radial sensory nerve. The extensor retinaculum is exposed (Fig. 4.9B). The extensor pollicis longus (EPL) tendon is identified and retracted radially with the use of a blunt self-retaining retractor (Fig. 4.9C). The wrist capsule is incised longitudinally between the interval of EPL and extensor digitorum communis (EDC) tendons (Fig. 4.9D). Care must be taken to protect the SLIL, which lies directly deep to the capsule. The capsule overlying the waist of the scaphoid and distally should not be violated to preserve the blood supply to the scaphoid. Once the joint is entered, the self-retaining retractor is placed deeper and proximal pole of the scaphoid is exposed (Fig. 4.9E).

The fracture is irrigated to remove hematoma and any intervening synovium is debrided. Reduction is performed with the wrist held in flexion, pronation and ulnar deviation over a bump of towels. Again, K-wires may be placed as joysticks into the fracture fragments to assist with the reduction. The reduction is provisionally held with a K-wire that is directed along the ulnar border of the scaphoid under fluoroscopic guidance. Using a cannulated screw system, the guidewire is placed at the apex of the proximal pole and directed along the long axis toward the base of the thumb. The position of the guidewire and reduction of the fracture are verified and length of the screw is measured. The screw length should be typically 2–4 mm shorter than the measured length to allow for compression and subchondral placement. The appropriate length screw is inserted and reduction of the fracture and position of the screw are confirmed (Fig. 4.10). Again, the head of the screw must be buried deep to the articular surface as seen on fluoroscopy and confirmed with direct visualization. The provisional guidewire is removed and the wound is copiously irrigated. The tourniquet is released, meticulous hemostasis is achieved, and the capsule is closed with absorbable interrupted sutures. The skin is reapproximated with nylon sutures and a thumb spica splint is applied.

Postoperatively, a thumb spica splint is applied for the first 2 weeks until suture removal. Once the sutures are removed, the patient is encouraged to work on active digit and wrist motion. Patients are allowed to return to work light duty, with a removable orthoplast thumb spica splint. Heavy manual work or contact sports are not allowed for at least 6 weeks or until evidence of radiographic fracture union. Radiographs are typically obtained at 6 and 12 weeks postoperatively.

DORSAL ORIF OF SCAPHOID FRACTURES: Pearls and Pitfalls

- Open the dorsal capsule with caution to avoid injury to the SLIL
- Place an antirotational guidewire to prevent rotational displacement of the fracture
- Position the screw guidewire central along the axis of the scaphoid, aiming distally in line with the thumb
- Select a 4 mm shorter cannulated screw than the measured guidewire length to adequately bury the screw below the articular surface

Technique 3: Volar Percutaneous Fixation of Scaphoid Fractures

The volar percutaneous screw fixation technique is indicated primarily for minimally and nondisplaced scaphoid waist fractures (Figs 4.11A to D). Displacement of more than 1 mm and comminution is an indication for open reduction to obtain anatomical alignment.

Surgical Technique

Although a tourniquet should be placed on the arm, it typically does not need to be inflated for percutaneous fixation. Two rolled towels are used under the supinated wrist to allow for adequate dorsiflexion. The guidewire for the cannulated screw system is placed through the volar scaphoid tuberosity and directed proximally, dorsally and ulnarly with the wrist hyperextended and slightly ulnarly deviated (Fig. 4.11A). Image intensification is used in multiple planes to ensure that the wire is placed accurately across the fracture site and that the proximal entry site

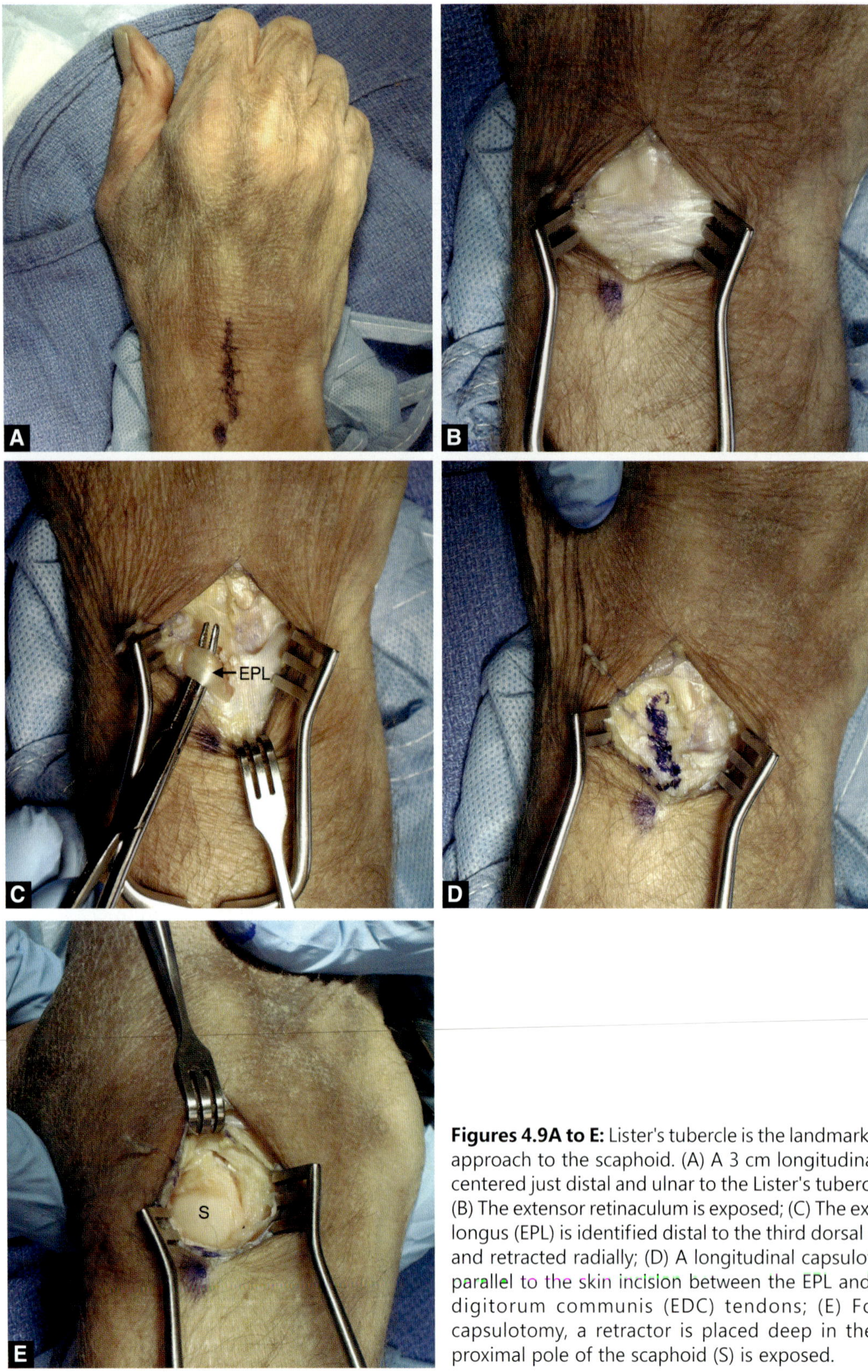

Figures 4.9A to E: Lister's tubercle is the landmark for the dorsal approach to the scaphoid. (A) A 3 cm longitudinal approach is centered just distal and ulnar to the Lister's tubercle (blue spot); (B) The extensor retinaculum is exposed; (C) The extensor pollicis longus (EPL) is identified distal to the third dorsal compartment and retracted radially; (D) A longitudinal capsulotomy is made parallel to the skin incision between the EPL and the extensor digitorum communis (EDC) tendons; (E) Following the capsulotomy, a retractor is placed deep in the wound and proximal pole of the scaphoid (S) is exposed.

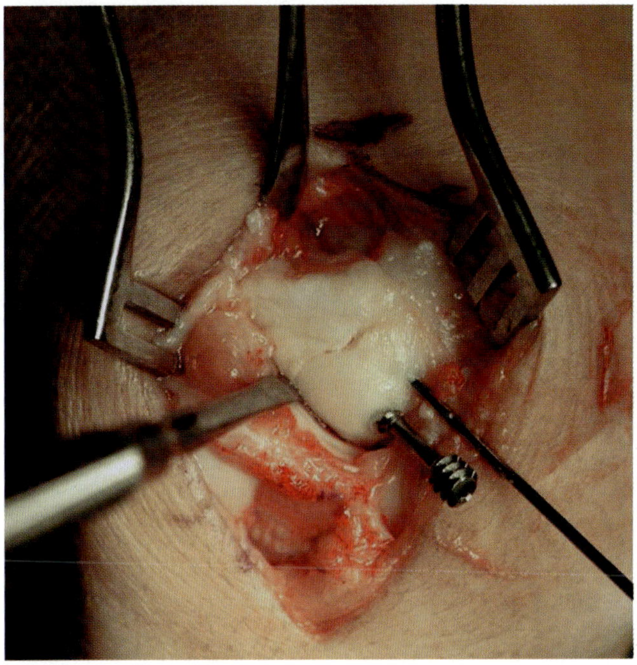

Figure 4.10: Dorsal approach and fixation of a proximal pole fracture of the scaphoid. Note that the fracture is reduced and a headless compression screw is being advanced over a guidewire. The second wire serves as an antirotational pin maintaining the reduction as the screw is advanced but is removed following definitive placement of the screw.

has enough bone volarly to support the screwhead (Fig. 4.11B). Dorsiflexion of the wrist assists in translating the trapezium dorsally out of the path of the wire. If necessary, the guidewire can be directed through a part of the trapezium, or alternatively a part of the overriding trapezium may be excised to gain access to the scaphoid tubercle. Furthermore, ulnar deviation increases flexion of the scaphoid volarly to aid in access for the guidewire. A second guidewire is placed parallel to the first guidewire for antirotation (Fig. 4.11C). Screw length can be measured with the measuring device available in the screw set or, alternatively, indirectly with a second guide pin. It is important to subtract 2–4 mm from the measured length of the guidewire, as the screw should be completely buried within the scaphoid. Once the guidewires are satisfactorily placed, a 3 mm incision is made around the guide pin to allow drill and screw passage. The scaphoid is then drilled with the cannulated drill with depth monitored by fluoroscopy. The cannulated screw is placed with fluoroscopic guidance. The antirotational wire is removed and final fluoroscopic images are obtained (Fig. 4.11D). The wound is irrigated and closed with a nylon suture, and a well-padded, short-arm thumb spica splint is applied.

Postoperatively, a thumb spica splint is applied for the first 2 weeks until suture removal for comfort. Once the sutures are removed, the patient is encouraged to work on active digit and wrist motion. Patients are allowed to return to work light duty, with a removable orthoplast thumb spica splint. Heavy manual work or contact sports are avoided for at least 6 weeks or until evidence of radiographic fracture union. Radiographs are typically obtained at 6 and 12 weeks postoperatively.

VOLAR PERCUTANEOUS FIXATION OF SCAPHOID FRACTURES: Pearls and Pitfalls

- Hyperextension and ulnar deviation of the wrist maximizes volar exposure of the scaphoid tuberosity
- Central position of the guidewire is crucial and must be confirmed on multiple views
- The overlying trapezium may be excised to gain access to the scaphoid tuberosity
- An antirotational wire is best placed prior to drilling and screw placement
- The screw placement is aided by making a small incision and bluntly dissecting down to the scaphoid tubercle

Technique 4: Dorsal Percutaneous Fixation of Scaphoid Fractures

The dorsal percutaneous screw fixation technique is indicated primarily for minimally and nondisplaced scaphoid waist fractures (Figs 4.12A to D).[9] Displacement of more than 1 mm and comminution is an indication for open reduction to obtain anatomical alignment.

Surgical Technique

By pronating, flexing and ulnarly deviating the wrist, the scaphoid can be viewed with fluoroscopy as a cylinder (Fig. 4.12A). A guidewire that is introduced down the center of this cylinder will be placed along the central anatomical axis of the scaphoid (Fig. 4.12B). The wire is advanced across the scaphoid fracture site under fluoroscopy. Once satisfied with the fracture reduction and wire position, the guidewire may either be left in place or

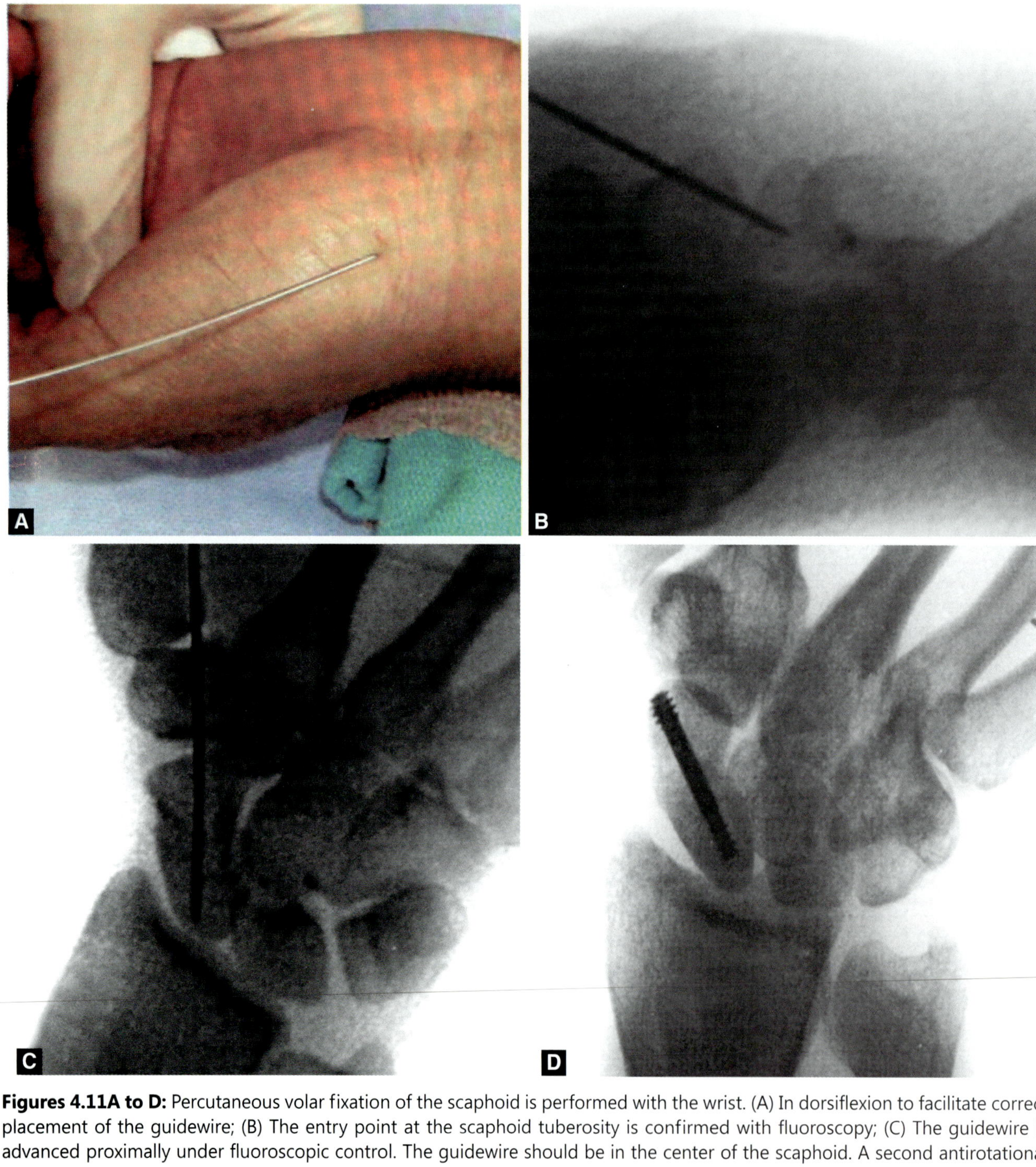

Figures 4.11A to D: Percutaneous volar fixation of the scaphoid is performed with the wrist. (A) In dorsiflexion to facilitate correct placement of the guidewire; (B) The entry point at the scaphoid tuberosity is confirmed with fluoroscopy; (C) The guidewire is advanced proximally under fluoroscopic control. The guidewire should be in the center of the scaphoid. A second antirotational wire is placed parallel to the guidewire; (D) Final view which shows the central placement of the screw and the anatomical reduction of the fracture.

advanced through the volar skin and withdrawn up to the radiocarpal joint. The latter allows the wrist to be freely extended without being blocked by the guidewire. Alternatively, if the fracture is displaced, the guidewire is further advanced into only the distal portion of the scaphoid. The fracture is manipulated and the distal pole is joysticked with the wire. Once the fracture is reduced, the wire is advanced retrograde from a volar to dorsal direction back

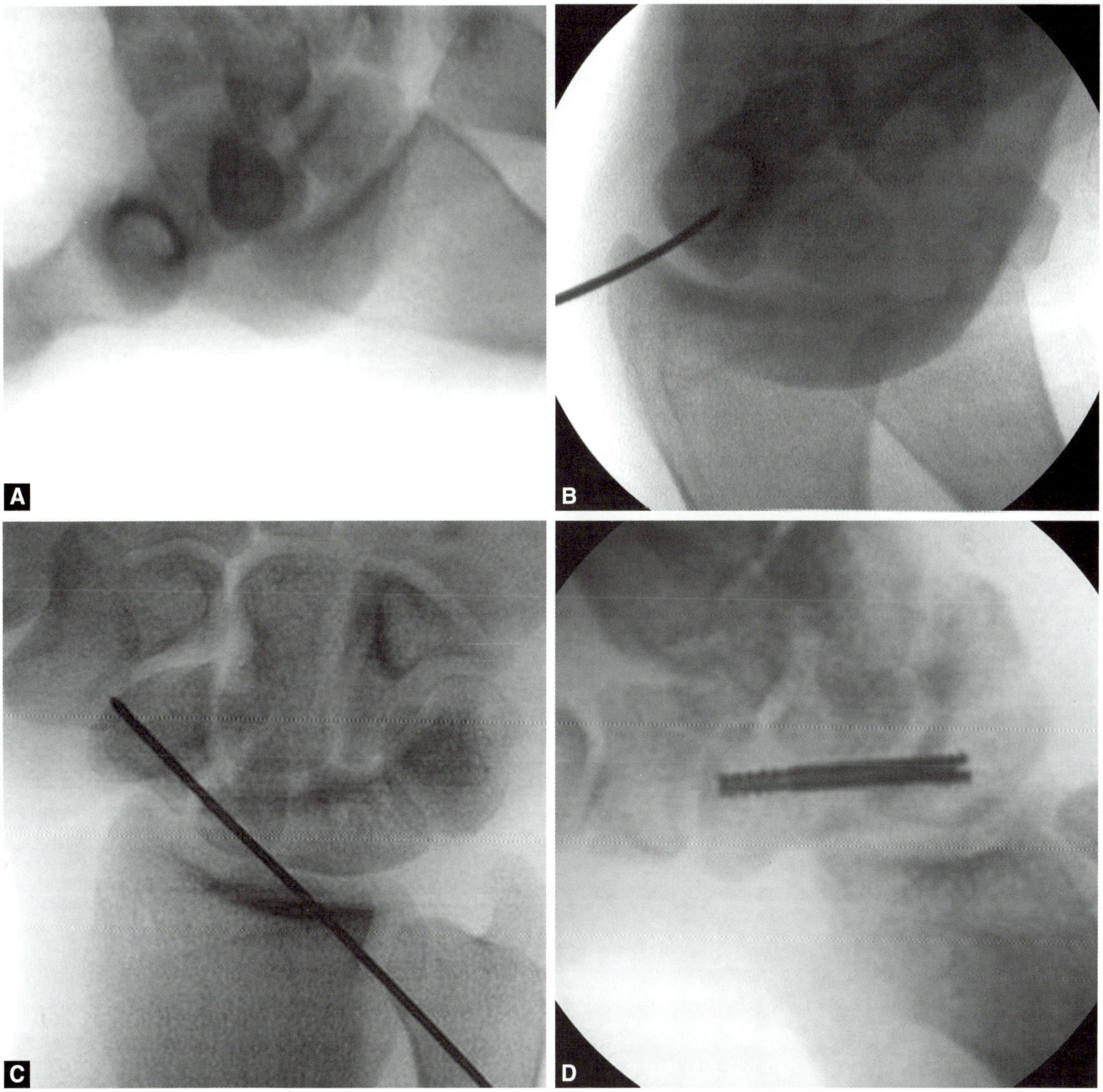

Figures 4.12A to D: Percutaneous dorsal fixation of the scaphoid is performed with the wrist in flexion. (A) With the wrist held in pronation, flexion and ulnar deviation, the scaphoid is seen under fluoroscopy as a circle; (B) Under fluoroscopic guidance, the tip of the guidewire is placed in the center of the circle and then the wire is advanced distally; (C) The guidewire should be placed along the central anatomical axis of the scaphoid. A second guidewire is placed parallel to the first guidewire for antirotational control; (D) The screw is placed in the center of the scaphoid and the reduction is checked with fluoroscopy.

into the proximal pole of the scaphoid. Next, a second guidewire is placed parallel to the first guidewire for antirotational control (Fig. 4.12C).

A 3 mm incision is made around the guide pin to allow drill and screw passage. The scaphoid is then drilled with the cannulated drill, with depth monitored by fluoroscopy. The scaphoid is drilled within 2 mm of the distal pole cortex, and screw length is measured with an appropriate depth gauge. It is important to subtract 2–4 mm from the measured length of the guidewire, as the screw should be completely buried within the scaphoid. The cannulated screw is then placed under fluoroscopic guidance. The antirotational guidewire is removed and final fluoroscopic images are obtained (Fig. 4.12D). The wound is irrigated and closed with a nylon suture, and a well-padded, short-arm thumb spica splint is applied.

Postoperatively, a thumb spica splint is applied for the first 2 weeks until suture removal for comfort. Once the sutures are removed, the patient is encouraged to work on active digit and wrist motion. Patients are allowed to return to work light duty, with a removable orthoplast thumb spica splint. Heavy manual work or contact sports are avoided for at least 6 weeks or until evidence of radiographic fracture union. Radiographs are typically obtained at 6 and 12 weeks postoperatively.

DORSAL PERCUTANEOUS FIXATION OF SCAPHOID FRACTURES: Pearls and Pitfalls

- The wrist is pronated and flexed until the scaphoid is seen as a circle. The center of the circle is the target point for insertion of the guidewire
- Use caution when extending the wrist with the guidewire in place dorsally as it may bend
- The central position of the guidewire in the scaphoid is the key
- Advance the guidewire aiming toward the tip of the thumb

Outcomes

Scaphoid fractures have traditionally been managed nonoperatively. However, nonoperative treatment requires prolonged immobilization and time away from work activities. Currently, there has been a growing trend toward early surgical fixation of scaphoid fractures, either open or percutaneous, in order to achieve a quicker return to work and activities.

The surgical treatment of nondisplaced and minimally displaced scaphoid fractures has resulted in better functional outcome, satisfaction, grip strength, shorter time to union, and earlier return to work.[10] In terms of treatment cost, it has been reported that the cost of nonoperative treatment for a nondisplaced scaphoid fracture is much higher than for operative treatment due to prolonged immobilization and lost productivity. Furthermore, the period of immobilization and lost productivity is significantly shorter with operative treatment, particularly for laborers.[11]

A union rate of approximately 95% can be achieved after rigid screw fixation of acute scaphoid fractures, either through a volar or dorsal approach. However, screw malpositioning can result in nonunion. The position of the implant near the central axis of the scaphoid is important for healing. For scaphoid waist fractures, clinical studies have shown a higher union rate, and cadaveric studies have shown a greater resistance to failure under bending loads for screws placed in the central third of both the proximal and distal poles.[12,13] Biomechanical testing of proximal pole fractures has shown that fixation from proximal to distal provides greater resistance to bending failure, probably because of the ability of the screw to engage more of the small proximal pole.[14]

The percutaneous technique had been recommended for nondisplaced or minimally displaced scaphoid fractures, but this technique has recently been used even for displaced scaphoid fractures, with reduction under fluoroscopic or arthroscopic control.[9,15] The reported union and complication rate with the percutaneous technique ranges from 94% to 100% and from 0% to 30% respectively, which is comparable with open technique.[16] In a landmark study, Bond et al. prospectively randomized 25 military personnel with nondisplaced scaphoid fractures to cast immobilization or percutaneous screw fixation. The time until union and return to work was significantly shorter for the percutaneous fixation group. However, at 2 years, there were no significant differences in function or satisfaction between groups.[18]

Complications

Complications are uncommon following internal fixation of the scaphoid, provided that satisfactory fracture reduction and fixation has been achieved at the time of surgery. Most complications are the consequences of delayed diagnosis and/or inadequate treatment resulting in nonunion and/or AVN.

Nonunions

Scaphoid nonunion occurs in 5–25% of cases (Fig. 4.13).[17] Factors contributing to nonunion include displacement

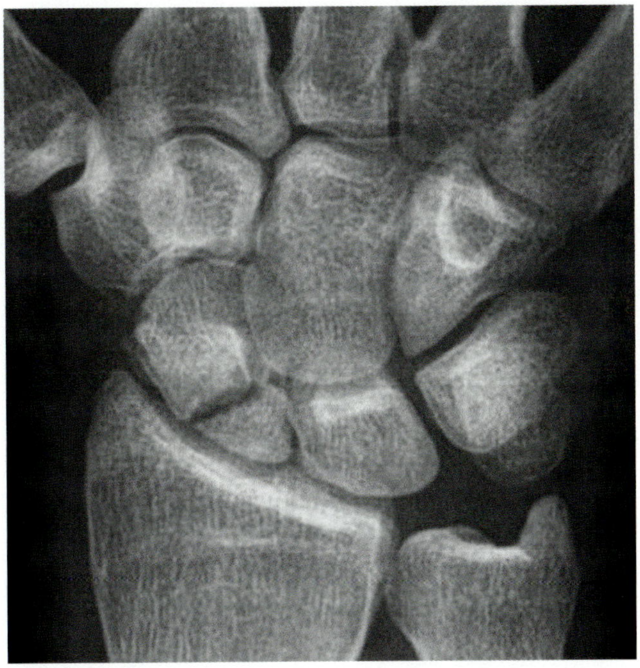

Figure 4.13: Nonunion of a scaphoid waist fracture. Note the lack of bridging bone, sclerosis and widening of the fracture line indicating chronicity of the injury.

greater than 1 mm, delay in diagnosis/immobilization greater than 4 weeks, location at the waist or proximal pole and a history of smoking.[18] Because of the strong relationship between nonunion with the development of post-traumatic arthritis of the wrist, surgery is recommended for most young, healthy patients even if they are currently symptom-free.[1]

Once the decision for surgical treatment of a scaphoid nonunion has been made, the surgeon should perform a careful preoperative plan to evaluate the characteristics of the nonunion. Magnetic resonance imaging is best indicated to assess the vascularity of the proximal pole of the scaphoid and assess for possible AVN (Figs 4.14A to E). Computerized tomography scanning of the scaphoid in longitudinal axis is the preferred technique to determine the presence of a humpback deformity and to evaluate for carpal alignment. Moreover, scaphoid nonunions often have significant bone loss and carpal collapse, along with volar rotation of the distal pole, which produces an apex dorsal humpback deformity which is best assessed by CT scan (Fig. 4.6).

Avascular Necrosis

Avascular necrosis can occur in approximately 30% of undertreated waist fractures and in nearly 100% of the proximal pole fractures (Figs 4.14A to E).[19] The proximal pole of the scaphoid is predisposed to AVN because of its distal location from the main nutrient vessels and the retrograde pattern of intraosseous blood supply.

The presence or absence of a humpback deformity and vascular status of the proximal fragment will dictate the surgical procedure. Generally, scaphoid nonunions with severe collapse and humpback deformity, and a viable proximal pole, must be approached through a volar approach with interposition of an intercalary bone graft and internal fixation.[20] In case of AVN, a VBG from the distal radius is our preferred method of treatment.[21] Vascular bone grafts theoretically provide restore vascularity that permits fracture union. Most series of VBGs report union between 6 weeks and 12 weeks following surgery. Merrell et al. in a meta-analysis, found an overall union rate of 88% with VBGs in patients with scaphoid nonunion and proximal pole necrosis as compared with 47% with the use of conventional grafts.[22] In another meta-analysis, Munk and Larsen reported that the use of VBGs led to a union rate of 91% in patients with prior failed surgery and/or proximal pole necrosis.[23] The high union rate reported with VBGs, and the fact that a failed conventional bone grafting operation makes the outcome of a revision surgery unpredictable, suggests that the use of VBGs should be the first treatment choice in scaphoid nonunion surgery even in the absence of AVN. Selection of a specific graft type depends on the location of the nonunion and presence or absence of significant deformity.

Arthritis

Untreated scaphoid nonunions result in carpal malalignment and wrist arthritis (Fig. 4.15). This pattern of arthritis consists of a predictable pattern of carpal collapse, the so-called scaphoid nonunion advanced collapse (SNAC) (Figs 4.16A to D). Radiographic findings of arthritis usually seen with scaphoid nonunion include radioscaphoid narrowing, capitolunate narrowing, cyst formation and pronounced DISI (Table 4.3). The radiolunate joint is usually spared in early stages, but may show degenerative changes as arthritis becomes more diffuse.

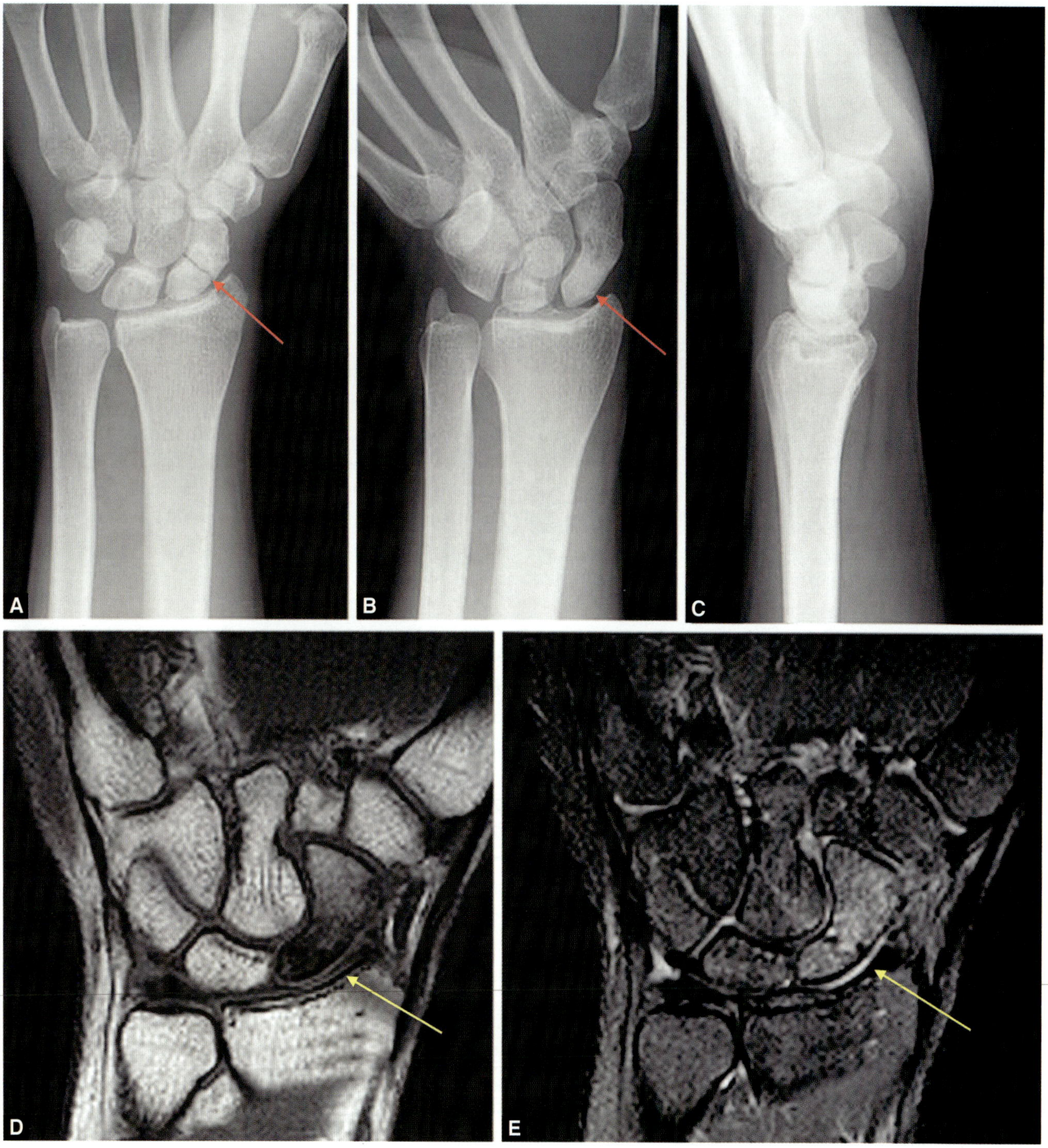

Figures 4.14A to E: Nonunion of the scaphoid with proximal pole avascular necrosis (AVN) as evidenced by sclerosis (red arrow) of the proximal pole on (A) posteroanterior (PA); (B) ulnar deviation, and (C) lateral radiographic views. The MRI findings correspond depending on imaging technique; (D) The coronal T1-weighted image shows a hypointense proximal pole which is characteristic for AVN; (E) The coronal T2-weighted image demonstrates edema around the nonunion site and a hypointense proximal pole (yellow arrows).

Table 4.3: Scaphoid nonunion advanced collapse stages (Figs 4.16A to D)

Stage I	Arthritis localized to the distal scaphoid and radial styloid
Stage II	Radioscaphoid plus scaphocapitate arthritis, but preservation of the lunocapitate joint
Stage III	Periscaphoid arthritis involving radiostyloid, distal scaphoid, scaphocapitate and lunocapitate joints
Stage IV	Diffuse arthritis of carpus and radiolunate fossa involvement

Although bone healing is needed for nonunions without arthrosis, but in cases where arthritis has already begun, additional procedures or salvage operations may be required. The optimal surgical management of SNAC wrists depends on several factors including patient's age, activity level, occupation and stage of degeneration (Figs 4.17A to H).

- Stage I SNAC wrist: Radial styloid excision and scaphoid nonunion repair

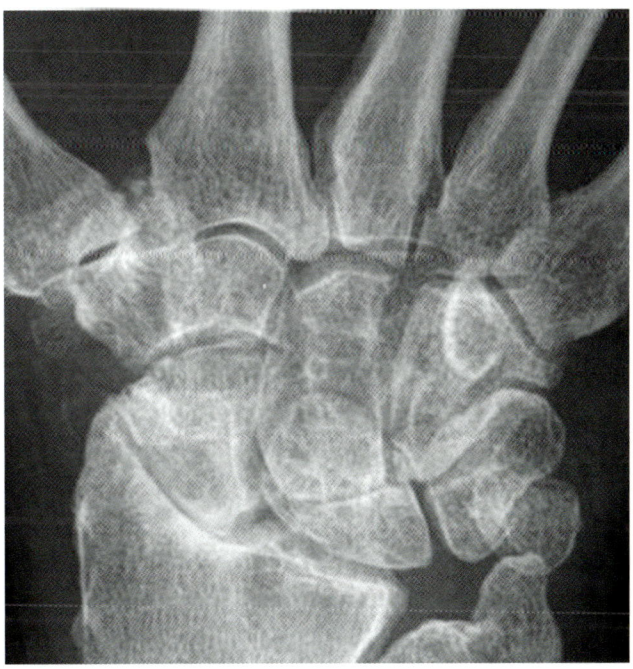

Figure 4.15: Untreated scaphoid nonunions result in a predictable pattern of carpal malalignment and wrist arthritis known as scaphoid nonunion advanced collapse (SNAC). Note the old scaphoid fracture and the subsequent pancarpal arthrosis.

- Stage II SNAC wrist: Proximal row carpectomy or four-corner intercarpal fusion with scaphoid excision. Generally, we recommend four-corner intercarpal fusion with scaphoid excision for younger patients, laborers and individuals with high activity level
- Stage III SNAC wrist: Four-corner intercarpal fusion with scaphoid excision or total wrist arthrodesis. Proximal row carpectomy is not an option for SNAC stage III because of involvement of the midcarpal joint and specifically the capitolunate joint (Fig. 4.18)
- Stage IV SNAC wrist: Total wrist arthrodesis

Authors' Preferred Management of Select Complications

Case 1: Proximal Pole Scaphoid Fracture Nonunion with Avascular Necrosis

A 30-year-old right hand dominant machinist presents with the chief complaint of left radial-sided wrist pain. He had a work related injury 4 months ago, when he fell backwards on his outstretched hand. He was diagnosed with a scaphoid fracture and was placed in a long-arm cast for a few weeks after which it was replaced with a short-arm cast. He was casted for a total of 10 weeks. The patient returned to his work and continued to have wrist pain and decreased grip strength. On physical examination, he had 70° of wrist extension and 60° of wrist flexion with pain at extremes of motion, marked tenderness over the anatomical snuff box, and pain with longitudinal compression of the thumb. Plain X-rays taken in the office showed a scaphoid nonunion as well as proximal pole AVN (Fig. 4.19A). Magnetic resonance imaging of the left wrist confirmed the diagnosis of proximal pole AVN (Fig. 4.19B).

Scaphoid proximal pole nonunions accompanied with AVN have been treated successfully with VBGs (Figs 4.19C and D). Several grafts are available for the treatment of this challenging problem and the choice of graft depends on the location and deformity of nonunion. In this particular case with no humpback deformity and no carpal malalignment, we prefer to use the capsular based VBG from the dorsal distal radius. This graft is technically straightforward and may be transferred to the scaphoid with minimal rotation (Fig. 4.20A). The graft is nourished

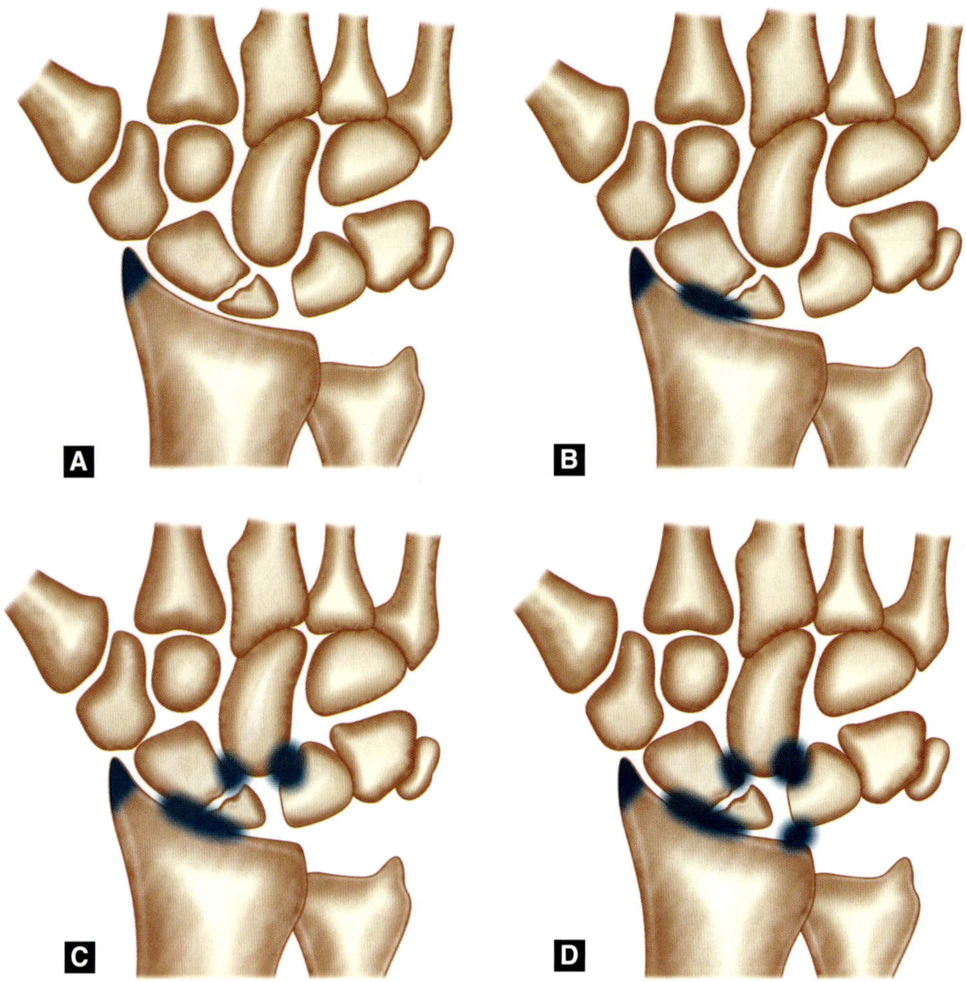

Figures 4.16A to D: Scaphoid nonunion advanced collapse (SNAC) follows a predictable pattern of carpal arthrosis. (A) Stage I consists of the development of radioscaphoid arthrosis localized between the distal pole of scaphoid and radial styloid; (B) Stage II includes scaphocapitate arthrosis; (C) Stage III includes progression into the midcarpal joint to include the lunocapitate joint; (D) Stage IV progresses to include the radiolunate joint resulting in pancarpal arthrosis.

by the fourth extensor compartmental artery (4th ECA) (Fig. 4.20B). The main advantage of the capsular based VBG is the convenient position of graft allowing easy access to the proximal scaphoid pole, with a short arc of rotation and low risk of nutrient vessel kinking.[21]

Technique

The procedure is performed under regional or general anesthesia and under tourniquet control and loupe magnification. A 4 cm straight dorsal incision centered just ulnar to the Lister's tubercle is placed. Dissection is carried through the subcutaneous tissue. The fourth dorsal compartment is partially released to expose the wrist capsule and the distal radius. The EPL tendon is identified and retracted radially, and the EDC tendons are retracted ulnarly. Next, the capsular based vascularized distal radius graft is outlined with a skin marker on the dorsal wrist capsule (Fig. 4.21A). The flap is trapezoidal in shape: the length is 2 cm and it widens from 1 cm at the bone block to 1.5 cm at its distal base. The bone block for the graft measures 1 × 1 cm and is harvested from the distal aspect of the dorsal radius just ulnar and distal to the Lister's tubercle. The depth of the bone graft is 7 mm and it includes the dorsal ridge of the distal radius. Two to three millimeters of the distal radius cortex is left intact to minimize the risk of propagation into the articular cartilage

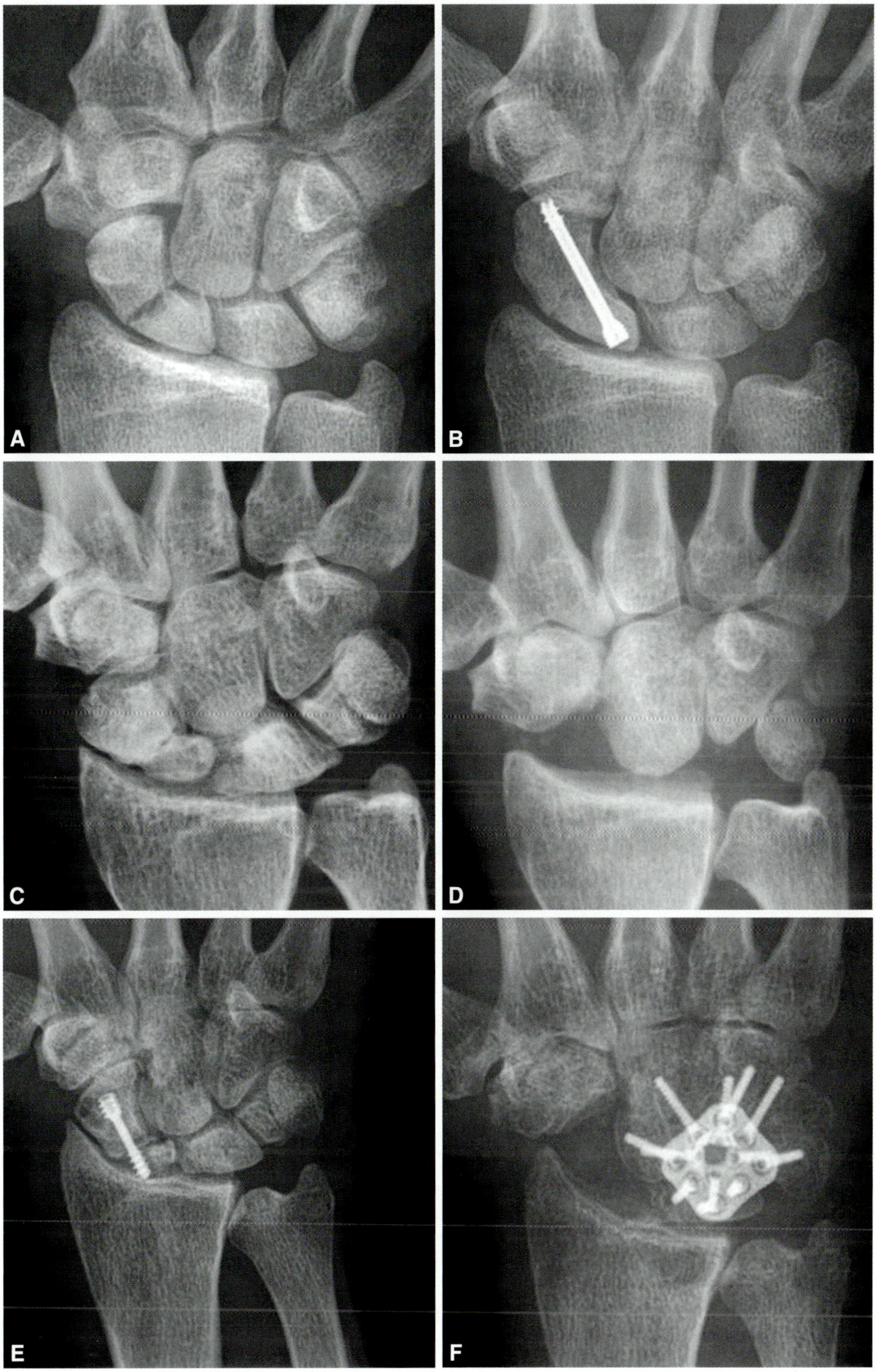

Figures 4.17A to F

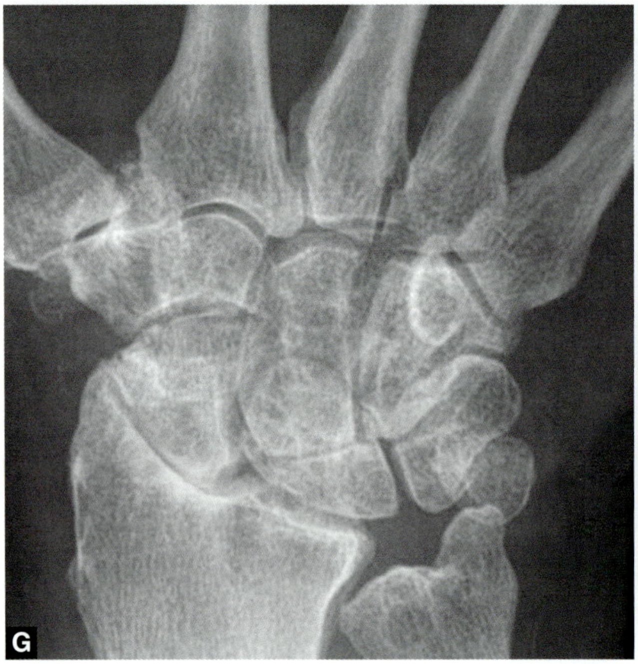

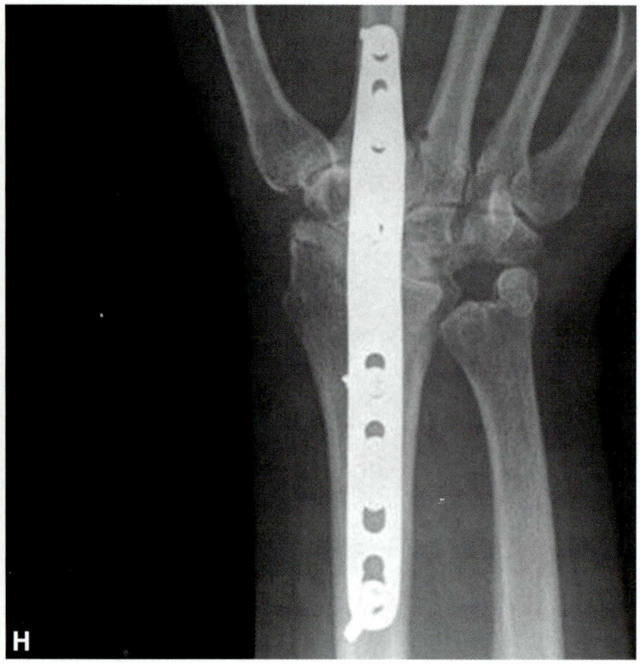

Figures 4.17A to H: The surgical management of scaphoid nonunion advanced collapse (SNAC) dependent upon the stage of disease. (A and B) Stage I SNAC treated with repair of the nonunion; (C and D) Stage II SNAC treated with a proximal row carpectomy; (E and F) Stage III SNAC treated with a four-corner intercarpal fusion and scaphoid excision; (G and H) Stage IV SNAC treated with a wrist fusion.

Courtesy: Asif M Ilyas

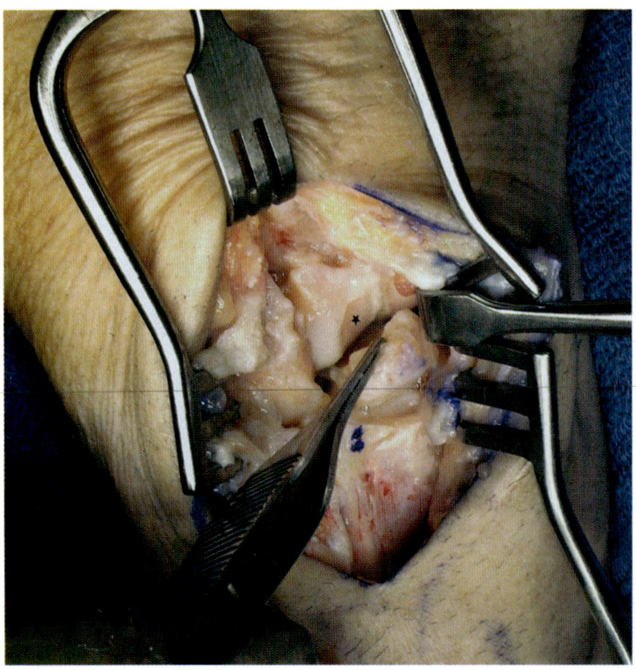

Figure 4.18: Note the intraoperative findings of stage III scaphoid nonunion advanced collapse (SNAC) wrist procedure. The asterisk marks the capitolunate joint, which is clearly arthritic, thereby contraindicating a proximal row carpectomy.

of the radiocarpal joint. The bone graft is outlined on the distal radius cortex with multiple drill holes by using a 1 mm side-cutting drill bit. A thin osteotome is then used to gently elevate the bone graft, with care not to violate the joint. The capsular flap is outlined sharply with a knife and is elevated along with the bone graft from the underlying tissues in a proximal to distal direction (Fig. 4.21B). Care should be taken to prevent detachment of the dorsal SLIL. The tourniquet is released to verify the vascularity of the bone graft.

Once the flap is elevated, attention is directed toward the scaphoid. Wrist flexion is often necessary to expose the proximal pole. If pseudarthrosis is present with disruption of the cartilage shell, the nonunion is cleaned with a dental pick and small curettes. It is important not to destabilize the nonunion site before scaphoid fixation because taking down the nonunion site can make fixation extremely challenging. If the cartilage shell is not grossly disrupted, the nonunion site is not violated. Fixation of the nonunion is performed under fluoroscopic control. Two 1 mm smooth wires are inserted from the proximal pole of the scaphoid oriented toward the base of the

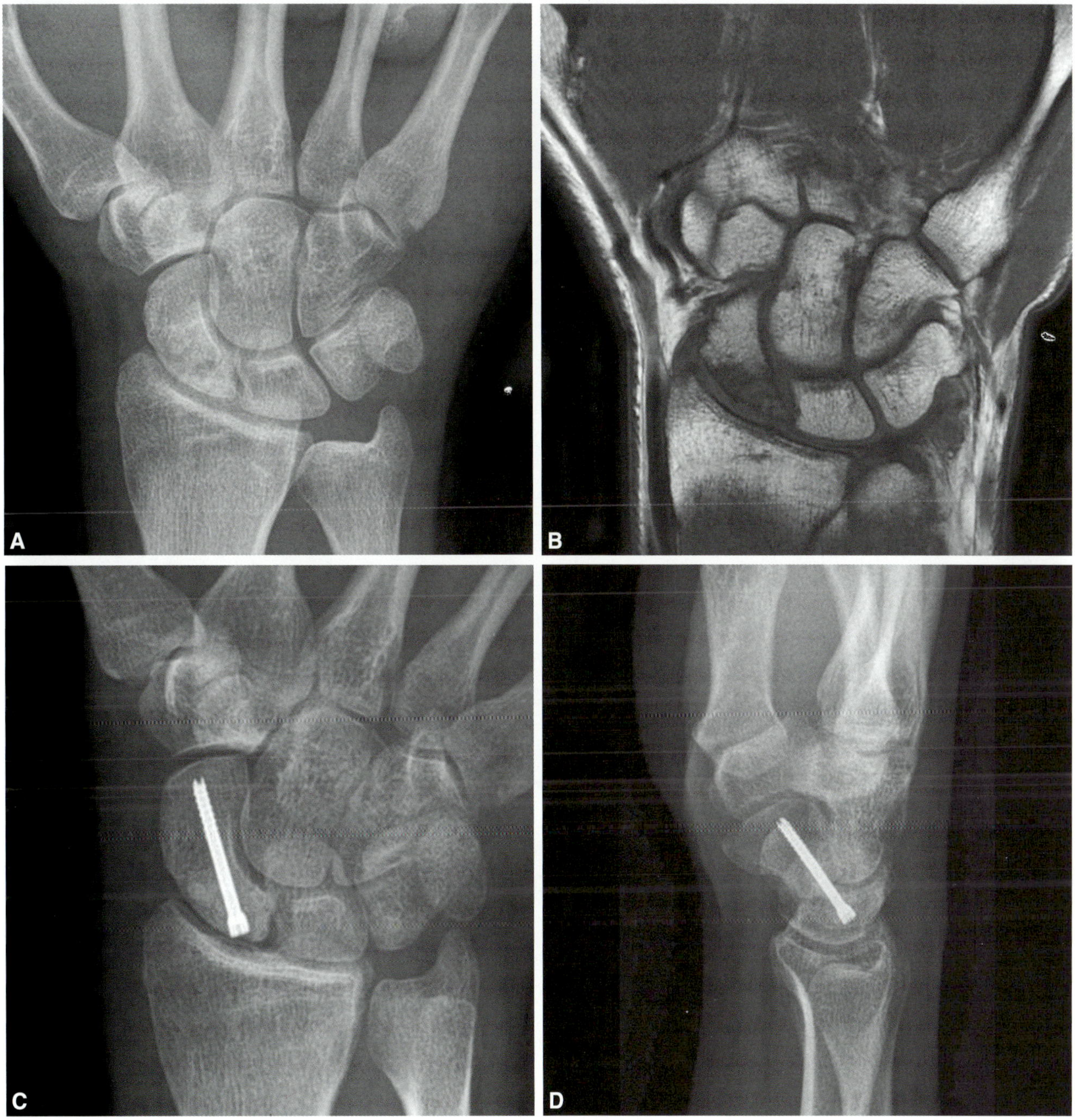

Figures 4.19A to D: A 30-year-old male laborer who incurred a proximal pole scaphoid fracture and was treated with cast immobilization for 10 weeks. Despite returning to work, he continued to have persistent wrist pain. (A) Plain radiograph showing scaphoid nonunion as well as proximal pole avascular necrosis (AVN); (B) MRI confirmed AVN of the proximal pole; (C and D) The patient underwent vascularized bone grafting from a dorsal approach with a headless compression screw.

Courtesy: Asif M Ilyas

thumb, with the wrist in extreme flexion (Fig. 4.21C). One of these serves as a guidewire for a cannulated screw and the other serves as an antirotational wire. Care should be taken to place the guidewire for the screw perpendicular to the fracture site and as volar as possible, while maintaining sufficient purchase of the proximal and distal

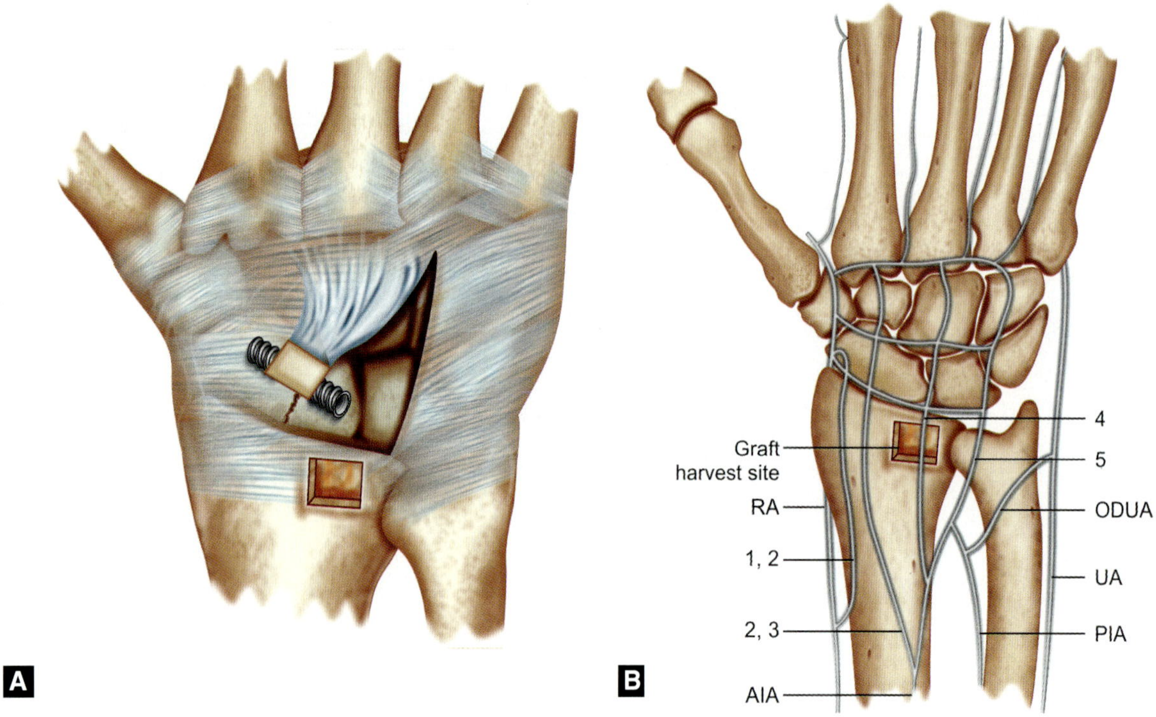

Figures 4.20A and B: (A) Transfer of the bone graft to the graft site with minimal rotation of the capsular flap; (B) The vascular supply of the dorsal wrist and vascularized graft. The capsular-based bone graft is an axial graft based on the artery of the fourth extensor compartment. (RA: Radial artery, UA: Ulnar artery, AIA: Anterior interosseous artery, PIA: Posterior interosseous artery, ODUA: Oblique dorsal ulnar artery, 1,2: 1,2 intercompartmental supraretinacular artery, 2,3: 2,3 intercompartmental supraretinacular artery, 4: Fourth extensor compartmental artery, 5: Fifth extensor compartmental artery).

Source: Sotereanos DG, Darlis NA, Dailiana ZH, et al. A capsular-based vascularized distal radius graft for proximal pole scaphoid pseudarthrosis. J Hand Surg Am. 2006;31(4):580-7.

fragments. The length of the screw is determined by measuring it next to an intact wire, followed by drilling and insertion of a cannulated screw. The screw is buried underneath the articular surface by 2 mm and the antirotational wire is removed (Fig. 4.21D).

Once the scaphoid is secured, the nonunion site is debrided with a small curette and a dorsal trough is created across the nonunion site with a side-cutting burr (Fig. 4.22A). The size of the trough is determined by the size of the VBG. At this point, the proximal pole fragment should be assessed to determine its vascularity. When the proximal pole fragment is too small to accommodate a trough, it is possible to position the graft in the excavated cavity of the proximal fragment. The authors prefer to secure the VBG with the placement of a small bone suture anchor. This bone anchor, which is loaded with two sutures, is placed at the floor of the trough (Fig. 4.22B). The VBG is then gently inserted into the scaphoid trough and is secured with a mattress stitch through the perimeter of the graft periosteum (Figs 4.22C and D). This must be tied over the graft in such a way so as not to compress the pedicle. Hemostasis is obtained, the wound is irrigated, and the skin incision is closed with 3-0 nylon sutures.

A short-arm thumb spica splint with the wrist in neutral position is applied for the first 2 weeks, followed by a short-arm thumb spica cast for another 4 weeks. Radiographs are obtained with the cast removed in 6 weeks and monthly thereafter to assess union progression. A removable forearm-based thumb spica splint may be used for protection in patients who have delay in union. Return to full activities is permitted only after solid union occurs.

Case 2: Scaphoid Nonunion without Avascular Necrosis

A 32-year-old male police officer who fell on his outstretched hand on duty incurred a nondisplaced scaphoid waist fracture. He was treated with cast

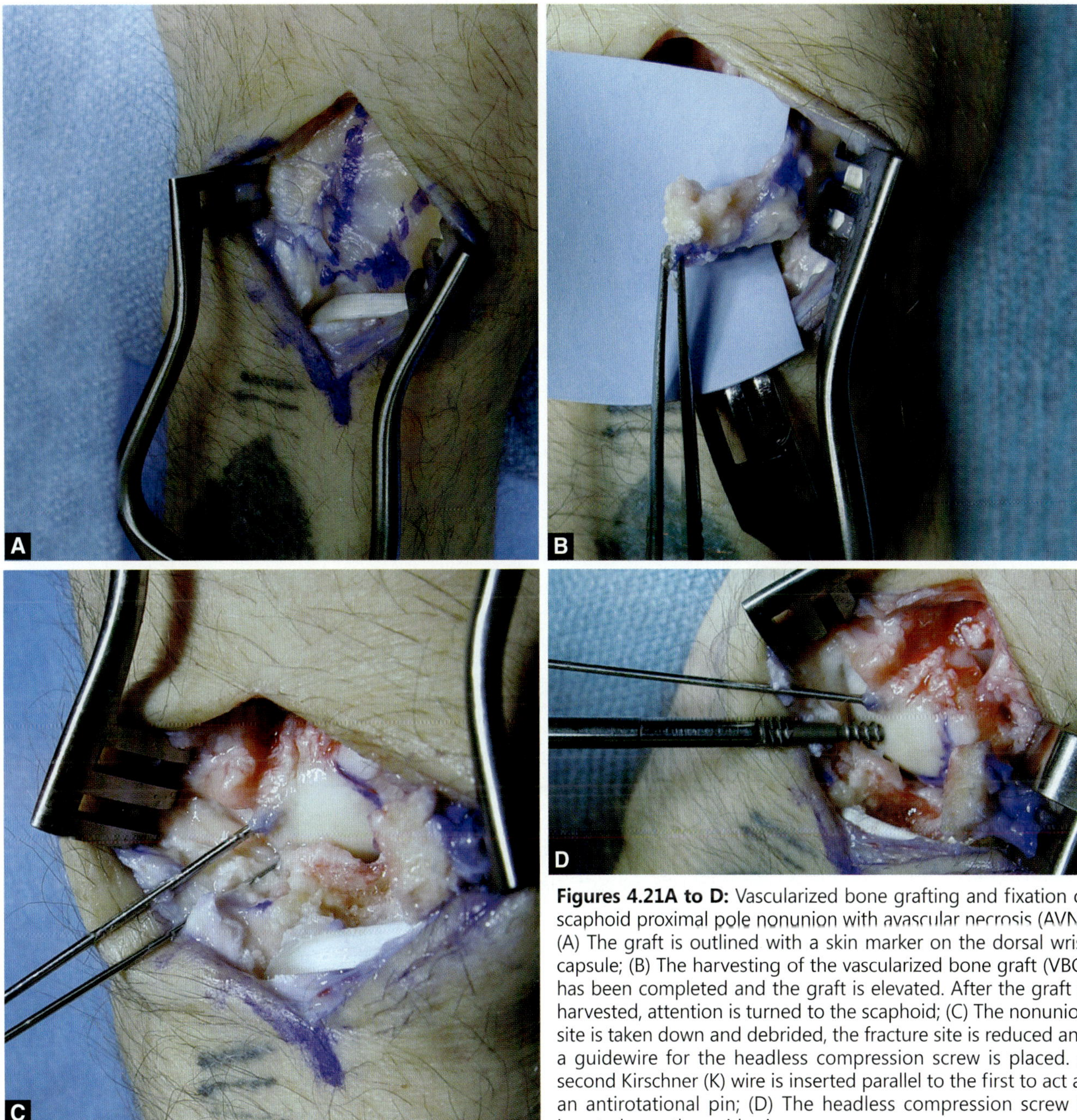

Figures 4.21A to D: Vascularized bone grafting and fixation of scaphoid proximal pole nonunion with avascular necrosis (AVN). (A) The graft is outlined with a skin marker on the dorsal wrist capsule; (B) The harvesting of the vascularized bone graft (VBG) has been completed and the graft is elevated. After the graft is harvested, attention is turned to the scaphoid; (C) The nonunion site is taken down and debrided, the fracture site is reduced and a guidewire for the headless compression screw is placed. A second Kirschner (K) wire is inserted parallel to the first to act as an antirotational pin; (D) The headless compression screw is inserted over the guidewire.

immobilization for 12 weeks. At radiographic reevaluation at 12 weeks, persistence of the fracture line was confirmed (Fig. 4.23A). Magnetic resonance imaging evaluation confirmed viability of the proximal pole of the scaphoid.

Scaphoid nonunion occurs in 5–25% of cases.[17] Factors contributing to nonunion include displacement greater than 1 mm, delay in diagnosis/immobilization greater than 4 weeks, location at the waist or proximal pole, and a history of smoking.[19] Because of the strong relationship between nonunion with the development of post-traumatic arthritis of the wrist, surgery is recommended for most young, healthy patients even if they are currently symptom-free.[1] Prior to surgical intervention, fracture displacement, angulation and vascularity is examined to direct the surgical approach.

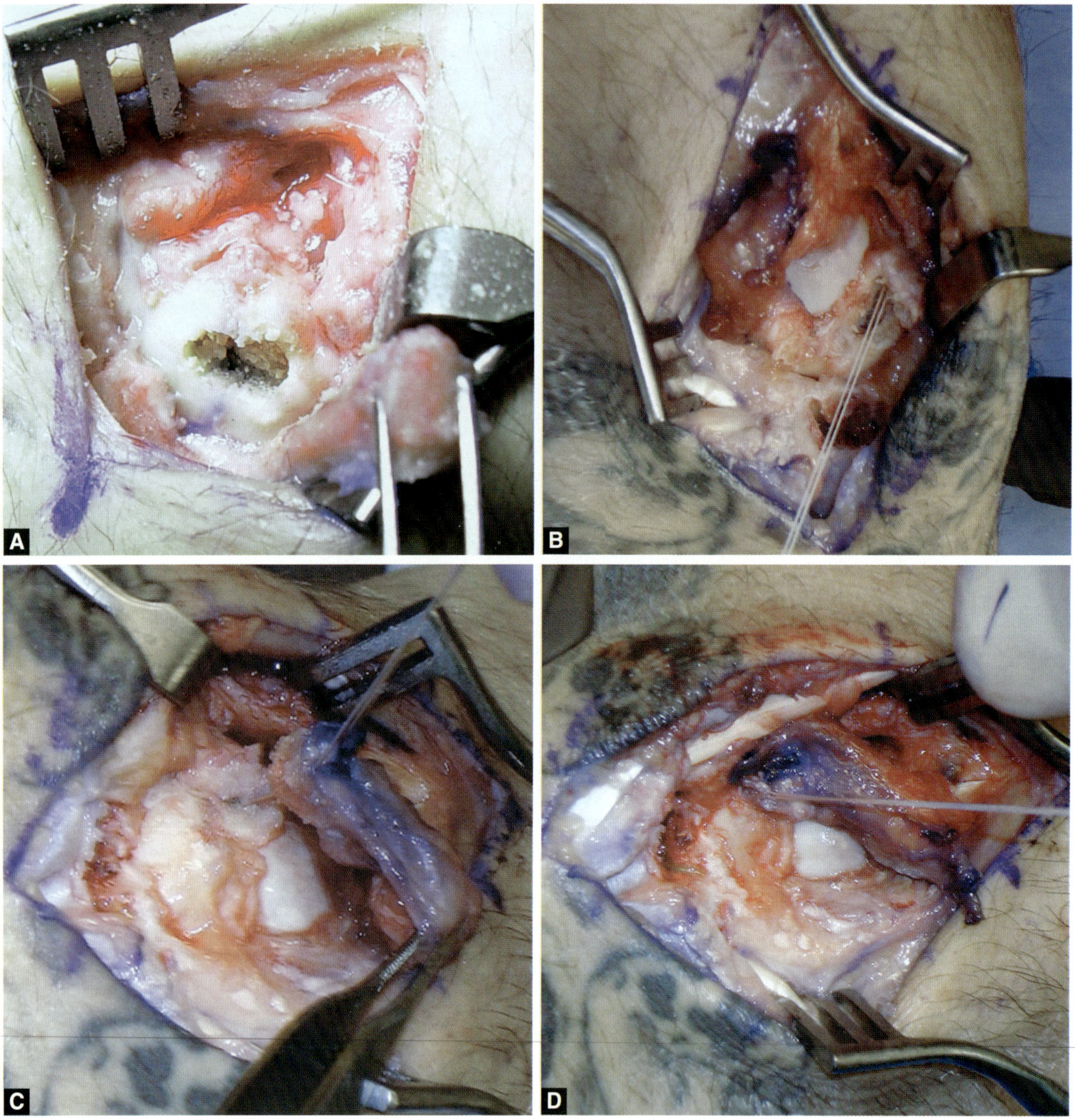

Figures 4.22A to D: Following nonunion debridement and fixation, attention is turned back to the vascularized bone graft (VBG). (A) A dorsal trough is created across the nonunion site; (B) A small bone suture anchor, loaded with two nonabsorbable sutures is placed deep into the trough; (C and D) The VBG has been inserted into the scaphoid trough and is secured with a mattress stitch through the perimeter of the graft periosteum.

Technique

The procedure is performed under regional or general anesthesia and under tourniquet control and loupe magnification. A longitudinal incision is placed just ulnar to the Lister's tubercle (Fig. 4.23B). The EPL tendon is identified and retracted. A capsulotomy is performed between the third and fourth dorsal compartments in an inverted-T fashion (Fig. 4.23C). Care should be taken not to violate the SLIL deep to the capsule. The scaphoid is exposed and the nonunion site is identified (Fig. 4.23D). Often the nonunion

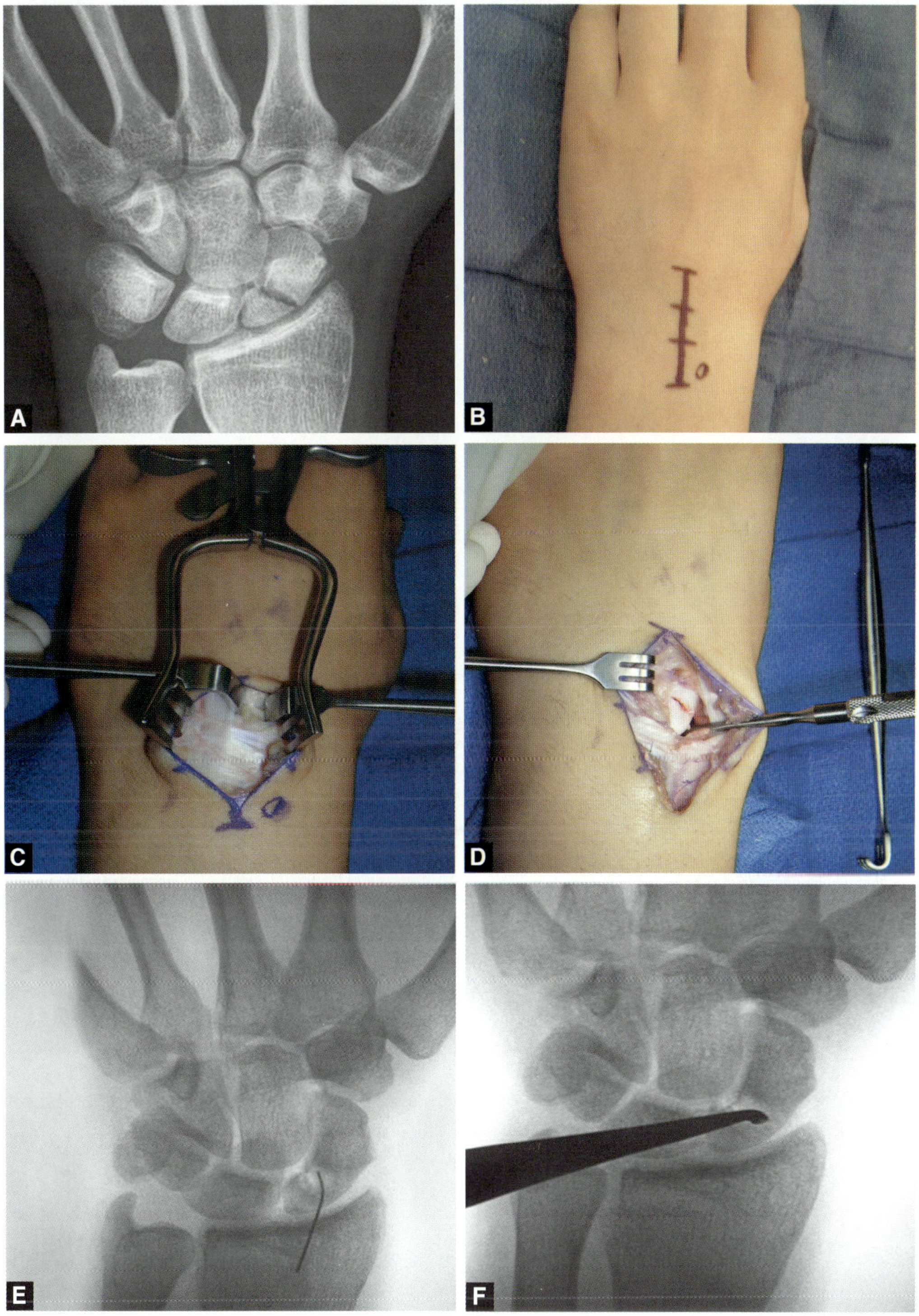

Figures 4.23A to F: A 35-year-old male who incurred a scaphoid waist fracture treated with cast immobilization for 12 weeks without evidence of fracture union. (A) Radiographs confirmed a nonunion of the fracture. Once viability of the scaphoid was confirmed by MRI, surgical correction was initiated through a (B) dorsal approach; (C) A capsulotomy is performed between the third and fourth dorsal compartments; (D) The scaphoid is exposed and the nonunion site is identified; (E) If not directly evident, a 25-gauge needle can be used to identify the nonunion site with fluoroscopy; (F) The nonunion site is debrided with curettes.

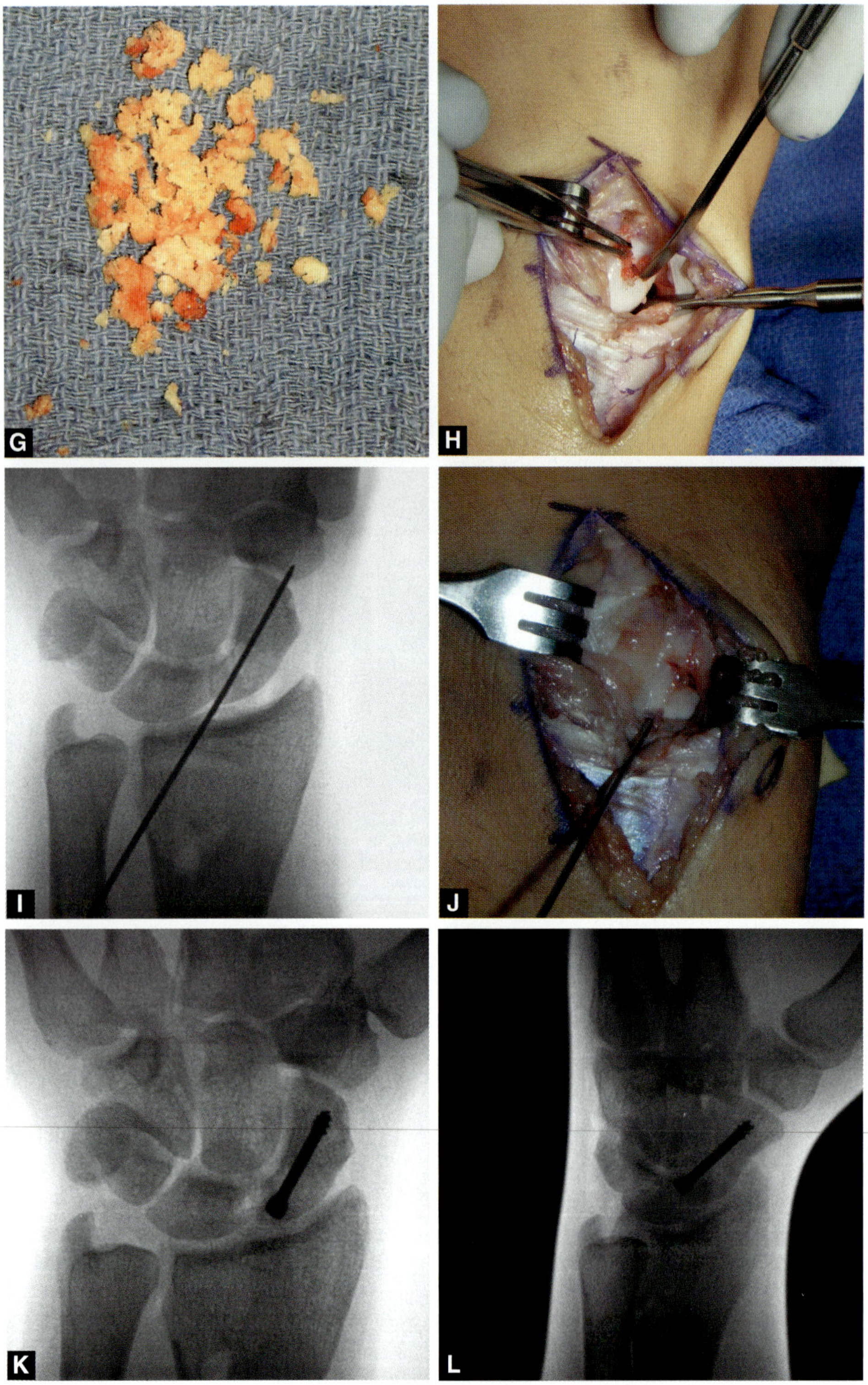

Figures 4.23G to L: (G) Autogenous cancellous bone graft is harvested from the distal radius through the proximal aspect of incision; (H) The nonunion site is packed with bone graft; (I and J) The fracture is reduced and provisionally fixed with a guidewire that will be used for placement of the headless compression screw. A second wire is placed for antirotational control; (K and L) A headless compression screw is placed.

Courtesy: Asif M Ilyas

site will not be directly evident and a 25-gauge needle can be used to identify the nonunion site with fluoroscopy (Fig. 4.23E). Once identified, the nonunion site is debrided with curettes (Fig. 4.23F). Autogenous cancellous bone graft is harvested from the distal radius through the proximal extent of incision (Fig. 4.23G). The dorsal cortex of the distal radius is exposed subperiosteally below the EDC tendon proximal to extensor retinaculum. The dorsal cortex is opened with osteotomes and cancellous bone graft is harvested from the distal radius metaphysis.

Attention is turned back to the scaphoid. The nonunion site is packed with bone graft (Fig. 4.23H). The fracture is reduced and provisionally fixed with a guidewire that will be used for placement of the headless compression screw. A second wire is placed for antirotational control (Figs 4.23I and J). The guidewire is measured and advanced into the base of the trapezium to hold it in place while the wire is overdrilled with the cannulated drill. A headless compression screw of adequate length is placed to obtain fixation within the subchondral bone, yet short of the articular cartilage on both ends of the scaphoid (Figs 4.23K and L).

Hemostasis is obtained, the wound is irrigated and the dorsal capsule is closed with 4-0 absorbable sutures in a figure of eight fashion. The skin incision is closed with 3-0 nylon horizontal mattress sutures. A thumb spica splint is applied for 2 weeks. At 2 weeks, sutures are removed and the patient is placed in a thumb spica splint for an additional 4 weeks at minimum until fracture union is confirmed. Computerized tomography scanning can be utilized to confirm fracture union.

Case 3: Scaphoid Nonunion Advanced Collapse Wrist: Four Corner Fusion with Scaphoid Excision

A 48-year-old right hand dominant man, who works as a carpenter, presented with a 3-year history of gradually increasing pain, swelling and loss of mobility in his right wrist. He recalled a wrist injury several years ago for which he never sought medical attention. A wrist splint, nonsteroidal anti-inflammatory medication and steroids injections did not relieve his symptoms. On physical examination, he had marked swelling over the radial aspect of his wrist with marked pain on palpation. Wrist motion was significantly decreased as compared to the contralateral side. He had approximately 30° of flexion and 5–10° of extension. X-rays taken in the office showed a stage III SNAC wrist (Figs 4.24A and B).

In stage III SNAC wrist, the capitolunate and scaphocapitate joints are involved, while the radiolunate articulation is spared. Surgical measures should be considered when wrist pain is refractory to conservative measures. Surgical options include an intercarpal fusion or a wrist arthrodesis. Proximal row carpectomy is a relative contraindication in stage III because of the presence of capitolunate arthrosis (Fig. 4.18). The biomechanical principle behind scaphoid excision and a four-corner fusion is that wrist motion occurs through preserved radiolunate and ulnocarpal joints. Wrist range of motion after four-corner fusion has been reported around 60% of the opposite wrist and grip strength approximately 80%.[24] The overall nonunion is between 4% and 8%.[25] Contraindications of four-corner fusion include radio-lunate articular degeneration and ulnar carpal translation (usually resulting from long radiolunate ligament insufficiency), which disrupts the normal congruity of the radiolunate joint and hastens its degeneration. Total wrist arthrodesis is the procedure of choice in these cases.

Technique

The procedure is performed under regional or general anesthesia and under tourniquet control and loupe magnification. Transverse incision provides a more cosmetic scar, but we prefer a longitudinal incision allowing for extensile exposure (Figs 4.24A to I). Dorsal soft tissue dissection is performed carefully with care to preserve dorsal nerves and veins.

Exposure may be obtained either through the fourth dorsal extensor compartment or via subperiosteal dissection in the interspace between the third and fourth compartments. The posterior interosseus nerve is identified in the floor of the fourth dorsal compartment and neurectomy is performed. The EPL is retracted radially, while EDC tendons are retracted ulnarly. A straight dorsal longitudinal capsulotomy, in line with the skin incision, is performed (Fig. 4.24C). Upon exposure of the wrist, the integrity of the lunate fossa is assessed. If the lunate fossa articular surface is not intact, the four-corner fusion is aborted for a total wrist fusion.

Once the radiolunate joint space has been confirmed to be preserved, the scaphoid is excised. Typically, the

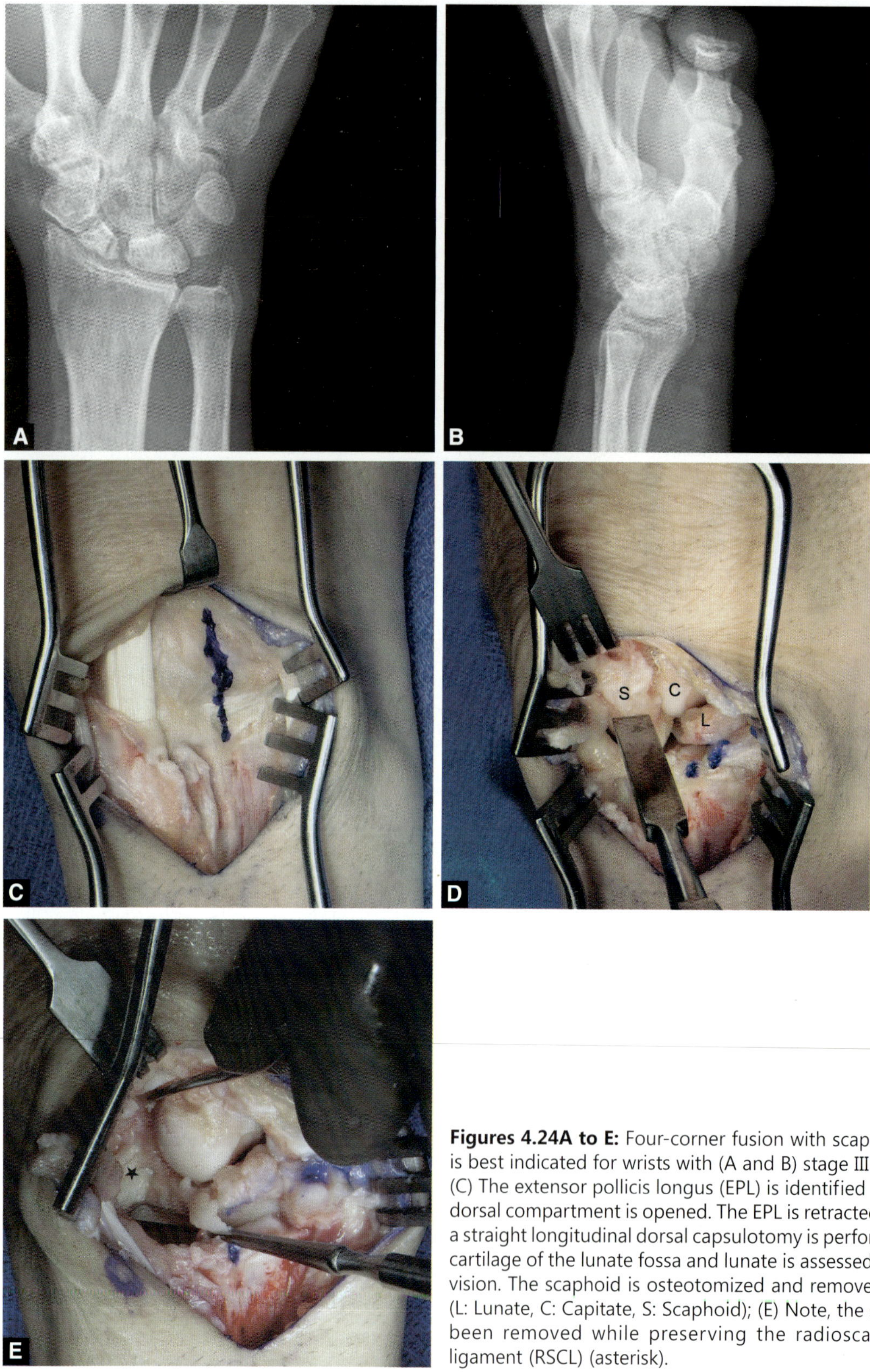

Figures 4.24A to E: Four-corner fusion with scaphoid excision is best indicated for wrists with (A and B) stage III SNAC wrists; (C) The extensor pollicis longus (EPL) is identified and the third dorsal compartment is opened. The EPL is retracted radially and a straight longitudinal dorsal capsulotomy is performed; (D) The cartilage of the lunate fossa and lunate is assessed under direct vision. The scaphoid is osteotomized and removed piecemeal. (L: Lunate, C: Capitate, S: Scaphoid); (E) Note, the scaphoid has been removed while preserving the radioscaphocapitate ligament (RSCL) (asterisk).

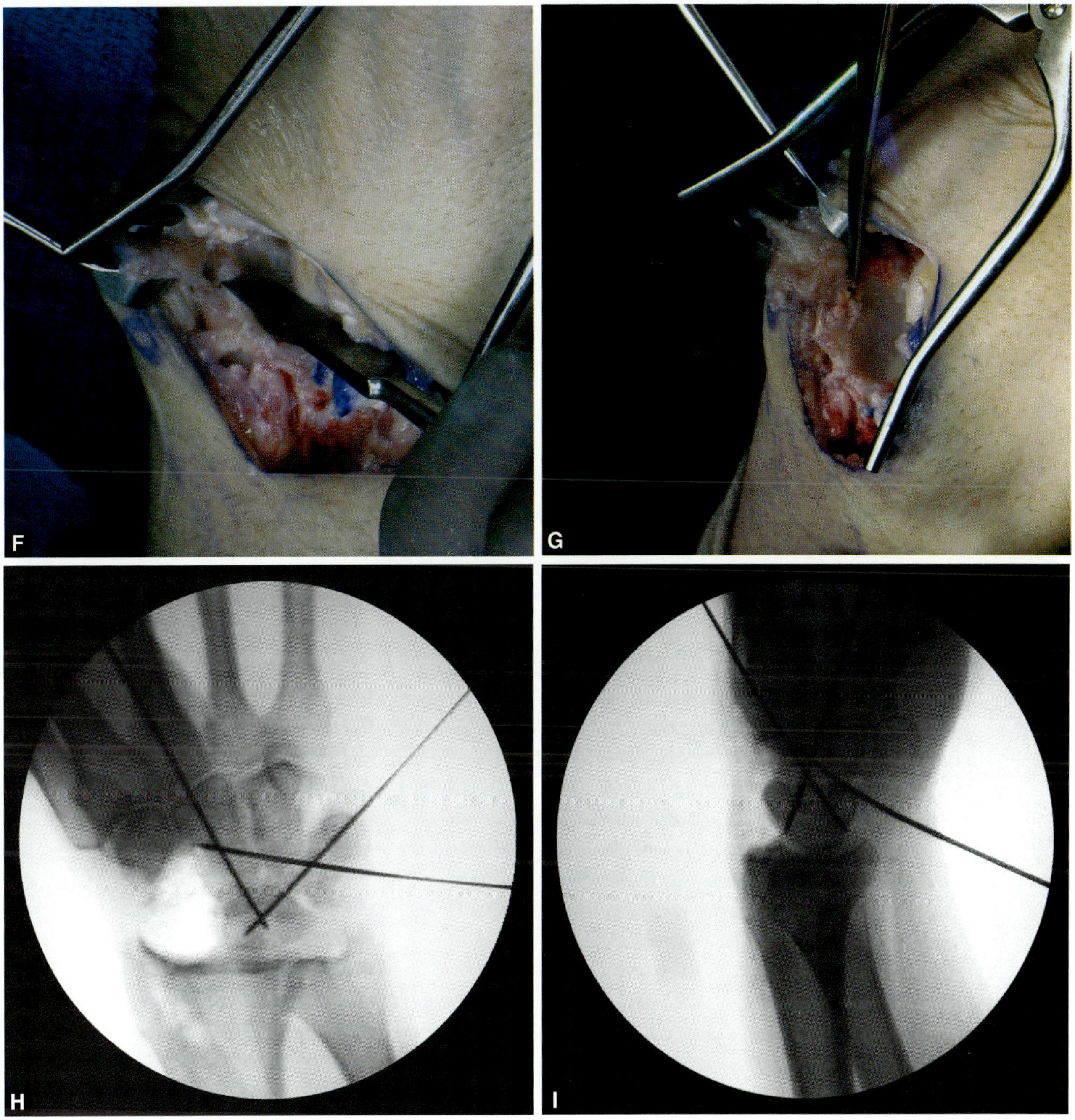

Figures 4.24F to I: (F) A radial styloidectomy is performed with a thin osteotome; (G) Cancellous bone graft can be harvested from the distal radius through styloidectomy with a small curette and from the resected scaphoid. The cartilage from the articular surfaces of capitate, lunate, triquetrum and hamate is removed up to subchondral bone. The intercarpal spaces are filled with bone graft and pinned in a triangular pattern to maintain the stability of the four-corner fusion as depicted on the (H) posteroanterior (PA) and (I) lateral views, which also confirms a well reduced lunate in the lunate fossa.

scaphoid fragments are osteotomized and are removed piecemeal (Fig. 4.24D). Care must be taken to preserve the RSCL which provides restraint to ulnar translation of the carpus (Fig. 4.24E). If the ligament is injured during the procedure, there is risk of ulnar translation post-operatively. In SNAC wrists, the distal pole of the scaphoid is volar flexed and may be difficult to excise. We find that the use of an elevator placed within the scaphotrapezial joint allows us to partially reduce the volar flexion and assist with scaphoid excision. In addition, the distal pole of the scaphoid may be palpated volarly and the residual scaphoid may be presented into the surgical field with volary to dorsally directed digital pressure. Then, we routinely perform a radial styloidectomy with careful preservation of the origin of RSCL in order to prevent impingement between the radial styloid and trapezium (Fig. 4.24F). This ligament originates from radial styloid and stabilizes the capitate preventing ulnar translocation. With the use of a small curette, we harvest cancellous bone graft from the distal radius through styloidectomy (Fig. 4.24G). The harvested graft from the distal radius in combination with the graft that can be extracted from the resected scaphoid gives adequate amount of graft for the fusion.

The next step is to expose the articular surfaces of lunate, capitate, hamate and triquetrum. Longitudinal traction on the fingers may prove helpful in providing access to the intercarpal joints. A rongeur or curette is used to remove the cartilaginous articulations between lunate, capitate, hamate and triquetrum down to cancellous matrix. Reduction of the carpal bones and correction of any carpal instability pattern (typically DISI) is then followed. Kirschner wires may be used as joysticks in correcting DISI deformity. After achieving neutral alignment between the radius and lunate, a 0.0625 inch wire is drilled through the dorsal distal radius into the lunate. Fusion of the lunate in slight flexion relative to the capitate may provide greater wrist extension. After reducing any carpal instability, a wire is advanced across the capitate and lunate under fluoroscopic control. If the reduction of the lunate is sufficient, cancellous bone is interposed between joint surfaces to enhance fusion. The stability of the four-corner is achieved by placing a K-wire between the triquetrum and lunate, and one more between the triquetrum and capitate, in a triangular fashion (Figs 4.24H and I). Further bone graft is added after the placement of the K-wires. The wires are then cut and buried under the skin. Alternatively, the intercarpal fusion may be performed with staples, headless compression screws or a dorsal plate.

Hemostasis is obtained, the wound is irrigated and the dorsal capsule is closed with 4-0 absorbable sutures in figure of eight fashion. The extensor retinaculum is closed typically after transposition of the EPL. The skin incision is closed with 3-0 nylon horizontal mattress sutures. Patients are splinted in slight dorsiflexion for 10–14 days after surgery and digital motion is begun immediately postoperatively. At the first postoperative visit, sutures are removed and the wrist is casted or splinted for a total of 6 weeks. The authors typically use a cast; however, some will receive a custom molded splint, primarily in an effort to assist with care and hygiene. The pins are removed between 6 weeks and 8 weeks in the operating room under local anesthesia, assuming the fusion mass seems well healed. Formal hand therapy begins after pin removal, first with gradual range of motion exercises and then progressive strengthening follows. Return to full activities is permitted only after solid union occurs.

Summary

Scaphoid fractures are commonly seen in young and active individuals. Prompt diagnosis and treatment is the key for successful management. Thus, it is advisable to treat all suspected injuries as fractures until proven otherwise. Although nonoperative treatment with casting is the standard of care for nondisplaced scaphoid fractures, there is a general agreement that unstable, displaced fractures or fractures susceptible to AVN, such as proximal pole fractures, should be treated surgically. The surgeon should be familiar with the operative treatment of those fractures and should be able to perform the fixation through a volar or dorsal approach, depending on the fracture pattern. Percutaneous fracture fixation is a reasonable option for nondisplaced fractures when the patient requests a rapid return to work or sports activities.

The healing rate of scaphoid fractures is high either with casting or operative treatment, as long as they have been diagnosed early and immobilized adequately. In case of delayed presentation or failed treatment, the authors should be prepared to treat the complications of scaphoid fractures, which can be extremely challenging. Scaphoid nonunions require stable fixation and bone grafting to heal and if the nonunion has been complicated by AVN, a VBG is needed. Long-standing scaphoid nonunions result in carpal malalignment and can lead to arthrosis. Salvaging surgical techniques have been developed for SNAC providing good pain relief and satisfactory wrist range of motion and function.

References

1. Duppe H, Johnell O, Lundborg G, et al. Long-term results of fracture of the scaphoid. A follow-up study of more than thirty years. J Bone Joint Surg Am. 1994;76(2):249-52.
2. Parvizi J, Wayman J, Kelly P, et al. Combining the clinical signs improves diagnosis of scaphoid fractures. A prospective study with follow-up. J Hand Surg Br. 1998; 23(3):324-7.
3. Hunter JC, Escobedo EM, Wilson AJ, et al. MR imaging of clinically suspected scaphoid fractures. AJR Am J Roentgenol. 1997;168(5):1287-93.
4. Smith M, Bain GI, Turner PC, et al. Review of imaging of scaphoid fractures. ANZ J Surg. 2010;80(1-2):82-90.
5. Herbert T, Fisher W. Management of the fractured scaphoid using a new bone screw. J Bone Joint Surg Br. 1984;66-B(1):114-23.
6. Cooney WP, 3rd. Scaphoid fractures: current treatments and techniques. Instr Course Lect. 2003;52:197-208.
7. Berger RA. The anatomy of the ligaments of the wrist and distal radioulnar joints. Clin Orthop Relat Res. 2001;383: 32-40.
8. Gelberman RH, Menon J. The vascularity of the scaphoid bone. J Hand Surg Am. 1980;5(5):508-13.
9. Slade JF, 3rd, Grauer JN, Mahoney JD. Arthroscopic reduction and percutaneous fixation of scaphoid fractures with a novel dorsal technique. Orthop Clin North Am. 2001; 32(2):247-61.
10. Buijze GA, Doornberg JN, Ham JS, et al. Surgical compared with conservative treatment for acute nondisplaced or minimally displaced scaphoid fractures: a systematic review and meta-analysis of randomized controlled trials. J Bone Joint Surg Am. 2010;92(6):1534-44.
11. Ram AN, Chung KC. Evidence-based management of acute nondisplaced scaphoid waist fractures. J Hand Surg Am. 2009;34(4):735-8.
12. Trumble TE, Gilbert M, Murray LW, et al. Displaced scaphoid fractures treated with open reduction and internal fixation with a cannulated screw. J Bone Joint Surg Am. 2000; 82(5):633-41.
13. McCallister WV, Knight J, Kaliappan R, et al. Central placement of the screw in simulated fractures of the scaphoid waist: a biomechanical study. J Bone Joint Surg Am. 2003; 85-A(1):72-7.
14. Gutow AP. Percutaneous fixation of scaphoid fractures. J Am Acad Orthop Surg. 2007;15(8):474-85.
15. Chen AC, Chao EK, Hung SS, et al. Percutaneous screw fixation for unstable scaphoid fractures. J Trauma. 2005; 59(1):184-7.
16. Bushnell BD, McWilliams AD, Messer TM. Complications in dorsal percutaneous cannulated screw fixation of non-displaced scaphoid waist fractures. J Hand Surg Am. 2007; 32(6):827-33.
17. Bond CD, Shin AY, McBride MT, et al. Percutaneous screw fixation or cast immobilization for nondisplaced scaphoid fractures. J Bone Joint Surg Am. 2001;83-A(4):483-8.
18. Haisman JM, Rohde RS, Weiland AJ. Acute fractures of the scaphoid. J Bone Joint Surg Am. 2006;88(12):2750-8.
19. Inoue G, Sakuma M. The natural history of scaphoid nonunion. Radiographical and clinical analysis in 102 cases. 1996;115(1):1-4.
20. Fernandez DL. A technique for anterior wedge-shaped grafts for scaphoid nonunions with carpal instability. J Hand Surg Am. 1984;9(5):733-7.
21. Sotereanos DG, Darlis NA, Dailiana ZH, et al. A capsular-based vascularized distal radius graft for proximal pole scaphoid pseudarthrosis. The Journal of Hand Surgery. 2006;31(4):580-7.
22. Merrell GA, Wolfe SW, Slade JF, 3rd. Treatment of scaphoid nonunions: quantitative meta-analysis of the literature. J Hand Surg Am. 2002;27(4):685-91.
23. Munk B, Larsen CF. Bone grafting the scaphoid nonunion: a systematic review of 147 publications including 5,246 cases of scaphoid nonunion. Acta Orthop Scand. 2004; 75(5):618-29.
24. Cohen MS, Kozin SH. Degenerative arthritis of the wrist: proximal row carpectomy versus scaphoid excision and four-corner arthrodesis. J Hand Surg Am. 2001;26(1): 94-104.
25. Siegel JM, Ruby LK. A critical look at intercarpal arthrodesis: review of the literature. J Hand Surg Am. 1996;21(4): 717-23.

Chapter 5

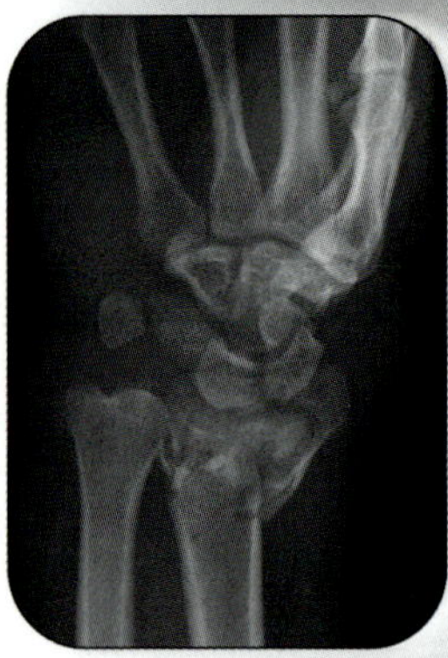

Distal Radius Fractures

Wendy Bruinsma, Frank Peters, Jesse Jupiter

Chapter Outline

Introduction
Diagnosis
Classification
Surgical Indications
- Closed Reduction and External Fixation
- Closed Reduction and Internal Fixation
- Open Reduction and Internal Fixation

Surgical Anatomy, Positioning and Approaches
- Positioning
- Approaches

Surgical Techniques
- Technique 1: Kirschner Wire Fixation
- Technique 2: External Fixation
- Technique 3: Intramedullary Nailing
- Technique 4: Volar Plating
- Technique 5: Dorsal Plating

Outcomes
Complications
- Complications of Kirschner Wire Fixation
- Complications of External Fixation
- Complications of Intramedullary Nailing
- Complications of Volar Plating
- Complications of Dorsal Plating

Authors' Preferred Management of Select Complications
- Case 1: Intra-articular Screw Placement
- Case 2: Loss of Reduction

Summary

Introduction

Distal radius fractures are one of the most common fractures treated in the emergency room, representing approximately one-sixth of all upper extremity fractures in emergency departments in the US.[1] The typical bimodal age distribution can be explained by the mechanism of injury, most commonly being a fall in majority of patients. In young adults, majority of cases are the result of high-energy trauma; whereas, in the elderly, most cases occur from low-energy trauma (Figs 5.1A and B and 5.2A and B). Furthermore, postmenopausal women are more prone to fractures due to a predilection toward osteoporosis.

Often referred to as a Colles fracture for Abraham Colles (1773–1843), who almost two centuries ago differentiated these common injuries as fractures and not dislocations of the wrist. Since then a number of classifications have been presented for distal radius fractures. But, controversy persists regarding appropriate treatment, classification and anticipation of functional outcomes. However, some consensus has been attained that there is a direct negative correlation between late

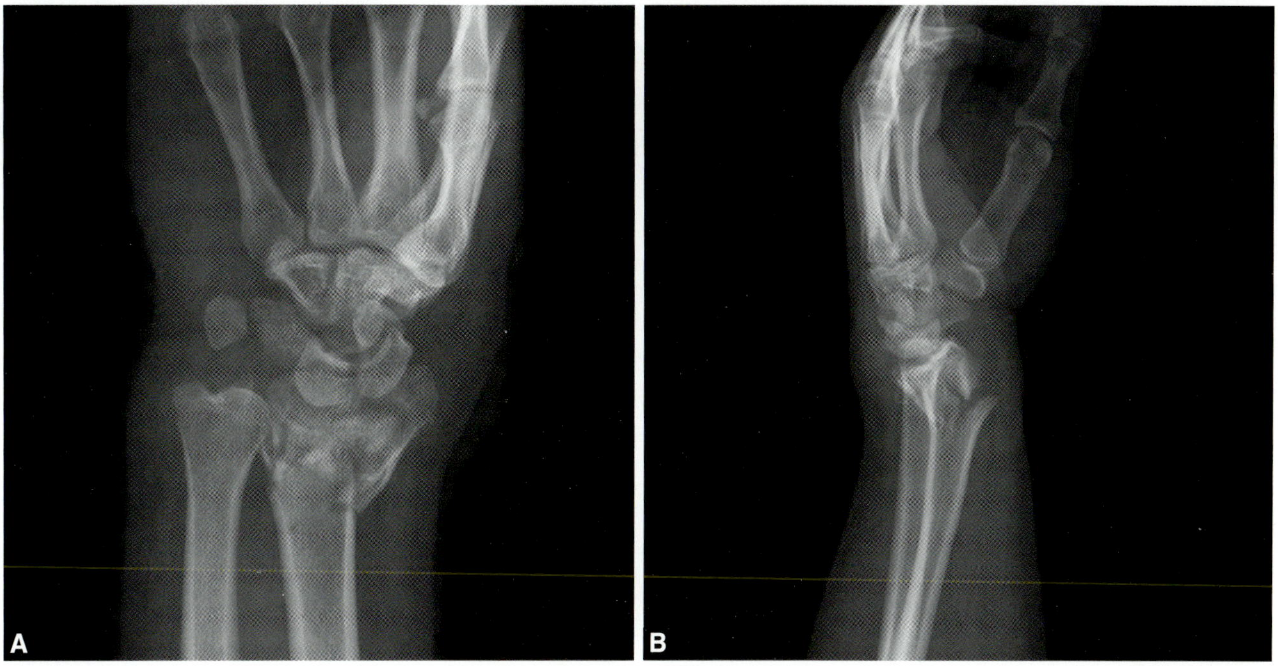

Figures 5.1A and B: Standard radiographs of a 30-year-old male, involved in a high-speed motor vehicle accident. (A) Anteroposterior (AP) view. Note the normal bone quality, but high level of comminution and displacement. The patient presented with severe pain and paresthesias necessitating urgent surgical decompression of the carpal tunnel and fracture fixation; (B) On the lateral view, note the large proximal volar cortical spike with dorsal angulation and displacement of the distal fragment. This extent of displacement can predispose to median nerve injury or compression.

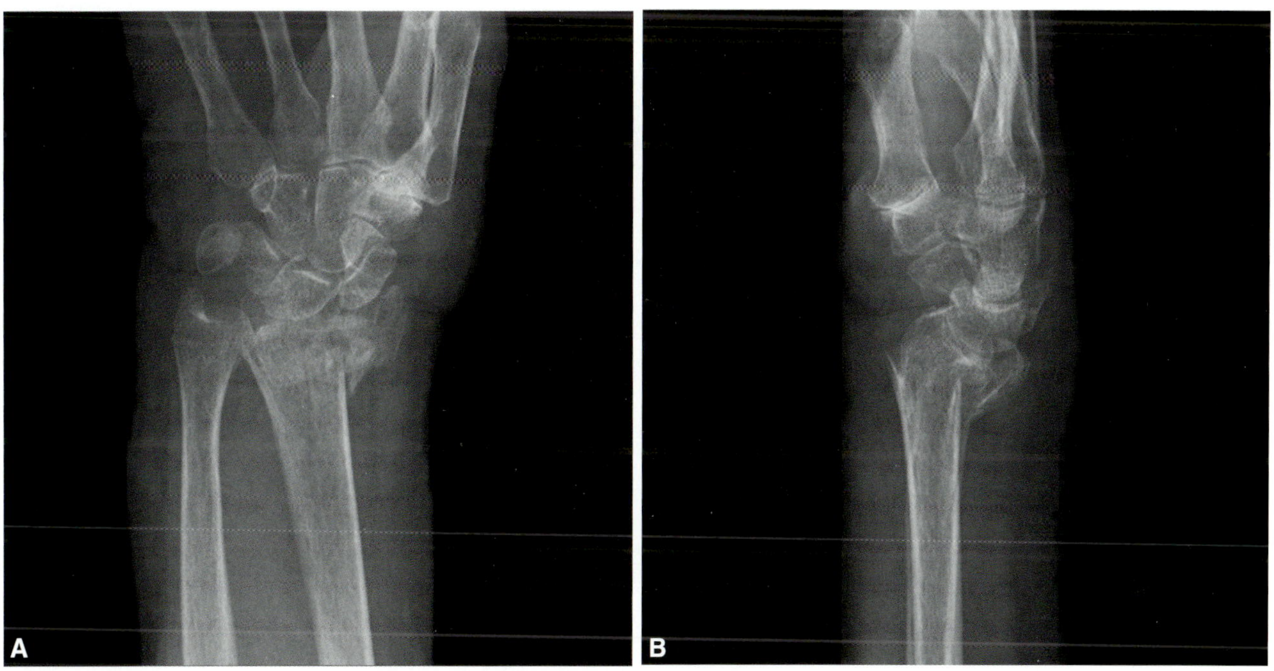

Figures 5.2A and B: Standard radiographs of an 80-year-old female, involved in a fall from standing. This otherwise low-energy injury resulted in a highly comminuted fracture due to underlying osteoporosis. (A) Anteroposterior (AP) view and (B) Lateral view.

functional results and residual deformity and it is increasingly appreciated that treatment of these fractures should focus on reconstructing the articular surface, recapturing normal alignment and minimizing deformity.[2,3]

Nonoperative reduction by manipulation and traction may not restore distal articular congruity. In addition, the collapse of these fractures due to inherent instability after primary reduction is not uncommon. Consequently, there is a tendency to make more frequent use of surgical fixation. This is strengthened by ongoing innovation and research in surgical techniques. Many operative techniques are used to treat displaced or unstable distal radius fractures. These techniques include Kirschner (K) wire fixation, use of external fixators and open reduction and internal fixation (ORIF) of the fracture. Also, different bone grafting techniques may be used to fill large structural loss or support unstable defects.

Treatment of unstable and displaced distal radius fractures may depend; however, on fracture classification, patient characteristics and preference of the surgeon. Available fracture fixation options include percutaneous pinning, external fixation, dorsal plating, volar plating, intramedullary nailing and fragment specific fixation. Although, an expanding variety of surgical techniques might optimize the chance of optimal alignment and functional outcomes, there is still no consensus on the best choice of treatment. Furthermore, more frequent and diverse use of invasive procedures also means a changing pallet of complications. Complications of surgical treatment include infection, loss of fixation (malunion/nonunion), iatrogenic nerve injuries, postoperative carpal tunnel syndrome, complex regional pain syndrome, post-operative tendon irritation, rupture or adherence to plating and articular damage due to malpositioning or failure of hardware.

Diagnosis

A history of injury may provide clues about the severity of injury and trauma mechanism. A thorough patient history should focus on relevant factors, such as age, hand dominance, occupational or recreational demands, medication use, history of prior injury to the injured limb, carpal tunnel syndrome and osteoporosis. This information may be of predictive value for the outcome as well as possible complications.

Pain, swelling, deformity and loss of function are the main physical symptoms following distal radius fractures. The absence of deformity or provoked pain with axial pressure; however, is not a proof of absence of fracture. The very elderly and young children require particular vigilance as fractures might not present in a standard fashion in these age groups.

Neurovascular function is essential and should be compared to the contralateral side. In particular, reassessment of neurovascular functions should be performed after any closed reduction maneuver. The most common associated injury is acute carpal tunnel syndrome or acute compression of the median nerve due to swelling resulting in pain and paresthesias in the median nerve distribution of the hand. This diagnosis warrants prompt surgical decompression of the median nerve followed by fracture fixation. Fractures associated with greater displacement may put the nerve on greater stretch increasing the chances of nerve injury (Figs 5.1A and B). Although uncommon, compartment syndrome of the forearm can develop following a distal radius fracture associated with a high-energy injury.

Soft tissue examination is crucial for the choice of surgical treatment. Open fractures and lacerations of the wrist may complicate primary ORIF, although there is substantial evidence that after early debridement of the wound, internal fixation is a safe method of treating open distal radius fractures.[4] Moreover, extensive swelling could be a reason to postpone the operative treatment until swelling has reduced to optimize surgical dissection, fracture reduction and wound closure.

Standard anteroposterior (AP) and lateral radiographs form the basis for the diagnosis of a fractured wrist, and together with patient's history, are essential in determining a treatment plan. The radiograph is scrutinized for multiple variables including location of the fracture, articular involvement, extent of displacement, amount of comminution and the presence of associated injuries. Measurements of the radiographs will help in fracture analysis, but is predicated on appropriate orthogonal views and understanding normal radiographic anatomy (Figs 5.3A and B).

On the AP view, we measure three basic aspects:

1. *Radial inclination:* Radial inclination is defined as the angle between 2 lines; one is drawn perpendicular to the long axis of the radius at the ulnar corner of lunate

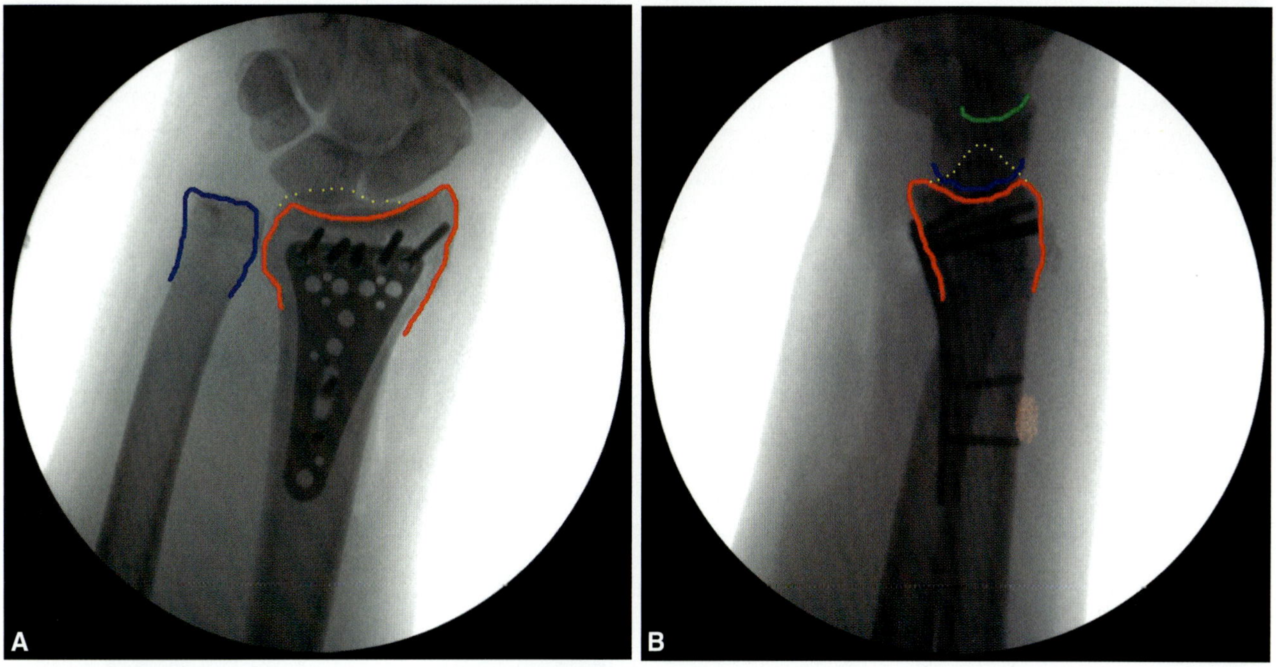

Figures 5.3A and B: Appropriate interpretation and measurements of distal radius radiographs are dependent upon standardized views and understanding of normal radiographic anatomy. (A and B) Radiographs must be orthogonal and consist of a true anteroposterior (AP) view that allows visualization across the distal radioulnar joint (DRUJ) and a true lateral view that demonstrates complete overlap of the radius and ulna. Note on the AP view, the outline of the volar articular rim of the distal radius marked with a red line versus the dorsal articular rim marked with a yellow dotted line. On the lateral view, note the relationship of the "Cs" stacked concentrically one on the other: base of the capitate marked with a green line, base of the lunate marked in a blue line, and the distal radial articular surface marked with a red line. The radial styloid, marked in a yellow dotted line, is typically superimposed on a true lateral view.
Courtesy: Asif M Ilyas

fossa and other between that point in the lunate fossa and the tip of radial styloid (Fig. 5.4A).

2. *Radial height:* Radial height is defined as the distance between two parallel lines drawn perpendicular to the long axis of the radial shaft; one from the tip of radial styloid and other from the ulnar corner of lunate fossa (Fig. 5.4B).
3. *Ulnar variance:* Ulnar variance is defined as the measurement of relative lengths of radius and ulna at the wrist. It is measured by determining the distance between two parallel lines drawn perpendicular to the long axis of the radius at the distal articular surface of the ulna and distal articular surface of the radius at the lunate fossa. Sixty percent of the population has a neutral position. The best way to determine whether there is a normal physiological situation to compare the measurement to previously taken radiographs or, if unavailable, radiographs of the contralateral side.

On the lateral view, we measure:

Lateral inclination: Lateral inclination, also known as volar tilt, is defined by the angle between 2 lines; one is drawn perpendicular to the long axis of the radius and other between the dorsal and palmar lips of the distal radial articular surface (Fig. 5.4C).

Despite the availability of standard values, a prior radiograph or radiograph of the contralateral uninjured side remains the best reference. To maximize the visualization of articular surfaces, specific views should be utilized (Figs 5.5A and B). The dorsal lunate fossa facet or dorsomedial facet can be better judged on a mostly supinated oblique AP view and the radial styloid is specifically assessed on a partially pronated oblique AP view. Unclear intra-articular extension or displacement on standard lateral and AP radiographs can be visualized on oblique views (Fig. 5.6A). Complex fractures can also be well visualized by use of computerized tomography scans and additional three-dimensional (3D) imaging techniques (Figs 5.6B and C).

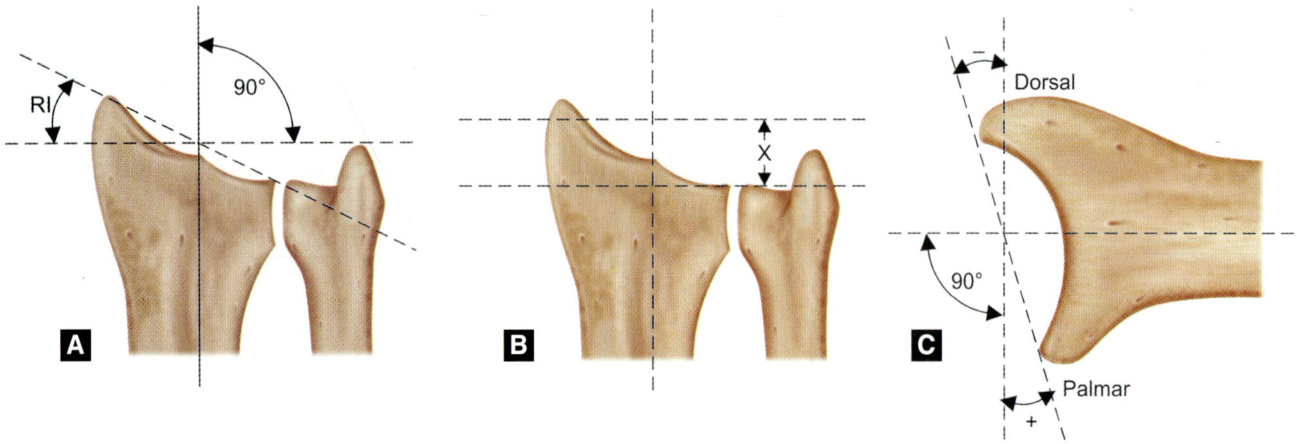

Figures 5.4A to C: Standard radiographic measurements of the distal radius include. (A) Radial inclination of approximately 20–23°; (B) Radial height of approximately 11–13 mm, and (C) Volar tile of 10–12°.

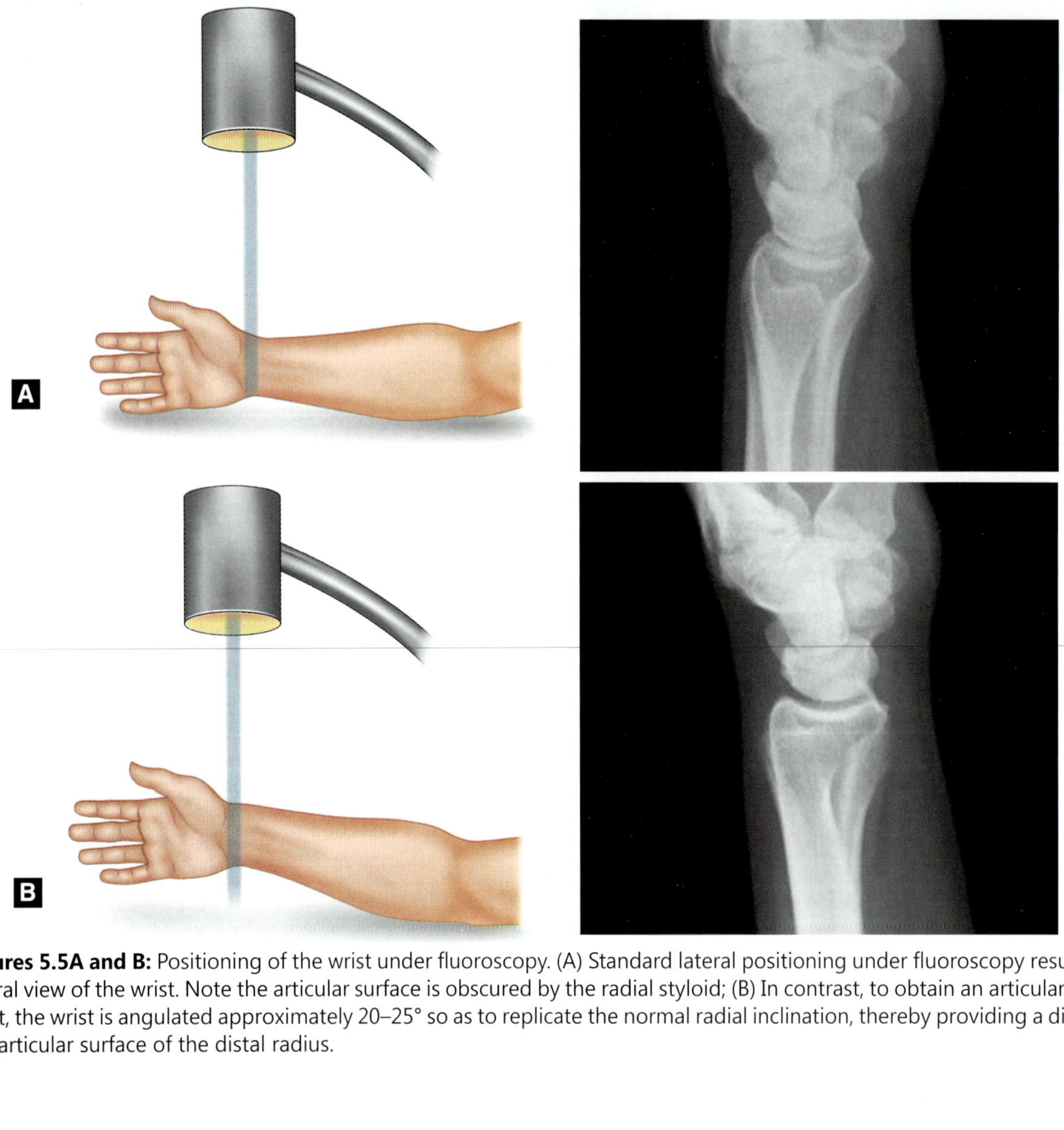

Figures 5.5A and B: Positioning of the wrist under fluoroscopy. (A) Standard lateral positioning under fluoroscopy results in a true lateral view of the wrist. Note the articular surface is obscured by the radial styloid; (B) In contrast, to obtain an articular view of the wrist, the wrist is angulated approximately 20–25° so as to replicate the normal radial inclination, thereby providing a direct view of the articular surface of the distal radius.

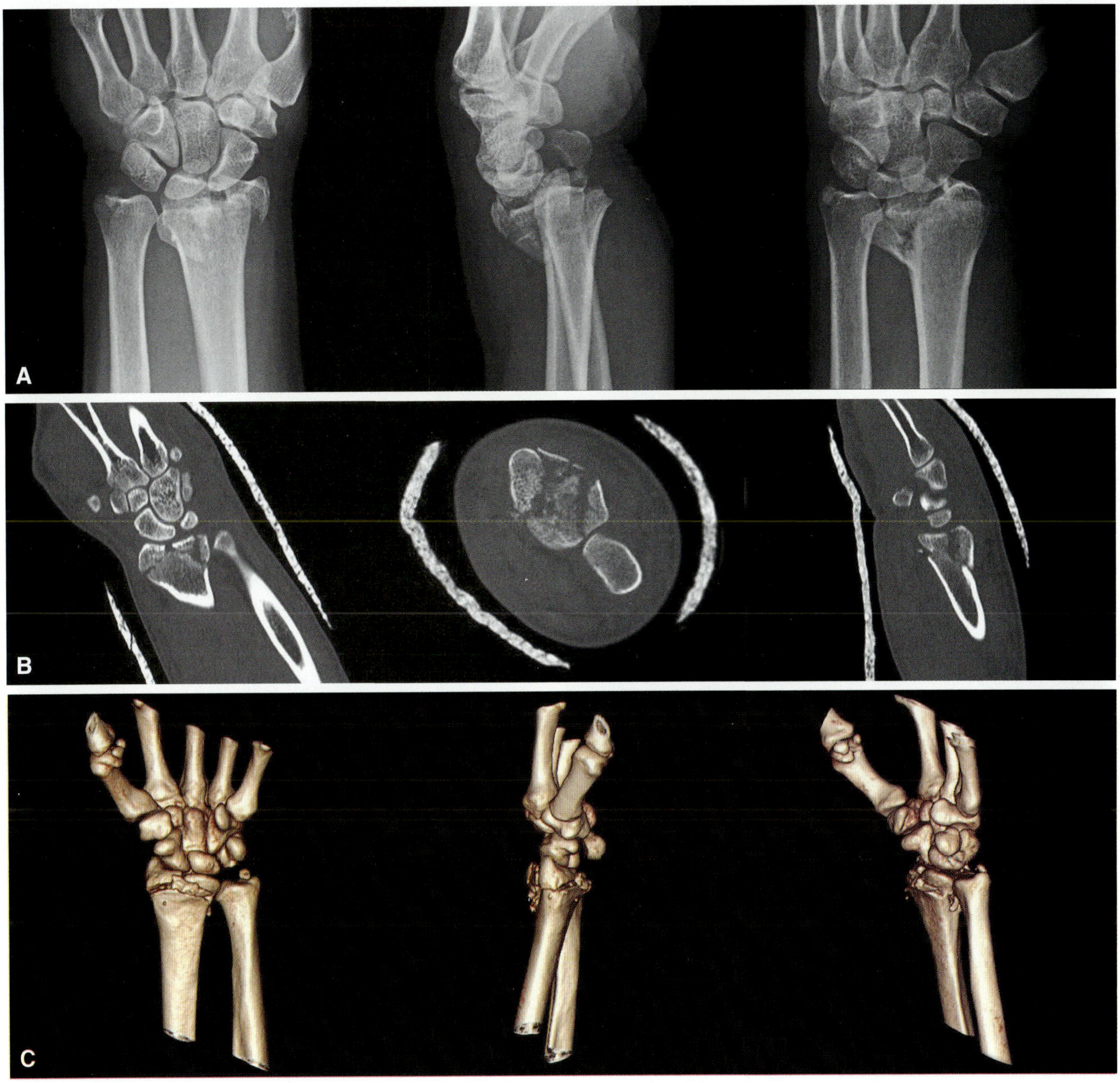

Figures 5.6A to C: (A) Note the standard radiographs of a 42-year-old male, who fell off of a truck resulting in a displaced intra-articular distal radius fracture resulting in severe swelling requiring urgent fasciotomy and fracture fixation; (B and C) The fracture was further analyzed with standard two-dimensional (2D) CT views and three-dimensional (3D) CT reconstructions.

In addition, a magnetic resonance imaging (MRI) scan may be indicated to evaluate for possible ligamentous or occult carpal injuries such as triangular fibrocartilage complex (TFCC) tear, intercarpal ligament injuries or scaphoid fractures. Of note, scapholunate ligament (SLL) injuries are common following intra-articular fractures that exit between the scaphoid and lunate facets. Lastly, some fractures of the distal radius are associated with pericarpal injuries and require particular mention here as radiographic assessment is central to accurate diagnosis and appropriate management. Radiocarpal dislocations are commonly associated with an avulsion fracture of the distal radius and can often be confused with a Barton's or articular shearing fracture of the distal radius (Figs 5.7A to C). It should be noted that

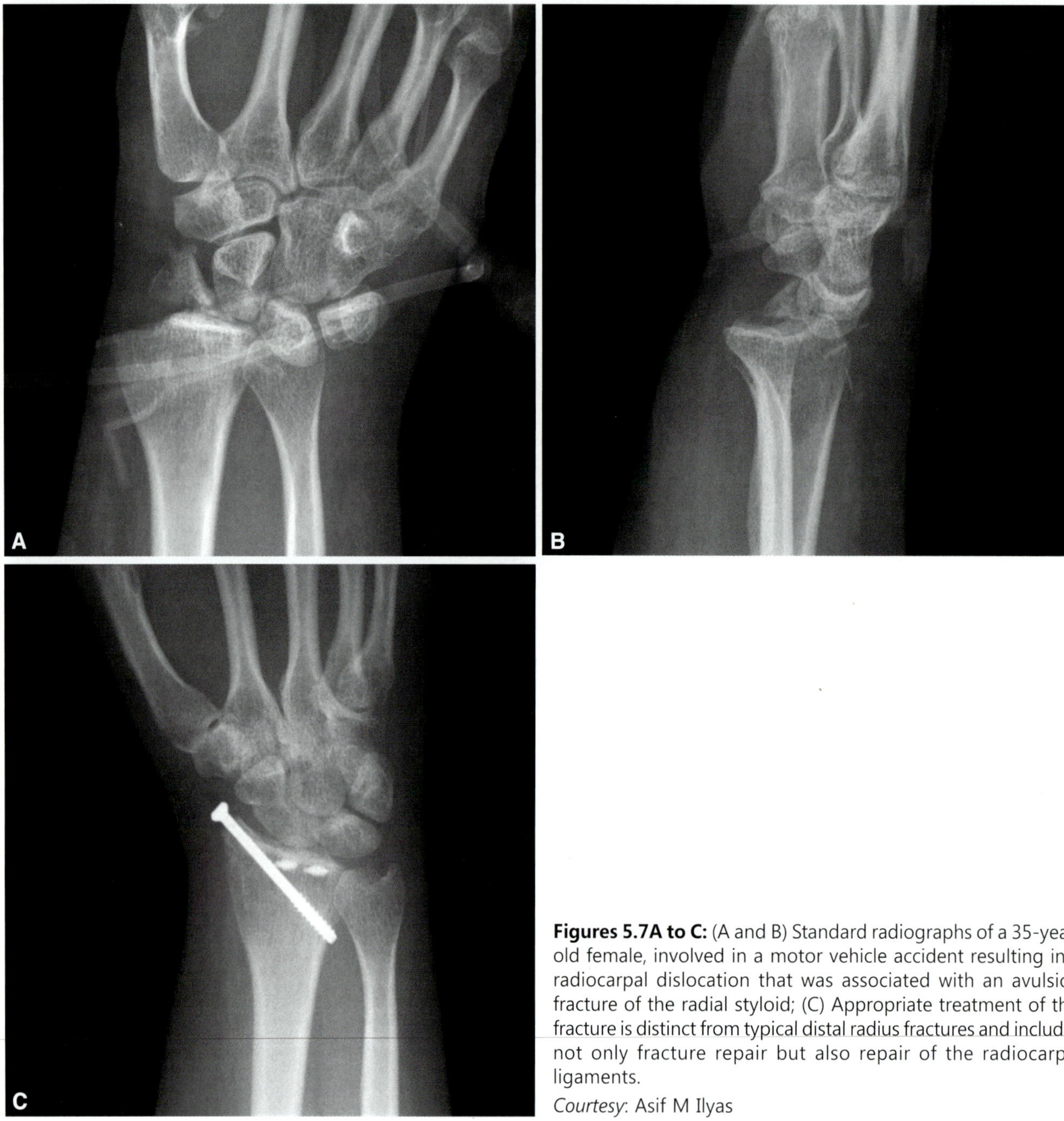

Figures 5.7A to C: (A and B) Standard radiographs of a 35-year-old female, involved in a motor vehicle accident resulting in a radiocarpal dislocation that was associated with an avulsion fracture of the radial styloid; (C) Appropriate treatment of this fracture is distinct from typical distal radius fractures and includes not only fracture repair but also repair of the radiocarpal ligaments.

Courtesy: Asif M Ilyas

radiocarpal dislocations are avulsion injuries and typically leave most of the articular surface behind as the carpus dislocates away (Figs 5.8A and B). Similarly, greater arc perilunate dislocations may be associated with fractures of the distal radial styloid as the carpus dislocates dorsally (Figs 5.9A and B).

DISTAL RADIUS FRACTURES DIAGNOSIS: Pearls and Pitfalls

- Neurological injury, particularly of the median nerve, is common following distal radius fractures and must be carefully assessed. The risks increase with greater energy and fracture displacement

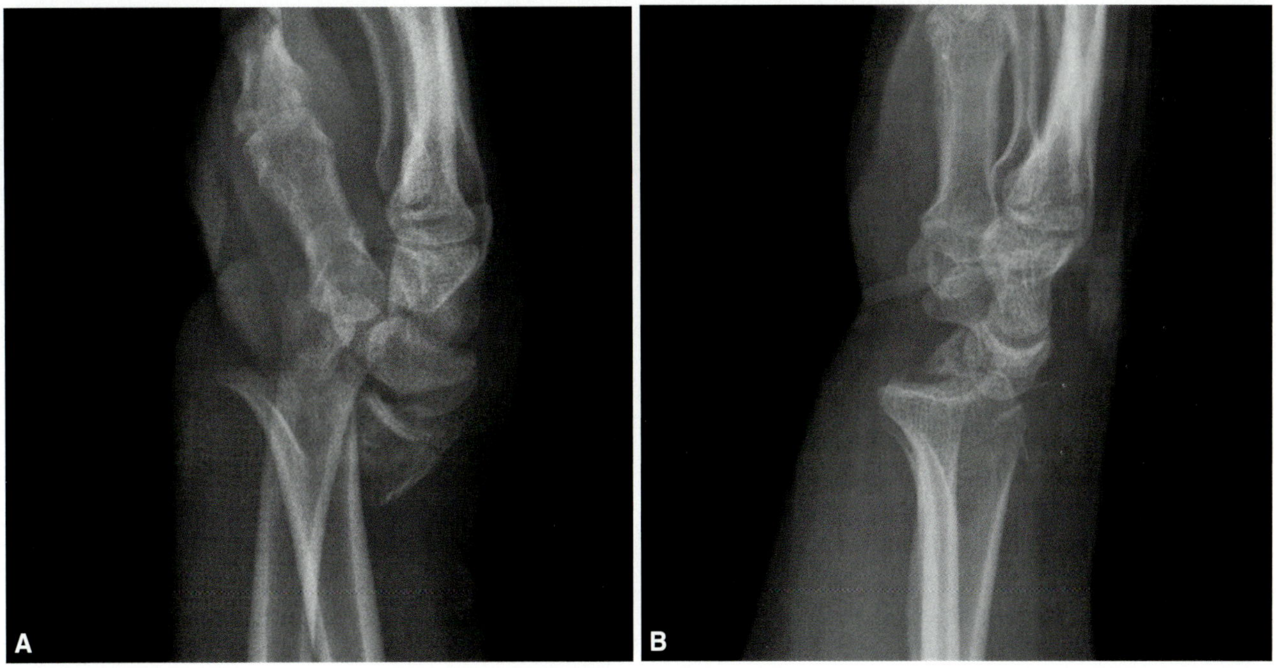

Figures 5.8A and B: Differentiating between a (A) dorsally displaced distal radius fracture and a (B) dorsally dislocated radiocarpal fracture-dislocation may be difficult. Note the maintenance of most of the articular surface with the radiocarpal fracture-dislocation.

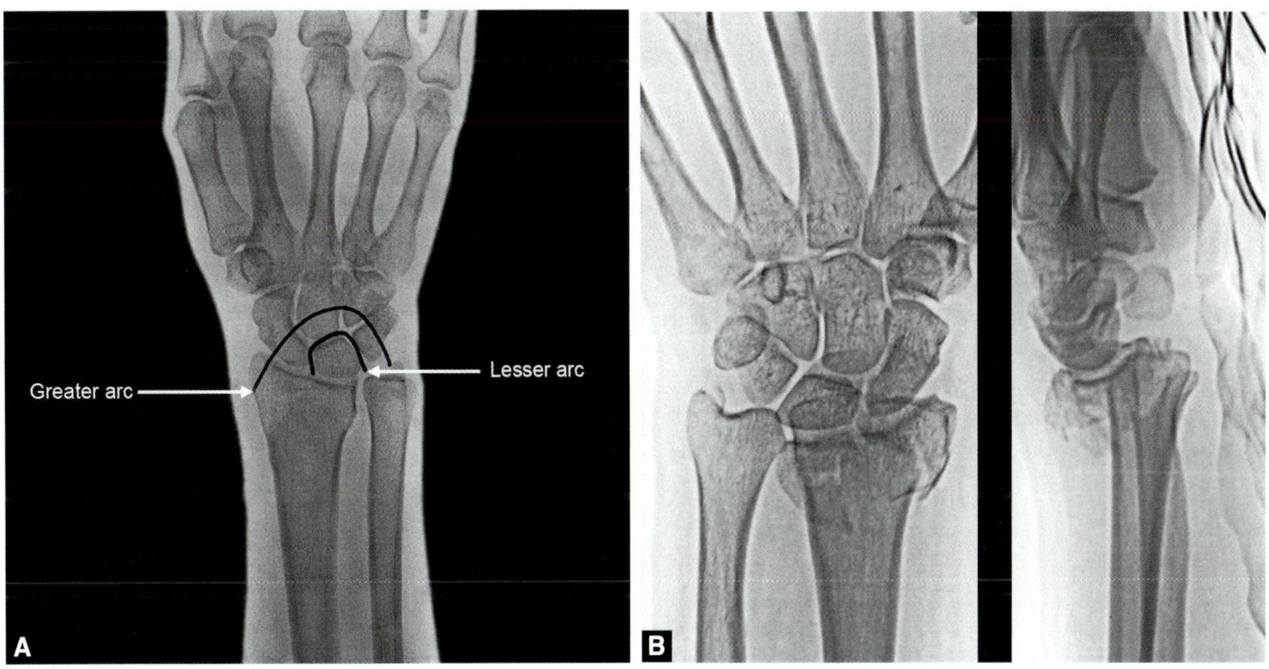

Figures 5.9A and B: Perilunate dislocations may be all soft tissue (lesser arc) or associated with fractures of the distal radius and/or scaphoid (greater arc).

- Standard radiographs can readily provide the diagnosis but must be scrutinized for associated injuries, such as SLL injuries or variant injuries, such as radiocarpal or perilunate dislocations

Classification

The classification of distal radius fractures has been in evolution for almost 200 years. The early eponymous classifications named after those who have first described these fractures are still well-known and are used amongst clinicians today. Colles, Barton and Smith were surgeons of historical significance and eponymous fame, who have described one or more specific fractures based on clinical evaluation and cadaveric studies. Since these early days of fracture categorization, different classifications have focused on different aspects, such as displacement direction, radiographic appearance, injury mechanism, articular surface involvement and degree of comminution. Frykman's classification was the most popular until the end of the last century and is noteworthy for identifying the importance of both intra-articular fracture extension and the association of ulnar styloid fractures. However, it lacks the assessment of displacement, radial shortening and comminution.

The AO classification is the most detailed current classification, identifying 27 fracture patterns, and has good reliability and consistency (Fig. 5.10).[5] Due to its comprehensive nature, it is particularly useful in clinical research. It has an increasing alphabetical scale correlating to the proportion of the articular surface involved and is numerically subdivided into increasing morphological severity.

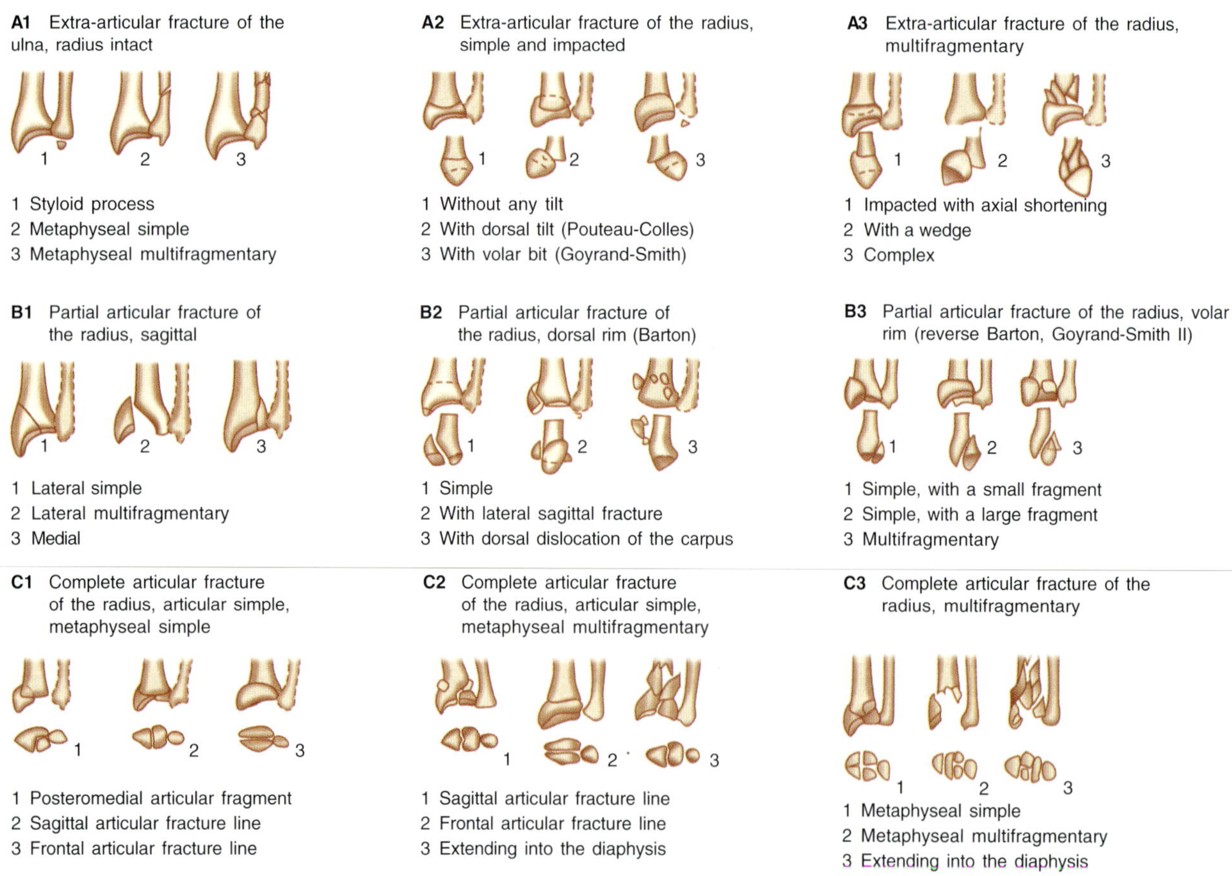

Figure 5.10: The AO classification of distal radius fractures includes 27 total types, but is broadly divided into three types: Type A consists of extra-articular fractures, Type B consists of partial-articular fractures and Type C consists of intra-articular fractures. Each of these is further subdivided, followed by another layer of subdivision yielding 27 total types.

Clinically, we find the Fernandez's classification (Fig. 5.11) to be the most useful because it addresses the mechanism of injury and the consequent treatment options.[6] It organizes fractures into 1 of 5 groups based on the direction and degree of force applied to the radius at time of injury (Figs 5.12A to E).

The three-column theory supports a concept aiding in the understanding of common fracture patterns and planning of internal fixation. It divides the wrist in three columns: (1) the radial column consisting of radial styloid and scaphoid facet, (2) the intermediate column consisting of lunate facet and sigmoid notch and (3) the ulnar column consisting of ulnar head, ulnar styloid and TFCC (Fig. 5.13). Based on cadaveric and *in vivo* studies on load transmissions,[7,8] load transmission theories have been formulated for each column. The radial column serves primarily as a carpal stabilizer by blocking radial translation by an osseous buttress and ulnar translation by radiocarpal ligaments originating from it. The intermediate column serves primarily for load transmission. Both the lunate and proximal pole of the scaphoid transmits their load directly to this column. The ulnar column sees very little load and it is transmitted mostly or entirely through TFCC. However, it primarily serves as a stabilizing pivot for the distal radius. Based on this theory, the aim of treating these fractures is to make sure that all three columns are stable.

Surgical Indications

Treatment indications for distal radius fractures continue to evolve. The propensity for surgical management of distal radius fractures has grown steadily over the past two decades with the advent of a myriad of implants along with the growing understanding of the benefits of articular reduction, restoration of proper length and rotation and early motion. In general, surgical indications for distal radius fractures can be broadly divided into four categories:

1. Patient factors
2. Fracture pattern
3. Fracture stability
4. Associated injuries

Patient factors include assessment of the patient's age, hand dominance, occupational demands, recreational expectations, preinjury functional level and comorbidities. Patients with higher demands and expectations may benefit from surgical treatment in order to optimize alignment, minimize late arthrosis and hasten return to activities. In contrast, patients with lower demand may be better managed nonsurgically even in light of residual malalignment.[9,10]

Fracture pattern analysis includes evaluation of the extent of fracture alignment, displacement, and comminution. Acceptable parameters for closed management are controversial, but typically include articular incongruity of less than 2 mm, radial inclination of greater than 15°, radial height greater than 5 mm, ulnar variance of at least 0 mm and lateral tilt of less than 20° dorsal angulation. Depending on the patient's age, needs and comorbidities, these radiographic patterns can be titrated up and down.

Fracture stability represents radiographic variables that indicate the risk for loss of reduction following closed treatment of a distal radius fracture.[11,12] Instability risk factors include volar cortical comminution, dorsal comminution greater than 50%, initial fracture displacement greater than 1 cm, initial radial shortening greater than 5 mm, the presence of an associated ulnar neck or shaft fracture, or severe osteoporosis. These variables can be taken into account in determining whether the fracture reduction will be maintained or if operative stabilization is indicated as well.

Associated injuries that may indicate a distal radius fracture to be treated surgically include open fractures, neurovascular injuries or additional extremity injuries. All open fractures warrant surgical debridement and qualify for fracture fixation, assuming the wound is acceptable. All neurological injuries including direct nerve injury, acute carpal tunnel syndrome or compartment syndrome warrant surgical decompression and fracture management. Additional extremity injuries as in the case of bilateral fractures or polytrauma situations warrant surgical fixation to facilitate patient mobilization.

Once surgery has been indicated, a number of surgical techniques exist that can be utilized. Each technique has specific fracture indications (Fig. 5.14). These techniques can be divided into three main categories (Figs 5.15A to F):

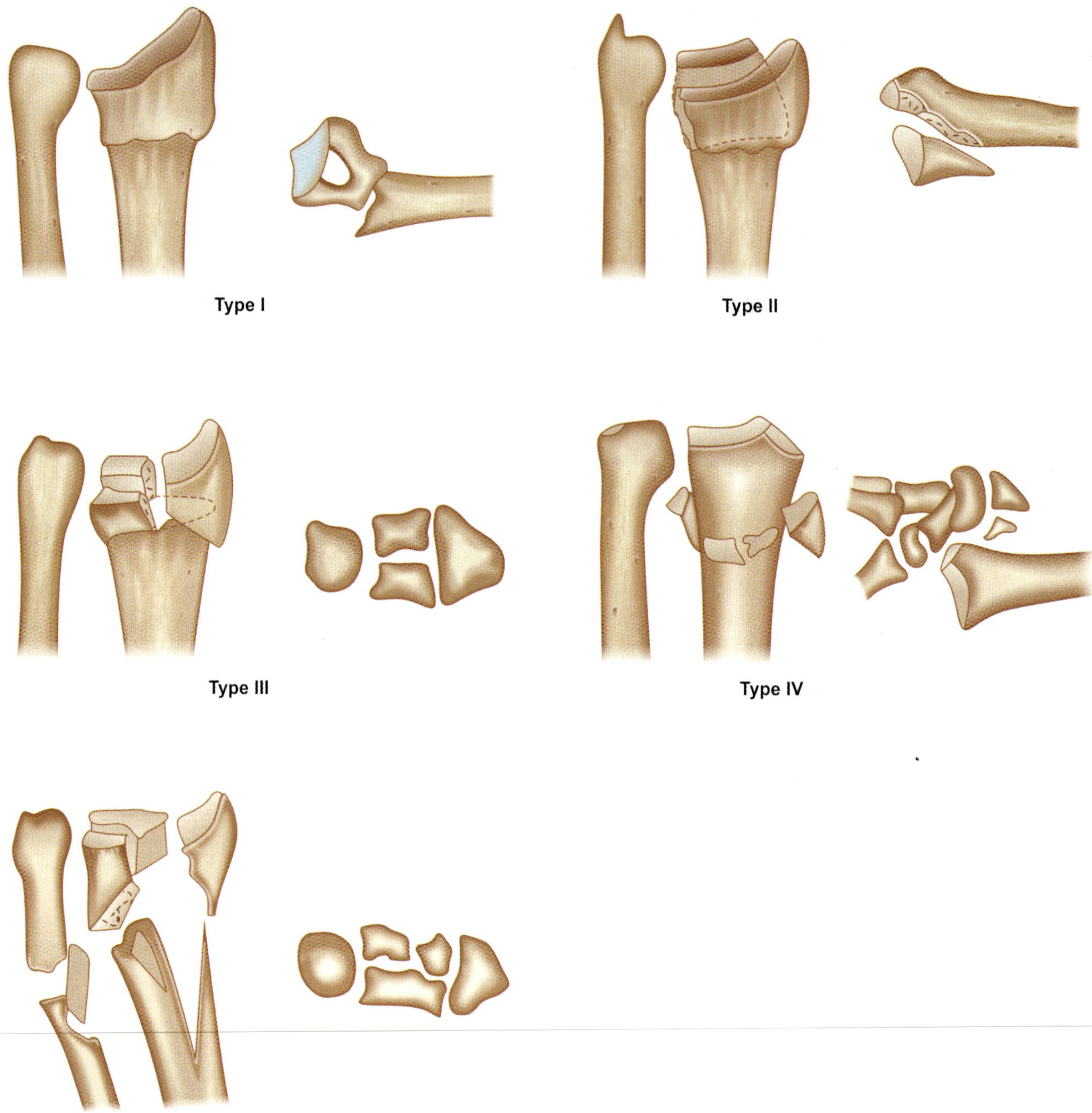

Figure 5.11: The Fernandez's classification is a mechanism-based classification consisting of Type I: Bending extra-articular fractures, Type II: Intra-articular marginal shearing fractures, Type III: Intra-articular compression fractures, Type IV: Avulsion fractures and Type V: Combination patterns.

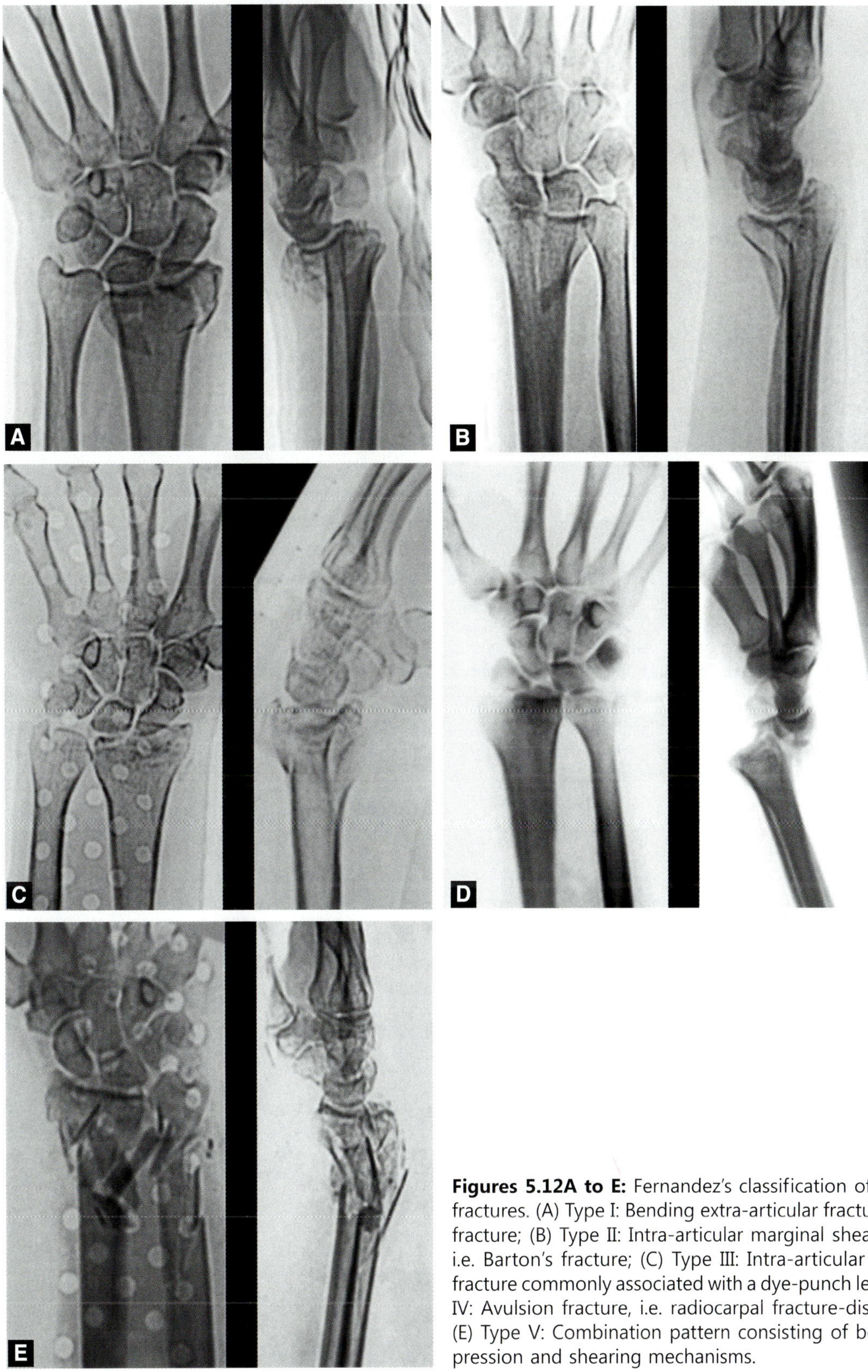

Figures 5.12A to E: Fernandez's classification of distal radius fractures. (A) Type I: Bending extra-articular fracture, i.e. Colles' fracture; (B) Type II: Intra-articular marginal shearing fracture, i.e. Barton's fracture; (C) Type III: Intra-articular compression fracture commonly associated with a dye-punch lesion; (D) Type IV: Avulsion fracture, i.e. radiocarpal fracture-dislocation; and (E) Type V: Combination pattern consisting of bending, compression and shearing mechanisms.

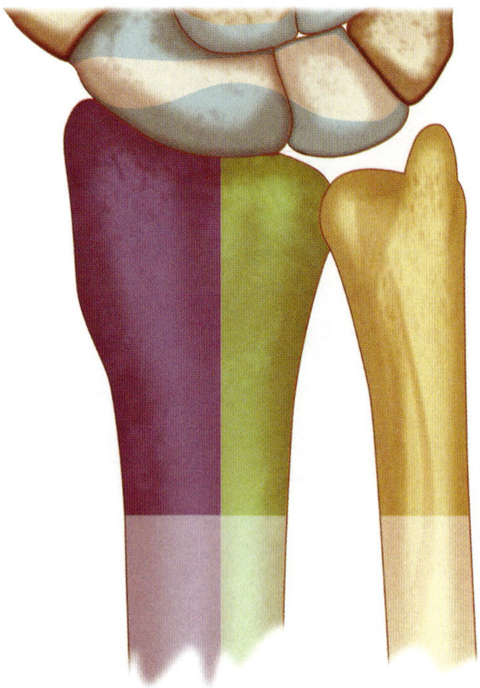

Figure 5.13: The 3-column theory to distal radius fracture includes a radial column, intermediate column and ulnar column. This theory focuses on role of each column in transmitting forces and maintaining stability. As per the theory, appropriate fracture management relies on restoring stability to all 3 columns.

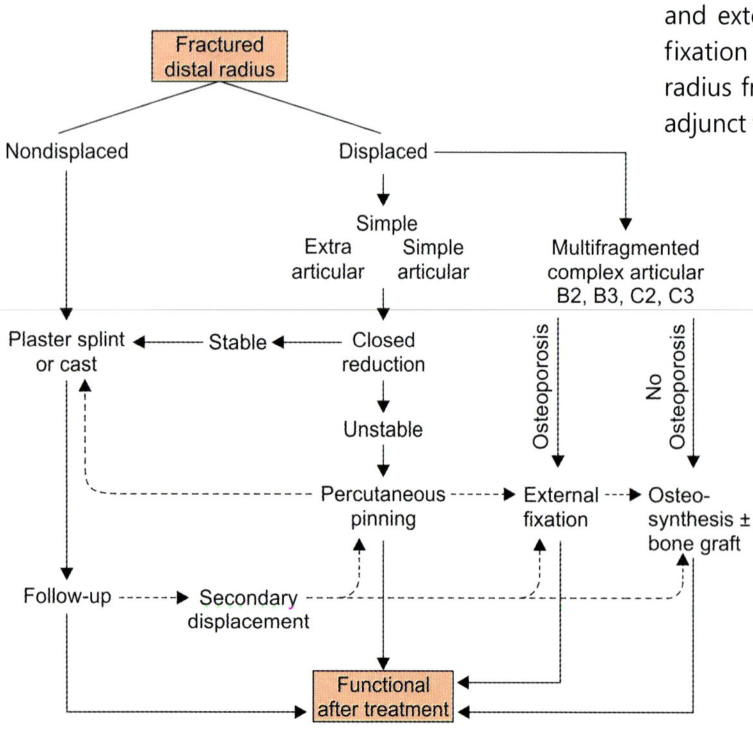

Figure 5.14: An algorithm for distal radius fracture management is outlined predicated initially on fracture displacement followed by fracture stability to help guide treatment and fixation.

1. Closed reduction and external fixation
   a. External fixators
2. Closed reduction and internal fixation
   a. K-wire fixation
   b. Percutaneous screw fixation
   c. Intramedullary nailing
3. Open reduction and internal fixation
   a. Volar, dorsal or radial plating
   b. Fragment specific fixation

Closed Reduction and External Fixation

External Fixator

Closed reduction and external fixation may be indicated for any unstable distal radius fracture. Reduction is achieved indirectly by ligamentotaxis and therefore, direct fracture reduction, in particular intra-articular fracture reduction, may be difficult to secure. However, externally fixed distal radius fracture may be augmented with K-wire fixation. Subsequently, and in light of advances in open plating techniques, the indications for external fixation has evolved to focus on distal radius fractures, where internal fixation may be contraindicated such as cases with severe comminution, advanced osteoporosis and extensive soft tissue damage (Fig. 5.15A). External fixation can also be used to temporarily stabilize distal radius fractures in the setting of a polytrauma or as an adjunct to other fixation techniques.

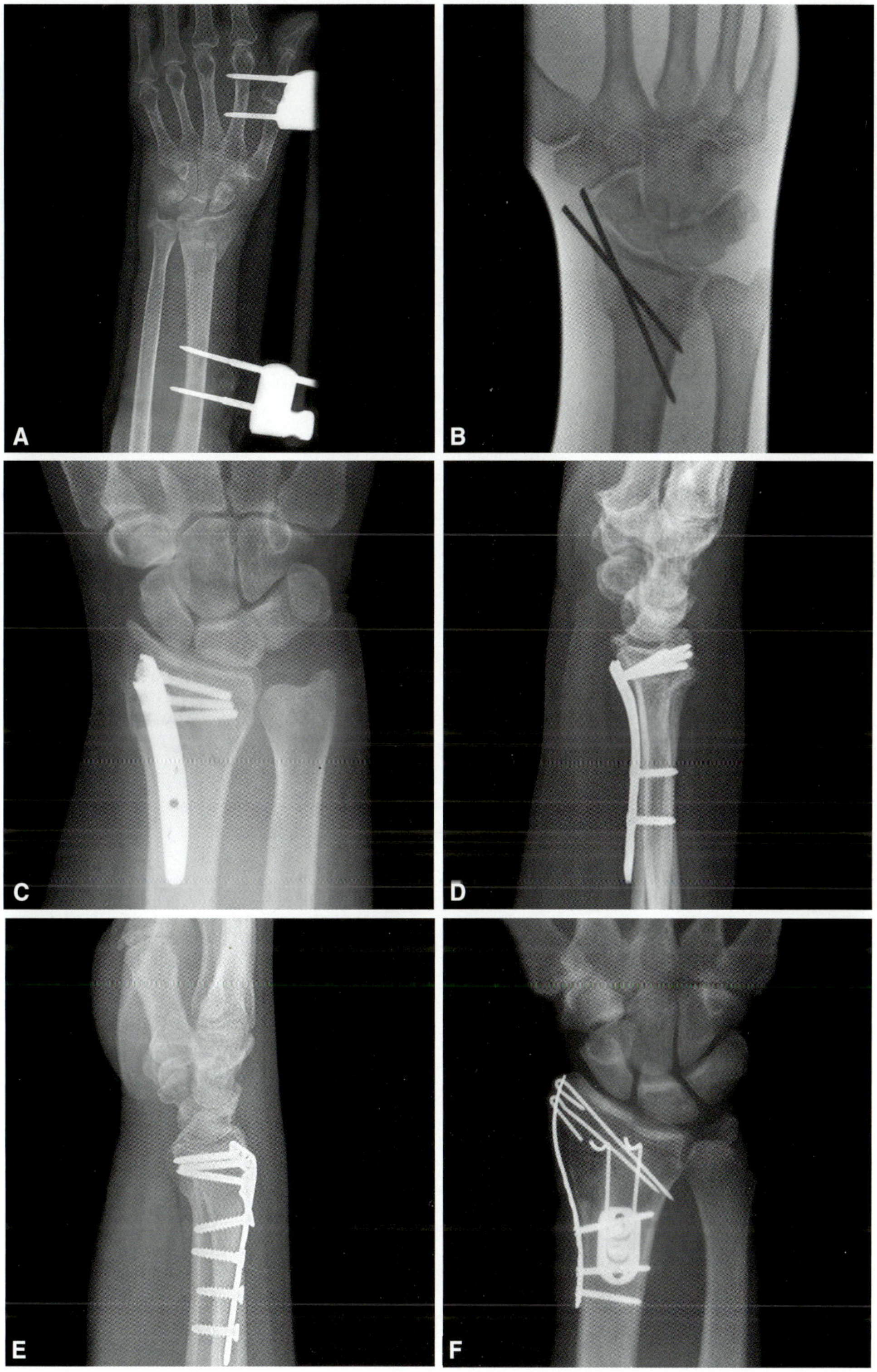

Figures 5.15A to F: Multiple surgical techniques and implants are available for fixation of distal radius fractures once indicated for surgery. Techniques can be broadly categorized as (A) Closed reduction and external fixation; (B) Closed reduction and internal fixation with percutaneous Kirschner (K) wire fixation; (C) With intramedullary nailing; (D) Open reduction and internal fixation (ORIF) with volar plating; (E) With dorsal plating, and (F) With fragment specific fixation.

Courtesy: Asif M Ilyas

Closed Reduction and Internal Fixation

Kirschner Wire Fixation

Closed reduction and K-wire fixation is indicated for extra-articular as well as intra-articular fractures (Fig. 5.15B). Relative contraindications include fractures with extensive intra-articular incongruity, severe fracture comminution or severe osteoporosis. Following fixation, the fracture may remain prone to shortening or collapse and therefore, typically require immobilization until fracture union.

Percutaneous Screw Fixation

Fractures with a simple configuration, minimal displacement and minimal articular congruity may be percutaneously fixed with screws.

Intramedullary Nailing

Distal radius fractures with extra-articular or simple intra-articular may be treated with intramedullary nails (Fig. 5.15C). Fixation is predicated upon closed or limited open fracture reduction and nail insertion. Contraindications to this technique include displaced intra-articular or dorsal/volar shear fractures.

Open Reduction and Internal Fixation

Volar Plating

The indications for volar plating has traditionally been intra-articular volar shear fracture or volar "Barton" fractures and volarly displaced extra-articular fracture or "Smith" fractures. However, with the advent of locking technology, volar locked plating has quickly become the primary implant of choice, when open reduction of the fracture is required (Fig. 5.15D). Locking screws allow for fixation of articular fragments and metaphyseal comminution without necessitating bicortical fixation (Fig. 5.16). Furthermore, the stiffness of the volar plate provides necessary fixed-angle subchondral support to prevent displacement and facilitate fixation in osteoporotic bone and early motion.

As such, most displaced and unstable distal radius fractures are indicated for fixation with volar locking plates. A potential limitation for volar locking plates are AO Type B2 fractures or dorsal shear or dorsal "Barton" fractures that may still potentially be successfully treated with a volar locking plate but would be better served with dorsal fixation.

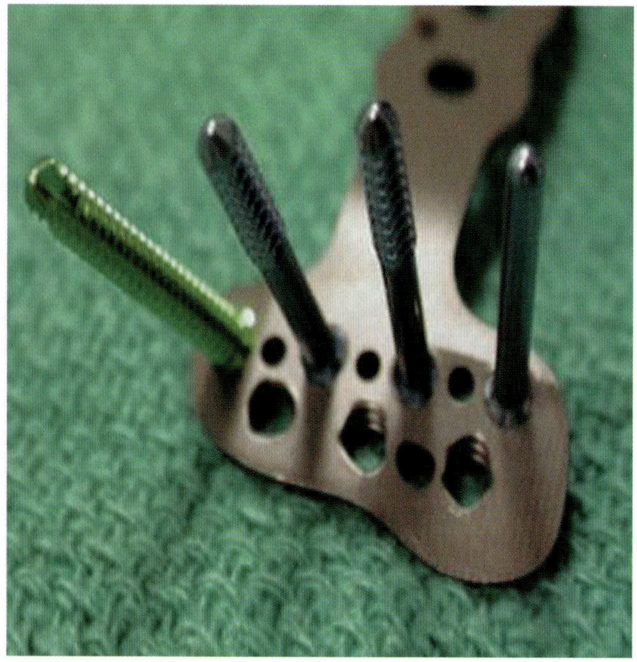

Figure 5.16: A volar locking plate. Note the fixed-angle locking screws that provide strong subchondral support and creates a fixed-angle device.

Dorsal Plating

The indications for dorsal plating are dorsally displaced fractures of the distal radius (Fig. 5.15E). Dorsal plate fixation provides a good view of the dorsal articular surface and dorsal comminution. Subsequently, a dorsal approach and plating is particularly useful in managing intra-or extra-articular dorsal fracture comminution, "die-punch" lesion or dorsal shear "Barton" fractures. The utilization of dorsal plates must be tempered against the propensity for soft tissue irritation of the extensor tendons.

Fragment Specific Fixation

Indications for fragment specific fixation include displaced intra-articular distal radius fractures (Fig. 5.15F). The technique may be employed exclusively or in conjunction with dorsal or volar plating. Although, effective in achieving articular fracture fixation, the technique may be cumbersome as multiple incision and small implants require manipulation and implantation.

Surgical Anatomy, Positioning and Approaches

The distal radius articulates with the ulna, scaphoid and lunate, and is part of a mechanism enabling pronation/supination, flexion/extension and radial/ulnar deviation at the wrist.

Wrist rotation with supination and pronation occurs at the distal radioulnar joint (DRUJ). This joint is formed by the circular head of distal ulna rotating within the concave semicircular sigmoid notch of the distal radius (Fig. 5.17A). This relationship of the DRUJ is important while assessing reduction and stability of the DRUJ, as well as during screw fixation during volar or dorsal plating. Screws placed too ulnar may traverse the DRUJ and could result in joint arthrosis or obstruct wrist rotation.

The articular surface of the distal radius includes the lunate fossa and scaphoid fossa (Fig. 5.17A). The articular surface has an average radial inclination of 22° and an average palmar tilt of 11°. The radial height averages 12 mm. The dorsal surface of the distal radius is irregular and the cortex is thin, leaving it most vulnerable to fractures with dorsal angulation and comminution (Fig. 5.17B). One of the irregularities on the dorsal side of the distal radius is Lister's tubercle (Fig. 5.17B). This tubercle acts as a pulley for the extensor pollicis longus (EPL) tendon but can also serve as a source for autologous bone graft. The volar cortex of the distal radius consists of stronger bone and is less prone to fracture. It represents the tensile side during fracturing. The distal extent of the volar cortex is the origin for the radiocarpal ligaments and also communicates closely with the finger flexor tendons. The lunate facet is particularly thin, but is prominent aspect of the volar cortical rim. The lunate facet is the origin of the important joint stabilizing radiolunate ligament (Fig. 5.18). Fractures of the lunate facet may be subtle but inadequate fixation can lead to late radiocarpal subluxation (Figs 5.19 A to C).

The dorsal side of the distal radius is directly covered by all of the extensor tendons. In contrast, the volar side is covered by the pronator quadratus (PQ) muscle. Only the distal most extent of the volar cortex communicates with the finger flexor tendons, particularly the flexor pollicis longus (FPL) and the flexor digitorum profundis (FDP).

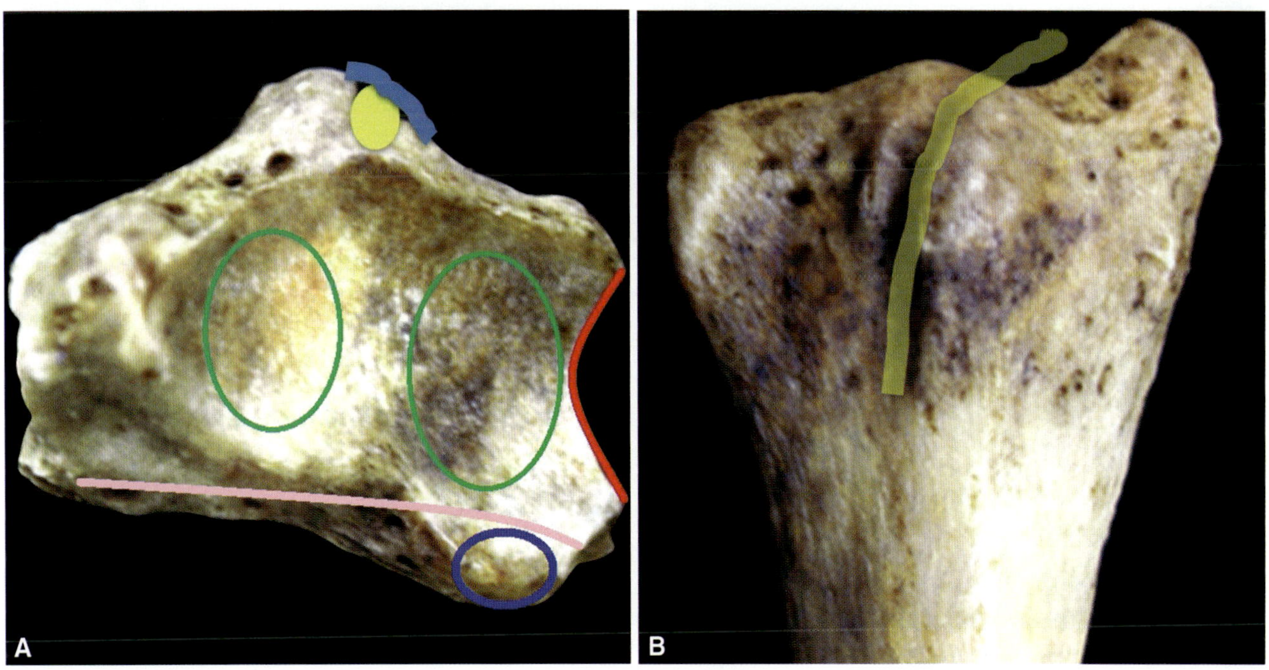

Figures 5.17A and B: The distal radius. (A) The articular surface has two articular facets: the scaphoid and lunate facets (in green), the ulna articulates with the sigmoid notch of the distal radius (in red), the distal volar cortex corresponds to the pink line, but note how the lunate facet (in blue) projects further volarly. The distal dorsal cortex includes the prominent Lister's tubercle that acts as a pulley for the extensor pollicis longus (EPL) tendon (in yellow); (B) On the dorsal view, note the thin dorsal cortex and the path of the EPL tendon (in yellow) wrapping around the Lister's tubercle.

Hardware placed dorsally is always prone to extensor tendon irritation due to intimate association of the extensor tendons and the dorsal cortex. However, hardware placed on the volar side is relatively free of soft tissue irritation when appropriately centered on the radius and positioned below the PQ, unless positioned too distally or angled too volarly (Fig. 5.20). Otherwise, the hardware may irritate the FPL and FDP tendons.

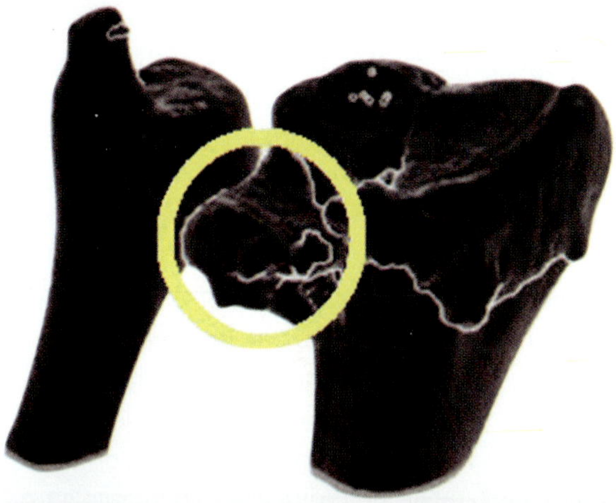

Figure 5.18: The lunate facet (in yellow) fracture in a three-dimensional CT reconstruction of an intra-articular fracture of the distal radius.

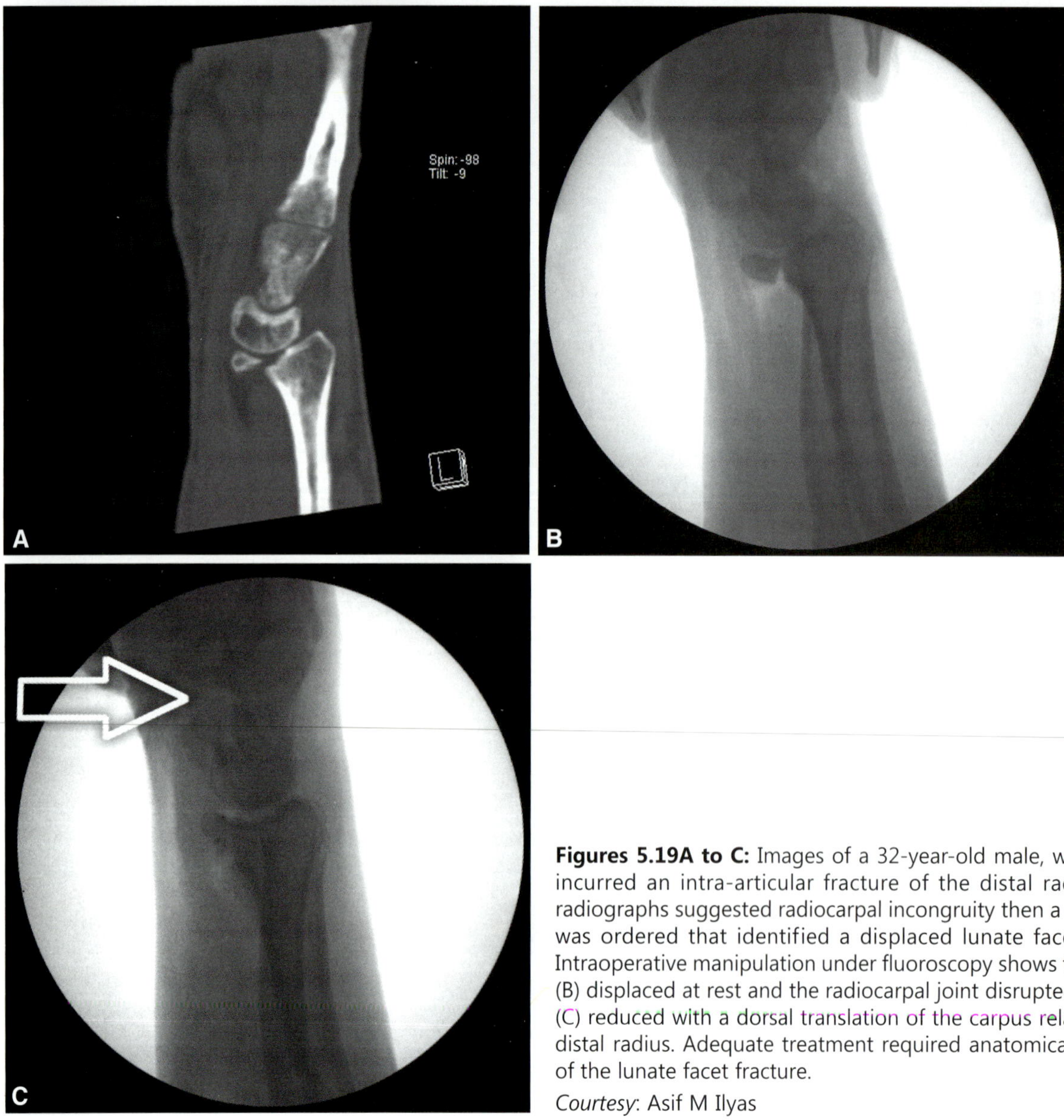

Figures 5.19A to C: Images of a 32-year-old male, who fell and incurred an intra-articular fracture of the distal radius. Initial radiographs suggested radiocarpal incongruity then a (A) CT scan was ordered that identified a displaced lunate facet fracture. Intraoperative manipulation under fluoroscopy shows the fracture (B) displaced at rest and the radiocarpal joint disrupted, and then (C) reduced with a dorsal translation of the carpus relative to the distal radius. Adequate treatment required anatomical reduction of the lunate facet fracture.

Courtesy: Asif M Ilyas

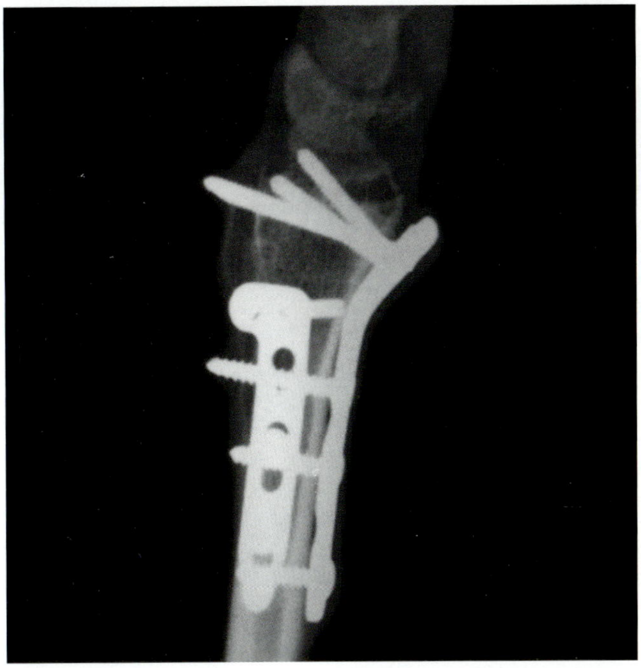

Figure 5.20: Note the prominence of the distal end of the volar plate. This patient complained of discomfort with thumb flexion and eventually presented with spontaneous loss of thumb flexion. The plate was angled too volarly and positioned too distally, thereby irritating the overlying flexor tendons. Furthermore, note the dorsal prominence of the subchondral screws that puts the extensor tendons at risk for attritional rupture.

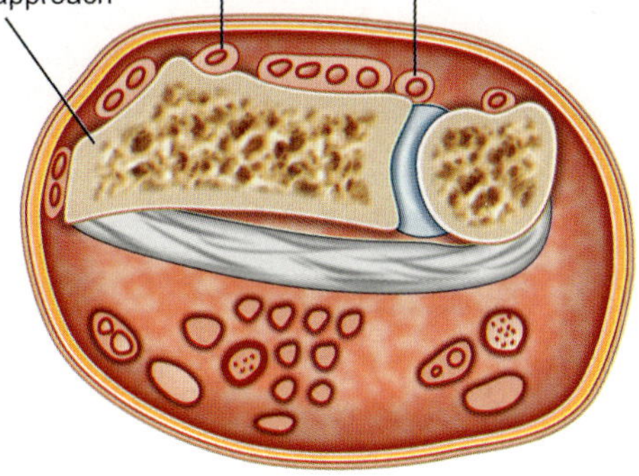

Figure 5.21: The dorsal approach to the distal radius involves navigating various extensor tendons of the distal radius. The standard trans-extensor pollicis longus (trans-EPL) or midradial approach involves opening the third dorsal compartment to facilitate the dorsal exposure of the distal radius.

Positioning

The authors prefer the patient in a supine position, using a hand table at all times. The image intensifier should be positioned for easy access throughout the case. A tourniquet is applied for hemostasis. For volar approaches, the forearm is supinated. For dorsal approaches, the forearm is pronated. Rotation through the wrist is minimized to avoid displacing the fracture site.

Approaches

Dorsal Approach

The dorsal approach provides access to the dorsal aspect of the distal radius and DRUJ by navigating through various extensor tendon compartments (Fig. 5.21). Generally, the dorsal approach can be divided in four separate approaches depending on which structures need to be exposed (Fig. 5.22). The standard or midradial dorsal approach to the distal radius involves placing a longitudinal incision just ulnar to the Lister's tubercle. The third dorsal compartment containing the EPL tendon is opened and the tendon is released and retracted radially. The dorsal surface of the distal radius is then exposed by raising the surrounding second and fourth dorsal compartments subperiosteally. Lister's tubercle is rongeured as necessary for access to the fracture site, bone graft or plate placement. Upon closure, the extensor retinaculum is closed over the site of third dorsal compartment while exteriorizing the EPL tendon outside the retinacular closure.

Radial Approach

A longitudinal skin incision is made over the radial wrist beginning from the level of the radial styloid or anatomical snuffbox and continuing proximally. Branches of the radial sensory nerve must be identified and protected. The radial cortex of the distal radius is exposed, thereafter either by opening the first dorsal compartment or elevating between the first and second dorsal compartments in a subperiosteal fashion. The insertion of the brachioradialis should, thereafter be visualized and released as necessary.

Volar Approach

The volar approach to the distal radius can be accomplished through three different intervals: (1) Transflexor

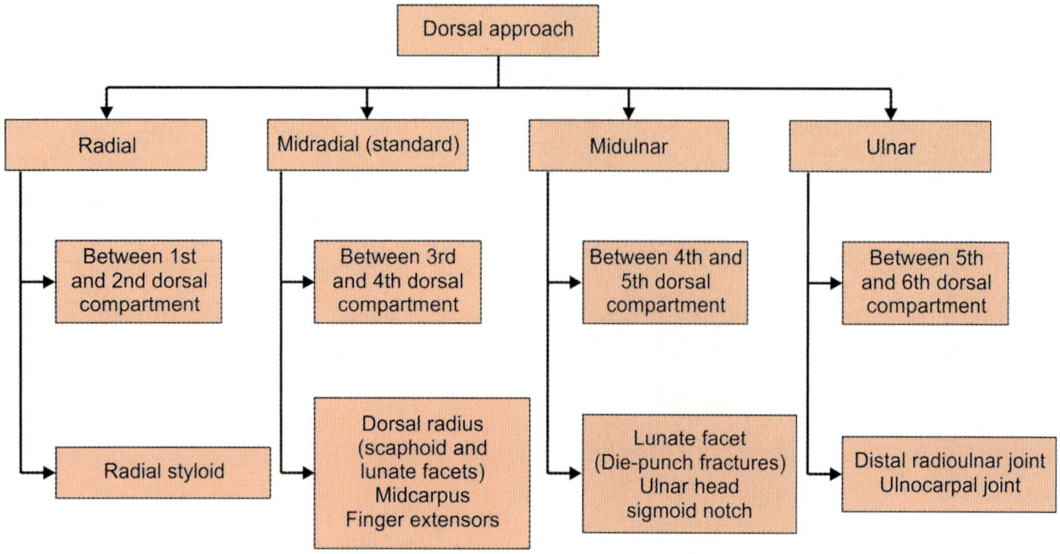

Figure 5.22: The dorsal approaches can be broadly broken down into four major intervals: radial, midradial, midulnar and ulnar.

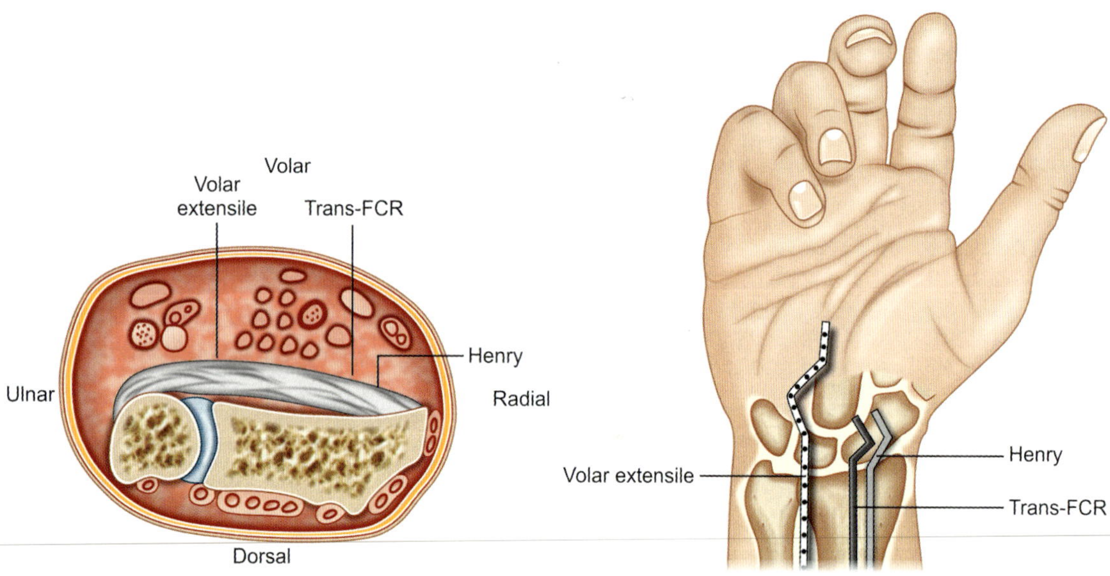

Figure 5.23: The volar approaches to the distal radius include the transflexor carpi radialis (trans-FCR), modified Henry and extensile volar-ulnar approaches.

carpi radialis (FCR), (2) Modified Henry, and (3) Extensile volar-ulnar approaches (Fig. 5.23).

Trans-flexor carpi radialis approach: The trans-FCR approach provides a safe and reliable approach to the volar distal radius (Figs 5.24A to F). A longitudinal incision is made over the FCR tendon beginning at the distal wrist crease and extending proximally 6–8 cm. Blunt dissection is performed down to the FCR tendon sheath. The radial artery lies just radial to the tendon and must be protected. The FCR sheath is opened and the tendon is retracted ulnarly. The floor of the tendon sheath is then opened facilitating access to the deep volar compartment. The FCR tendon and all of the finger flexor tendons are

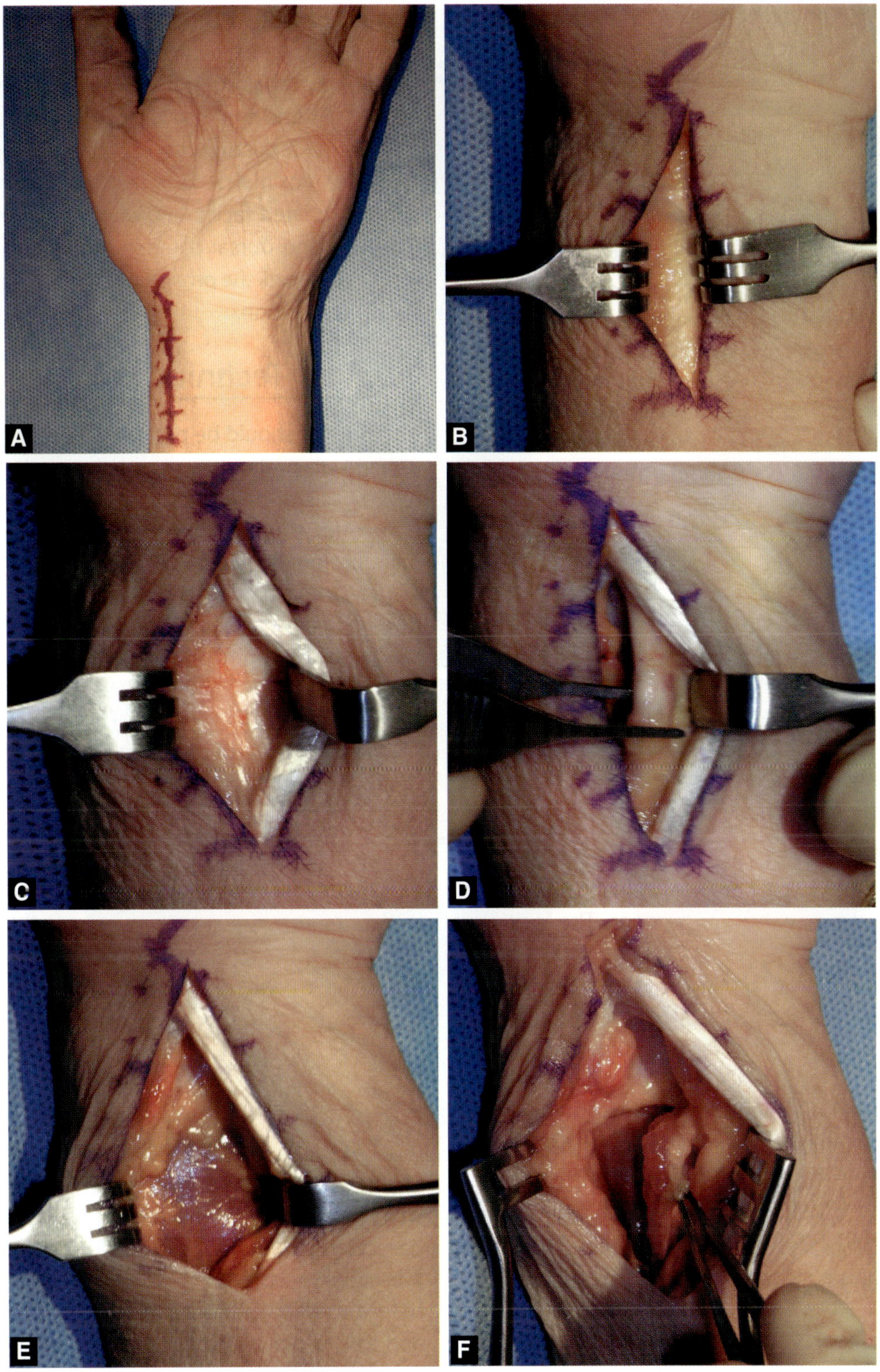

Figures 5.24A to F: (A) The standard transflexor carpi radialis (FCR) approach begins with a longitudinal incision; (B and C) The FCR tendon is exposed and the sheath is opened and retracted exposing the floor of the tendon sheath; (D) The flexor pollicis longus (FPL) tendon (held by the forceps) and finger flexor tendons are retracted ulnarly; (E and F) The pronator quadratus (PQ) is exposed and raised subperiosteally, thereby exposing the volar surface of the distal radius.

Courtesy: Asif M Ilyas

radial K-wires. The wires can be cut below the skin or bent and capped above the skin.

KIRSCHNER WIRE FIXATION: Pearls and Pitfalls

- Percutaneous K-wire fixation is predicated on adequate closed or limited open reduction of the fracture
- Branches of the radial sensory nerve are prone to injury along the radial styloid. Making small incisions and spreading down to the bone can help avoid injury. Alternatively, the wires may be advanced while "oscillating" versus "drilling"
- K-wires should be placed in oblique angles and at least two wires should be utilized to fix the fracture

Technique 2: External Fixation

Closed reduction is performed under fluoroscopy using traction. K-wires may be used to assist in reduction or augment fixation. In particular, as external fixation provides only indirect reduction, K-wires allow direct fracture reduction and provisional fixation (Figs 5.26A and B).

We prefer starting with insertion of the metacarpal pins in the index metacarpal. The first incision should be made from the base of the index metacarpal to about 1 cm distal. A 0.5 mm incision is placed first and blunt dissection is performed down to the bone to avoid the extensor tendon and branches of the superficial radial nerve. The pins are placed obliquely to maximize strength and spread of the construct and minimizing the risk of pull out (Figs 5.27A and B). The proximal pin is inserted by hand into a predrilled hole in the shaft near the base of the metacarpal with the use of a soft tissue protector. A small groove can be palpated that confirms the correct location for the pin insertion. The distal pin is inserted in the same fashion as the proximal pin, into the shaft near the head of the metacarpal, where a small groove may also point out the right location. Avoid pinning of the extensor tendon hood with the distal pin by flexing the second metacarpophalangeal joint at the moment of pin insertion to shift the extensor hood dorsally.

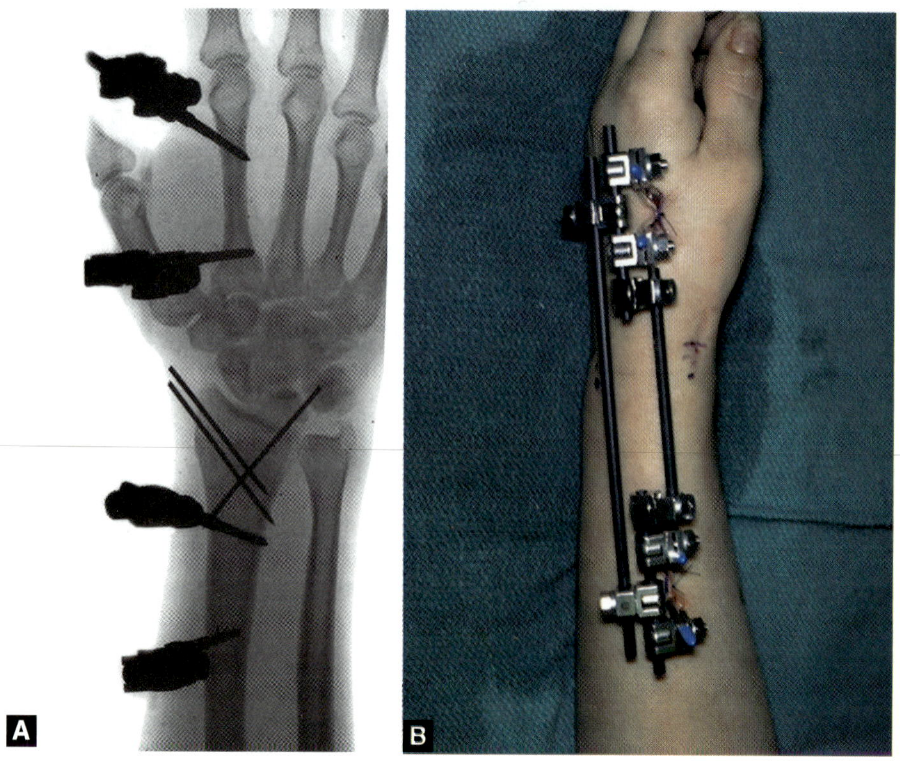

Figures 5.26A and B: A 41-year-old female, who fell and incurred a dorsally angulated and displaced distal radius fracture with simple intra-articular reduction of the dorsoulnar corner (AO Type C1). (A and B) She was treated with closed reduction and external fixation but was augmented with percutaneous K-wire fixation to improve articular reduction.

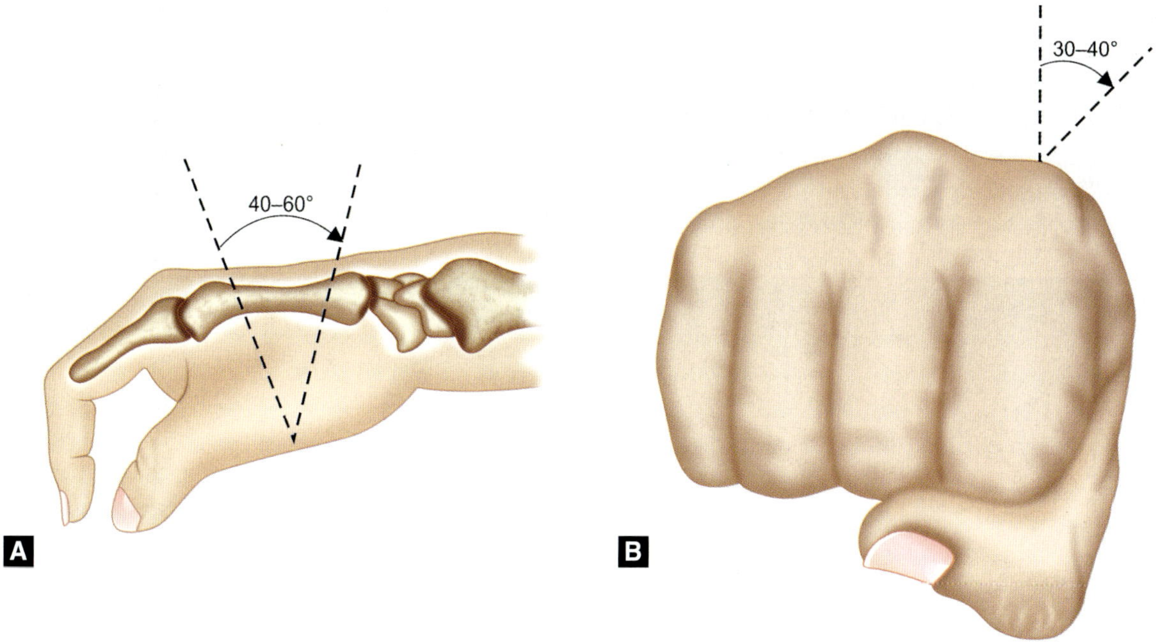

Figures 5.27A and B: The metacarpal ex-fix pins are placed obliquely to maximize strength and spread of the construct, while simultaneously minimizing the risk of pull out.

The radial cortex of the radial midshaft can be readily palpated through the skin. This is a safe and preferred zone to make small incisions and insert the 2 proximal pins, but again, care must be taken to avoid the radial sensory nerve and its superficial branches. Mark the skin where the two pins will be placed that are consistent with the type of fixator being used. Two 1 cm skin incisions, or a single 3–4 cm skin incision is made with diligent blunt dissection down to the bone. Predrill the hole using a soft tissue protector. The pins should be carefully placed, thereafter in a bicortical fashion. When their position is acceptable, excess skin can be closed around the pin insertion sites using 4-0 nylon sutures. Using pin-to-clamp or pin-to-bars, one or two carbon fiber rods are positioned but not tightened. The fracture is then reduced manually under traction and the reduction is checked using fluoroscopy. Once satisfactory reduction is confirmed by fluoroscopy, the bars are tightened with the wrist in slight palmar flexion and ulnar deviation. Excess palmar flexion can result in carpal tunnel syndrome and excessive distraction can result in cutaneous nerve injury.

EXTERNAL FIXATION: Pearls and Pitfalls

- Avoid overdistraction of the wrist joint. This can be seen radiographically by disproportionate widening at the radiocarpal or midcarpal joints
- If necessary, additional K-wires can be used to further stabilize and fix fracture fragments
- The patient should be instructed to keep the pin sites clean to prevent infection
- In case of an open wound, an external fixator can be used to avoid the placement of deep hardware and subsequent infection

Technique 3: Intramedullary Nailing

This technique has recently been described in the literature.[14] This technique is predicated on successful closed reduction and allows early motion and has subsequently resulted in good results in the management of extra-articular or simple intra-articular distal radius fractures.

The first step involves fracture reduction under fluoroscopy. When this has been achieved, the fracture is percutaneously fixed with a K-wire along the dorsal ulnar column of the distal radius (Figs 5.28A to H). This will maintain fracture reduction during placement of the nail. When there is a dorsal impaction or involvement of the volar cortex, a limited dorsal incision can be made to facilitate direct open reduction of the fracture. This same dorsal incision will later be used to place the proximal interlocking screws.

After the fracture is reduced and pinned, a 2–3 cm incision along the distal radial column of the radius is developed. Branches of the superficial radial sensory nerve should be identified and protected when performing blunt

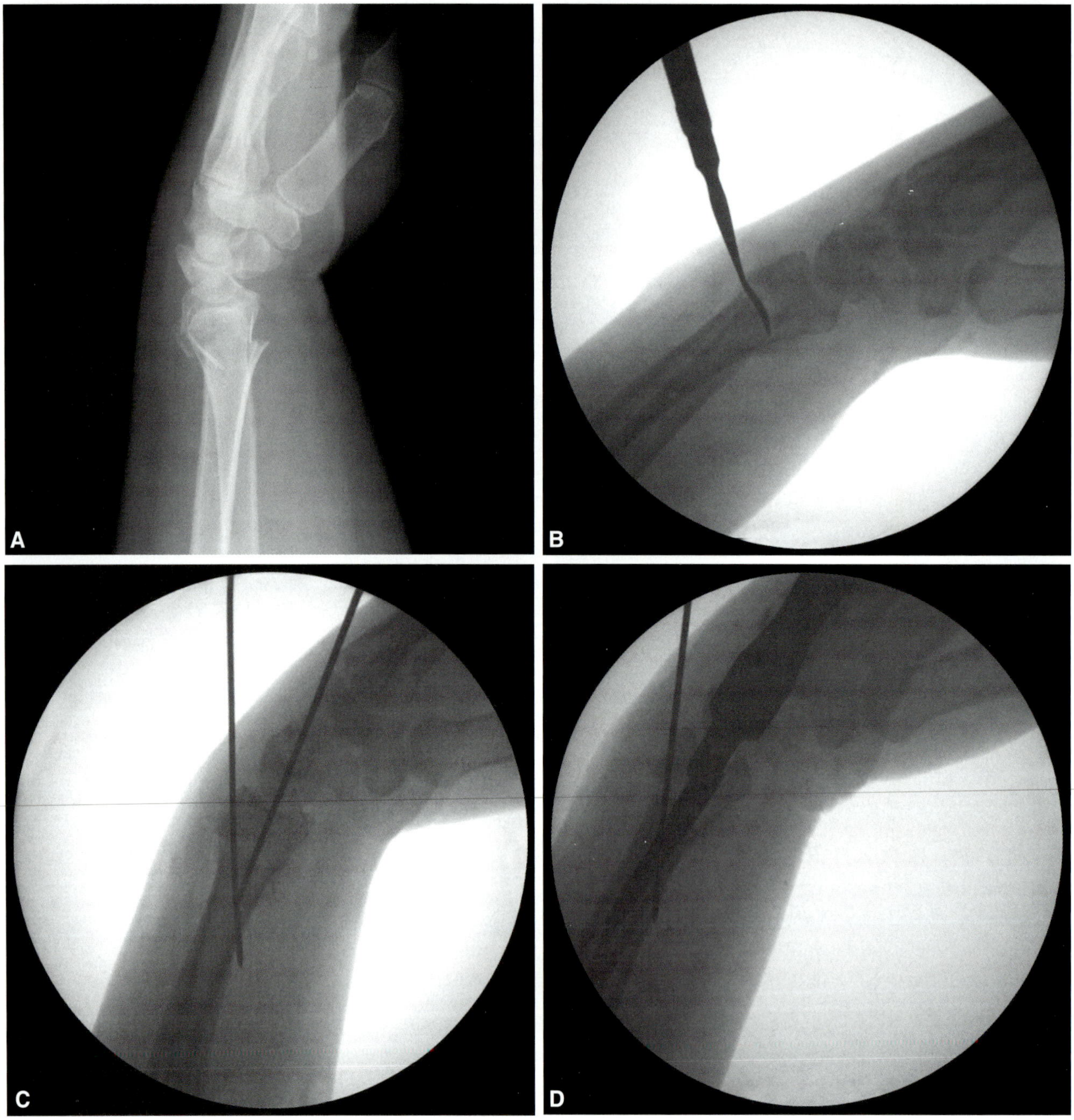

Figures 5.28A to D

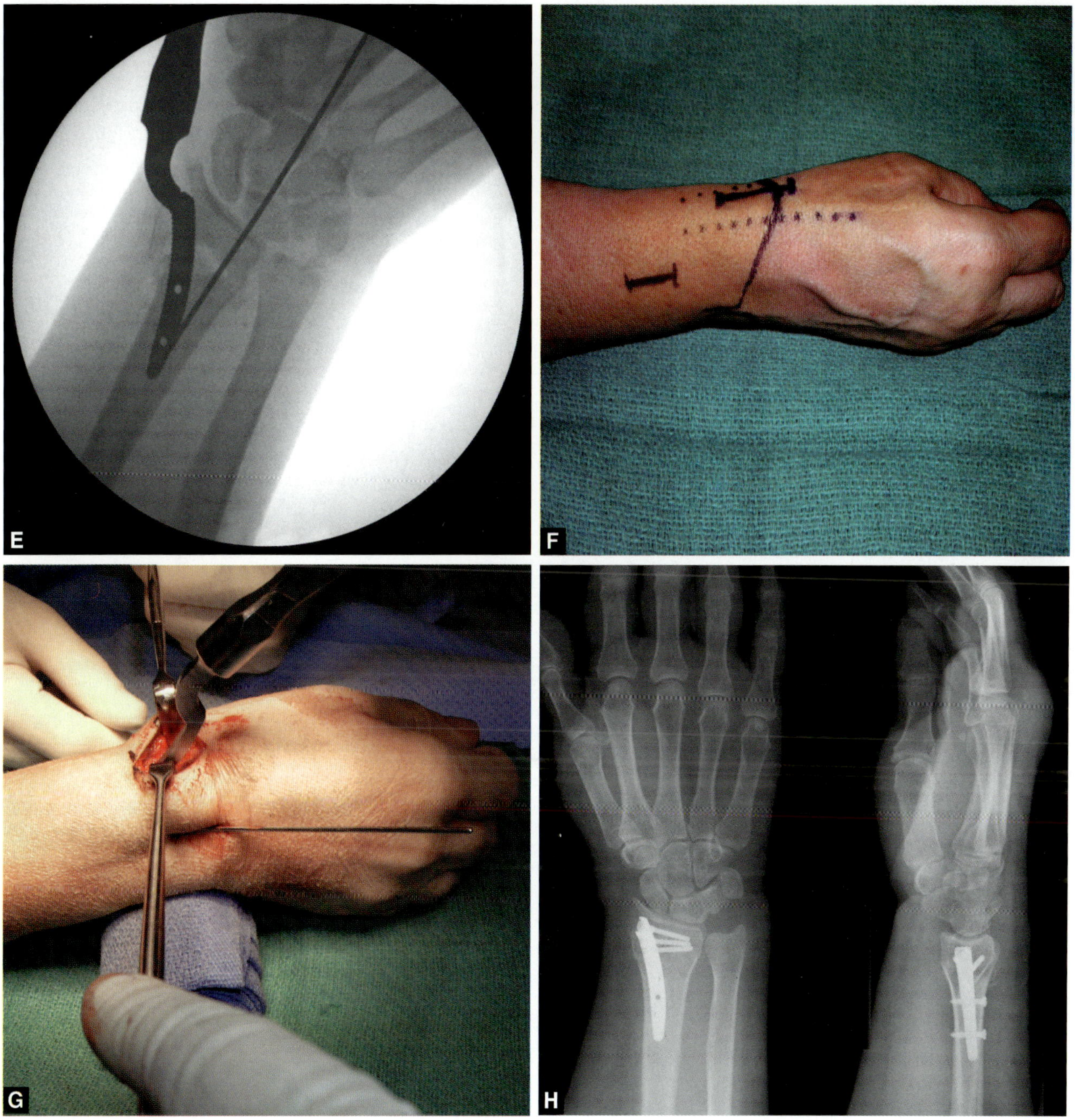

Figures 5.28A to H: This is a case of a 36-year-old female, who fell and incurred a dorsally angulated extra-articular distal radius fracture (AO Type A2). She initially underwent closed reduction but experienced a (A) loss of reduction in her cast and was subsequently offered intramedullary nailing. The procedure involves (B) percutaneous or limited open reduction, (C) provisional K-wire fixation; (D and E) broaching across the reduced fracture followed by nail insertion; (F) Note the location of the incisions to be placed relative to the radial sensory nerve (marked on the skin with a dashed line); (G) Following broaching of the distal radius, the nail is inserted and then (H) locked distally and proximally.

Courtesy: Asif M Ilyas

dissection down to the bone. The interval between the first and second dorsal compartments is developed in a subperiosteal fashion. A guidewire and reamer are placed to open the radial aspect of the distal radius. An awl is placed in the intramedullary canal of the distal radius through the radial-sided opening. Afterward, the canal is broached across the fracture until a good fill of the radius is achieved with the broach without a tight fit. The radius is trialed and an implant is selected. When the implant is sufficiently seated, place the divergent fixed-angle locking subchondral screws through the insertion jig. After the nail is locked distally, a 2 cm incision is placed approximately 1 cm proximal to the Lister's tubercle and the interval between the second and third dorsal compartments is developed to expose the dorsal cortex of the radius. The proximal bicortical screws are placed through the dorsal cortex. Close the skin incisions with 4-0 nylon sutures.

INTRAMEDULLARY NAILING: Pearls and Pitfalls

- The intramedullary nail should be limited to primarily displaced extra-articular fractures
- Adequate fracture reduction must be achieved prior to nail insertion, as further fracture reduction after nail insertion is not possible
- The superficial radial sensory nerve should be identified and protected, as it is highly susceptible to injury
- Use the fluoroscope meticulously during screw placement to prevent intra-articular screw placement. The distal radioulnar joint is the most susceptible
- Employ early wrist motion after surgery

Technique 4: Volar Plating

The authors recommend either a trans-FCR or the modified Henry approach to access and expose the volar surface of the distal radius (Figs 5.29A to D and 5.30A to D). Following elevation of the PQ, the fracture will come into view. Good exposure of the fracture is important. To maximize exposure, the wound should be irrigated and fracture hematoma or callus should be removed. Retractors should be placed along both sides of the radial shaft, and the volar cortex should be subperiosteally exposed. It is helpful to identify the radiocarpal joint either by fluoroscopy or by placing a hypodermic needle in the joint space. This permits maximizing exposure of the fracture while avoiding inadvertent violation of the origin of the radiocarpal ligaments. The fracture fragments, geography and articular alignment should be carefully identified. Particular attention should be paid for the presence of articular step-off, "die-punch" lesions, lunate facet fractures and DRUJ incongruity.

Reduction and fixation of the fracture can be accomplished in four general techniques (Figs 5.29A to D):

1. Direct fracture reduction followed by plate application
2. Indirect plate-assisted fracture reduction
3. Distal fracture fragment fixation to the plate followed by reduction to the shaft
4. Distal fracture fragment fixation to the plate

The first two techniques represent traditional nonlocking volar plate application. In the first scenario, the fracture is directly reduced, provisionally held or pinned and then a plate is applied to hold the fragments in the reduced position. The second scenario, indirect reduction, represents the traditional treatment for volar shear "Barton's" fracture treatment where an undercontoured plate is applied to the volar surface of the radial shaft and as it is compressed to the shaft, the distal articular fragment is secondarily reduced. However, with the advent of locking technology, volar locking plates have become reduction tools. In the third scenario, the locking plate is applied to the distal fragment alone with locking screws in the appropriate position. The fracture is then reduced when the plate is applied to the shaft. This technique is the best suited for extra-articular fractures and is predicated upon accurate positioning of the plate on the distal fragment. In the fourth scenario, the plate is applied to the shaft and then the distal fragment is reduced directly to the plate with distraction and volar flexion followed by locking screw fixation. In reality, a combination of these four scenarios is typically utilized to achieve optimum fracture reduction and fixation.

A preliminary reduction is typically achieved with traction, exaggeration of the deformity, direct dorsal pressure on the distal fragment and reconstitution of volar cortical alignment. If articular step off is present, the step-off should be reduced through the fracture site prior to reducing the volar cortices. Liberal use of K-wires can help reduce fragments as well as hold provisional reduction.

The goal of fixation is stable anatomical fixation that permits early motion. Final plate fixation should typically consist of minimum 2–3 cortical nonlocking shaft screws and 3–5 subchondral locking screws. Vigilance should be paid to avoid inadvertent screw placement in the radiocarpal joint or DRUJ. Similarly, the subchondral

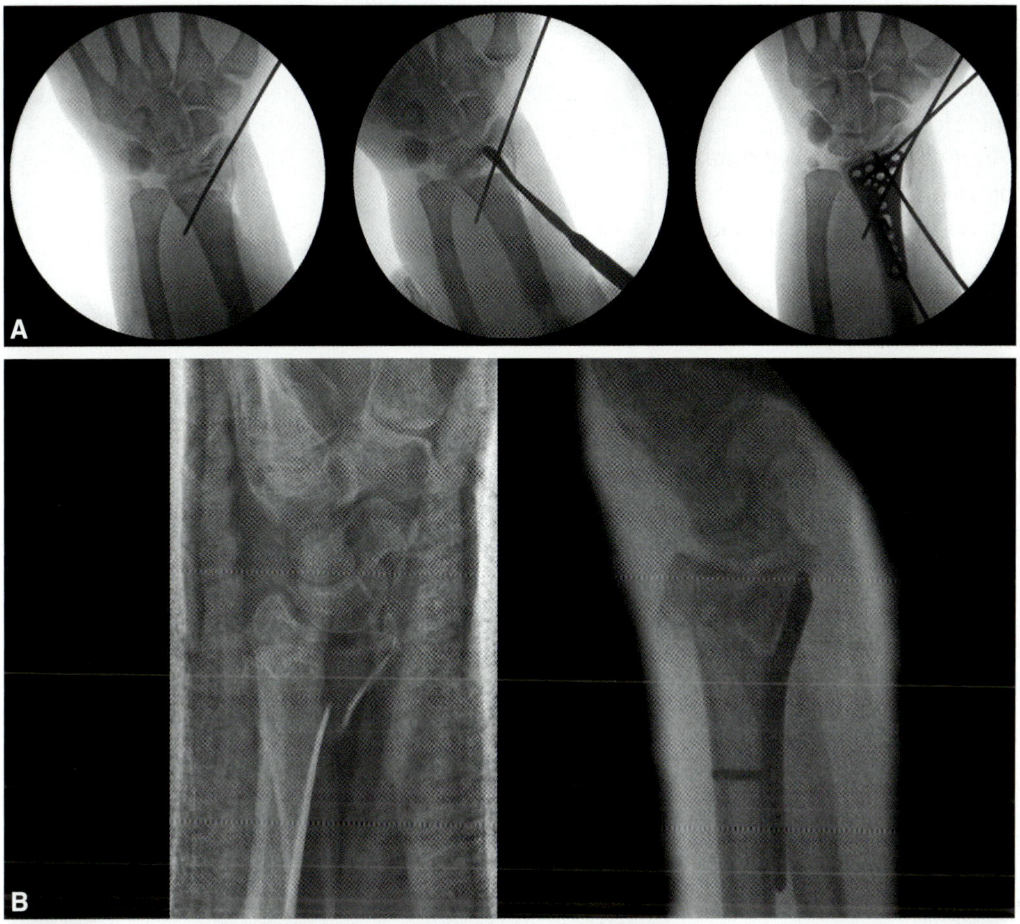

Figures 5.29A to D: Reduction and fixation of the fracture using a volar plate can be accomplished in four general techniques. (A) Direct fracture reduction followed by plate application; (B) Indirect fracture reduction by plate application; (C) Distal fracture fragment fixation to the plate followed by reduction to the shaft; (D) Distal fracture fragment reduction and fixation to the plate.

Courtesy: Asif M Ilyas

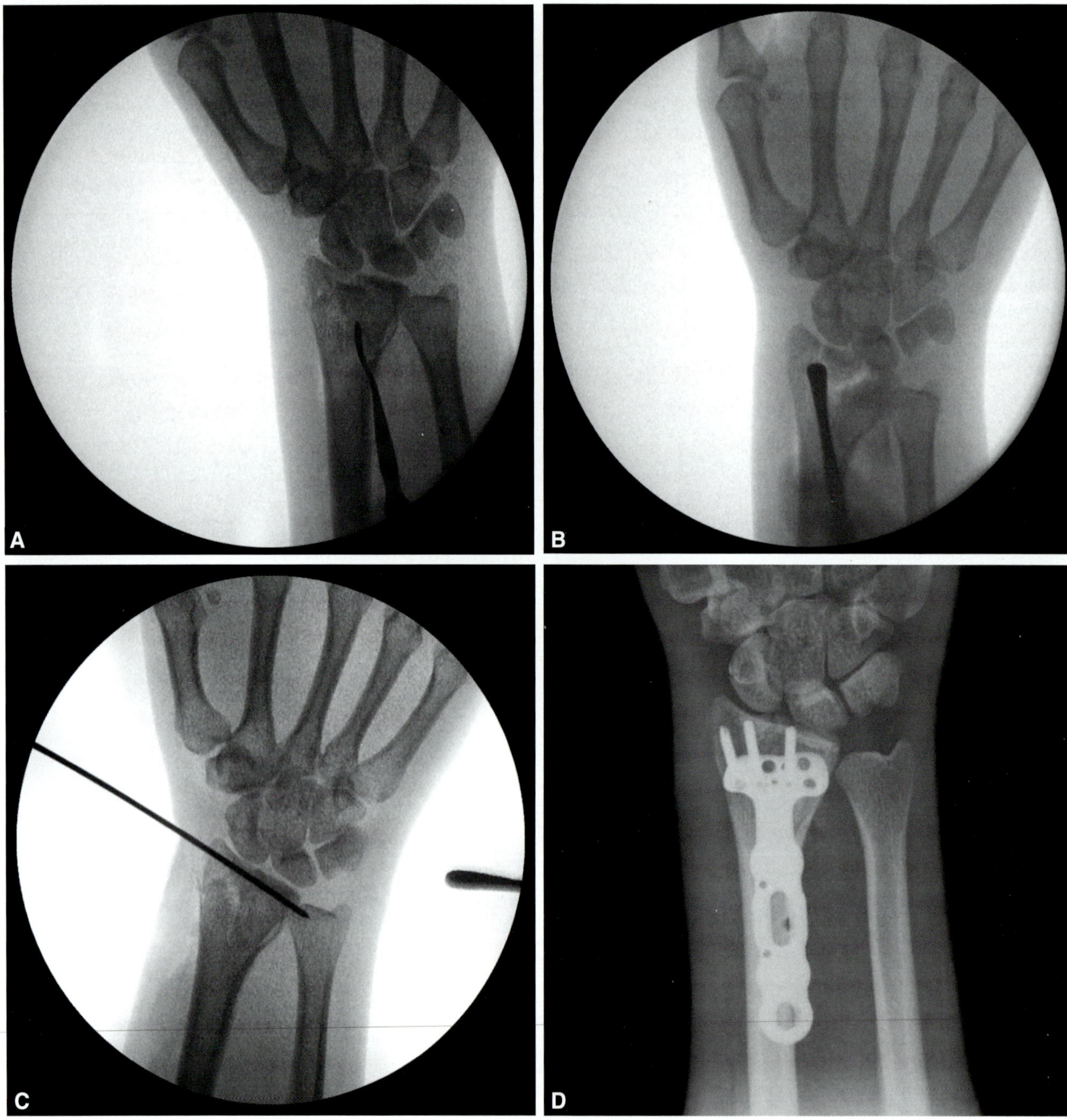

Figures 5.30A to D: This is a case of a 32-year-old female, who fell and incurred an intra-articular distal radius fracture with a "die-punch" lesion resulting in central depression of the articular surface. (A to D) Note the direct articular reduction through the fracture site followed by provisional pinning and volar plate fixation.

Courtesy: Asif M Ilyas

locking screws should be placed just short of the dorsal surface to avoid extensor tendon irritation. K-wires placed during the case may be kept. Bone grafting may also be considered, if there is a significant fracture void, although the utility of bone graft remains in question for acute fracture management.[15] Final intraoperative fluoroscopic images should be scrutinized for adequate fracture reduction, fixation stability and position of the hardware.

After fixation of all the fracture fragments, the stability of the DRUJ is assessed using a ballottement test with the forearm positioned in neutral, pronation and supination. An unstable DRUJ without an ulnar styloid fracture or a small avulsion should be splinted in supination. However, an unstable DRUJ with a large ulnar styloid fracture should be repaired with either screw fixation, plate fixation or a tension band construct.

The PQ may be repaired or allowed to simply drape back over the plate. The superficial fascial interval is reapproximated without sutures. The skin is closed in layers. Sterile dressings and a volar plaster splint is applied with the metacarpophalangeal joints and fingers free. Early motion is encouraged.

VOLAR PLATING: Pearls and Pitfalls

- Identifying the radiocarpal joint will assist in identifying the distal limit of exposure and plate position
- Releasing the brachioradialis can improve exposure of the radial column and also help restore radial inclination
- Articular fracture reduction may be performed through the fracture or by performing an extensile FCR approach by pronating the radial shaft out of the wound
- A volar plate can be used to hold a reduced fracture or aid in fracture reduction itself
- Distal subchondral locking screw positioning is critical and can often be difficult to assess fluoroscopically. Screws placed too long can result in dorsal extensor tendon injury. Screws placed inaccurately may violate the radiocarpal joint or DRUJ
- Lister's tubercle might conceal protrusion of the distal subchondral locking screws placing the EPL at particular risk for attritional rupture
- If a concomitant carpal tunnel release is indicated, avoid connecting the incision across the wrist as it may injure the palmar cutaneous branch of the median nerve. Rather, place a separate dedicated incision for the carpal tunnel release

Technique 5: Dorsal Plating

We recommend the standard dorsal approach through the third extensor compartment facilitating subperiosteal elevation of the dorsal surface of distal radius. The fracture site is visualized and irrigated clear of fracture hematoma and callus. The dorsal lip and articular surface is directly reduced. Radial styloid fractures and dorsoulnar fragments are reapproximated. K-wires should be used liberally to help reduce and provisionally fix fracture fragments. Articular incongruity can be reduced through the fracture site. Alternatively, unlike the volar side, where a capsulotomy is not recommended, a dorsal capsulotomy can be readily performed to directly visualize and reduce the articular surface. Like the volar side, a number of dorsal plates are available for application, including single unit plates versus complimentary 2 column plates meant to sit on each site of Lister's tubercle. Plate application is often facilitated with excision of Lister's tubercle. The goal of fixation is stable anatomical fixation that permits early motion. Final plate fixation should typically consist of minimum 2–3 cortical nonlocking shaft screws and 3–5 subchondral locking screws. Vigilance should be paid to avoid inadvertent screw placement in the radiocarpal joint or DRUJ. Bone grafting may also be considered, if there is a significant fracture void, although the utility of bone graft remains in question for acute fracture management. Final intraoperative fluoroscopic images should be scrutinized for adequate fracture reduction, fixation stability and position of the hardware.

Upon closure, the wrist capsule, if opened, is closed with 3-0 vicryl. The extensor retinaculum is repaired with 3-0 vicryl, while leaving the EPL outside of the repair. The skin is closed in layers. Sterile dressings and a volar plaster splint is applied with the metacarpophalangeal joints and fingers free. Early motion is encouraged.

DORSAL PLATING: Pearls and Pitfalls

- Soft tissue management is critical to avoid late hardware irritation. Skin flaps should be kept as full-thickness flaps. The dorsal surface should be exposed subperiosteally and should be repaired over the plate upon closure
- Unlike the volar side, radiocarpal capsulotomy and exposure of the articular surface can readily be performed on the dorsal side, while taking care to avoid inadvertent injury to the intercarpal ligaments
- Upon closure, leave the EPL outside of the extensor retinaculum to avoid tendon adhesion, constriction and attritional injury

Outcomes

Hundreds of studies have been published on the treatment of distal radius fractures. However, there is still no consensus on the best treatment of a distal radius fracture. The large amount of treatment options combined with many different fracture patterns makes it difficult to design one study that proves the best treatment in all situations. Studies comparing different modalities can give some insight in the cumulative risks and benefits of treatments over one another.

Handoll and Madhok's systematic review on distal radius fracture literature before 2000 suggests that external fixation and percutaneous pinning have better radiographic outcomes and may have improved functional outcomes as compared to closed reduction and casting.[16] The quality of the evidence was; however, suboptimal with many studies representing only small number of patients, lack of use of validated outcome measures and minimal allocation concealment.

Over the last decade study, methodology has improved significantly. However, the implants being used have also significantly changed. Newer studies have examined newer implants relative to their outcomes.[17-27] Wei et al. compared volar plating, dorsal radial column plating and external fixation.[27] The use of a locked volar plate led to better patient-reported outcomes in the first 3 months after fixation. However, at 6 months and 1 year, the outcomes of all three techniques evaluated in this study were found to be excellent, with minimal differences among them in terms of strength, motion and radiographic alignment. Several other studies have agreed with these results.

Open reduction internal fixation using fixed angle volar plating is becoming increasingly popular. Many different types of plates and plating techniques have been introduced the last decade. Unfortunately, evidence comparing the different techniques has not been published at the same pace. Ruch and Papadonikolakis published a level III case control study in which no difference was found in the disabilities of the arm, shoulder and hand scores between volar locked plating and dorsal nonlocked plating.[25] Koshimune et al. conducted a level II study concluding no clear radiographic advantage of volar locking plates over volar nonlocking plates.[23] However, a level I randomized clinical trial by Jakubietz et al. comparing locked dorsal with volar plating for distal radius fractures in the elderly focusing on early functional outcome identified improved motion, grip strength and pain in the volar plate group.[26]

Much has been published in all periarticular fracture management literature, on the association of intra-articular step-off and radiographic arthrosis. Kreder et al. demonstrated in their level I study that patients with residual articular step-off are 10 times more likely to develop radiographic arthrosis.[21,22] This confirms previous reports about this association.[3] However, the clinical impact of this arthrosis in the radiocarpal joint remains unclear. Different studies report discrepancies between radiological arthrosis and clinically symptomatic arthrosis. Goldfarb et al. demonstrated radiographic arthrosis was present in 13 out of 16 wrists, 16 years after a distal radius fracture.[24] However, despite the radiographic presence of arthrosis, clinically they demonstrated good function.

Complications

Complications are common following surgical management of distal radius fractures. Complications include soft tissue irritation, nerve injury, joint compromise and fracture problems. Discussion of complications will be presented relative to fixation techniques.

Complications of Kirschner Wire Fixation

Percutaneous K-wire fixation requires placing wires near essential structures like branches of the superficial radial nerve, radial artery and extensor tendons about the wrist. However, closed reduction and percutaneous pinning is considered to be relatively easy, minimally invasive and cost-efficient and it is a procedure that has been performed at length with few complications.[28-30] A recent Cochrane Review described no differences in terms of complications between ORIF or percutaneous K-wire fixation in the treatment of distal radius fractures.[31] Injury to structures during percutaneous K-wire placement can be minimized by placing small incisions and performing blunt dissection down to the bone. Similarly, K-wires may be placed by "oscillating" instead of "drilling" in order to avoid wrapping structures, such as cutaneous nerves, while advancing a wire.

Complications of External Fixation

Complications that may occur after external fixation include complex regional pain syndrome (CRPS), iatrogenic fracture at the pin sites, loss of reduction, injury to superficial branches of the radial nerve, or (most frequently) pin site infection. Iatrogenic nerve injury can be avoided by exposing the pin insertion site down to the cortical surface. Complex regional pain syndrome type 1 (also known as reflex sympathetic dystrophy) has been associated with external fixation, particularly when the fixator is used for prolonged periods and with excessive distraction. Similarly, CRPS type 2 (also known as causalgia) can result from direct injury to the radial sensory nerve. Loss of reduction in cases with extensive comminution is also possible following external fixation as reduction is a product of indirect reduction by ligamentotaxis. Fractures prone to secondary loss of reduction may benefit from augmentation with percutaneous K-wires. Pin tract infection is common and is best managed by predrilling pins to avoid loosening and thermal necrosis and diligent pin care postoperatively.

Complications of Intramedullary Nailing

Complications of intramedullary nailing of distal radius fractures include loss of reduction, inadvertent articular surface screw penetration, superficial radial sensory nerve injury and loss of motion. Risks for inadequate or loss of reduction is greatest with improper fracture selection. Use of an intramedullary nail should be limited to extra-articular of simple intra-articular fracture patterns and should be avoided in fractures with marginal rim or shear configurations, i.e. the volar or dorsal Barton's fractures and other AO type B patterns and in fractures with multiple and/or markedly displaced intra-articular fragments due to its limitations in fracture reduction and internal fixation.

Complications of Volar Plating

Complications of volar plating of the distal radius include loss of fixation, injury to the palmar cutaneous branch of the median nerve, postoperative carpal tunnel syndrome, extensor tendon rupture, flexor tendon injury, postoperative loss of motion and intra-articular screw placement. Loss of fixation is particularly serious when the volar lunate facet has not been adequately fixed. The result may be disruption and volar translation of the radiocarpal joint. When median nerve compression can be anticipated, for example in the case of preoperative symptoms of nerve compression or a predisposing high-energy mechanism of injury, a prophylactic carpal tunnel release should be readily performed. Preferably, a new incision should be made to accomplish this (except when an extensile volar ulnar approach is being used) to avoid inadvertent injury to branches of the palmar cutaneous branch of the median nerve. Extensor tendon injury may occur by subchondral locking screws placed too long dorsally. Flexor tendon injury may occur from prominence of the volar plate, particularly if the plate is placed too distal beyond the edge of the volar rim of the distal radius. Intra-articular screw placement in the radiocarpal joint and DRUJ can readily occur with poorly reduced fractures, careless screw placement and inadequate intra-operative radiographic assessment of the fracture and associated hardware.

Complications of Dorsal Plating

Even though reports of extensor tendon rupture were widespread with the first use of dorsal plates, the incidence of extensor tendon injury has decreased with improved technique and refined hardware. Other complications beyond extensor tendon injury following dorsal plating include loss of finger or wrist motion, loss of reduction and intra-articular screw placement. The same vigilant approach of assessing plate and screw positioning with fluoroscopy mentioned in the previous section on volar plate complications should also be upheld during dorsal plate fixation.

Authors' Preferred Management of Select Complications

Case 1: Intra-articular Screw Placement

A 62-year-old male, fell and incurred a simple intra-articular distal radius fracture (AO Type C1) with extensive osteopenia and dorsal comminution (Figs 5.31A to D). He underwent ORIF with a volar locking plate. Approximately 8 months postoperatively, he presented complaining of worsening pain and decreased range of motion. Plain radiographs demonstrated collapse of the fracture, a malpositioned volar plate and intra-articular screw placement.

Malpositioning of screws in volar plating for distal radius fractures is a relatively common complication.

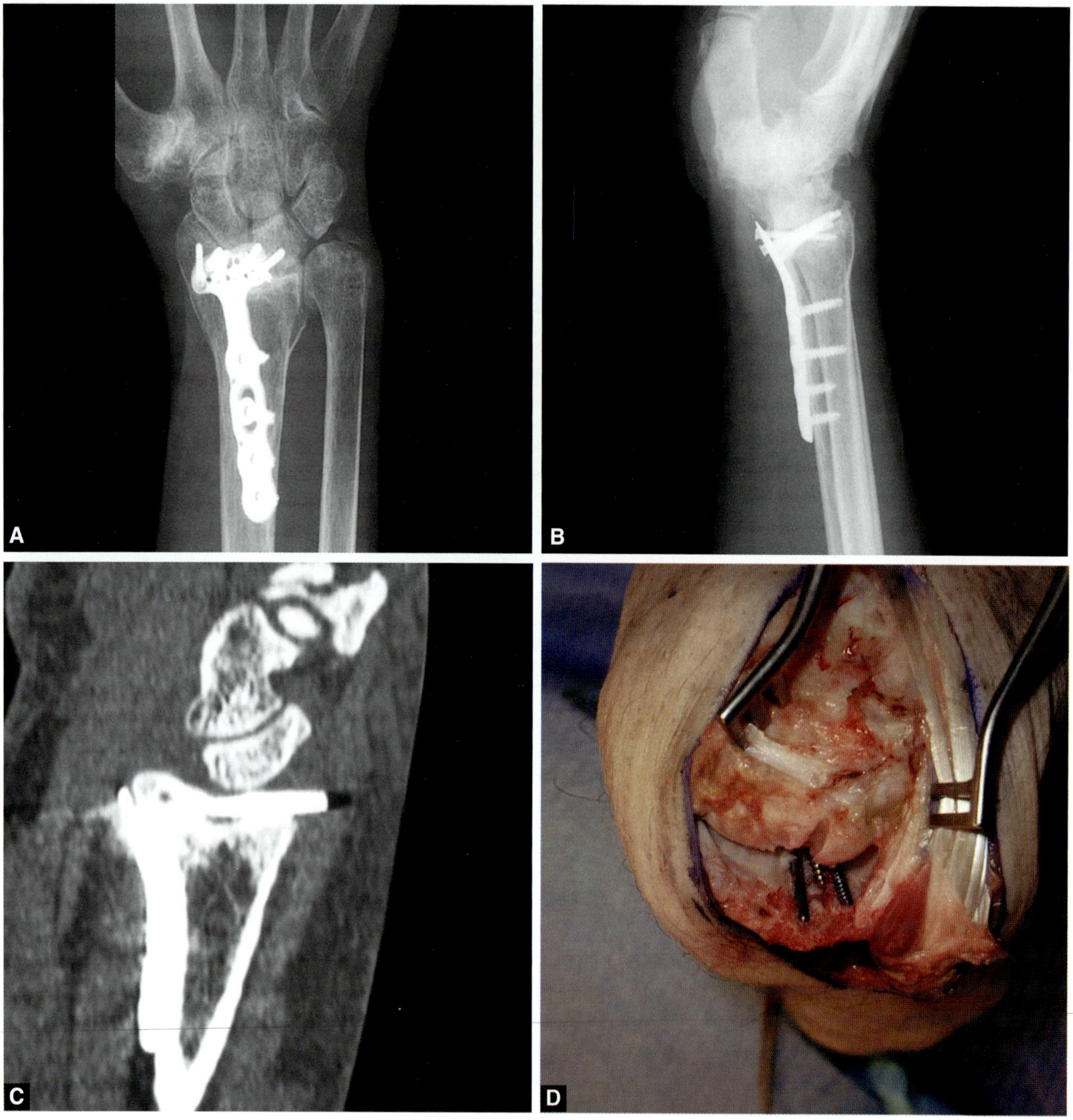

Figures 5.31A to D: A 62-year-old male fell and incurred a simple intra-articular distal radius fracture (AO Type C1) with extensive osteopenia and dorsal comminution. He underwent open reduction and internal fixation (ORIF) with a volar locking plate. Approximately, 8 months postoperatively, he presented complaining of worsening pain and decreased range of motion; (A and B) Plain radiographs demonstrated collapse of the fracture, a malpositioned volar plate and likely intra-articular screws. (C) CT scan confirmed the presence of intra-articular screw placement within the radiocarpal joint. The patient subsequently underwent removal of hardware and wrist arthrodesis; (D) Note the presence of screws in the radiocarpal joint and secondary joint destruction.

Soong et al. identified an incidence of malpositioned intra-articular hardware in 1.3% of cases.[32] Placement of screws in the joint can cause severe damage to the articular surface often leading to chronic pain and disability for the patient. Volar locking plates are currently available in fixed-angle and variable-angle versions. Fixed-angle versions are particularly prone to inadvertent intra-articular screw placement as appropriate screw placement is predicated upon appropriate positioning of the plate. If the plate is applied too distally, as in this case, screws may traverse the radiocarpal joint. If the plate is positioned too ulnarly, screws may traverse the DRUJ. Furthermore, if the fracture is inadequately reduced, the fixed-angle screws may again traverse a joint even if the plate is appropriately positioned on the volar cortex.

Vigilant intraoperative fluoroscopic evaluation of screw placement is central to avoiding intra-articular screw placement (Figs 5.32A to C). A true AP view should provide

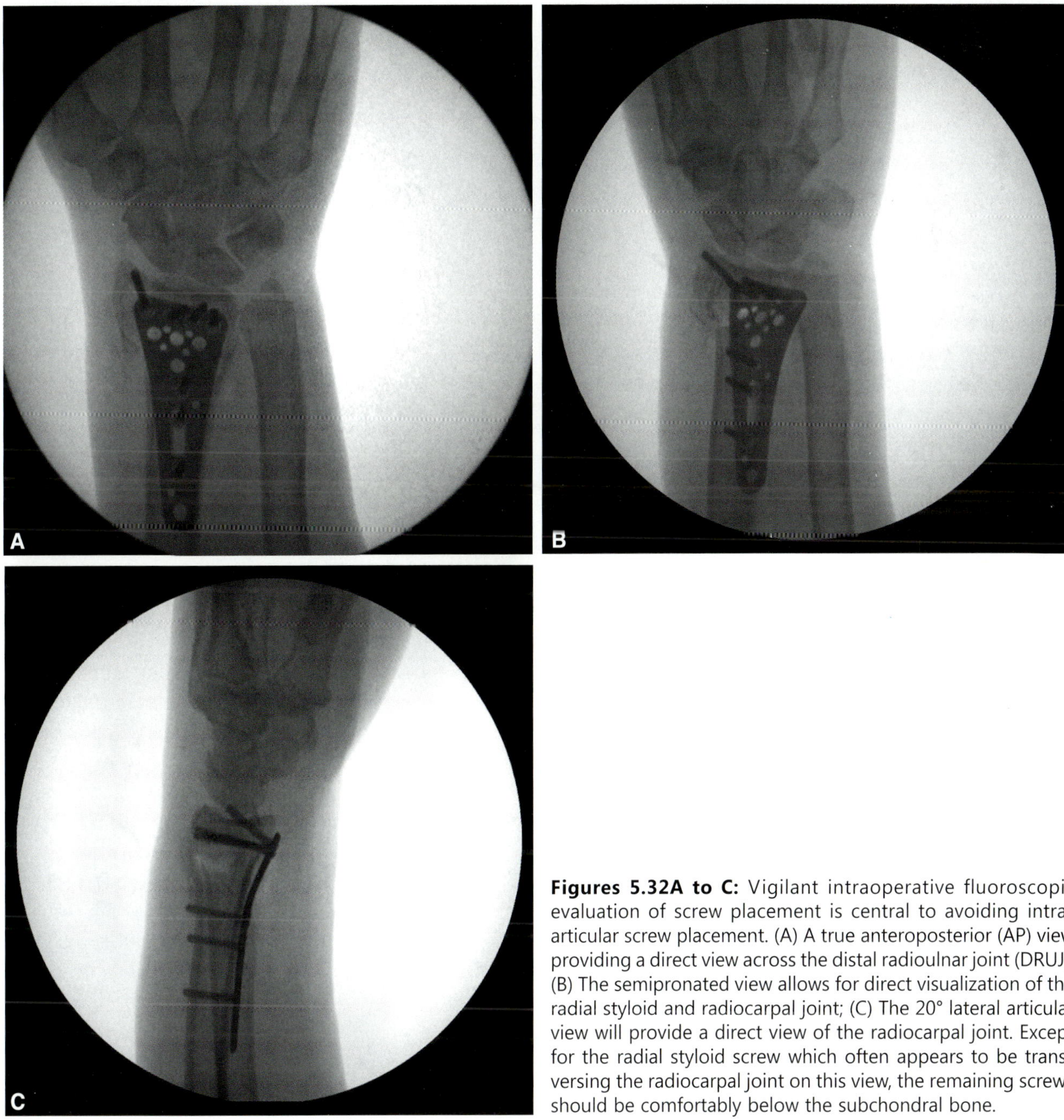

Figures 5.32A to C: Vigilant intraoperative fluoroscopic evaluation of screw placement is central to avoiding intra-articular screw placement. (A) A true anteroposterior (AP) view providing a direct view across the distal radioulnar joint (DRUJ); (B) The semipronated view allows for direct visualization of the radial styloid and radiocarpal joint; (C) The 20° lateral articular view will provide a direct view of the radiocarpal joint. Except for the radial styloid screw which often appears to be transversing the radiocarpal joint on this view, the remaining screws should be comfortably below the subchondral bone.

a clear view across the DRUJ. The DRUJ is semicircular and prone to subtle screw violation. Subsequently, the ulnar most screw should be positioned parallel or away from the DRUJ. The 20° lateral articular view will provide a direct view of the radiocarpal joint. Except for the radial styloid screw which often appears to be traversing the joint line, the remaining screws should be comfortably below the subchondral bone of the radiocarpal joint. The semipronated view allows for direct visualization of the radial syloid and radiocarpal joint. If suspicious persists, CT scanning can provide definitive evaluation of intra-articular screw placement.

In this case, three intra-articular screws were confirmed by CT. Also identified by CT and radiographs was the presence of extensive shortening of the distal radius and secondary radiocarpal arthrosis. Subsequently, the patient was offered removal of hardware and wrist arthrodesis.

Technique

The same volar incision was utilized to access the volar plate. Either the trans-FCR or modified Henry approach was utilized to access the deep volar compartment. The PQ was elevated, thereby exposing the volar plate. Screws were removed carefully making sure not to strip the screw heads. The universal screw removal system was available in case of stripped screws. The volar plate was elevated with a freer and carefully removed. The screw holes were debrided and the wound was washed. Next, attention was turned to the dorsal side and a formal wrist arthrodesis was performed.

Case 2: Loss of Reduction

A 36-year-old male, sustained a high-energy displaced and unstable volar shear fracture of the distal radius (AO Type B2) (Figs 5.33A to I). The fracture was treated with open reduction internal fixation using a volar locking plate. The patient was rehabilitated using the standard protocol including early motion until he returned 5 weeks postoperatively with an obvious deformity and decreased range of motion of the wrist. Standard radiographs demonstrated loss of reduction and volar displacement of the carpus.

The stability of comminuted distal radius fractures with volar fragmentation is not only determined by the reduction of the major fragments but also by the reduction of the small volar lunate facet fragment.[33] Understanding the articular fracture pattern is crucial in the treatment of these fractures. Often volar locking plates are placed too proximal for adequate fixation of lunate facet fractures. However, careful subchondral screw placement into the lunate facet fracture, either through or outside the plate, can stabilize this fragment or avoid late radiocarpal instability. Alternatively, a buttress pin or tension band fixation of the fragment can also secure stability (Figs 5.34A and B).

Technique

The same volar incision was utilized to access the volar plate. Either the trans-FCR or modified Henry approach is utilized to access the deep volar compartment. The PQ was elevated, thereby exposing the volar plate. The volar plate was carefully removed. The lunate facet fracture was identified and freed from the surrounding tissue. Reduction of the facet fracture was confirmed to result in reduction of the radiocarpal joint. The fragment was too small for screw fixation without any risk in intra-articular screw placement or possibly, blowing apart the fragment. Therefore, a buttress pin plate was selected and applied achieving excellent reduction of the lunate facet fracture fragment. Postoperatively, the wrist was placed in a splint and converted to a short arm cast. The patient was immobilized for 6 weeks until fracture union was confirmed.

Summary

Overall, distal radius fractures are most commonly treated nonsurgically. Surgical treatment goals are to restore articular alignment, minimizing deformity and early mobilization. Open reduction internal fixation using volar plating techniques is increasingly popular and has generally good clinical results. Advantages are earlier mobilization, less loss of function due to stiffness, less extensor tendon injury and less malunions. However, despite the increasing popularity, it is not proven to yield superior clinical results over other methods of internal fixation. More complex fractures, usually the result of a high-energy injury, often need a careful preoperative planning and a combination of operative techniques. Choosing the right treatment for each specific case remains a challenge, but should be predicated upon fracture pattern, fracture stability and patient needs. When properly performed, early treatment of unstable or

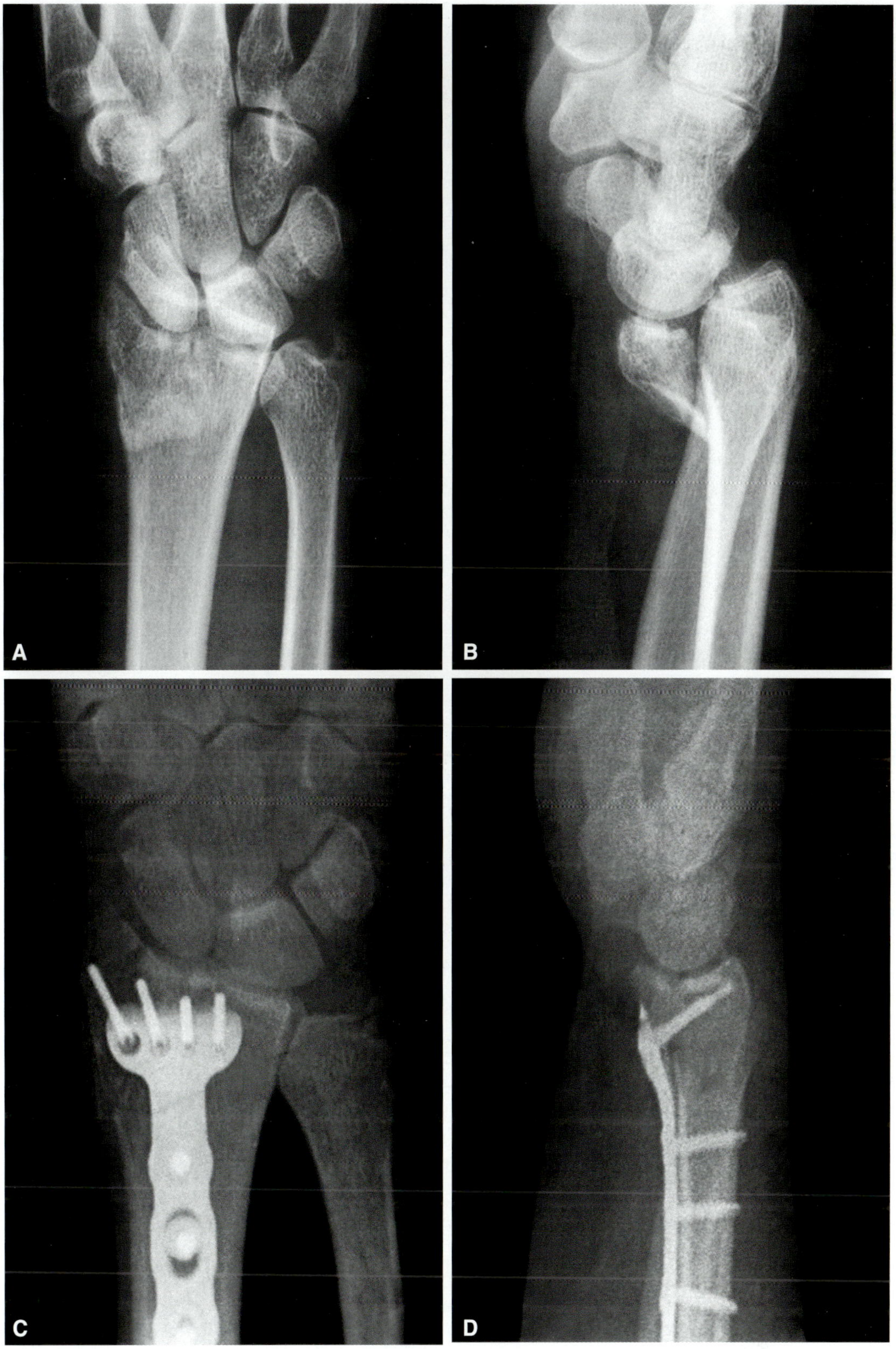

Figures 5.33A to D

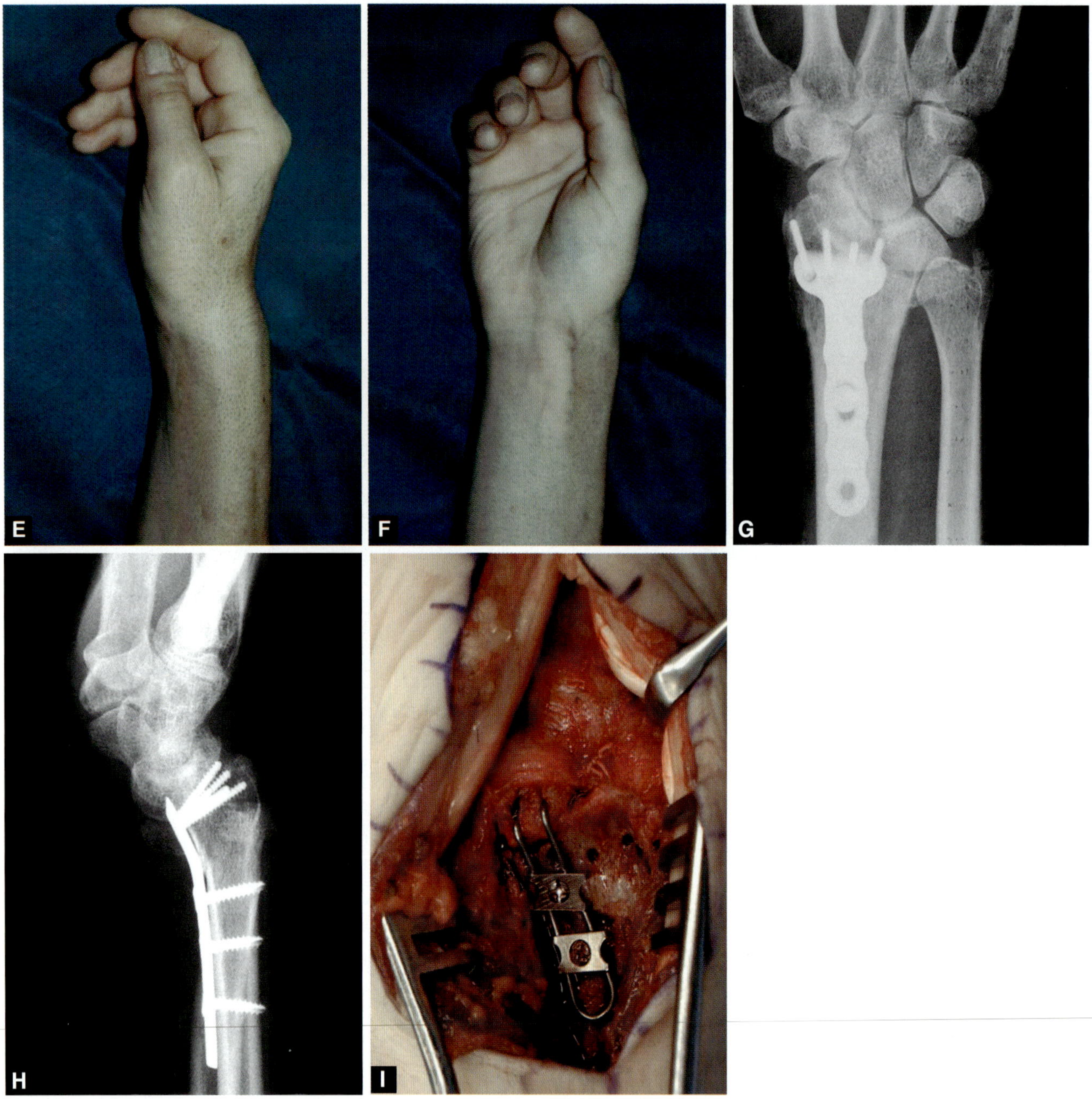

Figures 5.33A to I: This is a case of a 36-year-old male who sustained a high-energy (A and B) displaced and unstable volar shear fracture of the distal radius (AO Type B2), who underwent (C and D) open reduction internal fixation with a volar locking plate. Approximately, 5 weeks postoperatively, the patient returned with (E and F) an obvious deformity and decreased range of motion of the wrist; (G and H) Standard radiographs demonstrated loss of reduction and volar displacement of the carpus due to inadequate fixation of an unrecognized lunate facet fracture. The patient subsequently, underwent removal of the volar plate and (I) direct fixation of the lunate facet fragment with a buttress pin plate.

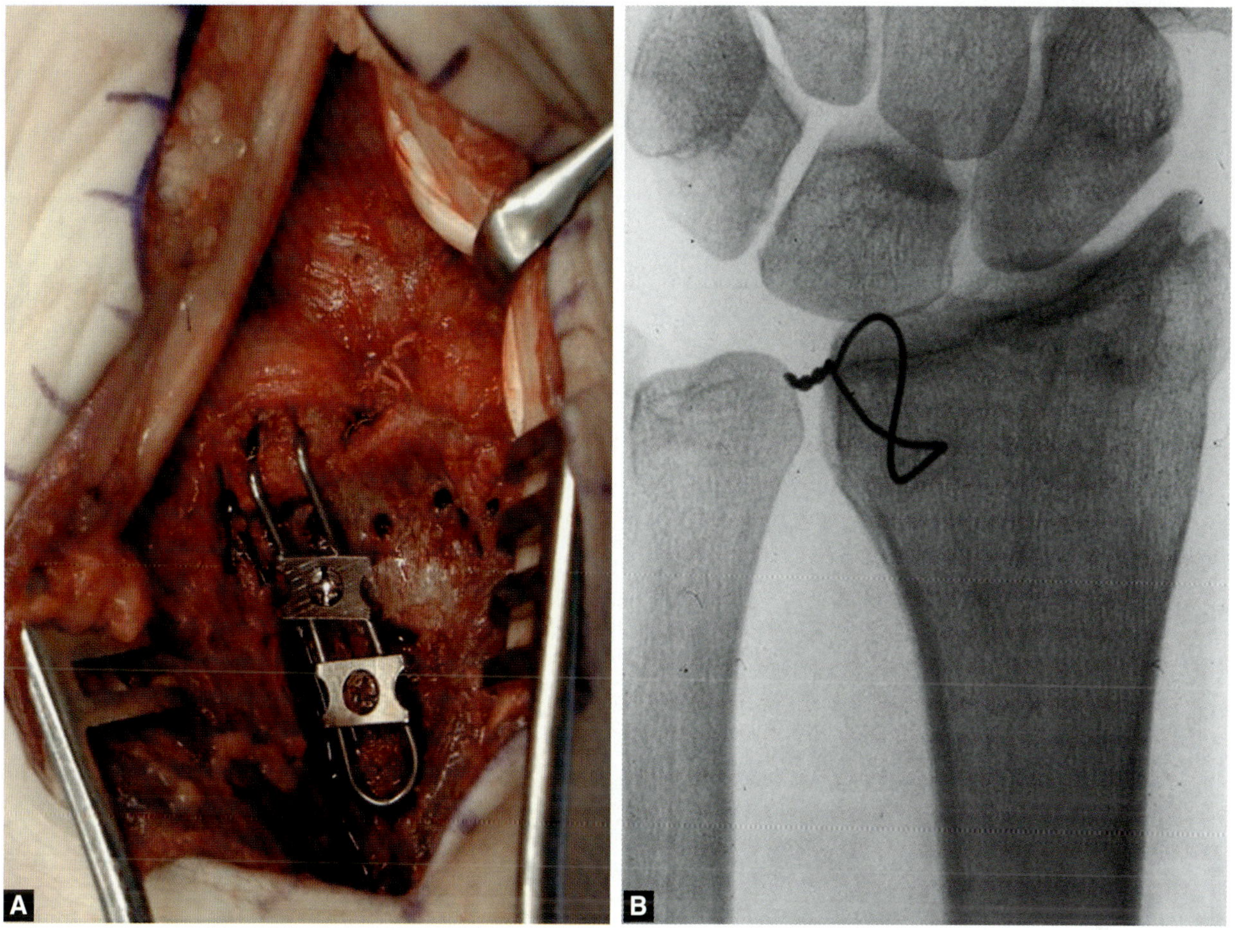

Figures 5.34A and B: Treatment options for lunate facet fractures include direct screw fixation either through or above the volar plate. Alternatively, the lunate facet may be fixed with a (A) buttress pin plate or (B) a tension band construct.

displaced distal radius fractures can yield good clinical results with a low complication rate.

References

1. Jupiter JB. Fractures of the distal end of the radius. J Bone Joint Surg Am. 1991;73(3):461-9.
2. Catalano LW 3rd, Cole RJ, Gelberman RH, et al. Displaced intra-articular fractures of the distal aspect of the radius. Long-term results in young adults after open reduction and internal fixation. J Bone Joint Surg Am. 1997;79(9):1290-302.
3. Knirk JL, Jupiter JB. Intra-articular fractures of the distal end of the radius in young adults. J Bone Joint Surg Am. 1986;68(5):647-59.
4. Moed BR, Kellam JF, Foster RJ, et al. Immediate internal fixation of open fractures of the diaphysis of the forearm. J Bone Joint Surg Am. 1986;68(7):1008-17.
5. Mueller ME, Nazarian S, Koch P, et al. The comprehensive classification of long bones. New York: Springer-Verlag. 1990;54-63.
6. Fernandez DL. Fractures of the distal radius: operative treatment. Instr Course Lect. 1993;42:73-88.
7. Rikli DA, Honigmann P, Babst R, et al. Intra-articular pressure measurement in the radioulnocarpal joint using a novel sensor: in vitro and in vivo results. J Hand Surg Am. 2007;32(1):67-75.
8. Viegas SF, Tencer AF, Cantrell J, et al. Load transfer characteristics of the wrist. Part II. Perilunate instability. J Hand Surg Am. 1987;12(6):978-85.
9. Jaremko JL, Lambert RG, Rowe BH, et al. Do radiographic indices of distal radius fracture reduction predict outcomes in older adults receiving conservative treatment? Clin Radiol. 2007;62(1):65-72.
10. Young BT, Rayan GM. Outcome following nonoperative treatment of displaced distal radius fractures in

low-demand patients older than 60 years. J Hand Surg Am. 2000;25(1):19-28.

11. Lafontaine M, Hardy D, Delince P. Stability assessment of distal radial fractures. Injury. 1989;20(4):208-10.
12. Mackenney PJ, McQueen MM, Elton R. Prediction of instability in distal radial fractures. J Bone Joint Surg Am. 2006;88(9):1944-51.
13. Orbay JL, Badia A, Indriago IR, et al. The extended flexor carpi radialis approach: a new perspective for the distal radius fracture. Tech Hand Up Extrem Surg. 2001;5(4):204-11.
14. Ilyas AM. Intramedullary fixation of distal radius fractures. J Hand Surg Am. 2009;34(2):341-6.
15. Tosti R, Ilyas AM. The role of bone grafting in distal radius fractures. J Hand Surg Am. 2010;35(12):2082-4.
16. Handoll HH, Madhok R. Surgical interventions for treating distal radial fractures in adults. Cochrane Database Syst Rev. 2003(3):CD003209.
17. Orbay JL, Fernandez DL. Volar fixed-angle plate fixation for unstable distal radius fractures in the elderly patient. J Hand Surg Am. 2004;29(1):96-102.
18. Grewal R, Perey B, Wilmink M, et al. A randomized prospective study on the treatment of intra-articular distal radius fractures: open reduction and internal fixation with dorsal plating versus mini open reduction, percutaneous fixation, and external fixation. J Hand Surg Am. 2005; 30(4):764-72.
19. Margaliot Z, Haase SC, Kotsis SV, et al. A meta-analysis of outcomes of external fixation versus plate osteosynthesis for unstable distal radius fractures. J Hand Surg Am. 2005; 30(6):1185-99.
20. Azzopardi T, Ehrendorfer S, Coulton T, et al. Unstable extra-articular fractures of the distal radius: a prospective, randomised study of immobilisation in a cast versus supplementary percutaneous pinning. J Bone Joint Surg Br. 2005; 87(6):837-40.
21. Kreder HJ, Agel J, McKee MD, et al. A randomized, controlled trial of distal radius fractures with metaphyseal displacement but without joint incongruity: closed reduction and casting versus closed reduction, spanning external fixation, and optional percutaneous K-wires. J Orthop Trauma. 2006;20(2):115-21.
22. Kreder HJ, Hanel DP, Agel J, et al. Indirect reduction and percutaneous fixation versus open reduction and internal fixation for displaced intra-articular fractures of the distal radius: a randomised, controlled trial. J Bone Joint Surg Br. 2005;87(6):829-36.
23. Koshimune M, Kamano M, Takamatsu K, et al. A randomized comparison of locking and non-locking palmar plating for unstable Colles' fractures in the elderly. J Hand Surg Br. 2005;30(5):499-503.
24. Goldfarb CA, Rudzki JR, Catalano LW, et al. Fifteen-year outcome of displaced intra-articular fractures of the distal radius. J Hand Surg Am. 2006;31(4):633-9.
25. Ruch DS, Papadonikolakis A. Volar versus dorsal plating in the management of intra-articular distal radius fractures. J Hand Surg Am. 2006;31(1):9-16.
26. Jakubietz RG, Gruenert JG, Kloss DF, et al. A randomised clinical study comparing palmar and dorsal fixed-angle plates for the internal fixation of AO C-type fractures of the distal radius in the elderly. J Hand Surg Eur Vol. 2008; 33(5):600-4.
27. Wei DH, Raizman NM, Bottino CJ, et al. Unstable distal radius fractures treated with external fixation, a radial column plate, or a volar plate. A prospective randomized trial. J Bone Joint Surg Am. 2009;91(7):1568-77.
28. Clancey GJ. Percutaneous Kirschner-wire fixation of Colles fractures. A prospective study of thirty cases. J Bone Joint Surg Am. 1984;66(7):1008-14.
29. Habernek H, Weinstabl R, Fialka C, et al. Unstable distal radius fractures treated by modified Kirschner wire pinning: anatomic considerations, technique, and results. J Trauma. 1994;36(1):83-8.
30. Mah ET, Atkinson RN. Percutaneous Kirschner wire stabilisation following closed reduction of Colles' fractures. J Hand Surg Br. 1992;17(1):55-62.
31. Handoll HH, Huntley JS, Madhok R. Different methods of external fixation for treating distal radial fractures in adults. Cochrane Database Syst Rev. 2008;(1):CD006522.
32. Soong M, van Leerdam R, Guitton TG, et al. Fracture of the distal radius: risk factors for complications after locked volar plate fixation. J Hand Surg Am. 2011;36(1):3-9.
33. Harness NG, Jupiter JB, Orbay JL, et al. Loss of fixation of the volar lunate facet fragment in fractures of the distal part of the radius. J Bone Joint Surg Am. 2004;86-A(9):1900-8.

Chapter 6

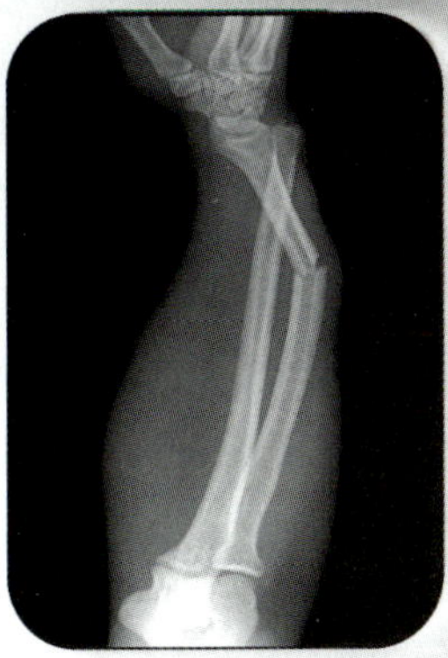

Forearm Fractures

Abtin Foroohar, River Elliott, Christina Endress, David Steinberg

Chapter Outline

Introduction
Diagnosis
Classification
Ulnar Shaft Fracture
Monteggia Fracture
Radial Shaft Fracture
Galeazzi Fracture
Both Bones Fracture
Surgical Indications
Ulnar Shaft Fracture
Monteggia Fracture
Radial Shaft Fracture
Galeazzi Fracture
Both Bones Fracture
Surgical Anatomy, Positioning and Approaches
Applied Anatomy
Positioning
Approaches
Surgical Techniques
Technique 1: Ulnar Shaft Fracture Fixation
Technique 2: Radial Shaft Fracture Fixation
Technique 3: Monteggia Fracture Fixation
Technique 4: Galeazzi Fracture Fixation
Technique 5: Both Bones Fracture Fixation
Technique 6: Intramedullary Fixation of Both Bones Fracture
Outcomes
Complications
Infection
Nonunion and Malunion
Synostosis
Authors' Preferred Management of Select Complications
Case 1: Nonunion
Case 2: Synostosis
Summary

Introduction

The forearm links the elbow to the wrist, but its critical function is the placement and maneuvering of the hand in space. It also enables rotation and power activities of the hand. Effective restoration of forearm function must be rooted in an appreciation of its anatomy. The focus of fracture management is protection of radial bow and ulnar length, as well as congruency of the proximal and distal radioulnar joints (PRUJ and DRUJ). The forearm is perhaps better viewed as a joint itself. Through its radioulnar articulations, proximally and distally, as well as its musculotendinous units, the forearm provides functional rotation by propelling the radius in an arc around the ulna. This arc of approximately 200° rotates around an axis from the center of the radial head proximally to the ulnar fovea distally (Fig. 6.1).[1] The ulna serves as the stable post of the forearm. The radius is the mobile segment and has a gentle dorsolateral bow that facilitates its rotation around the ulna. The interosseous membrane provides a dynamic link to each bone throughout its arc of motion or position. Preservation of the anatomic alignment of the ulna and radius, as well as stability of the PRUJ and DRUJ, is essential to successful recovery from forearm injuries.

The incidence of forearm fractures has varied according to different reports. McQueen et al. found only 5% of 2812 fractures to be pure diaphysial forearm injuries.[2] However, Chung et al. reported that radius and/or ulna fractures account for 44% of all forearm and hand fractures.[3]

The mechanisms of forearm injuries can be both low-energy injuries, such as fall on an outstretched hand to high energy, such as motor vehicle accidents and falls from heights. A subset of patients may suffer ballistic injuries to the forearm in which soft tissue and bony damage must also be carefully considered. Common injury patterns include isolated fractures of the radial shaft or ulnar shaft, both bone fractures, Galeazzi fractures and Monteggia fractures (Figs 6.2A to E).

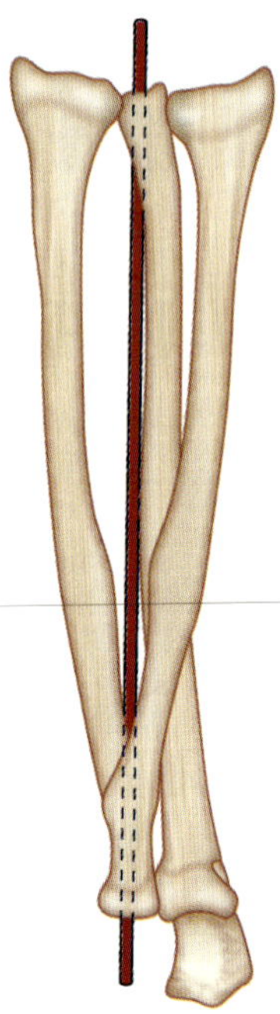

Figure 6.1: The forearm consists of the radius and ulna. The radius rotates around the ulna approximately 200° around an axis from the center of the radial head proximally to the ulnar fovea distally.

With the exception of minimally displaced ulnar shaft fractures, forearm fractures in the adult population typically require operative intervention. Early reports reviewing closed management of forearm fractures identified consistently poor outcomes including loss of rotation.[4,5] Knight and Purvis compared outcomes of conservative versus operative treatment in 100 forearm fractures. Of the nearly half which were treated conservatively, 71% had unsatisfactory results because of malunion and loss of motion.[5]

Diagnosis

Forearm fractures are typically the result of high-energy injuries and therefore, warrant a careful evaluation of the injured extremity, as well as an assessment of the overall patient. As such, grossly deformed and/or open fractures of the forearm should not serve as distractions from other life threatening injuries. Fractures of the forearm are readily evident by deformity of the forearm on exam and guarding of the extremity by the patient. The injured forearm should be closely inspected with attention to location of injury, degree of soft tissue damage, extent of swelling and for the possibility of an open fracture. Other than the tibia, forearm fractures have the highest ratio of open fractures. Because of the subcutaneous nature of the ulna and radius, all wounds should be scrutinized for the possibility of an open fracture.

A thorough neurovascular examination including motor function, sensibility and vascular status of the limb, is required. The forearm is particularly susceptible to the development of compartment syndrome. Pain level, as well as tension in forearm compartments should be vigilantly evaluated. Compartment pressures should be readily taken if suspicion exists. However, the diagnosis of compartment syndrome is a clinical one and if sufficient clinical suspicion exists then emergent fasciotomies should be undertaken. Moreover, in the noncompliant or obtunded patient, a low threshold for measuring intra-compartmental pressures of both the volar and dorsal forearm compartments must be maintained.

Diagnosis and fracture interpretation can be readily made with standard radiographs. Radiographic evaluation of the forearm should begin with anteroposterior (AP)

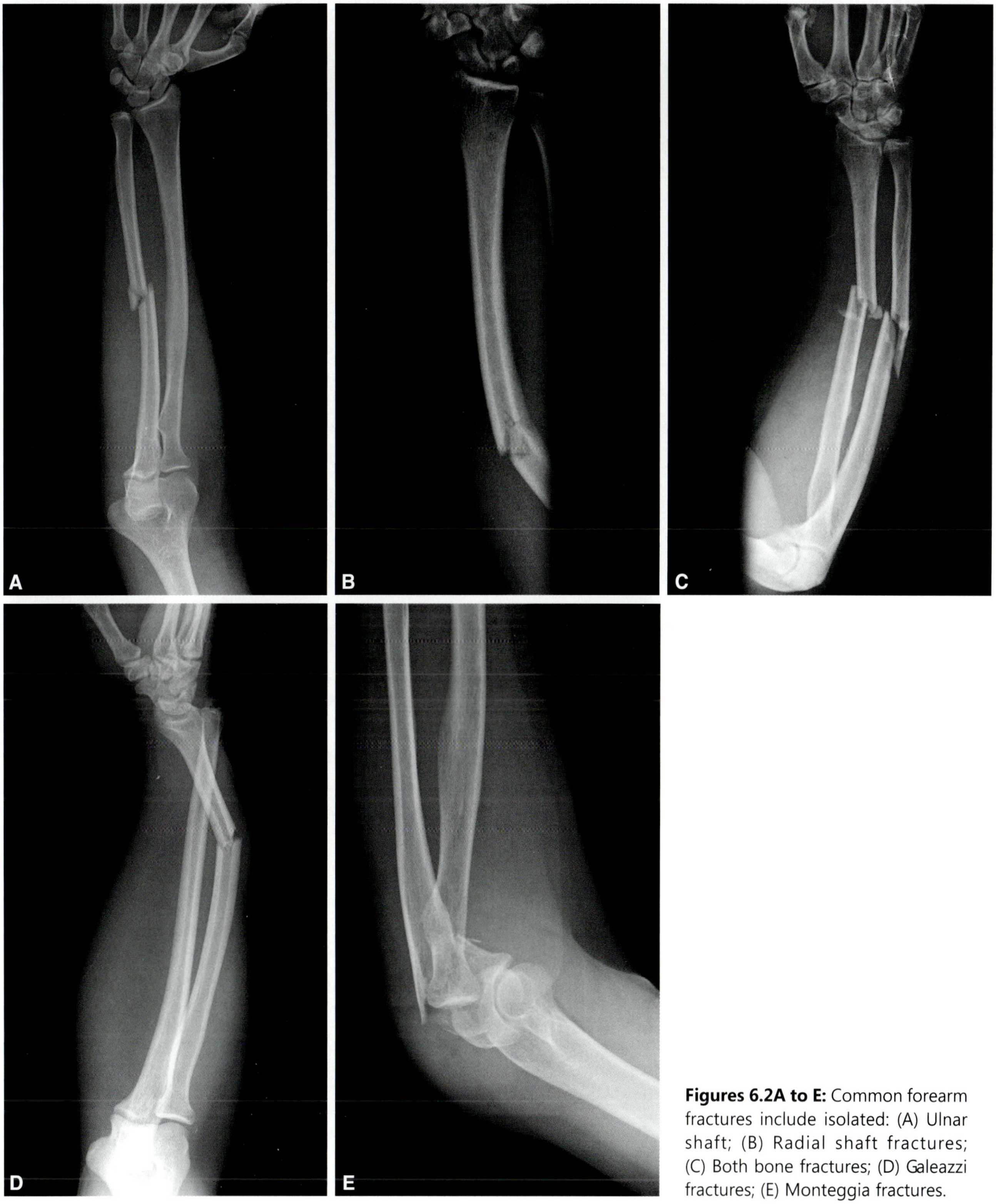

Figures 6.2A to E: Common forearm fractures include isolated: (A) Ulnar shaft; (B) Radial shaft fractures; (C) Both bone fractures; (D) Galeazzi fractures; (E) Monteggia fractures.

and lateral views of the forearm. In addition, dedicated AP and lateral views of both the wrist and elbow should be done to adequately examine the DRUJ and PRUJ, respectively. Advanced imaging is rarely indicated to make the initial diagnosis. A magnetic resonance imaging may be useful in the assessment of associated injuries, such as to the interosseous membrane. A computed tomography scan may be useful in assessing intra-articular injuries at the PRUJ and DRUJ.

Isolated fractures of the ulna represent the most common forearm fracture, and are often referred to as 'nightstick' fractures. On radiographs, they should be readily apparent. However, proximal ulnar shaft fractures must be scrutinized for any associated compromise of the PRUJ. In this case, a Monteggia fracture must be considered. Monteggia fractures are named after Giovanni Monteggia who prior to the advent of radiographs, described radiohumeral dislocation associated with proximal ulnar shaft fractures.[6] The ulna fracture associated with Monteggia fractures typically involve the proximal third of the ulnar shaft and should not involve the articular aspects of the olecranon process. Dedicated views of the elbow will assist in making the diagnosis.

In contrast, isolated radial shaft fractures have traditionally been considered to be uncommon and routinely warrant consideration for a Galeazzi injury. Galeazzi fractures, named after Ricardo Galeazzi, represent a fracture of the radial shaft with a concomitant disruption of the DRUJ.[7] Subsequently, any isolated shaft of the radius should be scrutinized for a possible injury to the DRUJ. However, isolated radial shaft fractures remain more common than a Galeazzi fractures, unless the radius fracture is within 7.5 cm of the DRUJ.[8] Dedicated views of the wrist will assist in making the diagnosis.

FOREARM FRACTURES DIAGNOSIS: Pearls and Pitfalls

- Open fractures are common warranting diligent physical examination of the forearm
- Compartment syndrome is common and any suspicion is sufficient to pursue emergent fasciotomy. However, if the pressures are in question or if the patient is obtunded, intracompartmental pressures should be obtained
- In addition to standard radiographic views of the forearm, dedicated views of both the wrist and elbow should be taken to assess both the PRUJ and DRUJ

Classification

Classification of forearm fractures can be done using the AO classification of fractures.[9] However, due to the cumbersome nature of this classification system and lack of value in directing treatment and indicating prognosis, the simple description of forearm fractures is often the best way to communicate these injuries.

Ulnar Shaft Fracture

The isolated ulnar shaft fracture, also known as a 'nightstick' injury, is usually caused by a direct blow to the ulna. Etiologies include blunt trauma and penetrating injuries. These fractures are most often described by fracture pattern and location. The forearm may be divided into proximal, middle and distal thirds. Comminution, displacement and rotation should also be noted.

Monteggia Fracture

Following the clinical description provided by the Italian physician Giovanni Monteggia (1762–1815), the fractures were further characterized by Jose Bado (1903-1977) radiographically by dividing them into 4 different patterns.[6] The Bado classification of Monteggia fractures is widely used to describe these injuries (Figs 6.3A to D):

Type I: Fracture of proximal or middle third of the ulna with anterior radial head dislocation

Type II: Fracture of proximal or middle third of the ulna with posterior radial head dislocation

Type III: Fracture of proximal or middle third of the ulna with lateral the radial head dislocation

Type IV: Fracture of the proximal or middle third of the ulna and radius with dislocation of the radial head.

Radial Shaft Fracture

Radial shaft fractures are described anatomically with emphasis on shortening, angulation, changes to the radial bow, as well as alterations to the DRUJ or PRUJ.

Galeazzi Fracture

Riccardo Galeazzi (1866–1952), also an Italian physician, worked extensively in orthopedic rehabilitation focusing on children and wounded soldiers from World War I. Galeazzi described a series of radial shaft fractures with

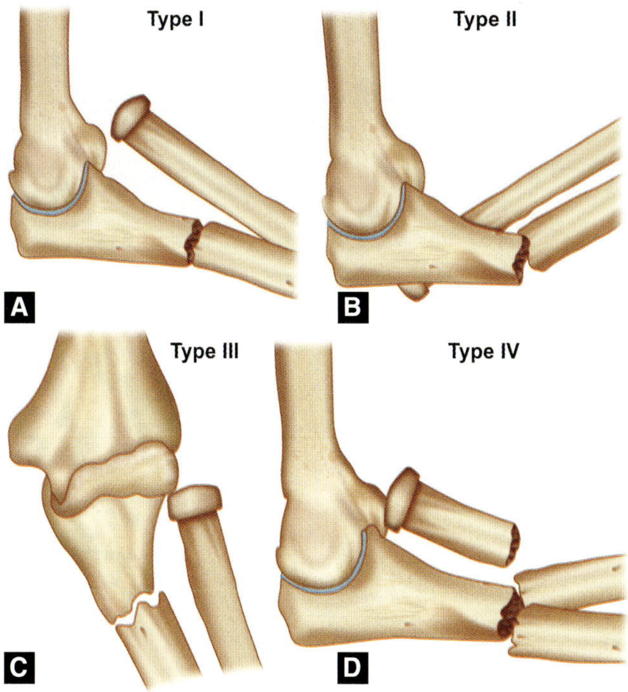

Figures 6.3A to D: The Bado classification of Monteggia fractures is based upon the status of the radial head. (A) Type I is an anterior dislocation of the radial head; (B) Type II is a posterior dislocation of the radial head; (C) Type III is a lateral dislocation of the radial head; and (D) Type IV involves a fracture of the proximal radius.

associated dislocation of the DRUJ.[10] The eponym continues to survive without further subclassification. The direction of the DRUJ dislocation occurs most commonly with the ulnar head dislocating dorsally and less commonly volarly. Any fracture of the radial shaft involving the junction of the middle and distal third should be scrutinized for possible concominant DRUJ instability. In particular, fractures involving the distal 7.5 cm of the radial shaft have the highest probability of an associated DRUJ injury than those occurring more proximally.[11]

Both Bones Fracture

Fractures of both the radial and ulnar shafts, often referred to as 'both bones fracture' are best described with descriptive terms. The forearm can be divided into proximal, middle and distal thirds with added assessments of comminution, angulation and displacement. The overall rotational integrity of the forearm, as well as any height or arc loss in the radius and ulna should also be assessed.

Surgical Indications

Operative treatment options for forearm fractures routinely involve open reduction and internal fixation. Plate fixation, affording anatomic reduction and early motion have consistently resulted in the best results.[12,13] Typically dynamic compression plates are utilized with three bicortical screws placed both above and below the fracture. In cases with osteopenia, locking screws may be utilized to increase rigidity of the construct. Alternatively, in cases with extensive comminution a bridge-plate construct may be utilized with or without locking screws.

Certain fracture patterns, most commonly isolated radius or ulnar shaft fractures or both bone fractures, can be treated with intramedullary fixation. This technique requires less surgical exposure and utilizes a straightforward fixation technique. Although anecdotally this technique has been associated with nonunions and synostosis, the available evidence indicates acceptable outcomes utilizing this technique with the appropriate indications.[14] We reserve the use of intramedullary fixation in cases with extensive soft tissue injury that would otherwise contraindicate surgical exposure and plate fixation of the fracture.

Ulnar Shaft Fracture

Isolated ulnar shaft fractures, unlike other forearm fractures, may reliably be treated nonoperatively.[15] Closed fractures of the distal two-thirds of the ulnar diaphysis with less than 50% displacement and 10° of angulation can be treated with approximately 4–6 weeks of immobilization. Various forms of immobilization have been described, all with similar outcomes.[16] Regardless of choice of immobilization, the elbow should not be immobilized for more than 3 weeks, particularly in the older patient.

In contrast, ulnar shaft fractures with greater than 50% displacement and greater than 10° of angulation are best treated with operative fixation. Fixation options include open reduction and dynamic compression plate fixation or intramedullary nailing. Fractures of the distal ulna, which are more susceptible to a concomitant DRUJ injury, are also best treated operatively.

Monteggia Fracture

Monteggia fractures should routinely be treated operatively. Anatomic reduction and fixation of the ulna is pivotal in securing a concentric and stable reduction of the radial head. In most cases, anatomic reduction of the ulna with plate fixation will facilitate indirect closed reduction of the radial head. However, in cases with an irreducible radial head, operative reduction of the radial head will be needed to clear any soft tissue interposition or button-holing through the capsule.

Radial Shaft Fracture

Unlike the ulna, isolated fractures of the radial shaft should routinely be treated operatively in order to restore the radial bow and length. The radius is vulnerable to extensive deforming forces. Shortening, excessive angulation and loss of radial bow have been associated with poor outcomes from compromised forearm rotation.[4,5] Fixation is best achieved with open reduction and plate fixation.

Galeazzi Fracture

Galeazzi fractures should routinely be treated operatively, requiring anatomic reduction of the radius to restore alignment of the DRUJ. Fixation is best achieved with plate fixation. Following fixation of the radius, stability of the DRUJ is assessed. If DRUJ stability is confirmed, early motion may be instituted. However if unstable, the forearm should be splinted in supination to reduce the DRUJ. Alternatively, open reduction and repair of the DRUJ may be necessary with or without associated pinning.

Both Bones Fracture

Both bones fracture, involving the shaft of both the radius and ulna, should routinely be treated operatively. Restoration of the radial bow and length, as well as stability of the ulnar shaft is central to achieving a successful outcome. Fixation options include open reduction and plate fixation or intramedullary fixation.

Surgical Anatomy, Positioning and Approaches

Applied Anatomy

A thorough understanding of forearm anatomy is essential for safe navigation and exposure of the radius and ulna. Both bones are covered with muscle and linked by the DRUJ distally, interosseous membrane in their midsubstance and the PRUJ proximally. Nerves susceptible to injury during exposure of the forearm includes the posterior interosseous nerve (PIN), the radial sensory nerve, the median nerve, the palmar cutaneous branch of the median nerve, the ulnar nerve and the dorsal ulnar sensory nerve. Vessels supplying the forearm include the radial artery and ulnar artery, which result from the bifurcation of the brachial artery in the proximal forearm.

The radial nerve travels between the brachioradialis and brachialis as it enters the forearm proximally. At the supinator, the radial nerve bifurcates into the radial sensory nerve and the PIN. The radial sensory nerve travels below the brachioradialis exiting superficially at the distal one third of the forearm and splitting into 2–4 branches. The PIN pierces the supinator before traveling with the posterior interosseous vessels along the interosseous membrane through the posterior compartment of the forearm. As the PIN traverses through the supinator, it travels directly over the posterior aspect of the proximal radial shaft. Here, the PIN is vulnerable to injury from dissection or placement of retractors or bone reduction forceps. The PIN can be protected during a lateral approach by pronating the forearm and avoiding placing retractors over the neck of the radius.

The median nerve travels with the brachial artery in the arm. After passing deep to the bicipital aponeurosis, the nerve travels between the two heads of the pronator teres to enter the volar proximal forearm. Distally the median nerve is located superficially beneath the palmaris longus tendon or ulnar and deep to the flexor carpi radialis (FCR) (if the palmaris longus is absent). The palmar cutaneous branch of the median nerve also runs between these two tendons, and typically branches from the median nerve 8.5 cm proximal to the distal wrist crease.

The ulnar nerve enters the forearm through the cubital tunnel. In the forearm, the nerve travels with the ulnar artery deep to the two heads of the flexor carpi ulnaris (FCU). Approximately 4 cm proximal to the ulnar styloid, the dorsal ulnar cutaneous nerve splits from the main nerve and crosses dorsally across the ulna to course superficially on its way to the dorsal hand. The dorsal ulnar sensory nerve is particularly susceptible to injury during dissection of the distal third of the ulna.

The brachial artery bifurcates into the radial and ulnar artery as it passes underneath the bicipital aponeurosis. In the proximal forearm, the radial artery travels deep to the muscle belly of the brachioradialis, while the ulnar artery travels deep to the muscle belly of the FCU with the ulnar nerve.

Positioning

For fractures of the forearm, the patient is typically placed in the supine position with the arm extended onto a hand table. Exposure of either the volar or dorsal surface of the radius can readily be achieved in this position. However, approaching the ulna in this position can sometimes be awkward but can be facilitated by using a bump or flexing the elbow. Use of a pneumatic tourniquet is essential to facilitate careful dissection.

Approaches

Henry Approach

The Henry approach is a safe and reliable approach to expose the distal two thirds of the volar surface of the radius. The incision is placed in line with the FCR tendon (Fig. 6.4A). Distally, the interval between the radial artery and the FCR tendon is developed. Proximally, the interval between the FCR and pronator teres muscle bellies and the brachioradialis is developed. The radial artery should be identified and carefully retracted radially throughout the exposure. Retraction of the flexor digitorum superficialis and profundus will provide direct exposure of the volar radius. Dissection below the brachioradialis must be done with care to avoid injury to the radial sensory nerve. Similarly, aggressive ulnar retraction can cause inadvertent injury to the median nerve.

The radius is covered with muscle along its entire length. The distal radius is covered by the pronator quadratus and exposure requires its release along its radial border. The middle third of the radius is covered by the pronator teres and exposure again requires its release along its radial border. The proximal third is covered by the supinator and exposure requires release along its ulnar border. However, due to the vulnerability of the PIN at this level during elevation of the supinator and the broad insertion of the biceps tendon, proximal third exposure of the radius is best achieved through a dorsal approach.

Thompson Approach

The Thompson approach provides reliable dorsal exposure to the radius. The incision is placed in line with Lister's tubercle and the lateral epicondyle (Fig. 6.4B). It utilizes the internervous plane between the radial nerve innervated extensor carpi radialis brevis and the PIN innervated extensor digitorum communis. In the mid-forearm, the interval can readily be identified by the crossing of the 'outcropping' extensor pollicis longus and abductor pollicis longus musculature. This approach is particularly useful for fractures of the proximal radial shaft as it permits direct identification of the PIN within the supinator.

Direct Ulnar Approach

Most fractures of the ulna may be exposed through a direct ulnar approach. This is a straightforward technique in which an incision is made over the subcutaneous border of the ulna (Fig. 6.4C) and the plane between the extensor carpi ulnaris (ECU) and the FCU is developed. The dorsal sensory branch of the ulnar nerve must be identified and protected during exposures of the distal third of the ulna.

Surgical Techniques

Technique 1: Ulnar Shaft Fracture Fixation

The patient should be placed supine on the operating room table. A nonsterile or sterile tourniquet can be placed above the elbow. With the patient in the supine position, approaching the ulna can be facilitated by positioning the arm in one of the three ways: (1) extended across the hand table, (2) held vertically with the elbow flexed or (3) placed across the patient's chest over a bump. The entire subcutaneous border of the ulna is palpable in most individuals. If not, a straight line drawn from the olecranon tip to the ulnar styloid will mirror its longitudinal axis (Fig. 6.4C). The planned surgical incision should be marked directly over the subcutaneous portion of the ulna according to the anticipated length needed for exposure and fixation. The approach to the ulnar shaft utilizes the internervous plane between the ECU and the FCU. The ECU is retracted dorsally and the FCU volarly. The ulnar neurovascular structures are potentially at risk during volar dissection of the FCU and are best protected by avoiding intramuscular dissection of the FCU. In addition, exposure

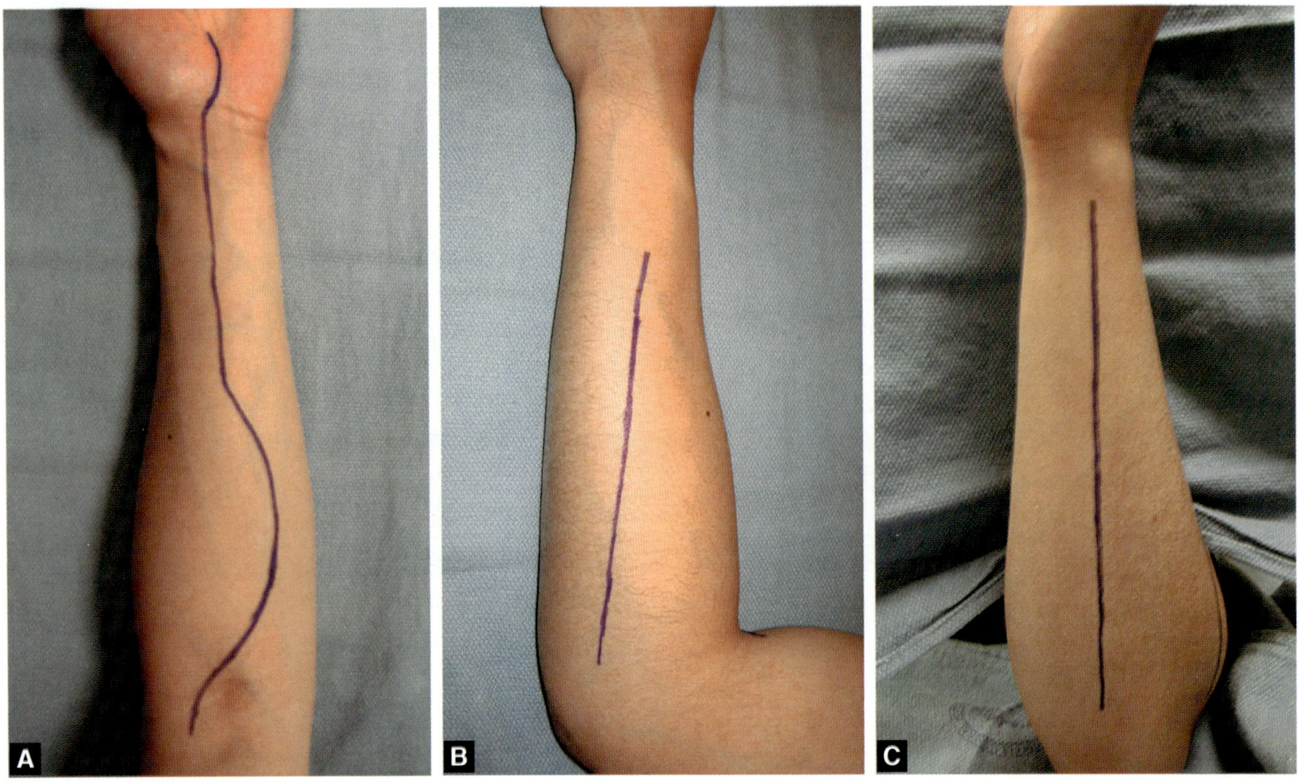

Figures 6.4A to C: Incision placement is dictated by the approach. (A) The volar Henry approach follows the flexor carpi radialis tendon; (B) The dorsal Thompson approach follows the line connecting the lateral epicondyle and Lister's tubercle; (C) The direct ulnar approach follows the subcutaneous border of the ulna and follows the line connecting the tip of the olecranon to the ulnar styloid.

of the distal third of the ulnar shaft should be done with care to avoid injury to the dorsal ulnar sensory nerve, which will cross the ulnar shaft approximately 6–8 cm proximal to the ulnar styloid.

Provisional fracture fixation may be achieved with reduction clamps or Kirschner (K) wires. Fractures with minimal comminution are directly reduced and fixed using small fragment dynamic compression plates (Figs 6.5A and B). Three bicortical screws should be placed on each side of the fracture. If obliquity of the fracture permits, the fracture may first be repaired with interfragmentary compression (lag) screws prior to plate application.

In comminuted fractures, smaller fragments with preserved soft tissue attachments may be lagged or provisionally approximated with K-wires to larger diaphyseal fragments prior to plate fixation, thus minimizing the number of fracture fragments to repair. However, in cases with extensive comminution that is not amenable to fixation, a bridge-plating technique can be employed where the comminution is bridged with a longer plate (Figs 6.6A and B). Furthermore, greater stability and rigidity of the construct can be obtained by utilizing locking plate and screws.

In smaller or thin individuals, where a dynamic compression plate may be too large, two one-third tubular plates may be stacked and fixed as a single unit. Furthermore, plate position should be considered as it can be applied straight ulnar, volar or dorsal. Ulnar placement of the plate allows for easier application but the plate may be palpable and potentially irritable to the patient. In contrast, both volar and dorsal placement offers more soft tissue coverage but require greater exposure and soft tissue dissection.

Prior to skin closure the reduction of the ulna, range of motion of the forearm and stability of both the DRUJ and PRUJ should be assessed. The skin is closed in layers. A splint may be applied; however is not necessary, assuming that stable fixation has been achieved.

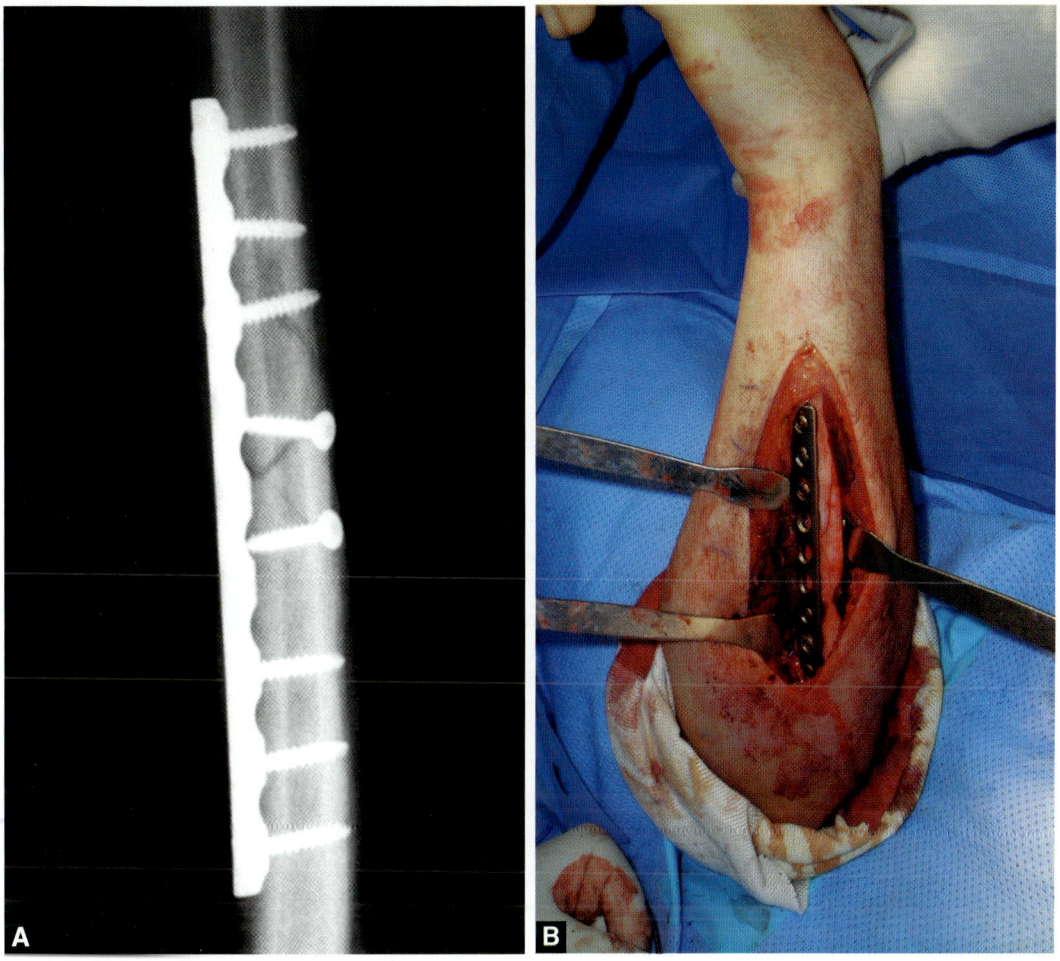

Figures 6.5A and B: This is a case of a displaced ulnar shaft fracture treated with a direct ulnar approach followed by (A) Lag screw fixation and dynamic compression plate fixation of the ulna; (B) Note the volar application of the plate to minimize hardware irritation.

Courtesy: Asif M Ilyas

ULNAR SHAFT FRACTURE FIXATION:
Pearls and Pitfalls

- With the patient in the supine position, approaching the ulna can be facilitated by positioning the arm in one of these three ways: (1) extended across the hand table, (2) held vertically with the elbow flexed or (3) placed across the patient's chest over a bump
- The ulnar neurovascular structures are potentially at risk during volar dissection and can be minimized by avoiding intramuscular dissection of the FCU
- Volar or dorsal placement of the plate minimizes hardware irritation
- In cases where a dynamic compression plate may be too large two one-third tubular plates may be stacked and fixed as a single unit
- In cases with excessive comminution or osteopenia, consider utilizing a locking bridge plate

Technique 2: Radial Shaft Fracture Fixation

For radial shaft fractures in the distal and middle thirds of the forearm, the authors recommend the volar Henry approach.[17] For proximal third fractures, a volar approach risks injury to the PIN as it branches off of the radial nerve proper and passes within the supinator muscle. For these

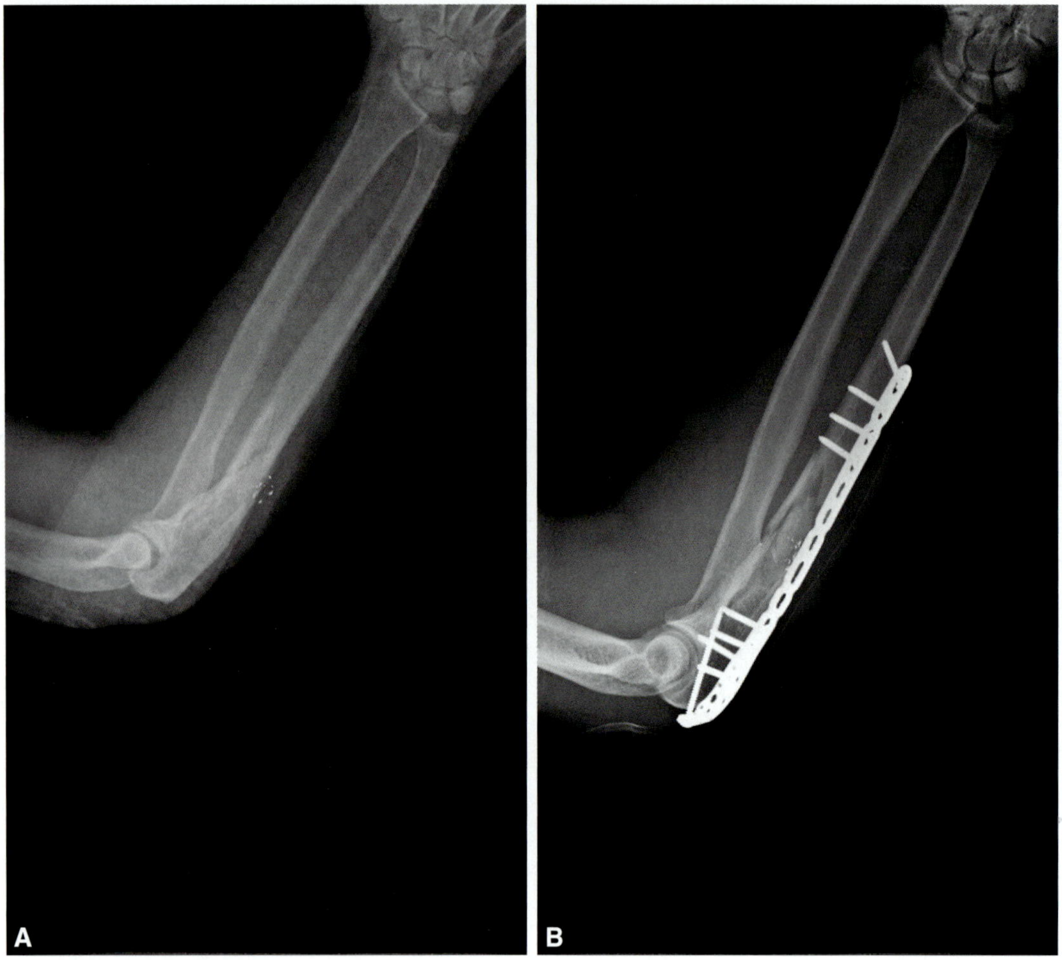

Figures 6.6A and B: This is a case of a (A) gunshot fracture of the ulnar shaft resulting in extensive comminution; (B) In order to provide stable fixation the fracture was treated with a locking bridge plate.

fractures, the authors recommend the dorsal Thompson approach.[18]

Volar Fixation of the Radius

Position the patient supine on the operating room table with the arm extended and supinated across a hand table. The incision is placed in line with the FCR tendon which should readily be palpable. Alternatively, the incision should be placed along a straight line placed from the lateral border of the biceps tendon proximally to the scaphoid tubercle distally. The Henry approach utilizes the internervous plane between the brachioradialis and the pronator teres proximally and the brachioradialis and FCR distally. Incise the forearm fascia over the FCR tendon. Identify the radial artery and retract it and the brachioradialis radially while the FCR and finger flexors are taken ulnarly. The interval is best developed bluntly. Branches from the radial artery may need to be cauterized for complete mobilization. Furthermore, radial dissection should be done carefully to avoid injury to the radial sensory nerve below the brachioradialis and the lateral antebrachial cutaneous nerve in the subcutaneous tissue. Similarly, the palmar cutaneous branch of the median nerve should be protected as it travels in the distal third of the forearm along the ulnar border of the FCR tendon. Deep dissection and exposure of the radius involve elevation of muscles directly covering the volar surface of the radius, including the pronator quadratus distally; the pronator teres over the middle third and the supinator proximally.

Provisional fracture fixation may be achieved with reduction clamps or K-wires. Fractures with minimal comminution are directly reduced and fixed using 3.5 mm small fragment dynamic compression plates (Figs 6.7A and B). Three bicortical screws should be placed on each side of the fracture. If obliquity of the fracture permits, the fracture may be first lagged using standard interfragmentary compression technique prior to plate application. In cases of osteopenia or extensive comminution, a locking plate may be utilized. Diligence must be paid to restore radial bow and avoid iatrogenic 'straightening' of the radius. Following plate fixation final alignment, radial bow, congruency of the DRUJ and PRUJ and overall forearm range of motion is assessed.

Dorsal Fixation of the Radius

The patient should be placed supine on the operating room table with the shoulder abducted and the forearm pronated on a hand table. The incision is placed along a line placed from the lateral epicondyle to Lister's tubercle. The internervous plan between the extensor carpi radialis brevis and the extensor digitorum communis is developed. Distally, the internervous plane continues between the extensor carpi radialis brevis and the extensor pollicis longus. Identification of the interval is facilitated with identification of the 'outcropping' muscles, abductor pollicis longus and extensor pollicis brevis, exiting between the internervous plane. These muscles are taken radially

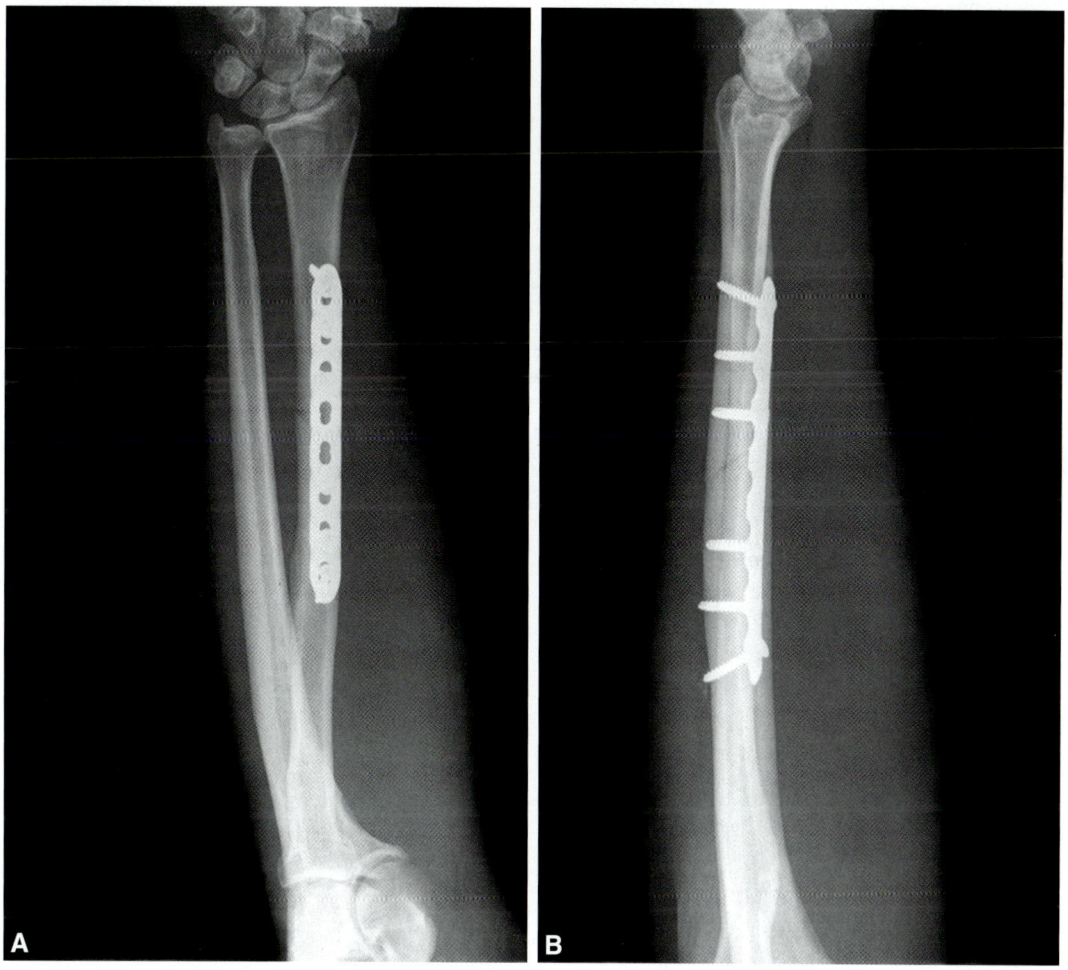

Figures 6.7A and B: This is a case of an isolated midshaft radius fracture without disruption of the distal radioulnar joints. (A and B) Fixation was achieved using a small fragment dynamic compression plate placed through Henry's volar approach to the forearm.

Courtesy: Asif M Ilyas

with the extensor carpi radialis brevis. Proximal dissection will reveal the supinator muscle. Prior to additional proximal exposure of the radius under the supinator, the PIN needs to be identified and protected. The PIN lies within the substance of the supinator muscle and emerges 1 cm proximal to the distal edge of the supinator. It runs perpendicularly to the direction of the supinator muscle fibers. With the nerve protected, the supinator can be detached from its insertion site by fully supinating the forearm and elevating the muscle along the radial-most border of the radius. Ulnar-sided dissection will be limited by the bicep's insertion into the radial tuberosity. Once the bone has been exposed, the fracture is reduced and stabilized in standard fashion.

RADIAL SHAFT FRACTURE FIXATION:
Pearls and Pitfalls

- For middle and distal third fractures use Henry's volar approach. For proximal third fractures use Thompson's dorsal approach
- 3.5 mm dynamic compression plates are the preferred method of fixation
- Hardware should be kept out of the interosseous space to avoid iatrogenic synostosis formation
- Carefully restore radial bow and avoid 'straightening' of the radius
- Confirm stability and congruency of the PRUJ and DRUJ following fixation

Technique 3: Monteggia Fracture Fixation

The surgical approach to the Monteggia fracture is similar to that of proximal ulnar shaft fracture described above. The most important factor in treating Monteggia fractures is achieving an anatomical reduction of the ulna (Figs 6.8A to D). This will typically lead to spontaneous reduction of the radial head. When the radial head is not readily reduced then interposition of soft tissue or buttonholing of the radial head through the posterior capsule must be suspected. Often interposed tissue, such as capsule, the common extensor origin or the anconeus may be preventing reduction. Once these structures are removed, given an anatomic reduction of the ulnar shaft, the radial head should readily reduce. To maintain stability, the torn collateral/capsular complex should be repaired. The forearm should be ranged to ensure stability throughout a functional range of motion. If despite removal of interposed tissue, appropriate fixation of the ulnar shaft and repair of injured collateral/capsular complex elbow is still unstable, a hinged external fixator may be applied.

MONTEGGIA FRACTURE FIXATION:
Pearls and Pitfalls

- Concentric reduction of the radial head is predicated upon anatomic reduction of the ulna
- Obstacles to reduction of the radial head, despite an anatomic reduction of the ulna, include buttonholing through the lateral ulnar collateral ligament complex, interposed capsule, common extensor origin or the anconeus musculature
- Associated fractures of the radial head are common and displaced or incarcerated fragments can also block reduction of the radiocapitellar joint

Technique 4: Galeazzi Fracture Fixation

Galeazzi fractures are approached through Henry's volar approach to the radius. Anatomic reduction of the radial shaft should readily lead to spontaneous and stable reduction of the DRUJ (Figs 6.9A to D). After fixation of the radius, the DRUJ should be ranged from full supination to full pronation to assess for stability. A preoperative examination of the contralateral hand can be very helpful in deciphering pathological versus normal laxity of the DRUJ for the patient. In the majority of cases, DRUJ remains stable and should be treated with closed immobilization for 4–6 weeks in supination to facilitate concentric reduction of the DRUJ, followed by mobilization. Alternatively, treatment with a Muenster cast in full supination for 4 weeks or a short-arm cast in neutral for 2 weeks followed by 4 weeks of functional bracing may also be utilized.

If the DRUJ is unstable, treatment options include prolonged immobilization, pinning, fixation of associated ulnar styloid fractures or direct repair of injured ligaments in an arthroscopic or open fashion (Figs 6.10A and B). Ulnar styloid fixation may be achieved with K-wires, screw or tension-band repair. If there is not an ulnar styloid fracture, the authors recommend percutaneous pinning of the DRUJ in neutral rotation with a 0.062 K-wire or larger K-wire across the DRUJ. Since there is a high-risk of pin breakage, the K-wire should be placed proud of both the radius and ulna to facilitate easy access and removal from either side.

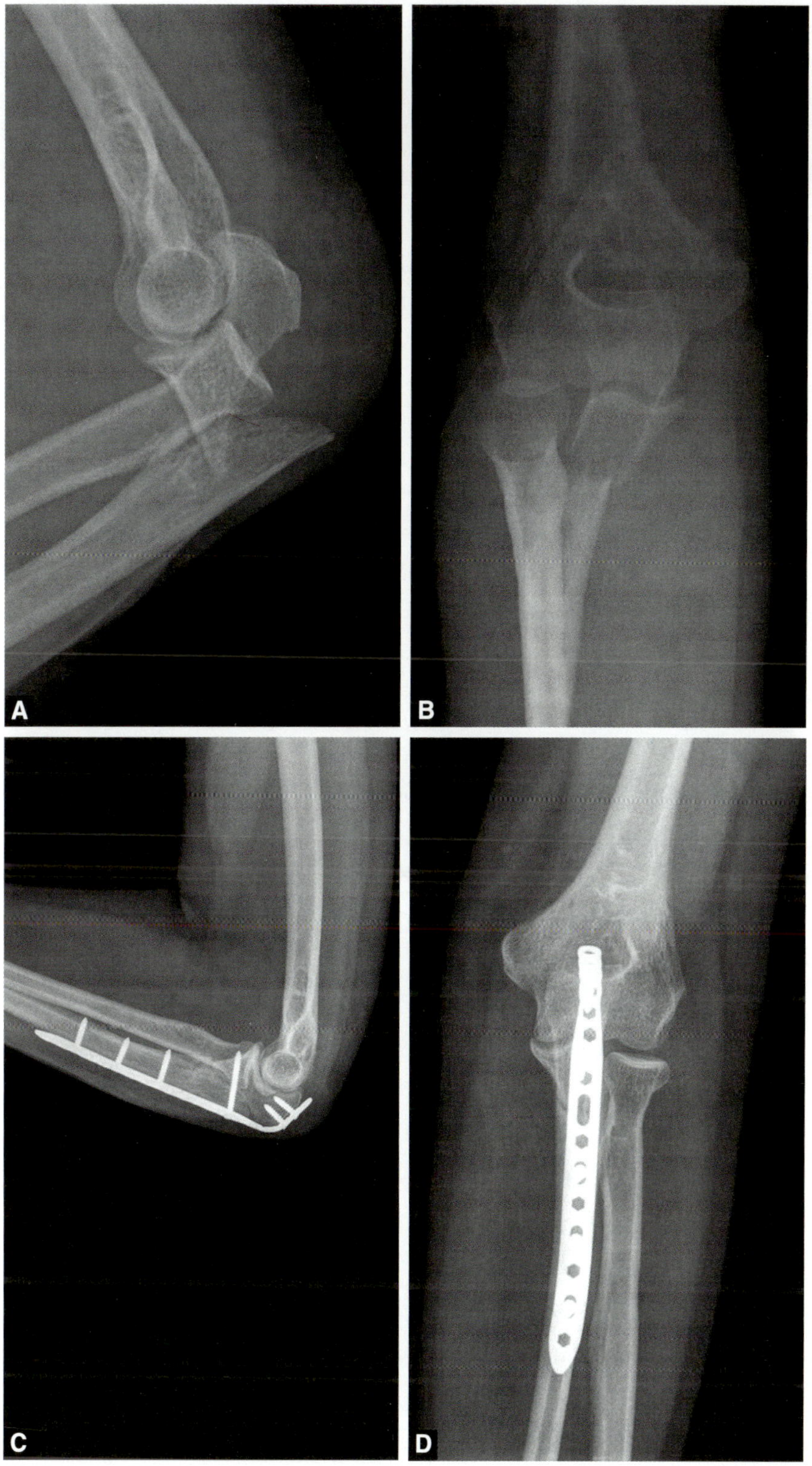

Figures 6.8A to D: This is a case of a (A and B) Monteggia fracture with a posterior dislocation of the radial head from a fall on the outstretched hand; (C and D) Fixation and reduction was achieved using a periarticular locking plate. Anatomic reduction of the ulna resulted in ready reduction of the radiocapitellar joint.

Courtesy: Asif M Ilyas

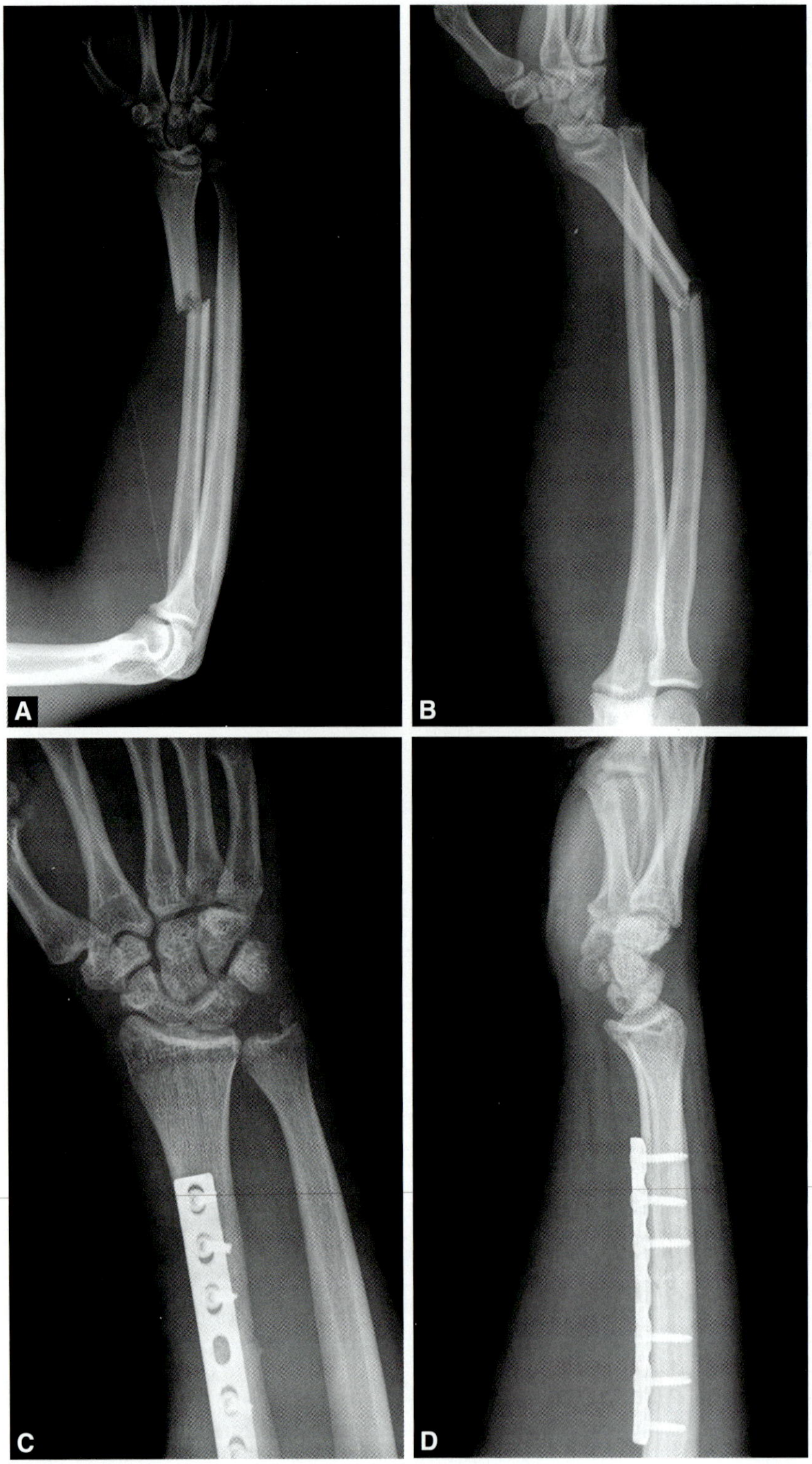

Figures 6.9A to D: This is a case of a 23-year-old male involved in a high-energy injury incurring a: (A and B) Galeazzi fracture. Note fracture of the radial shaft within 7 cm of the distal articular surface with concomitant dislocation of the distal radioulnar; (C and D) Following anatomic reduction and compression plate fixation of the radius the distal radioulnar joints assumed stable reduction.

Courtesy: Asif M Ilyas

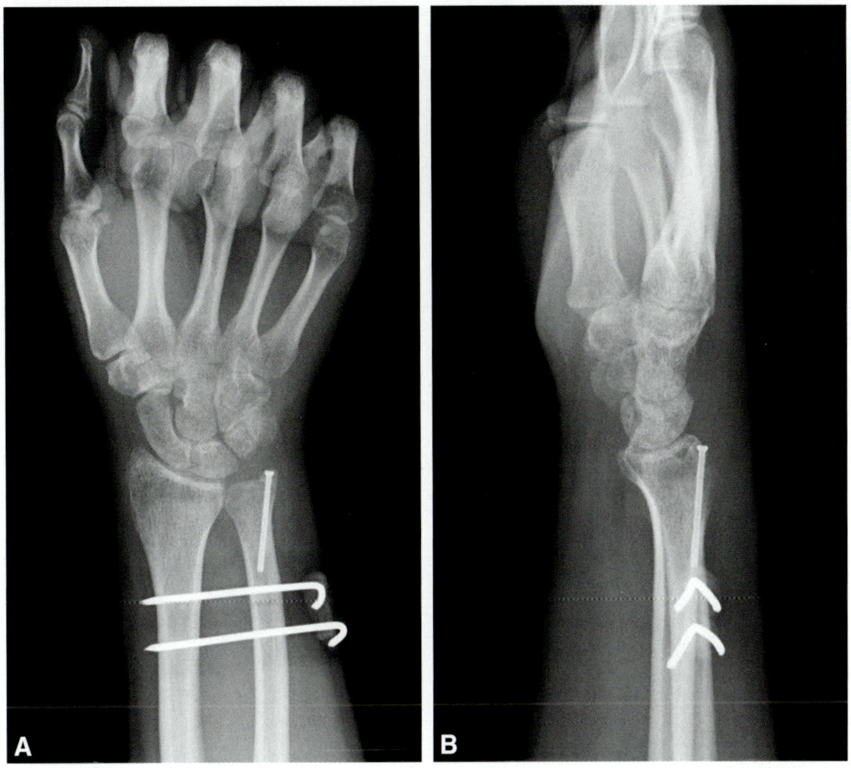

Figures 6.10A and B: In cases with persistent distal radioulnar joints (DRUJ) instability following stable anatomic fixation of the radius, treatment options include prolonged immobilization, pinning, fixation of associated ulnar styloid fractures or direct repair of injured ligaments in an arthroscopic or open fashion. (A and B) Note concentric reduction of the DRUJ following fixation of the ulnar styloid and pinning of the radius and ulna in a bicortical fashion with multiple K-wires.

In the case of an irreducible DRUJ, often the ECU or wrist capsule is interposed. The authors recommend approaching the wrist dorsally, opening the fifth extensor compartment and freeing any entrapped tendons. The dorsal cutaneous branch of ulnar nerve should be protected as it winds dorsally around the ulnar neck. Dissection should remain well radial to the ECU tendon sheath, which should be preserved. If a rent in the capsule is not encountered, a longitudinal arthrotomy is made just proximal to triangular fibrocartilage complex (TFCC). The TFCC and dorsal limb of the radioulnar ligament should not be violated. The joint is inspected and then reduced. The capsule is closed with nonabsorbable suture and tested for stability.

GALEAZZI FRACTURE FIXATION: Pearls and Pitfalls

- Patients with stable DRUJ reduction may be briefly immobilized followed by early motion. Alternatively, the forearm may be immobilized in supination for 4–6 weeks
- Persistent DRUJ instability after anatomic fixation of the radius may be addressed by fixation of an associated ulnar styloid fracture, repair of the radio-ulnar ligaments or pinning of the radius and ulna
- Pins placed across the DRUJ have a high risk of breakage and should be placed proud on both sides of the radius and ulna to facilitate easy access and removal

Technique 5: Both Bones Fracture Fixation

For concomitant fractures of the ulnar and radial shafts, the authors recommend open reduction and compression plate fixation through two separate incisions (Figs 6.11A to D). Both approaches are performed and the fractures exposed before definitive fixation is performed. Premature fixation of one bone may prevent anatomic reduction of the other.

The radial shaft fracture is exposed through the volar Henry approach. The ulnar shaft is exposed through the

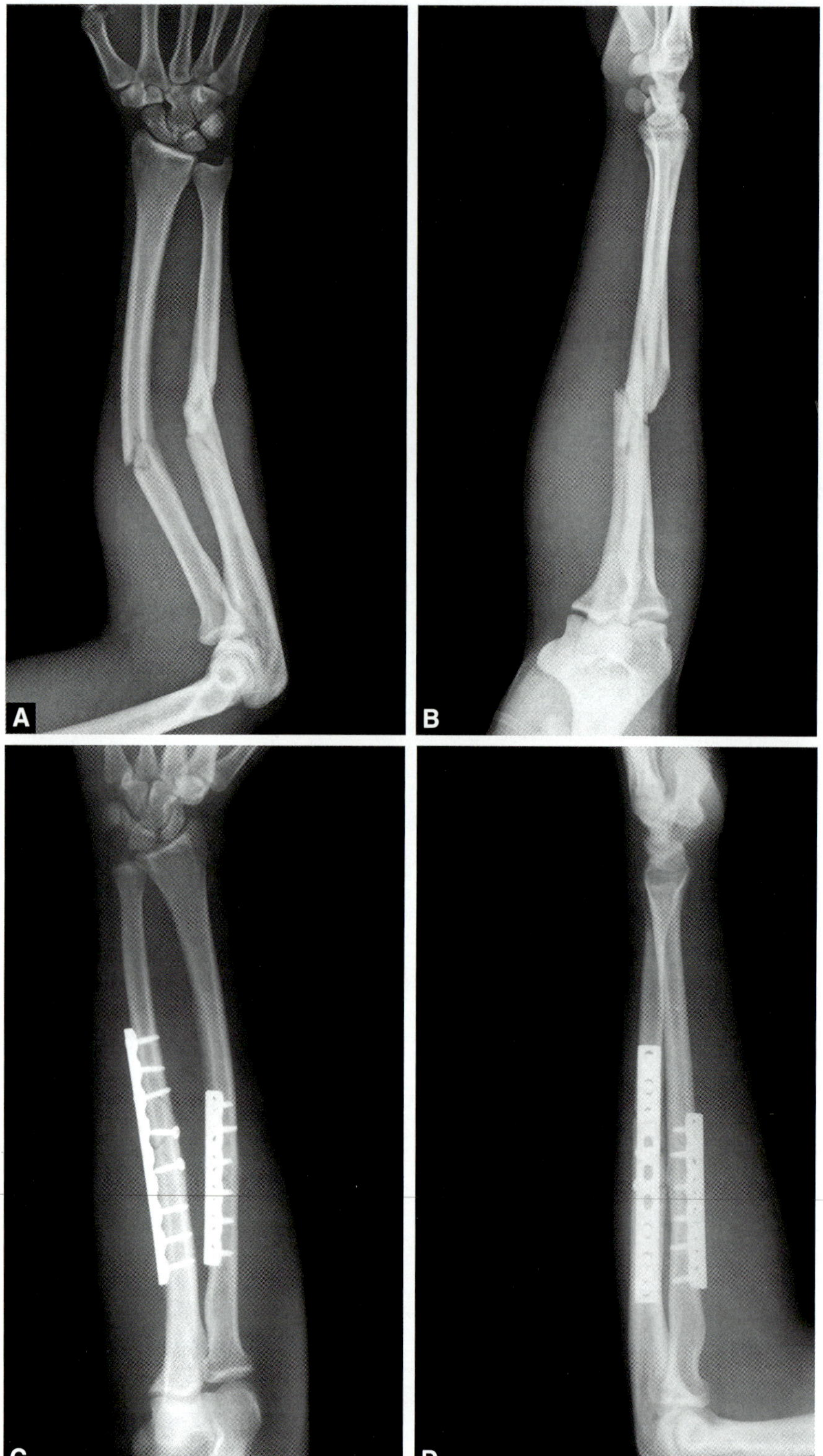

Figures 6.11A to D: This is a case of an 18-year-old male involved in a high-energy injury incurring a (A and B) both bones fracture of the forearm; (C and D) The patient was treated with open reduction and dynamic compression plate fixation of the radius and interfragmentary lag screw fixation of the ulna followed by neutralization plate application.

Courtesy: Asif M Ilyas

direct ulnar subcutaneous approach. Once the fractures are exposed, the less comminuted bone is provisionally fixed first, as this will more accurately restore normal length. Often this can be done with manual reduction and secure placement of reduction clamps. Then attention is turned to the other bone, making sure that it is still reducible. Dynamic compression plates are used to repair the fracture utilizing standard compression technique. Three 3.5 bicortical screws should be placed above and below each fracture. In cases with significant comminution compression, plate fixation should be avoided and bridging locked plate fixation be considered. Following fixation, the entire forearm should be evaluated fluoroscopically, ensuring satisfactory fracture fixation, congruency of the DRUJ and PRUJ and stable range of motion of the forearm.

BOTH BONES FRACTURE FIXATION: Pearls and Pitfalls

- Expose and provisionally reduce both the ulna and radius prior to definitive fixation of either bone
- Dynamic compression plates are the preferred method of fixation except in cases with extensive comminution
- Always check congruency and stability of the PRUJ and DRUJ following fixation
- Avoid hardware and dissection into the interosseous space in order to avoid secondary synostosis formation

Technique 6: Intramedullary Fixation of Both Bones fracture

Intramedullary fixation of both bones fractures has the potential advantages of a percutaneous technique with less soft tissue dissection. This technique may be particularly advantageous in cases with extensive soft tissue injury or segmental bony injuries where plating may be difficult or result in exposed hardware following fixation.

The patient should be placed supine on the operating room table with the forearm extended on a hand table. The radius is approached through a 2–3 cm longitudinal incision placed radial to Lister's tubercle. Blunt dissection is used to prevent injury to branches of the superficial sensory radial nerve. The extensor retinaculum is identified and incised longitudinally leaving the proximal third intact. The interval between the extensor carpi radialis brevis and the extensor pollicis longus is developed. The entry portal is located in line with the extensor carpi radialis brevis tendon, 5 mm proximal to the articular surface of the radius. Intramedullary techniques are predicated upon successful closed reduction of the fracture. During intramedullary fixation of the radius, restoration of the radial bow is critical. Awl entry, canal broaching and canal reaming should proceed as per the implant's manufacturer's technique. The nail length is measured, inserted and with the fracture reduced the nail is interlocked. The nail should be of adequate length but it typically will not cross proximally beyond the radial tuberosity.

The ulna is approached through the olecranon tip with a 1–2 cm longitudinal incision (Figs 6.12A to F). Dissection is carried through the subcutaneous tissues down to the triceps tendon. The entry portal for the ulna is located in the center of the olecranon and in line with its medullary canal. Awl entry, canal broaching and canal reaming should proceed as per the implant's manufacturer's technique. The nail is measured to the appropriate length, inserted and with the fracture reduced the nail is interlocked.

INTRAMEDULLARY FIXATION OF BOTH BONES FRACTURE: Pearls and Pitfalls

- Intramedullary nails may be used in cases of extensive soft tissue injury or segmental fracture patterns
- The contralateral arm may be template to determine nail length in cases of severe comminution
- Intramedullary nailing is predicated upon successful closed reduction of fractures and restoration of the radial bow

Outcomes

The outcomes of forearm fractures, since the advent of internal fixation, have been very good. Anderson et al. reviewed forearm fractures fixed with compression plating and reported a 97.9% rate of union for the radius, a 96.3% rate of union for the ulna and a 2.9 % rate of infection or nonunion.[12] They also presented a functional scale to assess outcomes.

Chapmen et al. evaluated 129 diaphyseal forearm fractures fixed with 3.5 mm compression plates.[13]

They found a 98% union rate and 92% rate of excellent and satisfactory results based on the Anderson forearm evaluation. They reported a 2.3% infection rate. Despite high rate of union, more recent studies have noted a moderate decrease in functional outcomes including forearm, wrist and grip strength.[19,20]

Complications

Complications following surgical fixation of forearm fractures are uncommon. The most common complications include infection, malunion, nonunion, nerve injury and synostosis formation.

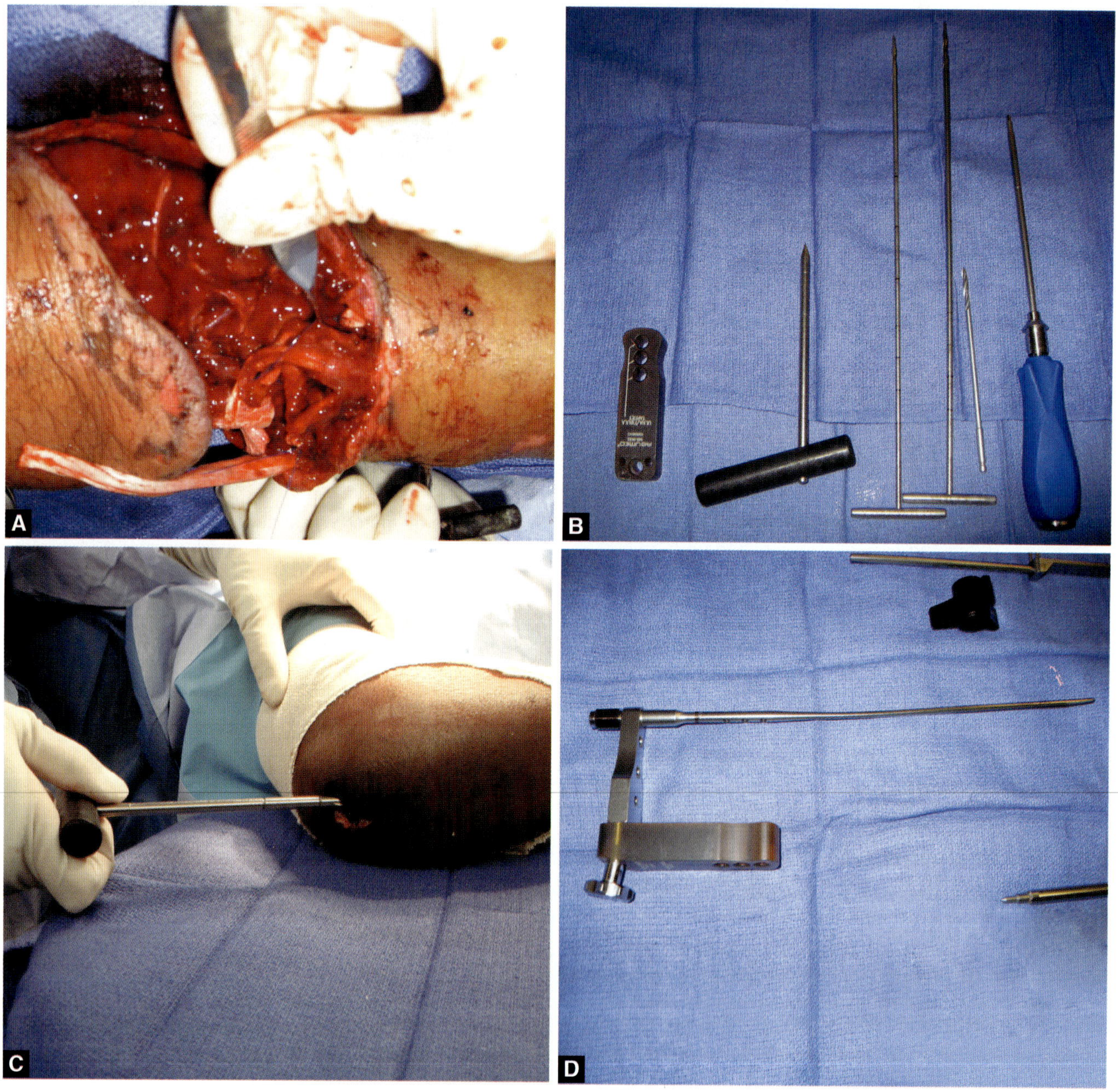

Figures 6.12A to D

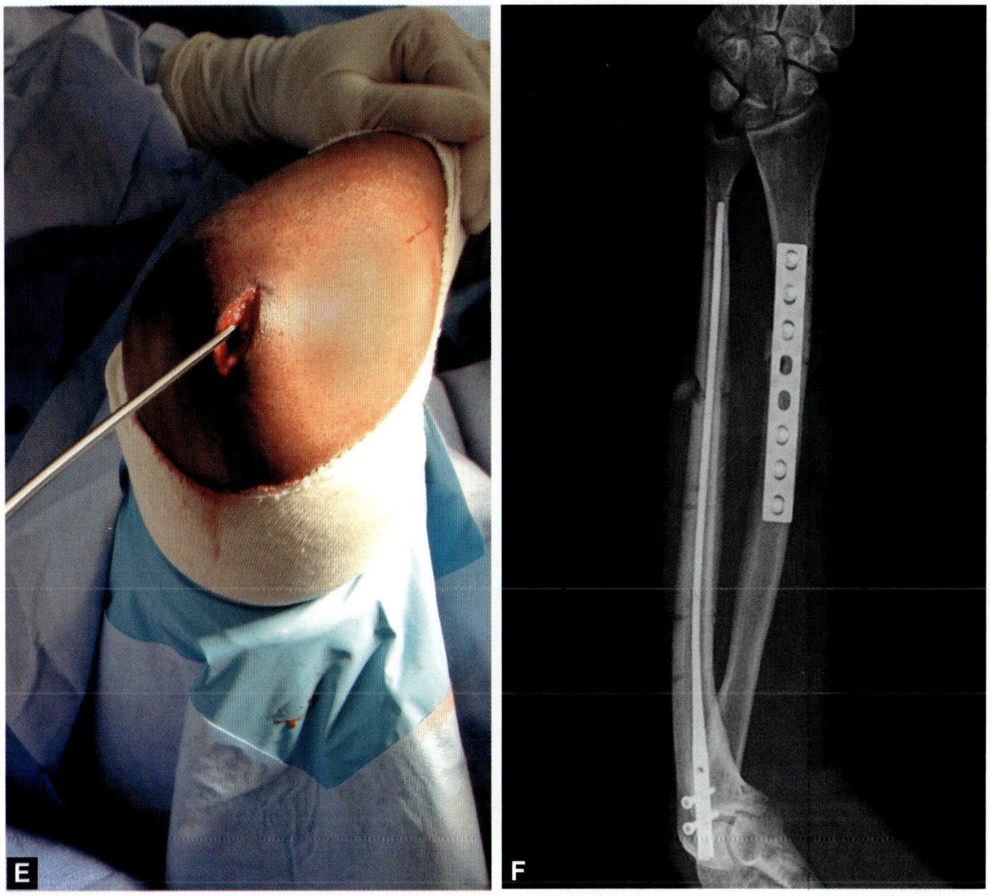

Figures 6.12A to F: This is a case of a 23-year-old male involved in a high-energy motorcycle accident resulting in a (A) mangled arm with an open and grossly contaminated both bones fracture of the forearm. The patient was initially treated with external fixation of the ulna followed by staged repair of the soft tissue injuries and skin coverage. Due to compromised soft tissue coverage of the ulna intramedullary fixation of the ulna was selected; (B) The necessary hardware is demonstrated including the starting awl, calibrated broach and interlocking screw jig, drill and screwdriver; (C) The ulna is entered posteriorly through the olecranon with a starting awl; (D) The assembled nail and insertion jig is shown; (E) The nail is inserted, the fracture reduced and the nail is interlocked under fluoroscopy; (F) Final radiograph confirm reduction and intramedullary fixation of the ulna.
Courtesy: Saqib Rehman

Infection

Infections after internal fixation in the forearm are uncommon.[12,21] Surgical technique, as well as host factors may affect the risk in a given patient. Treatment is determined by time or presentation of the infection relative to the original injury and fixation, extent of fracture healing and severity of infection.

Acutely, patients will present with erythema, induration or drainage. Fevers, chills, leukocytosis and elevated C-reactive protein and erythrocyte sedimentation rate may be expected. With time, infections will demonstrate changes on radiographs (Fig. 6.13). If an abscess or collection is suspected then incision, drainage, debridement of affected tissue and antibiotic treatment is required. If an infection can be controlled with debridement and antibiotics, then removal of hardware, especially in the face of an unhealed fracture is not recommended. Recent studies have shown that with early debridement and culture specific antibiotic treatment, fracture union can be achieved in a significant portion of patients with postoperative infections with the hardware retained.[22] For more extensive infections, hardware removal, aggressive debridement and placement of antibiotic impregnated beads may be required.

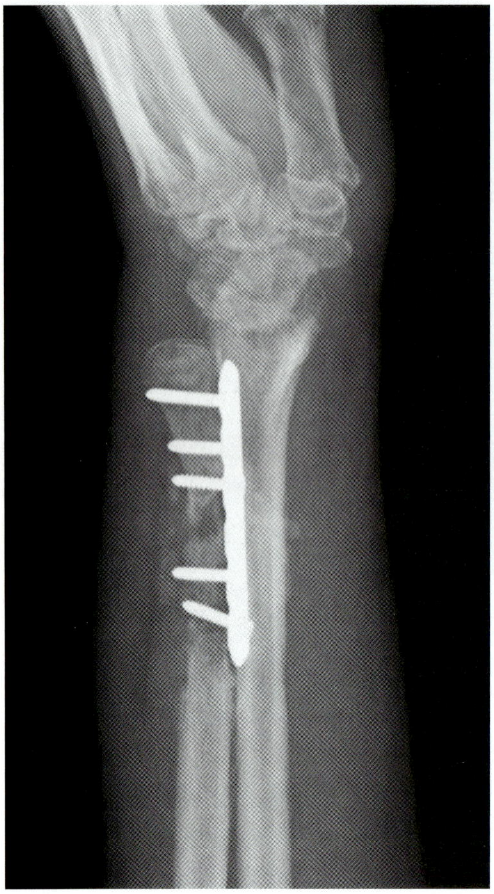

Figure 6.13: Acutely, infections typically do not reveal changes on radiographs. However, over time an infection will demonstrate bone absorption around the hardware and periosteal reaction as shown in the image.

Nonunion and Malunion

Nonunions of closed forearm fractures are uncommon but malunions can readily occur resulting in changes in radial and ulnar shaft length, secondary incongruency of the PRUJ and DRUJ, and subsequently rotational dysfunction of the forearm. Moreover, these changes may also alter the normal load bearing characteristics of the wrist and elbow, predisposing patients to arthritic changes. Nonunions are typically caused by compromise of the local fracture environment. Types and etiologies of nonunions include infected nonunion, hypertrophic nonunion (unstable fixation), hypotrophic nonunion (poor blood supply, extensive periosteal stripping, or bone loss) or delayed union (early motion, smoking and other host comorbidities). In contrast, malunions result from inadequate reduction or loss of reduction following surgical fixation.

While only a small percentage of both bones fractures of the forearm may progress to nonunion, there may be a higher incidence of nonunion in ulnar shaft fractures than has been previously appreciated. Previous studies have quoted a nonunion rate of 0–2% for closed treatment of minimally-displaced ulnar shaft fractures.[23] However, Szabo and Skinner identifed a 25% rate of nonunion in 28 diaphyseal fractures treated nonoperatively with the majority occurring in the proximal third of the forearm.[24] They found that middle and distal third fractures, if not displaced more than 5 mm, could be readily treated nonoperatively.

Synostosis

Forearm synostosis results from heterotopic ossification in the interosseous membrane and the soft tissues of the forearm, leading to impingement or a complete bony union between the radius and ulna. Although uncommon, it can result in significant loss of forearm rotation. Moreover, the forearm may lock in a poor position significantly compromising the use of the arm.

Forearm synostosis is typically a post-traumatic phenomenon resulting from either the initial injury or surgical intervention. More commonly, synostosis occurs in the setting of a high-energy fracture of both the radius and ulna (Figs 6.14A and B), with proximal third forearm fractures having a higher rate of synostosis.[25-27] Severe trauma, such as crushing injuries and those with significant soft tissue involvement, may predispose patients to forearm synostosis. Surgical risks for synostosis are decreased with the use of two incisions: early surgical fixation and by avoiding dissection of the interosseous membrane.

Authors' Preferred Management of Select Complications

Case 1: Nonunion

A 30-year-old male was involved in a motorcycle accident and incurred a both bones fracture that included an open ulna fracture (Figs 6.15A to C). The patient underwent emergent incision and debridement followed by plate fixation of the radius and intramedullary fixation of

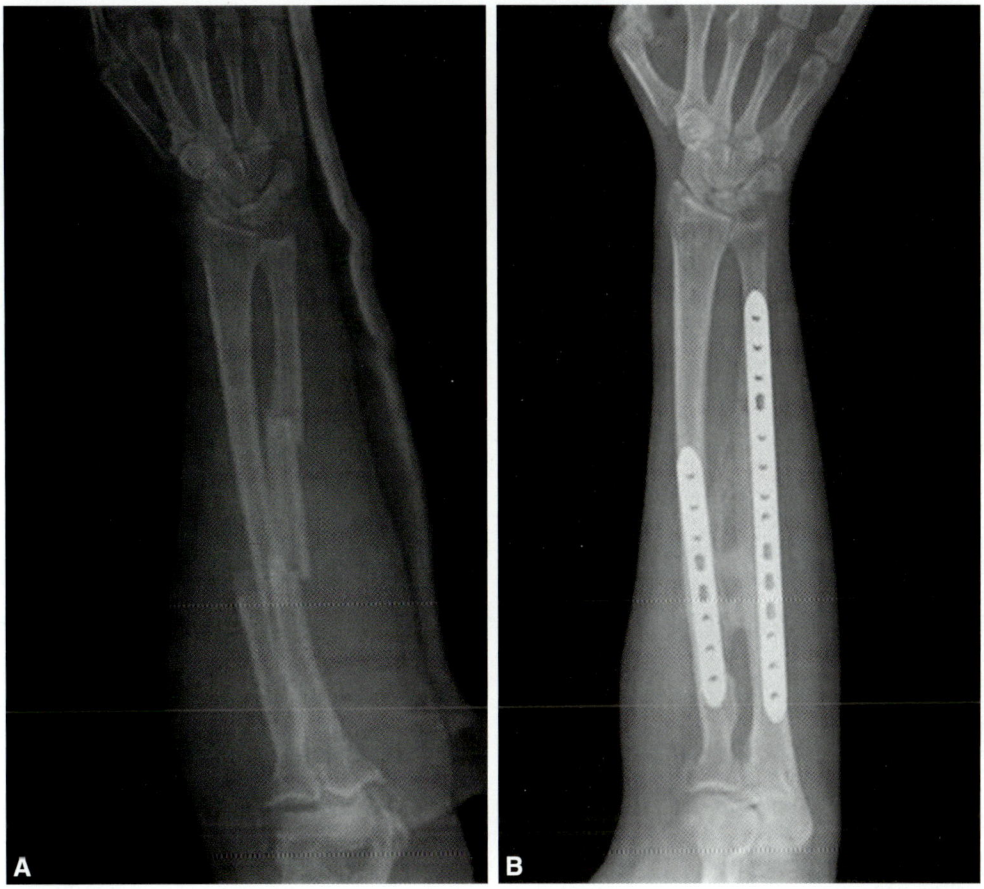

Figures 6.14A and B: This is a case of a 28-year-old female involved in a high-energy injury resulting in a (A) segmental open both bones fracture of the forearm complicated by compartment syndrome. The patient underwent emergent fasciotomies followed by plate fixation of both the radius and ulna. The patient returned 6 months postoperatively with loss of forearm rotation; (B) Radiographs demonstrated a complete synostosis formation between the radius and ulna.

the ulna. At 3 months postoperatively, the patient returned complaining of continuing pain at the ulnar fracture site. Radiographs taken at this time demonstrated good position of the hardware but persistence of the ulnar fracture line with associated distraction of the cortices and no evidence of bridging bone. The radius also demonstrated paucity of bridging bone but was clinically asymptomatic.

Forearm fractures generally achieve union in 2–3 months. Pain, loss of reduction, broken hardware and continued latency at the fracture may indicate a delayed union or nonunion. The etiology preventing a patient from reaching complete union is important to elucidate. It determines the treatment algorithm and decreases the chances of a recurrent or recalcitrant nonunion. Fractures with obvious forearm rotation deficiencies and bone loss with incongruence of DRUJ or PRUJ warrant corrective osteotomy with fixation and possible bone graft. In contrast, infection-mediated nonunion is approached differently (debridement, antibiosis) than a sterile hypertrophic nonunion (compression plating with grafting). Therefore, the authors' evaluation of a nonunion always includes white blood cell (WBC) count, erythrocyte sedimentation rate, C-reactive protein and possibly tissue cultures including a high power field WBC count to evaluate for infection first. If infection is found then treatment will begin with aggressive debridement, antibiotics and delayed reconstruction.

Technique

Surgical management of a forearm fracture nonunion following operative fixation begins with evaluation of a potential infection. Once a fracture is ruled out, treatment

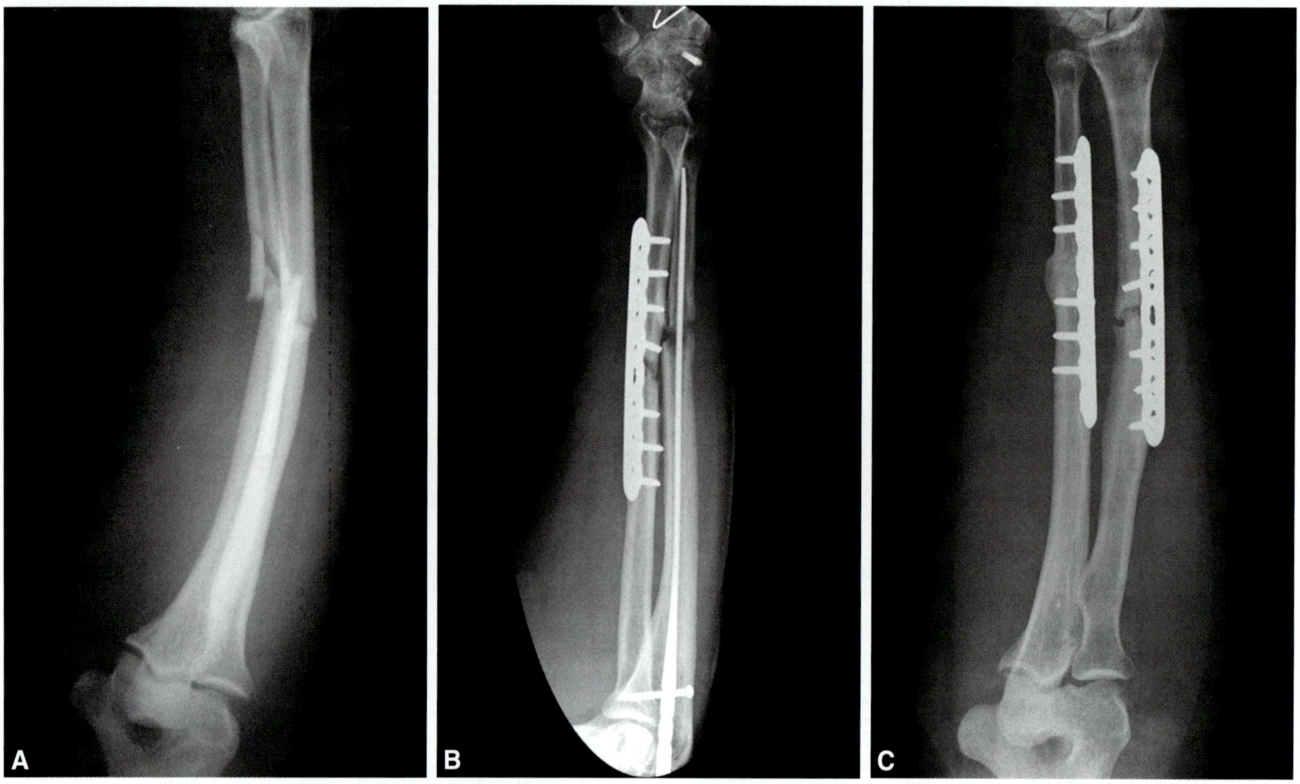

Figures 6.15A to C: This is a case of a 30-year-old male who incurred a (A) both bones fracture including an open ulna fracture. The patient underwent plate fixation of the radius and intramedullary fixation of the ulna. At 3 months postoperatively the patient complained of continuing pain at the ulna fracture site; (B) Radiographs demonstrated good position of the hardware but persistence of the ulnar fracture line with associated distraction of the cortices. The patient underwent removal of the hardware, open debridement of the fracture site and compression plate fixation with bone graft; (C) Radiographs taken 3 months following the second procedure confirmed union of the ulnar fracture.

is predicated upon current alignment of the bone and the type of hardware present. Whenever possible, removal of hardware, debridement to healthy bleeding bone and compression plating, with or without autologous bone graft is preferred. However, if an associated malunion is present with shortening, cortical incongruency or angulation correction of the deformity should simultaneously be undertaken. Autologous bone graft is preferable in nonunion cases. If angular correction or shortening is required then a cortical autologous graft can be obtained from the iliac crest. Fixation choices should preferably maximize stability and compression. The authors prefer the use of dynamic compression plates, with or without locking screws whenever possible.

In this case, the intramedullary nail was removed through its previous incisions. The nonunion site was then exposed through a direct ulnar approach. The nonunion site is debrided of fibrous tissue until bleeding bone is encountered on both ends. Compression plating was not possible due to the size of the defect. Therefore, autologous bone graft was harvested from the iliac crest to fill the defect and the ulna was then bridge plated across its ulnar border with a locking plate and screws.

Case 2: Synostosis

A 42-year-old male was involved in a motor vehicle accident incurring a head injury and an open both bones fracture of the forearm. Following stabilization, the patient underwent emergent irrigation and debridement followed by plate fixation of both the radius and ulna through two separate incisions. After a prolonged hospitalization course, the patient was discharged and returned for re-evaluation 2 months postoperatively as an outpatient with the complaint of loss of forearm rotation. Radiographs taken at this time demonstrated healed fractures but also a complete synostosis between the radius and ulna (Figs 6.16A to D).

Risk factors for the development of heterotopic ossification across the interosseous membrane resulting in a forearm synostosis include high energy injuries, severe soft tissue loss, dissection or exposure of the interosseous membrane, prolonged immobilization, and head injuries. Surgical management of a synostosis includes excision of the bridging heterotopic bone once the synostosis has "matured." Excision can be performed through one or both incisions and can be done leaving the hardware in place. In order to avoid recurrence a number of steps are taken, including interposition of soft tissue (Figs 6.17A and B), postoperative irradiation and the institution of immediate motion.

Technique

Surgical management of a forearm fracture resulting in a synostosis is performed through the previous incisions. The hardware may be removed but is preferably retained to avoid an iatrogenic refracture. After careful dissection of the soft tissue attachments the synostosis is removed with the use of osteotomes. Both the anterior and posterior interosseous neurovascular structures are at particular risk during synostosis excision and are best identified outside the zone of heterotopic bone for dissection and protection. Excision of the synostosis is performed until complete forearm rotation is restored without impingement of bone between the radius and ulna. In order to avoid recurrence, soft tissue interposition is performed by mobilizing the flexor carpi ulnaris and wrapping the ulna circumferentially. Care must be taken

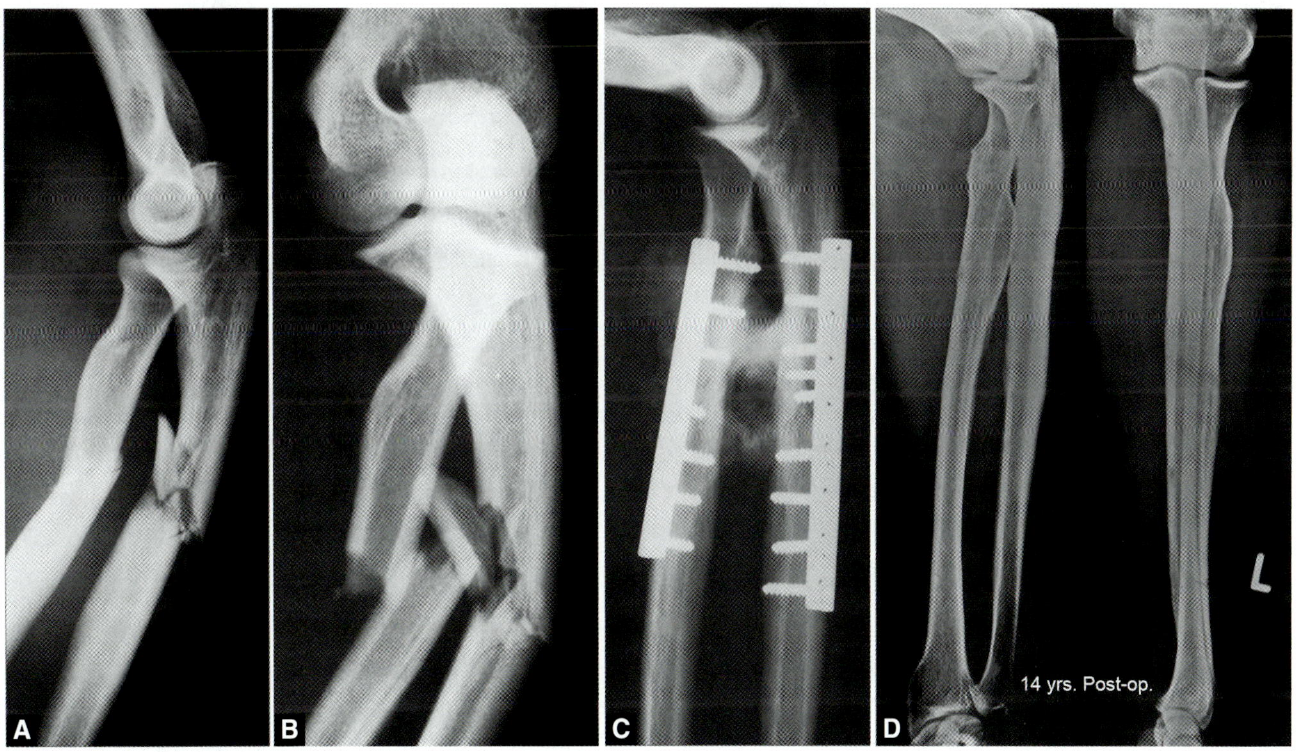

Figures 6.16A to D: This is a case of a 42-year-old male who incurred a high-energy injury resulting in a head injury and an (A and B) open both bones fracture of the forearm. The fracture was treated with emergent irrigation and debridement followed by plate fixation of both the radius and ulna through two separate incisions; (C) Radiographs taken 2 months postoperatively identified a forearm synostosis. The patient underwent excision of the heterotopic bone and removal of hardware with interposition of soft tissue resulting in restoration of forearm motion; (D) Radiographs taken over 10 years later confirmed no recurrence of the synostosis.

Courtesy: Jesse Jupiter

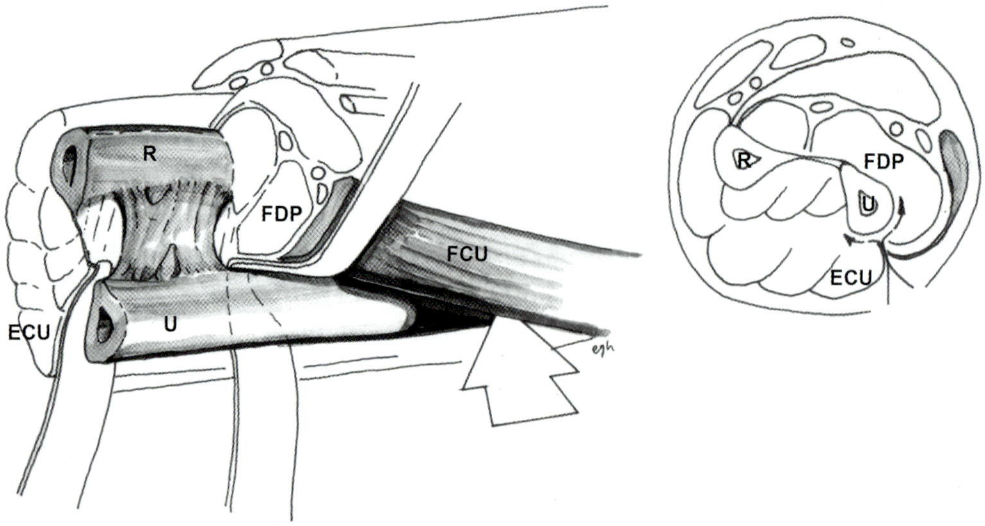

A

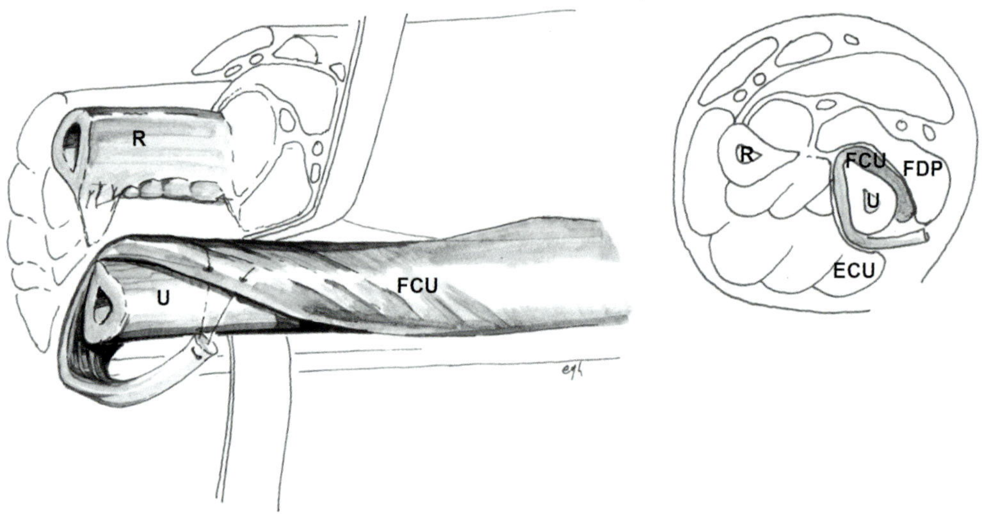

B

Figures 6.17A and B: Soft tissue interposition utilizing the flexor carpi ulnaris can minimize recurrence following surgical excision of the synostosis. (A) The flexor carpi ulnaris is released distally, mobilized and pulled proximally into the wound; (B) The tendon is then wrapped circumferentially in a volar to dorsal direction and sewn to itself along the ulnar border of the ulna.
Courtesy: Jesse Jupiter

to avoid secondary impingement of the ulnar neurovascular structures. Postoperatively the patient receives a single dose of radiation followed by immediate range of motion exercises.

Summary

Forearm fractures are comprised of a diverse spectrum of injuries, with varying etiologies and patterns. A large majority of these injuries require operative intervention to restore the anatomical relationship of the radius and ulna, and therefore allow for acceptable forearm function. Outcomes for forearm fractures treated operatively have traditionally been very good. It is important to maintain a high level of vigilance in seeking out associated injuries, selecting appropriately indicated implants and monitoring for potential complications. Although uncommon, complications including infection, malunion, nonunion and synostosis may be quite challenging. A systemic approach, with thorough preoperative planning, careful attention to surgical technique, consistent patient education and communication is recommended.

References

1. Means KR, Graham TJ. Disorders of the forearm axis. In: Green's Operative Hand Surgery, 6th edition. 2011. pp. 836-7.
2. McQueen MM. Epidemiology of fractures of the forearm. In: McQueen MM, Jupiter JB (Eds). Radius and Ulna. Oxford: Butterworth-Heinemann; 1997. pp. 1-11.
3. Chung KC, Spilson SV. The frequency and epidemiology of hand and forearm fractures in the United States. J Hand Surg Am. 2001;26(5):908-15.
4. Evans E Mervyn. Rotational deformity in the treatment of fractures of both bones of the forearm. J Bone Joint Surg Am. 1945;27:373-9.
5. KNIGHT RA, PURVIS GD. Fractures of both bones of the forearm in adults. J Bone Joint Surg Am. 1949;31A:755-64.
6. BadoJL. The Monteggia Lesion. Clin. Orthop Relat Res. 1967;50:71-86.
7. Sebastian SJ, Chung KC. A historical report on Riccardo Galeazzi and the management of Galeazzi fractures. J Hand Surg Am. 2010;35A:1870-7.
8. Ring D, Rhim R, Carpenter C, et al. Isolated radial shaft fractures are more common than Galeazzi fractures. J Hand Surg Am. 2006;31A:17-21.
9. Müller MF, Nazarian S, Koch P, et al. The Comprehensive Classification of Fractures of Long Bones, 1st edition. (1990) Berlin, Heidelberg, New York: Springer-Verlag. 1990.
10. Galeazzi R. Di una particolae sindrome traumatica dello scheletro dell' avambraccio. Attimem. Soc. Lombardi chir. 1934;2:12.
11. Rettig ME, Raskin KB. Galeazzi fracture-dislocation: a new treatment oriented classification. J Hand Surg Am. 2001; 26:228-35.
12. Anderson LD, Sisk D, Tooms RE, et al. Compression-plate fixation in acute diaphyseal fractures of the radius and ulna. J Bone Joint Surg Am. 1975;(3):287-97.
13. Chapman MW, Gordon JE, Zissimos AG. Compression-plate fixation of acute fractures of the diaphyses of the radius and ulna. J Bone Joint Surg Am. 1989;71(2):159-69.
14. Lee YH, Lee SK, Chung MS. Interlocking contoured intramedullary nail fixation for selected diaphyseal fractures of the forearm in adults. J Bone Joint Surg Am. 2008; 90:1891-8.
15. Sarmiento A, Latta LL, Zych G, et al. Isolated ulnar shaft fractures treated with functional braces. J Orthop Trauma. 1998;12(6):420-4.
16. Atkin DM, Bohay DR, Slabaugh P, et al. Treatment of ulnar shaft fractures: a prospective, randomised study. Orthopedics. 1995;18(6):543-7.
17. Henry AK. Extensile exposure, 2nd edition. Baltimore: Williams and Wilkins. 1970:100.
18. Thompson JE. Anatomical methods of approach in operations on the long bones of the extremities. Ann Surg. 1918; 68:309-29.
19. Droll KP, Perna P, Potter J, et al. Outcomes following plate fixation of fractures of both bones of the forearm in adults. J Bone Joint Surg Am. 2007;89(12):2619-24.
20. Goldfarb CA, Ricci WM, Tull F, et al. Functional outcome after fracture of both bones of the forearm. J Bone Joint Surg Br. 2005;87:374-9.
21. Bednar DA, Grandwilewski W. Complications of forearm-plate removal. Can J Surg. 1992;35(4):428-31.
22. Berkes M, Obremskey WT, Scannell B, et al. Maintenance of hardware after early postoperative infection following fracture internal fixation. J Bone Joint Surg. Am. 2010; 92(4):823-8.
23. Sarmiento A, Latta LL, Zych G, et al. Isolated ulnar shaft fractures treated with functional braces. J Orthop Trauma. 1998;12(6):420-4.
24. Szabo RM, Skinner M. Isolated ulnar shaft fractures. Retrospective study of 46 cases. Acta Orthop Scand. 1990; 61(4):350-2.
25. Bauer G, Arand M, Mutschler W. Post-traumatic radioulnar synostosis after forearm fracture osteosynthesis. Arch Orthop Trauma Surg. 1991;110(3):142-5.
26. Vince KG, Miler JE. Cross-union complicating fractures of the forearm. Part I: Adults. J Bone Joint Surg Am. 1987; 69A(5):640-53.
27. Stern PJ, Drury WJ. Complications of plate fixation of forearm fractures. Clin Orthop Relat Res. 1983;175:25-9.

Chapter 7

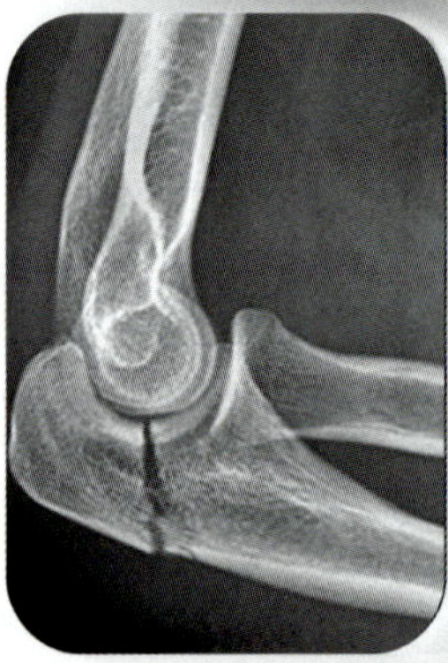

Olecranon Fractures

Brandon Steen, Andrew Jawa

Chapter Outline

Introduction
Diagnosis
Classification
Surgical Indications
- Tension Band Fixation
- Plate Fixation
- Intramedullary Screw
- Excision with Triceps Advancement

Surgical Anatomy, Positioning and Approaches
- Surgical and Applied Anatomy
- Positioning
- Surgical Approaches

Surgical Techniques
- Technique 1: Tension Band Fixation
- Technique 2: Plate Fixation
- Technique 3: Intramedullary Nailing
- Technique 4: Fragment Excision and Triceps Advancement

Outcomes
- Biomechanical Studies
- Clinical Studies

Complications
- Symptomatic Hardware
- Hardware Failure
- Malunion/Nonunion
- Stiffness
- Heterotopic Ossification
- Proximal Radioulnar Joint Injury
- Ulnar Neuropathy
- Infection

Authors' Preferred Management of Select Complications
- Case 1: Failure of Fixation
- Case 2: Proximal Radioulnar Joint Injury

Summary

Introduction

Fractures of the proximal ulna constitute a spectrum of injuries ranging from nondisplaced fractures of the olecranon to complex fractures resulting in both bony and ligamentous injury (Figs 7.1A and B). Injuries to the olecranon comprise approximately 10% of fractures about the elbow. Mechanisms of injury are quite variable and can occur from direct or indirect trauma. Direct injury usually arises from a fall or a blow to the subcutaneous point of the elbow. Indirect injuries result from forceful eccentric contraction of the triceps resulting in an avulsion of the proximal ulna while falling onto an outstretched hand. Associated injuries have been found in approximately 20% of olecranon fractures. Maintenance of the ulnohumeral articulation distinguishes olecranon fractures from complex elbow fractures that may also be associated with fractures of the radial head and coronoid process.

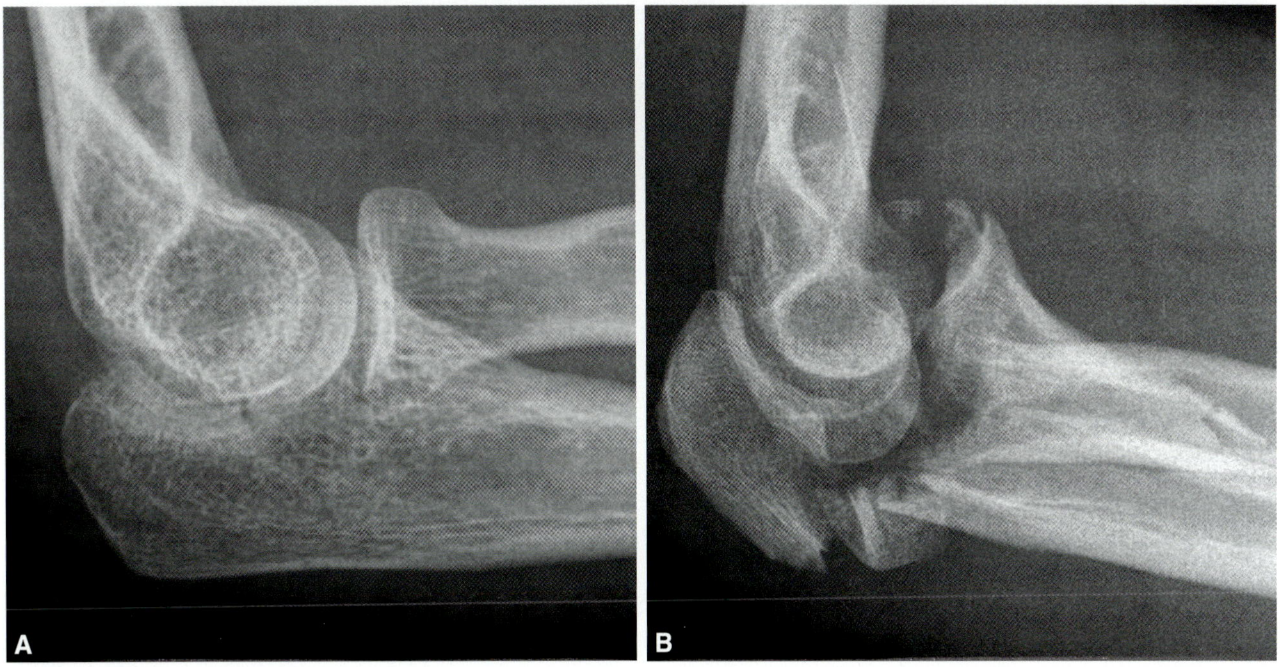

Figures 7.1A and B: Olecranon fractures involve the articular surface of the proximal ulna. (A) They may occur in isolation such as in this image of a nondisplaced olecranon fracture and (B) Olecranon fractures may occur as part of a more complex elbow fracture involving both bony and ligamentous injuries resulting in a dislocation and instability pattern.

Diagnosis

Diagnosis of an olecranon fracture can readily be established by physical examination and radiographic evaluation. On exam, swelling and ecchymosis of varying degrees will be present over the posterior aspect of the elbow. Hemorrhagic bursitis posteriorly is also commonly encountered. A palpable defect is often present in displaced fractures due to the subcutaneous nature of the olecranon. Due to the disruption of the extensor mechanism, loss or weakness of elbow extension can be expected.[1] Inability to extend the elbow against gravity in the absence of severe discomfort, is evidence of functional disruption of the extensor mechanism.

Standard radiographs, including anteroposterior and lateral views, will readily provide the diagnosis. If clinical suspicion warrants, radiographs of the humerus, forearm and wrist may be taken to rule out the presence of concomitant ipsilateral injuries. This is especially important if concomitant dislocation or subluxation of the elbow exists. Standard radiographs should be scrutinized for the extent of comminution and obliquity of the fracture line which are variables that will be important in deciding upon the type of treatment.

Distinguishing isolated olecranon fractures from complex elbow fracture-dislocation injuries is necessary and can usually be accomplished with careful evaluation of the radiographs (Figs 7.2A to D). Olecranon fractures are intra-articular injuries that involve the greater sigmoid notch. Congruence of the trochlea is maintained with the proximal and distal fragments in an olecranon fracture. However, if incongruity is present on the lateral radiograph a more complex pattern of injury should be suspected. In contradistinction, Monteggia type injuries are extra-articular fractures distal to the greater sigmoid notch and are associated with disruption of the radiocapitellar articulation but not the ulnohumeral articulation. Transolecranon fracture-dislocations may appear as simple olecranon fractures at first glance but will show incongruence of the ulnohumeral, and possibly also of the radiocapitellar, articulation on the lateral radiograph. Similarly, terrible triad complex elbow dislocations with a large coronoid process fracture can be confused with an olecranon fracture.

Computed tomography (CT) scans may also be useful in evaluating for an occult fracture, defining the extent of comminution, identifying fracture planes and diagnosing subtle associated injuries, such as distal humerus, radial

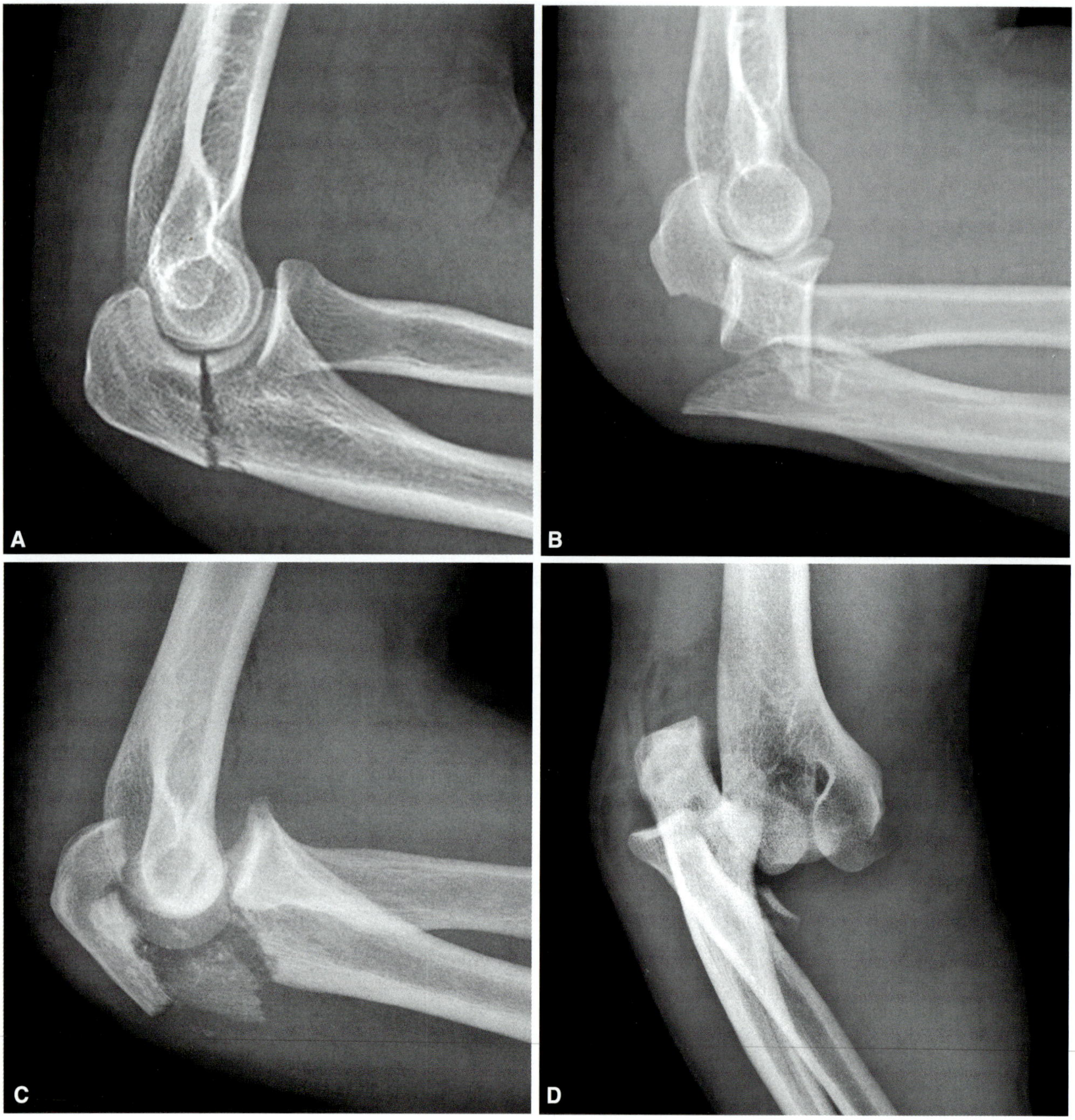

Figures 7.2A to D: Olecranon fractures can be confused for complex elbow fractures that are associated with additional bony and ligamentous injuries. (A) The proximal and distal fragments of an olecranon fracture will maintain congruity with the trochlea of the distal humerus regardless of displacement; (B) Monteggia-type injuries will present with a radiocapitellar disruption and a fracture of the proximal ulna that should not involve the ulnohumeral joint; (C) Transolecranon fractures can have variable presentations but will typically present with a comminuted olecranon fracture and disruption of both the ulnohumeral and radiocapitellar joints; (D) Terrible triad elbow dislocations may present with a large coronoid fracture but unlike with olecranon fractures there will be no violation of the posterior cortex of the proximal ulna.

Courtesy: Asif M Ilyas

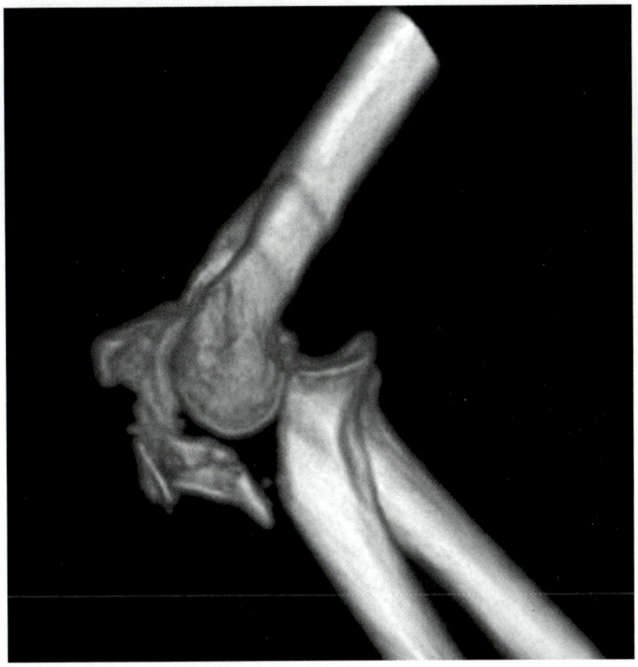

Figure 7.3: Computed tomography scan may be helpful in characterizing the fracture, quantifying fracture comminution, assessing for joint incongruency and evaluating associated or occult injuries.

head or coronoid fractures (Fig. 7.3). Assessment of the location of the fracture line, extent of displacement and the amount of comminution is necessary in determining treatment options.

OLECRANON FRACTURES DIAGNOSIS:
Pearls and Pitfalls

- Olecranon fractures can be distinguished from complex elbow fracture-dislocation injuries with proper plain radiographs. Maintained congruence of both the ulnohumeral and radiocapitellar joints is the defining difference from other fracture patterns
- It can be difficult to examine the elbow for ligamentous stability in the presence of an olecranon fracture
- If the fracture pattern is concerning for concomitant injuries, CT scans are valuable in identifying subtle joint incongruence that may be related to ligamentous incompetence
- Identification of fracture obliquity plays an important role in determining what type of fixation is the most suitable

Classification

Currently there are no universally accepted classification systems for olecranon fractures. However, olecranon fractures can be readily described by noting the direction of the fracture line, extent of displacement, degree of comminution and the presence or absence of associated ulnohumeral or radiocapitellar joint injury.

The first classification system was created by Colton.[2] Fractures were grouped based on location, obliquity, presence of comminution and associated collateral ligament injury. Type I fractures are nondisplaced, type II fractures are proximal avulsion, type III fractures are transverse, type IV fractures are oblique, type V fractures are comminuted, and type 6 fractures encompass the spectrum of fracture-dislocation injuries. Schatzker developed a classification system based on many of the same principles, but included a separate group for fractures with articular impaction.[3]

The Mayo classification describes fractures based on stability, displacement and comminution (Fig. 7.4). It simplifies the same concepts set forth by Colton and later by Schatzker. Fractures that do not involve the articular portion of the olecranon are excluded from the Mayo classification. Type I fractures are nondisplaced, type II fractures are displaced with a stable ulnohumeral joint, and type III fractures are displaced and unstable. Each group is then subdivided into A (noncomminuted) or B (comminuted).

Surgical Indications

Fractures of the olecranon are typically treated with operative fixation as they represent a discontinuity of the extensor mechanism of the elbow. Nonoperative management of olecranon fractures have consistently demonstrated decreased range of motion, decreased elbow extension strength, and a propensity to develop nonunions or fibrous unions.[4] Fractures displaced less than 2 mm at the fracture site may be amenable to nonoperative treatment. In these instances, it is possible the remaining soft tissue attachments are competent enough to allow active elbow motion without causing significant fracture gapping.[5] It should be understood that the chance of fracture displacement or late nonunion or fibrous union formation is high following nonoperative treatment.[4]

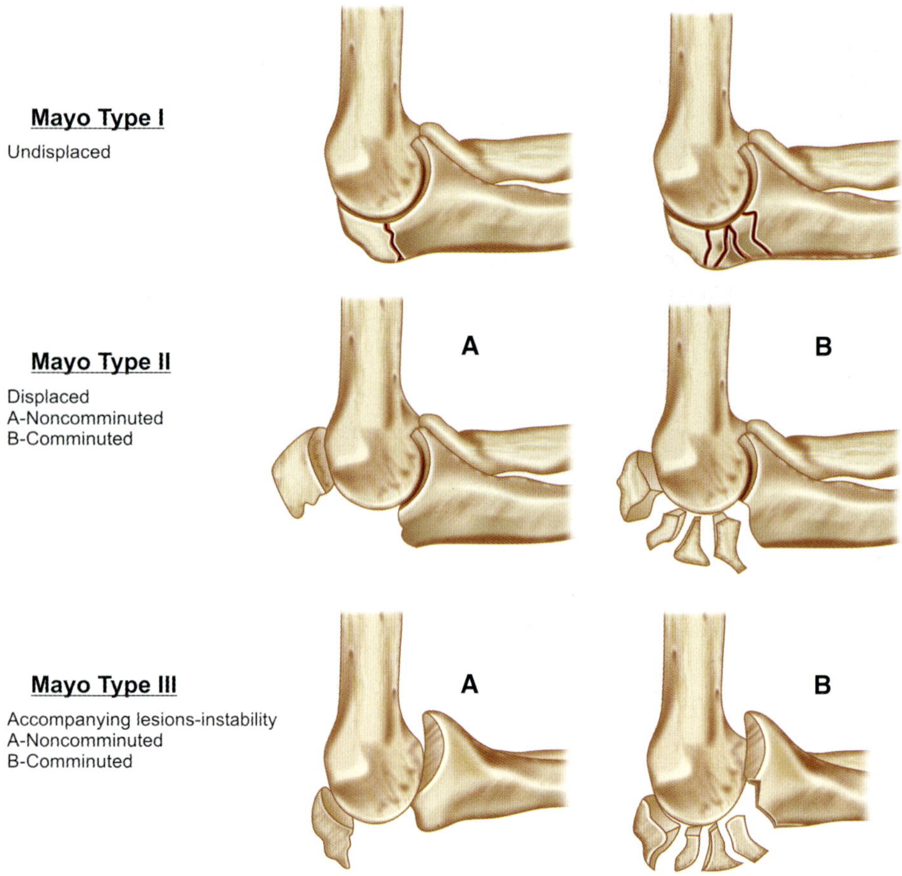

Figure 7.4: The Mayo classification for olecranon fractures.

The treatment is based on the fundamental principles of surgical fracture care: (1) anatomic reduction of the fracture and restoration of articular alignment, (2) placement of stable fixation and (3) institution of early motion.

Additional fracture management considerations with the olecranon include:

- Fractures that occur through a direct blow mechanism of injury commonly have articular comminution and depression of fragments within the greater sigmoid notch. When this type of injury pattern is identified, reduction of the articular fragments is vital and care must be taken not to narrow the trochlear groove.[2]
- Re-establishing stability and length of the proximal ulna provides the basis for treating complex elbow fracture-dislocation injuries with associated olecranon fractures. Ligamentous injuries often heal uneventfully if the joint congruency is properly restored.
- Rigid fixation of an olecranon fracture in the multiply injured patient is indicated to promote early range of motion of the elbow in an effort to limit fibrosis and posttraumatic contracture. Furthermore, in patients with lower extremity injuries, early fixation may enhance rehabilitation potential by allowing weight-bearing through the forearm with a platform type crutch. If stability of the fracture is in question postoperatively, the limb should not be used as a weight-bearing surface. Biomechanical studies have demonstrated that neither tension band, nor locked plating provide significant rigidity to withstand cyclical loading at levels equivalent to pushing up out of a chair.[6]

As with open fractures in other areas, treatment protocols are based on the severity of injury, degree of contamination, and viable soft tissue coverage. Open fracture rates up to 31% have been reported.[7] Simple grade I open injuries can be internally fixed immediately following thorough irrigation and debridement. Occasionally, staged procedures with splinting or external fixation can be utilized with contaminated fractures or fractures with severe soft tissue injury requiring coverage. In cases of open fractures with severe comminution, excision and triceps advancement is a reasonable treatment option. Injury to the LCL, coronoid or radial head must be ruled out prior to fragment excision or else postoperative ulnohumeral instability may ensue.

Surgical treatment options for olecranon fractures span a wide variety of techniques, each with its own advantages and disadvantages but are typically predicated upon the amount of fracture obliquity, extent of articular comminution, and the quality of the soft tissue envelope around the elbow. The most commonly employed methods of treatment include tension band wiring, intramedullary screw fixation, intramedullary nailing, compression plating, locked plating and fragment excision with triceps advancement.[5] Within each of these fixation types, there have been numerous technique modifications and a wide variety of implants that are currently available.

Tension Band Fixation

The biomechanical concept of the tension band construct is to convert tensile forces acting at the dorsal cortex to compression forces at the level of the joint (Figs 7.5A and B). Numerous variations of tension band constructs have been evaluated since the introduction of the technique by Weber in 1963.[8] The most studied and predictable construct consists of two parallel bicortical Kirschner wires (K-wires) with a figure of eight tension band construct looped over the K-wires deep to the triceps tendon.[9] In biomechanical studies, bicortical placement of the wires decreased the gap formation at the articular surface under physiologic tensile loads consistent with active range of motion. Also the use of a 2-wire tension band construct with two points of wire tensioning, medially and laterally, appears to improve the uniformity of wire tension and also reduce gapping.

Tension band constructs tend to provide adequate fixation in axially stable fractures without the presence of significant comminution or obliquity. Articular comminution is a contraindication to using the tension band technique as the principles of stability and compression requires the fracture to be stable axially, as well as angularly. Overcompression or apex dorsal malreduction will cause a decrease in the radius of curvature mismatch of the sigmoid notch that can result in ulnohumeral incongruency, arthrosis or instability.[7,10] Loss of fixation and significant fracture gapping has also been demonstrated, biomechanically and clinically with the use of tension band constructs in comminuted fractures.[11,12]

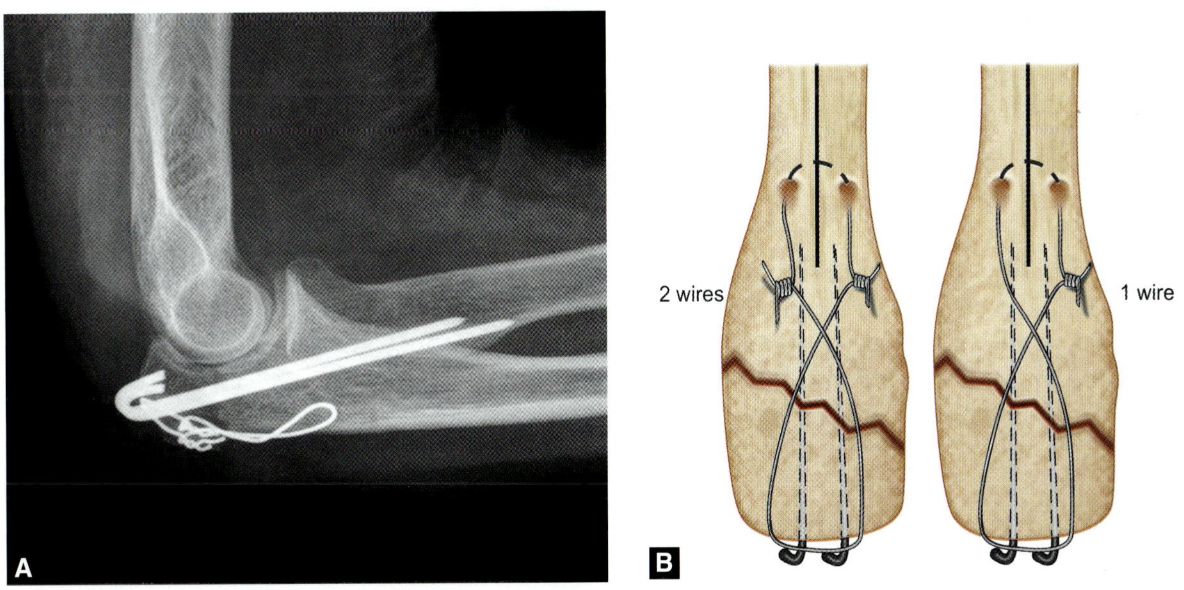

Figures 7.5A and B: The tension band construct is designed to convert tensile forces acting on the dorsal cortex to compression forces at the joint level. (A) The technique involves fracture reduction and placement of parallel K-wires bicortically across the fracture, followed by wire tensioning; (B) The technique can be employed with a single wire or two wires. The use of 2 wires has been found to provide more uniform compression.

Similarly, placement of a tension band construct in oblique fractures has been shown to lead to an unacceptable degree of fragment translation and is therefore, considered a relative contraindication.[9,11,13]

Plate Fixation

Zuelzer first described the use of a hook plate for the treatment of olecranon fractures in 1951.[14] Surprisingly, there was a relative paucity of early studies analyzing the use of plate osteosynthesis for olecranon fractures. Thirty-four years later, Fyfe et al. published the first biomechanical study comparing contoured plate fixation to tension band wiring in cadaveric extremities. Biomechanically, this construct was found to be equivalent or superior to tension band wiring in transverse, oblique and comminuted fracture patterns.[10] More recently, various plating methods have shown reasonable outcomes and are consistently superior to tension band techniques in biomechanical studies testing both physiologic loading and load to failure.[11,15-20]

Various plating techniques are available (Figs 7.6A to C). The use of a contoured one-third tubular hook plate with or without lag screws is consistently satisfactory for treatment of central one-third olecranon fractures including transverse and oblique. The presence of an intermediate articular fragment is not a contraindication to this technique, provided that the fragment can be adequately disimpacted and stabilized with a subchondral screw. Nonlocked one-third tubular plating has shown increased stiffness and less displacement in oblique and comminuted fracture patterns when compared to tension band fixation.[9,21,22] Nonlocked dynamic compression plate constructs can also be used effectively to treat most fracture patterns, except fracture-dislocation patterns and fractures with small proximal fragments. These patterns are best treated with locking plate constructs. Recently, several precontoured periarticular locking plates have become available. They can be utilized in all olecranon fracture patterns but their use must be tempered against their potential prominence on the subcutaneous border of the ulna. Periarticular locking plates are best indicated in the fixation of short segment proximal fragments, extensively comminuted fractures, distal fracture extension involving the shaft or coronoid and in cases with poor bone quality.

Intramedullary Screw

Intramedullary fixation can be achieved with partially threaded 6.5 mm or 7.3 mm screws or contoured

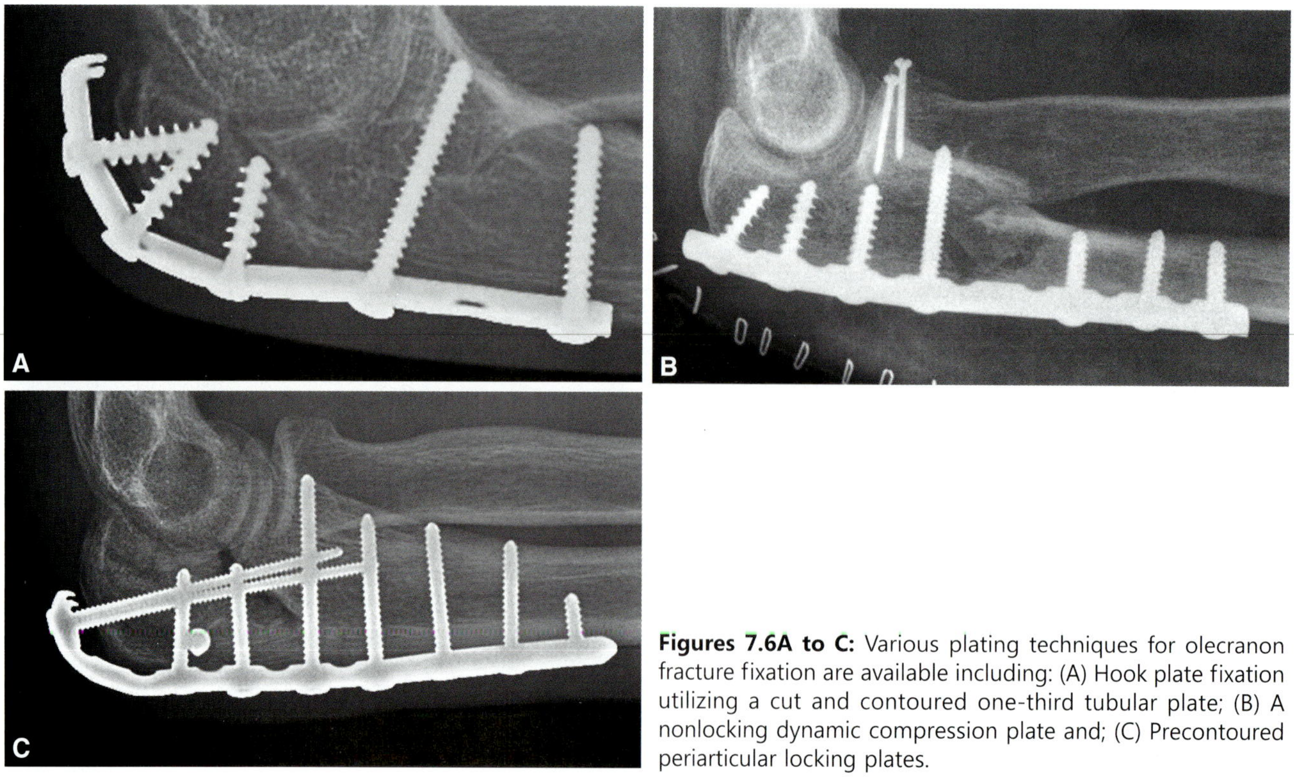

Figures 7.6A to C: Various plating techniques for olecranon fracture fixation are available including: (A) Hook plate fixation utilizing a cut and contoured one-third tubular plate; (B) A nonlocking dynamic compression plate and; (C) Precontoured periarticular locking plates.

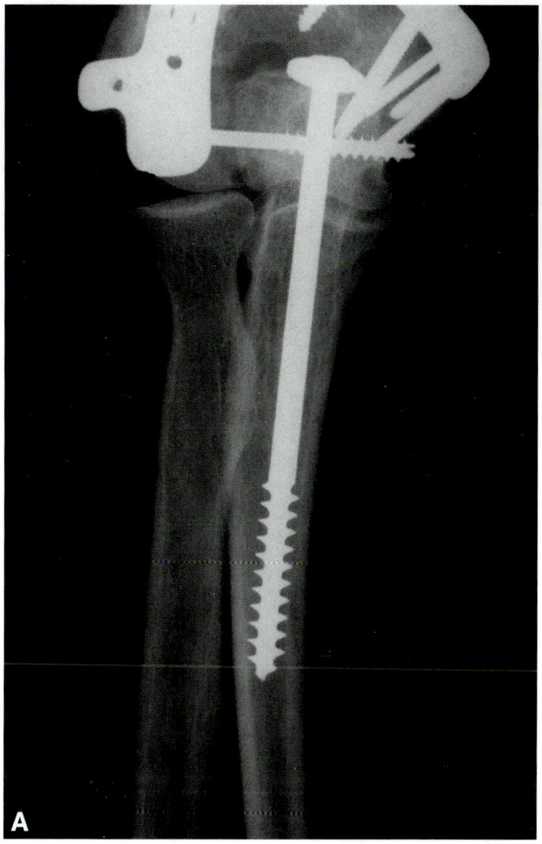

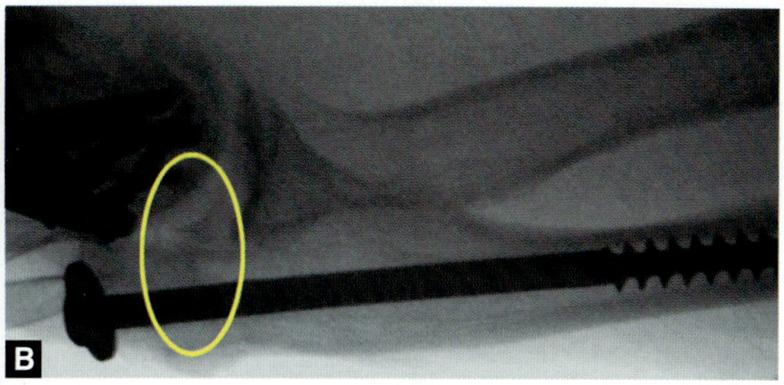

Figures 7.7A and B: Intramedullary screw fixation of olecranon fractures is best achieved with use of a 6.5 mm or 7.3 mm partially threaded screw and a washer. (A) Length of the screw will be limited by canal width and alignment of the ulnar shaft. There is normal varus angulation to the ulnar shaft which the screw should not be forced to cross. Appropriate screw length is best determined by tapping and measuring prior to screw placement; (B) Overcompression of the fracture site should be avoided in cases with articular comminution or poor bone quality. Note the secondary shortening and incongruency of the trochlear groove following overcompression of the fracture site.

Courtesy: Asif M Ilyas

intramedullary nails (Figs 7.7A and B and Fig. 7.8). Intramedullary screw fixation has demonstrated inconsistent results with fracture gapping and nonunions likely related to the variability of canal fill and bone quality potentially, compromising screw bone purchase.[9] Subsequently, intramedullary screw placement can be coupled with tension band wiring with the wire looped around the head of the screw instead of K-wires in order to increase the stiffness of the construct.

Contoured locked rigid nail fixation of olecranon fractures is a relatively new technique. There is no definitive evidence at this point to provide sound indications for intramedullary nail use. Purported benefits include less disruption of the soft tissue envelope and less hardware irritation. The use of locked nails for olecranon fractures is in its relative infancy and surgeons must be cognizant of the potential for anatomic mismatch. Fractures with significant comminution may be malreduced if the bone is forced to accommodate to the nail. In these instances, nail length and anatomic fit are essential to achieve the best outcome possible.[23] In simple transverse or oblique

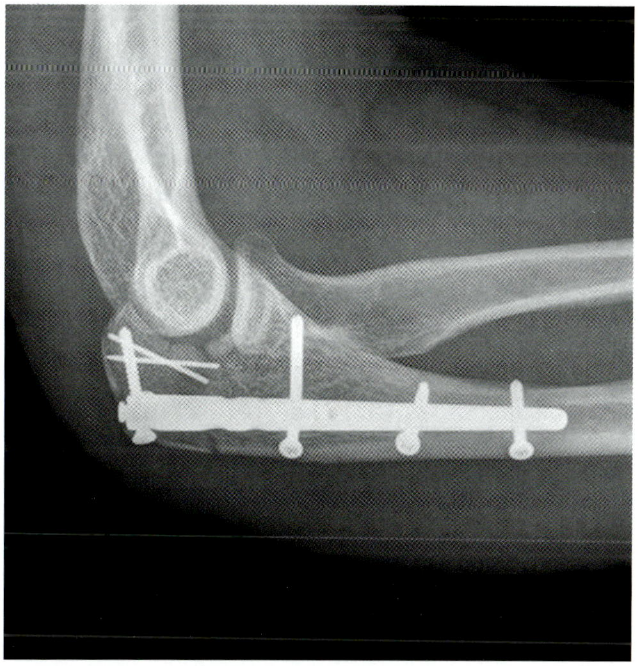

Figure 7.8: Intramedullary nail fixation of olecranon fractures has the potential advantages of a less invasive technique and less hardware irritation.

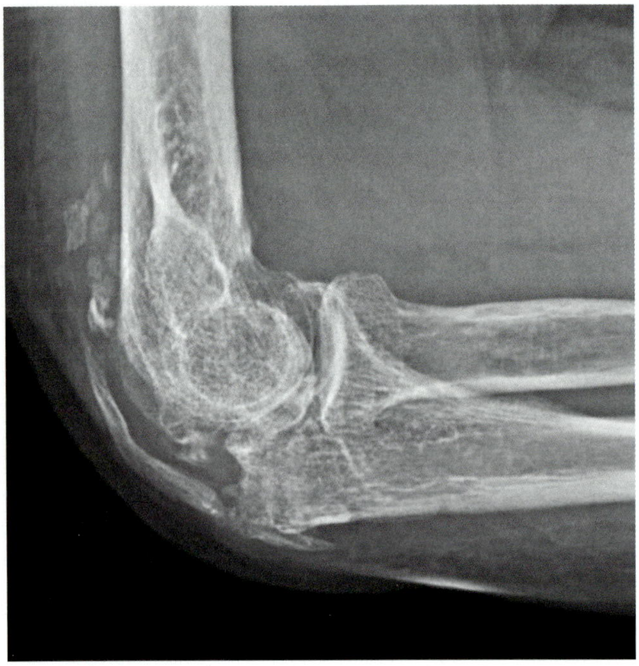

Figure 7.9: Fragment excision and triceps advancement is reserved for salvage cases to maintain elbow motion and extension strength.

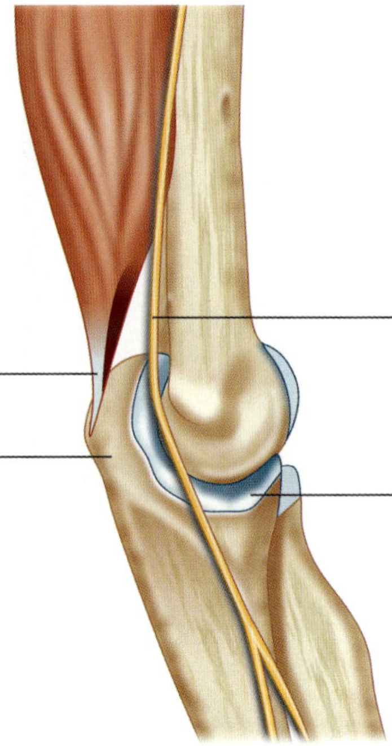

Figure 7.10: The olecranon is semilunar and provides an insertion site for the triceps and articulates with the trochlea of the distal humerus. The articular portion of the olecranon is known as the greater sigmoid notch. The dorsal surface of the olecranon is enveloped by the confluence of the triceps and anconeus insertions proximally and laterally, respectively, and by the extensor aponeurosis more distally. The extensor aponeurosis gives way to the muscular fascia of the extensor carpi ulnaris laterally and the flexor carpi ulnaris medially. Also medially, the ulnar nerve runs medial to the olecranon around the medial epicondyle.

patterns, this is less of an issue as appropriate reduction can be held with clamps while the nail is inserted.

Excision with Triceps Advancement

Primary excision with triceps advancement (Fig. 7.9) is rarely indicated for primary treatment of an olecranon fracture. Rather, this technique is usually reserved for salvage following infection or hardware failure. Even highly comminuted fractures can be effectively treated with the advent of locked plating. Occasionally, excision and advancement can be considered for primary treatment in low-demand patients with very proximal fractures.[24,25]

Surgical Anatomy, Positioning and Approaches

Surgical and Applied Anatomy

Displaced fractures of the olecranon are in essence, a disruption of the extensor mechanism of the elbow. The olecranon is semilunar and provides an insertion site for the triceps and articulates with the trochlea of the distal humerus (Fig. 7.10). The articular portion of the olecranon is known as the greater sigmoid notch. The highly contoured nature of the olecranon is congruent to the trochlea of the humerus and provides significant stability. A sagittal ridge runs longitudinally through the sigmoid notch further enhancing the bony stability of the ulnotrochlear joint. At the bottom of the sigmoid notch lies an area of subchondral bone that is devoid of articular cartilage known as the 'bare area.' The interdigitation of the coronoid and olecranon not only enhances stability of the elbow in terminal flexion and extension but also enhances the arc of motion. The lateral border of the proximal ulna contains the lesser sigmoid notch which articulates with the radial head. The articular portion of the olecranon is tilted posterior at an angle of approximately 30° with respect to the ulnar shaft. This arrangement allows for the elbow to come into full extension before the olecranon abuts the posterior aspect of the distal humerus. The normal elbow has a flexion-extension arc of 0–145° and a rotational arc of 180°. Functional range of motion to perform activities of daily living is 30–130° of flexion and approximately 50° of both pronation and supination.[6]

The proximal ulna is a subcutaneous structure making it especially vulnerable to direct injury. Overlying the proximal ulna is the olecranon bursa. The dorsal surface of the olecranon is enveloped in the confluence of the triceps and anconeus insertions proximally and laterally respectively and by the extensor aponeurosis more distally. The extensor aponeurosis gives way to the muscular fascia of the extensor carpi ulnaris (ECU) laterally and the flexor carpi ulnaris (FCU) medially. Medially, the ulnar nerve is identified through palpation and should remain protected by the medial soft tissue sleeve. Routine transposition of the ulnar nerve is unnecessary and may increase the risk of postoperative ulnar neuritis.[26] However, awareness of its proximity is important to prevent inadvertent injury with reduction forceps or K-wires that are placed too close to the medial soft tissue sleeve.

The proximal ulna has significant angulation in both varus and apex dorsal directions. The location and magnitude of these angulations are clinically relevant to fixation strategies of proximal ulna fractures. The varus bend in the proximal ulna occurs approximately 85 mm from the posterior tip of the olecranon with a variation of 45–110 mm, and the apex dorsal angulation occurs at a distance of approximately 50 mm from the tip of the olecranon. The degree of varus angulation is approximately 17° and the dorsal angulation approximately 6°. Failure to recognize the normal angulation of the ulna during fracture repair may lead to improper reduction and malunion. In cases of fracture dislocation in particular, failure to reconstruct the dorsal angulation may lead to persistent radiocapitellar instability.[4,27-29] Similarly, this normal varus angulation must be considered during intramedullary fixation.[4,27-30]

Positioning

Olecranon fractures are routinely approached posteriorly, but the patient can be positioned in several positions.

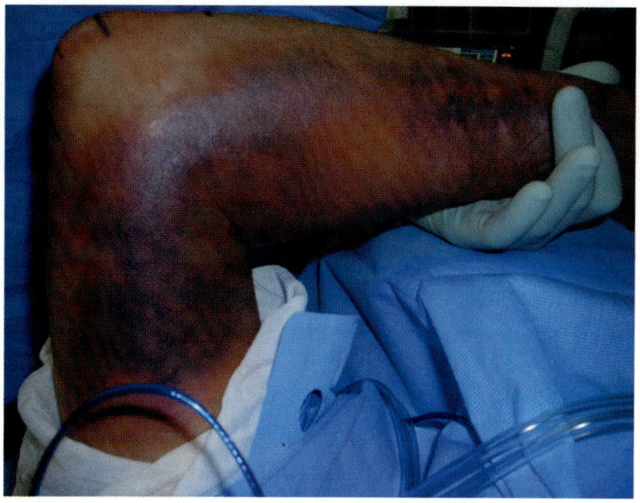

Figure 7.11: The authors prefer supine positioning with the arm suspended across the chest and prepped to the axilla. A sterile tourniquet is applied. A covered mayo stand or sterile bump on the chest can be use to drape the elbow across the chest allowing the surgeon to stand directly in front of the fracture. Alternatively, an assistant can hold the arm across the chest.

Supine

The authors prefer supine positioning on a regular operating room (OR) table (Fig. 7.11). The arm is suspended and prepped to the axilla. A sterile tourniquet is applied. A covered mayo stand or sterile bump on the chest can be use to drape the elbow across the chest allowing the surgeon to stand directly in front of the fracture. This facilitates easy access to image intensifier and also permits flexion and extension of the elbow when necessary to aid in fracture reduction. One disadvantage of this technique is the need for an assistant to hold and manipulate the arm during exposure, reduction and fixation.

Lateral Positioning

Lateral positioning of the patient affords the surgeon the benefit of gravity in positioning of the arm. The patient is placed in the standard lateral decubitus position with the use of trunk supports or a bean bag. The operative arm is draped over an arm board so that the forearm is hanging perpendicular to the floor. This provides adequate access to the posterior elbow and is the position of choice for some of the newer intramedullary devices. Imaging may be slightly easier in this position as the arm does not need to be moved from the arm board to obtain images.

Prone

The authors do not utilize prone positioning unless concomitant injuries to the humerus need to be addressed. The arm can be abducted and the elbow flexed to hang over the side of a fully retracted arm board.

Surgical Approaches

Posterior Approach

The olecranon is universally approached through a posterior midline incision (Figs 7.12A and B). The extent of the proximal exposure should be enough that the proximal fragment can be visualized and manipulated without putting tension on the overlying soft tissue envelope. The length of the distal incision is dependent upon the type of fixation that will be used. The incision can be either a straight midline centered over the tip of the olecranon or curved slightly laterally around the point of the olecranon to minimize tip sensitivity and wound complications. Sharp dissection is carried down through the bursa to the level of the triceps paratenon and the extensor fascia distally. The extensor fascia is sharply split longitudinally in a subperiosteal fashion over the triangular apex of the dorsal ulna. Elevation of the extensor mechanism is performed as necessary to expose and fix the fracture. However, elevation of the entire extensor mechanism off of the proximal fragment must be avoided. If necessary, the ECU and FCU musculature can be gently elevated to gain adequate exposure with care taken to avoid inadvertent injury to the ulnar nerve medially.

Surgical Techniques

Technique 1: Tension Band Fixation

Tension band fixation is best indicated for simple olecranon fractures with minimal articular comminution and minimal fracture obliquity.

Surgical Technique

The fracture is exposed through the standard posterior approach (Figs 7.13A to K). The fracture surfaces are cleaned of fracture hematoma and invaginating soft tissue. During reduction, the elbow is extended to relax the pull of the triceps. If difficulty in obtaining the reduction is encountered, a small tenaculum can be applied to the proximal fragment to aide in manipulation of the fracture. Once reduction is obtained, a large tenaculum is applied perpendicular to the fracture line reducing the fracture. Fixation can be achieved with 0.062 inch K-wires placed

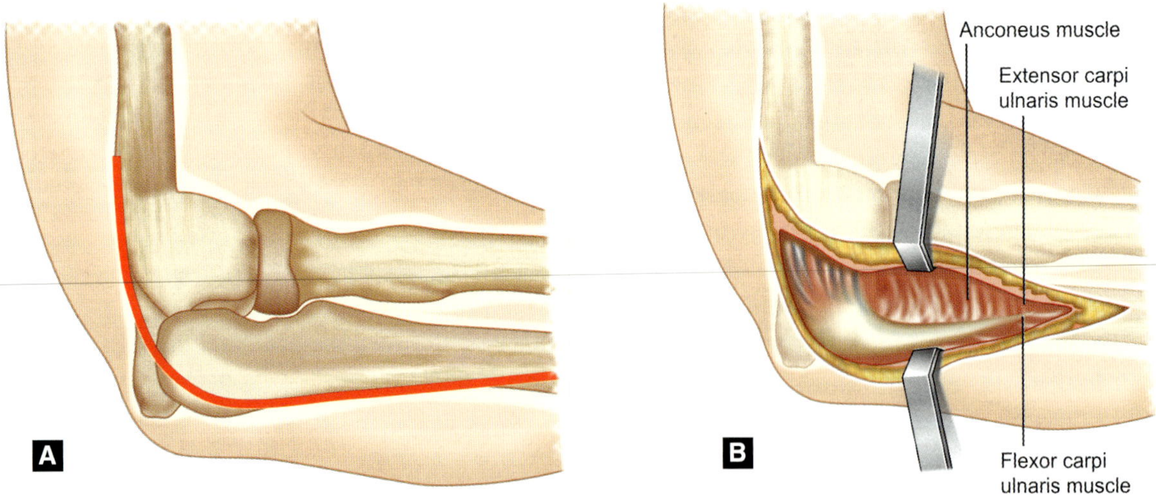

Figures 7.12A and B: The olecranon is universally approached through a (A) Posterior midline incision. The incision can be either a straight midline centered over the tip of the olecranon (as shown) or curved slightly laterally around the point of the olecranon; (B) The fracture site will typically demonstrate displacement interposed with fracture hematoma. The extensor aponeurosis inserting into the process fragment should be protected. The dorsal cortex of the ulna should be exposed subperiosteally between the extensor carpi ulnaris and the flexor carpi ulnaris.

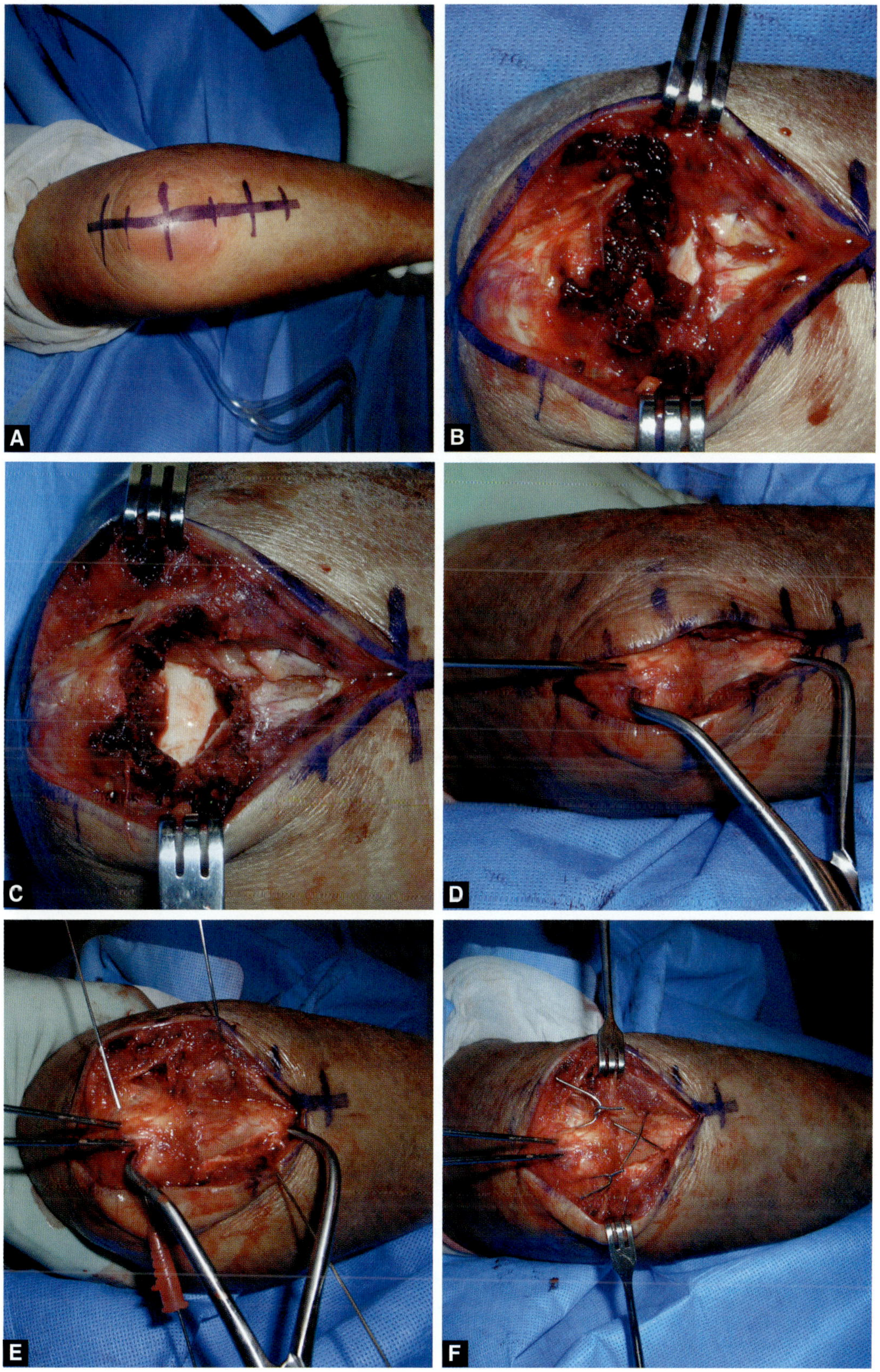

Figures 7.13A to F

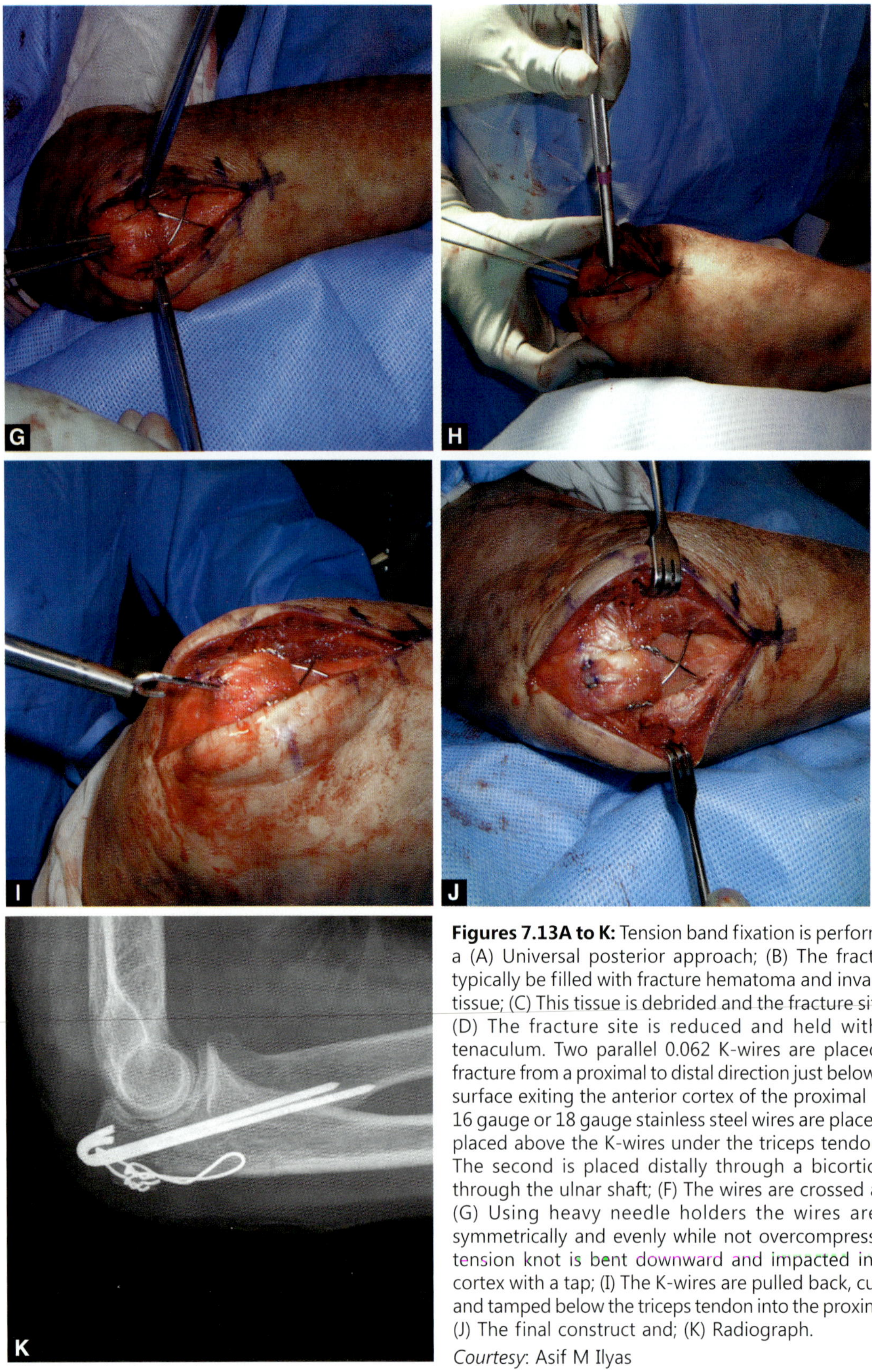

Figures 7.13A to K: Tension band fixation is performed through a (A) Universal posterior approach; (B) The fracture site will typically be filled with fracture hematoma and invaginating soft tissue; (C) This tissue is debrided and the fracture site examined; (D) The fracture site is reduced and held with a fracture tenaculum. Two parallel 0.062 K-wires are placed across the fracture from a proximal to distal direction just below the articular surface exiting the anterior cortex of the proximal ulna; (E) Two 16 gauge or 18 gauge stainless steel wires are placed. The first is placed above the K-wires under the triceps tendon proximally. The second is placed distally through a bicortical drill hole through the ulnar shaft; (F) The wires are crossed and knotted; (G) Using heavy needle holders the wires are tensioned symmetrically and evenly while not overcompressing; (H) The tension knot is bent downward and impacted into the ulnar cortex with a tap; (I) The K-wires are pulled back, cut short, bent and tamped below the triceps tendon into the proximal fragment; (J) The final construct and; (K) Radiograph.

Courtesy: Asif M Ilyas

across the fracture in a proximal to distal direction. The K-wires should be placed in parallel, cross just below the articular surface and exit the volar cortex of the ulna distal to the coronoid.[31] At this point the fracture site is stable enough so that the elbow can be gently manipulated and imaged under fluoroscopy to confirm reduction. A starting point should be chosen anterior enough that the wires pass close to the subchondral bone of the greater sigmoid notch. This improves stability at the articular surface.

Once the fracture is reduced and pinned the tension band is applied. A bicortical drill hole is then made through the dorsum of the proximal ulnar shaft distal to the fracture to pass the stainless steel wire. Alternatively, two drill holes may be placed for the passage of two wires creating a 'double tension band' construct. The drill hole should be placed anterior to the central axis of the ulna and a minimum of two centimeters distal to the fracture site or at least as far away as the length of the proximal fracture segment.[31,32] A 16 or 18 gauge stainless steel wire is then passed deep to the triceps tendon with the aid of an appropriate sized catheter. A second wire of the same gauge is placed through the distal drill hole and the two ends crossed over to create the figure of eight construct. The two wires are twisted together creating two knots. The medial and lateral knots should be tensioned in an alternating fashion to ensure uniform tensioning. The excess wire is then cut and the knots bent 180° to bury them in the underlying soft tissue and tamped into the bone surface to avoid prominence. The K-wires are then backed out slightly and cut to length. The proximal ends of the wires are bent 90–180° and advanced until buried underneath the triceps tendon. Care should be taken to avoid excessively long K-wires exiting the anterior cortex of the ulna as this has been implicated in cases of anterior interosseous nerve injury, development of heterotopic ossification, block to proximal radius rotation and radioulnar synostosis.[33-36]

Alternatively, an intramedullary screw can be used to create a tension band construct in place of the parallel K-wires. Intramedullary screw and K-wire tension band constructs have been found to be similar albeit slightly more rigid than conventional K-wire techniques.[4,9] Use of an intramedullary screw alone is not recommended as it has been shown to provide erratic compression at the fracture site.[9] While the use of an intramedullary screw provides the benefit of additional compression at the fracture site, it introduces the risk of complications not present with the use of K-wire tension band constructs. As stated previously, the anatomy of the proximal ulna is not that of a linear cylinder. The intramedullary canal diameter is variable along its length, and the canal has significant apex dorsal and varus bend in the proximal shaft.[28-30] If the appropriate length and diameter screw are chosen and inserted on the correct trajectory, they can provide sound fixation. However, the rigidity of the screw can lead to angular displacement at the fracture site if the screw insertion depth is not directed centrally down the medullary canal or is extended beyond the proximal bend of the ulna.[7] Typically, the canal will accept a 6.5–7.3 mm partially threaded screw. The proper depth of insertion can be determined by placing the corresponding drill to the appropriate depth under fluoroscopic guidance. Alternatively, proper depth can be ensured by tapping and measuring the appropriate length on the tap when good purchase has been achieved. Adequate purchase may not be gained in patients with larger medullary canals, however; it is rare that the medullary canal will accept a screw larger than 8 mm, and this should not be attempted. The screw can be placed over a washer to provide consistent compression across the proximal cortex and fracture site. With the screw placed but prior to compression, a 16 gauge or 18 gauge wire should be placed between the screw head or washer and the posterior cortex. The rest of the tension band wiring technique is applied as described previously.

Prior to closure final fluoroscopic images are taken to confirm fracture reduction and appropriate position of the hardware. The fascial interval is reapproximated covering as much of the wire construct as possible. The subcuticular layer is closed with interrupted absorbable suture and the skin is closed with skin staples or alternatively interrupted nylon stitches. Postoperatively, the patient may be placed into a posterior splint in 70° of flexion and neutral rotation for 1–2 weeks. Alternatively, a soft dressing may be applied facilitating immediate early motion. A straightforward protocol of progressive active and passive range of motion is begun. Strengthening exercises are delayed until radiographic union of the fracture.

TENSION BAND FIXATION: Pearls and Pitfalls

- Articular comminution is a contraindication to tension band wiring. Overcompression or apex dorsal malreduction will cause a decrease in the radius of curvature of the sigmoid notch that can result in ulnohumeral arthrosis or instability
- The fracture must be adequately reduced and fixed utilizing two parallel K-wires prior to tension banding
- K-wires placed too long exiting the anterior cortex of the ulna may cause a neurologic injury. Similarly, K-wires angulated laterally can interfere with rotation of the radius
- Intramedullary screw fixation is predicated on the placement of an appropriate length screw with adequate bone purchase. The reduced fracture should be drilled and then tapped to determine appropriate length
- A pair of single 16 gauge or 18 gauge or doubled-up 20 gauge or 22 gauge stainless steel wires may be utilized. The wires should be evenly tensioned by pulling upward and rotating the needle drivers holding the wire knot
- Avoid overtensioning at the fracture site in cases with poor bone quality that can lead to secondary incongruency at the ulnohumeral joint
- The need for hardware removal following tension band fixation is high and can be minimized by conscientious hardware positioning

Technique 2: Plate Fixation

Plate fixation is indicated for all displaced olecranon fractures, but particularly with fractures associated with articular comminution. Fixation can be achieved with a number of plating options including one-third tubular plates contoured into a hook plate, dynamic compression plate and a periarticular locking plate. Due to the advances in locking technology, the authors routinely utilize precontoured periarticular locking plates.

Surgical Technique

The fracture site is exposed through the universal posterior incision and debrided of fracture hematoma and interposed soft tissue (Figs 7.14A to G). The fracture is reduced with the aid of large tenaculums or K-wires. The locking plate is then positioned directly on the dorsal cortex of the ulnar shaft, not on the posteromedial or posterolateral surfaces. Two K-wires are then inserted through the posterior aspect of the plate to temporarily fix it to the bone. Some plates are designed to sit superficial to the triceps and have posterior tines to help provide fixation into the thick triceps tendon. Other plates are placed directly on the posterior olecranon by splitting the distal portion of the triceps tendon. A nonlocking screw or provisional fixation device is then placed distally to hold the fracture in a reduced position. When desired, the distal screw can be inserted through an eccentric drill hole to provide compression across the fracture site. However, compression should be applied with caution in cases with extensive comminution to avoid secondary articular incongruity.

With the fracture reduced with proximal K-wires and a distal bicortical screw placed, the elbow is typically quite stable and can be gently ranged and manipulated. Critical assessment of the fracture reduction and articular congruence is done at this point in time. Once satisfied with the reduction, a posterior intramedullary screw or proximal bicortical interfragmentary screw, exiting the anterior cortex of the ulna distal to the articular surface is inserted. Nonlocked bicortical screws can be used in the shaft if compression at the articular surface is desired, or locked screws can be placed to help support the overlying subchondral bone in cases of significant comminution. Our goal is to place at least three screws in the proximal fragment with the most proximal being either bicortical or intramedullary and the remaining being unicortical locking screws stopping below the articular surface. The distal segment is secured with three standard bicortical nonlocked screws. For stable fractures, three distal cortical screws are likely sufficient.

Alternatively, several nonlocked plating techniques include:

- A hook plate can be formed from a one-third tubular plate which is appropriately contoured to the posterior aspect of the ulna (Figs 7.15A and B). The proximal plate can be cut off transversely through the proximal-most hole. The remaining spikes can then be bent over 90° and used as tines to engage the triceps. Distally, the compression can be applied to the fracture site

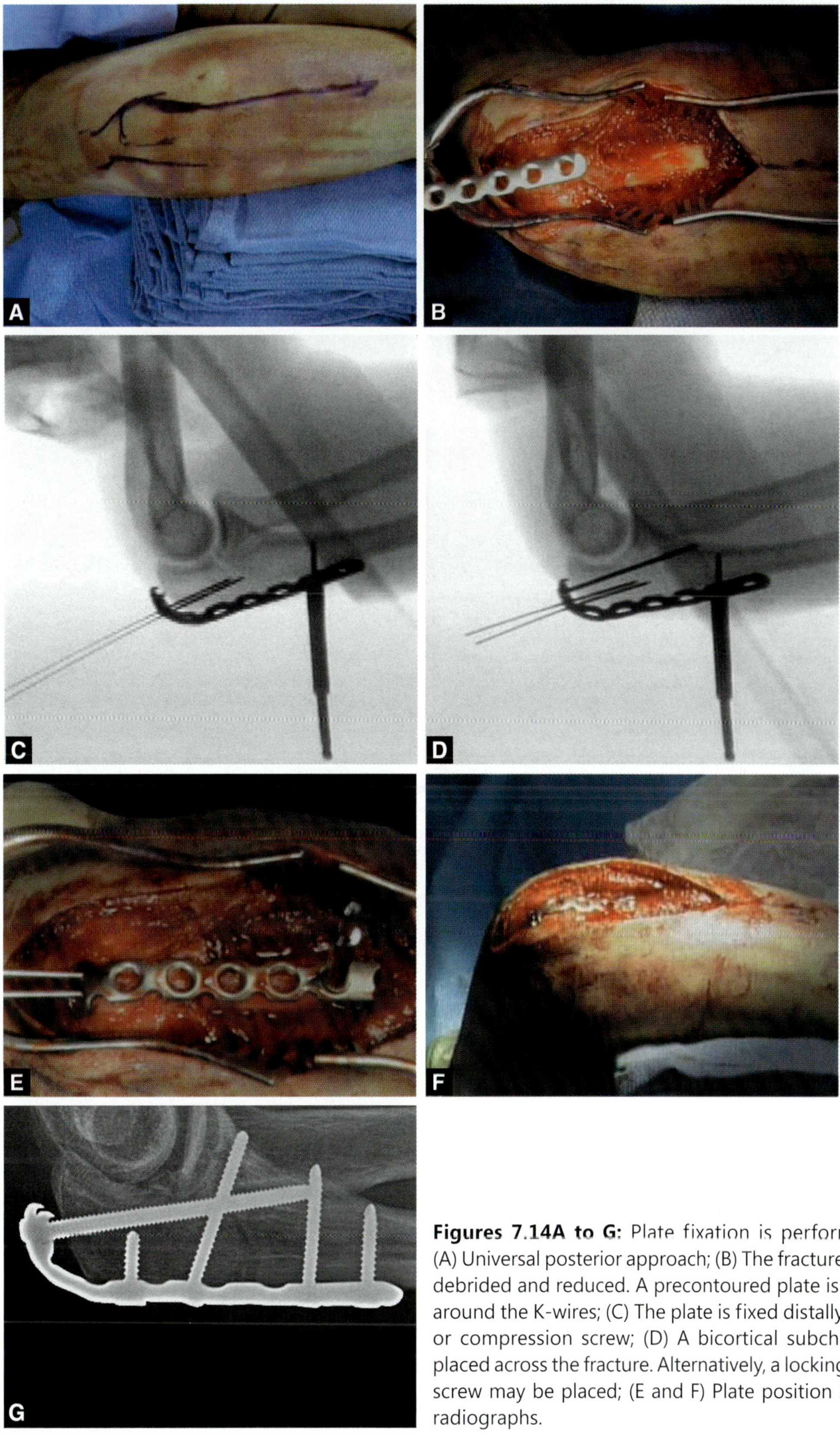

Figures 7.14A to G: Plate fixation is performed through a (A) Universal posterior approach; (B) The fracture site is exposed, debrided and reduced. A precontoured plate is applied over or around the K-wires; (C) The plate is fixed distally using a neutral or compression screw; (D) A bicortical subchondral screw is placed across the fracture. Alternatively, a locking intramedullary screw may be placed; (E and F) Plate position *in situ*; (G) Final radiographs.

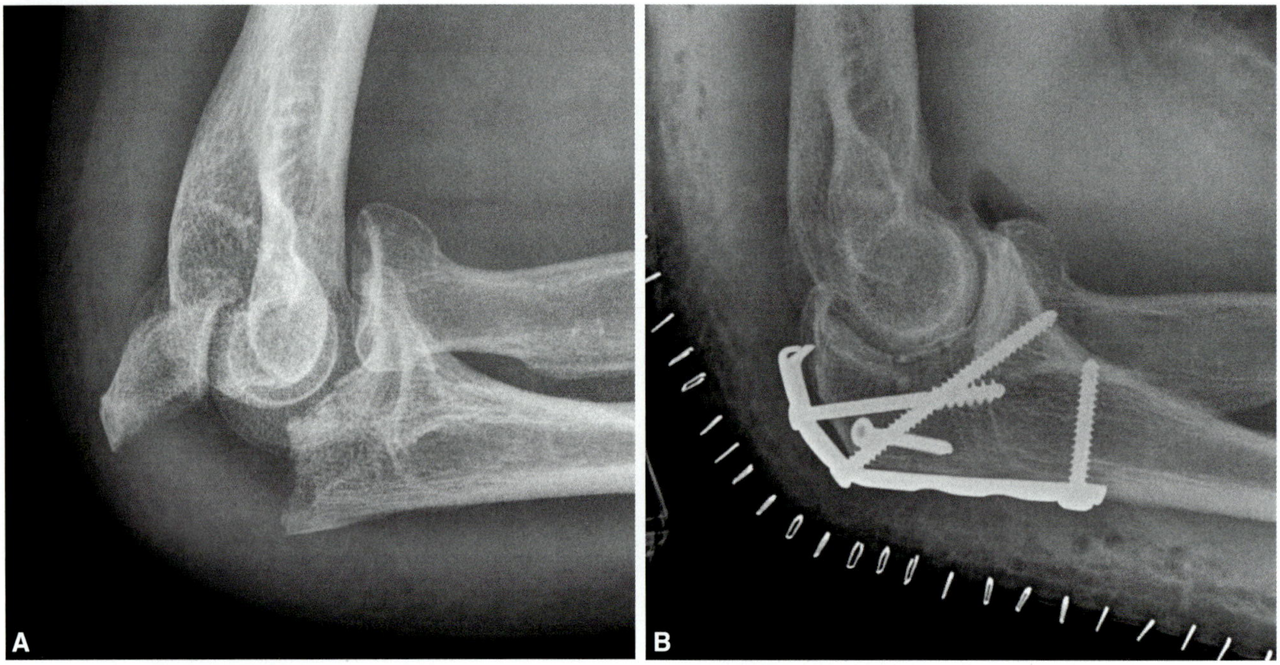

Figures 7.15A and B: A hook plate can be contoured from a one-third tubular plate. The proximal plate can be cut off transversely through the proximal most hole and bent 90° to create tines to engage the triceps.

with the use of a compression device or with a forcep placed in the distal most hole of the plate pulling it distally. Placement of a small drill hole with a 2.0 mm drill approximately 2 cm distal to the distal most hole allows a bone tenaculum to be used as a compression device. Once adequate compression is obtained, a bicortical screw is inserted into the distal fragment to maintain positioning.

- A dynamic compression reconstruction plate can be contoured and applied to the reduced olecranon fracture. Alternatively, a reconstruction plate can be contoured and applied to the medial surface of the ulna wrapping around posteriorly. This latter plate position affords the advantage of less potential hardware prominence at the tip of the elbow. However, it requires ulnar nerve dissection and mobilization. Moreover, diligence must be paid to avoid screw penetration and irritation of the proximal radioulnar joint.

Prior to closure final fluoroscopic images are taken to confirm fracture reduction and appropriate position of the hardware. Closure is similar for locked and nonlocked plates. The extensor aponeurosis is reapproximated distally to cover the plate. Typically, this will cover the distal two-thirds of the implant, reducing the subcutaneous prominence of the plate. The subcutaneous layer is closed with interrupted absorbable suture and the skin is closed with skin staples or nylon sutures. Postoperatively, the patient may be placed into a posterior splint in 70° of flexion and neutral rotation for 1–2 weeks. Alternatively, a soft dressing may be applied facilitating immediate early motion. A straightforward protocol of progressive active and passive range of motion is begun. Strengthening exercises are delayed until radiographic union of the fracture.

PLATE FIXATION: Pearls and Pitfalls

- Current precontoured locking plates are low profile and straightforward to use. A variety of hybrid constructs can be created to treat a wide variety of fracture patterns
- Advantages of locked plating include superior fixation for small proximal segments, comminuted fractures and fractures with articular depression
- Fractures with significant articular sided comminution benefit from the subchondral buttressing support provided by locking screws. The authors find this to be one of the most beneficial features of locked plates

- Patient discomfort can be reduced by limiting screw placement at the tip of the olecranon. The authors are very selective in placing a screw in this location as it is consistently the site of irritation in patients who have hardware complaints postoperatively. Meticulous soft tissue coverage of the plate can also help to reduce the incidence of hardware irritation
- As with many other locked plating constructs, reduction is not obtained by the plate and must be adequate prior to fixation otherwise malreduction may ensue

Technique 3: Intramedullary Nailing

Proposed benefits of intramedullary nailing include percutaneous insertion, rigid fixation, and less hardware irritation. Newer designs have evolved to provide multiaxial fixation, as well as compression across the fracture site. Like intramedullary nailing of other long bones, care must be taken to identify the correct insertion site, as the nail can malreduce the fracture if the nail is not directly aligned with the intramedullary canal. Unlike other long bones, intramedullary nailing of olecranon fractures requires articular reduction prior to nail insertion into the proximal ulna.

Surgical Technique

A longitudinal incision is made over the posterior olecranon beginning 1 cm proximal to the tip of the olecranon and extending far enough distally to obtain adequate reduction (Figs 7.16A to D). The fracture site is debrided of fracture hematoma and interposed soft tissue. The fracture is reduced and provisionally held with the use of large tenaculums. K-wires can be used to hold the reduction however they must be placed obliquely and away from the intramedullary canal as not to block the nail placement. Once reduction is obtained, the triceps tendon is incised longitudinally to aid in passage of the implant. Proper location of the starting portal is paramount in preventing malreduction. The proper starting point tends to be slightly inferior and lateral to the center point of the posterior surface of the olecranon to better align with the varus alignment of the ulnar shaft. This position allows for the most accommodation to the apex posterior and apex lateral bends of the normal ulnar shaft. The canal is reamed up to the appropriate diameter to except the chosen implant. The nail is inserted and locked distally. The currently available implants have extramedullary targeting devices for aiding in insertion of the locking screws. Once the nail is locked distally, the implant can be compressed or fixed in neutral depending upon the degree of fracture comminution. A compression device can be attached to the end of the nail that pulls the fixed distal segment proximally with tightening. Once the appropriate level of compression has been achieved, the proximal screws are placed and the targeting guide can be removed.

Prior to closure, final fluoroscopic images are taken to confirm fracture reduction and appropriate position of the hardware. As the technique is primarily percutaneous only simple closure is required. However, if open fracture reduction is undertaken standard closure is required including fascial closure followed by subcuticular and skin closure. Postoperatively, the patient may be placed into a posterior splint in 70° of flexion and neutral rotation for 1–2 weeks. Alternatively, a soft dressing may be applied facilitating immediate early motion. A straightforward protocol of progressive active and passive range of motion is begun. Strengthening exercises are delayed until radiographic union of the fracture.

INTRAMEDULLARY NAILING: Pearls and Pitfalls

- Potential benefits of intramedullary nailing include decreased hardware irritation and limited dissection
- Current nail designs vary widely in shape, bend and diameter. Preoperative planning is necessary to ensure that the nail will fit the patient's anatomy without displacing the fracture
- The fracture and articular surface must be reduced and held prior to nail insertion
- The proper starting point tends to be slightly inferior and lateral to the center point of the posterior surface of the olecranon to better align with the normal varus alignment of the ulnar shaft
- Following nail placement compression of the fracture site must be done with care in patients with articular comminution or poor bone stock

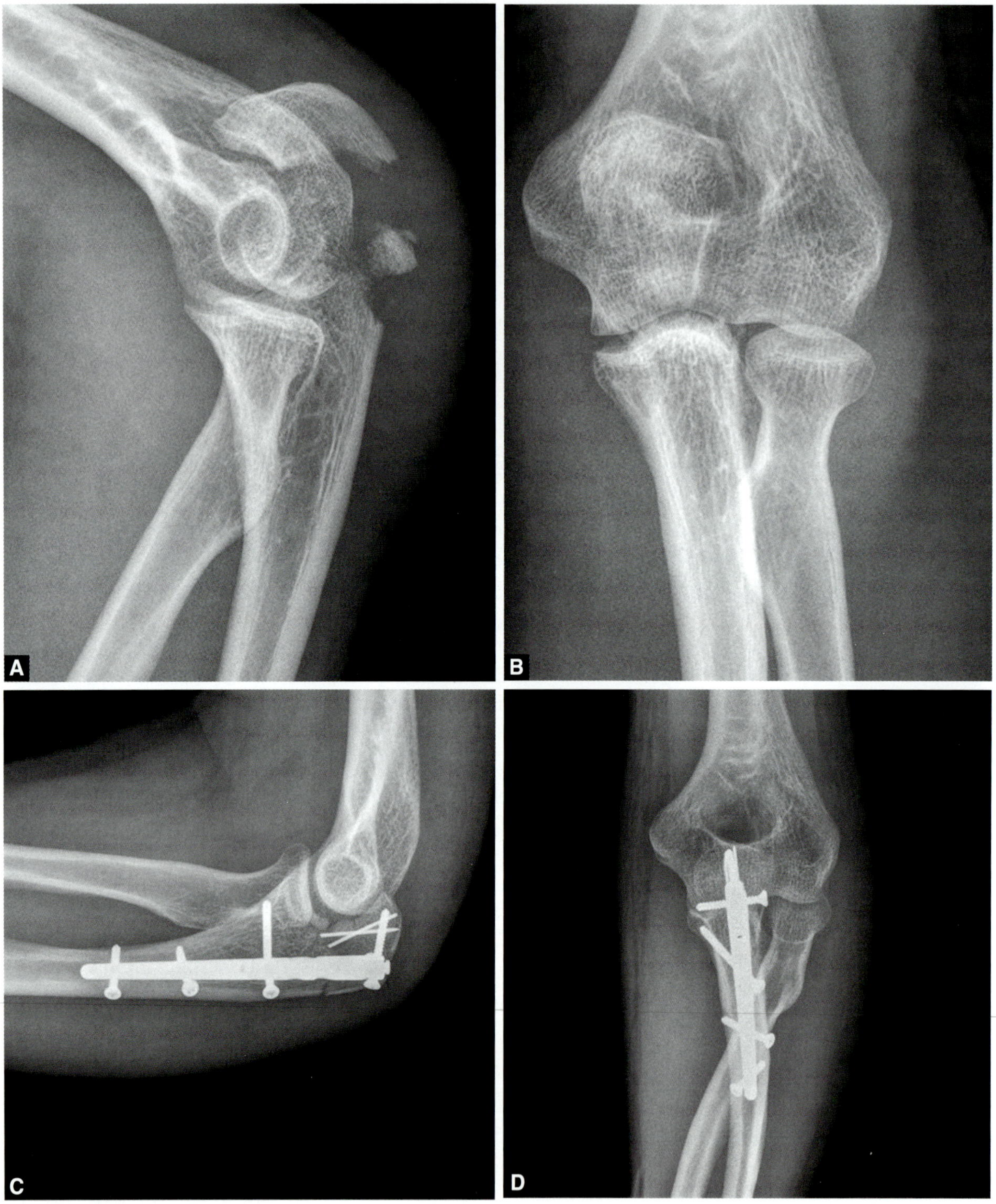

Figures 7.16A to D: Intramedullary nail fixation begins with a limited posterior approach extended distal enough to expose and reduce the fracture. (A and B) Particular attention is placed on the articular surface. Articular alignment may be provisionally or definitively supported with K-wires or screws; (C and D) Once the fracture is reduced the intramedullary nail is inserted using the manufacturer's technique. Diligence is paid to avoid secondary malreduction of the fracture during nail insertion and overcompression of the articular surface.

Technique 4: Fragment Excision and Triceps Advancement

With modern implant design, most fracture patterns can be reduced and adequately fixed with the use of locking plates and possibly intramedullary devices. However, fragment excision and triceps advancement is an option for primary treatment when the proximal fragment is extremely small, the wound is highly contaminated or when the functional demand of the patient is very low. It is also a useful technique as a salvage procedure following infection or hardware failure to re-establish the extensor mechanism and preserve stability of the elbow.[10,25,37] However, it is of utmost importance to confirm ligamentous stability of the elbow prior to excision and advancement. An intact coronoid, anterior capsule, lateral and medial collateral ligament are necessary to prevent chronic instability following fragment excision. Moreover, biomechanical studies have shown that as much as 60% of the greater sigmoid notch can be removed before instability ensues.[25]

Surgical approach is also through a posterior incision. The fracture is identified and the remaining fragments of the olecranon are sharply debrided off of the triceps tendon. Care should be taken to preserve as much of the tendon as possible. Once free from bone, the distal end of the tendon is sharply debrided perpendicular to the fiber orientation to prepare the tendon end for insertion into the remaining proximal ulna. Two 2.0 mm drill holes are placed through the fracture site just superficial to subchondral bone, exiting distally through the dorsal cortex of the ulna. A braided nonabsorbable suture is used to secure the distal tendon in a Krackow type fashion and the ends of the suture are passed through the drill holes. The suture ends are tied over the bony bridge on the dorsal cortex of the ulna and the wound is closed in appropriate layers. The patient is immobilized in 45–60° of flexion and motion is advanced slowly to allow the tendon to heal to the bone (Figs 7.17A and B).

The authors don't recommend using this technique in patients that have adequate bone stock to undergo an open reduction and internal fixation. However, as a salvage procedure following failed fixation or infections, the authors have had acceptable results.

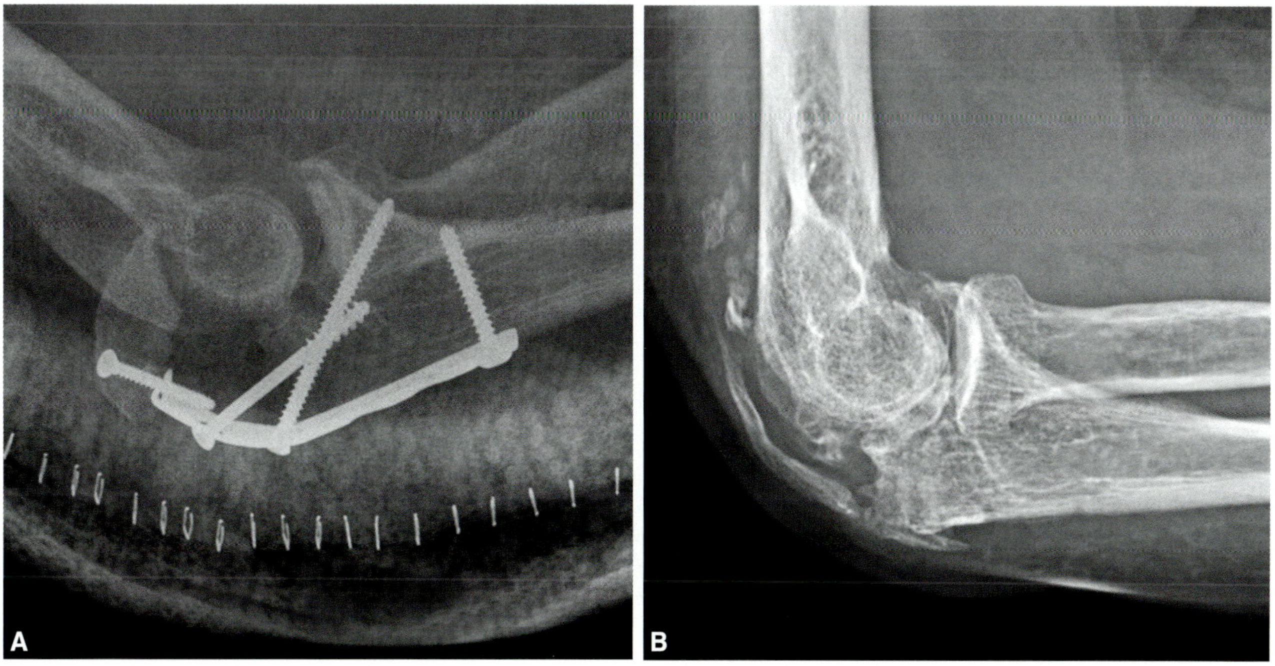

Figures 7.17A and B: This is a case of an open olecranon fracture treated with (A) Operative reduction and fixation with a hook plate following irrigation and debridement. However, the fixation failed with redisplacement of the fracture that was further complicated by a deep infection; (B) Elbow motion was salvaged with proximal fragment excision and triceps advancement. Radiographs taken 2 years postoperatively demonstrate maintenance of ulnohumeral stability.

FRAGMENT EXCISION AND TRICEPS ADVANCEMENT: Pearls and Pitfalls

- Ligamentous stability of the elbow should be confirmed prior to excision and advancement. An intact coronoid, anterior capsule, lateral and medial collateral ligament are necessary to prevent chronic instability following fragment excision
- The authors typically use a running locked stitch, with heavy braided nonabsorbable suture. The added strength of the suture provides more predictable security of the tendon
- It is important to space the drill holes on the distal cortex as wide apart as possible to prevent failure through the bony bridge between the drill holes
- The insertion point of the tendon should be close to the articular surface of the remaining olecranon, not the dorsal surface. This configuration provides a sling-like effect for the trochlea and theoretically improves the joint reaction forces on the remaining olecranon

Outcomes

The majority of studies published on treatment of olecranon fractures are comparative biomechanical studies and case series. Outcome data must be interpreted with caution because of the paucity of prospective comparative clinical investigations.

Biomechanical Studies

Initial studies compared variations in tension band constructs. Hutchinson et al. compared standard tension band constructs to compression screws with and without tension banding. They found that the degree of fragment displacement following simulated elbow range of motion and push up from a chair was significantly less with the use of an intramedullary screw than with a tension band.[4] This is the technique commonly employed by Morrey as anecdotally, there is less hardware migration leading to less need for hardware removal.[10] Similar studies have found somewhat different results. Fyfe et al. compared tension band wiring, compression screw fixation and plate fixation using a contoured one-third tubular plate. He found that plating had the most consistent resistance to gap formation under tensile stresses. Compression screw constructs showed high variability in resistance to gapping that was thought to be secondary to variable thread purchase. Of note, in comparing one knot versus two knot tension band techniques, they found that the two knot technique created more even compression across the fracture site and led to less gapping. One-third tubular plate fixation was superior in fixation of oblique and comminuted fracture patterns.[9]

The development of locking plates provided theoretical advantages for the fixation of olecranon fractures. Locking screws can help increase construct stiffness in comminuted fractures and improve fixation by allowing for insertion of unicortical screws. Bujize et al. looked at fracture displacement during cyclical loading and modes of failure with catastrophic loading of locked plating verses one-third tubular plating. They found no significant difference with respect to fracture site gapping or mode of failure. Failure occurred secondary to bone failure with both constructs. Locking plate constructs did prove to be significantly stiffer.[22] A recent study by Wilson et al. compared locking plates to tension band wiring and came to the interesting conclusion that tension band constructs do not provide compression across the fracture site with triceps loading. Locked plate constructs provided more than ten times the amount of compression across the fracture site, and maintained compression throughout elbow flexion and extension. The difference was even more pronounced at the articular margin of the fracture.[20]

With regards to intramedullary nailing, two studies have compared the stiffness, load to failure and fracture site gapping in comparison to tension band constructs. Molloy et al. found that intramedullary nails were twice as stiff and failed catastrophically under more than twice the loads of standard tension band constructs in a transverse fracture model. Nowak showed that fracture site gapping following intramedullary nailing was only 0.2 mm after 300 cycles of simulated physiologic loading compared to 1.5 mm in tension band constructs. All of these differences reached statistical significance.[23]

Clinical Studies

Clinical studies involving the treatment of olecranon fractures are for the most part, retrospective case series. The lack of prospective controlled trials comparing treatment methods creates a significant amount of controversy in determining treatment protocols. Evaluation of the available literature does reveal some consistent findings. Overall, patients that undergo surgical treatment of olecranon fractures tend to do well. Overall, clinical outcomes following fixation of olecranon fractures are difficult to assess because of the lack of consistent outcome criteria in the literature. The majority of clinical studies are retrospective case series with varying criteria for defining satisfactory results. Good and excellent outcomes are reported in 36–94% of patients undergoing tension band fixation or plating.[5,15,17,38,39] Postoperative loss of terminal flexion and extension is common finding regardless of the method of fixation used, however; functional range of motion is rarely lost. Overall complication rate, most notably stiffness, increases with the complexity of the fracture pattern. One consistent and somewhat surprising trend in the literature is hardware removal rate. The rate of hardware removal following tension band wiring approaches 85% in some studies.[25,38,40] This has not been mirrored in series of patients that underwent precontoured plating techniques.[15,19] Reported hardware removal rate following plating have been significantly lower than with tension band wiring. Anderson et al. recently reviewed 32 patients that underwent locked plating and found that only 4 of them required removal of hardware.[16] Range of motion and complication rate excluding hardware removal were similar to previous reports on tension band wiring. Hume et al. have published one of the only clinical trials to date comparing methods of fixation. He found significantly better clinical and radiographic outcomes in patients that underwent plating versus tension band wirings (86% vs 43%). He also found significantly less hardware irritation postoperatively in patients who received a plate when compared to those that received a tension band construct (42% vs 5%). Outcomes strongly favored plating, however it is somewhat concerning that their results for the tension band group were significantly worse than previous reports.[12] To further complicate interpretation of the literature, there is some evidence that simple fragment excision and triceps advancement lead to similar outcomes as internal fixation. Gartsman retrospectively reviewed patients over the age of sixty that underwent fragment excision, as well as patients that underwent internal fixation. They concluded that there were no significant differences in postoperative rates of arthrosis, strength and range of motion. Their conclusions question whether there is a need to attempt complex repairs in low demand patients.[25]

Overall, there are consistent trends that support the use of plate fixation in complex fracture patterns. While biomechanical studies routinely show superior stiffness, decreased gapping and load to failure in plate constructs compared to tension band constructs, the overall clinical results have not been substantially different following any fixation technique, including fragment excision. Because of the lack of solid evidence to support best practices, surgeons must evaluate their results critically and adopt different treatment strategies when necessary. To date, there is no evidence to support that plate fixation is inferior in treatment of any fracture patterns or patient population. Because of this, the authors have adopted precontoured periarticular plating as the mainstay for treatment for all fractures with any articular comminution and tension band construct for simple olecranon fractures.

Complications

Complications are common following fixation of olecranon fractures and include hardware complications, fixation failure, malunions, nonunions, stiffness, heterotopic ossification, proximal radioulnar joint injury and infection.

Symptomatic Hardware

Symptomatic hardware is unequivocally the most common complication following surgical treatment of olecranon fractures. The need for removal of hardware following tension band fixation is universally high regardless of the specific technique used. The majority of clinical studies show a 43–87% rate of reoperation for removal of painful or migrating hardware.[11,38,41-44] Numerous modifications to the various operative techniques have been trialed in an attempt to improve hardware removal rate. To date, no modification to tension band techniques has consistently reduced the hardware removal rate. The most common reason for hardware removal is patient discomfort. In our experience, virtually all patients complain of discomfort at the site of wire crossing on the subcutaneous border of the proximal ulna (Fig. 7.13J). Aside from this observation, outcome studies have been quite favorable with greater than 90% of patients having good or excellent outcomes following this technique.[38] Of note, reported hardware removal rate has been significantly less following plating techniques, with hardware removal in the range of 5–17%.[11,15,18,19] One prospective study exists that examines the rate of hardware irritation in fractures treated with tension band fixation or plate fixation. Consistent with other published case series, they found significantly higher rate of symptomatic hardware in the tension band group than in the plate group.[11]

Hardware Failure

Fixation failure rates are highly dependent upon the definition used to define failure. Numerous biomechanical and clinical studies have demonstrated that significant gapping of the fracture site can occur with the use of tension band fixation. When failure is defined as gapping greater than 2 mm post fixation, failure rates are as high as 83%.[11] Obviously, many of these patients go on to uneventful union despite some degree of loss of fixation. Reports of nonunions are rare (1–5%).[45,46] Despite gapping at the fracture site, clinical outcomes appear to be similar regardless of method of fixation. Few patients have significant loss of function or loss of range of motion greater than 15° regardless of fixation method.

Malunion/Nonunion

Malunion can occur from improper reduction or loss of reduction. Most commonly, compression at the level of the joint in comminuted fractures can result in a radius of curvature mismatch between the distal trochlea and the olecranon (Fig. 7.7B). Loss of the bare area following fixation is a worrisome sign that the olecranon has been fixed in an overly compressed position. The olecranon loses its inherent stability when its articular surface is incongruent with the distal trochlea. Other common pitfalls that lead to malunion include failure to recreate the normal ulnar shaft varus alignment. Similarly, the normal 6° apex dorsal bend in the proximal ulna may not be properly reconstructed in cases of comminution or when an improperly contoured rigid implant is used. Loss of this normal anatomic bend may be of most consequence when fracture dislocations are encountered. In these cases malunion of the proximal ulna can result in chronic radiocapitellar subluxation or dislocation. Also, loss of the normal dorsal angulation can represent improper contouring of the greater sigmoid notch, altering joint biomechanics and possibly increasing postoperative arthrosis.[28]

Nonunion is a worrisome complication that can stem from attempted nonoperative management of displaced olecranon fractures (Figs 7.18A and B). The constant pull of the triceps leads to a persistent displacement force across the fracture site. Nonoperative treatment of displaced injuries has been studied and the nonunion rate

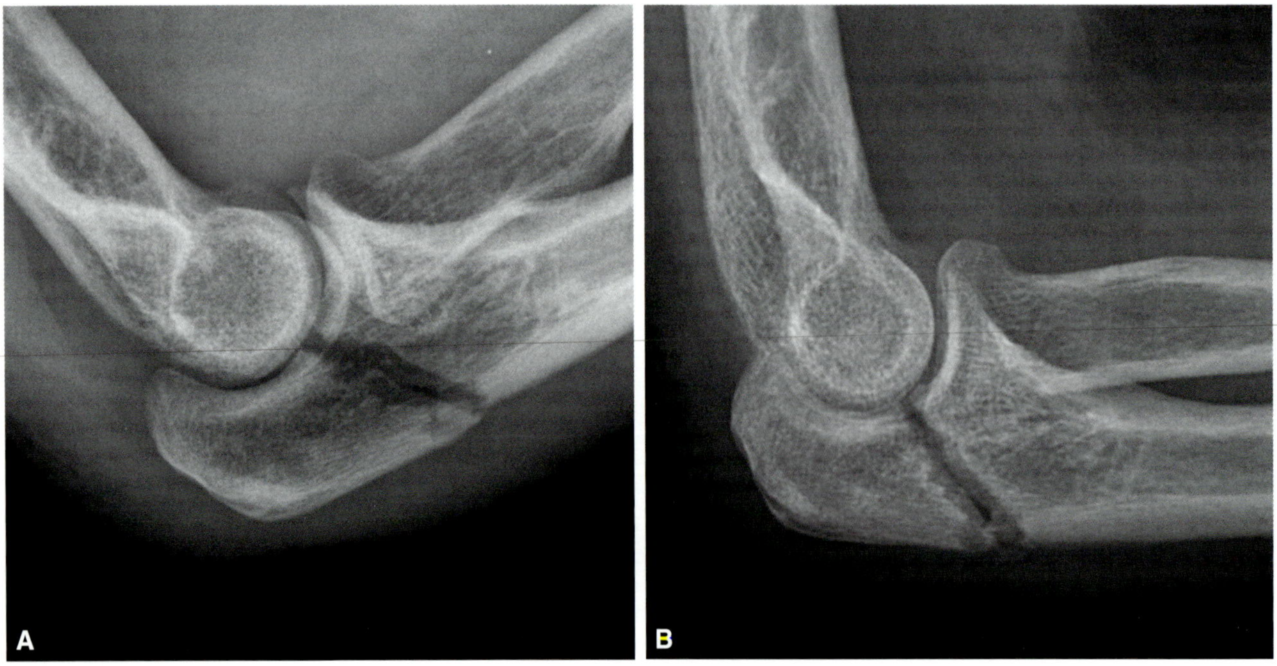

Figures 7.18A and B: This is a case of a patient who incurred a (A) minimally displaced olecranon fracture who also had multiple severe comorbidities contraindicating surgical intervention. The patient was treated nonoperatively in a cast for 3 weeks followed by progressive motion; (B) Radiographs taken 3 months later demonstrated a stable fibrous nonunion of the fracture. The patient was clinically asymptomatic and regained functional elbow motion.

is reported to be 75%, however functional outcomes do not correlate with radiographic union, as 67% of patients were pain free with minimal loss of range of motion.[7] Typically, the authors do not recommend treating displaced fractures conservatively unless the patient's health status contraindicates operative intervention. However, patients may occasionally present with a minimally displaced fracture where active extension against gravity is maintained without an extensor lag that can be treated nonoperatively with close radiographic follow-up to monitor for late fracture displacement.

Stiffness

Postoperative loss of range of motion is not the exception but the rule when operating on an elbow fracture. Typically, patients with isolated olecranon fractures regain excellent range of motion with the most common manifestation of stiffness being loss of 10–15° of terminal extension.[44] Postoperative range of motion tends to correlate with the severity of the presenting injury. Patients that sustain highly comminuted fractures or fracture-dislocations, tend to have predictably worse range of motion postoperatively.

Postoperative stiffness can be minimized with careful soft tissue handling, adequate fracture reduction and fixation, and aggressive postoperative therapy. Outcomes are dependent on the ability to begin range of motion exercises as early as possible. Because of this, the authors tend to err on the side of increasing the rigidity of fixation in order to begin aggressive early range of motion with 1–2 weeks postoperatively.

Heterotopic Ossification

Although an uncommon complication following olecranon fracture, heterotopic ossification (HO) commonly occurs around the elbow (Figs 7.19A to D). Rates are reported as high as 14%, however these series included olecranon fractures that were part of more complex injury patterns.[8,20] Patients typically present with a stepwise loss of function after uneventful fracture union. Loss of function typically precedes radiographic maturation of the ectopic bone. Heterotopic ossification is thought to occur secondary to cellular dysplasia in response to a severe soft tissue injury. While HO is not completely understood, it is thought that meticulous handling of the soft tissues can help prevent its development. Once clinical and radiographic signs of HO have developed, the best course of action is delayed excision. Physical therapy can and should be continued in attempts to prevent complete ankylosis, however the benefit is unknown. Excision of HO should be undertaken once maturation has been completed. This occurs typically 4–6 months postinjury. Commonly, anterior and posterior capsulectomy must be performed at the same time to reestablish motion of the elbow. Complications following HO excision include residual stiffness, nerve injury and recurrence of HO. Currently the evidence is unclear as to the efficacy of radiation therapy following olecranon fracture to prevent HO in the perioperative period. There is concern that postoperative radiation may increase nonunion rates and wound complications. However, radiation has been used successfully in preventing recurrence, following excision of HO and capsular releases.

Proximal Radioulnar Joint Injury

Although the likelihood of proximal radioulnar joint (PRUJ) injury is lessened with appropriate placement of precontoured locking plates, the radial head remains vulnerable as it intrudes significantly into the proximal ulna at the lesser sigmoid notch. There are two significant variables that need to be addressed with plating techniques to prevent chondrolysis and early arthrosis secondary to violation of the PRUJ. When custom contoured one-third tubular or dynamic compression plates are used, insertion of a posterior intramedullary screw alters the trajectory of subsequent screws in the proximal portion of the ulna. Angulation of the screws laterally to avoid impingement on the posterior intramedullary screw can result in inadvertent violation of the PRUJ (Figs 7.20A and B). This may not be readily recognizable unless careful fluoroscopic evaluation is used to confirm safe placement. Because of this risk, all screws inserted in the proximal ulna should be directed slightly medial to prevent impingement on the longitudinal posterior intramedullary screw. The introduction of precontoured locking plates has decreased this risk substantially by leaving the central intramedullary portion of the proximal ulna free for locking screws to be placed. The use of the appropriate drill guides allows for safe insertion of both the posterior screws and the proximal dorsal screws to be inserted without abutting one another. However, if the plate is misplaced or offset, the risk for inadvertent violation of the PRUJ is increased as the

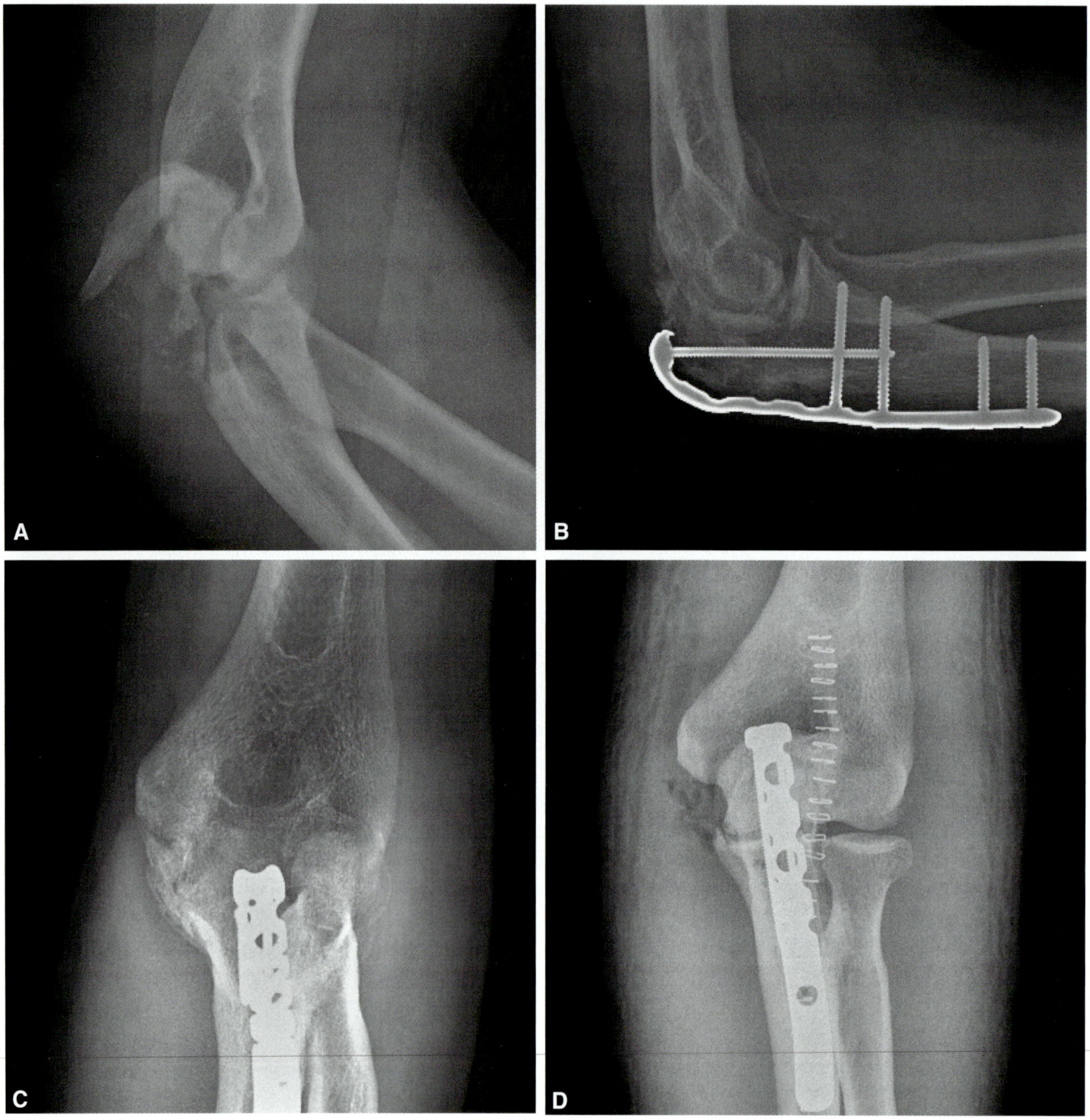

Figures 7.19A to D: This is a case of patient who incurred a (A) severely comminuted olecranon fracture. The patient also had a contralateral perilunate fracture-dislocation and transolecranon fracture after falling from a height. The patient underwent operative reduction and plate fixation with a precontoured periarticular locking plate. Despite a standard postoperative rehabilitation protocol including early motion and aggressive therapy the patient developed extensive heterotopic ossification (HO); (B and C) Radiographs taken 3 months postoperatively identified bridging HO across the anterior and posterior ulnohumeral joint; (D) Six months postoperatively the patient underwent excision of HO and capsular release. The patient also received a single dose of 700 cGy radiation treatment postoperatively. The patient ultimately regained functional range of motion including 20–100° of flexion and extension.

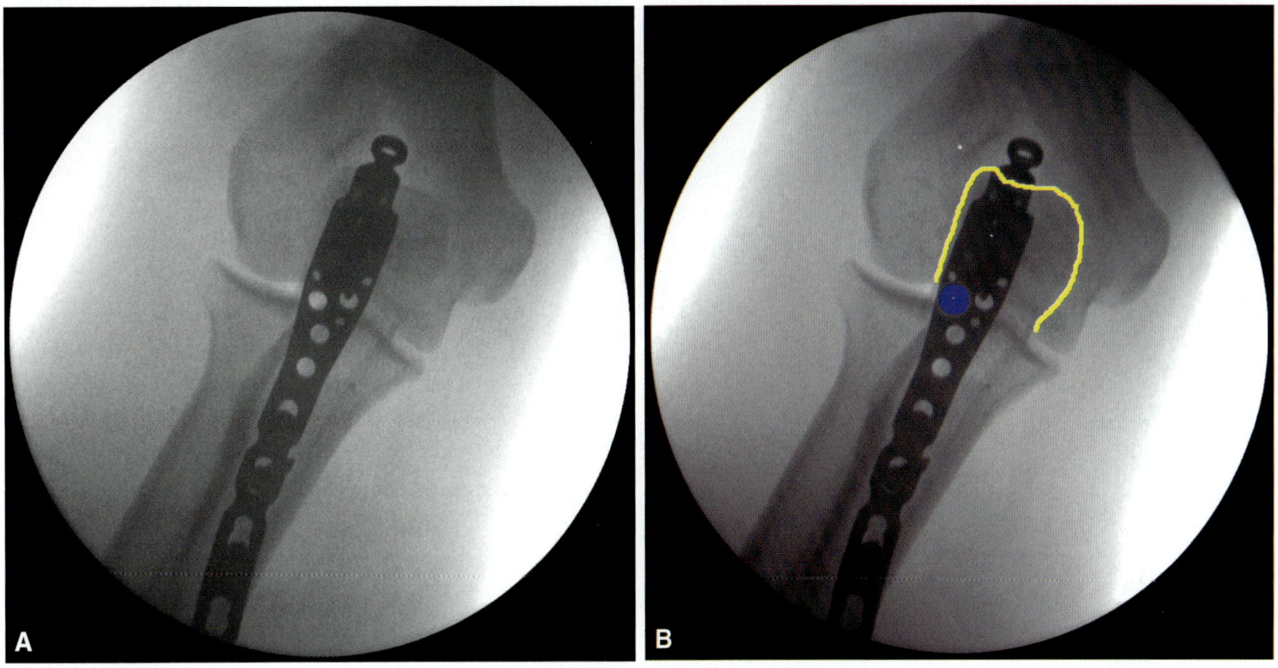

Figures 7.20A and B: The proximal radioulnar joint is susceptible to hardware irritation by screws placed too laterally or misapplied precontoured plates. Note how the plate depicted in the image is applied too laterally potentially risking proximal radioulnar joint violation if a screw was placed in the hole colored blue.

proximal screws will be inappropriately angled toward the radial head. Moreover, inadvertent PRUJ injury can be avoided by diligent evaluation of forearm rotation.

Ulnar Neuropathy

Postoperative ulnar nerve dysfunction is not a common complication but can have disastrous consequences on patient's functional outcomes. Ulnar neuropathy postoperatively has been reported to occur in up to 5% of patients.[11] Commonly injury is not secondary to operative technique but is associated with the severity of the injury at onset. Extrinsic compression secondary to fibrosis and scarring is thought to contribute to dysfunction postoperatively. For this reason the authors do not routinely identify the ulnar nerve when treating fractures of the olecranon. The authors feel that the added dissection of identifying the nerve may contribute to scarring and fibrosis and is not a beneficial step. While this has never been studied in fractures of the olecranon, leaving the ulnar nerve in place has been shown to decrease postoperative dysfunction in distal humerus fractures.[26] Care must be taken to recognize the ulnar nerve's location and avoid placing reduction forceps or K-wires near its vicinity. Often, its location can be felt readily with direct palpation.

Infection

Injuries to the upper extremity routinely have lower infection rate following fixation of both closed and open fractures in comparison to lower extremity injuries. This has been attributed to the rich vascularity and thick soft tissue envelope surrounding the underlying bones of the upper extremity. However, infections will inevitably occur. Based on published studies, infection rate following fixation of olecranon fractures ranges from 0–10%.[11,25,46] There are no studies that the authors are aware of to date that specifically address infection rate in open olecranon fractures. Treatment for postoperative infections should adhere to basic principles of aggressive and early irrigation and debridement with attempted maintenance of hardware until union is achieved.

Authors' Preferred Management of Select Complications

Case 1: Failure of Fixation

Patient is a 60-year-old male involved in a motor vehicle accident incurring a femoral neck fracture and an ipsilateral olecranon fracture (Figs 7.21A to E). The patient

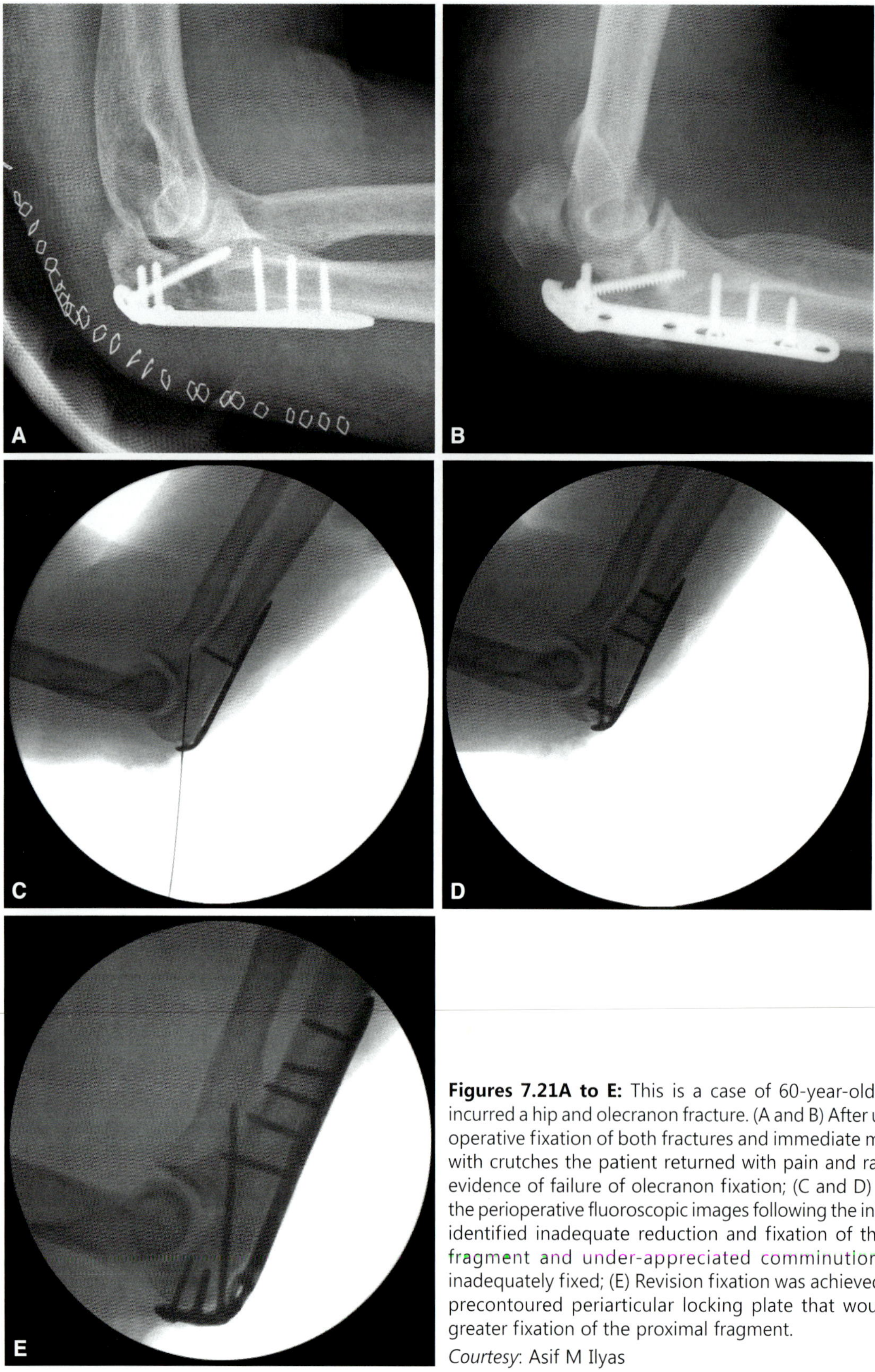

Figures 7.21A to E: This is a case of 60-year-old male who incurred a hip and olecranon fracture. (A and B) After undergoing operative fixation of both fractures and immediate mobilization with crutches the patient returned with pain and radiographic evidence of failure of olecranon fixation; (C and D) Analysis of the perioperative fluoroscopic images following the initial surgery identified inadequate reduction and fixation of the proximal fragment and under-appreciated comminution that was inadequately fixed; (E) Revision fixation was achieved utilizing a precontoured periarticular locking plate that would provide greater fixation of the proximal fragment.

Courtesy: Asif M Ilyas

was taken to the OR for operative fixation of both injuries. Open reduction and internal fixation utilizing a precontoured locking plate was performed for the olecranon fracture without incident. The patient immediately began weight-bearing with crutches using both the arms. The patient was re-evaluated 6 weeks postoperatively with a complaint of elbow pain and extension weakness. Radiographs identified loss of fixation and redisplacement of his olecranon fracture.

Fixation failures commonly occur when fixation techniques are not suited to the fracture pattern or when the fixation is inadequately applied. Biomechanical studies have shown that locked plating of olecranon fractures provide enough rigidity to safely allow for active range of motion, however; fixation failure can occur even with simple loads equivalent to pushing up from a chair. When sufficient bone stock remains, the authors advocate revision operative reduction and fixation. However, if there is inadequate proximal fragment bone stock and/or complicated by infection, the elbow can be salvaged with proximal fragment resection and triceps tendon advancement.

Technique

Preoperative evaluation of a failed fixation of an olecranon fracture begins with scrutinizing the injury and preoperative radiographs. The fracture lines, articular comminution and the quality of the proximal fragment are evaluated. In this case, the authors identified good bone quality and size of the proximal fragment but poor fixation. Subsequently, revision will require conversion to a plate that will provide better fixation of the proximal fragment.

The patient is positioned supine and the arm is prepped and draped across the chest. A sterile tourniquet is applied and assistant holds the arm. The fracture site is exposed through the same posterior incision. The previous hardware is removed and the fracture re-reduced with a large tenaculum. Fluoroscopy is used to confirm fracture reduction and restoration of the articular surface. Kirschner wires are placed to provisionally hold the fracture reduced. Various precontoured periarticular locking screws are available. A plate with adequate purchase of the proximal fragment is selected and first fixed distally. The proximal fragment is then fixed to the plate in a bicortical fashion. Additional unicortical locking screws are placed in the posterior aspect of the proximal fragment to avoid future redisplacement. At least three screws are placed bicortically in the shaft distally. Because of the prior history of failed fixation, the patient is mobilized slower under close supervision.

Case 2: Proximal Radioulnar Joint Injury

Patient is a 20-year-old male that presented with a displaced olecranon fracture. The patient underwent uneventful fixation utilizing a precontoured periarticular locking plate. Standard postoperative rehabilitation was initiated including early motion. The patient regained a flexion-extension arc of motion of 5–140° with no discomfort. However, he demonstrated marked limitation with attempted forearm rotation. He also noted a catching sensation when he attempted to supinate his wrist. Radiographs were repeated at that time which showed an area of osteolysis in the radial neck (Figs 7.22A to E).

The highly irregular contour of the proximal ulna and its complex articulations with the trochlea and the radial head at the PRUJ can make screw placement difficult at times. When standard plates are used for fixation, meticulous care must be taken to prevent placement of screws intra-articularly. Fluoroscopic views can be vexing when attempting to evaluate screw placement around the lesser sigmoid notch. Precontoured locking plates have largely decreased the risk of inadvertent screw penetration into the PRUJ, however; the risk is still present. Inadvertent placement of the plate slightly medial off the dorsal apex of the ulna may lead to angulation of the screws towards the PRUJ. Bicortical screws placed in this fashion will most certainly be placed intra-articularly. This is difficult to assess fluoroscopically because of the significant overhang of the anterolateral coronoid. Even with the use of fixed angle drill guides and careful fluoroscopic evaluation, it is imperative to perform a thorough examination through the entire arc of motion prior to leaving the OR. Any mechanical irregularities detected during range of motion should be investigated. Treatment involves removal or revision of hardware.

Summary

Fractures of the olecranon process are relatively common injuries that can present unique challenges. The powerful pull of the attached triceps, the subcutaneous nature of

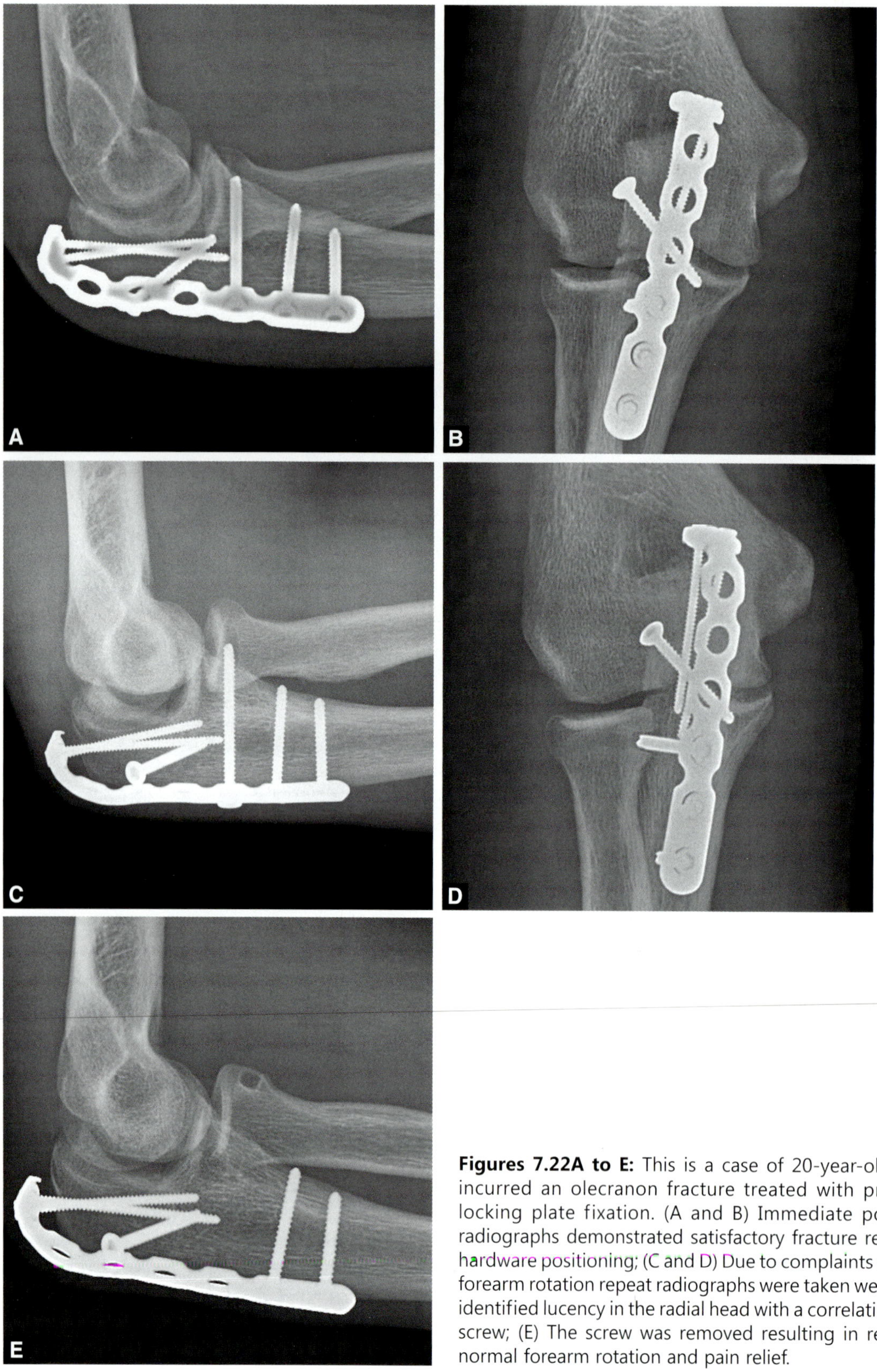

Figures 7.22A to E: This is a case of 20-year-old male who incurred an olecranon fracture treated with precontoured locking plate fixation. (A and B) Immediate postoperative radiographs demonstrated satisfactory fracture reduction and hardware positioning; (C and D) Due to complaints of decreased forearm rotation repeat radiographs were taken weeks later that identified lucency in the radial head with a correlating offending screw; (E) The screw was removed resulting in restoration of normal forearm rotation and pain relief.

the bone and the variety of fracture patterns that occur are common obstacles to recreating a stable and functional ulnohumeral joint. Tensile forces must be neutralized without excessive compression between the fragments, and this must be done with limited hardware secondary to the relative paucity of soft tissue covering this area.

Tension band wiring has been used with good success for over five decades. With the advent of alternative fixation strategies, the treating surgeon must be familiar with multiple methods of fixation, as well as their advantages and disadvantages. Numerous biomechanical studies are providing mounting evidence that the use of locked plates provide superior fixation in treating olecranon fractures with significant comminution, fracture-dislocation patterns, proximal injuries involving the coronoid process and fractures with small proximal fragments. With regards to secondary procedures for removal of hardware, there seems to be no advantage to tension band wiring in comparison to plating techniques. Uniformly, less displacement is seen following intramedullary nail techniques and plating in comparison to tension band wiring in biomechanical studies. While this has yet to infer any clinical advantage in comparison trials, it should be kept in mind when selecting an appropriate implant. The development of locking intramedullary implants may potentially improve the rate of secondary surgery due to the lack of external hardware to cause irritation. However, the use of these implants should be cautioned until clinical series confirm good outcomes.

Ultimately, the goal of treatment of these injuries is anatomic reduction, rigid fixation and early elbow motion. The complex nature of the elbow articulations and its surrounding anatomy can provide significant challenges to achieving good outcomes. However, adherence to sound techniques and indications can provide consistently strong outcomes.

References

1. Bryce CD, Armstrong AD. Anatomy and biomechanics of the elbow. Orthop Clin North Am. 2008;39(2):141-54.
2. Colton CL. Fractures of the olecranon in adults: classification and management. Injury. 1973;5(2):121-9.
3. Schatzker J, Tile M, Hu R. The Rationale of Operative Fracture Care Springer.
4. Hutchinson DT, Horwitz DS, Ha G, et al. Cyclic loading of olecranon fracture fixation constructs. J Bone Joint Surg Am. 2003;85(5):831-7.
5. Wolfgang G, Burke F, Bush D, et al. Surgical treatment of displaced olecranon fractures by tension band wiring technique. Clin Orthop Relat Res. 1987;(224):192-204.
6. Morrey BF, Askew LJ, Chao EY. A biomechanical study of normal functional elbow motion. J Bone Joint Surg Am. 1981;63(6):872-7.
7. Hak DJ, Golladay GJ. Olecranon Fractures: treatment options. J Am Acad of Othop Surg. 2000;8(4):266-75.
8. Weber BG, Vasey H. [Osteosynthesis in Olecranon Fractures]. Z Unfallmed Berufskr. 1963;56:90-6.
9. Fyfe IS, Mossad MM, Holdsworth BJ. Methods of fixation of olecranon fractures. An experimental mechanical study. J Bone Joint Surg Br. 1985;67(3):367-72.
10. Morrey BF. Current concepts in the treatment of fractures of the radial head, the olecranon and the coronoid. J Bone Joint Surg. 1995;77(2):316-27.
11. Hume M, Wiss D. Olecranon fractures. A clinical and radiographic comparison of tension band wiring and plate fixation. Clin Orthop Relat Res. 1992 dec(285):229-35.
12. Villanueva P, Osorio F, Commessatti M, et al. Tension band wiring for olecranon fractures: analysis of risk factors for failure. J Shoulder Elbow Surg. 2006;15(3):351-6.
13. Horner S, Sadasivan K, Lipka J, et al. Analysis of mechanical factors affecting fixation of olecranon fractures. Orthopedics. 1989;12(11):1469-72.
14. Weseley M, Barenfeld P, Eisenstein A. The use of the Zuelzer hook plate in fixation of olecranon fractures. J Bone Joint Surg. 1976;58(6):859-63.
15. Buijze G, Kloen P. Clinical Evaluation of Locking Compression Plate Fixation for Comminuted Olecranon Fractures. J Bone Joint Surg. 2009;91(10):2416-20.
16. Anderson ML, Larson AN, Merten SM, et al. Congruent elbow plate fixation of olecranon fractures. J Orthop Trauma. 2007;21(6):386-93.
17. Bailey C, MacDermid J, Patterson S, et al. Outcome of plate fixation of olecranon fractures. J Orthop Trauma. 2001; 15(8):542-8.
18. Siebenlist S, Torsiglieri T, Kraus T, et al. Comminuted fractures of the proximal ulna—Preliminary results with an anatomically preshaped locking compression plate (LCP) system. Injury. 2010;41(12):1306-11.
19. Simpson NS, Goodman LA, Jupiter JB. Contoured LCDC plating of the proximal ulna. Injury. 1996;27(6):411-7.
20. Wilson J, Bajwa A, Kamath V, et al. Biomechanical comparison of interfragmentary compression in transverse fractures of the olecranon. J Bone Joint Surg Br. 2011; 93(2):245-50.
21. Tejwani N, Garnham I, Wolinsky P, et al. Posterior olecranon plating: biomechanical and clinical evaluation of a new operative technique. Bull Hosp Jt Dis. 2002;61(1-2):27-31.

22. Buijze G, Blankevoort L, Tuijthof G, et al. Biomechanical evaluation of fixation of comminuted olecranon fractures: one-third tubular versus locking compression plating. Arch Orthop Trauma Surg. 2010;130(4):459-64.
23. Molloy S, Jasper LE, Elliott DS, et al. Biomechanical evaluation of intramedullary nail versus tension band fixation for transverse olecranon fractures. J Orthop Trauma. 2004;18(3):170-5.
24. Bell TH, Ferreira LM, McDonald CP, et al. Contribution of the olecranon to elbow stability: an in vitro biomechanical study. J Bone Joint Surg. 2010;92(4):949-57.
25. Gartsman G, Sculco T, Otis J. Operative treatment of olecranon fractures. Excision or open reduction with internal fixation. J Bone Joint Surg. 1981;63(5):718-21.
26. Chen RC, Harris DJ, Leduc S, et al. Is ulnar nerve transposition beneficial during open reduction internal fixation of distal humerus fractures? J Orthop Trauma. 2010;24(7):391-4.
27. Veras Del Monte L, Sirera Vercher M, Busquets Net R, et al. Conservative treatment of displaced fractures of the olecranon in the elderly. Injury. 1999;30(2):105-10.
28. Rouleau DM, Faber KJ, Athwal GS. The proximal ulna dorsal angulation: a radiographic study. J Shoulder Elbow Surg. 2010;19(1):26-30.
29. Wang A, Mara M, Hutchinson D. The proximal ulna: An anatomic study with relevance to olecranon osteotomy and fracture fixation. J Shoulder Elbow Surg. 2003;12(3):293-6.
30. Windisch G, Clement H, Grechenig W, et al. A morphometrical study of the medullary cavity of the ulna referred to intramedullary nailing. Surg Radiol Anat. 2006;29(1): 47-53.
31. Rowland SA, Burkhart SS. Tension band wiring of olecranon fractures. A modification of the AO technique. Clin Orthop Relat Res. 1992;(277):238-42.
32. Paremain GP, Novak VP, Jinnah RH, et al. Biomechanical evaluation of tension band placement for the repair of olecranon fractures. Clin Orthop Relat Res. 1997;(335):325-30.
33. Thumroj E, Jianmongkol S, Thammaroj J. Median nerve palsy after operative treatment of olecranon fracture. J Med Assoc Thai. 2005;88(10):1434-7.
34. Velkes S, Tytiun Y, Salai M. Proximal radio-ulnar synostosis complicating tension band wiring of the fractured olecranon. Injury. 2005;36(10):1254-6.
35. Parker JR, Conroy J, Campbell DA. Anterior interosseus nerve injury following tension band wiring of the olecranon. Injury. 2005;36(10):1252-3.
36. Finlayson D. Complications of tension-band wiring of olecranon fractures. J Bone Joint Surg Am. 1986;68(6): 951-2.
37. Bell JE. Advances in elbow fracture management. Curr Orthop Pract. 2010;21(5):478.
38. Karlsson MK, Hasserius R, Karlsson C, et al. Fractures of the olecranon: a 15- to 25-year followup of 73 patients. Clin Orthop. 2002;403:205-12.
39. Akman S, Erturer RE, Tezer M, et al. [Long-term results of olecranon fractures treated with tension-band wiring technique]. Acta Orthop Traumatol Turc. 2002;36(5):401-7.
40. Murphy DF, Greene WB, Gilbert JA, et al. Displaced olecranon fractures in adults. Biomechanical analysis of fixation methods. Clin Orthop Relat Res. 1987;(224):210-4.
41. Holdsworth B, Mossad M. Elbow function following tension band fixation of displaced fractures of the olecranon. Injury. 1984;16(3):182-7.
42. Macko D, Szabo RM. Complications of tension-band wiring of olecranon fractures. J Bone Joint Surg Am. 1985; 67(9):1396-401.
43. Edwards SG, Varecka TF, Cohen MS. Surgeon perceptions of patient outcomes regarding proximal ulna internal fixation. 2010.
44. Rommens PM, Küchle R, Schneider RU, et al. Olecranon fractures in adults: factors influencing outcome. Injury. 2004;35(11):1149-57.
45. Mayer PJ, Evarts CM. Nonunion, delayed union, malunion and avascular necrosis. In: Epps CH Jr (Ed). Complications in orthopaedic surgery; 1978. pp. 159-75.
46. Papagelopoulos PJ, Morrey BF. Treatment of nonunion of olecranon fractures. J Bone Joint Surg Br. 1994;76(4):627-35.

Chapter 8

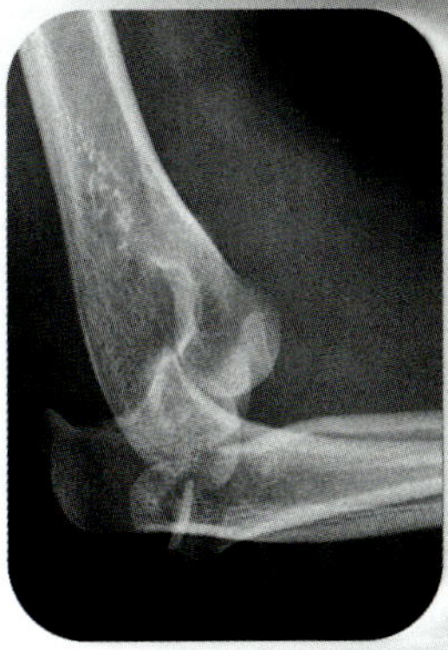

Radial Head Fractures and Terrible Triad Injuries

John Fowler, Joseph Thoder

Chapter Outline

Introduction
Diagnosis
Classification
Surgical Indications
Surgical Anatomy, Positioning and Approaches
- Applied Anatomy
- Positioning
- Approaches

Surgical Techniques
- Technique 1: Radial Head Fixation
- Technique 2: Radial Head Arthroplasty
- Technique 3: Terrible Triad Repair

Outcomes
Complications
- Heterotopic Ossification
- Elbow Stiffness
- Radial Head Malunion/Nonunion
- Essex-Lopresti Injury/Longitudinal Instability of the Forearm
- Elbow Instability

Authors' Preferred Management of Select Complications
- Case 1: Longitudinal Forearm Instability
- Case 2: Elbow Instability

Summary

Introduction

Radial head fractures are a common injuries, accounting for 1.7–5.4% of all fractures and up to one third of elbow fractures.[1] These fractures occur most often in patients 20–60 years of age with a female predominance of 3:2.[2] The most common mechanism of injury is a fall onto an outstretched hand with the forearm pronated and elbow flexed between 35–80°.[3,4] The combination of axial, valgus and external rotatory forces leads to the anterolateral rim of the radial head being driven into the capitellum resulting in fracture. Radial head fractures can occur in isolation; however, associated fractures and ligamentous injuries are common and have important ramifications when determining treatment options. Several classification systems have been proposed but the most important aspect in any treatment algorithm is the distinction between stable and unstable fractures and those resulting in a mechanical block to motion.[5] Radiographic parameters to define displacement have been an unreliable indicator of instability, although, the presence of greater than three fragments appears to predict poor results with attempts at open reduction and internal fixation (ORIF) (Fig. 8.1A).[5] Moreover, radial head fractures associated with elbow

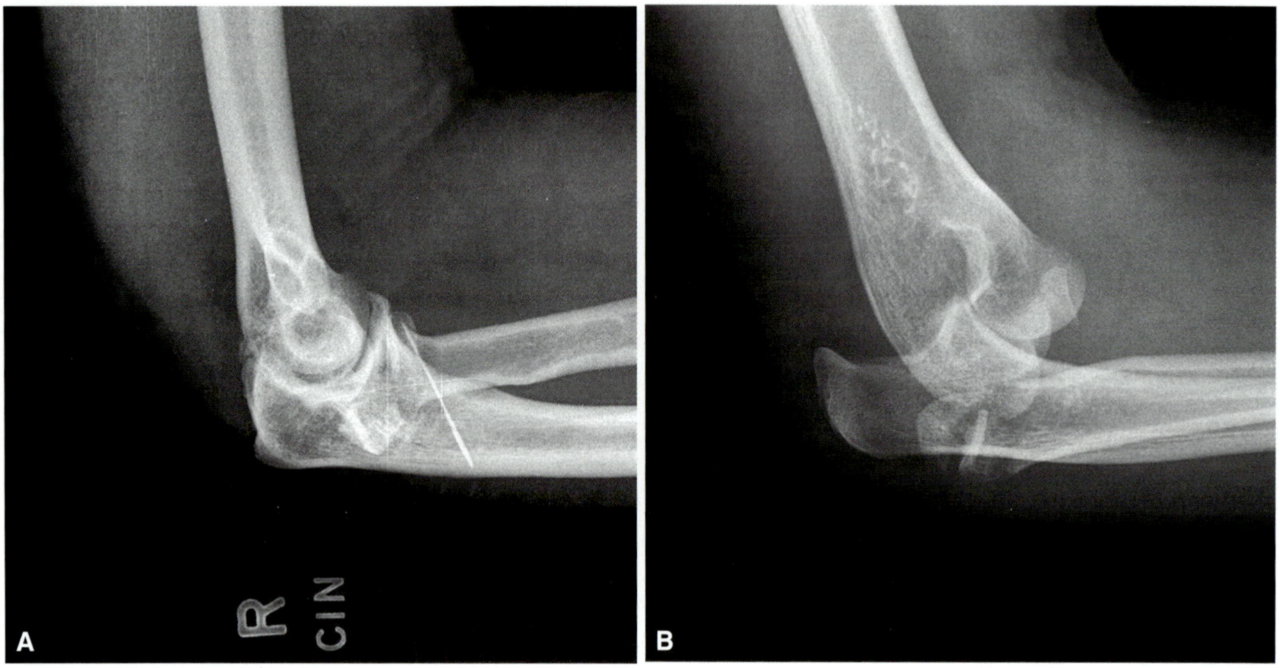

Figures 8.1A and B: Radial head fractures may occur in (A) Isolation or as part of a (B) Complex elbow instability pattern.

dislocations, also known as complex elbow dislocations should alert the surgeon to associated fractures and ligamentous injuries (Fig. 8.1B).[6]

Complex elbow dislocations consist of both ligamentous and bony injuries and are particularly prone to recurrent instability and arthrosis.[7] The most common bony injures are radial head and coronoid process fractures but can also include associated olecranon and distal humerus fractures. Effective treatment requires three steps: (1) concentric reduction of the ulnohumeral and/or radiocapitellar dislocation; (2) fracture repair; and (3) collateral ligament repair. The types of complex elbow dislocations include:

- Radial head fractures with a collateral ligament injury
- Isolated coronoid process fractures
- Terrible triad injuries
- Posterior monteggia fracture-dislocations
- Transolecranon fracture-dislocations

This chapter will focus on isolated radial head fractures and complex elbow dislocations consisting of a radial head and coronoid fracture, known as 'terrible triad' injuries.

Diagnosis

Patients with radial head fractures will typically present with complaints of pain and decreased elbow range of motion. Inspection may reveal swelling and ecchymosis along the dorsal aspect of the proximal forearm. Direct palpation of the radial head elicits pain and is often most notable anteriorly. Associated injuries are common with radial head fractures. Tenderness to palpation of the lateral epicondyle may indicate an occult lateral ligament complex injury. Alternatively, tenderness of the medial epicondyle may signify ulnar collateral ligament injury. The distal radioulnar joint (DRUJ) should also be examined for instability to rule out an associated Essex-Lopresti type injury with concomitant injury to the interosseous injury and subsequent longitudinal forearm instability.

Elbow range of motion including flexion and extension, as well as forearm rotation should be noted; however, pain and crepitus may limit participation. If forearm rotation is limited, joint aspiration and injection of a local anesthetic may be performed to determine if the limitation is due to pain or a true mechanical block. However, limitation of elbow flexion and extension is the most often due to an associated hemarthrosis. The lateral pivot shift maneuver, performed by applying a valgus stress to the supinated forearm as the elbow is flexed 40°, can be used to test for posterolateral rotatory instability or laxity of the lateral ulnar collateral ligament (LUCL) complex. However, this maneuver again may be limited by pain.

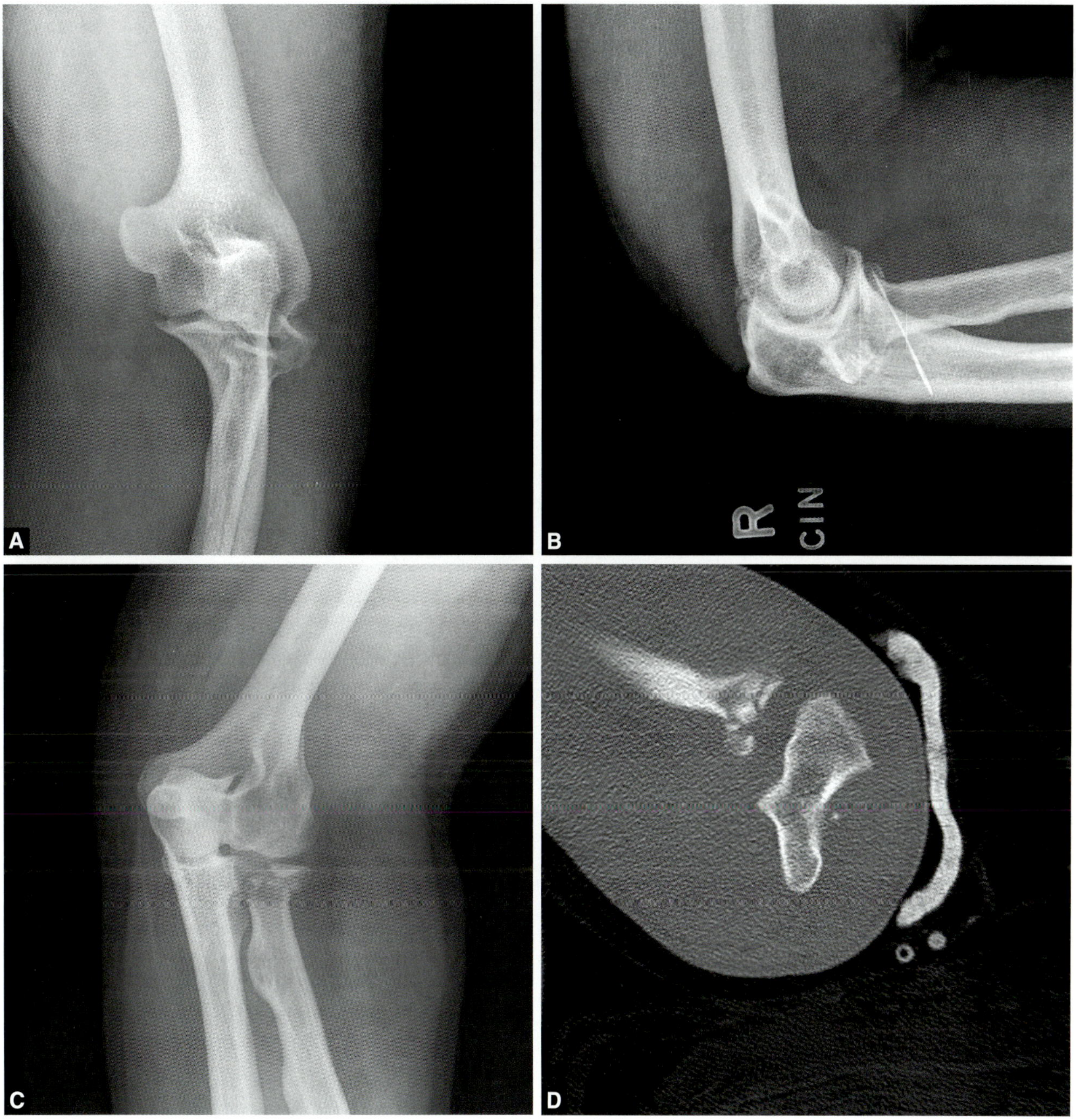

Figures 8.2A to D: (A to C) Standard radiographs of the radial head include anteroposterior, lateral and oblique views; (D) Further fracture characterization is best achieved with CT evaluation.

Most fractures of the radial head can readily be identified with standard imaging including anteroposterior, lateral and oblique radiographs of the elbow (Figs 8.2A to D). In the setting of an occult radial head fracture, the lateral view may demonstrate a 'fat pad sign' due to the hemarthrosis along the cortex of the distal humerus. The oblique view of the elbow performed in the lateral position with the tube angled 45° cephalad allows improved visualization of the radiocapitellar joint. Posteroanterior radiographs of the bilateral wrists can also be examined in patients with wrist pain to evaluate for potential DRUJ disruption. Stress radiographs may also be performed to evaluate for posterolateral rotatory instability. Computed tomography (CT) is useful in providing greater fracture characterization. Magnetic resonance imaging may also be considered, if there is suspicion for associated ligamentous injury or interosseous membrane disruption.

Radial head fractures occurring in the setting of an elbow dislocation typically represent a complex instability pattern with several associated bony and ligamentous injuries. Elbow dislocation with a radial head fracture and coronoid fracture has been termed the 'terrible triad' due to difficulty in management and its penchant for recurrent elbow instability and early arthrosis (Figs 8.3A to E). On evaluation, the most common direction of dislocation that will be encountered is either posterior or posterolateral. Patients will present with pain, swelling and decreased range of motion. Furthermore, open injuries and associated neurovascular compromise is common follow complex elbow dislocations. Once a reduction has been performed, the elbow is often unstable in extension and to valgus stress.

RADIAL HEAD FRACTURES AND TERRIBLE TRIAD INJURIES DIAGNOSIS: Pearls and Pitfalls

- Maintain a high index of suspicion for associated ligamentous injuries with isolated radial head fractures, as a spontaneous reduction of a concomitant elbow dislocation may have occurred
- Plain radiographs may underestimate fracture comminution and displacement. Consider obtaining a CT scan if better fracture characterization is necessary
- Intra-articular injection of a local anesthetic may be helpful in differentiating loss of motion from fracture pain versus a true mechanical block

Classification

Mark Mason, in 1954, defined the first widely used classification system for radial head fractures.[1] In his classification scheme, Mason identified three types of fracture: Type I fractures are nondisplaced; Type II fractures are displaced partial head fractures and Type III fractures are displaced fractures that involve the entire radial head. Mason used the classification system to guide treatment. Type I fractures were treated nonoperatively; Type II fractures were treated with fixation or excision of the fracture fragment and Type III fractures underwent excision of the entire radial head. Johnston added a fourth type to the Mason classification, defined as a fracture of the radial head with associated elbow dislocation.[8] Broberg and Morrey[9] further modified the Mason classification (Fig. 8.4). A Type I fracture was defined as less than 2 mm of displacement. A Type II fracture had more than or equal to 2 mm displacement and/or involved more than or equal to 30% of the joint surface. A Type III fracture was a comminuted fracture and a Type IV fracture was any of the above types with a concomitant elbow dislocation.

Hotchkiss modified the Mason classification in an attempt to better guide operative treatment.[10] Type I fractures were defined as nondisplaced fractures or minimally displaced marginal lip fractures (< 2 mm displacement) that do not block motion and can be treated nonoperatively. Type II fractures were displaced fractures (usually > 2 mm) that may have a mechanical block to motion or are incongruous without comminution. Type II fractures are often amenable to ORIF. Type III fractures are comminuted fractures that are unable to be repaired and are excised or undergo radial head arthroplasty. Ring[5] noted that in the Hotchkiss classification, there are no radiographic or intraoperative criteria to determine the specific fracture type and that fracture type is essentially determined by the treatment rendered.

As radial head fractures are often associated with fractures of the coronoid process, a review of the Regan and Morrey[11] classification of coronoid fractures is also warranted. They divided their scheme into three types. Type I fractures involve only a small fleck of bone representing a shear fracture that occurs during elbow subluxation or dislocation. Type II fractures involve 50% of the height of the coronoid or less and Type III fractures involve more than 50% of the height. Hotchkiss coined the term 'terrible triad' to describe an elbow dislocation with coronoid and radial head fractures, given its history of poor outcomes.[10] Elbow dislocations are classified based on the direction of the distal segment (posterior, anterior, posterolateral, etc).

Surgical Indications

Patient factors such as age, comorbidities and functional demands must be taken into consideration when

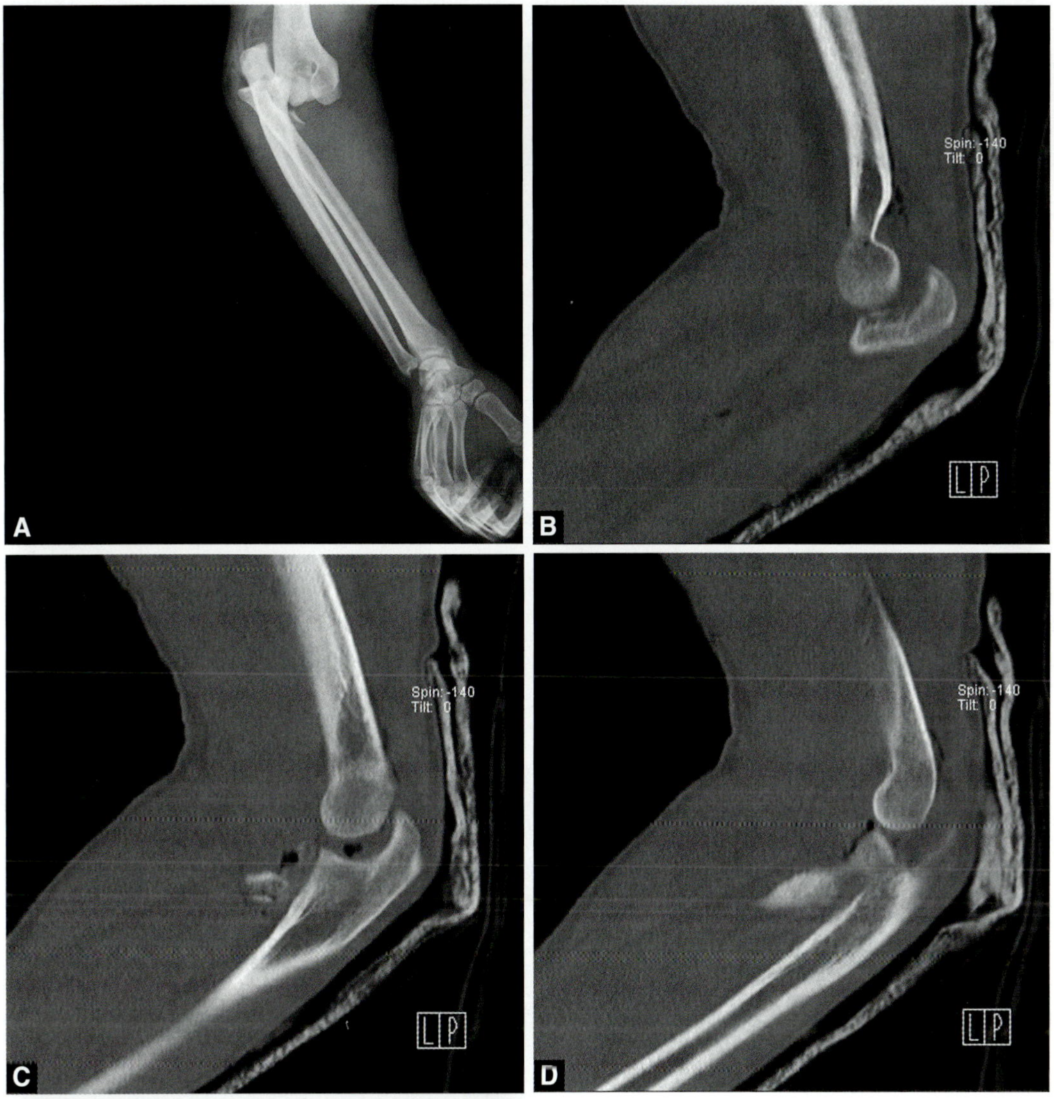

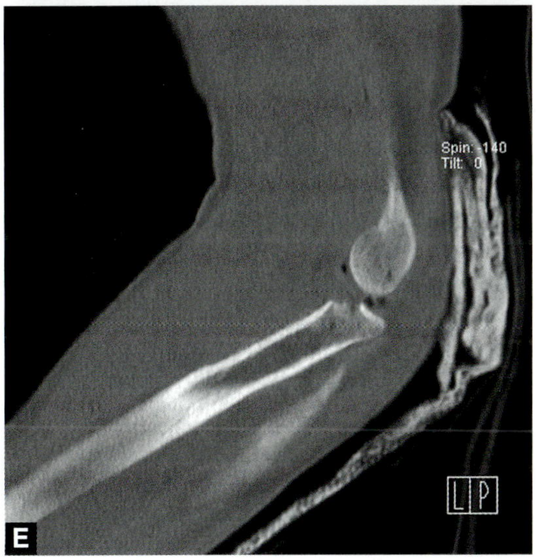

Figures 8.3A to E: Complex elbow dislocations consist of disruption of the ulnohumeral joint and associated fractures about the elbow. A scout radiograph of an injured elbow and subsequent CT scans identify a terrible triad injury which consists of a posterolateral dislocation of the elbow with associated fractures of the radial head and coronoid process. Initial examination should also consist of evaluation of associated neurovascular injury and open wounds. Provisional closed reduction will often result in persistent instability or subluxation of the elbow joint.

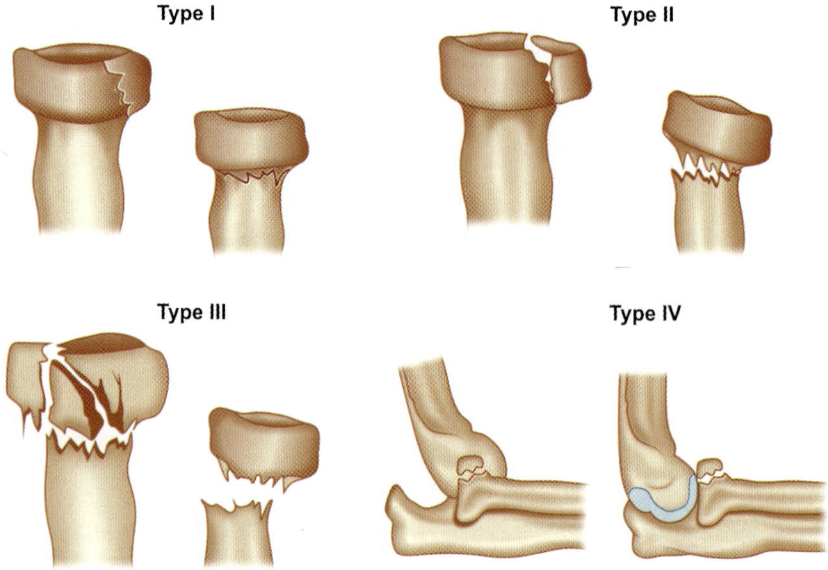

Figure 8.4: The Broberg-Morrey modification of the Mason classification of radial head fractures: Type I fractures have less than 2 mm of displacement. Type II fractures have more than or equal to 2 mm displacement and/or involve more than or equal to 30% of the joint surface. Type III fractures are comminuted. Type IV fractures consist of any of the above types with a concomitant elbow dislocation.

considering operative management of radial head fractures and elbow dislocations. Radial head fractures can be treated nonoperatively. Indications for nonoperative treatment include nondisplaced or minimally displaced fractures of the radial head without a mechanical block to motion. This includes fractures involving less than one third of the diameter of the radial head with less than 2 mm displacement.

A mechanical block to motion is an indication for operative treatment, regardless of fracture displacement or the amount of radial head involvement. Small fragments incarcerated within the proximal radioulnar joint are also an indication for operative treatment. Fractures with displacement of more than or equal to 2 mm and/or a fracture involving more than one third of the radial head are relative surgical indications. Open reduction internal fixation of the radial head fracture is indicated, if technically achievable. Alternatively, radial head arthroplasty is indicated for 'nonreconstructable' radial head fractures.

Operative treatment is indicated for elbow dislocations with radial head and coronoid fracture (terrible triad injuries) to restore a stable and functional elbow. Treatment requires addressing three components: the radial head, the coronoid process, and the collateral ligaments. The radial head should not be excised in these injuries as the radial head provides longitudinal forearm stability and secondary valgus stability to the elbow. Similarly, fixation of the coronoid process is indicated as it provides primary ulnohumeral stability to the elbow. Lastly, repair or reconstruction of the collateral ligaments is also necessary as they provide primary varus/valgus stability to the elbow.

Controversy exists over the indications for open reduction internal fixation versus radial head arthroplasty for comminuted radial head fractures. Historically, excision of the radial head was indicated in comminuted radial head fractures that were deemed nonreconstructable. However, the high predilection of an associated inter-osseous membrane injury or an Essex-Lopresti lesion, and secondary longitudinal forearm instability has limited the role of primary radial head excision for acute radial head fractures. Moreover, excision of the radial head is also contraindicated in instances of coronoid fracture and ligamentous injury, as the radial head assumes a role as the primary stabilizer to valgus in this circumstance.[6]

The indications for radial head arthroplasty include an acute comminuted fracture in which satisfactory reduction and stable fixation cannot be obtained. Radial head replacement may also be considered in patients with complex elbow injuries that involve greater than 30% of the articular rim of the radial head, which cannot be reconstructed. Radial head arthroplasty should also be considered in patients with three or more fragments or significant comminution. Patients who present in a delayed manner with persistent pain and instability from radial head resections, malunions or post-traumatic arthritis are also candidates for radial head arthroplasty.[12]

Surgical Anatomy, Positioning and Approaches

Applied Anatomy

The elbow is one of the most stable joints in the human body, with three primary constraints to instability: the ulnohumeral articulation, the medial collateral ligament (MCL) and the LUCL complex[6] (Figs 8.5A to C). The articular surfaces of the elbow are both highly irregular but also highly congruent providing strong osseous stability.[13] The congruent articulation of the ulnohumeral joint alone has been shown to be responsible for 50% of elbow stability.[13] The trochlea is centered over the distal humerus in line with the long axis of the humeral shaft. The medial ridge of the trochlea is more prominent than the lateral ridge, resulting in 6–8° of valgus angulation with the elbow fully extended. The lesser sigmoid notch articulates with the radial head while the coronoid process locks into the coronoid fossa in flexion, adding to bony stability.[13] The flexion axis of the elbow is oriented in 3–5° of internal rotation in relation to the plane of the medial and lateral condyles and in 4–8° of valgus in relation to the long axis of the humerus.[13] The normal range of motion of the elbow is 0–140° in flexion-extension and a rotation arc of motion of 160–180° (80–90° of both pronation and supination, each). Most activities of daily living require 30–130° of flexion extension and 100° of forearm rotation (50° pronation and 50° supination). The coronoid process is the key aspect of the ulnohumeral articulation due to its role as an anterior buttress and by serving as the attachment site of the anterior band of the MCL.[6] The trochlea and capitellum serve as the

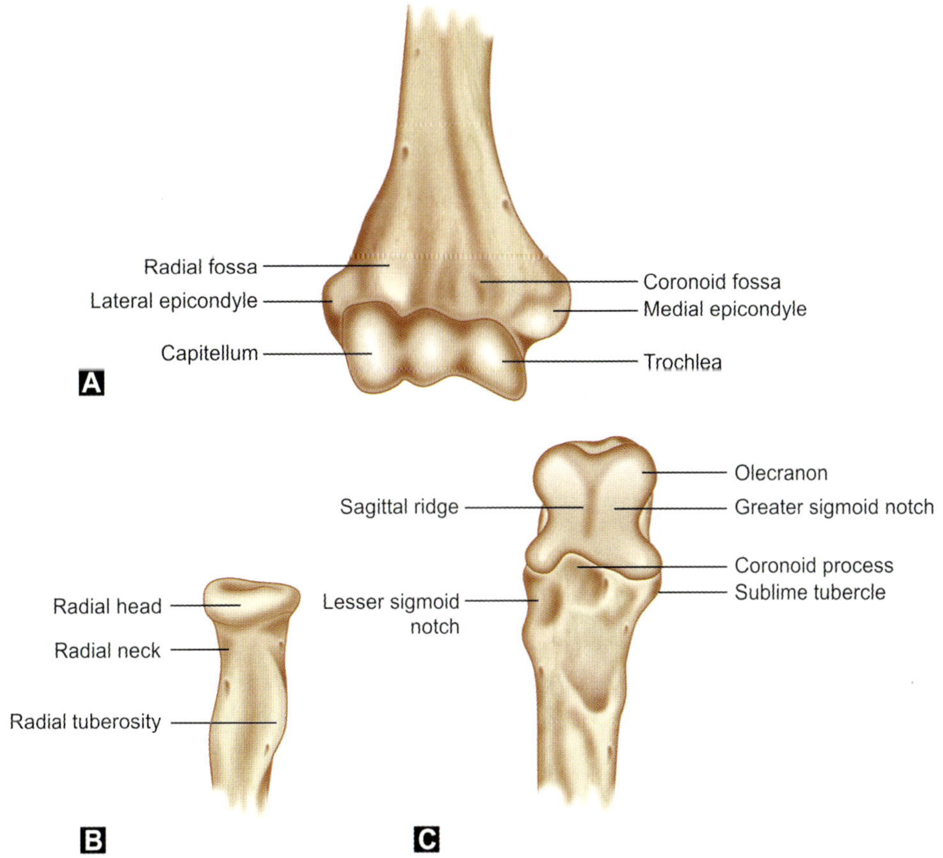

Figures 8.5A to C: The elbow is one of the most stable joints of the body. The articular surfaces of the distal humerus, proximal ulna and proximal radius are both highly irregular and highly congruent yielding great stability throughout the arc of motion.

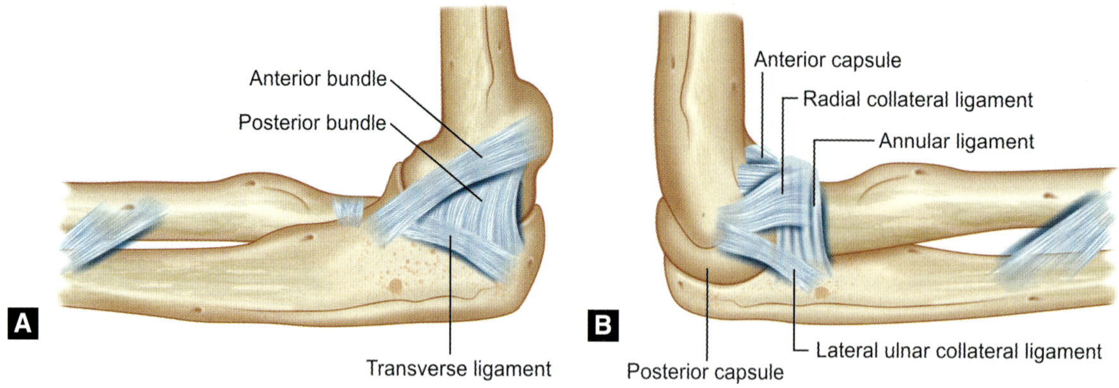

Figures 8.6A and B: The ligamentous stabilizers of the elbow include (A) The medial collateral ligament complex including the anterior bundle which is the primary stabilizer against valgus stress; (B) The lateral collateral ligament complex with the lateral ulnar collateral ligament being the primary stabilizer against varus stress.

proximal articular surface of the elbow. The concave surface of the radial head articulates with the capitellum and the rim of the radial head articulates with the lesser sigmoid notch.[13] The radial head has been recognized as an important valgus stabilizer of the elbow, especially in association with collateral ligament injuries and coronoid fractures.[6]

Beyond the congruent bony articulations, there are various soft tissue restraints to stability.[6] The primary dynamic stabilizers include the anconeus, triceps and brachioradialis. The anconeus helps prevent posterolateral displacement of the elbow. The MCL of the elbow is the primary restraint against valgus instability of the elbow. It consists of three components: an anterior bundle, posterior bundle and transverse ligament (Fig. 8.6A). The MCL originates at the anteroinferior surface of the medial epicondyle. The anterior bundle inserts onto the anteromedial aspect of the cornoid process at the sublime tubercle and acts as the primary restraint against valgus force. The posterior bundle is a capsular thickening that inserts on the medial olecranon. The transverse ligament, consisting of horizontally oriented fibers confluent with the capsule, runs between the coronoid and the tip of the olecranon.

The lateral collateral ligament (LCL) complex of the elbow consists of four distinct structures: The radial collateral ligament, LUCL, annular ligament and accessory collateral ligament (Fig. 8.6B). The LCL complex originates along the inferior surface of the lateral epicondyle. The annular ligament attaches to the lesser sigmoid notch and the radial collateral ligament inserts into the annular ligament and onto the crista supinatoris.[13] The LUCL inserts onto the crista supinatoris, serving as one of the primary constraints to varus and posterolateral instability.

The posterior interosseous nerve (PIN) branches off of the radial nerve at the proximal edge of the supinator and dives deep crossing over the radial neck approximately 4 cm distal to the radiocapitellar joint. The PIN provides most of the motor innervation to all the finger and thumb extensor. It can be kept away from the surgical field by keeping the forearm pronated.

Positioning

During the surgical management of radial head fractures the patient is best positioned in the supine position (Fig. 8.7). Alternatively, the patient may be positioned lateral or prone to also facilitate exposure of the ulna and distal humerus. With the patient in a supine position, the entire arm is draped into the surgical field and it can be either extended onto a hand table or positioned across the chest. Either position allows excellent access to the lateral and posterior aspect of the elbow. Furthermore, the supine position also permits access to the medial side of the elbow, if necessary. The image intensifier should be readily accessible and positioned on the ipsilateral side. A tourniquet should be applied sterile in the surgical field, if necessary to maximize access to the draped arm. Other advantages of the supine position include ease of access for the anesthesia team, readily available imaging and the ability to obtain bone graft, if needed.[14]

Approaches

The location of the pathology and extent of exposure required will dictate the optimal surgical approach. Various lateral approaches are available that provide reliable

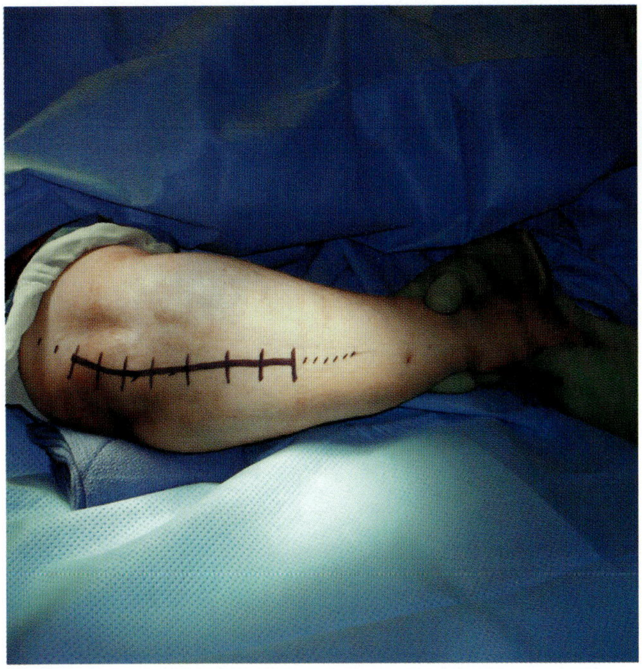

Figure 8.7: The patient is positioned supine with the flexed elbow placed across a hand table. Alternatively, the arm may be placed across the chest. This position provides excellent access to all the aspects of the elbow. Note placement of a sterile tourniquet to maximize access to the arm.

access to the radial head. Exposure of the elbow for complex fractures involving ligamentous injuries or terrible triad fractures requires use of the universal posterior skin incision. This incision allows circumferential access to both medial and lateral exposures of the elbow as necessary.

Kocher Approach

A common approach for radial head fixation, excision and/or arthroplasty is the Kocher approach (Fig. 8.8A). An incision is made along the subcutaneous border of the ulna, running obliquely across the posterolateral aspect of the elbow, ending just proximal to the lateral epicondyle. The interval between the anconeus and the extensor carpi ulnaris is identified and entered. The capsule is incised along the anterior border of the LUCL, about 1 cm above the supinator crest. If the radial head is to be excised, the extensor carpi ulnaris and a small portion of the supinator are dissected free of the capsule and retracted anteriorly. The LCL is very vulnerable to injury during this approach and should be preserved by carefully dissecting along the anterior border of the LUCL without excessive posterior dissection in order to avoid destabilizing the elbow. Distally, the PIN is at risk as it crosses the radial neck approximately 4 cm distal to the radiocapitellar joint. Keeping the forearm pronated moves the PIN further from the operative field. The Kocher approach can be extended both proximally by elevating the common extensor tendon off the supracondylar ridge.[14]

Kaplan Approach

The Kaplan approach affords excellent exposure of the radial head while minimizing inadvertent injury to the LCL (Fig. 8.8B). It utilizes the superficial interval between the extensor digitorum communis (EDC) and the extensor carpi radialis longus and brevis. With the elbow at 90° of flexion, the skin incision is begun at the tip of the lateral epicondyle and is extended distally approximately 3–4 cm toward Lister's tubercle. The interval between the digitorum communis and the extensor carpi radialis musculature is developed at the anterior portion of the lateral epicondyle and extended distally toward the anterior radial neck. At the deep level, the incision splits the lateral annular ligament complex but remains anterior to the LUCL and is carried along the equator of the radiocapitellar joint. The exposure can be extended proximally by elevating the common extensor tendon off the supracondylar ridge.

Midaxial Approach

The midaxial or EDC splitting approach splits the common extensor interval to gain access to the radial head (Fig. 8.8C). The midaxis of the radiocapitellar joint is palpated and the fascia and deep muscle overlying it is split down to the joint. Posterior dissection is avoided as to not compromise the LCL complex.

Medial Coronoid Approach

In the management of complex elbow instability cases including 'terrible triad' injuries, access to both the medial and lateral aspects of the elbow joint may be necessary. Lateral exposure will facilitate repair of a radial head fracture and/or repair of the LCL. Medial exposure will facilitate fixation of a coronoid fracture and/or repair of the MCL (Figs 8.9A and B).

A midline posterior skin incision is made in a longitudinal fashion, starting approximately 5 cm proximal to the tip of the olecranon and carried approximately 5 cm

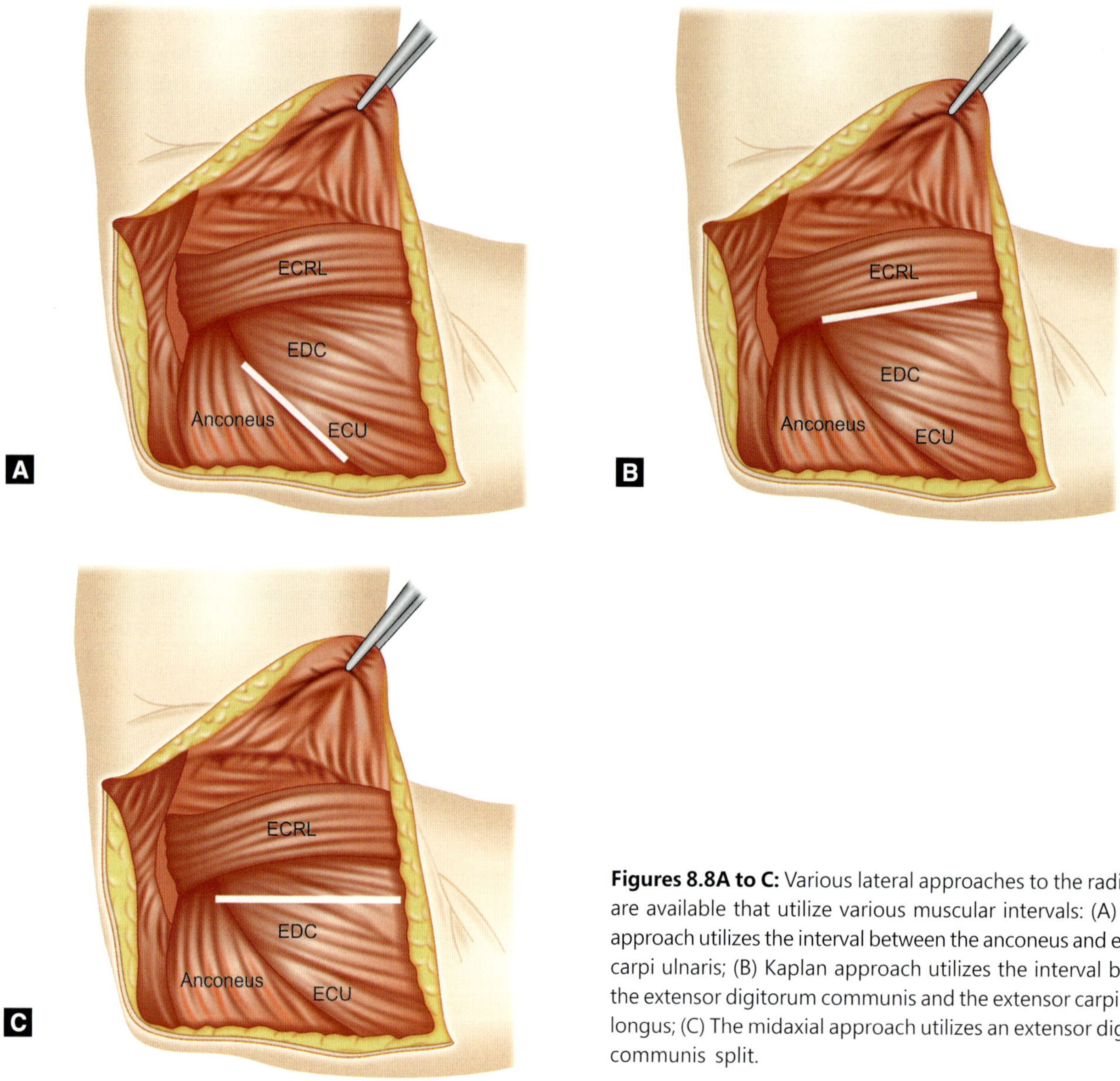

Figures 8.8A to C: Various lateral approaches to the radial head are available that utilize various muscular intervals: (A) Kocher approach utilizes the interval between the anconeus and extensor carpi ulnaris; (B) Kaplan approach utilizes the interval between the extensor digitorum communis and the extensor carpi radialis longus; (C) The midaxial approach utilizes an extensor digitorum communis split.

distally (Fig. 8.7). Dissection is carried out down to the level of the triceps fascia. Full-thickness flaps are developed both medially and laterally.[15] Once the flaps have been raised, a lateral approach can be performed, as described above, as needed for access to the radial head. A coronoid process fracture is approached medially through the floor of the cubital tunnel. The ulnar nerve is first identified behind the medial epicondyle by releasing the cubital tunnel retinaculum. The ulnar nerve is dissected distally as it dives between the two heads of flexor carpi ulnaris. The two heads are split and the anterior half is retracted anteriorly while the posterior half with the ulnar nerve is retracted posteriorly. The anterior band of the MCL lies deep to the ulnar nerve and the flexor carpi ulnaris musculature.[14] Depending on the size of the coronoid fracture, the anterior band may still be inserting on the coronoid fracture at the sublime tubercle. Exposure can be increased proximally by elevating the anterior head of the flexor carpi ulnaris and the remainder of the flexor pronator musculature off the medial epicondyle.

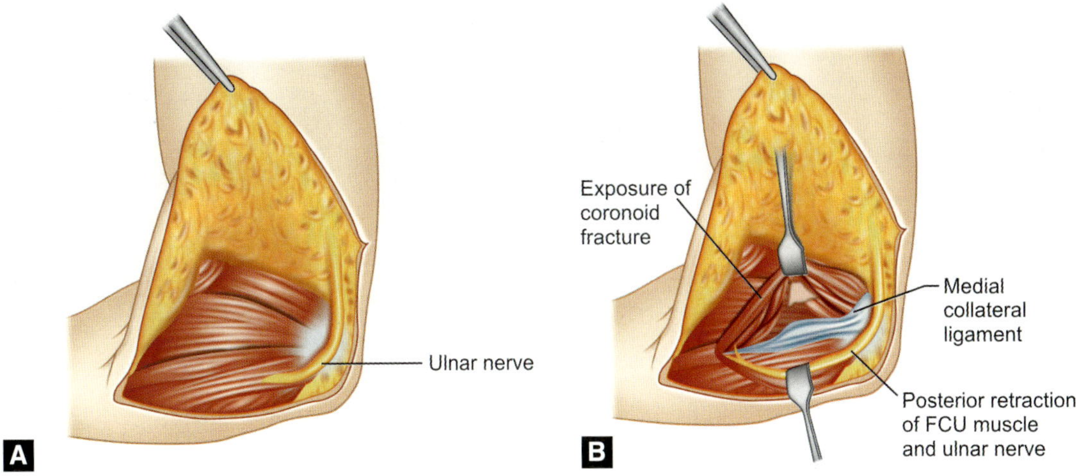

Figures 8.9A and B: The medial coronoid approach is performed by identifying and releasing the ulnar nerve medially through the cubital tunnel. As the nerve enters the two heads of the flexor carpi ulnaris the muscle is split exposing the coronoid. The anterior bundle of the medial collateral ligament may be attached to large coronoid fractures through its insertion at the sublime tubercle.

Surgical Techniques

Technique 1: Radial Head Fixation

The location of the incision for fixation of a radial head fracture is critical and is determined on whether only exposure of the radial head is necessary or will other aspects of the elbow need to be accessed also, as would be the case in a terrible triad injury repair. If the latter is a possibility, a posterior incision should be placed thereby permitting easy access to both the medial and lateral aspects of the elbow. Otherwise, a direct lateral incision can be placed with blunt dissection down to the fascia overlying the lateral epicondyle and the extensor mass origin. The authors recommend a midaxial approach to the radial head as it is the most straightforward approach and involves placing the split incision directly at the midline of the radiocapitellar axis without having to identify true muscular intervals. However, all lateral approaches are effective in obtaining adequate exposure of the radial head for fixation. No dissection is taken posteriorly in order to avoid injury to the LUCL. The midaxis of the radiocapitellar joint is palpated and the fascia and deep muscle overlying on it is split down to the joint. The radial head is exposed up to but not beyond the radial neck to avoid inadvertent injury to the PIN. The forearm is kept pronated to maximize the distance of the PIN from the surgical field.

The radial head fracture is reduced under direct visualization with emphasis being placed on restoration of the articular surface (Figs 8.10A to D). Articular depression is common and its elevation will be necessary. In our opinion, the need for bone grafting is uncommon in the management of radial head fractures. Fixation of the fracture can typically be achieved with mini-fragment or modular hand headed screws, headless compression screws or with a radial head plate. Use of a plate is our last choice as the risk for hardware irritation is highest with a plate during forearm rotation. The authors prefer to utilize headless compression screws as they can be placed over a guidewire that can initially be used for fracture reduction. In addition, they achieve excellent reduction and compression in a single step while avoiding articular cartilage prominence and secondary proximal radioulnar joint irritation. Reduction and fixation is the best confirmed under direct visualization with evidence of full unrestricted motion in flexion-extension and supination-pronation. If screws alone cannot achieve adequate reduction, a radial head plate is placed in the 'safe zone' of the radial head which correlates to the area between the radial styloid and Lister's tubercle.

Prior to closure, the radiocapitellar joint is irrigated and any loose bodies are debrided. The capsule and fascia are closed in a single layer. A sling is provided for comfort. Early protected motion is encouraged.

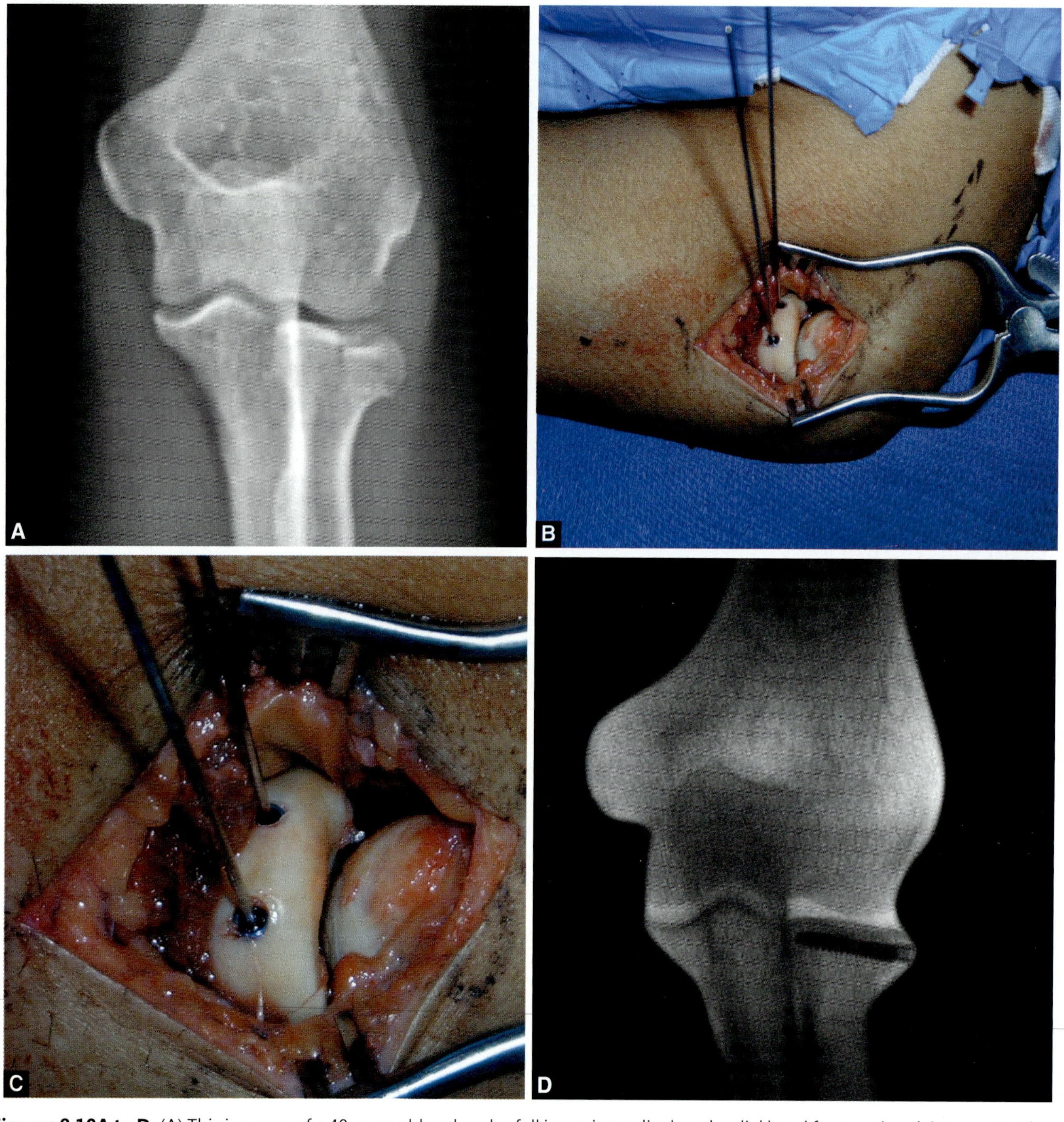

Figures 8.10A to D: (A) This is a case of a 40-year-old male, who fell incurring a displaced radial head fracture involving greater than a third of the radial head; (B) A mid-axial approach was utilized exposing the radial head followed by direct fracture reduction; (C) The fracture was reduced utilizing headless screw guidewires. Once satisfied with the reduction, headless compression screws were placed over the guidewire; (D) Final radiographs confirm reduction of the fracture and good position of the hardware. Range of motion confirmed restoration of full elbow motion without a block to motion or hardware impingment.

Courtesy: Asif M Ilyas

RADIAL HEAD FIXATION: Pearls and Pitfalls

- Computed tomography scan may be necessary to accurately determine the amount of radial head involvement and fracture displacement. Seemingly, minimally displaced fractures on plain radiographs may be found to have significant displacement and radial head surface involvement on CT
- Avoid excessive posterior dissection and indavertant LCL injury
- Keep the forearm pronated to protect the posterior interosseous nerve
- Hardware should be placed either below the articular surface or within the 'safe zone' to avoid hardware irritation during forearm rotation

Technique 2: Radial Head Arthroplasty

Comminuted or nonreconstructable radial head fractures should not be excised, but rather treated with prosthetic replacement. Any of the previously described lateral approaches can be used to access the radial head. The elbow is kept pronated at all times to protect the posterior interosseous nerve. Once the fracture is exposed, the radial head is exposed down to the radial neck (Figs 8.11A to D). The head may be removed piecemeal or by osteotomizing the radial head with an oscillating saw through the junction of the head and neck. The fragments are reassembled on the back table to replicate the native radial head anatomy to determine the normal size of the head. While choosing a radial head prosthesis that is too small may lead to instability; overstuffing the radiocapitellar joint has been shown to cause accelerated wear and erosion of the radiocapitellar joint. A modular radial head system will allow for mixing and matching various head, neck and stem sizes to optimize proper fit and tension. In general, it is preferable for the diameter and thickness of the prosthesis to be slightly undersized than oversized.

The specific implant's manufacturing technique guide should be followed for proper implant placement. A starting broach is placed into the canal and a radial neck reamer is used to flatten out the remains of any irregularity of the radial neck. Broaches are placed by hand and increased stepwise until good fit is achieved. For non press-fit prostheses, the final stem size selected should be one size smaller than the size of the final broach (the broach that began to achieve cortical chatter). The radial head arthroplasty is then trialed and the elbow is taken through a full arc of motion to assess for tracking and the relationship between the radial head and capitellum. One must avoid instability with too small a prosthesis while also avoiding 'over-stuffing' with too large a prosthesis. Ideally, there should be less than 1 mm of space between the prosthetic radial head and capitellum throughout the arc of motion. Once satisfied with the fit of the trial components, the wound is irrigated and the final radial head prosthesis is inserted. The interval is closed with interrupted sutures. At this time, the competence of the LCL complex should be evaluated and repaired if necessary. A sling is provided for comfort and early motion is initiated.

RADIAL HEAD ARTHROPLASTY: Pearls and Pitfalls

- When the LCL complex is injured, there is an increased risk for 'over-stuffing' the joint with too large a prosthesis
- Approximately 1 mm of space should be maintained throughout the arc of motion between the radius and capitellum
- Upon closure, the integrity of the LCL complex must be assessed and repaired if incompetent

Technique 3: Terrible Triad Repair

The overall goal of operative treatment of terrible triad injuries is to address both soft tissue and bony injuries to restore elbow stability and functional range of motion. The patient is placed supine and a sterile tourniquet is applied to allow for proximal exposure, if necessary. A midline posterior incision is used to allow access to both the medial and lateral aspects of the elbow. Full-thickness lateral flaps are elevated. The authors recommend repairing the injured structures in the following order: (1) radial head; (2) LCL complex; (3) coronoid and the (4) MCL complex (Figs 8.12A to K).

The lateral elbow is approached first. In cases of complex elbow dislocations, the LCL complex is typically already avulsed. This avulsion results in a bare spot over the lateral capitellum facilitating easy access to the radial head by utilizing this defect. The radial head is also often

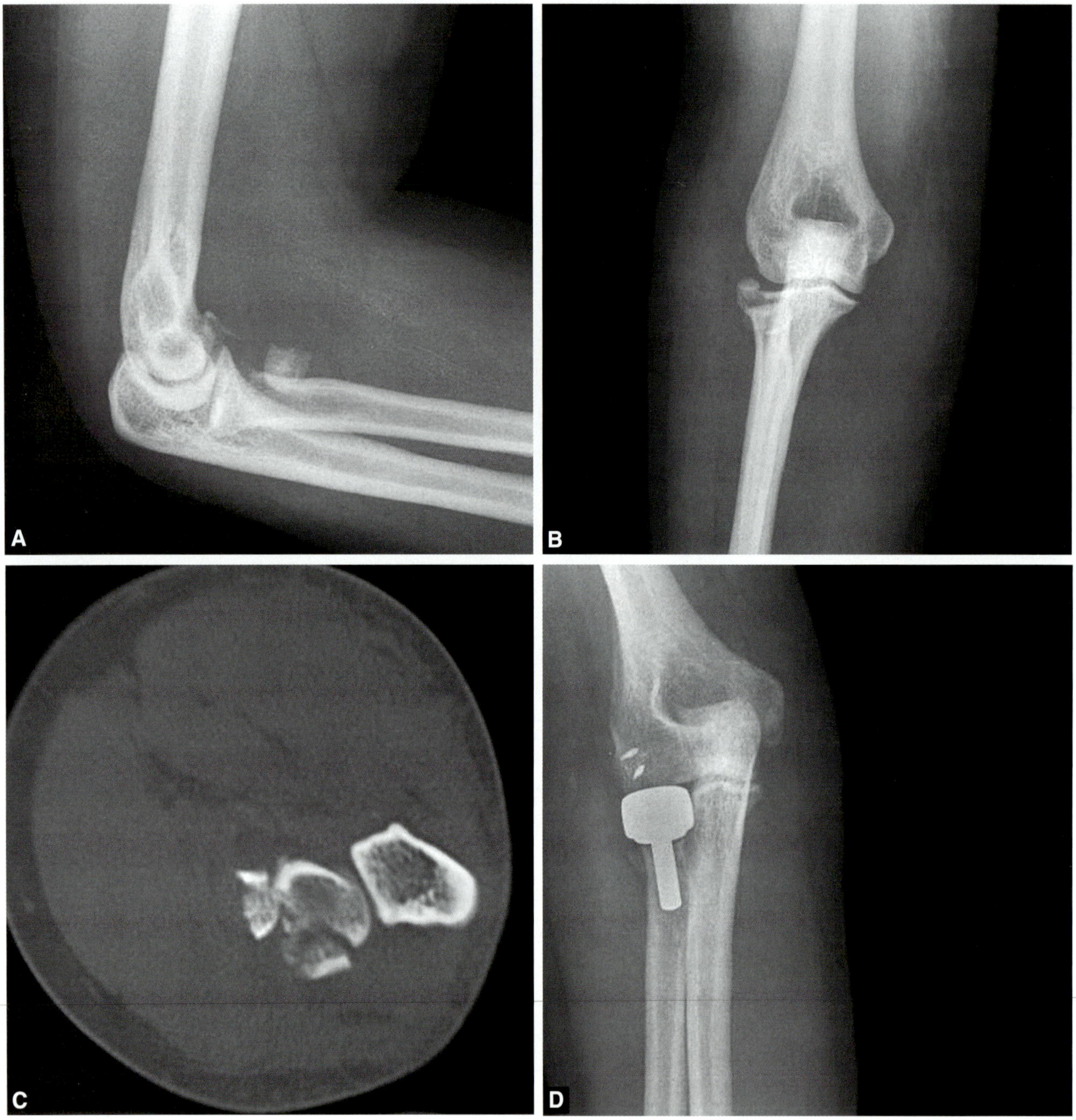

Figures 8.11A to D: (A and B) This is a case of a 55-year-old female, who fell incurring a radial head fracture; (C) Preoperative CT evaluation identified a comminuted fracture of the radial head considered to be nonreconstructable. The elbow was approached laterally utilizing the Kaplan approach and a radial head arthroplasty was performed. Upon closure the lateral collateral ligament was found to be incompetent and was subsequently repaired back to the lateral distal humerus with suture anchors; (D) Final radiographs confirmed concentric reduction of the elbow.

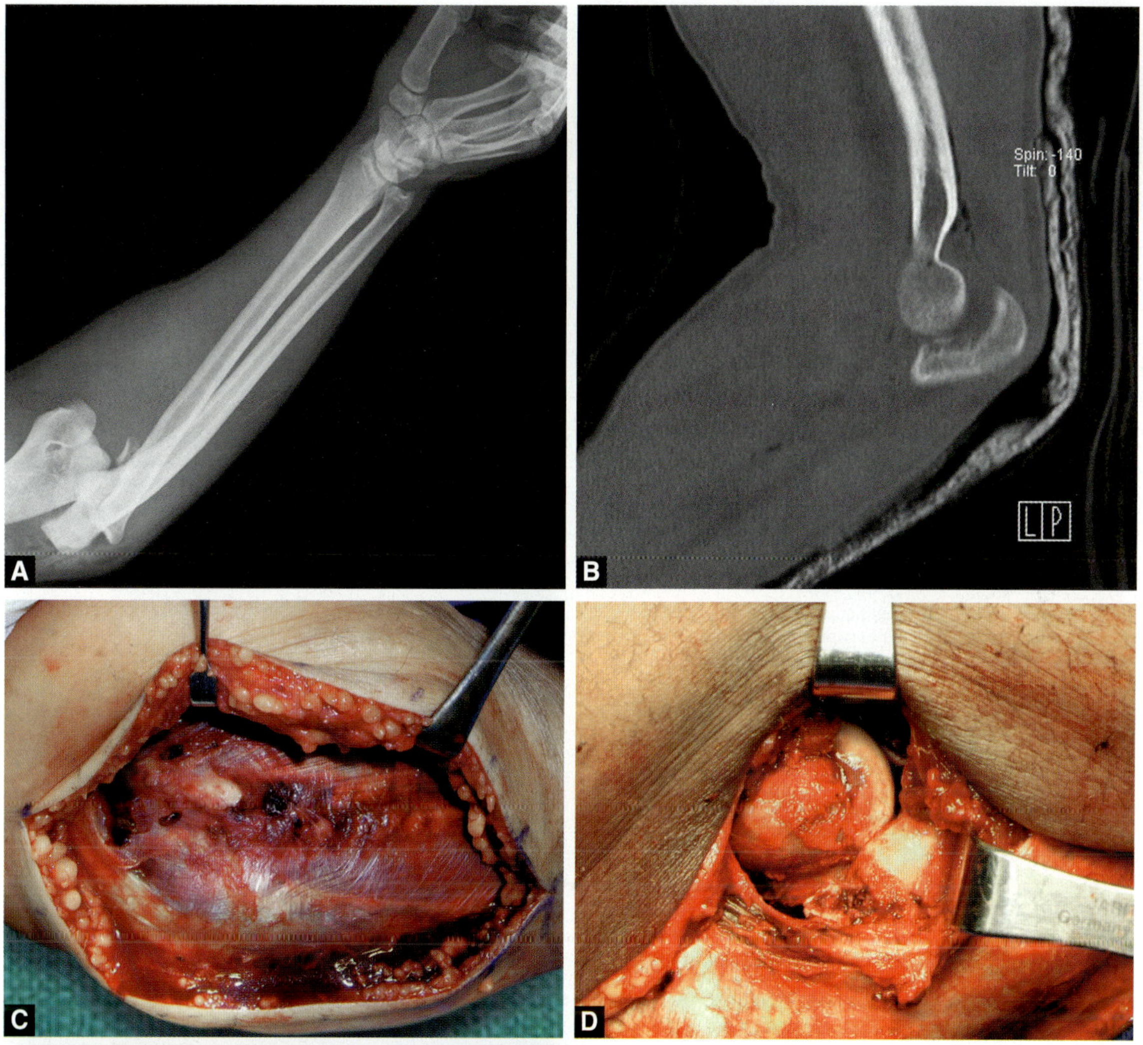

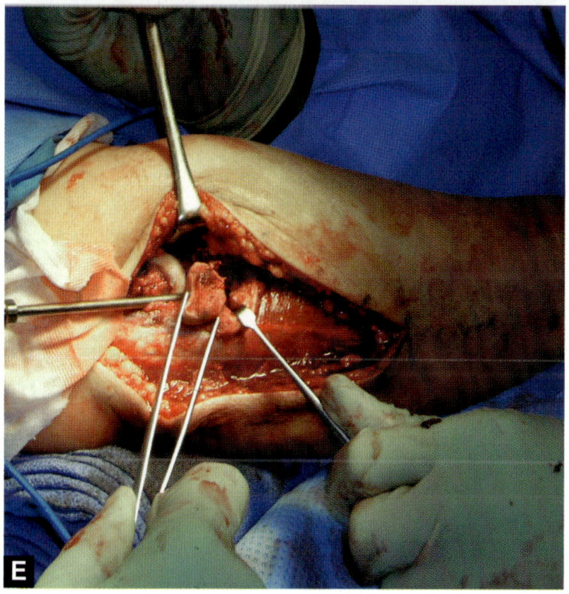

Figures 8.12A to E: (A) This is a case of a 29-year-old male involved in a high energy injury incurring a complex elbow dislocation; (B) Following provisional reduction CT scanning confirmed a terrible triad injury with an associated coronoid fracture and residual subluxation of the ulnohumeral joint; (C) A posterior skin incision was placed and lateral exposure was developed revealing a large lateral soft tissue defect which was utilized to expose the elbow joint laterally; (D) The lateral collateral ligament (LCL) complex was found to be avulsed off of the lateral capitellum and persistent radiocapitellar dislocation and a comminuted fracture of the radial head. First step in repair of a complex elbow dislocation is management of the radial head; (E) Due to comminution of the radial head, it was replaced; repaired structures and preserve elbow stability, the elbow was placed in a hinged external fixator and early protected motion was initiated. The fixator was removed after 6 weeks.

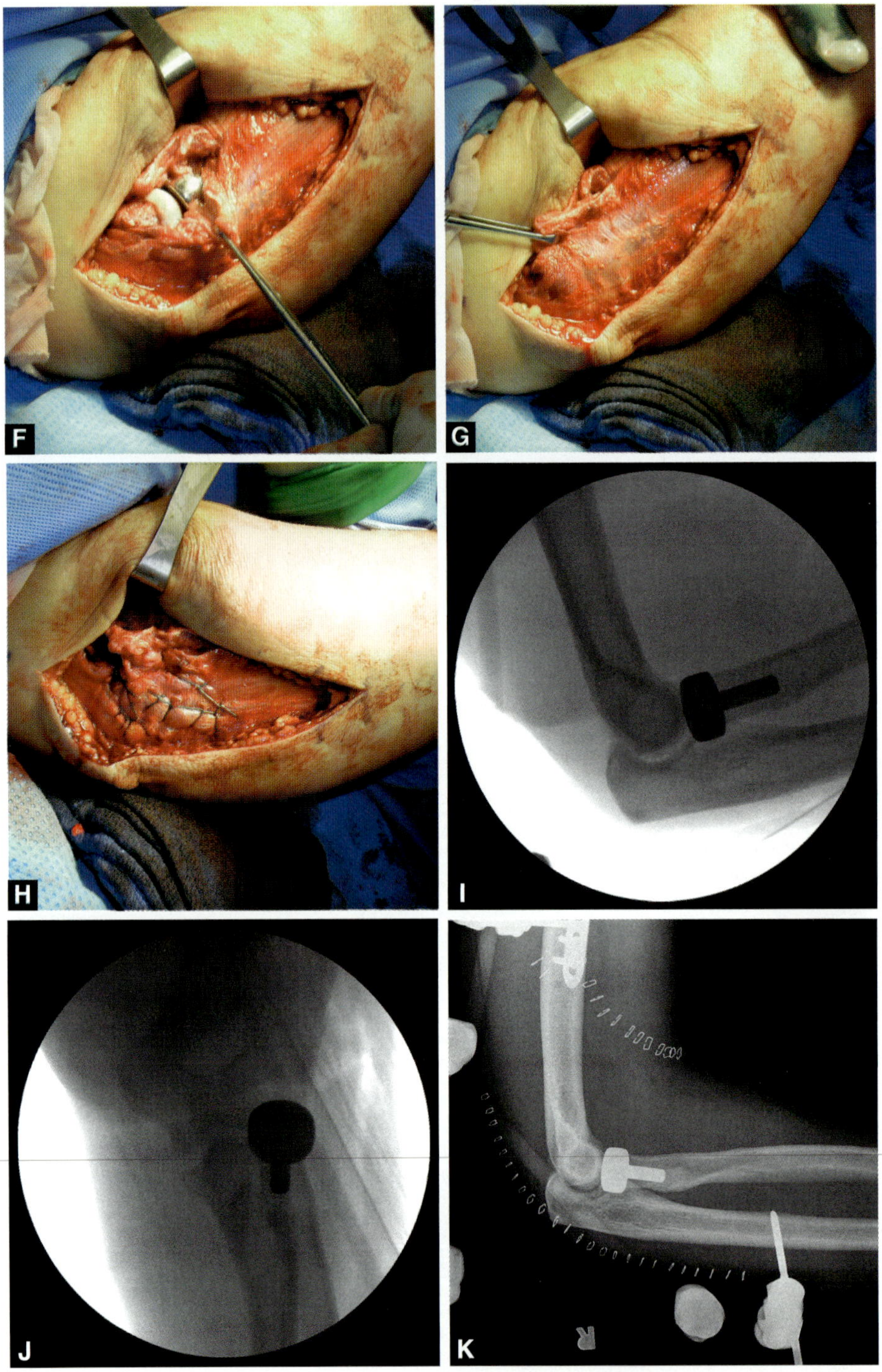

Figures 8.12F to K: (F and G) The second step in repair is identification and repair of the LCL complex; (H) Repair was performed with bio-absorbable suture anchors placed in the lateral capitellum with the sutures placed in a locking fashion recreating the path of the lateral ulnar collateral ligament; (I) Lateral radiographs subsequently demonstrated good reduction of the elbow joint; (J) Anterposterior radiographs demonstrated valgus instability with widening of the medial ulnohumeral joint. The third and fourth steps of repair consisted of coronoid fracture and medial collateral ligament (MCL) complex repairs, respectively, through a medial approach. As the coronoid fracture fragment was too small for hardware, a suture repair was performed. Next, the MCL complex was also repaired with suture anchors; (K) In order to protect the repaired structures and preserve elbow stability, the elbow was placed in a hinged external fixator and early protected motion was initiated. The fixator was removed after 6 weeks.

Courtesy: Asif M Ilyas

found to be subluxed. However, if the lateral soft tissue structures are intact, any of the lateral approaches can be used to expose the radial head. Once exposed, the radial head may be repaired or replaced. Excision of the radial head is absolutely contraindicated in complex elbow dislocation cases.

The LCL complex is treated second. If avulsed or compromised, the ligament is repaired using two suture anchors placed in the lateral capitellum which represents the axis off the elbow joint (Figs 8.13A to C). A locking stitch using a nonabsorbable suture is run distally and back proximally replicating the path of the LUCL. If LCL repair is not possible, an LCL reconstruction can be performed. The lateral interval is then closed using absorbable sutures.

The coronoid process is treated third. The ulnar nerve is freed behind the medial epicondyle by releasing the cubital tunnel retinaculum. The two heads of the flexor carpi ulnaris is split and separated thereby exposing the coronoid. A coronoid fracture may be repaired in several ways including suture fixation, screw fixation and plate fixationdepending on the size of the fragment (Figs 8.14A to C). Suture repair can be performed utilizing braided sutures passed over the top of a small coronoid fragment capturing the capsule, pulled out through drill holes posteriorly in the ulna, and then tied over the posterior ulnar cortex.[6] The reduction should be confirmed once tension is placed on the sutures. For larger coronoid fragments, fixation is achieved using either screws or periarticular coronoid plates specifically sized and contoured for this application.

The MCL complex is repaired last if residual elbow instability persists. Persistent valgus instability is uncommon following repair of the radial head, coronoid and LCL complex. However, if valgus instability persists, the MCL complex can be repaired with suture anchors or reconstructed if necessary.

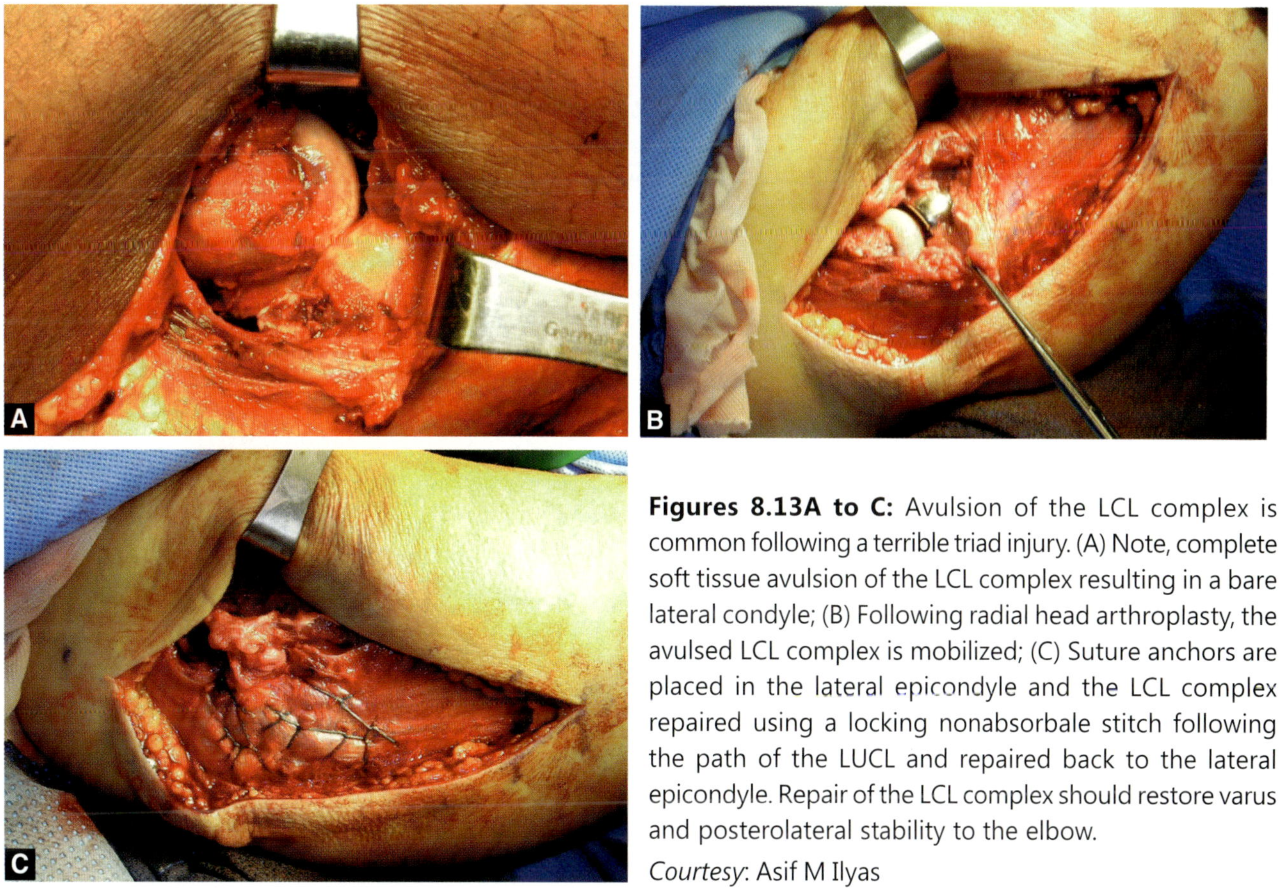

Figures 8.13A to C: Avulsion of the LCL complex is common following a terrible triad injury. (A) Note, complete soft tissue avulsion of the LCL complex resulting in a bare lateral condyle; (B) Following radial head arthroplasty, the avulsed LCL complex is mobilized; (C) Suture anchors are placed in the lateral epicondyle and the LCL complex repaired using a locking nonabsorbale stitch following the path of the LUCL and repaired back to the lateral epicondyle. Repair of the LCL complex should restore varus and posterolateral stability to the elbow.

Courtesy: Asif M Ilyas

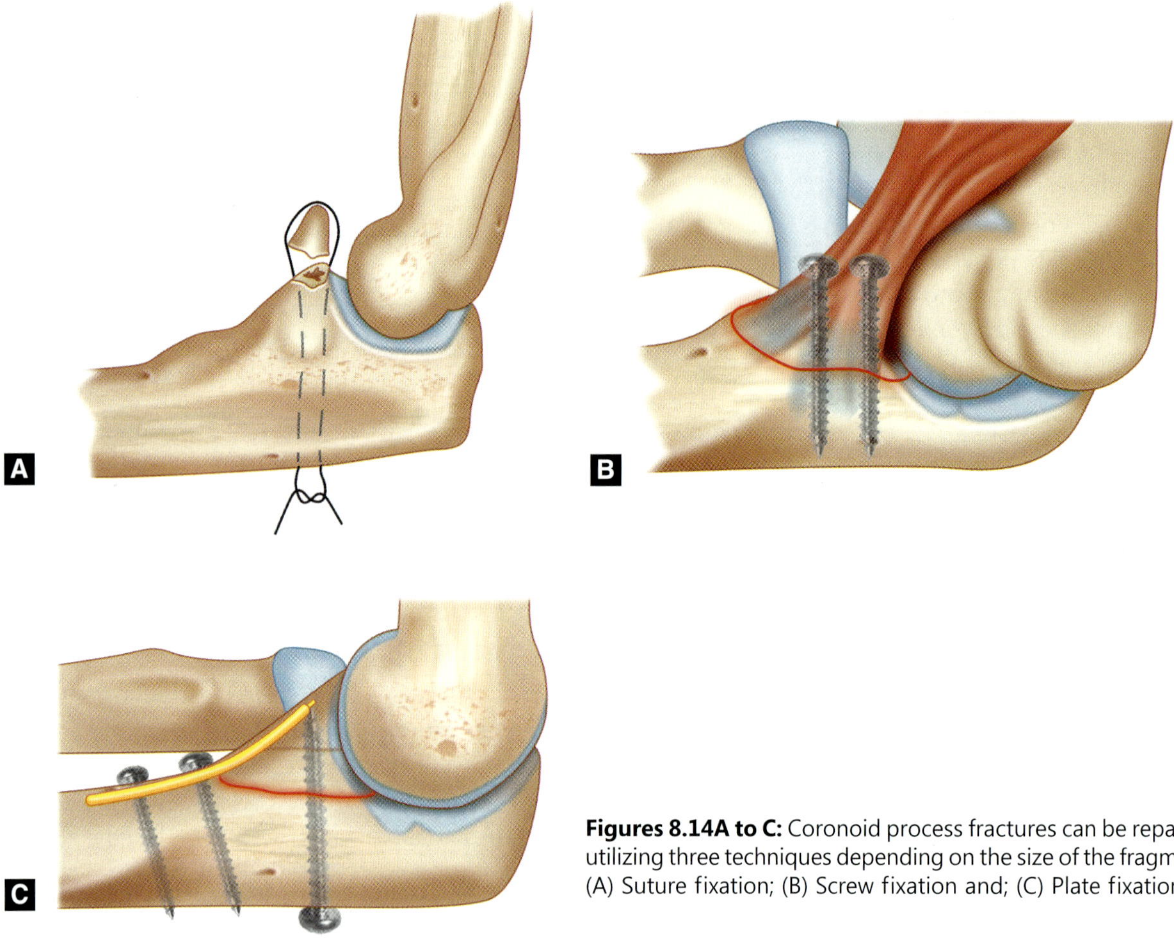

Figures 8.14A to C: Coronoid process fractures can be repaired utilizing three techniques depending on the size of the fragment: (A) Suture fixation; (B) Screw fixation and; (C) Plate fixation.

Prior to skin closure, it is paramount to confirm concentric reduction of the ulnohumeral and radiocapitellar joints. The elbow is tested for stability by placing the elbow in extension with the forearm in neutral and checking a lateral radiograph using image intensification. If there is residual subluxation or instability, competency of the repaired structures must be reassessed. In addition, a static or hinged external fixator may be applied to reinforce elbow stability and protect the repaired structures.

The fascial intervals are closed with interrupted absorbable sutures and the skin is closed. The elbow is immobilized at 90° with the forearm in neutral rotation. Finger motion is encouraged immediately; however, the rate of mobilization of the elbow motion depends greatly on the adequacy of fixation. If good intraoperative stability was achieved, range of motion can be started as soon as the patient is comfortable. If fixation is tenuous, range of motion may need to be delayed accordingly.

TERRIBLE TRIAD REPAIR: Pearls and Pitfalls

- Complex elbow dislocations result in injuries to both medial and lateral structures. Repair the injured structures in the following order: (1) radial head; (2) LCL complex; (3) coronoid and the (4) MCL complex
- The type of fixation chosen depends on the size of the coronoid fragment: suture fixation is preferred for small fragments and lag screw fixation for large fragments
- The addition of a hinged external fixator should be considered if fixation is felt to be tenuous or some degree of instability persists after repair of all injured structures

Outcomes

There is near universal agreement that the treatment of Mason Type I (nondisplaced) fractures should consist of a brief period of immobilization and early range of motion. Wesley and colleagues[16] noted 95% good or excellent outcomes in 329 Mason Type I fractures treated nonoperatively. Radin and Riseborough[17] confirmed the generally good results with nonoperative treatment of Mason Type I radial head fractures, but found less promising results in the subgroup of Type I fractures in which greater than one third of the radial head was involved. This finding is reflected in the Broberg and Morrey modification of the Mason classification, which classified this subgroup as a Type II fracture.[9]

The outcomes for nonoperative treatment of Mason Type II fractures are more variable. Some of this variation is likely due to the reliability of the classification systems used and the interobserver variation. In a retrospective series by Wesley et al.[16] 33/50 (66%) of patients with a Mason Type II fracture had excellent results and an additional 16/50 (32%) were rated as a good result. Khalfayan et al. using mechanical block to motion as an indication for surgery, contradicted those results by demonstrating 90% good or excellent outcomes in 10 patients treated with ORIF compared to 44% good or excellent outcomes in 16 patients treated nonoperatively.[18] The authors also found a significant difference in the Mayo Elbow scores between operative and nonoperative treatment. Lindenhovius et al.[19] reported on the long-term outcomes of ORIF of stable displaced partial articular radial head fractures (Mason Type II) at a mean follow-up of 22 months. The authors found an average flexion arc of 129° and average forearm rotation arc of 166°. Based on the Mayo Elbow Performance Index, 9/16 (56%) achieved an excellent result, 4/16 (25%) a good result, 2/16 (13%) a fair result and 1/16 (6%) a poor result. The authors noted that the operative treatment of stable displaced partial articular radial head fractures (Mason Type II) offered no significant advantage over nonoperative treatment when compared to previous reports.

While Mason Type II fractures with little displacement have been treated successfully with ORIF, several studies have found three or more displaced articular fragments as a predictor of worse outcomes when treated with internal fixation. King and colleagues.[20] found 33% good or excellent outcomes in Mason III fractures treated with ORIF compared to 100% good or excellent outcomes in Mason II fractures. Ring and Jupiter[21] retrospectively reviewed their experience with radial head fractures treated with ORIF and noted that all Type II fractures achieved a satisfactory outcome while 13 of 14 patients with a Type III fracture, consisting of three or more fractures, had an unsatisfactory outcome. These series suggest that ORIF of comminuted radial head fractures with three or more displaced articular fragments results in suboptimal results.

Although radial head fractures are common, radial head fractures associated with elbow dislocations are much less common. The relative rarity of this injury pattern accounts for the small numbers of patients in reported series. Ring and Jupiter.[22] reported on eleven patients with terrible triad injuries, followed for a minimum of 2 years. The radial head fracture underwent ORIF in five patients and excision in four patients. The LCL complex was only repaired in three patients and no coronoid fractures underwent internal fixation. The authors noted that seven elbows redislocated in a splint and five elbows redislocated after operative treatment, including all four treated with radial head excision. Overall, treatment was rated as unsatisfactory in 7 or 11 patients. Grewal and colleagues[23] reported outcomes on 26 patients with non-reconstructable radial head fractures and associated elbow injuries. Twenty-two of the twenty-six patients in the series had an associated elbow dislocation and thirteen of those twenty-two had an associated coronoid fracture. Based on the Mayo Elbow Performance Index, 50% of the patients had an excellent outcome, 17% a good outcome, 25% a fair outcome and 8% a poor outcome. The two patients with a poor outcome had a terrible triad injury.

Complications

Heterotopic Ossification

Heterotopic ossification (HO) is a common problem in elbow dislocations with concomitant bony and ligamentous injuries. The extent of HO is related to the extent of the soft tissue injury. Grewal[23] reported on 26 patients with comminuted radial head fractures that underwent radial head arthroplasty. Nearly one-quarter (6 of 26) of patients developed varying degrees of HO. Risk factors for the development of HO include: traumatic brain injury, spinal cord injury, male gender, young age and prolonged coma. Traumatic brain injury is a major risk factor for the development of HO with 20% of patients developing HO.[24] Indomethacin or postoperative radiation (700 cGy) can be used to prevent the development of HO in high risk patients. Limited active and passive range of motion is the hallmark of HO of the elbow. Plain radiographs are used to determine the location of the ectopic bone and also the extent. Computed tomography scans are also helpful in identifying the location and extent.

Not all patients with HO require surgical intervention. However, patients whose HO limits functional range of motion, the ability to perform activities of daily living, and causes significant pain, should be considered for surgery. The timing of surgical intervention is controversial. Traditionally, HO excision was reserved for when the ectopic bone had 'matured.' However, the authors advocate excision once the HO begins causing significant dysfunction for the patient followed by the use of prophylaxis in order to restore elbow function.

Voila et al.[25] have extensively reviewed the treatment of HO about the elbow. The exact surgical interventions required by each of the many different presentations of HO are beyond the scope of this text. However, Voila defined the essential steps of HO excision and capsular release that can guide treatment. The location of previous incisions, need for nerve decompression, direction of contracture, and the location of the HO must be taken into account during preoperative planning. Incisions are applied as needed to facilitate adequate resection of the heterotopic bone. Nerves caught in the heterotopic bone should be identified and decompressed. The anterior and/or posterior joint capsules should be excised while taking great care not to violate the collateral ligaments. Both the coronoid and olecranon fossae must be cleared of bone and scar tissue.[25]

Elbow Stiffness

Elbow stiffness is a common complication after radial head fracture and elbow dislocations. The most common finding is loss of terminal extension. The etiology of the stiffness may include capsular contracture, HO, impinging hardware, hemarthrosis or retained fragments. Ring et al.[19] reported on both short and long-term outcomes of surgically treated Mason Type II radial head fractures. At 1-year follow-up, the average elbow flexion was 132° and average flexion contracture was 10°. At long-term follow-up, the average elbow flexion improved to 134° with a flexion contracture of 6°. The length of postoperative immobilization appears to be directly correlated to postoperative stiffness, with poor results occurring in patients immobilized for longer than 3–4 weeks.[26] Management of stiffness is related to timing. In the early stages, treatment includes passive stretching exercises and/or progressive static splinting. Later or recalcitrant stiffness can be managed with open or arthroscopic capsular release.

Radial Head Malunion/Nonunion

Malunions are often due to inappropriate initial treatment, unstable fracture fixation or collapse secondary to avascular necrosis (AVN). Patients often present with pain, decreased range of motion, clicking and crepitus. In younger patients, osteotomy may be an option; however, in elderly individual, excision or radial head arthroplasty is preferred. Nonunion is most commonly associated with AVN and displaced radial neck fractures. Asymptomatic nonunions are treated conservatively while symptomatic nonunions are managed with revision ORIF, radial head excision or radial head arthroplasty.

Horne reviewed the following factors contributing to nonunion: open fracture, infection, segmental fractures, comminuted fractures, inadequate internal fixation and distraction at the fracture site.[27] Horne felt that comminuted intra-articular fractures were especially at risk because the comminution left the fragments without a vascular supply and these patients are often subjected to early range of motion to prevent postoperative stiffness. There is little published in the literature related to the rate of radial head nonunion; only sporadic case series exist. Faraj et al. reported on three cases of radial neck nonunion.[28] Two of the patients in their series had nondisplaced fractures that went on to nonunion. The authors suggested that increasing age, high energy injuries with associated instability, alcohol abuse and history of smoking may be risk factors for radial neck nonunion. Ring hypothesized that healing problems may occur due to a tenuous blood supply. In their series of five patients, four were asymptomatic despite radiographic evidence of a nonunion. The blood supply to the radial head is similar in anatomy to that of the femoral head, with vessels coursing along the radial neck and the majority of blood supply coming from intraosseous vessels, making it susceptible to compromise following a fracture.[30]

Essex-Lopresti Injury/Longitudinal Instability of the Forearm

An Essex-Lopresti injury is defined as a fracture of the radial head with disruption of the interosseous membrane and associated disruption of the DRUJ. The injury was named for Peter Essex-Lopresti who described two cases in 1951. This is an uncommon injury but can have serious consequences if not recognized. It most commonly occurs after a fall on an outstretched hand in which the energy is transmitted from the wrist, through the interosseous membrane to the radial head which fractures. It is estimated that 0.3–5% of all radial head fractures have an interosseous membrane injury, although the injury is frequently missed at the initial evaluation as patients do not commonly have wrist symptoms at the initial presentation.[30] After several weeks, patients may begin complaining of wrist pain and a block to forearm rotation. An unrecognized injury can be exacerbated by treatment of a radial head fracture with excision alone. Management of longitudinal instability of the forearm is restoration of length and the normal relationship at both the proximal and DRUJ.

Elbow Instability

Elbow instability after both operative and nonoperative treatment can occur in the setting of missed ligamentous injuries and/or improper or inadequate fixation. The goal of managing complex elbow instability is to obtain a concentric and stable reduction of the elbow that allows a functional range of painless motion. Addressing both bony and ligamentous injuries is critical to achieving this goal.

The radial head functions as a secondary valgus stabilizer to the elbow, providing up to 30% of valgus stability.[7] Biomechanical studies have demonstrated that the effect of excision of the radial head in the setting of otherwise normal anatomy has little effect on elbow stability.[7] However, in the setting of either coronoid fracture or injury to the medial collateral ligament, excision of the radial head can lead to gross elbow instability. An intact or prosthetic radial head adequately restores elbow stability even with release of the anterior band of the MCL. Furthermore, the ulnar band (LUCL) of the LCL and the radial head work act in concert to provide posterolateral stability. The radial head maintains the necessary tension in the LCL which in turn prevents the radiocapitellar joint and the ulnohumeral joint from dislocating posterolaterally. In elbows with a disrupted LCL, radial head replacement will improve but cannot entirely restore kinematics and stability. As such, an LCL repair is essential even with radial head replacement. These findings, as well as clinical series, have demonstrated that a radial head fracture in the setting of complex elbow instability should either undergo ORIF or arthroplasty.

Fracture of the coronoid process has been recognized as an important factor in the development of recurrent elbow instability. Fixation of the coronoid process restores the anterior capsule as a secondary stabilizer. Historically, fixation of coronoid process fractures was recommended if more than 50% of the process was involved. However, in the setting of complex elbow instability, the surgeons now advocate fixation of coronoid fractures regardless of size.

Despite fixation of fractures and repair of ligamentous injuries, elbow instability may persist. External fixation is utilized in these situations to achieve stability. Static and dynamic external fixators are available. Dynamic external fixators have the advantage of permitting controlled elbow range of motion, but are more technically challenging to apply. Indications for temporary external fixation include persistent instability despite ligamentous repair and for protection of fixation for comminuted radial head and/or coronoid fractures.[7]

Authors' Preferred Management of Select Complications

Case 1: Longitudinal Forearm Instability

A 30-year-old right hand dominant male fell from a height landing on his outstretched left arm. He had pain in the elbow with swelling and decreased range of motion (Figs 8.15A to K). Radiographs demonstrated a comminuted left radial head fracture. The radial head was

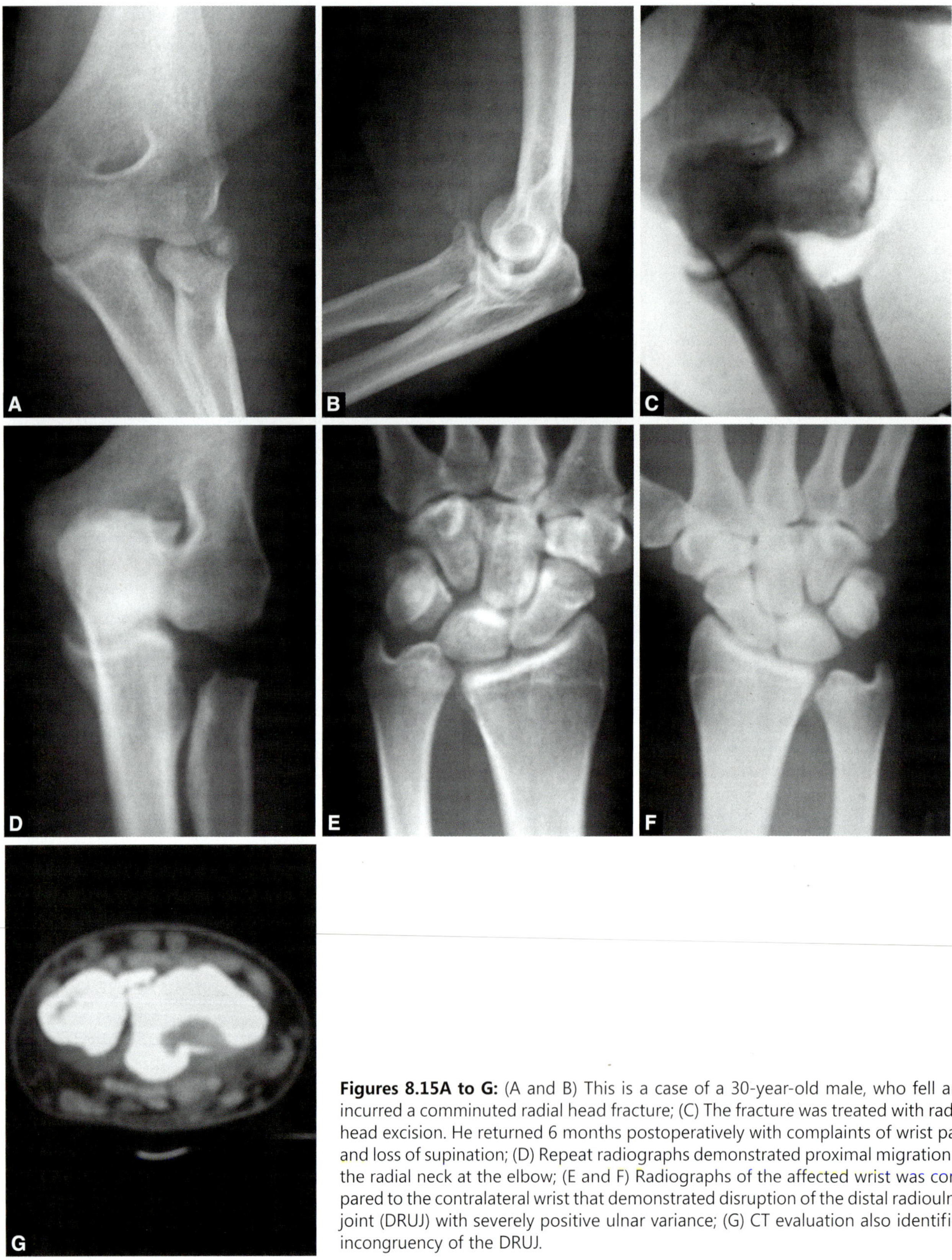

Figures 8.15A to G: (A and B) This is a case of a 30-year-old male, who fell and incurred a comminuted radial head fracture; (C) The fracture was treated with radial head excision. He returned 6 months postoperatively with complaints of wrist pain and loss of supination; (D) Repeat radiographs demonstrated proximal migration of the radial neck at the elbow; (E and F) Radiographs of the affected wrist was compared to the contralateral wrist that demonstrated disruption of the distal radioulnar joint (DRUJ) with severely positive ulnar variance; (G) CT evaluation also identified incongruency of the DRUJ.

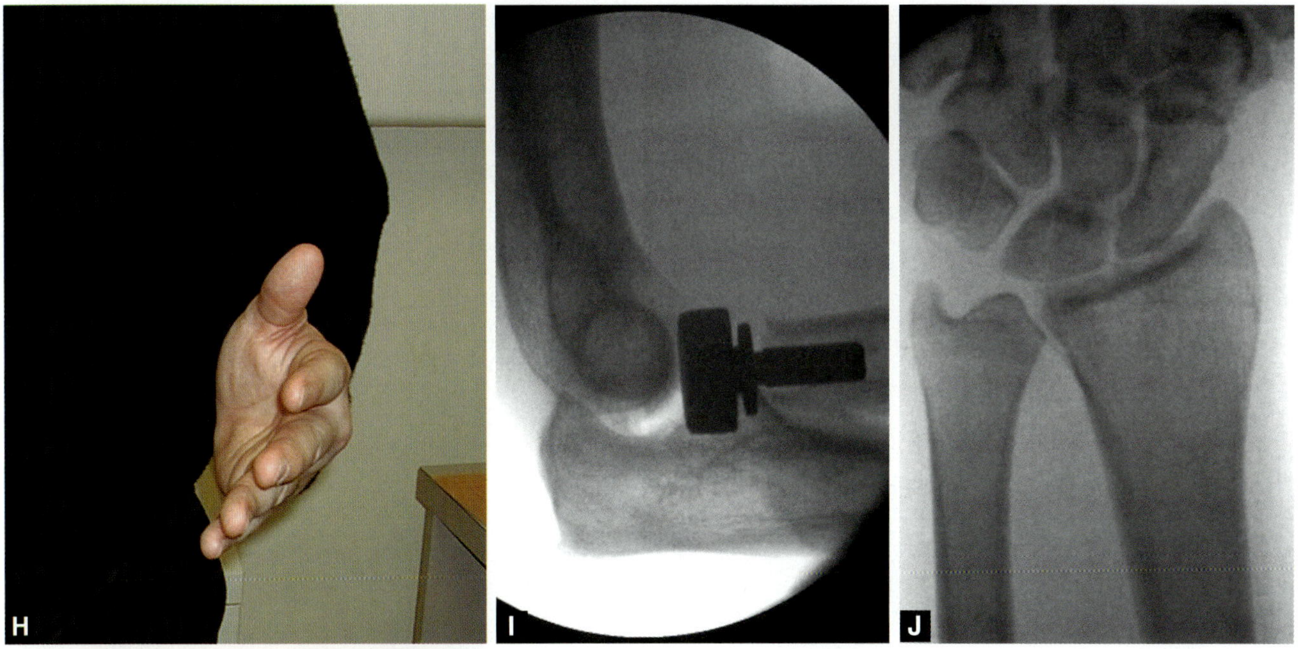

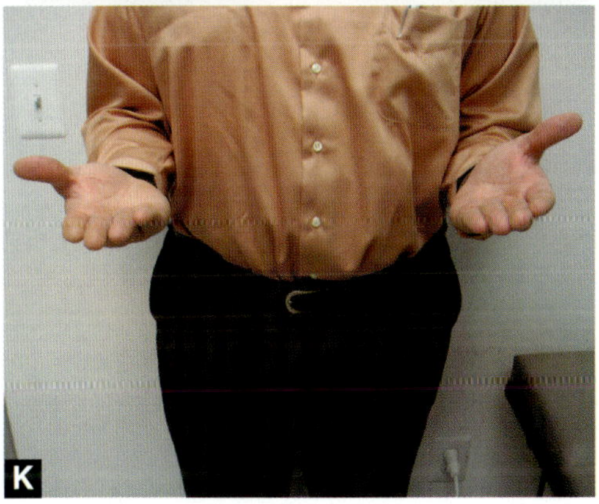

Figures 8.15H to K: (H) Physical examination identified limited supination; (I and J) The patient subsequently underwent radial head arthroplasty with the aim to restore radial length and longitudinal forearm stability and subsequently DRUJ congruency; (K) Postoperative clinical images confirmed restoration of supination.

considered 'nonreconstructable' and it was excised. The patient was immobilized for two weeks postoperatively in a posterior splint and then allowed to begin range of motion. Six months postoperatively, the patient presented for evaluation of wrist pain and limited supination. Patient's initial postoperative radiographs were compared to the latest radiographs taken on the re-evaluation that noted progressive longitudinal forearm instability with DRUJ disruption and proximal migration of the radial neck. The affected wrist had +10 mm of ulnar variance versus neutral ulnar variance of his contralateral uninjured wrist. Furthermore, clinical examination noted loss of supination.

Longitudinal forearm instability can occur following radial head fractures with concomitant interosseous membrane injury (Essex-Lopresti lesion). As such, anything that shortens the radius, including excision, radial head fixation with shortening or undersizing a radial head replacement, can result in proximal migration of the radius with incongruity of the proximal and DRUJ. Options to restore the length of the radius and congruity of the proximal and DRUJ include: shortening of the ulna or lengthening of the radius. Following a radial head excision, the surgeons recommend radial head arthroplasty to restore length of the radius.

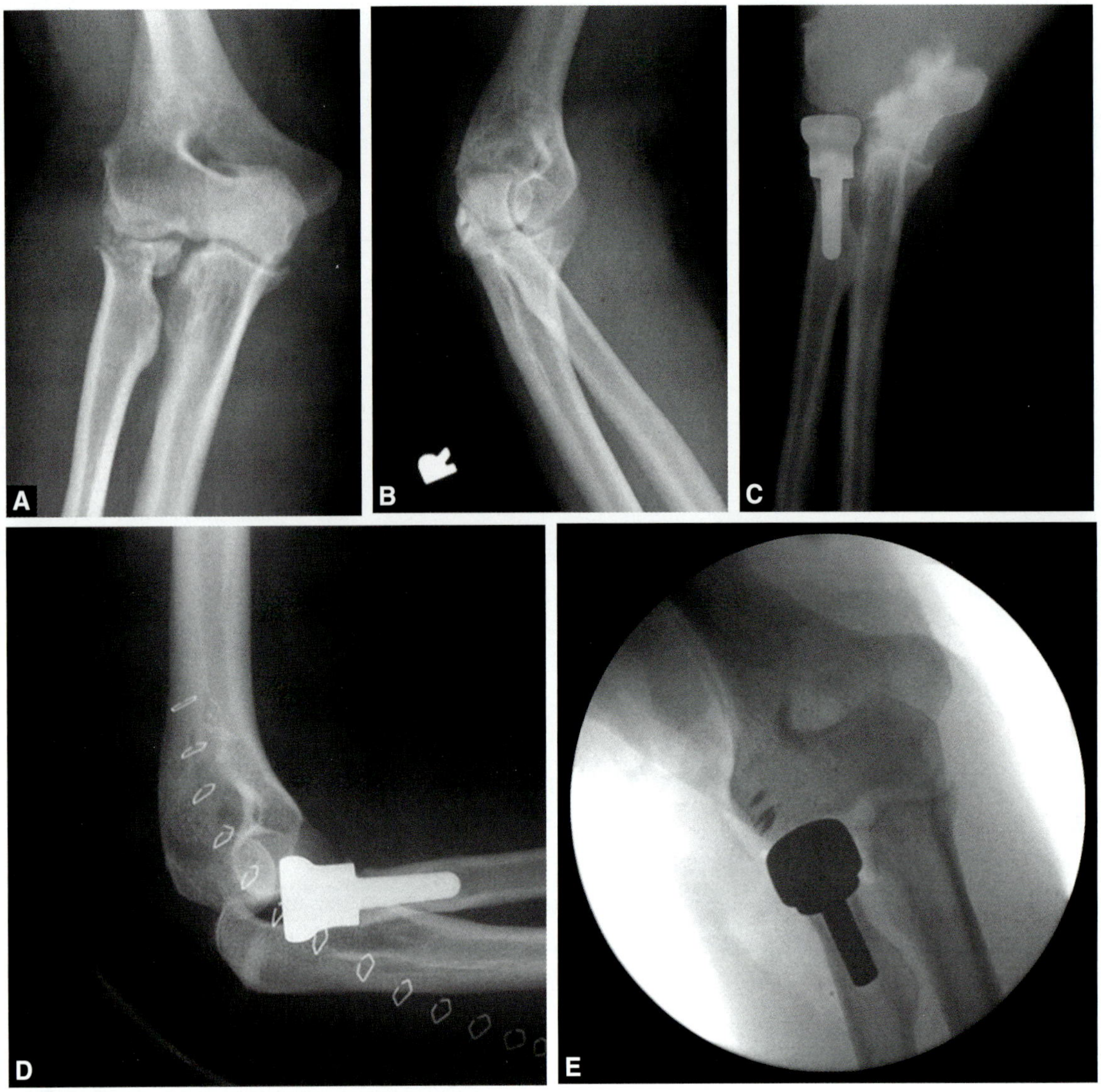

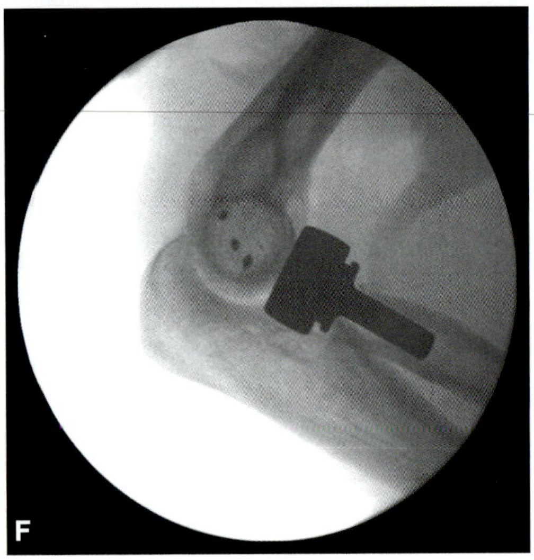

Figures 8.16A to F: (A and B) This is a case of a 52-year-old male who fell and incurred a comminuted radial head fracture treated with an arthroplasty; (C and D) The patient returned with complaints consistent with persistent posterolateral instability that was confirmed by radiographs that identified incongruency of both the radiocapitellar and ulnohumeral joints. The patient was offered surgical repair. Intraoperatively, the prosthesis was found to be undersized and revised accordingly. The lateral collateral ligament (LCL) complex was found to be avulsed off of the lateral capitellum but was suitable for repair; (G and H) Suture anchors were placed and the LCL, repaired under tension with the radiocapitellar joint concentrically reduced restoring joint stability.

Technique

The previous incision and approach is used to expose the radiocapitellar joint and identify the proximal radial shaft. A tensioning device, such as a lamina spreader or Gelpi is placed to distract the radiocapitellar space longitudinally and prepare for radial head prosthesis. Fluoroscopy is used to confirm restoration of radial length and reduction of the DRUJ. The tensioning device is then removed and radial head arthroplasty performed with an implant size that will restore radial length and DRUJ congruency. Following insertion of the radial head prosthesis, the DRUJ is examined for reduction and restoration of normal forearm rotation. Postoperatively, the patient is immediately mobilized.

Case 2: Elbow Instability

A 52-year-old right hand dominant male fell from a height and sustained a comminuted radial head fracture (Figs 8.16A to F). He underwent radial head arthroplasty for a 'nonreconstructable' radial head fracture. He presented several months after surgery, complaining of persistent elbow pain and a sense of 'giving way.' By examination and radiographs, the patient was found to have posterolateral instability of the elbow.

The patient demonstrates persistent posterolateral instability from her index elbow injury. While the radial head fracture was appropriately treated with prosthetic replacement, the injury to the LCL complex was not recognized. Options for management of persistent elbow instability include open ligament repair versus reconstruction. Furthermore, the size and fit of the radial head prosthesis must concomitantly be assessed and adjusted accordingly, if either undersized or overstuffed.

Technique

The previous incision is utilized and the lateral capitellum exposed, which is often found to be bare since the LCL complex had already avulsed off. The radial head prosthesis is assessed for size and fit, and revised accordingly. The LCL is inspected to determine if direct repair is possible or if reconstruction will be necessary. Assuming the LCL complex can be repaired, the isometric point is identified laterally and 2–3 suture anchors are placed. The LCL complex is repaired under tension with the elbow at 90° and the radiocapitellar joint concentrically reduced. The elbow is taken through a full range of motion and stability confirmed both clinically and fluoroscopically. If residual instability is identified, a hinged external fixator may be applied. Protected range of motion can be initiated within 2 weeks postoperatively.

Summary

Successful management of radial head fractures and terrible triad injuries depends on recognition and repair of all injured structures. Isolated radial head fractures with Mason Type I or Type II fractures can be readily treated with nonoperative or operative treatment in the form of an ORIF. Mason Type III or comminuted radial head fractures are best treated with radial head arthroplasty. Excision is no longer recommended. Terrible triad elbow dislocations are assessed and repaired in the following order: (1) concentric reduction of the ulnohumeral joint; (2) radial head repair; (3) coronoid repair; and (4) lateral and/or medial collateral ligament repair. Common complications include: HO, elbow stiffness, radial head malunion/nonunion, longitudinal forearm instability, and elbow instability.

References

1. Mason ML. Some observations on fractures of the head of the radius with a review of one hundred cases. Br J Surg. 1954;42(172):123-32.
2. Kaas L, van Riet RP, Vroemen JP, et al. The epidemiology of radial head fractures. J Shoulder Elbow Surg. 2010;19(4): 520-3.
3. Morrey B (Ed). Radial head fracture, 3rd edition. Philadelphia: WB Saunders; 2000. pp. 43-60.
4. Amis AA, Miller JH. The mechanisms of elbow fractures: an investigation using impact tests in vitro. Injury. 1995; 26(3):163-8.
5. Ring D. Displaced, unstable fractures of the radial head: fixation vs. replacement—what is the evidence? Injury. 2008;39(12):1329-37.
6. O'Driscoll SW, Jupiter JB, King GJ, et al. The unstable elbow. Instr Course Lect. 2001;50:89-102.
7. Tashjian RZ, Katarincic JA. Complex elbow instability. J Am Acad Orthop Surg. 2006;14(5):278-86.
8. Johnston GW. A follow-up of one hundred cases of fracture of the head of the radius with a review of the literature. Ulster Med J. 1962;31:51-6.

9. Broberg MA, Morrey BF. Results of treatment of fracture-dislocations of the elbow. Clin Orthop Relat Res. 1987;(216):109-19.
10. Hotchkiss RN. Displaced Fractures of the Radial Head: Internal Fixation or Excision? J Am Acad Orthop Surg. 1997;5(1):1-10.
11. Regan W, Morrey B. Fractures of the coronoid process of the ulna. J Bone Joint Surg Am. 1989;71(9):1348-54.
12. Monica JT, Mudgal CS. Radial Head Arthroplasty. Hand Clin. 2010;26(3):403-10.
13. Bryce CD, Armstrong AD. Anatomy and biomechanics of the elbow. Orthop Clin North Am. 2008;39(2):141-54.
14. Cheung EV, Steinmann SP. Surgical approaches to the elbow. J Am Acad Orthop Surg. 2009;17(5):325-33.
15. Hoppenfeld S, deBoer P, Buckley R, et al. Surgical exposures in orthopaedics: the anatomical approach, 4th edition. Philadelphia: PA-Lippincott; 2009.
16. Weseley MS, Barenfeld PA, Eisenstein AL. Closed treatment of isolated radial head fractures. J Trauma. 1983;23(1):36-9.
17. Radin EL, Riseborough EJ. Fractures of the radial head. A review of eighty-eight cases and analysis of the indications for excision of the radial head and non-operative treatment. J Bone Joint Surg Am. 1966;48(6):1055-64.
18. Khalfayan EE, Culp RW, Alexander AH. Mason type II radial head fractures: operative versus nonoperative treatment. J Orthop Trauma. 1992;6(3):283-9.
19. Lindenhovius AL, Felsch Q, Ring D, et al. The long-term outcome of open reduction and internal fixation of stable displaced isolated partial articular fractures of the radial head. J Trauma. 2009;67(1):143-6.
20. King GJW, Evans DC, Kellam JF. Open reduction and internal fixation of radial head fractures. J Orthop Trauma. 1991;5(1):21-8.
21. Ring D, Quintero J, Jupiter JB. Open reduction and internal fixation of fractures of the radial head. J Bone Joint Surg Am. 2002;84(10):1811-5.
22. Ring D, Jupiter JB, Zilberfarb J. Posterior dislocation of the elbow with fractures of the radial head and coronoid. J Bone Joint Surg Am. 2002;84(4):547-51.
23. Grewal R, MacDermid JC, Faber KJ, et al. Comminuted radial head fractures treated with a modular metallic radial head arthroplasty. Study of outcomes. J Bone Joint Surg Am. 2006;88(10):2192-200.
24. Cipriano CA, Pill SG, Keenan MA. Heterotopic ossification following traumatic brain injury and spinal cord injury. J Am Acad Orthop Surg. 2009;17(11):689-97.
25. Viola RW, Hastings H 2nd. Treatment of ectopic ossification about the elbow. Clin Orthop Relat Res. 2000;370:65-86.
26. Jackson JD, Steinmann SP. Radial head fractures. Hand Clin. 2007;23(2):185-93.
27. Horne G, Sim P. Nonunion of the radial head. J Trauma. 1985;25(5):452-3.
28. Faraj AA, Livesly P, Branfoot T. Nonunion of fracture of the neck of the radius: a report of three cases. J Orthop Trauma. 1999;13(7):513-5.
29. Ring D, Psychoyios VN, Chin KR, et al. Nonunion of nonoperatively treated fractures of the radial head. Clin Orthop Relat Res. 2002;(398):235-8.
30. Jungbluth P, Frangen TM, Arens S, et al. The undiagnosed Essex-Lopresti injury. J Bone Joint Surg Br. 2006;88(12):1629-33.

Chapter 9

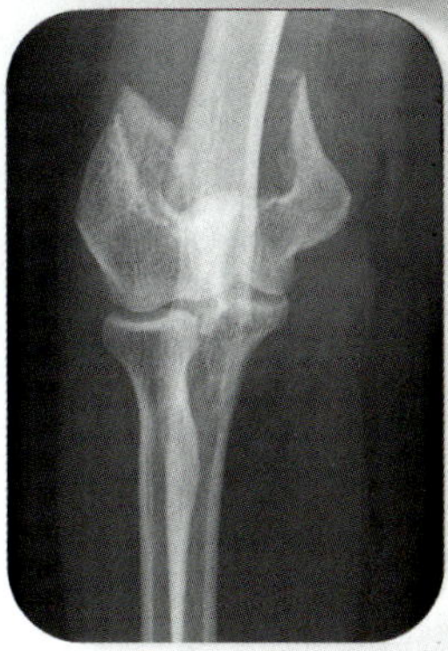

Distal Humerus Fractures

Asif Ilyas, Saqib Rehman

Chapter Outline

Introduction
Diagnosis
Classification
Surgical Indications
Open Reduction and Internal Fixation
Elbow Arthroplasty
External Fixation
Surgical Anatomy, Positioning and Approaches
Applied Anatomy
Positioning
Approaches
Surgical Techniques
Technique 1: ORIF of Distal Humerus Fracture
Technique 2: Total Elbow Arthroplasty of Distal Humerus Fracture
Technique 3: ORIF of Capitellum Fracture
Outcomes
Complications
Post-traumatic Elbow Stiffness
Heterotopic Ossification
Nonunion
Ulnar Neuropathy
Authors' Preferred Management of Select Complications
Case 1: Elbow Stiffness/Heterotopic Ossification
Case 2: Ulnar Neuropathy
Case 3: Nonunion
Summary

Introduction

Distal humerus fractures make up 0.5–2% of all fractures, but up to 30% of elbow fractures.[1] These fractures remain a challenging injury to manage, particularly as the population ages and the prevalence of osteopenic fractures grows.[2] Palvanen et al. identified more than a two-fold increase in the age-adjusted incidence of distal humerus fractures in Finnish women older than 60, between 1970 and 1995, and predicted a three-fold increase by the year 2030.[3] In adults, most distal humerus fractures are intra-articular, and involve both the medial and lateral columns. The distribution of distal humerus fractures follows a bimodal age distribution. High-energy injuries tend to occur among younger patients, while low-energy injuries are more common in older patients. Several variables are important in the successful management of these fractures, including restoration of articular congruity, secure bony fixation, achievement of bony healing, maintenance of a functional range of motion and avoidance of complications, such as heterotopic ossification and ulnar neuropathy.

Diagnosis

The important aspects of physical examination include a thorough evaluation of neurovascular status and the soft tissues. Peripheral pulses and capillary refill should be checked and compared with the contralateral limb to assess perfusion. The proximity of the brachial artery to the distal humerus places it in jeopardy with fractures of the distal humerus. Similarly, the radial, ulnar and median nerves are at risk for concomitant injury. When in doubt, additional imaging, such as ultrasound duplex or arteriography, may be warranted with distal humeral fractures and a careful sensorimotor neurologic examination is critical for adequate assessment. Neurovascular examination should be repeated after any closed reduction maneuvers, and the hand and wrist should be accessible for additional repeat examinations.

The soft tissues should be examined at the time of initial injury and regularly thereafter. Surgical management decisions will hinge upon the status of the soft tissues. Open fracture wounds are common and typically present posteriorly. Significant swelling and subsequent blistering around the elbow can potentially jeopardize open surgical management methods, such as open reduction and internal fixation (ORIF), as well as arthroplasty.

Diagnostic imaging begins with radiographic evaluation including standard anteroposterior and lateral views (Figs 9.1A and B). Due to frequent shortening and flexion of the elbow, visualization of the fracture is often improved with a traction radiograph (Figs 9.2A and B). Radiographs must be scrutinized for the presence of concomitant radial head, olecranon or coronoid fractures. In particular, capitellar-trochlear shear fractures may show a characteristic "double-arc" sign on lateral radiographic views (Fig. 9.3).

Due to the occasional difficulty with standard radiographs to adequately characterize distal humerus fracture patterns and with the increasing availability of advanced imaging modalities, we recommend routine use of computed tomography (CT) with three-dimensional (3D) reconstructions to assess complex intra-articular fractures (Figs 9.4A and B). Digital subtraction of the radius and ulna will improve characterization of the fracture pattern. Intra-articular loose bodies are also well identified on CT imaging (Fig. 9.5). The typical resting position of the elbow in a CT scanner, however, often leads to off-axis axial, coronal and sagittal tomographic images, which can be difficult to evaluate without 3D reformatting. Newer multidetector CT scanners can also obtain 2D imaging in the correct planes despite suboptimal patient positioning

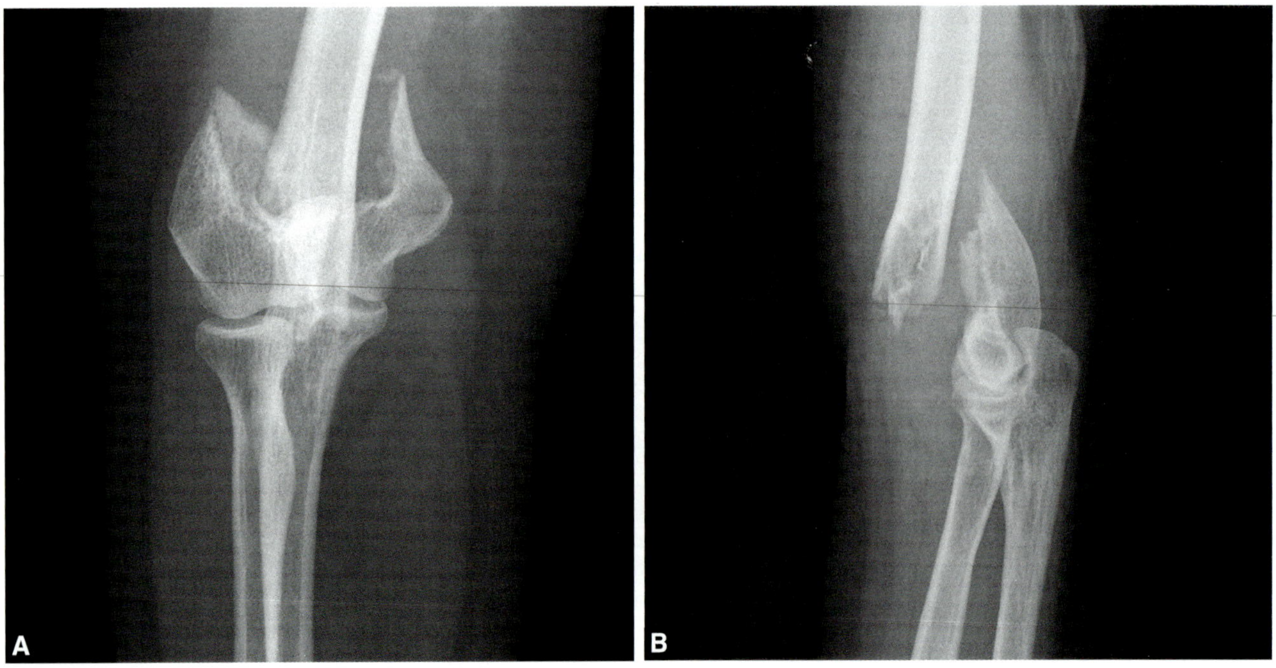

Figures 9.1A and B: (A) Anteroposterior and (B) Lateral radiographs of a distal humerus fracture.

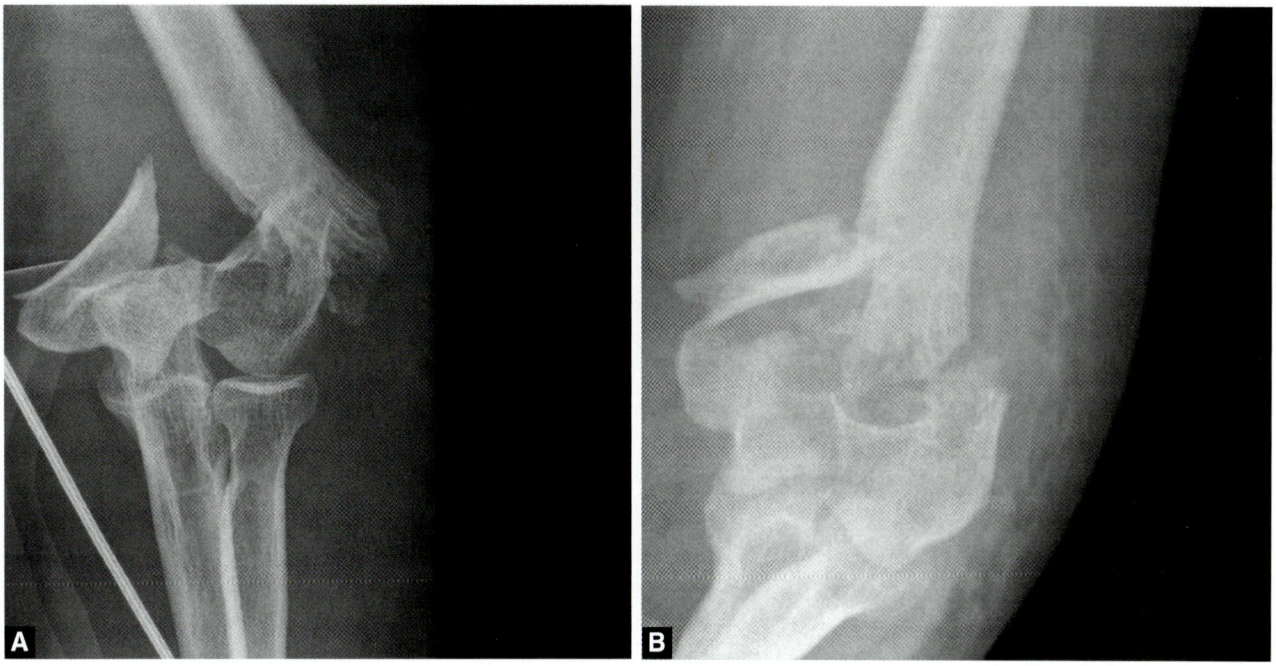

Figures 9.2A and B: Traction radiographs of a distal humerus fracture demonstrating improved fracture characterization. (A) Pretraction radiograph; (B) Post-traction radiograph.

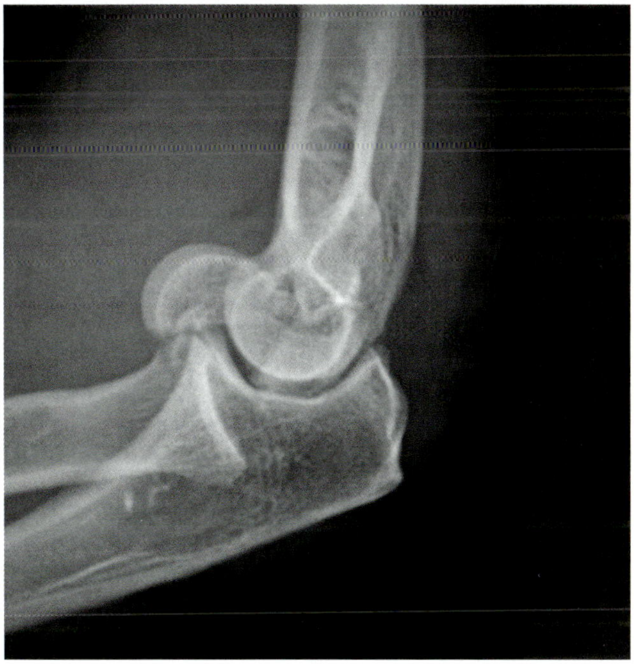

Figure 9.3: The "double-arc" sign of a displaced capitellar-trochlear shear fracture.

if the surgeon informs the CT technician of the desired imaging planes.

DISTAL HUMERUS FRACTURES DIAGNOSIS: Pearls and Pitfalls

- Open wounds and nerve injuries are common and should be vigilantly evaluated
- Initial radiographs are often difficult to interpret and traction radiographs can improve fracture characterization
- Computed tomography evaluation is important in fracture characterization and preoperative planning

Classification

The traditional classification of distal humerus fractures has centered around the terminal ends or the condyles of the humerus. When discussing distal humerus, the term "condyle" is converted to "columns" for the sake of classification. Single column fractures in adults are uncommon

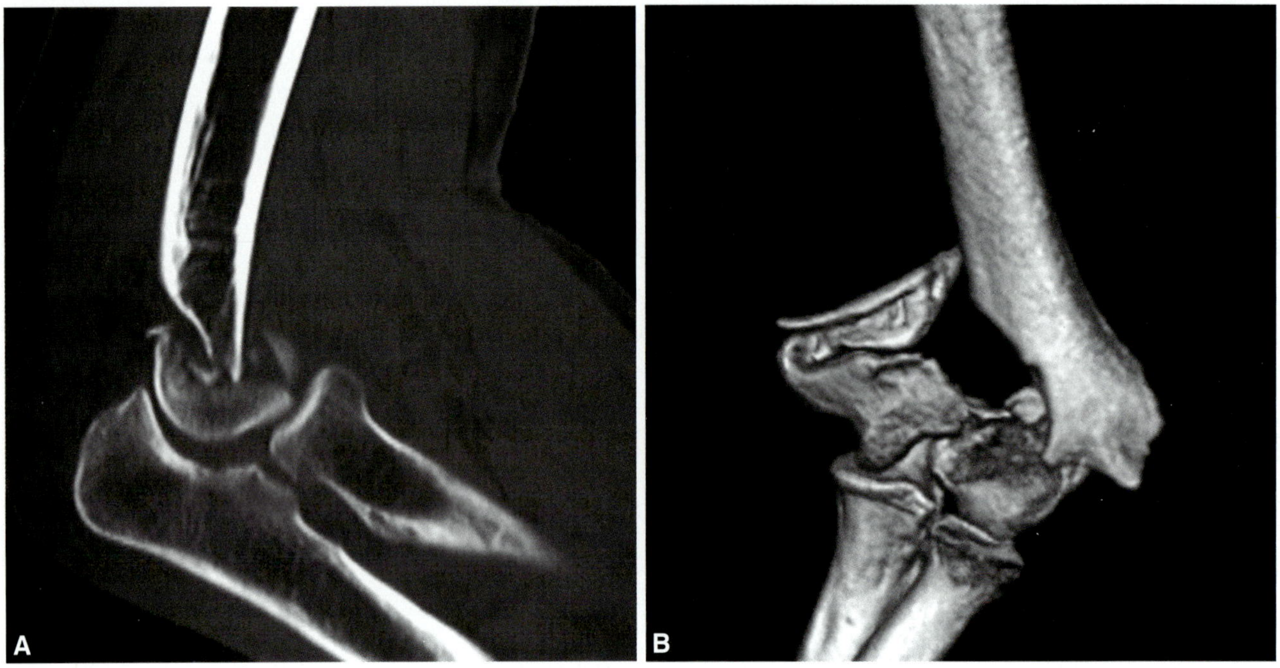

Figures 9.4A and B: (A) Standard two-dimensional and (B) three-dimensional CT evaluation of a distal humerus fracture.

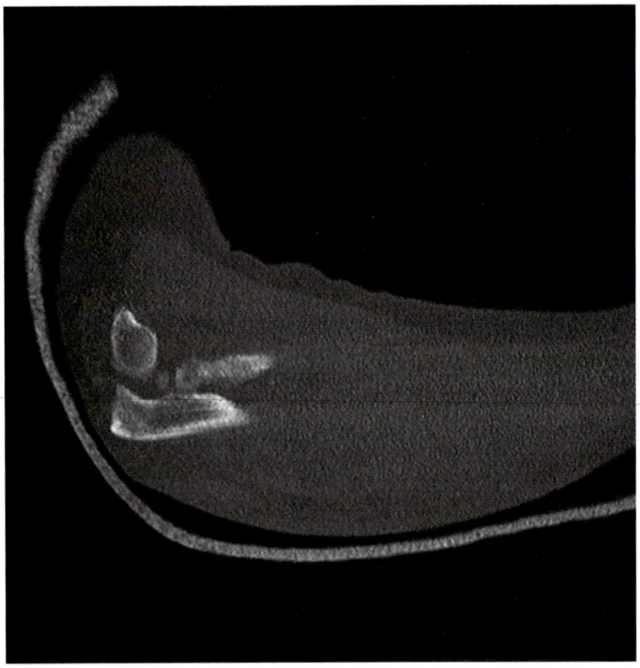

Figure 9.5: Sagittal-reformatted CT image of the elbow demonstrates a small intra-articular osteoarticular fragment after reduction of an elbow dislocation. This finding can be missed with routine radiographic imaging.

and when present generally involve the lateral column. Both column fractures on the other hand are more common.

Several classification systems for intra-articular both column fractures of the distal humerus have been proposed and predicated primarily on the positions of the articular fragment. Historical classifications include Reich, Riseborough and Radin, and Jupiter and Mehne.[4-6] We recommend the AO Classification of Fractures which is categorized into three main types: Type A (extra-articular), Type B (partial articular) and Type C (complete articular). Subtypes are given thereafter for further fracture characteristics.[7]

Capitellum fractures are divided into Type I to III. Type I fractures, also known as "Hahn-Steinthal" fragment, consist of a large fragment consisting of both articular cartilage and subchondral bone. Type II fractures, also known as "Kocher-Lorenz" fragment, consists of primarily articular cartilage. Lastly, Type III fractures represent a comminuted capitellum fracture.

Surgical Indications

Most fractures of the distal humerus in adults are routinely managed operatively. These injuries are typically articular, displaced, and unstable and therefore are poorly managed by casting and bracing methods. Nonoperative methods can be considered for stable extra-articular and minimally displaced intra-articular fractures, as well as fractures in very low-demand patients. However, nonoperative methods can lead to deformity, stiffness, instability and post-traumatic arthrosis of the elbow joint. Moreover, due to the unforgiving nature of the elbow with regard to post-traumatic stiffness, nonoperative methods which do not permit early motion, often result in significant loss of range of motion. Therefore, if nonoperative methods are chosen, a brief period of immobilization followed by protected range of motion exercises can potentially achieve acceptable results. The "bag of bones" method which consists of a brief period of immobilization followed by an early range of motion, can be selected in patients with osteoporosis and highly comminuted fractures. Although some return of function and range of motion can be achieved, alignment and stability are typically compromised.

Patients with distal humeral fractures are indicated for surgical management in most cases and particularly in cases with open fractures, vascular injury, multiply traumatized patients and displaced intra-articular fractures. Contemporary surgical management techniques may be divided into three main categories, including rigid with plates and screws, elbow arthroplasty and joint-spanning external fixation.

Open Reduction and Internal Fixation

This method is employed most frequently in the surgical management of distal humerus fractures. Open reduction and internal fixation affords versatility and the ability to restore anatomical relationships, as well as facilitate early range of motion. Fixation can be difficult in the distal humerus due to its limited cortical bone, predominance of thin metaphyseal bone, close proximity to articular cartilage and anatomical constraints imposed by the coronoid and olecranon fossae. These challenges are compounded in cases of osteoporosis and low transarticular comminuted fractures. Newer technologies, however, including locking technology and dual plating methods have arguably improved fixation in cases where rigid fixation had been previously difficult to obtain.

Elbow Arthroplasty

Elderly patients with osteoporosis can present challenges with ORIF, particularly in the distal humerus. Similarly, low transarticular distal humeral fractures are a particular example in which insufficient rigidity after ORIF can preclude early motion (Fig. 9.6A). Primary elbow arthroplasty of a distal humerus fracture may be indicated in cases of extensive articular comminution, low transarticular fractures, advanced osteoporosis and low demand elderly patients (Fig. 9.6B).

External Fixation

Joint-spanning external fixation is occasionally indicated as a temporary treatment in cases in which definitive treatment, such as ORIF, is not immediately indicated but skeletal stability is required. Patients with severe soft tissue injuries and lack of skin coverage can benefit from temporary joint-spanning external fixation rather than splinting. This can restore skeletal length, allow access to the skin and soft tissues, and prevent further injury from instability. Cases of vascular injury requiring repair and fasciotomies are also good indications for temporary external fixation in order to protect the vascular repair and allow access for wound care, which can be difficult with splints and braces.

Surgical Anatomy, Positioning and Approaches

Applied Anatomy

Understanding the anatomy of the distal humerus is critical to the effective treatment of distal humerus fractures. Divergent medial and lateral columns of bone, support the distal humeral articular surface in an inverted-Y configuration. The medial column diverges from the central humeral axis at an angle of 45°, and the lateral column at an angle of 20° (Figs 9.7A and B).

The trochlea lies in the center and links the two columns and articulates with the olecranon. Stability of the elbow is a product of bony articulations, soft tissue tension and the musculotendinous forces acting across it. The central sulcus of the trochlea interdigitates with the corresponding articular ridge on the olecranon providing significant bony

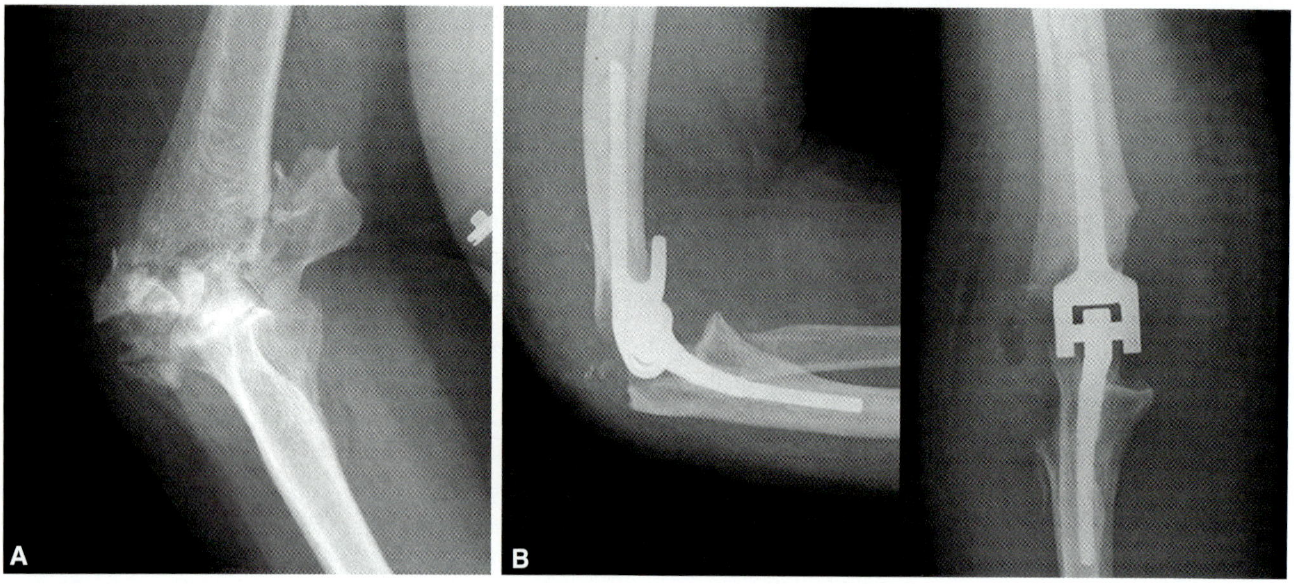

Figures 9.6A and B: (A) Anteroposterior radiograph of a distal humeral fracture in an elderly, low demand patient with significant articular comminution, particularly involving the lateral column; (B) Primary total elbow arthroplasty was chosen for definitive management of this injury.

stability to the elbow through this highly congruent articulation. The trochlea is covered by articular cartilage over an arc of almost 300° and subsequently permits a broad range of motion at the ulnohumeral joint. Compromise of the trochlea in the form of shortening, bone loss or residual incongruity can translate into the significant loss of elbow motion and stability.

The capitellum resides on the lateral column and provides 180° of articulating area. In contrast to the trochlea, the posterior aspect of the lateral column is nonarticular and allows for posterior placement of implants without risk of injury to cartilage or impingement with flexion and extension.

The distal articular surface lies in 4–8° of valgus and is externally rotated 3–4° relative to the central axis of the humerus. The capitellum and trochlea are translated anteriorly relative to the humeral diaphysis, creating an angle between the central humeral axis and the distal articular segment of 30–40° (Figs 9.7A and B). The lateral column and epicondyle follow this anterior translation, whereas the medial column and epicondyle are in line with the humeral shaft. Compromise of these dimensions during treatment can risk the loss of elbow motion.

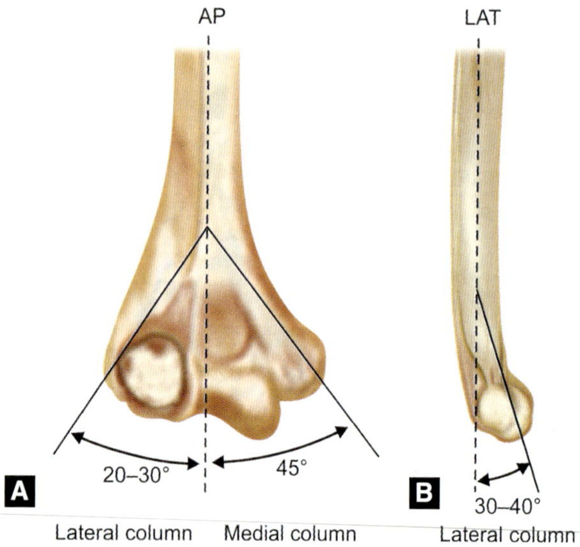

Figures 9.7A and B: Illustration of the divergent nature of both columns of the distal humerus and the anterior translation of the distal articular segment. Note on (A) the anteroposterior view that the medial column diverges from the central humeral axis at an angle of 45° and the lateral column at an angle of 20°; (B) On the lateral view, the capitellum and trochlea translate anteriorly relative to the humeral diaphysis, creating an angle between the central humeral axis and the distal articular segment of 30–40°.

There are some general principles for most surgical approaches to the distal humerus. A posterior skin incision should be utilized, in general. This takes advantage of the rich blood supply to the posterior elbow and decreases the risk for skin necrosis and painful postoperative neuroma formation. In cases of isolated capitellum or capitellar-trochlear shear fractures, a lateral approach may be utilized.

Full-thickness flaps are raised medially and laterally. Prior to deep dissection, the ulnar nerve must be identified and protected throughout the case. At the end of the procedure, the ulnar nerve may either be decompressed in situ along its entire length or transposed anteriorly as per the preference of the surgeon. If transposed, the overlying arcade of Struthers, medial intermuscular septum and the fascia between the two heads of the flexor carpi ulnaris must be adequately released. Similarly, during transposition devascularization of the nerve should be avoided.

The medial and lateral collateral ligament complexes should be protected throughout the procedure and not inadvertently released. The medial collateral ligament has its proximal attachment along the anteroinferior aspect of the medial epicondyle and has its distal attachment along the medial aspect of the ulna immediately distal to the coronoid process. The lateral collateral ligament complex has its proximal attachment at a point along the lateral epicondyle that marks the axis of the ulnohumeral joint and attaches to the lateral ulna along a broad base while coalescing with fibers of the annular ligament complex.

The blood supply of the distal humerus is segmental and depends on the status of the surrounding soft tissue. The capitellum is perfused along its posterior border and is at risk for devascularization with posterior approaches. The trochlea and the rest of the distal humerus are supplied both medially and laterally, and possess a watershed region in the center. Too extensive soft tissue dissection can compromise perfusion of the distal humerus. But, by maintaining the collateral ligaments and origin of the flexor-pronator mass sufficient collateral circulation should remain to avoid devascularization of the capitellum during standard posterior approaches.

Positioning

Although the patient may be positioned supine or prone, lateral positioning with the operative limb supported on a padded radiolucent bolster is recommended (Fig. 9.8). This allows comfortable positioning of the elbow directly in front of the surgeon, dependent positioning of the arm that indirectly aids in reduction, easier access for the image intensifier, convenient approach to the hip if autologous bone harvesting is planned, and quicker access (than prone positioning) to the patient's airway if necessary. In the cases of isolated capitellum fractures, supine positioning with a hand table is preferable. A sterile pneumatic tourniquet is routinely used.

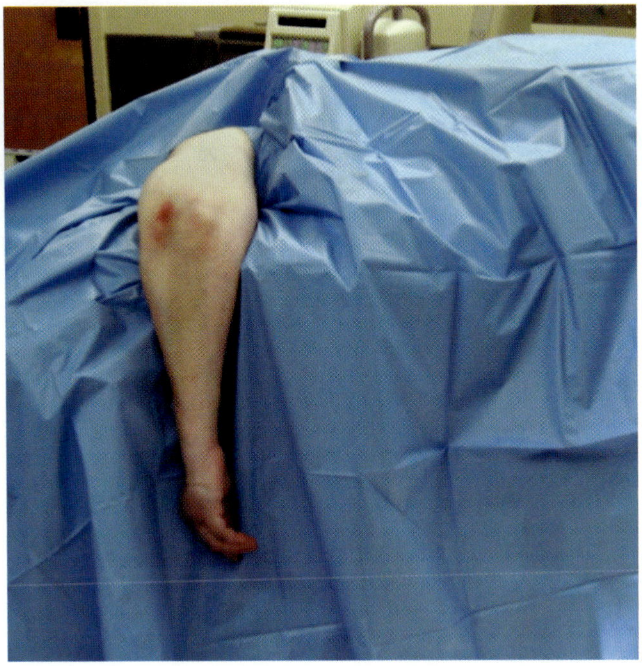

Figure 9.8: Lateral positioning of the patient on a radiolucent table and utilization of a radiolucent rectangular bolster allows both excellent support for the limb during the procedure and excellent intraoperative fluoroscopic imaging when needed. In this image, the patient's head is to the left and feet are to the right. The fluoroscope is brought from the opposite side of the table. A sterile tourniquet can also be utilized during the procedure.

Approaches

The Campbell approach, also known as the "triceps-splitting" approach, involves splitting the triceps longitudinally through the midline of the triceps aponeurosis down to the humerus followed by subperiosteal elevation of the triceps medially and laterally. The triceps split extends distally onto the olecranon. Proximally, the radial nerve limits the extent of dissection. This approach is useful in extra-articular distal humeral shaft and supracondylar fractures of the distal humerus. Full exposure of the articular surface of the distal humerus is not possible with this approach.

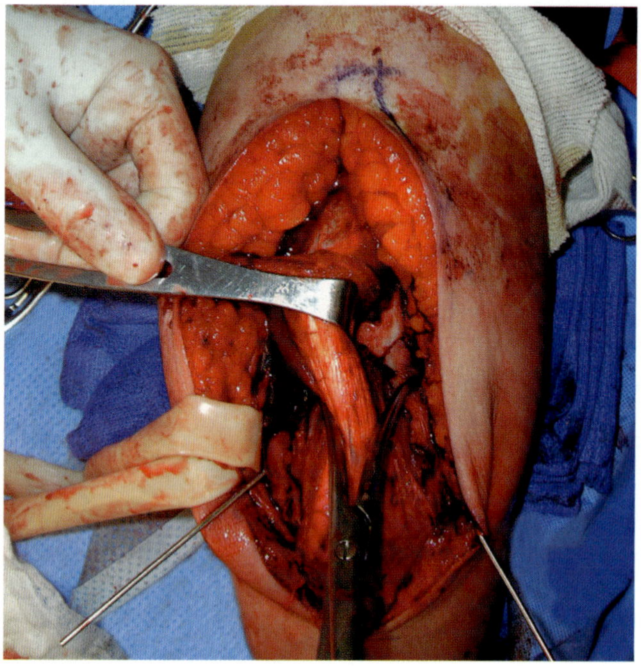

Figure 9.9: Triceps-sparing approach to the distal humerus. The triceps musculature is reflected off the medial and lateral intermuscular septums and subsequently raised subperiosteally off the humerus but its distal insertion into the olecranon is maintained.

The Alonso-Llames approach, or also known as the "triceps-sparing" approach, involves raising the triceps entirely off the distal humerus while maintaining its distal attachment in the olecranon (Fig. 9.9). The triceps musculature is reflected off the medial and lateral intermuscular septums and subsequently raised subperiosteally off the humerus. Like the triceps-splitting approach, exposure of the articular surface is limited.

The Bryan and Morrey approach provides access to the medial elbow that involves raising the triceps and extensor mechanism as a full subperiosteal sleeve from the posterior humerus and proximal ulna. Reflection of the sleeve of extensor mechanism results in exposure of the entire elbow joint. This requires meticulous technique to avoid violating the continuity of the extensor mechanism during dissection and can be difficult in an elbow that has recently experienced significant trauma.

The olecranon osteotomy has been the "workhorse" for approaching the distal humerus and is our preferred approach for the management of intra-articular fractures. It provides the best visualization and access to the articular surface of the distal humerus. After identification and mobilization of the ulnar nerve, a small sponge is placed from medial to lateral through the ulnohumeral joint (Fig. 9.10A). A chevron osteotomy is made along the posterior ulna so that the osteotomy enters within the trochlear notch, an area relatively devoid of articular cartilage. The osteotomy is performed incompletely with an oscillating saw. The osteotomy is then completed by an osteotome, resulting in an irregular border that will allow interdigitation of the osteotomy during repair, as well as minimize bone loss. The olecranon is then reflected proximally along with the attached posterior elbow capsule and triceps revealing excellent exposure of the articular surface (Fig. 9.10B). At the end of the procedure, the osteotomy is repaired with a tension band wire technique using two 0.045 or 0.062 inch K-wires or a 6.5 mm screw and 20 or 22 gauge stainless steel wire. Alternatively, a plate or intramedullary device may be used to repair the osteotomy site.

For isolated capitellum fractures, a lateral approach to the elbow may be utilized. The lateral approach to the elbow has multiple intervals that can be exploited. Traditionally, the Kocher approach has been advocated that utilizes the interval between the extensor carpi ulnaris and the anconeus and affords greater protection of the posterior interosseous nerve. This is a relatively posterior approach and although providing good access to the radial head it affords limited access to the distal humeral articular surface. Alternatively, the Kaplan approach utilizing the more anterior interval between the extensor carpi radialis brevis and extensor carpi digitorum communis or the extensor digitorum communis (EDC)-splitting approach (Fig. 9.11) both provide excellent exposure of the radiocapitellar approach while affording the ability to increase the exposure by extending the incision proximally along the lateral supracondylar ridge, if necessary. To avoid inadvertant injury to the lateral ulnar collateral ligament complex, dissection should not be taken posterior to the midaxis of the radiocapitellar joint. Lastly, there is often a capsular violation created by the initial injury that may be exploited to access the joint laterally without having to create a second soft tissue defect.

To increase exposure laterally, such as in the case of capitellar fractures, the lateral epicondyle may be osteotomized thereby taking down the lateral ulnar

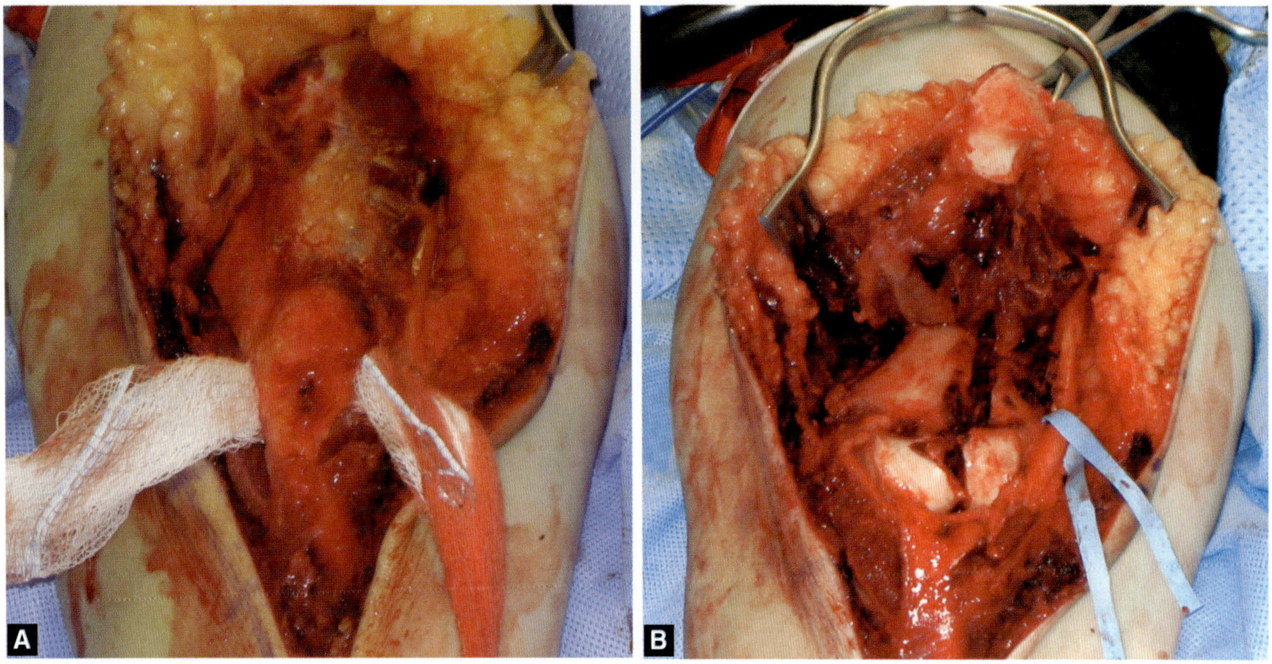

Figures 9.10A and B: Olecranon osteotomy can maximize exposure of the distal humeral articular surface. (A) The triceps mechanism is exposed and the ulnar nerve is mobilized. The proposed site for the chevron osteotomy is depicted with a "V" configuration with the apex pointing distally. Prior to making the cut a sponge is placed across the joint to protect against inadvertent articular injury to the distal humerus; (B) The completed osteotomy proximal ulna fragment with triceps mechanism attachment is reflected proximally towards the top of the photo. The distal humeral fracture fragments are shown clearly and the ulnar nerve is kept in the surgical field.

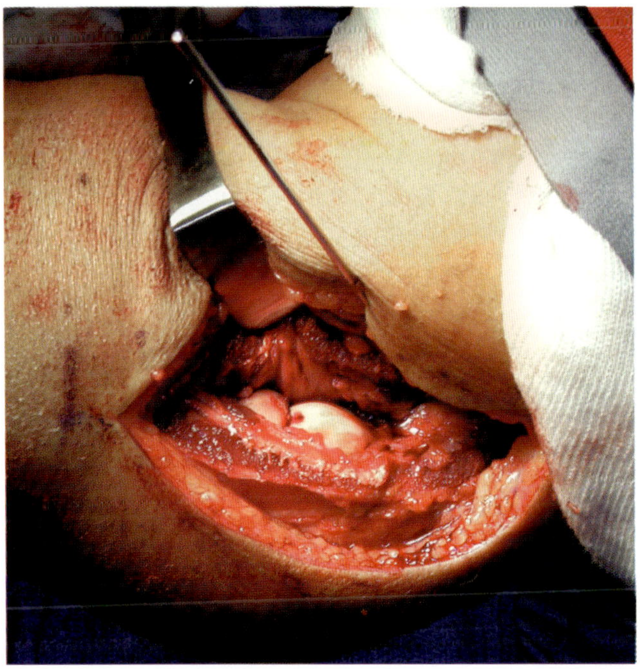

Figure 9.11: Extensor digitorum communis-splitting approach to the lateral elbow provides excellent exposure to the radiocapitellar joint. To increase exposure and access to the joint, the lateral extensor mass can be carefully raised off the supracondylar ridge proximally. To avoid inadvertent injury to the lateral ulnar collateral ligament or elbow instability, dissection should not be taken posterior to the midaxis of the radiocapitellar joint.

collateral ligament complex and allowing the elbow to hinge open on the medial collateral ligament with varus stress. The osteotomy site should be repaired with a plate and screws upon closure.

Surgical Techniques

Technique 1: ORIF of Distal Humerus Fracture

Instrumentation and implants to consider having on hand during the case include fluoroscopy, fracture reduction tools, Kirschner (K) wires, headless compression screws and small fragment instrumentation. Traditionally, small fragment reconstruction plates have been utilized. In order to maximize the strength of the construct the plates are contoured and applied in an orthogonal (90–90) alignment: the medial plate is applied directly medial while the lateral plate is applied along the posterior surface of the lateral column.[8]

More recently, periarticular locking plates have grown in popularity and availability that provide both contoured designs and locking technology. Locking plates provide the advantage of improved fixation in osteoporotic bone or unicortical fixation, where bicortical purchase is not always an option. The plate is fixed proximally with standard bicortical screws and therefore with locking screws distally. To maximize fixation and rigidity of the construct, as many screws as possible are passed through the plate and the distal humerus. Fixation may be reinforced with threaded K-wires cut flush to the bone or with headless compression screws. In addition, locking plates have made plate application more versatile by facilitating both orthogonal, as well as parallel plating.[9] The latter allows both locking plates to be applied directly medially and laterally (Figs 9.12A and B).

If an olecranon osteotomy is planned necessary equipment, such as K-wires or 6.5/7.3 mm partially threaded compression screws, stainless steel wiring or plate should be selected. More recently, olecranon osteotomy nails have become available that are placed prior to osteotomy creation that facilitates osteotomy repair at the end of the case.

For all distal humerus fractures, a posterior midline incision is placed and full-thickness flaps are raised medially and laterally. The ulnar nerve is identified and released at least 8 cm proximal and 6 cm distal to the medial epicondyle. A moistened unclamped half-inch penrose drain is placed around the nerve to gently facilitate its manipulation. It is protected throughout the case and we recommend routine anterior transposition at the end of the case.

For extra-articular fractures, we recommend a triceps-sparing approach by developing medial and lateral paratricipital windows (Figs 9.9 and 9.13A to N). However, for intra-articular fractures either the Bryan and Morrey extensile medial approach or an olecranon osteotomy can be utilized. We recommend an olecranon osteotomy for maximal exposure of the articular surface (Figs 9.10 and 9.14A to E).

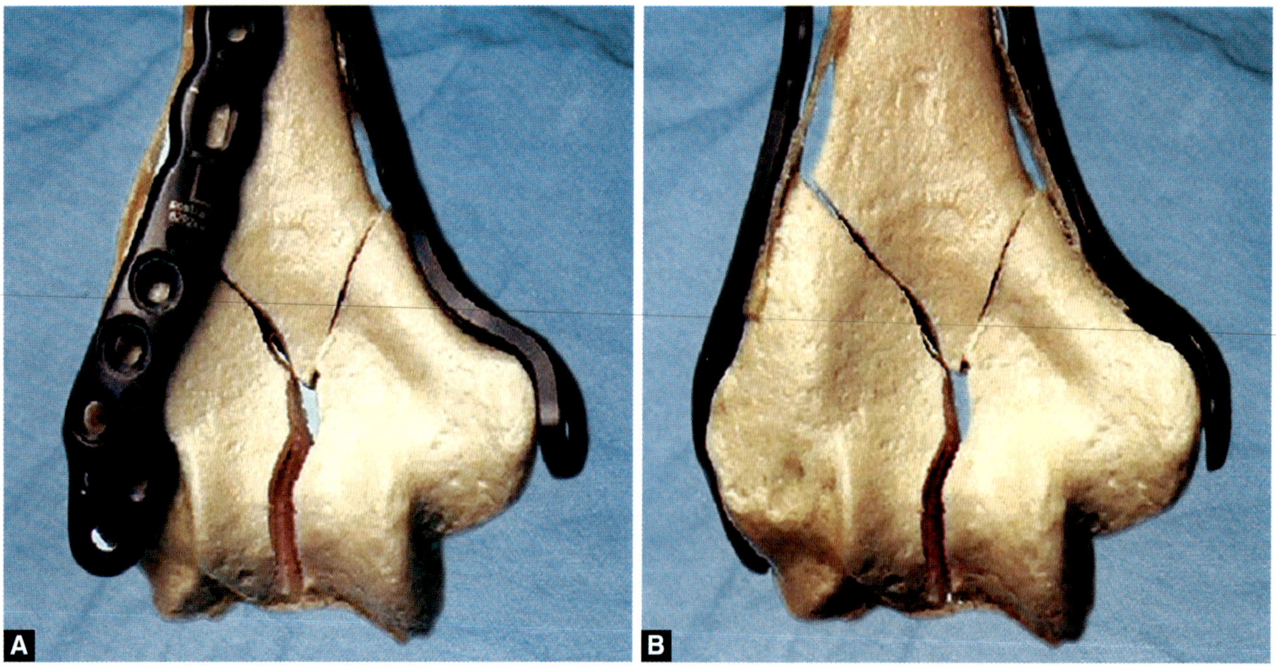

Figures 9.12A and B: Locked periarticular locking plates in the standard (A) Orthogonal and (B) Parallel plating configuration.

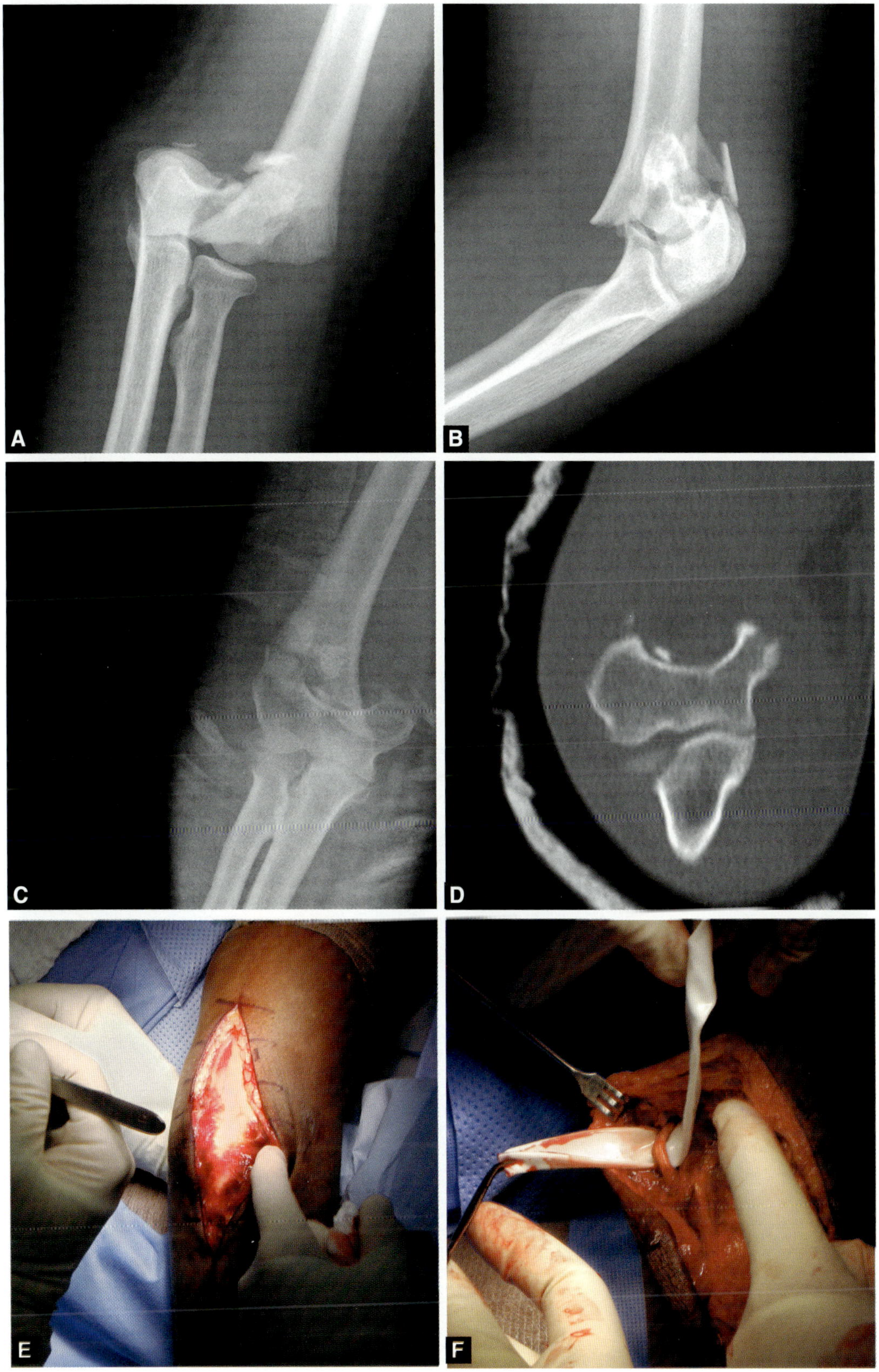

Figures 9.13A to F

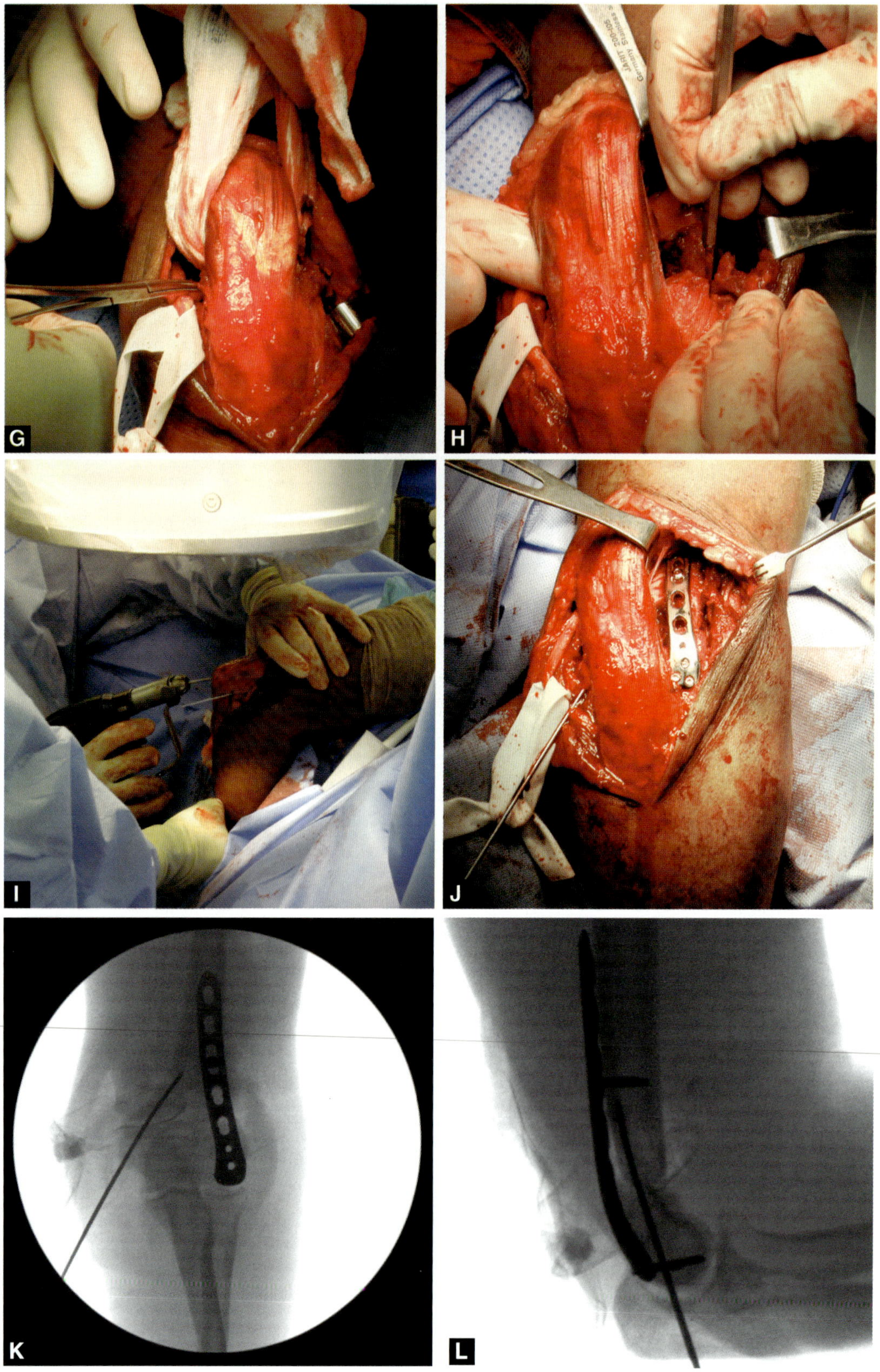

Figures 9.13G to L

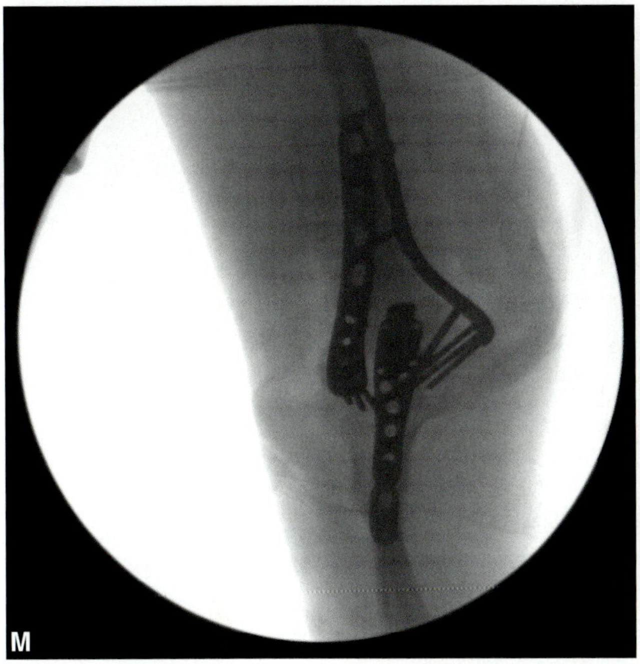

M

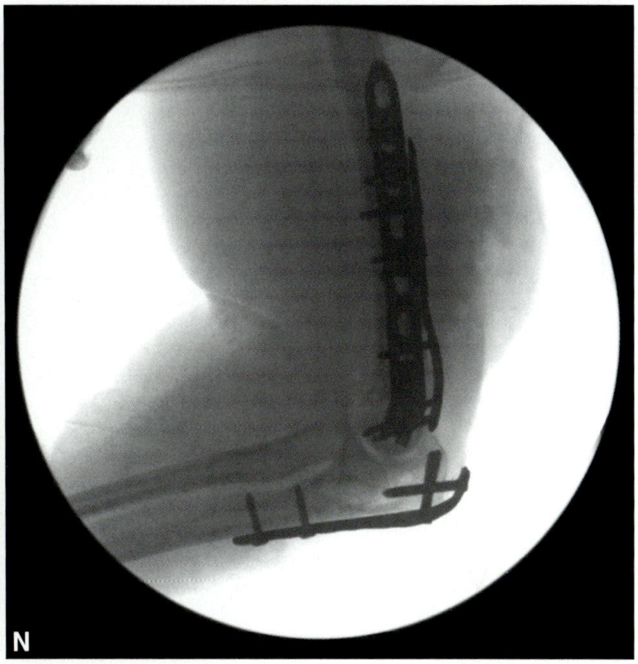

N

Figures 9.13A to N: ORIF of an extra-articular distal humeral fracture with medial and lateral paratricipital approaches without olecranon osteotomy. Preoperative (A) Anteroposterior (AP); (B) Lateral radiographs before closed reduction and splinting; (C) AP radiograph and (D) CT scan image after closed reduction confirm that there is no intra-articular involvement of the fracture; (E) After lateral positioning of the patient, a straight posterior midline incision is made, exposing the extensor mechanism; (F) The ulnar nerve is now identified and carefully protected throughout the procedure. Care is taken to avoid traction on the penrose drain placed here; (G) Dissection is now made on the medial and lateral borders of the triceps mechanism down to the humerus. A sponge is then placed as shown; (H) The fracture fragments are now exposed, reduced using forceps; (I) Provisionally pinned; (J) Fixation is performed posterolaterally with compression plating also seen on; (K) Anteroposterior; (L) Lateral fluoroscopic imaging. Fixation is completed with compression plating medially with care to ensure that the nerve is not draped directly over the edge of the medial plate. Final (M) Anteroposterior; (N) Lateral images demonstrate final orthogonal compression plating medially and posterolaterally.

Prior to performing the osteotomy, we recommend predrilling and tapping for a 6.5 mm or 7.3 mm cannulated screw that will be placed at the end of the procedure with a washer. Predrilling and preparing for eventual screw placement facilitates expeditious and accurate osteotomy repair at the end of the case. Alternatively, tension band wiring, olecranon plate or nail may be placed.

The olecranon osteotomy is typically done with a chevron cut along the posterior ulna centered at the trochlear notch. The osteotomy is performed incompletely with an oscillating saw and then completed by hand or an osteotome. This last step creates an irregular fracture at the articular surface, facilitating reduction at the time of osteotomy fixation. The olecranon tip is then wrapped in a wet sponge and reflected proximally by dividing the joint capsule. The triceps is freed medially and laterally parallel to the humerus along with the intermuscular septum.

Release of the triceps must be undertaken carefully. The ulnar nerve sits medial to the triceps. The radial nerve sits laterally along the humerus and crosses the posterior humerus approximately 11–14 cm proximal to the articular surface. The nerve can be kinked or stretched with overzealous proximal retraction of the extensor mechanism after osteotomy.

The fracture fragments are examined and debrided. Soft tissue attachments are left intact whenever possible. Care must be taken not to drop any loose fragments on the floor. Fracture reduction can be performed in a number of sequences depending upon fracture alignment and comminution. Our preference is to first restore the distal articular surface. Most commonly an intra-articular split will occur between the trochlea and capitellum, which can be reduced under direct visualization and reduced with a small fragment screw or cannulated screw. This is

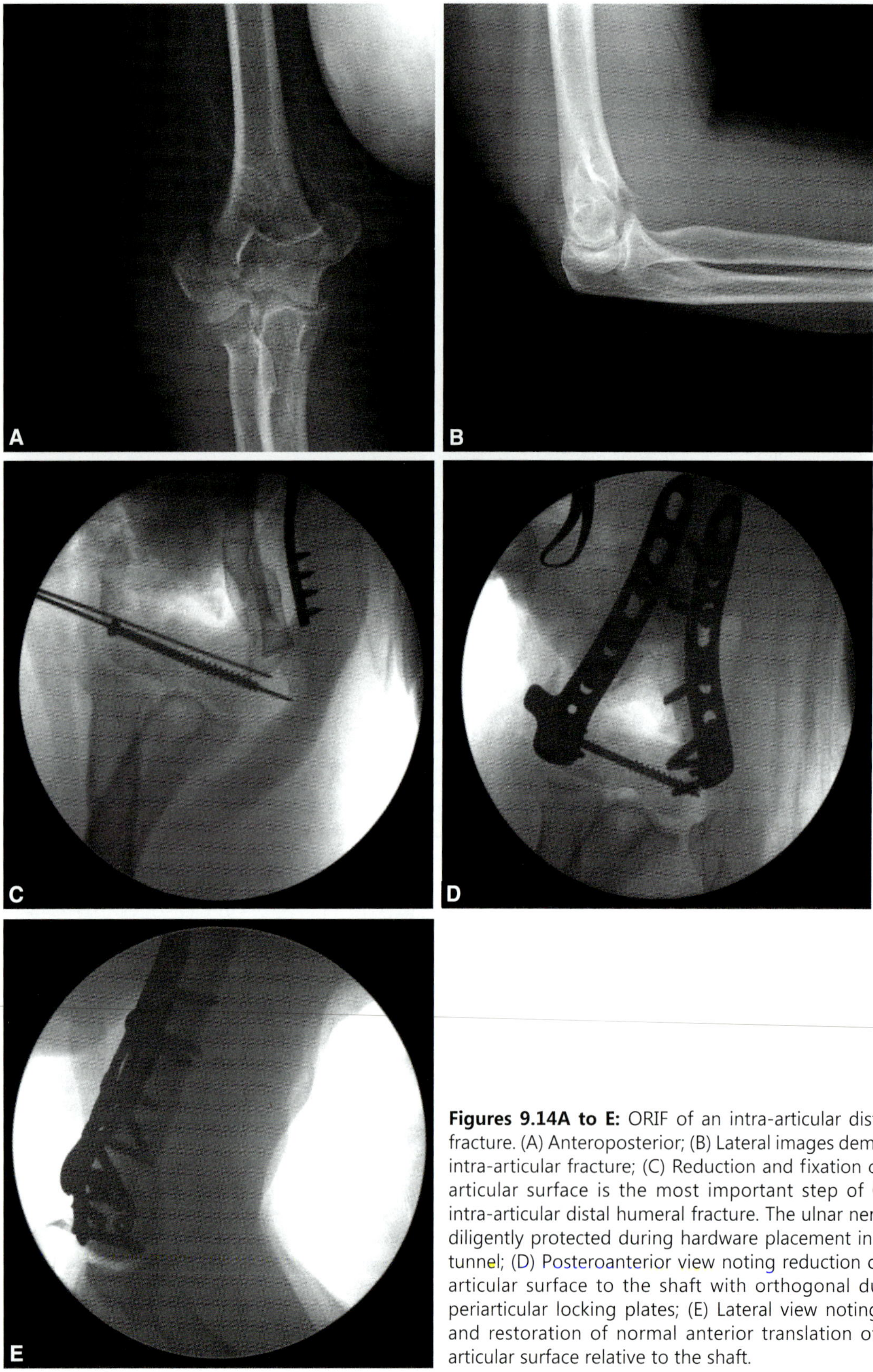

Figures 9.14A to E: ORIF of an intra-articular distal humeral fracture. (A) Anteroposterior; (B) Lateral images demonstrate an intra-articular fracture; (C) Reduction and fixation of the distal articular surface is the most important step of ORIF of an intra-articular distal humeral fracture. The ulnar nerve must be diligently protected during hardware placement in the cubital tunnel; (D) Posteroanterior view noting reduction of the distal articular surface to the shaft with orthogonal dual column periarticular locking plates; (E) Lateral view noting reduction and restoration of normal anterior translation of the distal articular surface relative to the shaft.

preferably performed from a medial to lateral direction to avoid intraoperative, as well as late ulnar nerve injury. If performed from a lateral to medial direction, the ulnar nerve must be protected and preferably transposed out of the cubital tunnel. Do not overcompress the articular surface in order to avoid shortening of the articular surface. Additional articular fragments may be reapproximated with K-wires for later fixation once the plates are applied or repaired primarily with headless compression screws. Screw placement in the distal humeral fragment is challenging and diligence must be paid to avoid injury of articular cartilage or overpenetration of either the coronoid or olecranon fossae.

Reduction of the distal articular surface to the shaft may be accomplished using either locking periarticular orthogonal or parallel plates. Although fracture fixation and articular surface reconstruction is done under direct visualization, image intensifier is utilized to confirm hardware position and fracture reduction. Beyond anatomic reduction of the articular surface, reduction of the distal humeral fragment to the proximal shaft may be equally challenging. The distal articular surface normally lies in 4–8° of valgus and is externally rotated 34° relative to the central axis of the humerus. The capitellum and trochlea are translated anteriorly relative to the humeral diaphysis, creating an angle between the central humeral axis and the distal articular segment of 30–40°. The lateral column and epicondyle follow this anterior translation, whereas the medial column and epicondyle are in line with the humeral shaft.

The olecranon osteotomy may be repaired by placement of a 6.5 mm/7.3 mm screw with washer or the olecranon nail as described previously. Alternatively, a tension-band wiring repair may be performed with two 0.045 or 0.062 inch K-wires directed from the posterior olecranon across the reduced osteotomy site into the anterior cortex of the proximal ulna. Avoid crossing the articular surface. A single or a double-looped 20 or 22 gauge stainless steel wire is looped in a Figure-8 fashion and positioned through a drill hole located distally at approximately the same distance from the osteotomy apex as is the tip of the olecranon. It is then passed behind the K-wires directly on the bone. This may be facilitated with a 14-gauge angiocatheter. The wire is tightened by evenly twisting the opposite arms of the figure-8 wire construct. The K-wires are bent over 180°, cut sharply and impacted firmly into the bone. Once the fracture is internally fixed the elbow is taken through a full range of motion to confirm joint reduction, fracture stability and no errant hardware placement.

The ulnar nerve is transposed anteriorly in a subcutaneous fashion. Throughout the release and transposition devascularization of the nerve must be avoided. The nerve is released proximally along its entire length behind the arcade of Struthers. The intermuscular septum is released distally off the medial epicondyle and a 1–2 cm distal portion is excised. Osborne's ligament is released completely and the release is taken distally between the two heads of the flexor carpi ulnaris musculature. The nerve is transposed anteriorly and a fascial sling is created off the flexor-pronator mass to avoid re-subluxation of the nerve posteriorly. Extreme diligence must be paid to confirm that the nerve is under no tension or compression in its new position in both flexion and extension of the elbow.

The skin is closed in layers and a hinged elbow brace is applied. We routinely immobilize the elbow in 90° of flexion locked for 10–14 days to allow the wounds to heal followed by aggressive range of motion under the supervision of a therapist. We avoid any restrictions on motion whenever possible. Alternatively, the elbow may be placed in the brace unlocked or in full extension. The rationale for the latter is to take tension off the nerve and posterior wound while also placing the anterior capsule on stretch to potentially avoid the loss of terminal extension.

ORIF OF DISTAL HUMERUS FRACTURE: Pearls and Pitfalls

- The patient should be warned preoperatively of a possible transient or prolonged ulnar nerve palsy
- Shortening or malreduction of the articular surface will result in elbow incongruence and loss of motion
- Dual column locked plating provides the strongest construct. Either orthogonal or parallel plating may be employed and the plate configuration should be selected that optimizes fracture reduction
- Stability of the construct is enhanced by maximizing the number of screws passing across the distal fragment
- The articular surface should be inspected to confirm that no screws violate the articular surface or fill the olecranon or coronoid fossae
- Using calibrated drill bits and self-tapping screws increase operative efficiency

Technique 2: Total Elbow Arthroplasty of Distal Humerus Fracture

We recommend routine use of a cemented semiconstrained total elbow prosthesis in the management of distal humerus fractures being treated primarily with arthroplasty. Primary elbow arthroplasty of a distal humerus fracture may be indicated in cases of extensive articular comminution, low transarticular fractures, advanced osteoporosis, and low demand elderly patients. (Figs 9.15A to D). Arthroplasty is contraindicated in cases of prior infection, neurologic dysfunction, and compromised skin or soft tissue.

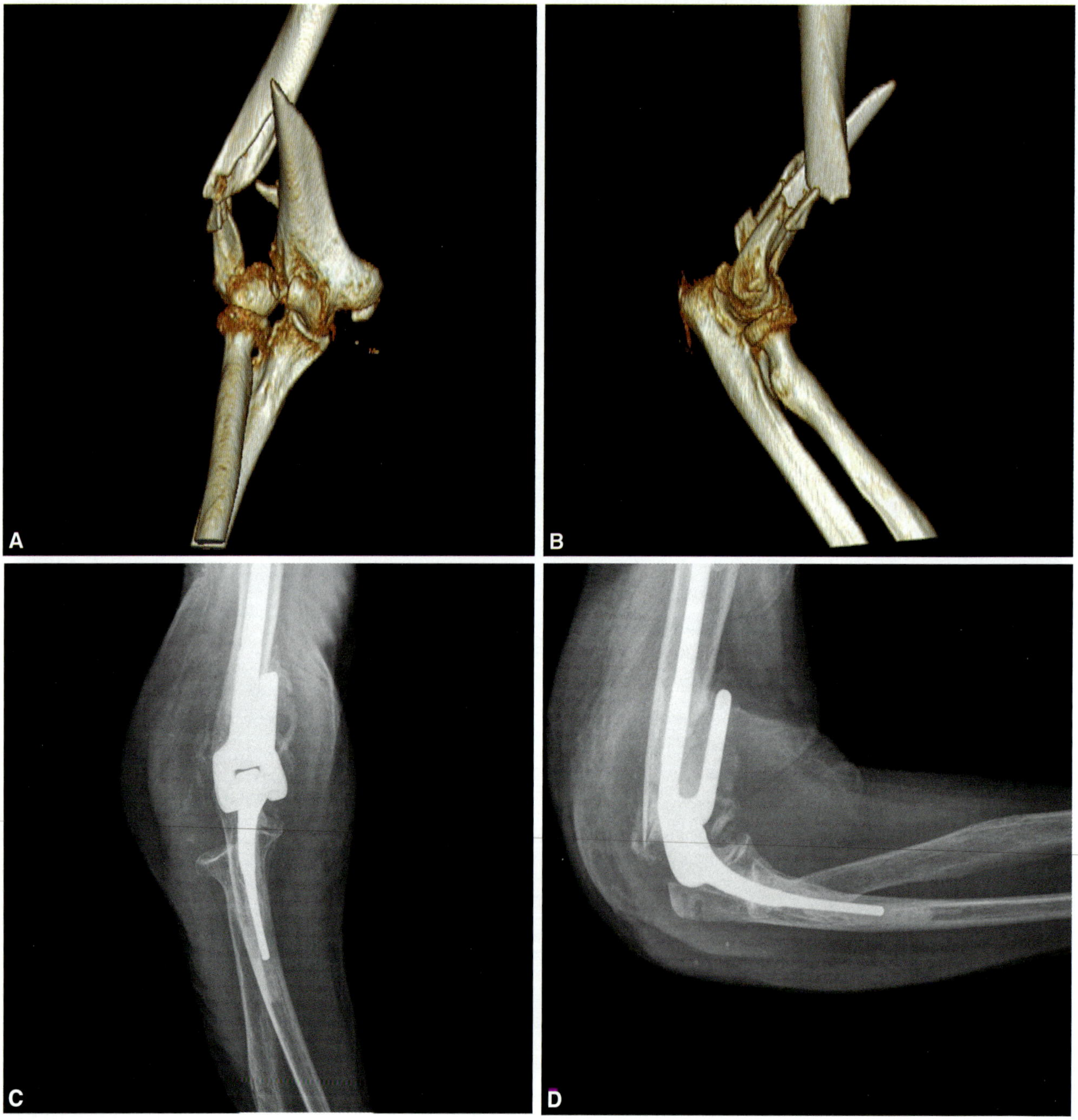

Figures 9.15A to D: Total elbow arthroplasty of a distal humerus fracture in an elderly patient. (A and B) Preoperative three-dimensional CT scanning demonstrated a comminuted intra-articular fracture of the distal humerus. (C and D) Postoperative radiographs following arthroplasty. Note the use of a cemented semiconstrained prosthesis. All fractured fragments, including the entire articular surface and the fractured condyles, were removed.

Necessary implants and technique should follow the instructions from the implant's manufacturer. We recommend supine or lateral positioning and concomitant use of an image intensifier during the case. As the columns of the distal humerus are typically fractured in cases indicated for primary arthroplasty, we recommend routine removal of all distal fracture fragments, including the condyles, and preparation of the humeral shaft alone for the humeral component. The ulna is prepared in standard fashion as per the manufacturer's instructions.

Following arthroplasty, the elbow is immediately mobilized in a supervised physical therapy regimen. A permanent weight restriction of 5 pounds is placed on the operative limb.

Technique 3: ORIF of Capitellum Fracture

Position of the incision depends on whether the capitellum fracture (Fig. 9.16) is an isolated injury or part of a more complex injury. For the latter a posterior incision is recommended. For isolated fractures, a 5–6 cm incision is placed obliquely across the lateral epicondyle beginning from the supracondylar ridge down to the radial neck.

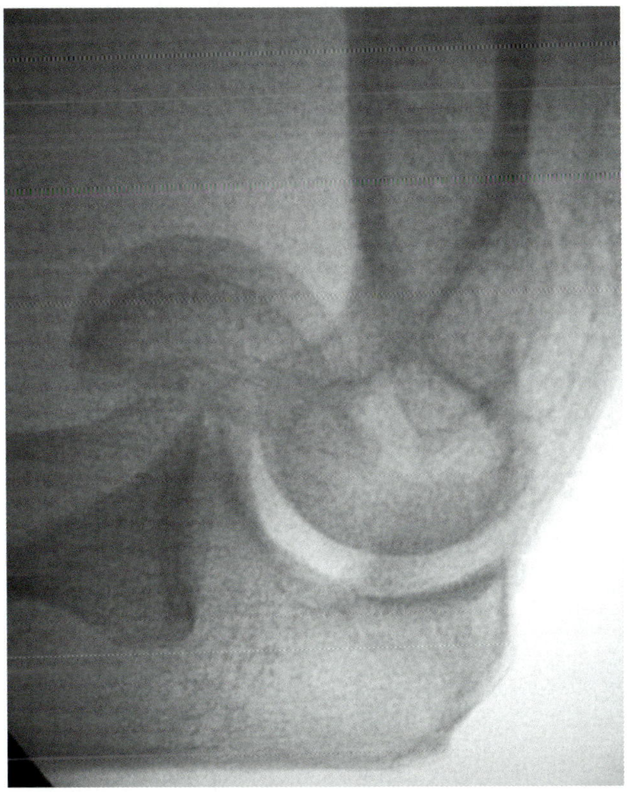

Figure 9.16: Preoperative lateral radiograph identifying an isolated displaced capitellar fracture.

Unless there is a large soft tissue or capsular defect, a lateral Kocher approach between the anconeus and extensor carpi ulnaris interval or Kaplan approach between the extensor carpi radialis brevis and extensor digitorum comminis may be developed. We recommend a direct lateral or EDC-splitting approach centered over the radio-capitellar joint (Fig. 9.11) To increase exposure, the common extensor origin is raised proximally off the lateral epicondyle and reflected anteriorly to expose the lateral elbow joint. Care must be taken to avoid damage to the radial nerve traveling between the brachialis and brachioradialis. Similarly, traction injury to the posterior interosseous nerve is protected by keeping the forearm pronated and avoiding placement of retractors anterior to the radial neck.

The lateral ligamentous complex may be avulsed from the distal aspect of the humerus with or without some aspect of the lateral epicondyle. This ligamentous violation may be exploited to improve exposure by hinging open the joint on the medial collateral ligament with varus stress. Alternatively, to increase exposure the lateral epicondyle may be osteotomized thereby taking down the lateral ulnar collateral ligament complex and the elbow hinged open on the medial collateral ligament with varus stress.

The capitellar fracture fragment is usually devoid of any soft tissue attachments and is typically displaced proximally and rotated (Fig. 9.17). The fragment is reduced under direct visualization and held with reduction tenaculums and provisionally fixed with 0.045 inch K-wires from an anterior-to posterior direction. Inability to anatomically reduce the fracture may represent fracture impaction and require either disimpaction and/or bone grafting.

Internal fixation options include fixation from posterior-to-anterior with cancellous screws or from either direction with headless compression screws (Figs 9.18A and B) Cancellous screws are best for fragments with a large subchondral component. Headless compression screws are best for fragments with less subchondral bone. Excision of fracture fragments may be considered in cases with small or thin articular pieces or extensive comminution that is not amenable to internal fixation.

Fragment reduction and hardware position should be confirmed by image intensifier. Unrestricted forearm rotation and elbow flexion-extension without mechanical block or catching should be confirmed intraoperatively.

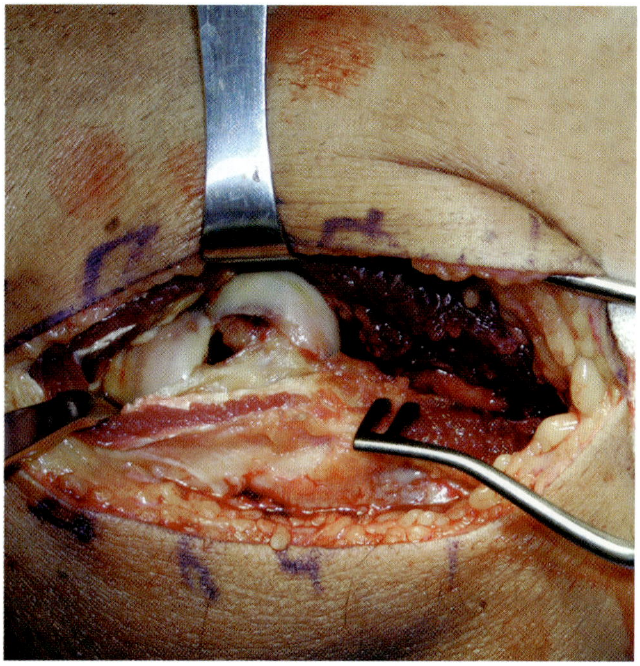

Figure 9.17: Lateral view of the radiocapitellar joint through an EDC-splitting approach. Note the capitellar fragment is displaced proximally and extruded out of the radiocapitellar joint.

If the lateral collateral ligament was found to be avulsed, it should be repaired back to the lateral epicondyle with drill holes and nonabsorbable suture or suture anchors. If the lateral epicondyle was osteotomized it should be replaced with plates and screws. The capsule, extensor origin and extensor origin are closed in layers.

ORIF OF CAPITELLUM FRACTURE:
Pearls and Pitfalls

- Lateral exposure can be enhanced by raising the common extensor origin off its origin along the lateral epicondyle and supracondylar ridge of the humerus
- Be wary of subchondral impaction of the capitellar fragment. Disimpaction and/or bone grafting may be required to obtain adequate reduction
- Prior to closing confirm that the lateral ulnar collateral ligament complex is intact and/or adequately repaired

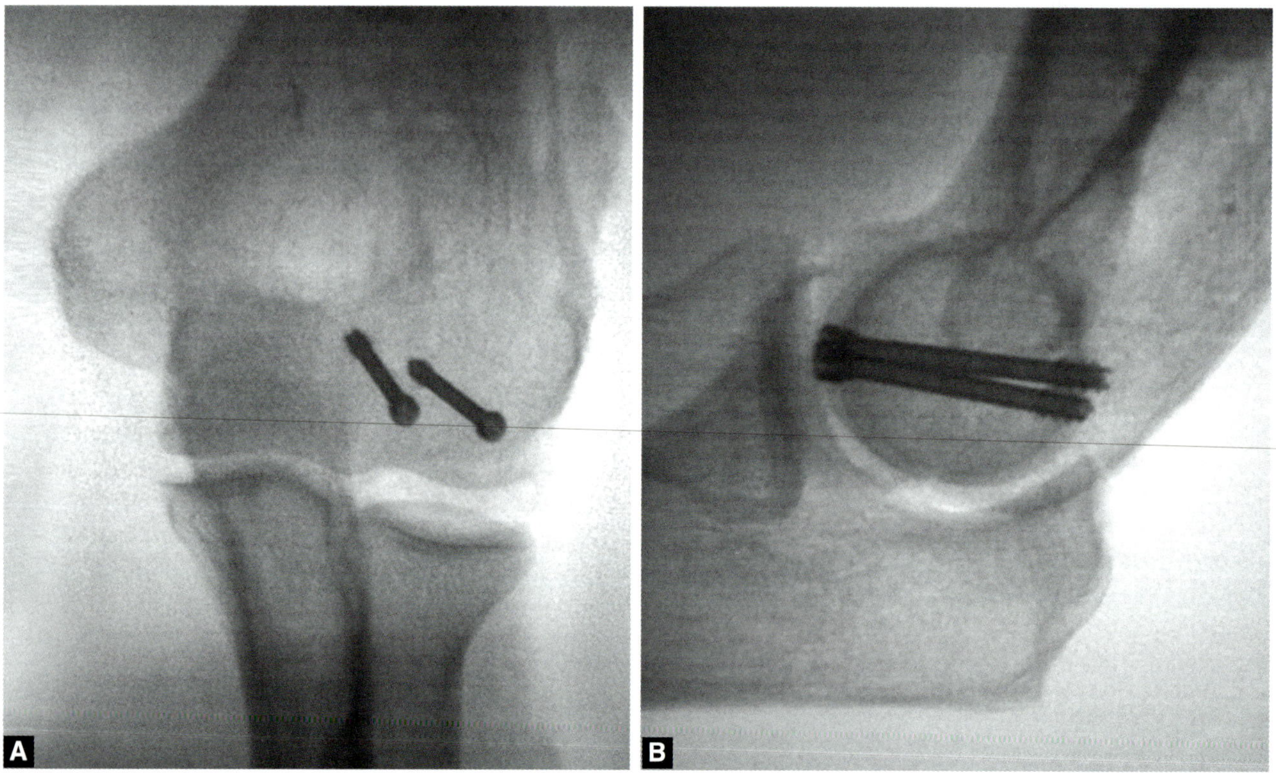

Figures 9.18A and B: (A) Anteroposterior and (B) lateral fluoroscopic images identifying a reduced capitellar fracture with headless compression screws placed in an anterior-to-posterior direction.

Outcomes

The goal of surgery for distal humerus fractures is to regain motion and strength of the elbow. Invariably, some stiffness will result in loss of terminal flexion and extension and patients should be warned of this preoperatively.[9-17] McKee et al. reported on a series of distal humerus fractures treated with ORIF at an average follow-up of 37 months and identified an average flexion contracture of 25° and an average arc of motion of 108°. They also identified an average 25% loss of strength.[14] A mean disability of the arm, shoulder and hand (DASH) score of 20 was also found indicating mild impairment. In a later report, similar results were reported by O'Driscoll et al. with 75% strength and a pain-free arc of motion of 105°.[15] Whereas both of these studies involved many cases involving olecranon osteotomies, Ek et al. more recently reported on nine patients treated with ORIF through a triceps sparing approach at a mean of 35 months with a mean arc of motion of 90° and DASH score of 17.9.[17] While most studies have employed 90–90 orthogonal plating, parallel plating methods of ORIF have also demonstrated similar.[9] Sanchez-Sotolo et al. achieved a 99° arc of motion and mostly good and excellent results. Thirty-one of thirty-two patients went on to union with five patients undergoing additional surgery for elbow stiffness.

Long-term results after ORIF of distal humeral fractures are similar to those in the short term, suggesting durable results. Doornberg reported on 30 patients at an average of 19 years after ORIF of intra-articular distal humeral fractures.[18] Twenty patients underwent olecranon osteotomies and all had fixation with plates, screws and Kirschner wires. The average arc of motion was 106°, DASH score was 7 points and average satisfaction score was 8.8 on a 0–10 point visual analog scale.

Although modern techniques of ORIF for complex intra-articular fractures of the distal humerus have yielded satisfactory results, difficulties with achieving fixation in comminuted low articular fractures in osteoporotic patients has led to the popularity of total elbow arthroplasty (TEA) as a treatment alternative. McKee et al. reported on a multicenter, randomized controlled trial in 2008 of 42 patients older than 65 years who sustained displaced, comminuted fractures of the distal humerus.[19] Treatment was either ORIF or primary semiconstrained TEA. Overall, TEA led to more predictable and improved 2-year outcomes compared with ORIF based on the Mayo Elbow Performance Score. The DASH scores were better in the short term, although not different at 2-year follow-up. Operative time was shorter in the TEA group and although reoperation rates were not statistically different, five patients randomized to the ORIF group actually had to be converted to TEA intraoperatively because the fracture could not be satisfactorily reconstructed.

Complications

Complications are common in the management of distal humerus fractures and include elbow stiffness, heterotopic ossification, nonunions, neuropathies and infections.

Post-traumatic Elbow Stiffness

Stiffness can arise from both intrinsic and extrinsic sources.[20] Intrinsic causes of stiffness include joint adhesions, synovitis, articular incongruity and intra-articular loose bodies. Extrinsic causes include capsular contractures and heterotopic ossification. Loss of some motion is expected after distal humerus fractures, particularly terminal extension. Post-traumatic elbow stiffness is best managed by avoidance and aggressive postoperative rehabilitation. During the early postoperative period motion should be instituted expeditiously and edema minimized. Early splinting in full extension should be considered as this position tensions the anterior capsule decreasing contracture formation, compresses posterior structures and relaxes the ulnar nerve.

Heterotopic Ossification

Heterotopic bone formation is common following elbow fractures, especially after distal humerus fractures treated surgically.[9-19] Susceptible patients include those with brain or spinal cord injury, severe trauma or open injuries and a history of prior heterotopic ossification. At-risk patients should receive radiation and/or medical prophylaxis. In cases where heterotopic bone is blocking elbow motion, surgical excision should be considered. Traditionally, confirmation of radiographic maturation of the heterotopic bone is done, typically by 12–18 months, prior to attempting excision.[21] However, the recurrence rate after early excision, such as 3–6 months postoperatively, combined with external beam radiation has been shown to be no higher than that for delayed excision and as such is becoming the favored approach.[22] Early excision also provides the advantage of minimizing capsular and ligamentous contracture, muscular atrophy and articular degeneration from restricted motion.

Nonunion

This is uncommon but a well-recognized complication of distal humerus fractures treated with ORIF. Risk factors include comminution, bone loss and inadequate fixation. Treatment options include revision ORIF with bone graft or total elbow arthroplasty in older low-demand patients with poor bone stock. Helfet et al. reported their series of 52 patients with delayed union or nonunion of the distal humerus that were treated with revision ORIF.[16] They achieved a 98% union rate after reoperation, utilizing autogenous bone graft in 88% of cases.

Ulnar Neuropathy

Ulnar neuropathy can occur from the initial injury, iatrogenically during surgery or secondarily from postoperative scarring. In situ release and/or subcutaneous transposition of the ulnar nerve at the time of surgery can reduce the risk of future neuropathy. Despite adequate release, with or without transposition, irritation and transient sensory changes have occurred in up to 50% of patients in some series.[10,14,15] McKee et al. found that neurolysis and transposition resulted in significant symptomatic relief and functional improvement for patients with postoperative ulnar neuropathy.[23] However, improvement in motor strength is often incomplete and may take several years.

Authors' Preferred Management of Select Complications

Case 1: Elbow Stiffness/Heterotopic Ossification

A 68-year-old male fell down a flight of stairs incurring an AO Type C3 distal humerus fracture of his dominant arm. The patient underwent primary total elbow arthroplasty (Fig. 9.19). The patient was initiated with early mobilization under the supervision of a therapist. By 1 month postoperatively, the patient demonstrated elbow

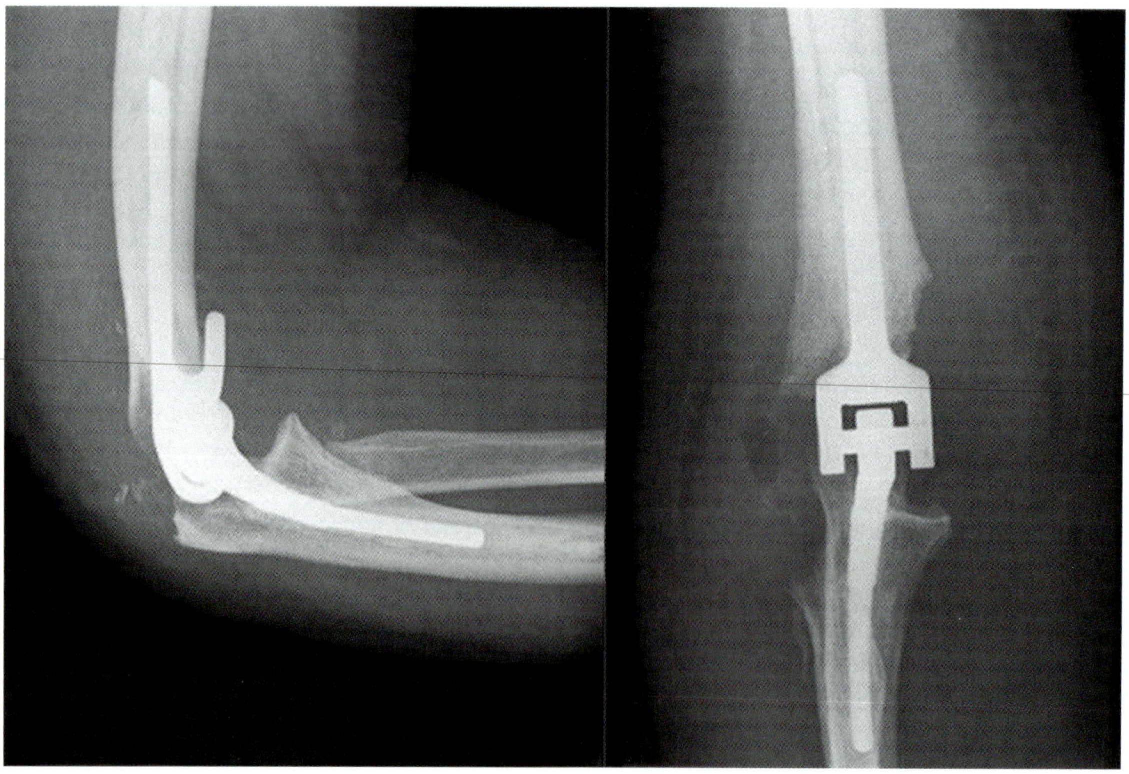

Figure 9.19: Radiographs demonstrating primary total elbow arthroplasty following a distal humerus fracture.

range of motion from 20° short of full extension to 120° of flexion, with full forearm supination and pronation. However, by the 6 month postoperative visit, the patient's range of motion had decreased to 45° short of full extension to 95° of flexion. In particular, the patient noted inability to bring food to his mouth and touch his head with his hands. Radiographs demonstrated the development of heterotopic bone (Fig. 9.20).

Elbow stiffness following a fracture of the distal humerus is common. The elbow is a highly congruent joint and is highly susceptible to developing stiffness. Risk factors for elbow stiffness are multifactorial and include joint arthrosis, malunion, nonunion, heterotopic bone formation and soft tissue contracture about the elbow joint. Moreover, even total elbow arthroplasty following distal humerus fracture fixation is not immune to the development of stiffness and heterotopic bone formation. Early mobilization can theoretically prevent stiffness by minimizing edema and limiting soft tissue contracture formation. However, heterotopic bone formation is associated with concomitant head trauma and extensive soft tissue trauma. Heterotopic bone may potentially be avoided with postoperative irradiation with 700 cGy and/or medical prophylaxis with nonsteroidal anti-inflammatory drugs.

If post-traumatic elbow stiffness and/or heterotopic bone formation occurs despite nonoperative efforts, such as early mobilization and static or dynamic splinting, surgical intervention can be considered. Surgical indication for release of post-traumatic elbow stiffness is highly individualized and can be entertained for any contracture of at least 30° once the fracture is healed. Surgical options include both arthroscopic, as well as open releases through a number of approaches. Our preference is to perform an elbow release using the previous posterior incision facilitating access to all aspects of the joint. The ulnar nerve is routinely identified, neurolysed and transposed anteriorly. In addition, assuming the fracture is healed, we recommend routine removal of the hardware to eliminate a nidus for infection and future scar formation.

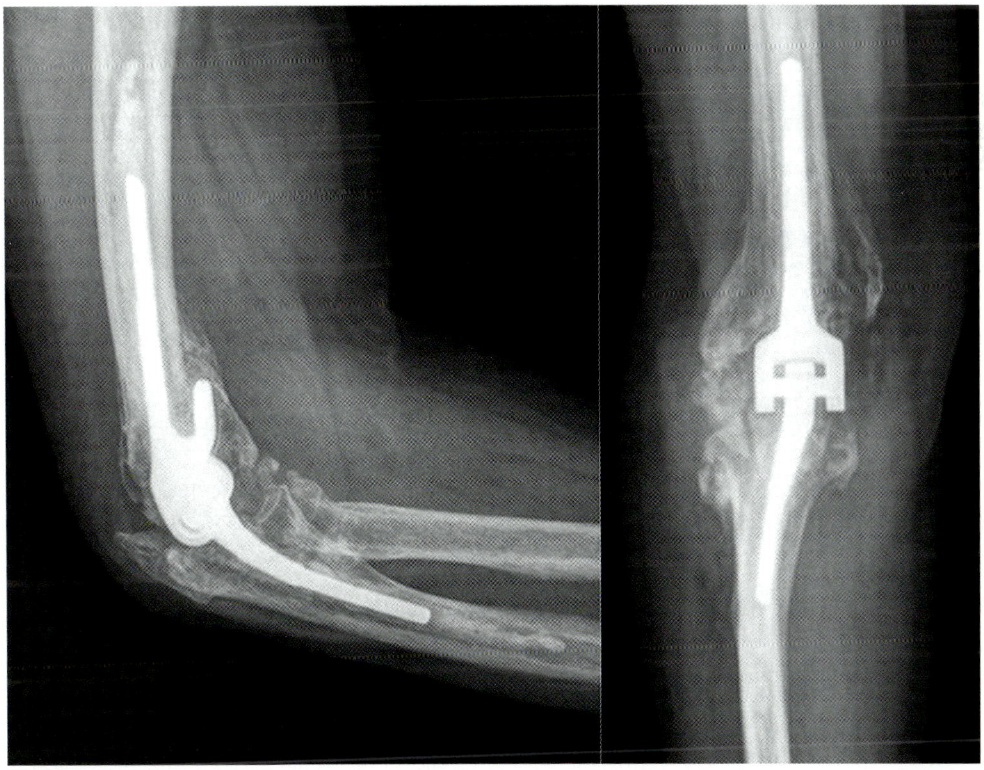

Figure 9.20: Radiographs taken 6 months postoperatively identifying heterotopic bone formation resulting in substantial loss of motion resulting in compromise in use of the arm and activities of daily living.

Technique

Following the development of full thickness medial and lateral flaps through the previous posterior incision, identification of the ulnar nerve and removal of hardware is first performed. Locating the ulnar nerve may be difficult and prior operative reports should be reviewed to determine whether the nerve was transposed or not. Once identified, it should be carefully freed from the surrounding scar tissue and diligently protected throughout the case. We recommend beginning the release on the lateral site. The supracondylar ridge is identified by raising the common extensor origin. The anterior capsule will then become evident. It should be carefully released off the anterior surface of the supracondylar humerus. Thereafter, the joint should be visualized, loose bodies removed, osteophytes debrided and the coronoid fossa cleared of debris and scar. Posterolaterally, the exposure will be limited by the lateral ulnar collateral ligament complex. The ligament complex may be managed by a number of options including sparing it, releasing it or osteotomy. We recommend sparing and protecting it whenever possible to avoid late posterolateral instability. However, either releasing or osteotomizing it off the lateral epicondyle with bone should be performed in order to achieve adequate exposure and a good release. Posteriorly, the lateral triceps is elevated off of the posterior aspect of the humerus and the anconeus off the ulna. With the elbow brought into extension, the posterior capsule is excised, the olecranon fossa is cleared of debris and scar, and the proximal ulna debrided of osteophytes. Along the medial side, with the ulnar nerve protected, dissection is initiated along the medial supracondylar ridge and taken distally to the flexor pronator mass origin. The origin may either be split and the anterior half dissected anteriorly or the entire origin may be elevated off the medial epicondyle. The medial collateral ligament complex deep to the flexor-pronator mass is identified and protected.

Resection of heterotopic bone is only necessary when it causes a mechanical block to motion. Heterotopic bone formation occurs most commonly anteriorly below the brachialis musculature but superficial to the joint capsule. The surgical approach for resection of heterotopic bone follows the same as outlined above. Central to successful resection is protection of neurovascular structures. In particular, the ulnar nerve and radial/posterior interosseous nerves are particularly susceptible to injury during resection, and must be identified and protected throughout the case. In contrast, the median nerve is protected by the brachialis muscle as it travels anterior to it. Resection should be limited to the sites causing the mechanical block. Heterotopic bone can readily be resected by identifying the interval between normal cortex and heterotopic bone. This interval is best developed with either an osteotome or rongeur. Heterotopic bone should be resected until the blocks to motion are eliminated (Fig. 9.21).

Following release, the elbow is immediately mobilized. If splinting is utilized for pain control or wound healing it is utilized very briefly and applied with the elbow in full extension. Postoperative continuous passive motion may also be utilized. On postoperative day 1, the elbow is irradiated with a single dose of 700 cGy to avoid recurrence of heterotopic bone formation.

Case 2: Ulnar Neuropathy

A 28-year-old male fell and incurred a displaced comminuted distal humerus fracture, consistent with an AO Type C3 classification. He had undergone ORIF through a posterior olecranon osteotomy with dual plate fixation. His fracture went on to heal uneventfully. However, he returned with complaints of numbness and weakness in his hands approximately 12 months after surgery. Physical examination identified advanced intrinsic atrophy of the hand (Fig. 9.22). An electrodiagnostic study identified marked slowing of motor and sensory conduction velocity of the ulnar nerve across the elbow with chronic denervation of the ulnar-innervated muscles of the hand and forearm.

Ulnar neuropathy following distal humerus fracture fixation is a recognized but an underappreciated phenomenon. It can result from the insult of the initial injury, intraoperative nerve management or later from scarring and compression. Symptoms can range from mild sensory paresthesias to advanced intrinsic atrophy of the hand. During surgery we recommend at minimum preliminary identification, in situ release, and protection of the nerve throughout the procedure. Final ulnar nerve placement following fracture fixation depends upon the nerve's new

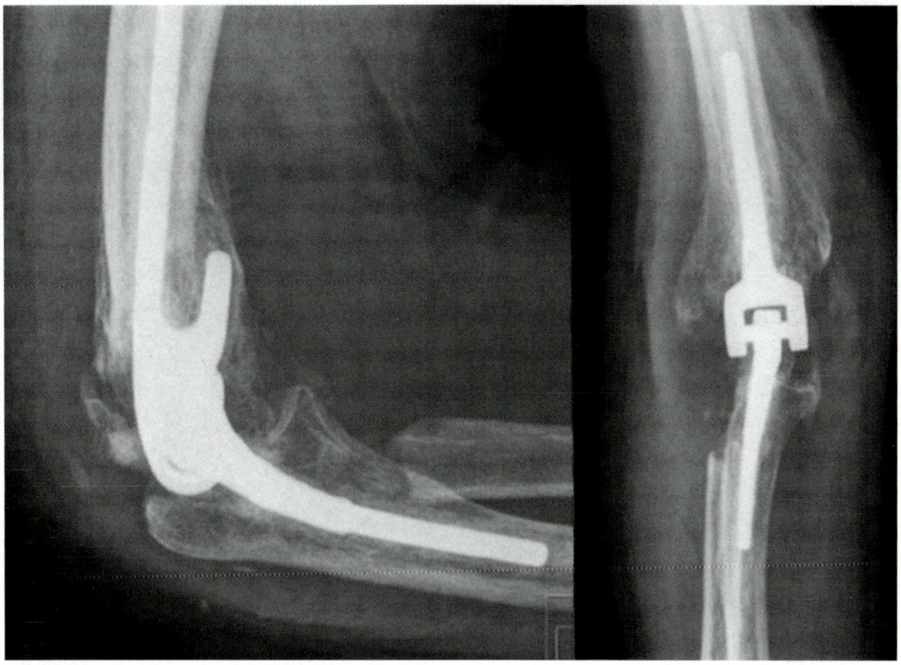

Figure 9.21: Radiographs taken following excision of heterotopic bone. Note the elimination of heterotopic bone in the medial and lateral gutters. Also note excision of the radial head which was performed to restore forearm rotation.

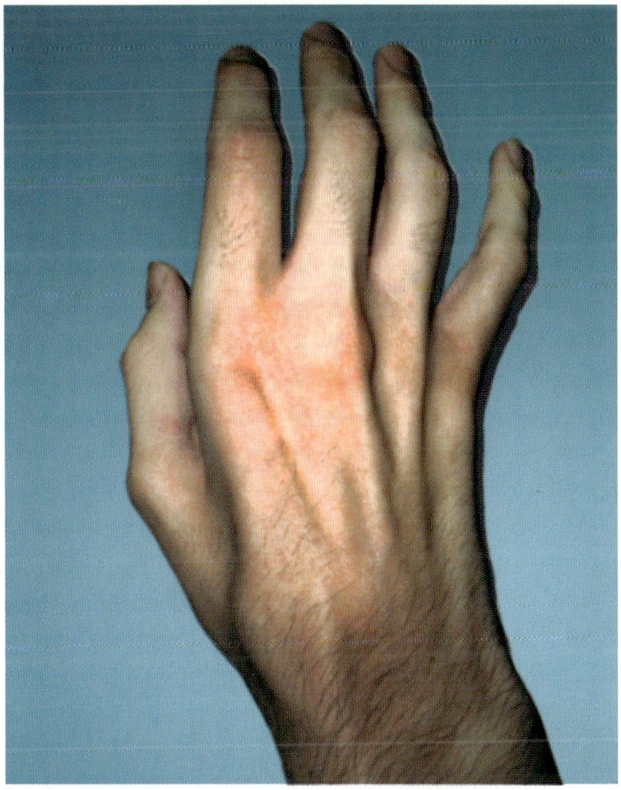

Figure 9.22: Intrinsic atrophy of the hand due to chronic ulnar neuropathy following ORIF of a distal humerus fracture.

local environment. We prefer maintaining the ulnar nerve within the cubital tunnel following fracture fixation whenever possible. However, if there is any tension and/or hardware present in the cubital tunnel we will perform a formal anterior subcutaneous transposition of the ulnar nerve. It is important to perform this diligently with the complete release of the nerve along its entire length using formal transposition techniques. The temptation to perform an anterior transposition of the ulnar nerve without releasing constricting structures, such as the arcade of Struthers or the intermuscular septum, may be high following a long difficult fracture procedure, but must be fought.

In this case with a late ulnar neuropathy, a formal surgical decompression of the nerve is warranted. Review of the previous operative report may provide clues as to the current location of the ulnar nerve. Our preference is to convert a previous in situ release or submuscular transposition to a formal anterior subcutaneous transposition. Similarly, a previous anterior subcutaneous transposition that is symptomatic is revised with diligent neurolysis and elimination of all potential offending structures (Fig. 9.23).

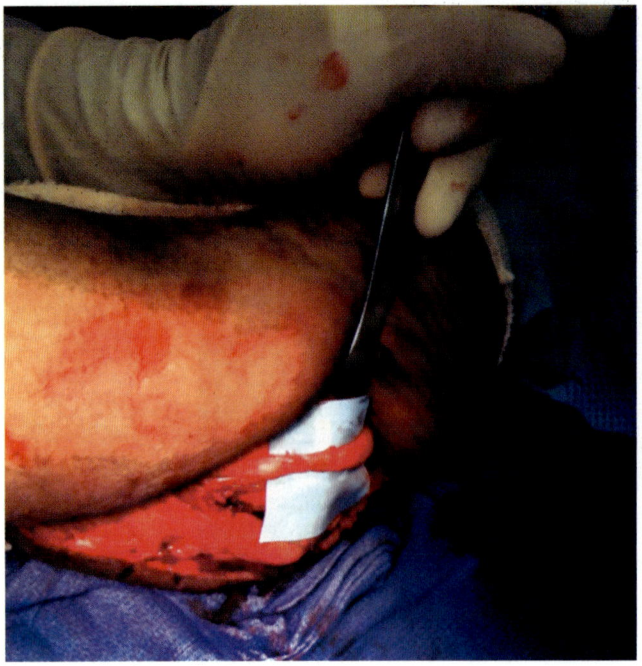

Figure 9.23: Intraoperative finding of compression and fibrosis of the ulnar nerve previously treated with in situ management following ORIF of a distal humerus fracture. The ulnar nerve was thoroughly decompressed and transposed anteriorly.

Technique

The same posterior incision should be utilized and large full thickness flap raised medially but with great care as the position of the ulnar nerve can be highly variable. Locating the ulnar nerve may be difficult and prior operative reports should be reviewed to determine whether the nerve was transposed or not. Once identified, the ulnar nerve is carefully dissected free from the surrounding tissue. A formal neurolysis is performed starting proximally at least 8 cm above the medial epicondyle where the ulnar nerve crosses the intermuscular septum posteriorly, across the arcade of Struthers and the fibers of the triceps muscle, through Osborne's ligament, and past the two heads of the flexor carpi ulnaris muscle. Vessels traveling with the nerve should be maintained whenever possible. The intermuscular septum is released sharply off the medial epicondyle and a 2 cm distal segment is excised to avoid a secondary compression. The ulnar nerve is then transposed anteriorly. A 1 cm fascial sling is formed from the flexor pronator mass with the pedicle based off the medial epicondyle and sewn carefully to the subcutaneous tissue to avoid late subluxation of the nerve. However, care must be taken not to place excessive tension and cause a secondary compression on the nerve. Our preference is to perform a subcutaneous transposition whenever possible but if the patient is thin, the flexor-pronator mass too bulky or if the nerve is placed under excessive tension with the elbow extended a submuscular transposition can be performed instead. Postoperatively, the patient is immediately mobilized without restriction.

Case 3: Nonunion

A 59-year-old male fell and incurred a displaced intra-articular distal humerus fracture, consistent with an AO Type C2 pattern, that was treated with an ORIF through a posterior approach and olecranon osteotomy utilizing nonlocked orthogonal plate fixation. The patient underwent early mobilization; however, he noted ongoing pain of his elbow and decreased range of motion. Radiographs taken approximately 6 months after surgery identified a hypertrophic nonunion in the supracondylar region of the distal humerus with failure of the hardware (Figs 9.24A and B).

Nonunions are an uncommon but well-recognized complication of distal humerus fractures. Risk factors include comminution, bone loss and inadequate fixation. Traditional plate fixation following distal humerus fractures includes orthogonal plate fixation with small fragment reconstructive plates contoured and applied to the posterior aspect of the lateral column and medially on the medial column. Bone stock, in particular cortical bone, is limited in the distal humerus. In addition, extensive articular cartilage surrounds the distal humerus. As such, plate fixation is often tenuous. The advent of locking technology has resulted in greater fixation options and stability of fracture fixation. The management of nonunions of the distal humerus follows the traditional principles of nonunion management including takedown of the nonunion, debridement to healthy bleeding bone, restoration of normal rotation and alignment, compression plating, and stable fixation (Figs 9.25A to E). Bone graft is applied based on surgeon preference and fracture needs. Graft options include iliac crest bone graft, allograft bone and synthetic bone substitutes.

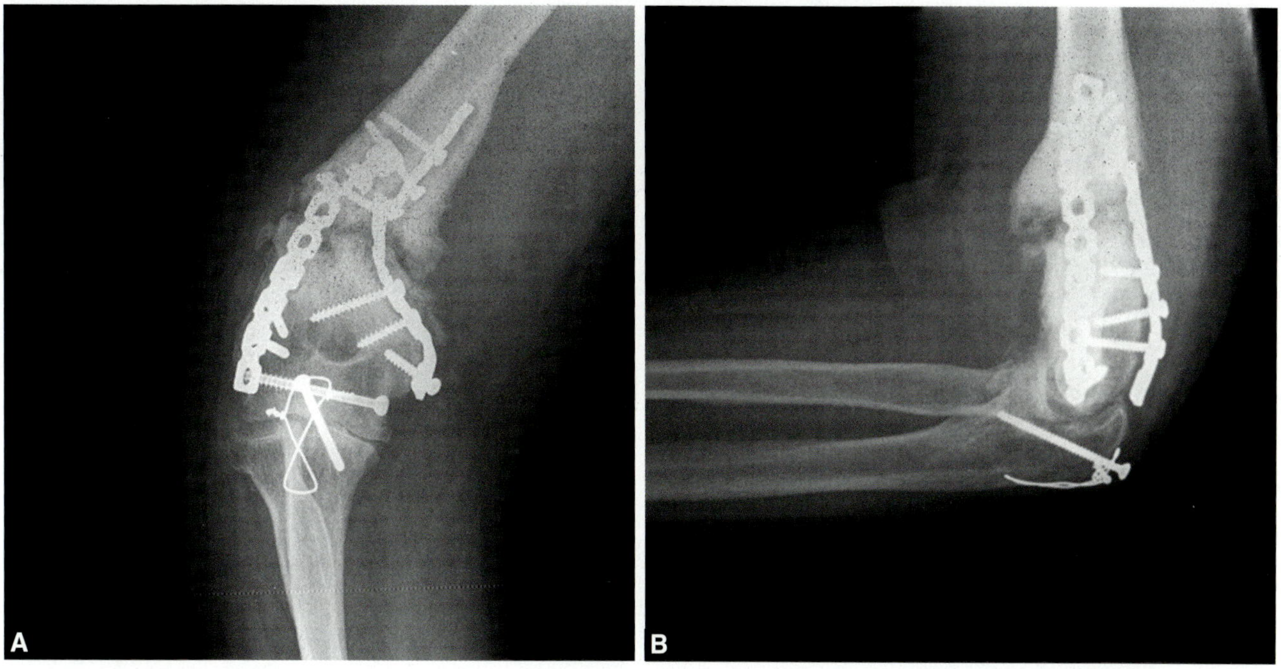

Figures 9.24A and B: (A) Anteroposterior and (B) Lateral radiographs demonstrating a distal humerus fracture treated by ORIF with orthogonal nonlocking plate fixation through an olecranon osteotomy that went on to a hypertrophic nonunion and fatigue failure of the hardware.

Technique

Following the development of full thickness medial and lateral flaps through the previous posterior incision, identification of the ulnar nerve and removal of hardware is first performed. Locating the ulnar nerve may be difficult and prior operative reports should be reviewed to determine whether the nerve was transposed or not. Once identified it should be carefully freed from the surrounding scar tissue and diligently protected throughout the case. An olecranon osteotomy is performed and the triceps musculature is retracted proximally. The nonunion site should be identified by gross inspection or with the assistance of fluoroscopy if necessary. The surrounding scar tissue and fibrous union is taken down to bleeding bone with the help of rongeurs and curettes. The fracture site is reconstituted and restored in a step fashion to facilitate alignment and maximize surface area for bony healing. Sagittal saws are avoided as they can result in secondary thermal necrosis of the bone which can compromise healing. The intramedullary canal above and below the fracture site is reconstituted with drills. The fracture site is rereduced and realigned to restore normal rotation and alignment of the distal humerus and provisionally fixed with K-wires along both the medial and lateral columns of the distal humerus. Locking pre-contoured plates are selected and applied. The plates are initially fixed with locking screws distally. In order to compress the fracture site, the proximal shaft screws are applied in a nonlocking fashion initially using standard compression technique. Adequate fixation consists of at least four screws both above and below the fracture site on each plate. If necessary, the fracture site can be back filled and reinforced with bone graft. Alternatively, shortening of the humeral shaft is well tolerated and can be performed during nonunion site debridement and subsequent compression during fixation. Our preference is to use utilize iliac crest bone graft draped out from the ipsilateral hip if necessary. Postoperatively, the elbow is placed in a hinged elbow brace and protected early range of motion is initiated.

Summary

Most fractures involving the distal part of the humerus in adults are treated surgically with the exception of minimally

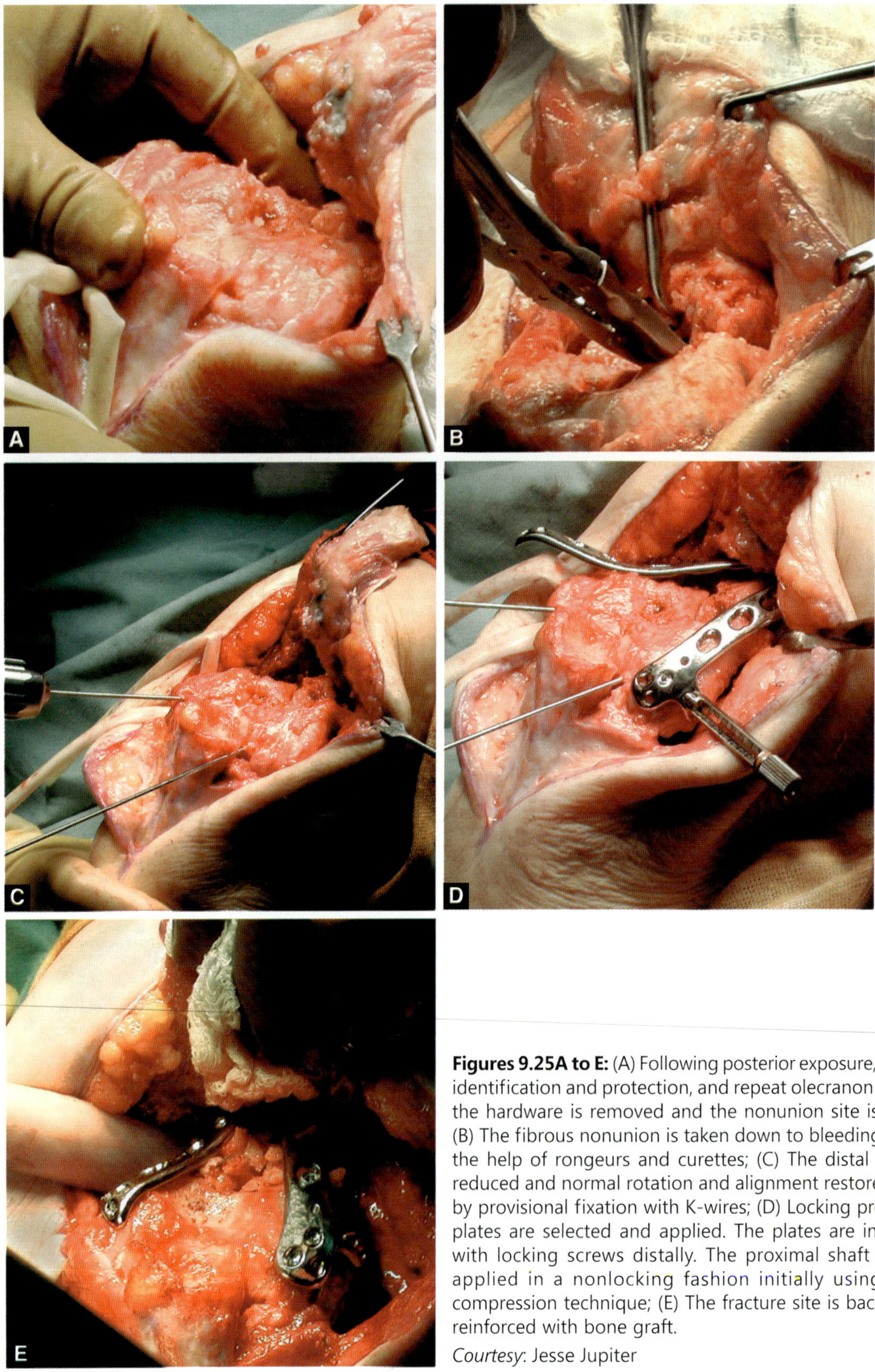

Figures 9.25A to E: (A) Following posterior exposure, ulnar nerve identification and protection, and repeat olecranon osteotomy, the hardware is removed and the nonunion site is identified; (B) The fibrous nonunion is taken down to bleeding bone with the help of rongeurs and curettes; (C) The distal humerus is reduced and normal rotation and alignment restored followed by provisional fixation with K-wires; (D) Locking precontoured plates are selected and applied. The plates are initially fixed with locking screws distally. The proximal shaft screws are applied in a nonlocking fashion initially using standard compression technique; (E) The fracture site is back filled and reinforced with bone graft.

Courtesy: Jesse Jupiter

or nondisplaced fractures. ORIF with either orthogonal plating or parallel plating techniques have resulted in generally satisfactory outcomes. Nevertheless, some loss of motion is to be expected, with even good results demonstrating no more than approximately a 100° arc of motion and about 75% of normal strength. Total elbow arthroplasty has been shown to be a viable option in elderly patients with comminuted distal humeral fractures in which fixation can be particularly difficult.

Complications are common after the surgical management of distal humerus fractures and include elbow stiffness, heterotopic ossification, and ulnar neuropathy. Although some of these complications can be avoided with attention to careful surgical technique and diligent postoperative rehabilitation, the surgeon should be prepared to deal with these problems should they arise.

References

1. Ali A, Douglas H, Stanley D. Revision surgery for nonunion after early failure of fixation of fractures of the distal humerus. J Bone Joint Surg Br. 2005;87(8):1107-10.
2. Court-Brown CM, Caesar B. Epidemiology of adult fractures: A review. Injury. 2006;37(8):691-7.
3. Palvanen M, Kannus P, Niemi S, et al. Secular trends in the osteoporotic fractures of the distal humerus in elderly women. Eur J Epidemiol. 1998;14(2):159-64.
4. Reich RS. Treatment of intercondylar fractures of the elbow by means of traction. J Bone Joint Surg. 1936;(18):997-1004.
5. Riseborough EJ, Radin EL. Intercondylar T fractures of the humerus in the adult. A comparison of operative and non-operative treatment in twenty-nine cases. J Bone Joint Surg Am. 1969;51(1):130-41.
6. Jupiter JB, Mehne DK. Fractures of the distal humerus. Orthopedics. 1992;15(7):825-33.
7. Muller M, Nazarian S, Koch P, et al. The Comprehensive Classification of Fractures of Long Bones. New York: Springer-Verlag; 1990.
8. Helfet DL, Hotchkiss RN. Internal fixation of the distal humerus: a biomechanical comparison of two methods. J Orthop Trauma. 1990;4:260-4.
9. Sanchez-Sotelo J, Torchia ME, O'Driscoll SW. Complex distal humeral fractures: internal fixation with a principle-based parallel plate technique. J Bone Joint Surg Am. 2007;89:961-9.
10. Gabel GT, Hanson G, Bennett JB, et al. Intraarticular fractures of the distal humerus in the adult. Clin Orthop Relat Res. 1987;(216):99-108.
11. Holdsworth BJ, Mossad MM. Fractures of the adult distal humerus. Elbow function after internal fixation. J Bone Joint Surg Br. 1990;72(3):362-5.
12. Henley MB, Bone LB, Parker B. Operative management of intraarticular fractures of the distal humerus. J Orthop Trauma.1987;1:24-35.
13. Helfet DL, Schmeling GJ. Bicondylar intraarticular fractures of the distal humerus in adults. Clin Orthop Relat Res. 1993;292:26-36.
14. McKee MD, Wilson TL, Winston L, et al. Functional outcome following surgical treatment of intra-articular distal humeral fractures through a posterior approach. J Bone Joint Surg Am. 2000;82-A(12):1701-7.
15. O'Driscoll SW, Sanchez-Sotelo J, Torchia ME. Management of the smashed distal humerus. Orthop Clin North Am. 2002;33(1):19-33.
16. Helfet DL, Kloen P, Anand N, et al. Open reduction and internal fixation of delayed unions and nonunions of fractures of the distal part of the humerus. J Bone Joint Surg Am. 2003;85-A(1):33-40.
17. Ek ETH, Goldwasser M, Bonomo AL. Functional outcome of complex intercondylar fractures of the distal humerus treated through a triceps-sparing approach. J Shoulder Elbow Surg. 2008 17(3):441-6.
18. Doornberg JN, van Duijn PJ, Linzel D, et al. Surgical treatment of intra-articular fractures of the distal part of the humerus. J Bone Joint Surg Am. 2007;89:1524-32.
19. McKee MD, Veillette CJH, Hall JA, et al. A multicenter, prospective, randomized, controlled trial of open reduction-internal fixation versus total elbow arthroplasty for displaced intra-articular distal humeral fractures in elderly patients. J Shoulder Elbow Surg. 2009;18(1):3-12.
20. Morrey B. The Elbow and its disorders, 2nd ed. Philadelphia: WB Saunders; 1993. O'Driscoll SW, Jupiter JB, Cohen MS (Eds). Difficult elbow fractures: Pearls and pitfalls. Instr Course Lect. 2003;52:113-34.
21. Jupiter JB. Heterotopic ossification about the elbow. Instr Course Lect. 1991;40:41-4.
22. McAuliffe JA, Wolfson AH. Early excision of heterotopic ossification about the elbow followed by radiation therapy. J Bone Joint Surg Am. 1997;79(5):749-55.
23. McKee MD, Jupiter JB, Bosse G, et al. Outcome of ulnar neurolysis during post-traumatic reconstruction of the elbow. J Bone Joint Surg Br. 1998;80(1):100-5.

Chapter 10

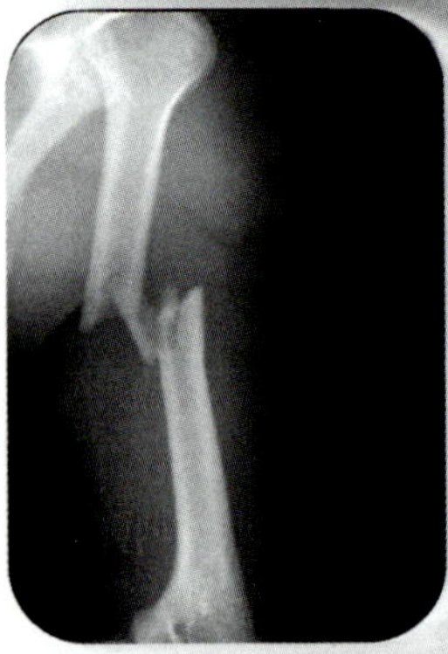

Humeral Shaft Fractures

Richard Tosti, Asif Ilyas

Chapter Outline

Introduction
Diagnosis
Classification
Surgical Indications
- Open Reduction and Internal Fixation
- Intramedullary Nailing

Surgical Anatomy, Positioning and Approaches
- Applied Anatomy
- Positioning
- Approaches

Surgical Techniques
- Technique 1: Open Reduction and Internal Fixation
- Technique 2: Intramedullary Nailing

Outcomes
- Open Reduction and Internal Fixation
- Intramedullary Nailing
- Plates Versus Nails
- Antegrade Versus Retrograde Nails

Complications
- Radial Nerve Injury
- Insertion Site Morbidity
- Nonunion
- Iatrogenic Fracture Extension

Authors' Preferred Management of Select Complications
- Case 1: Radial Nerve Injury
- Case 2: Humerus Nonunion

Summary

Introduction

A humeral shaft fracture is defined as a mechanical failure of bone between the superior border of the pectoralis major insertion and the supracondylar ridge (Fig. 10.1). Humeral shaft fractures comprise 20% of fractures of the humerus and are reported to affect an overall 14.5 per 100,000 people per year.[1,2] Epidemiologic studies report a bimodal distribution with respect to age, with a minor peak occurring in the third decade of life and the major peak in the seventh to eighth decade (Fig. 10.1).[2,3] However, a higher proportion of humeral shaft fractures are observed in young patients in areas where high-energy injuries are more prevalent.[4] Tytherleigh-Strong et al. and Ekholm et al. noted prominent high-energy injuries or sports-related injuries among young males, while falls from standing height are foremost in the elderly. Open fractures may account for 2–6% of cases.[2,3] Pathologic fractures of the humerus have a reported overall incidence of 6.0–8.5%, and metastases from breast or prostate cancer are the most common (Fig. 10.2).[2,3,5] As with any fracture, the goal of treatment is

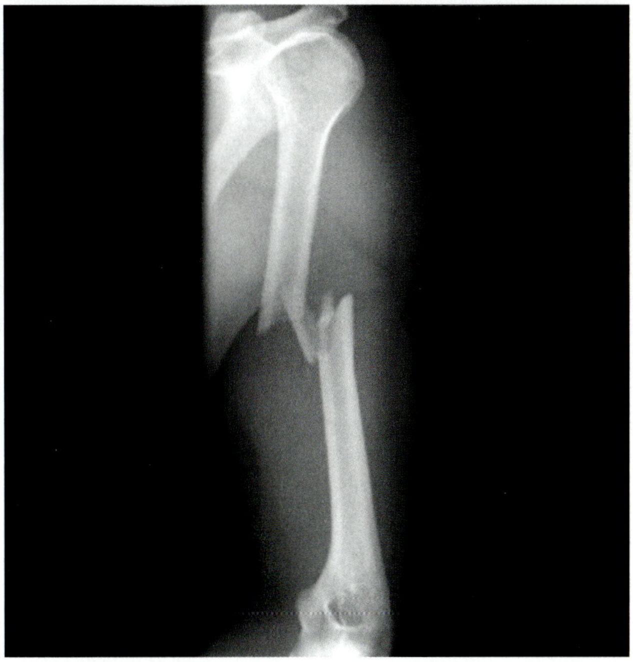

Figure 10.1: Anteroposterior radiographic view of a mid-shaft humerus fracture.

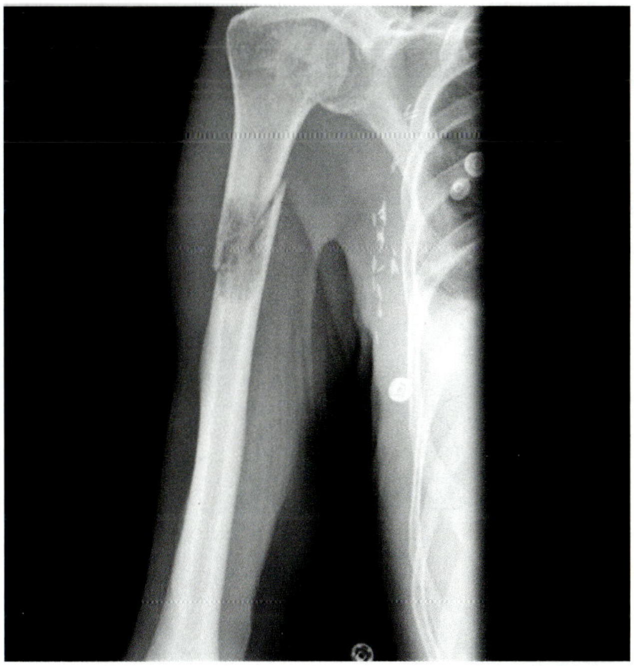

Figure 10.2: Anteroposterior radiographic view of pathologic humeral shaft fracture from metastatic prostate cancer. Note the 'moth-eaten' appearance of the lesion with cortical thinning.

restoration to pre-injury functional status. The humeral shaft is unique in that this goal can often be achieved with nonoperative management. Even in the presence of a malunion, a broad range of motion at the shoulder and elbow can overcome excessive fracture angulation.[6-8]

Diagnosis

The humerus is covered with a dense soft tissue envelope that often conceals its deformity following an injury. Similarly, the intimate association of this soft tissue envelope, including its associated neurovascular anatomy, makes fractures of the humerus prone to associated neurovascular injury. Evaluation should begin with a detailed history. Examination findings of a humeral shaft fracture are similar to most long bone fractures and include pain, deformity, swelling and guarding. The mechanism of injury is usually falling or twisting onto an outstretched hand or direct blunt or penetrating trauma. A thorough inspection should proceed noting any deformities, ecchymoses, wounds, lacerations or gross bleeding. Open fractures typically result from high-energy injuries but can also occur from low-energy trauma.[2,3] Palpation of the limb may reveal crepitus, tenderness or loss of sensation. Inspection, palpation and range of motion testing should be performed gently at the shoulder and elbow to evaluate associated injuries. Suspicion for abuse or a pathologic fracture should arise, if the mechanism of injury does not correlate with the fracture pattern. The humeral shaft is a common site of injury in domestic abuse and the most commonly involved upper extremity bone in metastatic disease.[5]

A thorough neurovascular examination is necessary with particular emphasis on the radial nerve and the profunda brachii vessels, which are particularly susceptible to injury following humeral shaft fractures. The radial nerve is a continuation of the posterior cord of the brachial plexus and courses with the profunda brachii as it bifurcates high in the posteromedial arm. Both structures pass through the posterior compartment of the arm and run distally between the medial and lateral heads of the triceps. After innervating the triceps, the radial nerve travels through the radial groove, turns anteriorly and pierces the lateral intermuscular septum just below the deltoid insertion (Fig. 10.3). At this point, the radial nerve and profunda brachii are at the highest risk of entrapment and tethering,

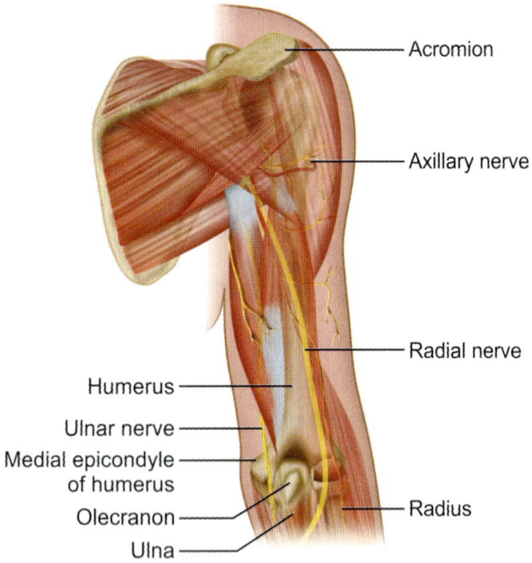

Figure 10.3: Note the path of the radial nerve as it traverses around the humerus. It bifurcates high in the posteromedial arm off of the posterior cord of the brachial plexus. It passes through the posterior compartment of the arm running between the medial and lateral heads of the triceps before contacting the posterior humerus through the spiral groove and then crossing into the anterior compartment of the arm by piercing the lateral intermuscular septum. Thereafter, it travels between the brachialis and biceps brachii before entering the forearm between the brachioradialis and brachialis.

either traumatically or iatrogenically (Figs 10.4A and B). Evaluation of the radial nerve should focus on wrist extension strength and sensation to the first dorsal web space of the hand. Finger extension can be used to assess radial nerve function, but must be carefully scrutinized as cursory examination may yield a false negative, as the intrinsic muscles of the hand will extend the interphalangeal joints of the hand, which can be misinterpreted as normal finger extension. If a detailed neurologic examination is not possible, as in the case of an unresponsive or intubated patient, inability to obtain this information should be clearly documented. Likewise, if a reduction is attempted, neurologic function should be documented prior to manipulation. Distal vascular examination can be performed by direct palpation, capillary refill and Doppler examination. The presence of poor distal pulses, hemodynamic instability and associated fractures of the clavicle and scapula warrant consideration of possible scapulothoracic dissociation.

Radiographic evaluation should begin with anteroposterior and lateral views at orthogonal angles. Each view should include the shoulder and elbow joints. The orthogonal views should be taken by rotating the patient and not the arm to avoid rotation at the fracture site (Figs 10.5A and B). If X-ray is not available, ultrasound can be a viable alternative. CT scan, MRI and bone scans are

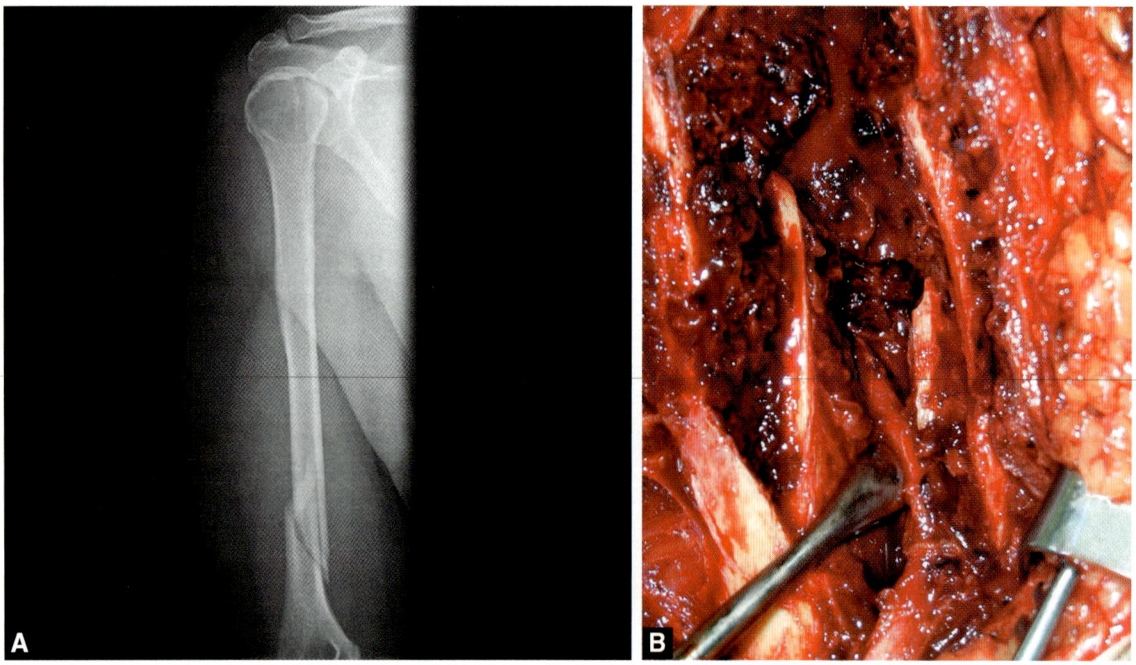

Figures 10.4A and B: (A) Anteroposterior radiographic view demonstrating a long spiral fracture at the junction of the middle and distal third of the humeral shaft. These fracture patterns are most prone to radial nerve injury and have been commonly referred to as Holstein-Lewis fractures; (B) Intraoperative image of the same patient, who had a preoperative radial nerve palsy, treated with plate osteosynthesis. Note how the radial nerve, identified by the cob, has subluxed between the fracture fragments.

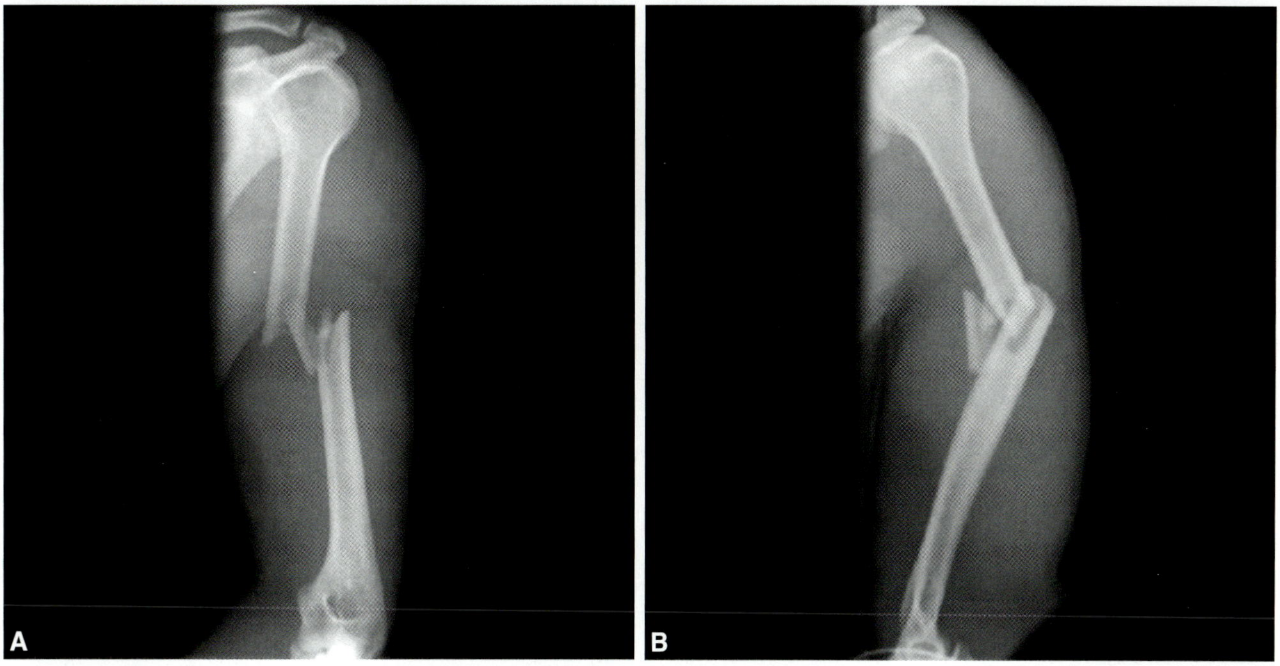

Figures 10.5A and B: (A) Anteroposterior and (B) lateral radiographs of a midshaft humerus fracture. Note that the images were taken by rotating the arm and not by preferably rotating the patient or the imaging equipment. As such, the distal fragment has rotated 90° relative to the proximal fragment.

seldom indicated; however, they may be useful in preoperative planning of pathologic fractures. CT scan may also be useful if intra-articular extension is suspected.

HUMERAL SHAFT FRACTURES DIAGNOSIS:
Pearls and Pitfalls

- Mechanism of injury and fracture pattern mismatch may herald abuse or pathologic fracture
- Neurologic examination, particularly of the radial nerve, should be performed in all patients and clearly documented. If nerve function cannot be determined due to the patient's medical status, this fact should also be documented
- Radial nerve function is best assessed by active wrist extension or finger extension at the metacarpophalangeal joint
- Carefully examine for associated injuries including intra-articular extension and injuries to the shoulder above and elbow below
- In high-energy polytraumatized patients with hemodynamic instability the shoulder girdle should be scrutinized for possible scapulothoracic dissociation

Classification

No single fracture pattern is used universally in classification of humeral shaft fractures. However, the AO comprehensive classification of fractures remains a well-accepted classification system and is also most useful in clinical research[9] (Fig. 10.6). Humeral shaft fractures are designated as number 12 and are subsequently classified into Types A, B and C. Type A fractures represent a simple fracture pattern; Type B a wedge fracture; and Type C is a complex fracture. The fractures are further subdivided by fracture orientation. For simple Type A fractures, group 1 are spiral patterns; group 2 are oblique patterns; and group 3 are transverse patterns. For Type B wedge fractures, group 1 are spiral wedge; group 2 are bending wedge; and group 3 are fragmented wedge. For Type C complex fractures, group 1 are spiral; group 2 are segmental; and group 3 are irregular. The AO/ASIF classification system is then further subdivided by segment within the shaft, i.e. proximal zone, middle zone, and distal zone.

Open fractures are not uncommon among humeral shaft fractures and are most often classified by the Gustilo-Anderson classification.[10] Type I fractures are low-energy injuries with an open wound less than 1 cm. Type II fractures

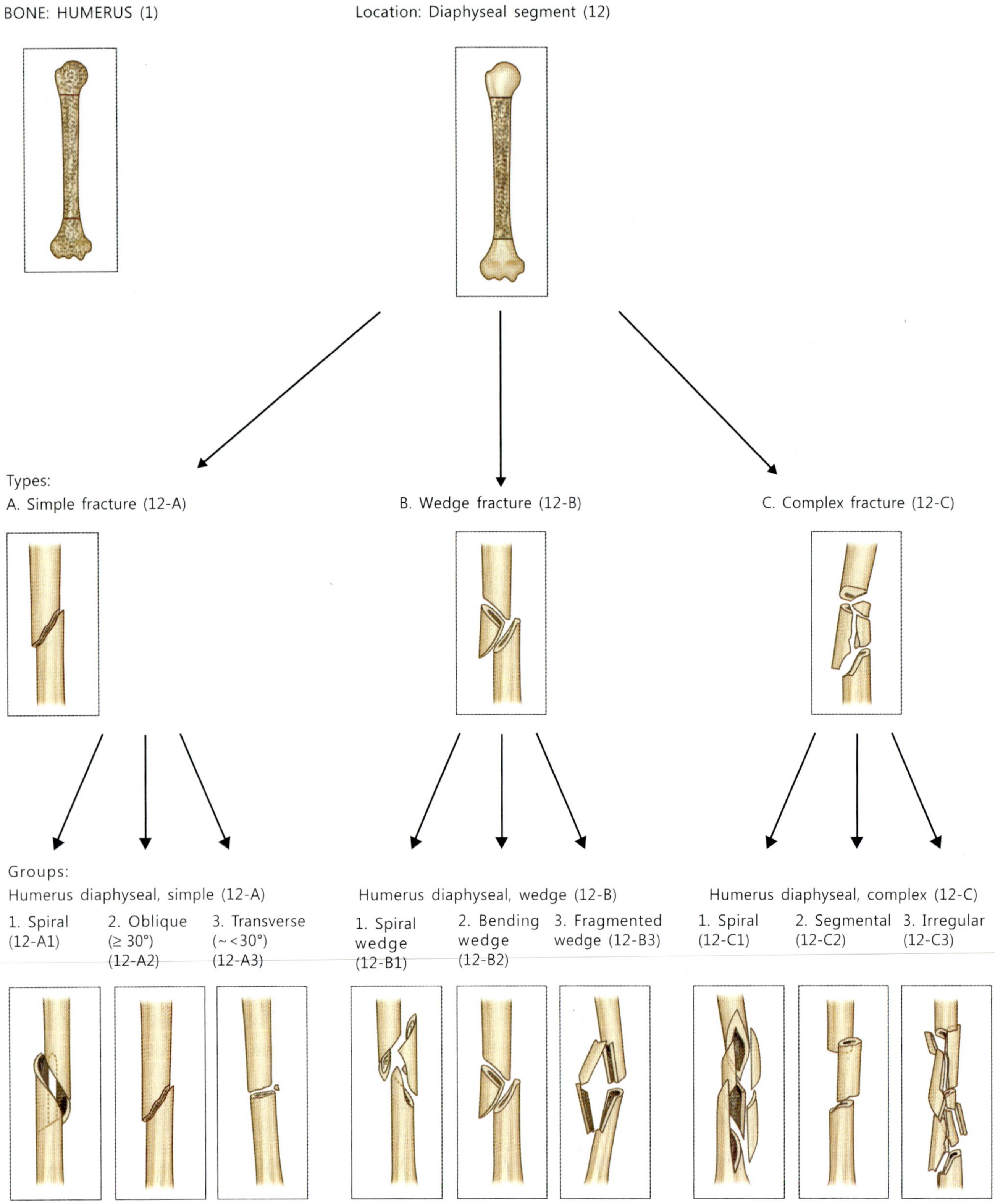

Figures 10.6: The AO classification designates humeral shaft fractures as number 12, with further fracture subclassification depicted above.

are low-energy injuries with an open wound greater than 1 cm, but no extensive soft tissue damage. Type III injuries are high-energy or contaminated injuries subdivided into three groups. Group IIIA is a high-energy, high comminution injury with extensive soft tissue damage, but the soft tissue is adequate for closure. Group IIIB is a high-energy injury in which the soft tissue is inadequate for closure and necessitates either local or free flaps for closure. Group IIIC is any open fracture associated with a vascular injury that requires repair regardless of the degree of soft tissue injury.

Surgical Indications

Fractures of the humeral shaft are largely managed nonoperatively, as high rates of union have been achieved with functional bracing, hanging arm casts and coaptation splints.[6-8] Generally, a coaptation splint is applied for 1 week until the swelling subsides, and then the splint is exchanged for a compressive fracture brace. Using this method, Sarmiento noted a union rate greater than 98%.[8] Nonoperative management is successful, largely as a result of the rich blood supply and stout soft tissue envelope surrounding the humeral shaft. Although perfect reduction is seldom achieved with closed methods, the extensive range of motion at the shoulder and elbow can generally accommodate up to 20° of anterior angulation, 30° of varus angulation, 30° of malrotation and 3 cm of shortening.[6]

Surgical indications for humeral shaft fractures can be broken down into fracture criteria, associated injuries and patient variables (Table 10.1). In terms of radiographic alignment, fracture alignment outside of 20° anterior angulation, 30° varus angulation, 30° malrotation and 3 cm of shortening can be indicated to surgical reduction and fixation of the humerus. Additional surgical indications include a segmental fracture of the humerus, intra-articular extension, and pathologic fractures. The presence of associated injuries such as open wounds, neurovascular compromise, forearm fractures (a floating elbow), shoulder girdle fractures (a floating shoulder), or patients requiring immediate upper extremity weight bearing (e.g. polytrauma or paraplegia) would also be indicated. Patient factors indicating surgical fixation include morbid obesity, Parkinsonism, and inability to tolerate nonoperative treatment.

Table 10.1: Surgical indications for humeral shaft fractures

Fracture Criteria
- Radiographic malalignment
  - >20° anterior angulation
  - >30° varus angulation
  - >30° malrotation
  - >3 cm of shortening
- Segmental fracture
- Intra-articular fracture
- Pathologic fracture

Associated Injuries
- Open wounds
- Neurovascular compromise
- Forearm fracture (floating elbow)
- Shoulder girdle fracture (floating shoulder)
- Polytrauma

Patient Variables
- Requirement for upper extremity weight bearing
- Morbid obesity
- Parkinsonism
- Inability to tolerate nonoperative management

Generally, techniques for operative fixation fall into two categories: open reduction internal fixation (ORIF) versus intramedullary (IM) nailing. External fixation is also a treatment option but typically reserved for complex fractures associated with soft tissue and neurovascular injuries.[11]

Open Reduction and Internal Fixation

Open reduction and internal fixation with plate osteosynthesis is the most popular method of fixation; as the rates of union are high, immediate mobilization and weight bearing are possible and the complication profile is acceptable (Fig. 10.7).[12-16] An ORIF is indicated for any of the above surgical indications and especially for patients with contraindications to IM nails, such as pre-existing shoulder pathology, open growth plates, small medullary canals and a requirement for immediate upper extremity weight bearing.

Intramedullary Nailing

Intramedullary nailing is considered a ready alternative to ORIF and may be particularly indicated in cases with

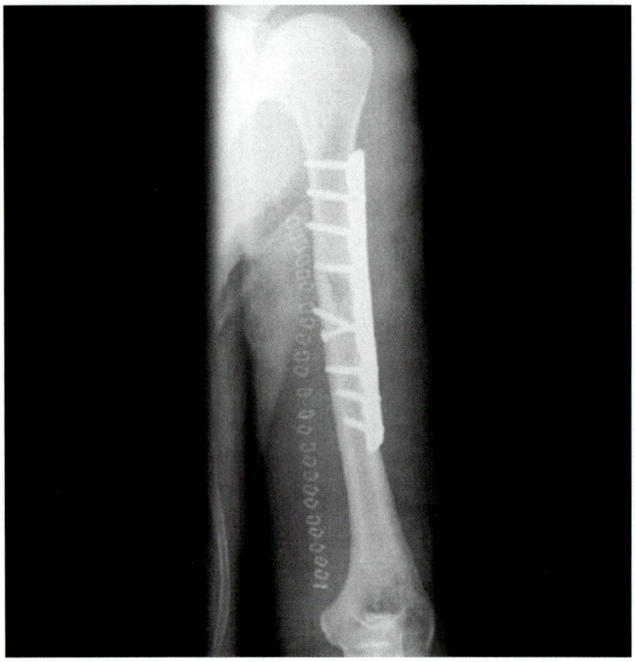

Figure 10.7: Open reduction internal fixation with plate osteosynthesis of a mid-shaft humerus fracture.

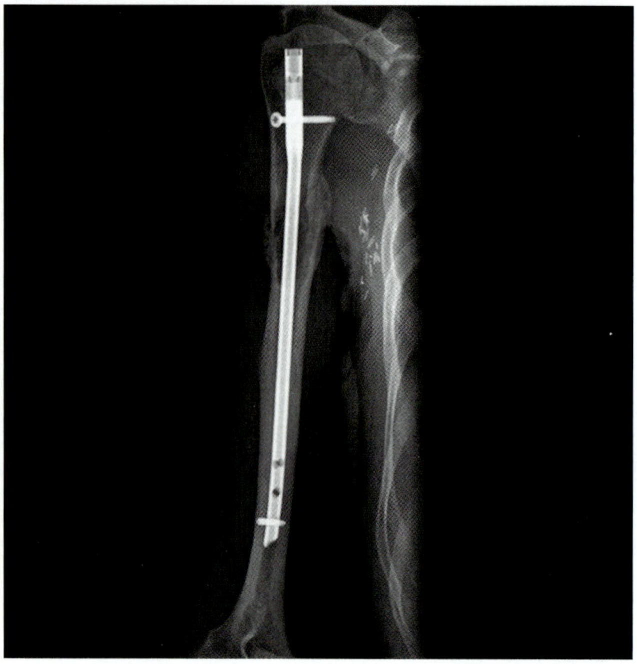

Figure 10.8: Intramedullary nailing of a pathologic humerus fracture.

segmental fractures, pathologic fractures and fractures with associated skin compromise; such as with burns or abrasions (Fig. 10.8). Advantages include limited dissection, ease of insertion and potentially shorter operative time. Intramedullary nailing can be performed antegrade or retrograde. Antegrade nailing is usually performed with reamed or nonreamed static locked nails and are best indicated for fractures of the proximal or middle third of the humeral shaft. The most common complication associated with antegrade IM nailing is shoulder pain, which is assumed to be secondary to rotator cuff injury during nail insertion and/or later nail irritation.[17] Retrograde IM nailing is best indicated for fractures of the distal third of the humeral shaft. Fractures of the middle third are also amenable to retrograde nailing and could avoid the potential for shoulder pain. However, risk of supracondylar fracture, elbow pain, heterotopic ossification and triceps weakness has been identified with retrograde IM nailing.[17]

Surgical Anatomy, Positioning and Approaches

Applied Anatomy

Prior to surgical exposure of the humerus a proficient knowledge of the anatomy of the brachium is an essential prerequisite, as neurovascular structures cross the anterior and posterior compartments intimately about the humerus. The skin is innervated by spinal nerve roots C5–T2. Although some dermatomal overlap exists, the proximal lateral half is innervated by the axillary nerve and the distal lateral half is innervated by terminal branches of the radial nerve, i.e. the distal lateral brachial cutaneous nerve and the posterior brachial cutaneous nerve of the arm. Proximal medial sensation is provided by the intercostobrachial nerve, which is a branch of the second intercostal nerve from the ventral ramus of T2. The distal medial arm is supplied by the medial cutaneous nerve of the arm, which is a direct branch of the medial cord of the brachial plexus. Two major superficial veins course in the anterior brachium are:

1. The cephalic vein ascends the lateral arm from the cubital fossa to the deltopectoral groove where it joins the axillary vein.
2. The basilic vein ascends from the medial cubital fossa and pierces the fascia in the distal medial arm and joins the brachial vein at the mid-brachium.

In the coronal plane, the arm is separated into anterior and posterior compartments by the medial and lateral intermuscular septum. The anterior compartment contains the major arm and minor shoulder flexors: biceps brachii, brachialis and coracobrachialis. The posterior compartment is chiefly occupied by the triceps muscle. The muscles of the anterior compartment are innervated by the musculocutaneous nerve, while the posterior compartment is innervated by the radial nerve. Both compartments are perfused by branches and collaterals of the brachial artery and the profunda brachii (also known as the deep brachial artery or deep artery of the arm).

Safe surgical dissection is predicated upon navigating the neurovascular structures of the brachium. The radial nerve is the most commonly injured nerve associated with humeral shaft fractures secondary to its close proximity to the bone as it travels through the spiral (radial) groove and tethering at the lateral intermuscular septum. The radial nerve is a continuation of the posterior cord of the brachial plexus, which courses with the profunda brachii as it bifurcates high in the posteromedial arm. The structures then pass through the triangular interval entering the posterior compartment of the arm and running distally between the medial and lateral heads of the triceps. After giving branches to the triceps, the radial nerve travels through the spiral (radial) groove, turns anteriorly, and pierces the lateral intermuscular septum just below the deltoid insertion. As mentioned previously, these are the most common sites of entrapment or laceration. Distally, the nerve will emerge between the brachialis and brachioradialis before bifurcating into the superficial radial nerve and the (deep) posterior interosseous nerve at the leading edge of the supinator.

The ulnar nerve courses along the medial side of the brachial artery in the anterior compartment until the mid-brachium where it pierces the medial intermuscular septum, passes through the arcade of Struthers and enters the posterior compartment. At the lower border of the axilla, behind the pectoralis minor and the insertion of the latissimus dorsi, the axillary artery becomes the brachial artery. Also at this point, the median nerve originates from the brachial plexus and both structures continue in tandem along the length of the anteromedial brachium. The medial antebrachial cutaneous nerve traverses closely with this bundle as well. The musculocutaneous nerve, the terminal branch of the lateral cord of the brachial plexus, pierces the coracobrachialis and continues between the brachialis and biceps brachii until it emerges distally from the lateral border of the biceps becoming the lateral antebrachial cutaneous nerve.

In summary, three of the five terminal nerves of the brachial plexus will remain in their respective compartments of origin; however, in the mid-brachium, the radial nerve crosses from posterior to anterior, while the ulnar nerve crosses from anterior to posterior relative to their respective intermuscular septums.

Muscular attachments in the upper arm are many and result in significant deforming forces in humeral shaft fractures. The pectoralis major insertion is superior and medial to that of the deltoid. In fractures above this level, fragments behave like two-part Neer fractures in that the humeral head will assume an externally rotated, abducted position via a pull from the rotator cuff, while the shaft displaces medially and proximally from the pectoralis major. Fractures between the deltoid and pectoralis insertion will assume a nearly opposite configuration, as the proximal fragment displaces medially from the pectoralis major and the distal fragment displaces laterally from the deltoid. Fractures distal to the deltoid tuberosity will produce an abducted proximal fragment and a medially displaced distal fragment.

Positioning

The choice of positioning is directed by the choice of approach and technique. For an anterior or anterolateral approach, a supine position with a hand table is preferred, as the arm is readily abducted at least 60° for exposure (Fig. 10.9). Generally, the surgeon will face the lateral arm, and the assistant is seated opposite. To enhance exposure, a small bump may be placed under the scapula. A sterile tourniquet is preferred if necessary, as a non-sterile tourniquet will limit the surgical field. For posterior or lateral approaches, a lateral decubitus position or a prone position are both acceptable. These positions are also appropriate for retrograde IM nailing (Fig. 10.10). In the lateral decubitus position, the patient's affected arm is placed over a padded draped Mayo or arm holder, while the patient's body is supported with a sandbag or Stulberg positioners. For antegrade IM nailing, the supine position, as described above, or a beach chair setup may be chosen (Fig. 10.11).

Approaches

The anterolateral approach is the most popular approach for ORIF (Figs 10.12A to C), as it allows deep dissection to

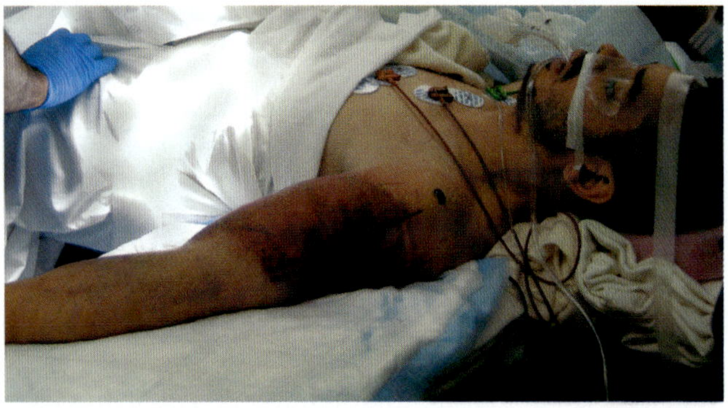

Figure 10.9: Supine positioning of the humerus to accommodate either an anterolateral or medial approach to the humerus.

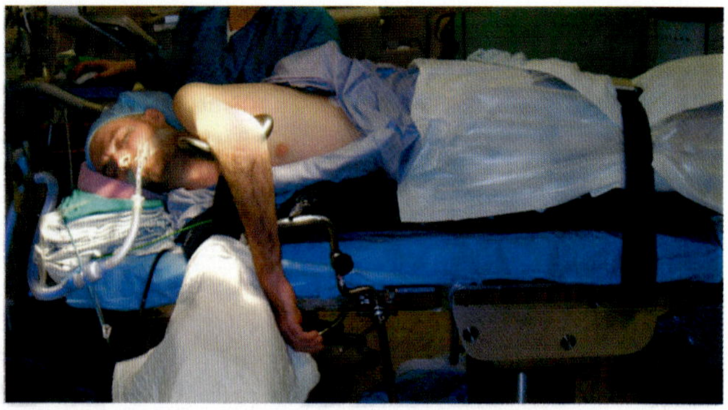

Figure 10.10: Lateral decubitus positioning of the humerus to facilitate the posterior approach to the humerus or for retrograde intramedullary nailing.

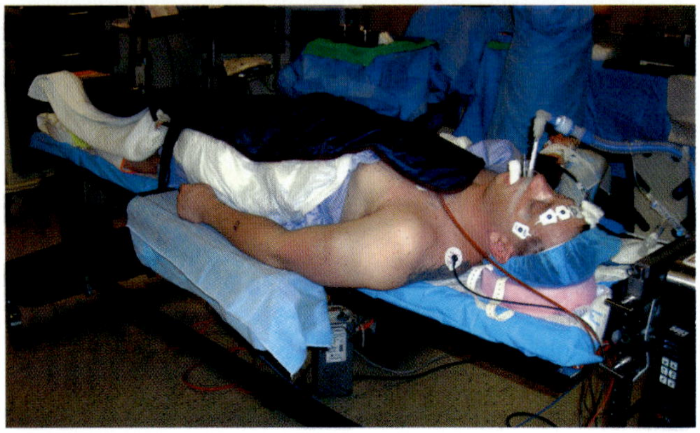

Figure 10.11: Supine positioning of the patient on a radiolucent table for antegrade intramedullary nailing of the humerus. Fluoroscopy can be brought in from the ipsilateral or contralateral side. Note the shoulder and arm is translated off of the table. The arm board is left on to support the elbow and forearm.

the humerus, can be readily extended both proximally and distally, and facilitates excellent access to the radial nerve. This approach is best indicated for shaft fractures of the proximal or middle thirds (Fig. 10.13A). Exposure of the distal third of the shaft, particularly for intra-articular fractures, is limited with the anterolateral approach. An incision is made over the lateral border of the biceps from just above the elbow flexion crease to about 10–15 cm proximally. The deep fascia of the arm is incised in-line with the skin to expose the biceps muscle, which is then retracted medially. The lateral antebrachial cutaneous nerve emerges from the plane between brachialis and the biceps and care should be taken not to injure it. After retracting the biceps, the interval between the brachialis and brachioradialis should then be visible. Since the radial nerve innervates the lateral brachialis and the brachioradialis, a true internervous plane does not exist. Furthermore, the radial nerve emerges from this interval, so development of the intermuscular plane should be performed bluntly and gently. However, routine identification of the radial nerve is recommended above the elbow between the interval of the brachialis and brachioradialis. Proximal dissection of the radial nerve thereafter will concomitantly develop the plane between the brachialis and triceps to the level of the spiral groove of the humerus. At this point, the anterolateral humerus is exposed and the fracture site should become visible. The humerus can be exposed subperiosteally by elevating the brachialis. Posterior exposure should be performed with care as the radial nerve may be tethered in the spiral groove. If proximal extension is required, the plane between the biceps and the deltoid is developed becoming continuous with the deltopectoral interval. If distal extension is required, the plane between the brachioradialis and the pronator teres may be developed. However, this extension would create an internervous plane between the radial and median nerves, and place the lateral antebrachial cutaneous nerve at risk.

The posterior approach is best indicated for humeral shaft fractures in the middle or distal thirds of the shaft (Fig. 10.13B). It is particularly advantageous for fractures with distal intra-articular extension. An incision is made starting 8–10 cm below the acromion and extending distally to the olecranon fossa. The deep fascia of the arm is incised in-line with the skin incision exposing the triceps. Once the triceps is exposed, the posterior humerus can be accessed by either a triceps-splitting or triceps-sparing

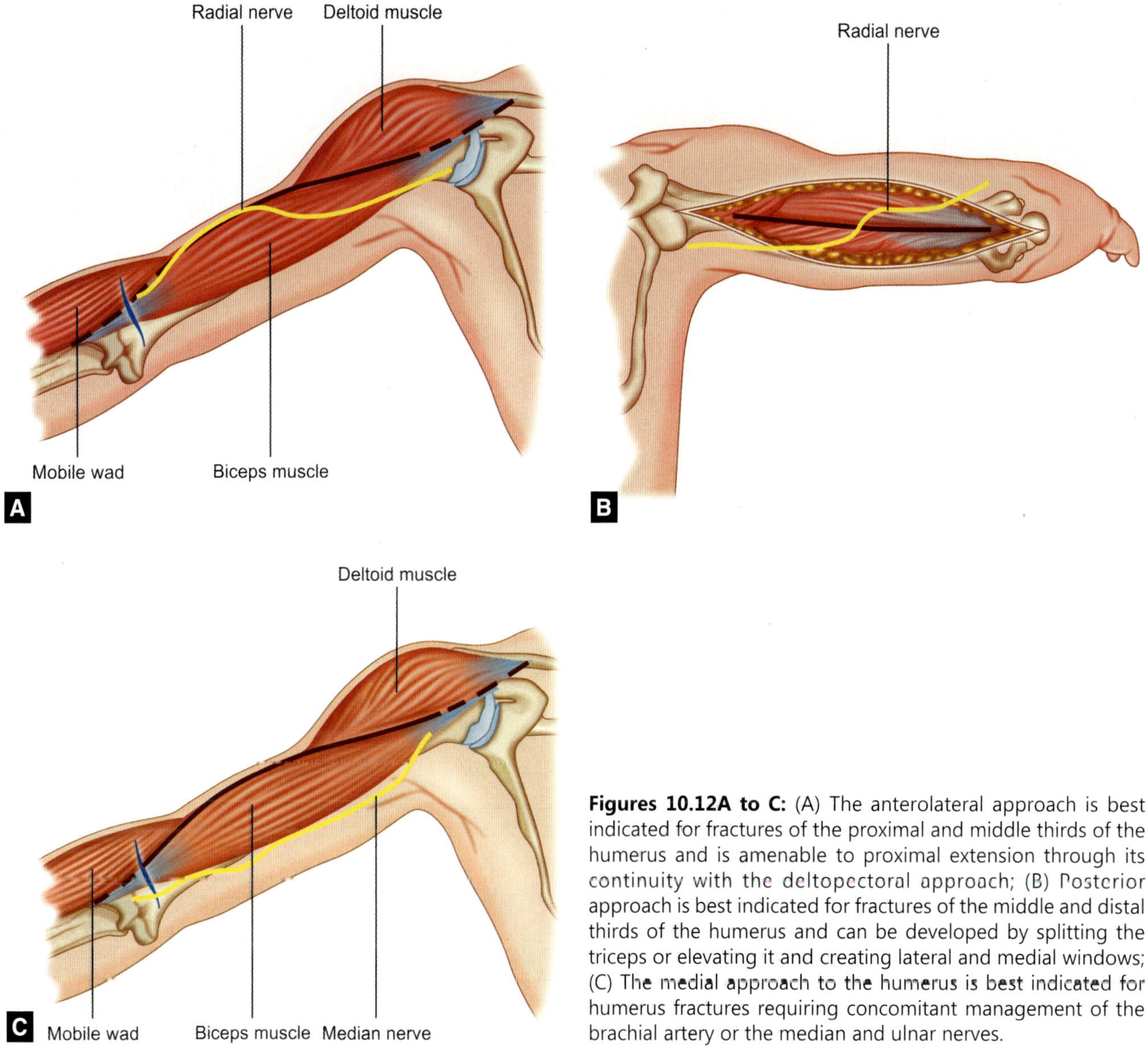

Figures 10.12A to C: (A) The anterolateral approach is best indicated for fractures of the proximal and middle thirds of the humerus and is amenable to proximal extension through its continuity with the deltopectoral approach; (B) Posterior approach is best indicated for fractures of the middle and distal thirds of the humerus and can be developed by splitting the triceps or elevating it and creating lateral and medial windows; (C) The medial approach to the humerus is best indicated for humerus fractures requiring concomitant management of the brachial artery or the median and ulnar nerves.

(also known as a paratricipital) approach. The triceps-splitting approach provides direct access to the humerus but is proximally limited by the radial nerve in the spiral groove found approximately, 10–13 cm proximal to the articular surface and potentially risks denervating the triceps musculature. The triceps-sparing approach involves developing 'windows' medially and laterally between the triceps and the intermuscular septum down to the level of the olecranon. The triceps-sparing approach provides an extensile approach to the humerus along the lateral side but necessitates identification and protection of the radial nerve as it exits the spiral groove. After the lateral head is retracted laterally and the long head medially, the radial nerve and profunda brachii in the spiral groove should become visible. Care should be taken, if dissection proceeds medially, as the ulnar nerve enters the posterior compartment deep to the medial side of the medial head of the triceps. If medial exposure is necessary, the ulnar nerve should be identified in the cubital tunnel behind the medial epicondyle, and dissected and protected proximally, thereby facilitating medial exposure of the humerus. Proximal medial extension is generally not possible safely

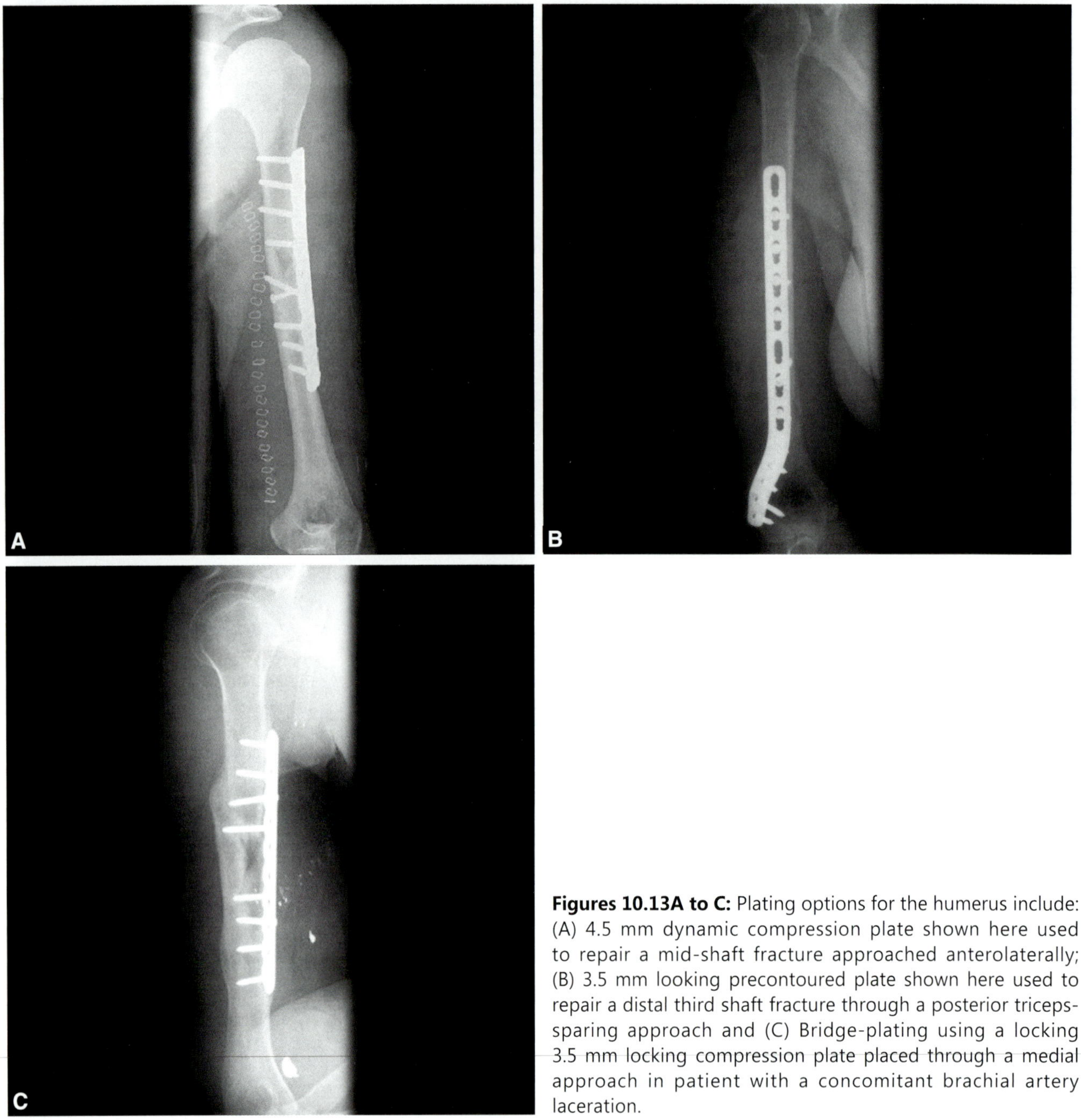

Figures 10.13A to C: Plating options for the humerus include: (A) 4.5 mm dynamic compression plate shown here used to repair a mid-shaft fracture approached anterolaterally; (B) 3.5 mm looking precontoured plate shown here used to repair a distal third shaft fracture through a posterior triceps-sparing approach and (C) Bridge-plating using a locking 3.5 mm locking compression plate placed through a medial approach in patient with a concomitant brachial artery laceration.

above the level of the spiral groove, as the neurovascular bundle is endangered.

The medial approach is seldom chosen, due to the close proximity of the brachial artery. However, this proximity may become an advantage when concomitant exploration of neurovascular structures is warranted (Fig. 10.13C). In such a case, the incision is made at the medial epicondyle and extends along the posteromedial biceps. The ulnar nerve is identified and retracted posteromedially; the median nerve and brachial artery are identified and retracted anterolaterally. The interval between the coracobrachialis (reflected anteriorly) and the triceps (reflected posteriorly) can be developed to expose the humerus. In the proximal incision, care must be taken not to injure the intercostobrachial nerve and the medial cutaneous nerve of the arm as well.

Surgical Techniques

Technique 1: Open Reduction and Internal Fixation

Open reduction and internal fixation by plate osteosynthesis of the humeral shaft may be performed with a variety of plating options. Traditionally, a large fragment 4.5 mm broad compression plate has been recommended (Fig. 10.13A). Alternatively, two 3.5 mm dynamic compression plates may be applied orthogonally. More recently, with the advent and popularization of locking plates, a single 3.5 mm limited contact dynamic compression plate may be used (Fig. 10.13B). In particular, locking plates may be better indicated in osteoporotic bone, as pullout strength is higher and the screws may theoretically be placed unicortically, or when fracture comminution must be bridged (Fig. 10.13C). Necessary implants beyond the plating systems noted above should also include fracture reduction clamps and a long bone distraction system.

Technique

The surgical approach and subsequent position of the plate depends on the location of the fracture. The anterolateral approach and plate fixation is desirable for fractures in the proximal or middle thirds of the humerus. The posterior approach is desirable for fractures in the middle or distal thirds of the humerus. The medial approach is seldom chosen, but may be indicated for complex reconstruction or if vascular exploration is concurrently warranted. The authors recommend routine identification and protection of the radial nerve throughout fracture reduction and fixation (Figs 10.14A to D). The radial nerve is susceptible to injury in the fracture site during fracture exposure, reduction, and plate fixation. As such, diligent protection of the radial nerve is paramount to successful fracture fixation.

Basic steps following exposure of the fracture, as detailed in the previous section include irrigation and aggressive debridement of the fracture site if it was open. Provisional fracture reduction may be accomplished with Weber reduction clamps or K-wires (Fig. 10.15A). If manual traction results in inadequate reduction, distraction with a long bone distractor or an external fixator may be employed. Once the fracture is reduced and normal rotation confirmed, the humerus is ready for plate osteosynthesis. The degree of comminution and fracture pattern will guide the type of plating technique: compression, neutralization and bridge plating are the various methods typically employed to internally fix the humeral shaft.

For simple, long oblique or spiral fractures (AO type A1 or A2), an interfragmentary compression screw or lag screw can provide the initial fixation, and a plate may then be applied in neutralization mode (Fig. 10.15B). The lag screw can tentatively hold the reduction and provide compression of the fracture but is not sufficient to withstand normal physiologic torsion and bending alone. Thus, the plate is applied over the lag screws to 'neutralize' these forces (Fig. 10.15C). Classically, six cortices of screw purchase above and below the fracture line is indicated, but longer plates or greater comminution may require 8 cortices SP.

For transverse or short oblique fractures with minimal comminution, dynamic compression plate fixation may be used. After provisional reduction of the fracture, the plate is applied and fixed using standard compression technique. Again, 6–8 cortices should be purchased above and below the fracture.

For comminuted or segmental fractures (AO type B or C), a bridge plate can span the fracture site and serve as an internal splint. The bridge plate will align and fix the two large fragments, but exclude the interposed comminution. Again, a minimum of 6–8 cortices should be purchased above and below the fracture site being bridged and the plate should not be applied in compression. Moreover, a bridge plate presents a strong indication for utilizing a locking plate to improve stiffness of the construct, and decrease the risk of screw pull out. Due to the lack of cortical contact during bridge plating of the fracture site, humeral length and rotation must be carefully determined prior to plate application.

Once definitive fixation is achieved, and reduction and hardware position confirmed by fluoroscopy (Fig. 10.15D), wound closure is performed. The patient's arm is placed in a sling for comfort and early motion is encouraged. Weight bearing depends on the security of fixation and

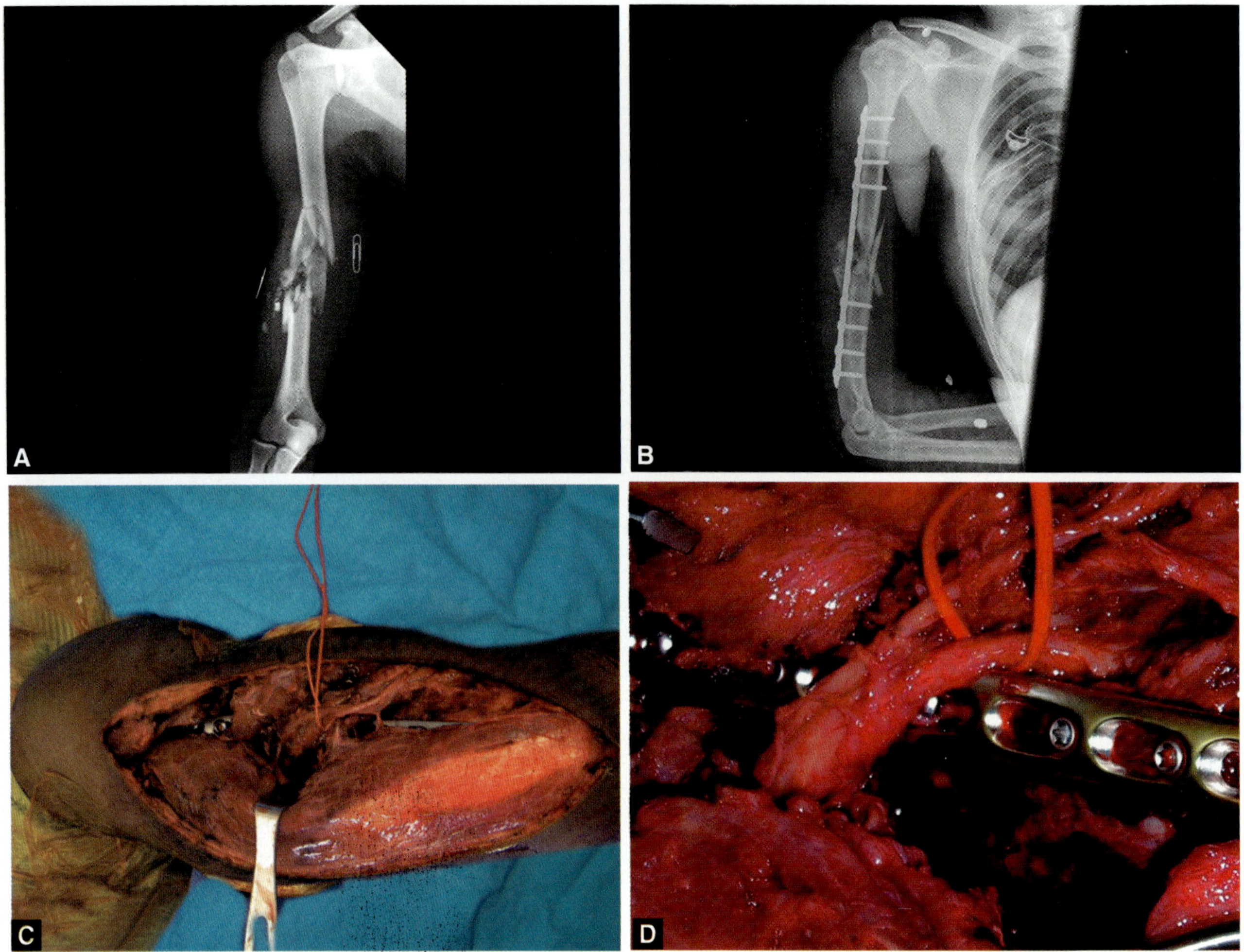

Figures 10.14A to D: Open reduction and internal fixation with plate osteosynthesis exposed through a posterior approach with concomitant identification and protection of the radial nerve. (A and B) Note the pre- and postoperative radiographs identifying a comminuted mid-shaft fracture of the humerus treated with a bridge-plate; (C) A posterior triceps-sparing lateral paratricipital approach was utilized with concomitant radial nerve exploration, which is typically identifed 11–13 cm proximal to the distal articular surface as it traverses the spiral groove of the humerus; (D) Note how the radial nerve was carefully dissected free and elevated allowing plate application below it. In order to avoid excessive tension on the radial nerve, careful dissection and release of the nerve proximally and distally is performed to increase its mobility.

Courtesy: Saqib Rehman

density of bone. Generally, the advantage to plating is immediate weight bearing; however, this may be contraindicated in osteopenic patients and in those treated with a bridge plate technique.

OPEN REDUCTION AND INTERNAL FIXATION: Pearls and Pitfalls

- Plating options include a broad 4.5 mm dynamic compression plates, two 3.5 mm dynamic compression plates applied orthogonally, or a locking 3.5 mm dynamic compression plates alone
- Anterolateral approach is indicated for proximal or middle third shaft fractures, while the posterior approach is indicated for middle and distal third fractures of the humeral shaft
- Routine radial nerve identification and protection is recommended during plate osteosynthesis

Technique 2: Intramedullary Nailing

A number of IM nailing options exist for the humerus, but a static interlocking nail would be the IM implant of choice.

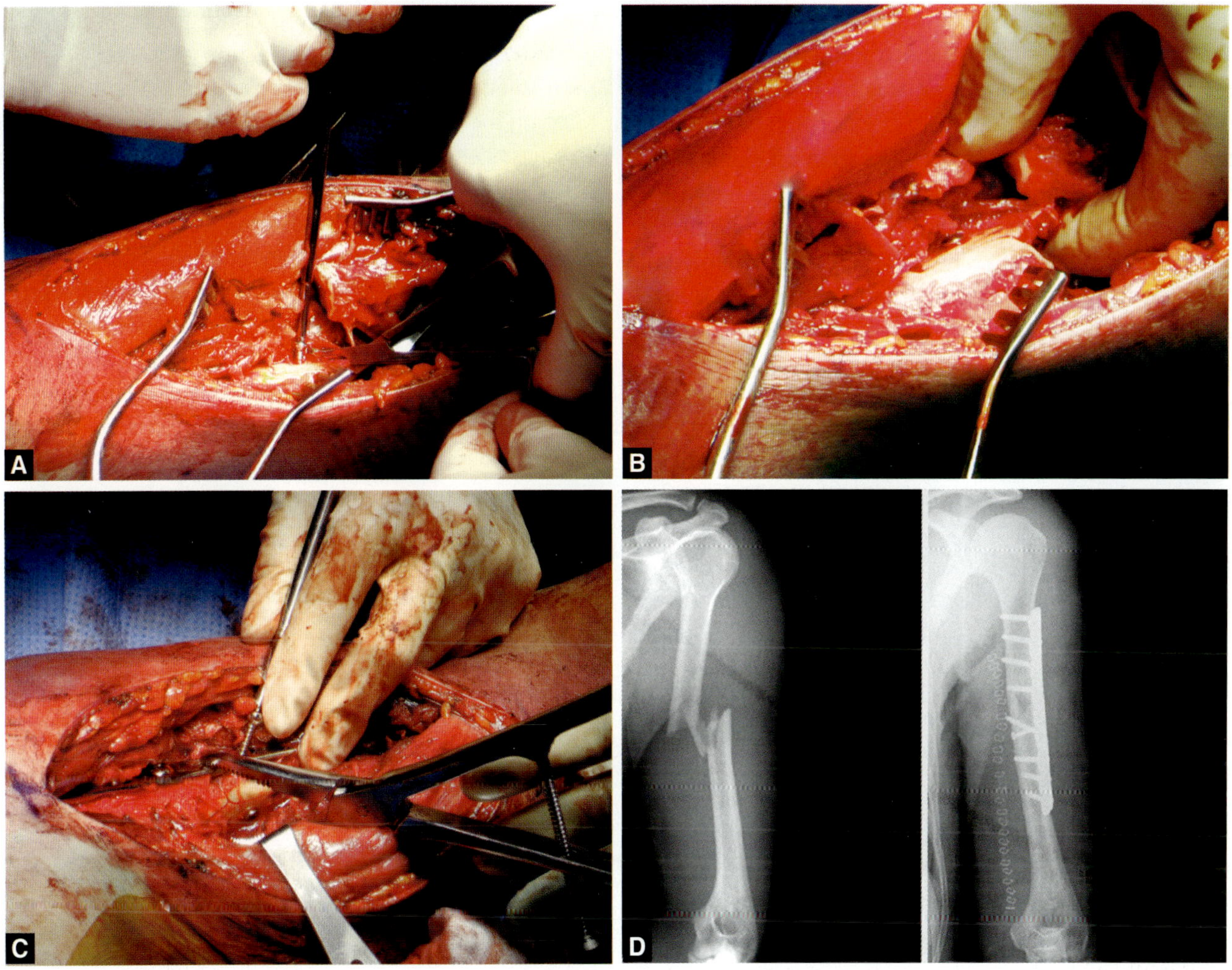

Figures 10.15A to D: Open reduction internal fixation with plate osteosynthesis exposed through an anterolateral approach. (A) Provisional fracture reduction of the humerus achieved with reduction clamps; (B) Initial fracture fixation achieved with an interfragmentary screw; (C) The compressed fracture is thereafter neutralized with a 4.5 mm plate; (D) Preoperative and postoperative anteroposterior radiographs.

Formerly, larger, straight, nonlocking or flexible implants were used, such as the Seidel, Rush or Ender nails, but these yielded high complication rates including nonunions and rotational instability. Consequently, smaller diameter, curved, static interlocking nails have replaced the earlier generation of humeral nails. An interlocking IM nail will provide rotational, axial and bending support and is considered a load-sharing device. The IM nail has several advantages over a plate: bending loads are smaller because the nail reapproximates the mechanical axis and the stress shielding that occurs from plates is not encountered. Furthermore, the type of fracture is not as critical with nails as it is with plates, as all AO fracture types of the humeral shaft can be treated with IM nails (Fig. 10.16A). However, the approach of the nail will depend on the location of the fracture. Fractures of the proximal and middle thirds of the humeral shaft are best treated using an antegrade approach, while middle and distal third fractures are best treated with a retrograde approach.

Antegrade Technique

With the patient positioned in the supine or beach chair position, the C-arm fluoroscopy is brought in from either the ipsilateral or contralateral side (Fig. 10.16B). A 5 cm anterolateral incision is made in-line with the lines of Langer anterolateral to the tip of the acromion (Fig. 10.16C). The raphe between the anterior and middle heads of the deltoid is spilt down to the sub-deltoid bursa. The deltoid split should be limited to no more than 2.5–3.0 cm from the acromion to avoid injury to the axillary nerve. The bursa may be split or excised to facilitate visualization of the greater tuberosity. The rotator cuff is sharply split longitudinally down to the greater tuberosity, but the insertion is not elevated. Under fluoroscopic guidance, the humeral head is opened with either a guide wire or an awl at the junction of the greater tuberosity and the articular cartilage (Fig. 16D). Depending on the nail design, the IM nail may be cannulated allowing it to be directed over a guide wire. Assuming the former, a ball-tipped guide wire is introduced through the proximal humerus and advanced across through the fracture site under fluoroscopic guidance. Orthogonal views should be taken to confirm reduction of the fracture with the guide wire. In addition, the fracture site should be manipulated with care during fracture reduction in order to avoid iatrogenic radial nerve injury. If reaming is deemed necessary, it should also be undertaken with care over the guide wire. Moreover, reaming should proceed slowly with the aid of fluoroscopy to avoid thermal necrosis, eccentric reaming or soft tissue injury. Alternatively, the nail may be inserted without reaming and without a guide wire.

Prior to nail insertion, the diameter and length must be judged and a nail selected accordingly taking into account that the nail be countersunk proximally (Fig. 10.16E), that the fracture site is not distracted, and that the medullary canal ends approximately 5 cm proximal to the olecranon fossa (Fig. 10.16F). The nail should be gently inserted into the canal and tapped to its endpoint while the reduction is held. Cortical gaps are not well-tolerated in the humerus, so repeated 'back-slapping' and rotation to eliminate gapping is advised. Through the insertion jig, the nail is first interlocked proximally. Attention should be paid not to violate the articular surface of the proximal humerus medially with the drill or screws (Fig. 10.16G). Once satisfied with fracture reduction, gap minimization and restoration of normal humeral rotation, the distal interlocking screws are placed. Typically, a freehand technique with fluoroscopy is used and a Mayo stand can be brought in to extend the arm and aid in stabilizing and visualizing the distal locking hole fluoroscopically. Once this hole is perfectly centered under fluoroscopy, a skin incision is made, and blunt dissection with a Kelly clamp is performed down to the anterior cortex of the humerus. Keeping the Kelly clamp spread to protect the surrounding soft tissue the drill bit is delivered down to the anterior cortex and drilled. The distal interlocking screw is measured and inserted anterior to posterior to avoid damage to the radial and ulnar nerves (Fig. 10.16H). As the drill hole is difficult to visualize, the distal interlocking screw is prone to getting lost in the soft tissue. To avoid losing the screw, an absorbable suture is tied around the head of the screw to serve as a leash, if the screw is lost or displaces off of the screwdriver. Prior to closure, final fluoroscopic images should be taken to confirm fracture reduction and appropriate position of the hardware (Fig. 10.16I). If desired, an endcap may be placed in the proximal end of the nail. The rotator cuff is closed with interrupted nonabsorbable sutures, and then the skin is closed. A sling is applied for comfort. Postoperatively, immediate mobilization of the arm is encouraged.

Retrograde Technique

The skin is incised longitudinally starting approximately 1–2 cm proximal to the tip of the olecranon along the posterior distal arm. The triceps is exposed, split and retracted. The proximal aspect of the olecranon fossa is exposed, and a 3.5 mm opening is placed in the distal cortex of the distal humerus approximately 2.5 cm proximal to the olecranon fossa. Once the IM canal of the humerus is accessed through a distal retrograde fashion the remaining steps are equivalent as outlined above in the anterograde fashion.

INTRAMEDULLARY NAILING: Pearls and Pitfalls

- Intramedullary nails are available in cannulated and non-cannulated forms
- The diameter of the IM canal is highly variable and should be carefully templated preoperatively. If reaming is deemed necessary it should be performed carefully and preferably over a guide wire
- Prior to interlocking the nail, proper rotation of the humerus must be confirmed. After interlocking the nail, the arm should demonstrate approximately 45–60° of passive external rotation. Compare to the contralateral limb for the patient's normal motion

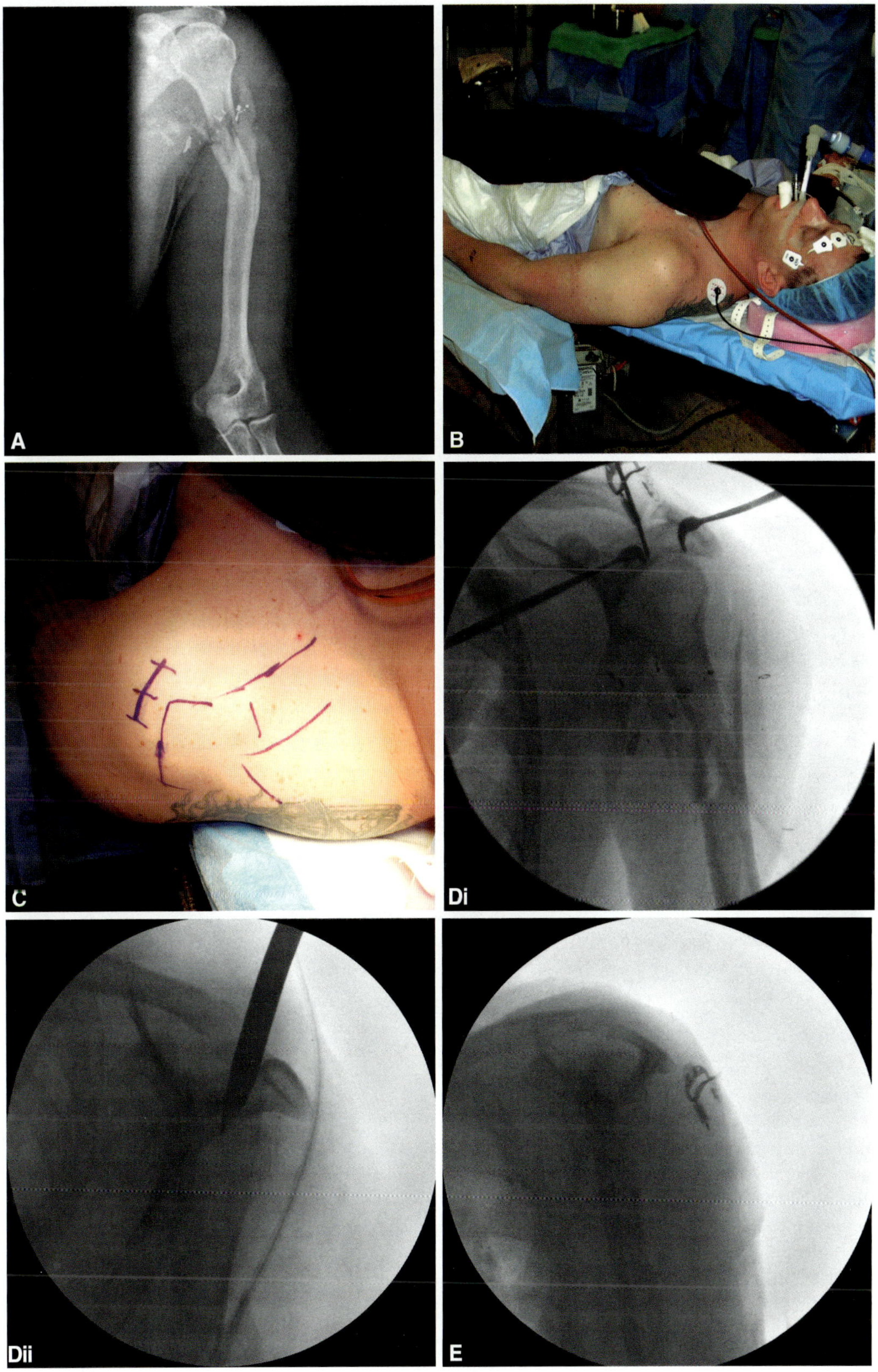

Figures 10.16A to E

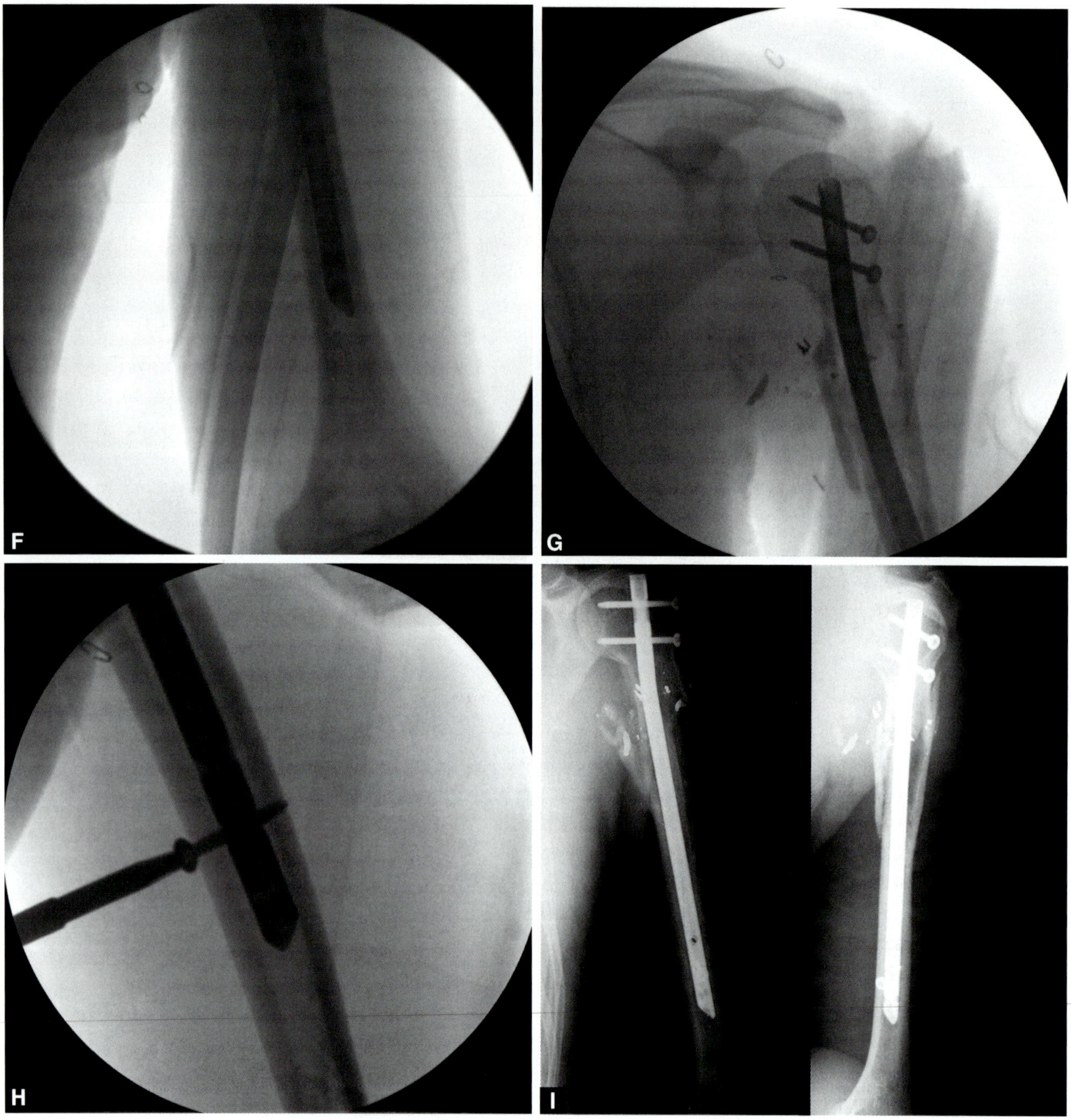

Figures 10.16A to I: Intramedullary nailing of humeral shaft can be performed regardless of fracture type. (A) Note the comminution of the proximal humeral shaft caused by a gunshot injury; (B) The patient is positioned supine on a radiolucent table with the operative arm translated off of the table; (C) An incision is placed anterolateral to the acromion; (D) The humeral head may be opened over a guidewire or with an awl; (E) Proximally, the nail must be countersunk below the articular surface; (F) Distally, the nail typically ends approximately 5 cm proximal to the olecranon fossa; (G) The proximal interlocking screws are placed through the insertion jig and should be placed short of the articular surface; (H) The distal interlocking screws are placed freehand; (I) Postoperative radiographs confirm reduction of the fracture and appropriate position of the hardware.

- After the proximal interlocking screws are placed but prior to placing the distal interlocking screws, back slapping can reduce fracture gapping.
- During freehand interlocking screw placement, an absorbable suture should be placed around the head of the screw to serve as a leash if the screw is lost off of the screwdriver into the soft tissue

Outcomes

Common parameters for the measurement of success after fixation of humeral shaft fractures include rates of union, functional scores, and rates of reoperation. The absence of complications such as nonunions, radial nerve palsy, shoulder pain and iatrogenic fracture extension are generally also included as benchmarks.

Open Reduction and Internal Fixation

Humeral shaft fractures treated with ORIF have a reported union rate of 94–100%.[13-17] Early case series reporting on outcomes after plate osteosynthesis reported a rate of union of 97% in two series each consisting of 34 patients and no permanent nerve damage was noted in either study. Although these studies lacked randomization and controls, they were the first to exclusively highlight the advantages of plate internal fixation, such as protection of soft tissue damage, early mobilization (preventing contracture), and easier nursing transfers.[13,14] More recently, McKee et al. reported on 114 patients treated with a limited contact dynamic compression plate and found a union rate of 97%.[15] Plate osteosynthesis has also been shown to be the method choice in open fractures. A recent retrospective review of 46 patients treated with immediate (most within 8 hours) plate fixation yielded a union rate of 100% with no iatrogenic nerve palsies or deep infections.[16] Finally, Tingstad et al. compared outcomes of immediate versus protected weight bearing following ORIF of humeral shaft fractures, excluding those with metaphyseal or intra-articular extension. Reporting an overall union rate of 94%, they showed that immediate weight bearing had no significant difference on the rate of union, alignment, hardware failure or reoperation. There were three cases of nonunions and two hardware failures necessitating subsequent operative treatment.[17]

Intramedullary Nailing

Success in the treatment of femoral and tibial fractures with IM nailing led to the early enthusiasm in studies evaluating IM nails for humeral shaft fractures. However, subsequent studies reported increased rates of complications such as rotational instability, nonunion, iatrogenic fractures and decreased shoulder function.[17-20] Robinson et al. reviewed 18 of 30 fractures treated with locked Seidel nails (Howmedica, Rutherford, New Jersey) over a 6-month follow-up and found that 13 patients reported moderate to severe shoulder pain and 8 required hardware removals.[19] Similarly, rates of nonunion have been controversial, as they range from 0–29% in the literature.[17] On the other hand, as the technology and technique of the locking nails improved by reducing the nail diameter and adding multiple locking screws, more recent studies have shown improved clinical results.[21-23] Ikpeme reported a 100% union rate at 2-year follow-up for 25 patients treated with antegrade Russell-Taylor (Smith and Nephew Richards, Inc., Memphis, Tennessee) nails. However, 6 patients complained of shoulder pain. This group also demonstrated migration or prominence of the proximal interlocking screws. Five of these patients subsequently underwent removal of the screws and noted relief of their symptoms.[21] Crates and Whittle also reported on outcomes following antegrade Russell-Taylor nail fixation and reported a union rate of 94%, full shoulder function in 90%, and reoperation for shoulder pain in 4% of patients.[22] Fernandez et al. reported a case series of 47 patients at follow-up after retrograde unreamed antegrade humeral nailing (Synthes, Paoli, Pennsylvania) and reported a union rate of 96% and good to excellent shoulder or elbow scores were found in 95% and 91% of patients respectively.[23]

Plates Versus Nails

Following years of debate on the most appropriate treatment for humeral shaft fractures, a number of prospective randomized controlled trials were published comparing outcomes of plating versus nailing humeral shaft fractures.[24-28] Many of these trials were small, and as a response, a series of meta-analyses emerged.[29-31] The meta-analysis by Bhandari et al. concluded that the risk of reoperation and shoulder pain was significantly higher in the nailing group. However, the rates of nonunion, infection and radial nerve palsy were not statistically different.[29] Heineman et al. published an updated meta-analysis measuring the total complication rate defined as any adverse outcome, such as pain, nonunion, infection etc. Ultimately, they concluded that nails had a significantly higher rate of complications than plates.[30,31] Although it seems that overall the outcomes following humeral shaft fixation may favor plating, each case must be individually assessed, as no single treatment has been proven superior in all cases.

Antegrade Versus Retrograde Nails

Few clinical trials have compared antegrade and retrograde nailing outcomes prospectively; however, a recent trial by Cheng and Lin did compare these techniques in a total of 92 patients and found comparable rates of complications and union (95% antegrade and 93% retrograde) in each group.[32] Significant differences included longer operative times in the retrograde approach but also less shoulder dysfunction. No differences were seen in Mayo elbow performance scores. Currently, it appears that both techniques can yield reasonable results, but the data support retrograde nailing in patients with pre-existing shoulder pathology. Antegrade nailing is recommended in critically ill patients, as the operative time and technical demands are reduced.

Complications

Radial Nerve Injury

Radial nerve palsy is the most common nerve palsy following any long bone fracture. Management of acute or iatrogenic palsies is controversial. Shao et al. performed a systematic literature review of 1,045 patients and found the overall incidence of radial nerve palsy was 11.8%. Fracture patterns associated with a higher risk of nerve palsies were those at the middle or distal thirds of the humeral shaft with transverse or spiral patterns, which includes the Holstein-Lewis pattern.[33] Generally, unless the fracture is open or is otherwise indicated for operative repair, observation of the palsy is the first step. They identified an overall 88% chance of nerve recovery, of which 70% represented spontaneous recovery. Furthermore, they identified no significant difference in recovery in those treated initially with observation versus those treated with early exploration. Their treatment algorithm states that an ultrasound should be performed at 3 weeks to determine whether operative repair is warranted, for example if there was a lacerated or entrapped nerve. Otherwise, observation should be utilized; however, the optimal waiting time before exploration is not defined. Most surgeons would agree this time is between 2 months and 6 months. Green et al. recommends calculating a time based on nerve regeneration at 1 mm/day plus 30 days. A measurement can be taken from the site of the fracture to 2 cm proximal to lateral epicondyle (brachioradialis innervation), which estimates the distance required for axonal regeneration.[34] In contrast, nerve palsies following fracture manipulation or operative fixation without perioperative nerve exploration, repeat surgery for nerve exploration is warranted.

Insertion Site Morbidity

Shoulder pain is the greatest challenge following IM nailing of the humerus. It can represent either direct rotator cuff injury during nail insertion versus secondary hardware irritation. Several suggestions of different sites of insertion, mini-incisions and repairs have been made but the risk of shoulder injury has not been eliminated. Currently, it is recommended to make a careful rotator cuff incision and to bury the nail below the humeral head to prevent impingement. In the event of severe functional deficit, the hardware may be removed at 12 months.

Nonunion

The diagnosis of a nonunion of the humerus should be considered if there is a lack of healing with bridging bone at 6 months. Generally, nonunions are the result of fracture distraction, soft tissue interposition, inadequate fixation or implant failure. General patient factors, such as nutritional status and smoking, are also contributory. Cortical gapping can be prevented when nailing by locking the proximal screws first and then back-slapping to compress the fracture prior to placing the distal screws. The gold standard for treatment of nonunions in the humerus is ORIF with bone graft. Exchange nailing has not been shown to achieve equal success.

Iatrogenic Fracture Extension

Generally, iatrogenic fractures occur during nail insertion and have a reported incidence of 1.8–6.0%. Retrograde approaches are more at risk especially, if the canal is small.

Most iatrogenic fractures are nondisplaced and do not cause fixation failure. Insertion of smaller diameter nails has reduced the rate of iatrogenic comminution, and some surgeons suggest using an olecranon fossa starting point rather than a supracondylar for straighter insertion and less bending moments.

Authors' Preferred Management of Select Complications

Case 1: Radial Nerve Injury

A 43-year-old male incurred a mid-shaft fracture of the humerus that underwent closed IM nailing. Preoperatively, the patient had intact radial nerve function. However, postoperatively the patient demonstrated a radial nerve palsy with no active finger or wrist extension. The patient was managed initially with expectant observation; however, there was still no evidence of nerve recovery at 3 months.

There are multiple causes of a postoperative radial nerve palsy including, but not limited to, direct nerve injury/laceration, excessive retraction/tension and direct compression by the hardware or in the fracture site (Figs 10.17A and B). The management of radial nerve palsy following fracture fixation depends upon three variables:

1. Radial nerve function preoperatively
2. Whether the nerve was visualized intraoperatively
3. Type of internal fixation utilized

In cases of radial nerve palsy preoperatively, continued postoperative palsy is expected. However, in such cases, if operative fixation is selected, IM nailing is a relative contraindication, ORIF with plate osteosynthesis should be the fixation of choice and the radial nerve must be carefully exposed, examined and vigilantly protected throughout the procedure. In this manner, the radial nerve is given the best chance of recovery while also excluding the question of whether the nerve has been secondarily injured or compressed in the fracture or fixation.

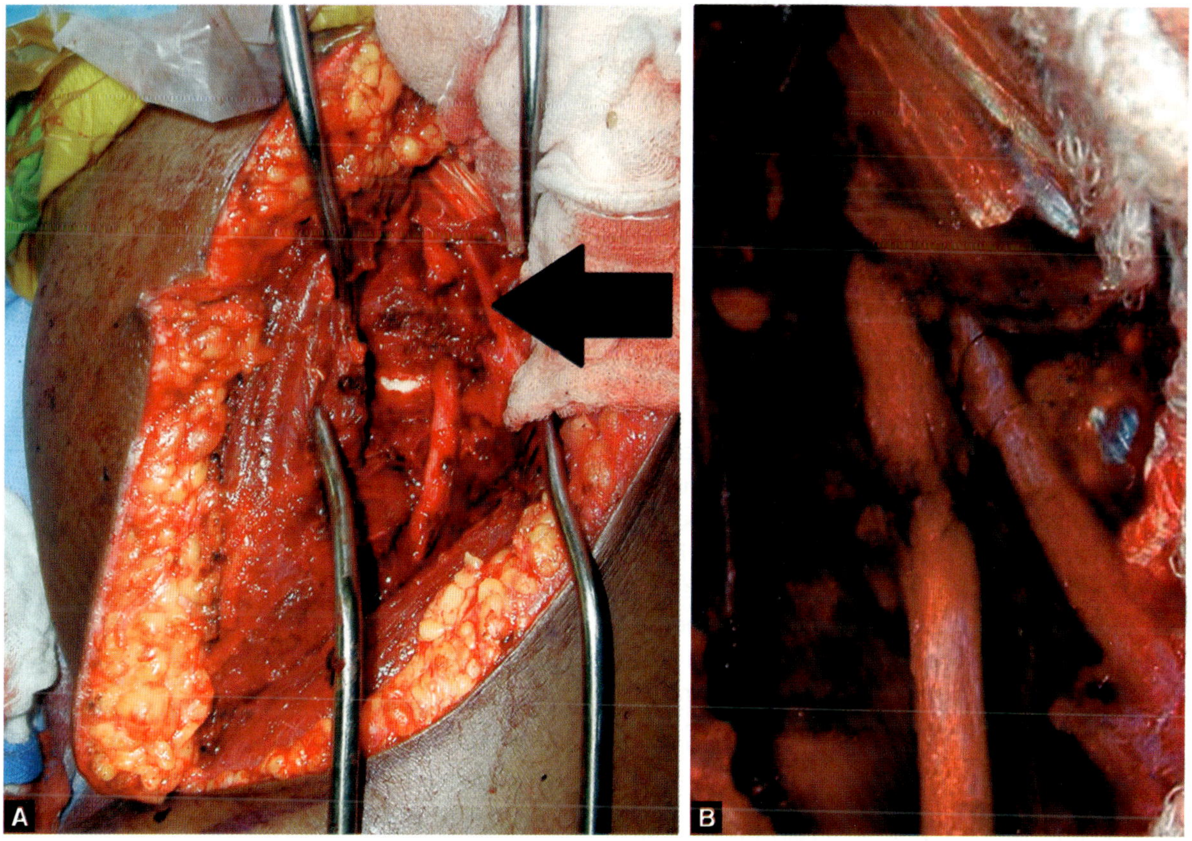

Figures 10.17A and B: Postoperative radial nerve palsy following humeral fracture fixation can result from direct iatrogenic nerve injury, excessive retraction/tension, and direct compression of the nerve by the hardware or within the fracture site. Note in Figure (A) an inadvertent but direct nerve laceration that had occurred during initial exposure of the humerus for plate osteosynthesis identified during re-exploration; (B) the radial nerve underwent primary epineural repair using standard microsurgical technique.

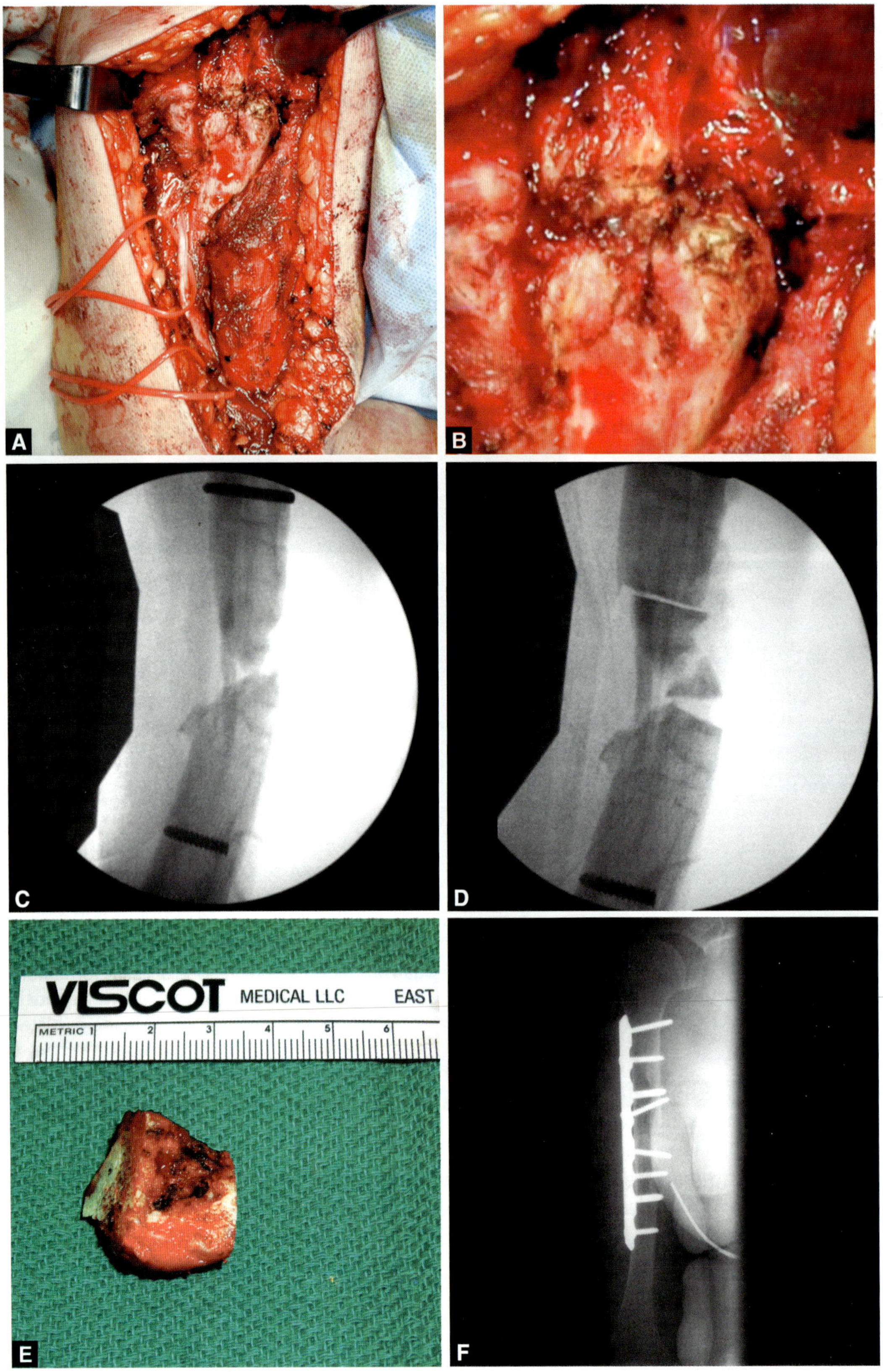

Figures 10.19A to F

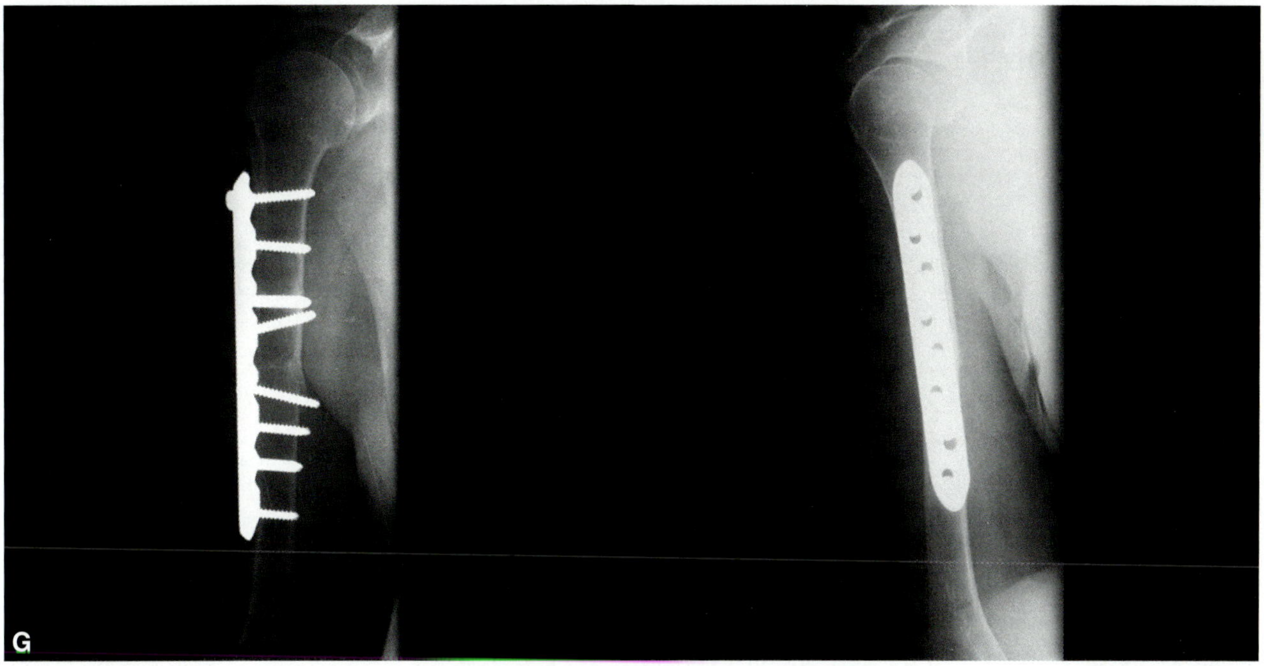

Figures 10.19A to G: During a nonunion repair, (A) the radial nerve should be identified first and protected throughout the procedure; (B) exposure of the nonunion site may reveal a pseudarthrosis with fibrous scar tissue enveloping the bone ends; (C) fluoroscopy should be used to confirm the nonunion site; (D) a microsagittal saw is used to excise the unhealthy bone ends along with the pseudarthrosis in a single resection; (E) note the nonunion segment with bony sclerosis and loss of the medullary canal which should now be restored with drill bits on both ends of the humeral shaft; (F) compression plating is then performed with a large fragment locking plate. First nonlocking screws are placed using standard AO compression technique, followed thereafter with locking screws if desired and (G) radiographs taken 3 months postoperatively confirm healing across the nonunion site.

Technique

In order to have adequate access to the previous hardware, the surgical approach used during the first surgery should be utilized again. As always careful dissection and meticulous protection of the radial nerve should be performed throughout the case. The previous hardware should be removed. The nonunion site and its two sclerotic ends are typically encased in a pseudarthrosis joint capsule. Sharp dissection down to bone and elimination of all soft tissue between the ends is paramount. Following exposure of the nonunion site, takedown of unhealthy bone, restoration of the medullary canals, reduction with proper rotation and alignment of the humeral shaft, and compression plating should be performed. The ends will be typically sclerotic and should be debrided down to healthy bleeding bone with either a rongeur or a an oscillating saw. In order to maximize bony contact and healing a step cut or oblique cut may be performed; however, proper rotation must be confirmed first. Starting with a 2.5 mm drill bit, the medullary canal is restored at both fractured ends. The canal can be serially drilled from larger diameter up to 4.5 mm in diameter, if desired. Restoring the medullary canal provides a conduit for delivery of the necessary factors for bone healing. Plate fixation is best achieved with a locking large fragment compression plate or a broad large fragment compression plate. Alternatively, two small fragment compression plates may be applied in an orthogonal manner. If a locking plate is selected, the plate should first be applied in compression using standard AO compression technique prior to placing any locking screws. Furthermore, the plate may be prebent to increase compression and apposition. Preferably, 6–8 cortices should be purchased both above and below the nonunion site.

In nonunion cases of the humeral shaft following IM nailing, reamed exchange nailing can be considered. However, we recommend removal of the nail followed by open takedown of the nonunion and compression plating as just described. In our opinion, open treatment of the nonunion increases the odds of successful healing.

Summary

Humeral shaft fractures are common injuries, generally, resulting from high-energy trauma in young patients and low-energy falls in the elderly. Open and pathologic fractures are common varieties. The initial assessment in a stable patient should focus on the neurovascular examinations, open wounds and associated injuries of the ipsilateral shoulder, and forearm. Radial nerve palsy is the most common associated injury and should be assessed by first dorsal web space sensation and wrist extension. The physical findings should be documented before and after any reduction maneuver, and preoperatively and postoperatively. Generally, orthogonal views of the humerus with the shoulder and elbow in view are sufficient. CT scans should be reserved for defining intra-articular extension. Classification is guided by the AO classification system.

Nonoperative management has a high rate of union with functional bracing, and the humerus can theoretically tolerate a malalignment of up to 20° of anterior angulation, 30° of varus angulation, 30° of malrotation and 3 cm of shortening. Surgical indications include fracture criteria, associated injuries and patient variables (Table 10.1). Surgical options include ORIF versus IM nailing. ORIF is most commonly utilized, but IM nailing has advantages for pathologic fractures, segmental fractures, or patients in whom shorter operative times are required. Recent comparative trials have shown similar rates of union for both procedures. Recent meta-analyses have shown the risk of complications, and reoperation is higher with IM nailing.

References

1. Rose SH, Melton LJ 3rd, Morrey BF, et al. Epidemiologic features of humeral fractures. Clin Orthop Relat Res. 1982;168:24-30.
2. Ekholm R, Adami J, Tidermark J, et al. Fractures of the shaft of the humerus. An epidemiological study of 401 fractures. J Bone Joint Surg Br. 2006;88(11):1469-73.
3. Tytherleigh-Strong G, Walls N, McQueen MM. The epidemiology of humeral shaft fractures. J Bone Joint Surg Br. 1998;80(2):249-53.
4. Mast JW, Spiegel PG, Harvey JP Jr, et al. Fractures of the humeral shaft: a retrospective study of 240 adult fractures. Clin Orthop Relat Res. 1975;112:254-62.
5. Frassica FJ, Frassica DA. Metastatic bone disease of the humerus. J Am Acad Orthop Surg. 2003;11(4):282-8.
6. Klenerman L. Fractures of the shaft of the humerus. J Bone Joint Surg Br. 1966;48(1):105-11.
7. Sarmiento A, Zagorski JB, Zych GA, et al. Functional bracing for the treatment of fractures of the humeral diaphysis. J Bone Joint Surg Am. 2000;82(4):478-86.
8. Koch PP, Gross DF, Gerber C. The results of functional (Sarmiento) bracing of humeral shaft fractures. J Shoulder Elbow Surg. 2002;11(2):143-50.
9. Marsh JL, Slongo TF, Agel J, et al. Fracture and dislocation classification compendium—2007: Orthopaedic Trauma Association classification, database and outcomes committee. J Orthop Trauma. 2007;21(10 Suppl):S1-133.
10. Gustilo RB, Merkow RL, Templeman D. The management of open fractures. J Bone Joint Surg Am. 1990;72(2):299-304.
11. Mostafavi HR, Tornetta P 3rd. Open fractures of the humerus treated with external fixation. Clin Orthop Relat Res. 1997;337:187-97.
12. Bell MJ, Beauchamp CG, Kellam JK, et al. The results of plating humeral shaft fractures in patients with multiple injuries. The Sunnybrook experience. J Bone Joint Surg Br. 1985;67(2):293-6.
13. Vander Griend R, Tomasin J, Ward EF. Open reduction and internal fixation of humeral shaft fractures. Results using AO plating techniques. J Bone Joint Surg. 1986;68(3):430-3.
14. McKee MD, Seiler JG, Jupiter JB. The application of the limited contact dynamic compression plate in the upper extremity: an analysis of 114 cases. Injury. 1995;26(10):661-6.
15. Connolly S, McKee MD, Zdero R, et al. Immediate plate osteosynthesis of open fractures of the humeral shaft. J Trauma. 2010;69(3):685-90.
16. Tingstad EM, Wolinsky PR, Shyr Y, et al. Effect of immediate weight bearing on plated fractures of the humeral shaft. J Trauma. 2000;49(2):278-80.
17. Farragos AF, Schemitsch EH, McKee MD. Complications of intramedullary nailing for fractures of the humeral shaft: a review. J Orthop Trauma. 1999;13(4):258-67.
18. Riemer BL, Foglesong ME, Burke CJ 3rd, et al. Complications of Seidel intramedullary nailing of narrow diameter humeral diaphyseal fractures. Orthopedics. 1994;17(1):19-29.
19. Robinson CM, Bell KM, Court-Brown CM, et al. Locked nailing of humeral shaft fractures. experience in Edinburgh over a two-year period. J Bone Joint Surg Br. 1992;74(2):558-62.

20. Bain GI, Sandow M, Howie DW. Treatment of humeral shaft fractures with the Seidel intramedullary nail. Aust NZJ Surg. 1996;66(3):156-8.
21. Ikpeme JO. Intramedullary interlocking nailing for humeral fractures: experiences with the Russell-Taylor humeral nail. Injury. 1994;25(7):447-55.
22. Crates J, Whittle AP. Antegrade interlocking nailing of acute humeral shaft fractures. Clin Orthop Relat Res. 1998;(350):40-50.
23. Fernandez FF, Matschke S, Hulsenbeck A, et al. Five years' clinical experience with the unreamed humeral nail in the treatment of humeral shaft fractures. Injury 2004;35:264-71.
24. Chapman JR, Henley MB, Agel J, et al. Randomized prospective study of humeral shaft fracture fixation: intramedullary nails versus plates. J Orthop Trauma. 2000; 14(3):162-6.
25. McCormack RG, Brien D, Buckley RE, et al. Fixation of fractures of the shaft of the humerus by dynamic compression plate or intramedullary nail. A prospective, randomised trial. J Bone Joint Surg Br. 2000;82(3):336-9.
26. Changulani M, Jain UK, Keswani T. Comparison of the use of the humerus intramedullary nail and dynamic compression plate for the management of diaphyseal fractures of the humerus. A randomised controlled study. Int Orthop. 2007;31:391-5.
27. Putti AB, Uppin RB, Putti BB. Locked intramedullary nailing versus dynamic compression plating for humeral shaft fractures. J Orthop Surg (Hong Kong). 2009;17(2):139-41.
28. Singisetti K, Ambedkar M. Nailing versus plating in humerus shaft fractures: a prospective comparative study. Int Orthop. 2010;34(4):571-6.
29. Bhandari M, Devereaux PJ, McKee MD, et al. Compression plating versus intramedullary nailing of humeral shaft fractures—a meta-analysis. Acta Orthop. 2006;77(2):279-84.
30. Heineman DJ, Poolman RW, Nork SE, et al. Plate fixation or intramedullary fixation of humeral shaft fractures. Acta Orthop. 2010;81(2):216-23.
31. Heineman DJ, Bhandari M, Nork SE, et al. Treatment of humeral shaft fractures—meta-analysis reupdated. Acta Orthop. 2010;81(4):517.
32. Cheng HR, Lin J. Prospective randomized comparative study of antegrade and retrograde locked nailing for middle humeral shaft fracture. J Trauma. 2008;65(1):94-102.
33. Shao YC, Harwood P, Grotz MR, et al. Radial nerve palsy associated with fractures of the shaft of the humerus: a systematic review. J Bone Joint Surg. 2005;87(12):1647-52.
34. Green DP, Hotchkiss RN, Pederson WC. Green's Operative Hand Surgery, Vol 2, 4th edition. New York: Churchill Livingstone; 1999. pp. 1492.

Chapter 11

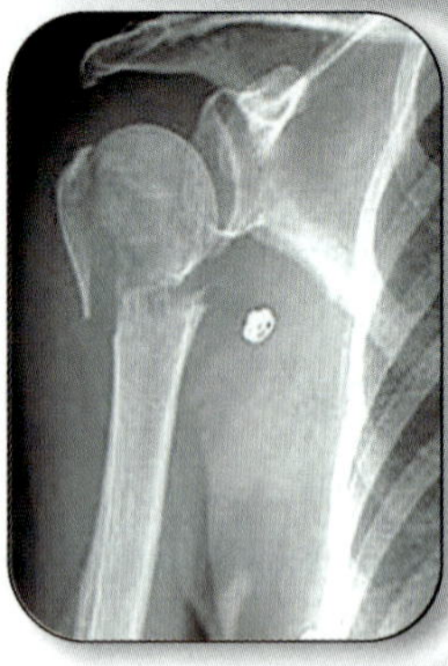

Proximal Humerus Fractures

David Wellman, Dean Lorich, David Helfet

Chapter Outline

Introduction
Diagnosis
Classification
Surgical Indications
Surgical Anatomy, Positioning and Approaches
- Surgical Anatomy
- Positioning
- Approaches

Surgical Techniques
- Technique 1: Open Reduction Internal Fixation
- Technique 2: Intramedullary Nailing
- Technique 3: Hemiarthroplasty

Outcomes
Complications
- Malunion
- Infection
- Avascular Necrosis
- Hemiarthroplasty—Specific Complications

Authors' Preferred Management of Select Complications
- Case 1: Failure of Fixation followed by Revision of Fixation
- Case 2: Failure of Fixation followed by Hemiarthroplasty
- Case 3: Open Reduction and Internal Fixation followed by Infected Nonunion

Summary

Introduction

Proximal humerus fractures are challenging to treat, as even low-energy mechanisms of trauma may yield complex fracture patterns, especially in the elderly population. Overall, proximal humerus fractures represent about 6% of fractures in the orthopedic literature.[1] Unlike fractures of the humeral shaft, proximal humerus fractures display a unimodal distribution in the population with the incidence of fractures increasing sharply in the aging male and female populations.[1] Seventy percent of proximal humerus fractures occur in women;[1] this highlights the need for coordination of osteoporosis evaluation and management in this patient population.

Treatment of proximal humerus fractures ranges from conservative to operative with varying fixation techniques and approaches described in the literature. With approximately 20% of cases requiring operative management,[2] appreciation for the anatomy, familiarity with exposures and an understanding of fixation options are paramount in treating these injuries.

Diagnosis

Diagnosis of a proximal humerus fracture begins with a thorough patient history. The examining physician should pay close attention to the mechanism of injury, as high-energy traumatic events often include associated injuries, such as dislocations and neurovascular injuries. The overall state of health should be assessed along with the patient's baseline functional demands as these help guide ultimate surgical management.

Physical examination begins with careful inspection of the soft tissue. Often, ecchymosis and edema obscure bony detail. Skin should be inspected for previous incisions and acute damage. Open fractures are exceedingly uncommon due to the extensive soft tissue envelope surrounding the proximal humerus. A thorough neurovascular check should be performed as 21–45% of fractures and dislocations have associated nerve injuries, most commonly of the axillary nerve.[3] Potential vascular issues are first assessed through palpation and comparison of pulses of both upper extremities. Any concern of arterial injury warrants further evaluation and a vascular surgical consultation. Range of motion (ROM), while usually fundamental in assessing shoulder injuries, is usually too painful for an awake and alert patient to tolerate. One should note the positioning of the arm, keeping in mind that fracture dislocations are often more masked than pure dislocations. As always, detailed preoperative documentation of the exam is essential, and the examination should be repeated after all interventions including reduction attempts.

The next step in evaluating a patient with a potential proximal humerus fracture is radiographic imaging. Initially, three views of the shoulder should be obtained on plain films. The ideal series include the true anteroposterior (AP) of the shoulder (30° oblique to the AP plane), the axillary lateral and the scapular Y view (Figs 11.1A to D). These images are often the only radiological studies needed to formulate a treatment plan. If an axillary view is difficult to position secondary to pain, a Velpeau view is an acceptable alternative. Displacement and angulation of fracture fragments, as well as subluxation/dislocation of the humeral head (best seen on the axillary lateral), should be noted at this stage.

When faced with complex, intra-articular fracture patterns, computerized tomography (CT) scan examination should be considered, as overlapping bony anatomy obscures the true fracture patterns and often limits ability to plan surgery (Figs 11.2A to C). Furthermore, CT scans can improve fracture fragment definition and allow for better assessment of articular injuries, such as the case of impaction injuries and head-splitting patterns (Figs 11.3A and B). However, Foroohar et al. showed that the addition of CT and 3D technology did not significantly improve the reproducibility of fracture classification or agreement in choice of treatment.[4]

FRACTURES OF THE PROXIMAL HUMERUS DIAGNOSIS: Pearls and Pitfalls

- Do not miss an occult neurological or vascular injury on initial exam
- Scrutinize plain film radiographs for evidence of dislocation
- Computerized tomography imaging can aide in fracture characterization

Classification

Classification of proximal humerus fractures should be performed with caution, as the most widely used classification systems cannot always be depended upon to assist with surgical decision making. The Neer system is the most commonly used classification system in practice (Fig. 11.4). Displacement of 1 cm or angulation of 45° defines a unique part.[5] A fracture of the proximal humerus that does not produce a single fragment meeting those criteria is termed a "1-part" fracture, regardless of the number of fracture lines present. A 2-part fracture occurs when a single fragment from the proximal humerus is displaced greater than 1 cm or angulated greater than 45°. Fractures classified as 3- and 4-part are defined by the number of fragments meeting these criteria. Criticisms of the Neer classification system include the arbitrary definition of a "part" and the fact that interpreting plain film displacement and angulation in the face of overlapping bony detail is difficult. Fracture-dislocations of the proximal humerus are typically described by noting the direction of displacement of the humeral head, as well as the number of distinct fracture parts.

The AO/OTA classification system[6] may also be somewhat limited at guiding decision making and ultimate treatment. It uses classic AO numerical grading and is divided into 27 subtypes (Fig. 11.5). This classification system is especially helpful as a research instrument and in clinical registries.

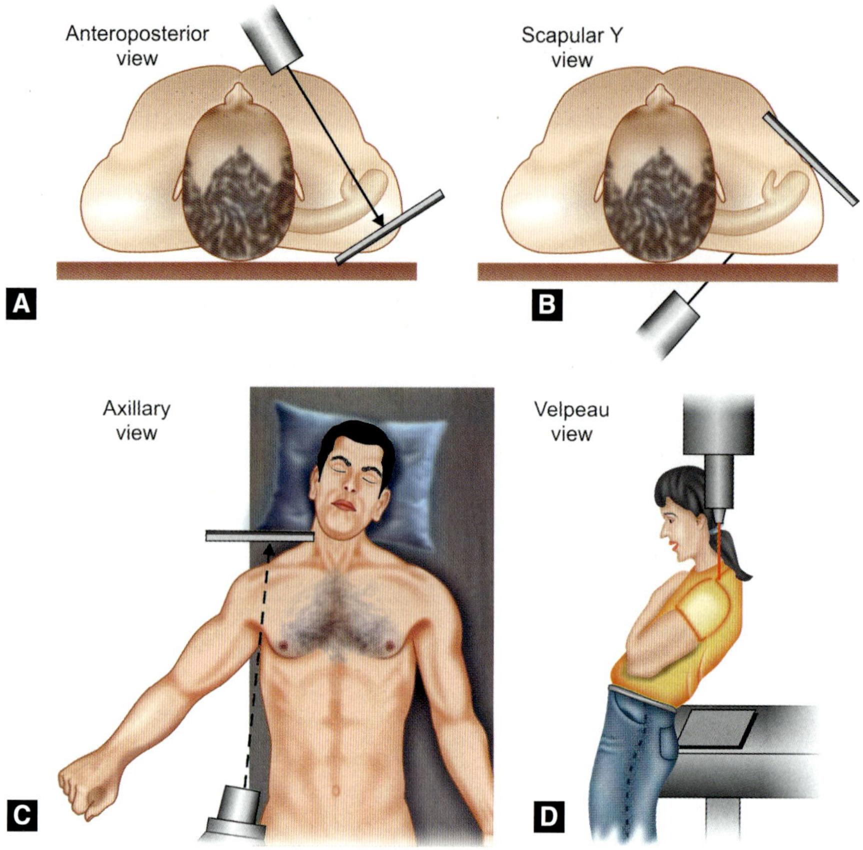

Figures 11.1A to D: (A) Radiographic examination of a proximal humerus fracture includes the standard views of the shoulder including an anteroposterior (AP); (B) lateral scapular-Y and (C) an axillary view. However, due to fracture pain abduction of the arm and positioning for the axillary view may not be possible; (D) Alternatively, a Velpeau view may be taken. The AP view is taken 30° obliquely to bring the image intensifier in line with the plane of the scapula. Similarly, the scapular Y view is taken 45° obliquely in the opposite direction to bring the image intensifier tangential to the plane of the scapula.

Surgical Indications

Proximal humerus fractures present a unique challenge to surgeons as surgical indications are poorly defined in the literature. Historically, studies are complicated by a lack of comparison groups and nebulous definitions of surgical indications. At this time, it is not clearly defined exactly which patient and fracture type perform better with surgical intervention.[7] Surgeons should always consider the patient and their expectations prior to recommending surgery, as satisfactory results have been shown from conservative care even in the face of displacement and comminution.[8]

Many fixation techniques have been described, including:

- Closed reduction and percutaneous pinning (CRPP)
- Suture fixation
- Tension band constructs
- Intramedullary nailing
- Open reduction and internal fixation (ORIF) with plate and screws
- Arthroplasty

As there is a lack of comparison studies using modern implants in the literature, evidence-based recommendations of one technique over another are not possible

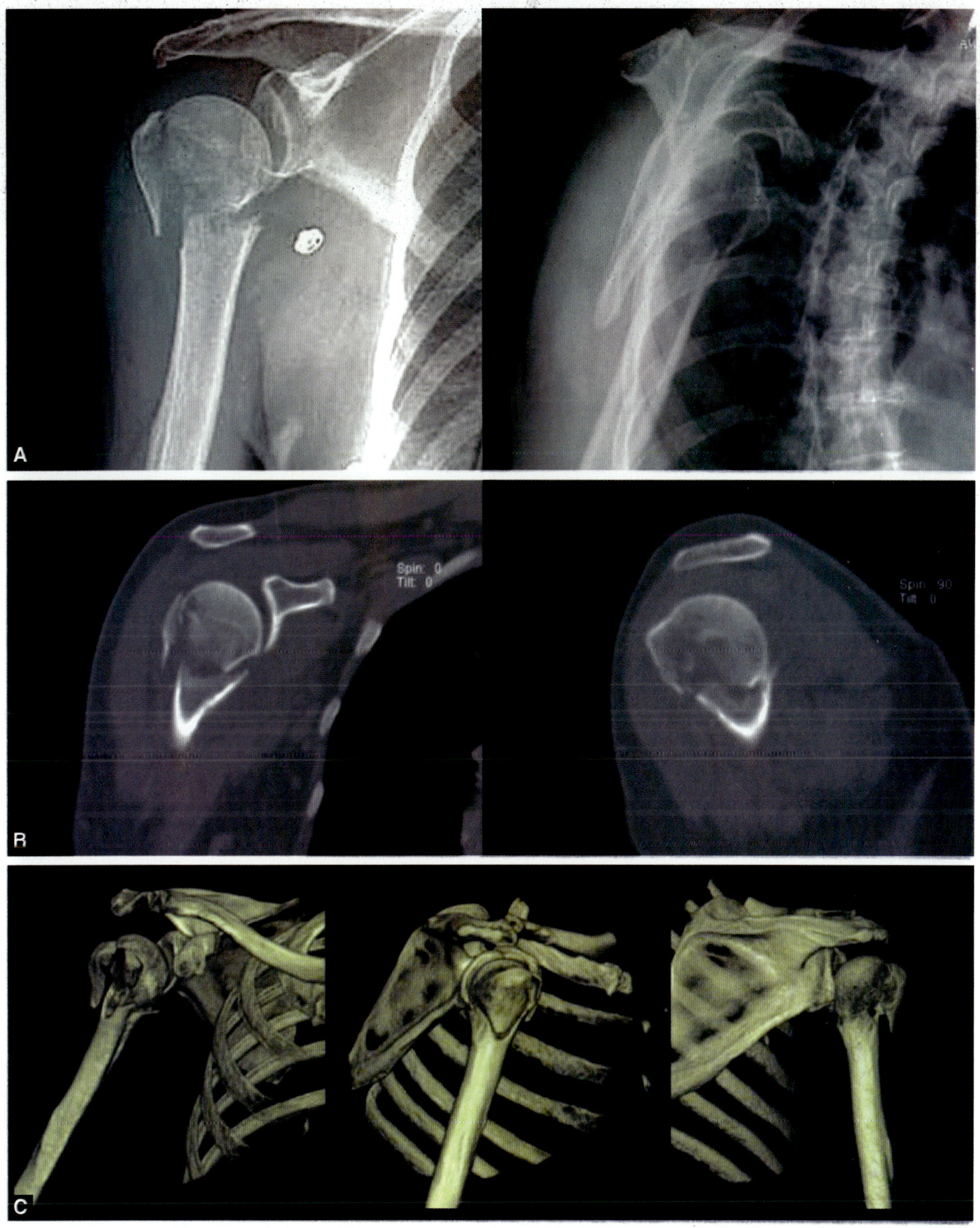

Figures 11.2A to C: When radiographic evaluation is unable to fully define the fracture, advanced imaging can improve its characterization. Note the (A) plain radiographs and the subsequent (B) standard (2D) CT images and (C) 3D CT reconstructed images.

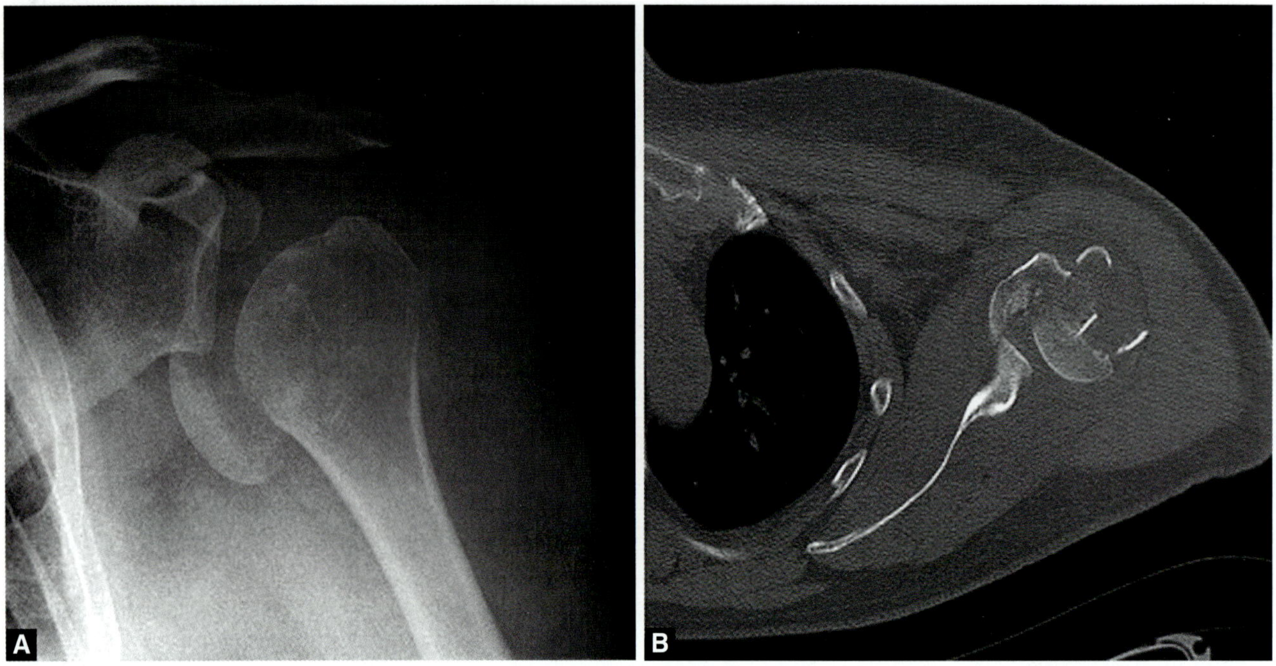

Figures 11.3A and B: Computed tomographic (CT) scans are particularly useful in articular fracture characterization. This is a 'head-splitting' proximal humerus fracture otherwise not evident with standard radiographs that was identified by CT scan.

at this time. Familiarity with several techniques and the associated pitfalls are recommended before pursuing operative intervention.

Displacement and instability are often cited as indications for surgical intervention in the literature with good outcomes reported using a multitude of techniques. Appreciation for the anatomy of the proximal humerus beyond what defines a "part" is necessary for determining surgical candidacy, selecting an implant and preoperative planning. When evaluating whether to perform surgery, one must first begin with an assessment of overall bone quality. Cortical thickness is an acceptable method of assessing the bone density of the proximal humerus.[9] This measurement is made by obtaining the average of the cortical thickness (medial and lateral) at two levels, 2 cm apart in the proximal humerus (Fig. 11.6).[9] While cortical thickness of less than 4 mm is suggestive of low density, there are no specific guidelines of what thickness is needed to tolerate implants, and surgeons must interpret the measurements along with other patient factors before making a decision on operative approach.

After assessing bone quality, the surgeon must next scrutinize the fracture pattern. Strict adherence to Neer's definition of a part can be risky; this is especially true for tuberosity fractures. It has been found that even 5 mm of superior displacement of the greater tuberosity leads to biomechanical alterations in abduction forces and 1 cm of displacement leads to abutment with the acromion.[10] Therefore, tuberosity displacements of greater than 5 mm, especially superiorly are commonly cited as surgical indications.

Simple fracture patterns have been shown to be adequately treated with a variety of techniques, including sutures alone, percutaneous pinning, locked nailing and plating. Minimally invasive techniques have been employed to counter deforming forces while minimizing surgical trauma. Using CRPP, several authors have demonstrated promising results. Many 2, 3 and 4-part fractures can be treated with this technique but contraindications exist. Fractures of the anatomic neck and head-split patterns are generally not amenable to CRPP.[11] Magovern and Ramsey recommend the following requirements to be met prior to attempting percutaneous surgery: (1) a stable closed reduction; (2) good bone stock; (3) minimal comminution; (4) an intact calcar and (5) a cooperative patient.[11]

In more complex fractures, minimally invasive techniques are not capable of maintaining reductions.

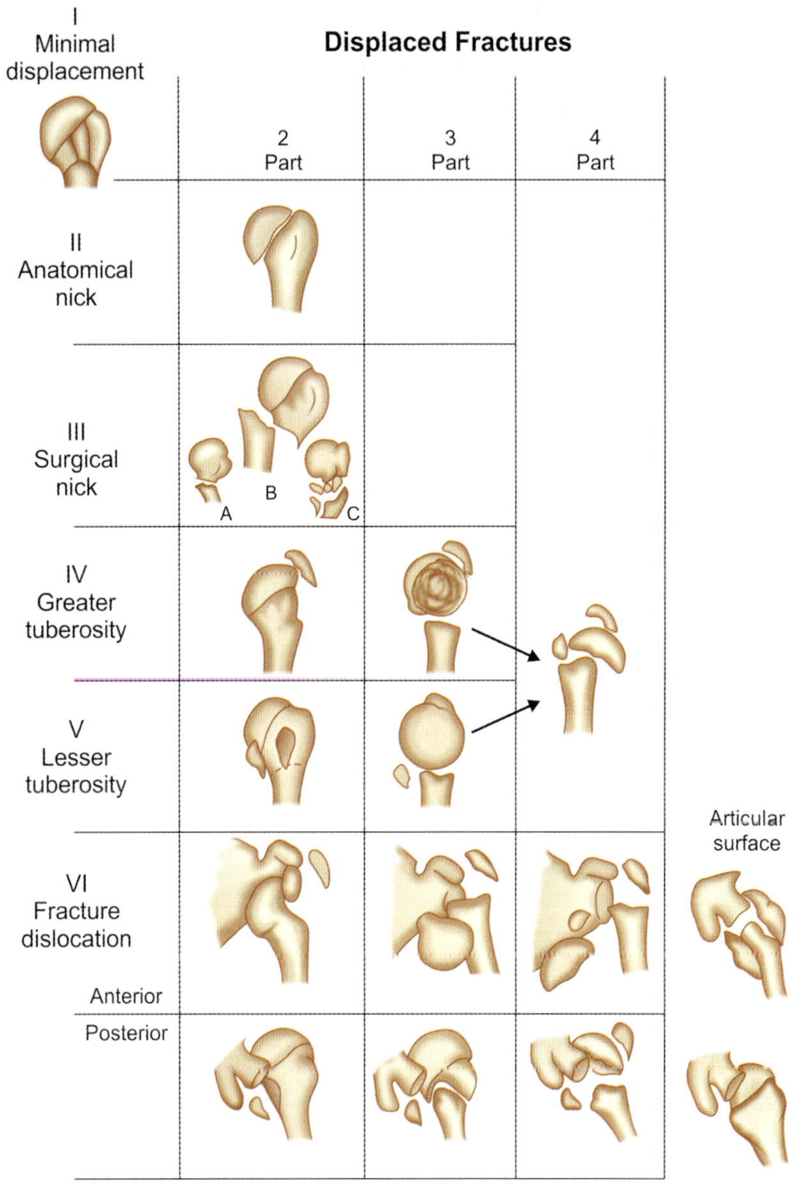

Figure 11.4: The Neer classification system for fractures of the proximal humerus; a part is identified as having more than 1 cm displacement or more than 45° of angulation.

Source: Neer CS. Displaced proximal humeral fractures. I. Classification and evaluation. J Bone Joint Surg Am. 1970;52(6):1077-89.

The most difficult question when treating these cases is whether ORIF or arthroplasty should be chosen. Classically, inability to achieve and maintain anatomic reduction and fear of avascular necrosis (AVN) has driven surgeons toward arthroplasty for complex fracture patterns. Understanding the risk factors for loss of fixation and AVN, as well as the outcomes of these complications, is important before an informed decision can be made.

As avoidance of fixation failure is critical, locked plates are the implants of choice when ORIF is chosen for severe fracture patterns. In the literature, maintenance of the reduction of greater tuberosity and reconstruction of the medial calcar are associated with improved outcomes,[12,13] and locked plates provide the best fixation strength in osteoporotic bone. While it is generally recommended ORIF be attempted if indications are met,[14] certain fracture

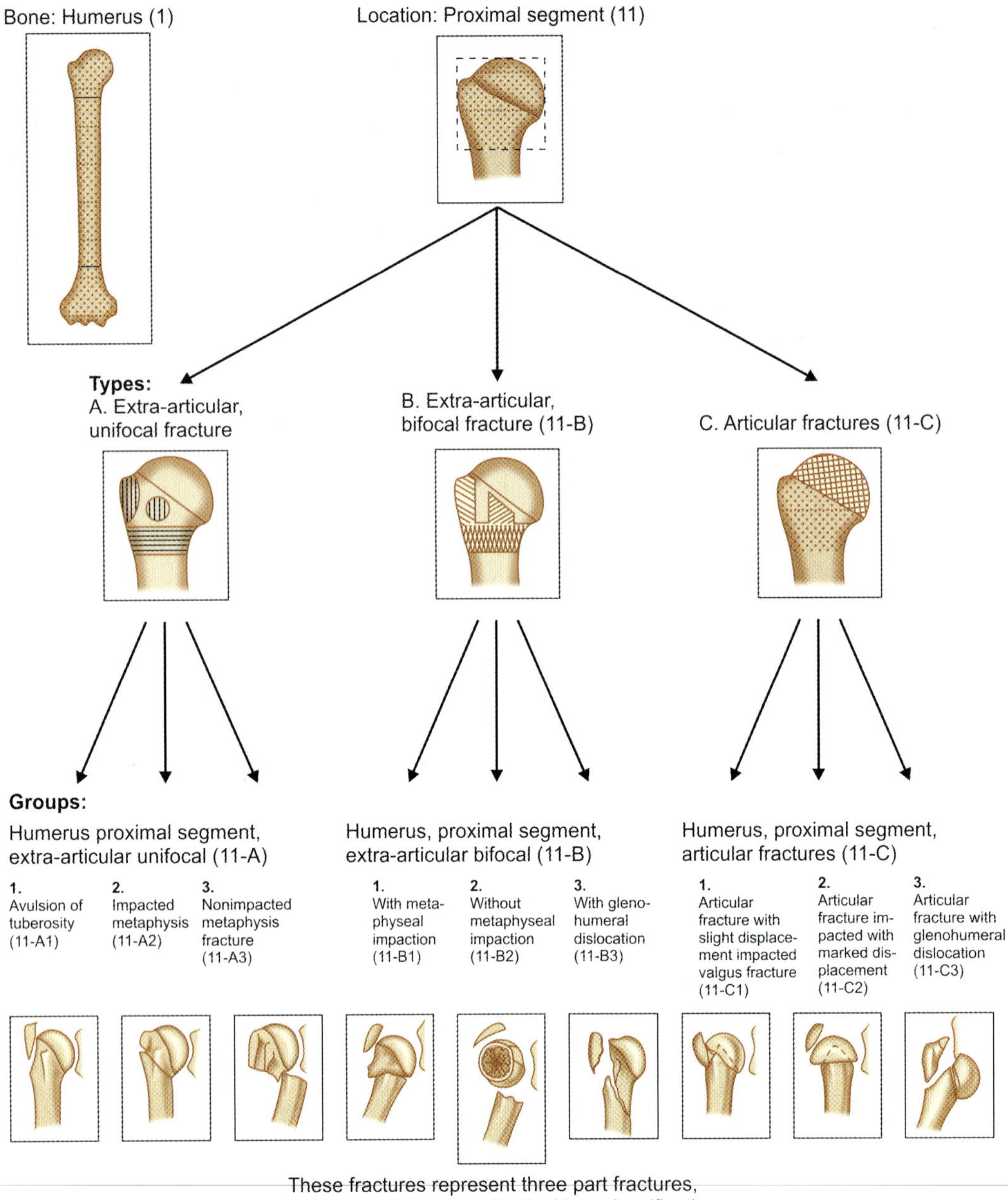

Figure 11.5: AO/OTA classification system; the humerus is designated as "1." The proximal aspect of the bone is then designated as "1." A, B, and C are assigned based on if the fracture is "unifocal", "bifocal" or "articular." Further subclassification leads to the 27 possible fracture patterns.

Source: Müller ME, Nazzarin S, Koch P. Classification AO des fractures. 1. Les os longs. New-York: Springer-Verlag; 1987.

patterns should be considered for arthroplasty. These fracture patterns include fracture-dislocations in the elderly with an anatomic neck fracture or head-splitting component. In a younger patient, however, every effort should be made to perform ORIF. Other relative contraindications to ORIF include inability to participate in therapy or dementia. As, these patients perform equally poorly with arthroplasty, the surgeons consider nonoperative modalities in these situations.

Unfortunately, no comparison studies currently exist in the literature evaluating the outcome of hemiarthroplasty as compared to modern ORIF techniques. Surgeons

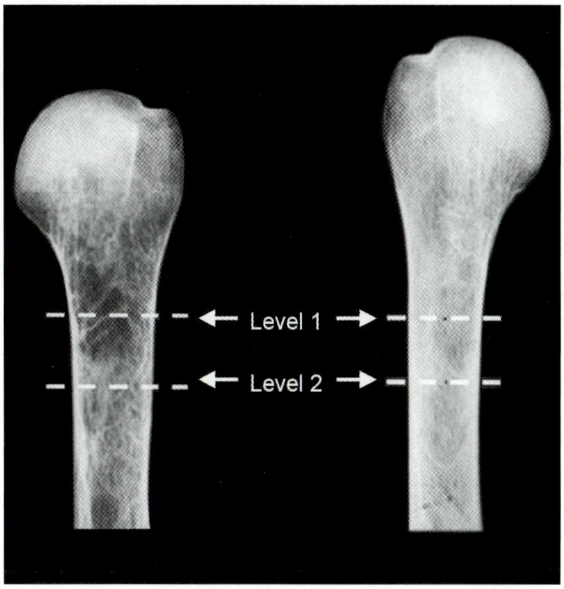

Figure 11.6: Measurement of the cortical thickness begins at the most proximal level where the endosteal surfaces of the medial and lateral cortices are still parallel before flaring into metaphyseal bone. The second measurement level is 2 cm distal to this landmark. The combined thickness is defined as the mean of the medial and lateral cortical thicknesses at the two levels.
Source: Tingart MJ, Apreleva M, von Stechow D, et al. The cortical thickness of the proximal humeral diaphysis predicts bone mineral density of the proximal humerus. J Bone Joint Surg Br. 2003;85(4):611-7.

should be aware of fracture patterns which will not allow ORIF to be performed optimally. However, careful scrutiny of the patient and the fracture should be made before proceeding with hemiarthroplasty, as the procedure can lead to marked functional limitations.[15] Contraindications to performing hemiarthroplasty include active infection, massive irreparable rotator cuff tears and paralysis of rotator cuff musculature.

Avascular necrosis is another issue that historically has influenced the choice of implant. In the literature, many fracture attributes have been implicated in AVN, including patient age, varus/valgus displacement/angulation, fracture classification, dislocation, metaphyseal extension and integrity of the medial cortex. However, no conclusive evidence has been reported on the specific fracture characteristics that reliably predicts AVN.[16] Therefore, in the active patient with sufficient bone quality for fracture reduction and fixation, ORIF should be recommended regardless of the risk of AVN.[17] This includes intra-articular fracture patterns.[17]

Occasionally, multipart proximal humerus fractures in the elderly will present with very poor soft tissue and bone stock. In these cases, the compromised tissues may prevent implanting a hemiarthroplasty secondary to the inability to repair the tuberosities and/or lack of a functioning rotator cuff. A reverse shoulder arthroplasty can be performed in this setting as a last resort.[18]

Surgical Anatomy, Positioning and Approaches

Surgical Anatomy

A thorough understanding of the osseous anatomy of the proximal humerus and the resulting fracture planes from trauma is essential prior to surgical intervention. Often, exposures do not afford complete visualization of all fragments, and a comprehensive understanding of the surrounding soft tissue envelope and bony anatomy is key to overcoming deforming forces on fracture fragments and choosing stable points of fixation. The head shaft angle of the proximal humerus is 130°. Lack of restoration of this angle will result in a varus malunion and predispose the shoulder to decreased abduction moment and potential hardware impingement if repaired.

The standard four "parts" of the proximal humerus include the head, greater tuberosity, lesser tuberosity and the humeral shaft (Fig. 11.7). Each part is susceptible to well recognized deforming patterns. When fractured through the anatomic neck, the head is often free floating and can displace out of the glenohumeral joint. The greater tuberosity typically displaces superiorly and posteriorly due to the pull of the supraspinatus and infraspinatus. The lesser tuberosity typically will displace medially due to the pull of the subscapularis. The shaft typically displaces medially due to the pull of the pectoralis major, latissimus dorsi and teres major.

Hertel describes five basic fracture planes creating 12 basic fracture patterns.[19] The planes are as follows: between the greater tuberosity and the head, between the greater tuberosity and the shaft, between the lesser tuberosity and the head, between the lesser tuberosity and the shaft, and between the lesser and greater tuberosities.[19] Surgical reduction and fixation not only require approximation of these parts along their fracture planes,

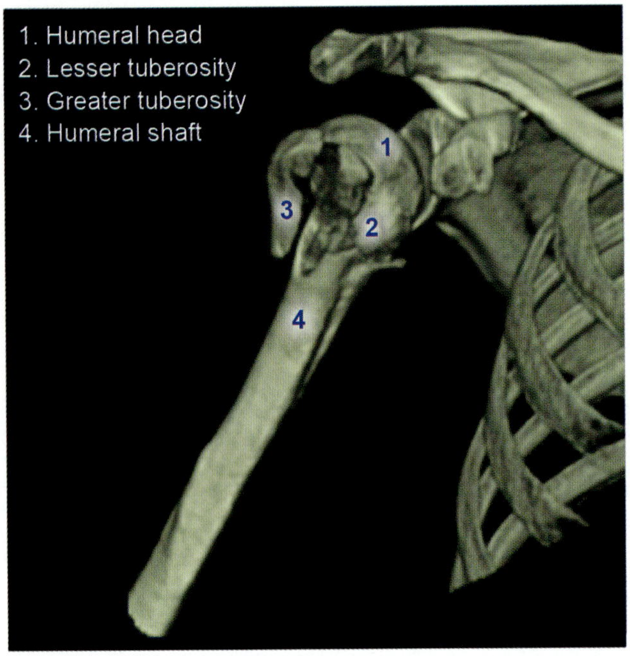

Figure 11.7: The standard parts of the proximal humerus include the head, greater tuberosity, lesser tuberosity and humeral shaft. Equally important is recognizing the calcar of the proximal humerus. The calcar represents the medial cortex of the proximal humeral shaft below the articular surface.

but also reapproximation of the calcar of the proximal humerus. The calcar represents the medial cortex of the proximal humeral shaft below the articular surface. Reapproximation of this calcar is necessary to stable fracture reduction and to avoid collapse and varus malunion of the fracture (Figs 11.8A to C).

As viability of the humeral head and tuberosity fragments is fundamental to healing, surgeons must also appreciate the vascular anatomy of the proximal humerus. The anterior and posterior humeral circumflex arteries arise as branches from the axillary artery. Occasionally, they share a common trunk.[20] The anterolateral branch of the anterior humeral circumflex artery arises from the anterior humeral circumflex artery and gives perforating branches to the proximal humerus. Older literature stressed the importance of the anterolateral branch of the anterior humeral circumflex artery saying that it provided most of the blood supply to the proximal humerus. If this was true, a far higher incidence of osteonecrosis would be expected than is evidenced, as the artery is torn in the majority of proximal humerus fractures. Rather, current evidence has suggested that the vascularity of the proximal humerus is

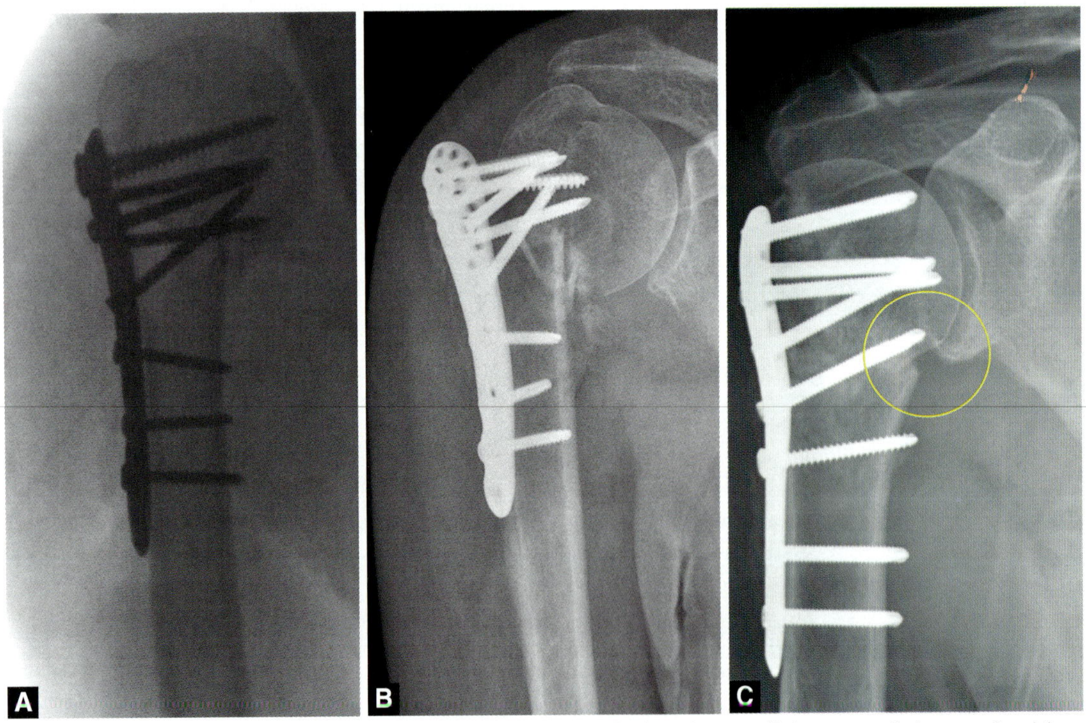

Figures 11.8A to C: The calcar of the proximal humerus is the weight-bearing medial cortex of the proximal humeral shaft. Reapproximation of this calcar is necessary to stable fracture reduction and avoidance of collapse and varus malunion of the fracture. (A and B) The images represent a case of a proximal humerus fracture repaired with low positioning of the screws in the head and poor reduction of the calcar resulting in varus collapse and redisplacement of the fracture; (C) In contrast, note in this image restoration of the calcar and appropriate position of the calcar locking screws to reinforce the construct.

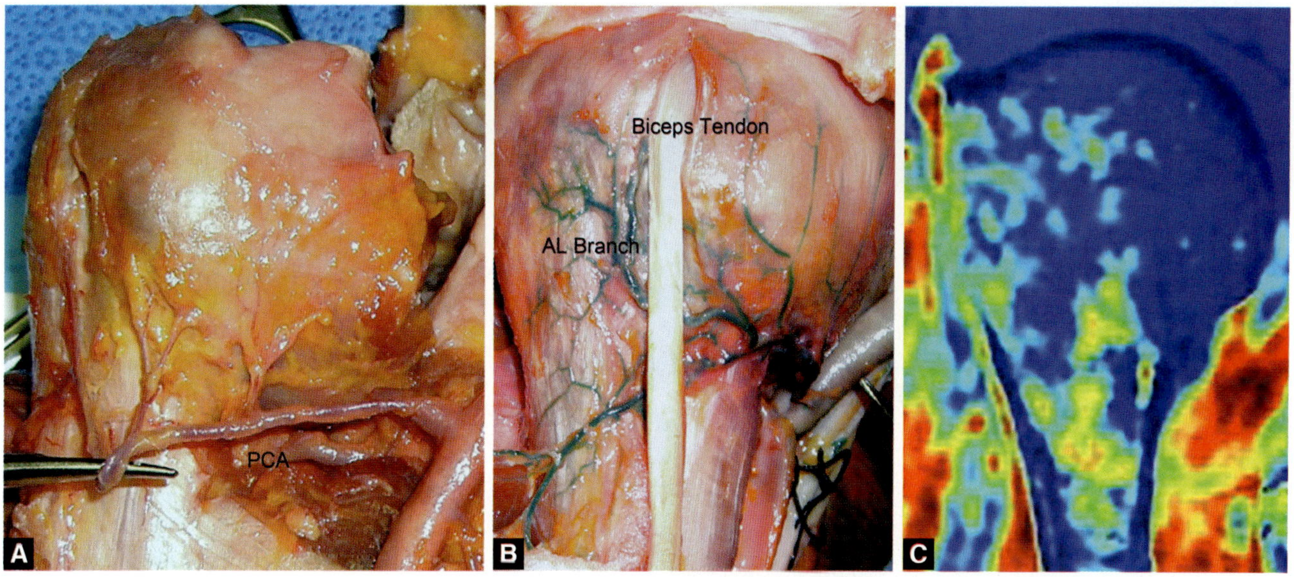

Figures 11.9A to C: The primary vascular sources for the proximal humerus consist of the anterior circumflex and the posterior circumflex vessels. (A) Posterior circumflex artery is shown branching off the axillary artery; (B) The anterior circumflex artery is shown branching off the axillary artery. The anterolateral branch is highlighted; (C) Sagittal MRI image showing posterior circumflex arterial perfusion with the anterior circumflex ligated.

increasingly dependent on the posterior humeral circumflex artery.

A recent cadaveric study using gadolinium enhanced magnetic resonance imaging (MRI) to quantify blood flow contribution found that the posterior circumflex artery supplied 64% of the blood flow to the humeral head and was the dominant blood supply to three of four humeral head quadrants (Figs 11.9A to C).[20] This may account for patterns of osteonecrosis seen clinically.[20] Care should be taken when exposing posteriomedially, and surgeons should avoid soft tissue stripping, as it may devascularize fragments from their critical blood supply.

Positioning

Multiple positioning options are available and are best selected based upon the planned surgical approach and the surgeon's preference. The deltopectoral approach is best performed utilizing a supine or beach chair position (Fig. 11.10). The anterolateral acromial approach is best performed utilizing a lateral or sloppy lateral position (Fig. 11.11). In all cases, the entire arm should be draped into the surgical field up to the neck. In addition, attention to ease of access for the image intensifier during the case should be considered regardless of position selected.

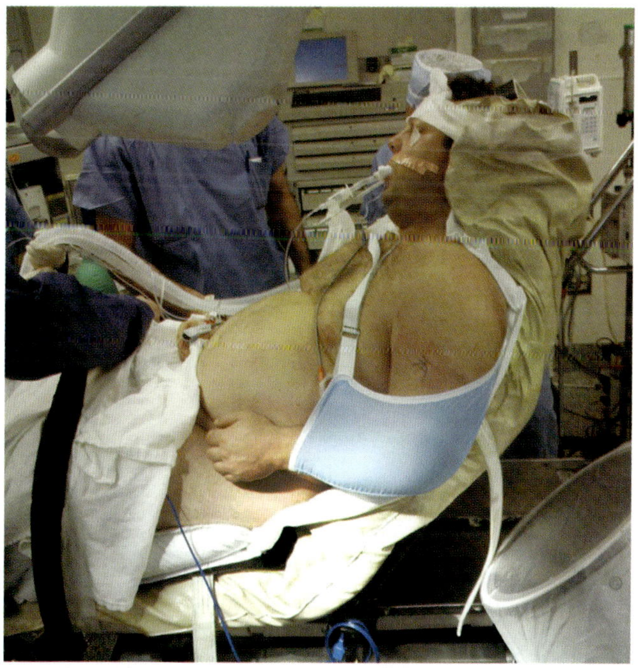

Figure 11.10: The Beach Chair position facilitates the deltopectoral approach. The patient is shown positioned as far lateral as possible on the table with a 45° torso elevation and the C-arm positioned ipsilterally. As pictured, a bean bag is helpful to assist holding a larger patient in position. The C-arm is placed as shown and draped sterilely into the case so that the machine movement interferes minimally when imaging is needed.

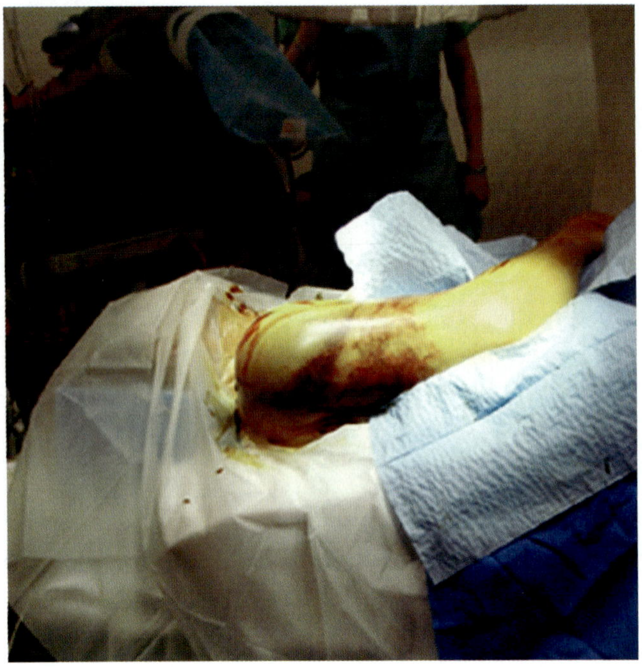

Figure 11.11: The lateral position is best indicated for the anterolateral approach. The authors prefer the 'sloppy lateral' position shown here with the patient positioned short of a full lateral position and imaging is brought in from the contralateral side of the table (seen in the background of the picture). Simple rotation of the c-arm facilitates anteroposterior and scapular-Y fluoroscopic views without moving the affected arm.

There are two major surgical approaches to the proximal humerus for fracture surgery: (1) the deltopectoral approach (Figs 11.12A to E) and (2) the anterolateral acromial approach (Figs 11.13A to C).

Approaches

The Deltopectoral Approach

The deltopectoral approach begins between the coracoid and clavicle, extending toward the insertion of the deltoid muscle while staying 1 cm lateral to the coracoid. The patient can be positioned either supine on a radiolucent table or in a beach chair position (Fig. 11.5). Small towels are placed behind the medial border of the scapula to elevate the operative shoulder from the table and improve access. The skin is divided and dissection is carried down to the cephalic vein which marks the deltopectoral interval. The vein is taken either medially or laterally depending on the surgeon's preference, and the interval is bluntly split. The clavipectoral fascia is next encountered and divided. It is advantageous to spend extra time developing the subacromial and subdeltoid spaces, thereby increasing visibility and ability to manipulate fracture fragments. If additional exposure is mandated, the rotator interval can be opened and the superior aspect of the pectoralis major insertion can be released. Further exposure can be obtained by releasing a portion of the deltoid insertion. Abduction helps to relax the deltoid and facilitate retractor placement for visualization. The long head of the biceps is a useful landmark to identify the lesser and greater tuberosity fragments.

One must be always cognizant of the musculocutaneous and axillary nerves during this exposure. The axillary nerve dives inferior to the subscapularis towards the quadrangular space at the inferomedial aspect of the humeral neck. The musculocutaneous nerve travels with the conjoined tendon and dissection should always be performed lateral to this structure and the coracoid. Careful retraction of the conjoined tendon can be performed, as long as the nerve does not undergo undue traction.

DELTOPECTORAL APPROACH: Pearls and Pitfalls

- Dissection medial to the conjoined tendon or medial retractor placement can result in inadvertent injury to the axillary artery and brachial plexus
- Medial exposure can be increased with an osteotomy of the coracoid. The coracoid process should be predrilled prior to osteotomy to facilitate repair upon closure. Note, the musculocutaneous nerve travels through the conjoined tendon and can be injured with excessive traction or retraction of the conjoined tendon
- A hemorrhagic bursa overlying the proximal humerus is common with fractures and should be excised to improve visualization
- Homan retractors are best placed in the subacromial space and lateral to the greater tuberosity
- The biceps tendon is often subluxed out of the bicipital groove with fractures and should be identified and tagged
- Exposure can be enhanced with partially releasing the deltoid and pectoralis major off of the humeral shaft. Furthermore, shoulder abduction will decrease deltoid tension

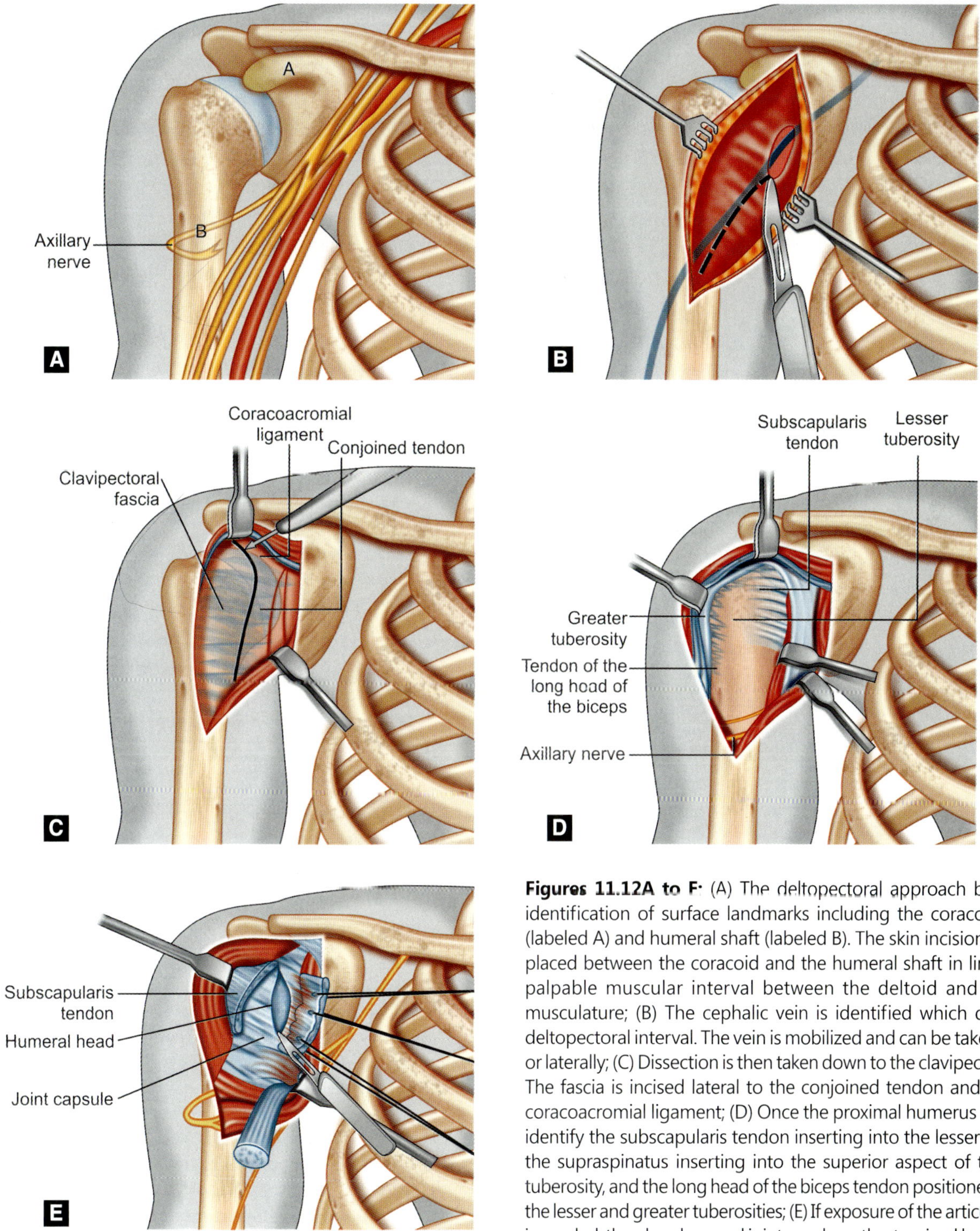

Figures 11.12A to F: (A) The deltopectoral approach begins with identification of surface landmarks including the coracoid process (labeled A) and humeral shaft (labeled B). The skin incision should be placed between the coracoid and the humeral shaft in line with the palpable muscular interval between the deltoid and pectoralis musculature; (B) The cephalic vein is identified which defines the deltopectoral interval. The vein is mobilized and can be taken medially or laterally; (C) Dissection is then taken down to the clavipectoral fascia. The fascia is incised lateral to the conjoined tendon and below the coracoacromial ligament; (D) Once the proximal humerus is exposed, identify the subscapularis tendon inserting into the lesser tuberosity, the supraspinatus inserting into the superior aspect of the greater tuberosity, and the long head of the biceps tendon positioned between the lesser and greater tuberosities; (E) If exposure of the articular surface is needed, the glenohumeral joint may be arthrotomized longitudinally after the subscapularis is released, tagged and reflected off of the lesser tuberosity. Furthermore, the coracoid process can be osteotomized and reflected distally.

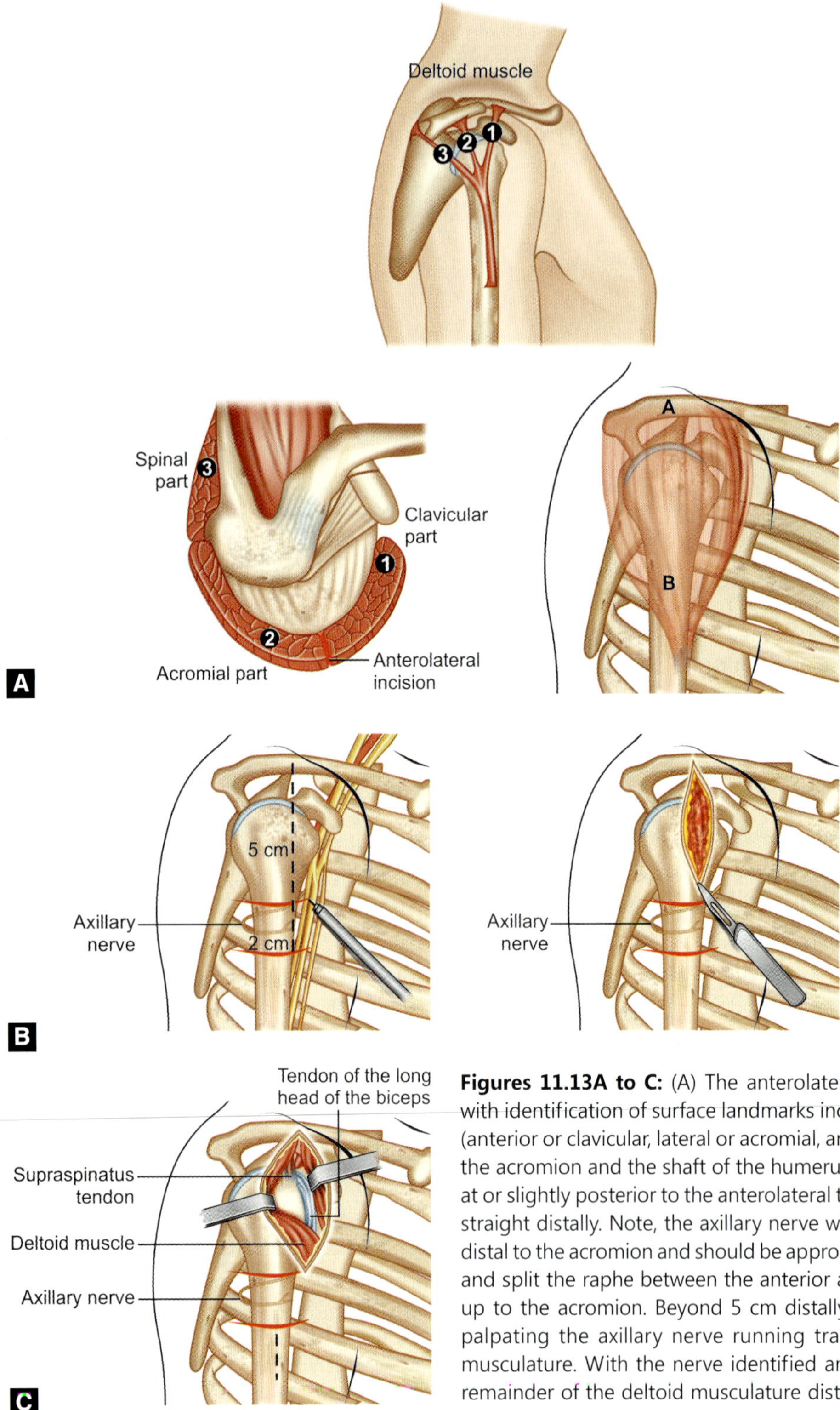

Figures 11.13A to C: (A) The anterolateral (acromial) approach begins with identification of surface landmarks including the heads of the deltoid (anterior or clavicular, lateral or acromial, and posterior or spinal), the tip of the acromion and the shaft of the humerus; (B) The skin incision is placed at or slightly posterior to the anterolateral tip of the acromion and directed straight distally. Note, the axillary nerve will reside approximately 5–7 cm distal to the acromion and should be appropriately marked out; (C) Develop and split the raphe between the anterior and lateral heads of the deltoid up to the acromion. Beyond 5 cm distally, identify the axillary nerve by palpating the axillary nerve running transversely deep to the deltoid musculature. With the nerve identified and protected, carefully split the remainder of the deltoid musculature distally. The axillary nerve will then be in the field crossing at the level of the surgical neck of the humerus.

The Anterolateral (Acromial) Approach

An alternative to the deltopectoral approach is the anterolateral acromial approach.[21] The patient may be placed in a supine, sloppy lateral or in beach chair position. The authors' choice is the sloppy lateral position with the c-arm positioned on the opposite side of the table (Fig. 11.11). The incision is marked starting 1 cm posterior to the anterolateral border of the acromion and proceeds, distall in line with the humeral shaft for about 10 cm. Soft tissues are divided to the level of the deltoid fascia. Here, the raphe between the anterior and lateral heads of the deltoid is identified and the interval is bluntly split. This raphe can be palpated and identified at the most lateral aspect of the anterior border of the acromion. In the proximal aspect of the wound, the bursa is identified beneath the deltoid fascia and divided. One must remain mindful that the axillary nerve crosses within the deltoid about 5–7 cm distal to the acromion. Once the proximal split has been developed, a finger is then used to palpate the axillary nerve running transversely deep in the deltoid tissue. The nerve then can be freed on its deep surface from the humerus with a blunt tipped instrument, and distally the deltoid can be safely divided below the nerve along the shaft, making sure to stay within the interval between the anterior and middle heads. Skeletonizing the nerve is not necessary (Fig. 11.14).

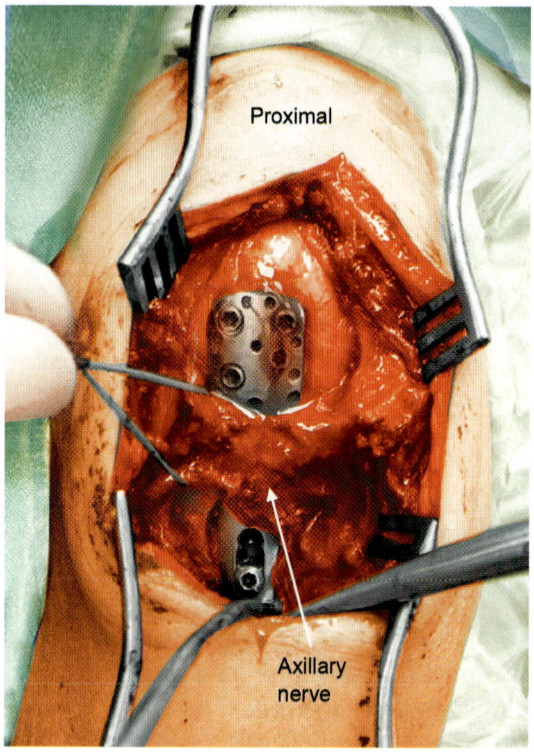

Figure 11.14: Excellent visualization can be obtained from the anterolateral approach as shown. A vessel loop has been passed around the axillary nerve that has not been skeletonized. A plate can be easily positioned under the nerve after it has been appropriately mobilized.

ANTEROLATERAL APPROACH: Pearls and Pitfalls

- This approach is useful for both plate and intramedullary fixation of proximal humerus fractures
- Dissection beyond 5 cm distal to the acromion should be taken with care and the axillary nerve should be directly identified and protected
- A hemorrhagic bursa overlying the proximal humerus is common with fractures and should be excised to improve visualization
- Exposure can be enhanced by partially releasing the deltoid insertion off of the humeral shaft

Surgical Techniques

Technique 1: Open Reduction Internal Fixation

Preoperative Planning

Prior to initiating fracture surgery, a thorough understanding of the fracture pattern, bone quality and surrounding anatomy should be attained. Often, complex proximal humeral fracture patterns are difficult to interpret on plain films alone, and a CT scan examination facilitates the planning phase of the case. CT scans are particularly useful in the evaluation of articular injuries.

In terms of fracture pattern, the location of the individual fragments has implications during a case. Far posterior displacement of the greater tuberosity and posterior humeral head dislocations can be proved extremely challenging to address from a deltopectoral approach alone. The dissection and manipulation required to address these issues are not only technically difficult but also potentially dangerous to the underlying bone stock and its vascularity. Therefore, the deltopectoral approach is not always the best choice for exposure and one must be familiar with alternate approaches, such as the anterolateral approach.

It is also important to assess overall bone quality preoperatively. As discussed in the surgical indication section of this chapter, cortical thickness provides a reasonable estimation of overall bone density.[9] Bony fragments must be able to tolerate alignment maneuvers and provisional fixation in order to achieve acceptable reductions prior to definitive fixation. In the face of small bone fragments and poor bone stock, pointed reduction clamps should not be used in favor of soft tissue sutures to achieve reduction and ultimate fixation.

In addition to addressing the above issues, preoperative planning includes preparing for instruments and equipment which may be required during the case. Fixed angle locking plates provide optimal stability for the proximal humerus. Precontoured locked periarticular plates are the authors' implant of choice when open reduction is required in this area of the body. Blunt retractors, nonabsorbable sutures and small *Kirschner* wire (K-wires) should also be made available prior to the case, and their utility will be described in detail below.

Finally, as these patients are often elderly with multiple medical problems, attention must be directed toward prevention and management of potential perioperative complications. A metabolic bone evaluation is helpful to address underlying bone health, as osteoporosis is common in this patient cohort.

Technique

Preoperative antibiotics are infused within 1 hour of skin incision and either a regional block or general anesthetic is administered. The authors prefer the anterolateral acromial approach because it affords superior access to displaced fragments and offers ease of plate placement, as the approach brings the surgeon directly onto the lateral aspect of the humerus. The surgeons' position of choice is a "sloppy lateral" with contralateral c-arm positioning (Fig. 11.11). The deltopectoral approach (Figs 11.12A to E) is the most commonly used approach for this procedure and is equally acceptable and best performed supine or in a beach chair position.

A 10 cm incision is made starting from the anterolateral corner of the acromion. The standard anterolateral approach, as previously described (Figs 11.13A to C), is performed down to the subdeltoid bursa. The bursa is carefully resected as not to injure the underlying rotator cuff tissue. This part of the exposure takes place in the superior 2–3 cm of the raphe to ensure that the axillary nerve is safely crossing distally. Blunt dissection, distally with a finger easily identifies the nerve on the deep surface of the deltoid. Once the nerve is identified, dissection can be progressed distal to the nerve with blunt instruments, staying within the interval between the anterior and lateral heads of the deltoid.

Attention is then directed towards identifying and freeing the individual fracture fragments. One of the benefits of the anterolateral acromial approach is that it provides direct exposure to the tuberosities and the shaft. Large nonabsorbable tag sutures can then be placed in the subscapularis, supraspinatus and infraspinatus insertions to assist with mobilization and reduction while preserving the often poor underlying bone stock of the tuberosities. Access to the head fragment can then be gained through retraction of the tuberosities posteriorly and anteriorly. Elevator instruments can then be used to bring the head out of varus or valgus. At this stage, liberal use of provisional K-wires for joysticks and temporary fixation is valuable. As quality of reduction has been associated with improved outcomes, time should be spent on this stage of the case to optimize fragment position and restore the calcar alignment. Orthogonal fluoroscopic confirmation of reduction is essential at this stage as the shaft is often still aligned in an apex-anterior position. Shoulder abduction and anterior pressure on the humerus assist in reducing this deformity.

The plate may now be brought into the field and slid under the axillary nerve (Fig. 11.14). One should be familiar with the subtle design differences between different plating systems to ensure that plate position is optimized; plates placed too proximally can lead to impingement. Provisional K-wires through the plate into the proximal segment assist in keeping the plate aligned as preparation for screw placement commences. It is beneficial to bring the limbs of the tag sutures through plate holes at this stage, as it is often difficult once screws have been placed. Fluoroscopy again should be used to confirm reduction. The first screw placed is typically a cortical screw through the slotted hole distal to the fracture. This maneuver turns the locking plate into a reduction tool as the screw is sealed. Attention should be paid to the tuberosity and calcar reduction again at this stage, as the shaft can be pulled too far laterally with this step.

After confirmation of plate positioning and fracture reduction, locking screws can then be placed into the head

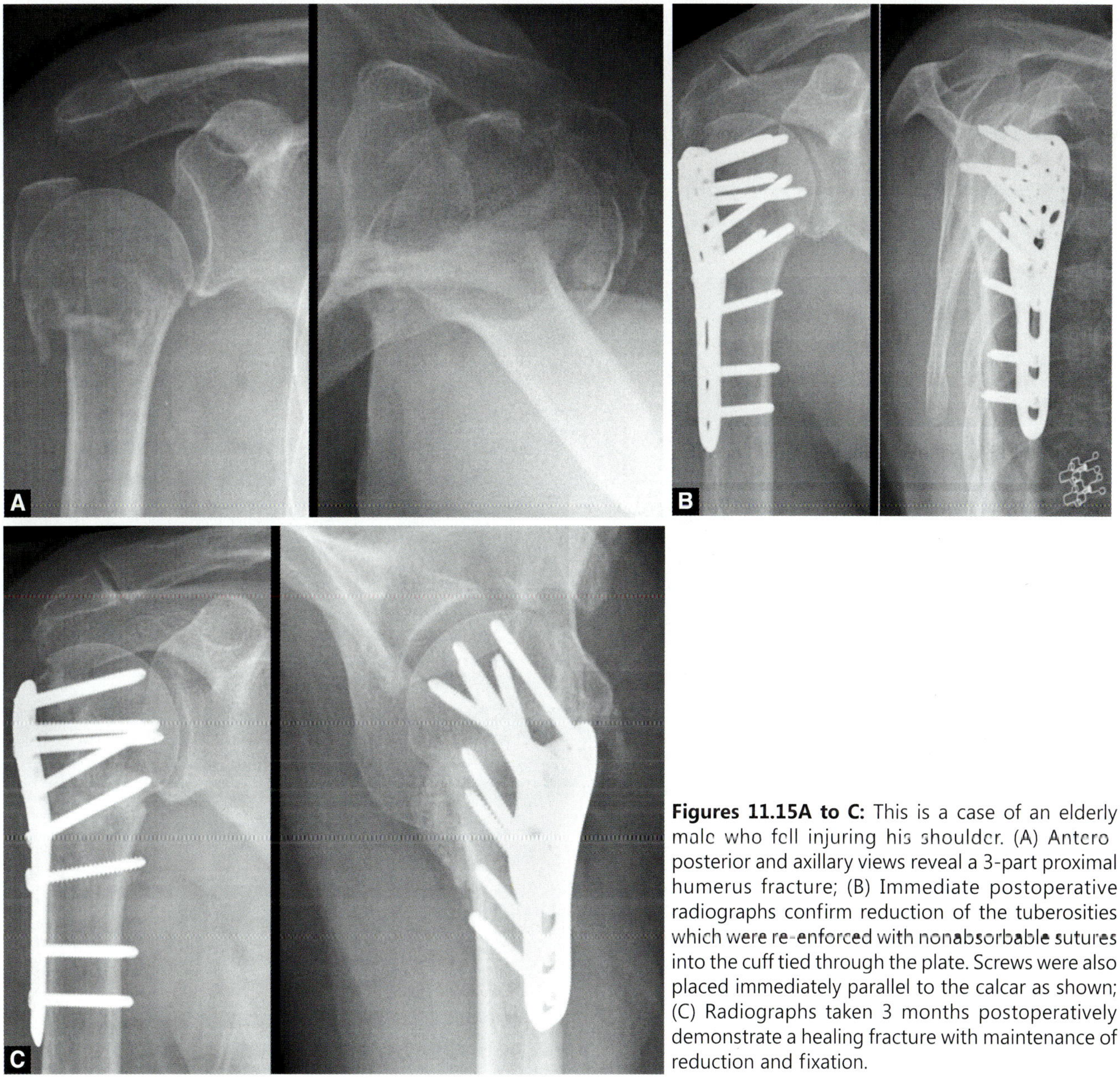

Figures 11.15A to C: This is a case of an elderly male who fell injuring his shoulder. (A) Antero posterior and axillary views reveal a 3-part proximal humerus fracture; (B) Immediate postoperative radiographs confirm reduction of the tuberosities which were re-enforced with nonabsorbable sutures into the cuff tied through the plate. Screws were also placed immediately parallel to the calcar as shown; (C) Radiographs taken 3 months postoperatively demonstrate a healing fracture with maintenance of reduction and fixation.

segment (Figs 11.15A to C). The most important of these screws is the one placed obliquely along the calcar, especially if this area is comminuted. Restoration of this medial buttress has been associated with improved outcomes and is an essential aspect of ORIF.[22] Once screws have been placed, the tag sutures are tied over the plate, further fixing the tuberosity fragments.

In the face of poor bone stock, bone graft substitutes have been used to enhance stability and encourage bone ingrowth. When bone quality is in question or if there is comminution of the medial calcar, the authors' preference is to augment the construct with a structural fibular allograft (Figs 11.16A to D). This can be impacted medially to re-enforce the calcar and held in position with screws through the plate. Fine tuning of the position of the allograft can be done with a push screw or a joystick K-wire inserted into the allograft piece. Biomechanical studies evaluating this technique have found reduced intercyclic motion, fragment migration and plastic deformation when compared to plating alone.[23] In a clinical series of 34 patients treated with an endosteal implant, only one loss of reduction was noted (2.8%) and only one patient went on to have partial AVN (2.8%).[24]

Proximal humerus fractures with associated articular fractures should be assessed with advanced imaging preoperatively. In cases with displaced articular fractures, as in the case of a "head-split" fracture, a deltopectoral approach (Figs 11.12A to E) should be considered as it provides greater access to the articular head and the glenohumeral joint (Figs 11.17A to F). With articular fractures, the articular surface is reduced and fixed prior to fixation of the tuberosities and shaft. The articular fracture repair can then be reinforced with application of a standard locking plate. However, in cases with two or

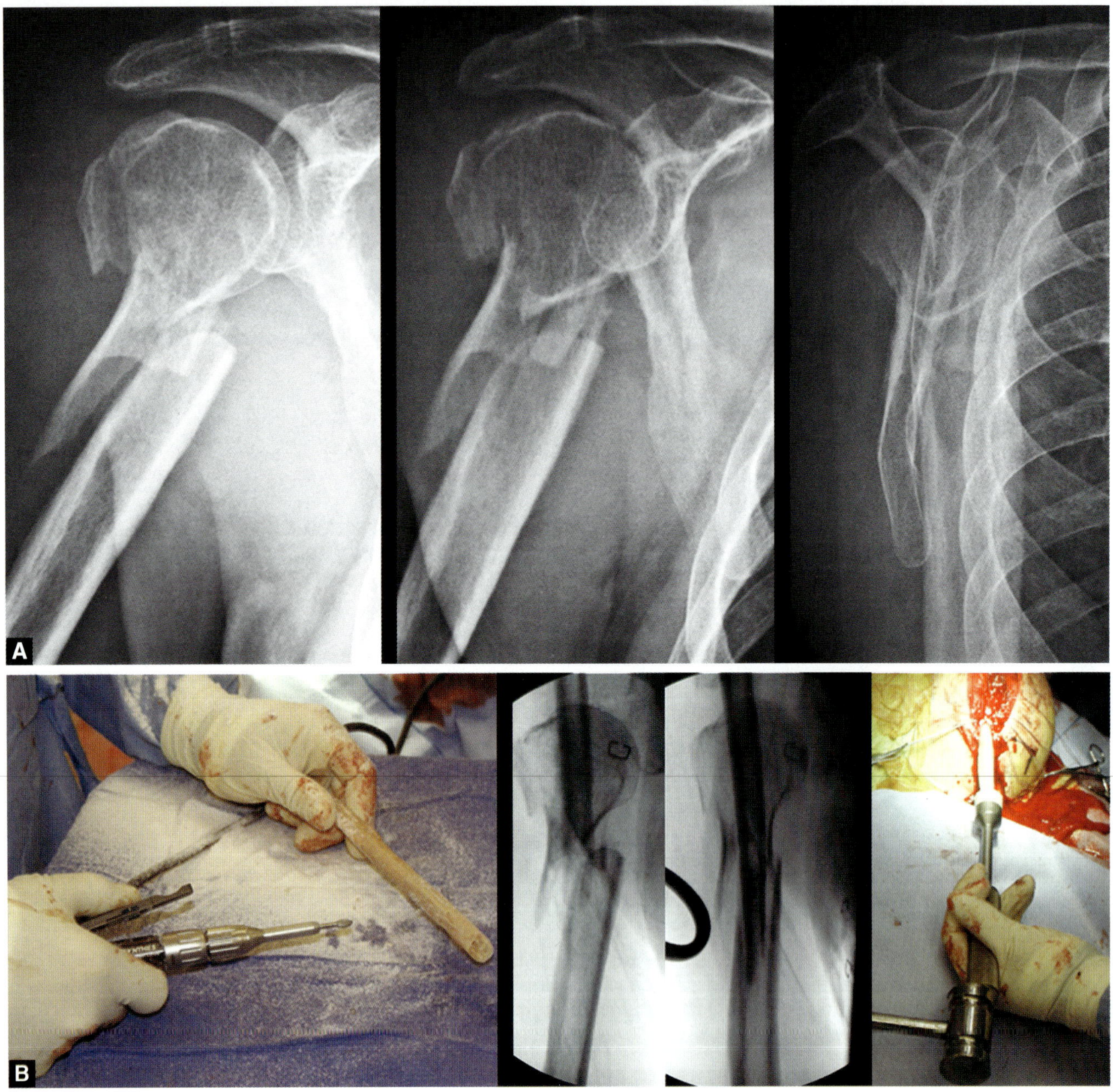

Figures 11.16A and B

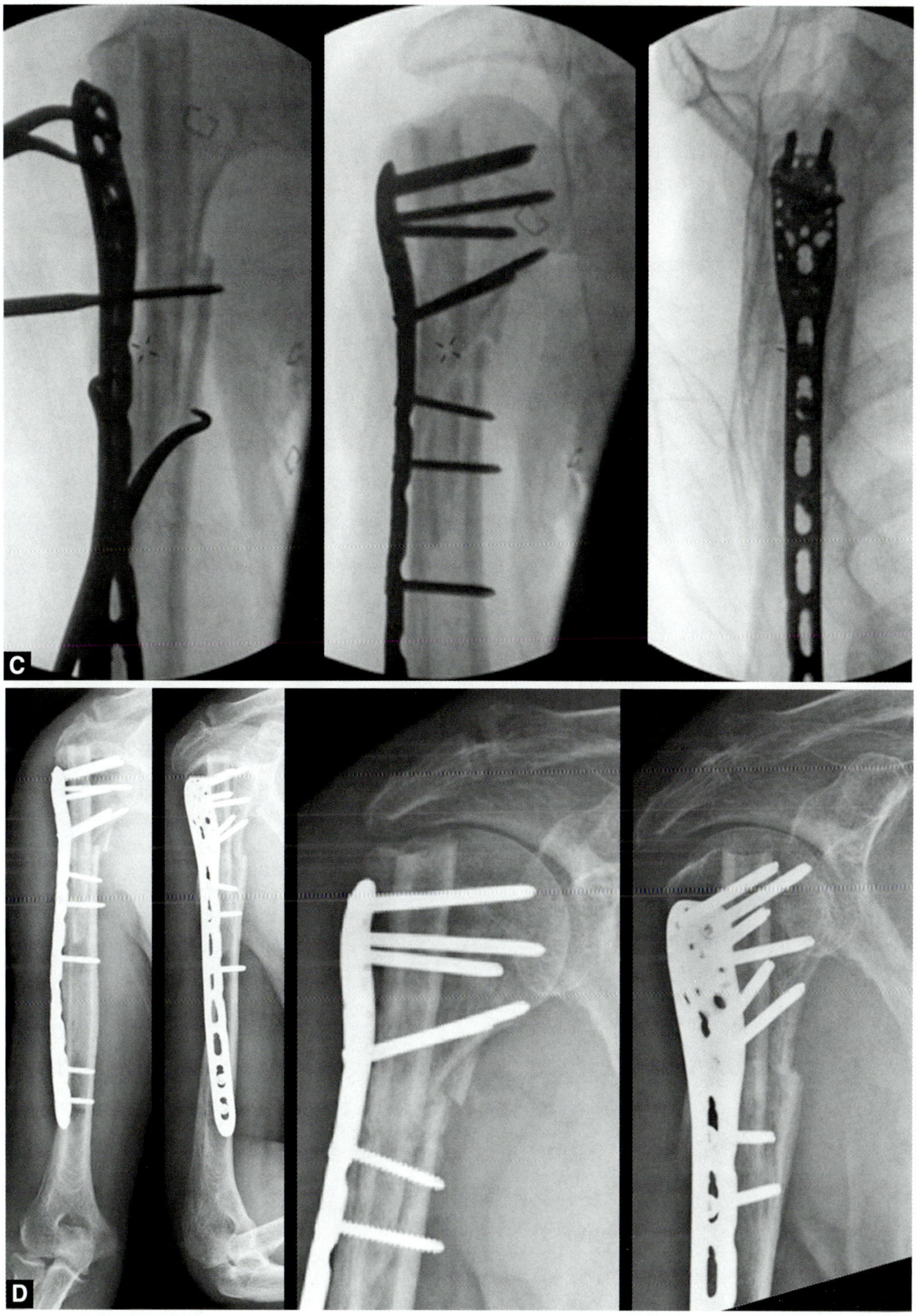

Figures 11.16A to D: This is a case of an elderly female with a history of osteoporosis who fell injuring her shoulder. (A) Radiographs demonstrate a comminuted fracture of the proximal humerus with poor bone quality; (B) To augment the strength of the construct, a fibular allograft is contoured with a burr and impacted through the fracture site into position along the medial calcar. Threaded pins can be inserted into the fragment acting as joysticks during the tamping process to assist with positioning. If the fracture has been perfectly reduced prior to the decision to place the graft, the starting point for allograft entry should be similar for that of a humeral nail at the top of the humeral head; (C) Intraoperative fluoroscopic imaging of clamps and a cortical screw in the distal segment (through the fibula) dialing in the reduction. Intraoperative anteroposterior and scapula Y view of the final construct with screws through the fibula and along the calcar; (D) Postoperative radiographs illustrating the final construct.

more articular fragments or articular comminution, hemiarthroplasty should be considered instead for management of the fracture.

Closure is then performed over a deep suction drain. Several interrupted sutures are placed in the superficial deltoid fascia to reapproximate the raphe and cover the plate. The superficial skin layer is closed with buried 3-0 interrupted absorbable sutures and 4-0 nylon on the outer skin layer.

Rehabilitation orders must be made with the fracture pattern in mind. Pendulum and light active-assisted modalities are begun immediately postoperatively. In the scenario of lesser tuberosity repair, active internal and passive external ROM exercise should be limited. Greater tuberosity repair

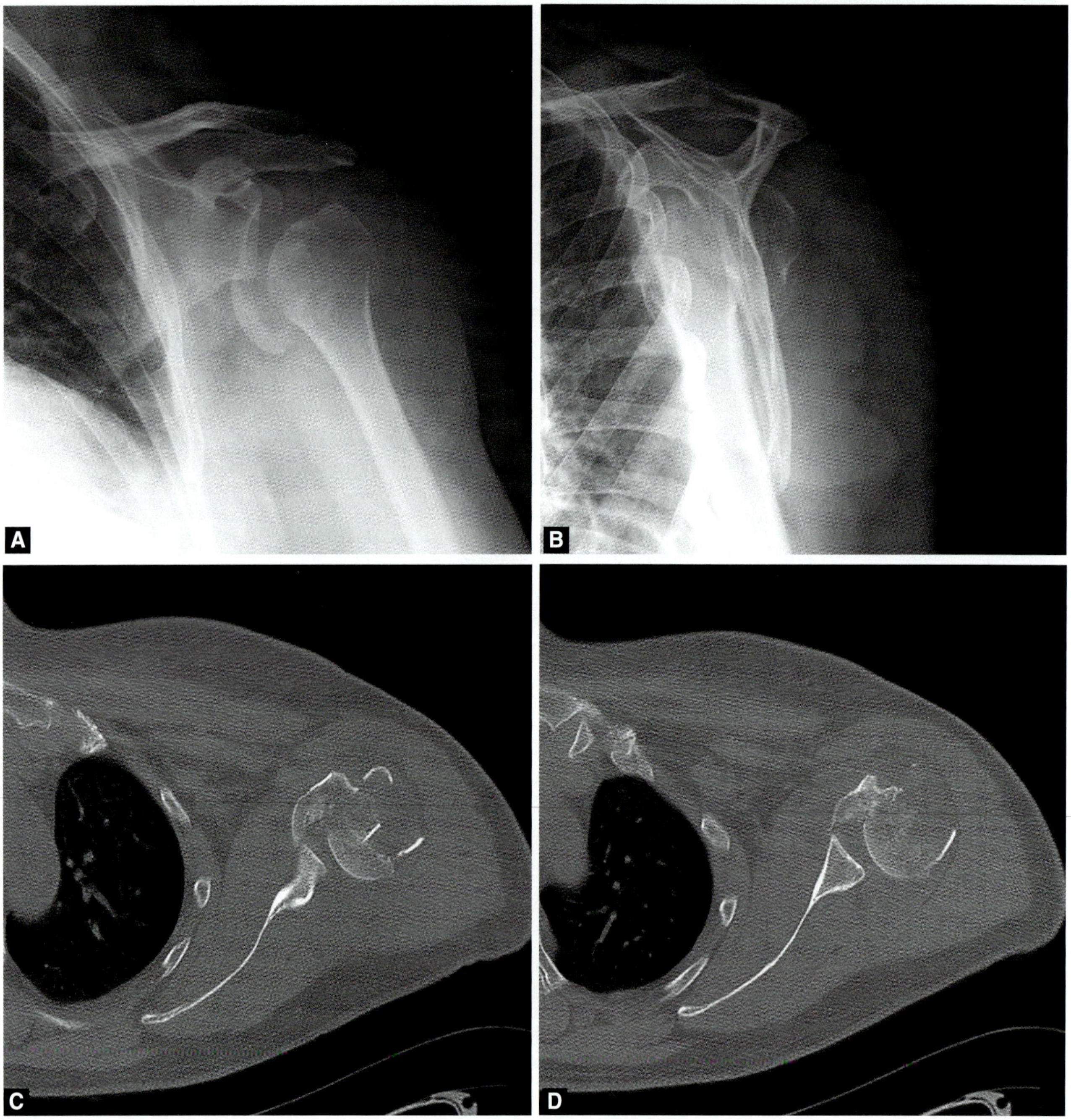

Figures 11.17A to D

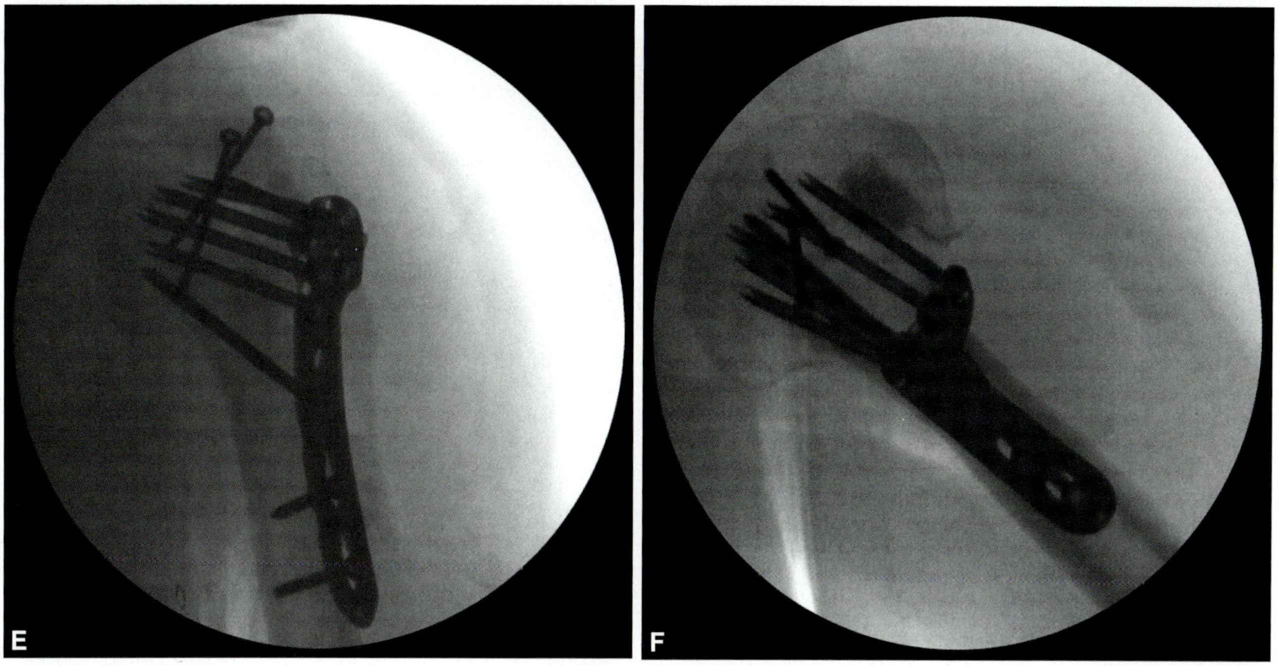

Figures 11.17A to F: This is a case of a young female involved in a high energy injury who incurred a "head-splitting" proximal humerus fracture. (A and B) Standard radiographs demonstrated a proximal humerus fracture with a displaced articular head fragment through the anatomic neck; (C and D) CT scanning confirmed a displaced "head-split" fracture with minimal comminution. The fracture was subsequently approached with a deltopectoral approach. The glenohumeral joint was arthrotomized and the articular head-split was reduced directly and repaired with screws. The head was then reduced to the shaft and tuberosities and repaired using a standard locking plate; (E and F) Intraoperative c-arm imaging confirms reduction of the articular fracture, tuberosities, shaft, appropriate position of the calcar screw, and restoration of the 130° neck-shaft angle of the proximal humerus.
Courtesy: Saqib Rehman

requires limitation of active abduction and external rotation. Typically, active ROM can be initiated at 6 weeks, and progressive resistance exercise can be initiated at 12 weeks.

ORIF: Pearls and Pitfalls

- Know the "personality" of the fracture prior to surgery. Obtain CT scans if necessary, particularly if articular involvement is suspected
- Confirm adequate orthogonal fluoroscopy prior to draping
- Avoid large clamps in favor of K-wire joysticks and cuff tag sutures for reduction
- Pay close attention to reduction of the calcar and tuberosities and restoration of the normal neck shaft angle of 130° prior to plate and screw placement
- The plate should be positioned lateral to the biceps tendon and bicipital groove and below the level of the greater tuberosity. Too proximal placement will result in hardware impingement with shoulder abduction. Too distal placement of the plate will result in inferior placement of the locking screws
- Consider augmenting the construct with a structural fibular allograft if poor bone stock or calcar comminution are encountered

Technique 2: Intramedullary Nailing

Preoperative Planning

A thorough understanding of the fracture pattern, bone quality and surrounding anatomy should be attained. The authors recommend the use of intramedullary fixation only with 1 or 2-part proximal humerus fractures involving the surgical neck. However, this technique may be utilized with care in cases with associated tuberosity fractures that are non or minimally displaced. Furthermore, the fracture must be amenable to closed reduction if intramedullary fixation is to be utilized. However, appropriate equipment for plate fixation should be available during the procedure in case adequate closed reduction of the fracture cannot be achieved. The authors recommend utilizing a mini anterolateral acromial approach limited to exposure of the humeral head superior to the axillary nerve. If conversion to plate fixation is necessary the approach can be extended in standard fashion.

Various intramedullary nails can be utilized and the specific insertion guide should follow the manufacturers' instructions. Both short and long intramedullary nails can be used. The nail should pass below a minimum length of at least two bicortical lengths.

Technique

Either a beach chair or supine position can be chosen for nail insertion (Figs 11.18A and B). The incision is placed anterolateral to the acromion in either a transverse or longitudinal fashion. The deltoid is split through the raphe between the anterior and lateral heads of the deltoid. The split should be limited to no more than 5 cm to avoid inadvertent injury to the axillary nerve. The subacromial bursa overlies the greater tuberosity and is often hemorrhagic. It should be excised with care to expose the greater tuberosity and rotator cuff.

Once adequate fracture reduction has been achieved, a longitudinal split is placed in the rotator cuff and a guidewire or awl is introduced into the humeral head (Figs 11.19A to F). While maintaining diligent fracture reduction the canal is reamed to the adequate size of the nail as per the manufacturer's guide. The canal length is measured and the nail assembled on the jig is inserted. Once adequately countersunk, the nail is fixed proximal to the fracture with screw placement into the humeral head. Humeral fracture length and rotation is then fixed by placing a bicortical interlocking screw distal to the fracture into the humeral shaft.

Closure is initiated with diligent repair of the rotator cuff split using nonabsorbable zero suture. Several 2-0 interrupted absorbable sutures are then placed in the superficial deltoid fascia to reapproximate the raphe and cover the plate. The superficial skin layer is closed with buried 3-0 interrupted absorbable sutures and 4-0 nylon on the outer skin layer.

Rehabilitation orders must be made with the fracture pattern in mind. Typically early motion is initiated when intramedullary fixation is utilized. Pendulum and light active-assisted modalities are begun immediately postoperatively. Typically, active ROM can be initiated at 6 weeks, and progressive resistance exercise can be initiated at 12 weeks.

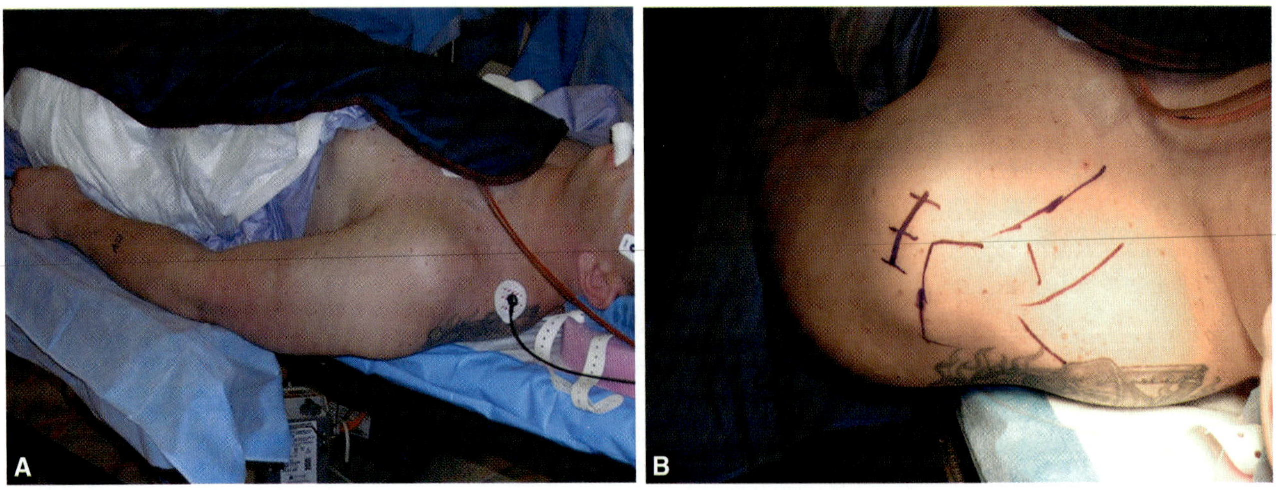

Figures 11.18A and B: Intramedullary fixation can be performed in either a beach chair or supine position. (A) A supine position is selected here with a radiolucent table. A large c-arm is placed on the opposite side to provide orthogonal imaging during the case; (B) The skin incision correlates to the anterolateral approach to the humerus. In this case a transverse incision is utilized but a longitudinal incision can also be utilized and affords easier extension to a full anterolateral approach for potential conversion to plate fixation.

Courtesy: Asif M Ilyas

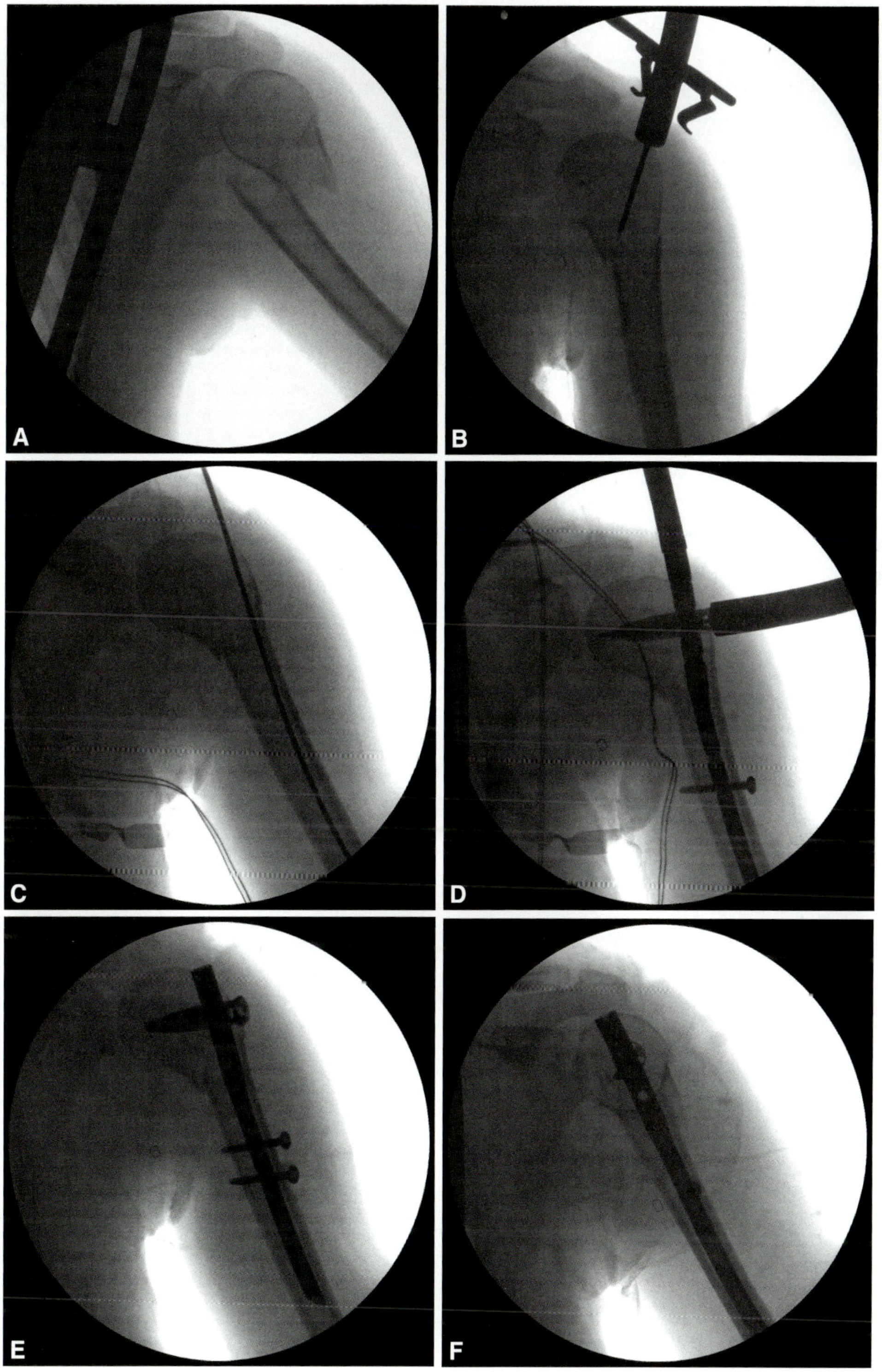

Figures 11.19A to F: (A) This is a case of a young female who fell from a height incurring a displaced 2-part fracture through the surgical neck with an associated nondisplaced greater tuberosity fracture. After a standard anterolateral approach to the proximal humerus a guidewire is placed into the reduced humeral head; (B) The head is then opened with a cannulated drill or awl; (C) A guidewire is placed across the reduced fracture; (D) Once adequately countersunk, screws are placed above and below the fracture line to lock in rotation, length and alignment; (E and F) Final intraoperative radiographs confirm fracture reduction and hardware position.

Courtesy: Asif M Ilyas

INTRAMEDULLARY NAILING: Pearls and Pitfalls

- Intramedullary nail fixation is best indicated for 1 or 2-part fractures involving primarily the surgical neck
- Positioning should afford for ease of orthogonal c-arm imaging during the case
- The fracture must be adequately reduced closed prior to nail insertion
- The deltoid split should be limited to 5 cm distal to the acromion. A stay suture can be placed at that level to avoid inadvertent injury to the axillary nerve
- The nail must be adequately countersunk to avoid hardware impingement

Technique 3: Hemiarthroplasty

Preoperative Planning

As described above, a thorough understanding of the fracture pattern, bone quality and surrounding anatomy should be attained. We make all attempts to perform ORIF but occasionally, elderly patients with fracture-dislocations and an anatomic neck component or head-split prevent ORIF. Hemiarthroplasty is chosen only when a patient is not a candidate for ORIF as hemiarthroplasty is often associated with poor functional results and low outcome scores.

Prior to the procedure, the contralateral shoulder should be imaged if possible to assist with templating. Head height, angulation and offset can be mapped from the intact shoulder films. Templates from the planned implant should be used to facilitate these measurements. These measurements can be difficult in the setting of tuberosity comminution and displacement, and preoperative imaging of the contralateral shoulder can be quite useful.

It is beneficial to choose a fracture stem that can be easily converted into a reverse shoulder arthroplasty stem in the situation of a non-reconstructable failure following a hemiarthroplasty.

Technique

The beach chair position is typically chosen. Towels are placed behind the medial border of the scapula. Prophylactic antibiotic administration should be performed within 1 hour of skin incision. For hemiarthroplasty, a deltopectoral approach is typically chosen. The incision begins between the coracoid and the clavicle, extending toward the insertion of the deltoid muscle staying 1 cm lateral to the coracoid, as described in the previous section. If additional exposure is needed, the rotator interval can be opened and the pectoralis major and deltoid insertions can be partially released. Care must be taken to preserve the biceps tendon and the coracoacromial ligament. As described in the previous section, one must protect the musculocutaneous and axillary nerves during this exposure. Blunt retraction of the deltoid and conjoined tendon is performed carefully to prevent damage to these nerves. Next, the head fragment is removed and measured on the back table to estimate the size of the prosthesis.

Nonabsorbable tag sutures are then placed into the subscapularis and supraspinatus tendon insertions adjacent to the bone to assist with retraction without compromising the often-poor bone stock of the tuberosities. A full inspection of the rotator cuff should be performed, as large, irreparable rotator cuff tears are a contraindication to performing a hemiarthroplasty. The shaft is then delivered into the wound for inspection via extension, adduction and external rotation. Small fractures of the shaft should be fixed anatomically, and a full inspection of bone quality should be performed. Typically, remaining bone stock is not sufficient for press-fit stems, and cemented stems are chosen.

Drill holes are now placed into the tuberosities and the humeral shaft for future suture repair (Fig. 11.20). This step in the case is very important as it sets the stage for a successful tuberosity repair once the implant is fully seated. All sutures should be placed prior to final stem placement to prevent a struggle once the cement has hardened.

Attention is now directed toward preparing the canal and trialing the stem (Figs 11.21A and B). Reaming and broaching should be performed according to the technique guide for the chosen implant system. The most important measurements to recreate with the final prosthesis include head height, head size, offset and retroversion. Head size can be estimated from the preoperative templates or the head fragment removed from the case. Head height can be estimated using a number of different techniques. Initial templating provides

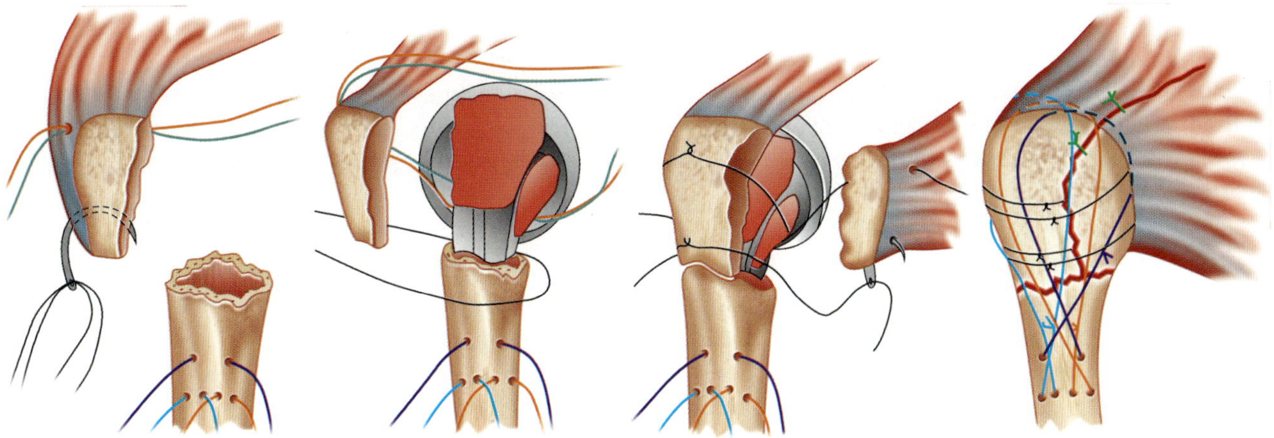

Figure 11.20: Suture configuration for tuberosity fixation is shown. Two sutures are placed around both the greater and lesser tuberosity (a total of four sutures). These are passed through the fracture stem and to the other tuberosity. Three sutures are then placed into the humeral shaft through six separate drill holes. These will be used to tie three separate tension band constructs to the cuff after reduction is obtained. The final suture is placed in cerclage fashion around the medial neck of the stem and tied into the supraspinatus insertion.

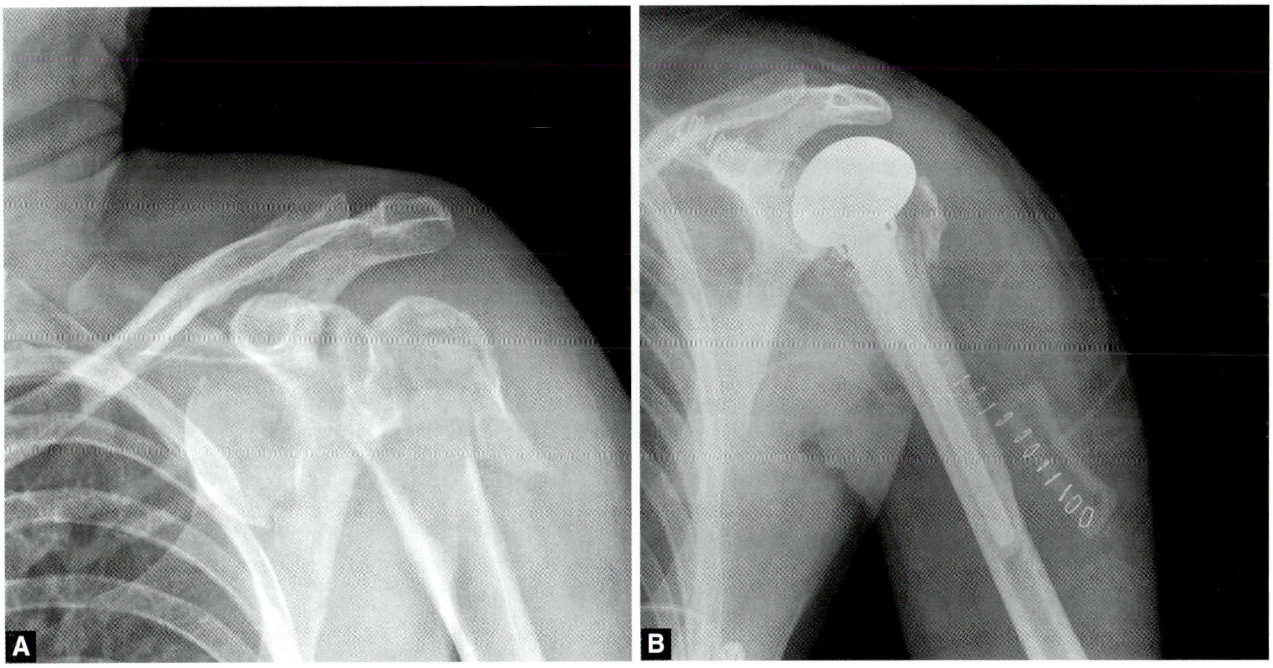

Figures 11.21A and B: (A) This is a case of a middle-aged man involved in a high-speed motorcycle accident incurring several injuries including a displaced 4-part proximal humerus fracture with dislocation of the humeral head; (B) Cemented hemiarthroplasty was performed with suture repair of the tuberosities to be the stem.

a reliable estimate. During the case, the tension on the biceps tendon and the distance from the pectoralis insertion to the top of the humeral head serve as estimates. The top of the humeral head is reliably 5–6 cm from the insertion of the pectoralis tendon.[25] Options for modularity depend on the design of the implant chosen. Modularity in the medial offset is beneficial, as a wide range of offsets are seen in the population.[26] Modularity in the neck shaft angle is less useful, as less variability exists in the population (mean of 137°).[26] Retroversion is difficult to reproduce, as there is a wide range seen in the general population; generally about 30° is chosen. Once the trial stem is in place, ROM in internal and external rotation is used to assess reduction stability anteriorly and posteriorly. Changes in version can be made to accommodate any imbalances. The final implant should then be cemented in place according to the final position of the trial prosthesis. Bone graft from the removed head fragment is then placed around the fin.

Next and most importantly, the tuberosities should be fixed into their anatomic position. Using the previously placed drill holes in the bone and suture holes in the proximal aspect of the final prosthesis, a systematic reduction and fixation of the tuberosities should be undertaken. First, the greater and lesser tuberosities should be fixed to the stem through heavy, nonabsorbable suture. Next, the tuberosities can be sutured to each other and the humeral shaft. Cerclage suture around the neck of the prosthesis is also a useful augmentation (Fig. 11.20).

A deep drain is placed and the wound is copiously irrigated. The rotator interval, pectoralis insertion and deltoid insertion should be repaired if released earlier in the case. Several absorbable sutures are used to close the deltopectoral interval paying close attention to the location of the cephalic vein. The superficial skin layer is closed with buried 3-0 interrupted absorbable sutures and 4-0 nylon is used on the outer skin layer.

Patients are initially placed in a sling with instructions to perform ROM exercises for the elbow and pendulum motion for the shoulder. At the 2-week follow-up visit, active assist ROM is begun at the shoulder in a very limited fashion with no forced passive ROM exercises. At 6 weeks, active ROM is allowed, and at 3 months, progressive resistance exercises are encouraged if tuberosity healing has been demonstrated radiographically.

HEMIARTHROPLASTY: Pearls and Pitfalls

- Obtain films of the contralateral arm to assist with templating
- Diligent recreation of head size, height, offset and retroversion are keys when placing the trial prosthesis
- Systematic suture repair of the tuberosities with a detailed plan should be performed prior to placement and cementing of the final implant

Outcomes

Outcomes from the proximal humerus fracture literature must be interpreted carefully as comparison studies are lacking and suboptimal classification systems can be a limiting factor.

Many fixation techniques have been described in the literature with promising results. Minimally invasive methods, such as CRPP strive to counter deforming forces while minimizing surgical trauma. While biomechanically weaker than formal plating techniques, Constant Scores from 74–84 have been reported in the recent literature; this includes patients with 3- and 4-part fractures.[11] Forward flexion of more than 140° and external rotation of more than 50° are reported in some series.[11] Familiarity with closed reduction techniques and adherence to surgical indications for CRPP are recommended before attempting to address more complex fracture patterns.

Locked plating is the most recent advancement in treatment for proximal humerus fractures. In patients meeting criteria for ORIF, outcome scores favor ORIF in comparison to hemiarthroplasty.[14] In the most recent systematic literature review, Constant scores were found to be 77.4 for 2-part fractures, 73.4 for 3-part fractures and 67.7 for 4-part fractures.[14] In a case series with 70% 3- and 4-part fractures, Ricchetti et al. observed 130.1° of forward flexion and 27.7°of external rotation.[27] While ROM and Constant scores are expected to decrease with increasing fracture severity, outcomes still remain favorable when compared to hemiarthroplasty.

Closer analysis of patients undergoing ORIF reveals several surgeon-controlled factors associated with improved outcomes. Prospectively collected data in a recent study confirm the findings of Gardner et al. that ensuring medial calcar stability is a central factor in optimizing functional outcomes.[12,22] Screw cutout from fracture collapse, a major cause of reoperation, may be prevented with attention to the medial calcar.[22] Avoidance of varus head malreduction and attention to tuberosity position have also been associated with improved outcome scores.[12,28]

Outcomes from hemiarthroplasty surgery highlight several areas of concern. However, one must keep in mind that this procedure is typically performed in the face of difficult to treat fractures with poor bone stock, and direct comparisons to other interventions are not always possible, as these patients are usually poor candidates for ORIF. A recent systematic review of the literature[15] cites average forward flexion of 105.7°, abduction of 92.4° and external rotation of 30.4°. Patients reported no pain or mild pain in 85% of cases. The most widely utilized outcome score in this population is the Constant score, and an average of 56.6 is observed in these patients. Forty-two percent of patients considered their outcomes unsatisfactory.[15] Surgeons must pay attention to restoring the humeral head height and minimizing medial calcar offset; both have been linked to improved Constant scores.[28]

Robinson et al. recently evaluated 163 consecutive patients treated with hemiarthroplasty with 138 available at 1 year follow-up. The 1 year modified Constant score was 64, and factors found to significantly affect the score were neurological deficit, age, tobacco and alcohol use, migration of the center of the prosthetic head, tuberosity displacement and need for reoperation.[29] Similar to other studies, pain relief was good, but function, ROM and power scores were low.[29]

Noyes et al.[30] followed 47 hemiarthroplasty patients out to 5 years and noted significant deteriorations in the patient population between 2 years and 5 years. Thirteen patients required revision to reverse shoulder arthroplasty. Significant superior humeral migration, tuberosity osteolysis and a decrease in outcome scores (Constant score dropped from 61–50) were noted during the follow-up period. Secondary to the poor outcomes they observed authors caution against using the hemiarthroplasty when possible.[30]

Occasionally, complex fractures in the elderly present with inadequate tuberosity bone stock for hemi-arthroplasty and a reverse shoulder arthroplasty is chosen. Outcomes from this procedure have no comparison in the literature, as the procedure is typically undertaken in a patient who is not a candidate for any other fixation method. Constant scores are understandably lower in this patient population. Long-term follow-up of reverse shoulder arthroplasties shows that Constant scores drop from 55–53 between 1 year and 6 years.[18]

Complications

Surgeons who decide to treat proximal humerus fractures operatively should be prepared to deal with associated complications. For this discussion, ORIF and hemi-arthroplasty will be addressed separately.

In a large, systematic review of proximal humerus locking plate use in the literature, Sproul et al. found an overall complication rate of 48.8%, resulting in a reoperation rate of 13%.[14] The most common complication was varus malunion (16.3%) followed by AVN (10.8%), screw perforation (7.5%), subacromial impingement (4.8%) and infection (3.5%).[14] The overall union rate was 96.6%.[14]

Malunion

Varus malunion is an important topic, as the complication is not just related to poor bone quality; but technical aspects of the surgery play a large role. First and foremost, anatomic reduction must be achieved in the operating room. Once obtained, the surgeon must evaluate the medial stability at the calcar, as the presence of medial support has been linked to preservation of reduction and improved outcome scores.[13,22] Medial support can be obtained from adequate bony reduction, fracture impaction or placement of an oblique screw along the calcar.[13] Furthering medial support can be augmented with a structural allograft. Preservation of reduction leads to less varus malreduction, less screw cutout and less subacromial impingement. Screw perforation and subacromial impingement are typically treated with removal of the offending hardware.

Infection

Infection management depends on timing and fracture healing. If the fracture is fresh, incision, debridement and initiation of antibiotics followed by late removal of hardware when union has been achieved preclude removing the implants early when the fracture is still unstable.

Avascular Necrosis

Avascular necrosis is a controversial subject. It can arise years after surgery but does not signify a failure of treatment or necessitate conversion to arthroplasty. While Constant scores are lower in patients with AVN compared to those without, often their function is still superior to that of a patient with a hemiarthroplasty. Conversions to arthroplasty in the face of AVN should be considered on a case-by-case basis and performed only after the patient fully understands the potential risks, benefits and functional limitations of a hemiarthroplasty.

Hemiarthroplasty—Specific Complications

Patients undergoing hemiarthroplasty face a different risk profile. Complications from hemiarthroplasty include tuberosity malunion/nonunion (11.2%), heterotopic ossification (8.8%), proximal migration of the humeral head (6.8%) and deep infection (0.6%).[15] Other complications include stem loosening and periprosthetic fracture.

Many of these problems require surgical management. Tuberosity healing issues are typically addressed with a return to the OR for revision of fixation. Development of glenohumeral arthritis can be managed with revision to a total shoulder construct. Rotator cuff tears and proximal migration are difficult problems to address as tissue quality is often poor; management options include repair or tissue transfer. Revision to a reverse prosthesis is also an option. Periprosthetic fractures can be managed with ORIF versus revision of the hemiarthroplasty; stem loosening requires a revision hemiarthroplasty.[31] Infection demands irrigation and debridement with implant revision depending on depth of infection and time from implantation. Non-reconstructable cases should be considered for conversion to reverse shoulder arthroplasty with an experienced shoulder surgeon.[31]

Authors' Preferred Management of Select Complications

Case 1: Failure of Fixation Followed by Revision of Fixation

A 72-year-old female fell from standing height onto her left shoulder. She was neurovascularly intact on examination with pain on ROM of the shoulder. X-rays and a CT scan were obtained with 3-D reconstructions to assist with diagnosis and surgical planning. A 4-part proximal humerus fracture was shown, and the decision was made to proceed with ORIF of the fracture with a locked plate through an anterolateral acromial approach (Figs 11.22A to F). A fibular strut graft was chosen to augment the patient's poor baseline bone stock and add stability to the construct.

Two weeks after surgery, the patient returned for a routine follow-up visit reporting continuing soreness about the shoulder. Plain radiographs showed loss of fixation and migration of the tuberosities with maintenance of fixation into the humeral head. Discussion was done with the patient regarding potential outcomes of surgical versus conservative management of the problem, and the decision was made to return for a revision ORIF.

Similar to primary fracture management, revision of fixation should be performed when the fracture fragments are stout enough to be held in position with new implants. As in the acute fracture setting, anatomic realignment and stable fixation of fractures should be performed to optimize outcome. In this case, the tuberosities had migrated more than 5 mm and surgery was planned to correct this deformity.

Attention should be paid to the status of the articular surface. Severe damage to the cartilage can be seen in the face of catastrophic hardware failure, and consideration should be made for hemiarthroplasty. The authors try to avoid hemiarthroplasty if at all possible secondary to the inferior outcomes in comparison to ORIF techniques, especially in young patients.

Technique

In this case, the previous incision was used to approach the fracture. Heavy, nonabsorbable suture had been used to fix the tuberosities to the plate during the index procedure, and these were found to be broken from both the greater and lesser tuberosity fragments.

Multiple new sutures were placed into the tuberosity fragments and an intraosseus suture was added for stability. As the patient had failed suture augmented repair already, the decision was made to add a second plate to the anterior aspect of the humerus for more stability to the comminuted lesser tuberosity. A 2.7 recon plate was chosen, and four screws were placed capturing the fibular graft. After tying the new sutures down through the plates, the shoulder was ranged and noted to be stable.

At the patient's 1 year follow-up from revision surgery, her forward flexion was equal to the contralateral side. External rotation lacked 15° of range compared to the right arm, and internal rotation was to T8. She had no signs of impingement and displayed 5/5 strength globally.

Case 2: Failure of Fixation Followed by Hemiarthroplasty

A 56-year-old male presented to the authors' clinic after sustaining a fall down the stairs resulting in a proximal

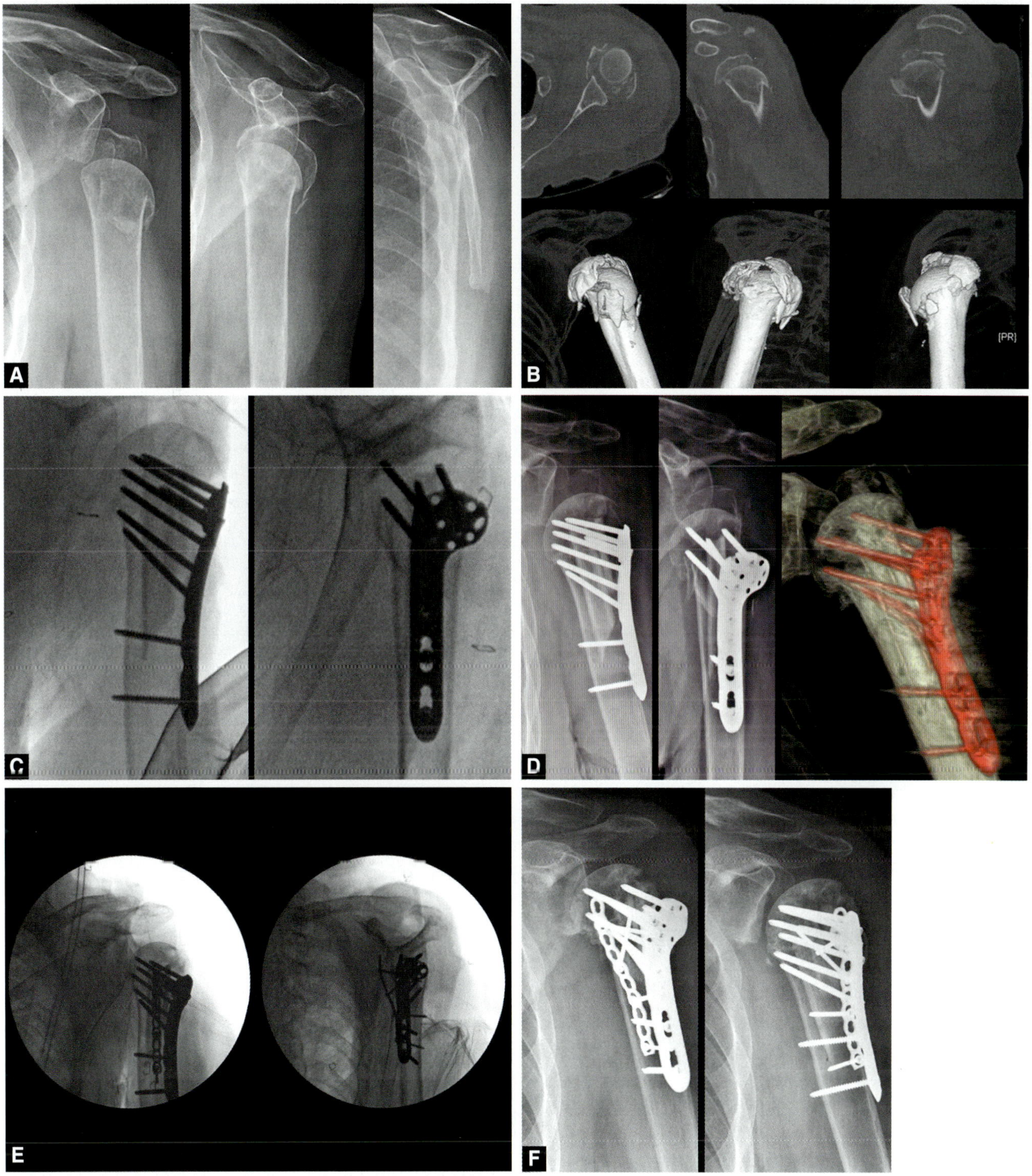

Figures 11.22A to F: This is a case of a failure of fixation following open reduction and internal fixation (ORIF) of a proximal humerus fracture treated with a revision ORIF. (A) Initial injury radiographs reveal a comminuted and displaced proximal humerus fracture with poor underlying bone quality; (B) Standard and 3D CT scan reconstructions provide further fracture pattern delineation; (C) Intraoperative fluoroscopic images after index procedure demonstrating acceptable reduction following ORIF using a fibular strut allograft to augment fixation; (D) Images taken after 2 weeks postoperatively demonstrate loss of fixation of the tuberosities; (E) Intraoperative fluoroscopic images following revision ORIF. The 2.7 mm recon plate has been contoured around the lesser tuberosity, augmenting the fixation; (F) Radiographs taken at 1 year postoperatively confirming a healed fracture.

humerus fracture that was initially treated with ORIF at an outside institution. Two weeks postoperatively he presented with severe pain and radiographs demonstrated failure of fixation. He was referred to the authors' institution for further management (Figs 11.23A to C).

Work up revealed screw cutout from the humeral head with gross loss of alignment. Magnetic resonance imaging images confirmed marked areas of osteonecrosis and collapse of the articular surface. Secondary to fixation concerns in the humeral head with poor quality cartilage, the authors decided to proceed with hemiarthroplasty. This was performed 5 weeks after the index procedure.

Unlike the previous complication case, this patient had poor bone quality in the remaining humeral head, severely limiting the likelihood of obtaining stable fixation. In addition, MRI revealed osteonecrosis and collapse of the articular surface. Despite the lower outcome scores of the procedure, hemiarthroplasty was chosen, as ORIF would be unlikely to be successful in the face of articular collapse.

Case 3: Open Reduction and Internal Fixation Followed by Infected Nonunion

A 70-year-old female presented to the authors' clinic following a failed trial of nonoperative treatment for a

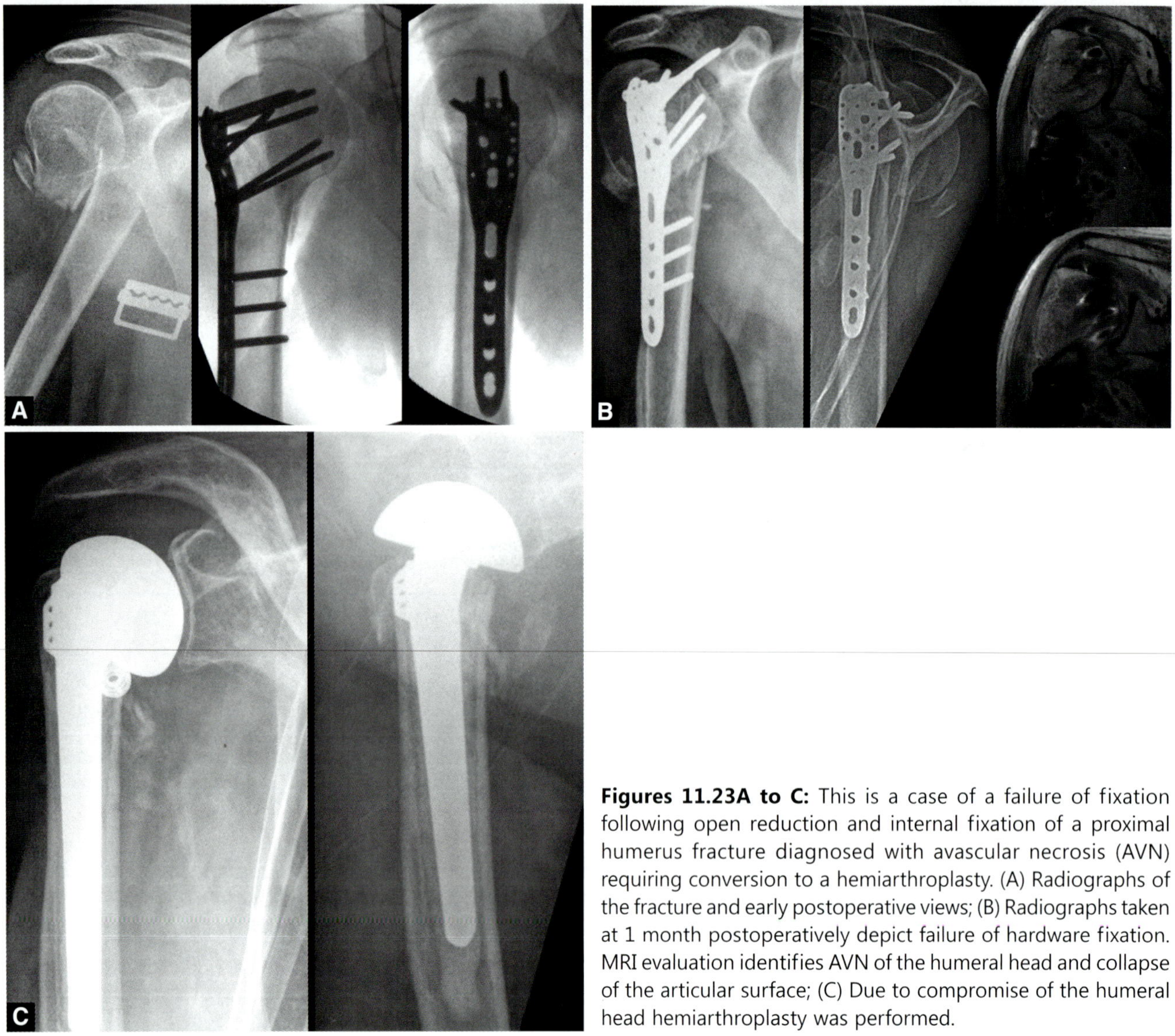

Figures 11.23A to C: This is a case of a failure of fixation following open reduction and internal fixation of a proximal humerus fracture diagnosed with avascular necrosis (AVN) requiring conversion to a hemiarthroplasty. (A) Radiographs of the fracture and early postoperative views; (B) Radiographs taken at 1 month postoperatively depict failure of hardware fixation. MRI evaluation identifies AVN of the humeral head and collapse of the articular surface; (C) Due to compromise of the humeral head hemiarthroplasty was performed.

proximal humerus fracture and subsequent ORIF for nonunion at an outside institution 4 months prior to this evaluation. The patient was complaining of night sweats, drainage and swelling. Physical exam revealed gross motion at the fracture site, and joint aspiration identified an enterococcal infection (Figs 11.24A to C).

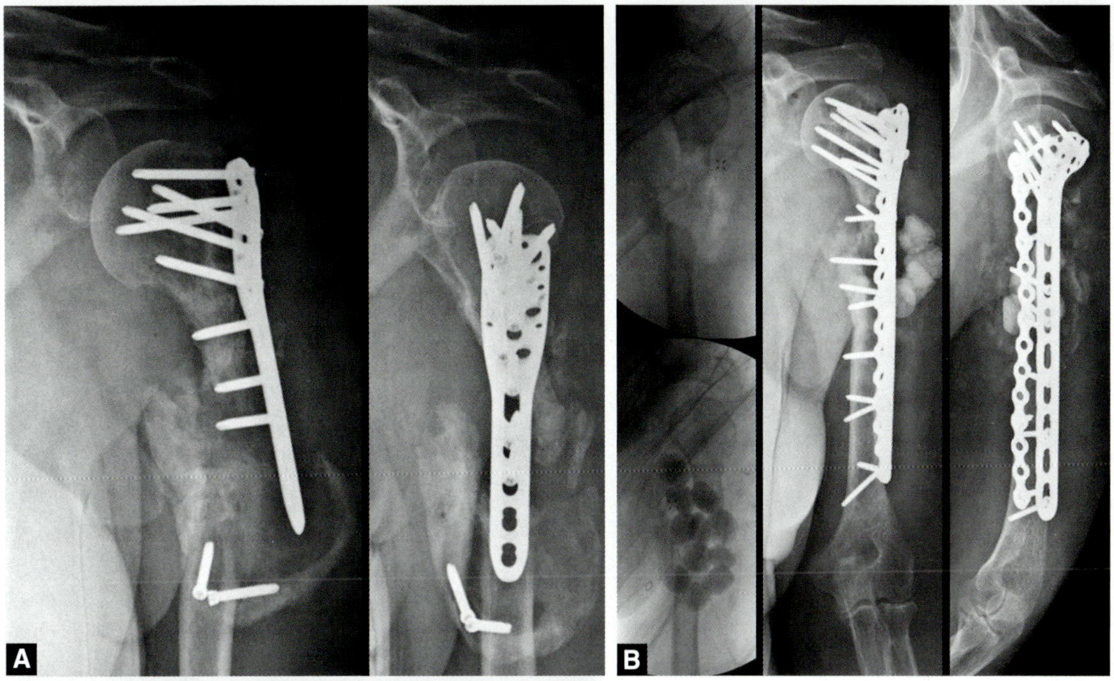

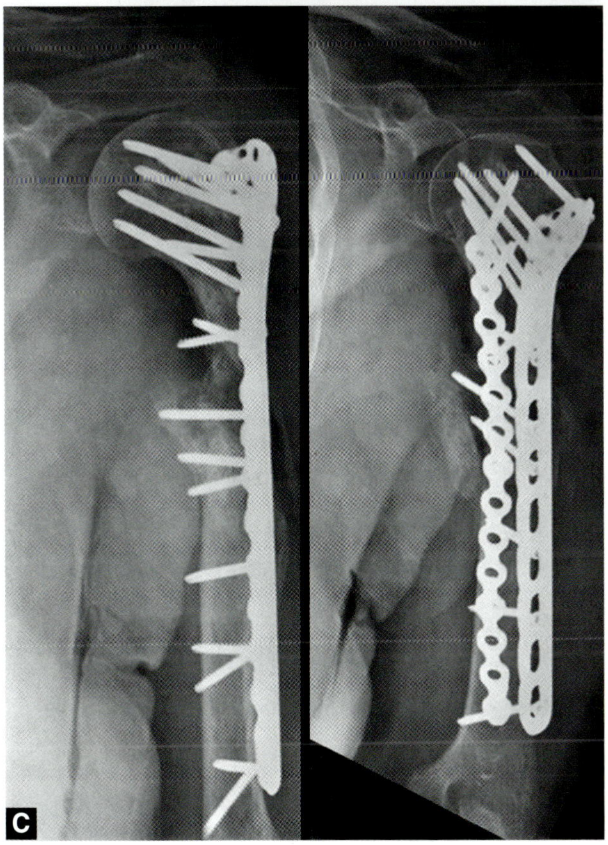

Figures 11.24A to C: This is a case of an infected nonunion following open reduction and internal fixation (ORIF) of a proximal humerus fracture with shaft extension. (A) Radiographs taken at the time of presentation to our institution demonstrate evidence of an infected nonunion; (B) Series of intraoperative fluoroscopic views obtained after removal of hardware and debridement of the fracture performed during the first trip to the operating room (OR) including antibiotic bead placement, followed by revision ORIF on the third trip to the OR. In between there was a second trip to the OR for a repeat debridement. Note the antibiotic beads were revised after all three cases and also kept following the revision ORIF. The patient returned to the OR 6 weeks postoperatively for removal of the antibiotic beads and repeat bone grafting with autograft; (C) Radiographs taken at 4 months postoperatively confirm a healed fracture.

Surgical management of the patient's infected humeral nonunion was undertaken initially with a removal of hardware, I & D of the wound, debridement of devitalized/infected tissue and placement of antibiotic beads. Repeat I & D and bead exchanges were performed 4 days and 6 days later. At the last washout/bead exchange surgery, no purulent material was noted and arrangements were made to proceed with definitive fixation. At 12 days after the first surgical debridement, the patient was taken back to the OR for repeat I & D, revision ORIF and placement of new antibiotic beads.

Early presentations of infection can often be treated by I & D, antibiotics, and close follow-up without removing the hardware from the index case. Once the fracture has healed, the hardware can be removed if deep colonization is expected.

Technique

This was not possible in this case secondary to the chronicity of the patient's complaints, the loose hardware and the development of an infected nonunion. Long standing infections in the face of nonunion require a removal of hardware as a part of the debridement stage of treatment, as the fracture is unlikely to go on to union with less invasive procedures. The authors prefer to address these difficult complications with removal of hardware, multistage debridements and antibiotic beads supplemented with intravenous antibiotic therapy. Once the tissue appears clean and healthy, the authors then perform an open reduction with revision of fixation and new antibiotic beads with a planned return to the OR for removal of the antibiotic beads and open bone grafting in 6 weeks. Patients should be counseled that they can expect multiple surgeries and a prolonged treatment course when a deep infection is diagnosed. In the worst of scenarios, a resection arthroplasty may be needed to control the infection and allow the patient to return to his or her life, albeit with significant disability.

For the definitive fixation portion of this case, the previous deltopectoral incision was advanced into an anterolateral approach to the humerus. The lateral brachial cutaneous nerve and the radial nerve were protected. After thorough debridement of the nonunion was completed, double plating of the fracture with interfragmentary compression was then performed with a proximal humeral locking plate and a 3.5 mm recon plate. Antibiotic beads were then placed and the wound was closed in standard fashion.

Summary

Fractures of the proximal humerus are difficult to treat, not only because of the technical issues involved but also because of a lack of definitive literature guiding the surgeon down the optimal treatment path. Each case should be evaluated individually, and surgeons should have a thorough understanding of the anatomy and fixation options prior to undertaking surgical management. Optimal outcomes in the setting of ORIF are achieved when the anatomy is restored and fixed in a rigid, stable fashion. Complications, such as screw cutout, varus collapse, impingement, infection and AVN, are common and surgeons should be prepared to treat each of these issues.

Management of fractures with hemiarthroplasty should be done on a very limited basis. In cases where a contraindication to ORIF is not present, it appears that outcome scores favor ORIF in comparison to hemiarthroplasty. Other concerns include declining function in patients treated with hemiarthroplasty over time. Unfortunately, fracture patterns exist where ORIF is precluded and hemiarthroplasty is required as a salvage procedure. Surgeons should be familiar with modern techniques of restoring height, offset, head size and retroversion. Tuberosity fixation is fundamental to optimizing results, and a detailed plan for suture management should be reviewed prior to each case. Complications, such as tuberosity malunion/nonunion, humeral head migration, stem loosening and periprosthetic fracture, are not uncommon, and surgeons should be familiar with management techniques including when to arrange for revision to a reverse arthroplasty system.

References

1. Court-Brown CM, Caesar B. Epidemiology of adult fractures: A review. Injury. 2006;37(8):691-7.
2. Nho SJ, Brophy RH, Barker JU, et al. Management of proximal humeral fractures based on current literature. J Bone Joint Surg Am. 2007;89 Suppl 3:44-58.
3. de Laat EA, Visser CP, Coene LN, et al. Nerve lesions in primary shoulder dislocations and humeral neck fractures. A prospective clinical and EMG study. J Bone Joint Surg Br. 1994;76(3):381-3.

4. Foroohar A, Tosti R, Richmond JM, et al. Classification and treatment of proximal humerus fractures: inter-oberserver reliability and agreement across imaging modalities and experience. J Ortho Surg Res. 2011;6:38.
5. Neer CS 2nd. Displaced proximal humeral fractures. I. Classification and evaluation. J Bone Joint Surg Am. 1970; 52(6):1077-89.
6. Müller ME. The comprehensive classification of fractures of long bones. New York: Springer-Verlag; 1990.
7. Lanting B, MacDermid J, Drosdowech D, et al. Proximal humeral fractures: a systematic review of treatment modalities. J Shoulder Elbow Surg. 2008;17(1):42-54.
8. Hanson B, Neidenbach P, de Boer P, et al. Functional outcomes after nonoperative management of fractures of the proximal humerus. J Shoulder Elbow Surg. 2009 18(4): 612-21.
9. Tingart MJ, Apreleva M, von Stechow D, et al. The cortical thickness of the proximal humeral diaphysis predicts bone mineral density of the proximal humerus. J Bone Joint Surg Br. 2003;85(4):611-7.
10. Bono CM, Renard R, Levine RG, et al. Effect of displacement of fractures of the greater tuberosity on the mechanics of the shoulder. J Bone Joint Surg Br. 2001;83(7):1056-62.
11. Magovern B, Ramsey ML. Percutaneous fixation of proximal humerus fractures. Orthop Clin North Am. 2008;39(4): 405-16.
12. Thanasas C, Kontakis G, Angoules A, et al. Treatment of proximal humerus fractures with locking plates: a systematic review. J Shoulder Elbow Surg. 2009;18(6):837-44.
13. Gardner MJ, Weil Y, Barker JU, et al. The importance of medial support in locked plating of proximal humerus fractures. J Orthop Trauma. 2007;21(3):185-91.
14. Sproul RC, Iyengar JJ, Devcic Z, et al. A systematic review of locking plate fixation of proximal humerus fractures. Injury. 2011;42(4):408-13.
15. Kontakis G, Koutras C, Tosounidis T, et al. Early management of proximal humeral fractures with hemiarthroplasty: a systematic review. J Bone Joint Surg Br. 2008;90(11): 1407-13.
16. Bastian JD, Hertel R. Initial post-fracture humeral head ischemia does not predict development of necrosis. J Shoulder Elbow Surg. 2008;17(1):2-8.
17. Gerber C, Werner CM, Vienne P. Internal fixation of complex fractures of the proximal humerus. J Bone Joint Surg Br. 2004;86(6):848-55.
18. Cazeneuve JF, Cristofari DJ. The reverse shoulder prosthesis in the treatment of fractures of the proximal humerus in the elderly. J Bone Joint Surg Br. 2010;92(4):535-9.
19. Hertel R, Hempfing A, Stiehler M, et al. Predictors of humeral head ischemia after intracapsular fracture of the proximal humerus. J Shoulder Elbow Surg. 2004;13(4): 427-33.
20. Hettrich CM, Boraiah S, Dyke JP, et al. Quantitative assessment of the vascularity of the proximal part of the humerus. J Bone Joint Surg Am. 2010;92(4):943-8.
21. Gardner MJ, Boraiah S, Helfet DL, et al. The anterolateral acromial approach for fractures of the proximal humerus. J Orthop Trauma. 2008;22(2):132-7.
22. Yang H, Li Z, Zhou F, et al. A prospective clinical study of proximal humerus fractures treated with a locking proximal humerus plate. J Orthop Trauma. 2011;25(1):11-7.
23. Osterhoff G, Baumgartner D, Favre P, et al. Medial support by fibula bone graft in angular stable plate fixation of proximal humeral fractures: an in vitro study with synthetic bone. J Shoulder Elbow Surg. 2011;20(5):740-6.
24. Nevaiser AS, Hettrich CM, Dines JS, et al. Rate of avascular necrosis following proximal humerus fractures treated with a lateral locking plate and endosteal implant. Arch Orthop Trauma Surg. 2011;131(12):1617-22.
25. Murachovsky J, Ikemoto RY, Nascimento LG, et al. Pectoralis major tendon reference (PMT): a new method for accurate restoration of humeral length with hemiarthroplasty for fracture. J Shoulder Elbow Surg. 2006;15(6):675-8.
26. Hertel R, Knothe U, Ballmer FT. Geometry of the proximal humerus and implications for prosthetic design. J Shoulder Elbow Surg. 2002;11(4):331-8.
27. Ricchetti ET, Warrender WJ, Abboud JA. Use of locking plates in the treatment of proximal humerus fractures. J Shoulder Elbow Surg. 2010;19(2 Suppl):66-75.
28. Solberg BD, Moon CN, Franco DP, et al. Locked plating of 3- and 4-part proximal humerus fractures in older patients: the effect of initial fracture pattern on outcome. J Orthop Trauma. 2009;23(2):113-9.
29. Robinson CM, Page RS, Hill RM, et al. Primary hemiarthroplasty for treatment of proximal humeral fractures. J Bone Joint Surg Am. 2003;85-A(7):1215-23.
30. Noyes MP, Kleinhenz B, Markert RJ, et al. Functional and radiographic long-term outcomes of hemiarthroplasty for proximal humeral fractures. J Shoulder Elbow Surg. 2011; 20(3):372-7.
31. Levy J, Frankle M, Mighell M, et al. The use of the reverse shoulder prosthesis for the treatment of failed hemiarthroplasty for proximal humeral fracture. J Bone Joint Surg Am. 2007;89(2):292-300.

Chapter 12

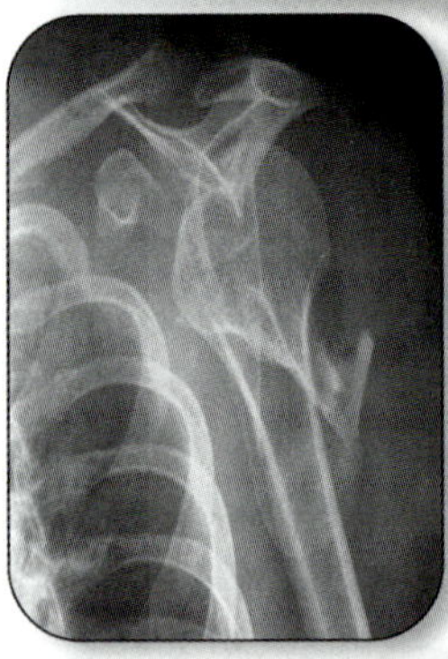

Glenoid and Scapula Fractures

Samuel Popinchalk, Neil MacIntyre

Chapter Outline

Introduction

Diagnosis

Classification

- Scapular Body Fractures
- Scapular Neck Fractures
- Glenoid Fractures
- Coracoid Process Fractures
- Acromion Process Fractures

Surgical Indications

- Scapular Body Fractures
- Scapular Neck Fractures
- Glenoid Fractures
- Coracoid Fractures
- Acromial Fractures

Surgical Anatomy, Positioning and Approaches

- Anterior Approach to the Scapula
- Posterior Approach to the Scapula

Surgical Techniques

- Technique 1: Scapular Body Fractures
- Technique 2: Scapular Neck Fractures
- Technique 3: Glenoid Fossa Fractures
- Technique 4: Coracoid Fractures

Outcomes

- Scapular Body Fractures
- Scapular Neck Fractures
- Glenoid Fractures
- Acromion Process Fractures
- Coracoid Process Fractures

Complications

- Malunion
- Iatrogenic Nerve Injury
- Compartment Syndrome
- Intrathoracic Scapular Impaction

Authors' Preferred Management of Select Complications

- Case 1: Glenoid Fossa Malunion
- Case 2: Scapular Neck Malunion with Glenoid Medialization

Summary

Introduction

Scapular fractures are relatively uncommon injuries, comprising 1% of all fractures.[1] They most commonly occur through high-energy mechanisms, which account for almost 90% of cases.[2-4] Scapular fractures are typically the product of high-energy injures and are typically present in the fourth decade of life. Moreover, males constitute more than 80% of injuries.

Scapular fractures are seldom isolated injuries. In the setting of life-threatening concomitant injuries, it often goes undetected initially or receives a low priority relative to other injuries. The scapular fracture itself seldom requires emergent intervention beyond immobilization with a sling and swath. The importance of a meticulous trauma evaluation and adequate resuscitation cannot be overemphasized. Key to the successful management of these fractures is an understanding of the anatomy and associated deforming forces acting on the fracture fragments.

Diagnosis

Complaints of pain about the shoulder region as a result of high-energy direct trauma to the shoulder should raise suspicion of a potential scapular fracture. The patient may demonstrate ecchymosis, crepitus and limited active shoulder range of motion in the setting of an acute injury. Similarly, hemorrhage into the rotator cuff musculature can mimic an acute rotator cuff tear with pain, weakness and decreased range of motion referred to as a "pseudo-rotator cuff rupture".[5]

Due to the high-energy mechanism of injury, 80–95% of patients with scapular fractures present with concomitant injuries.[3,6-9] Trauma to the head, cervical spine, ipsilateral chest wall and lungs constitute potentially life-threatening injuries and should be evaluated and treated according to Advanced Trauma Life Support (ATLS) guidelines. One series of 56 patients with 58 scapular fractures reported a 14.3% mortality rate with an average of 3.9 concomitant major injuries.[10] The incidence of concomitant injuries have been reported to include 53% with pulmonary contusions, 50% with thoracic injuries, 44–53.5% with rib fractures, 16–66% with pneumothorax or hemothoraces, 44–50% with ipsilateral upper extremity injuries, 26% with clavicle fractures, 24% with skull fractures, 20% with cerebral contusions, 12.5% with brachial plexus injuries, 12.5% with upper extremity vascular injuries and 10% with spine fractures.[5,7,9,11,12] Overall mortality is reported at 10–15% with the most common etiologies being head injury and pulmonary complications.[7,9]

A thorough neurological evaluation is mandatory. Neurologic injury with ipsilateral scapular fracture is present in approximately 12.5% of cases. Among scapular fractures, acromial fractures have the highest correlation with neurologic injury.[5] The mechanism, by which acromial fractures occur often involves depression of the shoulder with contralateral neck flexion resulting in traction to the brachial plexus.

Scapular fractures are particularly difficult to diagnose upon initial evaluation. The supine anteroposterior (AP) chest radiograph routinely obtained during initial trauma assessment is often inadequate to make the definitive diagnosis of scapular fracture. A retrospective review of 100 chest radiographs with identifiable scapular fractures revealed only 57, which were recognized by the radiologist at first reading.[13] Three dedicated views of the scapula (true AP, lateral and glenohumeral axillary) should be attained to assess the scapular body, scapular spine, acromial, coracoid and glenoid processes and the scapulothoracic, glenohumeral and acromioclavicular (AC) articulations. Injuries to the AC joint can be revealed on a weighted AP view of the shoulder. Whenever possible, the weight should be hung from the wrist rather than grasped by the patient, as gripping the weight can cause involuntary contraction of the trapezius, counteracting the weight.

Little debate exists regarding the utility of computed tomography (CT) and three-dimensional (3D) reconstructions in evaluating scapular fractures.[14-18] While fractures of the scapular body, spine and acromion can be identified with the three dedicated radiographic views, several more specialized views (stryker notch view, West Point lateral and apical oblique view) would be required to assess all anatomic regions of the scapula. Thoracic CT scans are often obtained during trauma assessment and dedicated scapular reconstructions can be readily obtained. Such reconstructions are vital to characterize the fracture pattern and, in most clinical settings, have replaced the aforementioned specialized views. Although two-dimensional (2D) CT scans have low sensitivity in detecting scapular neck and spine fractures, 3D CT scan reconstruction is the only tool proven to be the most sensitive in detecting fractures in all anatomic regions of the scapula.[19,20]

GLENOID AND SCAPULA FRACTURES DIAGNOSIS: Pearls and Pitfalls

- Almost 95% of patients with scapular fractures present with concomitant injuries
- Due to the high predilection of head, neck and chest injuries associated with scapular fractures, ATLS protocol should be followed if a scapular fracture is suspected

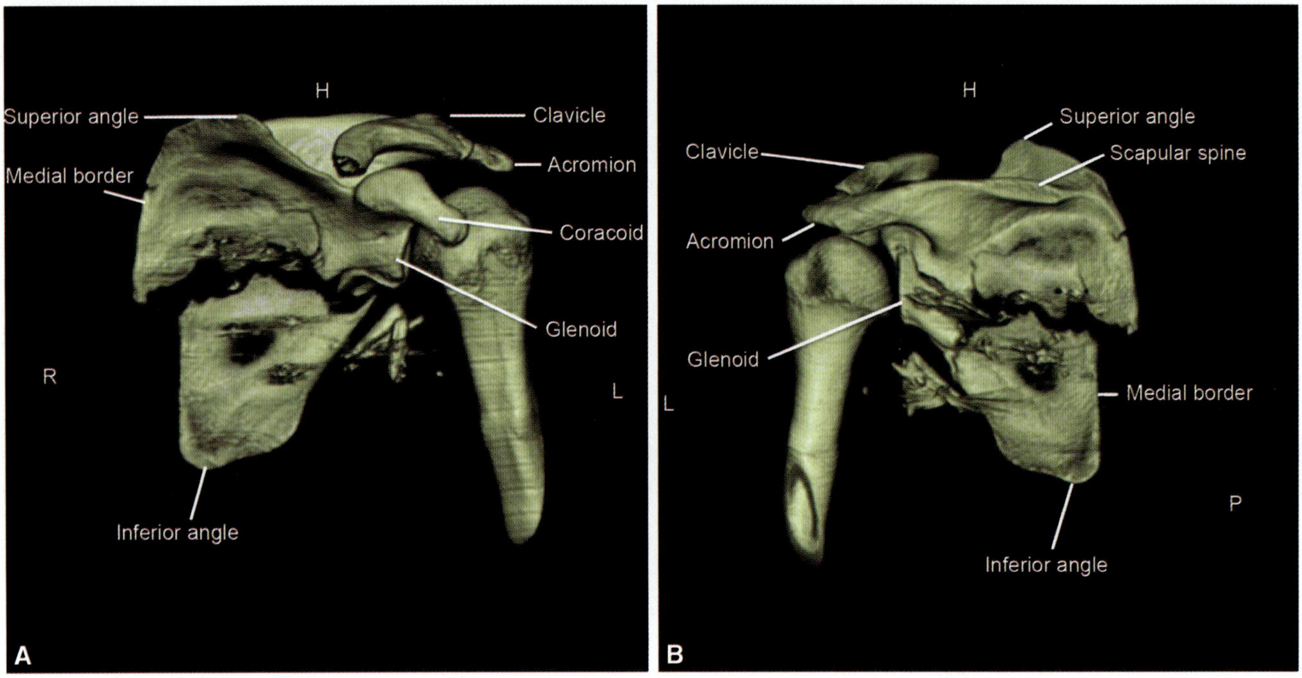

Figures 12.1A and B: Anatomic landmarks of the scapula identified on a three-dimensional (3D) reconstruction of scapula body fracture on (A) Anterior; (B) Posterior views.

- Three-dimensional CT scan reconstructions are highly sensitive in detecting fractures in all anatomic regions of the scapula

Classification

Scapular fractures are described by the anatomical region (Figs 12.1A and B). Fractures involving the body or spine comprise 50% of all scapular fractures. Fractures of the glenoid neck make up 25% and the glenoid cavity 10%. Finally, 7% of fractures involve the acromion process and another 7% involves the coracoid process.[3,5,17,20,21]

Several classification systems have been proposed to characterize scapular fractures. The AO classification is commonly utilized and represents an alphanumerically coded fracture compendium that identifies the scapula with the number 14.[20] In this system, fractures are classified based on their articular involvement. Type A fractures are extra-articular, Type B fractures are partial articular fractures involving the glenoid fossa and Type C fractures are articular fractures involving the scapular neck (Table 12.1). These types are further subdivided by fracture extension locations and extent of comminution.

Table 12.1: AO classification of scapular fractures

AO/OTA Type	*Fracture*
14-A1	Acromion
14-A2	Coracoid
14-A3	Body
14-B1	Anterior rim of glenoid fossa
14-B2	Posterior rim of glenoid fossa
14-B3	Inferior rim of glenoid fossa
14-C1	Extra-articular scapular neck (includes both anatomic and surgical neck)
14-C2	Intra-articular with scapular neck
14-C3	Intra-articular with scapular body

Various comprehensive classification schemes have been proposed in several large case series. In 1977, Wilber and Evans[21] reported 52 fractures in 41 scapulae and classified them in two groups: Group I (body, neck and spine) with 38 patients, all of whom regained full motion regardless of treatment versus Group II (acromion, coracoid and glenoid) with 10 patients, only 1 of which regained full glenohumeral motion.

Table 12.2: Ada and Miller classification of scapular fractures

Region	*Hardegger/Ada Type*	*% Total*
Acromion	IA	12
Spine	IB	11
Coracoid	IC	5
Neck	IIA, IIB, IIC	27
Glenoid	III	10
Body	IV	35

Scapular Body Fractures

Scapular body fractures make up at least 50% of all scapular fractures and do not have a dedicated classification scheme. They are the most common type of scapular fractures and often result from a direct blow of significant force. Scapular body fractures are represented by the AO/OTA type 14-A3 and Hardegger type IV. Ada and Miller, based on an analysis of 148 fractures in 116 scapulae (Table 12.2), further subdivided the Hardegger classification (Fig. 12.2).[22,23]

The glenopolar angle (Fig. 12.3) is a useful measurement to evaluate either lateralization of the scapular body or medialization of the glenoid neck. Muscle tension relationships are disrupted when the scapular body is displaced. The glenopolar angle is calculated by first drawing a line from the superior aspect of the glenoid to the inferior portion. Next, a line is drawn from the superior glenoid to the most inferior portion of the scapular body. This angle should measure between 30° to 45°. High or low angles, which fall out of this measurement, should be evaluated more closely, especially with a 3D CT scan.

Scapular Neck Fractures

Fractures of the scapular neck account for 25% of all scapular fractures. By definition, scapular neck fractures enter the lateral border of the scapula and exit the superior border, and therefore, are extra-articular. Anatomic neck fractures exit lateral to the coracoid process and surgical neck fractures exit medial to the coracoid process. Goss organized scapular neck fractures into two types: Type I fractures are non or minimally displaced and Type II fractures have displacement, defined as greater than or equal to 1 cm or 40° angular displacement.[13]

The mechanisms known to produce this fracture include direct trauma to the anterior, superior or posterior shoulder, or a fall on an outstretched arm. These fractures have potential for significant displacement with the long head of triceps acting as the major deforming force.

Glenoid Fractures

Fractures of the glenoid cavity comprise 10% of all scapular fractures. Ideberg proposed a classification system based on review of 300 glenoid rim and fossa fractures treated over a 10-year period.[24,25] Goss further distinguished glenoid cavity fractures to facilitate discussions of

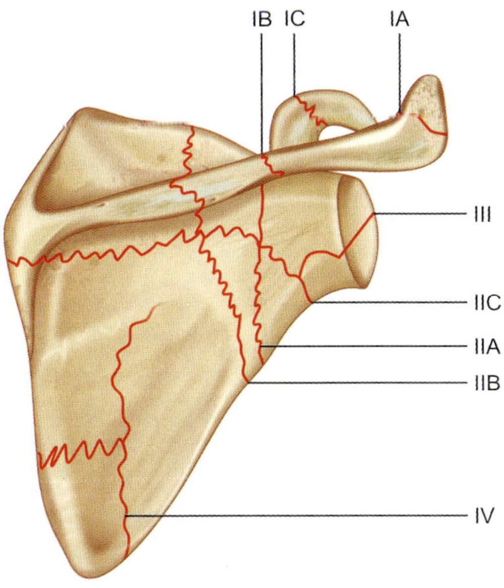

Figure 12.2: The Ada and Miller classification of scapular body fractures.

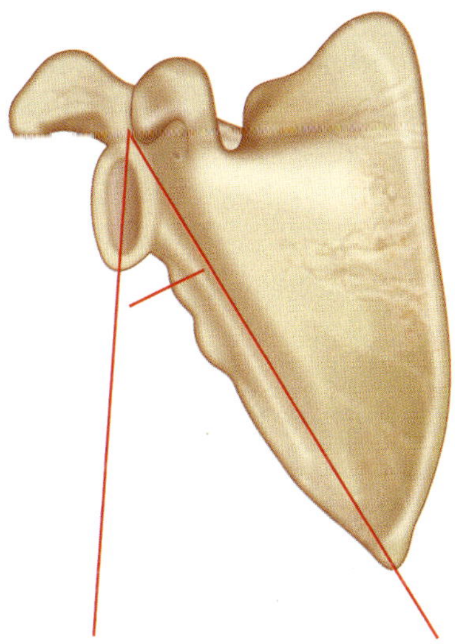

Figure 12.3: The glenopolar angle defines the relationship of glenoid to scapular body. This angle is useful in evaluating either lateralization of the scapular body or medialization of the glenoid neck.

operative management.[26] In their scheme, true fractures of the glenoid rim (Type I) are differentiated from small avulsion fractures associated with glenohumeral dislocations. True fractures result from the humeral head impacting the glenoid rim by a medially directed force, as opposed to small avulsion fractures, which result from a dislocating humeral head placing excessive tension on the capsulolabral complex. Glenoid rim fractures are subdivided by the involvement of the anterior (Type IA) or posterior rim (Type IB). Types II–VI involve the glenoid fossa and result from direct impact of the humeral head into the glenoid cavity from a medially directed force. Type II fractures result from an inferiorly directed force, with a fracture line entering the glenoid fossa and exiting the lateral border of the scapular body. Type III fractures result from a superiorly directed force and involve the superior articular surface of the glenoid including the coracoid process. Type III fractures can be associated with disruption of the superior suspensory complex of the shoulder. Type IV fractures result from a centrally directed force leading to a transverse split that exits along the medial border of the scapular body creating a smaller superior fragment and a larger inferior fragment. Type V fractures are combinations of Types II, III and IV fractures. Type V fractures result from even greater forces than isolated Types II, III and IV fractures. Type Va combines Type II and IV fractures; Type Vb combines Types III and IV; and Type Vc combines Types II, III and IV.

While the classification systems for glenoid fossa fractures of Ideberg and Goss are widely accepted, Mayo et al.[27] proposed a further refinement to fully capture the extent of scapular body involvement and provided consistent guidance for choosing a surgical approach (Figs 12.4A and B). Types I–III do not involve the scapular body. Type IV fractures involve the inferior glenoid fossa with extension into the body, and Type V fractures consist of a Type IV fracture pattern with the additional involvement of one of the scapular processes.

Coracoid Process Fractures

Coracoid process fractures account for approximately 7% of scapular fractures. Several classification systems have been proposed. Based on a review of 67 patients with coracoid process fractures, Ogawa classified coracoid fractures based on their relationship to the coracoclavicular ligament attachment—Type I being posterior and

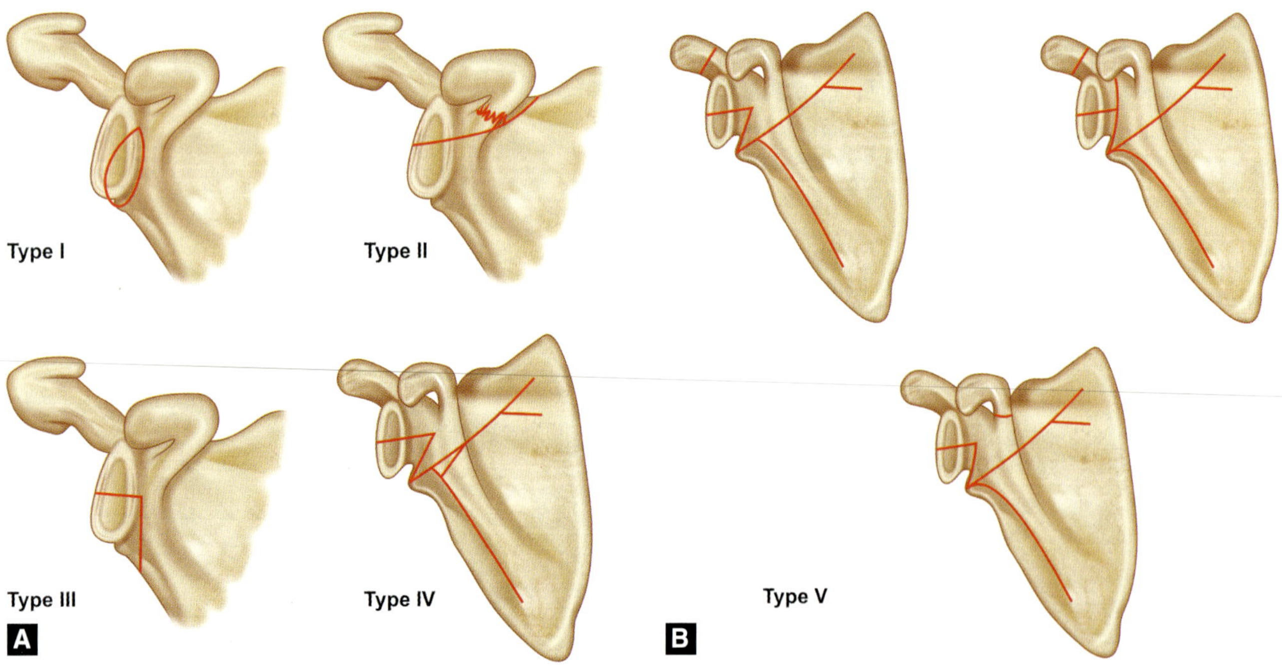

Figures 12.4A and B: The Mayo modification of the Ideberg classification of glenoid fossa fractures. It helped define the common associations between scapular body and process fractures. (A) Note that the Type I–III patterns do not involve the scapular body, while Type IV does involve the inferior glenoid fossa with extension into the body; (B) In contrast, Type V fractures consist of Type IV fracture patterns with the additional involvement of one of the scapular processes.

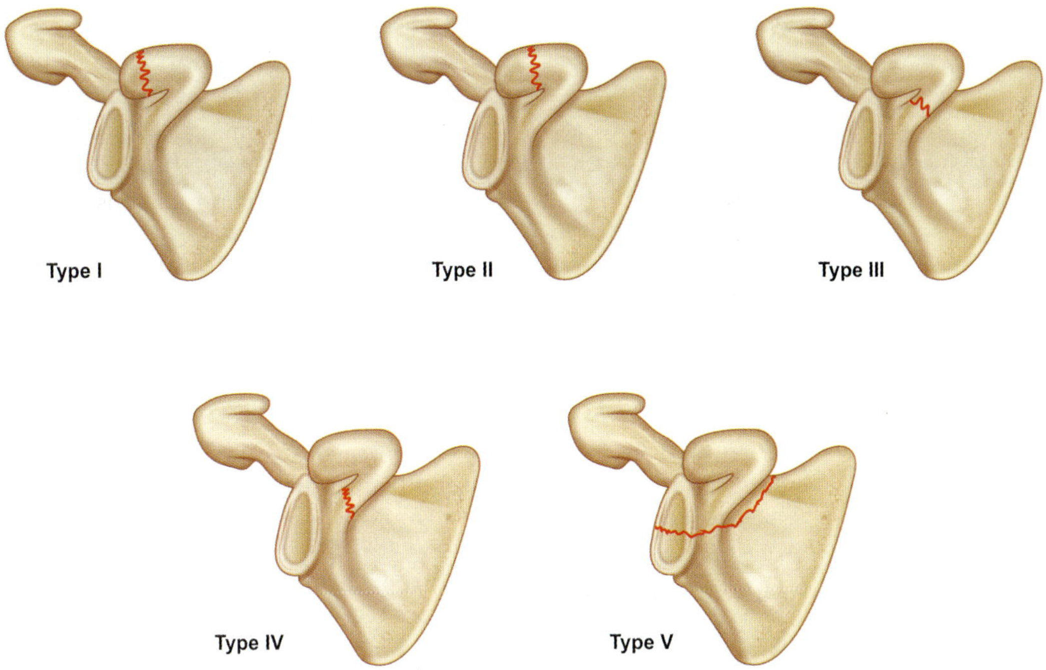

Figure 12.5: The Eyres classification of coracoid fractures—Type I: tip (epiphyseal) fracture; Type II: mid-process; Type III: basal fracture; Type IV: involving the superior body of scapula; Type V: involving the glenoid fossa.

Type II being anterior.[28] Type I fractures accounted for approximately 80% of all fractures and potentially could result in disruption of the scapuloclavicular connection.

Eyres et al. reviewed 12 fractures of the coracoid process and distinguished five fracture patterns (Fig. 12.5). Traction forces applied through attached ligaments or tendons cause Type 1 (tip or epiphyseal fracture), Type 2 (mid-process) and Type 3 (basal) fractures. Type IV (superior body of scapula) and Type V (extension into glenoid cavity) fractures result from shearing forces as the scapula translates medially or when the clavicle contacts the coracoid directly.[29] Each fracture type is then given an A or B modifier representing respectively, the presence or absence of associated AC joint injury. The Ideberg Type III glenoid cavity fracture also involves the coracoid. The fracture enters the glenoid cavity, follows the physeal scar and exits through the superior border of the scapula.

Acromion Process Fractures

Acromion process fractures account for 7% of all scapular fractures. Acromial fractures largely occur via two mechanisms: (1) a direct blow from a significant force or (2) from a forceful superior translation of the humerus. Kuhn et al. proposed a classification system of acromion process fractures based on review of 27 fractures (Fig. 12.6).[30] Type I fractures are nondisplaced and are subdivided into avulsion (Type Ia) and true fractures (Type Ib). Type II fractures are displaced superiorly; therefore, resulting in no reduction of the subacromial space. Type III fractures result in reduction of the subacromial space either through inferior displacement or in association with a superiorly displaced scapular neck fracture.

Surgical Indications

Scapular Body Fractures

Due to the enveloping musculature, the majority of scapular body fractures are non or minimally displaced and are routinely treated nonoperatively. The systematic review by Zlowodzki et al.[31] revealed 99% of all isolated scapular body fractures treated nonoperatively, achieving excellent or good results in 86% of cases. The surgical management of scapular body fractures is best indicated with combined injuries, such as, scapular body fractures associated with fractures of the glenoid neck and/or floating shoulder injuries.

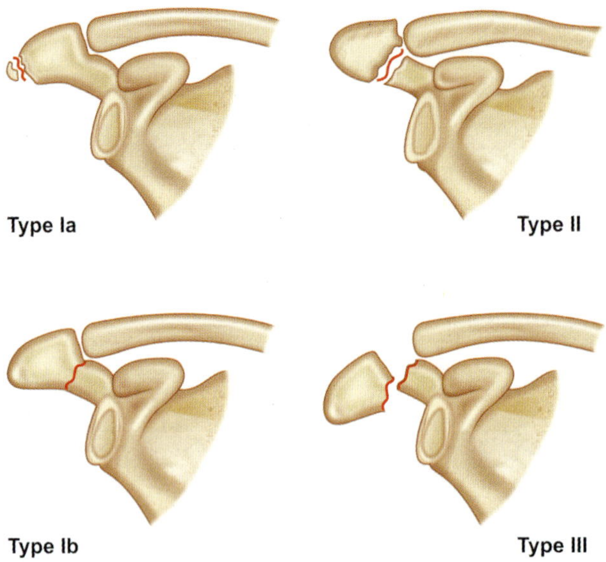

Figure 12.6: The Kuhn classification of acromion fractures—Type Ia: avulsion fracture; Type Ib: true nondisplaced acromial body fracture; Type II: superior displacement causing no reduction in subacromial space; Type III: inferior displacement causing reduction in subacromial space.

Scapular Neck Fractures

Indications for surgical treatment of scapular neck fractures remain controversial. Generally, surgical indications have originated with Ada and Miller's case series that identified displacement of greater than 1 cm or angulation greater than 40° as indicated for surgical fixation.[26] Ada and Miller found that patients with displaced scapular neck fractures had residual pain in 50% and residual weakness in 40% of cases. The authors concluded the complaints of pain and weakness resulted from rotator cuff dysfunction secondary to scapular neck fractures. As the glenoid cavity displaces, the normal lever arm of the rotator cuff is distorted. Furthermore, they noted that the normal compressive force of the rotator cuff would be transformed to shear force, when the tilt angle of the glenoid cavity reached 40–45° leading to subacromial impingement.

Glenoid Fractures

Operative intervention is indicated for all glenoid fractures resulting in articular incongruity greater than 2 mm, subluxation of the humeral head or glenohumeral instability. Ideberg Type I fractures displaced greater than 1 cm and involving greater than 25% of the articular surface anteriorly or 33% of the articular surface posteriorly can result in glenohumeral instability and therefore, operative fixation is indicated. Surgery is also indicated for Ideberg Types II, III and IV fractures displaced more than 2 mm or more, or with subluxation of the humeral head. Type V fractures are combinations of Types II, III and IV fractures and therefore, share the same indications for surgical intervention. Type VI fractures are characterized by extensive comminution, and therefore, surgery is not indicated even if fragments are significantly displaced.[23]

Coracoid Fractures

Coracoid fractures have a particularly high association with concomitant ipsilateral shoulder injuries. Ogawa reported an associated AC joint injury in 60 of 67 patients with coracoids fractures.[27] Operative fixation is indicated for all Ogawa Type I and Eyres Types IV and V fractures, as they are proximal to the coracoclavicular ligamentous attachment.

Acromial Fractures

Acromial fractures usually occur secondary to a direct blow to the lateral shoulder or significant superior displacement of the humeral head. One must, however, be aware of an os acromial, which occurs in up to 2.7% of the population and may mimic a fracture. Acromial fractures are most commonly minimally or nondisplaced, in which case conservative management yields good results. Kuhn Type III fractures result in inferior displacement and subsequent decrease in the subacromial space and are indicated for operative reduction and fixation to avoid impingement. It should be noted that the acceptable amount of displacement has not been well defined.

Surgical Anatomy, Positioning and Approaches

From Latin meaning "shoulder", the scapula is a flat and triangular bone, whose 18 muscular attachments and clavicular and thoracic articulations link the upper extremity with the axial skeleton (Fig. 12.7). The scapular body is thin to the point of translucency in the central portions of the supraspinatus and infraspinatus fossae,

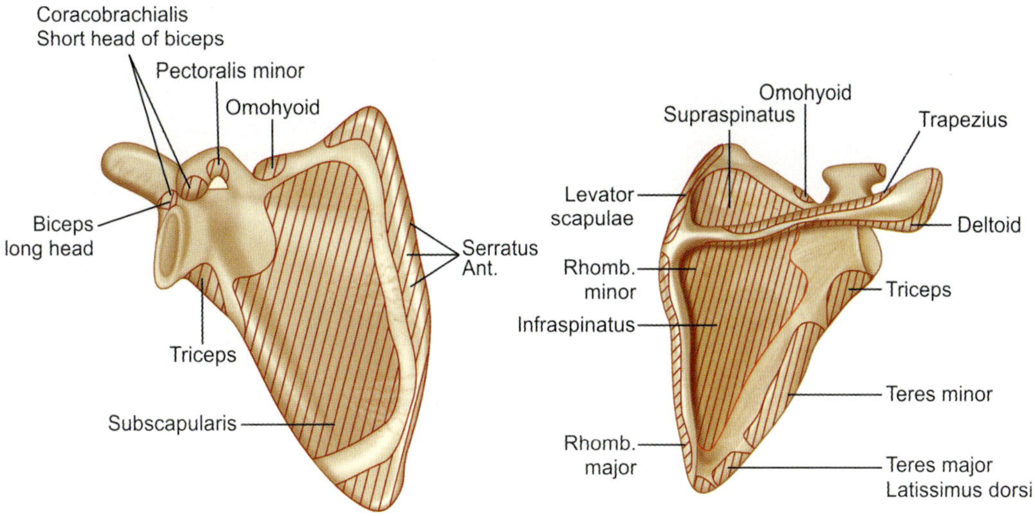

Figure 12.7: Note the sites of various muscular attachments to the scapula.

and is bordered by thicker peripheral bone. The anterior concave undersurface parallels the convex surface of the thorax, and is occupied by broad origin of the subscapularis muscle. Posteriorly, the scapular spine serves as a partition to the supraspinatus and infraspinatus fossae, from which originate their so named muscles. Medially, the scapular spine separates the superior and inferior angles of scapula and courses superolaterally, terminating as the acromion process. The acromion overhangs the head of the humerus and its overlying rotator cuff and subacromial bursa. The deltoid originates from this process. The trapezius inserts along the scapular spine and acromion anteriorly. Scapular protraction is achieved by the serratus anterior, which courses deep to the subscapularis to its insertion along the medial border of the scapula. The rhomboid muscles retract the scapula through their insertion on the medial border.

Approaches to the scapula can be divided into anterior and posterior approaches. The anterior approach is indicated for displaced intra-articular glenoid fractures involving anterior and/or inferior rim, coracoid fractures and scapular neck and body fractures with glenoid involvement not readily visualized by posterior approach alone (combined anterior and posterior approach). The posterior approach is indicated for scapular neck and body fractures, posterior glenoid rim fractures and posterior fracture dislocation of the glenohumeral joint.

Anterior Approach to the Scapula

Positioning

The patient is positioned in the semi-fowler position (30° elevation of the head of bed) with all bony prominences kept well padded. A rolled towel is placed along the medial border of the scapula to slightly elevate the involved shoulder. We typically use a pneumatically powered arm positioner to allow complete intraoperative range of motion of the shoulder. With an arm positioner, the surgeon can also stand freely in the axilla enhancing visualization and surgeon comfort. However, in the absence of previously mentioned arm positioner, a floating arm board attached to the side of the bed is more than adequate. The need for intraoperative fluoroscopy is minimal as the vast majority of the procedure is carried out under direct visualization. Still, we typically ensure that a single AP projection of the glenohumeral joint can be obtained by bringing the c-arm in "over the top" prior to prepping and draping.

Approach

With the arm held in neutral rotation and slight abduction, surface anatomy is palpated and the proposed incision is marked from a point directly superior to the coracoid at the anterior edge of clavicle to a point at the most anterior edge of humeral insertion of the deltoid. This line is slightly lateral to the axillary fold or deltopectoral groove, but

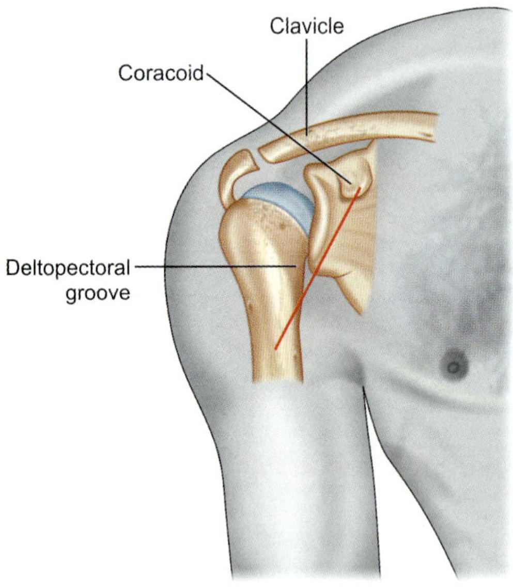

Figure 12.8: Note the incision placement for the anterior deltopectoral approach.

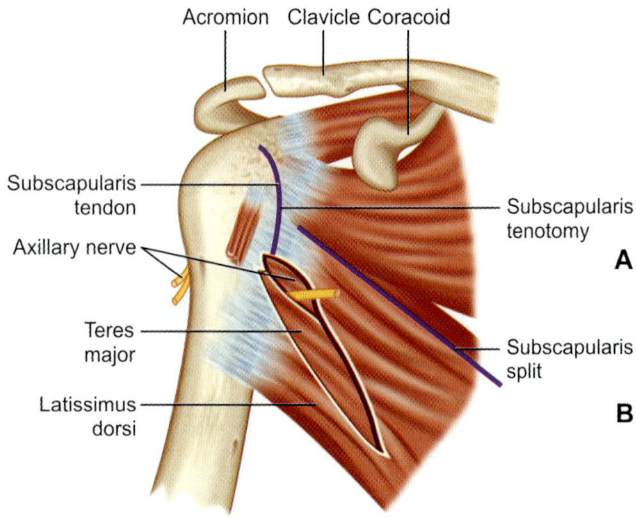

Figure 12.9: Exposure of the glenoid fracture or glenohumeral joint can be achieved by way of either (A) a subscapularis tenotomy placed 1 cm medial to its insertion onto the lesser tuberosity or (B) a longitudinal muscle split at the border of the superior two-third and inferior one-third along the length of its muscle fibers.

placement of the skin incision at this level will typically aid in lateral retraction of the deltoid. A skin incision is made along this line beginning at the most proximal extent and extending distally 10–20 cm dependent on the size of the patient and severity of injury (Fig. 12.8). The deltopectoral fascia is identified and full thickness cutaneous flaps are developed medially and laterally. Development of these flaps will again aid in deep retraction later in the case. The cephalic vein is then identified, and the interval between the deltoid and pectoralis major is developed by a combination of sharp and blunt dissection. It is typically easiest to identify the cephalic vein proximally, where a fat plane exists between the deltoid and pectoralis. Blood loss is decreased and the integrity of the cephalic vein is better maintained with retraction of the vein laterally with the deltoid. The subdeltoid space is developed and mobilized by blunt manual dissection from the clavicle over the humeral head and down to the deltoid insertion. Next, the clavipectoral fascia, which lies over the conjoined tendon and subscapularis, is incised up to the level of the coracoacromial ligament. A deltoid retractor is placed laterally, and the subscapularis insertion is identified. Gentle rotation of the shoulder will aid in identification of the subscapularis insertion as the tendon tightens in external rotation. Next, the subscapularis must be split or taken down with a tenotomy to allow access to the anterior capsule and glenoid (Fig. 12.9). Tagging sutures should be placed to aid in later repair. It is important to note that long-term outcome is highly dependent on subscapularis competence and function after surgery predicating the need for meticulous repair of subscapularis upon closure.[32,33]

Subscapularis Split Technique

Isolated anterior glenoid rim fractures with minimal comminution can typically be approached through a subscapularis split. This is a limited exposure without access to the extra-articular scapula, but the subscapularis footprint is not significantly compromised.[34,35] The superior and inferior borders of the subscapularis are initially defined. The axillary nerve should be palpated inferior to the subscapularis and should be protected. A longitudinal split is created at the junction between superior two-thirds and inferior one-third of the muscle belly. The split is taken down to, but not through the underlying anterior capsule. The capsule blends with the subscapularis tendon laterally near its insertion into the lesser tuberosity making identification of the plane between the two easier at a more medial location.

Traction sutures are placed in the superior and inferior aspects of the subscapularis, and further mobilization of the capsule is performed with a Cobb elevator. In the setting of trauma, the underlying capsule will often be violated and the fracture should be approached through a rent in the capsule. If intact, the anterior capsule should be opened sharply to identify the underlying glenoid rim. When possible, the capsule is closed with a 2-0 nonabsorbable braided suture. The subscapularis split is closed with a running absorbable suture. If the entirety of the case is performed through a subscapularis split alone, we allow full passive external rotation of the arm as tolerated postoperatively.

Subscapularis Tenotomy Technique

In contrast to the subscapularis split, the tenotomy technique yields greater exposure of the glenohumeral capsule and joint. However, postoperatively, the repaired tendon is ranged cautiously until the tendon has healed. With this technique, the superior extent of the subscapularis is identified and the rotator interval is opened sharply in a horizontal fashion. The subscapularis tendon is divided 1 cm medial to the bicipital groove with the arm held in neutral rotation. The tendon is reflected medially and is further elevated from the underlying capsule as previously described. The anterior circumflex humeral vessels lie at the inferior margin of the subscapularis, just superior to the axillary nerve. Care should be taken with inferior release of the subscapularis. At closure of the case, the subscapularis tendon is repaired back to the lateral cuff with nonabsorbable sutures. Alternatively, the subscapularis repair can also be released with suture anchors or other transosseous techniques. Postoperatively, external rotation is limited to neutral for a minimum of 6 weeks to allow adequate time for healing.

Posterior Approach to the Scapula

Positioning

The posterior approach to the scapula can be performed in prone or lateral decubitus position (Fig. 12.7). We prefer the lateral decubitus position for two reasons. First and most importantly, the anterior aspect of the shoulder is prepped into the surgical field allowing for access to the anterior approach if necessary. Similarly, an accessory anterior incision or arthroscopic portal can be established to aid in reduction and fixation of the intra-articular glenoid. Second, the lateral decubitus position allows greater mobility of the arm and shoulder girdle if significant manual manipulation is required to achieve anatomic reduction. The entire affected extremity from fingertip to neck is prepped and draped to allow access to the anterior and posterior aspect of the shoulder and appropriate access for manipulation. The arm is rested across the body on a sterile Mayo stand or large bump. Once positioned, the bed can be rotated 10–20° to bring the scapula up and into a more comfortable operative position. If significant intra-articular comminution exists and an arthroscopically assisted approach is planned, a commercially available lateral traction device is attached to the foot of the table and 10–15 pounds of weight are available intraoperatively. We do not advocate suspending the arm in traction for the entirety of the case, as this may increase the risk of neurologic injury in an already significantly traumatized extremity.

Approach

Surface anatomy and the planned incision are marked with a sterile marker (Figs 12.10A to C). The Judet posterior approach is created as a large L-shaped incision beginning at the posterolateral corner of the acromion, running medially along the superomedial border of the scapula, and then turning in a caudad direction along the medial vertebral border of the scapula.[36,37] An incision is made sharply along these lines and full thickness cutaneous flaps are developed. During preoperative planning, a decision should have been made to proceed with a full open or modified Judet approach. The full Judet approach involves complete detachment and elevation of all muscular attachments off the infraspinatus fossae. The modified Judet approach utilizes limited windows to access the posterior glenoid, medial and lateral borders. An extensile approach is typically indicated with more extensive fracture patterns exiting the medial scapular border at multiple locations.

This large skin flap is then dissected with an extrafascial plane laterally to expose the lateral aspect of the scapula. The deltoid is now easily identified and a nonabsorbable suture is placed on its most medial attachment to the spine.

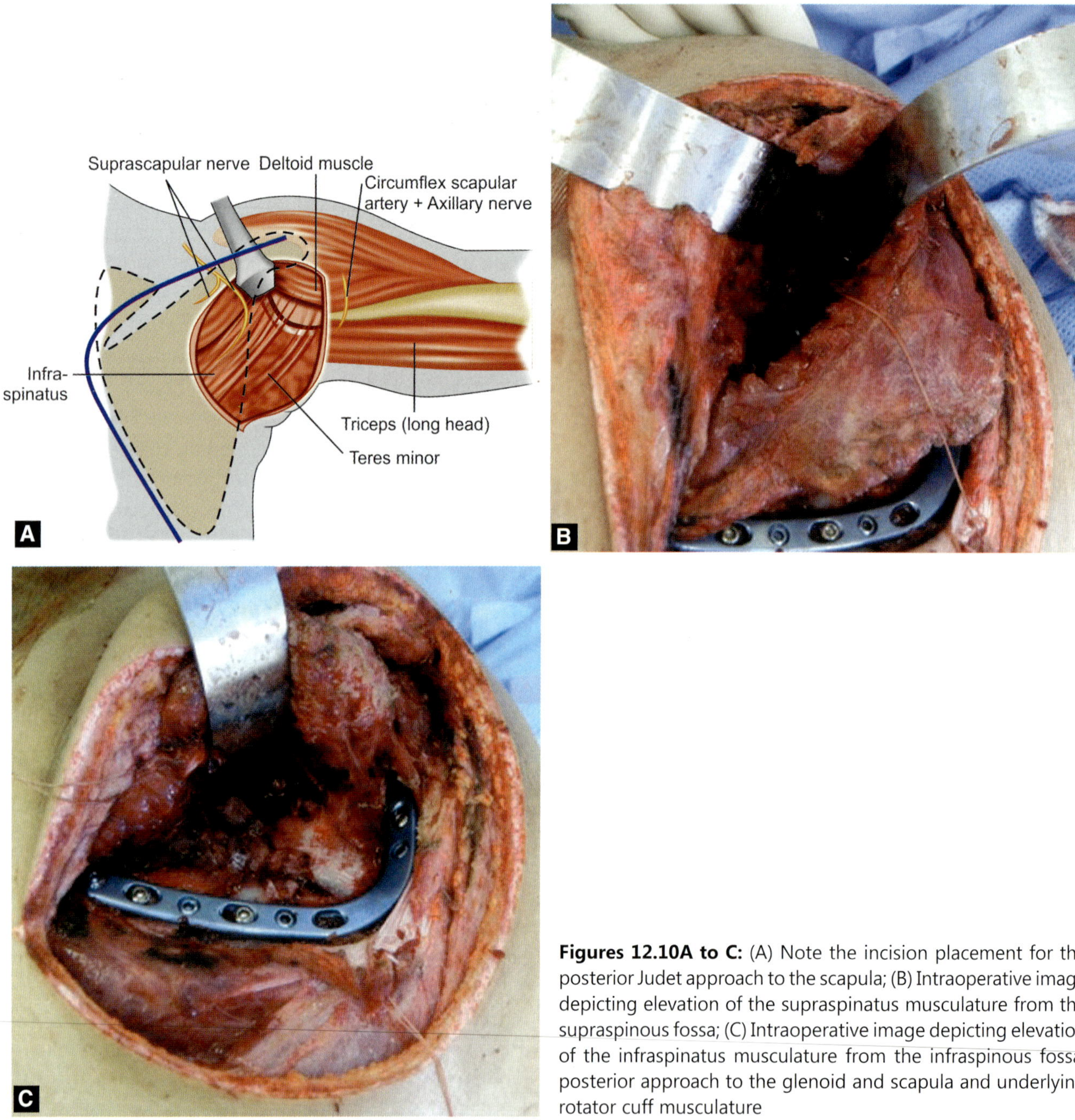

Figures 12.10A to C: (A) Note the incision placement for the posterior Judet approach to the scapula; (B) Intraoperative image depicting elevation of the supraspinatus musculature from the supraspinous fossa; (C) Intraoperative image depicting elevation of the infraspinatus musculature from the infraspinous fossa, posterior approach to the glenoid and scapula and underlying rotator cuff musculature

This will serve as a reference point for reattachment at the end of the case. The deltoid is then retracted laterally with blunt dissection off the infraspinatus and sharp dissection off the spine. With the deltoid elevated laterally, the supraspinatus, infraspinatous and teres minor are now easily visualized. The internervous plane is between infraspinatus (suprascapular nerve) and teres minor (axillary nerve). If the fracture is easily identified through this interval, reduction should proceed with small pointed reduction clamps and kirschner (k-) wire fixation.

Malunited fractures or partially healed fractures (>2–3 weeks) may require an extensile approach to remove fracture callus and to allow mobilization of fracture fragments (Figs 12.10A to C).

Surgical Techniques

Technique 1: Scapular Body Fractures

Preoperative Planning

Operative interventions for scapular body fractures are extremely rare, with Zolowdzki[31] reporting that 99% of these fractures are treated nonoperatively. In the circumstance in which operative fixation is favored, a thorough evaluation of the patient is paramount. Associated injuries such as rib fractures, pneumothorax and visceral injuries must not be overlooked. Moreover, adequate imaging with an AP, lateral and stryker notch views are needed. It is our practice to always obtain a CT with 3D reconstructions.

Available implants should include 2.0, 2.4, 2.7 and 3.5 reconstruction plates with a locking screw option. The locking screw option aids in fixation because the scapular body is thin and bicortical purchase can be difficult. Fluoroscopy and a radiolucent table should be utilized.

Technique

For isolated scapular body fractures, the patient is positioned in a lateral position with the arm draped free. A large bump is placed under the operative arm or a radiolucent platform is used under the drapes for support. The aseptic field is brought down to the midline of the back, midline of the chest and to the inferior neck region to maximise the surgical field. A posterior approach is used. It is our practice to utilize the modified Judet approach (Figs 12.11A to H).[38] As described, the superior aspect of the "L-shaped" incision parallels the horizontal plane of the scapular spine, and upon reaching the medial border of the scapula, incisions makes a 90° turn inferiorly. This large skin flap is then dissected with an extrafascial plane laterally to expose the lateral aspect of scapula. The deltoid is now easily identified and a nonabsorbable suture is placed on its most medial attachment to the spine. This will serve as a reference point for reattachment at the end of the case. The deltoid is then retracted laterally with a blunt dissection off the infraspinatous and sharp dissection off the spine. With the deltoid elevated laterally, the supraspinatous, infraspinatous and teres minor are now easily visualized. The internervous plane is between the infraspinatous (suprascapular nerve) and the teres minor (axillary nerve). If the fracture is easily identified through this interval, reduction should proceed with small pointed reduction clamps and k-wire fixation. A contoured 2.7 reconstruction plate sits well at the inferolateral portion of the scapula. Adjunct use of locking screws may help with stability if cortical screw purchase is poor. If the fracture is not well visualized, the infraspinatous can be elevated off of its fossa. Care must be taken; however, to prevent over retraction, which may result in suprascapular nerve palsy. Anteroposterior and scapular "Y" views are used during the case to assess fracture reduction and evaluate screw length. Overpenetration of screws can cause pain with scapulothoracic motion.

Upon closure, the supraspinatus and infraspinatus is placed back in the fossa and the deltoid is retracted back into position with the previously mentioned marking suture. The deltoid is reattached to the scapular spine with drill holes and nonabsorbable suture. A drain is placed. The skin and subcutaneous tissue are closed in layers.

Postoperatively, pendulum exercises are immediately started. Formal active, active-assisted and passive range of motion begins once the drains have been removed and the patient's pain is tolerable.

SCAPULAR BODY FRACTURES: Pearls and Pitfalls

- The patient should be positioned in the lateral decubitus position with the anterior shoulder draped into the surgical field
- A stay suture in the medial deltoid allows for anatomic realignment of the deltoid upon closure
- Overzealous retraction of the infraspinatous can cause suprascapular nerve palsy
- Overpenetration of the far cortex with screws can cause pain with scapulothoracic motion
- Early motion is favored as tolerated

Technique 2: Scapular Neck Fractures

Preoperative Planning

Extra-articular scapular neck fractures account for 25% of all scapular fractures. Rotator cuff dysfunction, shoulder girdle dysfunction and impingement are late sequelae that result from malunited or nonunited fractures. It is therefore, our protocol to operatively treat extra-articular scapular neck fractures with greater than 1 cm displacement and/or 40° of angulation in any plane.

Preoperative X-rays include AP, lateral Y and stryker notch views. Computerized tomography scans with 3D recons are invaluable. If the fracture line exits medial to the coracoid or through the body and the shoulder suspensory complex is intact, nonoperative management

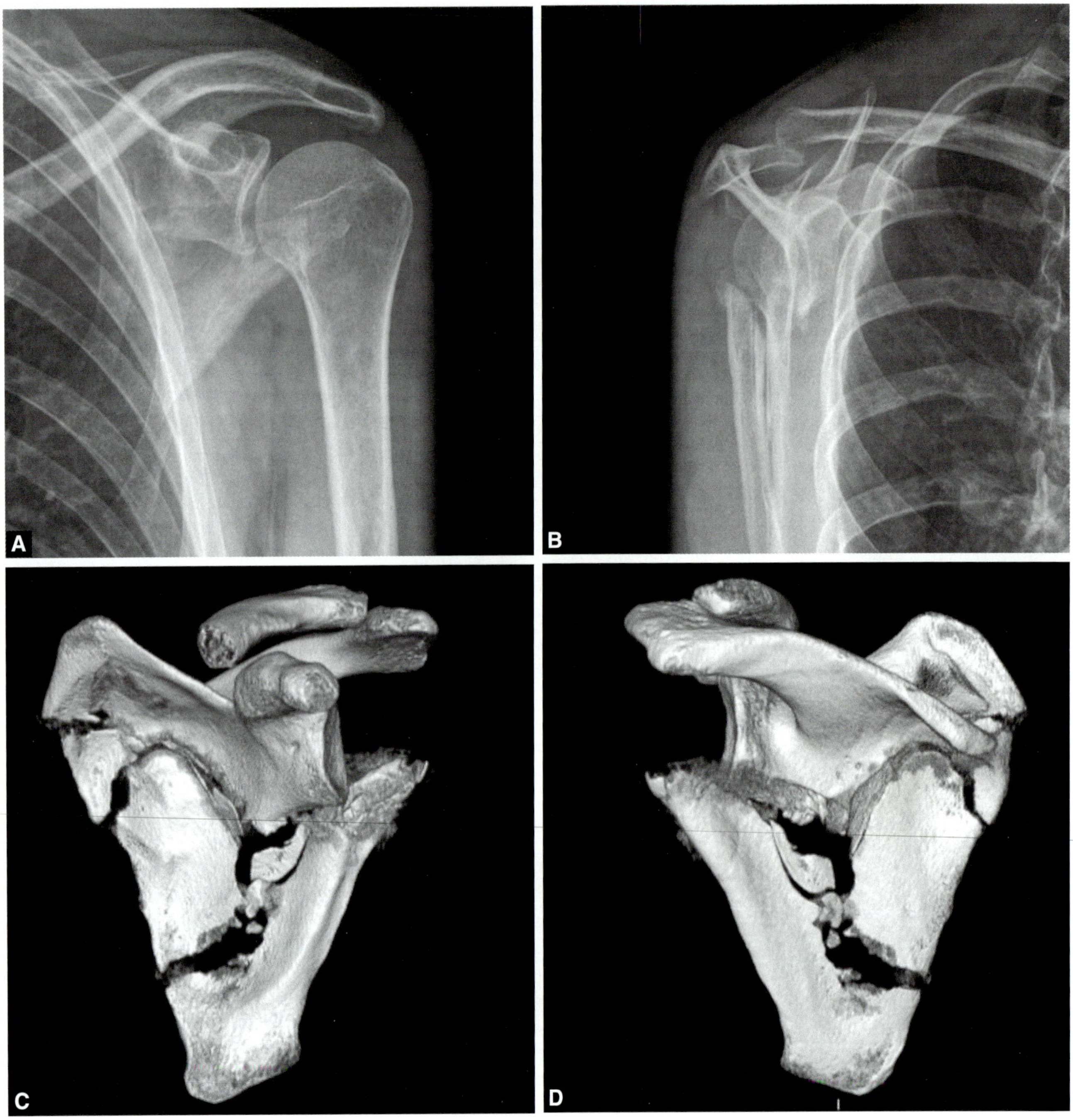

Figures 12.11A to D

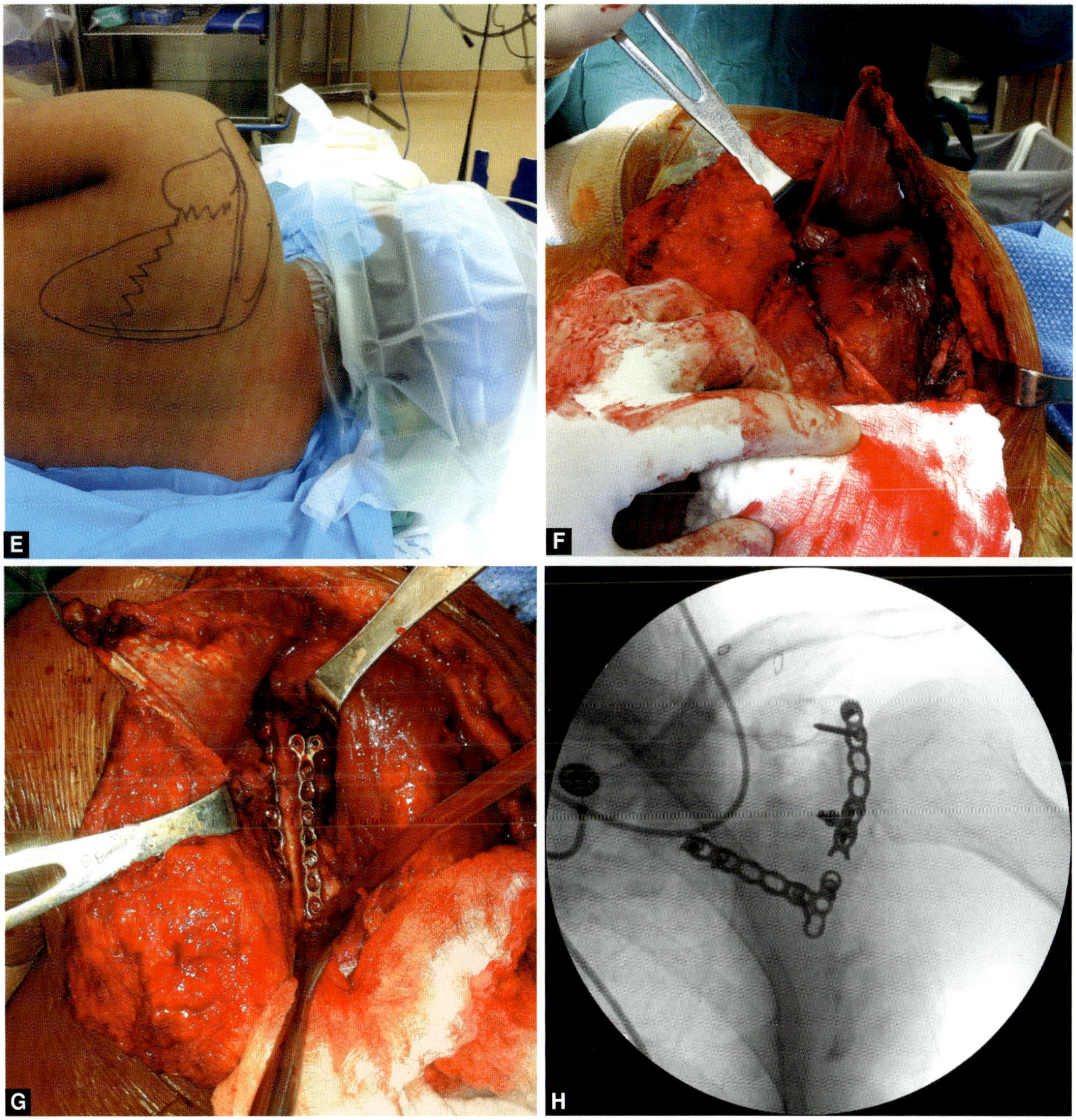

Figures 12.11A to H: This is a case of a 32-year-old male involved in a high energy motor vehicle accident, who incurred a number of injuries including a scapula fracture requiring open reduction and internal fixation (ORIF). (A and B) Radiographs demonstrated a comminuted and displaced scapular fracture; (C and D) Three-dimensional CT reconstructions demonstrated extensive comminution of the scapula body with shortening and displacement of the glenoid; (E) The patient is positioned in the lateral decubitus position draping the entire upper trunk and ipsilateral arm to the neck; (F) A Judet approach was utilized. Note the elevation of deltoid off the scapula revealing the supraspinatus muscle and scapular spine; (G) Deep dissection involves elevation of the supraspinatus and infraspinatus muscles off the scapula followed by reduction and plate fixation; (H) Postoperative radiographs following ORIF.

may be adequate if closed reduction restores the anatomy within the nonoperative protocol. If the fracture exits lateral to the coracoid, closed reduction will fail as ligamentotaxis is insufficient to hold the reduction.

Instrument we recommend include 2.0, 2.4, 2.7 and 3.5 reconstruction plates with the locking option. Moreover, headless compression screws, k-wires and small fragment reduction tools are very useful. A radiolucent table and fluoroscopy should also be utilized. Locking plates and nonlocking orthogonal (90-90) plating are techniques that we commonly utilize while fixing scapular neck fractures. Locking screws are advantageous because bicortical purchase is not always an option and osteoporotic bone will lead to screw fixation failure.

Technique

For glenoid neck fractures, we recommend a posterior approach. The patient is positioned in the lateral position with the arm draped free. A large bump is placed under the operative arm or a radiolucent platform is used under the drapes for support. The aseptic field is brought down to midline of the back, midline of the chest and to the inferior neck region to aid in exposure.

If the fracture exits medial to the coracoid, a posterior approach utilizing a modified Judet approach is used as previously described (Figs 12.12A to H). If the fracture exits lateral to the coracoid, a vertical posterior approach is used. The incision starts at the tip of the posterolateral acromium and follows the posterior axillary fold inferiorly. The deltoid is split in line with its fibers with limited lateral detachment of its origin. The internervous plane is between the infraspinatous (suprascapular nerve) and the teres minor (axillary nerve). In order to gain adequate exposure of the glenoid neck and rim, either a split of the infraspinatous or partial detachment of the insertion may be performed. The joint capsule and neck are now easily visualized. Reduction is accomplished with pointed reduction clamps or k-wires used as joysticks. Care must be taken to preserve all soft tissue attachments in order to preserve blood supply. After fluoroscopic assisted reduction is achieved, the fracture is held reduced with k-wires. Two reconstruction plates are contoured and are applied along the neck in an orthogonal manner. The locking option in the glenoid fragment is beneficial because it eliminates inadvertent intra-articular screw penetration. Cannulated screws are helpful if a large fragment is present that allows for lag screw fixation. During the reduction, one should be aware of the suprascapular nerve as it passes through spinoglenoid notch. It passes 2 cm medial to the glenoid rim at the level of supraglenoid tubercle and 1 cm medial to the level of scapular spine. The axillary nerve is inferior to the teres minor and remains out of the trajectory of implant insertion.

Upon closure, the infraspinatous is reattached with nonabsorbable suture. Similarly, the deltoid split is repaired. A drain is placed. The subcutaneous layer and skin are closed in layers.

Postoperatively, pendulum exercises are immediately started. Formal active, active-assisted and passive range of motion begins, once the drains have been removed and the patient's pain is tolerable.

SCAPULAR NECK FRACTURES: Pearls and Pitfalls

- Careful attention must be paid to the anatomic location of the suprascapular nerve
- The posterolateral deltoid may be liberally split or taken down to gain access to the scapular neck
- The use of locking screws allows for fixed angle fixation in the glenoid component
- Orthogonal 90-90 plating allows for a stronger construct to counter torque resistance

Technique 3: Glenoid Fossa Fractures

Preoperative Planning

Glenoid fossa fractures can result in joint incongruity, secondary glenohumeral instability and progressive joint degeneration. These fractures result from direct impaction of the glenoid fossa. Moreover, these injuries are distinctly different from avulsion fractures that occur with glenohumeral dislocations. Each fracture pattern utilizes a different approach and implants, and thus, will be described according to the Ideberg and Goss fracture type with Type IA representing an anterior and Type IB representing a posterior glenoid fossa fracture.

Preoperative radiographs include AP, scapular Y, axillary and weight-bearing views. The CT scans with 3D reconstructions are very useful in preoperative templating.

Recommended implants include 2.0, 2.4, 2.7 and 3.5 reconstruction plates with locking screw options. Moreover, headless compression screws are very useful. Small fragment reduction tools and k-wires are also imperative to have available.

Technique: Type IA Glenoid Fractures

Type IA fractures involve the anterior glenoid surface. Our operative indications are at least 10 mm of displacement

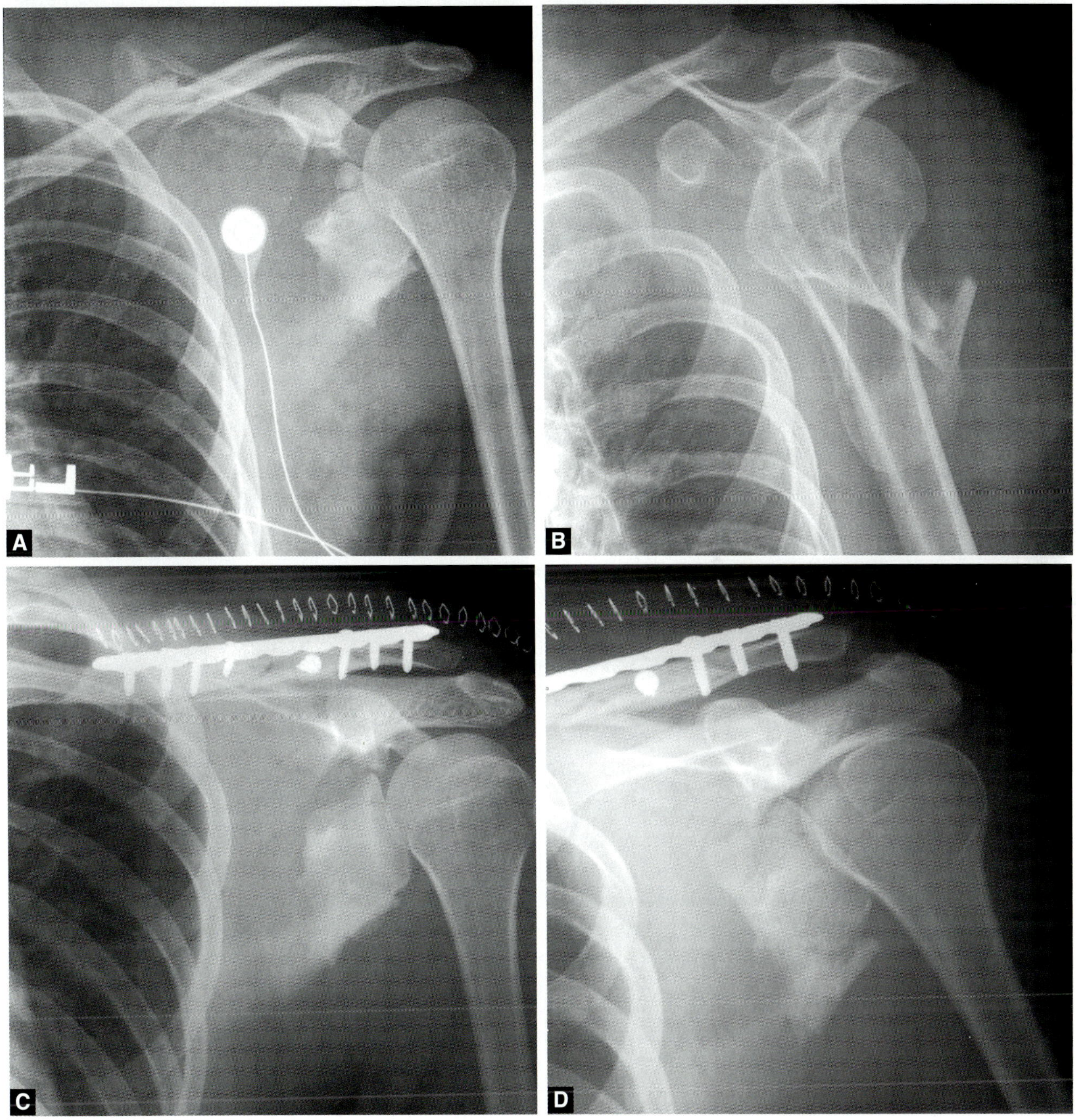

Figures 12.12A to D

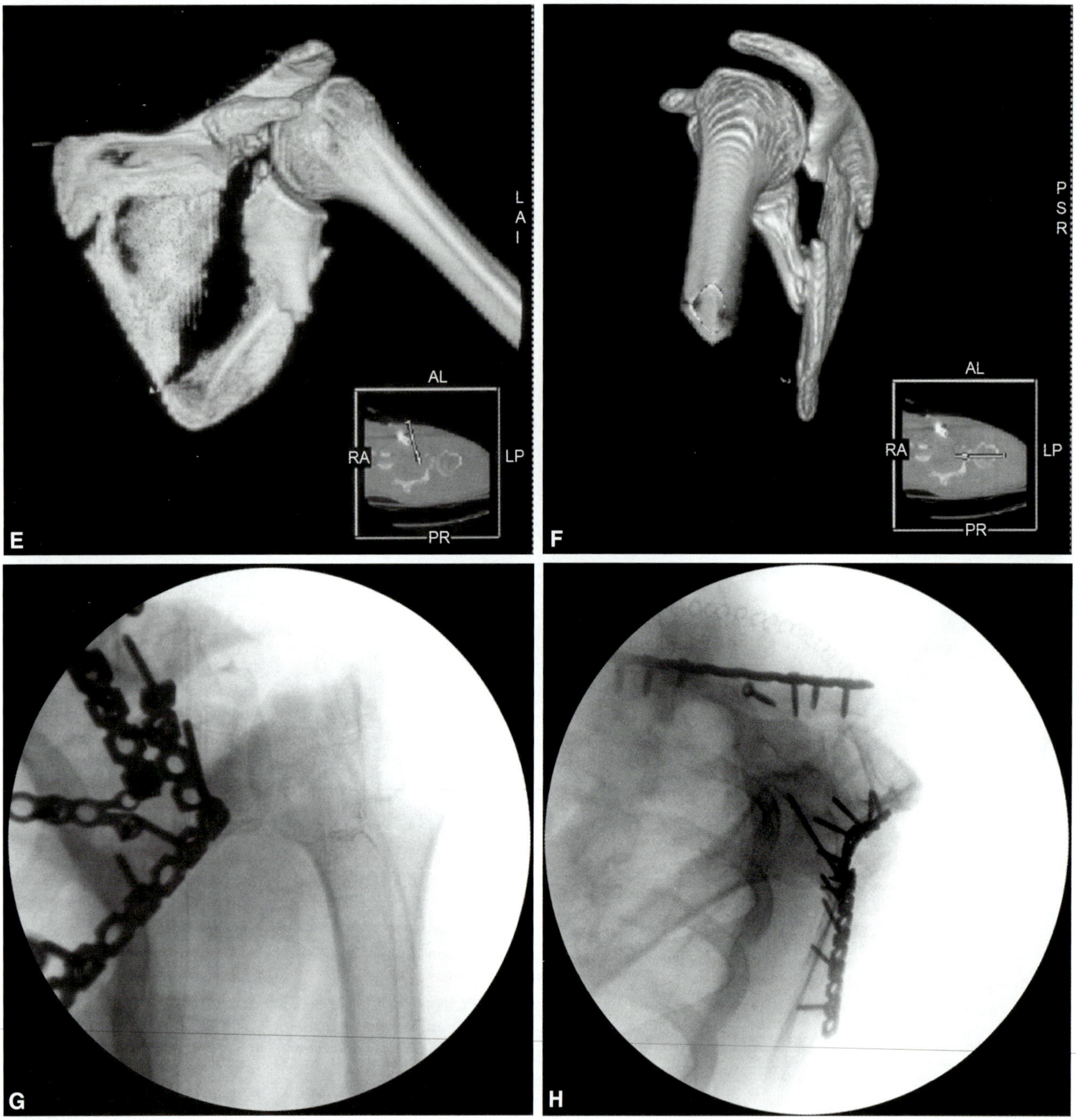

Figures 12.12A to H: This is a case of 29-year-old male, who fell from a height and incurred multiple injuries about the shoulder. (A and B) Standard radiographs of the shoulder demonstrated a concomitant fracture of the glenoid neck and clavicle; (C and D) The shoulder was stabilized with plate fixation of the clavicle; (E and F) Three-dimensional CT reconstructions demonstrated a glenoid neck fracture with displacement and medialization of the glenoid fragment. The patient underwent open reduction and plate fixation of the scapula through the posterior Judet approach; (G and H) Postoperative radiographs following open reduction and internal fixation.

or involvement of greater than one-fourth of the glenoid surface. It must again be emphasized that these fractures are distinctly different from Bankart lesions that occur during a glenohumeral dislocation.

The beach chair position is utilized to facilitate an anterior approach and to utilize an arthroscope to evaluate the glenohumeral joint. The upper extremity is draped from the midline anteriorly to a point medial to the scapula. The drapes extend beyond the base of the neck medially. We prefer to utilize the deltopectoral anterior approach (Figs 12.13A to D). During deep dissection, we utilize a subscapularis tenotomy. The subcapularis muscle

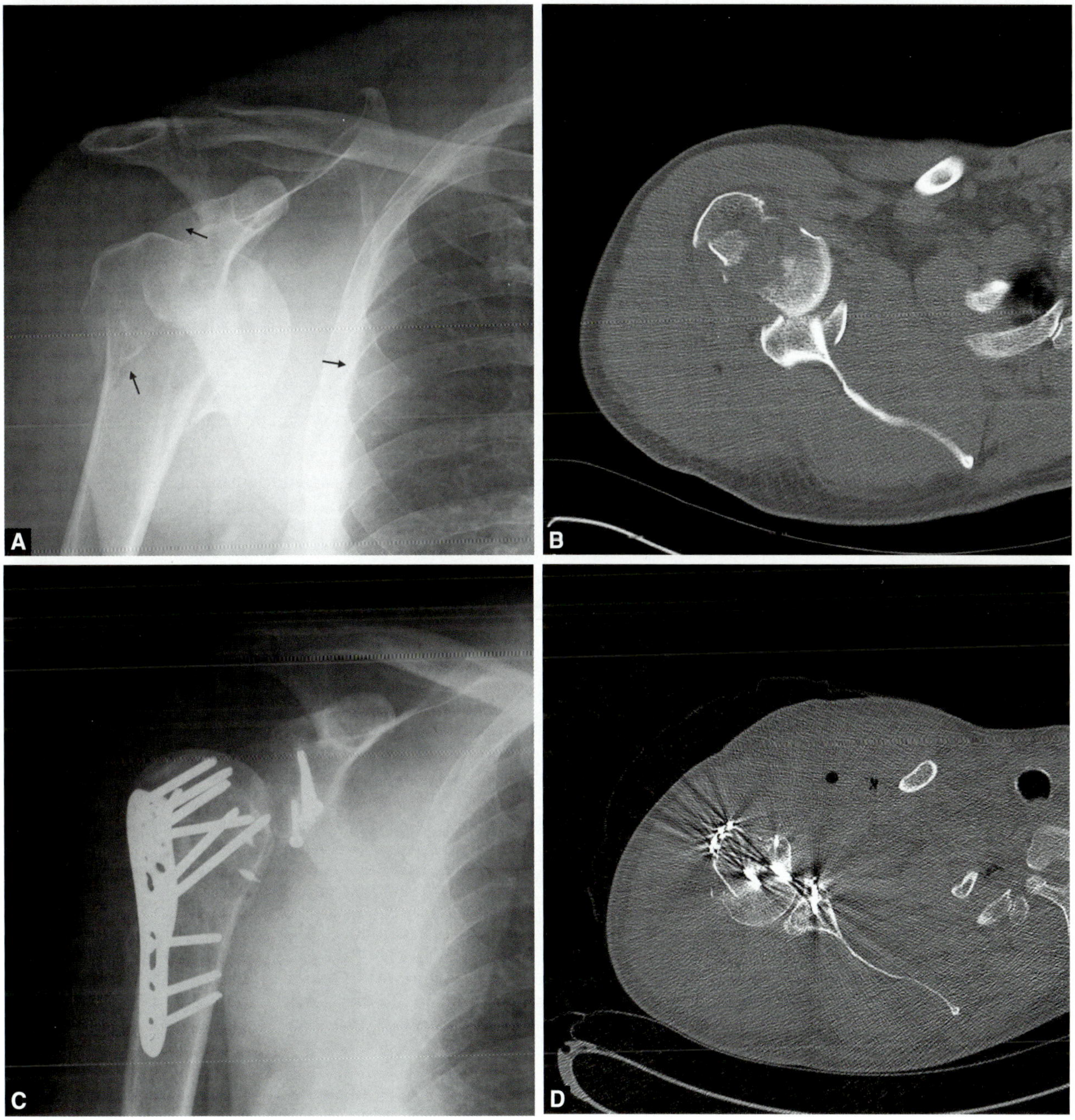

Figures 12.13A to D: This is a case of a 42-year-old male involved in a motor vehicle accident injuring his shoulder. (A) Radiographs demonstrated a proximal humerus fracture and a possible injury to the glenoid fossa; (B) CT scan examination of the shoulder joint confirmed the presence of a displaced anterior glenoid fracture. The patient was indicated for open reduction and internal fixation of the proximal humerus and glenoid through deltopectoral approach; (C) Postoperative radiographs and; (D) CT scans demonstrated a reduced glenohumeral joint and well positioned hardware.

is detached with a vertical incision leaving a substantial cuff of the tissue laterally to afford a sound repair, once the case is finished. The capsule is then identified and incised using a 15 blade. The fracture is exposed and debrided followed by direct reduction utilizing k-wires as joysticks and fracture reduction clamps. Fluoroscopic AP and scapular Y views are obtained to assess reduction. If the fragment is large enough, we recommend using 3.5 mm cortical screws for fixation. If the fragment is small or screw placement must be intra-articular, consider utilizing headless compression screws. Mini-fragment plates with locking constructs can also aid in fracture stabilization.

With the fracture reduced and glenohumeral joint congruity restored, the closure is initiated. The capsule is closed with a braided absorbable suture. The subscapularis is repaired with a braided nonabsorbable suture. The interval between the deltoid and pectoralis muscle is closed in a running fashion. A deep drain is placed. The subcutaneous tissue and skin are closed in layers.

Postoperatively, passive range of motion including pendulum exercise is instituted immediately. Active and passive range of motion begins as tolerated. Active-assisted motion is delayed until 6 weeks in order for fracture healing to occur. Torque resistance exercises are strictly forbidden until 3 months.

Technique: Type IB Glenoid Fractures

Type IB fractures involve the posterior glenoid surface. Our operative indications are at least 10 mm of displacement or involvement of greater than one-fourth of the glenoid surface.

We again prefer the beach chair position to facilitate the posterior approach but also to allow for access to the anterior approach and/or utilize an arthroscope to evaluate the glenohumeral joint. Alternatively, the lateral decubitus position may be utilized. The upper extremity is draped from the midline anteriorly to a point medial to the scapula. The drapes extend beyond the base of the neck medially. We prefer a deltoid splitting posterior approach, but the Judet approach is also effective. The incision starts at the tip of the posterolateral acromion and follows the posterior axillary fold inferiorly. The deltoid is split in line with it fibers along with limited lateral detachment of the deltoid. In order to achieve adequate exposure of the glenoid neck and rim, either a split of the infraspinatous or partial detachment of the insertion is performed. The joint capsule and neck should now be readily visualized. Reduction is accomplished with pointed reduction clamps and k-wires used as joysticks. Care must be taken to preserve all soft tissue attachments in order to preserve blood supply. Following provisional k-wire fixation of the reduced fracture, fluoroscopic AP and scapular Y views are taken to assess the reduction. If the fragment is large enough, we recommend using 3.5 mm cortical screws in a lag screw fashion. If the fragment is large enough, we recommend using 3.5 mm cortical screws for fixation. If the fragment is small or screw placement must be intra-articular, consider utilizing headless compression screws. Mini-fragment plates with locking constructs can also aid in fracture stabilization.

With the fracture reduced and glenohumeral joint congruity restored, closure is initiated. The capsule is closed with a braided absorbable suture. The subscapularis is repaired with a braided nonabsorbable suture. The interval between the deltoid and pectoralis muscle is closed in a running fashion. A deep drain is placed. The subcutaneous tissue and skin is closed in layers.

Postoperatively, passive range of motion including pendulum exercise is instituted immediately. Active and passive range of motion begins as tolerated. Active-assisted motion is delayed until 6 weeks in order for fracture healing to occur. Torque resistance exercises are strictly forbidden until 3 months.

GLENOID FOSSA FRACTURES: Pearls and Pitfalls

- Glenoid fractures must be distinguished from avulsion fractures associated with Bankart lesions following glenohumeral joint dislocation
- Arthroscopy can aid in fracture visualization and reduction
- Access to both the anterior and posterior glenohumeral joint must be available. Combined anterior and posterior approaches may be needed in select cases

Technique 4: Coracoid Fractures

Preoperative Planning

Isolated coracoid fractures are divided into two groups: (1) Type I fractures are proximal to coracoclavicular ligaments and (2) Type II fractures are distal to coracoclavicular ligaments. Type II fractures do not warrant surgical fixation unless they are preventing reduction of a glenohumeral joint dislocation. Indications for fixation of Type I injuries include displacement of coracoid base with involvement of glenoid fossa, brachial plexus compression, and/or fractures with a concomitant Type III or greater AC joint separation.

Preoperative evaluation should include AP, scapular Y and an anterior superior cephalic tilt view of 35°, axillary and weight-bearing views. Computerized tomography scans with 3D reconstructions are very useful in preoperative templating.

Recommended implants include 3.5 mm screws for the coracoids and 2.4, 2.7 and 3.5 reconstruction plates with a locking option for possible fixation of the AC joint. Small fragment reduction tools and k-wires should also be available.

The beach chair position with an anterior approach is utilized. The upper extremity is draped from the midline anteriorly to a point medial to the scapula. The drapes extend beyond the base of the neck medially. The coracoids may be approached through a deltopectoral approach. Alternatively, a direct superior approach may be utilized where the incision is started at the AC joint and is extended inferiorly over the coracoid. The AC joint is subcutaneous and is easily identified. Any disruption of the AC joint is first addressed. If displaced, the AC joint is reduced to its anatomic position and is held in place with either k-wires or plate fixation. Hardware placed across the AC joint will fatigue and fail over time and should, therefore, be removed in a timely manner once the injuries have healed.

The coracoid fracture is reduced and is provisionally fixed with guidewires for 3.5 or 4.5 cannulated screws. The guidewire is placed in an anterior to posterior direction. If a concomitant AC joint dislocation is present, the coracoid fracture will be displaced superiorly. Otherwise, the fracture is typically displaced inferiorly due to the pull of the conjoined tendon. Fracture manipulation should be done with care to avoid injury to the musculocutaneous nerve traveling through the conjoined tendon. A split of the subscapularis muscle is helpful to visualize reduction of the coracoid. Anteroposterior and lateral views are used to evaluate screw position. Fixation is achieved through placement of a 3.5 or 4.5 cannulated screw placed over the guidewire with a washer in an anterior to posterior direction.

The subcutaneous tissue and skin are closed in layers. Postoperatively, passive range of motion including pendulum exercise is instituted immediately. Active range of motion begins as tolerated. Active-assisted and passive motion is delayed until the fracture union is confirmed.

CORACOID FRACTURES: Pearls and Pitfalls

- Reduction of the AC joint is imperative for adequate reduction and fixation of the coracoids
- Fracture displacement may be difficult to assess preoperatively as the coracoclavicular distance will remain normal in the setting of an AC joint separation

Outcomes

Scapular Body Fractures

Long-term outcome studies have challenged the belief that the conservative management of scapular fractures yields uniformly good results. Nordqvist and Peterrson reported outcomes of fractures of the scapular body, spine and neck treated with sling immobilization and early range of motion.[18] Sixty-eight patients were followed for an average of 14 years. Thirty-two percent of patients with scapular neck fractures and 22% of patients with scapular body fractures had fair or poor outcomes, and radiographic deformity correlated to functional outcome. Zlowdowski et al. reviewed 520 scapular fractures from a thorough review of 22 level IV series reported in the literature. As stated earlier, 99% of scapular body fractures were treated nonoperatively; however, 14% of these patients went on to have a fair or poor result.[31] Whether it is lateralization of the scapular body or medialization of the scapular neck, a distinct sub-group clearly defines a cohort that would benefit from surgical fixation. Early ORIF, when possible, given comorbid conditions, can lead to improved outcomes. While combined reporting of outcomes of all scapular fractures is informative, fracture patterns of each anatomic region must be considered individually.

Scapular Neck Fractures

Although operative intervention is rarely undertaken, outcomes are encouraging with anatomic fixation.[38] Reports indicate that better results could be achieved with operative intervention. In one series of scapular neck fractures, 100% of patients had residual pain and 33% had residual weakness at 1-year postinjury following conservative management.[39] Importantly, none of these patients would have been indicated for ORIF based on the guidelines of 1 cm of displacement or 40° of angulation, suggesting that operative indications perhaps should be expanded.

Glenoid Fractures

Mayo et al. examined their experience treating 27 patients with a displaced glenoid fossa fracture with open reduction and internal fixation and identified 82% good and excellent results.[27] They concluded the key to success was anatomic fracture fixation and concentric joint reduction.

Acromion Process Fractures

Kuhn et al. reported excellent results with nonoperative management of all Type I–II fractures.[30] Early surgical intervention is indicated for all Type III fractures as any decrease of the subacromial space leads to significant loss of shoulder range of motion and pain.

Coracoid Process Fractures

On an average of 37 months following coracoid process fractures, Ogawa reported no significant difference between Types I and II fractures whether treated operatively or not.[28] All 53 Type I fractures were treated operatively and 9 of 11 Type II fractures were treated conservatively.

Complications

Zlowodzki et al.'s systematic review of 22 case series revealed that among 141 of 520 fractures treated operatively, there was a 16.5% rate of secondary surgical procedures.[31] The most common reason for return to the operating room was stiffness (8 of 141 requiring manipulation under anesthesia), followed by painful retained hardware (7 of 141 requiring hardware removal), infection (3 of 141 requiring irrigation and debridement), hematoma (2 of 141 requiring evacuation of hematoma) and failure of fixation (2 of 141 requiring revision fixation). One case requiring an arthrodesis for posttraumatic glenohumeral arthrosis was also reported. Furthermore, patients with concomitant head injury were at increased risk of heterotopic ossification.

Malunion

While nonunions are rare, malunions are common and can potentially lead to pain and dysfunction with shoulder function. Overall malunion of scapular body fractures is well tolerated, though occasionally, it can result in painful scapulothoracic crepitus. In contrast, malunions of scapular neck and glenoid fractures can result in glenohumeral instability and posttraumatic joint degeneration. Furthermore, shortening or translation of scapular neck can compromise rotator cuff function and shoulder kinematics.

Iatrogenic Nerve Injury

Iatrogenic nerve injury is best avoided by a thorough understanding of local anatomy and relevant surgical planes. The axillary and musculocutaneous nerves are susceptible to injury during the anterior approach to the shoulder. The suprascapular nerve is at risk during the posterior approach the scapular body. Anteriorly, the suprascapular nerve is vulnerable approximately 2 cm medial to the glenoid rim superiorly. Posteriorly, the suprascapular nerve is vulnerable to injury during surgical exposure of the spinous process as the nerve traverses the suprascapular fossa through the spinoglenoid notch into the infrascapular fossa.

Compartment Syndrome

Although rare, compartment syndrome of the periscapular musculature has been described.[40] Moreover, hemorrhage into the rotator cuff musculature can mimic an acute rotator cuff tear with pain, weakness and decreased range of motion referred to as a pseudorotator cuff rupture.[5] Given the high-energy mechanisms often causing these injuries, this hemorrhage can be significant. Landi et al. presented two cases demonstrating that the musculature surrounding the scapula is susceptible to compartment syndrome, one of which was directly related to a scapular body fracture.[40]

Intrathoracic Scapular Impaction

Four cases of intrathoracic scapular impaction have been reported from high-energy mechanisms of injury resulting in highly comminuted and displaced scapular fractures.[41-44] In each of these four cases, the inferior fracture fragment entered an intercostal space. This injury results from a sustained force that initially causes the scapular body fracture, then continues to exert enough force on the fractured fragment to then fracture one or more ribs and enter the thorax.

Authors' Preferred Management of Select Complications

Case 1: Glenoid Fossa Malunion

A 56-year-old male sustained an anterior glenoid fossa fracture in a motor vehicle accident. Preoperative radiographs and CT scanning confirmed that the fracture was confined to only the glenoid fossa and encompassed 40% of the glenoid surface. Greater than 1 cm of articular displacement was noted and glenohumeral instability was present on physical examination. The patient underwent ORIF through a deltopectoral approach in the beach chair position. Fixation was achieved with two headless compression screws placed in an anterior-to-posterior direction. Postoperatively, the patient was started in a supervised therapy regimen. The patient returned for re-evaluation 6 months postoperatively noting increasing pain and a sense of instability with shoulder motion. Radiographic and CT evaluation noted 5 mm of residual articular step off with evidence of post-traumatic arthritis of the glenohumeral joint.

Discussion

Management of a malunion of the glenoid fossa fracture is predicated upon the extent of residual articular step-off, the presence of instability, and the extent of glenohumeral arthrosis. Whenever possible, residual articular step-off of greater than 2–3 mm in the glenoid fossa comprising more than 25% of the glenoid surface, regardless of complaints of instability, is best treated with corrective osteotomy to restore articular alignment and deter the development of glenohumeral arthrosis. In cases complicated by instability, malunion correction may be augmented with capsular imbrication. However, in cases with established glenohumeral arthritis, total shoulder arthroplasty may be considered.

Technique

Because of the presence of advanced posttraumatic arthritis of the glenohumeral joint, a total shoulder arthroplasty was indicated. Preoperative rotator cuff examination indicated intact subscapularis, supraspinatous, infraspinatous, and teres minor. Deltoid function was also noted to be adequate. Given the fact the rotator cuff was competent, a standard arthroplasty was indicated. Alternatively, in the setting of rotator cuff deficiency, a reverse total shoulder should be considered by utilizing the biomechanical advantage of the deltoid muscle.

The deltopectoral approach was again utilized with the patient placed in the beach chair position. The subscapularis was taken down leaving a 5 mm cuff of tendon. Meticulous attention to the subscapularis integrity is imperative as the prior surgery may have compromised its insertion. The two headless screws were removed, and the total shoulder arthroplasty commenced. Although no augments were needed, a femoral head allograft was available if there was a need for glenoid augmentation. A standard total shoulder arthoplasty was placeed with a cemented glenoid component and a press-fit humeral component. The subscapularis was repaired using #2 ethibond. Physical therapy commenced on postoperative day number 1 per protocol.

Case 2: Scapular Neck Malunion with Glenoid Medialization

A 24-year-old female sustained a scapular neck fracture after a fall from height. Initial radiographs and CT scanning indicated 60° of posterior angulation, 100% displacement, and 2 cm of medial displacement. With the patient in the lateral decubitus position, a modified Judet approach was utilized using the interval between infraspinatous and teres minor. The fracture was reduced and secured with two 2.7 recon plates contoured to the scapular neck anatomy. Standard postoperative care was initiated with formal physical therapy starting on postoperative day number 2.

At her 6-month postoperative visit, she was noted to have made little progress with strength and range of motion. Abduction was 80°, forward flexion to 75°, internal rotation to 90°, and external roation to neutral. Examination of the rotator cuff indicated subscapularis muscle function with 5/5 strength; with the supraspinatous, infraspinatous, and teres minor being 4/5. A positive impingement sign was also noted.

Aggressive physical therapy continued but rotator cuff weakness and impingment were still present at the 1-year follow up visit. Repeat radiographs and CT scanning identified a malunion of the scapular neck with 40° of posterior angulation and 1 cm of medialization.

Discussion

Malunion of scapular neck fractures can result in pain and weakness stemming from rotator cuff dysfunction. The rotator cuff lever arm is altered with displacement of the glenoid fossa. This in turn transforms the normal compression forces of the rotator cuff into abnormal shear forces with neck angles greater than 40°. Impingement is also a common complaint. Management of a malunion of the scapular neck fracture is predicated upon the extent of glenoid medialization, residual malrotation, the presence of shoulder impingement, and the extent of glenohumeral arthrosis. Whenever possible, this is best treated with corrective osteotomy to restore neck length and alignment. The goal is to improve shoulder biomechanics, restore rotator cuff function, and deter the development of glenohumeral arthrosis. It was therefore determined that an osteotomy and revision ORIF would be indicated.

Technique

The modified Judet approach with the patient in a lateral decubitus position is utilized. The plane between the infraspinatous and teres minor is identified and developed. The previous hardware is identified and removed. Care is taken to avoid excess traction of the infraspinatous muscle in order to avoid iatrogenic injury to the suprascapular nerve. The malunited fracture was easily identified and the medialization was confirmed. Good fracture healing was noted. Two parallel K-wires were placed, one lateral and one medial to the proposed osteotomy site. Next, an oscillating saw was used to create the scapular neck osteotomy in the previously marked plane. The far cortex plane was completed using a small osteotome. Once mobilized, the malunion is corrected while using the previously placed K-wires as a guide. The osteotomy site is provisionally pinned in place followed by definitive plate fixation. The defect is filled with bone graft.

Summary

Traditionally, the mainstay of treatment for scapular fractures has been nonoperative care. More recently, however, a subgroup of these injuries has proven to benefit from surgical reduction and fixation. Disruption of the superior shoulder suspensory complex, rotator cuff weakness and painful malunions all appear to be the culprit that can lead to poor outcomes.

Anterior and posterior approaches to the scapula provide needed access to the scapula and glenohumeral joint, but they are not without pitfalls. Innovations in implant design, such as locking mini-fragment plates and headless compression screws allow for adequate fixation and early stable range of motion.

These injuries are difficult to treat. Current literature reflects the paucity of studies to help guide the surgeon with regard to indications and treatment options. Future research will hopefully better elucidate the fracture patterns and operative interventions that would be most beneficial to patients with scapular fractures.

References

1. Wilson PD. Experience in the management of fractures and dislocations (based on analysis of 4390 cases) by Staff of the Fracture Service MGH, Boston. Philadelphia: JB Lippincott; 1938.
2. Scavenius M, Sloth C. Fractures of the scapula. Acta Orthop Belg. 1996;62:129-32.
3. Imatani RJ. Fractures of the scapula: a review of 53 fractures. J Trauma. 1975;15:473-8.
4. Wilber MC, Evans EB. Fractures of the scapula. An analysis of forty cases and a review of the literature. J Bone Joint Surg Am. 1977;59:358-62.
5. Neviaser J. Traumatic lesions: injuries in and about the shoulder joint. Instr Course Lect. 1956;13:187-216.
6. McGahan JP, Rab GT, Dublin A. Fractures of the scapula. J Trauma. 1980;20:880-3.
7. Ideberg R, Grevsten S, Larsson S. Epidemiology of scapular fractures. Incidence and classification of 338 fractures. Acta Orthop Scand. 1995;66:395-7.

8. Armstrong CP, Van der Spuy J. The fractured scapula: importance and management based on a series of 62 patients. Injury. 1984;15:324-9.
9. Guttentag IJ, Rechtine GR. Fractures of the scapula. A review of the literature. Orthop Rev. 1988;17:147-58.
10. Thompson DA, Flynn TC, Miller PW, et al. The significance of scapular fractures. J Trauma. 1985;25:974-7.
11. Stephens NC, Morgan AS, Corvo P, et al. Significance of scapular fracture in blunt trauma patients. Ann Emer Med. 1995;26:439-42.
12. McLennan JG, Ungersma J. Pneumothorax complicating fracture of the scapula. J Bone Joint Surg Am. 1982;64:598-9.
13. Harris RD, Harris JH Jr. The prevalence and significance of missed scapular fractures in blunt chest trauma. AJR Am J Roentgenol. 1988;151:747-50.
14. Goss TP. Scapular fractures and dislocations: diagnosis and treatment. J Am Acad Orthop Surg. 1995;3:22-33.
15. Haapamaki V, Kiuru M, Koskinen S. Multidetector CT in shoulder fractures. Emerg Radiol. 2004;11:89-94.
16. Kopecky KK, Bies JR, Ellis JH. CT diagnosis of fracture of the coracoid process of the scapula. Comput Radiol. 1984;8:325-7.
17. Ng GP, Cole WG. Three-dimensional CT reconstruction of the scapula in the management of a child with a displaced intra-articular fracture of the glenoid. Injury. 1994;25: 679-80.
18. Nordqvist A, Petersson C. Fracture of the body, neck, or spine of the scapula. A long-term follow-up study. Clin Orthop Relat Res. 1992;283:139-44.
19. Tadros AM, Lunsjo K, Czechowski J, et al. Usefulness of different imaging modalities in the assessment of scapular fractures caused by blunt trauma. Acta Radiol. 2007;48: 71-5.
20. Marsh JL, Slongo TF, Agel J, et al. Fracture and dislocation classification compendium - 2007: Orthopaedic Trauma Association classification, database and outcomes committee. J Orthop Trauma. 2007;21(10 Suppl):S1-133.
21. Wilber MC, Evans EB. Fractures of the scapula. An analysis of 40 cases and a review of the literature. J Bone Joint Surg. 1977;59:358-62.
22. Ada JR, Miller ME. Scapular fractures. Analysis of 113 cases. Clin Orthop Relat Res. 1991;269:174-80.
23. Hardegger FH, Simpson LA, Weber BG. The operative treatment of scapular fractures. J Bone Joint Surg Br. 1984;66:725-31.
24. Ideberg R. Fractures of the scapula involving the glenoid fossa. In: Bateman JE, Walsh RP (Eds). Surgery of the Shoulder. Philadelphia: BC Decker; 1984. pp. 63-6.
25. Ideberg R. Unusual glenoid fractures: a report on 92 cases [Abstract]. Ada Orthop Scand. 1987;58:191-2.
26. Goss TP. Fractures of the glenoid cavity. J Bone Joint Surg Am. 1992;74:299-305.
27. Mayo KA, Benirschke SK, Mast JW. Displaced fractures of the glenoid fossa. Results of open reduction and internal fixation. Clin Orthop Relat Res. 1998;347:122-30.
28. Ogawa K, Yoshida A, Takahashi M, et al. Fractures of the coracoid process. J Bone Joint Surg Br. 1997:79:17-9.
29. Eyres KS, Brooks A, Stanley D. Fractures of the coracoid process. J Bone Joint Surg Br. 1995;77:425-8.
30. Kuhn JE, Blasier RB, Carpenter JE. Fractures of the acromion process: a proposed classification system. J Orthop Trauma. 1994;8:6-13.
31. Zlowodzki M, Bhandari M, Zelle BA, et al. Treatment of scapula fractures: systematic review of 520 fractures in 22 case series. J Orthop Trauma. 2006;20:230-3.
32. Ahmad CS, Wing D, Gardner TR, et al. Biomechanical evaluation of subscapularis repair used during shoulder arthroplasty. J Shoulder Elbow Surg. 2007 16 (3 Suppl): S59-64.
33. Armstrong A, Lashgari C, Teefey S, et al. Ultrasound evaluation and clinical correlation of subscapularis repair after total shoulder arthroplasty. J Shoulder Elbow Surg. 2006;15:541-8.
34. Jobe FW. Unstable shoulders in the athlete. Instr Course Lect. 1985;34:228-31.
35. Hinton M, Parker A, Drez D, et al. An anatomic study of the subscapularis tendon and myotendinous junction. J Shoulder Elbow Surg. 1994;3:224-9.
36. Brodsky JW, Tullos HS, Gartsman, GM. Simplified posterior approach to the shoulder joint. A technical note. J Bone and Joint Surg Am. 1987;69:773-4.
37. Leung KS, Lam TP. Open reduction and internal fixation of ipsilateral fractures of the scapular neck and clavicle. J Bone Joint Surg Am. 1993;75:1015-8.
38. Jones CB, Cornelius JP, Sietsema DL, et al. Modified Judet approach and minifragment fixation of scapular body and glenoid neck fractures. J Orthop Trauma. 2009;23:558-64.
39. Pace AM, Stuart R, Brownlow H. Outcome of glenoid neck fractures. J Shoulder Elbow Surg. 2005;14:585-90.
40. Landi A, Schoenhuber R, Funicello R, et al. Compartment syndrome of the scapula. Definition on clinical, neuro-physiological and magnetic resonance data. Ann Chir Main Memb Super. 1992;11:383-8.
41. Nettrour LF, Krufky EL, Mueller RE, et al. Locked scapula: intrathoracic dislocation of the inferior angle. A case report. J Bone Joint Surg Am. 1972;54:413-6.
42. Blue JM, Anglen JO, Helikson MA. Fracture of the scapula with intrathoracic penetration. A case report. J Bone Joint Surg Am. 1997;79:1076-8.
43. Schwartzbach CC, Seoudi H, Ross AE, et al. Fracture of the scapula with intrathoracic penetration in a skeletally mature patient. J Bone Joint Surg Am. 2006:88:2735-8.
44. Porte AN, Wirtzfeld DA, Mann C. Intrathoracic scapular impaction: an unusual complication of scapular fractures. Can J Surg. 2009;52:E62-3.

Chapter 13

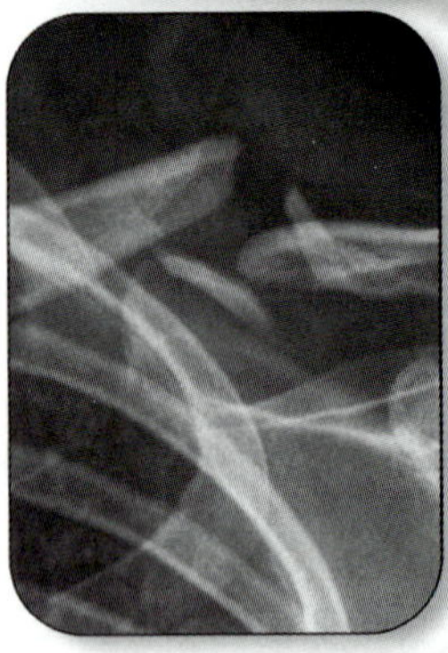

Clavicle Fractures

Roman Isaac, Meredith Osterman, Michael Rivlin, Neal Chen

Chapter Outline

Introduction
Diagnosis
Classification
Surgical Indications
- Midshaft Clavicle Fixation
- Distal Clavicle Fixation

Surgical Anatomy, Positioning and Approaches
- Anatomy
- Positioning
- Approaches

Surgical Techniques
- Technique 1: Plate Fixation of Midshaft Clavicle Fractures
- Technique 2: Rockwood Pin Fixation of Midshaft Clavicle Fractures
- Technique 3: Transarticular and Hook Plate Fixation of Lateral Clavicle Fractures
- Technique 4: Coracoclavicular Screw Fixation of Lateral Clavicle Fractures

Outcomes
- Midshaft Clavicle Fractures
- Lateral Clavicle Fractures

Complications
- Nonunion/Malunion
- Hardware Complications
- Thoracic Outlet Syndrome
- Brachial Plexopathy
- Wound Breakdown

Authors' Preferred Management of Select Complications
- Case 1: Clavicle Nonunion Repair
- Case 2: Clavicle Malunion Repair with Secondary Brachial Plexopathy

Summary

Introduction

Clavicle fractures are among the most common upper extremity fractures seen. Approximately, 80% involve the middle third of the clavicle. The management of clavicle fractures has evolved significantly over the last century. Historically, the operative management of clavicle fractures was considered a cosmetic procedure as the majority of fractures healed relatively uneventfully with only a small percentage of fractures failing to unite.[1] As such, the mainstay treatment has been nonoperative with a sling, even in widely displaced fractures. This therapeutic approach was based on reports of nonunion rates of 1% with conservative treatment.[2] However, there has been an increased interest toward surgical intervention as multiple recent studies have reported increased rates of nonunion and unsatisfactory patient outcomes with nonoperative treatment.

Hill et al. reported on 242 patients with nonoperatively treated clavicle fractures and identified 52 patients (15%)

with nonunions and 16 patients (31%) reporting unsatisfactory results with complaints of residual pain, brachial plexus irritation and cosmetic complaints.[3] Nordqvist et al. examined 225 patients with clavicle fractures treated nonoperatively. He found at final follow-up that 39 patients reported persistent pain, 53 patients had malunions and 7 nonunions.[4] McKee et al. evaluated muscle strength after nonoperatively treated midshaft clavicle fractures, comparing the injured arm to the uninjured arm and found only 67–85% of muscle strength as compared to the contralateral, uninjured arm. They also identified mean disabilities of the arm, shoulder and hand (DASH) scores of 24.6 points and mean constant shoulder scores (CSS) of 71 points, indicating residual disability despite radiographic union.[5] A multicenter, randomized clinical trial by the Canadian Orthopaedic Trauma Society compared operative vs nonoperative treatment of midshaft clavicle fractures. The results showed two nonunions in the operative group as compared to seven in the nonoperative group and no symptomatic malunions in the operative group as compared to nine in the nonoperative group. Patients undergoing open reduction internal fixation (ORIF) also reported more satisfactory results with regard to their shoulder appearance and general function.[6]

Over time, risk factors for nonunion of clavicle fractures treated nonoperatively have been identified. Lateral clavicle fractures have increased rates of nonunion of up to 30%. Nordqvist et al. reported on lateral clavicle fractures treated nonoperatively and found 43% complicated by nonunion.[7] In comparison, Eskola et al. identified only one nonunion among 23 lateral clavicle fractures treated operatively.[8] Moreover, there has been recent interest in clavicular malunion. Some patients have symptoms of early fatigue, thoracic outlet symptoms and more subtle limitations of shoulder function that may not affect activities of daily living, but may affect work or sports activities. This concern of clavicular malunion has prompted some surgeons to pursue operative intervention for fractures that may be less displaced than the historical criteria for operative treatment.

Operative treatment of clavicle fractures has yielded some reliable techniques to treat clavicle fractures including plating and intramedullary devices. These techniques continue to evolve; however, despite these technical advancements, structures at risk remain constant. However, the criteria for surgical treatment continues to change; and contemporary management requires an understanding of patient's activities and personal preferences as well as current evidence to help guide optimal patient management.

Diagnosis

The presentation of clavicle fractures can be quite variable, but typically results from falling onto the shoulder. Clavicle fractures are also common in polytrauma cases and can often be overlooked in the setting of more severe injuries as gross deformity is uncommon.

The physical examination of a patient with a clavicle fracture begins with an evaluation of the soft tissues. An open fracture or an impending open fracture should be readily identified as these warrant surgical intervention. Furthermore, small open wounds at the level of the fracture may represent an inside-out injury of an occult open fractures.

The distal extremity should be evaluated as well, taking care to assess the brachial, radial and ulnar artery pulses. If a pulse is not easily palpable, more advanced evaluation is warranted either by direct or indirect vascular or imaging studies. Vascular injuries may not always be apparent at initial evaluation and may manifest later in the form of aneurysms, pseudoaneurysms and thrombosis. A thorough neurological evaluation is also warranted as the brachial plexus may sustain an injury following a clavicle fracture. There are a number of major and minor neurovascular structures around the clavicle. The brachial plexus surrounds the second segment of the axillary artery and vein as they pass deep and inferior to the mid-clavicle. Also, in close proximity, is the lung and thoracic duct on the right side. Although, injury to these structures is infrequent, they oftentimes lie within millimeters of the fracture and should always be kept in mind. Superficially, a number of cutaneous supraclavicular nerves pass superficial to the platysma and the clavicle making them susceptible to injury.

Special attention should be paid to the brachial plexus in evaluation of a high-energy clavicle fracture. Horner's syndrome consists of ptosis, meiosis and anhydrosis. The ptotic eyelid is often times, a hallmark of a preganglionic lesion. If possible, the rhomboids and signs of scapular winging should also be assessed. Careful examination of the deltoid, rotator cuff and biceps can help detect injury to the upper trunk, while interosseous and thenar function of the head can help identify lower trunk injury. The complete evaluation of brachial plexus injuries lies outside the scope of this chapter, but the reader is encouraged to be particularly mindful of its examination when a brachial plexopathy is suspected.

In cases of nonunion or malunion, a hypertrophic callus can lead to thoracic outlet symptoms. Thoracic outlet syndrome can be evaluated with the Roos, Wright's and Adson's test as well as compressive maneuvers over the supraclavicular and infraclavicular plexus.

Often times, clavicle fractures are identified on chest radiographs. Dedicated imaging of the clavicle should begin with an anteroposterior (AP) radiograph of the clavicle. The radiograph should include the entire clavicle and the acromioclavicular (AC) and sternoclavicular (SC) joints. In patients with larger chests or greater soft tissue, radiographic evaluation of the clavicle can be improved by oblique views. We recommend routine oblique imaging including a 40° cephalad and 40° caudad views (Figs 13.1A to C). Imaging of the distal third of the clavicle is best achieved with the Zanca view, which consists of a 15° cephalad view centered over the AC joint. Imaging of the medial third of the clavicle is best achieved with the Serendipity view, which consists of a 40° cephalad view centered over the SC joint.

Cases with extensive comminution, malunions or nonunions are best evaluated with computed tomography (CT) scans using three-dimensional (3D) reconstructions. Magnetic resonance imaging (MRI) may be useful in the evaluation of pathological fractures. If neck pathology or pulmonary pathology is suspected, cervical spine or a chest radiograph should also be obtained. Furthermore, it is important to evaluate the scapula in a polytrauma situation with a concomitant clavicle fracture to ensure that a floating shoulder or an internal disarticulation is not overlooked.

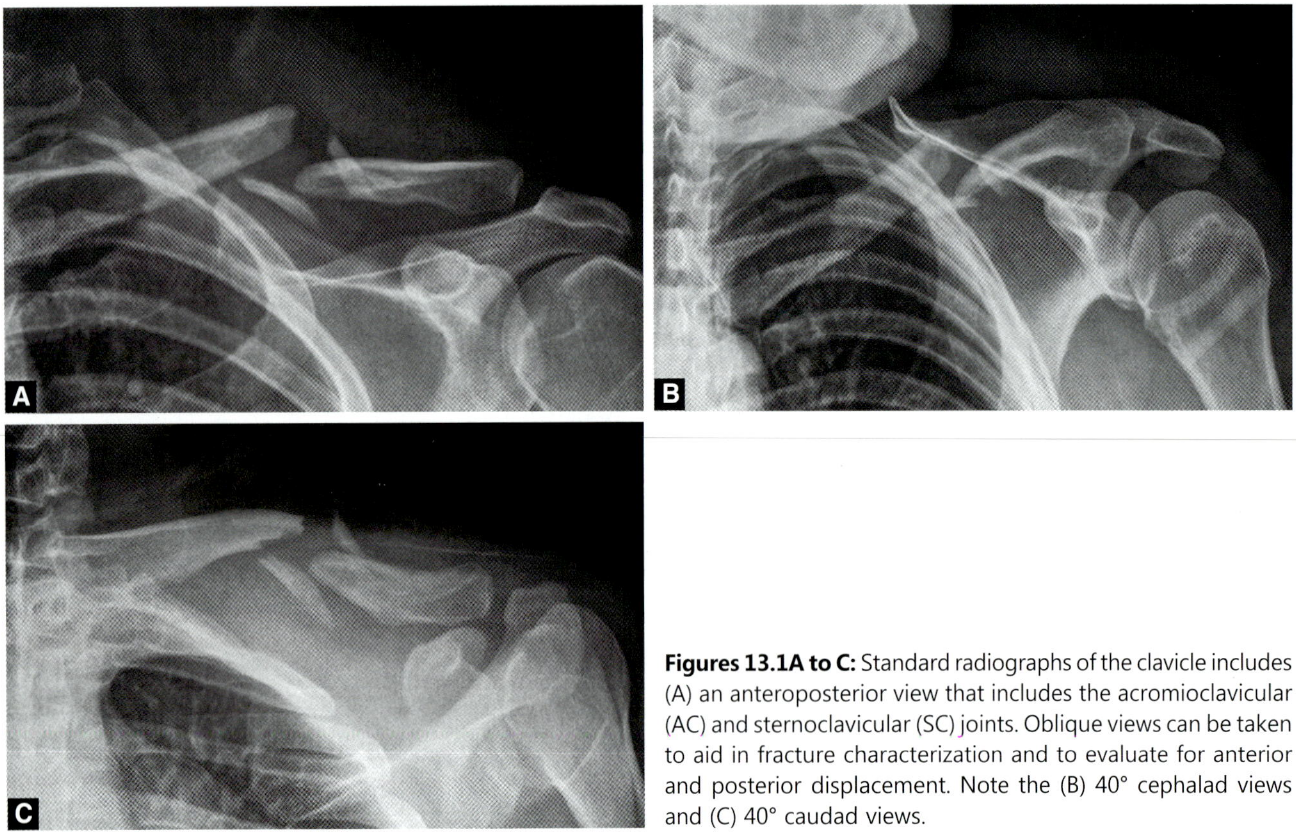

Figures 13.1A to C: Standard radiographs of the clavicle includes (A) an anteroposterior view that includes the acromioclavicular (AC) and sternoclavicular (SC) joints. Oblique views can be taken to aid in fracture characterization and to evaluate for anterior and posterior displacement. Note the (B) 40° cephalad views and (C) 40° caudad views.

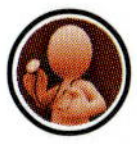

CLAVICLE FRACTURES DIAGNOSIS:
Pearls and Pitfalls

- Clavicle fractures may have a varied presentation with major trauma or relatively minor trauma
- Open or impending open fractures are common and careful evaluation of the skin integrity overlying the fracture is warranted
- A thorough neurovascular examination is paramount following clavicle fractures
- In the case of major trauma, be aware of the potential for an intrathoracic injury, a floating shoulder, or internal disarticulation

Classification

The utility of classifying clavicle fractures is limited. However, there are important radiographic features of clavicle fractures that aid in surgical decision making and are thereby used in its classification. The Allman system is the most common method of classifying clavicle fractures. It divides the clavicle fractures into three types (Fig. 13.2):

- Type I are midshaft fractures and make up approximately 80% of cases
- Type II are distal third fractures and make up approximately 15% of cases
- Type III are medial third fractures and make up approximately 5% of cases

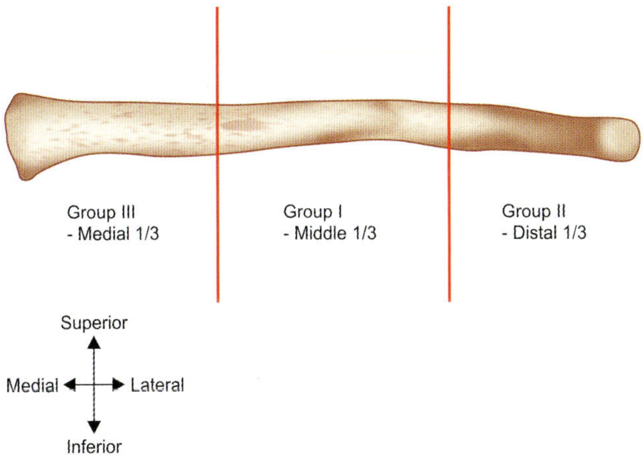

Figure 13.2: The Allman classification of clavicle fractures consists of Type I (midshaft), Type II (distal third) and Type III (medial third) fractures.

Neer further classified the distal third fractures based upon the relationship to and the integrity of the coracoclavicular (CC) ligaments (Fig. 13.3). The CC ligament has a conoid and a trapezoid component, which spans the distance of approximately 13 mm and terminates approximately 4 cm from the AC joint. Type I fractures are nondisplaced fractures that occur distal to the CC ligaments. Type IIA fractures consist of distal clavicle fractures that occur medial to the conoid ligament. Type IIB fractures consist of distal clavicle fractures that exit between the CC ligaments, often involving disruption of the conoid ligament. Type III fractures occur distal to the CC ligaments, but exit into the AC joint. Type IV fractures are pediatric fractures, which often involve metaphyseal disruption. Type V fractures occur when the CC ligaments are attached to a bony clavicular fragment in a comminuted fracture.

Surgical Indications

Surgical indications for the acute operative management of clavicle fractures include open fractures, pathological fractures, floating shoulders, scapulothoracic dissociation, polytrauma cases requiring weight bearing with assistive devices and cases with concomitant neurovascular injury. Relative indications include fractures in individuals, who desire an early return to work and weight bearing such as laborers, soldiers and athletes.

In midshaft clavicle fractures, the degree of displacement and shortening are predictive of union. Historically, union has been the primary determinant of the success of treatment. However, recent patient-rated outcomes and endurance measures suggest that despite the high incidence of union rate with nonoperative treatment, the presence of residual clavicular deformity can result in substantial disability.[5,6] Commonly used criteria for surgical intervention include 100% displacement of the fracture ends, shortening or overlap of greater than 2 cm and "Z" configuration fractures with a displaced vertical intercalary fragment (Figs 13.4A to C).

Unlike midshaft clavicular fractures, there has been a historical emphasis on early operative treatment of distal third clavicle fractures because of a suspected higher rate of nonunion. Type I and III fractures are typically minimally displaced and readily heal with nonoperative treatment. However, displaced fractures or fractures with concomitant disruption of the AC joint warrant operative treatment. In contrast, Type IIA and IIB fractures tend to present with greater displacement and a historically higher nonunion rate and therefore, are indicated for operative treatment.

Symptomatic nonunions and malunions are also indicated for operative correction to restore length, rotation and stability.

Midshaft Clavicle Fixation

Plate fixation is indicated for most cases involving a midshaft fracture (Fig. 13.5A). Plate fixation affords restoration of the normal anatomy of the clavicle and immediate weight bearing. In cases with thin or compromised soft tissue coverage, consideration should be given to avoid positioning the plate in a vulnerable position. Plates are

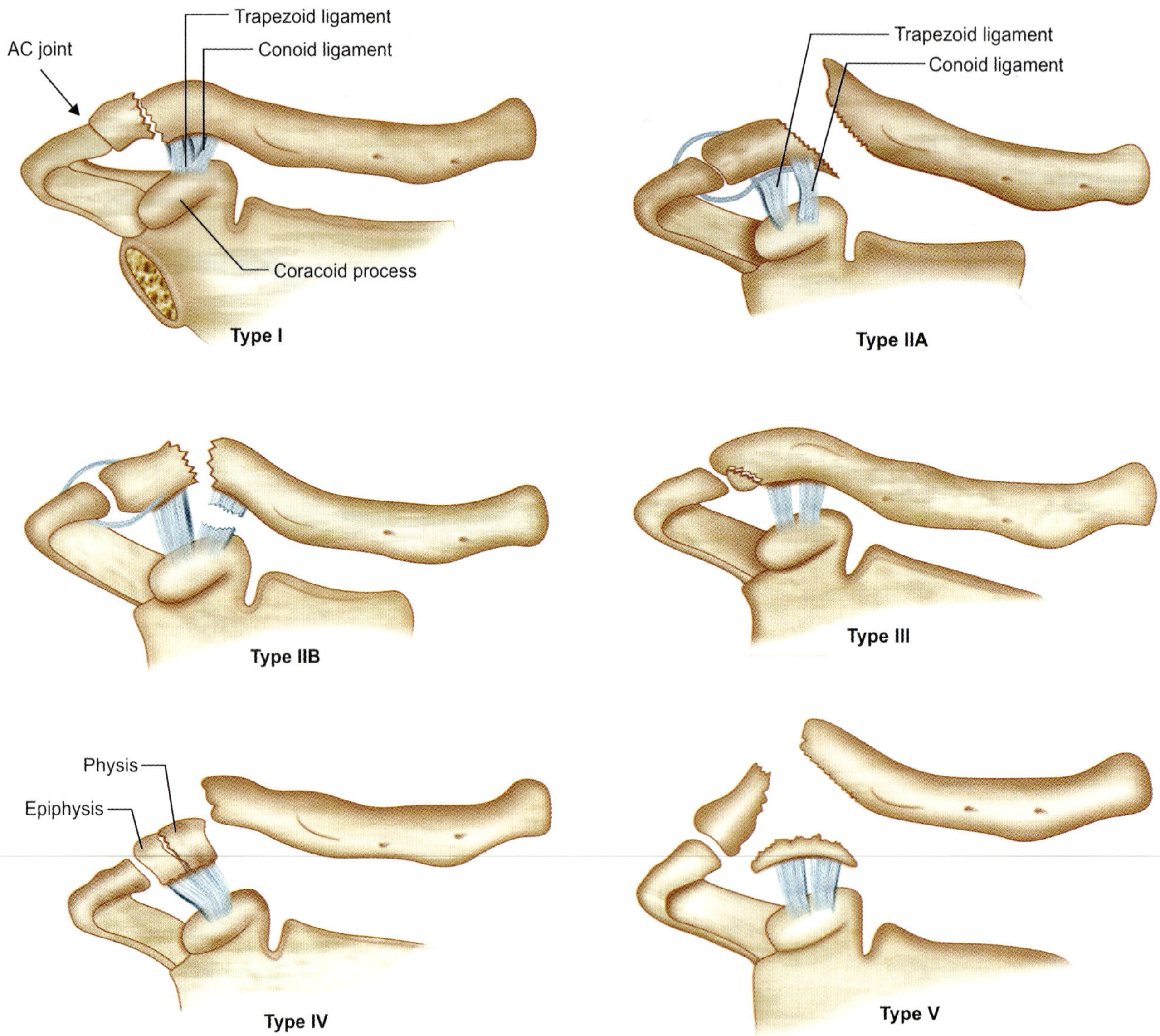

Figure 13.3: Neer classification of distal third fractures of the clavicle is defined by the fracture line's association with the coracoclavicular (CC) ligament. Type I fractures are nondisplaced fractures that occur distal to the CC ligaments. Type IIA fractures consist of a distal clavicle fracture that occurs medial to the CC ligaments. Type IIB fractures consist of a distal clavicle fracture that exit between the conoid and trapezoid ligaments. Type III fractures occur distal to the CC ligaments and exit into the acromioclavicular joint. Type IV fractures occur in the pediatric population through the distal physis. Type V fractures are comminuted.

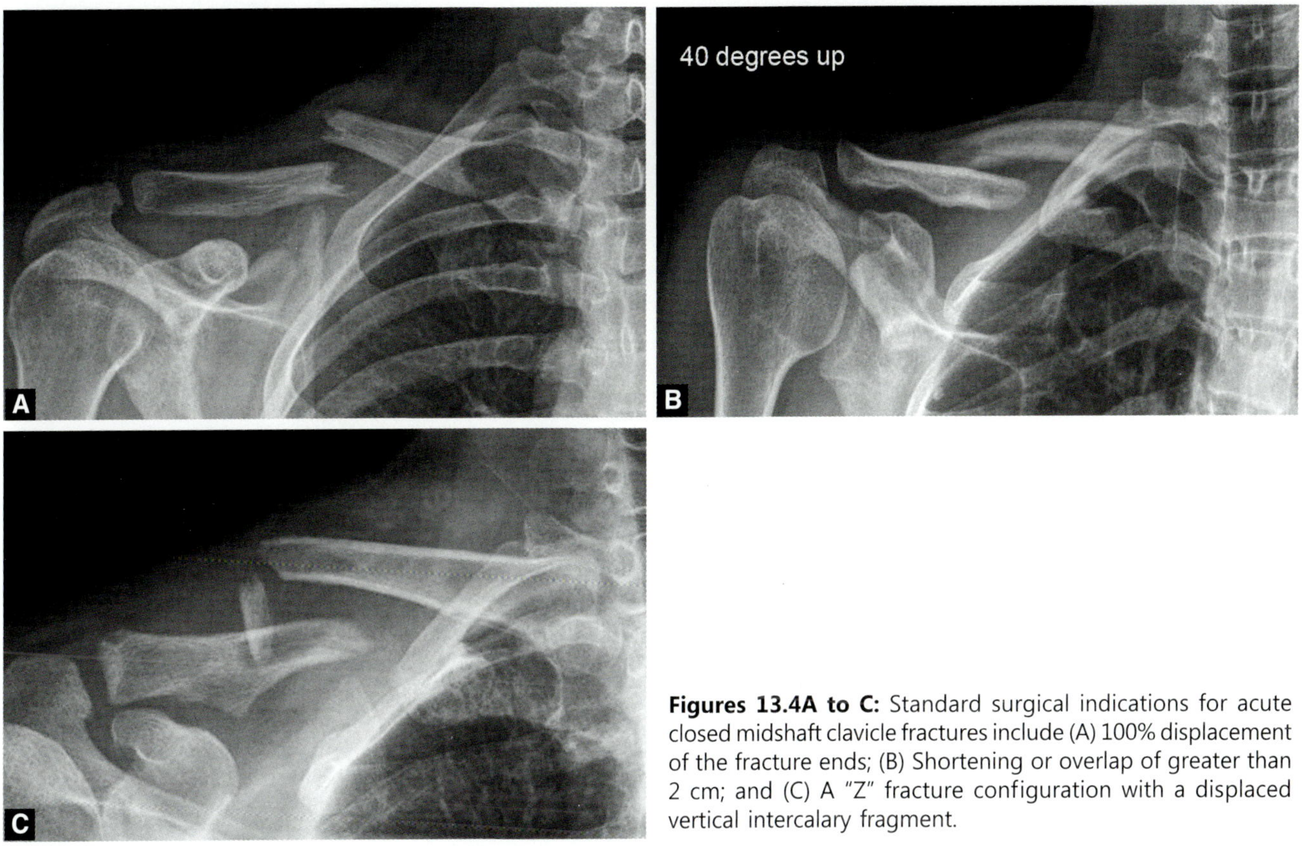

Figures 13.4A to C: Standard surgical indications for acute closed midshaft clavicle fractures include (A) 100% displacement of the fracture ends; (B) Shortening or overlap of greater than 2 cm; and (C) A "Z" fracture configuration with a displaced vertical intercalary fragment.

most readily applied superiorly, but may also be applied anteriorly or even anteroinferiorly. Alternatively, an intramedullary technique may be considered.

A plate may be applied in several techniques during clavicle fracture fixation including compression, bridge and neutralization. In cases with simple transverse patterns without comminution, compression plate fixation is the most appropriate. In cases with comminution, a bridge plate technique is utilized and should be reinforced with the utilization of locking screws. In cases with long oblique fractures, lag screws may be placed to fix the fracture and the plate may be applied to neutralize the fracture.

A number of intramedullary devices are available for fixation of the clavicle including the Rockwood pin, Hagie pin, Knowles pins, Herbert screws, Steinmann pins, elastic nails, flexible nails, cancellous screws and precontoured intramedullary nails. These implants are best indicated for midshaft clavicle fractures. To minimize the risks of hardware breakage or migration, the authors recommended the use of threaded implants such as the Rockwood pin (Fig. 13.5B) or precontoured nails (Fig. 13.5C) when intramedullary fixation is selected.

These techniques theoretically afford a less invasive technique that does not require extensive exposure of the clavicle while restoring alignment to the clavicle. These techniques also theoretically result in less hardware irritation and straightforward implant removal. Disadvantages include the risks of nonunion, implant breakage and migration.

Distal Clavicle Fixation

Distal clavicle fixation can be performed through a number of techniques, including transacromial kirschner (K) wire fixation, tension-band wiring, distal clavicle resection with modified Weaver-Dunn procedure, AC joint transarticular plate, a CC screw and a hook plate. The choice of implant is predicated upon surgeon preference and fracture alignment. Transarticular plate application is best indicated for Neer Type I or III fracture patterns as it allows bridging of a distal clavicle fracture with fixation being provided

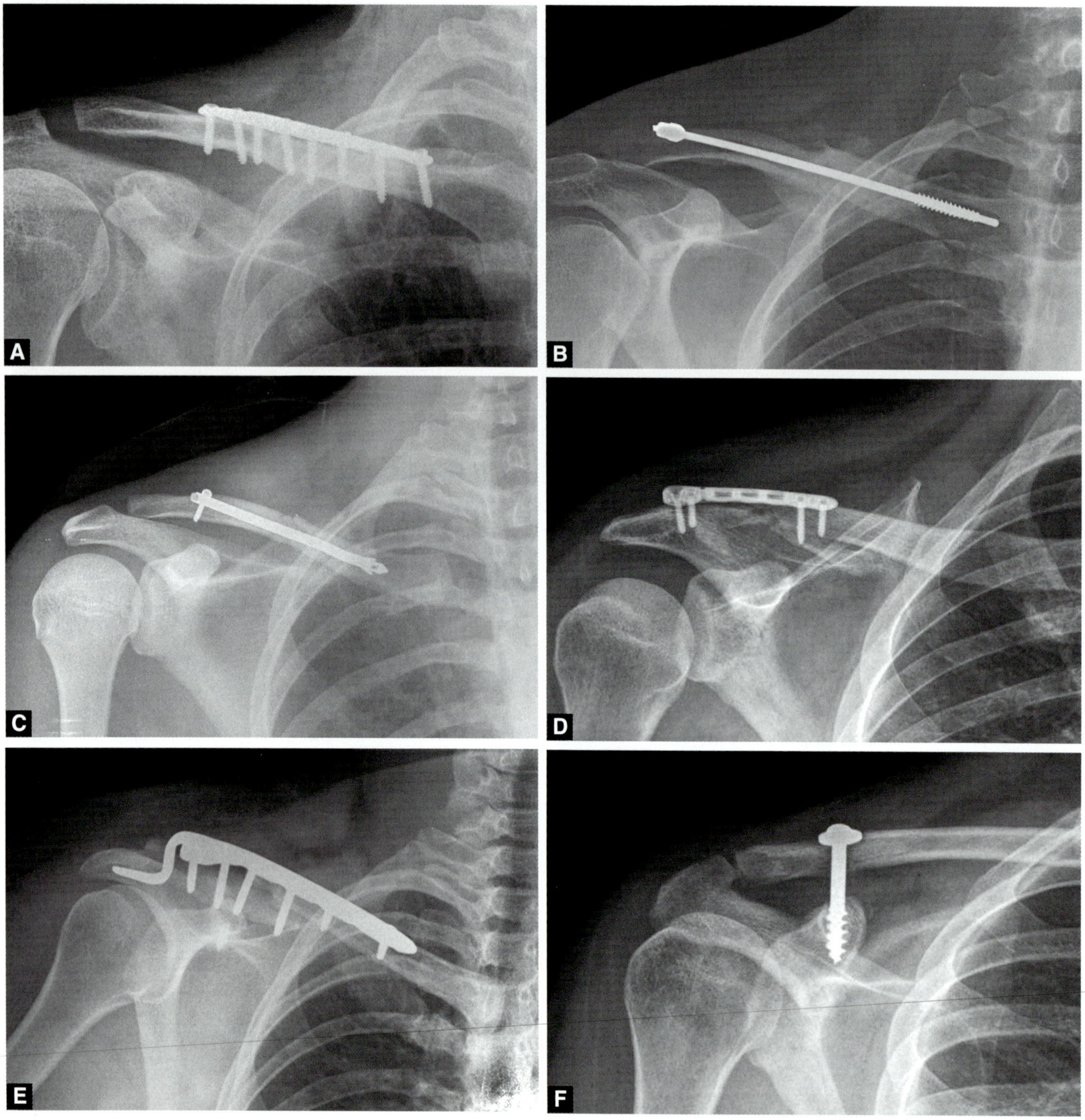

Figures 13.5A to F: Implant options for clavicle fracture fixation. (A) Plate fixation; (B) Rockwood pin fixation; (C) Intramedullary nail fixation; (D) Lateral clavicle transarticular plate fixation; (E) Hook plate fixation; (F) Coracoclavicular (CC) screw fixation.

by the midshaft clavicle and acromion (Fig. 13.5D). Upon fracture union, this plate is best removed to restore AC joint motion. Similarly, hook plate fixation is best indicated for Neer Type I or III fracture patterns as it also allows bridging the distal clavicle fracture and/or restores normal AC alignment (Fig. 13.5E). Upon fracture union, this plate is also best removed to restore AC joint motion and to avoid subacromial impingement. CC screw fixation, also used in the management of AC joint dislocations, is best indicated for Neer Type II fractures (Fig. 13.5F). Due to the high

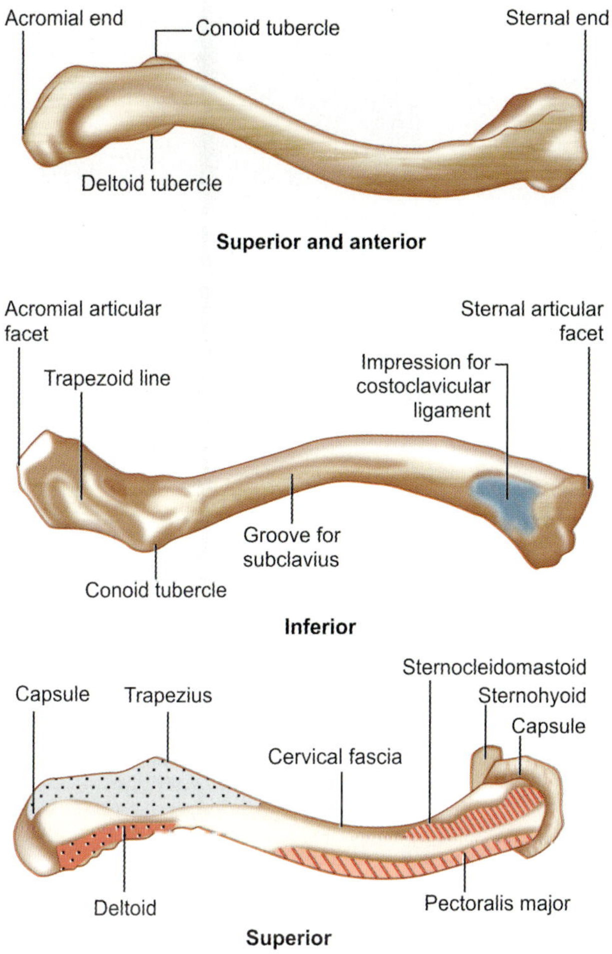

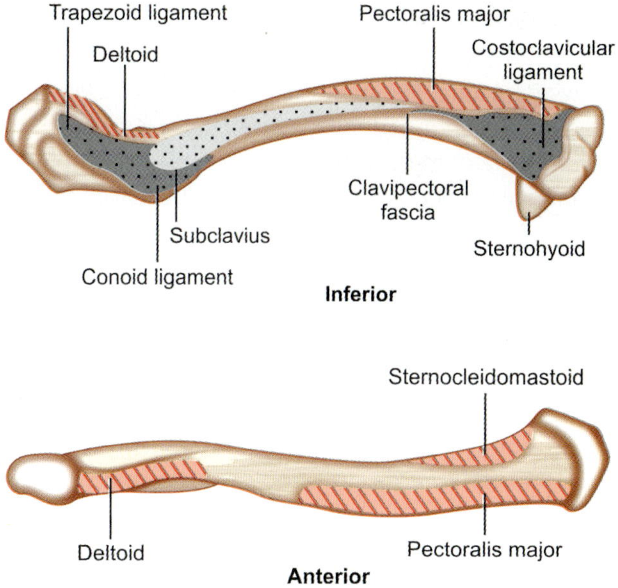

Figure 13.6: The clavicle is an S-shaped flat bone that articulates with the sternum medially and the acromion laterally. Note the sites of the attachment of several muscles inserting on the clavicle.

prevalence of fatigue failure, the authors do not recommend transacromial K-wire fixation or tension-band wiring.

Surgical Anatomy, Positioning and Approaches

Anatomy

The clavicle is a flat bone with an S-shaped anatomy that serves as a strut to connect the arm to the axial skeleton (Fig. 13.6). It also provides osseous protection to the underlying subclavian vessels and the brachial plexus. Viewed anteriorly to posteriorly, the clavicle is flat with a tubular middle third. However, viewed superiorly, the S-shaped clavicle is concave anterior on its medial end and concave posterior on its lateral end. Crossing anterior to the clavicle, are multiple supraclavicular nerves providing sensation to the anterior chest wall (Fig. 13.7).

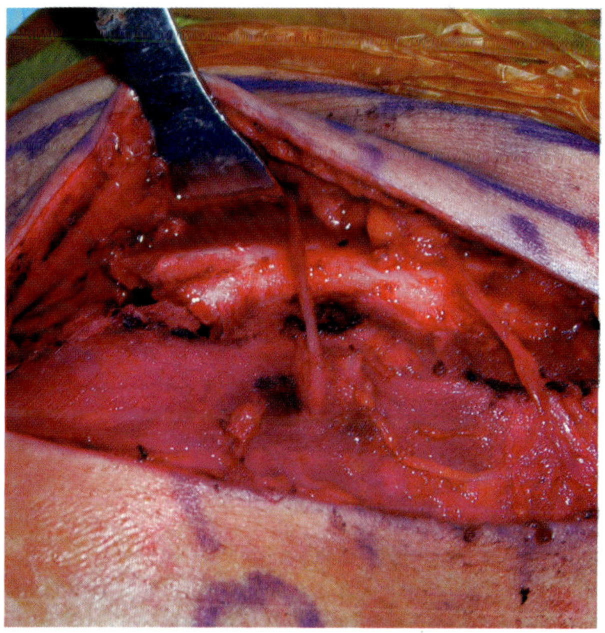

Figure 13.7: Supraclavicular nerves travel with the overlying platysma muscle and cross the anterior surface of the clavicle.

The clavicle has a number of muscular attachments that contribute to a predictable pattern of displacement following fracture. The sternocleidomastoid muscle inserts along the superior and medial aspect of the clavicle. The pectoralis major muscle inserts along the inferior, anterior and medial aspect of the clavicle. The subclavius muscle lies along its inferior border. The anterior deltoid originates along the anterior aspect of the lateral clavicle. In a typical midshaft clavicle fracture, the sternocleidomastoid muscle pulls the medial fragment superiorly, while the weight of the arm pulls the distal fragment inferiorly.

Stability of the ligament is provided by the surrounding ligamentous structures. Medially, the clavicle articulates with the sternum and is enveloped by the SC capsular ligaments. Laterally, the AC joint stabilizes the clavicle through the AC capsular ligaments and CC ligaments.

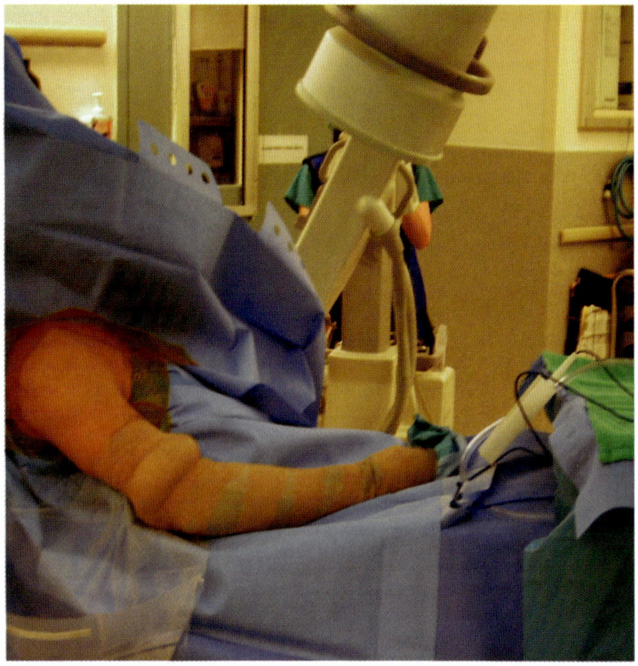

Figure 13.8: The patient is positioned in a beach-chair position with the image intensifier brought in from the contralateral side.

Positioning

Patient positioning options for clavicle fracture fixation includes either a supine position with the head of the bed elevated approximately 30° with a roll placed between the scapulae or in a formal beach chair position (Fig. 13.8). If bone graft harvesting will be needed from the ipsilateral pelvis, the supine position is preferred. Adequate intraoperative fluoroscopic visualization must be confirmed prior to start of the surgical case. We prefer utilizing a large c-arm that is brought in from the contralateral side. The arm is prepped and draped from the hand up to the neck.

Approaches

In general, a utilitarian approach to the clavicle is utilized through an anterosuperior approach. The skin is incised transversely just at the level of or below the clavicle. We prefer placing the incision slightly below the clavicle so that the closure does not occur directly over the hardware (Figs 13.9A and B). The subcutaneous fat and platysma is incised in line with the skin incision. Crossing supraclavicular branches are identified and protected to preserve cutaneous sensation (Fig. 13.7). The clavicle is exposed subperiosteally by splitting the pectoralis fascia and raising full thickness flaps, which will later be closed over the hardware. Circumferential stripping of the clavicle should be avoided in order to minimize healing complications and to prevent inadvertent injury of the underlying neurovascular structures.

SURGICAL POSITIONING: Pearls and Pitfalls

- If iliac crest bone graft harvesting is planned, the supine position with elevation of the head 30° is the most desirable
- Set up the fluoroscope before draping and ensure good images are able to be acquired
- The drape should allow access to the base of the neck and the sternoclavicular joint. The head may be positioned in slight axial rotation away from the field, if necessary
- Avoid circumferential stripping of the clavicle in order to prevent healing complications and deep neurovascular injury.

Surgical Techniques

Technique 1: Plate Fixation of Midshaft Clavicle Fractures

Plate fixation of a midshaft clavicle fracture is initiated with a standard anterior approach, incorporating any open wound if present (Figs 13.10A to E). The platysma is incised in line with the skin incision and crossing supraclavicular nerves are identified and protected. The clavicle is exposed subperiosteally along its anterior and superior surfaces. The fracture site is exposed and debrided of any interposed soft tissue. For a midshaft clavicle fracture, there is often central comminution with one or two major fragments. If present, these fragments are secured to the proximal or distal shaft, whenever possible, to create a two-fragment fracture pattern. Alternatively, the comminution may be bridged. The contralateral clavicle can be imaged for templating proper length and a bridge plate technique utilized. Typically, the fracture will be shortened and rotated. Lobster claw tenaculums are useful in securing the two major fragments and reducing the fracture, which can then be held with a pointed tenaculum. If fracture obliquity affords, interfragmentary lag screw fixation is performed to reduce the fracture. Preferably, two screws are placed to control rotation.

A number of plate fixation options exist including reconstruction plates, dynamic compression plates and precontoured plates. The plate is secured provisionally with tenaculum forceps proximally and distally with careful attention not to strip the soft tissue attachments and also to avoid injury to the underlying neurovascular structures. If a simple fracture pattern is present, screws may be placed in compression. However, some amount of fracture obliquity is common and therefore, compression plating should be performed with caution in order to avoid shortening or displacing the fracture. In cases with comminution, the plate may be applied to bridge the fracture. The plate is best applied with nonlocking screw medially and laterally and the remaining screws are applied in a locking fashion, if possible, to improve rigidity of the construct. If lag screws are reducing the fracture, the plate is applied in a neutral fashion with any combination of screws. During drilling and screw fixation, great care must be taken to avoid plunging and injuring the lungs or neurovascular structures. Consideration can be given to place a blunt retractor below the clavicle to protect the drill bit from injuring deep structures. A minimum of three bicortical screws should be placed medial and lateral to the fracture line.

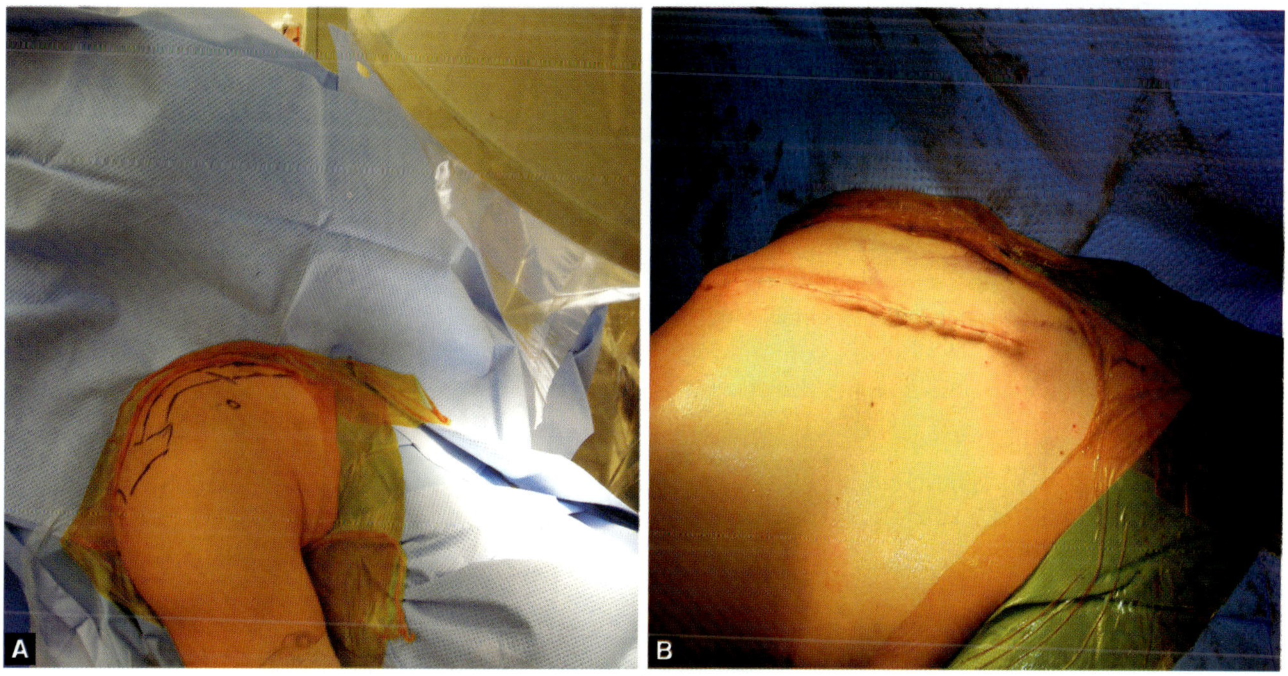

Figures 13.9A and B: Note the position of the incision placed inferior to the clavicle to avoid wound complications over the hardware.

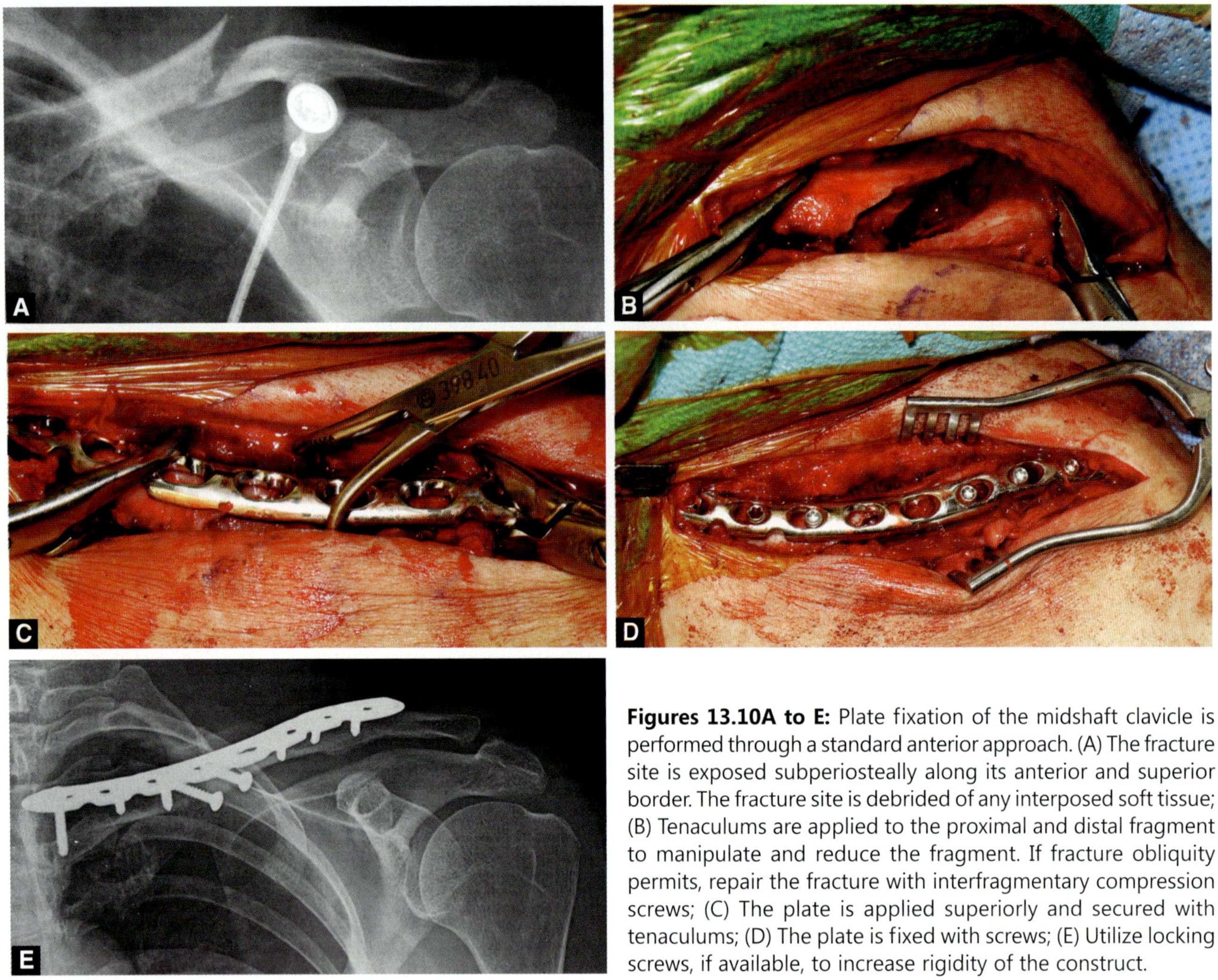

Figures 13.10A to E: Plate fixation of the midshaft clavicle is performed through a standard anterior approach. (A) The fracture site is exposed subperiosteally along its anterior and superior border. The fracture site is debrided of any interposed soft tissue; (B) Tenaculums are applied to the proximal and distal fragment to manipulate and reduce the fragment. If fracture obliquity permits, repair the fracture with interfragmentary compression screws; (C) The plate is applied superiorly and secured with tenaculums; (D) The plate is fixed with screws; (E) Utilize locking screws, if available, to increase rigidity of the construct.

Upon closure, the wound is irrigated. The pectoralis fascia is repaired over the plate. The platysma and subcutaneous tissues are closed in a single layer. The skin is closed in a subcuticular fashion. Active range of motion is initiated as soon as possible. However, concerns about fixation strength, initiation of motion may be delayed as dictated.

PLATE FIXATION OF MIDSHAFT CLAVICLE FRACTURES: Pearls and Pitfalls

- Avoid circumferential exposure of the clavicle and expose only the clavicle and fracture ends anteriorly and superiorly
- Comminution is common and any soft tissue attachment should be preserved
- The fracture will typically be shortened and rotated. Tenaculum control of each fragment will aid in fracture reduction
- If possible, repair comminuted fragments to the proximal or distal fragment
- When applying a plate, check to see if the proximal and distal most holes will lie on the bone prior to application and contour the plate further as needed
- When drilling, protect the inferior structures with a small smooth retractor
- Secure the proximal and distal most holes first utilizing nonlocking screws. To increase the rigidity of the construct, the remaining holes may be filled with locking screws

Technique 2: Rockwood Pin Fixation of Midshaft Clavicle Fractures

Rockwood pin fixation of midshaft clavicle fractures is initiated with a 3–5 cm transverse incision centered over the fracture (Figs 13.11A to E). The platysma is cut in line with the skin incision. The fascia and periosteum is typically disrupted at the fracture site. The fracture ends are exposed and mobilized. Leave associated comminuted fractures attached to their soft tissue attachments. The medial fragment is approached first. The canal is drilled, tapped and measured. The drill should be advanced carefully and allowed to follow the path of the canal. Care should be taken not to violate the anterior cortex. Next, the lateral fragment is approached. The canal is drilled through the fracture exiting out the posterolateral cortex. The lateral canal is tapped across its entire length exiting out the posterolateral cortex.

The pin is drilled retrograde through the lateral fragment with the nut removed and the trocar-end exiting through the drilled posterolateral cortex. A skin incision is placed and the trocar is directed out the incision. The drill is then placed on the trocar tip of the pin and drilled retrograde until the threads of the pin are within the lateral fragment. The fracture is then reduced and the pin is advanced into the medial fragment. With the fracture reduced and the pin seated medially, the pin is locked. The larger medial nut is spun down and advanced to the lateral cortex. The smaller lateral nut is then spun down and cold-weld against the larger medial nut. The pin is then cut lateral to the lateral nut.

Prior to wound closure, any butterfly fragment can be approximated to the clavicle with nonabsorbable sutures. The periosteum and fascial layer is closed over the fracture site. The skin is closed with a subcuticular repair. Immediate shoulder motion and weight bearing is permitted.

The authors recommend routine removal of the pin after 3–6 months, once the fracture is confirmed to be healed. Removal is performed by placing an incision over the previous lateral incision. Apply the extraction wrench over the larger medial nut and screw the pin out of the clavicle.

ROCKWOOD PIN FIXATION OF MIDSHAFT CLAVICLE FRACTURES: Pearls and Pitfalls

- Avoid penetration of the anterior cortex of the medial fragment
- Cold-weld the lateral nut to the medial nut and advance the two nuts down to the posterolateral fragment with careful compression of the fracture
- Butterfly or large comminuted fragments can be reapproximated to the fracture site with non-absorbable sutures

Technique 3: Transarticular and Hook Plate Fixation of Lateral Clavicle Fractures

The surgical technique and positioning for transarticular and hook plate begins similar to plate fixation of a mid-clavicle fractures. The lateral clavicle is approached superiorly. The incision may be placed slightly posterior on the clavicle to help preserve anterior soft tissue attachments. The fracture is exposed and if there is a ligamentous disruption of the AC joint capsule, these can be tagged with heavy, large gauge sutures and later incorporated into the repair. Large K-wires can be used for provisional fixation of the acromion to the clavicle. Transarticular plate fixation can be achieved with a reconstruction plate or a precontoured plate applied across the AC joint with screws placed in the clavicle medially and in the acromion laterally. Alternatively, a precontoured locking distal radius plate may be utilized. In contrast, the hook plate is first passed underneath the posterior acromion, any sutures supporting capsule can be passed through screw holes and the plate is fixed to the clavicle medially (Figs 13.12A and B).

TRANSARTICULAR AND HOOK PLATE FIXATION OF LATERAL CLAVICLE FRACTURES: Pearls and Pitfalls

- If the AC joint ligaments can be identified and tagged, incorporate them into the repair if possible
- K-wires can be used for provisional fixation across the AC joint during hook plate application
- Secure the most medial hole first to ensure proper plate positioning
- It is recommended that the plate should be removed after the distal clavicle is healed

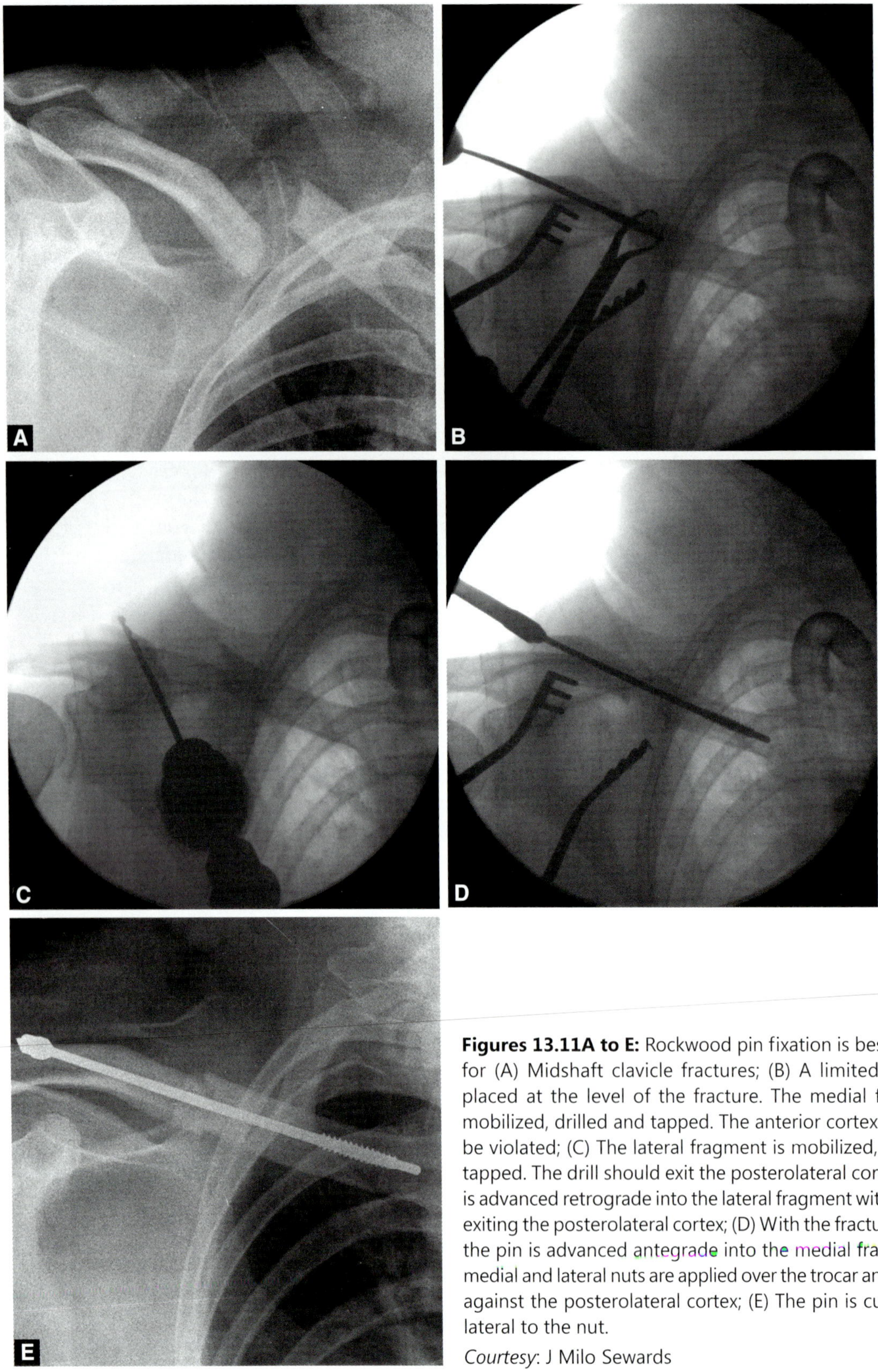

Figures 13.11A to E: Rockwood pin fixation is best indicated for (A) Midshaft clavicle fractures; (B) A limited incision is placed at the level of the fracture. The medial fragment is mobilized, drilled and tapped. The anterior cortex should not be violated; (C) The lateral fragment is mobilized, drilled and tapped. The drill should exit the posterolateral cortex. The pin is advanced retrograde into the lateral fragment with the trocar exiting the posterolateral cortex; (D) With the fracture reduced, the pin is advanced antegrade into the medial fragment. The medial and lateral nuts are applied over the trocar and advanced against the posterolateral cortex; (E) The pin is cut short just lateral to the nut.

Courtesy: J Milo Sewards

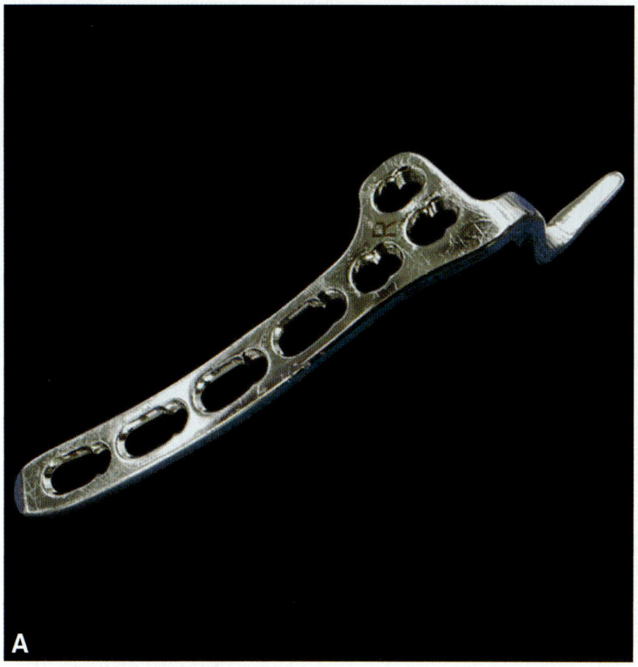

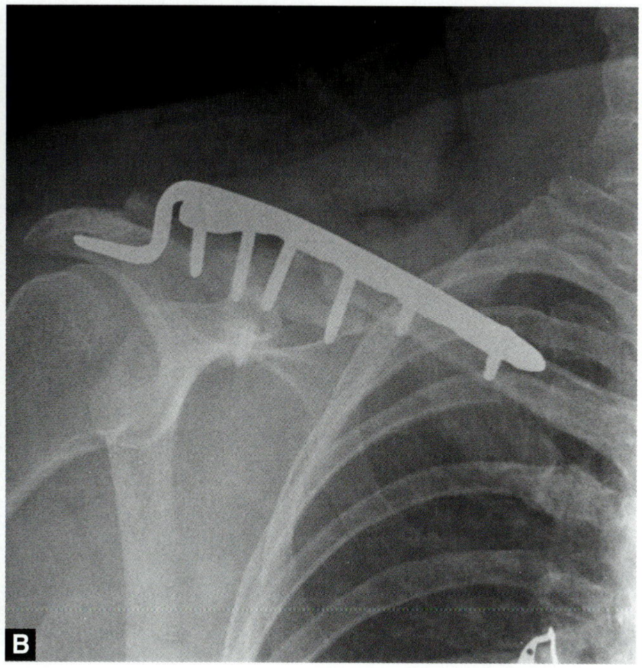

Figures 13.12A and B: Lateral clavicle fractures are best managed with a transarticular plate or (A) A hook plate; (B) Fixation of a comminuted lateral clavicle fracture with a hook plate. Note that the hook is first placed below the acromion and the plate bridges the comminution, while being fixed to the medial clavicle.

Technique 4: Coracoclavicular Screw Fixation of Lateral Clavicle Fractures

A vertical incision is placed centered over the coracoid process. The fascia joining the deltoid to the trapezius is divided at right angles to the skin incision. The clavicle is exposed subperiosteally at the level of coracoid. The coracoid is exposed with the care not to violate the conjoined tendon. The disrupted CC ligaments are identified and tagged with nonabsorbable sutures. After placing the clavicle in its anatomic position, it is provisionally fixed to the coracoid with a K-wire placed off center. Avoid plunging the K-wire through the second cortex of the coracoid, since the neurovascular bundle is in close proximity to its inferior border. A 3.2 mm hole is drilled centrally through the clavicle into the coracoid. Both cortices of the clavicle are overdrilled and a 6.5 mm cancellous bone screw is placed with a washer (Figs 13.13A to C). Subsequently, the K-wire is removed and the previously tagged sutures of the CC ligament are tied together. The wound is irrigated, followed by the closure of fascia and skin. The authors recommend routine removal of the screw at 3–6 months, once confirmed that the fracture is healed.

CC SCREW FIXATION OF LATERAL CLAVICLE FRACTURES: Pearls and Pitfalls

- A cancellous screw should be used and it must be placed bicortically through both the clavicle and coracoid
- Disrupted ends of the CC ligaments should be identified and repaired with nonabsorbable sutures once the screw has been placed

Outcomes

Midshaft Clavicle Fractures

Plate fixation of midshaft clavicle fractures has been successful with low rates of nonunion and symptomatic malunions and earlier return to function when compared to nonoperative treatment.[5,6,9] Kulshrestha et al. performed a prospective cohort study, where 73 patients were selected for either ORIF or conservative treatment of midshaft clavicle fractures.[9] There was 100% union of the fracture in the ORIF group as compared to eight nonunions in the nonoperative group. The nonoperative group also had 10 symptomatic malunions as compared to two in the operative group and the operative group had better CSS.

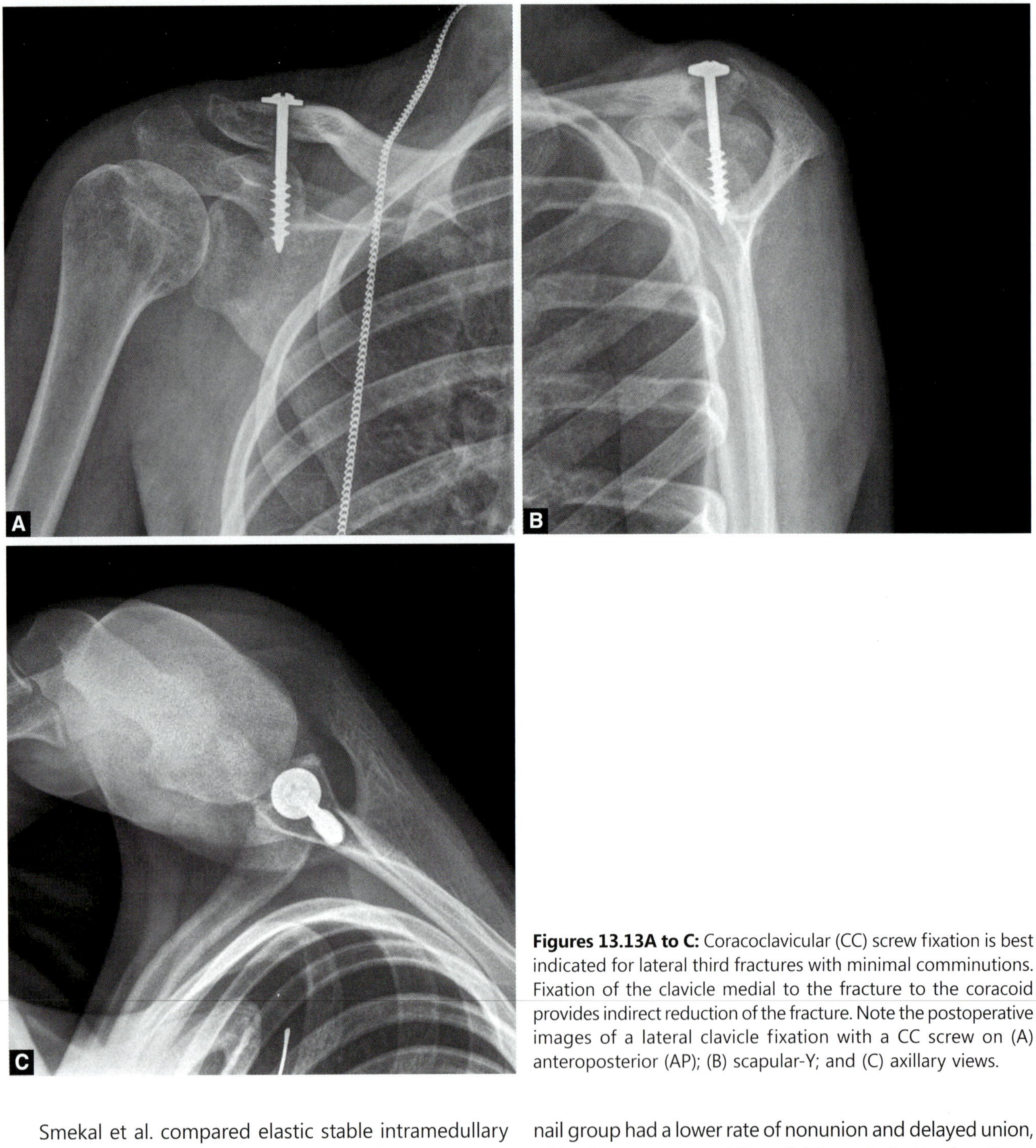

Figures 13.13A to C: Coracoclavicular (CC) screw fixation is best indicated for lateral third fractures with minimal comminutions. Fixation of the clavicle medial to the fracture to the coracoid provides indirect reduction of the fracture. Note the postoperative images of a lateral clavicle fixation with a CC screw on (A) anteroposterior (AP); (B) scapular-Y; and (C) axillary views.

Smekal et al. compared elastic stable intramedullary nailing (30 patients) with nonoperative treatment (30 patients) of fully displaced midshaft clavicular fractures in adults.[10] They were randomized to either operative or nonoperative treatment with a 2-year follow-up. Fracture union occurred in all patients in the operative group; nonunion occurred in three nonoperative patients. The nail group had a lower rate of nonunion and delayed union, with a faster return to daily activities and a better functional outcome. Clavicular shortening was significantly lower, and overall satisfaction was higher in the operative group. However, medial nail protrusion occurred in seven cases.

Ferran et al. performed a randomized clinical trial for clavicle fractures comparing plate and intramedullary fixation.[11] At a mean follow-up of 12 months, there was a 100% union rate in both groups and no statistical difference in terms of range of motion, CSS or Oxford scores. The primary difference was in the incidence of hardware complications. The intramedullary group required two nail removals and the plate group required eight plate removals.

Liu et al. performed a retrospective analysis of 110 cases treated with either a plate (59 cases) or intramedullary (51 cases) fixation.[12] They found no significant differences in functional outcome and nonunion rates between plate and nail fixation. However, the operative blood loss and surgical wound was significantly less in the nail group.

Lateral Clavicle Fractures

Lee et al. retrospectively reviewed a series of 52 patients treated with either hook plates or tension bands for lateral clavicle fractures.[13] In their study, hook plating was found to have lower rates of complication, less symptomatic hardware and an earlier return to work activity as compared to the tension band technique. In another retrospective review of 18 patients treated with hook plating for Neer Type II lateral clavicle fracture with a mean follow-up of 25 months, Tambe et al. identified two nonunions and five cases of acromial osteolysis.[14] Patients had good self-rated shoulder functions: 3 rated as normal, 11 as nearly normal and 1 as not normal. The authors also concluded that the plates need to be removed after union to prevent acromial osteolysis.

Coracoclavicular stabilization with a lag screw was first described by Bosworth in the 1940s. Its initial application was for the management of AC joint dislocations, but it has also been found to be effective in the management of lateral clavicle fractures. Ballmer and Gerber treated 5 consecutive Neer's type II lateral clavicle fractures using a temporary Bosworth-type screw.[15] There were no surgical complications and bone union occurred uneventfully within 9 weeks in all cases. Shoulder function was also restored to the preinjury level. Using the same technique, Yamaguchi et al. treated 11 consecutive Neer's type II lateral clavicle fractures and achieved a healed fracture within 10 weeks and shoulder function was restored to the preinjury level.[16] The strength of the CC screw is 80% greater than that of the original ligament, when it is placed bicortically as compared to only half in unicortical placement, which indicates the critical importance of correct screw placement.[17]

Complications

Complications following clavicle fractures are common and approach even 100% in some series. Common complications include cosmetic deformity, scar tenderness, wound complications, hardware prominence, hardware failure, hardware migration, nonunions, malunions, brachial plexus injury, subclavian vessel injury, thoracic outlet syndrome, adhesive capsulitis and pain.

Nonunion/Malunion

Traditionally, nonunions of clavicle fractures were thought to be the product of operative treatment, while nonoperative treatment resulting in a nonunion was exceedingly rare.[2] However, our current understanding of the literature coupled with the use of newer techniques has yielded a very low incidence of nonunion following primary operative fixation of clavicle factures. Moreover, the incidence of nonunions with nonoperatively treated fractures is now considered to be more common than previously reported. In an analysis of 581 nonoperatively treated clavicle fractures, an overall nonunion rate of 4.5% was identified.[18] A systematic review of the literature examining nonunions following the management of clavicular fractures identified a nonunion rate of 5.9% among nonoperatively treated fractures versus 2.2% among fractures treated with plate fixation and 2.0% among fractures treated with an intramedullary fixation.[20]

Clavicle fractures at an increased risk for nonunion are those with severe comminution and/or bone loss, displacement, increased patient age and female gender.[18] Nonunions after ORIF of midshaft clavicle fracture are uncommon in most recent series. Collinge et al. reported on 58 patients that underwent ORIF with precontoured 3.5 mm plate and found 95% union rate with one nonunion and one failure of fixation.[19] Similarly, the rate of nonunion is low after operative fixation of lateral clavicle fracture.[8] Treatment of a clavicle nonunion following ORIF consists of revision open reduction, takedown of the nonunion site, internal fixation and bone grafting. Fixation and stability can be augmented with double plating superiorly and inferiorly around the nonunion site. Furthermore, vascularized bone grafting can be utilized in the setting of recalcitrant atrophic nonunions and/or in cases with large segmental bone loss.

The definition of a malunion is not clear for clavicular fractures. Some authors have suggested that a clavicular malunion occurs when there is shortening greater than 15 mm, while others have defined malunion as a deformity resulting in shoulder symptoms.[20] Malunion may result in early shoulder fatigue or can cause symptoms of thoracic outlet syndrome. Initial treatment consists of scalene and pectoralis minor stretching, scapular and rotator cuff strengthening and postural training. If this is not helpful, clavicular osteotomy is an option. We recommend that symptoms of shoulder fatigue first should be treated with extensive therapy before considering clavicular osteotomy.

Hardware Complications

Hardware complications following clavicle fracture fixation are the most commonly reported complications in most reported series. These complications include hardware prominence and irritation, breakage and migration. All plating techniques are predisposed to prominence and irritation. The clavicle is relatively subcutaneous and has a thin soft tissue envelope, particularly along its lateral extent. Hardware breakage most commonly occurs with nonunions, where the plate fatigues over time. More common than breakage, hardware can migrate. Migration can be as simple as elevation of the plate on one end resulting in prominence, irritation or malunion formation. Or, migration can be more devastating as in the case of smooth intramedullary pins migrating into vital structures over time. Patients need to be made aware that hardware complications are common and are the most common reasons for secondary procedures following clavicle fixation.

Thoracic Outlet Syndrome

There are four variants of thoracic outlet syndrome: (1) arterial, (2) venous, (3) neural and (4) mixed. Most thoracic outlet symptoms consist of mixed symptoms. In the majority of cases, treatment begins with therapy. However, if the symptoms are primarily arterial resulting in microthrombi distally, earlier medical and surgical intervention may be warranted. Interventions range from anticoagulation in the acute period to clavicular osteotomy and thoracic outlet release in chronic cases.

Brachial Plexopathy

Brachial plexus neurapraxia has been reported with intramedullary pin fixation.[21] Late brachial plexopathy has also been described following clavicular nonunion and malunions.[22,23] These brachial plexopathies have been addressed by treatment of the clavicular deformity, resection of any space occupying lesion and neurolysis of the brachial plexus.

Wound Breakdown

Wound breakdown over a clavicle fracture can be problematic. Reasons for wound problems including compromised vascularity, infection or a previously irradiated surgical field. Infectious disease consultation is helpful for management of accompanying infection or control of bacterial colonization. Treatment options for coverage include vacuum dressings, synthetic biological tissue matrices or soft tissue flaps. Hartzell et al. described the successful use of latissimus flaps for wound coverage after clavicle sarcoma resection.[24]

Authors' Preferred Management of Select Complications

Case 1: Clavicle Nonunion Repair

A 25-year-old male fell onto his nondominant shoulder after a bicycling accident. He initially did not seek treatment and allowed his shoulder injury to heal without treatment. However, due to persistent pain and deformity to the shoulder for over 3 months following the injury, he sought treatment. Physical examination identified prominent swelling and pain over the clavicle. Shoulder exam demonstrated pain and decreased motion. Radiographs were taken that demonstrated a displaced, shortened and 'Z' configuration clavicle fracture that remained ununited (Fig. 13.14A).

The incidence of nonunions with nonoperatively treated fractures is now considered to be more common than previously reported. In an analysis of 581 nonoperatively treated clavicle fractures, an overall nonunion rate of 4.5%

was identified.[18] Clavicle fractures at increased risk for nonunion are those with severe comminution and/or bone loss, displacement, increased patient age and female gender. Treatment of a clavicle nonunion following ORIF consists of revision open reduction, takedown of the nonunion site, internal fixation and bone grafting. Fixation and stability can be augmented with double plating superiorly and inferiorly around the nonunion site. Furthermore, vascularized bone grafting can be utilized in the setting of recalcitrant atrophic nonunions and/or in cases with large segmental bone loss.

Technique

Preoperatively, the clavicle is templated by imaging the contralateral clavicle to anticipate the proper alignment following nonunion takedown. Bone graft options are determined preoperatively with options including local autograft from the clavicle intramedullary canal, ipsilateral iliac crest autograft and synthetic bone graft. Fixation is best achieved with locking plate fixation in order to maximize stability of the construct.

The patient is positioned supine with the head of the bed elevated 30°. The fluoroscope is positioned to ensure that adequate images can be obtained intraoperatively. Draping includes prepping in the arm and anterolateral shoulder and chest to the sternum. The ipsilateral hip should also be draped into the field if needed for bone graft.

The clavicle is exposed in standard fashion superiorly. Periosteal attachments are preserved whenever possible. The nonunion site is identified and debrided of fibrous tissue down to bleeding bone. Often, remnants of the fracture line can be identified that will allow recreation of the previous fracture. The freshened ends of the fracture are then controlled with bone holding forceps and the ends of the bone are recannulized with sequential reaming with progressively larger drill bits until reaching cortical interference and a bleeding cancellous bone surface.

If the fracture pattern permits, the clavicle fracture site may be initially repaired with an interfragmentary compression screw followed by plate fixation (Fig. 13.14B). Otherwise, the fracture fragments are realigned using indirect reduction with a superiorly applied locking plate. Diligence is paid not to overshorten or overlengthen the clavicle. Once satisfied with the reduction, the proximal and distal most holes are secured first with nonlocking screws to ensure appropriate plate position. The remaining holes are filled with locking screws. Bone graft is placed into the fracture site until the defect is densely filled on radiographs. The wounds are closed in standard fashion. Pendulum exercises are begun postoperatively. Active range of motion is initiated based on the quality of fixation.

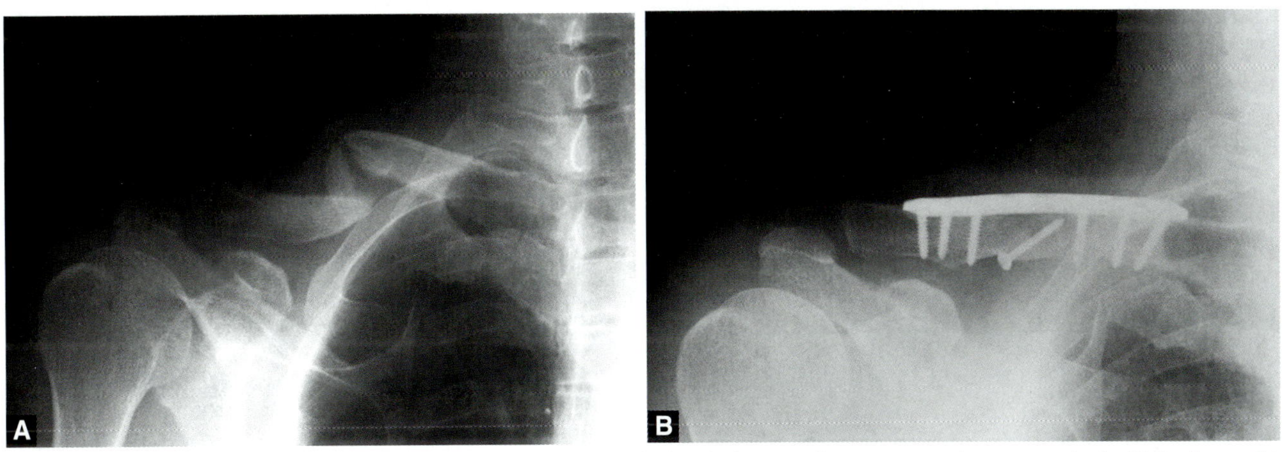

Figures 13.14A and B: A 25-year-old male who incurred a midshaft clavicle fracture that was treated nonoperatively. (A) Radiographic reevaluation at 3 months post injury, identified a clavicle nonunion; (B) Repair was performed with nonunion takedown, plate fixation and bone grafting.

Courtesy: Saqib Rehman

Case 2: Clavicle Malunion Repair with Secondary Brachial Plexopathy

A 45-year-old male fell from a height onto his dominant shoulder. Radiographs revealed a midshaft clavicle fracture. He was treated nonoperatively with a sling followed by progressive range of motion. Reevaluation at 8 weeks post injury confirmed a healed fracture. However, the patient returned 6 months post injury with decreased shoulder range of motion and strength. Radiographs demonstrated a well-healed clavicle fracture with approximately 5 cm of shortening as compared to the contralateral clavicle. In order to restore normal shoulder kinematics, malunion repair with an osteotomy and iliac crest bone graft was undertaken (Fig. 13.15A). Postoperatively, the patient noted significant weakness of the ipsilateral extremity with complete loss of finger, thumb and wrist extension. Electrodiagnostic testing identified a brachial plexus injury (Fig. 13.15B).

A clavicle malunion is typically defined when there is shortening greater than 15 mm. However, a more general definition of clavicle malunion is any fracture deformity resulting in shoulder symptoms and altered shoulder kinematics.[20] Malunion correction can result in brachial plexus injury from direct trauma to the underlying neurovascular structures or from traction following lengthening of the clavicle during repair. Treatment of an iatrogenic brachial plexopathy includes release of the tension following hardware removal and exploration and neurolysis, with possible repair of the brachial plexus (Fig. 13.15C). In cases with residual neurological deficits, nerve or tendon transfers can be entertained.

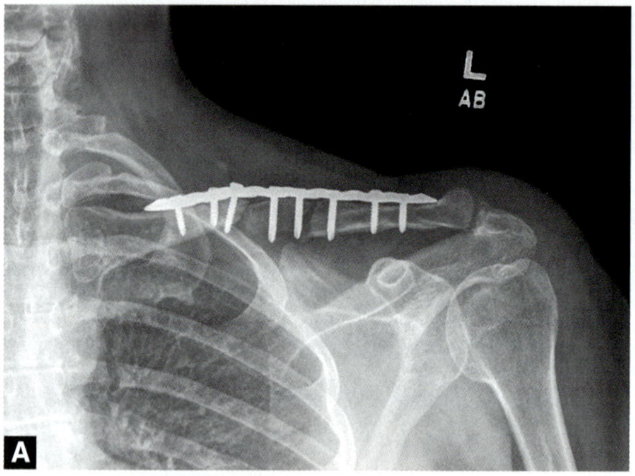

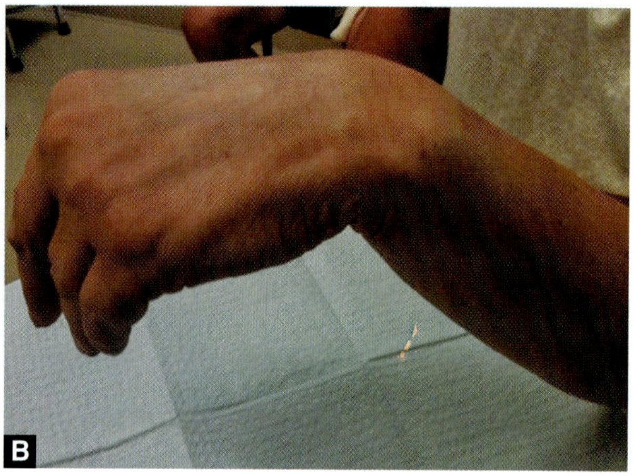

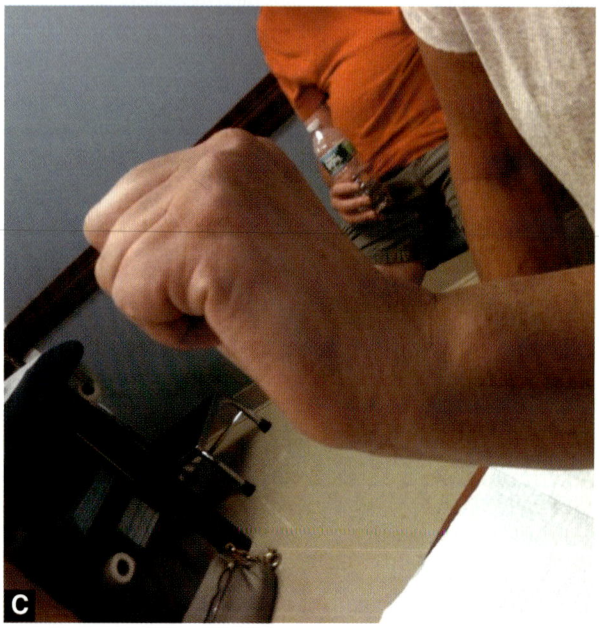

Figures 13.15A to C: A 45-year-old male incurred a midshaft clavicle fracture that healed with a malunion consisting of shortening of 5 cm. (A) The patient underwent malunion correction with an iliac crest interposition graft to restore length; (B) However, postoperatively, the patient developed a traction brachial plexopathy. The patient underwent removal of hardware and neurolysis of the brachial plexus; (C) Due to persistence of a partial plexopathy with residual loss of finger and wrist extension, the patient underwent tendon transfers in the form of pronator teres to the extensor carpi radialis brevis to restore wrist extension, flexor carpi radialis to the extensor digitorum communis to restore finger extension, and palmaris longus to the extensor pollicis longus to restore thumb extension.

Courtesy: Asif M Ilyas

Summary

Clavicle fractures are most commonly treated non-operatively. Considerations as to when operative repair should be undertaken include fracture location, feature alignment condition of the overlying skin, associated injuries and activity of the patient. There are various fixation options including plate fixation and intramedullary devices. Complications following clavicle fixation include malunions, nonunions, hardware irritation, wound dehiscence, thoracic outlet syndrome and brachial plexopathy.

References

1. McKee MD. Clavicle fractures in 2010: sling/swathe or open reduction and internal fixation? Orthop Clin North Am. 2010;41(2):225-31.
2. Neer CS. Nonunion of the clavicle. J Am Med Assoc. 1960;172:1006-11.
3. Hill JM, McGuire MH, Crosby LA. Closed treatment of displaced middle-third fractures of the clavicle gives poor results. J Bone Joint Surg Br. 1997;79(4):537-9.
4. Nordqvist A, Petersson CJ, Redlund-Johnell I. Mid-clavicle fractures in adults: end result study after conservative treatment. J Orthop Trauma. 1998;12(8):572-6.
5. McKee MD, Pedersen EM, Jones C, et al. Deficits following nonoperative treatment of displaced midshaft clavicular fractures. J Bone Joint Surg Am. 2006;88(1):35-40.
6. Canadian Orthopaedic Trauma Society. Nonoperative treatment compared with plate fixation of displaced midshaft clavicular fractures. A multicenter, randomized clinical trial. J Bone Joint Surg Am. Jan 2007;89(1):1-10.
7. Nordqvist A, Petersson C, Redlund-Johnell I. The natural course of lateral clavicle fracture. 15 (11-21) year follow-up of 110 cases. Acta Orthop Scand. 1993;64(1):87-91.
8. Eskola A, Vainionpaa S, Patiala H, et al. Outcome of operative treatment in fresh lateral clavicular fracture. Ann Chir Gynaecol. 1987;76(3):167-9.
9. Kulshrestha V, Roy T, Audige L. Operative versus non-operative management of displaced midshaft clavicle fractures: a prospective cohort study. J Orthop Trauma. 2011;25(1):31-8.
10. Smekal V, Irenberger A, Struve P, et al. Elastic stable intramedullary nailing versus nonoperative treatment of displaced midshaft clavicular fractures: a randomized, controlled, clinical trial. J Orthop Trauma. 2009;23(2): 106-12.
11. Ferran NA, Hodgson P, Vannet N, et al. Locked intramedullary fixation vs plating for displaced and shortened mid-shaft clavicle fractures: a randomized clinical trial. J Shoulder Elbow Surg. 2010;19(6):783-9.
12. Liu HH, Chang CH, Chia WT, et al. Comparison of plates versus intramedullary nails for fixation of displaced midshaft clavicular fractures. J Trauma. 2010;69(6):E82-7.
13. Lee YS, Lau MJ, Tseng YC, et al. Comparison of the efficacy of hook plate versus tension band wire in the treatment of unstable fractures of the distal clavicle. Int Orthop. 2009; 33(5):1401-5.
14. Tambe AD, Motkur P, Qamar A, et al. Fractures of the distal third of the clavicle treated by hook plating. Int Orthop. 2006;30(1):7-10.
15. Ballmer FT, Gerber C. Coracoclavicular screw fixation for unstable fractures of the distal clavicle. A report of five cases. J Bone Joint Surg Br. 1991;73(2):291-4.
16. Yamaguchi H, Arakawa H, Kobayashi M. Results of the Bosworth method for unstable fractures of the distal clavicle. Int Orthop. 1998;22(6):366-8.
17. Harris RI, Wallace AL, Harper GD, et al. Structural properties of the intact and the reconstructed coracoclavicular ligament complex. Am J Sports Med. 2000;28(1):103-8.
18. Robinson CM, Court-Brown CM, McQueen MM, et al. Estimating the risk of nonunion following nonoperative treatment of a clavicular fracture. J Bone Joint Surg Am. 2004;86-A(7):1359-65.
19. Collinge C, Devinney S, Herscovici D, et al. Anterior-inferior plate fixation of middle-third fractures and nonunions of the clavicle. J Orthop Trauma. 2006;20(10):680-6.
20. Khan LA, Bradnock TJ, Scott C, et al. Fractures of the clavicle. J Bone Joint Surg Am. 2009;91(2):447-60.
21. Ring D, Holovacs T. Brachial plexus palsy after intramedullary fixation of a clavicular fracture. A report of three cases. J Bone Joint Surg Am. 2005;87(8):1834-7.
22. Chen CE, Liu HC. Delayed brachial plexus neurapraxia complicating malunion of the clavicle. Am J Orthop (Belle Mead NJ). 2000;29(4):321-2.
23. Krishnan KG, Mucha D, Gupta R, et al. Brachial plexus compression caused by recurrent clavicular nonunion and space-occupying pseudoarthrosis: definitive reconstruction using free vascularized bone flap—a series of eight cases. Neurosurgery. 2008;62(5 Suppl 2):ONS461-469; discussion 469-70.
24. Hartzell TL, Hornicek FJ, Austen WG. Latissimus dorsi flap closure of the irradiated clavicular wound. J Shoulder Elbow Surg. 2008;17(6):875-80.

Chapter 14

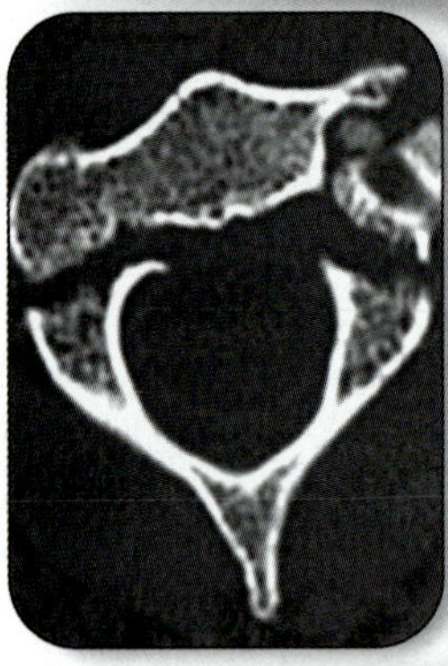

Cervical Spine Fractures and Dislocations

S Rajasekaran, Rishi Kanna, Ajoy Prasad Shetty

Chapter Outline

Introduction

Diagnosis
- Clinical Evaluation in the Emergency Department
- Radiographic Evaluation of Spine Injured Patient
- Clearing the Spine in Trauma Patients

Classification
- Occipital Condyle Fractures
- Occipitocervical Dislocation
- Atlas Fractures
- Odontoid Fractures
- Traumatic Spondylolisthesis of C2 (Hangman's Fracture)
- Subaxial Cervical Fractures

Management and Surgical Indications
- Fractures of the Atlas
- Fractures of the Odontoid Process
- Traumatic Spondylolisthesis of C2 (Hangman's Fracture)
- Subaxial Cervical Fractures

Surgical Anatomy
- Upper Cervical Spine
- Lower Cervical Spine

Surgical Approaches
- Anterior Approach to the Subaxial Cervical Spine
- Posterior Approach to the Cervical Spine

Surgical Techniques
- Technique 1: Direct C1 Posterior Fixation
- Technique 2: C1–C2 Fusion
- Technique 3: C2 Odontoid Fixation
- Technique 4: C2 Pars Fixation
- Technique 5: Subaxial Anterior Corpectomy and Fusion
- Technique 6: Lateral Mass Screw Fixation

Outcomes

Complications
- Complications related to the Injury
- Complications due to Lateral Mass Fixation
- Complications due to Anterior Fixation

Complication Cases
- Case 1: Conservatively Treated Odontoid Fracture Resulting in Nonunion
- Case 2: Neglected C2–C3 Fracture
- Case 3: Prominent Lateral Mass Screws with Cervical Radiculopathy

Introduction

Cervical spine injuries occur secondary to high-energy mechanisms, including motor vehicle accident (45%) and fall from a height (20%) and less commonly during athletic participation (15%).[1] Forced flexion or extension resulting from unrestrained deceleration forces is the most common mechanism for cervical spine injuries. Neurological injury occurs in 40% of patients with cervical spine fractures and is more frequently associated with lower cervical spine injuries.[1] Cervical spine fractures occur commonly at two levels. Thirty percent of cervical vertebral fractures occur at the level of C2, and 50% of injuries occur at the level of C6–C7. The most frequent level of spinal cord injury is C5.[2] Most fatal cervical spine injuries occur at the upper cervical levels, either at the craniocervical junction, C1 or C2 since it affects the vital functions of a person.[3]

Most deaths associated with spinal cord injury occur during the first 24 hours after hospitalization. These injuries are more commonly seen in males than females and are more frequently observed in young and middle-aged people.[4] The age distribution of patients presenting with lower cervical spine and spinal cord injuries is bimodal. Most patients with a cervical spine injury are young and they incur cervical spine injuries as a result of a high-energy trauma, such as motor vehicle accidents, accidents resulting from sporting activities, or violence.[5] In elderly patients, the injuries are relatively uncommon and the associated degenerative changes influence the outcome. These people sustain injuries from low-energy trauma, such as falling from standing or seated height.

Cervical spine injuries can be classified according to the level of injury, the mechanism of the trauma, morphology, or instability of the fracture. The exact mechanism of trauma in many patients often remains uncertain. The assessment of spinal stability is essential in deciding the correct choice of treatment in each specific type of cervical spine injury. The radiological evaluation of a patient with suspected cervical spine injury, clearing the cervical spine and role of computed tomography (CT) and magnetic resonance imaging (MRI) section have been explained in the subsequent sections. However, some important points have been reiterated below (Table 14.1 and Figs 14.1 and 14.2).

Table 14.1: Important points to observe while assessing plain radiographs of the subaxial cervical spine

- Continuity of radiographic lines: anterior vertebral line, posterior vertebral line, spinolaminar line and spinous process line
- Widening or narrowing of disc spaces
- Increased distance between spinous processes or facet joints
- Any fracture lines in the bodies or in the posterior elements
- Any displacement of the spinous process on the antero-posterior (AP) film
- Any antero- or retrolisthesis on the lateral roentgenogram
- Acute kyphosis or loss of lordosis
- Any increase in the width of the retropharyngeal space in front of the vertebral bodies (> 4 mm at C3, C4, > 15 mm at C5, C6, C7)
- Radiographic markers of cervical spine instability (on the lateral view) include the following:
  - Compression fractures with > 25% loss of height
  - Angular displacements > 11° between adjacent vertebrae
  - Translation > 3.5 mm on flexion-extension view

Diagnosis

Motor vehicle accidents are the most frequent causes of upper cervical spine injuries; however, falls, diving accidents, and gunshot wounds are also common mechanisms. In addition, congenital or developmental abnormalities, arthritic conditions, especially rheumatoid arthritis and tumors can predispose or complicate an upper cervical spine injury. Patients with an upper cervical injury may have an associated head injury which can interfere with an accurate history and physical examination. By thumb rule, all patients who sustain significant polytrauma and/or head trauma should be assumed to have a cervical spine injury and undergo appropriate stabilization maneuvers and screening radiographic studies.

Important aspects of the history are the mechanism of injury, whether the patient was restrained, and whether transient neurological symptoms or deficits occurred immediately after the injury at the scene of the accident. Patients often complain of neck pain, nuchal pain or occipital headache. Routine advanced trauma life support (ATLS) procedures of maintenance of airway, breathing, and circulation should be the first priority. A careful, complete physical examination of the entire spine should follow.

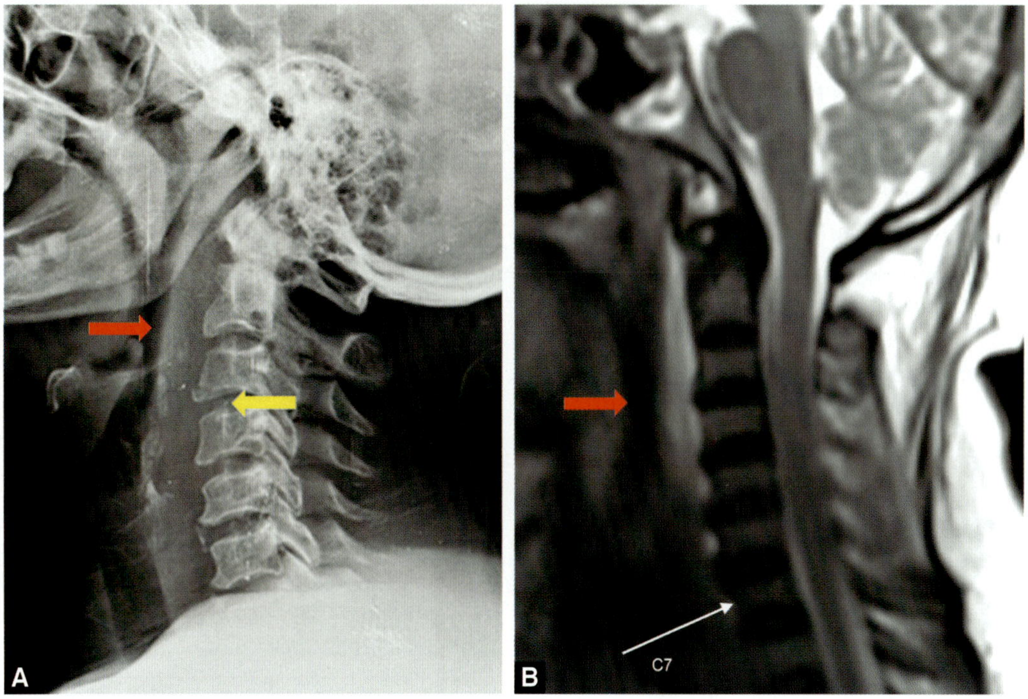

Figures 14.1A and B: (A) Lateral radiographs and (B) sagittal MRI of a 50-year-old patient with a stable C3 fracture (yellow arrow). Lateral radiograph shows a widened prevertebral space due to hematoma (red arrow), which is clearly demonstrated in the MRI.

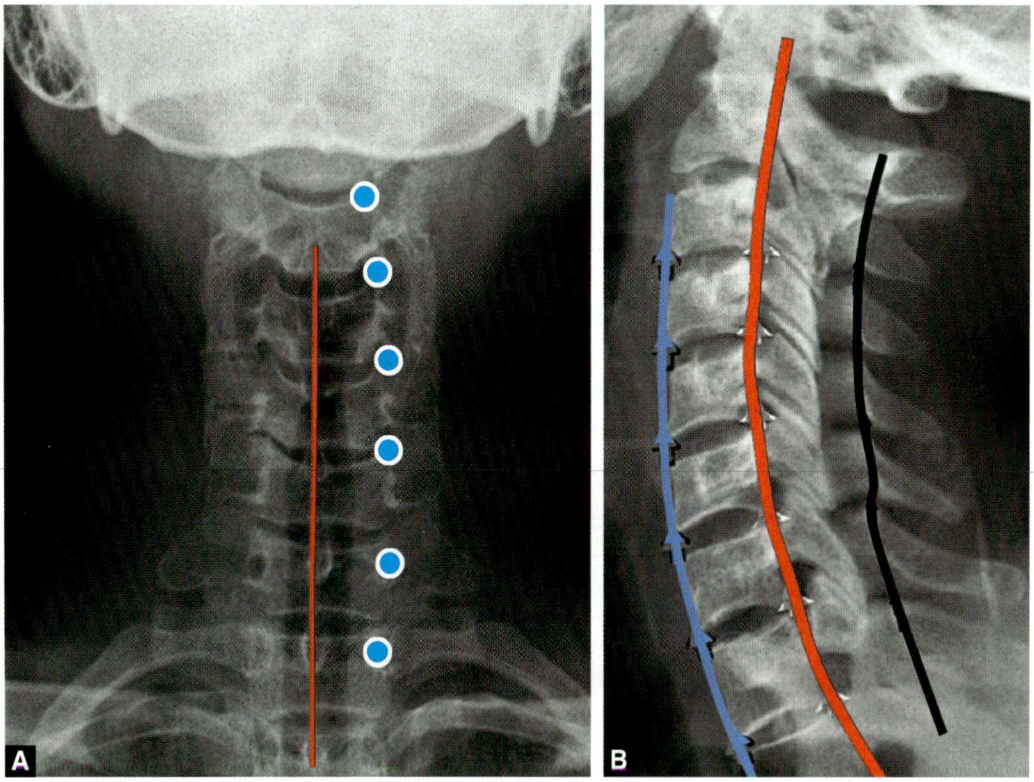

Figures 14.2A and B: (A) Anteroposterior (AP) and (B) lateral radiographs of a normal cervical spine. The entire cervical region is visualized in the lateral view. In the AP view, the spinous processes are in a straight line and the pedicles are well aligned. In the lateral view, the anterior and posterior vertebral borders, and the spinolaminar line is well aligned.

Inspection, palpation, and neurologic evaluation are performed while the head and neck are stabilized with collar and side supports. Neurologic examination should include testing of the cranial nerves as well as motor function, sensation, and reflexes in the extremities as explained in the following sections [American Spinal Injury Association (ASIA) assessment form]. Cranial nerve injury to the VI, VII, IX, XI, and XII nerves can result from upper cervical injuries and should not be overlooked.

Clinical Evaluation in the Emergency Department

General Evaluation

A patient with suspected spinal injury should have preliminary evaluation as per the ATLS guidelines to rule out serious systemic injuries such as abdominal, chest and head trauma.[1] Central nervous system evaluation is done as per the Glasgow Coma Scale. Injuries should be addressed in order of priority. Although life-threatening injuries such as chest, abdominal injuries and active bleeding limb injuries must be managed first, suspected vertebral injury should be temporarily stabilized and protected during these procedures. A quick history should include mechanism of injury, local symptoms of pain as well as subtle or overt symptoms of neurologic dysfunction ranging from tingling or numbness of an extremity to obvious paralysis.

Local Examination

The spine is then examined in detail. The patient is rolled on his or her side with a "log-roll" maneuver. Inspection should include looking for abrasions, lacerations or "seat-belt" injuries. The attitude of the patient's head and body should be observed. Each spinous process is palpated from cervical spine to lumbosacral spine. Any tenderness is suggestive of spinal injury. Ligament injury may be detected by noting palpable defects between the spinous processes or hematomas. A step-off may indicate the presence of a dislocation. Once gross unstable spinal injuries have been ruled out, the examiner should ask the patient to gently move his head from side to side if possible, and any painful movements should be noted. Forced testing of movements should be avoided. The vertebral injury can also occur at multiple non-contiguous levels in 15–20% of patients sustaining a spinal injury. Calenoff found a 5% incidence of multiple non-contiguous vertebral injuries with half of the secondary lesions having been initially missed.[6] Therefore, it is mandatory to evaluate other regions of the spine to look for tenderness, abrasions and interspinous widening.

Patients with cervical and thoracic spinal cord injuries can present with hypotension and bradycardia due to neurogenic shock secondary to sympathetic outflow disruption ("functional sympathectomy") with resultant unopposed vagal (parasympathetic) tone. Initial tachycardia and hypertension immediately after injury are followed by hypotension accompanied by bradycardia and venous pooling. Hypotension from neurogenic shock may be differentiated from cardiogenic, septic and hypovolemic shock by the presence of bradycardia, as opposed to tachycardia. Recognizing neurogenic shock as distinct from hemorrhagic shock is critical for safe initial resuscitation of a trauma patient (Table 14.2). Intravenous replacement therapy should maintain systolic blood pressure of atleast 100 mmHg. Treatment of bradycardia should begin with atropine 0.2–0.5 mg intravenously. Volume expansion is used judiciously to increase intravascular supply and stroke volume. If hypotension persists, vasopressors such as dopamine or dobutamine can be used.

Neurologic Examination

Approximately half of the patients with an acute spinal cord injury have a complete injury with no preservation of motor or sensory function in the sacral cord segments. Presently, the patient's neurological status after the period of spinal shock is the only factor that can predict the chances of neurological recovery. Any patient who remains to have a complete neurological deficit at the end of 72 hours after the injury has very poor chances of neurological recovery. Therefore, an accurate and detailed neurological evaluation of the motor power, sensory and reflex function should be performed at the time of

Table 14.2: Differentiating neurogenic from hypovolemic shock

Neurogenic shock	*Hypovolemic shock*
Hypotension	Hypotension
Bradycardia	Tachycardia
Warm extremities	Cold extremities
Normal urine output	Low urine output

initial evaluation. This examination should be repeated at intervals and documented. An important element of neurological examination is the evaluation of sacral sparing. Sacral sparing is represented by the presence of perianal sensation, voluntary rectal motor function, and great toe flexor activity; it indicates at least partial continuity of spinal cord tracts. It signifies an incomplete cord injury, with the potential for a greater return of cord function following resolution of spinal shock.

In approximately 50% of patients immediately after injury, there occurs a brief period of physiologic spinal cord "shutdown" in response to injury. This phase is described as the "spinal shock" characterized by a state of flaccid paralysis, areflexia, and lack of sensation below the level of injury. This occurs most commonly in cervical and upper thoracic injuries. Resolution of spinal shock may be recognized when reflex arcs caudal to the level of injury begin to function again, usually within 24–48 hours of injury. These caudal reflex arcs include the bulbocavernosus reflex (S3–S4) and the anal wink (S2–S4). The bulbocavernosus reflex refers to contraction of the anal sphincter in response to stimulation of the trigone of the bladder with either a squeeze on the glans penis, a tap on the mons pubis, or a pull on a urethral catheter. The anal wink is a contraction of the external anal sphincter in response to a perianal pinprick. The absence of these reflexes indicates the phase of spinal shock. The return of these reflexes generally within 24–48 hours of the initial injury hallmarks the end of spinal shock. The absence of motor or sensory function below the level of injury after spinal shock has resolved indicates a complete injury with a poor prognosis for neurological recovery. The sacral reflexes however are not prognostic for lesions involving the conus medullaris or the cauda equina.

Guidelines for the assessment of a spinal injured patient have been laid down by International Standards for Neurology and Functional Classification of Spinal Cord Injury patient (Fig. 14.3) and are known as American Spinal Injury Association (ASIA) guidelines. The elements of

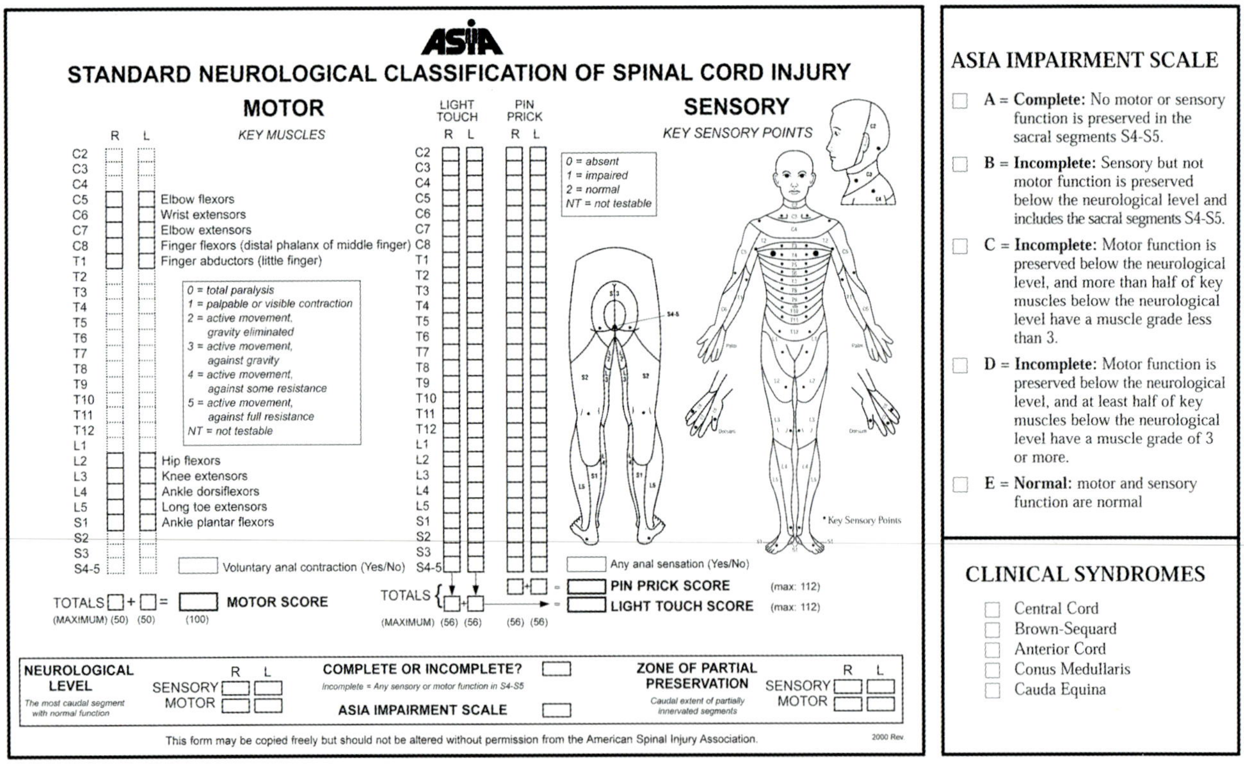

Figure 14.3: American Spinal Injury Association (ASIA) form for standard neurologic classification of spinal cord injury. For functional scoring, 10 key muscle segments corresponding to innervation by C5, C6, C7, C8, T1, L2, L3, L4, L5, and S1 are each given a functional score of 0 to 5 out of 5. For sensory scoring, both right and left sides are graded for a total of 100 points. For the 28 sensory dermatomes on each side of the body, sensory levels are scored on a 0- to 2-point scale, yielding a maximum possible pinprick score of 112 points for a patient with normal sensation.

Source: Used with permission from ASIA.

neurological examination have been chosen as the minimum necessary data-set for accurate communication, as well as for its reproducibility.

Neurological Examination of the Spinal Injured Patient

Neurologic examination consists of sensory examination and motor examination. This comprises certain required as well as optional elements. Required elements allow the determination of sensory, motor and neurologic levels, generation of sensory and motor index scores, determination of completeness of injury and classification of impairment. Rectal examination findings like deep anal sensation and voluntary anal contraction is part of required components of examination. Optional elements of examination include aspects of neurologic examination that may better describe the patient's clinical condition. These include proprioception and deep pressure sensation.

Sensory examination: There are 28 dermatomes included in the sensory examination. Each dermatome is tested separately for sharp and dull sensation with a disposable pin, and light touch using a cotton tip applicator on either sides of the body. Sensory examination results are graded on a three point scale 0 to 2, with the face as the normal control point. If the patient is able to distinguish between sharp and dull edge of the pin, 8 out of 10 times, correct answer is considered as accurate.[6] Accurate sensation is given a score of 2. Absent sensation, which includes the inability to distinguish between the sharp and dull edge of pin, yields a score of 0. A score of 1 (impaired) for pinprick testing is given when the patient is able to distinguish between the sharp and dull edge of the pin, but pin is not felt as sharp as on the face. Impaired score is also given if the patient reports altered sensation, including hyperesthesia.

For testing light touch, a cotton tip applicator is used and is stroked across the skin moving over a distance not exceeding 1 cm. When testing the digits for dermatomes C6–C8, the dorsal surface of the proximal phalanx should be tested. When testing the chest and abdomen, sensory testing should be performed in the midclavicular line. The sensation is compared to the face. When the sensation is the same as on the face, it is recorded as intact, and is scored as 2. Lesser sensation as compared to face is recorded as impaired and is graded a score 1. Absent touch sensation is scored as 0.

The rectal digital examination for deep anal sensation (S4–S5 dermatomes) is extremely important, since this represents the most caudal aspect of sacral spinal cord. The patient is asked to report any sensory awareness, touch or pressure, with firm pressure of the examiner's digit on the rectal walls. Deep anal sensation is recorded as either present or absent. "Sensory level" is the most caudal dermatome to have intact (2/2) sensation for both pinprick and light touch on both sides of the body. Sensory index scoring is calculated by adding the scores for each dermatome, for a total possible score of 112 (56 on each side of the body) for pinprick and for light touch.

If accurate sensory testing in any dermatome cannot be performed, NT (not tested) should be recorded, or an alternate location can be tested with a notation that an alternate site was chosen. Optional elements of the ASIA sensory examination are also important and include proprioception (joint position and vibration) and deep pressure sensations. These can be graded as absent, impaired or normal. These are useful to better describe the patients' neurologic condition.

Motor examination: The elements of ASIA motor examination include testing of 10 key muscles, five in upper limb and five in lower limb on each side of the body. These key muscles are chosen because of their consistency for being innervated primarily by the segments indicated and for their ease of testing in supine position. The muscles should be examined in rostral to caudal sequence, starting with the shoulder abductors and finishing with the ankle plantar flexors. Testing of all muscles during the initial and follow-up examinations are performed with the patient in the supine position and graded and recorded on a six point scale from 0 to 5. Testing the patient in supine position allows for a valid comparison of patients' scores obtained during the acute period to those obtained during the rehabilitation and follow-up phases of the care. Only whole number scores should be used when comparing the results (rather than pluses and minuses). If a particular muscle has grade 3/5 motor power, it is considered to have full innervation. For all practical purposes, a muscle with at least 3/5 motor power has antigravity strength and is considered useful for functional activities. The muscle should be tested by stabilizing the joint above and joint below. This is especially true if the muscle being tested does not have antigravity strength. This also excludes vicarious movements. For patients with severe pain or unstable spine, the muscles are tested isometrically. Testing is performed by asking the patient to move the limb against resistance without allowing movement.

"Motor Level" is defined by the lowest key muscle that has a motor strength of grade 3/5 and the muscle above the key muscle should have strength of 5/5. The clinical condition of the patient often prevents a complete and accurate clinical examination. These limiting factors could be such as pain and might present such that the motor only grades a 4/5 power. In such situations the muscle should be graded as 5 with an asterisk(*), referring to the factors which were preventing the examination. The patient's condition should be recorded as NT in place of a numeric score, when the patient presents with spasticity, uncontrolled clonus, severe pain, a fracture limiting examination, traumatic brain injury, comatose patient, injury to brachial plexus and lumbosacral plexus. If the limitation of range of motion following the fracture is less than 50%, the muscle should be graded through the available range and is subjected to the same Medical Research Council (MRC) grading scale 0 to 5. A muscle contracture limiting range of motion more than 50% of the normal range, should be graded as NT. Abbreviations and symbols like pluses and minuses are not considered for motor index scoring.

Motor index scoring: This is calculated by adding the muscle scores of each key muscle group. The total score obtained is 100, 25 each for each extremity.

Rectal examination: This is essential to complete the neurologic examination. The perianal skin is tested for pinprick and dull sensation with a gloved finger. Motor activity is tested by asking the patient to voluntarily contract the sphincter. Voluntary anal contraction is tested as part of the motor examination by sensing contraction of the external anal sphincter around the examiner's finger and graded as either present or absent. During this examination, one can again document the presence or absence of anal sensation.

Neurologic level of injury: It is the most caudal level at which motor and sensory modalities are intact on both sides of the body. For example if the motor level is C7, and sensory level is C8, then over all neurologic level of injury (NLI) will be C8. In situations like thoracic spine injuries, where specific muscles cannot be clinically tested to evaluate the spinal segment, the sensory level is used to determine the neurological level. Examinations may need to be repeated at intervals between 72 hours and 10 days following injury to accurately classify and prognosticate. Initial assessment may be fallacious due to shock, pain or intoxication. There may also be worsening within 72 hours due to cord swelling.

Skeletal level: It is defined as the spinal level at which the greatest vertebral damage has occurred as found by radiographic examination.

Classification and Scoring of the Spinal Injuries

Frankel and associates in 1969 described a five grade system of classifying traumatic spinal cord injury, with a broad division into complete and incomplete injuries. The extent of remaining sensory or motor function determined the specific Frankel classification.

Frankel Scale

A. Complete: Motor and sensory function below the segmental level was absent.
B. Sensory only: Implies some sensation present below the lesion but the motor paralysis was complete below that level. This does not apply when there is a slight discrepancy between the motor and sensory level but does apply to sacral sparing.
C. Motor useless: Some motor power present below the lesion but of no practical use to the patient.
D. Motor useful: Implies that there is some useful motor power below the level of the lesion. Some patients could move the lower limb, and many could walk with or without aids.
E. Recovery: Free of neurologic symptoms, that is, no weakness, no sensory loss, no sphincter disturbances. Abnormal reflexes may be present.

Since the motor scale was arbitrary without definitive quantification of neurological deficit, the Frankel scale was replaced by ASIA grading (Table 14.3 and Fig. 14.4).

American Spinal Injury Association Classification

American Spinal Injury Association in 1982, attempting to improve the communication and consistency among the

Table 14.3: American Spinal Injury Association (ASIA) definitions for neurological status following spinal injury

Term	*Definition*
Neurologic level	The most caudal segment with normal sensory and motor function on both sides
Sensory level	The most caudal segment with normal sensory function on both sides
Motor level	The most caudal segment with normal motor function on both sides
Skeletal level	Radiographic level of greatest vertebral damage
Sensory score	Numeric summary value of sensory impairment
Motor score	Numeric summary value of motor impairment
Incomplete injury	Partial preservation of sensory and/or motor function below the neurologic level and sensory and/or motor preservation of the lowest sacral segment
Complete injury	Absence of sensory and motor function in the lowest sacral segment
Zone of partial preservation	Dermatomes and myotomes caudal to the neurologic level that remain partially innervated. Only used in complete injuries

Source: ASIA Standards for Neurological Classification of Spinal Injury. Chicago: American Spinal Injury Association; 2006.

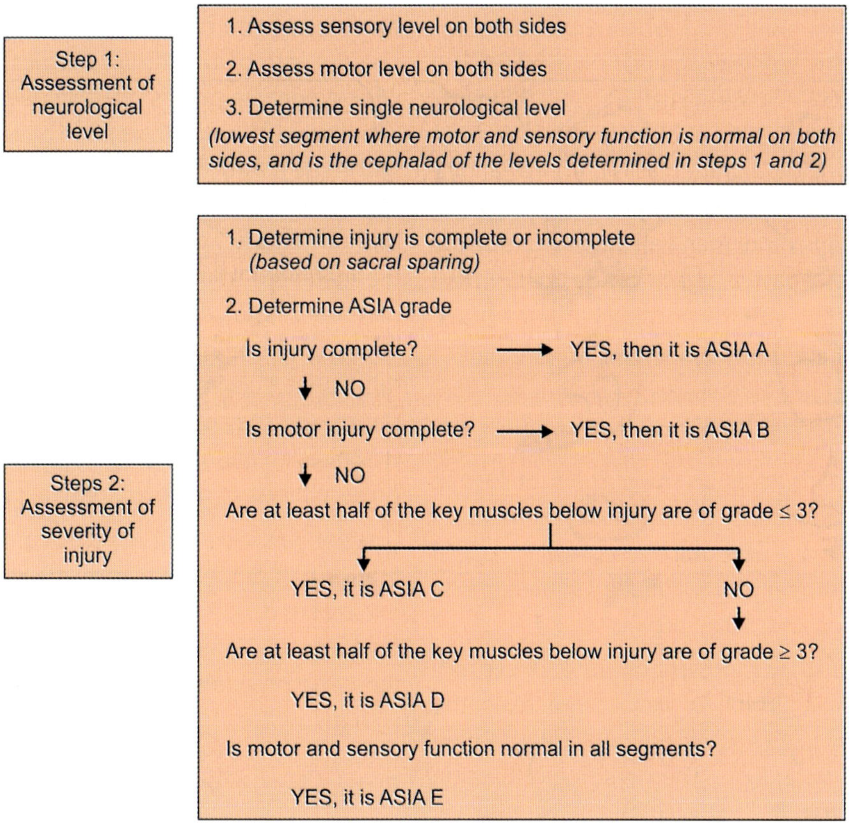

Figure 14.4: Steps in classifying spinal cord injury.

clinicians and researchers developed and published standards for neurological classification of spinal injured patients. The ASIA guidelines incorporated the Frankel grades A to E and motor scores described by Lucas and Austin. The sensory testing recommended included examination of 28 dermatomes. The sensory examination was scored on a three point scale, by Bracken and colleagues by testing each side of the body for light touch and pinprick. The ASIA guidelines also defined the neurologic level of injury, quadriplegia and paresis, paraplegia and paresis, complete and incomplete spinal injuries.

ASIA Impairment Scale

A. Complete: No motor or sensory function preserved in the lowest sacral segment, S4–S5.
B. Incomplete: Sensory function below neurological level and in S4–S5 but no motor function below the neurologic level.
C. Incomplete: Motor function is preserved below the neurologic level, and more than half the muscles below the neurologic level have a muscle grade less than 3/5.
D. Incomplete: Motor function is preserved below the neurologic level, and more than half the muscles below the neurologic level have a muscle grade greater than or equal to 3/5.
E. Normal: Sensory and motor functions are normal.

Other Important Definitions

Tetraplegia: This is defined as an impairment or loss of motor or sensory function in the cervical segments of spinal cord due to damage of neural elements within spinal cord. This results in impairment of function in the arms as well as the trunk, legs and pelvic organs.

Paraplegia: This refers to impairment of motor or sensory function in the thoracic, lumbar, or sacral segments of the spinal cord secondary to damage of neural elements within the spinal canal. In paraplegia, the neurologic function within the upper extremity is spared, but depending on the level of injury, the trunk, legs and pelvic organs may be involved. The term paresis describes the incomplete injury imprecisely.

Complete injury is defined as the absence of sensory or motor function below the level of injury including the lowest sacral segments.

Incomplete injury is defined as preservation of motor function or sensation below the neurologic level of injury that includes the lowest sacral segments, i.e. sacral sparing. This can be tested by checking light touch and pinprick sensation at the anal mucocutaneous junction (S4–S5 dermatome), on both sides, as well as by testing voluntary anal contraction and deep anal sensation. If any of these is present, the individual has an incomplete injury.

Clinical Syndromes of Incomplete Spinal Cord Injury (Table 14.4 and Figs 14.5A to D)

Central cord syndrome: It is the most common of the incomplete spinal cord injury syndromes. It is characterized by motor weakness in the upper limb greater than lower limb in association with sacral sparing. Other than motor weakness, there is also bladder dysfunction and varying sensory loss below the level of lesion. Although central cord syndrome occurs most frequently in older patients with cervical spondylosis and hyperextension injury, this syndrome may occur in patients of any age. The postulated mechanism of injury involves compression of the cord both anteriorly and posteriorly, with inward buckling of the ligamentum flavum during hyperextension in an already narrowed spondylotic spinal canal. The prognosis for this injury is fair, and 50–60% of patients have significant functional recovery. Bladder and bowel control is likely to return, and they would be able to walk with a spastic gait. However, the upper limbs lag behind in recovery, and fine functions of the hand remain permanently affected.

Cruciate paralysis: This is a syndrome with similar clinical features of upper extremity paresis or paralysis, with minimal to no lower extremity involvement. This occurs in fractures of C1 and C2, with neurologic compromise at the cervicomedullary junction. Here the lesion is higher with respiratory insufficiency seen in 25% of patients.

Brown-Sequard Syndrome

This involves a hemisection of the spinal cord. This accounts for about 2–4% of all traumatic spinal cord injuries. There is ispilateral loss of all sensory modalities

Table 14.4: Descriptions of incomplete cord injury patterns

Syndrome	*Lesion*	*Clinical presentation*
Brown-Sequard syndrome	Hemicord injury with ipsilateral motor, light touch sensation and proprioception loss, and contralateral pain and temperature sensory loss	• The result of a unilateral laminar or pedicle fracture, penetrating injury, or rotational injury resulting in a subluxation • The prognosis is good, with > 90% of patients regaining bowel and bladder function, and ambulatory capacity
Central cord syndrome	Incomplete cervical white matter injury The centrally located arm tracts in the cortical spinal area are the most severely affected, and the leg tracts are affected to a lesser extent	• Associated with an extension injury to an osteoarthritic spine in a middle-aged patient and presents with flaccid paralysis of the upper extremities and spastic paralysis of the lower extremities • Radiographs frequently demonstrate no fracture or dislocation, because the lesion is created by a pincer effect between anterior osteophytes and posterior infolding of the ligamentum flavum • The prognosis is fair, and more than 50% of patients have return of bowel and bladder control, become ambulatory, and have improved hand function
Anterior cord syndrome	The lesion involves the anterior gray matter with preservation of dorsal columns	• The patient presents with variable motor and pain/temperature loss with preserved light touch and proprioception • The prognosis is good if recovery is evident and progressive within 24 hours of injury
Posterior cord syndrome	This is rare injury with isolated involvement of the posterior column	• Loss of deep pressure, deep pain, and proprioception with full voluntary power, pain, and temperature sensation
Conus medullaris syndrome	This is seen in T12–L1 injuries and results in an areflexic bladder, bowel, and weak lower extremities	• A pure lesion involves a loss of voluntary bowel and bladder control with preserved lumbar root function. The irreversible nature of this injury to the sacral segments is evidenced by the absence of the bulbocavernosus reflex and the perianal wink
Cauda equina	Injury to the lumbosacral nerve roots within the spinal canal	• Bilateral radicular pain, numbness, weakness, hyporeflexia or areflexia in lower limbs, saddle anesthesia and loss of voluntary bowel and bladder function
Root injury	Avulsion or compression injury to single or multiple nerve roots (brachial plexus avulsion)	• Dermatomal sensory loss, myotomal motor loss, and absent deep tendon reflexes

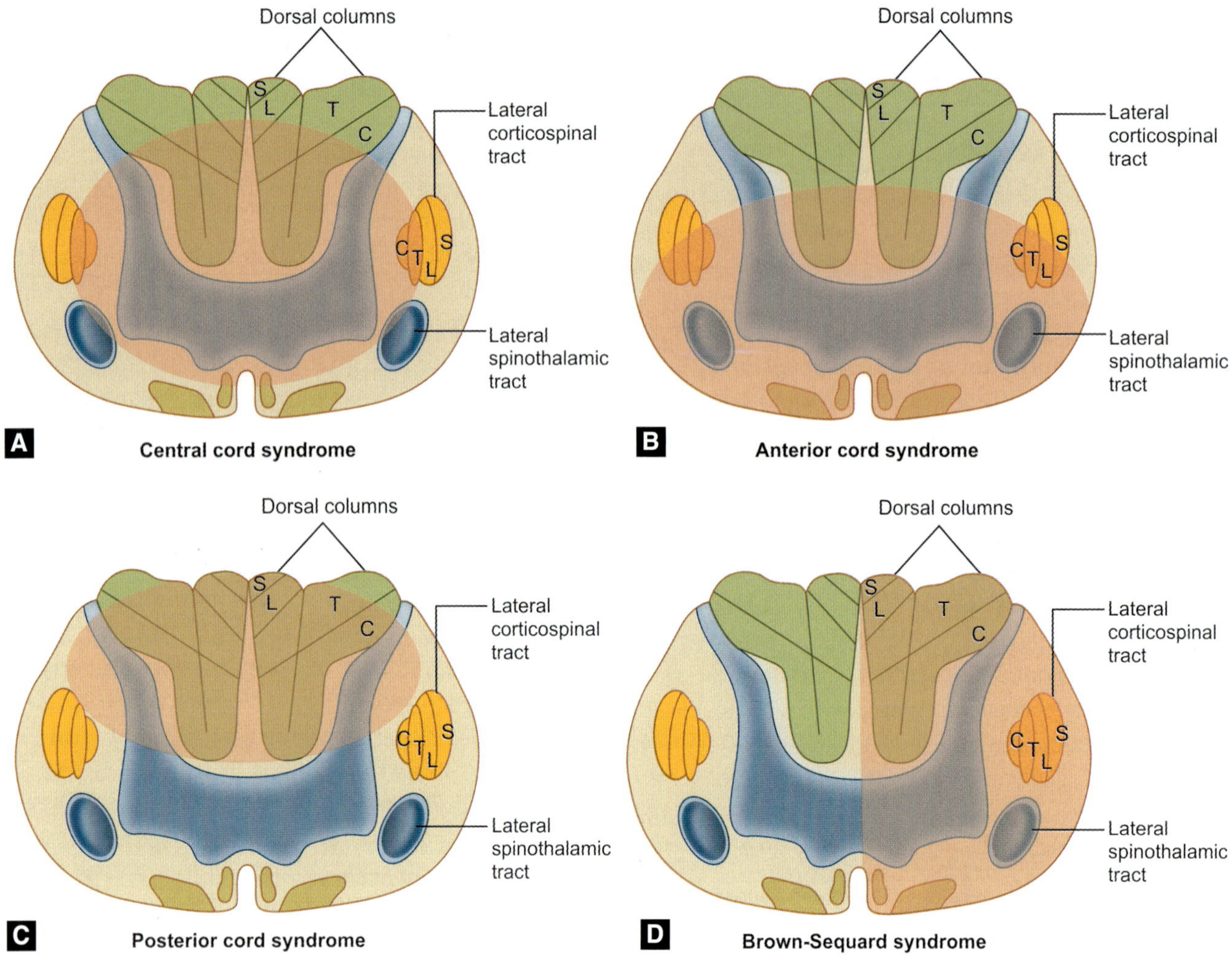

Figures 14.5A to D: Diagrammatic representation of cross-sections of the spinal cord. The various ascending and descending tracts of the spinal cord have been marked. The regions of the spinal cord injured in (A) Central cord syndrome; (B) Anterior cord syndrome; (C) Posterior cord syndrome; and (D) Brown-Sequard syndrome are shown in shaded pink zones.

at the level of the lesion, ipsilateral flaccid paralysis at the level of the lesion, ispilateral loss of position sense and sense of vibration below the lesion, contralateral loss of pain and temperature below the lesion, and ipsilateral motor loss below the level of the lesion. Neuroanatomically, this is explained by the crossing of the spinothalamic tracts in the spinal cord, as opposed to the corticospinal and dorsal columns which decussate in the brain stem. This injury has a good prognosis. More than 90% of the patients regain significant neurologic function.

Anterior cord syndrome: This involves lesion involving the anterior two-third of the spinal cord, with posterior spinal cord being preserved. Etiologies could be due to retropulsed disc or bone fragments, direct injury to the spinal cord, or lesions of the anterior spinal artery which provides blood supply to the anterior spinal cord. This presents with variable loss of motor and sharp pain, with relative preservation of light touch, proprioception, and deep pressure sensation. Prognosis is poor, with only 10–15% of patients showing functional recovery.

Posterior Cord Syndrome

This is the least common of the incomplete spinal cord injury syndromes. It is characterized by preservation of pain, temperature, and touch appreciation with motor preservation and absence of all dorsal column function such as proprioception, deep pain and deep pressure.

Radiographic Evaluation of Spine Injured Patient

The standard trauma series would include anteroposterior (AP), lateral, and open-mouth views. An open-mouth radiograph allows visualization of the atlas, odontoid process, and lateral masses of the axis. Although the lateral masses of the atlas normally articulate symmetrically with the axis, asymmetry between the dens and the lateral masses of the atlas is not always indicative of injury. For specific injuries, CT and MRI may yield additional diagnostic information.[7] Important points to consider in interpreting plain radiographs of the occipitocervical spine are shown in Table 14.5 and Fig. 14.6A to C.

The lateral view will detect up to 85% of significant cervical spine injuries provided that the occiput-C1, all seven cervical vertebrae and the C7–T1 junctions are visualized (Fig. 14.7). In patients with a short neck, it is necessary to obtain a "swimmer's view" to visualize the cervicothoracic junction. To obtain a "swimmer's view", the upper extremity proximal to the X-ray beam is abducted 180° with axial traction on the contralateral upper extremity, and the beam directed 60° caudad (Figs 14.8A to C). Stress flexion/extension radiographs rarely if ever should be performed if instability is suspected; they should be performed in the awake and alert patient only (Figs 14.9A and B). In a patient with neck pain, they are best delayed until spasm has subsided, which can mask instability. Passive flexion and extension stressing of the cervical spine, performed by an experienced physician under fluoroscopy, has a reported sensitivity of 92.3% and specificity of 98.8% for detecting significant ligamentous injuries and instability of the cervical spine.[8]

Table 14.5: Important landmarks, lines and angles to be observed in plain radiographs of the occipitocervical spine

- Wackenheim line is drawn as a continuation from the clivus caudally. The tip of the odontoid should be within 1–2 mm of this line.
- *Powers ratio*: The basion to posterior C1 arch distance divided by the anterior arch to opisthion distance (BD/AC) should be < 1. A ratio greater than 1 suggests possible anterior dissociation.
- The anterior cortex of the odontoid should be parallel to the posterior cortex of the anterior ring of the atlas. Any kyphotic or lordotic deviation may indicate an odontoid fracture or transverse atlantal ligament disruption.
- The atlas-dens interval (ADI) should be less than 3 mm in an adult (5 mm in a child).
- The space available for the cord (SAC) is measured as the distance from the posterior cortex of the odontoid to the anterior cortex of the posterior arch of the atlas and should amount to more than 13 mm.
- Widening of the prevertebral soft tissue (normal is < 10 mm at C1)

Computed tomography scanning can provide rapid and detailed assessment of the spine (Table 14.6). It is a cost-effective primary screening tool in patients at high or moderate risk for cervical injuries. It is valuable to assess the upper cervical spine or the cervicothoracic junction, especially if it is inadequately visualized by plain radiography and in intubated patients (plain films can miss up to 17% of injuries of the upper cervical spine).[8] Computed tomography scans with reconstructions may be obtained to characterize the fracture pattern and degree of canal compromise more clearly (Fig. 14.10). Magnetic resonance imaging is extremely sensitive and specific for evaluation of the paravertebral soft tissues, including the spinal cord, intervertebral discs and ligamentous structures. Patients with abnormal neurological findings, particularly incomplete injuries, should undergo MRI scanning of the relevant spinal segment(s) to visualize the spinal cord and nerve roots. It can also detect injuries in other regions of the spine since up to 12% of patients have multiple, non-contiguous spinal injuries (Figs 14.11 and 14.12). However, MRI is less sensitive, less specific and less cost-effective than the plain film series or screening CT for the identification and evaluation of cervical fractures.[7]

With a normal atlanto-occipital relationship, the clivus on lateral radiograph should point toward the tip of the odontoid, and the basion (tip of the clivus) should be within 5 mm of the odontoid vertically (Table 14.5, Figs 14.13 and 14.14). Retropharyngeal soft-tissue swelling greater than 5 mm at C3 is abnormal and should raise suspicion for the presence of an anterior arch fracture of the atlas. A diastasis greater than 2 mm between the occiput and atlas is also abnormal. Harris et al. described the rule of 12, which is superior to the Powers ratio for identifying occipitocervical dissociation.[9] The rule of

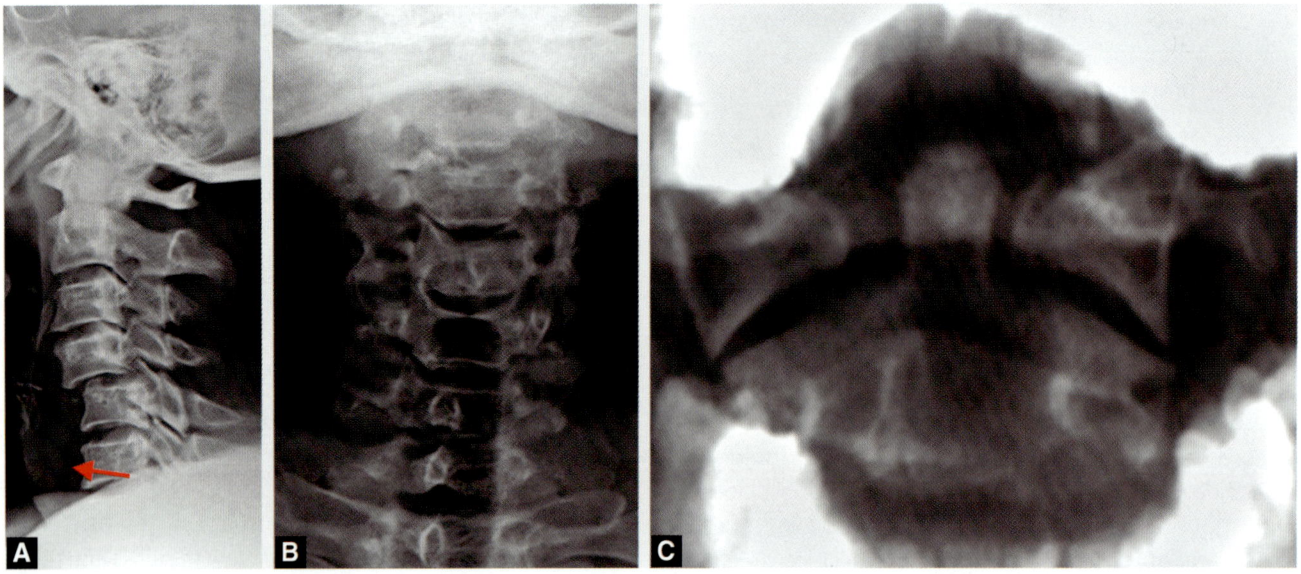

Figures 14.6A to C: (A) Lateral radiograph of a cervical spine injured patient shows subluxation at C4–C5. Note the enlarged prevertebral soft tissue shadow (red arrow); (B) Anteroposterior (AP) radiogarph of the same patient shows a change in the alignment of the spinous processes of the subaxial cervical spine indicating subluxation; (C) Transoral radiograph shows the odontoid and C1–C2 articulation.

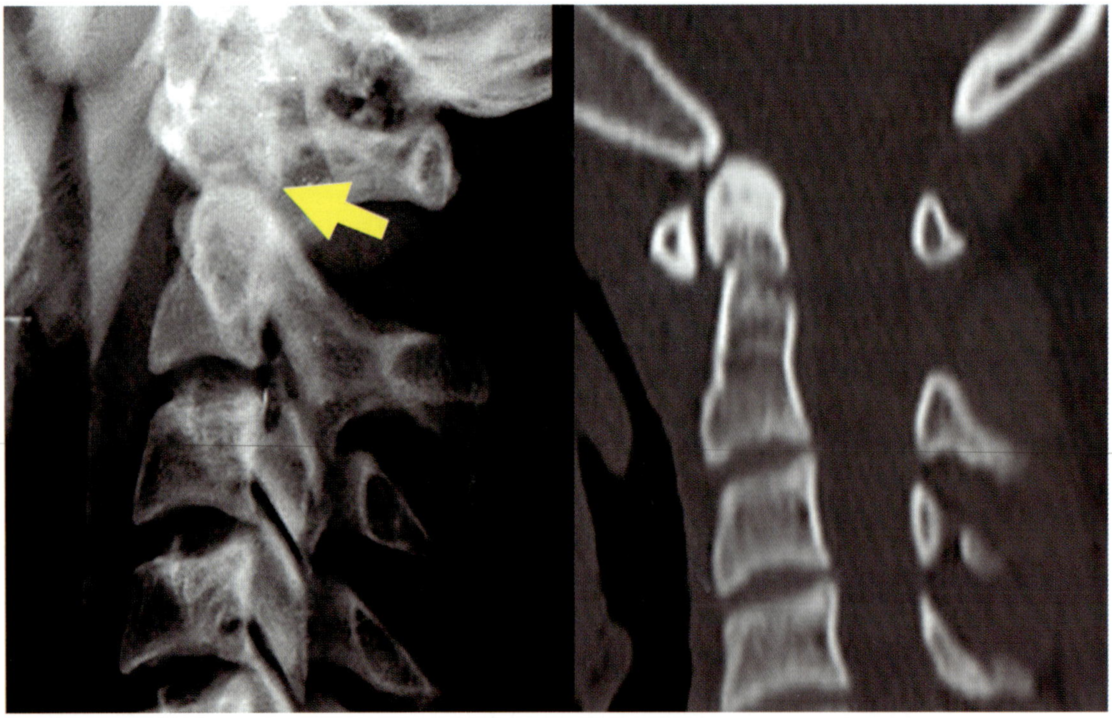

Figure 14.7: Preoperative lateral view of a patient with suspected odontoid fracture (yellow arrow). Sagittal CT scan of cervical spine images clearly show displaced fracture of odontoid process.

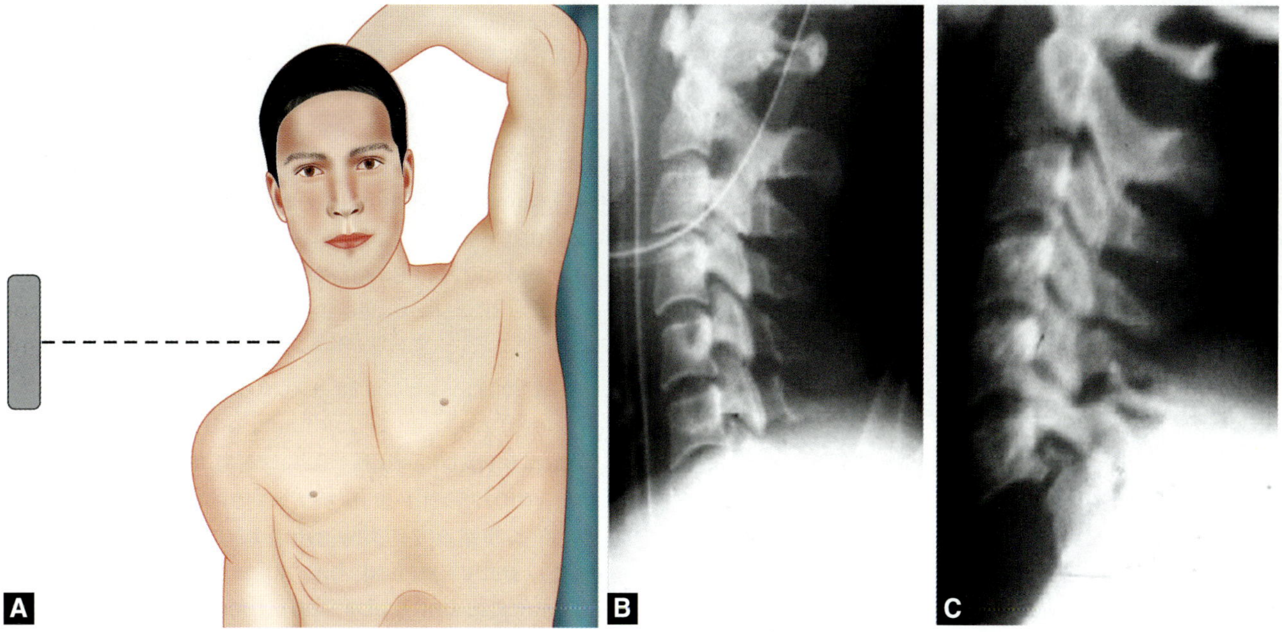

Figures 14.8A to C: Importance of visualizing the entire cervical spine: (A) Swimmer's view is performed by hyperabducting the arm close to the X-ray plate and by pulling the opposite arm down; (B and C) Lateral radiographs of a patient who presented with quadriplegia. (B) The cervical spine upto C6 is visualized and is normal; (C) Radiographs taken after pulling the arms down shows that there is C6–C7 dislocation.

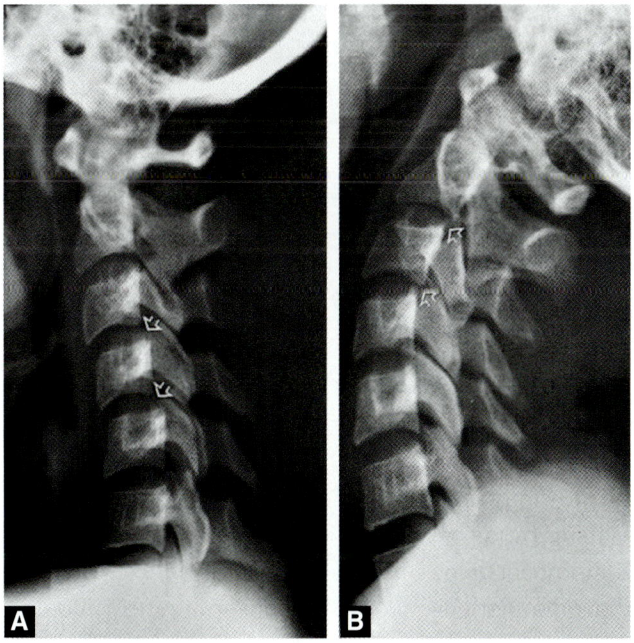

Figures 14.9A and B: Stress flexion-extension lateral radiograph views of a patient with post-traumatic neck pain. The flexion view (A) and extension view (B) show subtle instability at C3 and C4 although the posterior laminar line is intact. This indicates that there is no gross instability and the patient can be treated conservatively.

Table 14.6: Advantages of CT and MRI in spinal trauma

CT Scan

- Quick and detailed assessment of bony injury
- Three-dimensional knowledge about the fracture
- Useful in "hidden" regions like upper cervical, cervico-thoracic and thoracic spine (Fig. 14.7)
- Three-dimensional reconstructions provide better information for surgical planning.
- Degree of canal compromise is clearly evident.

MRI Scan

- Useful in patients with incomplete neurology and when neurological level does not correlate with X-ray features.
- Sensitive to assess the extent of cord edema and hemorrhage.
- Status of intervertebral discs, ligaments and posterior ligament complex is evident.
- Multiple spinal injuries can be detected.

12 uses three landmarks: the basion, the rostral tip of the odontoid, and the rostral extension of the posterior cortical margin of the axis (posterior axial line). The basion-axial interval is the distance between the basion and the posterior axial line; the basion-dental interval is the

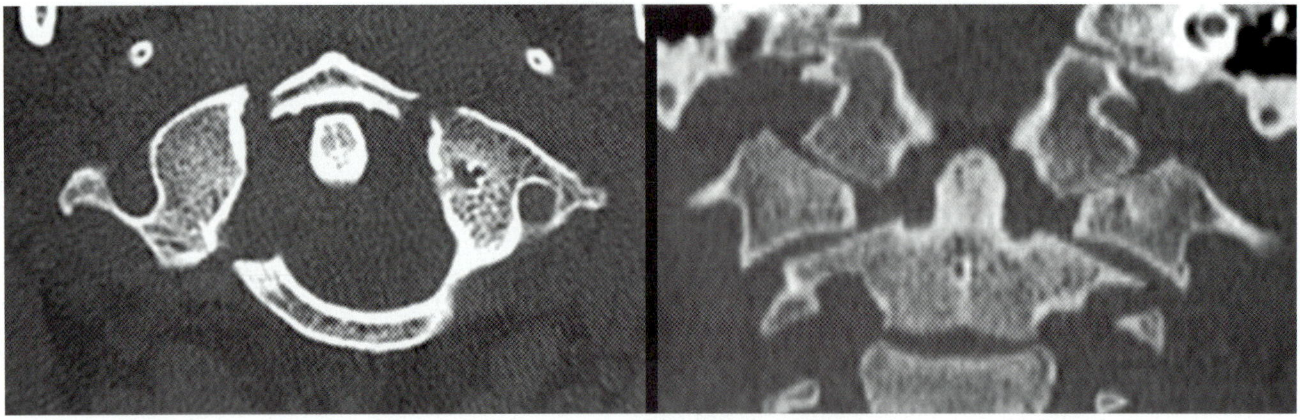

Figure 14.10: Axial CT scan of a patient with a C1 burst fracture. The coronal reconstructions indicate that the C1 lateral masses are displaced indicating complete transverse atlantal ligament injury. Here the combined lateral mass displacement on either side is more than 7 mm.

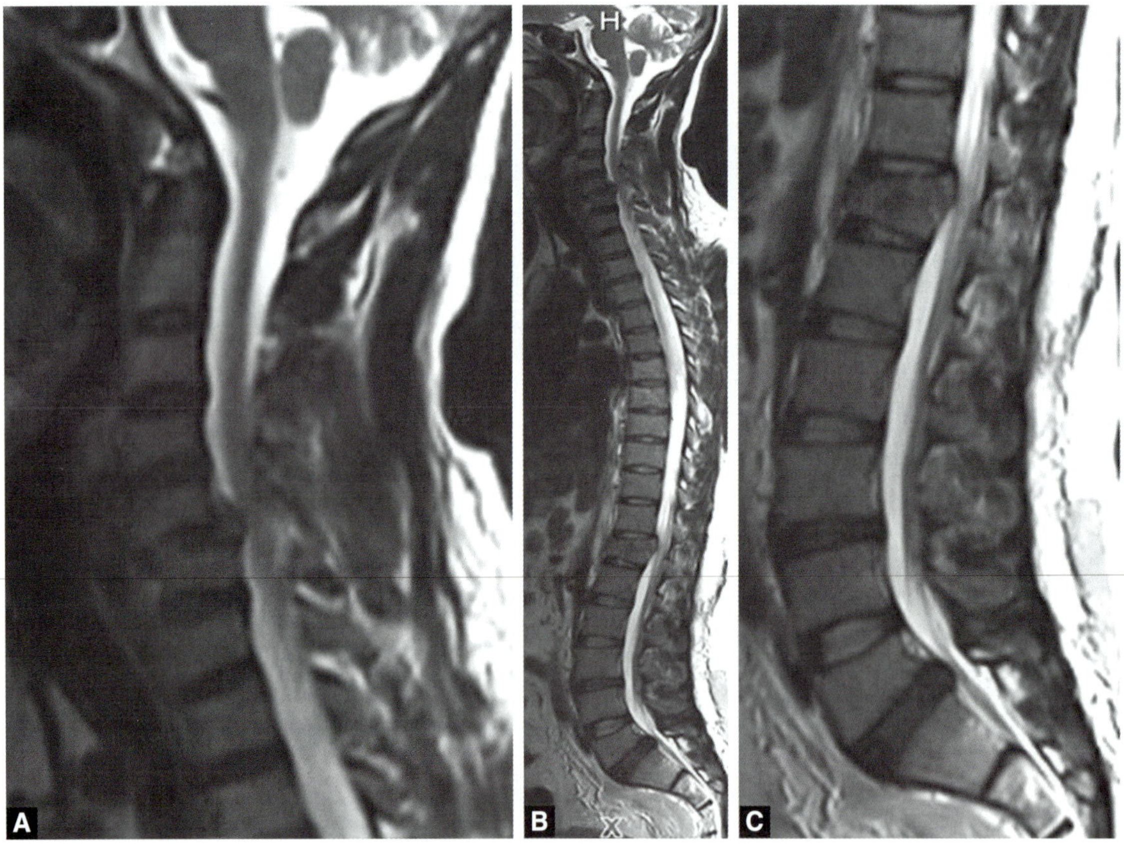

Figures 14.11A to C: Multilevel non-contiguous spinal injury. (A) Sagittal MRI sequences of a patient with cervical spine injury show the presence of a C5–C6 subluxation with spinal cord compression; (B and C) Whole spine mid-sagittal MRI sequence and thoracolumbar MRI indicates the presence of another wedge compression fracture at T12 level.

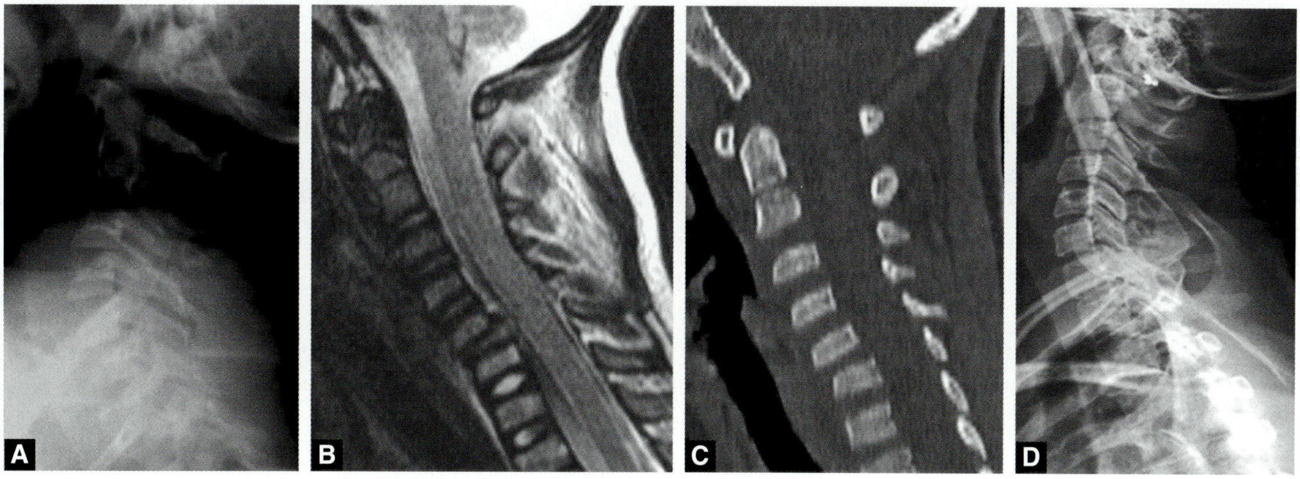

Figures 14.12A to D: (A) Lateral cervical radiograph of a child who presented with neck pain after a road traffic accident. The radiograph does not reveal any obvious pathology; (B and C) Sagittal MRI and CT images show subluxation at C5–C6 level with disc disruption and cord contusion; (D) In such situations, a "Swimmer's view", taken by hyperabducting one arm and pulling the other arm down, also helps in visualizing the lower cervical spine.

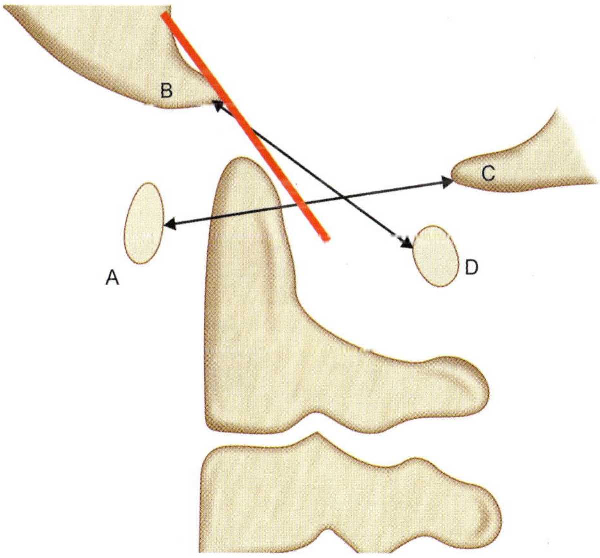

Figure 14.13: Powers ratio and Wackenheim's line (red). Powers ratio: The basion to posterior C1 arch distance divided by the anterior arch to opisthion distance (BD/AC) should be < 1. A ratio greater than 1 suggests possible anterior dissociation. Wackenheim line is drawn as a continuation from the clivus caudally. The tip of the odontoid should be within 1–2 mm of this line.

Source: Redrawn from Frymoyer JW, Wiesel SW, An HS, et al. (Eds). The Adult & Pediatric Spine, 3rd edition. Philadelphia, PA: Lippincott Williams & Wilkins; 2004.

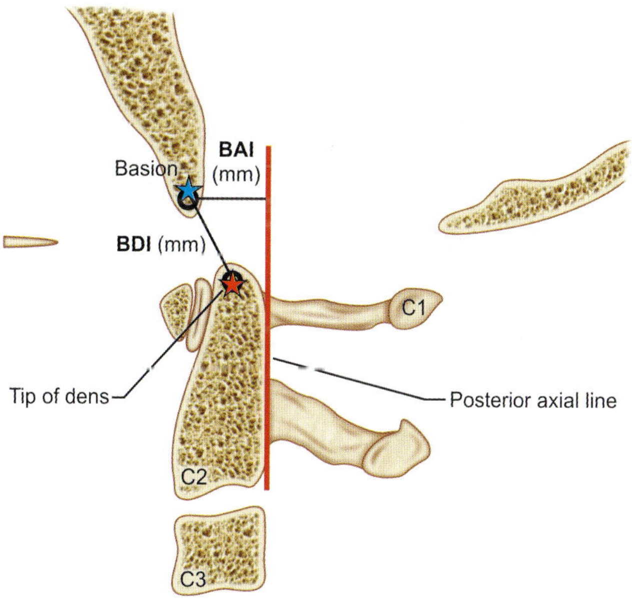

Figure 14.14: Occipitocervical dissociation demonstrating the rule of 12. The blue asterisk identifies the basion and the red asterisk indicates the dens. The distance between them is the basion-dental interval (BDI). The vertical line represents the posterior axial line. The distance between it and the basion is the basion-axial interval (BAI). If these distances are > 12 mm, it is abnormal.

distance between the basion and the tip of the odontoid. The method is applicable to adults and to children older than 13 years. Both intervals should be less than 12 mm in normal individuals.

Clearing the Spine in Trauma Patients

A "cleared spine" in a patient implies that spine evaluation is complete and the patient does not have a spinal injury requiring treatment. The necessary elements for a complete spine evaluation are a good history to assess for high-risk factors, a thorough physical examination to check for physical signs of spinal injury or neurological deficit and appropriate imaging studies based on initial evaluation.

Clinical Clearance

Although there are reports of bony or ligamentous injuries in asymptomatic patients, it is very uncommon for an asymptomatic patient to have an unstable cervical spine fracture or suffer neurological deterioration due to the injury. The cervical spine may be cleared clinically if the following preconditions are met: fully alert and orientated, no head injury, no drugs or alcohol, no neck pain, no abnormal neurology, no significant other "distracting" injury (another injury which may "distract" the patient from complaining about a possible spinal injury). Provided these preconditions are met, the neck may then be examined. If there is no bruising or deformity, no tenderness and a pain free range of active movements, the cervical spine can be cleared. Radiographic studies of the cervical spine are not indicated.

Conscious, Symptomatic Patients

Radiological evaluation of the cervical spine is indicated for all patients who do not meet the criteria for clinical clearance as described above (Fig. 14.15). Imaging the spine should not take precedence over life-saving diagnostic and therapeutic procedures. Imaging studies should be adequate and interpreted by experienced clinicians.

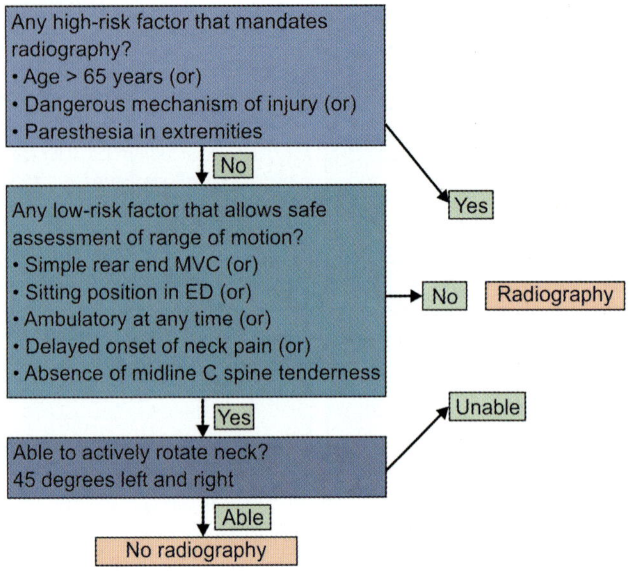

Figure 14.15: Canadian C-spine rules: For patients with trauma who are alert (as indicated by a score of 15 on the Glasgow Coma Scale) and in stable condition and in whom cervical spine injury is a concern, the determination of risk factors guides the use of cervical spine radiography. A dangerous mechanism is considered to be a fall from an elevation of greater than 3 ft or 5 stairs; an axial load to the head (e.g. diving); a motor vehicle collision at high speed (>100 km/hr) or with rollover or ejection; a collision involving a motorized recreational vehicle; or a bicycle collision. A simple rear-end motor vehicle collision excludes being pushed into oncoming traffic, being hit by a bus or a large truck, a rollover, and being hit by a high-speed vehicle.

The standard plain film radiograph series is the lateral, AP and open-mouth view. The lateral cervical spine film must include the base of the occiput and the top of the first thoracic vertebra. The lateral view alone will miss up to 15% of cervical spine injuries. The lower cervical spine from C6 may be difficult to examine and caudal traction on the arms should be used to improve visualization or a Swimmer's view can be performed. Repeated attempts at plain radiography are usually unsuccessful and waste time and resources. If the lower cervical spine is not visualized, a CT scan of the region is indicated. The AP view must include the spinous processes of all the cervical vertebrae from C2 to T1. The open-mouth view should visualize the lateral masses of C1 and the entire odontoid peg. The addition of two oblique views to the standard 3-view series does not increase the sensitivity of plain film evaluation.

Thin-cut (2 mm) axial CT scanning with sagittal and coronal reconstruction should be used to evaluate abnormal, suspicious or poorly visualized areas on plain radiology. With adequate studies and experienced interpretation, the combination of plain radiology and directed CT scanning has a low false negative rate. The scan should include a few vertebral bodies above and below the region of interest, as these must be undamaged for subsequent internal fixation.

A patient with normal radiological evaluation as described above who has persistent symptoms requires an evaluation of soft tissue injury with active flexion and extension imaging of the neck. Pure disc or ligamentous disruption can produce unstable cervical spine injuries and can usually be detected by such stress views. The movements are safe provided the patient performs them actively and halts if there is an increase in pain or neurological symptoms.

The role of a routine MRI in spinal injuries is controversial. Generally, an MRI scan of the spine is indicated in patients with an abnormal neurological examination. Patients who report transient neurological symptoms (the "stinger" or "burner") but who have a normal clinical examination must also undergo an MRI assessment of their spinal cord.

Unconscious, Intubated Patients

The standard radiological examination of the cervical spine in the unconscious, intubated patient is a lateral cervical spine film, AP cervical spine film and CT scan of the craniocervical junction. Thin-cut (2 mm) axial CT scanning with sagittal and coronal reconstruction should be used to evaluate abnormal or poorly visualized areas on plain radiology. The incidence of unstable spinal injury in adult, intubated trauma patients is around 10.2%. When doubtful, cervical spine clearance must not be given until the patient is fully conscious, or an evaluation by an MRI scan or CT scan or dynamic flexion-extension fluoroscopy has been performed.

Passive dynamic flexion/extension stressing of the cervical spine performed in an unconscious patient is potentially dangerous and many spinal surgeons are unwilling to perform this maneuver due to safety issues. Of 625 patients currently reported in the literature, dynamic fluoroscopy has a sensitivity of 92.3% and specificity of 98.8% with two cases of neurological deterioration including one complete quadriplegia.[8]

Full cervical spine CT for assessment of spinal injury seems to be the ideal imaging technique in the unconscious patient to rule out spinal injuries. There are several studies that have demonstrated the robustness of the full CT scan for the exclusion of significant spinal injury. Abnormal findings on the CT scan are evaluated by a spinal surgeon and additional modalities, such as MRI, can be employed. Helical or multislice CT scanning from the occiput to T1 is performed and sagittal and coronal reconstructions must be closely examined for indications of ligamentous instability.

Magnetic resonance imaging of ventilated patients is a significant undertaking requiring special non-ferromagnetic equipment and hence is performed only in special circumstances in an intubated patient. Magnetic resonance imaging is extremely sensitive at detecting soft tissue injuries without stressing the cervical spine. However, the significance of such injuries with regards to the clinical stability of the spine is not clear and the number of false positive examinations is high.

DIAGNOSIS OF CERVICAL SPINAL INJURIES: Pearls and Pitfalls

- A 5% incidence of multiple non-contiguous vertebral injuries has been identified in patients who present with spinal fractures. Half of the secondary lesions having been initially missed. Therefore, it is mandatory to evaluate other regions of the spine to look for tenderness, abrasions and interspinous widening and appropriate radiological evaluation.
- Presently, the patient's neurological status after the period of spinal shock is the only factor that can predict the chances of neurological recovery. Hence, an accurate neurological examination is necessary to prognosticate an injury.
- The standard trauma radiographs would include AP, lateral, and open-mouth views. An open-mouth radiograph allows visualization of the atlas, odontoid process, and lateral masses of the axis. An abnormal prevertebral shadow or loss of alignment either in the AP or lateral views mandates immediate immobilization and need for further investigation.

Classification

Occipital Condyle Fractures

Occipital condyle fractures should be considered as a marker for potentially lethal trauma, since there is an 11% mortality rate from associated injuries. The incidence of associated cervical spine injury at another level can be as high as 31%. The mechanism of injury usually involves compression and lateral bending; this causes either compression fracture of the condyle as it presses against the C1 facet or avulsion of the alar ligament on the contralateral side. Cranial nerve palsies may develop days to weeks after injury and most frequently affect cranial

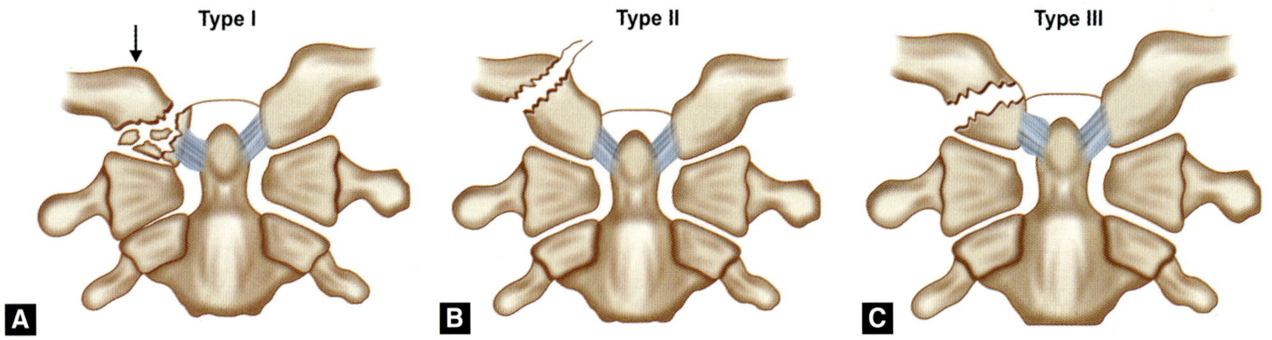

Figures 14.16A to C: Anderson and Montesano classification of occipital condyle fracture. (A) Type I: comminuted impaction fractures; (B) Type II: condyle fractures extending into the base of the skull; (C) Type III: avulsion fractures.

Source: Redrawn from Anderson PA. Injuries to the occipital cervical articulation. In: Clark CR, Dvorak J, Ducker TB, et al. (Eds). The Cervical Spine, 3rd edition. Philadelphia, PA: Lippincott-Raven; 1998. p. 391.

nerves IX, X and XI. The sensitivity of plain radiography for diagnosis can be as low as 3% and a CT scan is frequently necessary for diagnosis.

Occipital condyle fractures have been classified by Anderson and Montesano.[10] Type I fractures (3% of occipital condyle fractures) are comminuted impaction condyle fractures resulting from an axial load and are usually stable. Type II fractures (22%) involve extension of a basilar skull fracture into the condyle and these are also stable. Type III fractures (75%) are condylar avulsion fractures; they are potentially unstable and should raise clinical suspicion for an underlying occipitocervical dissociation injury mechanism (Figs 14.16A to C). Type I and II fractures are stable and can be managed nonoperatively in a rigid cervical collar or halo vest for 8 weeks. Type III fractures are unstable and immobilization for 12 weeks in a halo vest is recommended. After the period of immobilization, if instability is observed on flexion and extension films, an occipital-to-C2 fusion may be necessary.

Occipitocervical Dislocation

Occipitocervical dislocations are high-energy injuries resulting from a combination of hyperextension, distraction and rotation at the craniocervical junction. It is twice as common in children, owing to the inclination and shallowness of the condyles and the large head. Most instances of traumatic occipitocervical dislocation are lethal and survivors may demonstrate a wide range of neurological injuries with a 50% mortality risk.

Diagnosis of occipitocervical dislocation can be challenging because of the poorly visualized osseous detail on plain radiographs. The most frequently described measurement is the Powers ratio (Fig. 14.13). A ratio greater than 1 suggests possible anterior dissociation. The Harris rule of 12 is considered by some to be the most sensitive measurement. Overall, the sensitivity of plain radiographs for occipitocervical dislocation is approximately 57%. The sensitivity of CT and MRI has been estimated to be 84% and 86%, respectively, and one or both of these adjunctive studies is recommended for patients with suspected occipitocervical dissociation injuries. Occipitocervical dislocation injuries have been classified by Traynelis,[11] based on the position of the occiput in relation to C1 (Figs 14.17A to C). Immediate treatment includes halo vest application with strict avoidance of traction. Early surgical stabilization of the atlanto-occipital joint is recommended as ligamentous healing in a halo vest is unpredictable, and many of these injuries are so unstable that displacement may occur even in the halo vest.

Atlas Fractures

Fractures of the atlas constitute approximately 7% of cervical spine fractures and are rarely associated with neurological injury. This is because of the large amount of space available for the cord at this level. Fifty percent of these injuries are associated with other cervical spine fractures, especially odontoid fractures and spondylolisthesis of the axis. The mechanism of injury is axial compression with elements of hyperextension and asymmetric loading of the condyles causing variable fracture patterns.

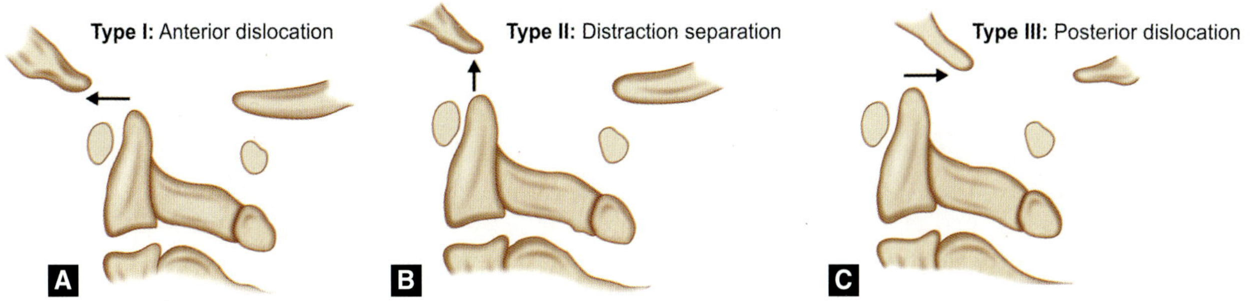

Figures 14.17A to C: Classification of occipitocervical dislocation. (A) Type I: Occipital condyles anterior to the atlas; most common; (B) Type II: Condyles longitudinally dissociated from atlas without translation (result of pure distraction); (C) Type III: Occipital condyles posterior to the atlas.

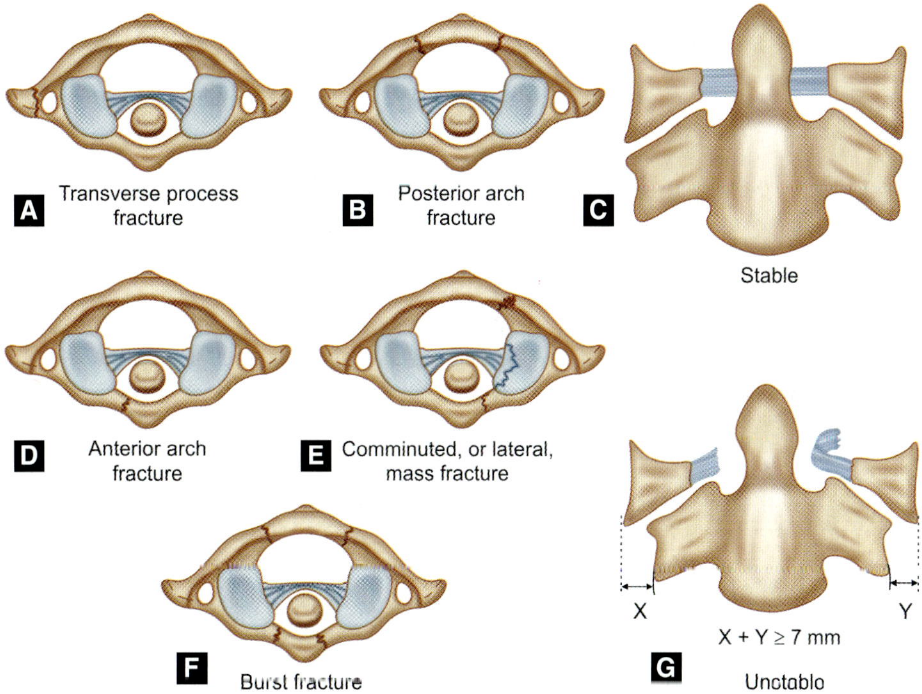

Figures 14.18A to G: Classification of atlas fractures. (A) Isolated transverse process fracture; (B) Isolated posterior arch fracture; (C) Isolated anterior arch fracture; (D) Comminuted or lateral mass fracture; (E) Burst fracture (Jefferson type); (F and G) Jefferson fractures. When a comminuted fracture of C1 shows bilateral overhang of the lateral masses that total 7 mm or more, rupture of the transverse ligament has probably occurred, rendering the spine unstable.

Source: Redrawn from Bucholz RW, Heckman JD, Court-Brown C, et al. (Eds). Rockwood and Green's Fractures in Adults, 6th edition. Philadelphia, PA: Lippincott Williams & Wilkins; 2006.

Clinical symptoms include headache and occipital pain with limitation of neck movement. Cranial nerve injuries and neurapraxia of the suboccipital and greater occipital nerves may be associated. Damage to the spinal cord is uncommon because a significant cord injury at this level causes immediate death. Uncommonly vertebral artery occlusion can cause symptoms of basilar insufficiency such as vertigo, blurred vision and nystagmus. Anteroposterior films, including an open-mouth view and a lateral view, and CT scanning are performed. The common fracture sites are the anterior arch, either midline or just lateral to the midline, and the posterior arch at its narrowest portion just posterior to each lateral mass.

Levine and Edwards (Figs 14.18A to G) classified atlas fractures into three types:[12] (1) isolated posterior arch fractures, (2) lateral mass fractures and (3) burst fractures

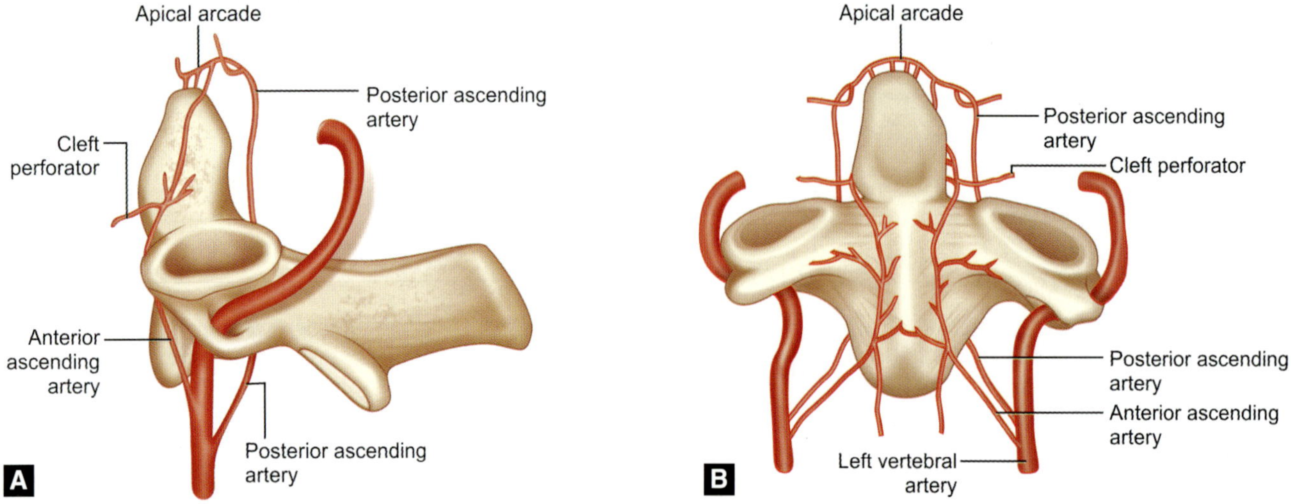

Figures 14.19A and B: Blood supply to odontoid: posterior and anterior ascending arteries and apical arcade. The blood flow from the apex is through a periapical plexus that is supplied by a branch of the basilar artery, and from the base through the vertebral artery with a watershed area in the neck of the odontoid.
Source: Redrawn from Campbell's textbook of Orthopaedics.

(Jefferson fracture). Other fractures that occur include: isolated transverse process fracture, isolated anterior arch fracture and anterior tubercle.

Fracture stability is based on the integrity of the transverse ligament. If the transverse ligament is disrupted, the C1 injury is considered unstable. It is important to recognize this instability as the management is different from other stable burst fractures. In open-mouth radiographs, if the combined lateral mass overhang is 7 mm or more, rupture of the transverse ligament has probably occurred. The integrity of the ligament can also be evaluated by measuring the atlantodens interval on the lateral view. An atlantodens interval greater than 3 mm in adults is indicative of a ligament insufficiency. Transverse ligament insufficiency may also be diagnosed directly by identifying bony avulsion on CT scan or ligament rupture on MRI.

Odontoid Fractures

Odontoid fractures constitute 8–18% of all cervical fractures, with neurological deficits occurring in 10–20% of cases. High-velocity trauma such as motor vehicle accidents account for most odontoid fractures in young adults, whereas low-velocity injuries such as falls account for the injuries in the elderly (osteoporotic fractures). The mechanism of injury includes avulsion of the apex of the dens by the alar ligament or lateral/oblique forces that cause fracture through the body and base of the dens. Posteriorly displaced fractures are the result of hyperextension whereas anteriorly displaced fractures are due to a hyperflexion force.

The vascular supply of the C2 vertebra is from the apex, via a periapical plexus that is supplied by a branch of the basilar artery, and from the base, via the vertebral artery with a watershed area in the neck of the odontoid (Figs 14.19A and B). This watershed area of poor vascularity, lack of periosteum and cancellous bone results in high nonunion rates of Type II odontoid fractures.

Odontoid fractures have been classified by Anderson and D'Alonzo[13] into three types with Hadley adding a fourth type – Type IIA (Table 14.7 and Figs 14.20 and 14.21).

Traumatic Spondylolisthesis of C2 (Hangman's Fracture)

Traumatic spondylolisthesis of C2 is characterized by bilateral fractures of the pars interarticularis with varying degrees of intervertebral disc disruption. It is commonly termed as Hangman's fracture.

The mechanism of injury includes motor vehicle accidents and falls with flexion, extension and axial loads. Hanging mechanisms involve hyperextension and

Table 14.7: Classification of odontoid fractures

Type/Incidence	*Fracture characteristics*	*Important facts*
Type I (5%)	Oblique avulsion fracture of the apex	Represents an avulsion of the alar and apical ligaments Rule out atlanto-occipital dislocation
Type II (60%)	Fracture at the junction of the dens with the body of C2	High nonunion rate Rule out associated transverse atlantal ligament injury
Type IIA (Hadley)	Comminuted injury extending from the waist of the dens into the body of the axis	Highly unstable
Type III (30%)	Fracture extending into the cancellous portion of the body of C2 and possibly involving one or both of the superior articular facets	High likelihood of union owing to the cancellous bed of the fracture site

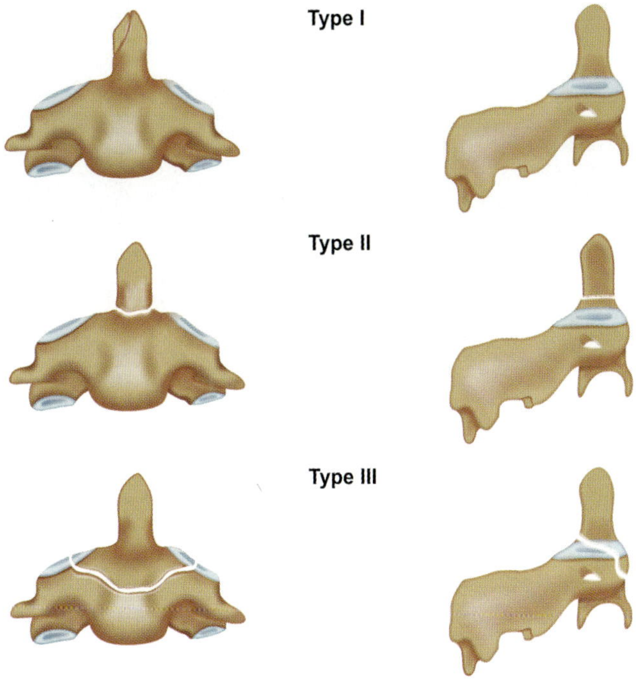

Figure 14.20: The Anderson and D'Alonzo classification of odontoid fractures.
Source: Redrawn from Anderson LD, D'Alonzo RT. Fractures of the odontoid process of the axis. Bone Joint Surg Am. 1974; 56(8):1663-74.

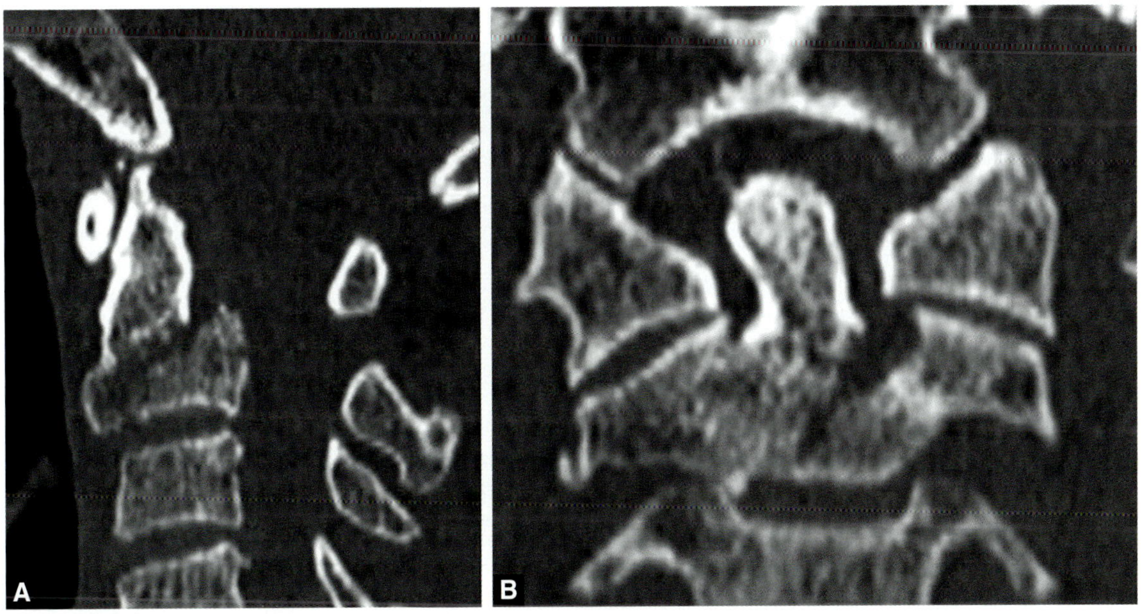

Figures 14.21A and B: Type III odontoid fracture. (A) Sagittal and (B) coronal CT images show that the fracture line is oblique and extends into the body of C2.

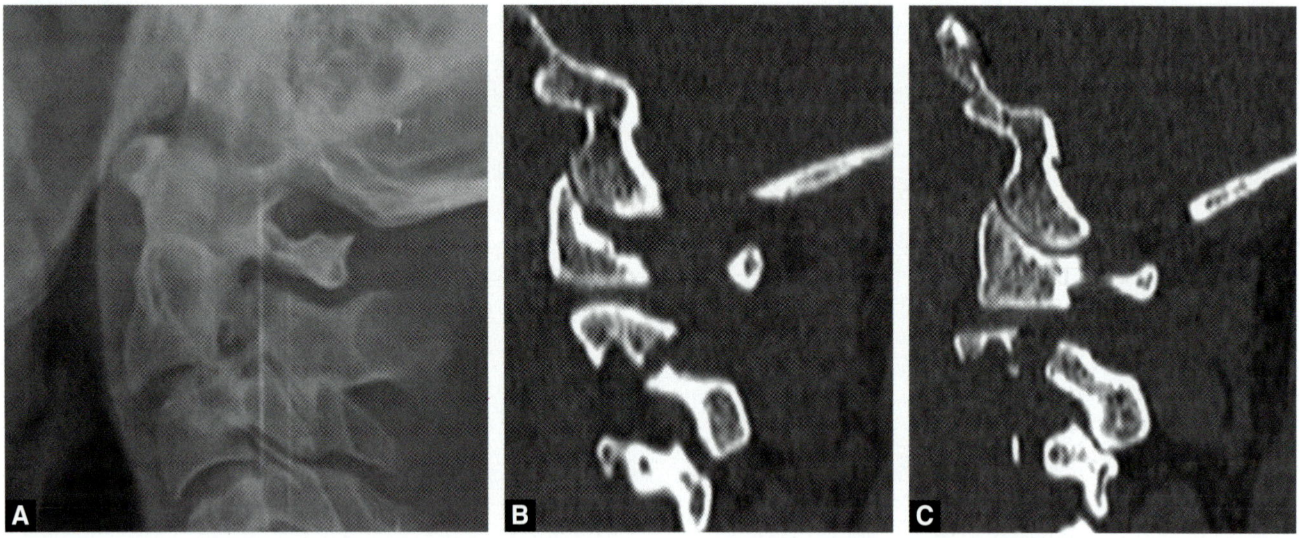

Figures 14.22A to C: (A) Lateral radiograph of a patient with Type II Hangman's fracture; (B) The parasagittal images indicate the break in the pars interarticularis bilaterally.

Table 14.8: Classification of traumatic spondylolisthesis of the axis

Type/Incidence	*Fracture characteristics*	*Stability*	*Mechanism of injury*
Type I (29%)	Nondisplaced or minimally displaced (translation < 3 mm) fractures with no angulation	Relatively stable as C2–C3 disc is intact and only minimal ligamentous injury	Result from hyperextension and axial loading with failure of the neural arch in tension
Type II (56%)	Type II fractures have more than 3 mm of anterior translation and significant angulation at C2–C3 disc. Predominantly vertical fracture line	Unstable as the C2–C3 disc is disrupted	Result from hyperextension and axial load followed by rebound flexion
Type IIA (6%)	Variant of Type II fractures that has severe angulation between C2 and C3 with minimal translation Usually have a more horizontal than vertical fracture line	Unstable due to extensive discoligamentous injury	Result from a flexion-distraction injury. Avulsion of entire C2–C3 intervertebral disc in flexion with injury to posterior longitudinal ligament, leaving the anterior longitudinal ligament intact
Type III (9%)	A pars interarticularis fracture with posterior facet injuries; severe angulation and translation with unilateral or bilateral facet dislocation of C2–C3	Unstable due to extensive discoligamentous and facet dislocation injury	Result from flexion-distraction followed by hyperextension; initial anterior facet dislocation of C2 on C3 followed by extension injury fracturing the neural arch

distraction injury, in which the patient may experience bilateral pedicle fractures and complete disruption of the disc and ligaments between C2 and C3.

Spinal cord injury and neurological deficits are relatively uncommon and the patients usually complain of local pain and stiffness. There is localised tenderness over the spinous process of C2. Anteroposterior and lateral radiographs and a CT scan are essential (Figs 14.22A to C). The retropharyngeal space may be widened on the lateral view. There is a 30% incidence of concomitant cervical spine fractures. The commonly used classification scheme is Levine and Edwards' modification of the Effendi and Francis classification[14] (Table 14.8 and Figs 14.23A to D).

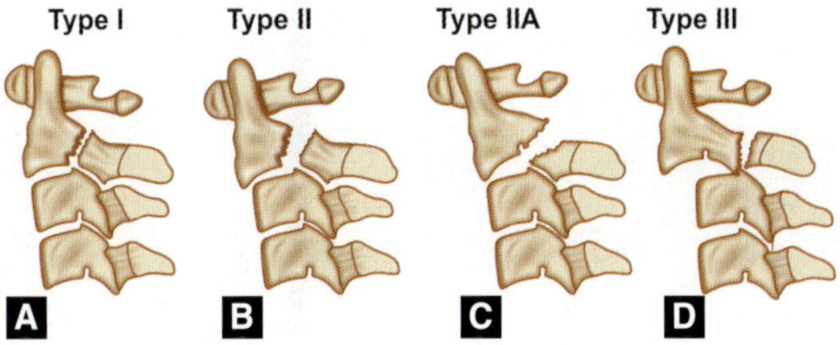

Figures 14.23A to D: Classification of traumatic spondylolisthesis of the axis (according to Effendi, modified by Levine). (A) Type I, nondisplaced fracture of the pars interarticularis; (B) Type II, displaced fracture of the pars interarticularis; (C) Type IIA, displaced fracture of the pars interarticularis with disruption of the C2–C3 discoligamentous complex; (D) Type III, dislocation of C2–C3 facets joints with fractured pars interarticularis.

Source: Adapted from Levine AM, Edwards CC. The management of traumatic spondylolisthesis of the axis. J Bone Joint Surg Am. 1985;67:217-26.

Subaxial Cervical Fractures

In 1982, Allen classified injuries based on the type of force causing the injury (compression/distraction) and the position of the head at the time of trauma (flexion/extension/neutral).[15] Six different injury types are broadly described and based on the severity, a spectrum of injuries is described within each type to aid surgical decision making. The six types are flexion compression, extension compression, vertical compression, flexion distraction, extension distraction and lateral flexion. Each phylogeny is subdivided into stages of progressive severity. Further details regarding fracture subclassification and morphology have been explained in the following section.

Management and Surgical Indications

Fractures of the Atlas

Avulsion injuries are treated symptomatically in a soft collar for 4–6 weeks. A posterior arch fracture is also a stable injury, and hence treated in a collar for 10–12 weeks. It has a high union rate. The anterior arch fracture may be accompanied by avulsion of the odontoid process by the apical and alar ligaments during extension and posterior translation of the head. Anterior arch fractures can be treated successfully in halo vests, with the neck slightly flexed, or by C1–C2 posterior fusion in selected cases with instability.

Treatment of burst and lateral mass fractures is based on the amount of lateral mass displacement or instability, determined by open-mouth radiograph. Minimally displaced fractures (< 7 mm total displacement) or significantly displaced fractures (≥ 7 mm) correspond to the integrity of the transverse ligament. Spence et al. demonstrated that combined displacement of greater than 6.9 mm occurs only with disruption of the transverse ligament. Nondisplaced and minimally displaced fractures can be immobilized in a collar; displaced fractures require more definitive treatment. A patient with a markedly displaced or unstable burst fracture is treated by anatomic reduction using traction, followed by either halo immobilization or surgery. Reduction generally will not be maintained with immediate mobilization; therefore, traction for 4–6 weeks is required before mobilization in a halo vest if treated nonsurgically. Periodic open-mouth radiographs should be performed to detect progressive lateral displacement of C1 lateral masses. Stabilization with C1–C2 transarticular screws and fusion after reduction can be a primary treatment of unstable burst fractures, allowing immediate mobilization. There are recent reports of posterior C1 osteosynthesis alone, sparing fixation to the occiput and the C2, and has been shown to provide good results. C1–C2 arthrodesis or occasionally occiput-C2 arthrodesis is indicated for progressive displacement after nonsurgical treatment, late C1–C2 instability, or symptomatic C1 nonunion.

Nonsurgical Management

Halo orthosis: Halo ring and vest orthotics offer the most stable form of external upper cervical spine immobilization. Another advantage of halo as compared to bracing is that the halo allows for some fracture manipulation. It can also be easily converted to a halo vest once initial fracture reduction is achieved with halo traction. However, secondary loss of reduction can occur. A phenomenon of fracture displacement inside the halo called "snaking" has been described where the fracture can displace between the supine and upright positions. As halo vests work based on tight fit of the vest over the torso, halo vests are poorly tolerated by elderly patients, patients with pulmonary compromise and thoracic injuries. In general, the halo-vest orthosis has been recommended as a definitive management system for patients with isolated occipital

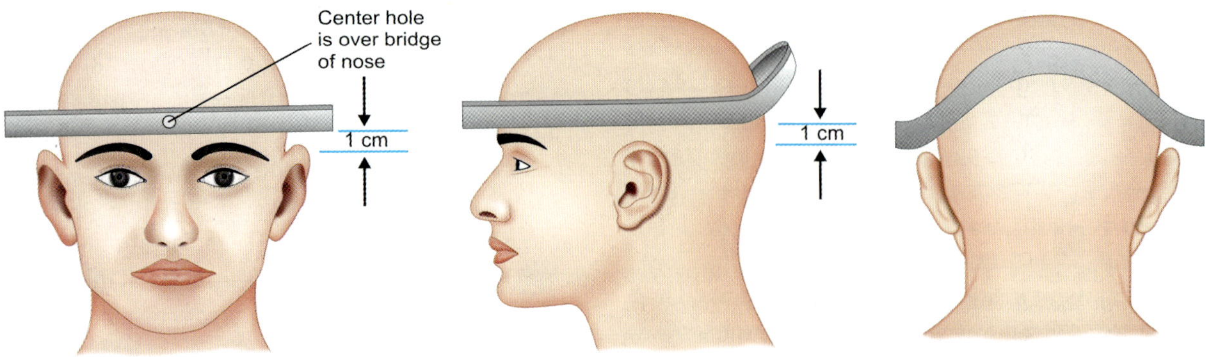

Figure 14.24: Technique of Halo ring application. When applying halo ring, the anterior pin sites should be 1 cm above lateral one-third of eyebrows avoiding the supraorbital and supratrochlear nerves and posteriorly the pins are placed 1 cm above the tops of ears in occipital area (mastoid area).

Source: Redrawn from Young R, Thomasson EH. Step-by-step procedure for applying halo ring. Orthop Rev. 1974;3:62.

condyle fractures, unstable atlas ring fractures, odontoid fractures, and displaced neural arch fractures of the axis. A preliminary period of halo traction to reduce the fracture followed by conversion to halo vest is recommended in displaced fractures. Check radiographs are taken initially every week for the first 3 weeks, then every 2 weeks and then every month till complete union is achieved. This can be approximately 10–12 weeks depending on the individual fracture.

The procedure can be done under local or general anesthesia. The patient is placed supine in the operating table. The head is kept at the edge of the table and held firmly by an assistant in neutral position. A small roll of towel is placed behind the occiput. An appropriate-sized ring with two finger breadth space between the head and the ring is selected. The proposed pin sites are prepped in sterile fashion with povidone iodine. The hair should be shaved from the posterior pin sites before sterile preparation. The optimal position of the anterior pins is 1 cm above the lateral third of the orbital rim (Fig. 14.24). This avoids injury to the supraorbital nerve and supra-trochlear nerves. Further lateral placement risks injury to the temporal artery and inserting the pins in the thin temporal bone provides poor bone fixation. It is important that the patient closes the eyes during pin insertion as keeping the eyes open prevents winking later on.

The posterior pins should be placed 1 cm above the helix of the ear. The pins or ring should not contact the ear, because even gentle pressure can lead to skin necrosis over time. Opposing pins should be tightened at the same time to avoid displacement of the ring. Optimal pin fixation is achieved if placed perpendicular to the bone. Tightening should be gradual, switching between the two pairs of opposing pins until the final torque of 8 inch-pounds is achieved. The lock nuts are then tightened to prevent pin loosening. Pins should be retightened once after 24–48 hours later. If a pin becomes loose with time, it can be retightened once to 8 inch-pounds if resistance is met. If not, then another pin should be placed in a new site and the loosened one removed. It is always better to remove a loose pin than to tighten it. Even with meticulous pin site care, complications occur in about 6% of cases. Once the ring has been secured, the longitudinal struts are attached and secured.

If the spine fracture has been reduced using the halo ring traction, the traction can remain in place till the vest is applied. For convenience, the posterior part of the vest can be placed first by log-rolling the patient, keeping in line cervical traction at all times. The anterior part of the vest can be then applied and secured using the straps and buckles. An appropriately fitted vest should extend down to the level of the xiphoid process and be secured enough to maintain its position while still allowing access to the underlying skin. Cervical X-rays can then be obtained and careful adjustments made to the device to optimize reduction and alignment.

Various complications have been reported with use of the halo device. Pin site problems, such as loosening, infection and bleeding can occur in 6–20% of cases.[16] Accidental dural punctures can also occur and are treated by pin replacement, prophylactic antibiotics and antiseptic dressing.

The rent usually seals in 4 days. Patients can report swallowing difficulty, which may be associated with the head and neck being hyperextended. Returning the neck to a neutral or slightly flexed position can relieve this in most cases. Pressure sores have been reported in 4–11% of patients and are usually associated with improper vest fit.[16] Meticulous skin care and frequent inspection can help avoid this complication.

Recumbent skeletal traction: Skeletal traction, with either the halo ring or the Gardner-Wells tongs, plays a significant role in acute fracture reduction. Once reduction of dislocation or fracture alignment is attained, cranial traction can be used to maintain spinal alignment and stability for extended periods to achieve initial consolidation of an unstable fracture. Subsequently, the patient can be mobilized with a halo vest or rigid brace. Although there are no fixed guidelines, suggested time frames for traction range from several days to weeks. However, prolonged recumbence carries an increased morbidity and mortality risk, and strict attention must be paid to care of the skin, bladder, and bowel and thromboembolism prophylaxis. The role of prolonged traction has diminished progressively as stabilization techniques have become more versatile and comprehensive.

Application of Gardner-Wells tongs. Gardner-Wells tongs are fixed to the skull through two cranially angulated fixation pins. Before application of skull traction, radiographs or a CT scan should be carefully inspected to rule out skull fractures. The optimal site of insertion is in line with the external auditory meatus, approximately 1 cm above the eyebrow (Figs 14.25A to C). This neutral pin position aligned with the external auditory meatus achieves longitudinal traction. By placing the pins slightly anterior or posterior to this point, extension or flexion moments can be delivered to help reduce kyphotic or hyperlordotic deformities, respectively. The skin over the pin site should be marked and prepared sterile with povidone iodine solution. It is not necessary to shave the scalp and the area is then anesthetized with a local infiltration of lidocaine in the subcutaneous region up to the underlying periosteum. Since the scalp is highly vascular, bleeding can occur during the injection and pin insertion, and it is essential to counsel the patient about this beforehand.

Next, the tongs are held in position and the pins are advanced through the skin until they engage the outer cortex of the cranium. Most tongs have a pin indicator on the pin ends which are usually depressed. As adequate torque is reached, the pin indicator pops out. Both the pins are tightened simultaneously so that the traction pulley is located in the center. It is important not to overtighten the pins, because they can penetrate the inner dipole of the skull, which might lead to intracranial injury. In contrast, pins that are insufficiently secured can be loosen and pull out from the skull, leading to substantial bleeding from scalp laceration. Brain abscess has also been described as a complication of cranial tongs.

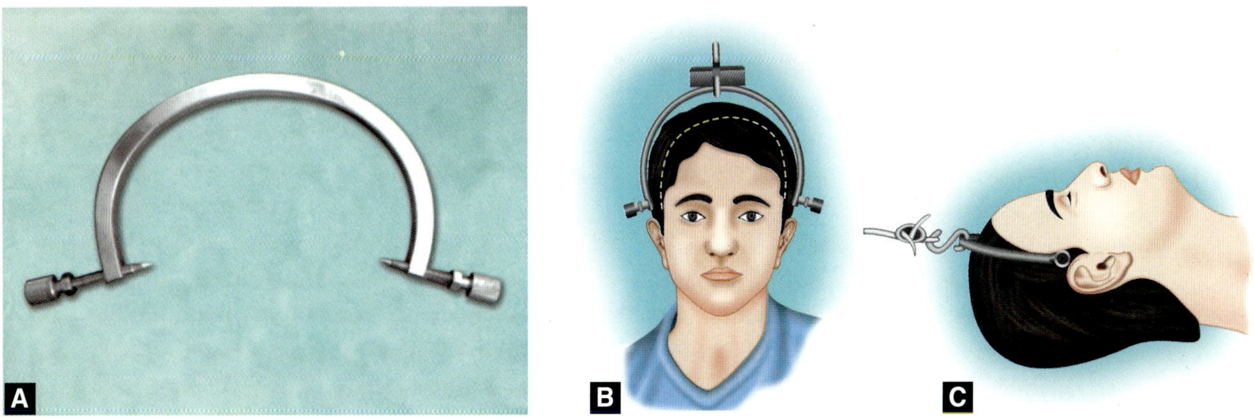

Figures 14.25A to C: (A) Gardner-Wells tongs; (B and C) It is placed just above ears, below the greatest diameter of skull. It is important to avoid placing the pins either too anteroinferior in the temporal bone (poor hold and potential risk to middle meningeal vessels) or too higher above the greatest diameter of skull.

Source: Reproduced from Stauffer ES. Surgical management of cervical spine injuries. In: Evarts CM, (Ed). Surgery of the musculoskeletal system. New York: Churchill Livingstone; 1983.

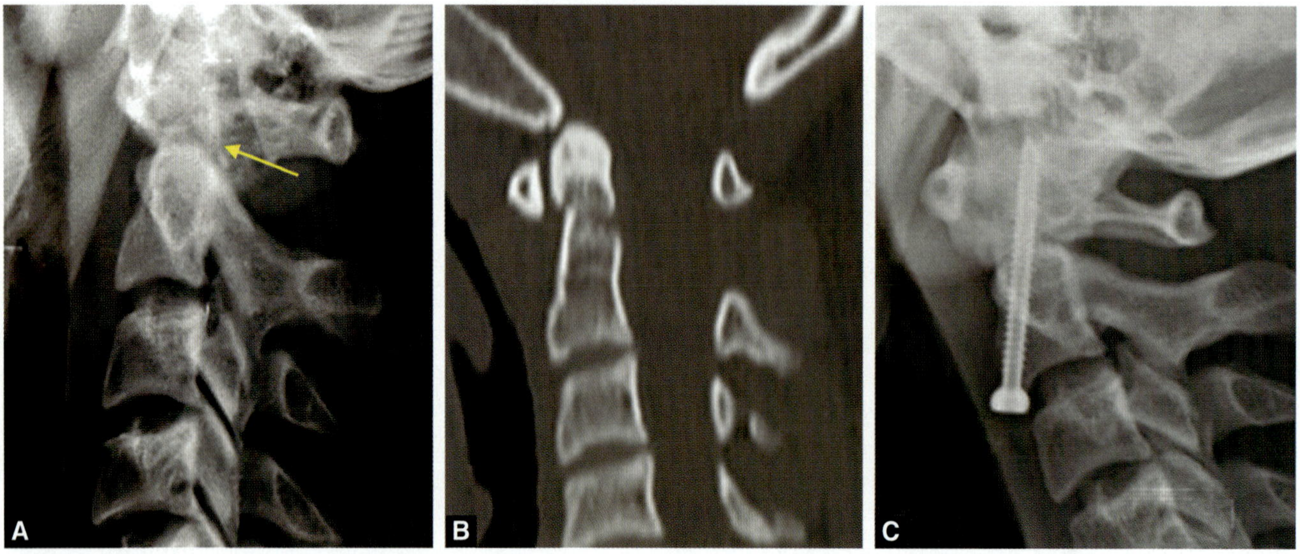

Figures 14.26A to C: (A) Preoperative lateral view and (B) sagittal CT scan of cervical spine showing displaced fracture of odontoid process; (C) Postoperative radiograph shows good reduction of the odontoid fracture and ideal position of a single screw inserted through an anterior approach.

Fractures of the Odontoid Process

Type I fractures can be immobilized in an external orthosis for 6–8 weeks. Type III fractures have been reported to have a sufficiently high healing rate with rigid external immobilization in a halo vest. Treatment of Type II fractures is controversial and depends largely on specific patient and fracture characteristics. Treatment options include halo-vest immobilization, anterior odontoid screw stabilization or a posterior C1–C2 fusion. While undisplaced or minimally displaced fractures that are easily reduced may be treated with halo-vest immobilization for 6–12 weeks, nonunion rates ranging from 10% to 77% have been reported for displaced fractures.

A number of risk factors associated with an increased incidence of nonunion for Type II odontoid fractures have been identified. These include initial fracture displacement of greater than 4 mm, greater than 10° angulation, posterior displacement, fracture comminution, elderly patients, delayed treatment, smoking and inability to achieve or maintain a reduction. Early surgical treatment is an option for patients with any of these risk factors. Elderly patients tolerate halo-vest immobilization poorly, demonstrate decreased healing rates and should be considered for early surgical management.

Anterior fixation is indicated for most Type II and shallow Type III fractures (Figs 14.26A to C). The procedure is contraindicated in fractures with an oblique pattern, disruption of the atlantal transverse ligament, nonunions, pathological fractures and osteoporosis. Patients with a short neck, a rigid neck or cervical kyphosis and thoracic kyphosis/barrel chest are not suitable for this procedure as there is a technical difficulty associated with passage of the screw. Posterior C1–C2 fusion (transarticular or individual C1–C2 screws) is then indicated (Figs 14.27A to H).

Traumatic Spondylolisthesis of C2 (Hangman's Fracture)

Type I injuries are stable and heal within 12 weeks of immobilization in a rigid cervical orthosis. Type II injuries usually require skull traction with slight extension of the neck over a rolled up towel for 3–6 weeks to maintain anatomical reduction. Serial radiographic confirmation of maintenance of reduction is required. The patient can be mobilized in a halo vest for the rest of the 3-month period. In Type IIA injuries, traction may exacerbate the condition; therefore, a halo vest with slight compression is applied under image intensification to achieve and maintain anatomical reduction for 12 weeks until union occurs. Anterior interbody fusion and plating of the C2–C3 interspace for a Type IIA injury may be performed as an alternative to halo immobilization. Bilateral C2 pars screw osteosynthesis is an option to stabilize Type II injuries after

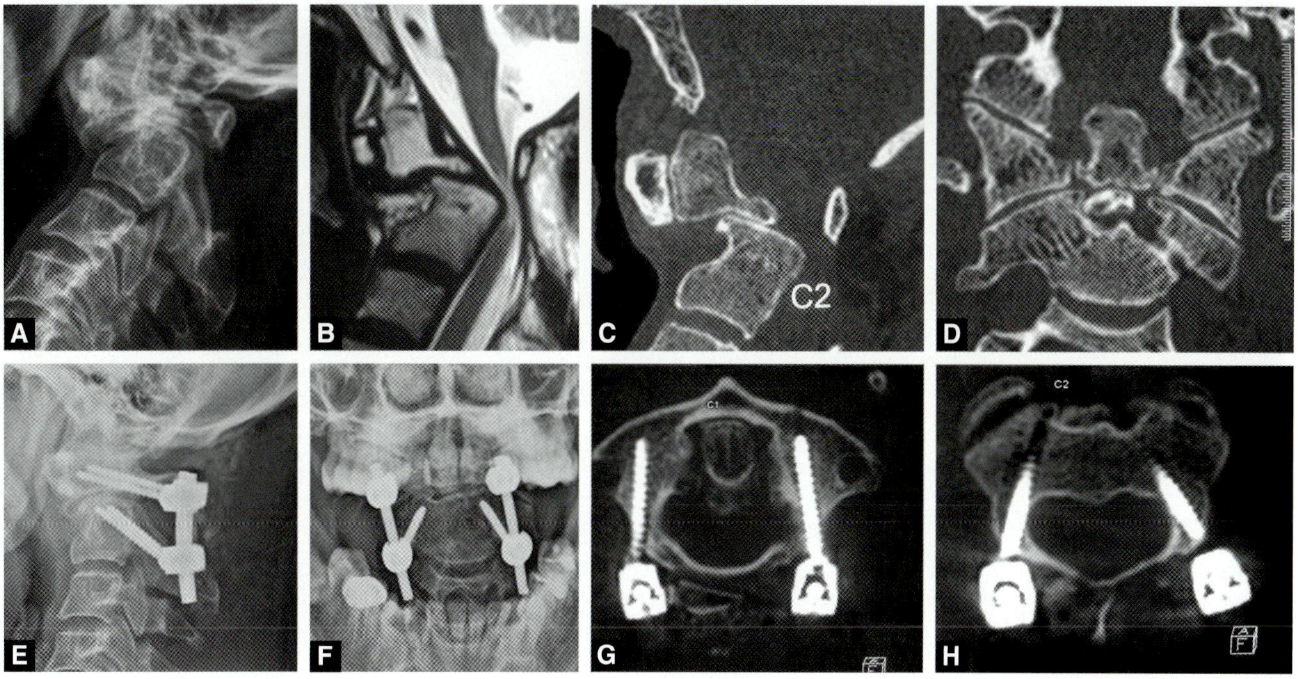

Figures 14.27A to H: Posterior fusion for an odontoid nonunion. (A to D) Preoperative lateral radiograph, CT and MRI scan images reveal odontoid nonunion with spinal instability and cord compression; (E and F) The patient was treated with posterior C1–C2 reduction and instrumented fusion through Goel-Harm's technique; (G and H) Axial CT images show good containment of screws and posterior spinal fusion.

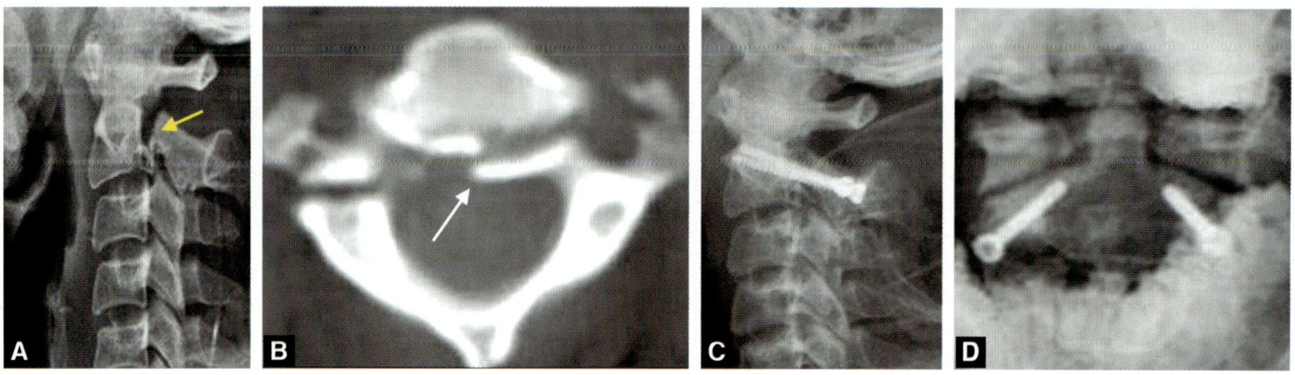

Figures 14.28A to D: (A and B) Preoperative lateral radiograph and CT scan showing bilateral fracture of pars interarticularis of C2 with extension into the vertebral artery foramen; (C and D) Postoperative anteroposterior (AP) and lateral radiographs showing good reduction of the fracture and bicortical purchase of the screws on both the pedicles.

reduction (Figs 14.28A to D). For Type III injuries, surgery is required because of the inability to obtain or maintain reduction of the C2–C3 facet dislocation. Initial halo traction is followed by open reduction and fusion. Surgical options include an anterior C2–C3 interbody fusion (Figs 14.29A to D) or a posterior C1–C3 fusion.

Subaxial Cervical Fractures

Management depends on the extent of injury to the stabilizing structures (anterior and posterior columns, posterior ligamentous complex), extent of instability and neurological injury. The most widely used classification system of lower cervical spine injuries that helps in

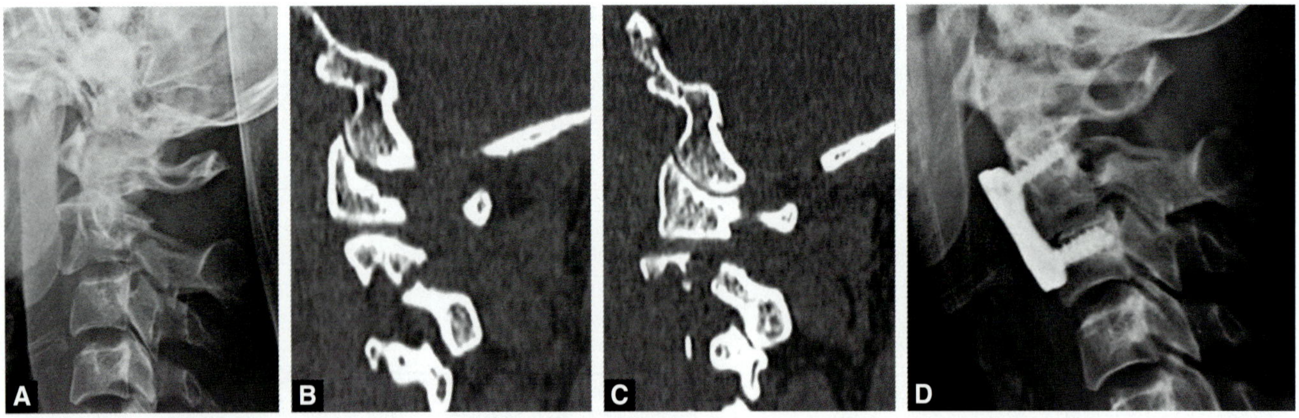

Figures 14.29A to D: (A) Lateral radiograph and (B and C) sagittal CT images indicating a Type III odontoid fracture with C2–C3 subluxation (D) treated by anterior C2–C3 fusion with bone grafting and plating.

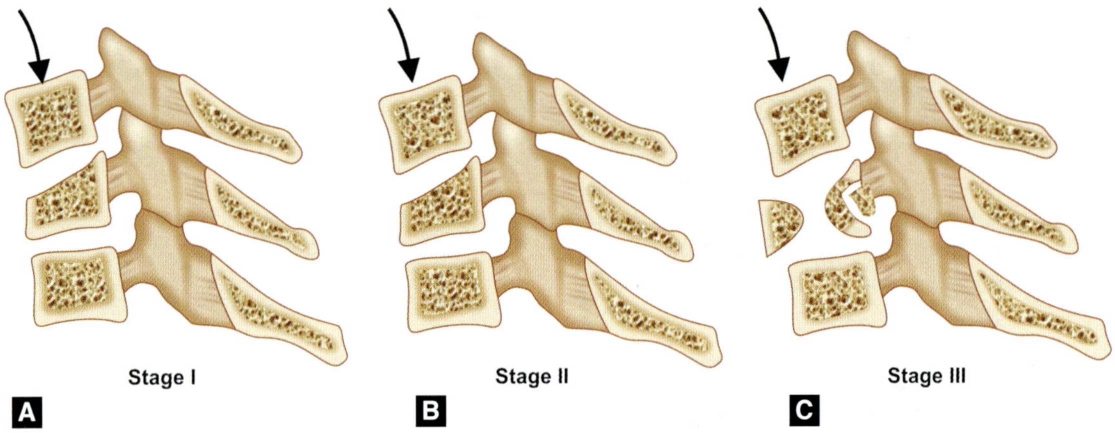

Figures 14.30A to C: The three stages of vertical compression (VC) injuries. (A) Stage I (VCS-I): Fracture through the superior or inferior endplate with no displacement; (B) Stage II (VCS-II): Fracture through both endplates with minimal displacement; (C) Stage III (VCS-III): Burst fracture; displacement of fragments peripherally and into the neural canal.

Source: Redrawn from Bucholz RW, Heckman JD, Court-Brown C, et al. (Eds). Rockwood and Green's Fractures in Adults, 6th edition. Philadelphia, PA: Lippincott Williams & Wilkins; 2006.

evaluating the extent of damage to the bone and ligaments is the mechanistic classification of Allen et al. Injuries are divided into six groups, each named according to the dominant force vector leading to failure and the position of the cervical spine at the time of injury. The groups include compressive flexion, vertical compression, distractive flexion, compressive extension, distractive extension, and lateral flexion. The three most common groups are compressive flexion, distractive flexion, and compressive extension. The least common are distractive extension and lateral flexion, with vertical compression falling between. Compressive indicates that compression accounts for the initial structural failure in a motion segment, whereas distractive indicates that tension is the dominant force. The use of flexion or extension denotes the position of the cervical spine at the time of injury.

Vertical Compression Injuries

An axial load applied with the spine in the neutral position results in loading of the anterior column leading to failure of either the intervertebral disc or the vertebral body. Failure of the disc may result in disc herniation. Depending upon the severity of the injury, a variety of fracture patterns are seen within the vertebral body (Figs 14.30A to C). Vertical compression (VC) stage I and II injuries represent a stable fracture of either the superior or inferior end plate or both end plates without any posterior ligament injury. Both the anterior and posterior vertebral wall height

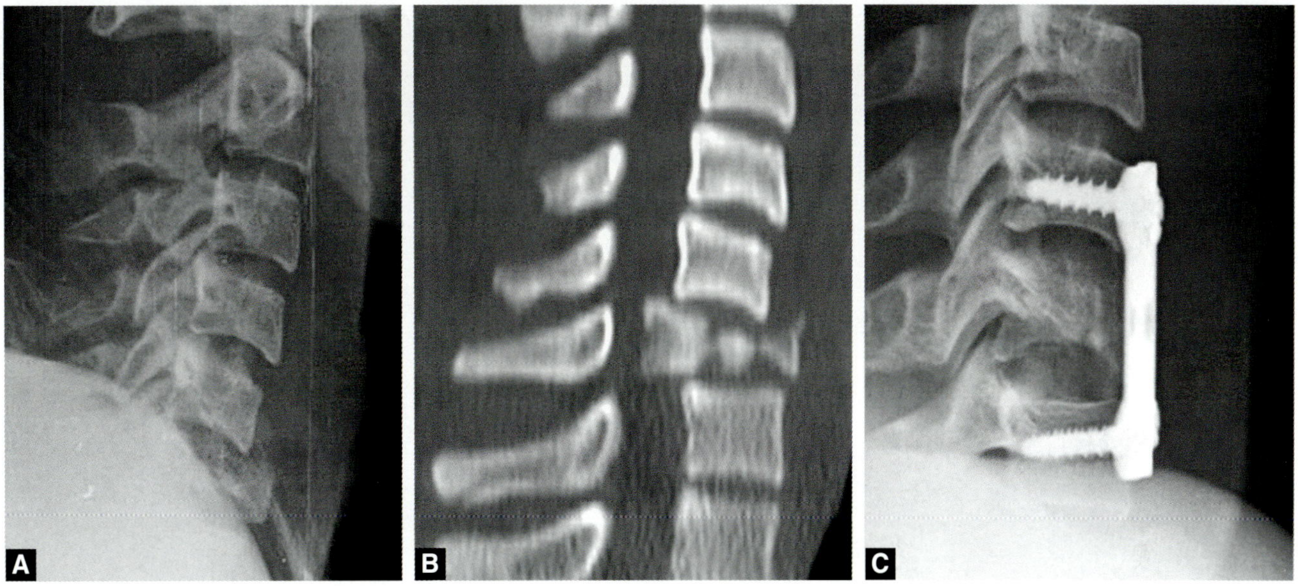

Figures 14.31A to C: (A and B) Lateral radiographs and CT scan of cervical spine showing burst fracture of C6 vertebral body with retropulsion of bony fragment into the canal; (C) Postoperative lateral radiographs shows complete corpectomy of C6 with anterior cervical plate and screws in good position.

is symmetrically reduced resulting in a cupping deformity of the vertebral body. Neurologic deficits are rare. Most such injuries are treated with external immobilization for 8–12 weeks.

Vertical compression stage III injuries are burst fracture of the vertebral body with variable comminution, collapse and displacement of fracture fragments that may result in spinal cord compression and neurological deficit. Often the neurologic injury is much worse than the compression observed on imaging because the maximum retropulsion occurs at the time of impact. Posterior ligaments may or may not be disrupted. In neurologically intact patients, without posterior ligament injury or significant kyphosis, halo-vest immobilization for 12 weeks may be sufficient. However, Koivikko[17] reported better sagittal alignment, fusion rates and neurological outcome following surgery compared to halo-vest immobilization for 69 patients with teardrop and burst fractures. The surgical procedure of choice is an anterior cervical corpectomy and instrumented fusion which allows decompression and provides mechanical stability (Figs 14.31A to C). In neurologically intact patients, a posterior lateral mass/pedicle screw stabilization restricts the fusion to a single motion segment and hence may be preferred over an anterior fusion.

Compressive Flexion Injuries

Compressive flexion (CF) injuries are commonly seen following either a fall from height or due to the fall of a heavy object on the head. A compression force applied to a flexed cervical spine initially results in a compression failure of the vertebral body. Further axial loading generates shear forces that are directed posteriorly across the intervertebral disc and may be followed by a posterior ligament failure in tension. The resultant injuries may range from a wedge compression fracture (CF stage I and II) where the posterior ligaments are intact to teardrop fractures and quadrangular fractures with a posterior ligament disruption (Figs 14.32A to E). Two-thirds of the patients will also have an associated sagittal split of the vertebral body and a bilaminar fracture. In a teardrop fracture, the severe forward-bending forces shear off a triangular piece of the anterior lip of the rostral vertebral body with varying degrees of retropulsion of the remaining body into the spinal canal and disruption of the posterior ligaments (CF stage III, IV and V). The quadrangular fracture is distinguished from the teardrop fracture, as an injury in which a larger piece of anterior vertebral lip is fractured off. Neurological deficit is seen in 25% of CF stage III, 38% of CF stage IV and 91% of CF stage V injuries due to retropulsion of bony fragments. A focal kyphosis is almost always present with circumferential soft tissue disruption.

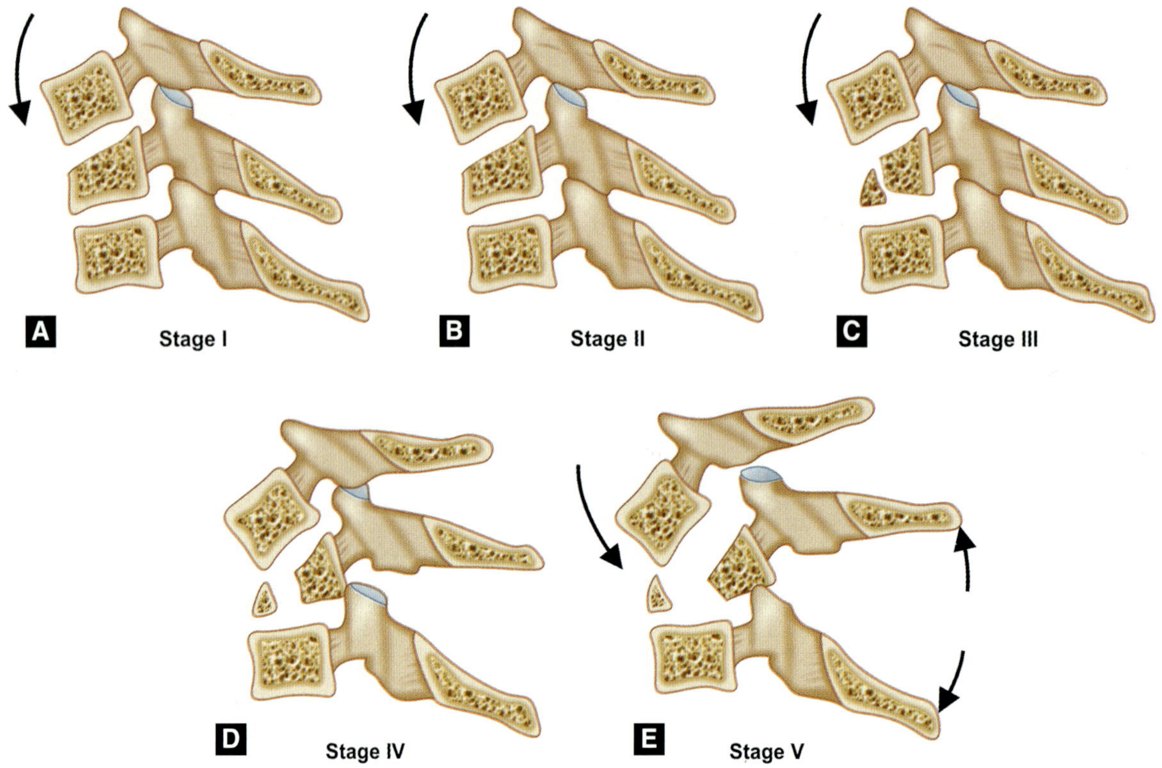

Figures 14.32A to E: The five stages of compression flexion (CF) injuries. (A) Stage I (CFS-I): Blunting of anterior body; posterior elements intact; (B) Stage II (CFS-II): "Beaking" of the anterior body; loss of anterior vertebral height; (C) Stage III (CFS-III): Fracture line passing from anterior body through the inferior subchondral plate; (D) Stage IV (CFS-IV): Deformation of the centrum and fracture of the beak with inferoposterior margin displaced less than 3 mm into the neural canal; (E) Stage V (CFS-V): "Teardrop" fracture; bony injuries as in stage III, but with more than 3 mm of displacement of inferoposterior margin into the neural canal.
Source: Redrawn from Bucholz RW, Heckman JD, Court-Brown C, et al. (Eds). Rockwood and Green's Fractures in Adults, 6th edition. Philadelphia, PA: Lippincott Williams & Wilkins, 2006.

Wedge compression fractures are treated with a cervical orthosis. Most teardrop and quadrilateral fractures are highly unstable and are best treated with anterior corpectomy and instrumented fusion. Additional posterior stabilization may be necessary to restore the tension band if there is severe posterior ligament injury or if multilevel anterior corpectomy has been performed. Fisher reported less kyphosis and instability at follow-up in teardrop fractures treated with surgery as compared to halo vest.[18] If the spine can be realigned easily with traction, then a posterior stabilization alone may be performed in neurologically intact patients.

Distractive Flexion Injuries

Distractive flexion (DF) injury is a hyperflexion injury and involves a distraction force that travels from posterior to anterior with the center of rotation lying anterior to the vertebral body. Initially the posterior ligamentous/osseous structures fail in tension. Sometimes a compression fracture of the vertebral body may occur secondarily. The spectrum of injuries can range from simple facet sprains and perched facets to unifacet or bifacet dislocations and spondyloptosis (Figs 14.33A to D). Facet sprains (DF stage I) involve posterior ligament and facet capsule disruption but are often dismissed as innocuous injuries when viewed on a lateral supine film where the spine is in a reduced position. MRI may show facet widening with increased T2-weighted signal intensity in the posterior ligaments. If missed or left untreated, these patients can later present with pain and instability (Figs 14.34A to D).

Unifacet (DF stage II)/bifacet dislocations (DF stage III and IV) are more severe injuries involving a tear of the

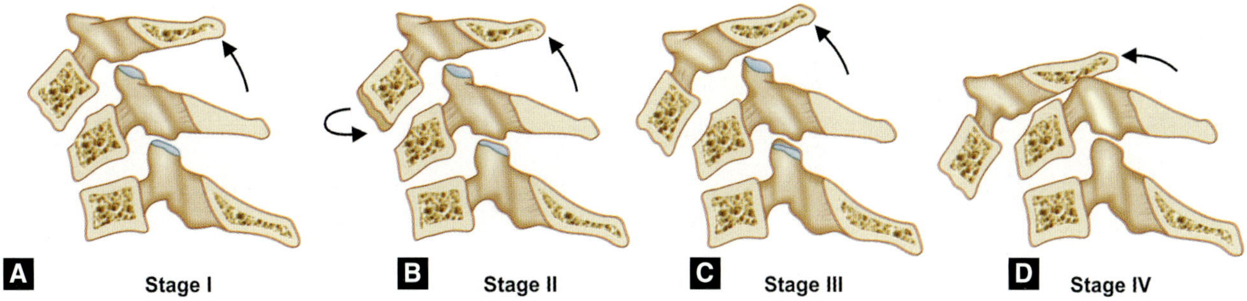

Figures 14.33A to D: The four stages of distraction flexion (DF) injuries. (A) Stage I: Failure of the posterior ligaments, divergence of the spinous processes and facet subluxation; (B) Stage II: Unilateral facet dislocation; translation always less than 50%; (C) Stage III: Bilateral facet dislocation; translation of 50% and "perched" facets; (D) Stage IV: Bilateral facet dislocation with 100% translation (giving the appearance of a "floating" vertebra).

Source: Redrawn from Bucholz RW, Heckman JD, Court-Brown C, et al. (Eds). Rockwood and Green's Fractures in Adults, 6th edition. Philadelphia, PA: Lippincott Williams & Wilkins, 2006.

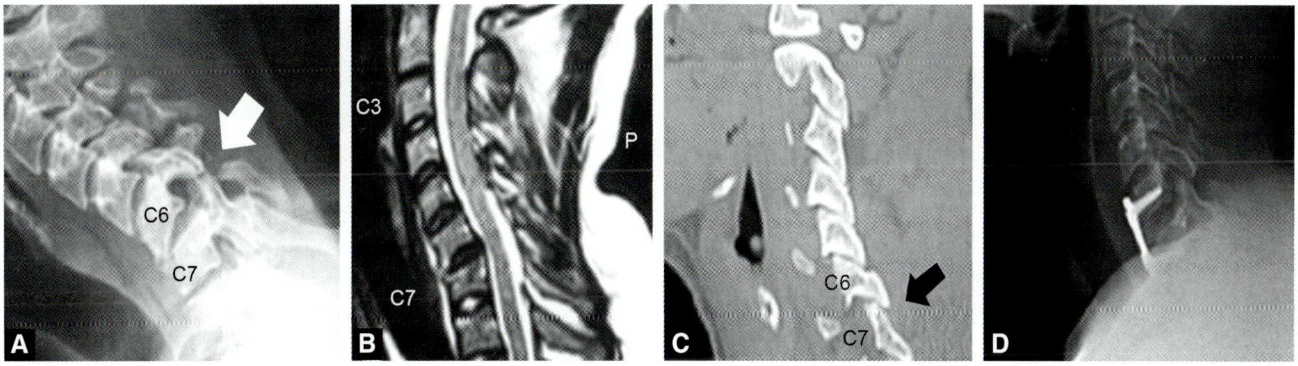

Figures 14.34A to D: (A) Lateral radiograph of cervical spine showing a perched C6–C7 facet due to flexion distraction injury; (B and C) Midsagittal T2WI of MRI and CT scan of the same patient show a C6 on C7 bifacetal subluxation; (D) Following an anterior cervical discectomy, complete reduction could be achieved. Stabilization by instrumented fusion with a tricortical iliac bone graft and locking plate was performed.

supraspinous and interspinous ligaments, the ligamentum flavum and the facet capsule. The posterior longitudinal ligament (PLL) may be disrupted or stripped off the posterior surface of the vertebral body. Varying degrees of intervertebral disc disruption are seen in almost 60% of patients. They are often associated with a facet fracture in the axial plane. The presence of a facet fracture reduces the chances for a successful closed reduction. Spinal cord or root injury is much more common with DF stages II, III and IV. Occasionally, the inferior lip of the inferior facet of the cranial vertebra locks onto the tip of the superior lip of the superior facet of the caudal vertebra resulting in significant kyphosis and distraction. This condition is known as perched facets.

Emergency treatment consists of obtaining quick realignment of the spine. Reduction of the dislocation reduces compression of the neural elements and the abnormal stretch of the ligaments and muscles. This in turn reduces the patient's severe pain and also produces a milieu that halts further neurologic injury and may promote neurological recovery. Closed reduction of the dislocation can be performed using either cervical traction or by manipulating the neck under sedation. In case of a failed closed reduction, open reduction is performed either anteriorly or posteriorly (Figs 14.35 to 14.37).

There are proponents for both anterior and posterior approaches for open reduction in case of failed closed reduction. Traditionally, posterior open reduction has been preferred. Through a posterior midline incision, the spine is exposed subperiosteally till the facet joints. Reduction can be achieved by manipulating the spinous processes with a towel clip and then extending the spine to obtain

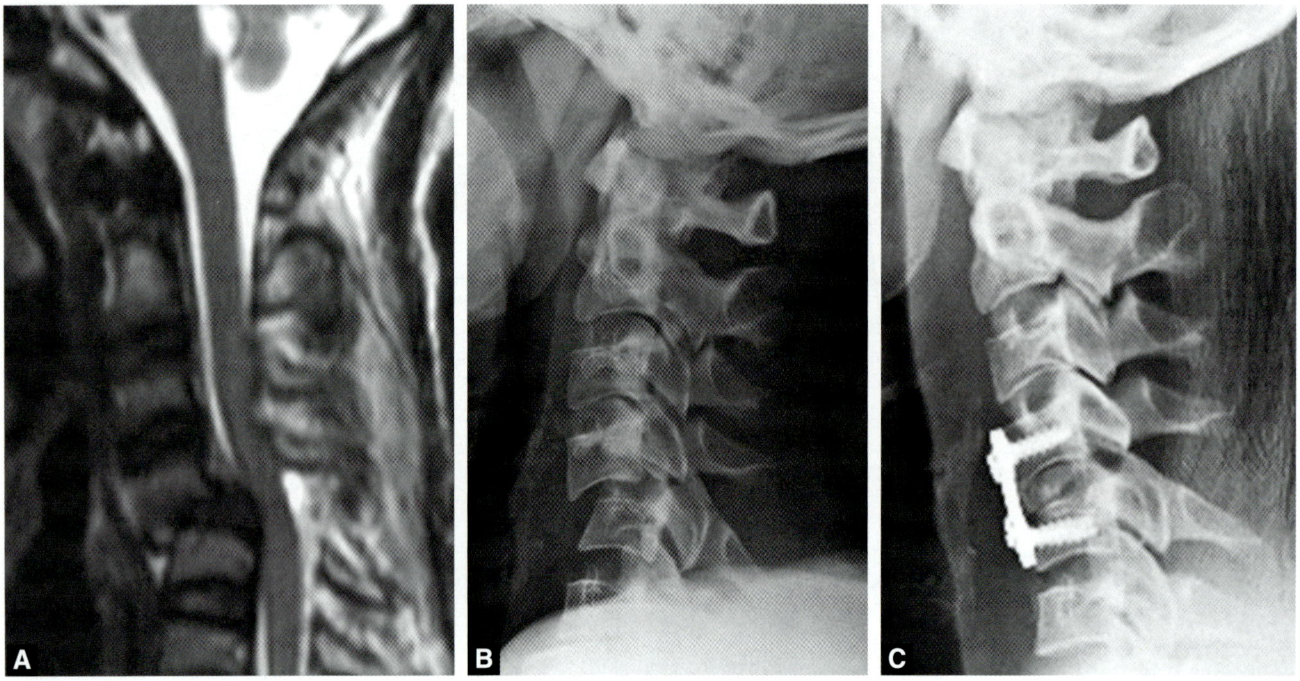

Figures 14.35A to C: (A) C4–C5 bifacetal dislocation with a disrupted disc. Manipulative reduction by traction can produce a neurological deficit in this patient; (B and C) An anterior cervical discectomy followed by reduction and anterior cervical plating is the treatment of choice.

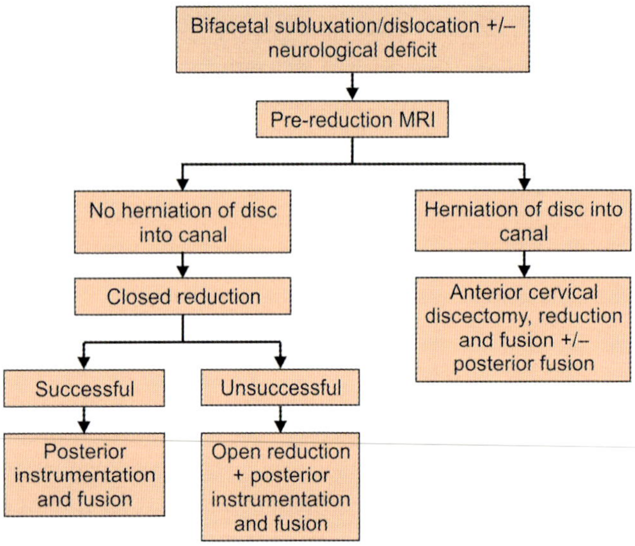

Figure 14.36: Treatment algorithm for bifacetal dislocations.

a reduction. Another safer and easier method is to excise the superior facet of the inferior vertebra which acts as a block to the reduction. Then by gentle levering the superior facets in combination with a lateral mass screw-rod assembly to pull the dislocated vertebra back into alignment. The posterior approach is familiar and is almost certain to allow reduction of the dislocation in an acute setting. However, turning the patient into a prone position with an unstable spine can cause neurological worsening. Posterior reduction also carries a small risk of displacing a disc fragment that may result in postoperative neurological deterioration and hence an MRI must be preferably done before any posterior open reduction. If it shows a displaced disc fragment, then an anterior discectomy must be done prior to reducing the dislocation.

Anterior open reduction (Figs 14.38A to F) involves the classical Smith Robinson approach to the spine. The intervertebral disc at the dislocated level is then excised and the neural elements are decompressed. Then by manipulation using a vertebral body distractor or a pin distractor, reduction can usually be achieved. In the rare event that the dislocation cannot be safely reduced, then it is advisable to turn the patient over and attempt a reduction from a posterior approach. The anterior open reduction is performed with visualization of the spinal cord and hence neurological deterioration due to displaced disc fragments is less likely.

Once reduced, either by closed or open techniques, surgical stabilization is the preferred definitive treatment. Both anterior and posterior approaches have shown good

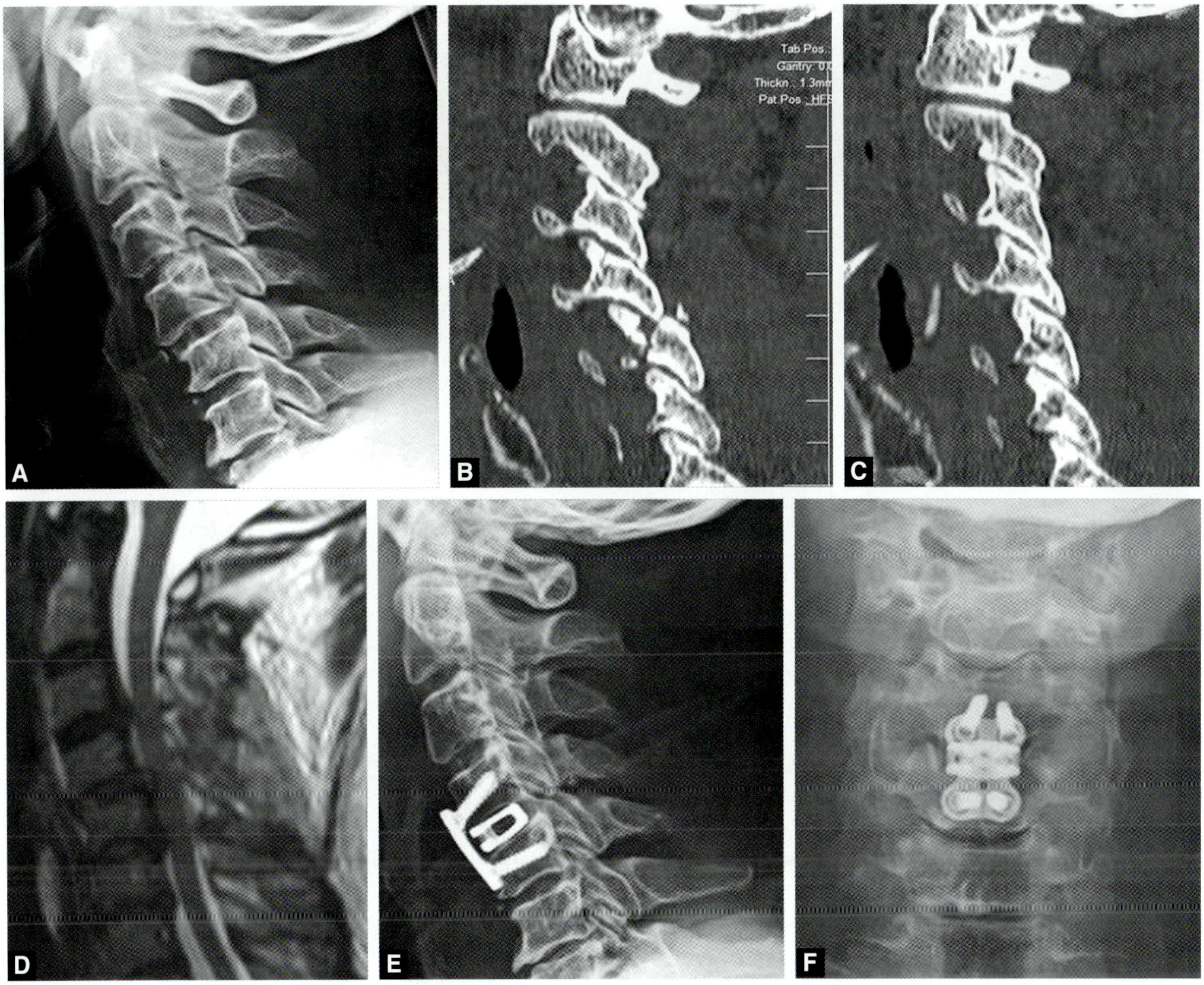

Figures 14.37A to F: A 56-year-old patient presented with C4–C5 unifacetal subluxation. (A to C) The X-ray and CT scan images show that on the right side, there is a facet fracture with subluxation with intact facets on the left side; (D to F) The patient was treated by anterior cervical discectomy and fusion with titanium cages and plate.

long-term results. Traditionally, posterior stabilization has been preferred because it helps to restore the posterior tension band that is lost due to disruption of the posterior ligaments and muscles. Biomechanical studies have shown that posterior stabilization allows a more rigid fixation than anterior plates. Besides the posterior approach is familiar, reduction is easy and instrumentation can be easily extended over multiple levels if required. In osteoporotic bone, posterior stabilization offers better fixation than anterior plating. Posterior stabilization can be achieved using either interspinous or laminar wires as well as with lateral mass screws and plates.

Compressive Extension Injuries

A fall from height or even domestic falls may result in a direct blow to the forehead or the face resulting in a compression force being applied to an extended cervical spine (Figs 14.39A to E). The axial loading of the posterior spinal elements results in unilateral [compressive extension (CE) stage I] or bilateral (CE stage II) fractures of the vertebral arch at one or more levels. These are stable injuries and are commonly treated nonoperatively with a rigid cervical orthosis for 12 weeks. Occasionally, unilateral fractures of both the pedicle and the lamina may occur resulting in a dissociation of the lateral mass

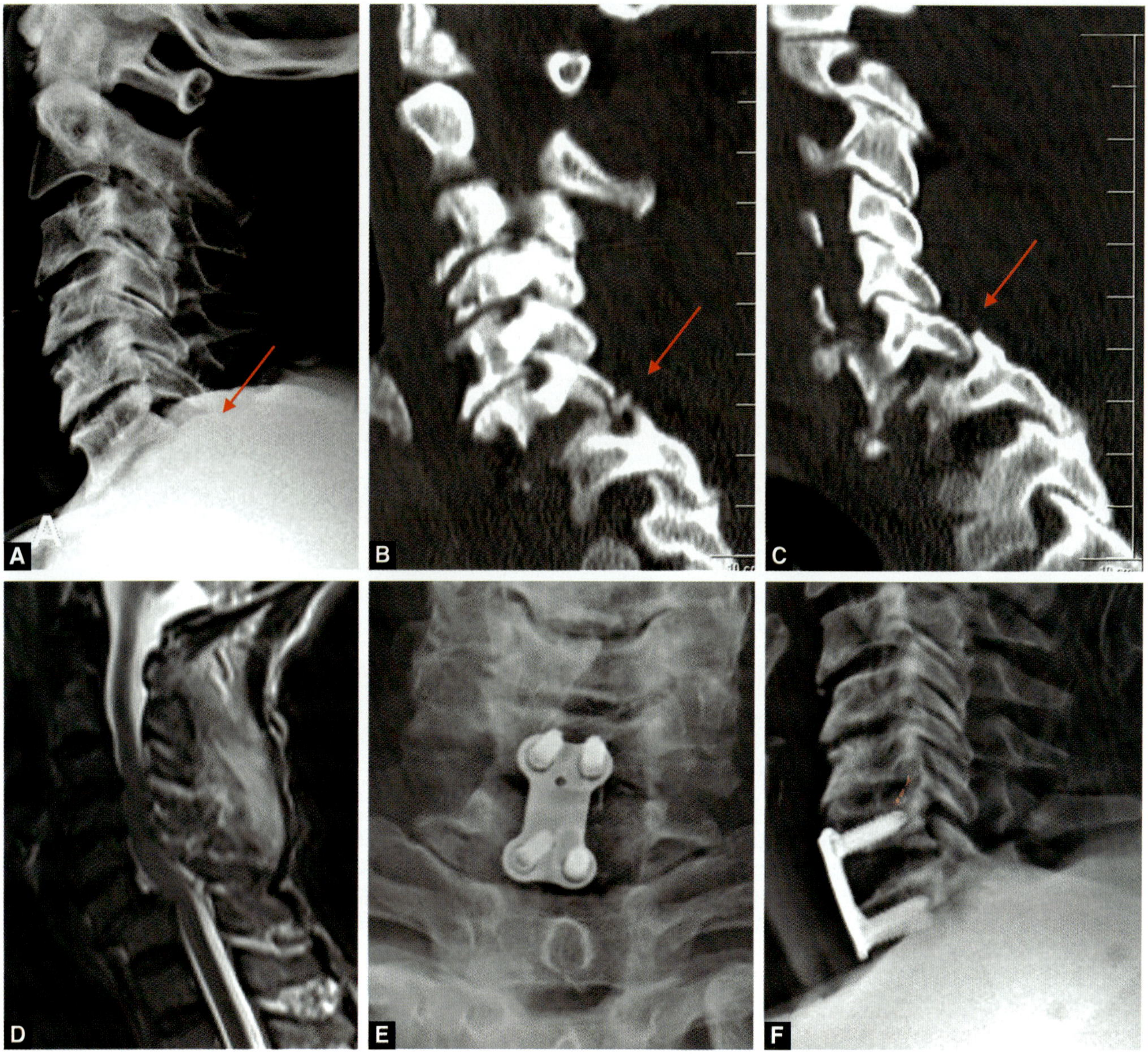

Figures 14.38A to F: (A to C) This patient presented with a bifacetal dislocation evident in the parasagittal CT images and (D) sagittal MR images also show spinal cord kink and deviation; (E and F) The patient was treated by anterior cervical discectomy, distraction, reduction and fusion with a bone graft and plate.

and a rotary listhesis which requires anterior or posterior stabilization.

With further extension or increased loads, the center of rotation of the extension moment shifts anteriorly and inferiorly resulting in a shear force that travels obliquely across the vertebral body or the disc, rendering the spine unstable. The spinal alignment is maintained in CE stage III but there is a progressive anterior translation of the cephalad spinal column in CE stage IV and V. This injury is most common in the lower cervical spine. In spite of the larger force required to cause the more severe injuries, the incidence of neurological deficit is low because of autodecompression resulting from separation of the anterior and posterior elements. Whilst stage III injuries can be managed nonoperatively in a halo vest, stage IV and V injuries require surgical stabilization to restore

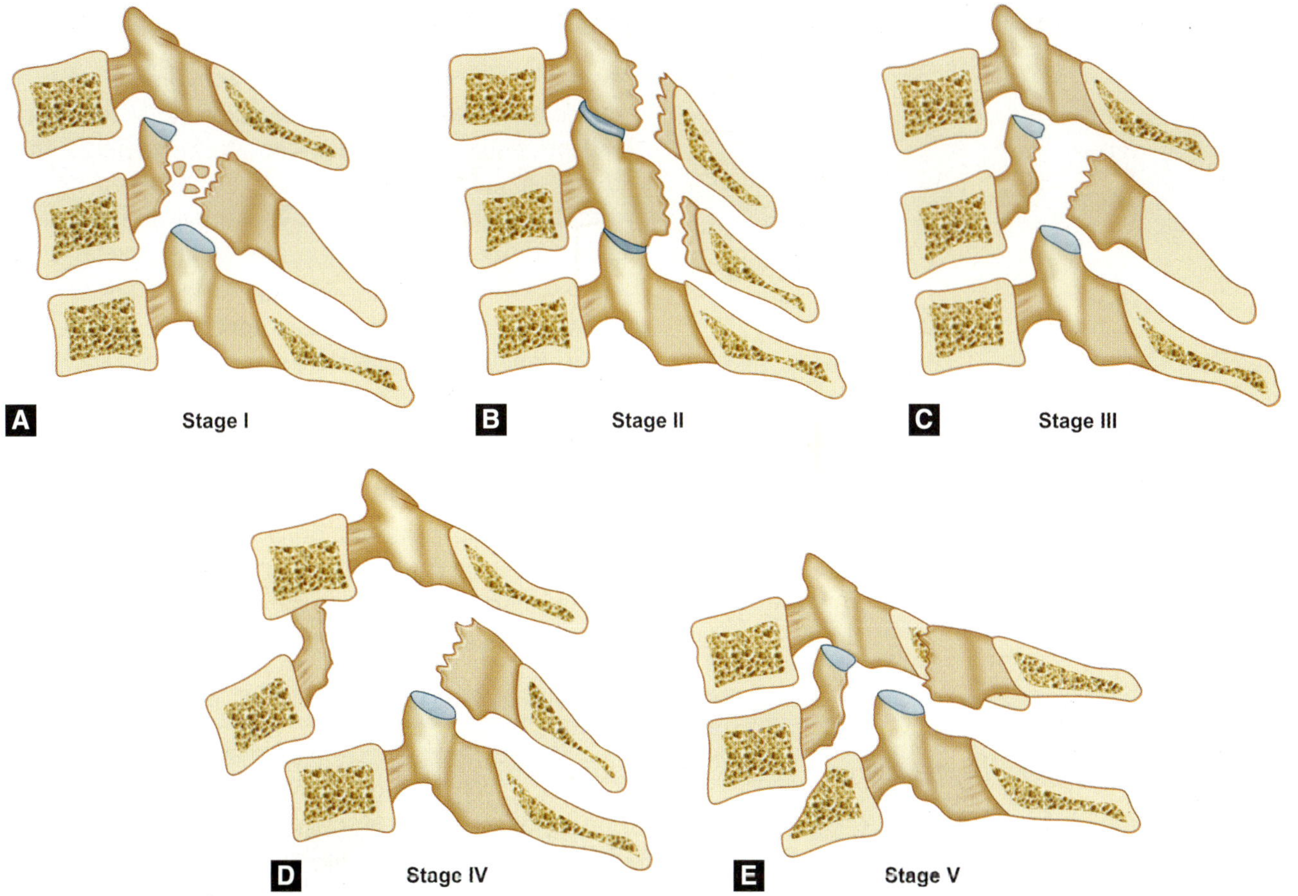

Figures 14.39A to E: The five stages of compression extension (CE) injuries. (A) Stage I (CES-I): Unilateral vertebral arch fracture with or without anterior rotatory vertebral displacement; (B) Stage II (CES-II): Bilateral laminar fracture without other tissue failure; (C) Stage III (CES-III) Bilateral vertebral arch fractures with fracture of the articular processes, pedicles, lamina or some bilateral combination without vertebral body displacement; (D) Stage IV (CES-IV) Bilateral vertebral arch fractures with partial vertebral body width displacement anteriorly; (E) Stage V (CES-V): Bilateral vertebral arch fracture with full vertebral body displacement anteriorly; ligamentous failure at the posterosuperior and anteroinferior margins.

Source: Redrawn from Bucholz RW, Heckman JD, Court-Brown C, et al. (Eds). Rockwood and Green's Fractures in Adults, 6th edition. Philadelphia, PA: Lippincott Williams & Wilkins; 2006.

spinal stability. Multilevel posterior lateral mass fixation is the preferred option. In case of significant vertebral body comminution, additional anterior reconstruction may be required to restore the load bearing mechanics. Anterior stabilization alone is inadequate to neutralize the large shear forces involved.

When extension injuries occur in elderly patients with pre-existing cervical spondylosis, there is a severe momentary compression of the spinal cord between the ligamentum flavum and the anterior osteophytes at the time of impact. This often results in a selective injury to the central spinal cord called the central cord syndrome where in the neurologic deficit is worse within the upper extremity as compared to the lower extremity. The prognosis for recovery is generally good although the patients may have significant residual hand dysfunction and variable spasticity. If there is any instability or malalignment, then surgical stabilization is indicated. The debate is whether a spinal canal decompression is necessary and if so the timing of decompression is also controversial. Guest reported that decompression within 24 hours of injury for traumatic central cord syndrome secondary to cervical fractures or acute disc prolapse is safe and promoted greater motor recovery than delayed decompression.[19] But if the central cord syndrome is associated with cervical spondylosis or stenosis, then the neurological recovery was not appreciable.

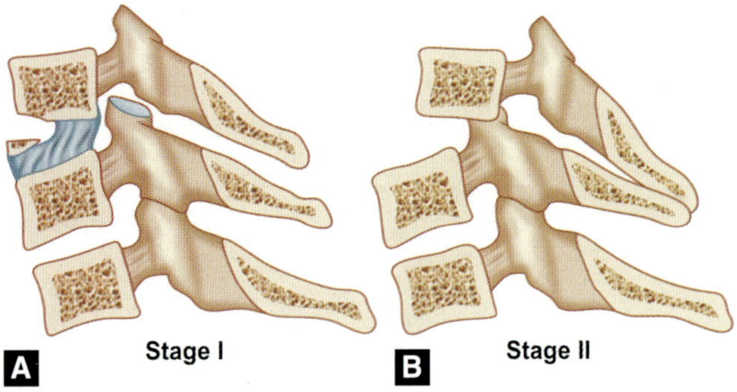

Figures 14.40A and B: The two stages of distraction extension (DE) injuries. (A) Stage I (DES-I): Failure of anterior ligamentous complex or transverse fracture of the body; widening of the disc space and no posterior displacement; (B) Stage II (DES-II): Failure of posterior ligament complex and superior displacement of the body into the canal.

Source: Redrawn from Bucholz RW, Heckman JD, Court-Brown C, et al. (Eds). Rockwood and Green's Fractures in Adults, 6th edition. Philadelphia, PA: Lippincott Williams & Wilkins, 2006.

Distractive Extension Injuries

Distractive extension (DE) injuries occur following high-velocity vehicular accidents or following trivial falls in patients with pre-existing ankylosing spondylitis, diffuse idiopathic skeletal hyperostotis (DISH) or severe cervical spondylosis (Figs 14.40 and 14.41). Facial injuries are common. The spinal injury is often highly unstable and may be associated with a significant neurologic deficit.

When a distraction force is applied to an extended cervical spine, the resultant injury progresses transversely from anterior to posterior resulting in sequential disruption of the anterior longitudinal ligament (ALL), the intervertebral disc followed by the PLL and in the end either a distraction failure of the posterior ligament complex or a fracture of the posterior bony elements (Figs 14.42A to C). DE stage I signifies an injury where the PLL is intact and the injury is confined to the anterior column without any retrolisthesis. The transverse disruption of the anterior

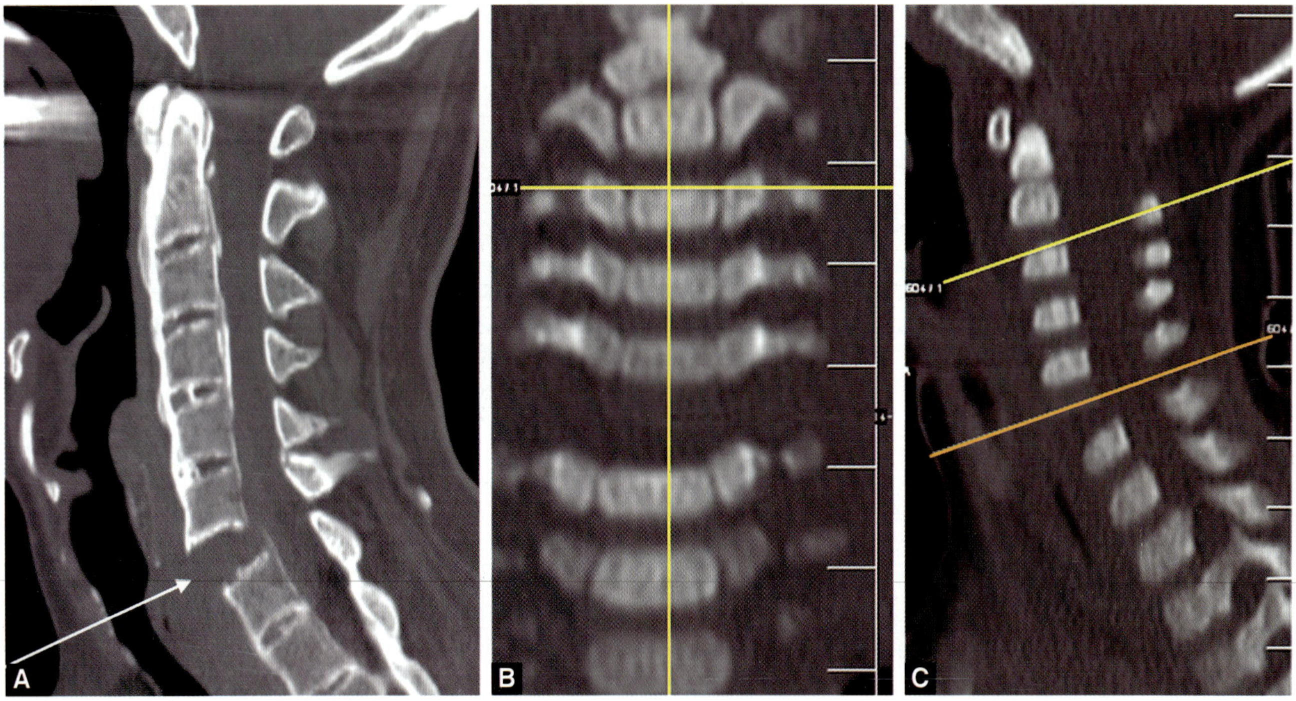

Figures 14.41A to C: Distraction injuries of cervical spine. (A) Sagittal CT image shows C6–C7 extension distraction three column injury in a patient with ankylosing spondylosis. This is a highly unstable injury with an increased risk of neurological deficit; (B and C) Coronal and sagittal CT images of a 6-month-old child who sustained spinal injury in a vehicular accident. She has sustained distractive injury at the level of C5–C6 vertebra evident by significant widening of C5–C6 intervertebral space. These are highly unstable injuries and traction is contraindicated in both these injuries.

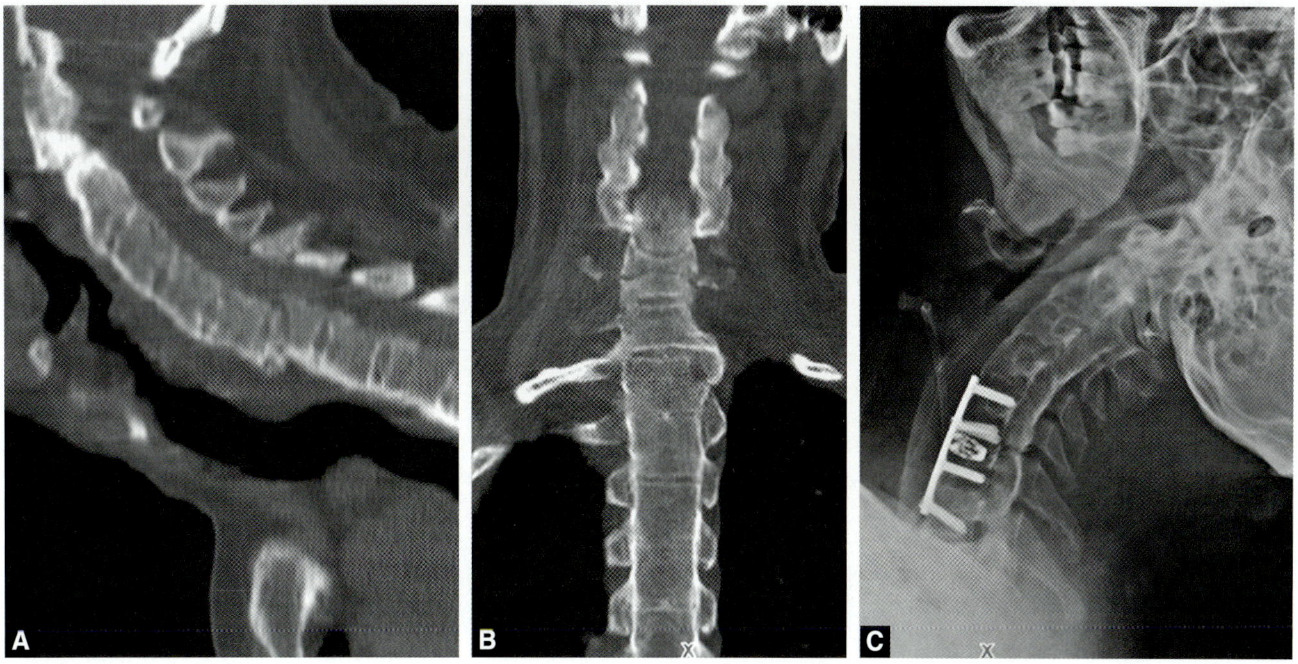

Figures 14.42A to C: Three column extension injury of the cervical spine in a patient with ankylosing spondylitis. The patient was treated with anterior long segment extended stabilization with titanium cage. In patients with fused spine, it is vital to have long fixation points to prevent implant failure.

column may traverse through the disc or may result in avulsion of the anteroinferior corner of the vertebra (extension teardrop fracture). A DE stage II injury is extremely unstable due to failure of the PLL with retrolisthesis of the cephalad vertebra which may result in spinal cord compression between the posteriorly displaced vertebra and the anterosuperior lamina of the next caudal vertebra. These injuries are stable in flexion and hence often missed when radiographs are obtained in a supine patient. The distorted anatomy in patients with ankylosing spondylitis or DISH also makes radiographic interpretation difficult.

When treating these injuries in patients with ankylosing spondylitis, the patient is propped up on pillows to recreate the preinjury spinal alignment rather than positioning them in hard collars which may cause further extension and result in a worsening of the neurologic deficit. Application of traction for realignment of the spine can result in over-distraction and worsening of the neurological deficit. The spine is best realigned in the flexed position.

Definitive treatment can be either a halo-vest immobilization or a surgical stabilization. In patients with significant pre-existing deformity, elderly patients and patients with a neurologic deficit, a halo vest is difficult to maintain. Hence surgery is usually preferred. For DE stage I injuries, anterior cervical fusion with plating is the treatment of choice, especially if the failure is purely discoligamentous. DE stage II injuries are highly unstable and require posterior reduction with stabilization followed by an anterior fusion if necessary. In patients with ankylosing spondylitis, anterior stabilization alone is avoided because the osteoporotic vertebral bone affords poor fixation. If the spine gets realigned with gentle traction applied to the flexed neck then multilevel posterior instrumentation may be adequate. However, if spinal realignment cannot be achieved, then posterior instrumentation is done along with an anterior decompression and instrumented fusion. Some surgeons recommend using the fracture to achieve deformity correction; however, this carries a significant risk of developing a neurologic deficit.

Lateral Flexion Injuries

With the head flexed to one side, any compression force applied would result in an asymmetric fracture of the vertebral body and a unilateral fracture of the posterior elements with the fracture line lying in the sagittal plane (LF1). Neurological injury is uncommon. Most LF1 injuries

A

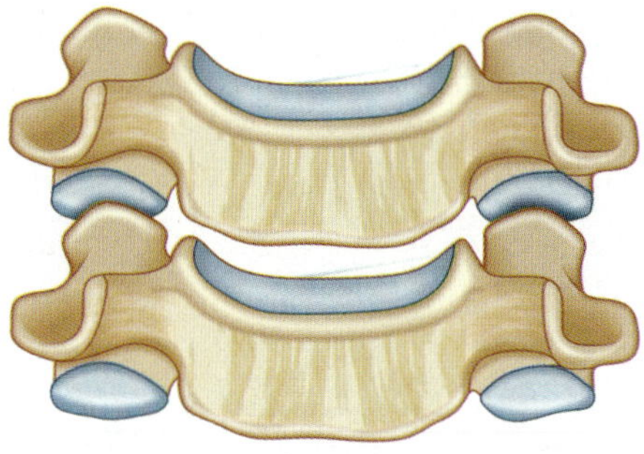

B

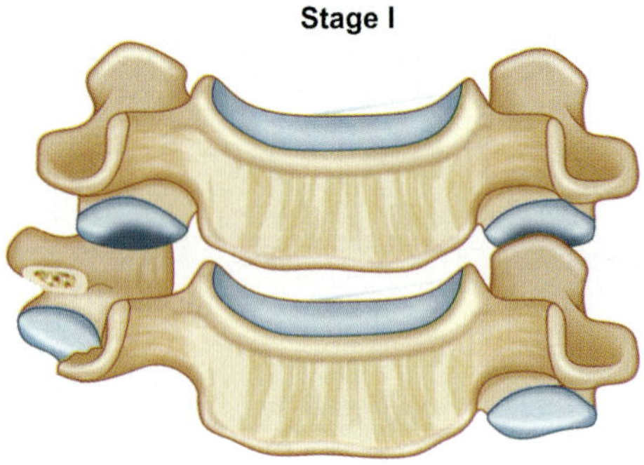

Figures 14.43A and B: Lateral flexion (LF) injuries. Blunt trauma from the side places the ipsilateral spine in distraction while compressing the contralateral spine. (A) Stage I injury, asymmetric centrum fracture with a unilateral arch fracture; (B) Stage II injury, with displacement of the body and contralateral ligamentous failure.

Source: Redrawn from Bucholz RW, Heckman JD, Court-Brown C, et al. (Eds). Rockwood and Green's Fractures in adults, 6th edition. Philadelphia, PA: Lippincott Williams and Wilkins; 2006.

are treated nonoperatively. A more severe lateral bending injury (LF2) would result in avulsion of the contralateral posterior ligaments which is seen as facet joint widening on the AP X-ray (Figs 14.43A and B). LF2 injuries are frequently associated with avulsion of nerve roots or the brachial plexus. For LF2 injuries, posterior stabilization can be done with the goal of fusing only one motion segment whenever possible.

Surgical Anatomy

The cervical spine is made up of seven individual vertebrae. The upper cervical vertebra includes the C1 and C2 (atlas and axis) respectively. C1 and C2 through their articulations provide a great degree of mobility for the skull. Approximately 50% of flexion-extension of the neck occurs between the occiput and C1 and predominant rotation of the neck happens between C1 and C2. The lower cervical or subaxial vertebrae (C3–C7) are similar in anatomy having a body, pedicles, laminae, spinous processes, and facet joints. The cervical spine is much more mobile than the thoracic or lumbar regions of the spine. A peculiar feature of the cervical spine is the presence of transverse foramina in each vertebra for the passage of vertebral arteries.

Upper Cervical Spine

Each bone of the upper cervical spine is anatomically unique with complex stabilizing structures (Fig. 14.44).

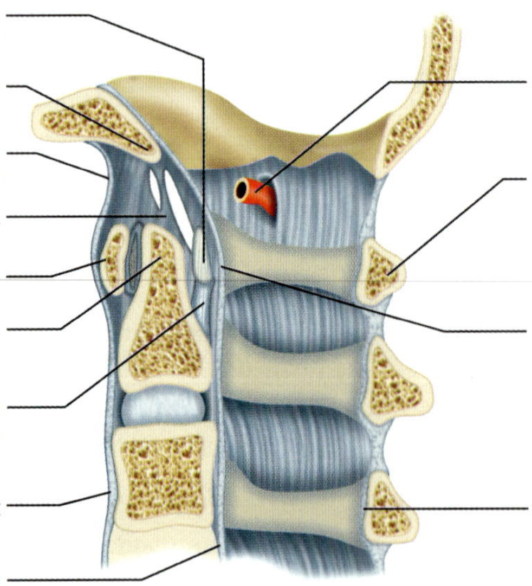

Figure 14.44: Pictorial representation of midsagittal view of the occipitocervical articulation showing the various ligamentous attachments of the upper cervical and craniocervical articulations.

Source: Redrawn from Jackson RS, Banit DM, Rhyne AL, et al. Upper Cervical Spine Injuries. J Am Acad Orthop Surg. 2002;10: 271-80.

The highly specialized anatomy allows weight transfer between the head and trunk, facilitates neck motion and protects the neurovascular structures. The occiput articulates with the atlas through paired synovial joints. The paired occipital condyles project inferiorly from the occiput at the antero-lateral margin of the foramen magnum. The concave atlantal lateral masses with the convex occipital condyles form the occipito-atlantal articulation. These joints are shallower and less well developed in children and therefore contribute to the higher incidence of atlanto-occipital injuries in the pediatric population.

The lateral masses of the atlas are connected by an anterior and a posterior arch. The anterior tubercle, located in the midline on the anterior arch, serves as the attachment site for the ALL and longus colli muscles. The posterior tubercle serves as the attachment site for the ligamentum nuchae. The odontoid process extends rostrally from the body of the axis to articulate with the posterior aspect of the anterior arch of the atlas. This joint and the laterally placed paired facet joints, through which the atlas and axis articulate, are synovial joints facilitating significant rotation movements at this level.

The craniocervical ligaments play a significant role in the stability of the spine (Figs 14.45A and B). The extrinsic ligaments include the ligamentum nuchae, which extends from the external occipital protuberance to the posterior aspect of the atlas and cervical spinous processes. The intrinsic ligaments provide most of the ligamentous stability. These ligaments form three layers anterior to the dura and include the tectorial membrane, the cruciate ligament, and the odontoid ligaments. The tectorial membrane connects the posterior body of the axis to the anterior foramen magnum and is the cephalad continuation of the PLL. The cruciate ligament lies anterior to the tectorial membrane, just behind the odontoid process. The transverse atlantal ligament is the strongest and connects the posterior odontoid to the anterior atlas arch inserting laterally on bony tubercles. Vertical bands extend from the transverse ligament to the foramen magnum and body of the axis. The alar and apical ligaments (collectively referred as the odontoid ligaments) are the most anterior of the ligamentous structures, connecting the odontoid to the occipital condyles.

The major stabilizing structures between the occiput and upper cervical spine are the tectorial membrane and alar ligaments. Flexion is limited by the bony anatomy, while extension is limited by the tectorial membrane. Rotation and lateral bending are restricted by the contralateral alar ligaments. Distraction is prevented by the tectorial membrane and alar ligaments.

Lower Cervical Spine

The five cervical vertebrae that make up the lower cervical spine are C3–C7. Each has an anterior vertebral body and

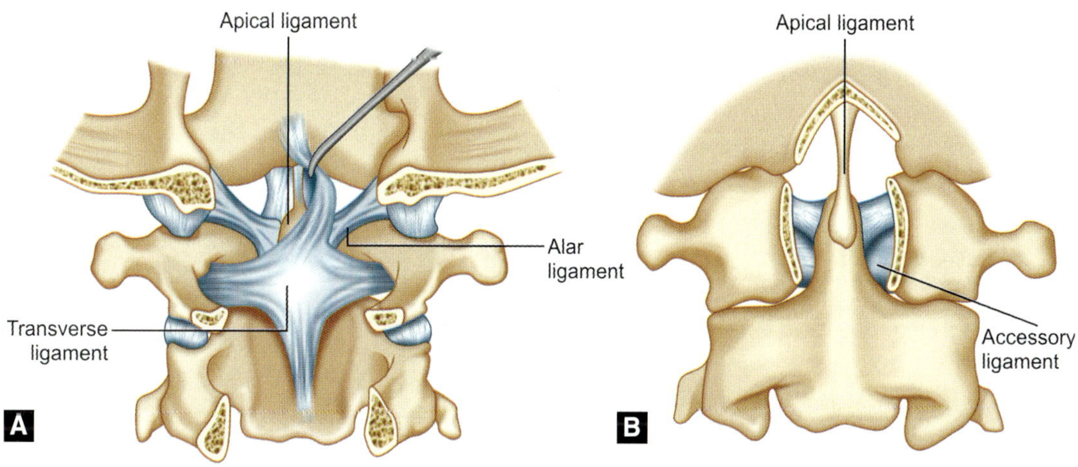

Figures 14.45A and B: Pictorial representations of the (A) posterior and (B) anterior views of the atlantoaxial articulation. The attachments of the apical ligament, transverse ligament, alar ligament and the accessory ligaments are clearly shown.

Source: Redrawn from Jackson RS, Banit DM, Rhyne AL, et al. Upper Cervical Spine Injuries. J Am Acad Orthop Surg. 2002;10: 271-80.

a posterior neural arch. The subaxial cervical spine can be divided into anterior and posterior columns. The anterior column consists of the typical cervical vertebral body sandwiched between supporting disks. The anterior surface is reinforced by the ALL and the posterior body by the PLL.

On the superolateral surfaces of the bodies are raised processes or hooks called uncinate processes, which articulate with a corresponding depressed area on the inferior lateral aspect of the superior vertebral body, called the anvil, forming the uncovertebral joint. Between two vertebral bodies lies the intervertebral disc. The disk is thicker anteriorly, contributing to normal cervical lordosis, and the uncovertebral joints in the posterior aspect of the body define the lateral extent of most surgical exposures.

The spinous processes of C3–C6 are usually bifid, whereas the spinous process of C7 is usually nonbifid and somewhat bulbous at its end. There are two facet joints on either side which provide the necessary stability and mobility for the lower cervical spine. The facet joints are oriented at a 45° angle to the axial plane, allowing a sliding motion. The joint capsules are more lax in the lower cervical spine than in other areas of the spine to allow gliding movements of the facets. Supporting ligamentum flavum, posterior, and interspinous ligaments also strengthen the posterior column. The longitudinal ligaments are vital for maintaining the integrity of the spinal column. Whereas the ALL and PLL maintain the structural integrity of the anterior column, the posterior column alignment is stabilized by a complex of ligaments, including the nuchal and capsular ligaments, and the ligamentum flavum. The interspinous ligament and the ligamentum flavum control excessive flexion and anterior translation. The ligamentum flavum also connects to and reinforces the facet joint capsules.

Surgical Approaches

Anterior Approach to the Subaxial Cervical Spine

The Smith-Robinson approach provides a comprehensive access to the vertebral bodies and discs of the subaxial cervical spine. Theoretically, the left-sided approach is preferable because of the lesser chances of injury to the recurrent laryngeal nerve as the anatomy of this nerve is constant on the left side but variable on the right side. Iatrogenic recurrent laryngeal nerve palsy can result in hoarseness of voice.

Position

Patient is positioned supine on the operating table with the head slightly rotated away from the operative side and strapped with a tape. A rolled sheet is placed between the scapulae to provide slight extension of the cervical spine. The shoulders are pulled down and strapped to the table to aid in adequate fluoroscopic view of the lower cervical spine. The intended level of surgery is marked with the aid of a fluoroscope and the line of incision is infiltrated with a mixture of local anesthetic and adrenaline to minimize blood loss and provide postoperative pain relief.

Procedure

A 3–5 cm transverse incision is made extending from the midline over the marked level till the medial border of sternocleidomastoid. In the subcutaneous layer, the platysma muscle is identified by the longitudinal and superomedially oriented muscle fibers. The platysma muscle is divided along the line of skin incision using an electrocautery to minimize bleeding. The anterior border of sternocleidomastoid is now identified by feeling for the muscle bulk between the thumb and index finger and by the direction of the muscle toward the ipsilateral mastoid process. A plane medial to it is developed by bluntly dissecting the superficial layer of deep cervical fascia. The strap muscles can be seen coursing over the carotid sheath deep to the sternomastoid muscle. The strap muscles are dissected bluntly toward the midline and held with a Langenbeck's retractor. The carotid pulse is identified by palpating with the left index finger and the middle layer of deep cervical fascia which lies medial to it is divided by blunt dissection. The trachea and esophagus lie medial to this plane. The carotid sheath with the sternocleidomastoid is gently retracted laterally. The anterior aspect of cervical spine can now be palpated with a finger and the trachea, esophagus with the strap muscles are retracted medially. The prevertebral fascia is then divided and elevated from the underlying bone to expose the anterior aspect of cervical spine. The two longus colli muscles lie along the lateral edges of the anterior aspect of the vertebral bodies. The medial border of longus colli muscles on either side is exposed completely to limit the level of deep dissection. The longus colli muscle is elevated from the vertebral body and the retractor blades of the self-retaining retractors are placed deep to the muscle. After the retractor blades have been distracted, the anesthetist deflates the endotracheal tube and inflates it again. This has been demonstrated to decrease the incidence of postoperative hoarseness of voice. Once the cervical bony procedure has been performed, meticulous hemostasis is achieved. The trachea, esophagus, carotid sheath and the strap muscles are allowed to fall back into position. The platysma is closed as a separate layer over a drain followed by the skin by subcuticular sutures.

Posterior Approach to the Cervical Spine

Upper Cervical Spine

The suboccipital approach provides access to the occiput, atlas and the axis to fix fractures pertaining to the craniovertebral region. Anterior approach to fractures in this region is difficult and complex. Further, the posterior approach also provides an extensive vascular bed for bone grafting for fusion in craniovertebral junction instabilities.

Position: The patient is positioned prone over two bolsters (one beneath the chest and another one beneath the iliac crests, with abdomen hanging free without any pressure). The cervical spine is positioned in neutral flexion-extension plane. The upper limbs are strapped by the sides of the body with aid of adhesive tapes. All the bony prominences are adequately padded.

Operative steps: The skin and subcutaneous tissue are infiltrated with a diluted solution of 1:500,000 epinephrine to provide hemostasis. A midline longitudinal skin incision is made extending from the occiput to C2. The incision is deepened in the midline through the avascular thin white median raphe which is usually wavy in nature. No spinal segments, other than necessary should be exposed, especially in children, to avoid spontaneous fusion at adjacent levels. The occiput is exposed subperiostially with periosteum elevators. Caudal to the occiput is the ring of C1 which lies deeper than the spinous process of C2. The posterior tubercle of C1 is identified in the midline, and subperiosteal dissection is done to expose the bone. Care should be taken to prevent inadvertent penetration of the atlanto-occipital membrane. Below C2, the lateral margins of the facet joints are the safe lateral extent of dissection. A large venous plexus is present around the atlantoaxial joint and can cause profuse bleeding during dissection of the C1–C2 joint. At this level, the dissection should not exceed more than 1.5 cm laterally on either side of the midline to prevent inadvertent injury to the vertebral arteries. The planned surgical procedure is then performed.

Lower Cervical Spine

Posterior cervical spine exposure is indicated for posterior cervical instrumentation, and fusion. This exposure utilizes the internervous plane between the paraspinal muscles in the midline which are supplied separately by the dorsal rami of the corresponding cervical roots on either side.

Position: The patient is positioned prone over two bolsters (one beneath the chest and another one beneath the iliac crests, with the abdomen hanging free without any pressure). The neck should be in mild flexion or neutral position and the head is strapped to the table to prevent change in position during surgery. The upper limbs are strapped to the side of the body and standard precautions are taken to prevent undue pressure in the eyes.

Operative steps: The skin and subcutaneous tissue is infiltrated with a diluted solution of 1:500,000 epinephrine to provide hemostasis. A midline skin incision is made from C2 to C7 spinous process and the subcutaneous tissue is incised along the same line. Frequent reapplication of self-retaining retractors at each level maintains the soft tissue tension and also aids in developing the plane of dissection. The deep dissection is carried out with electrocautery to reach the tip of the spinous processes. Stripping of the muscles should proceed from a distal to proximal direction because it can be stripped from the spinous process in the acute angle at their bony insertion and thus minimize bleeding. The deep dissection should stay along the wavy ligamentum nuchae which provides an avascular surgical plane. The paraspinal muscles are elevated from the spinous process subperiosteally with a Cobb elevator to expose the posterior elements on both sides. Lateral dissection is continued only till the lateral border of the facet joint and the articular mass should be completely exposed which facilitates lateral mass fixation.

SURGICAL APPROACH OF CERVICAL SPINE:
Pearls and Pitfalls

Anterior cervical exposure

- A nasotracheal tube should be used for anesthesia in cases where exposure above the level of C3 is needed.
- Self-retaining retractors should be applied under the medial edges of longus colli muscle carefully to avoid injury to the recurrent laryngeal nerve and the trachea-esophageal structures.
- It is advisable to relax the retractors intermittently in cases of longer duration of surgery to avoid inadvertent pressure over the neurovascular structures.

Posterior cervical exposure

- Dissection should proceed along the ligamentum nuchae to minimize bleeding.
- Try to preserve the ligamentous attachments at C2 and C7 spinous processes to prevent postoperative instability.
- While positioning for fusion surgeries, the cervical spine should be straight but head should be adequately flexed in a "military tuck" position as it facilitates separation of foramen magnum from C1 arch.
- The dissection should not exceed more than 1.5 cm laterally on either side to prevent damage to the vertebral arteries.

Surgical Techniques

Technique 1: Direct C1 Posterior Fixation

In the management of C1 burst fractures, primary posterior C1–C2 or C0–C2 fusion is advocated to restore the atlanto-occipital and atlantoaxial congruity and to avoid possible atlantoaxial instability. Both have the advantage of having a simpler approach with low complication rate albeit at the cost of restriction of cervical motion. Ruf et al. proposed anterior reduction and C1 osteosynthesis by transoral approach to avoid multisegmental fixations.[20] But this approach is associated with a high complication rate. Koller et al. in a recent cadaveric biomechanical analysis have demonstrated that under physiological loads, direct C1 osteosynthesis restores C1–C2 stability.[21] So when indicated, the authors prefer direct posterior C1 osteosynthesis and use computer navigation guided posterior polyaxial screws and a transverse rod.

Technique

With the patient in prone position over a carbon fiber radiolucent operating tabletop, skull traction is applied via tongs. Traction is applied with 5–10 pounds weight so that through ligamentotaxis, the displaced fracture fragments of C1 are reduced. Reduction is confirmed and considered to be acceptable when there is less than 7 mm combined lateral displacement/overhang of the lateral masses of the atlas over the axis. The achieved reduction is maintained with a 5-pound weight.

Through a standard posterior midline approach, the posterior elements of C1, C2 and C3 are exposed (Fig. 14.46). Use of intraoperative fluoroscopy in the AP and lateral views is necessary for safe screw insertion.

The entry point for the C1 lateral mass screws is located just beneath the posterior arch of C1 where it thins out and just above the midpoint of the C1–C2 facet joint. The vertebral artery arches just proximal to the posterior arch of C1 from lateral to medial and hence it is important to avoid a superior and lateral entry. The C2 nerve root ganglion is situated below the entry for screw insertion. An inferior entry can potentially injure the ganglion and is also associated with brisk venous bleeding from the venous plexus. A medial entry results in a weak screw and can potentially injure the spinal cord. Once the correct

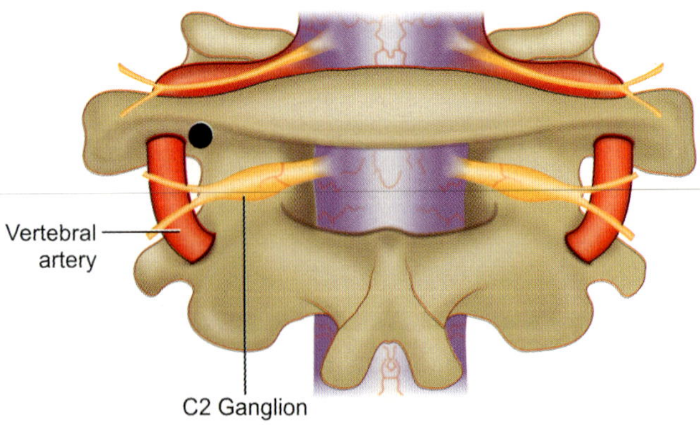

Figure 14.46: Anatomy of the posterior C1–C2 articulation indicating the close proximity of vital neurovascular structures and the safe entry zone for lateral mass screw insertion (black dot).

entry is identified, the entry hole is marked with a 2.5 mm diamond-tipped burr and further drilling is performed with a 2.7 mm drill bit. Drilling is performed slowly with frequent checks with a ball-tipped probe to assess the integrity of the walls of the screw track. The screw is directed 10–15° medially and in the lateral plane, it is directed toward the anterior arch of the atlas. This is confirmed with the use of fluoroscopy. No attempt should be made to intentionally breach the anterior cortex. Since there is potential for movement of the unsupported lateral masses, the entry point and the direction of the screw track must be executed without applying undue pressure. Drilling must be done in installments of 2–3 mm with repeated checking with the probe. Importantly both the screw holes must be drilled before commencing the screw insertion process as the force applied while screw insertion can cause interfragmentary movement. Polyaxial cervical lateral mass screws are inserted into the screw track (Figs 14.47A to F). The screws are connected with a contoured rod and compressed gradually in a controlled manner to reduce the lateral displacement and to compress the fractured fragments. In this technique, the use of intraoperative computer navigation increases the safety and accuracy of screw insertion and can also assess the accuracy of fracture reduction three dimensionally after screw insertion.

Technique 2: C1–C2 Fusion

Magerl's Technique

In 1986, Magerl described a posterior transarticular C1–C2 screw fixation technique which provided a biomechanically strong fixation.[22] The procedure is technically demanding and the surgeon must be well versed with the anatomy of the region and the morphometric dimensions of C2 pedicles, and the presence of a high-riding vertebral artery in each patient should be preoperatively assessed.

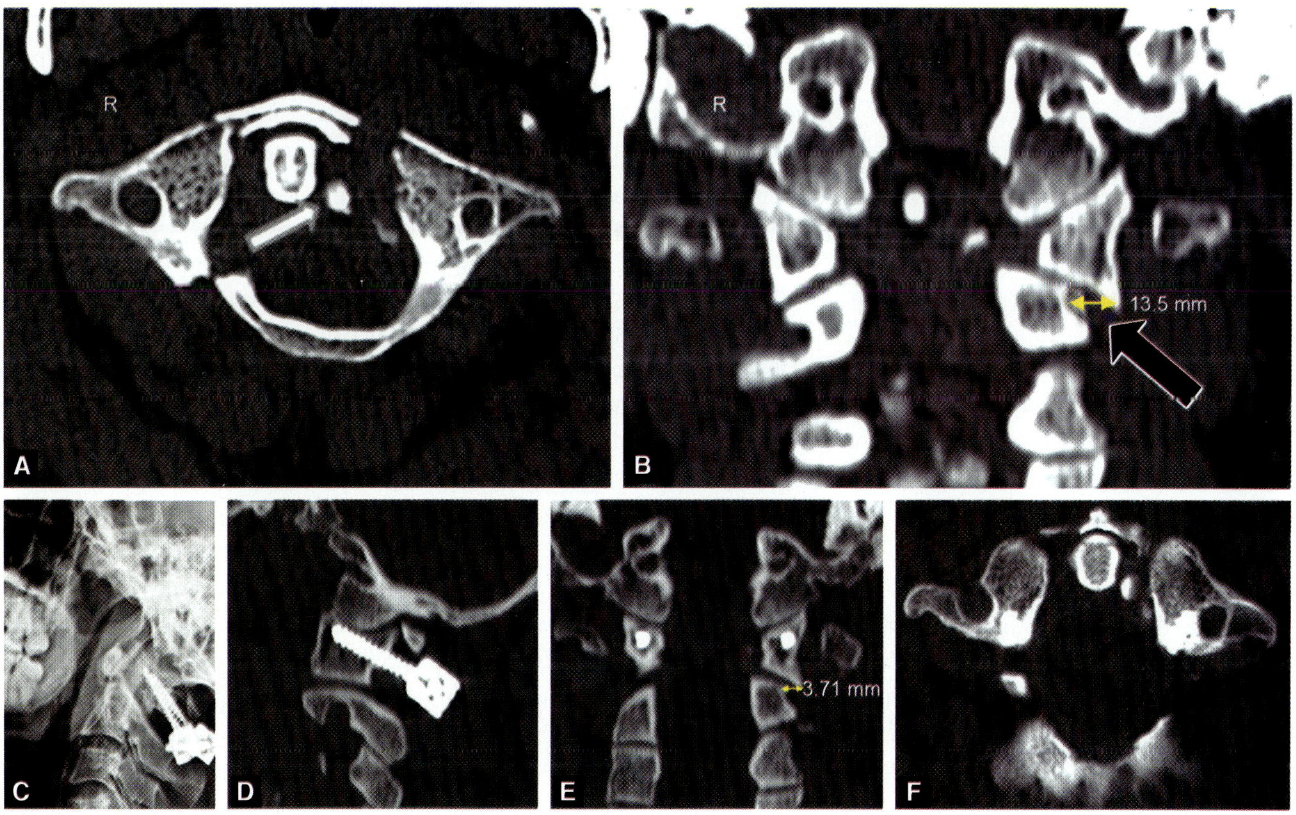

Figures 14.47A to F: (A and B) Axial and coronal CT scan images show an unstable Jefferson's fracture; (C) Postoperative lateral radiograph shows that the fracture has been reduced and stabilized by C1 lateral mass screws alone; (D to F) Sagittal, coronal and axial CT images show well-contained lateral mass screws.

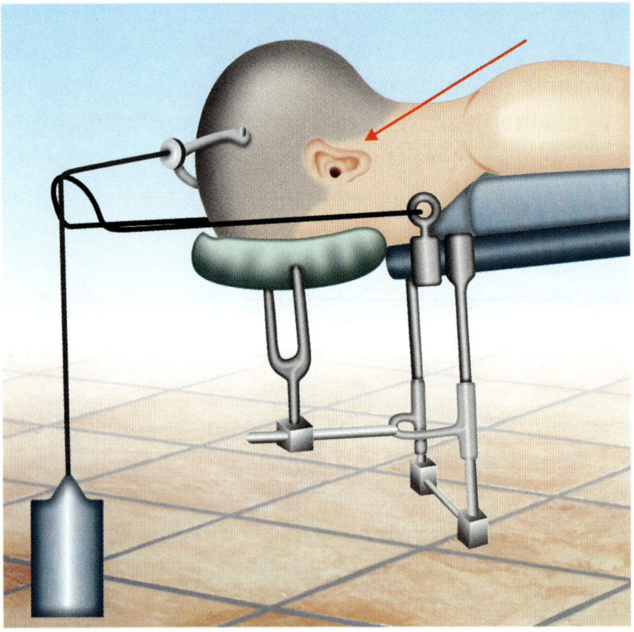

Figure 14.48: Patient is positioned prone on the Mayfield frame with traction. The neck is flexed slightly at the craniocervical junction and the subaxial spine is placed in a neutral position. This helps to attain an ideal screw trajectory (red arrow) without being hindered by the thorax.

Proper positioning of the patient is crucial to allow a safe screw trajectory. The patient is placed prone and the use of a Mayfield traction helps in proper positioning allowing reduction of the fractured fragments and free movement of the image intensifier around the cervical spine (Fig. 14.48). A mild flexion at the craniocervical junction will allow the drilling instrument to be placed appropriately and get a proper orientation of the drill.

A posterior midline incision is made from occiput to the midcervical region. The tip of the bifid C2 spinous process can be split in the midline to retain the muscular attachments of C2. The C2 lamina is then exposed subperiosteally up to the lateral border of C1–C2 facet joint. Care should be taken to avoid troublesome bleeding from the venous plexus between the C1 and C2 facets. The entry point for the screw is 2–3 mm cranial to the lower margin of C2 lamina and slightly medial to the midpoint of the facet joint (Figs 14.49A to F). Starting the drill hole with a burr will help to secure an accurate entry point and this can be further developed with a drill. Passage of the drill must be done carefully with C-arm monitoring in both the AP and lateral planes as the margin of safety is low. The direction of the screw track along the mediolateral plane must be controlled directly by palpating the medial border of the C2 isthmus with a probe. The drill should pass at least 2 mm laterally to this curved border, which represents the lateral boundary of the spinal canal. On the sagittal plane, the drill should be angulated either straight or just 10° medially so that it is always inside the bone between the vertebral artery laterally or the spinal canal medially. On the lateral plane, the position of the screw must be controlled on the image intensifier. The image on the screen should show a clear profile of the atlas and the axis. In the lateral C-arm image, the drill should be seen to start at the entrance to the C2 lamina, run through the C1–C2 joint in its posterior third and reach the upper half of the lateral portion of the anterior atlas ring, which should appear oval shaped on the screen. The drill should be passed slowly, progressing back and forth frequently in order to check that the drill is still inside the bone, i.e. to feel the resistance of the bone continuously. If there is no resistance at the tip of the drill bit, drilling must be stopped to avoid a potential injury to the vertebral artery. In patients who have fixed rotation between C1 and C2, monitoring the correct passage of the drill will be impossible and hence the procedure carries considerable risk.

Although the Magerl's technique provides a biomechanically sound fixation, long-term results depend upon obtaining a secure bony fusion between C1 and C2. In the original technique described by Magerl, this was achieved by a classical Gallie's fusion technique. Here a bicortical posterior iliac graft is harvested and placed on a bed of the posterior arch of C1–C2 which are carefully decorticated. The graft is fixed between the arch of the atlas and the C2 spinous process with wires or a nonresorbable suture. Postoperatively, a simple soft neck collar is worn for comfort and fusion is assessed by follow-up radiographs, which is expected at 10–12 weeks.

A preoperative CT scan will reveal details of the patient's anatomy and a reconstruction of the C2 isthmus on the sagittal plane will allow us to plan the appropriate screw size needed. If unilateral vertebral artery hypoplasia is observed, screw insertion should be limited to a unilateral fixation or an alternative technique used. A single screw can provide a satisfactory healing but rigid external immobilization is required for 2 months.

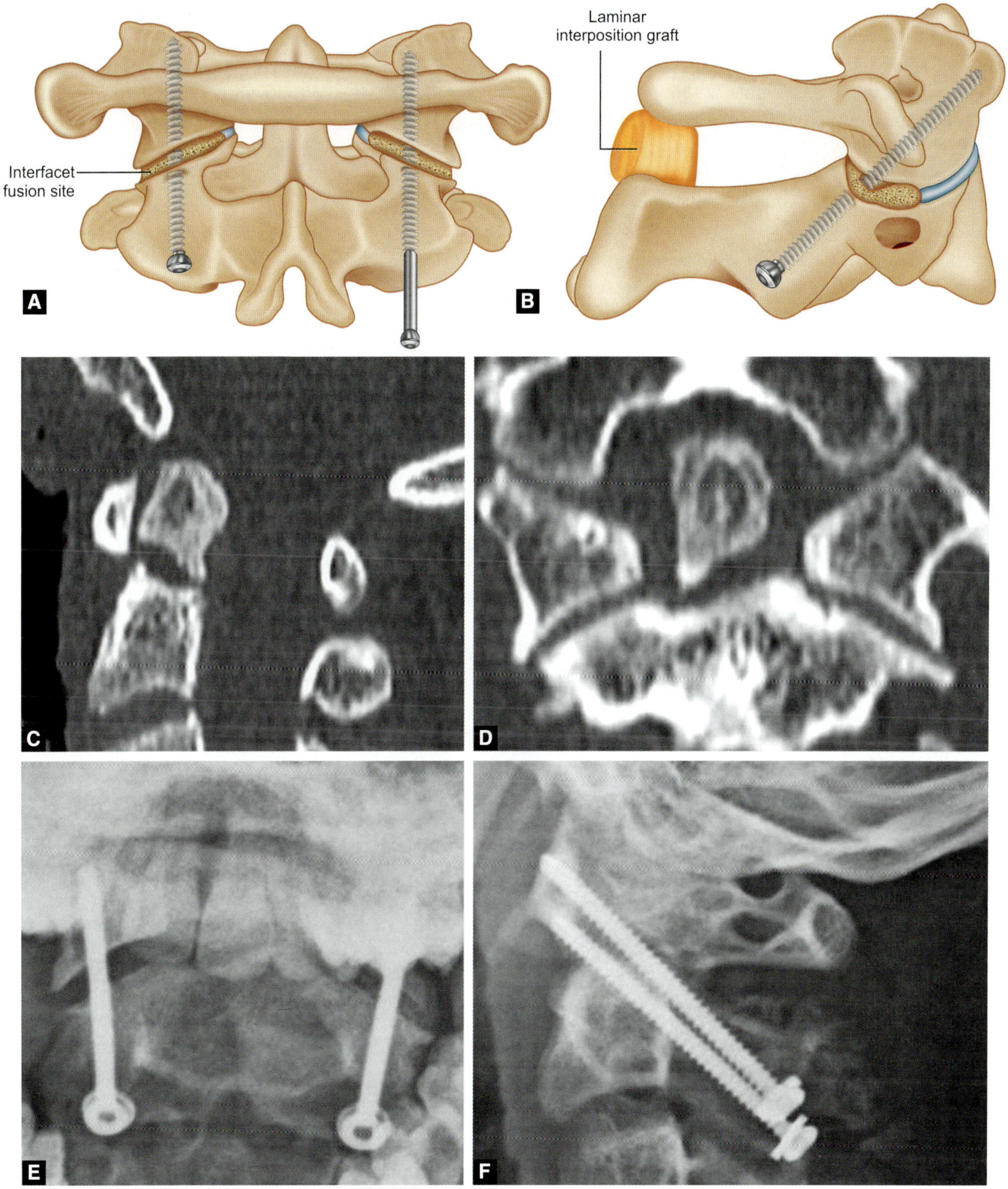

Figures 14.49A to F: (A and B) Pictorial diagrams representing Magerl's screw fixation in the coronal and sagittal planes; (C to F) Patient who presented with a 3-week old odontoid fracture was treated by Magerl's screw fixation. The sagittal and coronal CT images indicate the fracture. The AP and lateral radiographs indicate the screw entry and trajectory.

Patient positioning is of crucial importance. Flexion at the atlanto-occipital joint and extension of the subaxial cervical spine must be attempted. This position places the cervical spine in a favorable situation with respect to the rib cage. Thus, it is possible to angulate the drill sufficiently to insert the screw in an ideal position. In patients who are obese or who have marked thoracic kyphosis, the technique could be difficult to carry out and some other techniques of C1–C2 fusion should be tried.[23]

Special care must be taken while directing the screw in the mediolateral plane. Since at this level, the spinal canal provides ample space for the spinal cord on its medial aspect, placing the screw too laterally is comparatively dangerous, where the vertebral artery is traversing through the vertebral foramen. Hence it is preferred to place the screw in the medial-most portion of the isthmus simultaneously palpating the medial wall with a probe placed along the isthmus.

The presence of a massive hemorrhage after drilling into the isthmus could be indicative of an injury to the vertebral artery. As a first step, the screw can be inserted into the hole. If bleeding persists, arterial ligation may be attempted, but this is a highly technically demanding procedure where expertise and extensive bony resection would be needed. Hemorrhage outside the perforated hole may stem from the venous plexus surrounding the vertebral artery. In these cases screw insertion often provides adequate hemostasis. In patients with suspected vertebral artery injury, the contralateral screw must not be placed.

Goel-Harm's Technique

This technique involves placement of independent C1 lateral mass and C2 pedicle screws on either side.[24] Biomechanically these are strong constructs and also have potential advantages like ability to reduce a C1–C2 subluxation and also useful in patients with suspected vertebral artery anomalies.

Under general anesthesia, the patient is placed in the prone position and the neck is held in alignment by traction in Mayfield frame. The position of the C1–C2 complex is verified by use of an image intensifier. The cervical spine is exposed subperiosteally from the occiput to C3–C4. The C1–C2 complex is exposed to the lateral border of the C1–C2 articulation.

Bleeding typically arises from dissection around the epidural venous plexus along the C1–C2 joint. This is effectively controlled with a combination of bipolar electrocautery, Gelfoam with thrombin, and cotton pledgets. The C1–C2 joint is exposed and opened by dissection over the superior surface of the C2 pars. This joint is a key anatomic landmark for accurate placement of the C1 lateral mass screw. The dorsal root ganglion of C2 is retracted in a caudal direction to expose the entry point for the C1 screw, which is in the middle of the junction of the C1 posterior arch and the midpoint of the posterior inferior part of the C1 lateral mass (Fig. 14.50). This entry point is marked with a 1–2 mm high-speed burr to prevent slippage of the drill point. The pilot hole is then drilled in a straight or slightly convergent trajectory and parallel to the plane of the C1 posterior arch in the sagittal direction, with the tip of the drill directed toward the anterior arch of C1. The drilling is guided by intraoperative landmarks, preoperative fine-cut axial computed tomographic images, and lateral fluoroscopic imaging. The hole is tapped, and a 3.5 mm polyaxial screw of an appropriate length is inserted bicortically into the lateral mass of C1.

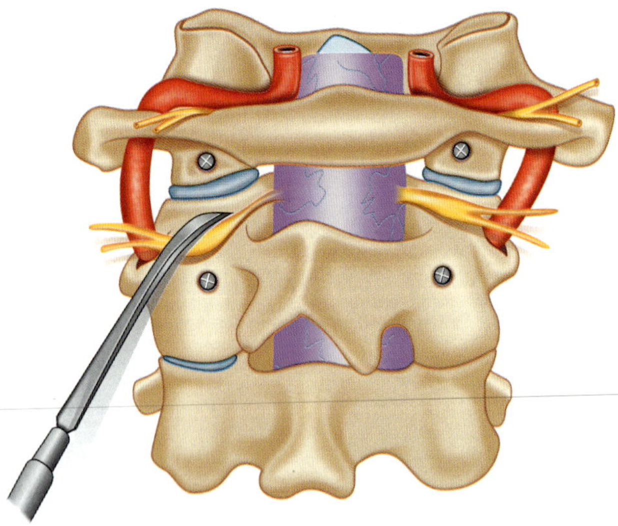

Figure 14.50: The entry point for the C1 screw is in the middle of the junction of the C1 posterior arch and the midpoint of the posterior inferior part of the C1 lateral mass. The entry point for C2 pedicle screw is in the cranial and medial quadrant of the isthmus surface of C2.

Source: Redrawn from Harms J, Melcher RP. Posterior C1–C2 fusion with polyaxial screw and rod fixation. Spine (Phila Pa 1976). 2001;26(22):2467-71.

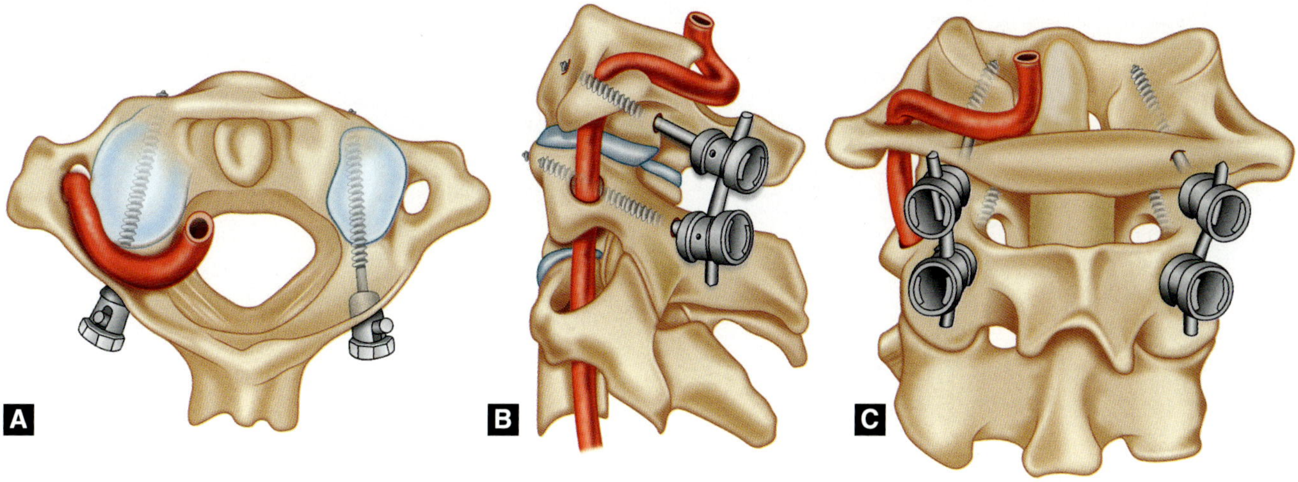

Figures 14.51A to C: Axial, lateral and posterior views of C1–C2 Harms-Goel construct.

Source: Redrawn from Harms J, Melcher RP. Posterior C1–C2 fusion with polyaxial screw and rod fixation. Spine [Phila Pa 1976]. 2001;26(22):2467-71.

The position of the screws is verified by an image intensifier. A number 4 Penfield dissector is used to delineate the medial border of the C2 pars interarticularis, and the entry point for placement of a C2 pedicle screw is marked with a high-speed burr. This is in the cranial and medial quadrant of the isthmus surface of C2 (Figs 14.51A to C). The pilot hole is prepared with a 2 mm drill bit, just perforating the opposite cortex. The direction of the bit is approximately 20–30° in a convergent and cephalad direction, guided directly by the superior and medial surface of the C2 isthmus, respecting individual anatomic variations.

The hole is tapped, and a 3.5 mm polyaxial screw of the appropriate length is inserted bicortically. If a definitive fusion is required, C1 and C2 are decorticated posteriorly, and cancellous bone taken from a small incision in the posterior iliac crest can be placed over the decorticated surfaces of C1 and C2. An articular fusion can also be performed by decorticating the joint surfaces under direct vision.

Gallie's Wiring Technique

There are two basic techniques of wiring for atlantoaxial fusion that have been described in the literature: the Gallie, and the Brooks & Jenkins techniques. The Gallie technique[25] has the advantage of using only one wire, which is passed beneath the lamina of C1 and in the Brooks technique, sublaminar wires are passed underneath both C1 and C2 laminae. In Gallie fusion, tightening of the wire can cause an unstable C1 vertebra to displace posteriorly and fuse in a dislocated position, which is disadvantageous. But the Brooks technique gives greater resistance to rotational movement, lateral bending, and extension. Presently due to the need for supplemental supports in the form of halo or Minerva casts and the risks of violating the spinal canal, other techniques like the Magerl's technique or the C1–C2 screw-rod constructs are preferred in most situations.

The patient is placed prone on padded bolsters and, the occiput and the upper cervical spine is exposed through a standard posterior midline approach. The posterior arch of the atlas and the laminae of C2 are exposed subperiosteally. Care should be exercised to restrict the dissection laterally along the atlas to not more than 2 cm from the midline, to prevent injury to the vertebral arteries and vertebral venous plexus that lie on the superior aspect of the ring of C1. Similarly the upper surface of C1 is exposed no farther laterally than 1.5 cm from the midline avoiding injury to the vertebral artery. An appropriate-sized wire (22 gauge to 18 gauge) depending on the age of the patient and the size of the spinal canal is bent as a wire loop and passed upward under the arch of the atlas. The free ends of the wire are passed through the loop, grasping the arch of C1 in the loop. A corticocancellous graft from the iliac crest is harvested and placed against the laminae of C2 and the arch of C1 beneath the wire (Figs 14.52A and B). One end of the wire is passed through

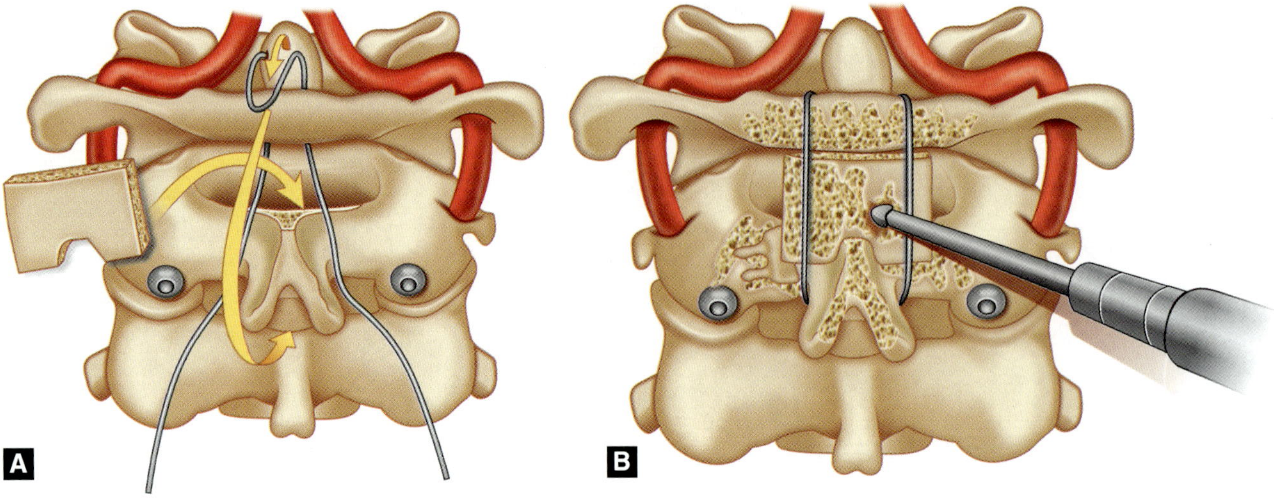

Figures 14.52A and B: Technique of Gallie's fusion. (A) A trimmed graft is placed in between C1 and C2 arches and (B) a sublaminar wire is tightened around the lamina incorporating the graft.

the spinous process of C2, and twisted on itself to secure the graft in place. The patient is immobilized in a Minerva cast, halo cast or vest. Immobilization usually is continued for 12 weeks.

Brooks and Jenkins' Wiring Technique

The occiput and upper cervical spine are exposed similarly. A Mersilene suture is passed from cephalad to caudad on each side of the midline under the arch of the atlas and then beneath the laminae of C2. This serves as a guide to introduce the stainless steel wires under the laminae of C1 and C2. The size of the wires used varies depending on the size and age of the patient. Two full-thickness bone grafts are harvested from the iliac crest, and fitted in the interval between the arch of the atlas and the lamina of the axis. The wires are tightened over the graft and twisted on each side (Figs 14.53A to D). The patient is provided with a Minerva cast or a halo vest as external support till fusion occurs.

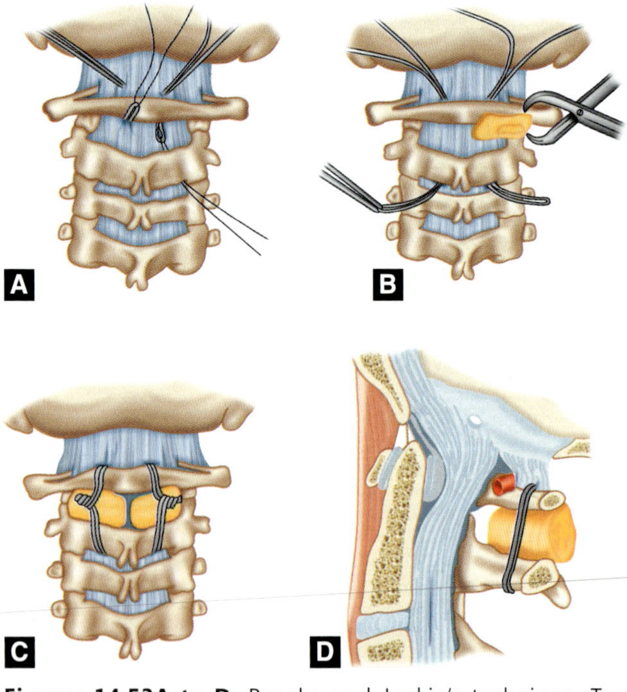

Figures 14.53A to D: Brooke and Jenkin's technique. Two separate sublaminar wires are passed around the lamina of C1 and C2 to hold two independent rectangular grafts placed in the interlaminar region.

Source: Redrawn from Brooks AL, Jenkins EB. Atlantoaxial arthrodesis by the wedge compression method. J Bone Joint Surg. 1978;60(3):279-84.

Technique 3: C2 Odontoid Fixation

Anterior odontoid screw fixation has the advantages of preserving atlantoaxial motion and is minimally invasive in terms of the exposure and muscle damage. It is imperative that anatomical closed reduction of the fracture should be achieved to consider direct fixation. If two fluoroscopes (biplanar fluoroscopy) are available, it makes the procedure simpler. Good visualization of the odontoid in both the planes is mandatory. The authors prefer to use a cannulated technique for anterior screw fixation.

Under fluoroscopic guidance, the patient is placed in the supine position with the neck extended. A radiolucent mouth gag is used to keep the mouth open to provide a transoral AP view. After fiberoptic intubation with in-line stabilization, the lateral C-arm fluoroscopy is brought into position with the arm passed under the operating table. Because biplanar C-arm fluoroscopy is required to perform this procedure, the second unit is put into the AP position to obtain simultaneous projections prior to preparation of the patient.

A small, transverse midcervical skin incision is made over the level of the cricothyroid junction (the C5–C6 interspace). Similar to a standard Cloward-type approach performed for anterior cervical discectomy, blunt dissection is performed down within the avascular plane to the prevertebral region and then extended cephalad to the C2–C3 disc space. The trachea and esophagus are retracted medially, and the sternocleidomastoid muscle and the carotid sheath are mobilized laterally by using a Cloward hand-held retractor. The dissection is then performed cephalad on the midline under fluoroscopic guidance to reach the C2–C3 interspace. The hand-held retractors are then replaced by sharp-toothed, transverse self-retaining retractor blades, which are placed at C5–C6 to obtain adequate exposure. The C2–C3 interspace level is verified using the lateral C-arm fluoroscopic view.

Using biplanar fluoroscopy, a 2 mm threaded K-wire is anchored into the midline of the anteroinferior edge of C2. By applying a prying motion with the K-wire anchored into C2 and levered on C3 in the dorsal-to-ventral direction, the C2 body is rocked slightly anteriorly, allowing for adequate trajectory to traverse the fracture line and incorporate the superior fragment (Figs 14.54A to F).

After the drill guide and K-wire are anchored and the trajectory is deemed adequate, the K-wire is then drilled through the fracture line into the distal portion of the fractured dens. The K-wire should be drilled approximately 1 mm beyond the distal odontoid fragment to incorporate the outer cortex. The inner guide tube is then removed, and the K-wire is left in place. A pilot hole is then drilled into the C2 body with the cannulated drill bit sliding over the K-wire across the fracture line and into the apical cortical surface of odontoid process.

Before the fracture line is crossed, additional head manipulation can be attempted to realign better the odontoid fracture prior to screw placement. Once the pilot hole is made, the depth of penetration of the drill can be determined by reading the markers on the drill bit or K-wire shaft. The drill is then withdrawn, and the drill hole is tapped over the K-wire to cut threads in the interface. A 4 mm non self-tapping, partially threaded titanium cannulated lag screw is then gradually inserted through the guide tube over the K-wire, under direct fluoroscopic view, and countersunk 2 mm into the C2 vertebral body. The tip of the screw should barely penetrate the apical cortex of the odontoid process, and it should be just adequately tightened to engage the distal odontoid fragment (Figs 14.55 and 14.56). It is important to choose a slightly shorter screw length than is measured by approximately 2 mm because the lag effect derives only from final tightening of the screw to increase compression and to approximate the fracture line. The neck is manually flexed and extended, and alignment and screw placement are verified on biplanar fluoroscopy.

Inadvertent penetration of the guidewire into the spinal canal should be avoided while drilling and tapping. Adequate precaution must be taken to prevent backing out of the guidewire while withdrawing the drill. The steps of drilling and tapping as well as removal should be done under fluoroscopy to ensure that the guidewire has not migrated.

Technique 4: C2 Pars Fixation

As the pathomechanism behind the fracture is the tensile forces along the pedicles, the logical treatment would be fixation of the fracture with compression lag screws. Bilateral transpedicular repair could be the most physiologic surgery as it spares the motion segments from fusion (Figs 14.57A and B). But pedicle screw fixation of the upper cervical spine is technically difficult, especially when there is fracture instability and displacement of fragments. Computer-assisted navigation helps improving accuracy in such demanding situations and allows accurate and safe placement of cervical pedicle screws.

Patient is positioned prone on a radiolucent operating table. The fracture is reduced by extension of the neck

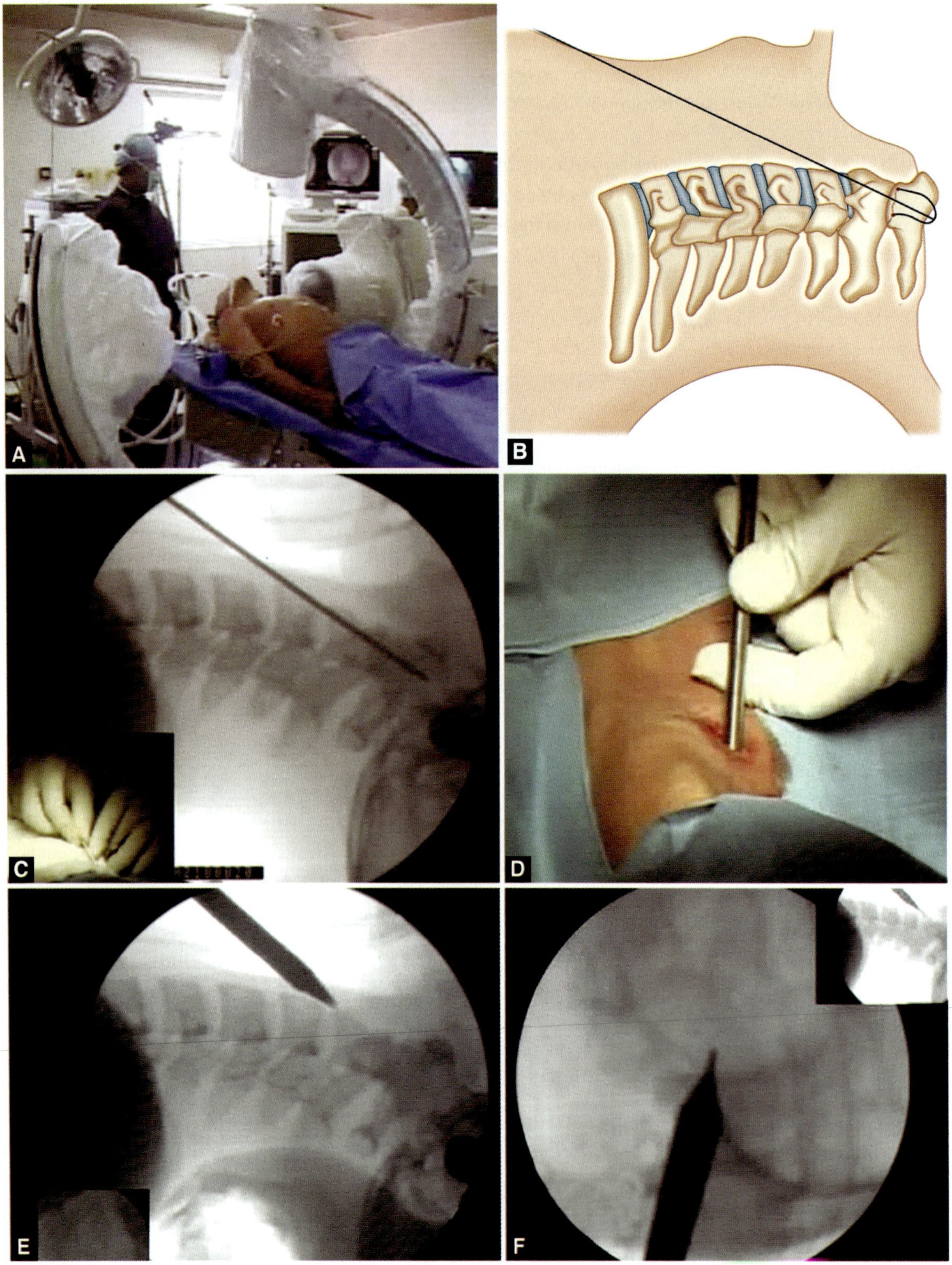

Figures 14.54A to F: (A) Positioning of two C-arms around the cervical spine; (B and C) The trajectory of the guidewire and the screw, and the skin incision are planned by placing it along the neck and checking it with the C-arm; (D to F) Through a standard Robinson approach at C5–C6, the drill sleeve is passed to reach the C2 base. This is confirmed in the AP and lateral fluoroscopy images.

and the reduction is assessed under fluoroscopic image. After achieving reduction, the head is strapped to the table with an adhesive tape to prevent movement of the head. Alternatively, the head and cervical spine can be stabilized in a Mayfield head rest. The line of skin incision from C1 to C4 in the midline is infiltrated with a mixture of local anesthetic and adrenaline.

A midline incision is made from C1 to C4 spinous process. Dissection is carried out in the midline through the ligamentum nuchae till the tips of the spinous process from C2 to C4. The paraspinal muscles are elevated subperiosteally from the spinous process and the lamina of C2 bilaterally till the tips of the lateral mass. A dissector is used to delineate the medial border of the C2 pars interarticularis, and the entry point for placement of a C2 pedicle screw is marked with a high-speed burr. This is in the cranial and medial quadrant of the isthmus surface of C2. The pilot hole is prepared with a 2.7 mm drill bit, just perforating the opposite cortex. The distal fragment is overdrilled with a 3.5 mm drill. The direction of the bit is approximately 20–30° in a convergent and cephalad direction, guided directly by the superior and medial surface of the C2 isthmus, respecting individual anatomic variations (Figs 14.38A to F). The drilling is performed in

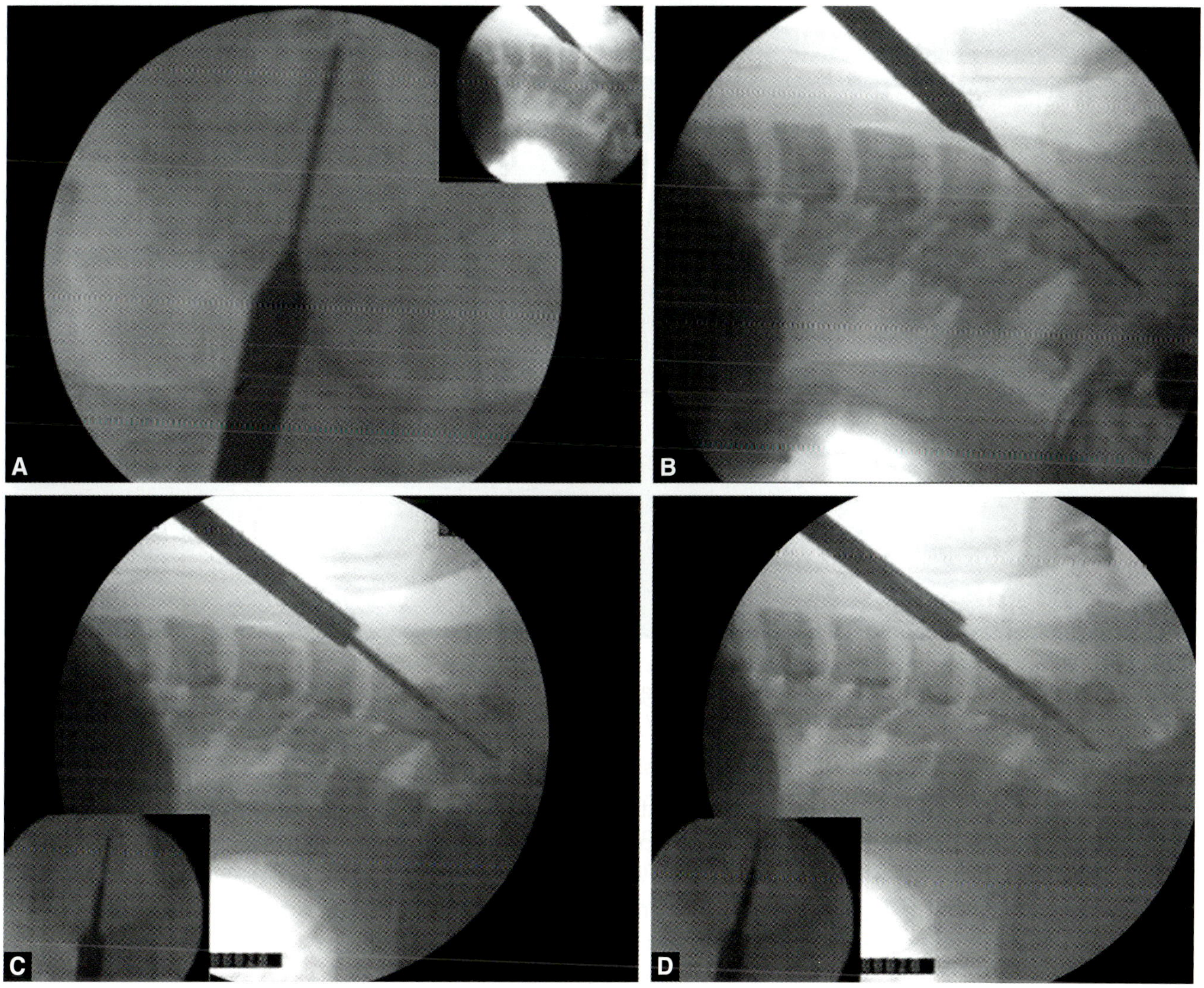

Figures 14.55A to D

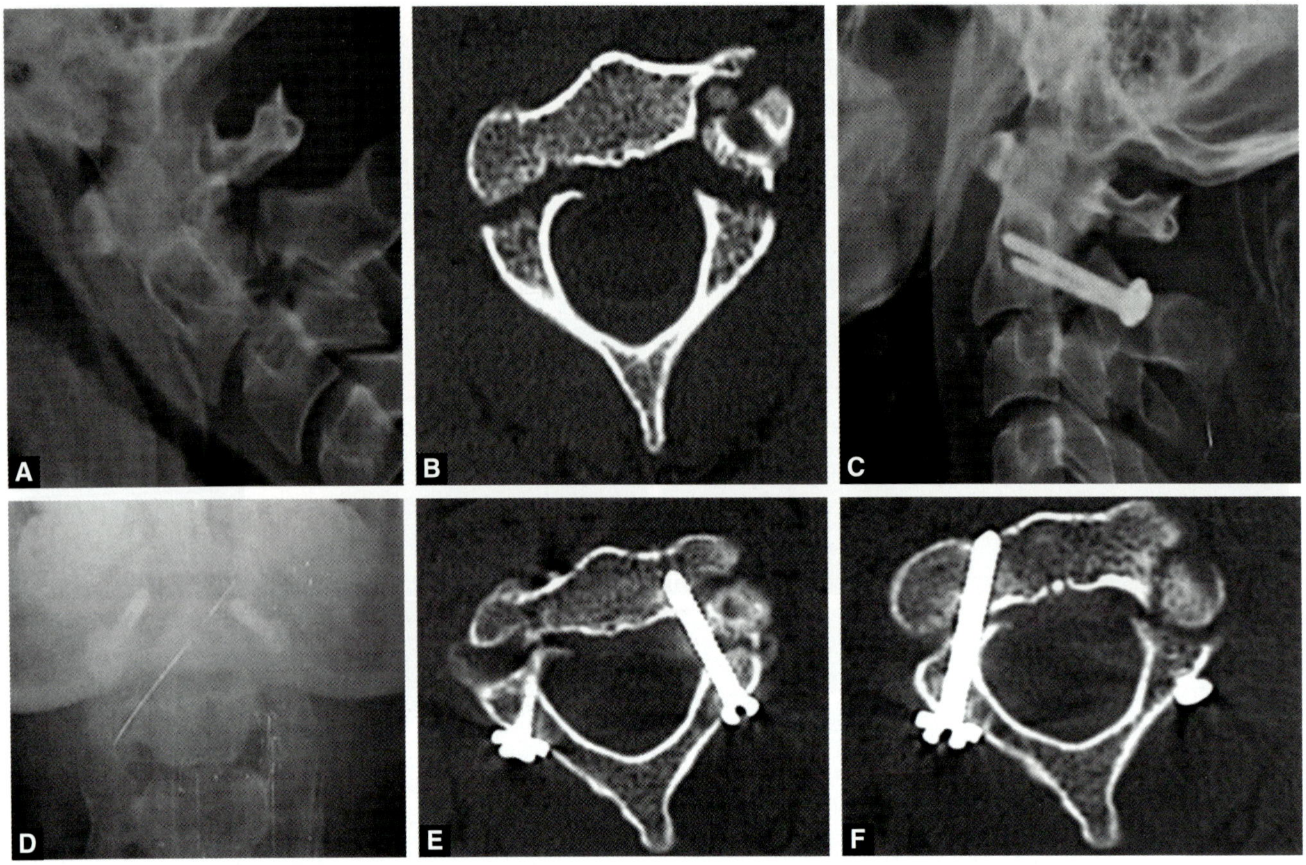

Figures 14.58A to F: (A) Lateral radiographs and (B) CT images indicate bipedicular pars fractures. (C and D) The fracture has been directly fixed with interfragmentary screws. (E and F) The axial images show good containment of the screws.

skin incision is made along the medial border of sternocleidomastoid centered over the involved level. The platysma splits in line with skin incision. The plane of dissection lies medial to the anterior border of sternocleidomastoid, between the carotid sheath laterally and the trachea and esophagus medially. The longus colli on either side are elevated from the vertebral bodies by gentle dissection. Self-retaining retractors are placed with the blades under the longus colli muscle. This facilitates the corpectomy while protecting the vital structures (Figs 14.59A to F).

Using an operative microscope, the discs cranial and caudal to the fractured vertebra are incised and removed. A rongeur may be used initially to remove large pieces of the comminuted vertebra in a piecemeal fashion. A small probe is used at regular intervals to assess the thickness of the remaining vertebra to complete the decompression. High-speed Rosen burrs, small-sized curettes and finally a diamond burr are used to thin the posterior cortex of the fractured vertebra. A 1 mm Kerrison's rongeur is then used to remove the wafer thin posterior cortical wall. The dura should be seen over the entire length of corpectomy defect devoid of any compression. Dissection lateral to the uncovertebral joints risks injury to the vertebral artery. Superior and inferior end plates are decorticated with high-speed Rosen burr and curettes to prepare a vascular bed for fusion. An appropriately-sized tricortical iliac crest graft is harvested for fusion. Preferably a titanium mesh cage of appropriate length filled with the bone graft saved during corpectomy can be used as it can avoid donor site morbidity. The cage/bone graft is tamped into position after traction is applied manually by the anesthetist. A titanium locking plate of adequate length is placed over the corpectomy site to secure it to the cephalad and

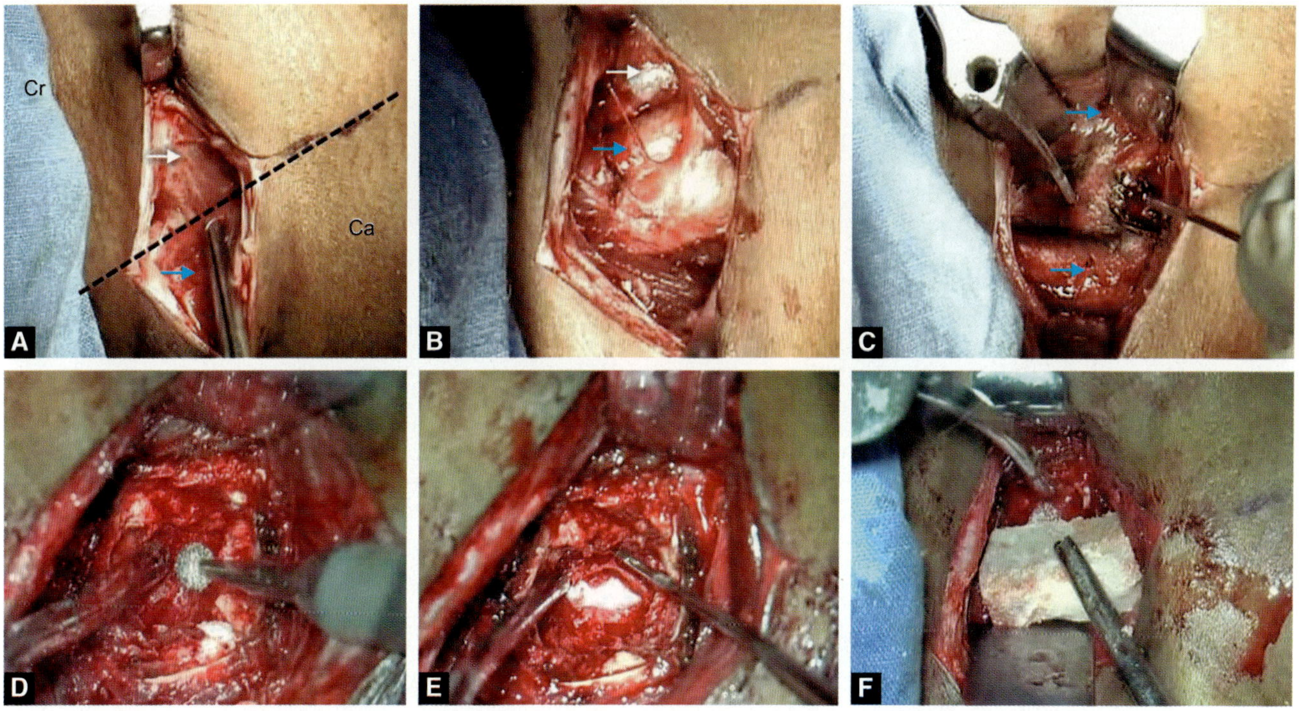

Figures 14.59A to F: Anterior cervical dissection for a corpectomy. (A) The midline is indicated by the solid black line. The dotted line indicates the anterior border of sternomastoid along which a vertical incision is made; (B) The plane between sternomastoid (blue arrow) and the strap muscles (white arrow) is identified. The next plane is developed between the carotid sheath (blue arrow) and the esophagus (white arrow); (C) The prevertebral fascia is opened between the two longus colli muscles (blue arrow) to expose the vertebra. The corpectomy is performed with burr and rongeurs to decompress the spinal cord; (D to F) An appropriate-sized tricortical iliac crest graft is harvested to reconstruct the defect (Cr: Cranial; Ca: Caudal).

caudad vertebra. A 2.5 mm drill bit is used to make drill holes to secure diagonally opposite screws under fluoroscopic guidance. The screws are tightened simultaneously till the rim of screw head is flush with the plate. Locking screws are placed after all the anchor screws are fully tightened. Final plate position is checked under image intensifier. Closure is completed routinely under a suction drain (Figs 14.60 and 14.61).

Technique 6: Lateral Mass Screw Fixation

Posterior plating utilizing lateral mass screw fixation has been widely accepted for treating the unstable cervical spine. Clinical studies have shown that posterior cervical plating results in a high rate of fusion. It provides comparable biomechanical stability when compared to anterior plating or traditional interspinous wiring techniques. A solid anatomic and radiographic knowledge may avoid or minimize anatomic complications during lateral mass screw insertion.

Several techniques of lateral mass screw placement have been developed. Each has its unique entrance point for screw insertion and screw trajectory (Figs 14.62A to F). The procedure is performed in the prone position, on bolsters with care taken to maintain normal cervical lordosis. The patient is preferably strapped in this position to prevent change in position during the procedure. The arms are taped by the side of the torso. Standard precautions to prevent pressure on the eyes and the superficial nerves must be taken.

Technique

Standard midline posterior exposure from C3 to C6 is carried out depending on the exact location of the fracture up to the lamina facet border taking care to preserve the muscular attachments to C2 and C7 spinous process. The dissection is carried out to expose the lateral border of the lateral mass. Levels are confirmed by fluoroscopy. The entry point is determined by the surgeon's preference

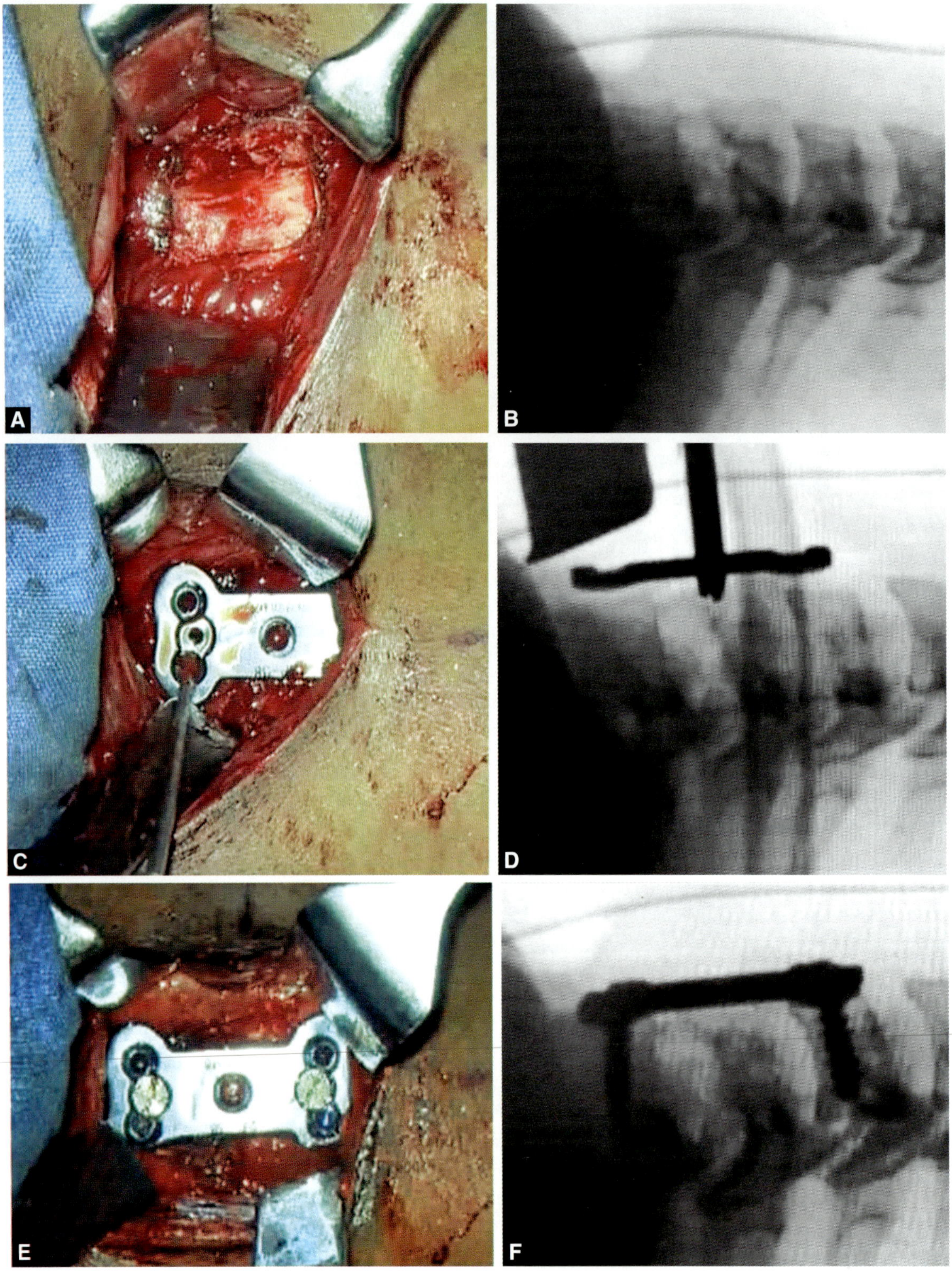

Figures 14.60A to F: (A and B) The graft has been used to reconstruct the anterior column defect; (C and D) An appropriate-sized locking plate is placed to check the length of the plate and screw dimensions; (E and F) The unicortical locking screws have been inserted into the superior and inferior vertebral bodies through the plate holding the graft in place.

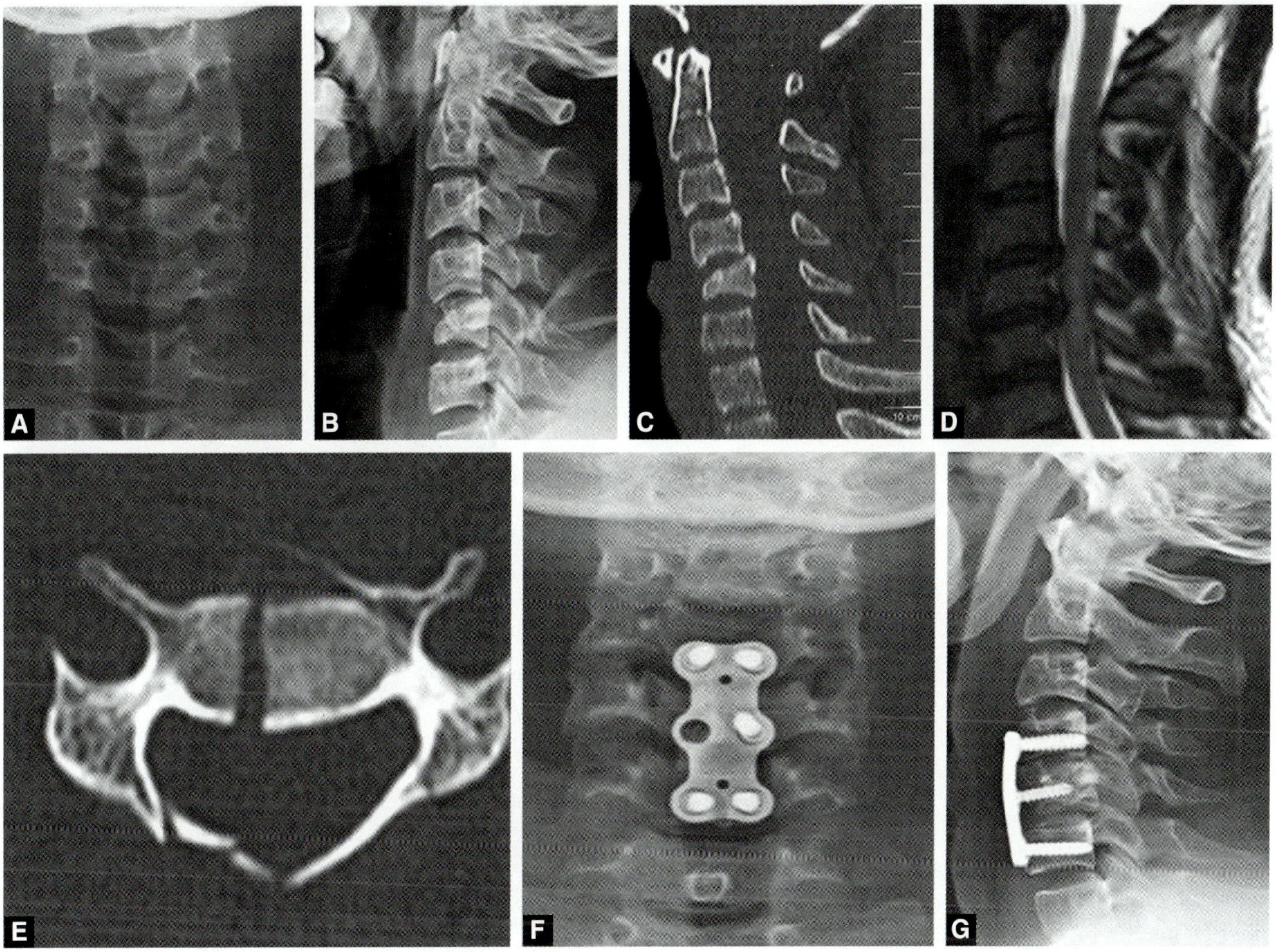

Figures 14.61A to G: (A) Anteroposterior (AP) and (B) lateral radiographs of a patient with split burst fracture of C5; (C) The sagittal, (D) axial CT images and (E) sagittal MR image show the extent of injury to the vertebral body and the presence of traumatic disc prolapse with cord edema; (F and G) The fracture has been stabilized through anterior cervical corpectomy, reconstruction with bone graft and stabilization with locking plates.

to the different techniques described in the literature (Figs 14.63 and 14.64). The author prefers the "An" technique of screw insertion. The entry point is located by a point 2 mm medial to the midpoint of a square defined by the lateral and medial borders of the lateral mass and the upper and lower articular facet. A small entry point is made using a 2 mm burr. A 2 mm drill with a drill guide having a drill-stop is then used to drill the screw hole. The drill is directed 15° superiorly and 30° laterally. The anterior cortex of the lateral mass need not necessarily be penetrated since unicortical screws have been shown to have equivalent biomechanical stability as that of bicortical screws. The screw is then measured and inserted. Longer screws can irritate the corresponding cervical nerve root. The lateral mass screws have to be parallel to the facet joint in the lateral image intensifier view. The direction of the screw can be ascertained by placing a Freer elevator into the corresponding facet joint. It may be necessary to probe and measure the screws but delay their insertion if decompression in the form of laminectomy is contemplated. This is advised because the screw heads tend to encroach on the operative field. The facet joints must then be prepared using a burr and can be grafted with bone graft from the spinous processes. The screws are now inserted into the pre-drilled tracks (Figs 14.65A to D). The rods are contoured to the cervical lordosis and tightened with nuts.

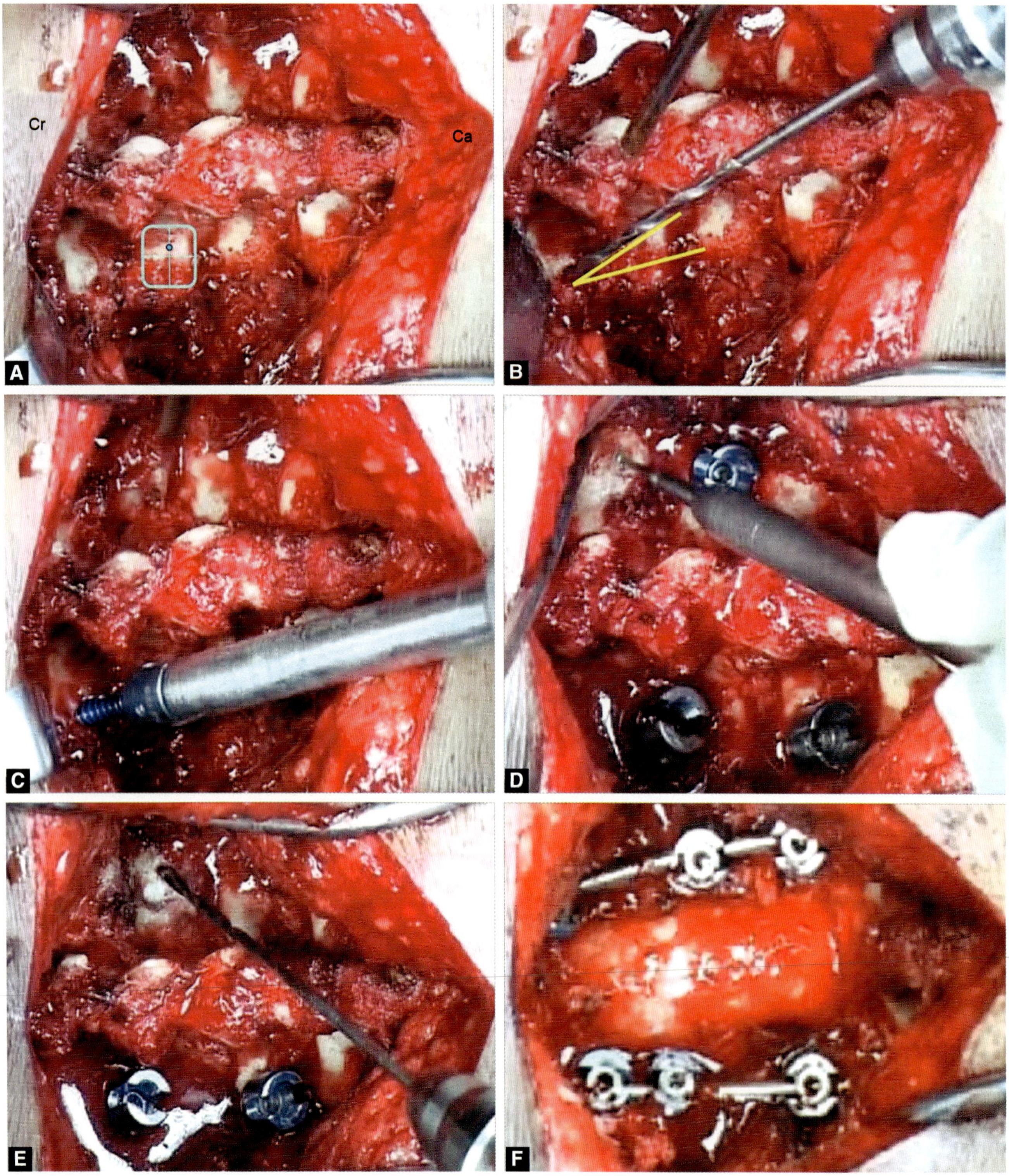

Figures 14.62A to F: Technique of lateral mass screw fixation. (A) The entry point for the lateral mass screw is in the medial inferior quadrant of the lateral mass (about 2 mm from the center) and is created with a burr; (B to F) The drill is guided about 15° cephalad and 30° laterally along the facet joint. An appropriate-sized screw is then inserted in the drilled track.

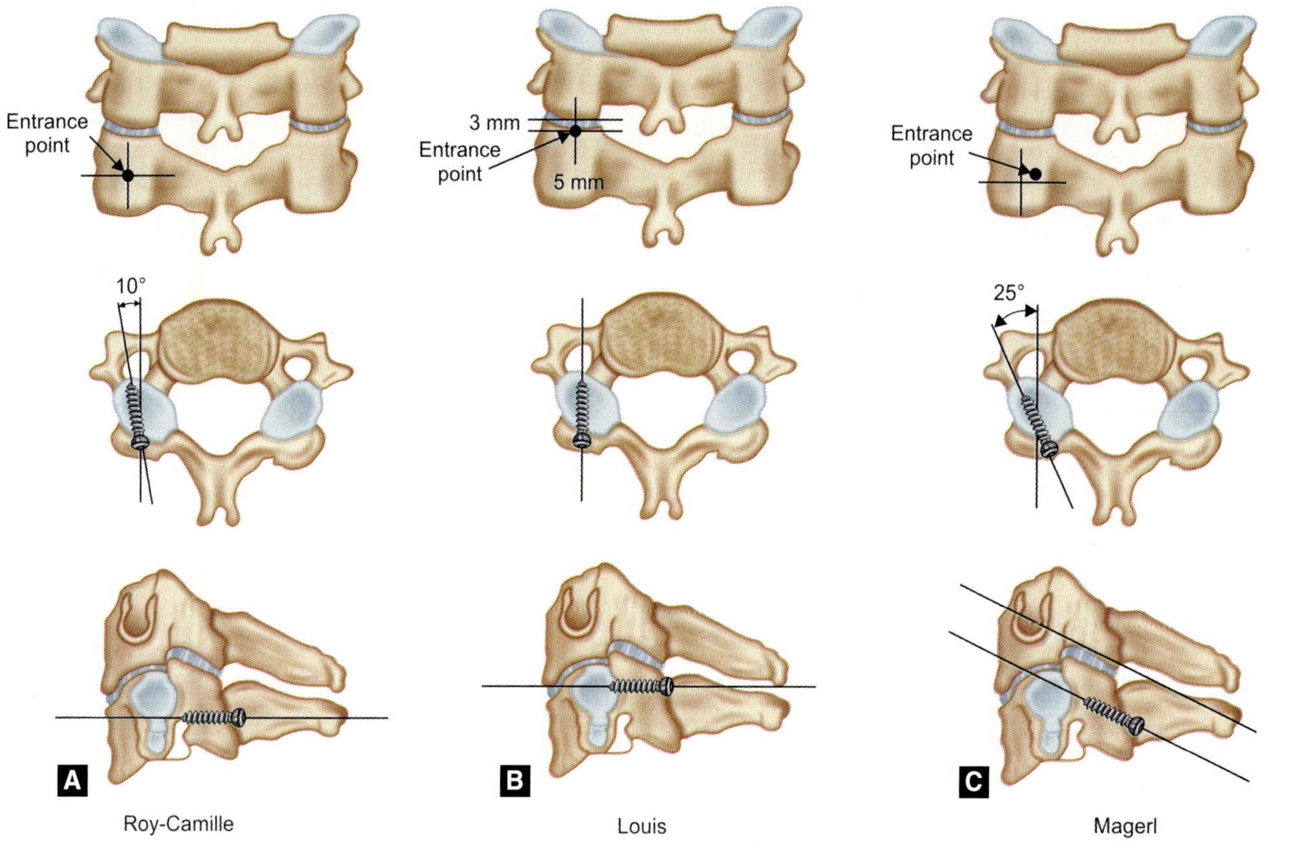

Figures 14.63A to C: Different techniques of lateral mass screw fixation: (A) Roy Camille: The entrance point for screw insertion should be located at the top of the lateral hill of the lateral mass, exactly at its midpoint. The entrance point is then drilled with a 2 mm bit, perpendicular to the vertebral plane and 10° lateral to the sagittal plane. The drill hole is further tapped with a 3.5 mm tap, and a contoured Roy-Camille cervical plate of appropriate length is secured with cortical screws of 3.5 mm diameter; (B) Louis: The starting point for screw insertion is situated at the intersection of a vertical line 5 mm medial to the lateral margin of the inferior facet and a horizontal line 3 mm below the inferior margin of the inferior facet. The screw hole is drilled with a 2.8 mm bit, and the drill bit is directed strictly parallel to both sagittal and axial planes of the vertebra. The screw should not penetrate the ventral cortex, otherwise the nerve roots directly anterior to the superior facet may be at increased risk; (C) Magerl: The screw entrance point is to be slightly medial and cranial to the posterior center of the lateral mass and the orientation of the screw be 20–30° lateral and parallel to the adjacent facet.

Source: Redrawn from Ebraheim N. Posterior lateral mass screw fixation: Anatomic and radiographic considerations. The University of Pennsylvania Orthopaedic Journal Univ Penn Ortho J. 1999;12:66-72.

MANAGEMENT OF CERVICAL SPINAL INJURIES: Pearls and Pitfalls

- The ATLS principles of management of a trauma patient should be followed during pre-hospital resuscitation and emergency room management.
- It is essential to maintain rigid cervical immobilization and keep the patient on a back board during initial evaluation.
- The transverse ligament is important for the stability of the atlantoaxial joint. Its integrity should always be evaluated in fractures of the atlas, dens and rotary subluxations.
- Traction is contraindicated for Type IIA spondylolisthesis injuries of C2, fractures in ankylosing spondylitis and distraction injuries of upper cervical spine.
- Patients with unilateral and bilateral facet dislocations require MRI before reduction to evaluate for a herniated disc. This is more important, especially if a patient is not awake and alert, and unable to cooperate with neurologic assessment during reduction maneuvers.

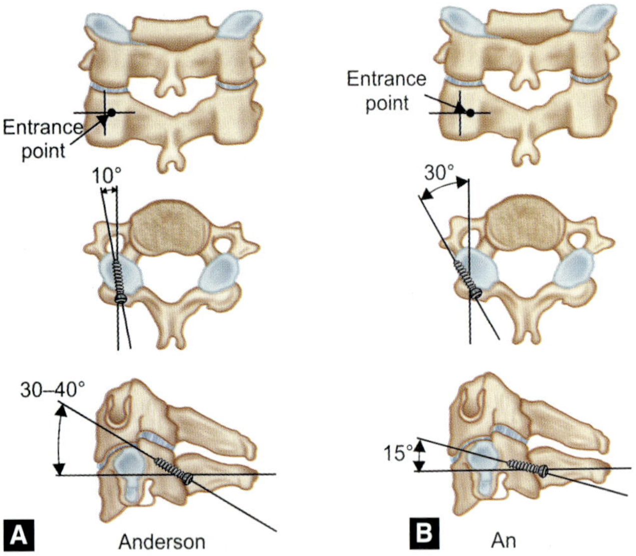

Figures 14.64A and B: Different techniques of lateral mass screw fixation. (A) Anderson's modification of Magerl's technique. The starting point for screw insertion is 1 mm medial to the center of the four boundaries of the lateral mass and screw direction should be 30–40° cephalad (parallel to the facet joint) and 10° lateral. The screw hole tapping should be limited to the dorsal cortex to achieve sound bicortical bony purchase; (B) An et al. The screw direction should be approximately 30° lateral and 15° cephalad starting 1 mm medial to the center of the lateral mass. *Source*: Redrawn from Ebraheim N. Posterior lateral mass screw fixation: Anatomic and radiographic considerations. Univ Penn Ortho J. 1999;12: 66-72.

Outcomes

Injuries of the upper cervical spine can be a major cause of morbidity and mortality. Mortality has decreased in the last two decades due to improvements in automobile safety measures and advances in spinal stabilization techniques. The anatomy of the upper cervical spine is unique with significant contributions from both bony and ligamentous structures contributing to the stability. Ligamentous injuries of the atlanto-occipital joint and the transverse atlantal ligament have a poor intention for spontaneous healing and hence would require surgical stabilization. Most bony injuries of the occiput and atlas tend to heal in 6–8 weeks even with nonoperative treatment methods. Specific unstable patterns like the Type II odontoid fracture, traumatic spondylolisthesis of axis with instability and Jefferson's fracture with transverse alar ligament (TAL) injury require surgical stabilization.

Forty percent of subaxial spinal injuries are associated with neurological deficits. Patients with incomplete neurological deficit have a better prognosis for neurological recovery. Except in patients with worsening neurology, there is no indication for emergency surgery. However, dislocations and subluxations are preferably reduced as early as possible with controlled and expedient traction to align the cervical spine and decrease the

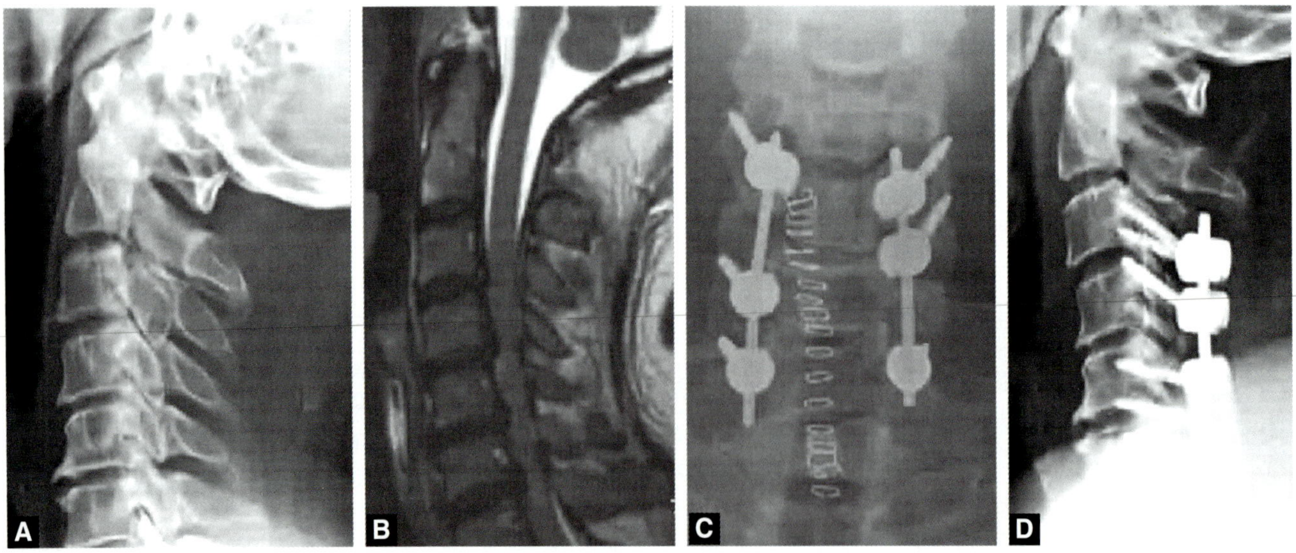

Figures 14.65A to D: This 57-year-old patient presented with neck pain, incomplete neurological deficit (ASIA C) following an injury. Lateral radiograph did not reveal any spinal fracture or instability. Sagittal MR image showed multilevel spondylotic changes with cord compression. The clinical presentation and radiological images were typical of central cord syndrome and hence treated with cervical laminectomy and posterior lateral mass screw fixation.

pressure on the spinal cord. Patients with complete neurological deficit have a poor prognosis for neurological improvement and survival. The purposes of surgical treatment in these patients are mainly vertebral stabilization for easier rehabilitation and providing a better milieu for the spinal cord to recover from the injury. Apart from the role played by primary injury mechanisms on the spinal cord damage, secondary injuries like hypoxia, oxidative stress, mitochondrial injury, and inflammation play a significant role in perpetuating the injury zone. Current research efforts are mainly focussed toward ameliorating the effects of secondary injury insults. The role of high-dose steroids in preventing these insults is still controversial and newer drugs like Riluzole are being experimentally studied. The role of stem cells in both the acute and chronic spinal cord injuries is still in experimental stages without any proven clinical benefit at present.

Complications

Complications related to the Injury

The most frequent complication following cervical spine injury is a missed diagnosis. A missed spine injury can have devastating long-term consequences and hence in all blunt trauma patients, a spine injury must be presumed until it is proven otherwise. A thorough clinical and radiological assessment must be performed to identify the cervical injury and also to rule out associated injuries.

Secondary neurological deterioration is reported in 6% of patients presenting with cervical spine trauma.[26] Continued spinal immobilization during emergency treatment, maintenance of oxygenation and reversal of systemic hypotension, early identification of the spinal injury and urgent restoration of spinal alignment are the key preventive measures.

Vertebral artery injuries occur in up to 11% of patients with cervical injury.[27] Flexion-distraction and flexion-compression injuries to the cervical spine are the frequent causes (19.7%) of vertebral artery injury.[28] Stretching or compression of the vertebral artery are the mechanisms by which this injury can occur. Most such injuries are asymptomatic and hence missed. Symptoms such as dysarthria, dizziness, diplopia, dysphagia, blurred vision and tinnitus may appear immediately or even upto 3 months following the injury. Magnetic resonance angiogram is used to diagnose this injury in a symptomatic patient. In patients with unifacet/bifacet dislocations when surgical procedures such as pedicle screw fixation are planned that may endanger the normal vertebral artery, a magnetic resonance anagiography (MRA) must be done. In asymptomatic patients, no formal treatment is recommended. In symptomatic patients, the treatment options range from fibrinolysis with streptokinase to anticoagulation with heparin and warfarin to surgical treatment.[29] When surgery is required for a dissecting vertebral artery, ligation of the injured artery proximal and distal to the site of lesion is recommended if there is adequate collateral blood flow.

Deep vein thrombosis and pulmonary embolism are seen in 14.5% and 5% amongst patients with spinal cord injury.[30] Diagnosis is often difficult due to the absence of presenting symptoms. Graduated compression stockings and sequential calf compression pumps must be started immediately. Anticoagulation is the mainstay of treatment but should be delayed until any paraspinal and epidural hematomas have settled and surgical intervention has been completed.

Complications due to Lateral Mass Fixation

The complications associated with lateral mass screw fixation include anatomical and biomechanical. Potential anatomic complications include injury to the spinal cord, vertebral artery, spinal nerves, and facet joints. Biomechanical complications involve screw loosening, screw pullout, or screw failure. Injury to the spinal nerve is the only reported neurological complication with lateral mass screw insertion. The reported incidence of spinal nerve injury with lateral mass screw insertion varies greatly in different studies. Levine et al. reported that 6 of 72 patients developed radicular symptoms following posterior lateral mass screw placement.[31] Based on a review of 72 cases, Heller et al. documented that the incidence of spinal nerve injury associated with posterior plating and lateral mass screw fixation was 0.6%.[32] Graham et al. reported a high (6.1%) incidence of nerve root complication with lateral mass screw insertion. They found that 10 of 164 lateral mass screws were misplaced in 21 consecutive patients.[33] Nerve root injury was attributed to improper placement of excessively long screws.

chronic injury, the traction was increased slowly to 15 pounds over 24 hours. The patient's neurological status was carefully and serially monitored. Lateral radiographs were taken which showed partial reduction of the fracture.

Now the options were either to do an anterior odontoid screw fixation or to do a posterior fusion. Since the fracture is only partially reducible, an anterior screw fixation is not possible technically. Hence the patient was planned for a posterior reduction and C1–C2 fusion. Under general anesthesia, the patient was placed prone on a Mayfield frame. Through a standard posterior midline approach, the posterior elements of C1 and C2 were exposed. Based on anatomical landmarks and image intensifier guidance, C1 lateral mass screws and C2 pedicle screws were inserted. The C1 screw head was placed slightly proud than C2 screws. This would help to correct the partial C1–C2 subluxation. Straight rods were placed over the screw heads and tightened with nuts. The position of the screws and the C1–C2 anatomy was checked in the lateral image intensifier. The posterior elements of C1 and C2 were decorticated and autograft harvested from the iliac crest was placed over the bed to aid in fusion (Figs 14.66A to F). The patient started showing neurological recovery after the surgery.

The important principles in this case are:

1. A Type II odontoid fracture is an unstable spinal injury with potential for displacement. Even in patients being treated conservatively, it is advisable to perform periodic radiographs to look for displacement. Patients with neurological deficit would benefit from early surgery.
2. In patients presenting late after the injury, a short period of skull traction would help to reduce the fracture.
3. In patients where a complete reduction can not be achieved, an anterior odontoid screw fixation can not be performed.

Case 2: Neglected C2–C3 Fracture

This 62-year-old gentleman had suffered a polytrauma with multiple injuries to the lower limb and pelvis. Three

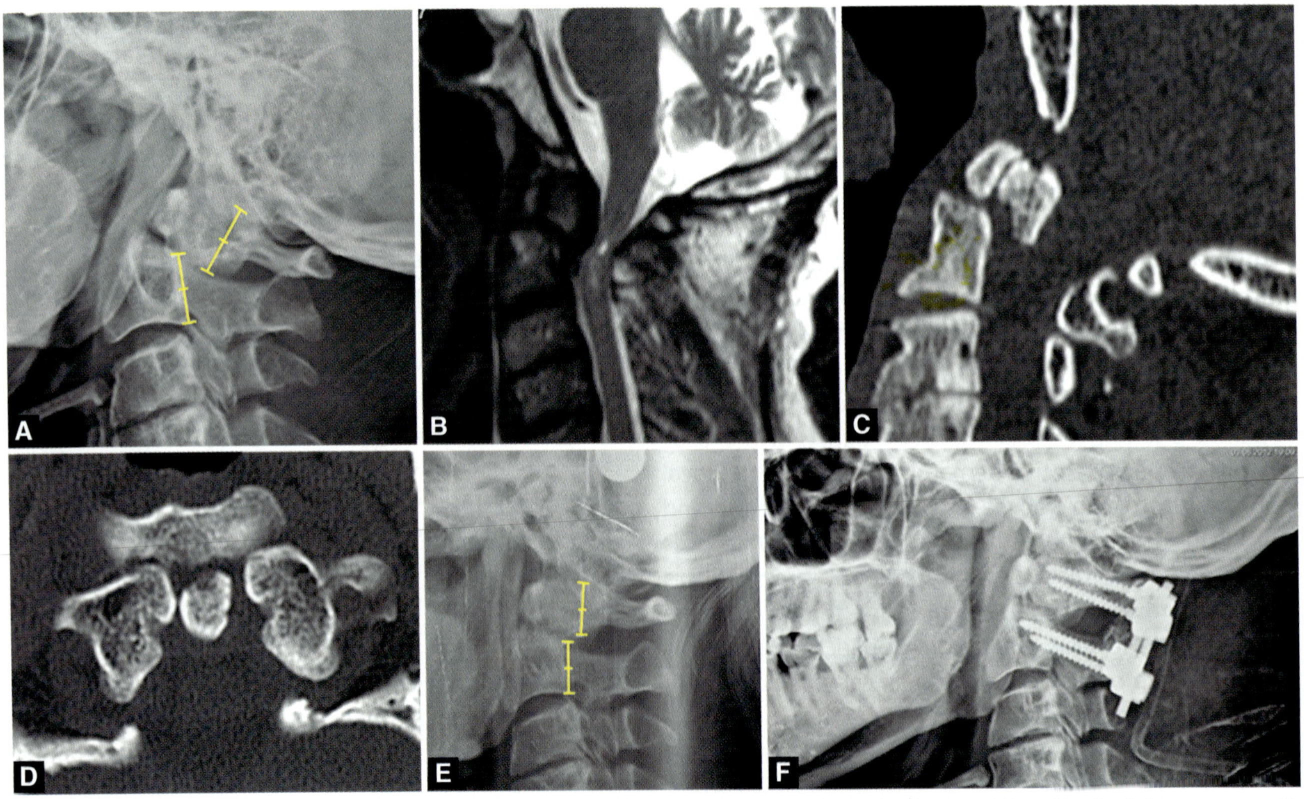

Figures 14.66A to F: (A to C) Lateral radiograph and sagittal images show a posteriorly displaced Type II odontoid fracture with cord compression; (D) The axial CT image indicates that the proximal fragment has been displaced posteriorly; (E) Lateral radiograph after applying traction indicates that the angulation and displacement of fracture has reduced significantly; (F) Postoperative lateral radiograph shows C1, C2 screws with partial reduction of fracture and fusion with bone grafting.

weeks after the injury, when the patient was mobilized gradually, he started developing pain in the neck. Lateral radiographs taken revealed a C2–C3 unifacetal subluxation with a resultant segmental kyphosis and "swan-neck" deformity. Computed tomography and MRI scan were performed which confirmed the findings. The patient was neurologically intact. He was treated by anterior cervical discectomy and fusion with plating. This was performed through a standard Smith Robinson approach through the right side. Technically it is difficult to access above the C2 base with this approach. However, with a vertical incision and proximally undermining the platysma , it is possible to reach the C2–C3 disc space. After discectomy with a microscope, appropriate-sized iliac crest graft was harvested from the right iliac crest, placed in the C2–C3 disc space, and a 26 mm locking plate was used to fix the fracture. The subluxation was only partially correctable because of the chronicity of the injury (Figs 14.67A to F). However, adequate bony approximation could be achieved between C2–C3 and hence the reduction was accepted.

The important learning points in this case are:

1. It is crucial to look for cervical injuries in patients with "polytrauma", especially with distracting injuries.
2. A standard Smith Robinson approach is adequate in most patients to access the C2–C3 disc space.
3. A partial reduction is acceptable if there is sufficient bone contact between the C2–C3 bones, especially if it is chronic.
4. An appropriate-sized bone graft or cage should be placed in the interbody space to correct the segmental kyphosis.

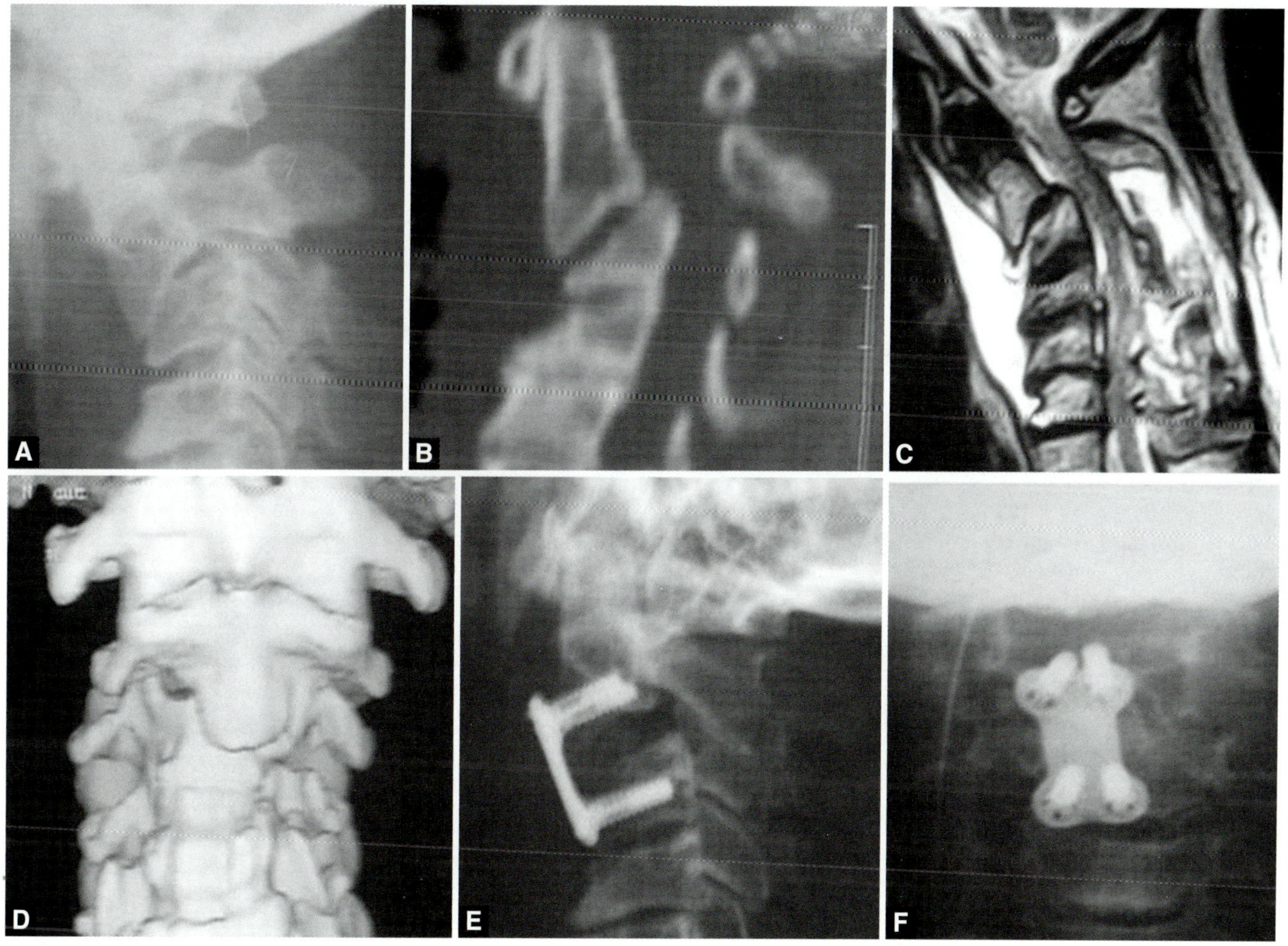

Figures 14.67A to F: (A and B) A 62-year-old gentleman presented with C2–C3 facetal dislocation 3 weeks after the injury; (C and D) MRI and CT scan—cord compression is seen on the MRI; (E and F) Initial skull traction led to partial reduction. The patient underwent an anterior C2–C3 discectomy, fusion and fixation with locking plate and screws. Note that the reduction could not be fully achieved.

Case 3: Prominent Lateral Mass Screws with Cervical Radiculopathy

This 63-year-old gentleman was admitted in the emergency department with difficulty in using the upper limbs after he sustained a fall in his home the previous day. The patient was apparently normal before the injury except for occasional neck pain and stiffness. Presently on clinical examination, he had grade 3 power in the upper limbs and normal power in the lower limbs. He had loss of manual dexterity in both the hands. Radiographs did not reveal any bony injury but there was a mild subluxation at C3–C4 level with extensive spondylotic changes.

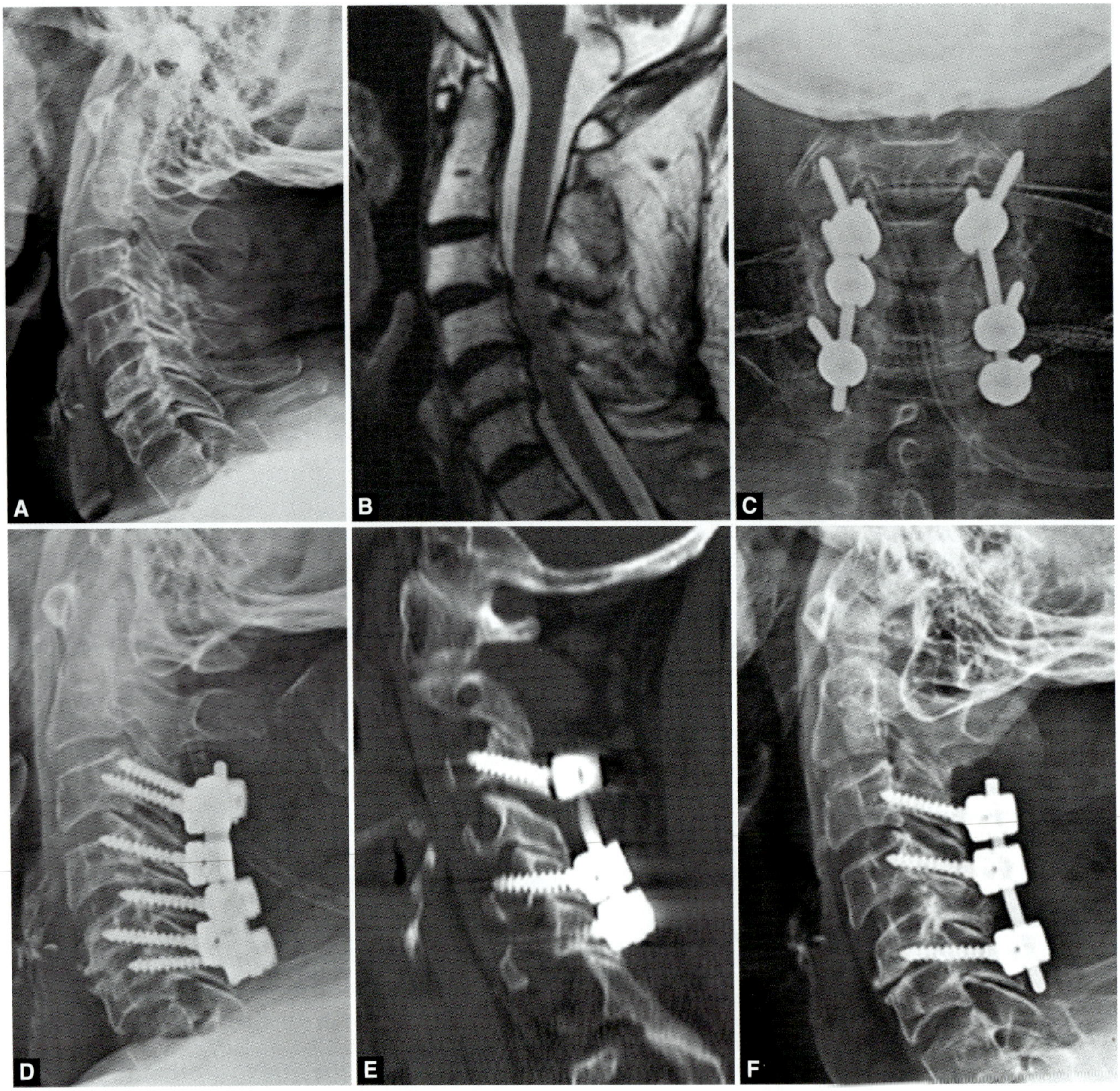

Figures 14.68A to F: (A and B) Lateral radiograph and sagittal MRI scan reveal a C3–C4 subluxation and spondylotic myelopathy with signal intensity changes suggestive of cord edema; (C and D) AP and lateral radiographs show lateral mass screw fixation; (E) Sagittal CT image shows that the right C5 screw has violated the neural foramina; (F) The right-sided lateral mass screws have been removed leaving the left side screws alone.

Magnetic resonance imaging revealed cervical spondylotic myelopathy from C3 to C5 with cord edema at C3–C4 level. The clinical presentation and radiological features are typical of central cord syndrome. The patient had sustained a hyperextension injury in the setting of cervical spondylotic stenosis with pinching of the cord at the level of C3–C4.

The problems in this patient were:

1. Cervical spondylotic traumatic myelopathy
2. Incomplete neurological deficit
3. Instability at C3–C4

The patient was treated by posterior cervical laminectomy from C3–C6 and lateral screw fixation at C3, C5 and C6 on the right side and C3, C4 and C6 on the left side. Postoperatively, the patient's neurological status improved gradually. He started developing neuropathic pain along the right C5 nerve root. By the end of 2 months, the radicular pain worsened significantly and hence a CT scan was performed. The CT images showed that the right C5 screw was long violating the neural foramina with resultant pressure on the C5 nerve root. Since it was 2 months after the surgery, it was decided to remove the screws on the right side. After removal of the screws, the patient's arm pain improved tremendously (Figs 14.68A to F).

References

1. Rajasekaran S, Rishi MK, Shetty AP. Spinal fractures. Mercer's Textbook of Orthopaedics and Trauma, 10th edition. UK: Hodder Arnold; 2012. pp. 439-66.
2. Prasad VS, Schwartz A, Bhutani R, et al. Characteristics of injuries to the cervical spine and spinal cord in polytrauma patient population: experience from a regional trauma unit. Spinal Cord. 1999;37(8):560-8.
3. Hahn YH. (2004). Cervical spine fractures. [online] Available from http://chorus.rad.mcw.edu/doc/00907.html [Accessed June 2012].
4. Braakman M, Braakman R. Hyperflexion sprain of the cervical spine. Follow-up of 45 cases. Acta Orthop Scand. 1987;58:388-93.
5. Jackson AB, Dijkers M, Devivo MJ, et al. A demographic profile of new traumatic spinal cord injuries: change and stability over 30 years. Arch Phys Med Rehabil. 2004;85: 1740-8.
6. Calenoff L, Chessare JW, Rogers LF, et al. Multiple level spinal injuries: importance of early recognition. AJR Am J Roentgenol. 1978;130:665-9.
7. Vaccaro AR, Kreidl KO, Pan W, et al. Usefulness of MRI in isolated upper cervical spine fractures in adults. J Spinal Disord. 1998;11:289-93.
8. Woodring JH, Lee C. Limitations of cervical radiography in the evaluation of acute cervical trauma. J Trauma. 1993; 34:32-9.
9. Harris JH, Carson GC, Wagner LK. Radiologic diagnosis of traumatic occipitovertebral dissociation. 1. Normal occipitovertebral relationships on lateral radiographs of supine subjects. AJR Am J Roentgenol. 1994;162:881-6.
10. Anderson PA, Montesano PX. Morphology and treatment of occipital condyle fractures. Spine (Phila Pa 1976). 1988; 13:731-6.
11. Traynelis VC, Marano GD, Dunker RO, et al. Traumatic atlanto-occipital dislocation. Case report. J Neurosurg. 1986;65:863-70.
12. Levine AM, Edwards CC. Fractures of the atlas. J Bone Joint Surg Am. 1991;73:680-91.
13. Anderson LD, D'Alonzo RT. Fractures of the odontoid process of the axis. J Bone Joint Surg Am. 1974;56:1663-74.
14. Effendi B, Roy D, Cornish B, et al. Fractures of the ring of the axis. A classification based on the analysis of 131 cases. J Bone Joint Surg Br. 1981;63:319-27.
15. Allen BL, Ferguson RL, Lehmann TR, et al. A mechanistic classification of closed, indirect fractures and dislocations of the lower cervical spine. Spine (Phila Pa 1976). 1982;7: 1-27.
16. Garfin SR, Botte MJ, Waters RL, et al. Complications in the use of the halo fixation device. J Bone Joint Surg Am. 1986;68:320-5.
17. Koivikko MP, Myllynen P, Karjalainen M, et al. Conservative and operative treatment in cervical burst fractures. Arch Orthop Trauma Surg. 2000;120:448-51.
18. Fisher CG, Dvorak MF, Leith J, et al. Comparison of outcomes for unstable lower cervical flexion teardrop fractures managed with halo thoracic vest versus anterior corpectomy and plating. Spine (Phila pa 1976). 2002;27: 160-6.
19. Guest J, Eleraky MA, Apostolides PJ, et al. Traumatic central cord syndrome: results of surgical management. J Neurosurg. 2002;97:25-32.
20. Ruf M, Melcher R, Harms J. Transoral reduction and osteosynthesis C1 as a function preserving option in the treatment of unstable Jefferson fractures. Spine (Phila Pa 1976). 2004;29:823-7.
21. Koller H, Resch H, Tauber M, et al. A biomechanical rationale for C1-ring osteosynthesis as treatment for displaced Jefferson burst fractures with incompetency of the transverse atlantal ligament. Eur Spine J. 2010;19:1288-98.
22. Magerl F, Seemann P. Stabile posterior fusion of the atlas and axis by transarticular screw fixation. In: Kehr P, Weidner

A (Eds). Cervical Spine. Strassbourg, Wien, New York: Springer Verlag; 1986. pp. 322-7.
23. Grob D, Jeanneret B, Aebi M, et al. Complications of atlantoaxial fusion with transarticular screw fixation. J Bone Joint Surg Br. 1993;75:972-6.
24. Harms J, Melcher RP. Posterior C1-C2 fusion with polyaxial screw and rod fixation. Spine (Phila Pa 1976). 2001; 26(22):2467-71.
25. Gallie W. Fractures and dislocations of the cervical spine. Am J Surg. 1939;46:495-9.
26. Harrop JS, Sharan AD, Vaccaro AR, et al. The cause of neurologic deterioration after acute cervical spinal cord injury. Spine (Phila Pa 1976). 2001;26:340-6.
27. Inamasu J, Guiot BH. Vertebral artery injury after blunt cervical trauma: an update. Surg Neurol. 2006;65:238-46.
28. Giacobetti FB, Vaccaro AR, Bos-Giacobetti MA, et al. Vertebral artery occlusion associated with cervical spine trauma. A prospective analysis. Spine (Phila Pa 1976). 1997; 22:188-92.
29. Deen HG Jr, McGirr SJ. Vertebral artery injury associated with cervical spine fracture. Report of two cases. Spine (Phila Pa 1976). 1992;17:230-4.
30. Merli GJ, Crabbe S, Paluzzi RJ, et al. Etiology, incidence and prevention of deep vein thrombosis in acute spinal cord injury. Arch Phy Med Rehabil. 1993;74:1199-205.
31. Levine AM, Mazel C, Roy-Camille R. Management of fracture separations of the articular mass using posterior cervical plating. Spine (Phila Pa 1976). 1992;17:S447-54.
32. Heller JG, Carlson GD, Abitbol JJ, et al. Anatomic comparison of the Roy-Camille and Magerl techniques for screw placement in the lower cervical spine. Spine (Phila Pa 1976). 1991;16:S552-7.
33. Graham AW, Swank ML, Kinard RE, et al. Posterior cervical arthrodesis and stabilization with a lateral mass plate: clinical and computed tomographic evaluation of lateral mass screw placement and associated complications. Spine (Phila Pa 1976). 1996;21:323-9.

Chapter 15

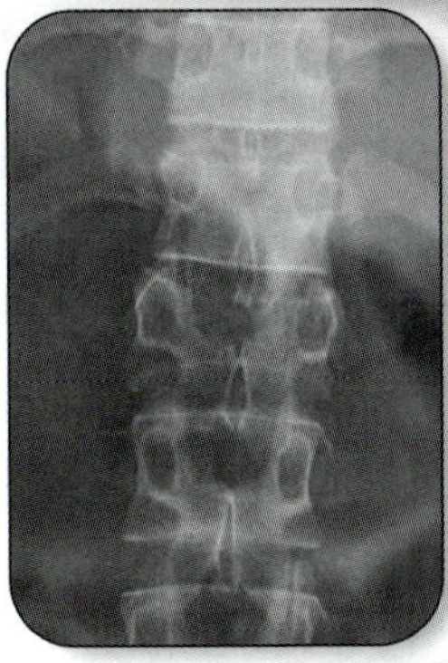

Thoracic and Lumbar Spine Fractures and Dislocations

S Rajasekaran, Rishi Kanna, Ajoy Prasad Shetty

Chapter Outline

Introduction

Classification

- Boehler's Classification
- Column Concept
- Denis Classification
- Allen-Ferguson Classification
- McAfee's Classification
- AO Classification
- Thoracolumbar Injury Classification System
- Load Sharing Classification
- Concept of Instability

Diagnosis

- Compression Fractures
- Burst Fractures
- Unstable Thoracolumbar Injuries

Management and Surgical Indications

- Compression Fractures
- Burst Fractures
- Unstable Thoracolumbar Injuries

Surgical Techniques

- Technique 1: Percutaneous Stabilization
- Technique 2: Anterior Decompression and Fixation
- Technique 3: Posterior Decompression and Fixation

Outcomes

Complications

- Posterior Approach
- Anterior Approach
- Chronic Complications

Complication Cases

- Case 1: Post-traumatic Kyphosis
- Case 2: Implant Failure with Worsening Kyphosis
- Case 3: Failure to Recognize Fracture Patterns
- Case 4: Missed Systemic Injury in a Polytrauma Patient

Summary

Introduction

Fractures of the thoracic and lumbar region constitute a spectrum of injuries ranging from undisplaced fractures to fracture dislocations (Figs 15.1A to D). Anatomically and functionally, the thoracic and lumbar spine can be divided into three regions—thoracic spine (T1–T10), thoracolumbar junction (T11-L2) and lumbar spine (L3–L5). The upper thoracic spine is relatively stiff due to the small intervertebral discs, coronal orientation of facet joints and the presence of the ribcage allowing only small amounts of motion. The rigidity of the upper thoracic spine requires high degrees of energy to produce fractures and dislocations and the narrow spinal canal in this region predisposes to spinal cord damage and neurological deficit. Since the thoracic spine is attached to the ribs and sternum, concomitant injuries of these structures are also common. The lumbar spine, on the other hand, allows flexion and extension movements due to the height of the discs, sagittal orientation of the facet joints and the absence of the rib cage. The relatively lesser incidence of neurological injury following lumbar fractures has been attributed to the large size of the neural canal and the greater resilience of the cauda equina nerve roots.

Injuries to the thoracolumbar spine are usually the result of high-energy blunt trauma. Sixty-five percent of thoracolumbar fractures occur due to motor vehicle injuries and fall from a height, with the remainder contributed by sports injuries and violence.[1] Approximately 50% of all thoracic and lumbar fractures occur at the thoracolumbar junction. The factors contributing to the higher incidence of fractures at the thoracolumbar junction are: (a) thoracolumbar junction is the transition point between the rigid thoracic rib cage and the more mobile lumbar spine, (b) change of sagittal alignment from kyphosis to lordosis resulting in more stress on the anterior and middle columns and (c) change in facet orientation from coronal in the thoracic spine to a sagittal alignment in the lumbar spine thus allowing for greater flexion and extension motion. Neurological injury complicates 15–20% of fractures at the thoracolumbar junction.[2]

Classification

Biomechanics of the load bearing and range-of-motion forms the basis of understanding the spinal injuries, and their classification systems. Biomechanics also form the basis of understanding instability, and surgical decision making regarding indications and appropriate methods for stabilization. The classification of thoracolumbar fractures has evolved over the years as our understanding of the biomechanical stability, mechanism of injury and identification of stability has improved.

Boehler's Classification

Boehler recognized five different injury categories which described the most common injury patterns affecting the thoracolumbar spine.[3] He delineated five categories as compression injuries, flexion-distraction injuries, extension fractures, shear fractures and rotational injuries. Watson-Jones first introduced the concept of instability and described that the integrity of the posterior ligamentous complex is essential for spinal stability.[4] He made additions to Boehler's work and proposed a modified classification system accounting for the concept of instability and its effect on the treatment of thoracolumbar injuries. He classified fractures into three major patterns with seven subtypes (the three major patterns were simple wedge fractures, comminuted fractures and fracture dislocations).

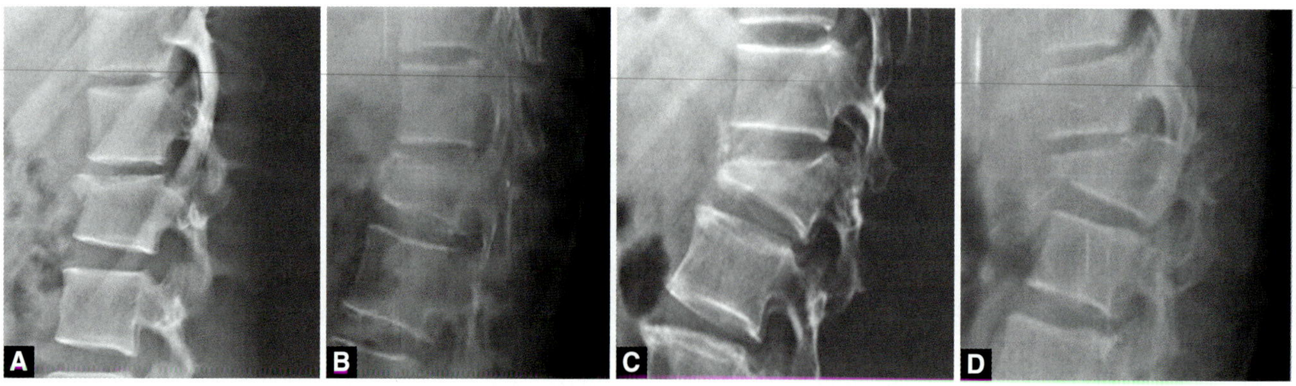

Figures 15.1A to D: The spectrum of thoracolumbar fractures. (A) Simple wedge compression fractures; (B) Burst fracture; (C) Flexion-distraction injury; (D) Fracture dislocation.

Column Concept

In 1949, Nicoll attempted to further define the concept of stability using an anatomical classification.[5] The concept of stability depending on the damage to anatomical structures was novel and he felt that the major determinant of stability was the integrity of the interspinous ligament. Holdsworth expanded Nicoll's system and revolutionized the thoracolumbar injury classification with the introduction of the 'column concept.' He divided the spine into two major columns, the anterior column, consisting of the vertebral body and intervertebral disc, and the posterior column, consisting of the facet joints and the posterior ligament complex (interspinous ligament, supraspinous ligament and ligamentum flavum).[6] Holdsworth was the first to introduce the concept of a "burst fracture." He reported that both burst and anterior compression fractures were inherently stable given that the posterior column was intact. His concept of stability was rather simplistic, i.e. if both the columns are injured, the fracture is considered unstable.

Denis Classification

In 1983, Denis reviewed CT scans of patients with thoracolumbar fractures and proposed the "three-column concept" in spinal injuries[7] (Figs 15.2A to D). According to the description by Denis, the anterior column is defined by the anterior longitudinal ligament (ALL), the anterior annulus fibrosis, and the anterior part of the vertebral body. The posterior column consisted of all structures posterior to the posterior longitudinal ligament (PLL) including the osseous posterior elements and the posterior ligament complex. The middle column was defined anatomically as the posterior half of the vertebral body, including the annulus fibrosus and the PLL.

Denis believed that the middle column is the key to the stability of the fracture. This concept was based on the understanding that the anterior third of the vertebral body or the anterior column normally transmits only 30% of the body weight, and posterior column transmits only 20% of the body weight. But, combined with the middle column, the anterior column resists 70–80% of the body weight in flexion, whereas together with the middle column, the posterior column may resist as much as 60% of body weight in extension.

Denis classified spine fractures into four distinct groups based on the three-column theory: (1) Compression fractures sustained secondary to the failure of the anterior column under compression; (2) Burst fractures were result of the failure of the anterior and middle

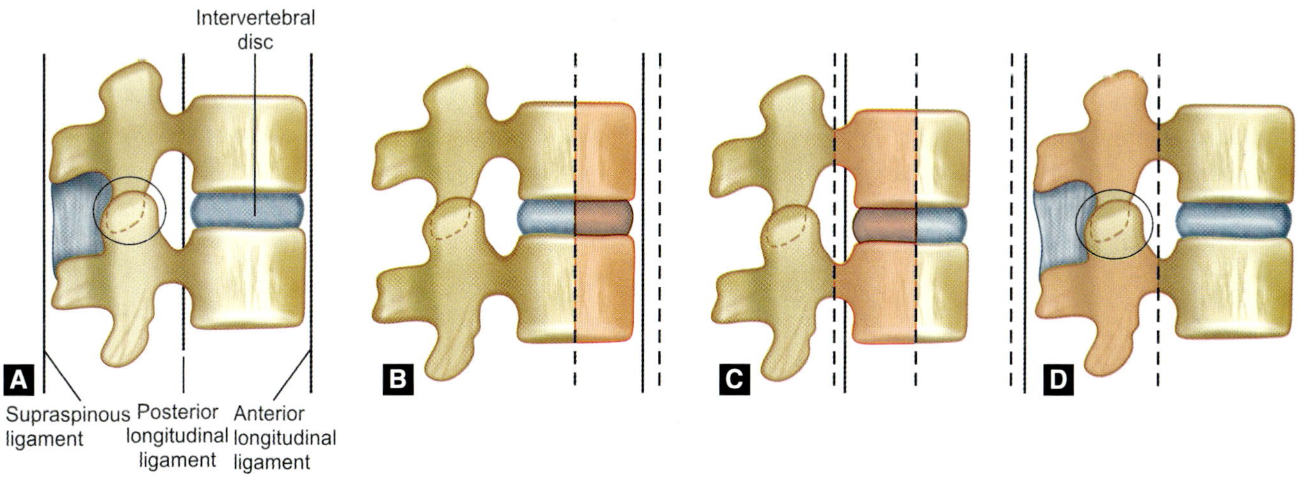

Figures 15.2A to D: The Three columns of the spine as described by Denis. The anterior column is defined by the anterior longitudinal ligament, the anterior annulus fibrosis and the anterior part of the vertebral body. The posterior column consisted of all structures posterior to the posterior longitudinal ligament including the osseous posterior elements and the posterior ligament complex. The middle column was defined anatomically as the posterior half of the vertebral body, including the annulus fibrosus and the posterior longitudinal ligament.

columns, resulting in fracture of the vertebral body under axial load; (3) Seat-belt injuries were sustained secondary to flexion-distraction forces and resulted in the failure of both the posterior and middle columns, and finally; (4) Fracture-dislocations were defined as injuries resulting from failure of all three columns.

Allen-Ferguson Classification

Ferguson and Allen contested the "column concept" advocated by Holdsworth and Denis.[8] Based on their more widely accepted cervical spine injury classification, they proposed a purely mechanistic classification of the thoracolumbar fractures and classified them as flexion-compression, axial compression, flexion-distraction, hyperextension-compression, hyperextension-distraction, and rotation-shear. But this did not gain much acceptance and popularity.

As the Denis' column concept was questioned by others, the relative role played by each of the three columns in contributing to the stability of the spine was evaluated. Panjabi et al. studied the multidirectional flexibility of the thoracolumbar spine in ten fresh cadaver spine specimens after creating burst fractures with high-speed axial trauma.[9] Compared to intact specimens, the flexibility increased after burst fracture by 202% in flexion-extension, 403% in axial rotation, 266% in lateral bending, and 462% in tension or compression. The neutral zone parameters of these motions were even more destabilized following burst fractures. James et al.[10] further studied the specific role of anterior, middle and posterior column by serial sections of the ligaments in these columns in cadaver spines. They found statistically significant increase in motion after anterior and posterior column disruption, but not for added middle column disruption. Both the studies pointed out that disruption of the posterior ligament complex is more important indicator of the instability than middle column disruption.

McAfee's Classification

The Holdsworth two-column concept and Denis three-column concept are based on purely morphological pattern of the fracture. The X-ray and CT scan identification of the location of the disruption is adequate to use these classification systems. McAfee[11] pointed out that one of the major deficiencies of the weight-bearing column concepts is that it does not consider the mechanism of failure of the columns. He proposed a further modification to the Denis classification by introduction of mechanism of failure of the middle column (Figs 15.3A to E). According to McAfee there were three modes of failure of the middle column: axial compression, axial distraction and translation.

McAfee's simplified system of classifying injuries to the thoracolumbar spine is as follows:

- Wedge compression fractures result from isolated failure of the anterior column due to forward flexion. They rarely are associated with neurological deficit except when multiple adjacent vertebral levels are affected.
- In stable burst fractures, the anterior and middle columns fail because of a compressive load, with no loss of integrity of the posterior elements (Figs 15.4A to D).
- In unstable burst fractures, the anterior and middle columns fail in compression, and the posterior column is disrupted. The posterior column can fail in compression,

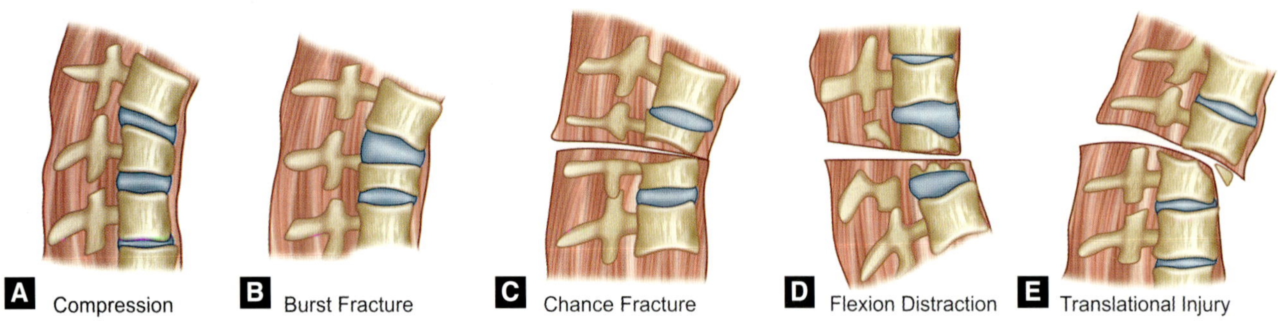

Figures 15.3A to E: McAfee's classification of thoracolumbar fractures.

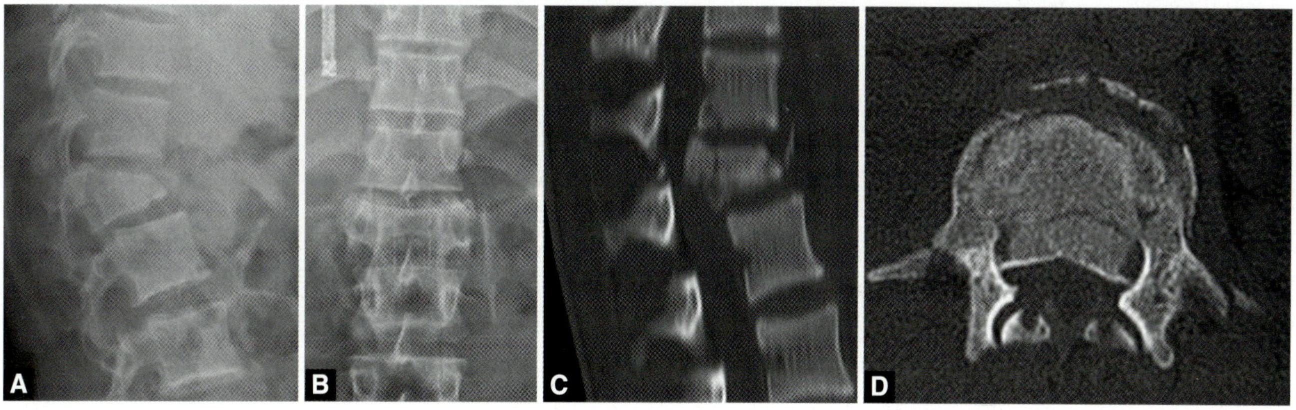

Figures 15.4A to D: (A and B) Anteroposterior and lateral radiographs and (C and D) sagittal, axial CT images of an unstable burst fracture. Factors indicative of instability in burst fractures included fragment retropulsion, more than 50% canal compromise, more than 15–25° of kyphosis and more than 40% loss of anterior body height.

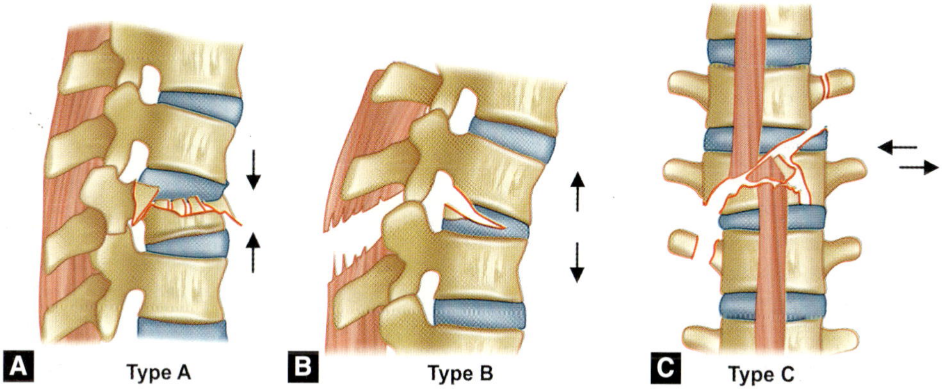

Figures 15.5A to C: AO classification of thoracolumbar injuries. (A) Compression; (B) Distraction; (C) Rotationally unstable injuries.

lateral flexion or rotation. There is a tendency for post-traumatic kyphosis and progressive neural symptoms because of instability. If the anterior and middle columns fail in compression, the posterior column cannot fail in distraction.

- Chance fractures are horizontal avulsion injuries of the vertebral bodies caused by flexion around an axis anterior to the ALL. The entire vertebra is pulled apart by a strong tensile force.
- In flexion-distraction injuries, the flexion axis is posterior to the ALL. The anterior column fails in compression, whereas the middle and posterior columns fail in tension. This injury is unstable because the ligamentum flavum, interspinous ligaments, and supraspinous ligaments usually are disrupted.
- Translational injuries are characterized by malalignment of the neural canal, which has been totally disrupted. Usually all three columns have failed in shear.

AO Classification

In 1994 Magerl analyzed 1,445 cases of thoracolumbar injuries and presented a comprehensive classification of thoracolumbar fractures based on mechanism of injury and morphological pattern of the fracture.[12] The classification implemented AO concepts that had been originally applied to extremity fractures, with categorization of the severity of the injury on a progressive scale from Type A to Type C, and has been adopted as the AO classification. The primary types of fracture depend on the injury-mechanism (Figs 15.5A to C). Type A involves compression, Type B results from distraction, and Type C due to rotation and/or shear.

Each of the three main fracture types is divided into three subtypes (1, 2 and 3), which in turn are separated into three subgroups, depending on injury-mechanism (flexion or extension) and morphology of the fracture. In designing the AO classification, Magerl et al. abandoned the three-column concept of Denis and adopted the older two-column concept of Holdsworth.

According to the AO classification, Type A1 indicate the most simple and Type C3 indicates most severe form of injury, and the magnitude of instability and the risk of neurological deficit increases with the ascending category of the fracture types. Despite being a comprehensive classification system, this system had two big deficiencies. AO classification system failed to offer a clear definition of instability. This system also did not consider presence of neurological deficit, which is often a very important determinant in clinical decision making.

As imaging modalities have enhanced our understanding of these complex injury patterns, newer information became available. Oner et al. described the MRI findings in 100 cases with thoracolumbar spine injuries and proposed a classification based on the ligament injury pattern.[13] The ALL, the PLL, posterior ligament complex, disk, end plate and vertebral body are each identified and scored separately for injury severity. This system has been independently validated and found to predict progression of deformity and pain.[14] Recent classifications by McCormick et al. and the TLICS are more helpful in guiding the type of management and also the surgical approach for each patient.[15]

Thoracolumbar Injury Classification System

The TLICS was created by an international group of spine surgeons referred as "The Spine Trauma Study Group". It is based on three major injury characteristics—mechanism of injury, integrity of the posterior ligamentous complex and neurologic status.[16] Based on the severity scores within these three categories, a total score is calculated that can be used to guide treatment (Fig. 15.6).

The mechanisms of injury in the TLICS system are identical to those proposed by the AO group (axial compression, distraction, rotation/shear) and these were scored with greater points for more unstable injury

Morphology of Injury

Type	*Points*
Compression	1
Burst	1
Translation	3
Distraction	4

Neurologic status

Involvement	*Points*
Intact	0
Root injury	2
Cord/Conus	
- Complete	2
- Incomplete	3
Cauda Equina	3

PLC status

Involvement	*Points*
Intact	0
Indeterminate	2
Distupted	3

Score < 3	Nonoperative management
Score = 4	Nonoperative or operative (Surgeon Preference)
Score > 5	Operative management

Figure 15.6: Thoracolumbar injury classification system

mechanism. Although it is a fracture severity score, the classification seeks to uniformly categorize injuries and indicate protocols for treatment (Table 15.1).

Load Sharing Classification

The concept of short segment posterior stabilization became a popular surgical method of stabilization of thoracolumbar fractures. Unfortunately, failure of fixation was common following short-posterior fixation. Because of reports of high failure rates after short-segment posterior fixation for thoracolumbar fractures, McCormack, Karaikovic, and Gaines introduced a scale to predict the risk of implant failure (Fig. 15.7). They identified three important factors in predicting posterior fixation failure: the degree of vertebral body comminution, apposition of fracture fragments, and the amount of sagittal plane deformity (kyphosis). Each factor was evaluated using McCormick's criteria and scored on a point system from 1 to 3, with a higher number indicating increased severity. Fractures with a total score greater than seven had a high risk of failure with posterior short-segment fixation alone. The advantage of McCormack and Gaines classification was that it could predict inadequacy of posterior fixation alone and identify need for anterior column reconstruction. Beyond this specific advantage, this classification is far too inadequate to consider other important aspects like neurological status or ligamentous stability.

Concept of Instability

One of the most important goals for classification of spinal injuries is to identify potentially unstable fracture, and provide indication for surgical stabilization, as well as

Table 15.1: The thoracolumbar injury classification system provides a guide to the approach for spinal decompression and stabilization based on the neurological status and injury to posterior ligamentous complex

	Posterior ligamentous complex	
Neurologic status	*Intact*	*Disrupted*
Intact	Posterior approach	Posterior approach
Root injury	Posterior approach	Posterior approach
Incomplete SCI or cauda	Anterior approach	Combined approach
Complete SCI or cauda equina	Posterior (anterior)* approach	Posterior (combined)* approach

*Aggressive decompression in ASIA A patients is practiced in many institutions to optimize any potential for neurologic recovery, reconstruct the vertebral support column, restore cerebrospinal fluid (CSF) flow to prevent syringomyelia, and allow for short-segment fixation.

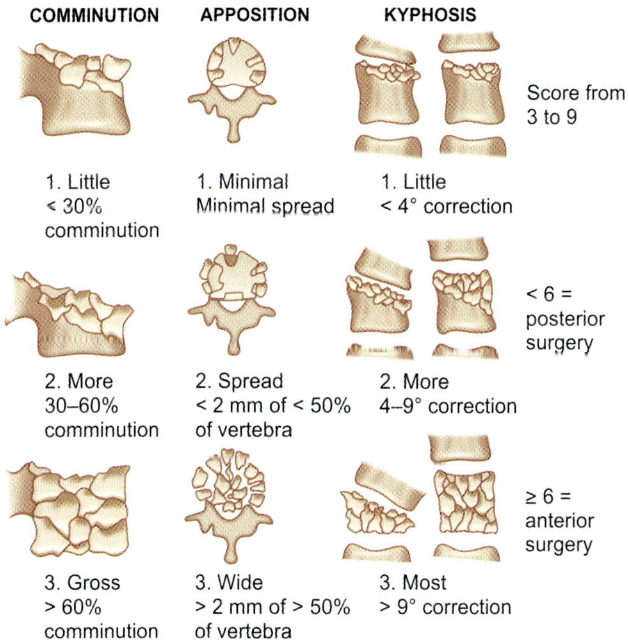

Figure 15.7: McCormack and Gaines classification depends on a scoring system based on the degree of comminution, and spread of fracture fragments as noted from sagittal and axial CT scans respectively, and the angle of kyphosis in lateral radiograph. On each factor, the score can vary from 1 to 3 and the maximum total score can be nine. Burst fractures with score six or more indicate significant comminution and need for surgical restoration of anterior column.

suggest methods of adequate stabilization. White and Panjabi[17] defined instability of thoracolumbar fracture as inability to maintain structural integrity under physiological load to prevent progression of neurological deficit or pain. It is important to remember that clinical instability in degenerative lumbar spine is an entirely different concept, which involves identification of the cause of back pain. Toward the extremes of the range of thoracolumbar fracture classification, instability is more clearly understood. Simple compression fractures are often stable, whereas distraction injuries and rotation/shear injuries are frequently unstable. Most of the controversies of stability surround the burst fractures. Differentiation of stable from unstable burst fractures remains difficult. It is generally accepted that a burst fracture may be considered unstable when it is associated with one or more of the following: (1) loss of anterior vertebral body height more than 50%, (2) kyphosis at the level of fracture more than 30°, (3) comminution of the vertebral bodies with encroachment inside the canal by 50% of the canal diameter, (4) associated injuries to the posterior ligament complex. Once a fracture is designated as unstable, it indicates need for surgical stabilization.

Diagnosis

Acute fractures present as axial, nonradiating back pain of stabbing or aching quality. Pain may not be midline in distribution and it can be referred to the ribs, hip, groin or buttocks. Inspection may reveal a kyphotic posture due to wedging of the vertebra. Midline tenderness corresponding to the radiographic level of injury is present in most of the cases. Most of these fractures are considered to be stable. However, in severe injuries, there may be disruption of the posterior column. Presence of a palpable gap in between spinous processes indicates rupture of the posterior osteoligamentous complex suggestive of an unstable injury. In these situations, the injury is classified as a flexion-distraction injury rather than as a compression injury. These fractures may heal in kyphosis without symptoms depending on the extent of kyphosis, status of adjacent vertebrae and bone quality. Patients with chronic compression fractures usually seek medical attention for persistent pain, progressive deformity or neurological deficit. Persistent pain in these situations is often multifactorial and can be attributed to loss of vertebral height, kyphotic deformity, alteration of sagittal balance, adhesions and fibrosis in the damaged muscles after immobilization, disruption of the endplates, facet joint subluxation, and excessive strain on the paraspinal muscles that puts them to a mechanical disadvantage.[18,19]

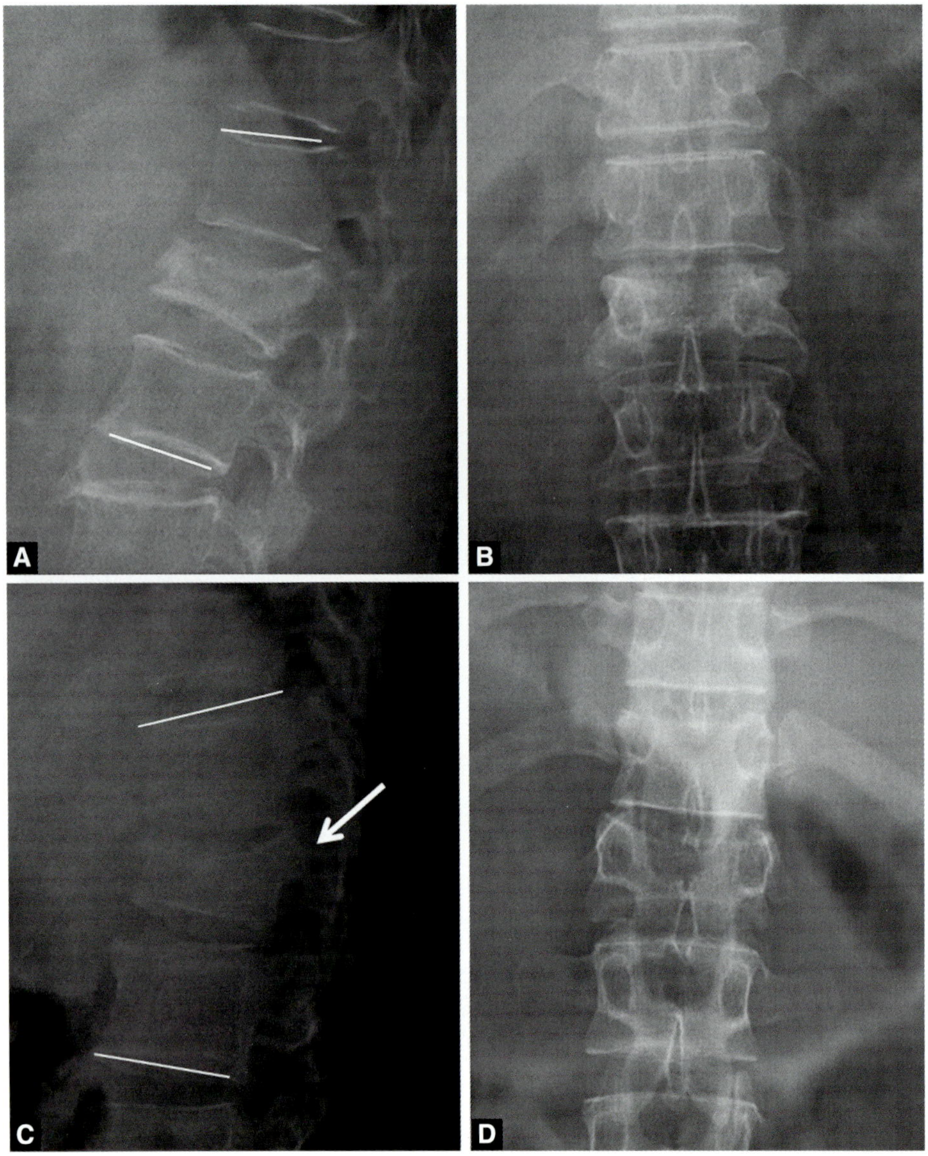

Figures 15.8A to D: (A and B) Anteroposterior and lateral radiographs of a stable burst fracture; (C and D) Anteroposterior and lateral radiographs of an unstable burst fracture. Factors indicative of instability in burst fractures included fragment retropulsion (white arrow), more than 50% canal compromise, more than 30° of kyphosis (measured between the proximal and distal vertebra white lines) and more than 50% loss of vertebral body height.

Standard radiographic evaluation includes anteroposterior (AP) and lateral radiographs. Radiographic evaluation should include assessment of the kyphosis angle, loss of anterior vertebral height and interspinous distance on lateral radiographs as well as rotation and translation on the AP radiographs as this provides information regarding the status of the posterior osteoligamentous complex (Figs 15.8A to D). Disruption of the posterior osteoligamentous complex implies a three-column injury; these are unstable injuries requiring surgical management (Table 15.2). The posterior vertebral angle and the posterior vertebral height help to differentiate

Table 15.2: Plain radiographic indicators of unstable injury

- AP view—translation of vertebra identified by drawing a line along the spinous processes, widened interpedicular distance
- Lateral view—translation of vertebra identified by drawing a line along the posterior vertebral body, vertebral body fracture more than 50%, widened interpedicular distance

between a compression fracture and burst fracture (Figs 15.9A and B). In an ambulatory patient, the difference in kyphus angle in sitting and standing gives an indirect evidence of posterior osteoligamentous complex injury in burst fractures.

CT scan of the injured area may be obtained to characterize the fracture further and evaluate the degree of canal compromise. CT scans provide finer detail of the bony involvement, the extent of canal compromise and occult posterior element fractures (Figs 15.10A and B).

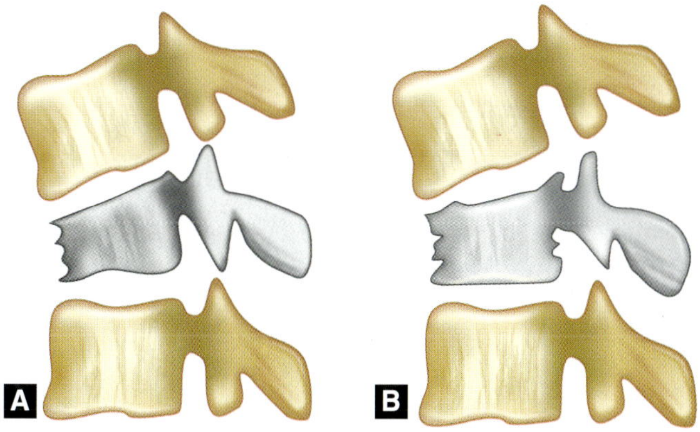

Figures 15.9A and B: In a wedge compression fracture, the posterior vertebral height is maintained whereas in the burst type, the posterior vertebral border collapses resulting in varying degrees of fragment retropulsion into the canal.

Approximately 25% of burst fractures are misdiagnosed as compression fractures if radiographs alone are evaluated; hence, it is important to evaluate significant thoracic and lumbar fractures with a CT scan.[20]

MRI is required for patients with a neurological deficit to identify possible spinal cord, cauda equina or root injury, cord edema and hemorrhage, or epidural hematoma (Figs 15.11A to C). The advantages of MRI are its ability to evaluate injury to the intervertebral discs and posterior osteoligamentous complex (Figs 15.12A to D) screening of the whole spine and evaluation of epidural hematoma and cord injury.

Compression Fractures

Lateral radiographs will typically show a decrease in the anterior height of the vertebral body, while the posterior height is normal (Figs 15.13A and B). There is no translation of the vertebral bodies. T12, L1 and L2 vertebrae are most commonly involved in that order. Multiple vertebral levels may also be affected. Quantification of loss of vertebral height and degrees of kyphosis on radiographs help to determine the stability of the fracture. Loss of over 50% vertebral height, more than 30° of kyphosis or any interspinous widening should arouse a suspicion of posterior osteoligamentous complex disruption. These are

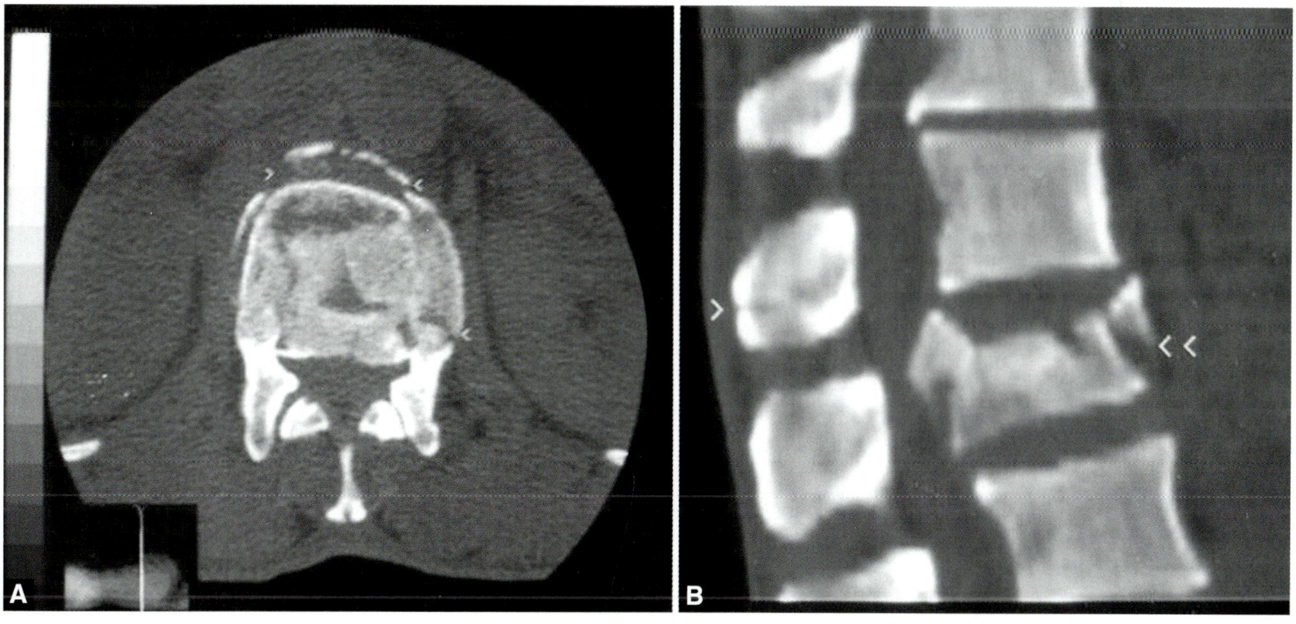

Figures 15.10A and B: CT scan of a patient with burst fracture. Axial CT image shows fracture of the vertebral body with splaying of the fragments. Part of the vertebral body is retropulsed into the canal. The sagittal image shows collapse of the vertebral body with canal compromise.

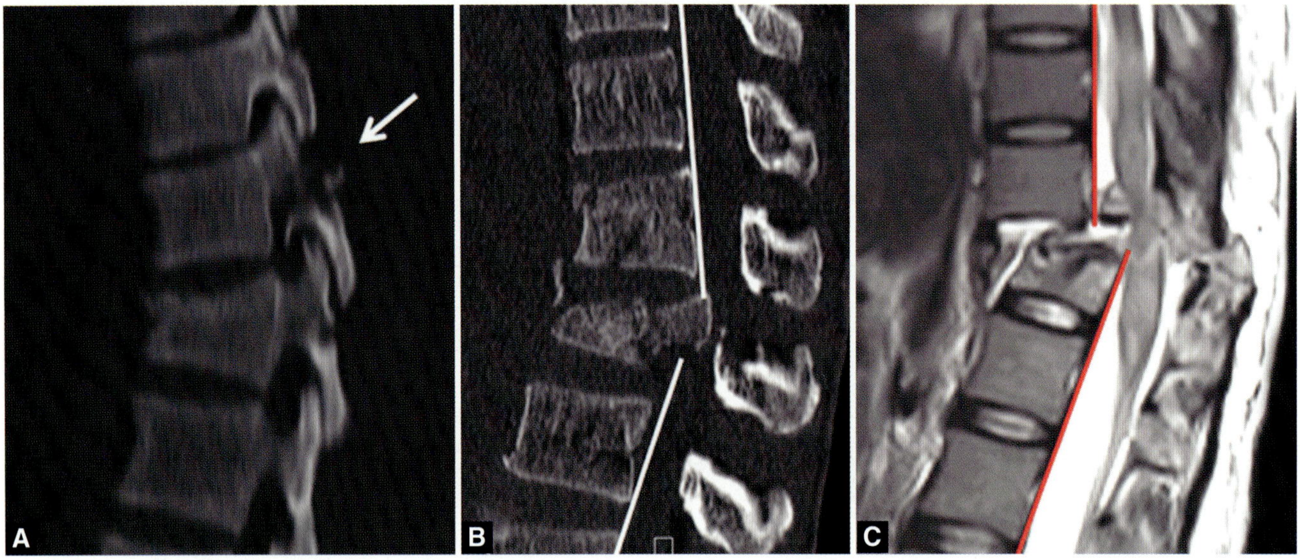

Figures 15.11A to C: Unstable spinal injuries. (A) Chance fracture. The sagittal CT image shows disruption of the lamina and fracture of the inferior vertebral body indicating disruption of all the three vertebral columns; (B) Sagittal image of a patient with flexion-distraction injury. The fulcrum is at the anterior column; the middle and posterior column fail in distraction. The vertebral collapse and retropulsion of fracture fragments into the spinal canal is clearly visualized; (C) Fracture dislocation. All the three columns have failed in translation by shear forces. This sagittal magnetic resonance image shows the cord compression and the extent of spinal cord damage.

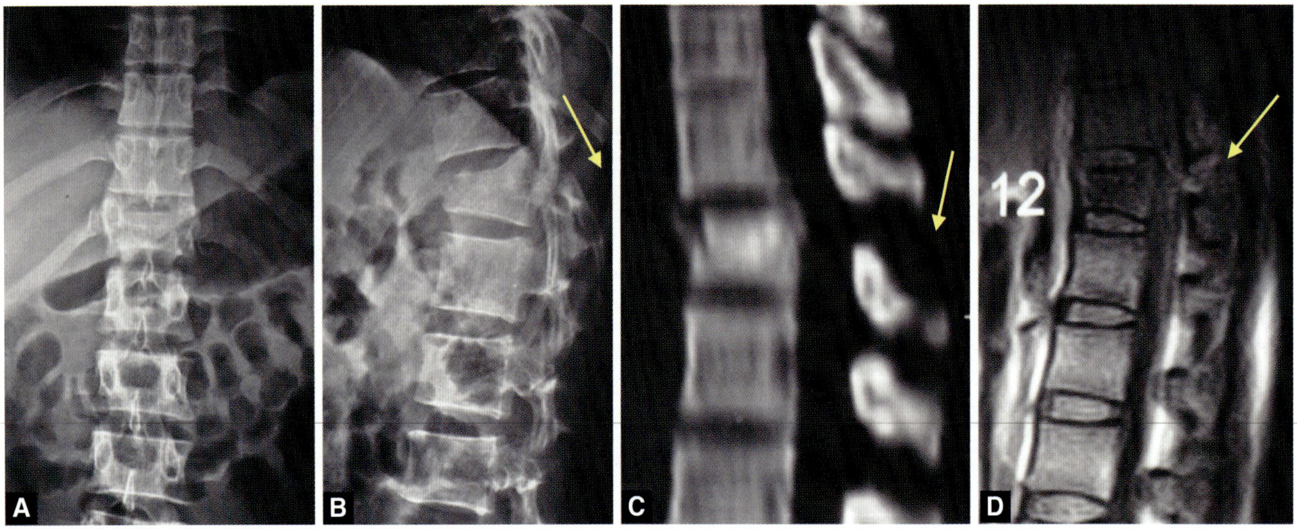

Figures 15.12A to D: Complete radiological evaluation of a patient with flexion-distraction injury. (A) Anteroposterior X-ray shows widening of the pedicle; (B) Lateral X-ray shows collapse of the vertebral body; (C) Sagittal CT image shows widening of the interspinous distance; (D) The magnetic resonance image shows disruption of the posterior ligamentous complex injury indicated by high signal intensity.

unstable injuries with a risk of progressive kyphotic deformity and neurological deficit. "Concertina" type of compression fractures are characterized by uniform compression of the whole vertebral body with little or no angular deformity. It occurs in the elderly patients with degenerative changes and an osteoporotic spine. A CT scan must be undertaken in doubtful cases to rule out a Chance fracture as it offers good visualization of the posterior elements. It also allows visualization

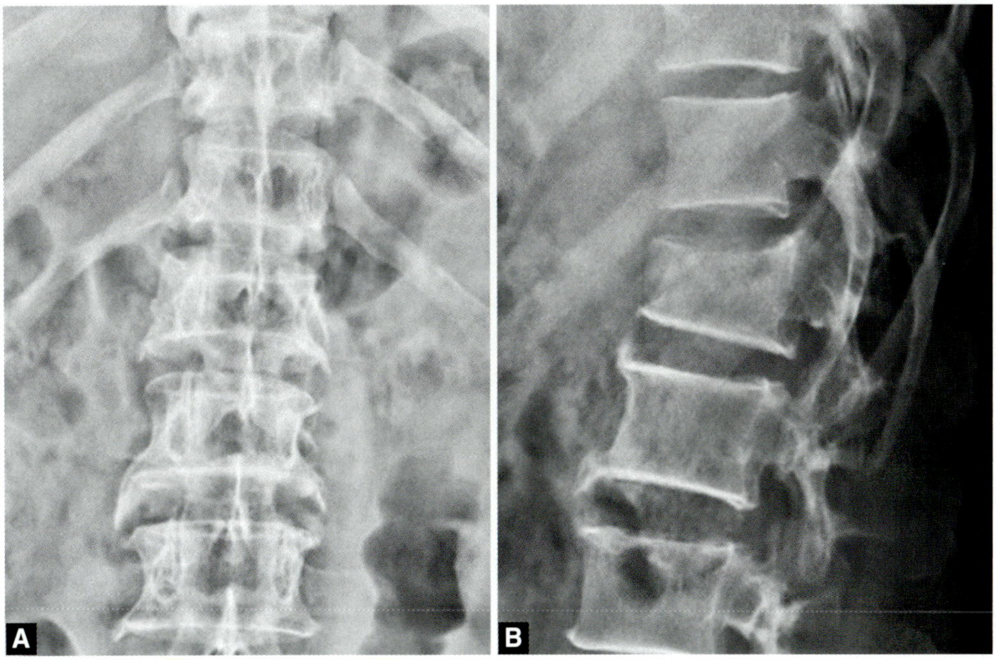

Figures 15.13A and B: Simple wedge compression fractures: Anteroposterior and lateral radiographs of a patient with wedge compression fracture. (A) In the AP view, the inter pedicular distance and the interspinous distance are maintained; (B) In the lateral radiograph, the anterior column is collapsed but the middle and posterior columns are intact.

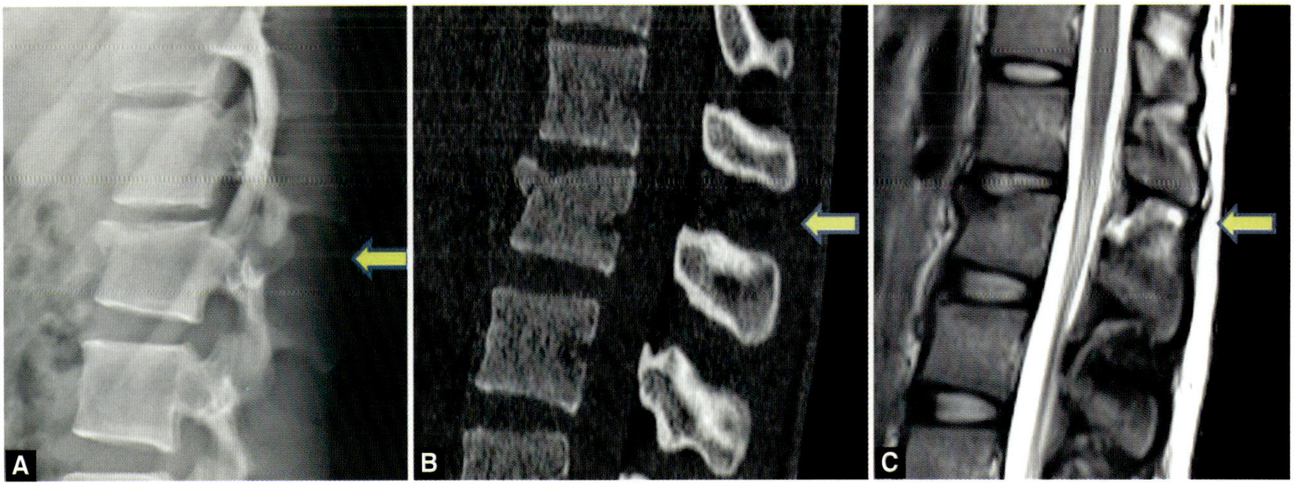

Figures 15.14A to C: Wedge compression fracture with posterior osteoligamentous complex injury: lateral radiograph of a patient with a wedge compression fracture. The middle column is intact. Note the widened interspinous distance in the (A) X-ray and (B) CT images. (C) The sagittal MR image shows disrupted posterior ligamentous complex.

of the spinal canal, degree of canal compromise, the degree of comminution and apposition of fragments in a burst fracture. MR imaging is not needed but can be useful to identify any injury to the intervertebral disc or the posterior osteoligamentous complex (Figs 15.14A to C).

Burst Fractures

The diagnosis can usually be made on plain radiology by a reduction in posterior vertebral body height and an increase in the anteroposterior diameter in the lateral view.

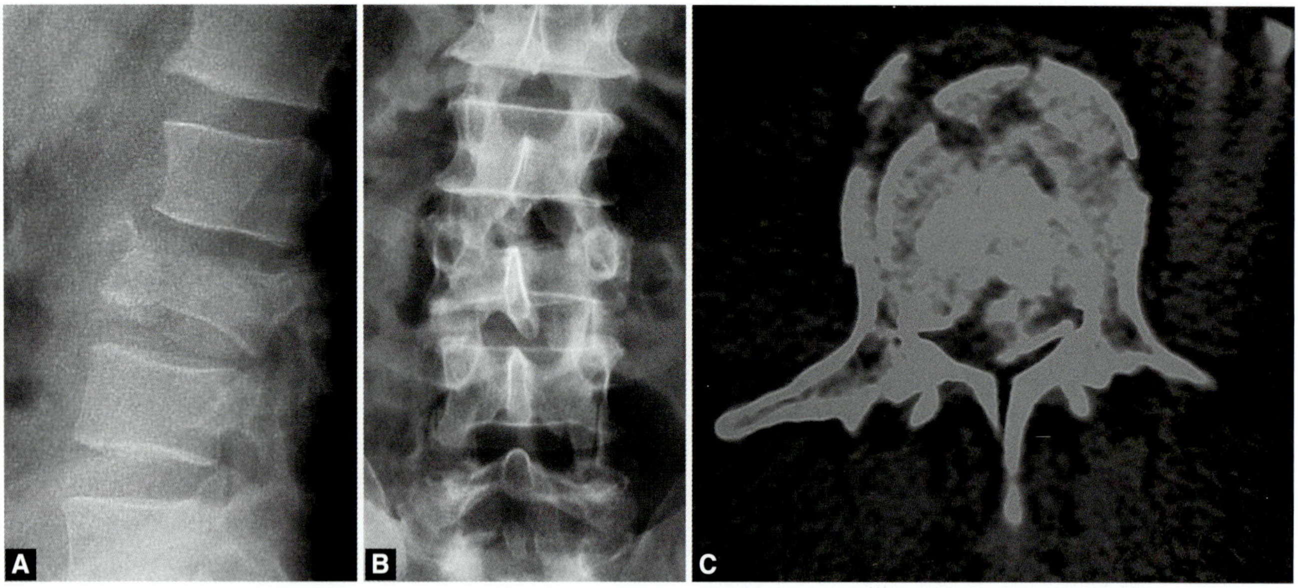

Figures 15.15A to C: Note typical features of a burst fracture on the anteroposterior, lateral radiographs and the axial CT images. The anterior and middle columns have failed in compression. The inter pedicular distance has increased in the anteroposterior view. The axial CT image shows displacement of fracture fragments and retropulsion of fragments into the canal.

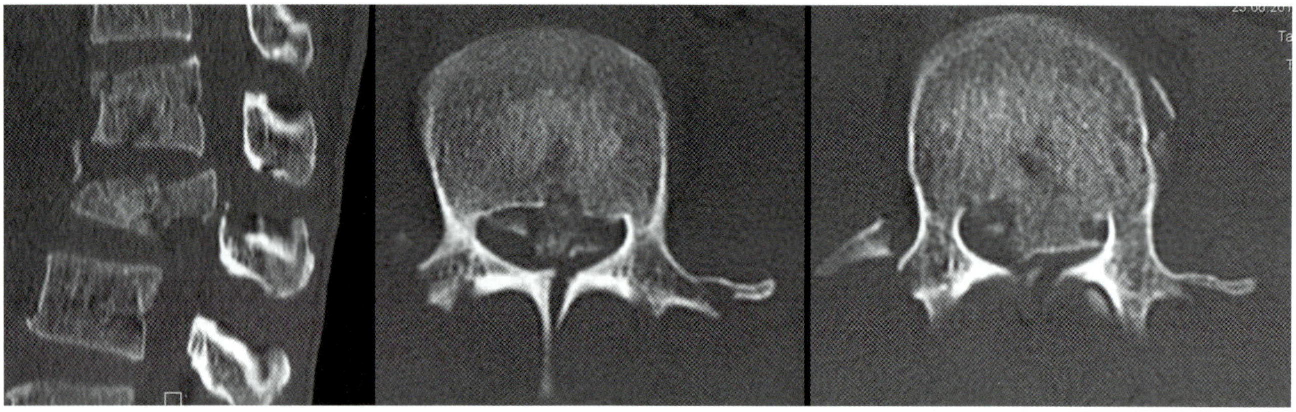

Figure 15.16: The sagittal and axial CT images show the extent of vertebral body destruction and the retropulsion of fragments into the canal. Note that the lamina is also fractured. This could probably protect the spinal canal contents by dissipating the energy and widening the spinal canal. During spinal decompression, the ruptured dura and the nerve roots could be entangled in the laminar fracture and could be potentially injured if the surgeon is unaware.

In the AP view, there is increased width of the body with increased interpedicular distance. CT scan shows scattering of the fractured fragments beyond the normal dimensions of the vertebral body in the axial plane. Retropulsion of fragments especially at the level of the pedicle and the extent of canal compromise are more accurately seen in the CT (Figs 15.15 and 15.16). However, many studies have failed to show any correlation between the extent of canal compromise in the CT and the degree of neurological damage or subsequent recovery.[21-23] Associated fractures of the rib heads and transverse process fractures are indicative of severe violence and possibility of instability and chest injuries. Often times a vertical laminar fracture is seen on the axial cuts of the CT in burst fractures. This may depict the energy dissipation through the posterior elements and is thought to protect the cord by transiently enlarging the canal. It has also been documented that the dura tends to get entrapped in the fracture line resulting

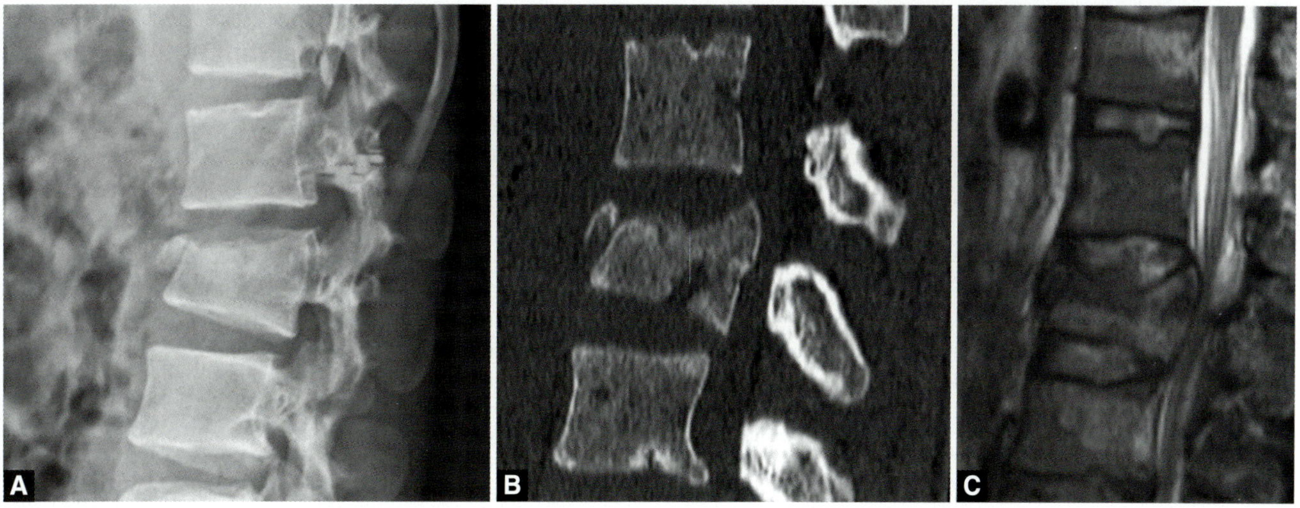

Figures 15.17A to C: Lateral radiograph and sagittal CT and MR images of a patient with unstable burst fracture. MRI provides additional information like bone edema, damage to the disc, retropulsion of fragment into the canal, cord compression, spinal cord edema and status of posterior ligamentous complex.

Table 15.3: Imaging characteristics of flexion-distraction injuries

Imaging technique	*Imaging plane*	*Imaging finding*	*Frequency of occurrence (percentage)*
Radiograph	AP	Empty body sign	100
Radiograph	AP	Pedicle radiolucency	66
Radiograph	AP	Wide interpedicular distance	18
Radiograph	Lateral	Fanning spinous processes	80
Radiograph	Lateral	Lateral pedicle radiolucency	73
CT Scan	Transaxial	Dissolving pedicle sign	76
CT scan	Transaxial	Naked facet sign	40
MRI scan	T2 weighted	Sandwich sign	100

Source: Bernstein MP, Mirvis SE, Shanmuganathan K. Chance-type fractures of the thoracolumbar spine: imaging analysis in 53 patients. AJR AMJ Roentgenal. 2006;187:859-68.

in tears when approaching this lesion unwarily (Fig. 15.16). Though laminar fractures indicate a higher grade of burst fracture, they do not necessarily indicate greater instability. MRI scans are helpful to diagnose soft tissue injuries, especially of the posterior ligament complex, associated disc injuries and the extent of spinal cord trauma (Figs 15.17A to C).

Unstable Thoracolumbar Injuries

This includes the flexion-distraction injuries, chance fractures and the fracture-dislocations of the thoracolumbar spine. These injuries are characterized by significant injuries to all the three columns of the spine and hence are unstable injuries. Radiological recognition of these injuries is mandatory for appropriate surgical stabilization.

Radiographs, CT scans and MRI scans, each with its advantages and disadvantages, provide maximum information of the bony and soft tissue components when used in combination (Table 15.3). MRI scans identify posterior ligamentous complex and intervertebral disc injury with implications on spinal stability and management. Additionally a screening MRI scan of the whole spine may help identify noncontiguous injuries. Thirty percent of AO Type B distraction fractures are misdiagnosed as Type A compression injuries when only plain X-rays and CT scans are used.[24]

As discussed earlier, flexion-distraction injuries lead to all three spinal columns failing in tension with either osseous or ligamentous disruption of the posterior elements (Fig. 15.18). The fulcrum differs in flexion-distraction and Chance fractures. In flexion-distraction injuries, the fulcrum is in the anterior column which fails in compression and the middle and posterior column fail in distraction. In Chance fractures, the fulcrum is in front of

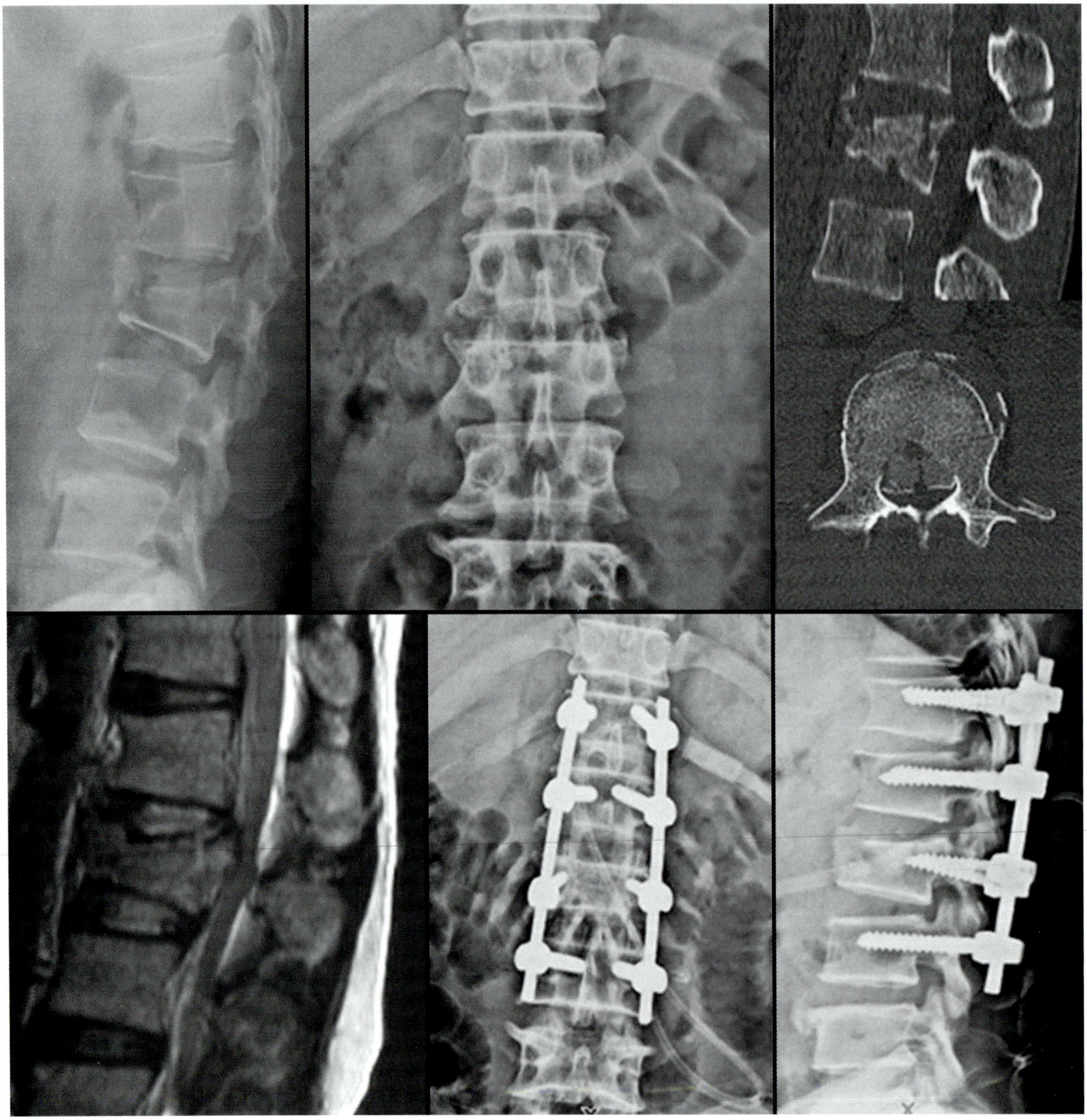

Figure 15.18: Lateral and anteroposterior radiographs of a patient with flexion-distraction injury. The sagittal and axial CT images show the fracture of L2 with retropulsion into the canal. The fracture has been fixed by posterior decompression and multisegmental stabilization.

the anterior column and all the three columns fail in distraction (Fig. 15.19). An increased interspinous distance results in a relative radiolucency over the involved vertebral body on anteroposterior radiographs referred to as the "empty vertebral body" sign.[25] A transverse fracture through the pedicles, increased intercostal spacing, horizontally oriented fractures across the transverse processes, laminae and articular processes are also noted. Lateral radiographs show fanning or distraction of the spinous processes and pedicle radiolucency.

Transaxial CT images of the thoracolumbar spine reveal uncovering of articular facets secondary to the vertical distraction of the posterior elements and is described as the naked-facet sign. Serial transaxial CT images reveal a gradual loss of definition of the pedicles, referred to as the "dissolving pedicle" sign. However, transaxial CT scans may occasionally miss horizontal fractures and fracture-dislocations if the image is in the same plane as the fracture. MRI scans reveal posterior ligamentous complex injury and surrounding soft tissue injury. The sandwich sign is characterized on T2-weighted MRI images by low-signal hemorrhage along the fracture line with flanking high-signal marrow edema. Table 15.3 highlights the various imaging findings in flexion-distraction injuries of the thoracic and lumbar spine.

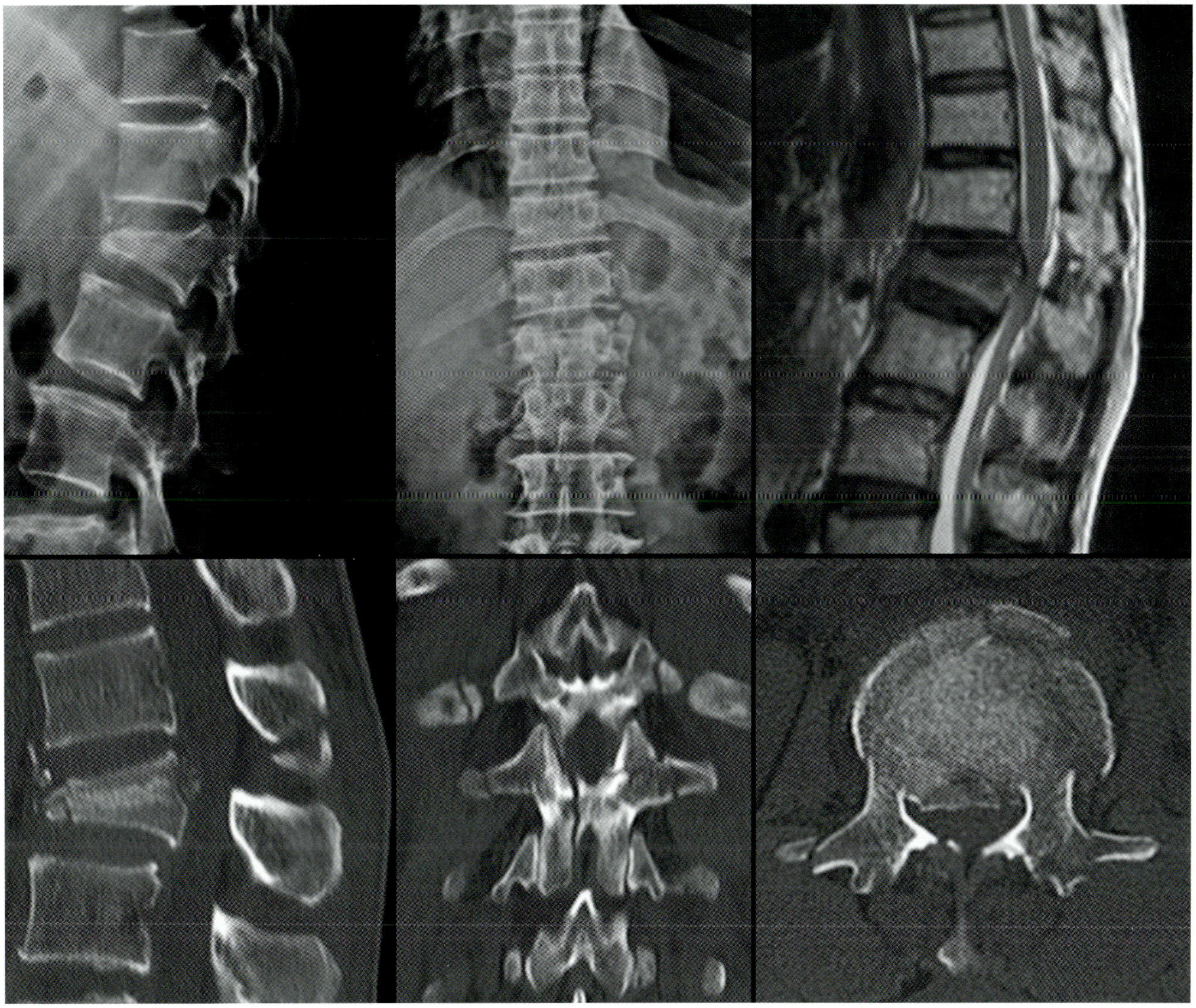

Figure 15.19: Imaging series of a patient with Chance fracture. The fulcrum is anterior to the anterior column and all the three columns have failed in distraction. In the sagittal and coronal CT images, the fracture line is seen to traverse through the spinous process and the lamina.

In vitro studies have shown that a kyphotic angle of the functional spinal unit more than or equal to 12° (impending instability) or more than or equal to 19° (total instability) on the lateral radiographs and an increase in interspinous process distance more than or equal to 20 mm (impending instability) or more than or equal to 33 mm (total instability) on the anteroposterior radiographs are signs of instability.[26]

Fracture-dislocations of the thoracic spine are severe injuries involving the three columns of the spine resulting in anteroposterior or lateral translation of one vertebra over another with associated fractures of the posterior elements and vertebral body. These injuries with loss of normal spinal column alignment are obvious on anteroposterior and lateral radiographs, CT scans and MRI scans, each providing different information relating to the bony, soft-tissue structures and spinal cord.

Management and Surgical Indications

Compression Fractures

Stable vertebral compression fractures are managed conservatively with analgesics and activity modification (avoidance of forward bending, ground level activities, prolonged sitting, lifting of heavy weights, and providing postural correction). Medical treatment however, cannot control the loss of height due to collapse of the vertebral body and the resulting kyphotic deformity. Severe kyphotic deformity may affect the pulmonary and gastrointestinal function. For every thoracic VCF, there may be a 9% loss of forced vital capacity.[27]

Controversy still exists regarding the role of bracing. A hyperextension orthosis or a thoracolumbar sacral orthosis (TLSO) is usually prescribed for these fractures, where it is believed to offer pain relief, correct posture and help immobilization of spine. However various authors have shown that external support has no mechanical stabilizing effect on the lumbar spine.[28,29] In a systematic review of studies, Giele et al. concluded that there is no evidence for the effectiveness of bracing in patients with traumatic thoracolumbar fractures. Standing lateral radiographs must be taken initially to assess any increasing vertebral collapse or widening of the interspinous distance, which would indicate that the injury is potentially unstable. Once the injury is considered stable enough to be treated conservatively, periodical standing lateral radiographs are performed to monitor the progress of healing, vertebral collapse, deformity and overall sagittal alignment of the spine.

Special mention must be made about these fractures in polytrauma patients. Here minimally invasive percutaneous stabilization using pedicular screws and rods is a useful alternative in patients where conservative treatment is not advisable. The screw-rod construct acts as an internal fixator that offers immobilization till the biological healing of the fracture takes place.[30]

The application of minimally invasive techniques in the surgical management of spine fractures reduces the approach-related morbidity associated with the conventional techniques including iatrogenic muscle denervation, ischaemia, pain and functional impairment. Minimally invasive surgery is an option in case of the polytrauma, venous disease or previous deep venous thrombosis, obesity and bronchopulmonary disease when conservative treatment is not advisable.

Burst Fractures

There are relatively few absolute indications for emergency surgery in burst fractures. These include progressively deteriorating neurology and open spine injures. In the absence of the above indications, the patient is to be nursed on a firm mattress with frequent log rolls to avoid pressure sores, and meticulous attention to bowel, bladder and skin care. There is no evidence that early surgery can improve neurological outcomes.[31] But in many centers, it is a standard practice to operate neurologically deficient patients on an emergent basis based on the premise that persistent compression of neural structures would reduce the chances of neurological recovery.

Most burst fractures are stable unless proven otherwise by one of the criteria for instability and may be treated conservatively. The usual protocol consists of ambulation with a brace support (an appropriate TLSO brace) worn for a period of 6–12 weeks. The fracture is monitored by serial radiographs to look for significant collapse. Hyperextension jackets are also effective, and preferred by some surgeons. Braces are worn between 6 weeks to 3 months and progressive spinal rehabilitation exercises are started thereafter.

There are two common indications for surgery in a burst fracture at the thoracolumbar region—neurological deficit and instability. In the former the priority is for decompression of the spinal cord and in the latter event it is stabilization of the unstable segments. Diagnosing neurological damage is essentially simple; however the same is not true for instability. Mechanical instability is an intangible quantum and is based on various morphological and clinical parameters. There is no consensus on what constitutes instability. White and Punjabi's work still forms one of the basic foundations on which instability is diagnosed.[18,26] Nonetheless this system has the disadvantage of being based on cadaveric spine models subjected to serial loading and therefore often is difficult to translate into clinical settings. The measured parameters are anatomical, clinical or social, making the scoring arbitrary. Once the decision has been made to perform a surgery, the following issues have to be addressed.

There is little evidence that emergency surgery has better outcomes than elective surgery in spine fractures.[32] Nevertheless it seems logical that in the presence of neurological deficit, specifically incomplete or progressing neurological change that can be attributed to the vertebral injury, decompression of the spinal cord on an emergent basis would yield better results. For American Spinal Injury Association (ASIA) grades A and E, surgery may be performed under more controlled environments.

Stabilization and fusion by posterior approach is the most popular and widely employed surgical management of a thoracolumbar burst fracture. The familiarity of approach, the ease of decompression and stabilization, and the decreased rate of complication make this approach a favored one for most surgeons. Short segment pedicle screw fixation allows preservation of as many motion segments as possible. Addition of a pedicle screw at the level of the fracture has also been found to increase stability, improve kyphosis correction and also reduce implant failure. In patients with significant collapse of the vertebral body with a load sharing score greater than seven, extended long column constructs are preferable. Alternatively reinforcement with kyphoplasty, calcium phosphate and transpedicular bone grafts can be used to maintain the anterior height. In patients with severe comminution of the vertebra, reconstruction with a titanium cage may also be necessary to prevent an anterior collapse.

Anterior decompression removes the bony compression on the spinal cord and aids reconstruction of the anterior column. Use of anterior instrumentation and cages has greatly improved postoperative spinal stability and also reduced donor-site morbidity from major bone graft harvesting techniques. Although combined anterior/posterior approaches seem better to retain kyphosis correction, it is not clear if this difference is clinically relevant. Indications for combined approaches include complete posterior ligamentous complex disruption, partial neurological injury and rigid post-traumatic kyphotic deformity as seen in injuries, which are more than 2-weeks-old. The advantages of combined surgical approaches are improved sagittal alignment, thorough spinal canal and neural decompression for optimum recovery of neural function and stabilization of the disrupted posterior ligamentous complex.

Unstable Thoracolumbar Injuries

These are unstable injuries involving all the three columns of spine and hence need surgical stabilization in most instances. A posterior approach is advisable when the neurology is intact or in the presence of a nerve root injury. However, in the presence of an incomplete spinal cord or cauda equina injury, a combined anterior and posterior approach is suggested. In the presence of a complete spinal cord or cauda equina injury, a posterior approach may be supplemented with an anterior approach to ensure complete neural decompression to optimize any potential for neurological recovery. However, in the absence of neurological and intra-abdominal injury, certain bony Chance fractures may be treated nonoperatively in a hyperextension brace.

There are two schools of thought regarding posterior instrumentation for spinal fractures, namely those that believe in long segmental constructs and those that believe in short constructs.[33] Long segment constructs refer to the old rule of "three-above, two-below" or more recently with the use of pedicle screws constructs "two-above, two-below" (Fig. 15.20). The thoracic spine is relatively immobile and tolerant of fusion, and extending the construct into these segments has little mechanical cost, while providing more extensive fixation. Extending fusion into the lower lumbar spine does alter segmental mechanics and

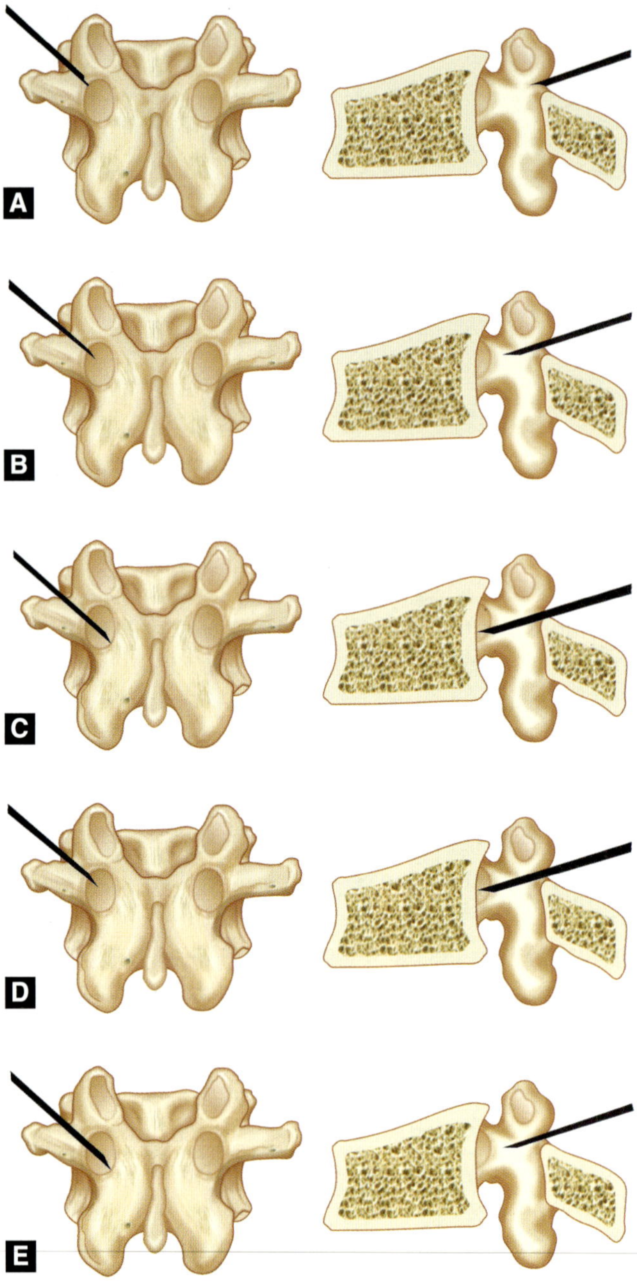

Figures 15.22A to E: Technique of vertebroplasty. (A to C) The ideal entry point is in the upper and lateral corner of the pedicle. The medial angulation is maintained as it traverses the pedicle. When it reaches the medial pedicle wall, it should have crossed the posterior vertebral border; (D) Possible error 1: The needle has been inserted with less medial angulation. In the AP view, it is still well away from the medial pedicle wall but in the lateral view, the tip is already beyond the posterior vertebral wall; (E) Possible error 2: The needle has been inserted with too much of medial angulation. In the AP view, the tip is touching the medial pedicle cortex but in the lateral view, the tip has not traversed the pedicle fully.

Once the needle position is confirmed to be in the ideal position (anterior one third of vertebra in lateral view and middle of the vertebra in the AP view), cementing can be started to perform a unipedicular VP. If the needle is lateralized in the AP view, then a bipedicular VP is performed to ensure adequate fill. In thoracic vertebrae, a unilateral, extra pedicular approach is performed by starting the needle entry at the rib facet joint junction. This reduces the chances of canal breach and also makes certain that the cement fill is adequate in the vertebra. Biopsy, if indicated, can be performed in case of suspected pathological fractures (Figs 15.23 and 15.24).

The cement [polymethylmethacrylate (PMMA)] is prepared and mixed until it becomes like toothpaste and then injected through the needle (3–6 ml) under continuous lateral fluoroscopic control in order to observe and prevent any cement leakage. By adjusting the position of the needle, one can avoid cement leakage into the disc space. Any suspected leakage into the canal should force the surgeon to stop cementing. The cement is allowed to set for some more time and the needle is redirected to start cementing. If there is any further leakage, then cementing should be abandoned. It is important to understand that VP in a fractured vertebral body should be performed with extreme caution as the chances of cement leakage are much higher than in other situations like pseudoarthrosis. Injecting a small amount of radio-opaque contrast before injecting the cement to look for posterior vertebral wall deficiencies, use of continuous fluoroscopy while injecting the cement and using the cement only when the consistency has become tooth paste-like are some of the measures that can reduce the chances of cement leakage. The cement diffuses into osseous space and after solidification, stabilizes the vertebral body. The mechanisms, by which adequate analgesia is obtained, are two: the first mechanism is based on the ability of PMMA to combine the individual bone fragments in a single block, avoiding the painful micro-movements of individual fragments between them. The second mechanism may be related to the exothermic process that accompanies the polymerization of PMMA and that would result in a "thermal neurolysis" of the nerve within the vertebral body. In addition, the PMMA results in a significant strengthening of osteoporotic bone, reducing the risk of subsequent fractures.

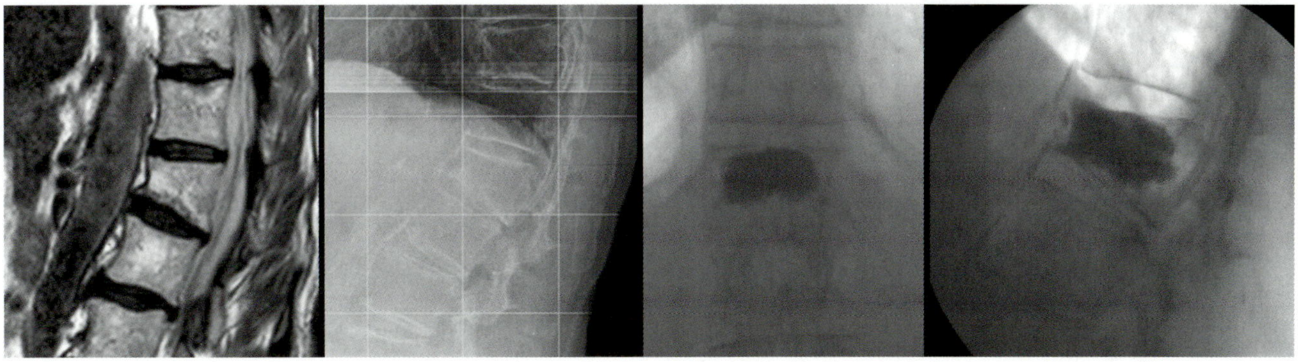

Figure 15.23: A patient with a partially healed wedge compression fracture evident by persistent edema in the vertebral body. Percutaneous vertebroplasty has been performed shown by good fill of the cement in the anteroposterior and lateral views.

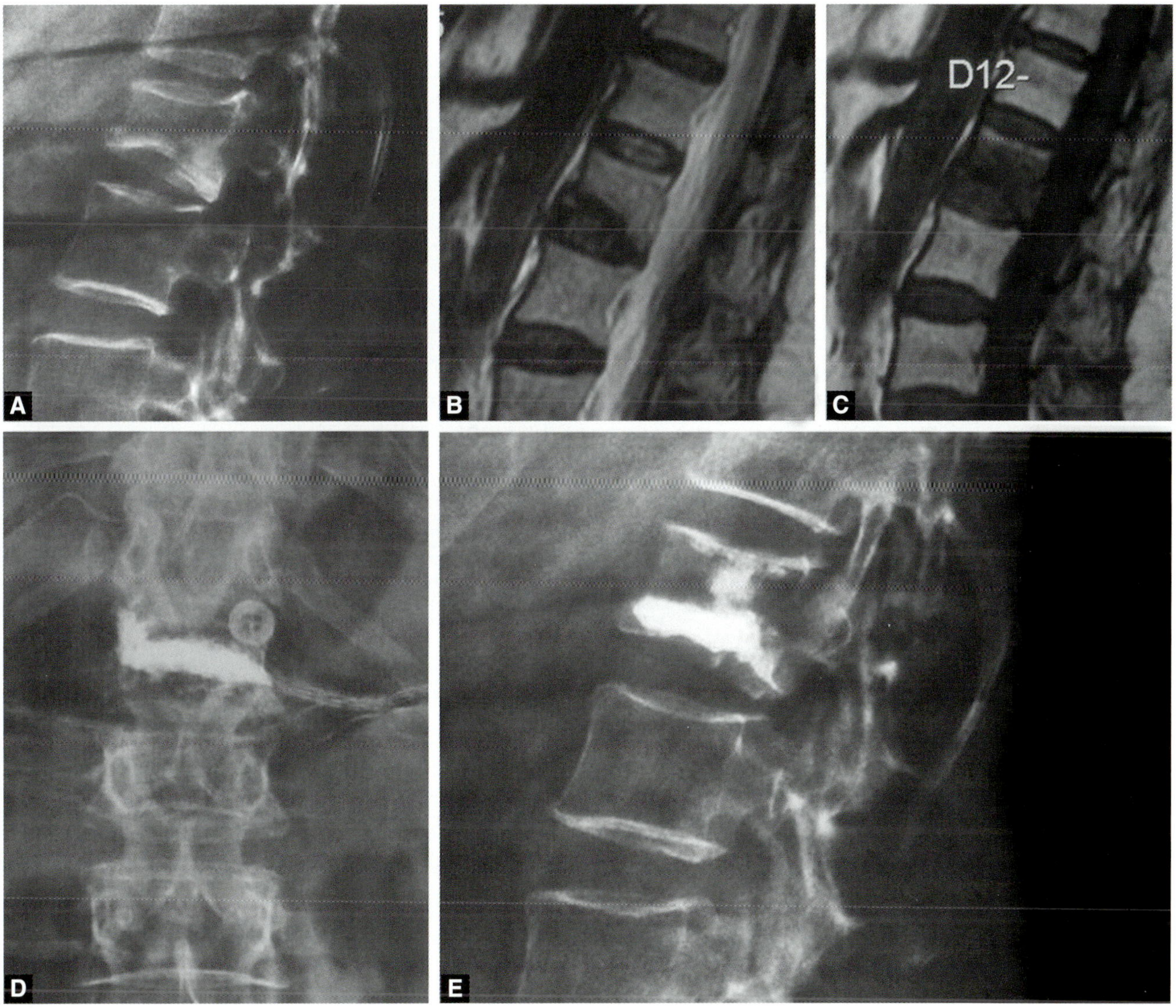

Figures 15.24A to E: (A) Lateral radiograph and (B and C) sagittal T1 and T2 MR images show marrow edema indicating a pseudoarthrotic cleft in a patient with old wedge compression fracture; (D and E) Anteroposterior and lateral radiographs indicate adequate cement fill into the cleft with some restitution of vertebral height.

The incidence of complications ranges from 1% to 3% in osteoporotic vertebrae.[39] The possible complications include bleeding at the site of needle insertion, rib fracture, transient fever, cement leaks into the disc or in paravertebral soft tissues, epidural space, paravertebral veins leading to pulmonary embolism, new fractures in adjacent vertebrae, infection and rarely cerebral embolism and even death.[40] The possible extrusion of cement in the spinal canal (which occurs with an incidence of around 3%) is a dangerous complication, requiring immediate surgical decompression in an attempt to limit the damage from spinal cord compression.[41] Cement can also leak into the disk space. After VP, it has been reported that a marked improvement in pain symptoms can occur in 90% of cases, but residual pain may persist in the early days in the area of needle insertion.[42]

Recently, Knavel et al. have shown that VP can be successfully used in management of traumatic VCFs, where conservative treatment has failed or as an alternative to more invasive spinal reconstruction techniques.[43] PMMA cement was used in his series. Though the procedure has been shown to be successful in the elderly patients, its use in young patients is not recommended since the long term effects of the PMMA cement mixture are not known. Resorbable calcium phosphate cement that gets substituted by new bone over a period of time may be an effective alternative to PMMA in young patients.[44]

Kyphoplasty

Kyphoplasty is similar to VP and can be performed in the thoracic and lumbar vertebrae. Beside the relief of pain secondary to the VCF, it is possible to obtain a partial recovery of the height of the vertebral body.[45] To restore vertebral anatomy after a fracture, the vertebral endplates must be reduced to their correct anatomic position. The reduction of the fractured vertebra reduces the kyphosis of the spine. Kyphoplasty involves the inflation of a percutaneously inserted balloon in the vertebral body. The balloon restores the vertebral body height in addition to creating the cavity. PMMA is injected into the cavity created by the balloon. The risk of cement extravasation is probably reduced as compared to VP due to containment produced by the newly created vertebral cavity.[46]

The technique of KP is similar to VP[47,48] (Figs 15.25 and 15.26). The Jamshidi needle is inserted till the middle third of the vertebral body. Then a special drill is gently advanced into the anterior third of the vertebral body to create a track for the balloon. It is essential that the needle is positioned in the middle of the vertebra in the lateral fluoroscopy view so that when inflated, the upper and lower end plates are pushed uniformly. The introducer with the collapsed balloon is inserted into the vertebra through the outer cannula. Once the balloon has crossed the needle tip, it is gently inflated by the pressurizing bulb. The balloon can hold 3–4 ml of saline after full inflation. While inflating the balloon, periodical breaks or pauses are given to allow the bone to stretch without breaking. Once fully inflated, the balloon is deflated and taken out. Cementing is performed to fill the cavity created by the balloon. Unlike in VP where considerable pressure is needed to inject the cement, in KP, cementing is performed through cement-filled cannulae which ensure smooth cementing without undue pressure.

In a study involving 300 patients who received KP treatment or non-surgical care, authors concluded that balloon KP was an effective and safe procedure for patients with acute vertebral fractures and could be used as an early treatment option.[49] Based on similar principle of support for the anterior column, Korovessis et al. reported successful use of minimally invasive short posterior instrumentation plus balloon kyphoplasty in severe compression lumbar fractures.[50]

Percutaneous Pedicle Screw-assisted Spinal Stabilization

The use of percutaneous pedicle screw-assisted spinal stabilization has become popular worldwide. Standard "open" techniques for pedicle screw placement have been associated with a long midline incision over the back, damage to paraspinal muscles with extensive blood loss and lengthy periods of hospitalization and costs. Minimally invasive posterior fixation, in which percutaneous screws and rods are used, minimizes paraspinous tissue trauma.

Percutaneous posterior fixation of the lumbar spine is performed under general anesthesia (Figs 15.27 and 15.28). The patient is positioned prone on top of bolsters with

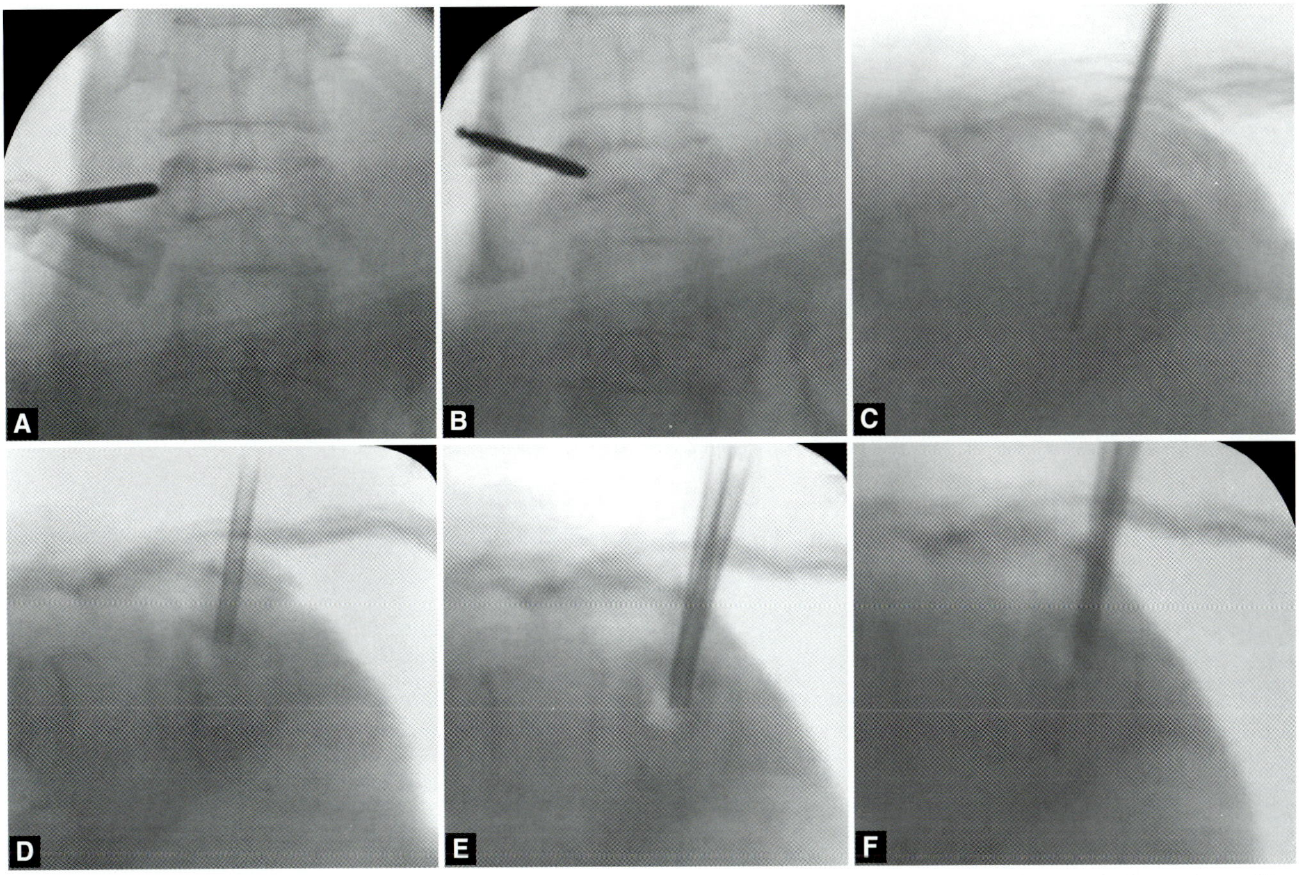

Figures 15.25A to F: The sequential operative steps of performing a kyphoplasty. After appropriately adjusting the image intensifier, the Jamshidi needle is inserted into the pedicle starting at the outer and lateral border of pedicle. Biopsy is taken preferably in all the patients. A guide wire is inserted over which the final working cannula is passed. Both the cannulas have been placed. The deflated balloon is now inserted through the working cannula.

the abdomen hanging free over a radiolucent table. A C-arm fluoroscopy device is used for guidance of percutaneous screw placement. It is important to determine whether adequate AP and lateral fluoroscopic images of the lumbar spine can be obtained before preparing and draping the patient.

The C-arm is adjusted appropriately in the cranio-caudal and mediolateral planes (as explained for VP) before starting the procedure. A 15 mm long incision is made at the skin entry point and extended into the underlying subcutaneous tissue. The Jamshidi needle is inserted till the anterior third of the vertebral body. Once the ideal location is confirmed in both AP and lateral views, a guide wire is inserted through the needle and fixed into the cancellous bone of the vertebra in its anterior third. Cannulated tapping instruments are used to create the screw path over the guide wire. Then a screw of appropriate size is inserted over the guide wire. Similarly screws are inserted on the other pedicle and at the two pedicles below the fractured vertebra. An appropriately contoured rod is then passed through the screw heads on each side and secured with nuts. The screws are distracted gently to achieve fracture reduction and the nuts are tightened.

Rarely, surgical treatment in the form of posterior stabilization using pedicular screws is indicated in painful compression fractures in young patients.[51,52] However, instrumentation breakage and/or loss of correction after

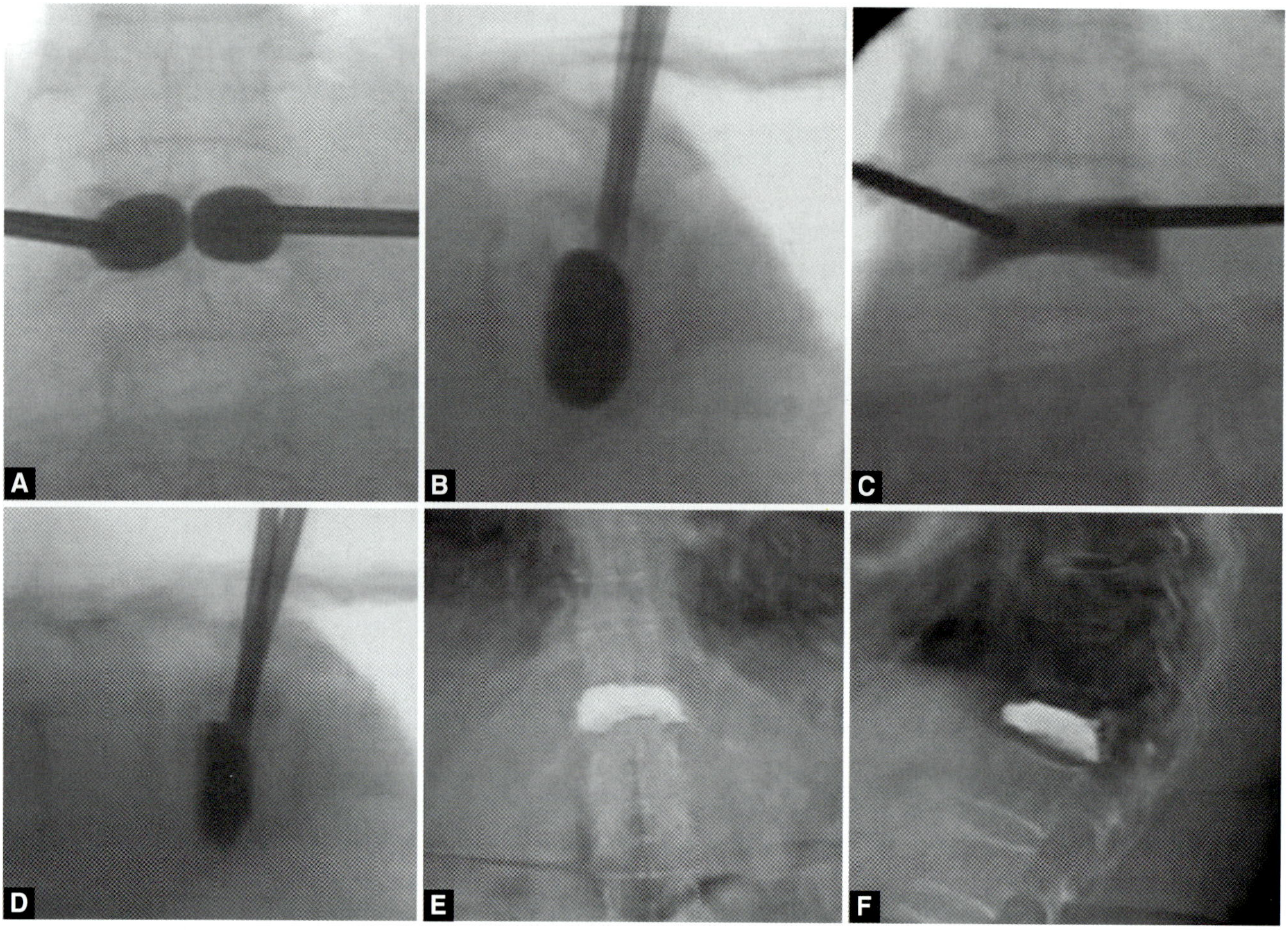

Figures 15.26A to F: (A and B) Both the balloons have been inflated now and are appropriately positioned in the anteroposterior and lateral views; (C and D) The balloons are deflated and the cement is injected into the vacuum created in the vertebra; (E and F) Final AP and lateral radiographs show that the kyphosis has been partially corrected and there is a good cement fill into the vertebra.

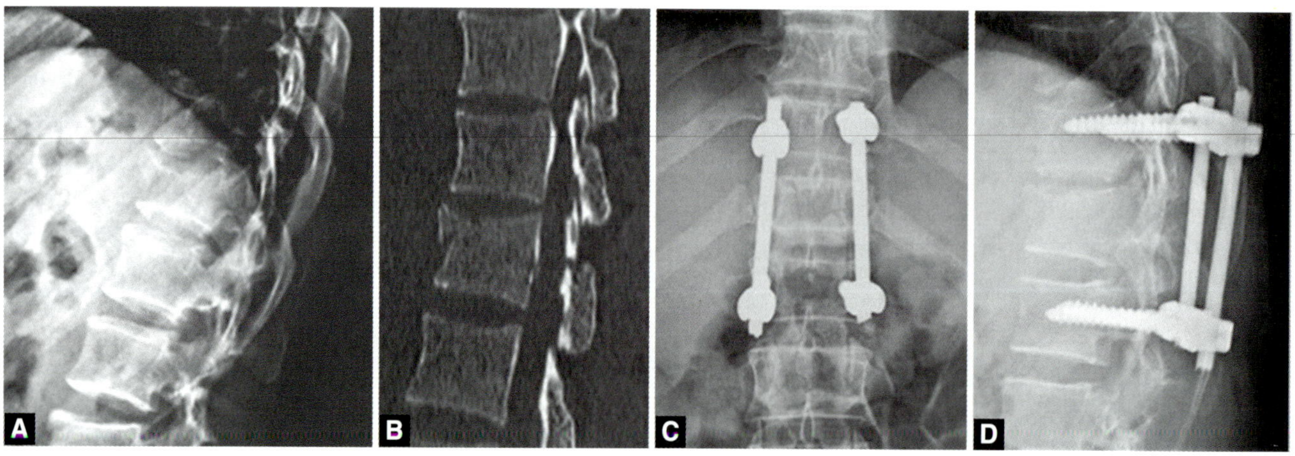

Figures 15.27A to D: (A and B) Lateral radiograph and sagittal CT image indicate three column Chance fracture; (C and D) The fracture has been stabilized with posterior percutaneous stabilization.

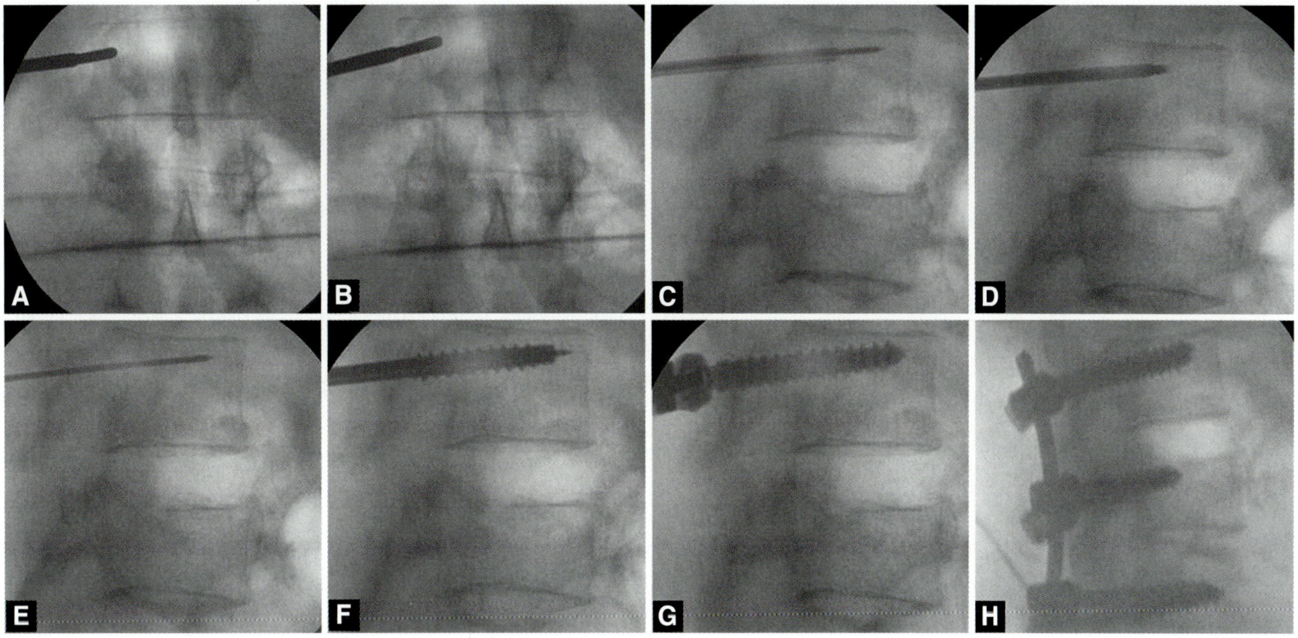

Figures 15.28A to H: The steps of performing a percutaneous pedicle screw fixation. The Jamshidi needle is placed at the lateral wall of the pedicle and passed through the pedicle. Once into the vertebral body, a guide wire is inserted through the needle. A cannulated reamer is passed over the guide wire and the appropriate length of the screw is measured. The cannulated screw is passed over the guide wire into the vertebra. Similarly screws have been inserted into fractured vertebra and the vertebra distal to it. An appropriately contoured rod is maneuvered percutaneously across all the three screws and fixed with nuts.

removal of the instrumentation has been reported from 0% to 45%.[53] A lack of anterior column support caused by a void in the vertebral body after height restoration is held responsible for these failures.[44]

Technique 2: Anterior Decompression and Fixation

Anterior Surgical Approaches

The main indication for anterior decompression is an incomplete neurological injury with a radiological evidence of canal compromise due to displaced bone and disc fragments. The goal of surgery is to provide an optimum environment for recovery by complete decompression of the neural tissue alongwith a stable reconstruction. As the compression is anterior, many surgeons favor an anterior approach as this will allow direct removal of the offending retropulsed bone and disc fragments. Access through the left side is preferred since the aorta is easy to mobilize and the liver is on the right side. The patient is positioned in a direct lateral position with the left side up, shoulders and hips perpendicular to the floor (Figs 15.29A to E). A kidney rest is placed at the apex of the thoracolumbar fracture to prevent the spine sagging between the chest and the pelvis. In this position, the abdomen of obese patients will also sag away from the spine. Generally the rib resected in the thoracotomy and thoracoabdominal incision should be two levels above the vertebra that will be instrumented proximally. It is generally easier to dissect from proximal to distal along the vertebra in anterior spinal approaches. Some variation may be required depending on the obliquity of the ribs and this should be assessed from preoperative lateral X-rays. If the exposure is not adequate, proximal or distal ribs may be osteotomized to improve the exposure. Fractures of T11 and above require thoracotomy only. Fractures of T12 to L1 generally require a thoracoabdominal approach and fractures of L2–4 can be managed through curvilinear infracostal incision that does not require opening of the chest. For thoracotomy approaches, the pleura is incised and the lung is either retracted or deflated to reach the spine. For thoraco-abdominal and abdominal approaches, a retroperitoneal approach to the spine is performed.

Anterior Approach to the Thoracic and Lumbar Spine

Thoracotomy for T4–T10: Thoracic spine can usually be approached by the excision of a rib corresponding to two levels above the level of pathology. Usually, three vertebral bodies and two disc spaces can be visualized well with the excision of a single rib.

The patient is placed in right lateral position with the left side facing upwards. Padded supports are placed beneath the shoulder and buttock. The skin incision is placed from about two finger breadths below the inferior angle of scapula, curving it anterior paralleling the rib to be resected till the anterior axillary line and extending it distally along the anterolateral abdominal wall lateral to the rectus abdominis muscle. The latissimus dorsi and serratus anterior are cut along the line of skin incision down to the ribs. This allows elevation of the scapula to incise the muscles in the back to expose the ribs. The periosteum is incised with the cautery along the surface of the rib and elevated from the rib. Care should be exercised to avoid damaging the intercostal neurovascular bundle that runs along the inferior border of the rib. The posterior three fourths of the rib are resected as far posterior as necessary. The periosteum is lifted with two Adson artery forceps and incised with a knife. The pleural cavity is entered now. A rib retractor is placed between the two adjoining ribs and retracted to enter the thoracic cavity. The lung is gently retracted with moist pads. The parietal pleura over the spine is incised and the disc and vertebrae to be fused are exposed. The segmental vessels in the mid portion of the vertebral body are identified, clamped and divided. The discs are identified as soft, rounded and protuberant area in contrast to the concave surface of the vertebral body. After the procedure has been performed, the lungs must be fully inflated by the anesthetist and checked for atelectasis. A chest tube is inserted and the intercostal muscles are closed by approximating the ribs with a towel clip. The deep muscles (latissimus dorsi, serratus anterior), subcutaneous tissue and skin are closed in layers.

Thoracolumbar Exposure from T11 to L1

Anterior thoracolumbar approach affords an excellent access to the entire thoracolumbar spine. Technically, it is a difficult procedure due to the presence of diaphragm and simultaneous exposure of thoracic and retroperitoneal space. Because of this, it is associated with a higher incidence of perioperative morbidity and careful patient selection is important.

A left-sided approach is usually preferred with the patient placed in a right lateral position. Padded supports are placed beneath the shoulder and buttock. A rolled towel placed under the area of pathology will allow better access to the field of interest but care must be taken to remove it before any instrumentation so that normal spinal contour can be achieved.

The thoracolumbar junction is usually approached through the bed of 10th rib. An oblique skin incision is made from the lateral border of erector spinae muscle to the costochondral junction of the selected rib and extended distally till the lateral border of rectus abdominis. The underlying subcutaneous tissue and muscular layer (latissimus dorsi and serratus anterior) are divided along the line of skin incision. The tenth rib is exposed and the periosteum is elevated with an Alexander elevator. The rib is separated from the underlying pleura with a Doyen retractor. The rib is cut with a rib cutter close to the costocartilage junction anteriorly and as far posteriorly as the dissection is needed. The underlying pleura is opened with a scissor or electrocautery. Identify the diaphragm, which is closely approximated to the thoracic wall, and care is taken while incising the pleura to prevent inadvertent injury to the edge of the lung. Blunt dissection is begun caudal to the diaphragm in the retroperitoneal fat. The parietal peritoneum is separated from the abdominal muscles anteromedially. The dissection is carried out posteriorly toward the diaphragm. The diaphragm is incised 2 cm away from its insertion and tagged with sutures for easier identification during closure. The incision follows the lateral contour of diaphragm and the underlying rib medially to its attachment to the vertebra. The prevertebral fascia is incised, and the segmental vessels that run along the middle of the vertebral bodies are ligated and divided. This provides adequate exposure of the thoracolumbar junction. If further exposure is needed distally, the incision is extended along the lateral border of rectus abdominis muscle and the vertebra can be exposed till L3.

Anterior Retroperitoneal Approach to the Lumbar Spine (L1–L5)

The retroperitoneal approach provides access to all vertebrae from L1 to the L5. The patient is placed on the operating table in the semilateral position. The left side is kept up for ease of retracting the aorta. The patient's body should be at about a 45° angle to the horizontal, facing away from the surgeon. This angle allows the peritoneal contents to fall away from the incision. The patient is fixed in this position throughout the surgery by placing sandbags under the hips and shoulders, and strapping to the table.

The image intensifier can be used to mark the incision by placing a radio-opaque instrument over the flank. Alternatively the 12th rib in the affected flank and the pubic symphysis in the lower part of the abdomen are palpated and the incision is placed between these boundaries depending on the level. The incision extends down from the posterior half of the 12th rib toward the rectus abdominis muscle. The subcutaneous fat is cut to expose the aponeurosis of the external oblique muscle. The aponeurosis of this muscle is in line with the skin incision and is split in the line of its fibers. The internal oblique muscle is identified and cut perpendicular to the line of its muscular fibers. Under the internal oblique muscle lies the transversus abdominis muscle. It is divided in line with the skin incision to expose the retroperitoneal space. Using blunt finger dissection, a plane is developed between the retroperitoneal fat and the fascia that overlies the psoas muscle. The peritoneal cavity and its contents are retracted medially with a Dever's retractor. The ureter, which is attached loosely to the peritoneum, is carried forward with it. The psoas fascia, is identified and the surface of the psoas muscle is followed medially to reach the anterior lateral surface of the vertebral bodies.

The aorta and vena cava effectively are tied to the waist of the vertebral bodies by the lumbar arteries and veins. These smaller vessels must be dissected individually on the involved vertebrae and tied so that the aorta and vena cava can be mobilized and the anterior part of the vertebral body reached. A needle is placed into the fractured lumbar vertebra and a radiograph is performed to identify the exact location.

Surgical Technique of Anterior Decompression and Stabilization

Once the spine is reached, the appropriate level is confirmed either by palpation to look for the fractured vertebra or by placing a needle into a disc space and checking with the image intensifier. Segmental vessels may need to be ligated over the fractured vertebra and proximal and distal vertebrae for instrumentation. The segmental vessel should be ligated at the midlateral level of the vertebral body. The surgical exposure should demonstrate the anterior and lateral side of the body (Figs 15.29 and 15.30). In the lumbar spine, the psoas muscle needs to be mobilized. It can be dissected off the vertebral body where it originates above and below each disc. The use of a Cobb elevator along the disc will allow the psoas to be gradually dissected away from its origin, allowing the concavity of the vertebral body wall to be displayed and the segmental vessels to be ligated. The psoas muscle may obstruct an adequate view of the vertebral body and the decompression. Once it has been mobilized, the muscle can often be held out of the way by a Steinmann pin inserted into the lower vertebra below the fracture. In the chest, the rib head of the relevant vertebral bodies should be resected so as to allow identification of the pedicle and the foramen, and to assist with anatomical landmark identification. Anteriorly the vertebral body should be displayed beyond the midline.

Firstly, the disc above and below the vertebra is resected back to the posterior portion of the disc. The vertebral body is then removed at the front and the left side back to the canal. Curettes and Kerrison rongeurs are used, or a high-speed burr is used to remove the fracture fragments. Dissection into the canal starts inferiorly and should be carried across to the opposite side so that the neural elements do not bulge out and obscure the view. The maximum compression of the neural elements is normally at the proximal level of the involved vertebral body. Dissection proceeds proximally to resect the fragment that is wedged between the two pedicles. This can be removed with curettes. The remainders of the discs above and below the fracture are resected to demonstrate the posterior longitudinal ligament and the dura.

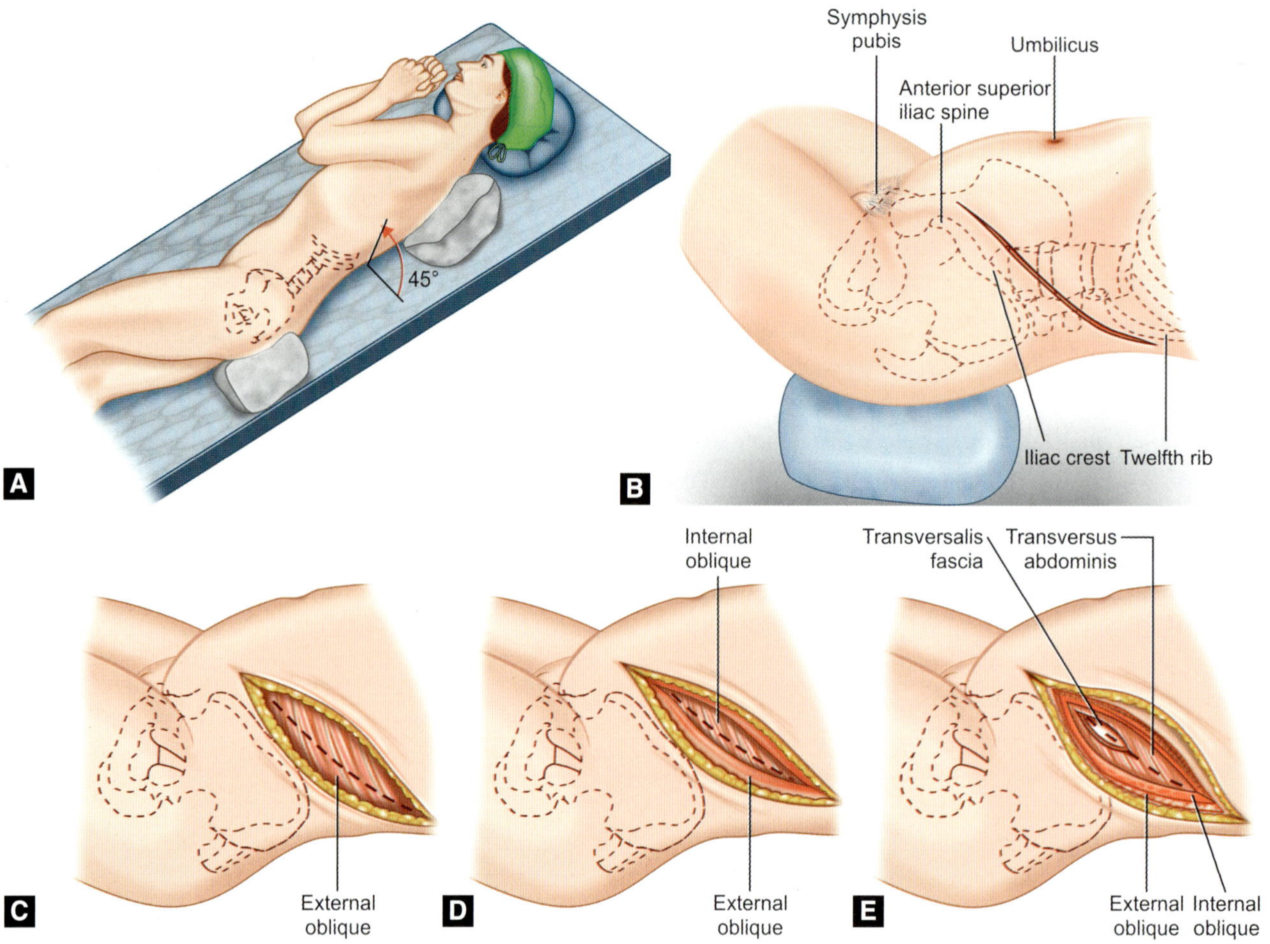

Figures 15.29A to E: For an anterior approach, the patient is positioned in the lateral decubitus position with appropriate supports. The incision is planned depending on the level of the fracture. The skin, subcutaneous tissue, external oblique, internal oblique and the transverses abdominis are all opened in the same line as that of the skin incision.

The pedicles on each side must be identified to identify the lateral extent of the decompression. The canal above and below the relevant disc should be palpated to confirm decompression. Dissection must be far enough across the vertebral body to the right side to allow proper seating of the cage. It is important to preserve the end plates of the adjacent vertebra. Hemostasis can be obtained with gel foam, surgical or bipolar diathermy in the canal.

The defect in the vertebral body can be filled up either by tricortical iliac crest graft, cortical allografts or by cages. Iliac crest autografts provide an ideal osteogenic environment for fusion but are associated with donor site morbidity. The disadvantages of allografts are delayed fusion, infection risks and availability. Cages offer an excellent option and can be sized to fill the corpectomy space. They must be filled with bone, usually that was obtained during the vertebral body resection, or augmented with rib graft. A cage should be placed anteriorly and centrally and must be clearly away from the canal.

If a posterior stabilization has been performed or planned for the patient, then a stand alone anterior vertebral reconstruction should suffice. However if an anterior reconstruction alone is planned, the patient requires supplemental stabilization with screws and rods. The screws of the stabilization device must be placed above and below the vertebra resected. They should be placed parallel to the relevant end plates. A needle can be inserted

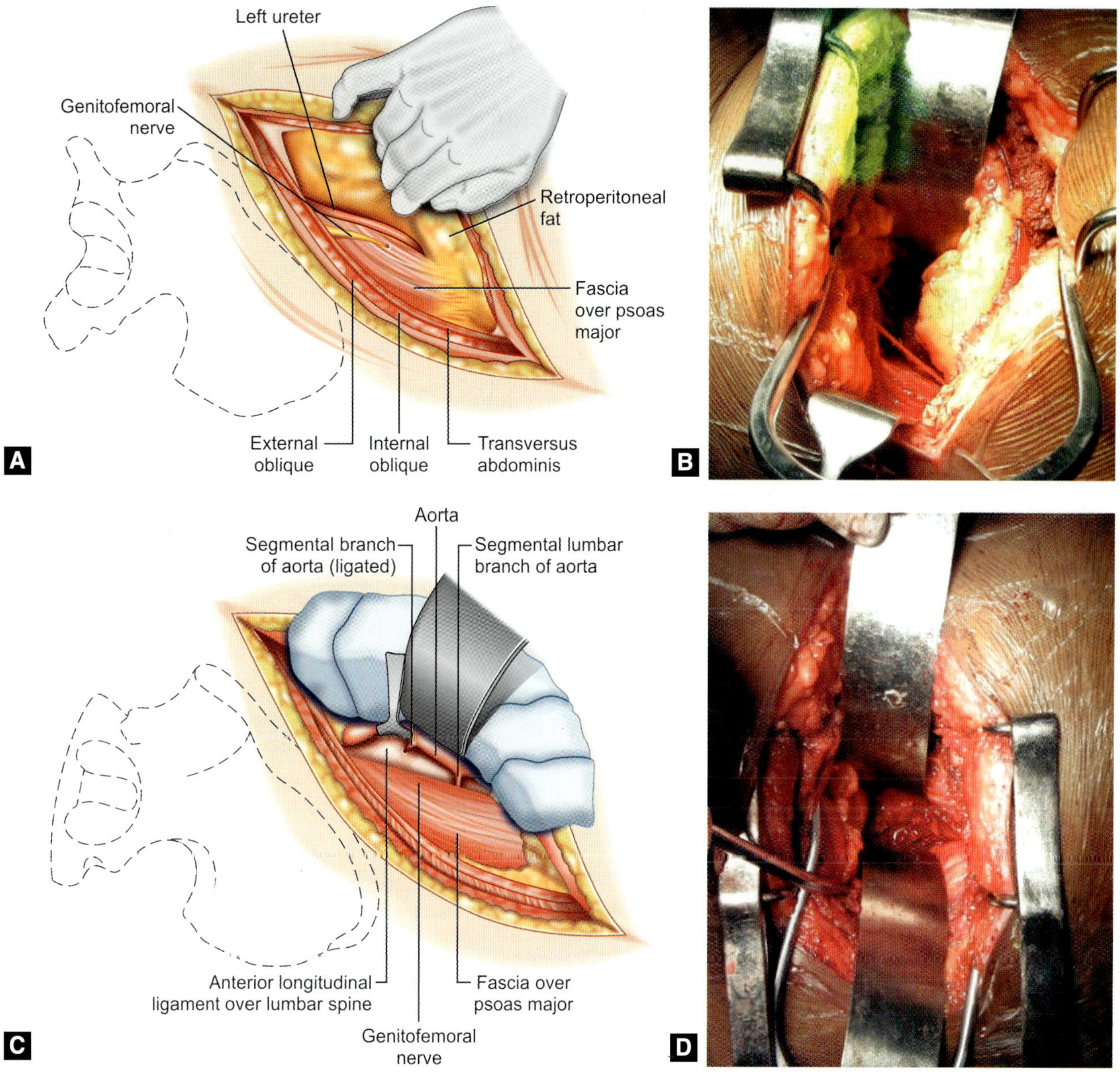

Figures 15.30A to D: The retroperitoneal space is identified by the fat pad and gentle blunt dissection is performed to reach the psoas muscle. The genitor femoral nerve is seen to traverse across the ilio psoas muscle. The psoas muscle is retracted laterally and the vertebral body is reached. The segmental vessels over the vertebral body are ligated and the anterior column reconstruction is performed.

into the adjacent disc space to guide the placement of screws parallel to the end plate. When screws are placed, it is important for the screws to be longer so that the opposite cortex of the body is engaged to obtain maximum biomechanical strength. The corpectomy site should be distracted and this is best done with vertebral body spreaders rather than overloading the screws. The screws can be used to stabilize the distraction when the reconstruction device is placed. Now a rod is connected to the two screws above and below the fractured vertebra. Chest drains are required if thoracotomy has been performed. Strong nonabsorbable sutures are used to reapproximate the ribs and they must be passed subperiosteally on the inferior side to avoid entrapment of the subcostal vessels and nerves. Local anesthetics injected along the intercostal interspaces are useful to assist with postoperative pain management. An intrapleural catheter can also be placed to allow ongoing post-operative analgesia.

The patient should be recovered supine and log rolled for comfort. The chest drains are removed when X-rays show that the lung is expanded and the drainage reduced.

Technique 3: Posterior Decompression and Fixation

Posterior Exposure of the Thoracic and Lumbar Spine

Stabilization by posterior approach is the most popular and widely employed surgical management of the thoracolumbar spine fracture. The familiarity of approach, the ease of decompression and stabilization, and the decreased rate of complication make this approach a favored one for most surgeons. Many forms of instrumentation, such as the sublaminar wire systems, the rod and hook system and more recently the pedicle screw systems, have all been utilized to achieve a stable reduction. The number of levels of vertebral instrumentation and the need for fusion are under debate (Figs 15.31 and 15.32). Unstable burst fractures without significant vertebral body destruction may be treated with short segment pedicle fixation devices but may require additional levels of instrumentation when hooks and sublaminar wires are used. Unstable thoracolumbar injuries like flexion-distraction injuries, fracture-dislocations, burst fractures with a load sharing score greater than seven, fractures associated with severe osteoporosis, and those in patients with ankylosing spondylitis require, long segment fixation, frequently extending to three segments above and three segments below the fractured site.

A significant disadvantage of the posterior approaches to the spine includes the fusion disease. Fusion disease includes denervation of paraspinal muscles and facet capsules, damage to the proximal facet joint, and weakening of other supportive structures, resulting in prolonged postoperative pain and disability.[54] Recently, to reduce the posterior-approach related complications, minimally invasive techniques, such as percutaneous pedicle screw fixation of thoracolumbar burst fractures, have become popular with improved clinical and functional results, shorter time of recovery and lower complication rates.[55]

Surgical Technique (Figs 15.33 and 15.34)

The posterior approach to the lumbar spine provides direct access to the spinous processes, laminae and facet joints at all levels. The approach is through the midline, and it can be extended proximally and distally as required. Laminectomy to decompress the spinal cord and pedicle screw fixation, and fusion of spinal fractures can be performed through this approach.

The patient is positioned prone on two bolsters with one underneath the sternum and the other beneath the pubis and anterior superior iliac spine. This allows the abdomen to be entirely free, thus reducing venous plexus filling around the spinal cord and decrease bleeding during the procedure.

The involved level is marked by marking the spinous process with a hypodermic needle. Accurate localization of the involved segment with an image intensifier in the operating room is important before proceeding with the skin incision and exposure. The skin and subcutaneous tissue are infiltrated with a 1: 500,000 epinephrine solution to minimize blood loss. A midline skin incision is made centered over the involved segment. The length of the incision depends on the number of levels to be explored. The dissection is carried down in the midline through the subcutaneous tissue and lumbodorsal fascia to the tips of the spinous processes. In a young patient, the tip of the spinous process is a cartilaginous apophysis; it can be split in the midline making subperiosteal muscle removal easier.

Self-retaining retractors are used to retract and maintain tension on soft tissues. The paraspinal muscles are elevated subperiosteally from the underlying laminae in distal to proximal direction, using a Cobb elevator. Dissection is done along the spinous process and lamina till the medial one third of the transverse process. Close to the facet joints in the area between the transverse processes, are the vessels supplying the paraspinal muscles on a segmental basis. These branches of the

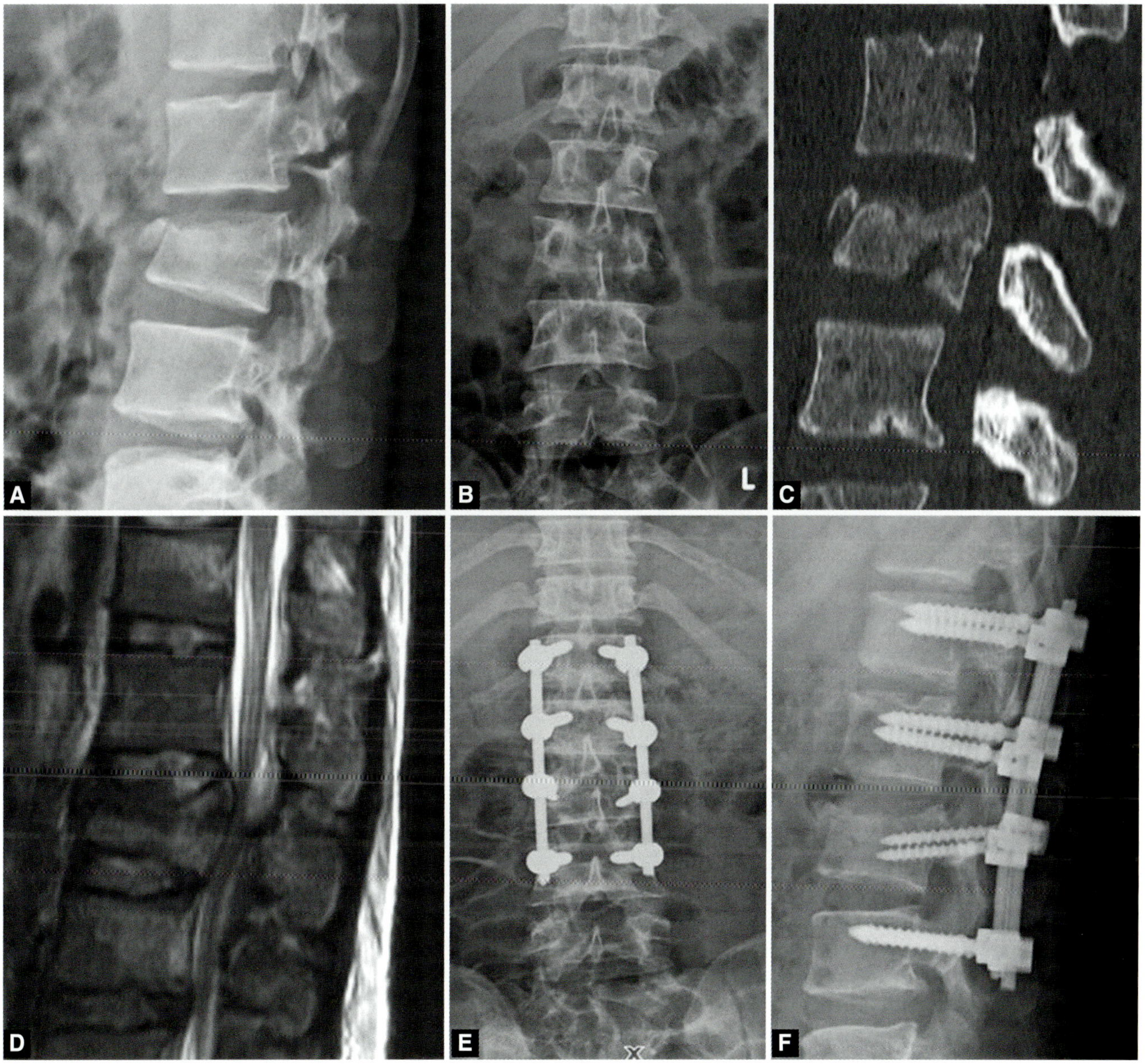

Figures 15.31A to F: An unstable burst fracture of L2 vertebra treated with decompression and multisegmental fixation.

lumbar vessels frequently bleed as the dissection is carried out laterally. Vigorous cauterization of these vessels may be necessary to stop the bleeding. The posterior primary rami of the lumbar nerves, which also supply the paraspinal muscles segmentally, run with these vessels. After completion of the desired spinal procedure, the wound is closed in layers.

Technique of Fracture Stabilization

Pedicle screws are inserted into the vertebra cephalad and caudal to the fracture. The authors use the following landmarks to insert the pedicle screws. In the thoracic spine, the entry point is located at the junction of a line drawn across the upper one third of the transverse

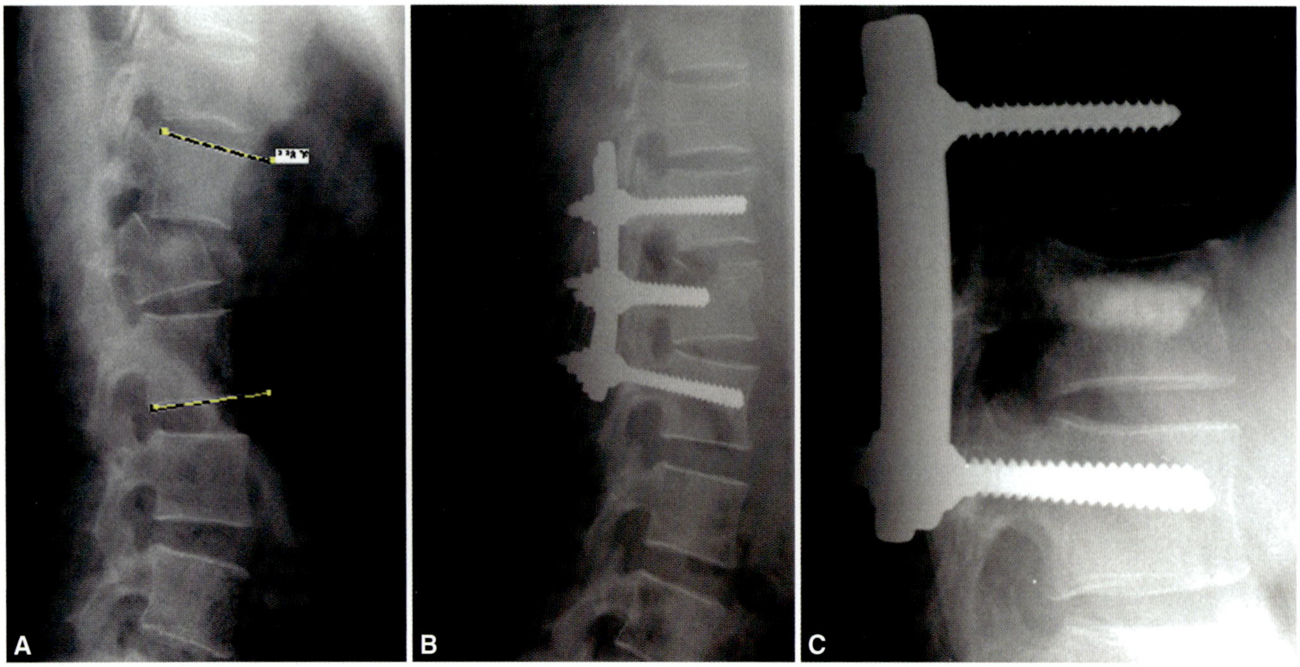

Figures 15.32A to C: Short-segment pedicle screw based posterior reduction and stabilization in neurologically intact B1.3 fracture with and without ceramic augmentation.

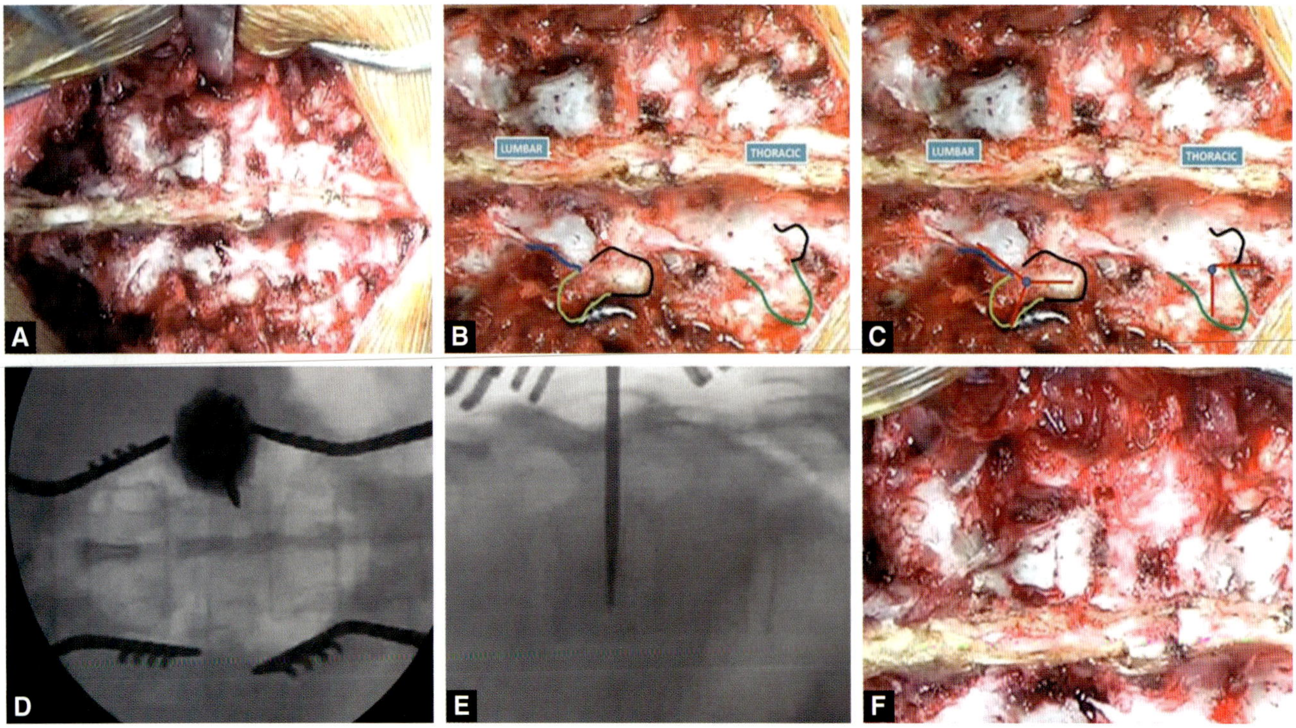

Figures 15.33A to F: (A) The posterior elements of spine have been exposed; (B) The T12 and L1 vertebral anatomy of the lamina, transverse process and the facet joint have been marked; (C) The ideal entry point for the screw at T12 and L1 vertebra has been marked. The pedicle awl has been passed through the pedicle and confirmed in (D) anteroposterior and (E) lateral views; (F) Usually bright red bleeding from the cancellous vertebral bone through the pedicle hole indicates correct pedicle track. This is confirmed by using a thin pedicle probe.

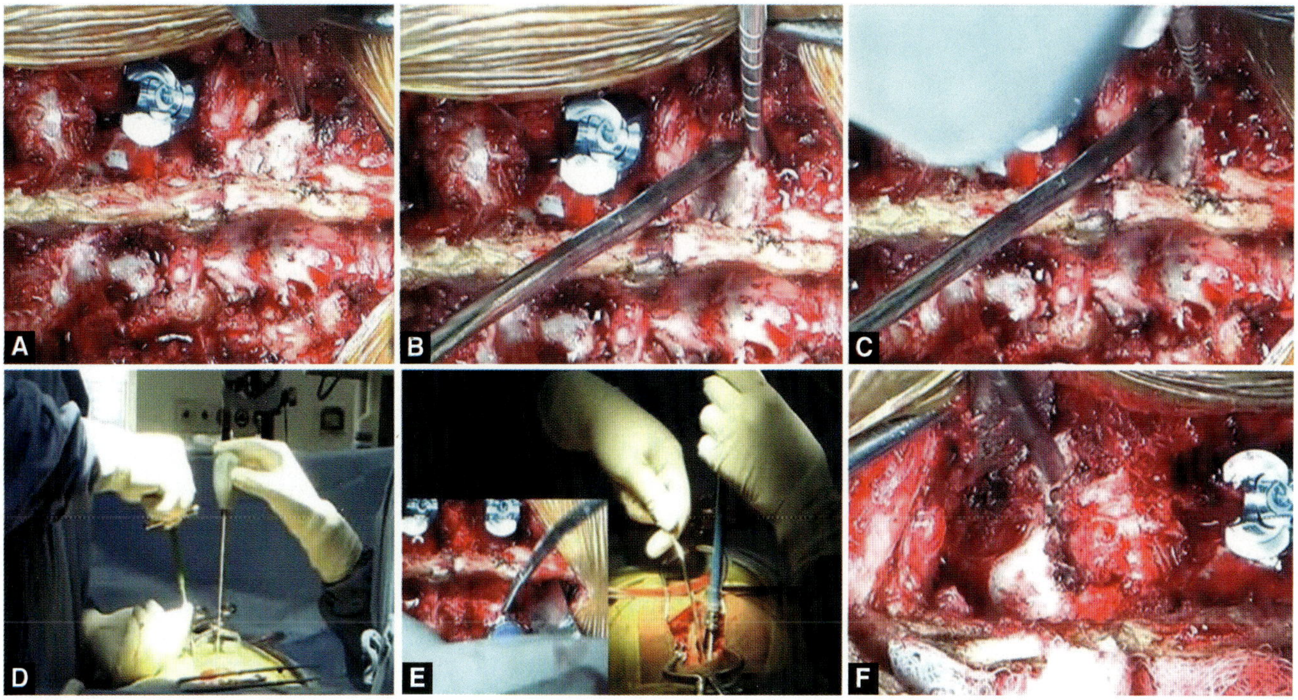

Figures 15.34A to F: Similarly screws are inserted into the T 12 pedicle first with an awl and then with a curved Lenke probe. The Lenke probe is initially turned laterally as it traverses through the pedicle and once it has reached the vertebral body, the probe is turned through 180° to face medially. This reduces the chances of pedicle fracture. The appropriate medial angulation of the pedicle screw at the L1 and T12 levels is demonstrated. At L2 level, the pedicle screw entry is at the junction of the upper one third of the transverse process and the lateral facet joint.

process and another line along the lateral aspect of the facet joint. An entry into the bone is made with a sharp awl. Then a pedicle probe is used to slowly pass through the pedicle by gentle rocking movements of the probe. The probe is angulated about 15–20° medially. The cephalocaudal angulation is decided by the sagittal orientation of the vertebra at each level. For example, the T1,T2 vertebra are at the top of the thoracic kyphosis and hence the probe is angulated about 20° to the floor. Once the probe enters into the vertebral body, it is removed and a thin pedicle feeler is used to check the integrity of all the pedicle walls and the floor. Any suspicious break or a soft non-bony feel is potentially dangerous and this is checked with an image intensifier. This technique is called the "free-hand technique" and the author prefers it. One can also use the image intensifier to decide the entry point and the pedicle path as is used for the percutaneous technique. The advantage would be a lesser risk of pedicle violation and the disadvantage is the larger radiation dose.

In the lumbar spine, the entry point is located at the junction of the following three lines ("Mercedes Benz Sign"): (1) one along the lateral border of the facet joint, (2) one along the middle of the transverse process and (3) one along the pars interarticularis. The rest of the procedure is the same as it is for thoracic spine. Once the pedicle tracks are created, appropriate sized screws are inserted. For short segment fracture stabilization, screws are inserted into the cephalad and caudad vertebra. Under fluoroscopic guidance, screws are also inserted into the pedicles of the fractured vertebrae (intermediate screws) and left proud compared to the screws inserted above and below (Figs 15.35A to D).

A lateral entry point is used to insert all the screws so as to avoid damaging the facet capsule and joint. Intermediate screws are inserted in both the pedicles of the fractured vertebra; however if a pedicle (as assessed on the CT scan) is fractured, no screw is inserted in to that pedicle. If both the pedicles are injured, then an extended

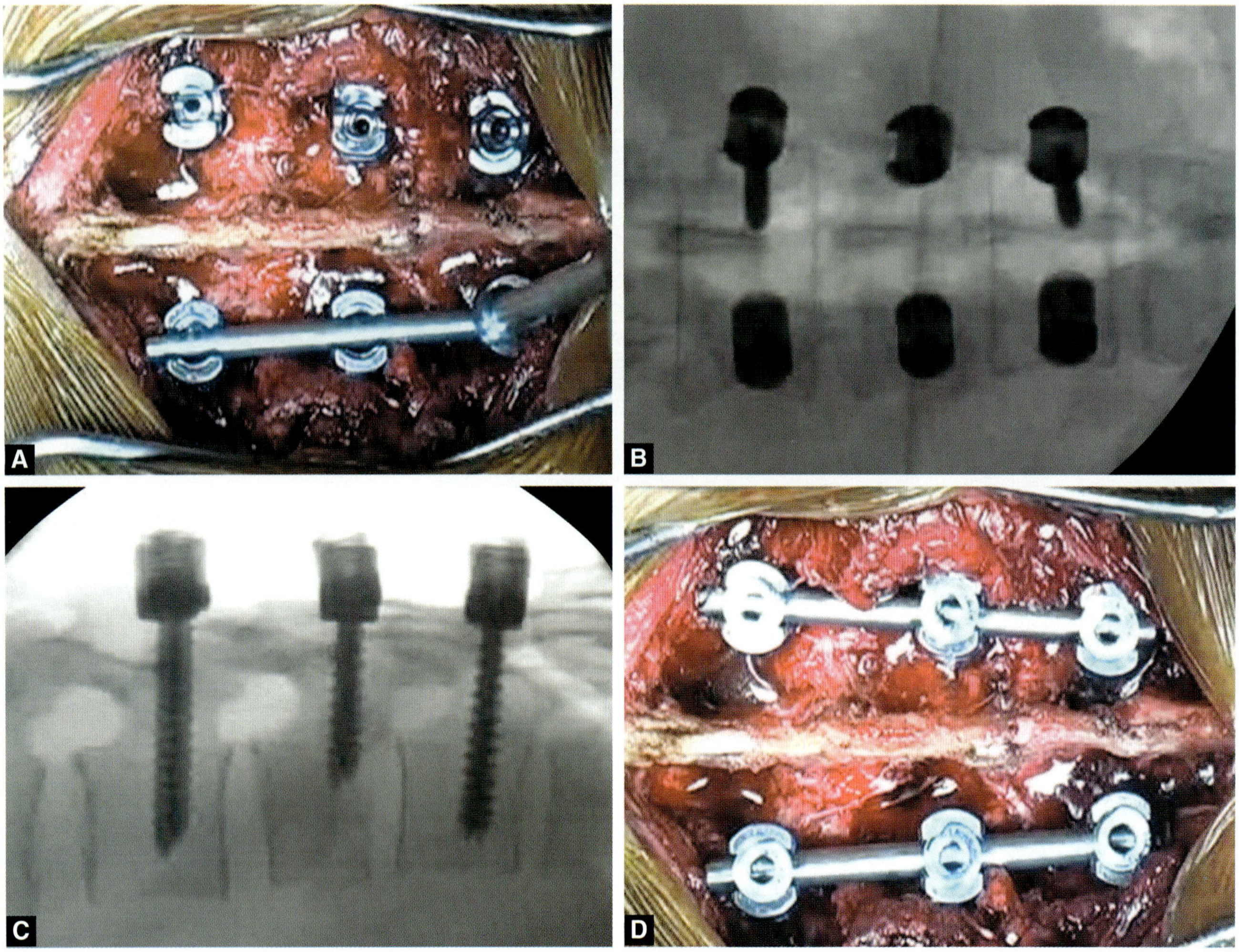

Figures 15.35A to D: The three pedicle screws have been inserted on either side and confirmed in the anteroposterior and lateral image intensifier views. Appropriately contoured rods are placed in the screws and fixed with nuts.

construct or a combined anterior procedure is performed. The length of the intermediate screws is generally kept short so that it just enters the vertebral body after crossing the pedicle. This serves two purposes: allows an anterior reconstruction on a later date if required without disturbing the posterior construct and also does not interfere with fracture healing. The screws are then connected by physiologically contoured rods. Attempt can be made at achieving complete reduction of kyphosis or restoring height to normal by rod over-contouring, compression or distraction. However in these cases, a significant restoration of the anterior vertebral height would mandate its reconstruction either by transpedicular bone grafting, cementing or an anterior procedure. In fractures with a significant lateral compression component, minimal distraction is performed on the ipsilateral side. In patients with neurological deficits or if the spinal canal compromise is greater than 40% in patients without deficit, a midline fenestration and decompression can be done at the level of the pedicles.

The wound is closed in layers over a suction drain. Postoperatively, patients are fitted with a thoracolumbar orthosis and mobilized on the 2nd or 3rd day based on comfort levels. As this is a motion preserving technique, the implants can be removed at 6–12 months, once the fracture has healed.

The degree of kyphosis correction and the position of screws can be assessed by the postoperative radiographs.

To assess features like the degree of indirect reduction of fracture and improvement in canal width, position and containment of screws, a postoperative CT scan is required.

THORACOLUMBAR EXPOSURE: Pearls and Pitfalls

Posterior exposure

- In burst fractures, the lamina could have been fractured with possible entrapment of thecal sac between the fracture fragments. An unwary surgeon can easily injure the nerve roots while performing the laminectomy.
- Blood vessels from the segmental arteries supplying the paraspinal muscles are situated close to the facet joints, in the area between the transverse processes. These branches of the lumbar vessels frequently bleed as the dissection is carried out laterally. Vigorous cauterization of these vessels may be necessary to stop the bleeding.

Anterior exposure

- The aorta and inferior vena cava are tethered to the anterior surface of the lumbar vertebrae by the lumbar segmental vessels. These smaller vessels must be ligated and cut to allow the aorta to be dissected off the lumbar vertebrae. It is important to dissect these vessels out carefully without cutting them flush with the aorta. If the vessels are cut flush, the bleeding may be extremely difficult to control.
- Mobilization of the venous structures should be undertaken very carefully because they are fairly fragile and easily traumatized. Damage to these vessels may result in thrombosis and hence, mobilization and retraction should be kept to a minimum.
- The sympathetic chain lies on the lateral aspect of the vertebral body and on the most medial aspect of the psoas muscle. It is easy to identify as the tissue is cleared from the front of the vertebrae. Injury to the sympathetic chain can result in flushing and warmth on the ipsilateral lower limb due to loss of sympathetic tone.
- The genitofemoral nerve lies on the anterior medial surface of the psoas muscle attached to its fascia. Injury to the nerve can result in numbness around the groin and perineum.

Outcomes

Thoracolumbar region is a common site for spinal injuries due to the transition from the rigid thoracic spine to the mobile lumbar spine. Many classification systems have been developed over the years to characterize the injury and to guide the surgeon regarding therapeutic decision making. With the diverse patterns of bony, ligamentous and spinal cord injury possible in spinal injured patients and with each injury component having potential significant contribution to the direct outcome of the patient, their involvement in decision making becomes important. Existing classification systems have their own pros and cons. Surgeons likely show better agreement if the choice of a treatment category has direct consequences for treatment. Reproducibility and interobserver reliability of classification systems also remains a key issue. As imaging modalities have enhanced our understanding of these complex injury patterns, the role of soft tissues have started gaining importance in assessment of injuries and management. The MRI findings in 100 cases with thoracolumbar spine injuries were analyzed and a classification based on the ligament injury-ALL, PLL, posterior ligament complex, the injuries to the disk, end plate, and vertebral body was proposed by Oner et al.[21] This system has been independently validated and found to predict progression of deformity and pain.[22] Also classifications by McCormick et al. and the TLICS have been observed to be helpful in guiding the type of management and surgical approach for each patient.[23] McCormick's load sharing classification guides the surgeon to decide on whether a particular patient would require anterior column reconstruction or not. Presently, among the different classification systems, TLICS seems to be the best system available for therapeutic decision-making for TL spine injuries. There is evidence that posterior ligament complex injury (which has been given significant weightage in TLICS) can be reliably detected by MRI and this has moderately correlated with the intraoperative findings. Though there is no strong evidence that MRI findings of posterior ligament complex disruption contributes significantly to surgical decision-making beyond what is determined by morphologic criteria using plain radiographs and CT, the presence of definite posterior ligament complex injury is considered as a strong indicator for surgical stabilization.

The exact timing and type of surgical treatment for thoracolumbar spinal injuries also remains controversial. Factors, such as the anesthetic and surgical burden to the patient, morbidity, complication rates, costs, and disutility should be taken into account in the choice of surgical approach. Regarding the timing of surgery, there is no evidence that early surgery can improve neurological outcomes.[31] But logically it is better to operate on neurologically deficient patients on an emergent basis based on the assumption that persistent compression of neural structures would reduce the chances of neurological recovery.

Stabilization by posterior approach is the most popular and widely employed surgical management of the thoracolumbar spine fracture. The familiarity of approach, the ease of decompression and stabilization, and the decreased rate of complication make this approach a favored one for most surgeons. Short segment pedicle screw fixation allows preservation of as many motion segments as possible. Addition of a pedicle screw at the level of the fracture has also been found to increase stability, improve kyphosis correction and also reduce implant failure.[56,57] In patients with significant collapse of the vertebral body with a load sharing score greater than seven, short segment fusions have the risks of loss of fracture reduction and increased kyphosis due to greater recollapse of the anterior column. Extended long column constructs, reinforcement with kyphoplasty, calcium phosphate and transpedicular bone grafts in this setting augment the anterior column, thus maintaining the anterior height.[58,59] In patients with severe communition of the vertebra, reconstruction with a titanium cage may also be necessary to prevent an anterior collapse.

Anterior decompression relieves the bony compression on the spinal cord and aids reconstruction of the anterior column. The degree of neurological recovery, rate of spinal fusion, sagittal spine alignment, and return to preinjury activities after anterior decompression appear more favorable compared to techniques that do not decompress the spinal canal.[60] Use of anterior vertebral plates, dual rod and screw systems, titanium mesh cages and expanding cages has greatly improved postoperative spinal stability and also reduced donor-site morbidity from major bone graft harvesting techniques.[61-65] In a study of 150 patients with thoracolumbar burst fracture and associated neurological injury treated with a single stage anterior decompression, instrumentation and fusion, the fusion rate was 93%, and improvement of at least 1 Frankel grade was observed in 142 patients. Fifty-six (72%) of the 78 patients with preoperative paralysis or dysfunction of the bladder recovered completely. One hundred twenty-five (96%) of the 130 patients who were employed before the injury returned to work after the operation, and 112 (86%) returned to their previous job without restrictions. Although combined anterior/posterior approaches seem better able to retain kyphosis correction, it is not clear if this difference is clinically relevant. Based on existing literature, there is no specific surgical approach that can be strongly recommended for a thoracolumbar fracture with incomplete neurologic deficit that has any advantage as far as neurologic recovery is concerned.

Relatively few studies compare anterior to posterior approaches for thoracolumbar burst fractures, and most of them show an advantage of the anterior approach. In his series, Gertzbein reported that bladder function significantly improved following anterior compared to posterior procedures.[66] Hitchon et al. showed that angular deformity was more successfully corrected and maintained when the anterior approach was used.[67] Others also showed that although both approaches are associated with a statistically significant initial improvement in sagittal alignment, the posterior approach was associated with increased loss of sagittal correction (8.1°) compared to the anterior approach (1.8°) at follow-up.[68] Minimal access and endoscopic approaches also offer significant advantages to the patient in terms of reduction of access related morbidity but tend to have larger learning curves, more complications, higher costs related to specialized implants and instruments, more radiation exposure, etc.

Select patients with thoracolumbar burst fractures may benefit from combined surgical approaches. Indications include complete posterior ligamentous complex disruption and partial neurological injury, and rigid post-traumatic kyphotic deformity as seen in injuries, which are more than 2-weeks-old. The advantages of combined surgical approaches are improved sagittal alignment, thorough spinal canal and neural decompression for optimum recovery of neural function, and stabilization of the disrupted posterior ligamentous complex. In a series of 20 consecutive patients with a single-level unstable thoracolumbar burst fracture treated by bisegmental posterior fixation followed by anterior corpectomy and titanium cage implantation 7–10 days later, 12 patients with initial neurological deficits recovered an average of 1.5 grades on the ASIA scale.[69] Two years postoperatively, the mean visual analog scale score for back pain was 1.6 points and the mean pain at the anterior approach site was 1.2 points. At 2 years after treatment, instrumentation failure did not occur; the mean loss of kyphosis correction was 3°. At a mean follow-up of 6 years, a comparative retrospective study of combined versus posterior-only fixation reported similar clinical outcome and neurological improvement, fusion rate and angle of kyphotic deformity in both groups. However, loss of reduction more than 5° and instrumentation failure were significantly higher in the posterior-only fixation.[70]

MANAGEMENT: Pearls and Pitfalls

- Radiographic evaluation should include assessment of the interspinous diastasis on lateral radiographs as well as rotation and translation on the AP radiographs as this provides information regarding the status of the posterior osseoligamentous complex. Disruption of this ligament complex implies a three-column injury and these are unstable injuries requiring surgical management.
- Approximately 25% of burst fractures are misdiagnosed as compression fractures if radiographs alone are evaluated and hence it is important to evaluate significant thoracic and lumbar fractures with a CT scan.
- Fractures with failed anterior column with a significant kyphosis and collapse would require anterior column reconstruction.
- In patients who are neurologically incomplete or with cauda equina injury due to pressure on neural elements by fracture fragments, an anterior decompression, reconstruction and stabilization are advocated.
- Patients with spinal fractures following a high velocity injury are at risk of having other multi system injuries like lung, pleural injuries, diaphragmatic injuries and solid organ injuries of the abdomen. Hence it is crucial to perform a critical systemic assessment to avoid missing serious organ injuries.

Complications

Posterior Approach

Since its first introduction by Harrington and Tullos in 1969[71] and further development by Roy-Camille et al.[72] pedicle screw fixation has become the mainstay of spinal instrumentation for fracture stabilization. Despite increasing experience and knowledge on the use of pedicle screws and technical advances, pedicle screw insertion is still associated with a certain degree of complications. The most commonly reported complication is screw malpositioning, with an overall incidence of 0–42% in the literature.[73-75] Most of them are asymptomatic without any major sequelae, and serious screw-related complications, such as neurological, visceral or vascular are very rare. A meta-analysis with 130 studies involving a total of 37,337 pedicle screws by Kosmopoulos and Schizas found a mean misplacement rate of 8.7%.[76] Thorough anatomical knowledge, respect for anatomical landmarks, careful evaluation of preoperative images and use of modern imaging systems in difficult cases can potentially reduce the risk of screw misplacement. Although minor misplacement poses little problem, a larger displacement (> 4 mm) out of the pedicle especially medial and inferior is associated with a high risk of injury to neighbouring vital structures. Perforations that are lateral or superior can result in a biomechanically weak construct.

Neurological Injury

The overall incidence of nerve root or spinal cord injury due to screw malpositioning is low, ranging between 0.6% and 11%.[77] An overall mean incidence of dural lesions of 0.18% per pedicle screw and an overall mean incidence of nerve root irritations of 0.19% per pedicle screw have been reported in a study.[78] Although a transient self-limiting neurapraxia in the form of numbness or mild weakness is more common, the incidence of a permanent neurological deficit is rare. A new neurological deficit or postoperative radicular pain requires evaluation by CT scan. The presence of a breach requires revision of the screw. A medial breach can result in spinal cord injury and this requires immediate removal of the screw as soon as it is identified.

If there is leakage of clear fluid indicating a CSF leak during pedicle screw insertion, it indicates that the screw is too medial or inferior. Although most CSF leaks may spontaneously resolve, direct visualization of the screw with relation to the neurological structures by laminectomy is ideal to identify and suture the dural injury. The removal of a screw placed too medially into the spinal canal is challenging because of potential neurological injury. Therefore, removal of the screw should always be done under direct visualization of the adjacent nervous structures.

Vascular Injury

Vascular injuries related to misplacement of screws are potential life and limb threatening complications that require early recognition with prompt repair of vascular lesions and screw repositioning. Several vascular structures can potentially be damaged during pedicle screw insertion depending on the anatomical level of the surgical procedure. This includes the azygos vein, intercostal artery, inferior vena cava, aorta for the thoracic spine and mainly the aorta and common iliac vessels for the lumbar spine. Injury to a major vessel is catastrophic and hence immediate recognition of a vascular injury is crucial. With the help of a vascular surgeon, a direct vascular suture or embolization can be performed in emergency situations after appropriate repositioning of the patient.

There is considerable debate regarding replacement of a misplaced screw, which is in close contact with a blood vessel in an asymptomatic patient.[79] There are proponents for both immediate removal versus observation.[80]

Visceral Injury

Visceral injuries related to pedicle screw insertions are very rare. The proximity of thoracolumbar vertebral bodies to structures like lung, pleura and esophagus can potentially result in pneumothorax, effusion or an esophageal injury if a too long pedicle screw has been used. Using the appropriate sized screws and image intensifier will avoid this complication.

Biomechanical Complications

A pedicle fracture can result if there is a mismatch between the screw size and the pedicle diameter making the right choice of screw size as of utmost importance. In patients with a hard cancellous bone, tapping is recommended before screw insertion. If a pedicle fracture occurs, the surgeon can either try to create a new pedicle track or choose an alternative method of fixation or extend the levels of fixation.

Screw pullout can result in patients with poor bone density (osteoporosis), excessive strain on the implant, defective screw hole preparation, high torque of insertion and a weak screw purchase. If a screw pullout occurs, the surgeon can opt to observe if there is reasonable fracture consolidation and acceptable local kyphosis or revise the implant if there is significant post-traumatic progressive kyphosis.

Screws can break when the fracture has not healed completely, deficient anterior column, progressive kyphosis and pseudoarthrosis. This is mainly attributable to metal fatigue due to excessive strain on the implant. In such cases, there is a need to revise the implant. Depending on the reason for failure, there may be need for anterior column reconstruction, augmentation with bone graft and extension of the fusion construct.

Anterior Approach

The abdomen contains many vascular structures, which are exposed during anterior surgeries, and hence at risk for injury. These include the aorta with its bifurcation, inferior vena cava with its major tributaries, segmental vessels, and numerous veins. Most anterior approaches to the spine are performed through the left side for the ease of retracting the aorta. The abdominal aorta bifurcation is usually situated at the level of the L4 vertebral body, while the confluence of the common iliac veins into the inferior vena cava is usually located at the level of the L4/5 intervertebral region. Most vascular injuries occur when operating at the L4/5 level due to the above mentioned anatomical reasons. Venous laceration is the most common vascular injury and usually occurs during manipulation and retraction of the great vessels. Vascular injury may also occur while performing the corpectomy, placing the graft, and inserting the screws. The veins most commonly injured are the left common iliac vein, inferior vena cava and iliolumbar vein. Manual compression or primary repair of the tear is generally effective at treating this complication. In a review of vascular injuries during anterior spinal approaches, Inamasu and Guiot found that the most common arterial injury occurring during anterior lumbar interbody fusion is left iliac artery thrombosis.[81] This complication occurs due to prolonged retraction of the common iliac arteries to the right, causing diminished arterial flow and subsequent left-sided thrombosis. Treatment of this complication is considered an emergency and involves thrombectomy and/or bypass surgery. Preventative strategies proposed include intermittent release of the retraction intraoperatively, and lower-extremity pulse oximetry during and after the procedure.

Adynamic postoperative ileus is a common complication after anterior spinal procedures and is a major determinant of length of hospital stay. In addition, postoperative ileus stands as a barrier to effective pain management in many of these patients as opioid analgesics are contraindicated in this group of patients. The possible pathogenic mechanisms of postoperative ileus include neurogenic, inflammatory and pharmacological. Experimental evidence suggests that reactive hyperactivity of the sympathetic nervous system overcomes normal parasympathetic-driven gastrointestinal smooth-muscle activity, diminishing normal gastrointestinal motility. The handling of bowel contents also makes the intestine sluggish in the immediate postoperative period. Though postoperative ileus is a common but self-limiting problem, other rare but serious complications like acute colonic pseudoobstruction, toxic megacolon and mechanical obstruction must be considered to avoid catastrophic complications. With persistent symptoms, a CT scan would be required to rule out these complications.

Retrograde ejaculation can complicate any abdominal surgery in male patients due to injury of the superior hypogastric plexus. This plexus lies beneath the peritoneum, courses anterior to the aorta, and crosses anterior to the left common iliac vein. Postoperative lymphocele or chyloretroperitoneum is an uncommon complication following anterior spine surgery. Lymph vessels and nodes are numerous around the spinal column, and persistent leakage can result in lymphedema, mechanical compression, nutritional deficiencies, immunosuppression, and sometimes death. Usually management includes observation and if persistent, ultrasonogram guided drainage can be performed.

Injuries to the peritoneum are very common but are easily repaired and do not lead to significant problems. Very rarely injury to the bowel or the ureter can happen. This is usually evident intraoperatively and requires the expertise of the general abdominal surgeon to repair. Experience, expertise and use of blunt surgical dissection would help in avoiding these injuries.

Chronic Complications

Chronic complications like pseudarthrosis and implant subsidence can be observed in anterior fusion technique. In a systematic review by Jacobs et al. the authors found a fusion rate ranging between 47% and 90% for anterior lumbar surgeries with most cited fusion rates approaching 90%.[82] Madan et al. compared 27 patients who received non-instrumented anterior fusion with graft only with 29 patients who received instrumented fusion. The authors found a significant difference in fusion rates between the two groups of 83.3% and 100%, respectively.[83] The use of biologics like bone morphogenetic protein has also increased the fusion rate in anterior spine surgery. Subsidence is defined as a decrease in the vertical height of the disc space prior to complete incorporation of the fusion mass. This can be problematic in patients with osteoporotic bone, fractures in the adjacent vertebral end plates and in those with a weak posterior tension band.

Complication Cases

Case 1: Post-traumatic Kyphosis

A 17-year-old female had sustained multiple injuries to the head and chest in a road traffic accident. Initially after the injury, her Glasgow Coma Scale was nine due to the head injury and had a pneumothorax following a rib fracture on the left side. She had been resuscitated and regained her full consciousness after 2 weeks. When she was mobilized, she complained of pain in the mid back region. She was referred to the authors about 6 weeks

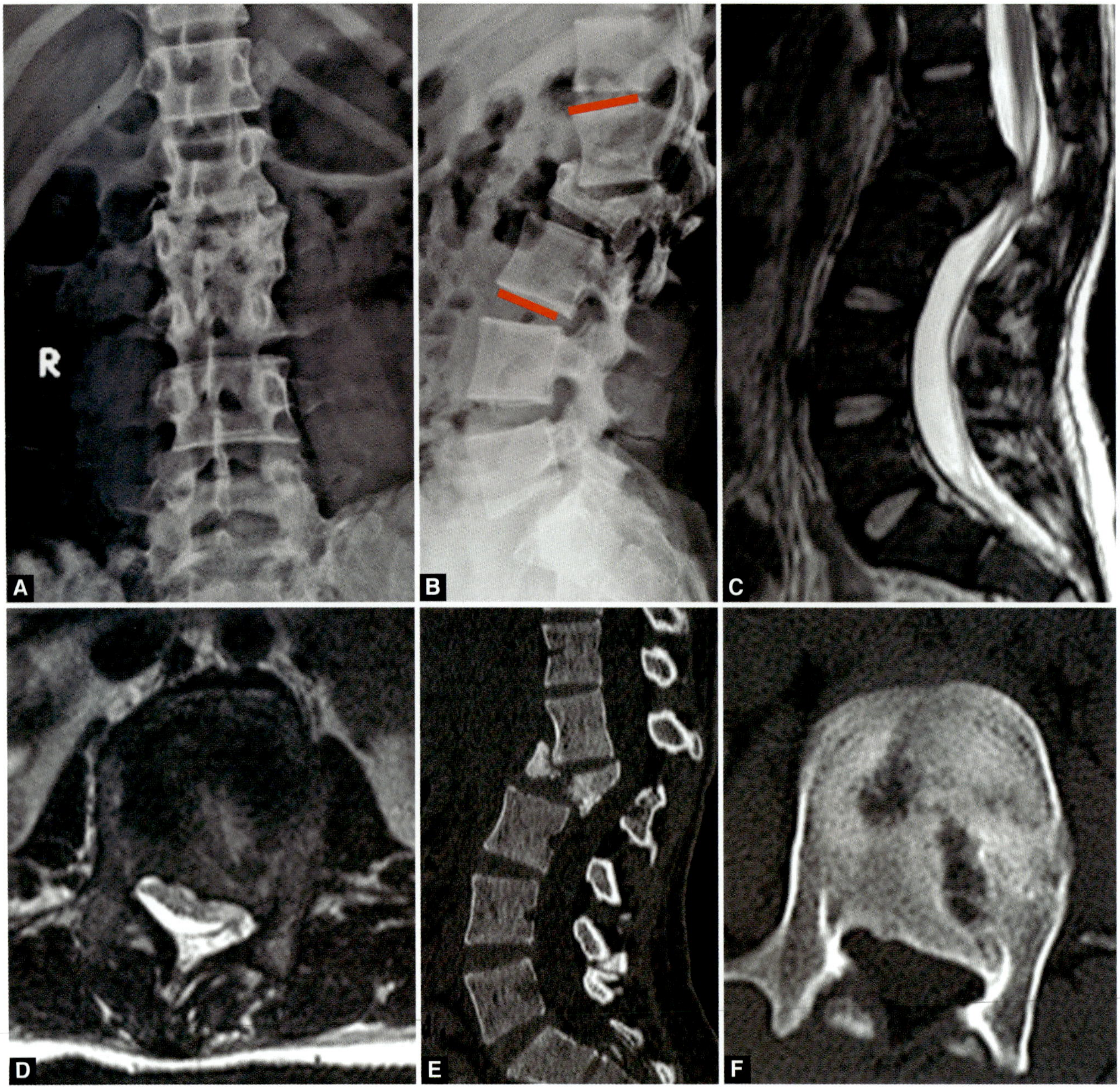

Figures 15.36A to F: (A and B) Anteroposterior and lateral radiographs of the thoracolumbar spine indicating a neglected flexion-distraction injury of the L2 vertebra; (C to F) Sagittal and axial MRI and CT images indicate the retropulsion of fragments into the canal with resultant compression on the conus.

after the injury with significant pain in the mid and low back region and difficulty in walking. On clinical examination, her cervical and thoracic spines were normal but she had a prominent sharp kyphosis in the thoracolumbar region. She had tenderness around the deformity and the spine was stiff. Neurological examination of both the lower limbs was normal. Radiographs of the lumbar spine revealed a missed fracture of the L2 vertebra (flexion-distraction injury) resulting in significant kyphosis of L2 and distracted posterior elements and a local kyphosis angle of about 32°. CT images showed that the vertebral collapse had healed partially with retropulsed bony fragments into the spinal canal. Corresponding MRI images showed that the thecal sac and distal conus being

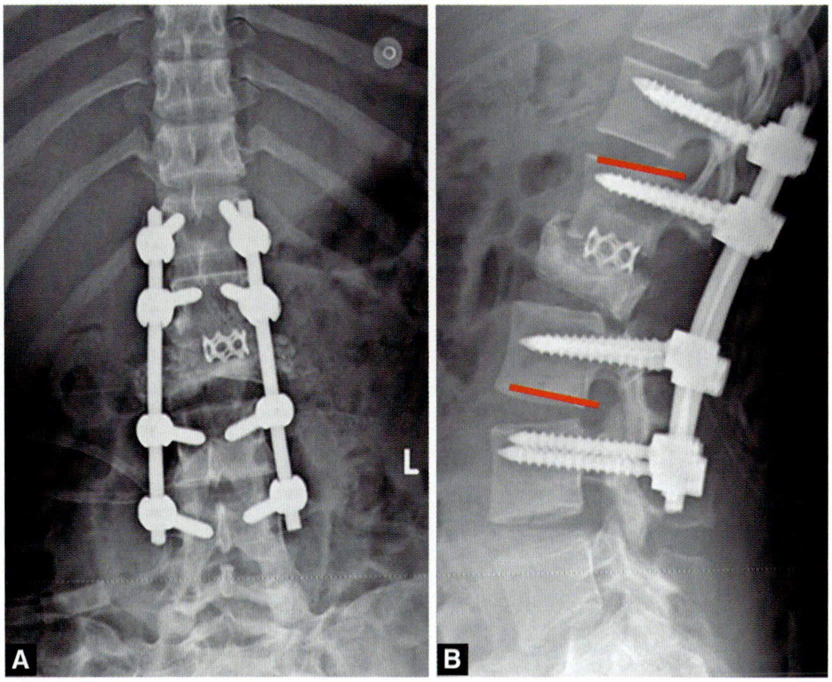

Figures 15.37A and B: (A) Postoperative AP and (B) Lateral radiographs depicting a pedicle substraction osteotomy at L2, L1–2 interbody fusion and posterior stabilization from T12–L4.

compressed by the bony fragments (Figs 15.36A to F). The deformity in this patient had a tendency to progress due to loss of anterior column and failed posterior tension band. Any kyphosis in the thoracolumbar region affects the sagittal balance of the spine and can result in muscle fatigue and distress. Progressive pressure over the neural elements would result in neurological deficits. Hence it was planned to correct the deformity, decompress the neural elements, provide anterior support and fuse the spine posteriorly through an all posterior approach.

The patient was placed in a prone position on a radiolucent table. Through a standard posterior midline approach, the posterior elements were exposed from T12 to L4 subperiosteally. Appropriate size pedicle screws were inserted bilaterally at T12, L1, L3 and L4. Laminectomy of L1 and L2 was performed. The pedicles of L2 was removed and through the pedicles, the L1–2 disc space was accessed and debrided thoroughly. The L1 and L2 nerve roots were protected on both side and the discs were completely excised and the retropulsed bony fragments were also removed. An appropriately contoured rod for the lumbar lordosis is placed on the T12 and L1 pedicle screws and slowly maneuvered into the L3 and L4 screws. This corrected the kyphotic deformity. A 10 mm rectangular titanium cage was placed into the L1–2 disc space. Another rod was placed on the other side over the pedicle screws and the screws between L1 and L3 were compressed to provide more lordosis. The posterior and lateral elements were decorticated using a thin osteotome and packed with bone grafts (Figs 15.37A and B). The wound was closed in layers.

The important principles of this case are:

- Do not miss a spinal injury in a poly trauma setting.
- Segmental kyphosis, especially in the thoracolumbar region can affect the global sagittal balance of the spine. This needs to be addressed by appropriate surgical techniques.
- Patients who require a pedicle substraction osteotomy will require interbody fusion to reduce the chances of pseudoarthrosis.

Case 2: Implant Failure with Worsening Kyphosis

This 22-year-old male had suffered a spinal injury following a fall from a height of about 10 feet. At the time of injury, he was neurologically intact and he had been treated by posterior short segment stabilization excluding the fractured vertebra. Six months after the surgery, he started developing significant back pain. When he presented to the authors, he had severe back pain, which was aggravated with movements like bending. On clinical examination, he had a prominent kyphosis over the operated site with tenderness around the scar. He had a normal neurological examination. Lateral radiographs revealed a healed L1 flexion-distraction injury with a prominent thoracolumbar kyphosis of about 72°. The index surgeon presumably had underestimated the extent of the injury and treated it with a laminectomy and short-segment fusion, which resulted in a vicious cycle of progressive kyphosis and implant breakage and further kyphosis. Originally this could have been probably avoided by one of the following strategies: anterior column reconstruction, fixation including the fractured vertebra or by an extended long column construct. Now the present problems are kyphosis and implant failure.

The thoracolumbar spine was exposed through the previous scar from T10 to L2. The implants were exposed and the extraosseous broken parts were removed. Pedicle screws were inserted at T10, T11, L1 and L2 levels. The posterior elements of T11 and T12 were removed completely and the disc space of T11–12 was prepared. The preoperative radiographs depict proximal junctional kyphosis and disc failure at T11–12 levels and hence it was planned to fuse at that level. Appropriately contoured rods were placed over the screws and the kyphosis was corrected over an interbody cage at T11–12. The postoperative kyphosis between T10 and L2 was 22° (Figs 15.38A and B).

The important principles in this case are:

- Patients with flexion-distraction injury or a failed anterior column will require either anterior column support or an extended posterior stabilization.
- It is important to recognize the location of failure (i.e. the origin of kyphosis) so that appropriate length of fixation and need for interbody fusion can be determined.

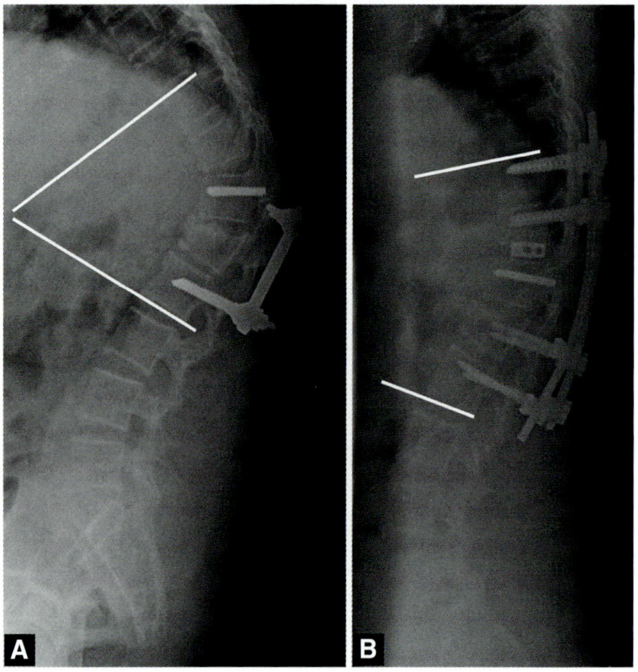

Figures 15.38A and B: (A) Post-traumatic kyphosis. This patient was treated surgically (posterior decompression and instrumentation) for an unstable burst fracture T12. Two years later he presented with progressive deformity, back pain and unsteady gait. The X-ray shows a kyphosis of 72°. Careful evaluation of the radiographs revealed a mobile kyphosis above the upper instrumented level; (B) Postoperative X-ray showing correction of the deformity to 22°.

Case 3: Failure to Recognize Fracture Patterns

This 35-year-old patient sustained injury in a road traffic accident. His lumbar spine radiographs were reviewed and he was diagnosed to have an upper end pale wedge compression fracture of L1 vertebra. Hence no further evaluation has been done and the fracture was treated conservatively in a brace. The patient subsequently developed worsening back pain and bladder symptoms suggestive of a neurogenic bladder. Radiographs were performed 2 months later, which revealed segmental kyphosis and retropulsion. Retrospective analysis of the previous radiographs revealed a flexion-distraction injury evident by widened interspinous distance and rotational component in the AP radiographs (Figs 15.39A to F). That was a three-column injury, which should have been treated by posterior stabilization and fusion.

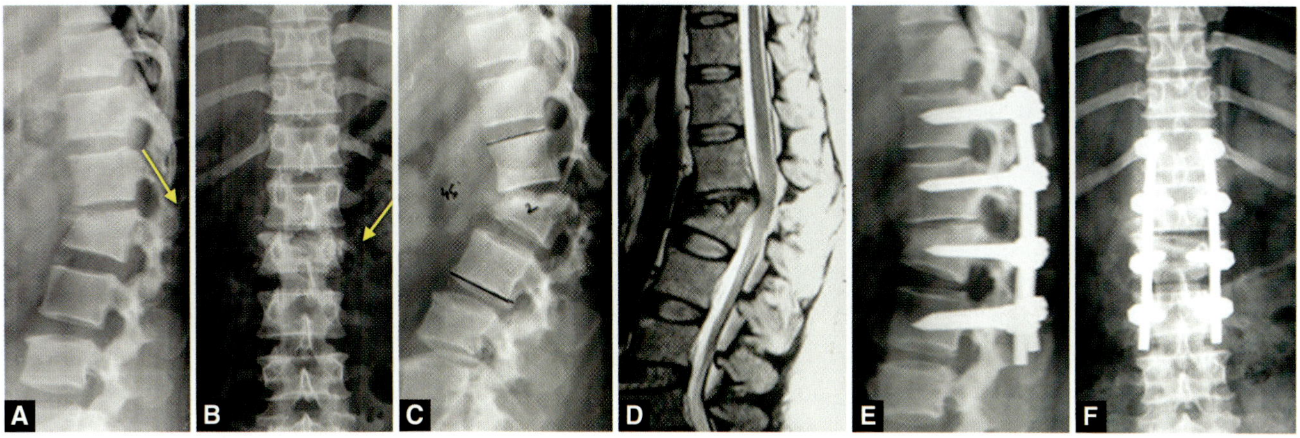

Figures 15.39A to F: (A and B) Lateral and anteroposterior X-rays of fracture L2 without neurological deficit. Note the increased interspinous distance at L1–2 and the rotation and lateral subluxation on the anteroposterior view suggesting that it is a three column injury); (C and D) He was treated conservatively and then he presented with paraparesis and severe pain. The X-rays show kyphotic deformity and the MRI reveals cord compression; (E and F) A posterior only approach with fusion was performed with posterior pedicle screw instrumentation.

To treat the patient's present problems of kyphosis and neurological deficit, it was planned to do a posterior spinal stabilization, decompression and fusion. The spine was exposed from T11 to L2 and pedicle screws were inserted at each level on either side. L1 laminectomy was done to decompress the neural elements. A straight rod was placed and the kyphotic deformity was corrected. The posterolateral elements were prepared for bone grafting and bone grafts were packed.

The important principles in this case are:

- Critical evaluation of anteroposterior and lateral views to assess posterior ligamentous complex injury and other elements of three-column injury and instability are essential to avoid disastrous complications.
- When in doubt, an MRI scan, CT scan or standing radiographs can help in assessing posterior instability.
- Correction of kyphosis will require long-segment stabilization and fusion with anterior reconstruction, if necessary.

Case 4: Missed Systemic Injury in a Polytrauma Patient

A 40-year-old male was brought in the emergency department room following a road traffic accident. On examination, the patient was conscious and oriented. His main complaints were severe mid-back pain. He was intact neurologically in both lower limbs. Systemic examination showed that he had tenderness in the left upper quadrant and decreased air entry on the left side. Though he was comfortable at rest, his respiratory rate was higher and the oxygen saturation on room air was 90%. Though the spinal fracture seeks attention and was the main complaint of the patient, it is crucial to remember that spine fractures are part of polytrauma injuries. In that patient, the anteroposterior radiographs of the chest showed that there was a radiolucent globular gas shadow within the left thoracic cavity obliterating the lung shadow. This indicates a rupture of the left hemidiaphragm with migration of intra-abdominal contents into the thorax. It was a surgical emergency and the patient was treated by emergency diaphragmatic repair. The spine fracture was also stabilized at the same sitting through a posterior approach (Figs 15.40A to D).

The important learning point in this case is:

- Remember that spine fractures are part of systemic injuries. Strict adherence to ATLS protocol is essential to avoid other serious systemic injuries.

Summary

After decades of treating spinal fractures with different methods and approaches, some questions still remain unanswered. The basic evaluation as in any other trauma patient should be followed to look for serious injuries first. Spinal immobilization is a priority during initial

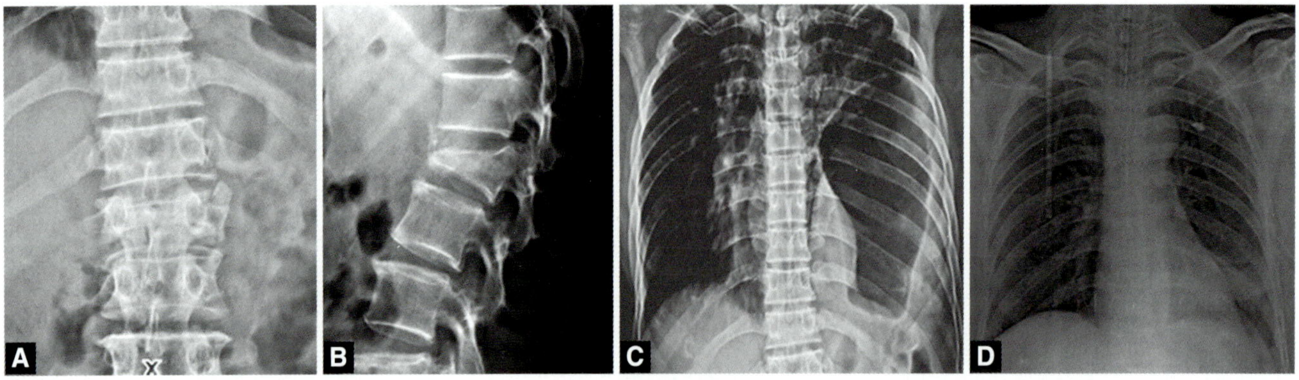

Figures 15.40A to D: (A and B) Anteroposterior and lateral radiographs of the thoracolumbar spine indicate an unstable spinal fracture at L1 level; (C) Anteroposterior radiograph of the thoracic spine indicates that there is a radiolucent globular shadow in the left thoracic cavity indicative of diaphragmatic fracture; (D) Postoperative chest anteroposterior radiograph indicates that the diaphragm has been repaired with normal appearance of the lung shadows.

assessment and evaluation. Radiographs and CT scan are sufficient in most patients to plan the management.

Treatment decisions in these patients require complete evaluation of the neurological status and identification of the presence of spinal instability. Compression fractures and stable burst fractures can be treated by nonoperative methods. The presence of neurological deficits and spinal instability require surgical treatment through the appropriate surgical approach.

Decompression in the form of laminectomy alone is contraindicated in spinal trauma. The only current indications for laminectomy are open fractures with rootlet prolapse (for inspecting and repairing the dural sac) and laminar fractures with dural entrapment (a limited laminotomy would suffice). Indirect decompression of the fractures may sometimes be possible through posterior pedicle screw stabilization with controlled distraction, especially when only one endplate of the vertebra is burst. But when both the endplates are burst or there is a sagittal/coronal split with retropulsion, one may have to resort to direct decompression through the anterior route.

The use of screws in the fractured vertebra when the pedicles are intact has several potential advantages like the lateral splaying of the vertebra is reduced, which can indirectly clear the canal; the load per screw on the construct is reduced thus reducing implant failure rates; it facilitates better elevation of the collapsed end plate and holds it in place till union occurs. Anterior approach is the access of choice when decompression of the spinal cord is the priority. After direct decompression, reconstruction of the load bearing column is performed by large autologous bone graft or cages.

References

1. Eastlack RK, Bono CM. Fractures and Dislocations of the Thoracolumbar Spine. In: Bucholz RW, Heckman JD, Court-Brown CM (EDs) et al. Rockwood and Green's Fractures in Adults: Vol 2. Philadelphia: Lippincott Williams and Wilkins, 2006; 1543-80.
2. Kraemer WJ, Schemitsch EH, McKee MD, et al. Functional outcome of thoracolumbar burst fractures without neurological deficit. J Orthop Trauma. 1996; 10(8):541-4.
3. Doo T, Shin D, Kim H, et al. Clinical relevance of pain patterns in osteoporotic compression fractures. Journal of Korean Medical Sciences. 2008;23:1005-10.
4. Liu J, Tang X, Xu N, et al. Preliminary results for the treatment of a pain-causing osteoporotic vertebral compression fracture with a sky bone expander. Korean J Radial, 2009; 9:420-5.
5. McAfee PC, Yuan HA, Fredrickson BE, et al. The Value of Computed Tomography in Thoracolumbar Fractures. J Bone Joint Surg, Am, 1983;65-A(4):461-73.
6. Vaccaro AR, Nachwalter RS, Klein GR et al. The significance of Spinal Canal size in spinal cord injury patients. Spine. 2001;26(4):371-6.
7. Hashomoto T, Kaneda K, Abumi K. Relationship between traumatic spinal canal stenosis and neurological deficits in thoracolumbar burst fractures. Spine. 1988;13(11): 1268-72.

8. Willen J, Anderson J, Toomoka K et al. The natural history of burst fractures at the thoracolumbar junction. J Spinal disord. 1990;3(1):39-46.
9. Rogers LF. The roentgenographic appearance of transverse or chance fractures of the spine: the seat belt fracture. Am J Roentgenol Radium Ther Nucl Med. 1971;111(4):844-9.
10. Bernstein MP, Mirvis SE, Shanmuganathan K. Chance-type fractures of the thoracolumbar spine: imaging analysis in 53 patients. AJR Am J Roentgenol. 2006;187(4):859-68.
11. Neumann P, Nordwall A, Osvalder AL. Traumatic instability of the lumbar spine. A dynamic in vitro study of flexion-distraction injury. Spine (Phila Pa 1976). 1995; 20(10):1111-21.
12. Boehler L. Die Techniek der Knochenbruchbehandlung im Grieden und im Kriegeed. Vienna, Auystria: Verlag von Wilheim, Maudrich, 1930.
13. Watson-Jones R. The results of postural reduction of fractures of the spine. J Bone Joint Surg Am, 1938;20: 567-86.
14. Nicoll EA. Fractures of the dorso-lumbar spine. J Bone Joint Surg Am, 1949;31B:376-94.
15. Holdsworth F. Fractures, dislocations, and fracture-dislocations of the spine. J Bone Joint Surg Am, 1970;52: 1534-51.
16. Denis F. The three column spine and its significance in the classification of acute thoracolumbar spinal injuries. Spine (Phila Pa 1976). 1983;8:817-31.
17. Ferguson RL, Allen BL, Jr. A mechanistic classification of thoracolumbar spine fractures. Clin Orthop Relat Res. 1984:77-88.
18. Panjabi MM, Oxland TR, Lin RM, et al. Thoracolumbar burst fracture. A biomechanical investigation of its multi-directional flexibility. Spine (Phila Pa 1976). 1994;19:578-85.
19. Oner FC, Ramos LM, Simmermacher RK, et al. Classification of thoracic and lumbar spine fractures: problems of reproducibility. A study of 53 patients using CT and MRI. Eur Spine J. 2002;11:235-45.
20. McAfee PC, Yuan HA, Fredrickson BE, et al. The value of computed tomography in thoracolumbar fractures. An analysis of one hundred consecutive cases and a new classification. J Bone Joint Surg Am. 1983;65:461-73.
21. Oner FC, van Gils AP, Dhert WJ et al. MRI findings of thoracolumbar spine fractures: a categorisation based on MRI examinations of 100 fracture. Skeletl Radiol. 1999; 28:433-43.
22. Oner FC, van Gils AP, Faber JA et al. Some complications of common treatment schemes of thoracolumbar spine fractures can be predicted with MRimaging: prospective study of 53 patientswith 71 fractures. Spine. 2002;27: 629-36.
23. McCormack T, Karaikovic E, Gaines RW. The load sharing classification of spine fractures. Spine (Phila Pa 1976), 1994;19:1741-4.
24. Magerl F, Aebi M, Gertzbein SD, et al. A comprehensive classification of thoracic and lumbar injuries. Eur Spine J. 1994;3:184-201.
25. Vaccaro AR, Lehman RA Jr, Hurlbert RJ, et al. A new classification of thoracolumbar injuries: the importance of injury morphology, the integrity of the posterior ligamentous complex, and neurologic status. Spine (Phila Pa 1976). 2005;30:2325-33.
26. Panjabi MM, Thibodieau LL, Crisco JJ, et al. What constitutes spinal instability? Clin Neurosurg. 1988; (34):313-9.
27. Silverman SL. The clinical consequences of vertebral compression fracture. Bone. 1992; 13(suppl):27.
28. Axelsson P, Johnsson R, Stromqvist B. Effect of lumbar orthosis on intervertebral mobility. A roentgen stereo-photogrammetric analysis. Spine. 1992;17:678-81.
29. Connolly PJ, Grob D. Bracing of patients after fusion for degenerative problems of the lumbar spine- yes or no? Spine. 1998;23:1426-8.
30. Palmisani M, Gasbarrini A, Barbanti Brodano G, et al. Minimally invasive percutaneous fixation in the treatment of thoracic and lumbar spine fractures. European Spine Journal. 2009;18(Supplement 1):71-4.
31. Krengel WF, Anderson PA, Henley MB. Early stabilization and decompression for incomplete paraplegia due to thoracic level spinal cord injury. Spine. 1993;18:2080-87.
32. Wessberg P, Wang Y, Irstam L, et al. The effect of surgery and remodeling on spinal canal measurements after thoracolumbar burst fractures. Eur Spine J. 2001;(10):55-63.
33. McLain RF. The biomechanics of long versus short fixation for thoracolumbar spine fractures. 2006;31(11 Suppl). S70-9; discussion S104.
34. Mathis JM, Barr JD, Belkoff SM, et al. Percutaneous Vertebroplasty: A Developing Standard of Care for Vertebral Compression Fractures . AJNR Am J Neuroradiol 2001; 22(2):373-81.
35. Taylor RS, Fritzell P, Taylor RJ. Ballon kyphoplasty in the management of vertebral compression fractures: an updated systematic review and meta-analysis. Eur Spine J. 2007;16:1085-1100.
36. Foley KT, Gupta SK, Justis JR et al. Percutaneous pedicle screw fixation of the lumbar spine. Neurosurg Focus 2001;10 (4):Article 10.
37. Galibert P, Deramond H, Rosat P et al. Preliminary note on the treatment of vertebral angioma by percutaneous acrylic vertebroplasty [in French]. Neurochirurgie. 1987;33(2): 166-8.

38. Deramond H, Depriester C, Galibert P et al. Percutaneous vertebroplasty with polymethylmethacrylate: technique, indications and results. Radiol Clin North Am. 1998; 36(3):533-46.
39. Lindsay R, Silverman SL, Cooper C, et al. Risk of a new vertebral fracture in the year following a fracture. JAMA. 2001;285(3):320-3.
40. Scroop R, Eskridge J, Britz GW. Paradoxical cerebral arterial embolization of cement during intraoperative vertebroplasty: case report. AJNR Am J Neuroradiol. 2002;23(5): 868-70.
41. Mathis JM. Percutaneous vertebroplasty:complication avoidance and technique optimization. AJNR Am J Neuroradiol. 2003;24(8):1697-1706.
42. Negri PD and Tirri T. Minimally Invasive Treatment of Vertebral Body Fractures. Osteoporosis. InTech. 32: 649-64.
43. Knavel EM, Thielen KR, Kallmes DF. Vertebroplasty for the treatment of traumatic nonosteoporotic compression fractures. AJNR Am J Neuroradiology. 2009;30: 323-7.
44. Verlaan JJ, van Helden WH, Oner FC, et al. Balloon vertebroplasty with calcium phosphate cement augmentation for direct restoration of traumatic thoracolumbar vertebral fractures. Spine. 2002;27(5):543-8.
45. Lieberman IH, Dudeney S, Reinhardt MK, et al. Initial outcome and efficacy of kyphoplasty in the treatment of painful osteoporotic vertebral compression fractures. Spine. 2001;26(4):1631-8.
46. Taylor RS, Fritzell P, Taylor RJ. Ballon kyphoplasty in the management of vertebral compression fractures: an updated systematic review and meta-analysis. Eur Spine J. 2007;16:1085-1100.
47. Garfin SR, Yuan HA, Reiley MA. New technologies in spine: kyphoplasty and vertebroplasty for the treatment of painful osteoporotic compression fractures. Spine (Phila Pa 1976). 2001;26(14):1511-5.
48. Groen RJM,du Toit DF, Phillips FM, et al. Anatomical and Pathological Considerations in Percutaneous Vertebroplasty and Kyphoplasty: a Reappraisal of the Vertebral Venous System. Spine. 2004;13:1465-71.
49. Wardlaw D, Cummings SR, Van Meirhaeghe J. et al. Efficacy and safety of balloon kyphoplasty compared with nonsurgical care for vertebral compression fracture: a randomised controlled trial. Lancet. 2009;373(9668):1016-24.
50. Korovessis P, Hadjipavlou A, Repantis T. Minimal invasive short posterior instrumentation plus balloon kyphoplasty with calcium phosphate for burst and severe compression lumbar fractures. Spine. 2008;33(6):658-67.
51. Bradford D, McBride G. Surgical management of thoracolumbar spine fractures with incomplete neurological deficits. Clinical Orthopaedics. 1987;218:201-15.
52. Denis F. Thoracolumbar Injuries. Instructional Course Lecture. 1988;230.
53. Kramer DL, Rodgers WB, Mansfield FL. Transpedicular instrumentation and short segment fusion of thoracolumbar fractures: a prospective study using a single instrumentation system. J Orthop Trauma. 1995;9:499-506.
54. Sihvonen T, Herno A, Paljarvi L, Airaksinen O, Partanen J, Tapaninaho A. Local denervation atrophy of paraspinal muscles in postoperative failed back syndrome. Spine (Phila Pa 1976). 1993;18(5):575-81.
55. Rampersaud YR, Annand N, Dekutoski MB. Use of minimally invasive surgical technique in the management of thoracolumbar trauma: current concepts. Spine (Phila Pa 1976). 2006;15:96-102.
56. Mahar A, Kim C, Wedemeyer M, et al. Short-segment fixation of lumbar burst fractures using pedicle fixation at the level of the fracture. Spine (Phila Pa 1976). 2007; 32(14):1503-7.
57. Qian BP, Qiu Y, Wang B, et al. Effect of posterolateral fusion on thoracolumbar burst fractures. Chin J Traumatol. 2006; 9(6):349-55.
58. Oner FC, Verlaan JJ, Verbout AJ, et al. Cement augmentation techniques in traumatic thoracolumbar spine fractures. Spine (Phila Pa 1976). 2006; 31(Suppl 11):89-104.
59. Ebelke DK, Asher MA, Neff JR, et al. Survivorship analysis of VSP spine instrumentation in the treatment of thoracolumbar and lumbar burst fractures. Spine (Phila Pa 1976). 1991; 16(8 Suppl):S428-32.
60. Kaneda K, Abumi K, Fujiya M. Burst fractures with neurologic deficits of the thoracolumbar-lumbar spine. Results of anterior decompression and stabilization with anterior instrumentation. Spine (Phila Pa 1976). 1984; 9(8):788-95.
61. Robertson PA. Anterior approaches for thoracolumbar fractures. ANZ J Surg. 2007; 77(Suppl 1):A54.
62. Kaneda K, Taneichi H, Abumi K, et al. Anterior decompression and stabilization with the Kaneda device for thoracolumbar burst fractures associated with neurological deficits. J Bone Joint Surg Am. 1997; 79(1):69-83.
63. Sasso RC, Best NM, Reily TM, et al. Anterior only stabilization of three-column thoracolumbar injuries. J Spinal Disord Tech. 2005; 18(Suppl):S7-S14.
64. Riska EB, Myllynen P, Bostman O. Anterolateral decompression for neural involvement in thoracolumbar fractures. J Bone Joint Surg Br. 1987;69(5):704-8.
65. Haas N, Blauth M, Tscherne H. Anterior plating in thoracolumbar spine injuries: Indication, technique, and results. Spine (Phila Pa 1976). 1991; 16(3 Suppl):S100-111.
66. Gertzbein SD. Scoliosis Research Society. Multi Center Spine Fracture Study. Spine (Phila Pa 1976). 1992; 17(5):522-40.

67. Hitchon PW, Torner J, Eichholz KM, et al. Comparison of anterolateral and posterior approaches in the management of thoracolumbar burst fractures. J Neurosurg Spine. 2006; 5(2):117-25.

68. Sasso RC, Renkens K, Hanson D, et al. Unstable thoracolumbar burst fractures: anterior-only versus short-segment posterior fixation. J Spinal Disord Tech. 2006; 19(4):242-8.

69. Payer M. Unstable burst fractures of the thoracolumbar junction: treatment by posterior bisegmental correction/fixation and staged anterior corpectomy and titanium cage implantation (published onlne ahead of print November 28, 2005). Acta Neurochir (Wien). 2006; 148(3):299-306.

70. Been HD, Bouma GJ. Comparison of two types of surgery for thoracolumbar burst fractures: combined anterior and posterior stabilization vs. posterior instrumentation only. Acta Neurochir (Wien). 1999; 141(4):349-57.

71. Harrington PR, Tullos HS, Reduction of severe spondylolisthesis in children. South Med J. 1969;62:1-7.

72. Roy-Camille R, Saillant G, Mazel C: Internal fixation of the lumbar spine with pedicle screw plating. Clin Orthop Relat Res. 1986;203:7-17.

73. Hicks JM, Singla A, Shen FH, et al. Complications of pedicle screw fixation in scoliosis surgery: a systematic review. Spine. 2010;(Phila Pa 1976)35:E465–E470.

74. Lonstein JE, Denis F, Perra JH, et al. Complications associated with pedicle screws. J Bone Joint Surg Am. 1999; 81:1519-28.

75. Merloz P, Tonetti J, Pittet L, et al. Pedicle screw placement using image guided techniques. Clin Orthop Relat Res. 1998;354:39-48.

76. Kosmopoulos V, Schizas C. Pedicle screw placement accuracy: a meta-analysis. Spine. 2007;(Phila Pa 1976)32: E111–E120.

77. Matsuzaki H, Tokuhashi Y, Matsumoto F, et al. Problems and solutions of pedicle screw plate fixation of lumbar spine. Spine. 1990;(Phila Pa 1976) 15:1159-65.

78. Gautschi OP, Schatlo B, Schaller K, et al. Clinically relevant complications related to pedicle screw placement in thoracolumbar surgery and their management: a literature review of 35,630 pedicle screws Neurosurg Focus. 2011; 31(4):E8,1-9.

79. Foxx KC, Kwak RC, Latzman JM, et al. A retrospective analysis of pedicle screws in contact with the great vessels. Clinical article. J Neurosurg Spine. 2010;13:403-6.

80. Vanichkachorn JS, Vaccaro AR, Cohen MJ, et al. Potential large vessel injury during thoracolumbar pedicle screw removal. A case report. Spine. 1997;(Phila Pa 1976) 22:110–13.

81. Inamasu J, Guiot BH. Vascular injury and complication in neurosurgical spine surgery. Acta Neurochir (Wien). 2006; 148:375-87.

82. Jacobs WC, Vreeling A, De Kleuver M. Fusion for low-grade adult isthmic spondylolisthesis: a systematic review of the literature. Eur Spine J. 2006;15:391-402.

83. Madan SS, Harley JM, Boeree NR. Anterior lumbar interbody fusion: does stable anterior fixation matter? Eur Spine J. 2003;12:386-92.

Index

Page number followed by *f* and *t* indicates figure and table respectively.

A

Acetabulum fracture 552–553
anterior column 566
anterior wall 565–566
case study
heterotopic ossification of hip 575, 577, 577*f*–578*f*, 579
infection, management of 575, 576*f*
classification 555–556, 556*t*
complications 553
DVT 573
heterotopic ossification 572–573
late instability after ORIF 575
late stage arthritis 574–575
malunion 574
nerve palsy 573
nonunions 574
pulmonary embolism 573
CT scan 556–557
epidemiology 553
hemitransverse 569–571
heterotopic ossification 572–573
obese patients and 553
percutaneous fixation 571–572
antegrade anterior column screw 571, 571*f*
ischial posterior column screw 572
LC-II screw 571
posterior column screw 572
retrograde anterior column screw 571–572
posterior column fractures 565
posterior wall fractures 564–565, 565*f*
radiographic evaluation 554
anteroposterior view 554, 554*f*
iliac oblique view 555, 555*f*
obturator-oblique view 554, 555*f*
roof-arc measurements 557, 557*f*
surgical management
anterior approach 560–563
extensile approaches 563–564, 564*f*
iliofemoral approach 561
ilioinguinal approach 561–562, 561*f*, 562*f*
indications for 557–558, 557*f*
Kocher-Langenbeck approach 558–560, 559*f*
modified Stoppa approach 562–563, 563*f*
posterior approach 558–560
trochanteric osteotomy 560, 560*f*
transverse fractures 566–567, 566*f*
T-type fractures 568–569, 569*f*–570*f*
ACL *see* Anterior cruciate ligament (ACL)
Acromioclavicular (AC) joint 360, 360*f*
Acromion process fractures 339, 340*f*
outcomes 354
surgical indications 340
Advanced trauma life support (ATLS) 335, 381, 581, 582
cervical spine injury 379
ALL *see* Anterior longitudinal ligament (ALL)
Alonso-Llames approach, distal humerus 256, 256*f*
American College of Radiology (ACR) 95
American Spinal Injury Association (ASIA)
impairment scale 386
spinal cord injury assessment form 382, 382*f*
spinal cord injury grading 384–386, 385*f*, 385*t*
Anatomy
ankle joint 903*f*
cervical spine 416–418, 416*f*, 417*f*
clavicle 365–366, 365*f*
distal femur fractures 741–742, 741*f*
distal humerus 253–255, 254*f*
elbow 229–230, 229*f*
femoral neck fractures 618–624
femoral shaft fractures 713
hand and wrist 69–72, 70*f*
humeral shaft fractures 282–283
intertrochanteric femur fractures 656–657
metacarpals 36–37, 36*f*
patellar fractures 770–771
phalangeal fractures 6–7, 6*f*
proximal humerus 309–311, 310*f*, 311*f*
proximal tibia fractures 794–795
scaphoid 99–100, 99*f*, 100*f*
scapula 340–341, 341*f*
subtrochanteric femur fractures 677, 678*f*
thoracic and lumbar spine 447–448
Ankle-brachial index 738
Ankle fractures
anteromedial approach 935–936
bimalleolar 931
classification system 928–931
AO/OTA 929
Danis-Weber 928–929, 931*f*
Lauge-Hansen 928, 930*f*

concomitant 959*f*
diagnosis 927–928
CT scan 928
MRI 928
physical examination 927
radiography 927–928
squeeze test 927
dime sign 937*f*
external fixation role 932
fracture blisters 927*f*
hardware fixation loss 945
infection 945
treatment 946–947
lateral approach 935
malunion 946
nonunion 946
open 932
ORIF 931, 936–944
fibular length restoration 937*f*, 938*f*
lateral ankle incision dehiscence 947*f*
overview 926–927
peroneal tendonitis 946
posterior malleolar fractures 931
posterolateral approach 935
surgery 931–944
applied anatomy 932–935
approaches 935–936
complications 945–951
indications 931–932
outcomes 944–945
positioning 935
techniques 936–944
syndesmotic injuries 931–932, 946
unstable 944
wound breakdown 945
Ankle syndesmosis *see* Syndesmotic injury, ankle
Antegrade femoral nailing
femoral shaft fractures 713–720, 714*f*–718*f*
Anterior cord syndrome 387*t*, 388, 388*f*
Anterior cruciate ligament (ACL) 789
Anterior ligamentous complex injury, pelvis 498, 499*f*
Anterior longitudinal ligament (ALL) 449, 451
Anterior sacroiliac (SI) ligaments 496, 498
Anterior superior iliac spine (ASIS) 561, 563, 564, 621
Anterolateral approach
distal tibia fractures 901, 904*f*–906*f*, 915
humeral shaft fractures 283–284, 285*f*, 286*f*
proximal humerus fractures 314*f*, 315
talar neck fractures 971–972
Anteromedial approach
ankle fractures 935–936
distal tibia fractures 901–902, 906*f*–907*f*, 915
talar neck fractures 970–971
Antibiotic cement-coated nails
femoral shaft fractures 724
AO/OTA classification system
acetabular fractures 556*t*
ankle fractures 929
distal femur fractures 739, 740*f*
distal tibia fractures 900*f*
femoral neck fractures 616*f*
femoral shaft fractures 710, 711*f*, 712*f*
intertrochanteric femur/hip fractures 655, 656*f*
proximal humerus fractures 303, 308*f*
proximal tibia fractures 791–792, 791*f*
scapular fractures 336*t*
subtrochanteric femur fractures 675, 676*f*
tibial shaft fractures 846–847, 847*f*
Arthritis
acetabulum fracture 574–575
femoral head fractures 601
hip dislocations 601
patellar fractures 778
proximal tibia fractures 836, 839–840
scaphoid fractures 111, 113, 113*f*, 113*t* *see also* Scaphoid fractures
talus fractures 975–977
Arthrodesis 948–951, 950*f*, 991, 1001*f*
Arthroplasty 618
elbow 253, 254*f*, 264–265, 264*f*, 268
phalangeal fractures 19, 19*f*, 20*f*
radial head 228–229
Articular fragments, reconstruction 611–613
ASIA *see* American Spinal Injury Association (ASIA)
ASIF *see* Swiss Association for the Study of Internal Fixation (ASIF)
ASIS *see* Anterior superior iliac spine (ASIS)
Atlas-dens interval (ADI) 389*t*
Atlas fractures 396 *see also* Cervical spine injuries
classification of 397–398, 397*f*
clinical symptoms 397
injury mechanism 396
management 401
Gardner-Well tongs 403, 403*f*
Halo ring and vest orthotics 401–403, 402*f*
skeletal traction 403
ATLS *see* Advanced trauma life support (ATLS)
Autologous bone graft 188
Avascular necrosis (AVN) 309, 612
femoral neck fractures 640 *see also* femoral neck fractures
proximal humerus fractures 327, 330, 330*f*
scaphoid fractures 111, 112*f*
talus fractures 972–975
Axial dislocations 61, 61*f*, 68

B

Bag of bones method 253
BAI *see* Basion-axial interval (BAI)
Bare area 200
Basicervical femoral neck fractures 618
Basion-axial interval (BAI) 391–392, 393*f*
Basion-dental interval (BDI) 393*f*
Beach-chair position 311, 311*f*, 351, 352, 366, 366*f*
Bennett's fractures 34, 34*f* *see also* Metacarpal fractures
Bicondylar fractures 791 *see also* Proximal tibia fractures
dual plating 812, 813*f*–815*f*

hybrid circular external fixation 815–822, 818*f*–820*f*
locked plating 812–815, 816*f*–817*f*
Bimalleolar ankle fractures 931
Biplanar fluoroscopy 717
Blade plate management, subtrochanteric femur fractures 691–694, 692*f*, 693*f*
Blocking screws 748
subtrochanteric femur fractures 680, 682*f*
Blunt dissection 621
BMP *see* Bone morphogenic proteins (BMP)
Bone block arthrodesis, talus fractures 966–981
Bone morphogenic proteins (BMP) 759, 825
Bone scan, subtrochanteric femur fractures 673
Both bone fractures 169*f*, 171 *see also* Forearm fractures
intramedullary fixation 183, 184*f*–185*f*
surgical fixation 181–183, 182*f*
surgical indications 172
Brachial artery 172, 173
Brachial plexopathy 621
Brachial plexus 359
neurapraxia 374
Brachium, anatomy of 282–283
Bridge plating 45, 46
comminuted fractures 865
midshaft clavicle fixation 363
proximal metaphyseal tibial fracture 869*f*–870*f*
Brodén's views, subtalar joint 967*f*
Brooke and Jenkin's technique, C1–C2 fusion 426, 426*f*
Brown-Sequard syndrome 386–388, 387*t*, 388*f*
Bryan and Morrey approach, distal humerus 256
Burst fractures 448*f*, 449, 457–458, 458*f* *see also* Thoracic and lumbar spine fractures
stable 450, 454*f*
surgical management 462–463
unstable 450–451, 453, 454*f*
Buttress pin plate 162, 164*f*, 165*f*

C

Calcaneus fractures 954–966 *see also* Talus fractures
classification 954–955
concomitant ankle fractures 959*f*
diagnosis 954
displaced intra-articular fractures 956
Essex-Lopresti technique 957
grades 955
intramedullary nail 966
lateral extensile approach 957–958, 958*f*, 959*f*
medial approach 958–960, 960, 960*f*
ORIF 961*f*
infection and loss of reduction 964*f*–966*f*
medial exposure 962*f*–963*f*
physical examination 954
soft tissue complications 966
surgery
anatomy 955–956
techniques 957–960
sustenacular displacement 959–960
tibiotalocalcaneal fusion 966
Calcar of proximal humerus 310, 310*f*
CAM fracture boot *see* Controlled ankle motion (CAM) fracture boot
Campbell approach, distal humerus 255
Canadian C-spine rules 394*f*
Canadian Orthopaedic Trauma Society 359, 821
Cannulated screw fixation
anatomic considerations 625, 625*f*, 627*f*
instrumentation, patient positioning 625–626
pearls and pitfalls 629
technique 626–627, 628*f*, 629*f*, 631*f*
Capitate fractures 60 *see also* Carpal fractures and perilunate dislocations
Capitellum fractures 256, 265–266, 265*f*, 266*f*
Capsular reinforcements, types 618, 620
Capsulotomy 621
role of 640
C-arm fluoroscopy 625
Carpal dislocations 67
Carpal fractures 53–54
capitate 60
carpal dislocations 61–63
classification 55–63
complications 81–85
management of, case studies on 85–92
diagnosis 54
CT scans 55
history examination 54–55
MRI 56, 58*f*
physical examination 55
radiographic 54*f*, 55, 56*f*, 57*f*
hamate fractures 60
incidence 54
injury mechanism 54
lunate fractures 59–60, 60*f*
open reduction and internal fixation
of other carpal bone fractures 77
of perilunate dislocations 77–80
of scaphoid fractures 74–76, 75*f*, 76*f*
scaphoid fractures 58–59, 58*f*, 59*f* *see also* Scaphoid fractures
surgical management
anatomy relevant to 69–72
dorsal midline approach 72–73, 73*f*
modified distal Henry approach 72
outcomes 80–81, 81*f*
patient positioning 72
techniques 74–80
trapezial fractures 59
triquetral fractures 59, 59*f*, 60*f*
Carpal instability 85
Carpometacarpal (CMC) joint, fracture-dislocations at 30–31, 34–35 *see also* Metacarpal fractures
CAS *see* Computer assisted surgery (CAS)
Cast immobilization, scaphoid fractures 94–95, 98

Causalgia 159
CBC *see* Complete blood count (CBC)
Central cord syndrome 386, 387*t*, 388*f*
Cephalomedullary nailing, subtrochanteric femur fractures 684–689, 685*f*–688*f*
Cerclage wire 771
Cervical spine injuries 379
  anatomy related to 416, 416*f*, 417*f*
    lower cervical spine 417–418
    upper cervical spine 416–417, 416*f*
  atlas fractures 397–398, 397*f*, 401–403, 402*f*, 403*f*
  case study
    lateral mass screws 444–445, 444*f*
    neglected C2–C3 fracture 442–443, 443*f*
    nonunion 441–442, 442*f*
  classification and scoring of 384–386
  cleared spine 394–395
  clinical evaluation 381
    local examination 381
    neurologic examination 381–384
  complications
    anterior fixation related 440–441, 440*t*
    due to lateral mass fixation 439
    injury-related 439
  CT scan 389, 391, 392*f*
  Hangman's fracture 398, 400–401, 400*f*, 400*t*, 401*f*, 404–405, 405*f*
  history/physical examination 379, 381
  incomplete 386–389
  injury mechanism 379
  lower 379
  motor examination 383–384
  MRI 380*f*, 389, 391, 392*f*
  occipital condyle fractures 395–396, 396*f*
  occipitocervical dislocation 396, 397*f*
  odontoid fractures 398, 399*f*, 399*t*, 404, 404*f*, 405*f*
  radiographic evaluation 379*t*, 380*f*, 389, 389*t*, 390*f*–391*f*, 393*f*
  rectal examination 384
  sensory examination 383
  subaxial cervical fractures 401, 405–416
  surgical management
    anterior approach 418–419
    anterior corpectomy and fusion 431–433, 433*f*, 434*f*, 435*f*
    C1–C2 fusion 421–426
    C2 odontoid fixation 426–427, 428*f*, 429*f*–430*f*, 431*f*
    C2 pars fixation 427, 429–430, 431*f*, 432*f*
    C1 posterior fixation 420–421, 420*f*, 421*f*
    lateral mass screw fixation 433, 435, 436*f*, 437*f*, 438*f*
    outcomes 438–439
    posterior approach 419
  upper 379
Chance fractures 451
Clavicle fractures 358–359
  anatomy related to 365–366, 365*f*
  case study
    nonunion repair 374–375, 375*f*
    nonunion repair with secondary brachial plexopathy 376, 376*f*
  classification
    Allman system 361, 361*f*
    Neer system 361, 362*f*
  complications 373
    brachial plexopathy 374
    hardware complications 374
    malunion 374
    nonunions 373–374
    thoracic outlet syndrome 374
    wound breakdown 374
  diagnosis 359–361
    CT scans 360
    MRI 360
    neurological evaluation 359
    physical examination 359
    radiographic evaluation 360, 360*f*
  distal third 361–362
  lateral 359, 369, 371, 371*f*, 372*f*, 373
  midshaft 359, 361, 361*f*, 362*f*, 367–369, 371–373
  nonoperative treatment 358–359
  surgical management
    approaches 366
    coracoclavicular screw fixation 371, 372*f*
    distal clavicle fixation 363–365, 364*f*
    indications for 361–365
    midshaft clavicle fixation 362–363, 364*f*, 367–368, 368*f*
    outcomes 371–373
    patient positioning 366, 366*f*
    plate fixation 362–363, 364*f*, 367–368, 368*f*
    Rockwood pin fixation 364*f*, 369, 370*f*
    transarticular and hook plate fixation 369, 371*f*
  treatment 358–359
Closed reduction and percutaneous pinning (CRPP)
  midfoot and forefoot fractures 990–991
  phalangeal fractures 4, 5*f*, 8, 10*f*, 13*f*
Cobb elevator 621
Cobra retractors 559
Colles fracture 128 *see also* Distal radius fractures
Comminuted fractures, bridge plating 865
Compartment syndrome
  bicondylar fractures 812
  foot 1013
    ORIF 1017
    treatment 1015–1018
  forearm 168
  leg, 887
    fasciotomy 890–891, 891*f*–892*f*
    management principles 891–893
    tibial shaft fractures and 846, 872
    treatment of 887–893, 891*f*–892*f*
  periscapular musculature 354
  proximal tibia fractures 786
  tibial plateau fractures 797–798
Complete blood count (CBC) 728
Complex elbow dislocations 224, 224*f*, 227*f*

Complex regional pain syndrome (CRPS) 159
Compression plate fixation 44–45, 46, 47*f*
Computed tomography (CT)
  acetabulum fracture 556–557
  ankle fractures 928
  carpal fractures and perilunate dislocations 55
  clavicle fractures 360
  distal femur fractures 739, 739*f*
  distal humerus fractures 250–251, 252*f*
  femoral head fractures and hip dislocations 582–583, 585*f*
  femoral neck fractures 612, 614*f*
  femoral shaft fractures 710
  forearm fractures 170
  metacarpal fractures 32, 33*f*
  midfoot and forefoot fractures 986
  Olecranon fractures 193, 195, 195*f*
  pelvic ring and sacral injuries 496
  proximal humerus fractures 303, 305*f*, 306*f*
  proximal tibia fractures 786
  scaphoid fractures 97
  subtrochanteric femur fractures 673, 683, 683*f*
  thoracic and lumbar spine fractures 455, 455*f*, 458*f*, 459, 461*f*
Computer assisted surgery (CAS) 683
  subtrochanteric femur fractures 683
Concomitant ankle fractures 959*f*
Condylar fractures, of phalanx 15, 15*f*
Constant shoulder scores (CSS) 359
Continuous passive motion (CPM) 777
Controlled ankle motion (CAM) fracture boot 997
Coracoclavicular (CC) ligaments 361, 362*f*
Coracoclavicular screw fixation, clavicle fractures 364*f*, 371, 372*f*
Coracoid process fractures 338–339, 339*f*
  operative technique 353
  outcomes 354
  surgical indications 340
Corona mortis 510, 510*f*, 562, 562*f*
Coronoid fracture 232, 239, 240*f*
Cortical ring sign 55, 57*f*
Cortical screw fixation 871
CPM *see* Continuous passive motion (CPM)
Craniocervical ligaments 417, 417*f*
C-reactive protein (CRP) 831
CRPP *see* Closed reduction and percutaneous pinning (CRPP)
Cruciate paralysis 386
Crush injury 846
CT *see* Computed tomography (CT)

D

Damage control orthopedics 726–727, 726*f*
  see also Femoral shaft fractures
Deep vein thrombosis (DVT) 694
  acetabulum fracture 573
  subtrochanteric femur fractures 695
Deltopectoral approach, proximal humerus fractures 312, 313*f*
Diaphyseal fibula fractures, ORIF 936–938
Dime sign 937*f*
Direct ulnar approach, forearm fractures 173, 174*f*
Disabilities of the arm, shoulder and hand (DASH) scores 359
Displaced femoral neck fractures
  instrumentation, implant and patient positioning 629, 632, 634*f*, 636*f*
  preoperative planning and anatomic consideration 629
  technique 632
Displaced intra-articular fractures, calcaneus 956
Dissolving pedicle sign 461
Distal femur fractures 737–738
  case study
    atrophic nonunion with stable implant 759, 761*f*, 762*f*
    chronic deep infection 759–764, 762*f*, 763*f*
    nonunion with implant failure 758–759, 760*f*
  classification 739
    AO/OTA Müeller's classification 739, 740*f*
  complications
    knee stiffness 756–757
    malunion 758
    nonunion 757–758
  diagnosis 738*f*
    CT scan 739, 739*f*
    MRI 739
    pearls and pitfalls 739
    X-rays 738, 739*f*
  outcomes 756
  surgical management
  acute knee arthroplasty 741
  anatomy 741–742, 741*f*
  external fixation 741
  intramedullary fixation 741
  lateral approach 742, 743*f*
  medial subvastus 743–745
  minimally invasive plate osteosynthesis plating 745, 746*f*
  positioning 742, 743*f*
  retrograde intramedullary nail 747–749, 747*f*
  type B fracture 751–753, 752*f*, 754*f*
  type C fracture 749–751, 750*f*, 751*f*
Distal fibular fractures
  ORIF 936–938
  posterior plating 937*f*
Distal humerus fractures 249
  anatomy related to 253–255, 254*f*
  case study
    elbow stiffness 268–270
    ulnar neuropathy 270–272
  classification 251–252
  complications 267
    elbow stiffness 267
    heterotopic ossification 267–268
    nonunion 268
    ulnar neuropathy 268
  diagnosis 250–251
    CT scan 250–251, 252*f*
    physical examination 250
    radiographic evaluation 250, 250*f*, 251*f*

incidence 249
nonoperative treatment 253
surgical management
approaches 255–257, 256*f*, 257*f*
elbow arthroplasty 253, 254*f*, 264–265, 264*f*
external fixation 253
indications for 252–253
open reduction and internal fixation 253, 257–263
outcomes 267
patient positioning 255, 255*f*
Distal interphalangeal (DIP) joint 7, 21
Distal radioulnar joint (DRUJ) 131*f*, 143, 143*f*, 154, 157, 161*f*, 162, 167, 168, 170–172, 178, 181, 224
Distal radius fractures 128–130
anatomy related to 143–144, 143*f*–145*f*
case study
intra-articular screw placement 159–162, 160*f*, 161*f*
loss of reduction 162, 163*f*–165*f*
classification 136–137, 136*f*
AO classification 136, 136*f*
Fernandez's 137, 138*f*, 139*f*
Frykman's 136
three-column theory 137, 140*f*
diagnosis 130–136
history examination 130
MRI scan 133
neurovascular functions assessment 130
physical examination 130
radiographic evaluation 129*f*, 130–131, 131*f*–133*f*
injury mechanism 128, 129*f*
intra-articular 160*f*
and perilunate dislocations 134, 135*f*
and radiocarpal dislocations 133–134, 134*f*, 135*f*
surgical management 137
closed reduction and external fixation 140, 141*f*
closed reduction and internal fixation 141*f*, 142
and complications 158–159
dorsal approach 145, 145*f*, 146*f*
extensile flexor carpi radialis approach 148
extensile volar-ulnar approach 148
modified Henry approach 148
open reduction and internal fixation 141*f*, 142, 142*f*
outcomes 158
patient positioning 145
radial approach 145
techniques 137, 140, 140*f*, 141*f*, 148–157
trans-FCR approach 145–148, 146*f*
volar approach 145–148
surgical techniques 148–157
dorsal plating 157
external fixation 150–151, 150*f*, 151*f*
intramedullary nailing 151–154, 152*f*–153*f*
Kirschner wire fixation 148–150, 149*f*
volar plating 154–157, 155*f*, 156*f*
treatment 130
unstable and displaced 130, 163*f*–164*f*
Distal tibia fractures 894–924
anterior and medial fixation 912*f*
anterolateral approach 901, 904*f*–906*f*, 915
anteromedial approach 901–902, 906*f*–907*f*, 915
aseptic malunion/nonunion, treatment 921–924
circular external fixation 902*f*
classification systems 898
AO/OTA classification 900*f*
Ruedi and Allgower 899*f*
closed 895*f*
complications 916–924
arthrosis 917
chronic osteomyelitis 916
malunion and nonunion 916–917, 923*f*–924*f*
management 917–924
soft tissue compromise 916
diagnosis 895–898
extra-articular 914–915
fibula fixation 911
fracture blisters 896*f*
infected nonunion, management 919–921
lateral approach 903
nonoperative management 888–889
nonunion repair, treatment 919
ORIF 899–901, 904*f*–907*f*, 915, 916
partial articular fracture 914*f*
overview 894–895
partial articular 913, 914*f*
posterolateral approach 902–903, 916
intraoperative image 908*f*
posterior shearing injury treatment 908*f*
postoperative care 913
recalcitrant nonunion, management 915–919, 922*f*
skin tenting 895*f*
soft tissue injury 896–897, 897*f*
special consideration 913–915
staged treatment 901–913, 915
first stage 903–911
second stage 911–913
spanning external fixation 910*f*
timing 911
surgical anatomy 901
surgical evolution 899–901
treatment outcomes 916
Dorsal extension block pinning, phalangeal fractures 15, 16*f*
Dorsal intercarpal (DIC) ligament 100, 100*f*
Dorsal plate fixation, distal radius fractures 142, 157, 159
Double-arc sign 250, 251*f*
Drill holes 324, 325*f*
DRUJ *see* Distal radioulnar joint (DRUJ)
DVT *see* Deep vein thrombosis (DVT)

Dynamic compression plate 182*f*, 183
humeral shaft fractures 287
olecranon fractures 198, 198*f*, 208
Dynamic external fixation, phalangeal fractures 15–16, 17*f*

E

East Baltimore lift 587 *see also* Femoral head fractures and hip dislocations
EDB *see* Extensor digitorum brevis (EDB)
Elbow 229–230, 229*f*
instability 243, 246*f*, 247
ligamentous stabilizers of 230, 230*f*
stiffness 242
Empty vertebral body sign 461
Erythrocyte sedimentation rate (ESR) 831
Essex-Lopresti injury 243
Exchange nailing, tibia infection treatment 876, 877*f*–879*f*
Extensile volar-ulnar approach 148
Extensor digitorum brevis (EDB) 991
Extensor pollicis longus (EPL) tendon 105, 106*f*, 143
Extensor tendon adhesions 51
External fixation
ankle fractures 932
distal radius fractures 140, 141*f*, 150–151, 151*f*, 159
phalangeal fractures 6
Extra-articular first-fifth metatarsal fractures 988
with dorsal plating 1004*f*
ORIF 1003–1006
preoperative planning 1003–1004
rehabilitation 1005
technique 1004–1005
wound closure 1005
surgical indications 990
surgical treatment of 993
Extra-articular metatarsal neck fractures, ORIF 1005*f*

F

Farabeuf/pelvic reduction clamp and screws, anterior pelvic fixation 511, 513*f*
Fasciotomy, leg compartment syndrome 890–891, 891*f*–892*f*
Fat pad sign 225
FCR *see* Flexor carpi radialis (FCR)
FDA *see* Food and Drug Administration (FDA)
Femoral circumflex artery
lateral 618
medial 618
Femoral head fractures and hip dislocations 581–582
Allis maneuver 587
case study
nonunion and osteonecrosis management 606–609, 607*f*, 608*f*
osteonecrosis management 605–606, 605*f*, 606*f*
classification 585, 585*f*–587*f*
Levin 585
Pipkin 585, 587*f*, 587*t*
Thomas and Epstein 585, 587*t*
complications
heterotopic ossification 602–603, 602*f*, 604*f*
osteonecrosis 601–602
post-traumatic arthritis 601
residual instability 603–604
retained loose bodies 603
sciatic nerve injury 603
diagnosis 582–583, 583*f*
CT scan 582–583, 585*f*
MRI 583
pearls and pitfalls 583, 585
radiographic evaluation 584*f*
X-rays 582
East Baltimore lift 587
incidence 581
Kocher-Langenbeck approach 592, 593
osteosynthesis 590
rehabilitation 600
Smith-Peterson incision 593
Stimson gravity technique 587
surgical management
anatomy 590–592
anterolateral approaches 593
arthroscopic excision 594–595
indications 585–590, 588*t*, 589*f*, 591*f*, 592*f*
Kocher-Langenbeck posterior approach 597–598, 597*f*, 598*f*
patient positioning 592
posterior approaches 593
Smith-Peterson approach 595–597, 595*f*, 596*f*
transtrochanteric approaches 593–594, 594*f*
trochanteric flip osteotomy 598–600
Watson-Jones incision 593
Femoral neck fractures 611–612
basicervical 618
case study
angled blade plate fixation 642–645, 646*f*–650*f*
loss of fixation 650–651
subtrochanteric femur fracture 645–650
total hip arthroplasty 640–642, 644*f*
classification 613–617, 616*f*
Garden 614, 617*f*
Pauwels 617, 617*f*
complications 641*f*
avascular necrosis 640
nonunion 639–640
diagnosis 612
CT scan 612, 614*f*
MRI 612, 615*f*
pearls and pitfalls 613
physical examination 612
radiographic evaluation 612, 613*f*
health care expenditures 611
outcomes 639
radiographs 613*f*
screw placement 629*f*
surgical management
anatomy and positioning 618–624
closed reduction/cannulated screw fixation 625–629
hemiarthroplasty 632–639

indications 618
ORIF of displaced 629–632
Femoral nerve palsy 573
Femoral shaft fractures 708–709
associated femoral neck fractures 727, 728*f*
case study
femur fracture infection 731–732, 731*f*, 732*f*
femur nonunion 730–731, 730*f*, 731*f*
classification 710
AO/OTA 710, 711*f*, 712*f*
Winquist-Hansen 710, 711*f*
complications
heterotopic ossification 730
infection 729
leg length discrepancy 729
malunion 728–729
nonunion 728
pudendal nerve palsy 730
damage control orthopedics 726–727, 726*f*
diagnosis
CT scan 710
history/physical examination 710
imaging 710
pearls and pitfalls 710
floating knee 727
gunshot wounds 725–726, 726*f*
open fractures 725
outcomes 725
surgical management
anatomy and positioning 713
antegrade femoral nailing 713–720, 714*f*–718*f*
antibiotic cement-coated nails 724
intramedullary nailing 712
plate fixation 712, 713*f*
retrograde intramedullary nailing 720–723, 720*f*, 721*f*
traction pin placement 723
vascular injuries 727
FHL tendon *see* Flexor hallucis longus (FHL) tendon
FiberWire 804
Fibula fixation, distal tibia fractures 911
Fibular length, restoration 937*f*, 938*f*
Fibular sesamoid fracture 986*f*
tangential sesamoid radiograph 986*f*
Finger alignment, metacarpal fractures and 31
Fixation failure, olecranon fractures 214, 217–219, 218*f*
Flexion distraction injuries, spine 451
Flexor digitorum profundis (FDP) 143
Flexor hallucis longus (FHL) tendon 934
Flexor pollicis longus (FPL) 143
Floating knee 727 *see also* Femoral shaft fractures
Food and Drug Administration (FDA) 825
Forearm fractures 167–168, 169*f*
anatomy related to 167–168, 168*f*, 172–173
both bones fractures 171, 172
case study
nonunions 186–188, 188*f*
synostosis 188–190, 189*f*, 190*f*
classification 170–171
complications 184
infection 185, 186*f*
malunion 186
nonunions 186
synostosis 186, 187*f*
diagnosis 168
CT scan 170
MRI 170
neurovascular examination 168
radiographic evaluation 168–170, 169*f*
Galeazzi fractures 170–172
incidence 168
injury mechanism 168
Monteggia fracture 170, 171–172, 171*f*
radial shaft fractures 170, 172
surgical management
direct ulnar approach 173
Henry approach 173, 174*f*
indications 171–172
outcomes 183–184
patient positioning 173
techniques 173–183
Thompson approach 173
ulnar shaft fracture 170, 171
Fracture blisters
ankle fractures 927*f*
associated with distal tibia fractures 896*f*
Frankel scale, spinal cord injury 384

G

Galeazzi fractures 169f, 170–171 *see also* Forearm fractures
surgical approach 178, 180*f*, 181, 181*f*
surgical indications 172
Gallie technique, C1–C2 fusion 425–426, 426*f*
Garden classification, femoral neck fractures 614, 617*f*
Gardner-Well tongs 403, 403*f*
Gerdy's tubercle 795
Gilula's lines 55, 56*f*
Glenohumeral joint 342*f*
Glenoid fractures 337–338, 338*f*
exposure of 342*f*
operative technique 348–349, 351–352, 351*f*
outcomes 354
surgical indications 340
Glenopolar angle 337, 337*f*
Goel-Harm's technique, C1–C2 fusion 424–425, 424*f*, 425*f*
Greater sigmoid notch 200
Guidewire placement, tibial shaft fracture 854, 855*f*
Gunshot wounds 725–726, 726*f* *see also* Femoral shaft fractures

H

Hallucal fracture-dislocations
ORIF 1008–1009
rehabilitation 1009
technique 1008–1009
wound closure 1009
preoperative planning 1008

Hallucal joint injuries 988–989
surgical approach 993
Hallucal sesamoid fractures 989
ORIF 1010–1011
preoperative planning 1010
rehabilitation 1011
technique 1010–1011
wound closure 1011
surgical approach 993–994
surgical indications 990
Halo ring 401–403, 402*f*
Halo vest 396, 401
Hamate fractures 60, 67
Hangman's fracture 398, 400–401, 400*f*, 400*t*, 401*f*, 404–405, 405*f*
Hardware complications, olecranon fractures 213–214
Hardware fixation, ankle fractures 945
Harris Hip Scores 639
Hemiarthroplasty
femoral neck fractures
instrumentation, implant and patient positioning 636
pearls and pitfalls 639
preoperative planning 632, 635–636
technique 636–637, 638*f*
proximal humerus fractures 324–326, 325*f*, 328
Hemi-hamate reconstruction, phalangeal fractures 18–19, 18*f*
Hemorrhagic blisters, ankle fractures 927*f*
Henry approach, forearm fractures 173, 174*f*
Henry approach, modified, volar distal radius 148
Herbert's classification system, scaphoid fractures 97, 98*t*
Heterotopic ossification (HO) 582, 602–603, 602*f*, 604*f*, 730
see also Femoral shaft fractures
acetabulum fracture 572–573
distal humerus fractures 267–270, 271*f*
elbow dislocations 241–242
olecranon fractures 215, 216*f*
Hindfoot fractures
calcaneus fractures 954–966
overview 953
talus fractures 966–981
Hip joint, ligaments 618, 620*f*
HO *see* Heterotopic ossification (HO)
Hoffa fracture 739, 739*f*, 753–756, 755*f*
see also Distal femur fractures
Hohmann retractor 749
Hook plate fixation
clavicle fractures 364, 364*f*
olecranon fractures 198, 198*f*, 206, 208, 208*f*
Horner's syndrome 359
Hospital for special surgery (HSS) 821
HSS *see* Hospital for special surgery (HSS)
Humeral shaft fractures 276–277, 277*f*
anatomy related to 282–283
case management
nonunion 296–300, 297*f*–299*f*
radial nerve injury 295–296, 295*f*
classification 279–281, 280*f*
complications
iatrogenic fracture extension 294–295
insertion site morbidity 294
nonunion 294
radial nerve palsy 294
diagnosis 277–279, 278*f*, 279*f*
neurovascular examination 277–278, 278*f*
physical examination 277
radiographic evaluation 278–279, 279*f*
nonoperative management 281
open fractures 279, 281
pathologic 276, 277*f*
surgical management
anterolateral approach 283–284, 285*f*, 286*f*
indications for 281, 281*t*
intramedullary nailing 281–282, 282*f*, 288–293, 291*f*–292*f*
medial approach 286–287
open reduction internal fixation 281, 282*f*, 287–288, 288*f*, 289*f*
outcomes 293–294
patient positioning 283, 284*f*
posterior approach 284, 286*f*
triceps-sparing approach 285
triceps-splitting approach 285
Humpback deformity 100, 101*f*, 111
Hypertrophic nonunion, tibia 883–886, 886*f*
Hypovolemic shock 381

I

Iliac crest pin 501, 502*f* *see also* Pelvic ring and sacral injuries
Iliofemoral ligament 620
Iliosacral screw insertion, retropelvic fixation 517–537, 518*f*–539*f*
prone technique 524–537, 527*f*–537*f*
imaging 524–527
insertion technique 527–529
sacral dysmorphism 531–533
sacral fracture style screws 530–531
sacroiliac style screws 530
sacroiliac *vs.* sacral style screws 529–530
S2 screws 533–535
transiliac-transsacral screws 535–536, 536*f*–538*f*
supine technique 517–524, 518*f*–524*f*
Iliotibial (IT) band 795
Ilizarov method 876
chronic osteomyelitis 880
Incisions
metacarpal fractures 37, 37*f*
olecranon 202, 202*f*
phalangeal fractures 7, 7*f*
Infections
forearm fractures 185, 186*f*
olecranon fractures 217
proximal humerus fractures 327
Interosseous ligaments 498
Interphalangeal (IP) joint 2, 7
Intertrochanteric femur/hip fractures
case study
lag screw cut-out 667, 668*f*
nonunion 667, 669f, 670*f*
classification 655
AO/OTA 655, 656*f*
complications 666–667

diagnosis 654–655
MRI 655
pearls and pitfalls 655
radiographic evaluation 655
incidence 654
outcomes 663–666
surgical management
anatomy and positioning 656–658, 657*f*, 658*f*
fracture reduction 658–659, 659*f*, 660*f*
indications 655
intramedullary nailing 661–663
ORIF 659–661
types of 655
Intramedullary devices, for midshaft clavicle fixation 363 *see also* Clavicle fractures
Intramedullary (IM) nailing
calcaneus fractures 966
distal radius fractures 141*f*, 142, 151–154, 152*f*–153*f*, 159
distal tibial metadiaphyseal fracture 863–871
humeral shaft fractures 281–282, 282*f*, 288–293, 291*f*–292*f*, 293
of intertrochanteric femur/hip fractures
pearls and pitfalls 663
preoperative planning 661–662
technique 662–663, 662*f*, 664*f*–665*f*
olecranon fractures 199–200, 199*f*, 209, 210*f*
proximal humerus fractures 321–324, 322*f*, 323*f*
subtrochanteric femur fractures 679
talus fractures 976–977
tibia 857*f*
tibial shaft fractures 849–871
acute infection treatment 873*f*–875*f*
patient assessment 850
portal preparation 852*f*
preoperative planning 849–850
proximal 858–863
reamed, locked 849–858
technique 850–858
Ischiofemoral ligament 620
IT band *see* Iliotibial (IT) band

J

Jersey finger fractures 20–21
Joint stiffness, after finger fracture fixation 27
Judet approach, scapula 343, 344*f*
Judet quadricepsplasty 757

K

Kaplan approach, radial head fractures 231, 232*f*
Kirschner (K) wires 4
distal femur fractures 745, 746*f*
distal radius fractures 141*f*, 142, 148–150, 149*f*, 158
femoral neck fractures 632
lateral clavicle fractures 369
olecranon fractures 202–206, 203*f*–204*f*
patellar fractures 771
proximal humerus fractures 316
proximal tibia fractures 801
scaphoid fractures 99, 101, 104*f*, 105
subtrochanteric femur fractures 691
Knee Society Pain Score 757
Knee Society Rating Scale (KSRS) 836
Kocher approach, radial head fractures 231, 232*f*
Kocher-Langenbeck approach 592, 593 *see also* Femoral head fractures
Koch's biomechanical study, subtrochanteric femur fractures 677
KSRS *see* Knee Society Rating Scale (KSRS)
Kyphoplasty 468, 469*f*, 470*f*

L

Lag screw fixation 44, 45–46, 46*f*
Lateral collateral ligament (LCL) 230, 230*f*, 231, 237*f*–238*f*, 239, 239*f*, 247, 789
Lateral malleolar fractures 931
Lateral mass screw fixation, cervical spine injuries 433, 435, 436*f*, 437*f*, 438*f*, 439
Lateral ulnar collateral ligament (LUCL) complex 224, 229, 229*f*
Lauge-Hansen classification system, ankle fractures 928, 930*f*
LCL *see* Lateral collateral ligament (LCL)
Leg length discrepancy 729 *see also* Femoral shaft fractures
Less invasive stabilization system (LISS) 756
Levin classification, femoral head fractures 585
Lisfranc fracture-dislocation 987*f*
classification systems 987–989
homolateral
complete 987*f*
incomplete 988*f*
midfoot arthrodesis 999–1003
preoperative planning 999–1000
rehabilitation 1002–1003
technique 1000–1002
wound closure 1002
ORIF 994–999
anatomical factors 994
instrumentation and implant 994–995
patient factors 995
preoperative planning 994–995
rehabilitation 997–999
technique 995–996
wound closure 996–997
ROM exercises 997
two-incision approach 1001–1002
Lisfranc injury 987*f*
diagnosis 986–987
ORIF radiographs 997*f*, 998*f*
Lisfranc ligament, neglected injury 1001*f*
LISS *see* Less invasive stabilization system (LISS)
Lister's tubercle 105, 106*f*, 143, 143*f*
LMWH *see* Low molecular weight heparin (LMWH)
Locked plates 307, 326
Log-roll maneuver 381
Long oblique fracture, reduction 851*f*

Long radiolunate (LRL) ligament 70, 70*f*
Low molecular weight heparin (LMWH) 827
Lunate dislocations 61
Lunate fractures 59–60, 60*f*, 143, 144*f*, 165*f*
see also Carpal fractures and perilunate dislocations
Lysholm scores 725

M

Magerl's technique, C1–C2 fusion 421–424, 422*f*, 423*f*
Magnetic resonance imaging (MRI)
ankle fractures 928
carpal fractures 56
clavicle fractures 360
distal femur fractures 739
distal radius fractures 133
femoral head fractures and hip dislocations 583
femoral neck fractures 612, 615*f*
forearm fractures 170
intertrochanteric femur fractures 655
midfoot and forefoot fractures 986 987
proximal tibia fractures 786
scaphoid fractures 96–97, 97*f*
subtrochanteric femur fractures 673
thoracic and lumbar spine fractures 455, 456*f*, 459–460
Malleolar ankle fractures 930*f*
lateral 931
posterior 931
Mallet fractures 21–22, 22*f*
Malunion
acetabulum fracture 574
ankle fractures 946
clavicle fractures 374
forearm fractures 186
metacarpal fractures 51
olecranon fractures 214
phalangeal fractures 23–26, 25*f*
proximal humerus fractures 327
radial head fractures 242
scapular fractures 354
talus fractures 975
Mayo scissors 621
Mayo stand cover 621
Medial collateral ligament (MCL) 229, 229*f*, 230, 789
Medial coronoid approach, radial head fractures 231–232, 233*f*
Medial femoral circumflex artery (MFCA) 583
Medial malleolus fractures 948*f*
nonunion, treatment 947–948
operative fixation 938–941
supination-adduction vertical shear type 940*f*
transverse 940
Medial open wound, open ankle fractures 932*f*
Medial wounds, open tibial fracture 896*f*
Median nerve 71, 172
compression of 130
Metacarpal fractures 30–31
anatomy related to 36–37, 36*f*
case study
finger stiffness 51, 51*f*
tendon rupture 51–52, 52*f*
classification 33–35, 33*t*, 34*f*
closed reduction, pinning 40–44, 41*f*–43*f*
Bennett fractures 47–48, 48*f*, 49*f*
Bouqet pinning 41*f*
cross pinning 40, 41*f*
crucifix pinning 40, 41*f*, 42*f*, 43
intramedullary pinning 41*f*, 43, 43*f*
transarticular pinning 41*f*, 44
transverse pinning 41*f*
complications 50
malunion 51
nonunion 51
stiffness 50–51
diagnosis 31–33
CT scan 32, 33*f*
physical examination 31, 31*f*
radiographic evaluation 31–32,32*f*
etiologies 30
fifth metacarpal neck fracture 30,31*f*
incidence 30
surgical management
approaches for 37–38, 37*f*, 38*f*, 39*f*
basal thumb metacarpal fractures 35–36
indications for 35–36
metacarpal shaft fractures 35
outcomes 50
patient positioning 37
pinning technique 40–44, 41*f*–43*f*, 47–48, 48*f*, 49*f*
plate and screw fixation 38–39, 49*f*, 44–47, 45*f*–47*f*, 48, 50*f*
Wagner approach 38, 39*f*
thumb 30, 32–33
Metacarpophalangeal (MP) joints 2, 6, 31
open wounds 31
stiffness 51
Metatarsophalangeal (MTP) joints 984
Methicillin-resistant *Staphylococcus aureus* (MRSA) 872
MFCA *see* Medial femoral circumflex artery (MFCA)
Midaxial approach, radial head fractures 231, 232*f*
Midfoot and forefoot fractures 983–1019
anatomy related to 984, 984*f*
classification systems 987–989
compartment syndrome 1013
treatment 1015–1018
diagnosis 985–987
computed tomography 986
imaging 986
MRI 986–987
physical examination 985
radiographs 986
soft tissue examination 985–986
hallucal joint injuries 988–989
management 1013–1018
midfoot fusion 991
nonunion 1012–1013
vs refracture 1015
ORIF 990, 994–999, 1003–1011
overview 983–985
postoperative infection 1012
post-traumatic arthritis 1012
treatment 1013
proximal fifth metatarsal fractures 985

proximal phalangeal fractures 988, 989*f*
standard dual-incision 992*f*
standard incision 993*f*–994*f*
surgery
anatomy 991–992
approaches 992–994
complications 1012–1018
indications 989–991
outcomes 1011–1012
positioning 992
techniques 994–1012
wounds 1012
Midfoot fusion 991
Minimally invasive plate osteosynthesis (MIPO) 745
proximal metaphyseal tibial fracture 869*f*–870*f*
Monteggia fractures 169*f*, 170 *see also* Forearm fractures
Bado classification 170, 171*f*
surgical approach 178, 179*f*
surgical indications 171–172
Moore classification, proximal tibia fractures 792, 792*f*, 793*f*
Morel-Lavallee lesion 496, 497*f*
Motor index scoring 384
MRI *see* Magnetic resonance imaging (MRI)
MRSA *see* Methicillin-resistant *Staphylococcus aureus* (MRSA)
MTP joints *see* Metatarsophalangeal (MTP) joints
Müeller's classification, distal femur fractures 739

N

Naviculocuneiform fusion 1001*f*
Nerve palsy, acetabulum fracture 573
Neurogenic shock 381
vs. hypovolemic shock 381
Neurovascular examination
forearm fractures 168
humeral shaft fractures 277–278, 278*f*
Nightstick fractures 170 *See also* Ulnar shaft fractures
Nonsteroidal anti-inflammatory drugs (NSAIDs) 835
Nonunion
acetabulum fracture 574
ankle fractures 946
clavicle fractures 359, 373–374
distal humerus fractures 268, 272–273, 273*f*, 274*f*
distal tibia
post-traumatic arthritis 918*f*
revision ORIF 921*f*
femoral neck fractures 639–640
femoral shaft fractures 728
forearm fractures 186–188, 188*f*
humeral shaft 294, 296–300, 297*f*–299*f*
intertrochanteric femur/hip fractures 667, 669*f*, 670*f*
medial malleolus fracture 947–948
midfoot and forefoot fractures 1012–1013
olecranon fractures 214–215, 214*f*
patellar fractures 777, 780*f*, 781*f*
proximal tibia fractures 831–836
radial head fractures 242–243
scaphoid fractures 95, 110–111, 111*f*
subtrochanteric femur fractures 696–697
NSAID *see* Nonsteroidal anti-inflammatory drugs (NSAIDs)

O

OA *see* Osteoarthritis (OA)
Obturator artery 618
Occipital condyle fractures 395–396, 396*f* *see also* Cervical spine injuries
Occipitocervical dislocations 316, 317*f* *see also* Cervical spine injuries
Odontoid fractures 398, 398*f*
classification of 399*f*, 399*t*
management 404, 404*f*, 405*f*
Type III 399*f*
Olecranon fractures 192, 192*f*
anatomy related to 200–201, 200*f*
case study
fixation failures 217–219, 218*f*
classification 195
Colton 195
Mayo 195, 196*f*
Schatzker 195
and complex elbow fractures 193, 194*f*
complications 213
fixation failure 214
hardware complications 213–214
heterotopic ossification 215, 216*f*
infection 217
malunions 214
nonunions 214–215, 214*f*
proximal radioulnar joint injury 215, 217, 217*f*, 219, 220*f*
stiffness 215
ulnar neuropathy 217
diagnosis
CT scans 193, 195, 195*f*
physical examination 193
radiographic evaluation 193
injury mechanisms 192
surgical management
excision with triceps advancement 200, 200*f*, 211–212, 211*f*
indications for 195–200
intramedullary nailing 198–200, 199*f*, 209, 210*f*
outcomes 212–213
patient positioning 201–202, 201*f*
plate fixation 198, 198*f*, 206–209, 207*f*, 208*f*
posterior approach 202, 202*f*
tension band fixation 197–198, 197*f*, 202–206, 203*f*–204*f*
Olecranon osteotomy 256, 257*f*
Open ankle fractures 932
dislocation with morbid obesity 933*f*
with medial open wound 932*f*
Open fractures 725 *see also* Femoral shaft fractures
Open reduction and internal fixation (ORIF) 16–17, 17*f*

ankle fractures 931
calcaneus fractures 961*f*
capitellum fracture 265–266, 265*f*, 266*f*
carpal bones and fragments 77, 77*f*
compartment syndrome, foot 1017
diaphyseal fibula fractures 936–938
of displaced femoral neck fractures
 instrumentation, implant and patient positioning 629, 632, 634*f*, 636*f*
 preoperative planning and anatomic consideration 629
 technique 632
distal femur fractures 740–741
 type B3/Hoffa 753–756, 755*f*
 type B/unicondylar 751–753, 752*f*, 754*f*
 type C 749–751, 750*f*, 751*f*
distal fibular fractures 936–938
distal humerus fractures 253, 257–263
 extra-articular 258, 259*f*–261*f*
 intra-articular 258, 262*f*
distal radius fractures 141*f*, 142, 142*f*, 158
distal tibia fractures 899–901
extra-articular first fifth metatarsal fractures 1003–1006
extruded talus 977, 978*f*–979*f*, 980*f*
of fibula 857*f*
hallucal fracture-dislocations 1008–1009
hallucal sesamoid fractures 1010–1011
humeral shaft fractures 281, 282*f*, 287–288, 288*f*, 289*f*, 293
of intertrochanteric femur/hip fractures
 pearls and pitfalls 661
 preoperative planning 659
 technique 659–660, 661*f*
Lisfranc fracture-dislocation 994–999
midfoot and forefoot fractures 990, 994–999, 1003–1011
open calcaneus fractures 961*f*–963*f*
partial articular fracture 914*f*
perilunate dislocations 77–80, 78*f*–79*f*
phalangeal fractures 5, 5*f*, 8, 14*f*, 15, 17, 26, 26*f*
proximal fifth metatarsal fractures 1006–1008
proximal humerus fractures 315–321, 317*f*, 318*f*–319*f*, 320*f*–321*f*
proximal metaphyseal tibial fracture 869*f*–870*f*
scaphoid fractures 74–76, 98
 dorsal approach 105, 106*f*, 107*f*
 volar approach 101–104, 102*f*–104*f*
tibial diaphyseal fracture 864–870
 indications 864–865
 technique 865
tibial shaft fracture 866*f*–868*f*
ORIF *see* Open reduction and internal fixation (ORIF)
Orthopaedic Trauma Association (OTA) 613, 767
Osteoarthritis (OA) 590
Osteomyelitis
 1A 872
 chronic, cure 877
 distal tibia fractures 916
 implants removal 876
Osteonecrosis 601–602 *see also* Femoral head fractures
OTA *see* Orthopaedic Trauma Association (OTA)

P

Palmaris longus (PL) 69
Paraplegia 386
Patellar fractures
 case study 778–784
  knee stiffness 778, 783–784
  partial or total patellectomy 778
  revision fixation 778
 classification 767–770
 complications
  arthritis 778
  hardware irritation 777
  infection 777, 779*f*, 780*f*
  knee stiffness 777–778, 782*f*, 783*f*
  loss of reduction 777
  nonunion 777, 780*f*, 781*f*
 diagnosis 766–767, 768*f*, 769*f*
  pearls and pitfalls 767
  physical examination 766–767
  radiographic evaluation 767
  saline load test 767
 management
  anatomy and positioning 770–771
  indications 770
  partial patellectomy 770
 outcomes 777
 surgical management
  partial patellectomy 773–776
  tension band technique 771–773
Patient positioning *see* Positioning, patient
Pauwels angle 629, 632
Pauwels classification, femoral neck fractures 617, 617*f*
PCL *see* Posterior cruciate ligament (PCL)
Pedicle fracture 484
Pelvic C-clamp 520–521
Pelvic instability 497 *see also* Pelvic ring and sacral injuries
Pelvic ring and sacral injuries 495–496
 anterior ligamentous complex injury 498, 499*f*
 classification 496–499, 499*f*
 complications, management of
  errant placement of anterior external fixation pins 541, 543, 543*f*
  nonunion of pelvis after anterior external fixation 544, 548–550, 548*f*–550*f*
  percutaneous treatment of pelvic fracture nonunion 543–544, 547*f*–549*f*
  unstable injury with malreduction of posterior ring 538–539, 540*f*–542*f*, 541

diagnosis 496
clinical evaluation 496, 497*f*
CT scan 496
radiographic evaluation 496, 498*f*
sacral fracture classification 499, 499*f*
surgical management 499–501, 500*f*, 501*f*
anterior iliac crest pin insertion 501–502, 502*f*–505*f*
anterior pelvic fixation 505, 507–517
external fixation of pelvis 501–505
iliosacral screw insertion 517–537, 518*f*–539*f*
medullary ramus screws 513–516, 516*f*
supra-acetabular pins insertion 502, 502*f*, 505, 506*f*–508*f*
symphyseal plate fixation 507–513, 510*f*–515*f*
unstable 500*f*, 501*f*
Perched facets 409
Percutaneous fixation
distal radius fractures 142
scaphoid fractures 98, 110
dorsal approach 107–110, 109*f*
volar approach 105, 107, 108*f*
Periarticular locking plates 258, 258*f*
olecranon fractures 198, 198*f*
Perilunate dislocations 54, 55, 57*f*, 61, 62*f*, 63*f*, 81 *see also* Carpal fractures
greater arc 134, 135*f*
Peroneal nerve palsy 621
Peroneal tendonitis, ankle fractures 946
Pfannenstiel approach, anterior pelvic fixation 508–511, 510*f*
Phalangeal fractures 1–2
anatomy related to 6–7, 6*f*
classification 2, 4
comminuted 2, 4
complications 23
malunion 23–26, 25*f*
stiffness 24, 26–27, 26*f*
condylar fracture 15, 15*f*
diagnosis 2
pearls and pitfalls 2
physical examination 2, 3*f*
radiograph evaluation 2, 4*f*
ultrasound 2
diaphyseal 11–12, 13*f*, 14*f*
distal 4, 20–21, 22*f*
extra-articular 4, 8, 10*f*
incidence 1
injury mechanisms 1
intra-articular 4, 12*f*, 15
Jersey finger fractures 20–21
mallet fracture 21–22, 22*f*
middle 4, 15–19, 16*f*–20*f*
nondisplaced 4
proximal 4, 8, 8*f*, 10–11, 10*f*, 11*f*, 12*f*
spiral 4
surgical management 7–8
CRPP 4, 5*f*
dorsal approach 8, 8*f*
external fixation 6
incisions placement 7, 7*f*
indications 4–6
midaxial approach 8, 9*f*
ORIF 5, 5*f*
positioning 7
techniques 8–21
volar approach 8, 9*f*
transverse 2
treatment 1–2
Physical examination
carpal fractures and perilunate dislocations 55
clavicle fractures 359
distal humerus fractures 250
distal radius fractures 130
femoral neck fractures 612
femoral shaft fractures 710
humeral shaft fractures 277
metacarpal fractures 31, 31*f*
olecranon fractures 193
patellar fractures 766–767
phalangeal fractures 2, 3*f*
proximal humerus fracture 303
proximal tibia fractures 786
scaphoid fractures 95, 95*f*
subtrochanteric femur fractures 673
Pilon fractures *see* Distal tibia fractures
PIN *see* Posterior interosseous nerve (PIN)
Pin tract infection 159
Pipkin classification, 585, 587*f*, 587*t*
Piriformis tendon 622
Plafond fracture, foot position and 898*f*
Plate and screw fixation
Bennett fractures 48, 50*f*
metacarpal neck fractures 44, 45*f*
metacarpal shaft fractures 44–47, 46f, 47*f*
midshaft clavicle fixation 362–363, 364*f*, 367–368, 368*f*
olecranon fractures 198, 198*f*, 206–209, 207*f*, 208*f*
PMMA *see* Polymethylmethacrylate (PMMA)
Pneumatic tourniquet 749
Poller screws 748
Polymethylmethacrylate (PMMA) 466, 468, 822, 875, 875*f*
Popliteal artery 738
Positioning, patient
ankle fractures 935
calcaneus fractures 955–956
distal femur fractures 742, 743*f*
femoral head fractures and hip dislocations 592
femoral neck fractures 618–622
femoral shaft fractures 713
forearm fractures 173
humeral shaft fractures 283, 284*f*
intertrochanteric femur fractures 657, 657*f*, 658*f*
metacarpal fractures 37
patellar fractures 770–771
phalangeal fractures 7
proximal humerus fractures 311–312, 311*f*, 312*f*
proximal tibia fractures 794–795
subtrochanteric femur fractures 677–678
talus fractures 970
tibial shaft fractures 848

Posterior cord syndrome 387*t*, 388–389, 388*f*
Posterior cruciate ligament (PCL) 789
Posterior interosseous nerve (PIN) 71, 172, 230
Posterior longitudinal ligament (PLL) 449
Posterior malleolar fractures 931
- anatomic reduction 941–942
- closed reduction 941*f*
- open reduction 942
- ORIF 941–942

Posterior malleolus 934
Posterior sacroiliac (SI) ligaments 498
Posterior superior iliac spine (PSIS) 564
Posterior vertebral angle 454–455
Posterior vertebral height 454–455
Posterolateral approach
- ankle fractures 935
- distal tibia fractures 902–903, 916

Post-traumatic arthritis 1012
- Lisfranc injury 1013, 1014*f*
- treatment 1013

Post-traumatic arthrosis
- loss of reduction 948–951, 949*f*–950*f*

Powers ratio 389*t*, 393*f*, 396
Pronator quadratus (PQ) muscle 143
Proximal femoral locking plate
- subtrochanteric femur fractures 679, 689–691, 690*f*

Proximal femur, anatomy 619*f*
Proximal fifth metatarsal fractures 985
- ORIF 1006–1008
- preoperative planning 1006
- rehabilitation 1005
- technique 1006–1007
- wound closure 1005

Proximal humerus fractures 302
- anatomy related to 309–311, 310*f*, 311*f*
- bone graft substitutes 317–318, 318*f*–319*f*
- case study
  - failure of fixation followed by hemiarthroplasty 328, 330, 330*f*
  - failure of fixation followed by revision of fixation 328, 329*f*
  - ORIF followed by infected nonunion 330–332, 331*f*
- classification 303, 307*f*, 308*f*
  - AO/OTA classification system 303, 308*f*
  - Neer classification 303, 307*f*
- complications 327–328
  - avascular necrosis 327
  - hemiarthroplasty-related 328
  - infection 327
  - varus malunion 327
- cortical thickness measurement 306, 309*f*
- diagnosis 302–303
  - CT scan 303, 305*f*, 306*f*
  - history examination 302–303
  - physical examination 303
  - radiographic imaging 303, 304*f*
- in elderly 309
- head-split 318, 320–321, 320*f*–321*f*
- incidence 302
- surgical management
  - anterolateral acromial approach 314*f*, 315, 316
  - deltopectoral approach 312, 313*f*
  - hemiarthroplasty 324–326, 325*f*
  - indications for 304, 306–309
  - intramedullary nailing 321–324, 322*f*, 323*f*
  - open reduction internal fixation 315–321, 317*f*–321*f*
  - outcomes 326–327
  - patient positioning 311–312, 311*f*, 312*f*
- treatment 302

Proximal interlocking, tibial shaft fractures 854
Proximal interphalangeal (PIP) joint 6, 15, 18–19, 20*f*, 21
Proximal phalangeal fractures 988, 989*f*
Proximal radioulnar joint (PRUJ) injury, olecranon fractures 215, 217, 217*f*, 219, 220*f*
Proximal tibia fractures 785
- case study
  - infection 830–831, 831*f*–833*f*
  - loss of fixation 827–830, 828*f*–830*f*
  - malunion and nonunion 831–836, 834*f*–835*f*, 837*f*–839*f*
  - post-traumatic arthritis 836–840
- classification
  - AO/OTA 791–792, 791*f*
  - Moore 792, 792*f*, 793*f*
  - Schatzker 790–791, 790*f*
- diagnosis
  - associated injuries 789–790
  - CT scan 786
  - imaging 786–787, 787*f*, 788*f*
  - mechanism of injury 787–789
  - MRI 786
  - pearls and pitfalls 790
  - physical examination 786
- surgical management
  - anatomy and positioning 794–796, 795*f*, 796*f*
  - bicondylar fractures 812–822
  - emergent treatment 796–799, 798*f*–800*f*
  - indications 792
  - lateral fracture dislocations 804, 804*f*
  - medial plateau fracture 805, 806*f*, 807*f*
  - posterolateral fracture 804–805
  - posteromedial fracture 805–811, 808*f*–811*f*
  - postoperative care 826–827
  - pure depression fracture 801, 803*f*
  - repair 794
  - split depression fracture 801, 802*f*
  - split fracture 799–801
  - tibial plateau fracture 822–826, 823*f*, 824*f*, 826*f*

Pseudorotator cuff rupture 335
Ptotic eyelid 359–360
Pubofemoral ligament 620
Pudendal nerve palsy 730
Pulmonary embolism, acetabulum fracture 573

Q

Quadricepsplasty 757
- Judet 757
- Thompson 757

R

Radial head fractures 223
  anatomy related to 229–230, 229*f*, 230*f*
  case study
    elbow instability 246*f*, 247
    longitudinal forearm instability 243–247
  classification 226, 228*f*
    Broberg and Morrey 226, 228*f*
    Hotchkiss 226
    Mason 226
  complications
    elbow instability 243
    elbow stiffness 242
    Essex-Lopresti injury 243
    heterotopic ossification 241–242
    longitudinal instability of forearm 243
    malunions 242
    nonunion 242–243
  diagnosis 224–226
    CT scan 226
    physical examination 224
    radiographic evaluation 225–226, 225*f*
  with elbow dislocations 223–224, 224*f* (*see also* Complex elbow dislocations)
  injury mechanism 223
  isolated 223, 224*f*
  nonoperative treatment 228
  surgical management 226, 228–229
    indications for 226, 228–229
    Kaplan approach 231, 232*f*
    Kocher approach 231, 232*f*
    medial coronoid approach 231–232, 233*f*
    midaxial approach 231, 232*f*, 233
    outcomes 240–241
    patient positioning 230, 231*f*
    radial head arthroplasty 235, 236*f*
    radial head fixation 233–235, 234*f*
    terrible triad repair 235–240, 237*f*–240*f*
  and terrible triad injuries 224
Radial sensory nerve 71, 172
Radial shaft fractures 169*f*, 170 *See also* Forearm fractures
  fixation 175–176
    dorsal fixation 177–178
    Henry's volar approach 176–177, 177*f*
  surgical indications 172
Radiocarpal dislocations 61, 61*f*, 67, 133, 134*f*, 135*f*
Radiographs
  acetabulum fracture 554–555, 554*f*, 555*f*
  clavicle fractures 360, 360*f*
  distal humerus fractures 250, 250*f*, 251*f*
  distal radius fractures 129*f*, 130–131, 131*f*–133*f*
  femoral neck fractures 612, 613*f*
  forearm fractures 168–170, 169*f*
  humeral shaft fractures 278–279, 279*f*
  intertrochanteric femur/hip fractures 655
  metacarpal fractures 31–32, 32*f*
  olecranon fractures 193
  patellar fractures 767
  pelvic radiographic triad 496, 498*f*
  phalangeal fractures 2, 4*f*
  proximal humerus fractures 303, 304*f*, 305*f*
  scaphoid fractures 95, 96*f*
  thoracic and lumbar spine fractures 454–455, 454*f*, 454*t*, 457*f*, 458*f*, 460*f*
Radioscaphocapitate ligament (RSCL) 95, 100, 100*f*
Radioscapholunate (ligament of Testut) ligament 70, 70*f*
Radius 168, 168*f*
Rami fractures, pubic 507
Range of motion (ROM) 785
  elbow 224
  hip and knee 997
Reamer irrigator aspirator (RIA) 706, 722
Reaming, tibial shaft fracture 854, 855*f*, 866*f*
Reconstruction nails, subtrochanteric femur fractures 679
Rectus femoris, heads 621
Reflex sympathetic dystrophy 159
Rehabilitation
  extra-articular first-fifth metatarsal fractures 1005
  hallucal fracture-dislocations 1009
  Lisfranc fracture-dislocation 997–999, 1002–1003
  proximal fifth metatarsal fractures 1005
Retrograde intramedullary nail
  distal femur fractures 747–749, 747*f*
  femoral shaft fractures 720–723, 720f, 721*f*
  pearls and pitfalls 722, 749
RIA *see* Reamer irrigator aspirator (RIA)
Rockwood pin fixation, clavicle fractures 364*f*, 369, 370*f*
Rolando's fractures 34, 34*f* *see also* Metacarpal fractures
ROM *see* Range of motion (ROM)
Roof-arc measurements 557, 557*f*
RSCL *see* Radioscaphocapitate ligament (RSCL)
Russell-Taylor classification, of subtrochanteric femur fractures 674–675, 675*f*

S

SA *see* Shear angle (SA)
Sacral sparing 382
Sacrum, fractures of 499, 499*f* *see also* Pelvic ring and sacral injuries
Saline load test, patellar fractures 767
Sandwich sign 461
Scaphocapitate ligament (SCL) 100, 100*f*
Scaphoid fractures 54, 54*f*, 94–95
  anatomy related to 99–100, 99*f*, 100*f*

case study
 nonunions without AVN 118–123, 121f–122f
 proximal pole nonunions with AVN 113–114, 116–118, 117f–120f
 stage III SNAC wrist 123–126, 124f–125f
classification 97–98, 98t
complications 95, 110
 arthritis 111, 113, 113f, 113t
 avascular necrosis 111, 112f
 delayed union 81
 malunion 83
 nonunion of scaphoid 81–83, 82f
 nonunions 110–111, 111f
 osteoarthritis 83, 83f, 84f
criteria for displacement and instability 98t
diagnosis 95
 bone scan 97
 CT scan 97
 MRI 96–97, 97f
 pearls and pitfalls 97
 physical examination 95, 95f
 radiographic evaluation 95, 96f
displaced 65–67
distal pole 98
Herbert's classification 58–59, 58f
incidence 94
management 94–95, 98
 headless compression screws 98–99
 nonoperative treatment 98
 ORIF 98
 percutaneous fixation 98
nondisplaced 63–65, 64f, 65f, 66f
ORIF of 74
 mini-open dorsal approach 76, 76f
 open volar approach 74, 76
 percutaneous volar technique 74, 75f
 postoperative management 76
outcomes 80–81, 81f
proximal pole 101, 105
Russe's classification 59, 59f
surgical indications 63–67
surgical management
 approaches to 101
 dorsal ORIF 105, 106f, 107f
 dorsal percutaneous fixation 107–110, 109f
 outcomes 110
 positioning 100–101
 volar ORIF 101–104, 102f–104f
 volar percutaneous fixation 105, 107, 108f
unstable 98, 101
Scaphoid nonunion advanced collapse (SNAC) 83, 83f, 84f, 111, 113, 113f
 stages 113, 113t, 114f
 surgical management 113, 115f–116f
Scapholunate interosseous ligament (SLIL) 99
Scapholunate ligament (SLL) 85, 133
Scapula and glenoid fractures 334–335
 anatomy related to 340–341, 341f
 case study
 glenoid fossa malunion 355
 scapular neck malunion 355–356
 classification 335–339
 complications 354
 compartment syndrome 354
 iatrogenic nerve injury 354
 intrathoracic scapular impaction 355
 malunion 354
 and concomitant injuries 335
 diagnosis 335
 surgical management
 anterior approach 341–343
 indications for 339–340
 outcomes 353–354
 posterior approach 343–344
 techniques for 345–353
Scapular body fractures 337
 operative technique 345, 346f–347f
 surgical indications 339
Scapular neck fractures 337
 operative technique 345–346, 348, 349f–350f
 surgical indications 340
Schanz screws 511
Schatzker classification, proximal tibia fractures 790–791, 790f
Sciatic nerve injury 603 *see also* Femoral head fractures and hip dislocations
Sciatic nerve palsy 573
SCL *see* Scaphocapitate ligament (SCL)
Screw fixation 265, 266f
 metacarpal head fractures 38–39, 40f
 olecranon fractures 199, 199f
 scaphoid fractures 98–99
Seinsheimer's classification, of subtrochanteric femur fractures 673–674, 674f
Sensory index scoring 383
Serous fracture blister 896f
Shear angle (SA) 812
Short Musculoskeletal Functional Assessment (SMFA) scores 944
Short radiolunate (SRL) ligament 70, 70f
SIGN nail *see* Surgical Implant Generation Network (SIGN) nail
Skin tenting, distal tibia fractures 895f
SLL *see* Scapholunate ligament (SLL)
Sloppy lateral position 311, 312f, 316
SMFA scores *see* Short Musculoskeletal Functional Assessment (SMFA) scores
Smith-Peterson incision 593 *see also* Femoral head fractures and hip dislocations
SNAC *see* Scaphoid nonunion advanced collapse (SNAC)
Space available for cord (SAC) 389t
Space of Poirier 70
Spinal fractures *see* Cervical spine injuries
Spinal shock 382
Spine evaluation, in trauma patients 394
 Canadian C-spine rules 394f
 clinical clearance 394
 conscious, symptomatic patients 394–395

SPN *see* Superficial peroneal nerve (SPN)
Steinmann pin 658
Sternoclavicular (SC) joint 360, 360*f*
Stiffness
  elbow 242, 267
  metacarpal fractures 50–51
  olecranon fractures 215
  phalangeal fractures 24, 26–27, 26*f*
Stimson gravity technique 587 *see also* Femoral head fractures and hip dislocations
Subaxial cervical fractures 401, 405–406 *see also* Cervical spine injuries
  compressive extension injuries 411–413, 413*f*
  compressive flexion injuries 407–408, 408*f*
  distractive extension injuries 414–415, 414*f*, 415*f*
  distractive flexion injury 408–411, 409*f*–412*f*
  lateral extension injuries 415–416, 416*f*
  vertical compression injuries 406–407, 406*f*, 407*f*
Subscapularis split technique 342–343
Subscapularis tenotomy technique 343
Subtalar fusion, talus fractures 975–976
Subtalar joint, Brodén's views 967*f*
Subtrochanteric femur fractures 672–673
  case study
    intertrochanteric femur fracture 698–701, 699*f*, 700*f*
    pertrochanteric femur fracture 701, 702*f*, 703*f*
    proximal femur locking plate 703–706, 704*f*, 705*f*
  classification
    AO/OTA 675, 676*f*
    Russell-Taylor 674–675, 675*f*
    Seinsheimer's 673–674, 674*f*
  complications and management
    DVT 695
    loss of fixation and malunion 695–696, 696*f*
    malrotation 697–698
    nonunion 696–697
  diagnosis
    bone scan 673
    CT scan 673
    diagnostic imaging 673
    MRI 673
    pearls and pitfalls 673
    physical examination 673
  occurrence 673
  outcomes 694–695
  surgical management 678–679
    anatomy 677, 678*f*
    95° angled plates 679
    blade plate 691–694, 692*f*, 693*f*
    CAS 683
    cephalomedullary nailing 684–689, 685*f*–688*f*
    clinical assessment 683
    CT scan 683, 683*f*
    definitive fixation 677
    fluoroscopic measurement 680
    intramedullary nails 679
    intraoperative assessment 683–684
    lesser trochanteric profile 680–681
    positioning 677–678
    postoperative protocol 694
    preoperative planning 679–680
    proximal femoral locking plate 679, 689–691, 690*f*
    reconstruction nails 679
    reduction technique 680, 681*f*, 682*f*
    temporizing measures 675–677
    trochanteric nails 679
Superficial peroneal nerve (SPN) 934
Supra-acetabular pin 501, 502*f*, 506*f*, 507*f* *see also* Pelvic ring and sacral injuries
Supraclavicular nerves 365, 365*f*
Supracondylar femur fractures 737
Suprascapular nerve, injury to 354
Surgical Implant Generation Network (SIGN) nail 850
Suture placement, proximal humerus fractures 324, 325*f*
Swimmer's view 389, 391*f*, 393*f*
Syndesmotic injury, ankle
  anatomy 934–935
  cotton test 932*f*, 938, 940
  late 946
  occult, diagnosis 929*f*
  open reduction and internal fixation 942–944
    preoperative planning 942–943
    technique 943–944
  repair 943*f*
Synostosis, forearm fractures 186, 187*f*, 188–190, 189*f*, 190*f*

T

TAD *see* Tip-apex distance (TAD)
Talar neck fractures *see also* Talus fractures
  anterolateral approach 971–972
  anteromedial approach 970–971
  Bohler's incision 971*f*
  Hawkins classification 967–968, 968*f*
  medial vascular structures 970*f*
  ORIF comminuted, displaced 973*f*–974*f*
  treatment 969
Talus fractures 966–981 *see also* Calcaneus fractures
  arthritis 975–977
  avascular necrosis 972–975
  chronic infection management 977
  classification 967–968
  malunion 975
  subtalar fusion 975–976
  surgery
    anatomy 969–970
    positioning 970
  tibiotalocalcaneal fusion 976–977
Tarsometatarsal (TMT) joints 983–984
  first-third 1001*f*, 1002*f*
  incongruity 987–988

irreparable cartilage 1001
midfoot fusion 991
Taylor Spatial Frame 758
Tension band technique, in patellar fractures *see also* Patellar fractures
closure 773
fracture reduction techniques 771–773, 772*f*–775*f*
instrumentation and implant consideration 771
pearls and pitfalls 773
rehabilitation 773
surgical approach 771
Terrible triad injuries 224, 226*f*, 227 *see also* Radial head fractures
Terry Thomas sign 55, 57*f*
Tetraplegia 386
TFCC *see* Triangular fibrocartilage complex (TFCC)
Thomas and Epstein classification 585, 587*t* *see also* Femoral head fractures and hip dislocations
Thompson approach, forearm fractures 173, 174*f*
Thompson quadricepsplasty 757
Thoracic and lumbar spine fractures 447–448
burst fracture 448*f*
burst fractures 457–459, 458*f*, 459*f*
case study
failure to recognize fracture patterns 488–489
implant failure 488
missed systemic injury 489, 490*f*
post-traumatic kyphosis 485–487, 486*f*, 487*f*
Chance fracture. 461*f*
classification 448
Allen-Ferguson 450
AO 451–452, 451*f*
Boehler's 448
column concept 449
Denis 449–450, 449*f*
load sharing 452
McAfee's 450–451, 450*f*
TLICS 452, 452*f*, 453*f*
complications
anterior approach 484–485
chronic 485
posterior approach 483–484
compression fractures 455–457, 457*f*
diagnosis 453
CT scans 455, 455*f*, 458*f*, 459, 461*f*
MRI 455, 456*f*, 459–460
radiographic evaluation 454–455, 454*f*, 454*t*, 457*f*, 458*f*, 460*f*
flexion distraction injury 448*f*, 459–461, 459*t*, 460*f*, 463–464
fracture dislocation 448*f*, 462, 464*f*
surgical management
anterior decompression and fixation 471–476, 474*f*, 475*f*
indications for 462–465
kyphoplasty 468, 469*f*, 470*f*
outcomes 481–483
percutaneous pedicle screw fixation 468–471, 470*f*, 471
percutaneous stabilization 466–471
percutaneous vertebroplasty (VP) 465–468, 465*f*, 466*f*, 467*f*
posterior decompression and fixation 476–481, 477*f*–480*f*
unstable thoracolumbar injuries 459–462, 460*f*, 461*f*
wedge compression fractures 448*f*
Thoracic outlet syndrome 360, 374
Thoracolumbar fractures 448 *see also* Thoracic and lumbar spine fractures
concept of instability 442–453
Thoracolumbar injury classification system (TLICS) 449, 452, 452*f*, 453*f*
Thoracolumbar junction 448
Thoracolumbar sacral orthosis (TLSO) 462
Thumb epibasal fractures 34, 34*f* *see also* Metacarpal fractures
Tibia 845
anteromedial aspect 848
nonunion of 871
aseptic, atrophic, treatment 882–883, 884*f*–85*f*
established infected, treatment 876–880, 887*f*–879*f*
hypertrophic, treatment 883–886, 886*f*
Tibial bone loss, acute
massive autogenous bone grafting 886–887, 888*f*–890*f*
Tibial shaft fractures 845–893
classification 846–848
AO-OTA 846–847
Gustilo and Anderson 847
Tscherne 847–848
compartment syndrome 846, 872
treatment of 887–893, 891*f*–892*f*
complications 871–872
infection 871
malalignment and malunion 871–872
management 872–893
nonunion of tibia 871
crush injury 846
diagnostic imaging techniques 846
guidewire placement 854, 855*f*
instrumentation and implant 849–850
intramedullary nailing 849–871
acute infection treatment 873*f*–875*f*
patient assessment 850
portal preparation 852*f*
preoperative planning 849–850
reamed, locked 849–858
technique 850–858
ORIF 868*f*
outcomes, treatment 871
overview 845–846
physical examination 846
positioning 848
proximal 858–863
proximal interlocking 854
surgery 848–871
anatomy 848–849
techniques 849–871
traction 848–849

Tibiotalocalcaneal (TTC) fusion
  calcaneus fractures 966
  talus fractures 976–977
Tip-apex distance (TAD) 659
TMT arthritis, surgical approach 992–993
TMT joints *see* Tarsometatarsal (TMT) joints
Total hip arthroplasty 642
Traction pin placement
  femoral shaft fractures 723
  pearls and pitfalls 723
Traction, tibial shaft fractures 848–849
Transarticular plate fixation
  lateral clavicle 364*f*, 369, 371*f*
Trans-flexor carpi radialis (trans-FCR) approach, volar distal radius 146–148, 147*f*
Transiliac-transsacral screws 535–536, 536*f*–538*f*
Translational injuries, spine 451
Transolecranon fracture-dislocations 193
Transverse dislocations 61, 68–69, 68*f*
Trapezial fractures 59 *see also* Carpal fractures and perilunate dislocations
Traumatic spondylolisthesis of C2 *see* Hangman's fracture
Triangular fibrocartilage complex (TFCC) 133, 181
Triceps-sparing approach, distal humerus 256, 256*f*
Tricortical iliac crest 976
Triquetral fractures 59, 59*f*, 60*f*, 67 *see also* Carpal fractures and perilunate dislocations
Trochanteric flip osteotomy 598–600, 599*f*
Trochanteric nails 662
  subtrochanteric femur fractures 679
Tscherne classification
  soft tissue injury, closed fractures 897*f*
  tibial shaft fractures 847–848
TTC fusion *see* Tibiotalocalcaneal (TTC) fusion

U

Ulna 168, 168*f*
Ulnar nerve 71, 172, 173, 201, 232
Ulnar neuropathy
  distal humerus fractures 268
  olecranon fractures 217
Ulnar shaft fractures 169*f*, 170 *see also* Forearm fractures
  fixation 173–175, 173*f*, 175*f*, 176*f*
  isolated 170
  surgical indications 171
Ulnocarpal ligaments 70, 70*f*
Ulnohumeral joint 229
Ultrasound, phalangeal fractures 2
Unicondylar fractures 751–753 *see also* Distal femur fractures
  pearls and pitfalls 753

V

Varencline 835
Vascularized bone graft (VBG) 101, 111, 113–114, 118, 118*f*
Vertebroplasty 465–468, 465*f*, 466*f*, 467*f*
Volar intercalated segment instability (VISI) 85
Volar locking plates 142, 142*f*, 161
Volar plate arthroplasty 19, 19*f*
Volar plate fixation
  distal radius fractures 141*f*, 142, 142*f*, 145*f*, 154–157, 155*f*, 156*f*, 159
    and malpositioning of screws 159–162, 160*f*, 161*f*

W

Wackenheim line 389*t*, 393*f*
Watson-Jones anterolateral approach 642
Watson-Jones incision 593 *see also* Femoral head fractures and hip dislocations
WBC *see* White blood cell (WBC)
Weber clamp application, anterior pelvic fixation 511, 512*f*
Wedge compression fractures 407–408, 448*f*, 450, 455–457, 457*f* *see also* Thoracic and lumbar spine fractures
  diagnosis 455, 457, 457*f*
  surgical management 462
Well-leg compartment syndrome 625
White blood cell (WBC) 831
Winquist-Hansen classification, femoral shaft fractures 710, 711*f*
Wounds
  breakdown, ankle fractures 945
  midfoot and forefoot fractures 1012

X

X-rays *see also* Radiographs
  distal femur fractures 738, 739*f*
  femoral head fractures and hip dislocations 582

Contemporary Surgical Management of Fractures and Complications

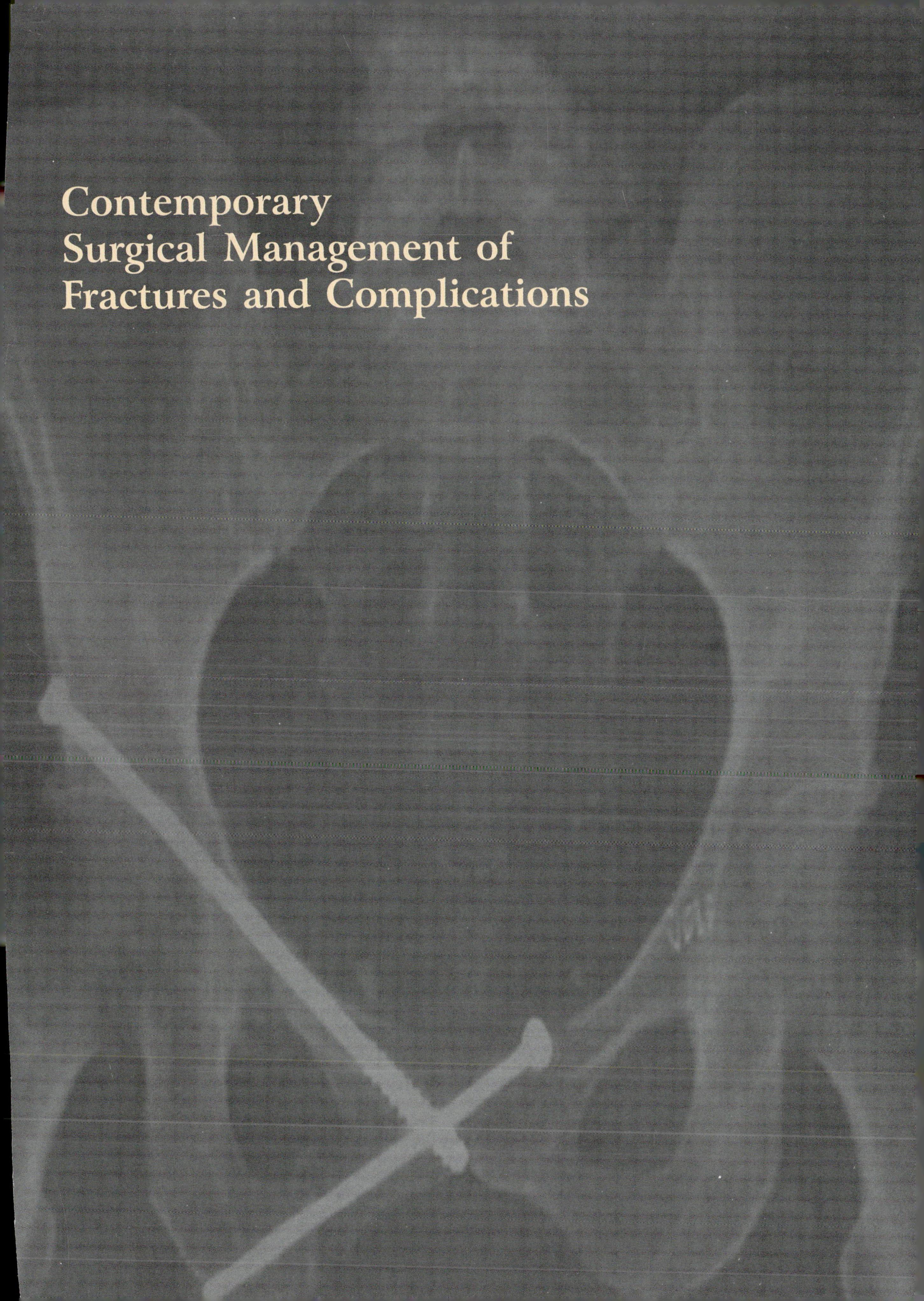

Volume 2: Pelvis and Lower Extremity

Contemporary Surgical Management of Fractures and Complications

Editors

ASIF ILYAS MD
Program Director of Hand and Upper Extremity Surgery Fellowship
Rothman Institute
Associate Professor of Orthopaedic Surgery
Thomas Jefferson University
Philadelphia, Pennsylvania, USA

SAQIB REHMAN MD
Director of Orthopaedic Trauma
Temple University Hospital
Associate Professor of Orthopaedic Surgery
Temple University
Philadelphia, Pennsylvania, USA

Foreword

JESSE B JUPITER MD

JAYPEE BROTHERS MEDICAL PUBLISHERS (P) LTD

New Delhi • Panama City • London • Philadelphia (USA)

Jaypee Brothers Medical Publishers (P) Ltd

Headquarters

Jaypee Brothers Medical Publishers (P) Ltd
4838/24, Ansari Road, Daryaganj
New Delhi 110 002, India
Phone: +91-11-43574357
Fax: +91-11-43574314
Email: jaypee@jaypeebrothers.com

Overseas Offices

JP Medical Ltd
83 Victoria Street, London
SW1H 0HW (UK)
Phone: +44-2031708910
Fax: +02-03-0086180
Email: info@jpmedpub.com

Jaypee-Highlights Medical Publishers Inc
City of Knowledge, Bld 237, Clayton
Panama City, Panama
Phone: +507-301-0496
Fax: +507-301-0499
Email: cservice@jphmedical.com

Jaypee Brothers Medical Publishers (P) Ltd
17/1-B Babar Road, Block-B, Shaymali
Mohammadpur, Dhaka-1207
Bangladesh
Mobile: +08801912003485
Email: jaypeedhaka@gmail.com

Jaypee Brothers Medical Publishers (P) Ltd
Shorakhute, Kathmandu
Nepal
Phone: +00977-9841528578
Email: jaypee.nepal@gmail.com

Website: www.jaypeebrothers.com
Website: www.jaypeedigital.com

Inquiries for bulk sales may be solicited at: jaypee@jaypeebrothers.com

Contemporary Surgical Management of Fractures and Complications

First Edition : **2013**

ISBN: 978-93-5025-964-1

Printed at: Ajanta Offset & Packagings Ltd., New Delhi

Dedicated to

My wife Erum and my children Dean, Amber and Sammy
for their inspiration to excel and their patience
with my ever-growing commitments.
My parents Qazi and Sajda Ilyas for their
commitment to my education and perfect guidance
through my personal and professional development.
And lastly, to my fellows and residents for continually challenging me
to better myself as a clinician and educator.

Asif Ilyas

The residents and fellows whom I have had the privilege to work with;
My mentors Drs William DeLong and Christopher Born as well as
the many other surgeons whom I have learned so much from;
My brother Asim, my wife Saadia, and
my children, Omar, Laila and Sofia for their support;
Omar, in particular, for reminding me that there is far more to life than work.
Most importantly, to my parents, Khalid and Sabeeha Rehman,
for being true role models and paving the way to help me achieve
my goals and aspirations.

Saqib Rehman

Contributors

Jamal Ahmad MD
Assistant Professor of
Orthopaedic Surgery
Thomas Jefferson University Hospital
Rothman Institute
Philadelphia, Pennsylvania, USA

Andrea Bauer MD
Orthopaedic Surgery Fellow
Massachusetts General Hospital
Boston, Massachusetts, USA

Stephen Becher MD
Orthopaedic Surgery Resident
Atlanta Medical Center
Atlanta, Georgia, USA

Pedro Beredjiklian MD
Chief, Hand Surgery Service
Rothman Institute
Associate Professor of
Orthopaedic Surgery
Thomas Jefferson University
Philadelphia, PA, USA

Christopher Born MD
Chief of Orthopaedic Trauma and
Director of the Weiss
Laboratory for
Orthopaedic Trauma Research
Rhode Island Hospital
Intrepid Heroes Professor of
Orthopaedic Surgery
The Apert Medical School of
Brown University
Providence, Rhode Island, USA

Wendy Bruinsma MD
Orthopaedic Surgery Fellow
Massachusetts General Hospital
Boston, Massachusetts, USA

Neal Chen MD
Assistant Professor of
Orthopaedic Surgery
Thomas Jefferson University
Philadelphia Hand Center
Philadelphia, Pennsylvania, USA

Peter Cole MD
Chief of Orthopaedic Surgery
Regions Hospital
Professor of Orthopaedic Surgery
University of Minnesota
St Paul, Minnesota, USA

Katharine Criner MD
Orthopaedic Surgery Resident
Temple University
Philadelphia, Pennsylvania, USA

William DeLong MD
Chief of Orthopaedic Surgery
St Luke's Health Network
Professor of Orthopaedic Surgery
Anatomy and Cell Biology
Temple University
Philadelphia, Pennsylvania, USA

River Elliott MD
Plastic Surgery Resident
University of the Pennsylvania
Philadelphia, Pennsylvania, USA

Christina Endress MD
Orthopaedic Surgery Resident
University of the Pennsylvania
Philadelphia, Pennsylvania, USA

Ryan Ficco MD
Orthopaedic Surgery Resident
University of Miami
Miami, Florida, USA

Abtin Foroohar MD
Orthopaedic Surgery Fellow
University of the Pennsylvania
Philadelphia, Pennsylvania, USA

John Fowler MD
Orthopaedic Surgery Resident
Temple University
Philadelphia, Pennsylvania, USA

Matthew Frank MD
Orthopaedic Surgery Resident
New Jersey Medical School
Newark, New Jersey, USA

Elie Ghanem MD
Orthopaedic Surgery Resident
Thomas Jefferson University
Philadelphia, Pennsylvania, USA

Melissa Gorman MD
Assistant Professor of
Orthopaedic Surgery
Louisiana State University
Health Science Center
New Orleans, Louisiana, USA

Steven Gross MD
Orthopaedic Surgery Resident
NYU-Hospital for Joint Diseases
New York, New York, USA

Christopher Haydel MD
Orthopaedic Trauma Fellow
Temple University Hospital
Philadelphia, Pennsylvania, USA

David Helfet MD
Director of Orthopaedic Trauma
Hospital for Special Surgery
Professor of Orthopaedic Surgery
Weill Medical College of Cornell
University
New York, New York, USA

Zhiyong Hou MD
Orthopaedic Research Fellow
Geisinger Medical Center
Danville, Pennsylvania, USA

Asif Ilyas MD
Program Director of Hand and Upper Extremity Surgery Fellowship
Rothman Institute
Associate Professor of Orthopaedic Surgery
Thomas Jefferson University
Philadelphia, Pennsylvania, USA

Kaan Irgit MD
Orthopaedic Research Fellow
Geisinger Medical Center
Danville, Pennsylvania, USA

Roman Isaac MD
Orthopaedic Surgery Resident
Thomas Jefferson University
Philadelphia, Pennsylvania, USA

Andrew Jawa MD
Assistant Professor of Orthopaedic Surgery
Boston University
Boston, Massachusetts, USA

Jesse Jupiter MD
Hansjorg Wyss/AO Professor of Orthopaedic Surgery
Harvard Medical School
Massachusetts General Hospital
Boston, Massachusetts, USA

Rishi Kanna MS
Consultant Spine Surgeon
Ganga Hospital
Coimbatore, Tamil Nadu, India

Stephen Kayiaros MD
Orthopaedic Trauma Fellow
Rhode Island Hospital
Providence, Rhode Island, USA

Emily Keener DO
Orthopaedic Surgery Resident
University of Medicine and Dentistry of New Jersey
Stratford, New Jersey, USA

Sanjit Konda MD
Orthopaedic Surgery Resident
NYU-Hospital for Joint Diseases
New York, USA

Stephen Kottmeier MD
Chief of Orthopaedic Trauma and Associate Chairman
Associate Professor of Orthopaedic Surgery
Stony Brook University Hospital
Stony Brook, New York, USA

Peter Krause MD
Director of Orthopaedic Trauma
Louisiana State University Public Hospital
Associate Professor of Orthopaedic Surgery and Residency Director
Louisiana State University Health Science Center
New Orleans, Louisiana, USA

Paul Lafferty MD
Assistant Professor of Orthopaedic Surgery
University of Minnesota
St Paul, Minnesota, USA

Charles Leinberry MD
Associate Professor of Orthopaedic Surgery
Thomas Jefferson University
Philadelphia, Pennsylvania, USA

Frank Liporace MD
Associate Professor of Orthopaedic Surgery
New Jersey Medical School
Newark, New Jersey, USA

Dean Lorich MD
Associate Director of Orthopaedic Trauma
Hospital for Special Surgery
Assistant Professor of Orthopaedic Surgery
Weill Medical College of Cornell University, New York, USA

Neil MacIntyre MD
Director of Orthopaedic Trauma
New Hannover Regional Medical Center
Wilmington, North Carolina, USA

Megan Manthe MD
Orthopaedic Surgery Resident
University of Florida, Shands
Jacksonville, Florida, USA

Jonas Matzon MD
Assistant Professor of Orthopaedic Surgery
Thomas Jefferson University
Philadelphia, Pennsylvania, USA

Matthew Mellon MD
Director of Orthopaedic Trauma
Total Orthopaedics and Sports Medicine
Massapequa, New York, USA

Matthew Mendez-Zfass MD
Orthopaedic Surgery Resident
University of Miami
Miami, Florida, USA

Chaitanya Mudgal MD
Interim Chief and Program Director of Orthopaedic Hand Service
Massachusetts General Hospital
Assistant Professor of Orthopaedic Surgery
Harvard Medical School
Boston, Massachusetts, USA

Valentin Neuhaus MD
Orthopaedic Surgery Research Fellow
Massachusetts General Hospital
Boston, Massachusetts, USA

Meredith Osterman MD
Orthopaedic Surgery Resident
Thomas Jefferson University
Philadelphia, Pennsylvania, USA

Frank Peters MD
Orthopaedic Surgery Fellow
Massachusetts General Hospital
Boston, Massachusetts, USA

Samuel Popinchalk MD
Orthopaedic Surgery Resident
Temple University
Philadelphia, Pennsylvania, USA

S Rajasekaran PhD
Chairman of Orthopaedic and
Spine Surgery, Ganga Hospital
Adjunct Professor of
Orthopaedic Surgery
Tamil Nadu Medical University
Coimbatore, Tamil Nadu, India

Saqib Rehman MD
Director of Orthopaedic Trauma
Temple University Hospital
Associate Professor of
Orthopaedic Surgery
Temple University
Philadelphia, Pennsylvania, USA

J Spence Reid MD
Chief, Division of Orthopaedic Trauma
Milton S Hershey Medical Center
Professor of Orthopaedic Surgery
Penn State University College of
Medicine
Hershey, Pennsylvania, USA

Michael Rivlin MD
Orthopaedic Surgery Resident
Thomas Jefferson University
Philadelphia, Pennsylvania, USA

ML Chip Routt Jr MD
Professor of Orthopaedic Surgery
University of Washington
Harborview Medical Center
Seattle, Washington, USA

Ajoy Prasad Shetty MS
Consultant Spine Surgeon
Ganga Hospital
Coimbatore, Tamil Nadu, India

Wade Smith MD
Professor of Orthopaedic Surgery
University of Colorado
Mountain Orthopaedic Trauma
Surgeons
Englewood, Colorado, USA

Dean Sotereanos MD
Professor of Orthopaedic Surgery
Drexel University College of Medicine
Allegheny General Hospital
Pittsburgh, Pennsylvania, USA

Brandon Steen MD
Orthopaedic Surgery Resident
Boston University
Boston, Massachusetts, USA

David Steinberg MD
Program Director of Hand
Upper Extremity and Microsurgery
Associate Professor of
Orthopaedic Surgery
University of the Pennsylvania
Philadelphia, Pennsylvania, USA

Michael Suk MD JD MPH FACS
Chairman, Department of
Orthopaedic Surgery
Geisinger Health System
Danville, Pennsylvania, USA

Nirmal Tejwani MD
Associate Director and Chief of
Orthopaedic Service
Bellevue Hospital
Professor of Orthopaedic Surgery
New York University Langone
Medical Center, New York, USA

Joseph Thoder MD
Chairman, Department of
Orthopaedic Surgery
Professor of Orthopaedic Surgery
Temple University
Philadelphia, Pennsylvania, USA

Richard Tosti MD
Orthopaedic Surgery Resident
Temple University
Philadelphia, Pennsylvania, USA

Uzoma Ukomadu MD
Orthopaedic Surgery Resident
Thomas Jefferson University
Philadelphia, Pennsylvania, USA

Aaron Venouziou MD
Orthopaedic Surgery Fellow
Allegheny General Hospital
Pittsburgh, Pennsylvania, USA

Fernando Vilella-Hernandez MD
Assistant Professor of
Orthopaedic Surgery
University of Miami
Jackson Memorial Hospital
Miami, Florida, USA

Barton Wax MD
Orthopaedic Surgery Resident
Louisiana State University Health
Science Center
New Orleans, Louisiana, USA

David Wellman MD
Instructor of Orthopaedic Surgery
Weill Medical College of Cornell
University, Hospital for Special
Surgery, New York, USA

Bruce Ziran MD
Director of Orthopaedic Trauma
Atlanta Medical Center
Atlanta, Georgia, USA

Foreword

It is a pleasure and honor to be asked by Dr Ilyas and Dr Rehman to write a foreword to their new fracture textbook. This is not just because I have had the true joy of seeing the growth in the academic career of Dr Ilyas since completing our Hand and Upper Limb Fellowship but also because that this is a text whose purpose is clearly defined and well achieved.

This is a twenty-first century text focusing less on historical highlights, background principles, and alternative treatments to internal fixation that formed the basis of what was considered standard formats for fracture texts in the past. Rather, the editors have decided to create a text that the practicing surgeon can have at his/her fingertips when faced with a clinical fracture problem. Accordingly, the reader will find a consistent format in each chapter emphasizing the surgical approaches, techniques of specific fracture fixation, as well as practical tips and "pitfalls". Complications and their management are to be found in each chapter. The chapters are well illustrated sprinkled throughout with excellent clinical examples.

What I found to be strength of this text is the list of contributing authors. While located throughout are the "usual suspects", the vast majority of contributors represent the "rising stars" of the next generation of thought leaders and fracture surgeons.

We are in the era of instant information, which will now be found in a variety of modalities from multiple websites, web-based how-to videos, industry educational sites or easy access journals. So too will the surgeon treating fractures find ready access to specific questions and techniques in *Contemporary Surgical Management of Fractures and Complications*.

Jesse B Jupiter MD
Hansjorg Wyss/AO Professor of Orthopaedic Surgery
Harvard Medical School
Massachusetts General Hospital
Boston, Massachusetts, USA

Preface

"The surgeon who has not had a complication has not done enough surgery."

We have all heard this quote at some point in our training or practice. Complications in fracture management are unfortunately a common occurrence. There are many reasons for the association of fractures with complications.

Patients can present at unpredictable times of the day, requiring urgent surgery by a surgeon who may be inexperienced in the necessary fracture management. Fracture surgery frequently utilizes bacteria-harboring implants which are placed in damaged soft tissue beds potentially inviting infections. Also, modern fracture management has witnessed a significant growth of new implants and biologics which are often quickly applied before their indications are well defined. Furthermore, there still exist significant deficits in our understanding of fracture healing. Why some fractures heal while others do not continue to elude us. And sometimes, the problem lies with the patient and subsequent lack of compliance with the prescribed postoperative regimen.

There are many outstanding textbooks which go to great lengths to describe proper techniques of fracture management. Nevertheless, complications will happen and correcting them can represent a significant challenge. Despite all the excellent references available to orthopaedic surgeons, it became apparent to us that there are few modern texts that actually focus on the management of complications at length. When we came together to discuss our aspirations and goals of this book, this deficit in our literature quickly came to the forefront.

What we have therefore set out to do was to present a concise, practical text for the orthopaedic surgeon who manages fractures on a regular or occasional basis. The goals of this book are to clearly describe the indications for surgery, provide appropriate surgical techniques, present tips for achieving good results, and offer an extensive case-based discussion on how to manage select complications. Whereas many other texts have given a more exhaustive review of the historical literature as well as basic principles of fracture management (including nonoperative management), we have chosen to go directly to the surgical management of fractures and their complications. Of course, this is not to downplay the importance of the basic principles of nonoperative fracture care or to imply all fractures be treated operatively. As such, this text should not be viewed as a comprehensive textbook of fracture management, but rather a practical and thorough text for the orthopaedic surgeon managing a fracture operatively and/or its complication.

This textbook contains several highlights. We have included focused "pearls and pitfalls" sections to allow the author to share important practical points on various surgical techniques with the reader. To this end, we have also tried to make generous use of figures and images to help illustrate the key concepts in each chapter. The section on "Author's preferred management of select complications" is what we feel is the most unique and important part of this textbook. Here we have included actual cases with complications such as nonunions, malunions and infections managed by the chapter contributors.

We sincerely hope that this textbook will be a useful addition to your library and that you will use it for years to come. Incurring a fracture is a significant event for a patient. Experiencing a subsequent complication from fracture management can further compromise a patient's outcome. As orthopaedic surgeons, it is our job not only to avoid these complications, but also to know how to effectively navigate through them when they occur. If this book helps you in this effort, then we have succeeded in our mission.

SAQIB REHMAN

ASIF ILYAS

Acknowledgments

First and foremost, this book would clearly not be possible without the generous contributions by an outstanding group of surgeons who authored the chapters. To these authors, we are sincerely grateful and appreciative of their efforts and for sharing their expertise with our readers. We have clearly learned much from them in the process of editing this text.

What would we be without our mentors who helped us start and mold our careers, showing us how to properly manage fractures, and most importantly, reminding us to "do the right thing" for our patients?

Although we consider ourselves educators, we have been fortunate to be surrounded by exemplary colleagues, residents and fellows who educate us on a daily basis through our exchanges, collaborations and daily clinical care. For this, and for their support with this project, we thank them.

We would also like to thank the wonderful people at Jaypee Brothers Medical Publishers (P) Ltd, New Delhi, India for their support throughout this process and particularly for letting us see our vision come to fruition.

Finally, it goes without saying that a project like this could not happen without the support of our wives and families. We sincerely thank them for their patience, understanding and encouragement throughout this process.

Contents

Volume 1: Upper Extremity and Spine
Asif Ilyas

1. **Phalangeal Fractures** 1
Jonas Matzon, Elie Ghanem, Pedro Beredjiklian

2. **Metacarpal Fractures and Carpometacarpal Fracture-Dislocations** 30
Charles Leinberry, Uzoma Ukomadu, Asif Ilyas

3. **Carpal Fractures and Perilunate Dislocations** 53
Valentin Neuhaus, Andrea Bauer, Chaitanya Mudgal

4. **Scaphoid Fractures** 94
Aaron Venouziou, Dean Sotereanos

5. **Distal Radius Fractures** 128
Wendy Bruinsma, Frank Peters, Jesse Jupiter

6. **Forearm Fractures** 167
Abtin Foroohar, River Elliott, Christina Endress, David Steinberg

7. **Olecranon Fractures** 192
Brandon Steen, Andrew Jawa

8. **Radial Head Fractures and Terrible Triad Injuries** 223
John Fowler, Joseph Thoder

9. **Distal Humerus Fractures** 249
Asif Ilyas, Saqib Rehman

10. **Humeral Shaft Fractures** 276
Richard Tosti, Asif Ilyas

11. **Proximal Humerus Fractures** 302
David Wellman, Dean Lorich, David Helfet

12. **Glenoid and Scapula Fractures** 334
Samuel Popinchalk, Neil MacIntyre

13. **Clavicle Fractures** 358
Roman Isaac, Meredith Osterman, Michael Rivlin, Neal Chen

14. **Cervical Spine Fractures and Dislocations** 378
S Rajasekaran, Rishi Kanna, Ajoy Prasad Shetty

15. **Thoracic and Lumbar Spine Fractures and Dislocations** 447
S Rajasekaran, Rishi Kanna, Ajoy Prasad Shetty

Volume 2: Pelvis and Lower Extremity

Saqib Rehman

16.	**Pelvic Ring and Sacral Injuries** *Stephen Kottmeier, ML Chip Routt Jr*	495
17.	**Acetabulum Fractures** *Bruce Ziran, Stephen Becher*	552
18.	**Femoral Head Fractures and Hip Dislocations** *Kaan Irgit, Zhiyong Hou, Wade Smith*	581
19.	**Femoral Neck Fractures** *Christopher Haydel, Saqib Rehman*	611
20.	**Intertrochanteric Femur Fractures** *Stephen Kayiaros, Christopher Born*	654
21.	**Subtrochanteric Femur Fractures** *Paul Lafferty, Emily Keener, Peter Cole*	672
22.	**Femoral Shaft Fractures** *Matthew Mendez-Zfass, Ryan Ficco, Fernando Vilella-Hernandez*	708
23.	**Distal Femur Fractures** *Matthew Mellon, William DeLong, Saqib Rehman*	737
24.	**Patellar Fractures** *Peter Krause, Melissa Gorman, Barton Wax*	766
25.	**Proximal Tibia Fractures** *J Spence Reid*	785
26.	**Tibial Shaft Fractures** *Saqib Rehman, Katharine Criner*	845
27.	**Distal Tibia Fractures** *Michael Suk, Megan Manthe, Saqib Rehman*	894
28.	**Ankle Fractures and Syndesmotic Injuries** *Nirmal Tejwani, Sanjit Konda, Steven Gross*	926
29.	**Hindfoot Fractures** *Frank Liporace, Matthew Frank*	953
30.	**Midfoot and Forefoot Fractures** *Jamal Ahmad*	983
	Index	*I-i-xx*

Chapter 16

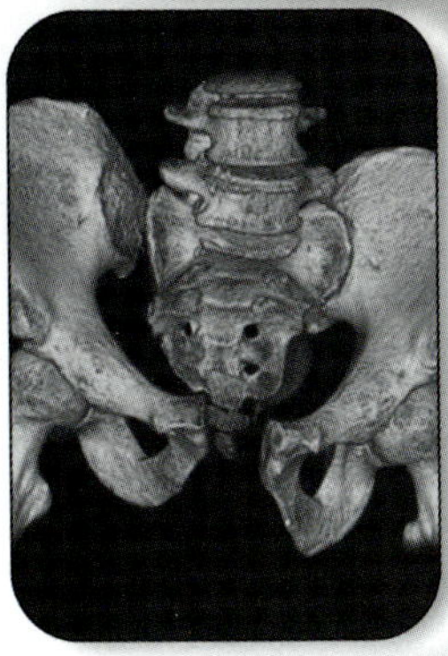

Pelvic Ring and Sacral Injuries

Stephen Kottmeier, ML Chip Routt Jr

Chapter Outline

Introduction
Diagnosis
Classification
Surgical Indications
Surgical Anatomy, Positioning and Approaches
Surgical Techniques
- Technique 1: External Fixation of the Pelvis
- Technique 2: Anterior Pelvic Fixation
- Technique 3: Iliosacral Screw Insertion

Authors' Preferred Management of Select Complications
- Case 1: Malreduction of Sacroiliac Joint Fracture Dislocation with Iliosacral Screws
- Case 2: Errant Placement of Anterior External Fixation Pins
- Case 3. Nonunion of Nondisplaced Pelvic Ring Fractures Treated with Percutaneous Compression Screws
- Case 4: Symptomatic Pelvic Nonunion after Routine External Fixation Treated with Anterior and Posterior Fixation

Summary

Introduction

The pelvis provides structural continuity between the axial skeleton and lower extremities. It affords protection and passage for genitourinary, gastrointestinal and neurovascular structures. Traumatic disruptions of the pelvic ring may be of soft tissue, osseous or combined origins. They may result from mechanisms of high energy and low energy. Elderly patients often present with concerning medical comorbidities while younger patients may have associated closed cavity, extremity and spinal injuries.

Acute pelvic ring disruption may precipitate life-threatening intrapelvic and retroperitoneal hemorrhage.[1,2] Pelvic stabilization secures bleeding cancellous fracture surfaces while decreasing available intrapelvic volume. Numerous methods, both invasive and noninvasive, afford satisfactory pelvic ring stabilization for purposes of acute life support and initial patient mobilization.[3] Intravenous fluid resuscitation, coagulopathy correction, mechanical pelvic stabilization and selective pelvic angiography are critical components toward efficacious patient resuscitation.[4]

Pelvic instability may be multiplanar and of varying degrees of severity. Its immediate impact and long-term consequences are not always appreciated during the course of treatment. Parameters of "acceptable" displacement and operative reduction are not firmly established. Closed or open reduction combined with internal fixation may facilitate patient mobilization offering stability and preventing deformity and functional consequences. Unstable pelvis fractures can be addressed with numerous surgical fixation options. Posterior pelvic ring injuries result in a wide spectrum of severity and instability of both osseous and ligamentous origins. Operative treatment can be complicated by fracture displacement and comminution, soft tissue and neurovascular compromise. Percutaneous and minimally invasive techniques continue to evolve. These contemporary fixation methods demand a thorough understanding of pelvic osteology, appreciation of soft tissue anatomy, pathoanatomy and "normal" anatomic variants.

Diagnosis

Diagnosis of pelvic injury begins with an adequate history and physical examination. The history in terms of mechanism of injury offers insight into the energy of injury sustained. Force application and magnitude dictate pelvic injury type and instability patterns in addition to type and frequency of associated injuries. Life-threatening massive hemorrhage, a complication of pelvic injury can be of arterial, venous plexus or fracture surface origins. The patient's age may impact both on physiologic reserve and bone quality. This dictates the hemodynamic response and energy required to generate certain osseous injury patterns. Pelvic ring disruption may be accompanied by concerning injuries to organs, vessels and nerves within the pelvis in addition to closed cavity lesions of the head, thorax and abdomen. Adherence to principles of resuscitation is of paramount importance followed by primary and secondary systemic and skeletal surveys.

Clinical evaluation includes observation for peripelvic soft tissue abrasions, contusions and closed soft tissue degloving injuries (Morel-Lavallee lesion) (Fig. 16.1A).[5] Lower extremity limb length inequality and malrotation deformities must be appreciated and origins discerned (Fig. 16.1B). Palpation and manual testing for pelvic instability may be pursued with caution. Open fracture variants or those with rectal or vaginal continuity must be identified and managed appropriately and expeditiously as they are associated with increased sepsis and mortality rate (Fig. 16.1C). The genitourinary region is inspected for regional hemorrhage. This implies a urethral tear in a male and a vaginal tear in a female. Lumboplexopathy may present in combination with sacral spinal canal or foraminal fractures.[6] Neurologic deficits must be identified and recorded during the course of evaluation and treatment.

Diagnostic imaging commences with an anteroposterior (AP) radiograph of the pelvis. This offers a static assessment of the pelvis. Both stability and instability can be implied radiographically but neither can be confirmed. In an unstable patient, the AP radiographic alone may be sufficient to initiate treatment (Fig. 16.2A). The pelvic radiographic "triad" consists of pelvic inlet and outlet views in combination with the AP radiograph. Axial and rotational displacements are best depicted on the inlet view (Fig. 16.2B). The outlet view demonstrates vertical displacement and sagittal plane deformity (Fig. 16.2C). Posterior pelvic displacement of more than 1 cm suggests posterior pelvic disruption. Symphyseal diastasis greater than 2.5 cm denotes compromised integrity to the anterior ligament complex [symphysis pubis, ischiosacral and anterior sacroiliac (SI) ligaments]. Additional radiographic clues implying vertical or rotational instability include sacrospinous ligament and iliolumbar ligament avulsions, displaced sacral fractures and SI diastasis. Computed tomography (CT) is a valuable adjunctive study. Posterior lesions are further characterized on cross-sectional axial images. Sacral foraminal, central canal and any posterior tension band involvement are scrutinized. Sacral fracture gapping as opposed to impaction may imply inherent instability.

PELVIC RING INJURIES DIAGNOSIS:
Pearls and Pitfalls

- Pelvic hemorrhage is life-threatening and the treating physician should consider this as a source of major bleeding in the patient with the pelvic fracture
- Careful attention to the soft tissues is important to recognize degloving injuries, such as the Morel-Lavallee lesion
- A thorough radiographic evaluation includes AP, inlet and outlet radiographs and a CT scan
- Additional concomitant injuries, particularly genitourinary, should be looked for and treated accordingly

Classification

Structural compromise to the pelvic ring may result from either low- or high-energy injury mechanisms. Low energy

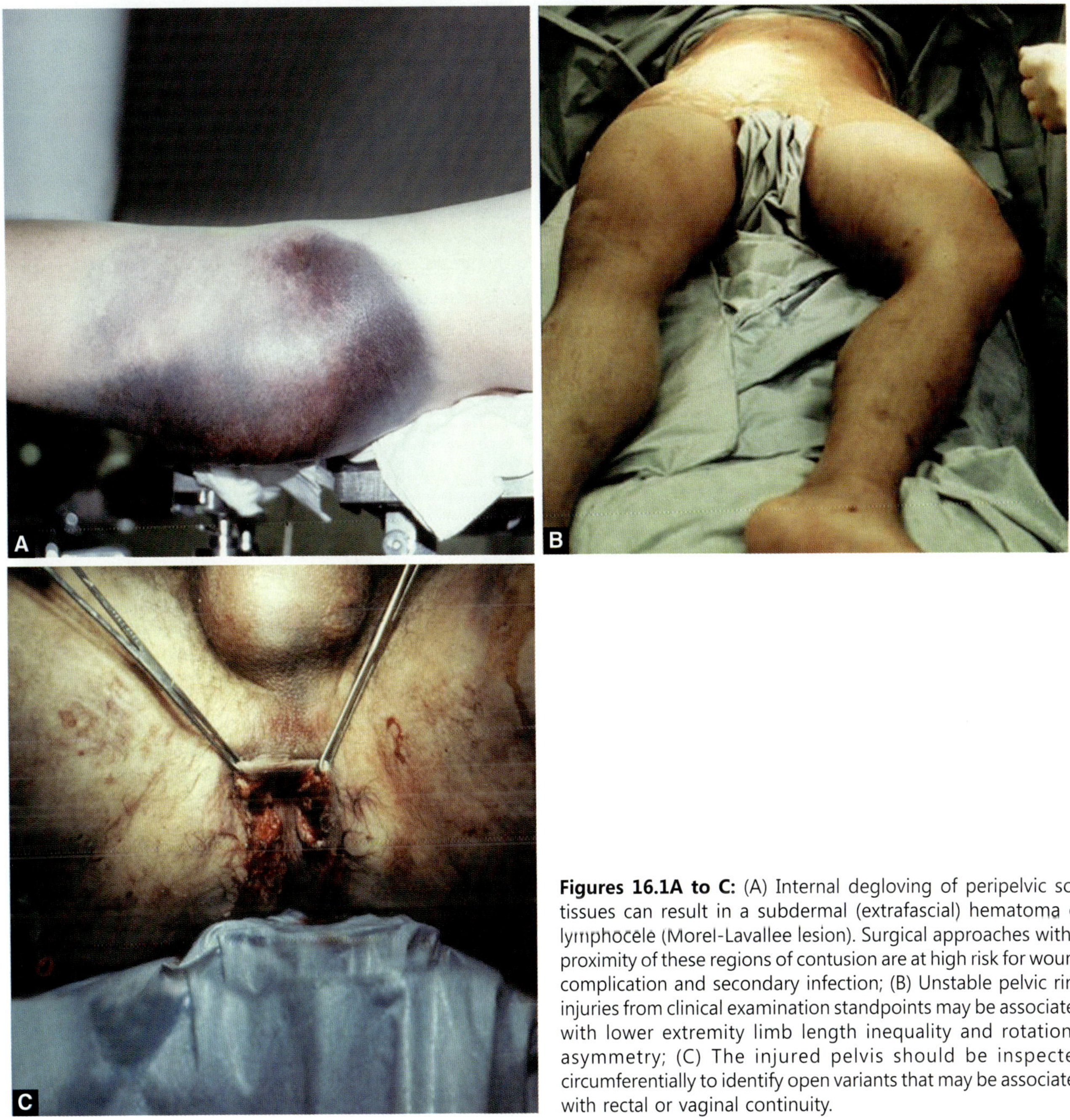

Figures 16.1A to C: (A) Internal degloving of peripelvic soft tissues can result in a subdermal (extrafascial) hematoma or lymphocele (Morel-Lavallee lesion). Surgical approaches within proximity of these regions of contusion are at high risk for wound complication and secondary infection; (B) Unstable pelvic ring injuries from clinical examination standpoints may be associated with lower extremity limb length inequality and rotational asymmetry; (C) The injured pelvis should be inspected circumferentially to identify open variants that may be associated with rectal or vaginal continuity.

injuries may result in fractures in senescent bone while higher energy injuries may present in a younger population. Similar fracture patterns in the two groups suggest a higher magnitude of injury in the younger group. This accordingly may be accompanied by additional injuries of concerning severity.

Pelvic instability is defined as the inability of the pelvis to assume physiologic loads without displacement and functional compromise. The anterior portion of the pelvic ring offers limited weight bearing function and confers little to pelvic ring stability. The osseous components of the pelvis include the paired innominate bones and the

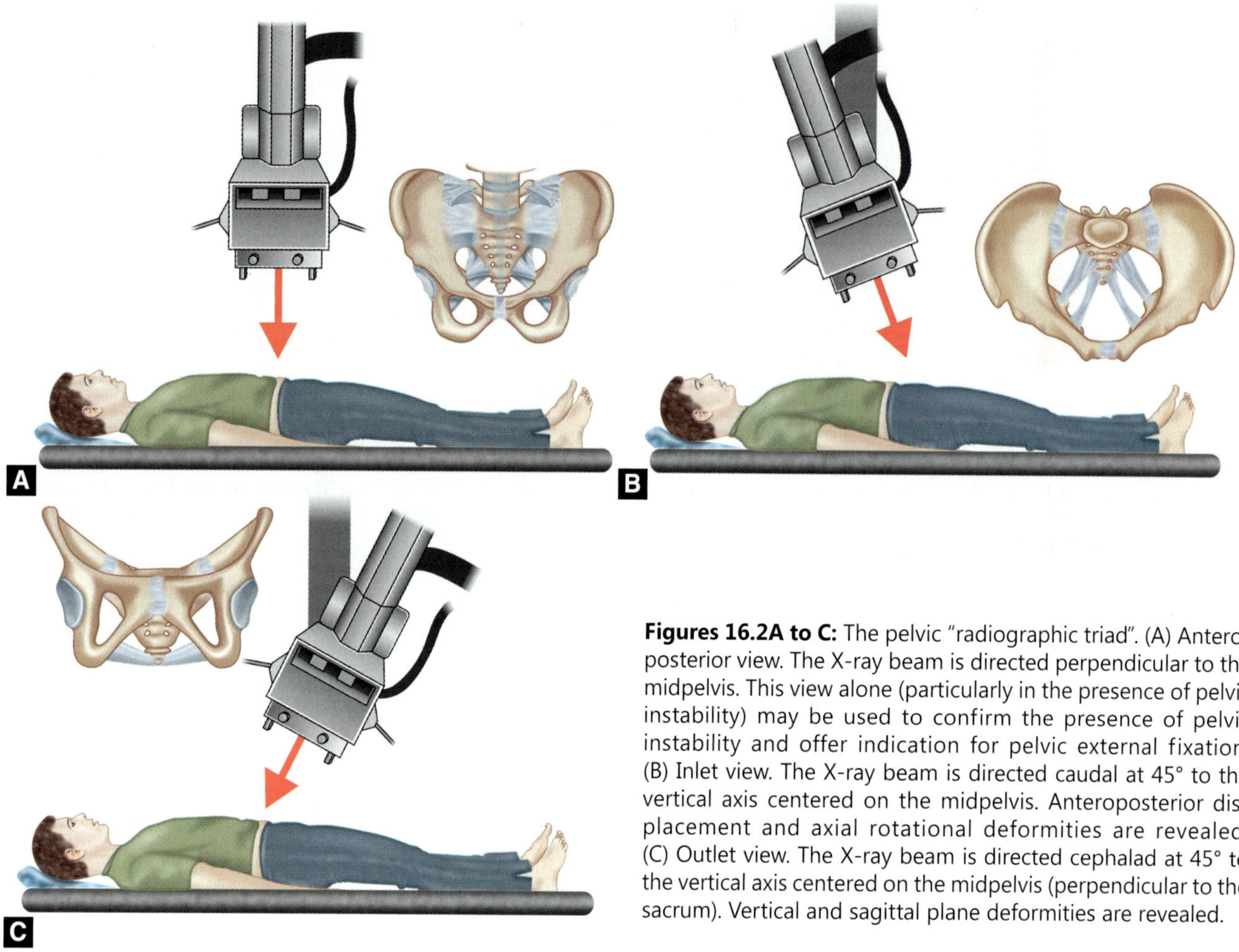

Figures 16.2A to C: The pelvic "radiographic triad". (A) Anteroposterior view. The X-ray beam is directed perpendicular to the midpelvis. This view alone (particularly in the presence of pelvic instability) may be used to confirm the presence of pelvic instability and offer indication for pelvic external fixation; (B) Inlet view. The X-ray beam is directed caudal at 45° to the vertical axis centered on the midpelvis. Anteroposterior displacement and axial rotational deformities are revealed; (C) Outlet view. The X-ray beam is directed cephalad at 45° to the vertical axis centered on the midpelvis (perpendicular to the sacrum). Vertical and sagittal plane deformities are revealed.

sacrum. Stability of the intact pelvis is dependent on the integrity of the posterior tension band of the SI complex. This is comprised of the anterior SI ligaments, interosseous ligaments and the posterior SI ligaments. The ligaments of the "pelvic floor" (sacrotuberous and sacrospinous) contribute to rotational stability. The osseous architecture of the pelvis contributes little to stability. Injury patterns (osseous or ligamentous) are determined by the direction, magnitude and site of force application. Applied forces in simplest terms can be described as anterocompression, lateral compression and vertical shear. The resultant instability patterns are commonly categorized as: (1) vertically and rotationally stable, (2) rotationally unstable and vertically stable, and (3) rotationally and vertically unstable.

Anteroposterior compression and resultant hemipelvic rotational forces may render the "anterior ligamentous complex" incompetent (Fig. 16.3A). Structural compromise (in increasing severity order and sequence) is sustained to the symphysis pubis, ischiosacral (sacrotuberous and sacrospinous) and anterior SI ligaments. The posterior tension band (posterior SI ligament) is, however intact and vertical stability is accordingly maintained.

Disruption of the posterior tension band of the pelvis may impart vertical instability (Fig. 16.3B). The lesion may be of osseous, ligamentous or combined origin. Traumatic compromise to the sacrospinous and sacrotuberous ligaments in the presence of an intact posterior tension band will result in rotational instability. Further division of the posterior ligaments of the SI complex will result in both vertical and rotational instability. In this scenario, the imparted deforming forces may demonstrate multiplanar (axial, sagittal and coronal) hemipelvic instability.

Depending on severity, lateral compression injuries may result in internal collapse of the pelvis. Ligaments,

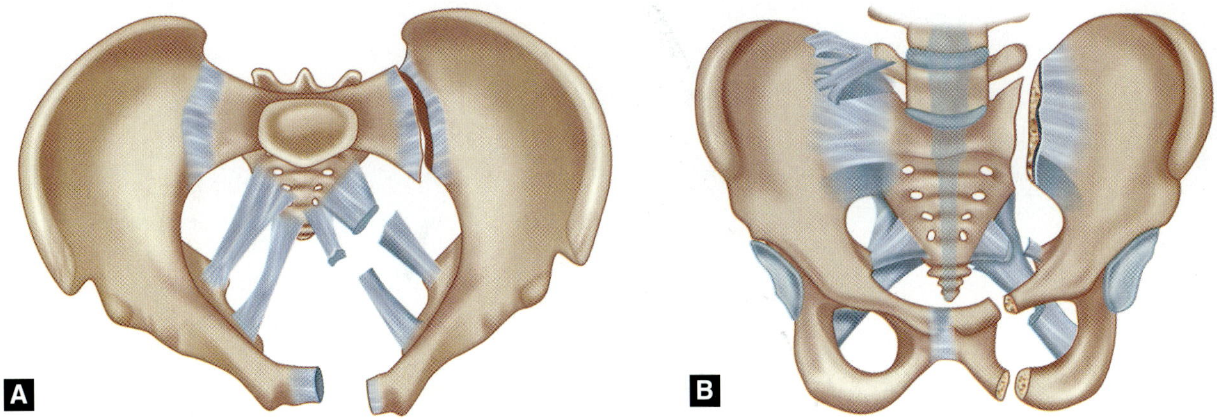

Figures 16.3A and B: (A) An external rotational injury (anteroposterior compression) resulting in "anterior ligamentous complex injury". Instability is rotational in character and demonstrated in the axial plane. The posterior tension band is intact and vertical stability is preserved; (B) A vertical shear injury. In addition to compromise to the "anterior ligamentous complex", the integrity of the posterior tension band is disrupted. The involved hemipelvis is unstable in all planes.

both anteriorly and posteriorly, are often intact and osseous injuries are typically of a stable impaction pattern. Infrequently, severe internal rotational instability and deformity may result and require operative intervention.

Any of the aforementioned injury mechanisms (anterocompression, vertical shear, lateral compression), if of sufficient magnitude, may result in complete (vertical and rotational) instability. The contribution of pelvic fractures (osseous compromise) toward pelvic ring instability may vary and must be evaluated carefully. Fractures of the pelvis frequently involve displaced and unstable injuries to the anterior and/or posterior pelvic ring. These injuries include fractures and fracture-dislocations of the SI joint, iliac wing fractures, parasymphyseal fractures and fractures of the sacrum. Fractures of the sacrum have been classified as occurring through three zones: zone 1 (alar), zone 2 (transforaminal), and zone 3 (sacral canal) (Fig. 16.4).

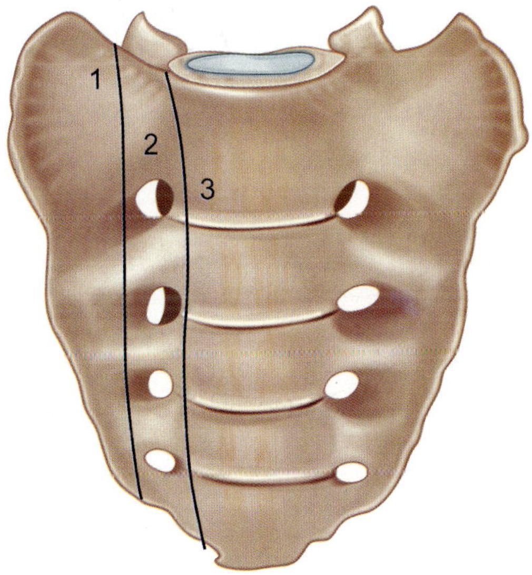

Figure 16.4: Sacral fracture classification (Denis). Zone 1: sacral ala, Zone 2: transforaminal, and Zone 3: sacral body.

Surgical Indications

The treatment goals for surgical and nonsurgical treatment do not differ. Common to both includes deformity correction or avoidance, preservation of stability and pain free function. Nonsurgical management is appropriate for lesions deemed clinically and is radiographically stable.

Pelvic external fixation can serve several different indications depending on hemodynamic and pelvic structural stability.[7] Early application during the resuscitative phase serves to control intrapelvic hemorrhage. In some injury patterns, it may offer sufficient stability to permit comfortable patient mobilization. With rotationally unstable yet vertically stable patterns, it may serve well as definitive care. In vertically unstable patterns, external fixation alone may prove inadequate toward treatment goals. In such scenarios, it may demonstrate an inability to achieve and maintain posterior reduction and stability (Figs 16.5A to C).

Posterior instability and displacement may result in concerning sequelae both short and long-term. Among

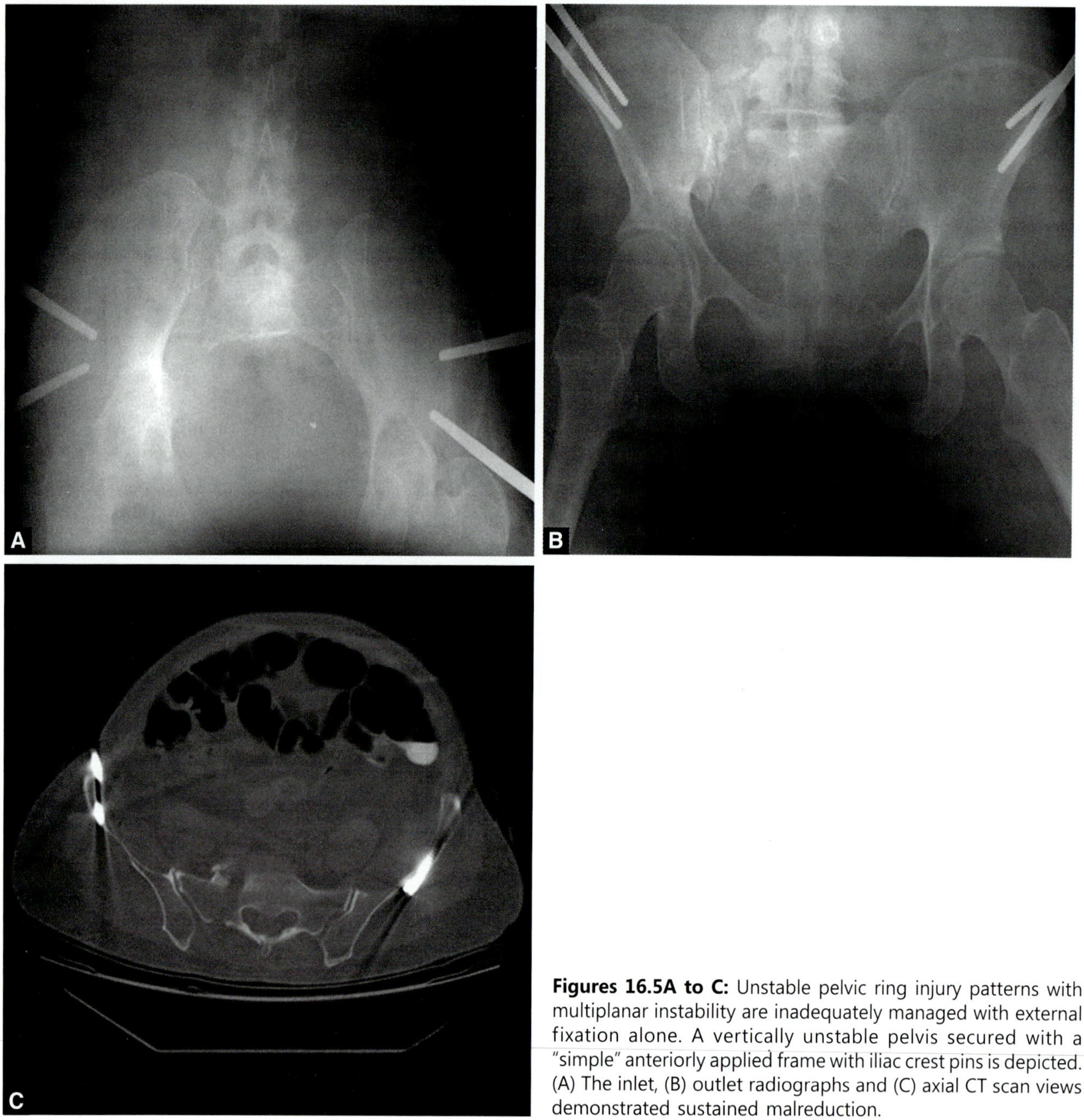

Figures 16.5A to C: Unstable pelvic ring injury patterns with multiplanar instability are inadequately managed with external fixation alone. A vertically unstable pelvis secured with a "simple" anteriorly applied frame with iliac crest pins is depicted. (A) The inlet, (B) outlet radiographs and (C) axial CT scan views demonstrated sustained malreduction.

these include painful nonunion, symptomatic malunion (anisomelia and sitting imbalance), acute and progressive lumbosacral plexopathy (Fig. 16.6). The advent and evolution of posterior pelvic reduction and fixation techniques continue to offer remedy but not without significant potential for complication. The surgeon must have a clear understanding of the limitations and attributes of various surgical exposures, reduction techniques and fixation devices. Much like a pretzel, the pelvis is a ring and if broken must be violated in two locations, one of which is often posterior. The pathoanatomy of the posterior lesion has considerable implication with regard to surgical indication and technique. Traumatized retropelvic soft tissues may be unreceptive to surgical insult. Patient

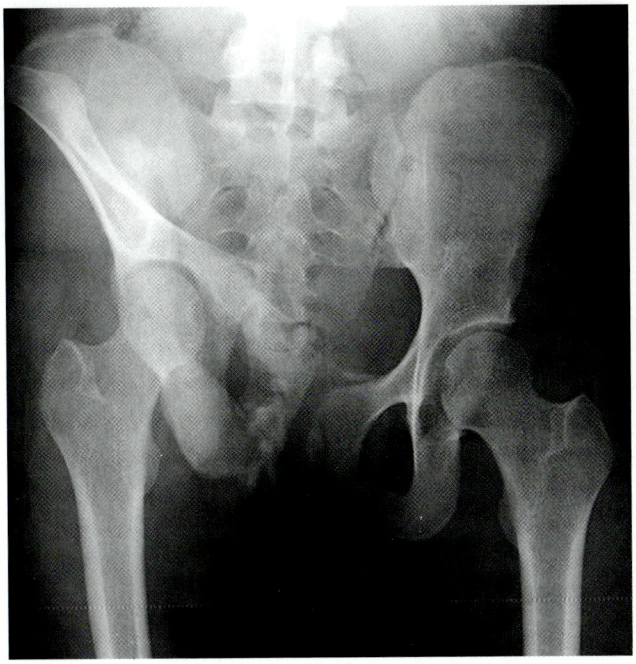

Figure 16.6: Unstable pelvic ring in injuries if inadequately managed can result in significant deformity. This can result in sitting imbalance, limb length inequality and neurologic deficits.

positioning (prone vs supine) and anterior ring status (reduced vs displaced) may aggravate or contribute to posterior pelvic reduction.

Surgical Anatomy, Positioning and Approaches

The treating surgeon characterizes the presence and type of pelvic instability. The intended purpose of fixation type, location and sequence must be predetermined. This is based on anticipated reduction maneuvers, methods and access routes for insertion of implants. Patient physiologic and neurologic, as well as regional soft tissue envelope status, may have impact on all of these. The herein described surgical techniques invoke unique and differing anatomy and exposure strategies. Accordingly, surgical anatomy, patient positioning and approaches will be discussed independently as they pertain to each other.

Surgical Techniques

Technique 1: External Fixation of the Pelvis

Prior to external fixation of the pelvis associated intrapelvic, vascular, urologic and gynecological comorbidities are identified. Any neurologic deficit is identified and documented. The soft tissue status of the pelvis circumferentially is determined. Pelvic stability is assessed and any instability characterized. The intended function of the external fixator is defined (resuscitation or provisional vs definitive stabilization). If applied for provisional stabilization purposes, the timing sequence and method of subsequent stabilization efforts must be considered. Frame design and pin location (anterior iliac crest, supra-acetabular) are selected based upon injury pattern, hemodynamic stability, available imaging and surgeon familiarity. Anterior pelvic external fixator pins may be placed in either the anterior iliac crest or in the supra-acetabular region (Figs 16.7A and B).[8] Pin placement within the iliac crest is more expeditiously performed and with lesser anatomic hazard. Placement in either location is also determined by regional fractures and soft tissue concerns within pin proximity (Fig. 16.8). Pins within the more inferiorly located dense bone of the anterior inferior iliac spine ("supra-acetabular pins") may offer enhanced fixation and improved abdominal access.[9] Insertion of these pin is more fluoroscopic dependent than those placed within the iliac crest.

Anterior Iliac Crest Pins

The patient is positioned supine on a radiographic table. An 8–10 cm oblique skin incision is established adjacent to the iliac crest anteriorly. To reduce tension on soft tissues, it is made in the anticipated site of the reduced hemipelvis (Figs 16.9A and B). Subjacent soft tissues are bluntly dissected revealing the underlying iliac crest. The inner table of the ilium is exposed by subperiosteal dissection of the external oblique (Fig. 16.10A). Similarly, subperiosteal elevation of the hip abductors exposes the outer table (Fig. 16.10B). Dissection on both sides is carried inferiorly to the depth of the surgeon's digit at which time the thick anterior pillar is identified (Fig. 16.10C). The surgeon's index digit positioned on the inner table confirms its inclination. Together the surgeon's thumb and index finger palpate the outer and inner tables, respectively (Fig. 16.10D). This aids in establishing proper pin orientation within the two tables. Alternatively, in an effort to limit dissection and retain intrapelvic tamponade, needles may be employed instead leaving periosseous muscular attachments undisturbed.

The initial pin is placed 1–2 cm posterior to the anterior superior iliac spine within the anterior portion of the pillar.

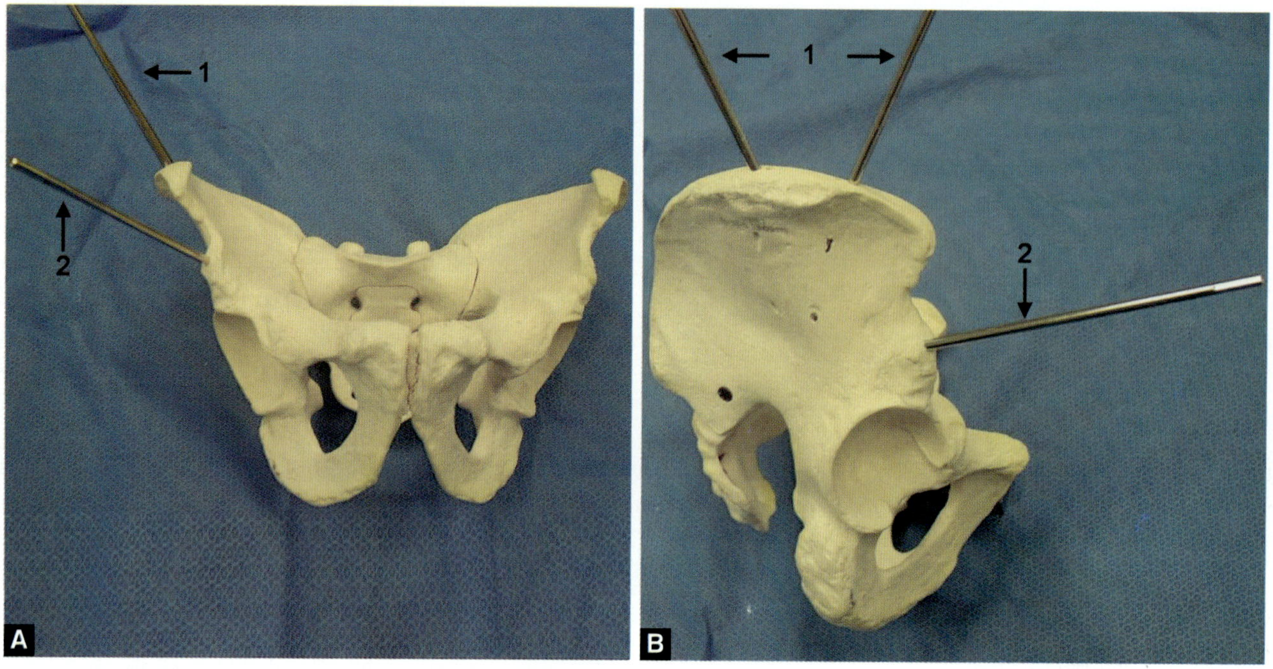

Figures 16.7A and B: Iliac crest pin (1) and supra-acetabular pin (2). (A) Frontal view; and (B) Side view.

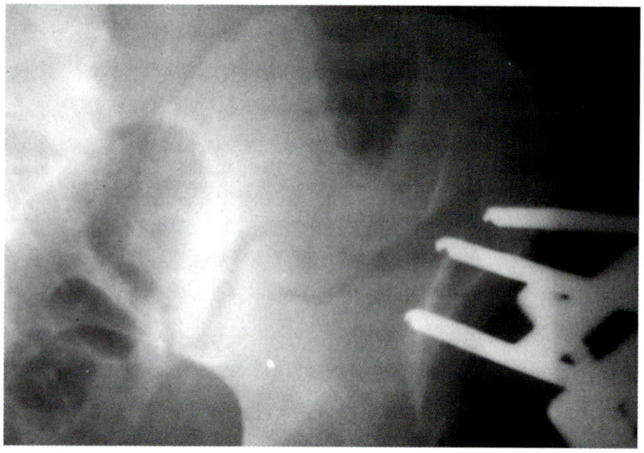

Figure 16.8: The surgeon must be aware of any fracture planes (depicted in this example) within proximity of the inserted external fixation pins.

The ideal starting point is at the medial third of the crest at the junction of the inner and middle thirds ("rule of thirds") (Fig. 16.11A). Owing to coronal plane asymmetry, pin introduction centrally or laterally will result in pin deviation from the desired intercortical path. A unicortical drill path is initiated no more than 1–2 cm deep. Pin introduction is guided by simultaneous digital palpation on both sides of the crest, as well as fluoroscopic control (Fig. 16.11B). Typical inclination is 25–40° medially and 1–15° caudal. The pin may be introduced through the established surgical wound or adjacent percutaneous wounds (Fig. 16.12). The pin is advanced within the osseous tables of the ilium. Additional pins as required are inserted posteriorly, approximately one finger breadth apart. The curved profile of the iliac crest does not allow for parallel pin insertion (Fig. 16.13A). The common target of each pin inferiorly is the supra-acetabular region of the anterior pillar (Fig. 16.13B). Final pin position can be assessed on a fluoroscopic obturator oblique outlet view (Fig. 16.13C). This will identify any misdirected pins exiting the intercortical path prematurely.

The technique described can be performed in percutaneous fashion. Perpendicularly oriented percutaneous wounds are preferred to limit pin tension and permit drill and pin trajectory modification (Fig. 16.14). Needles are introduced adjacent to the inner and outer pelvic tables to assist pin targeting. Serial fluoroscopic obturator oblique outlet views verify proper pin introduction, trajectory and final position.

Supra-Acetabular Pins

The patient is positioned supine on a radiolucent table. A vertical approach begins along the medial border of the

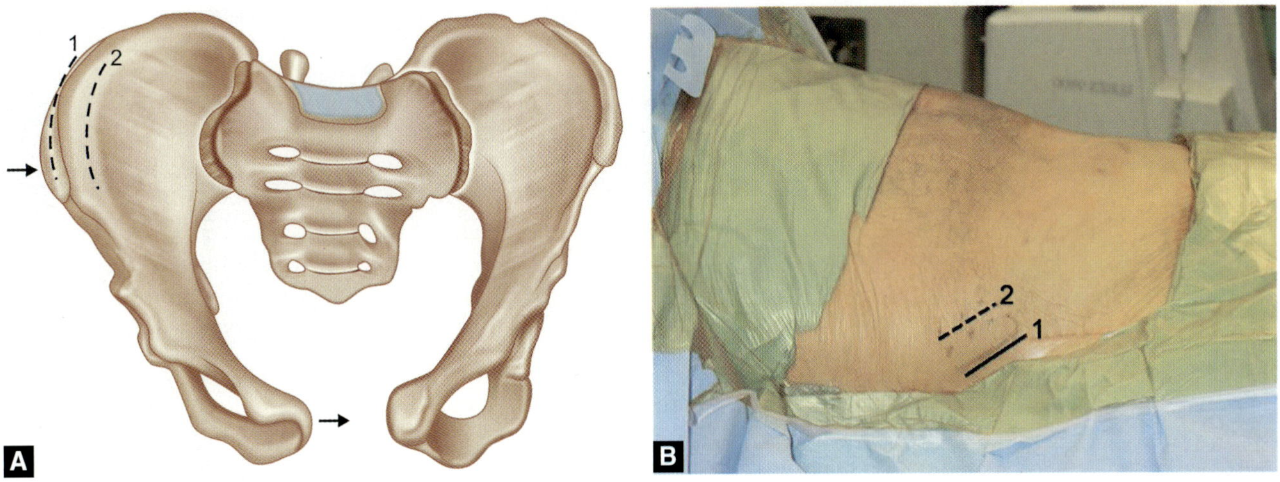

Figures 16.9A and B: Anterior iliac crest pin insertion—skin incision site. An 8–10 cm oblique skin incision is established in the anticipated site of the reduced hemipelvis (1) rather than its present displaced state (2). (A) Schematic; and (B) Operative case of right hemipelvis.

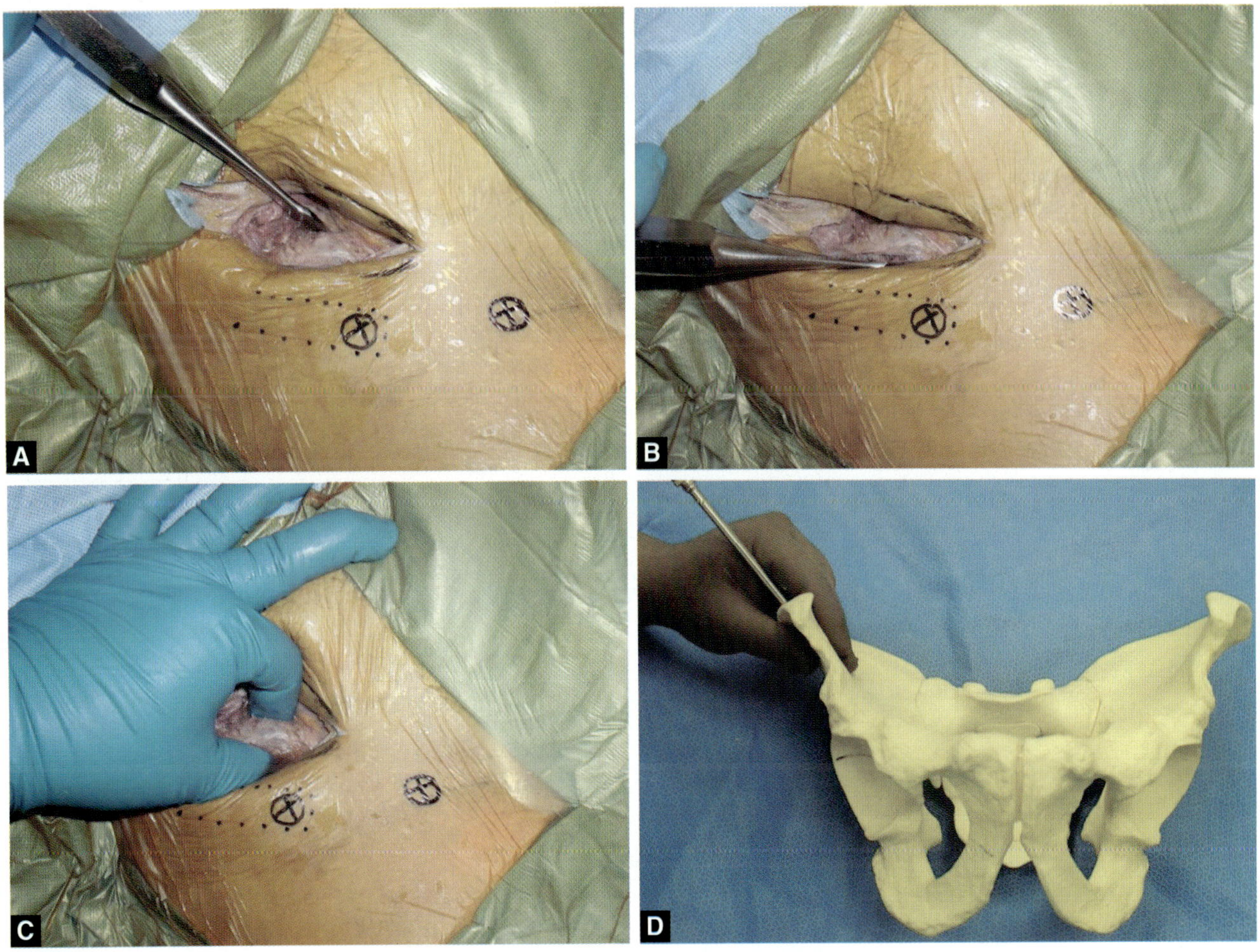

Figures 16.10A to D: Anterior iliac crest pin insertion. (A) The inner table is exposed by subperiosteal elevation of the external oblique; (B) The outer table is exposed by subperiosteal elevation of the hip abductors; (C) Dissection is carried down on both inner and outer tables to the depth of the surgeon's digit; (D) The surgeons thumb and index finger confirm pelvic inclination and drill/pin trajectory.

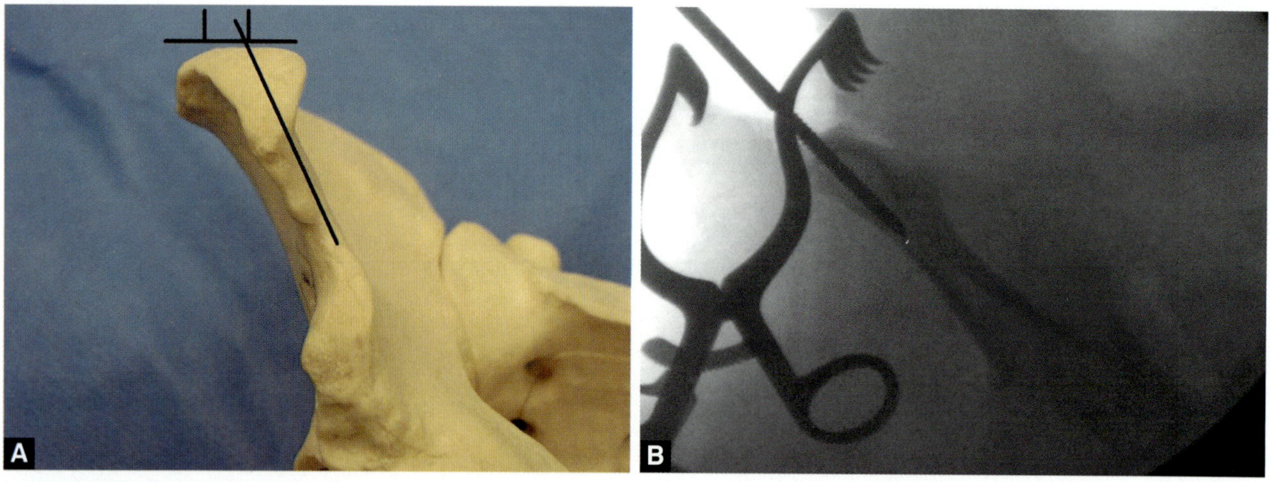

Figures 16.11A and B: Anterior iliac crest pin insertion ("rule of thirds"—ideal starting point). (A) Pin insertion should be at the junction of the inner and middle thirds of the iliac crest within the coronal plane; (B) This permits proper placement within the inner and outer tables of the pelvis (intercortical path).

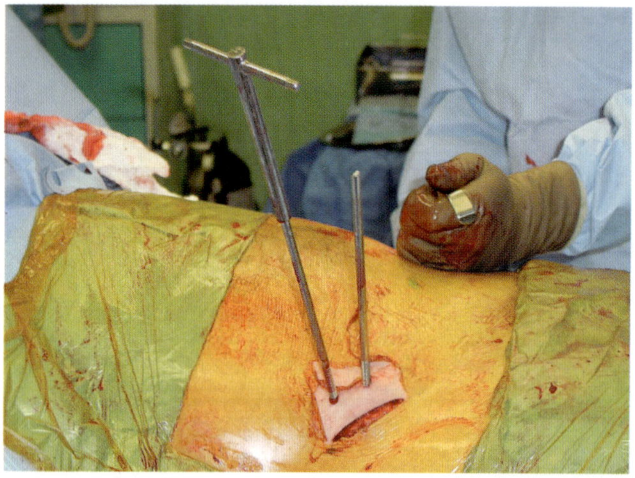

Figure 16.12: Anterior iliac crest pin insertion. Pins within the anterior iliac crest can be inserted through the established surgical wound or alternatively (depicted here) adjacent percutaneous wounds.

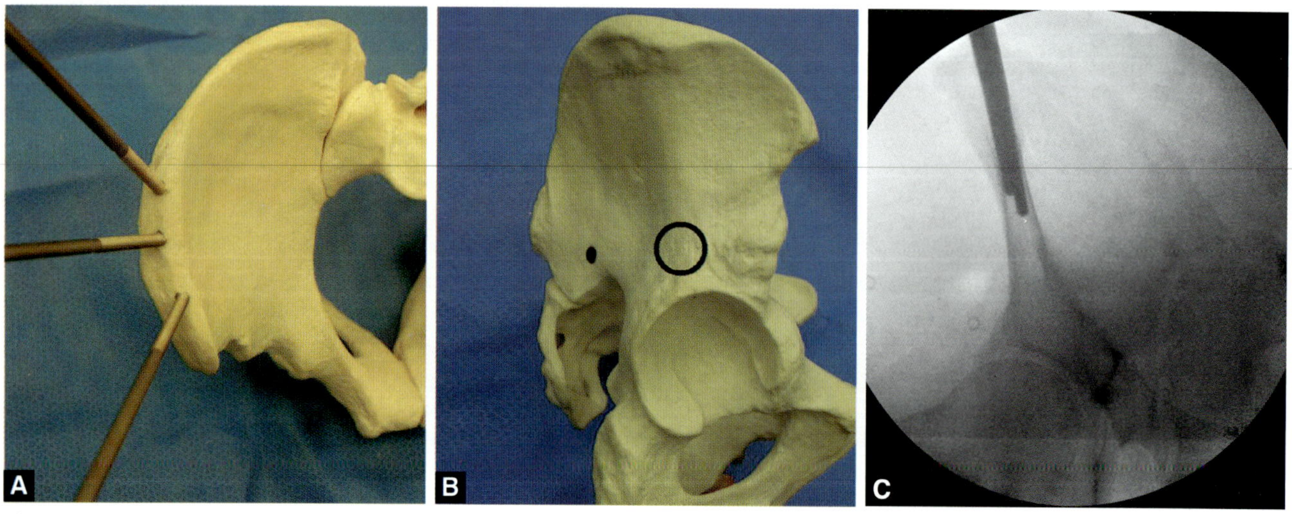

Figures 16.13A to C: Anterior iliac crest pin insertion. (A) The curved profile of the iliac crest does not permit linear or parallel pin insertion; (B) The common target of inserted pin is the supra-acetabular region of the anterior pillar (black circle); (C) Final pin insertion can be assessed on fluoroscopic obturator oblique outlet view (cephalad inclination with rotation toward affected side).

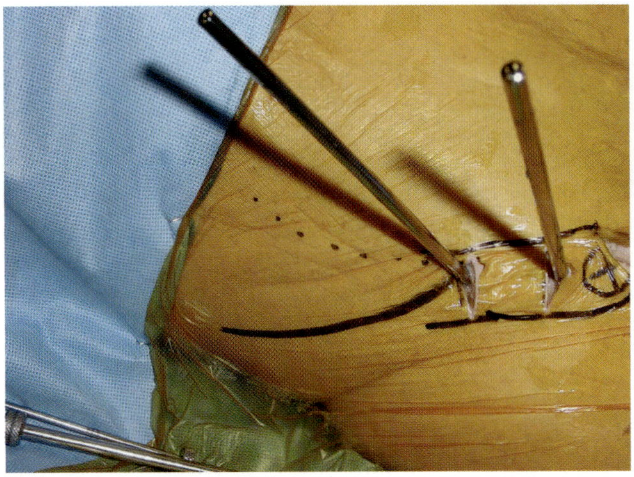

Figure 16.14: Anterior iliac crest pin insertion. Pins can be introduced under fluoroscopic guidance through perpendicularly oriented wounds.

anterior superior iliac spine extending distally to the level of the anterior inferior iliac spine (Fig. 16.15A). A transverse incision may offer less congestion of soft tissues upon reduction if significant prereduction deformity exists. Medial to the anterior superior iliac spine, the lateral femoral cutaneous nerve is sought (Fig. 16.15B).[10] Its course however, may be variable and within close proximity of the inserted pin. The interval between the sartorius and tensor fascia lata is identified and developed with blunt dissection to the level of the anterior inferior iliac spine. Protective drill sleeves limit regional soft tissue and neurologic injury. Supra-acetabular pins should be inserted no less than 2 cm proximal to the joint to avoid articular penetration as hip capsular extension may be up to 16 mm superiorly (Figs 16.16A and B).

An obturator oblique view with slight cephalad angulation (obturator oblique-outlet view) is first obtained. A metallic marker is positioned 2 cm proximal to the hip joint under fluoroscopic control (Fig. 16.17A). The cannulated drill sleeve assembly is positioned within the radiographic "tear drop" and the outer cortex drilled (Fig. 16.17B). The drill followed by the pin is advanced avoiding intra-articular penetration (Fig. 16.18A). Customary pin angulation is 20° medial from the vertical axis and slightly cephalad. An iliac oblique view with slight cephalad angulation (iliac oblique outlet view) demonstrates preferred pin position superior to the greater sciatic notch (30–45° in the sagittal plane) (Figs 16.18B and C). Intercortical pin orientation within the tables of the pelvis is monitored on an obturator-oblique inlet view (rollover view) (Figs 16.19A to C).

Frame Application and Reduction

Regardless of frame complexity, no anteriorly applied external pelvic fixator restores sufficient stability to vertically unstable injury patterns. Accordingly, simple constructs are adequate and preferred for resuscitation and patient mobilization purposes. Converging pins adequately positioned within the curvature of the iliac crest do not allow for parallel pin placement. Pin fixation clamps with independent ball joint design are best suited for this application concern. Clamps should be applied three finger breadths above skin surface level permitting proper pin tract care. The frame is fabricated with articulating couplings or universal ball joints. Anteroposterior compression injuries are reduced with midline directed compression. Lateral compression injuries require distracting force reduction maneuvers. For vertically displaced injury patterns, adjunctive lower extremity skeletal traction may prove necessary to limit vertical hemipelvic ascent and retropelvic displacement.

EXTERNAL FIXATION OF THE PELVIS:
Pearls and Pitfalls

- Be careful to insert iliac crest pins between the inner and outer tables of the pelvis. A fluoroscopic obturator outlet view will confirm proper placement
- Supra-acetabular pins should be placed no less than 2 cm proximal to the hip joint to avoid intra-articular penetration
- Remember that anterior external fixators do not restore sufficient stability to the posterior ring for vertically unstable injury patterns. Lower extremity skeletal traction may be required in addition

Technique 2: Anterior Pelvic Fixation

Plate fixation and anterior pelvic external fixation remain the primary forms of treatment when operative stabilization of the anterior pelvis is performed.[11-13] Pin-tract related complications and patient mobilization concerns may render external fixation disadvantageous. Plate fixation of symphyseal dislocation and pubic rami fractures

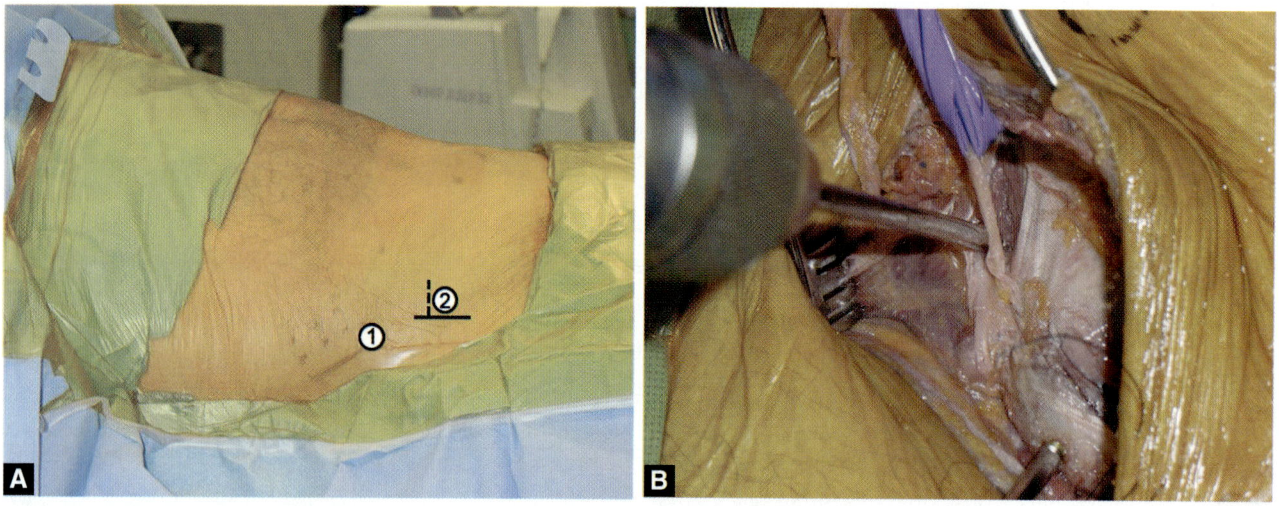

Figures 16.15A and B: Supra-acetabular pin insertion. (A) Vertical approach (2) is established along the medial border of the anterior superior iliac spine (1) extending distally to the level of the anterior inferior iliac spine (straight line). A transverse incision (dashed line) may be preferred to avoid "congestion" of soft tissues upon pelvic reduction; (B) The interval between the sartorius and tensor fascia lata is developed and the lateral femoral cutaneous nerve (depicted within elastic drain) protected.

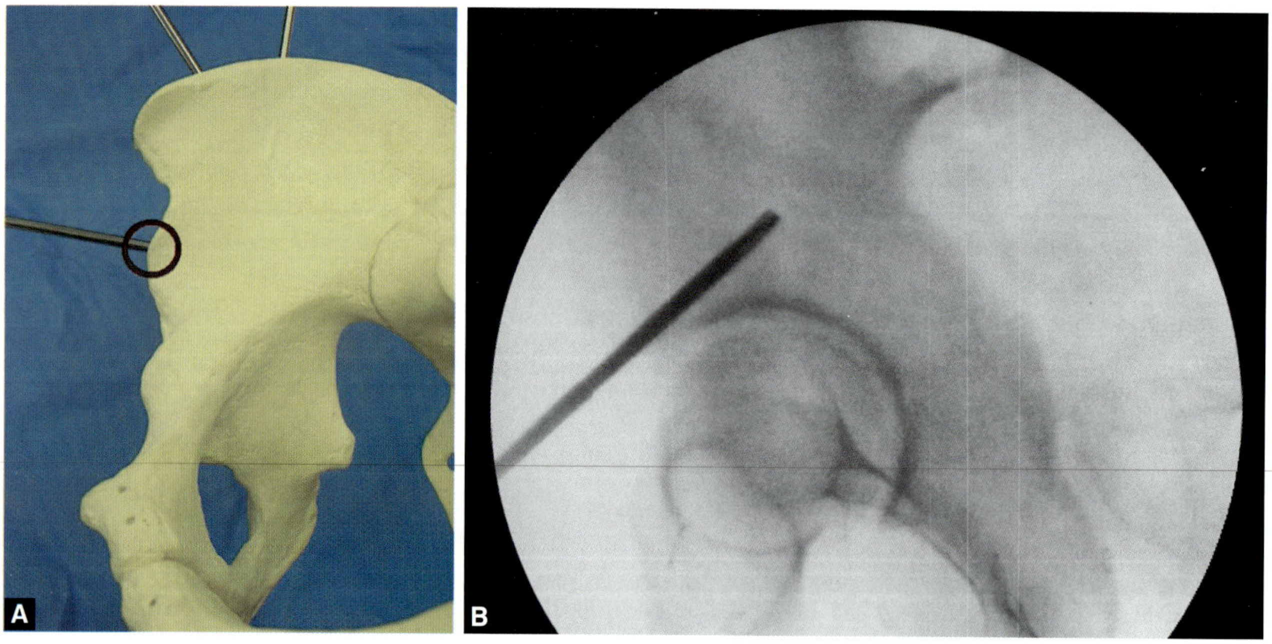

Figures 16.16A and B: Supra-acetabular pin insertion. (A) Pins should be inserted no less than 2 cm proximal to the hip joint to avoid intra-capsular penetration (circle); (B) Intraoperative fluoroscopic image. Pins placed within 2 cm of the hip joint (depicted here) are at risk for both intracapsular and intra-articular incursion.

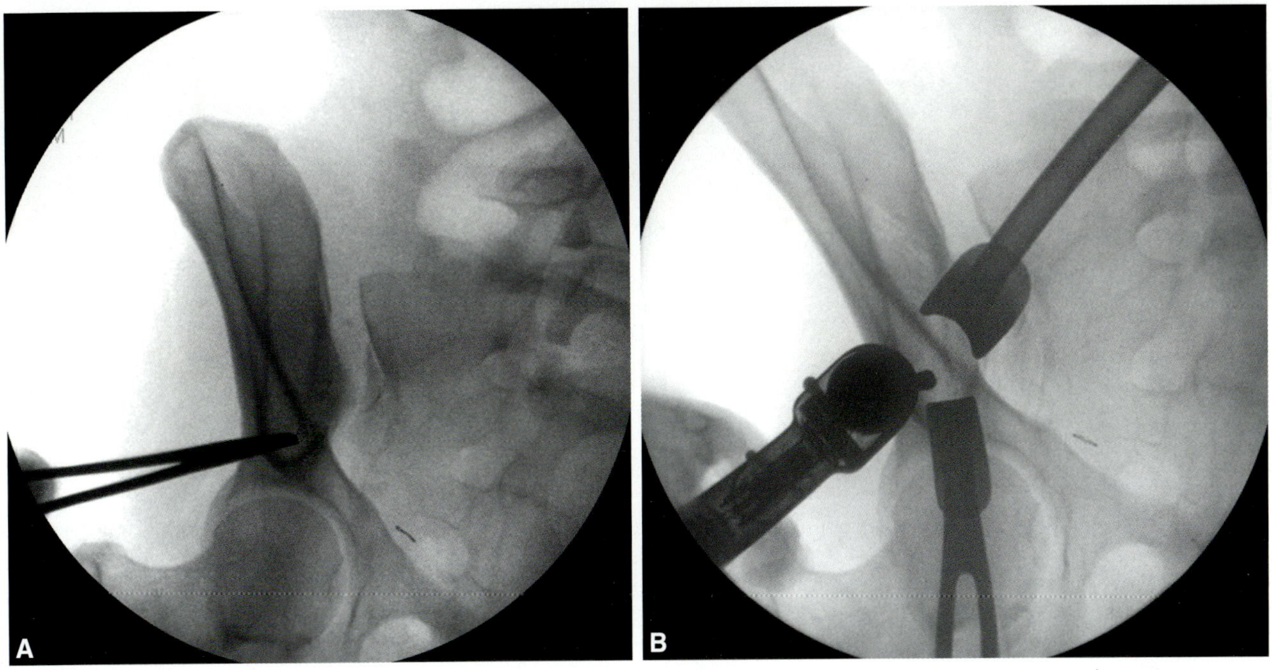

Figures 16.17A and B: Supra-acetabular pin insertion. (A) Metallic marker is positioned over the radiographic "tear drop" (obturator-oblique outlet view); (B) Drill with protective drill sleeve is advanced unicortically.

obviate these concerns. Additionally, reduction and fixation stability are more predictably achieved. Symphyseal diastasis greater than 2.5 cm implies injury to the anterior ligamentous complex imparting rotatory instability to the involved hemipelvis. In the presence of an intact posterior tension band, operative stabilization anteriorly is sufficient to restore pelvic stability.

Indications for operative treatment of pubic rami fractures and its impact on outcome and long-term results remain poorly defined. Most rami fractures are unlikely to displace further during the course of treatment. The consequences of rami fractures with regard to pelvic stability are uncertain and variable. Owing to robust adjacent soft tissues, fractures of the rami may not need operative intervention even if associated with an operatively managed symphyseal diastasis. Advances in the understanding of regional anatomy in combination with enhanced imaging techniques have made percutaneous methods of parasymphyseal fracture fixation increasingly attractive.

Vertically unstable pelvic injury patterns present with posterior pelvic discontinuity lesions. These may be osseous, ligamentous or combinations of both. Fixation of the anterior ring (symphysis pubis diastasis or rami fractures) may enhance posterior pelvic fixation stability. Regardless of the method elected, no form of anterior fixation will suffice for an inadequately fixed posterior pelvic construct. Anatomic reduction and fixation of the anterior ring component may improve posterior ring displacement. Anterior malreduction, however, may forbid it. Consequently, patient preparation, surgical reduction and fixation strategies may demand simultaneous anterior and posterior reduction efforts.

Urethral and bladder injuries are not prohibitive when managing anterior pelvic ring injuries with internal fixation. It must be performed in collaboration with a urologic consultant. Timing of urologic repair and osseous stabilization, as well as catheter placement (urethral or suprapubic cystostomy), must be considered. The patient's history and physical examination must ascertain the presence of previous regional operative procedures that may complicate the treatment.

Symphyseal Plate Fixation

The patient is placed supine on a radiolucent table with the pelvis suspended on several longitudinally oriented folded sheets. The adequacy of pelvic "tilt" views (40° cephalad

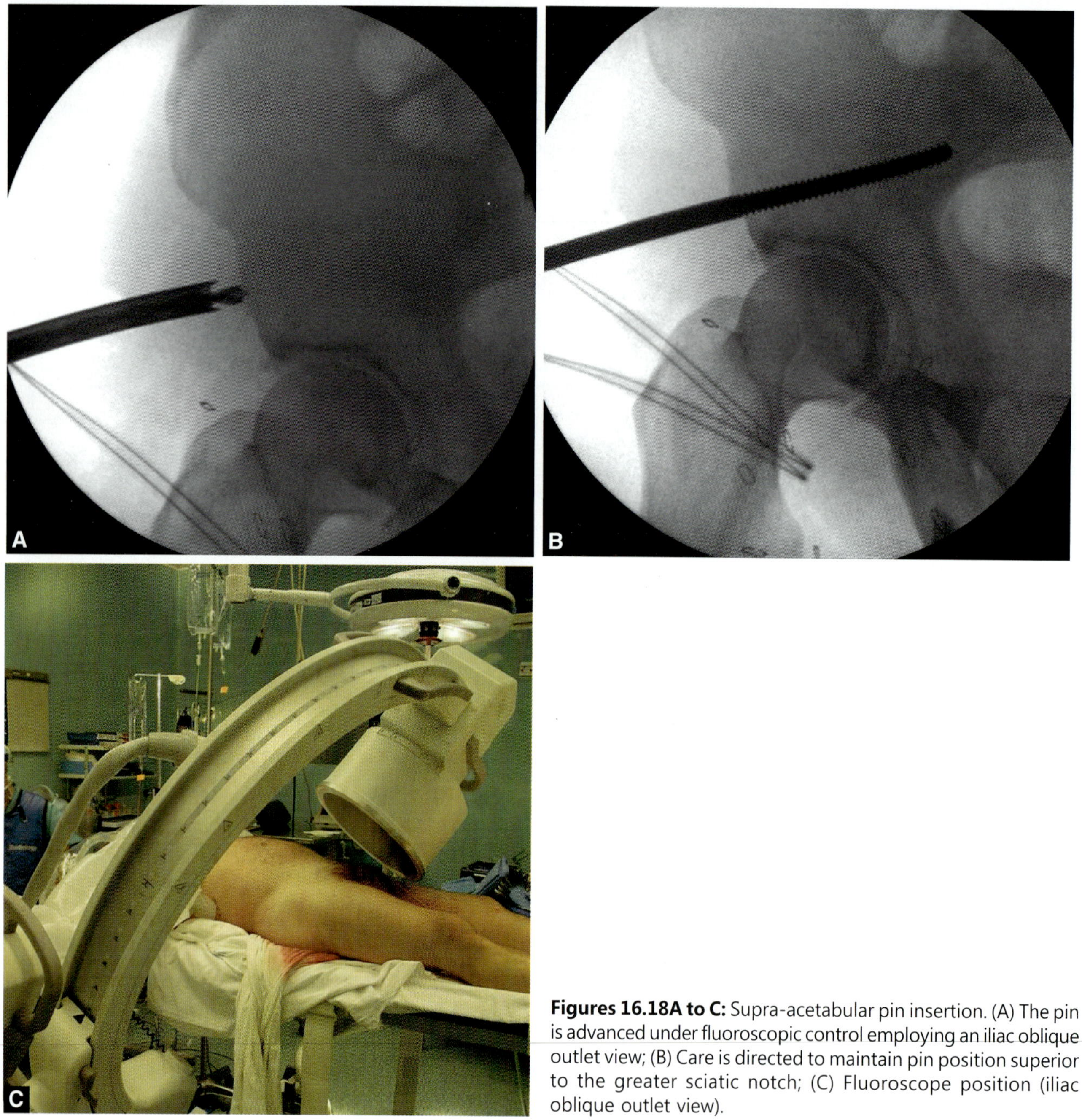

Figures 16.18A to C: Supra-acetabular pin insertion. (A) The pin is advanced under fluoroscopic control employing an iliac oblique outlet view; (B) Care is directed to maintain pin position superior to the greater sciatic notch; (C) Fluoroscope position (iliac oblique outlet view).

and caudal) is assessed and any conflicts resolved. Draping and surgical preparation should include the contralateral hemipelvis even if the operative strategy and injury are focused unilaterally (Fig. 16.20). This permits fixator assisted reduction techniques. Additionally, the operative field should permit pelvic access sufficient to allow percutaneous screw (ramus/iliosacral) or reduction aid instrumentation insertion. Surgical trauma consultants should be advised on the need for draping inferiorly to the level of the pubis during the course of midline laparotomy exposure preparation.

The Pfannenstiel approach begins with an incision, approximately 10–15 cm in length and 2 cm cranial to the palpable superior aspect of the pubis (Fig. 16.21). This approach offers excellent exposure to the symphysis and

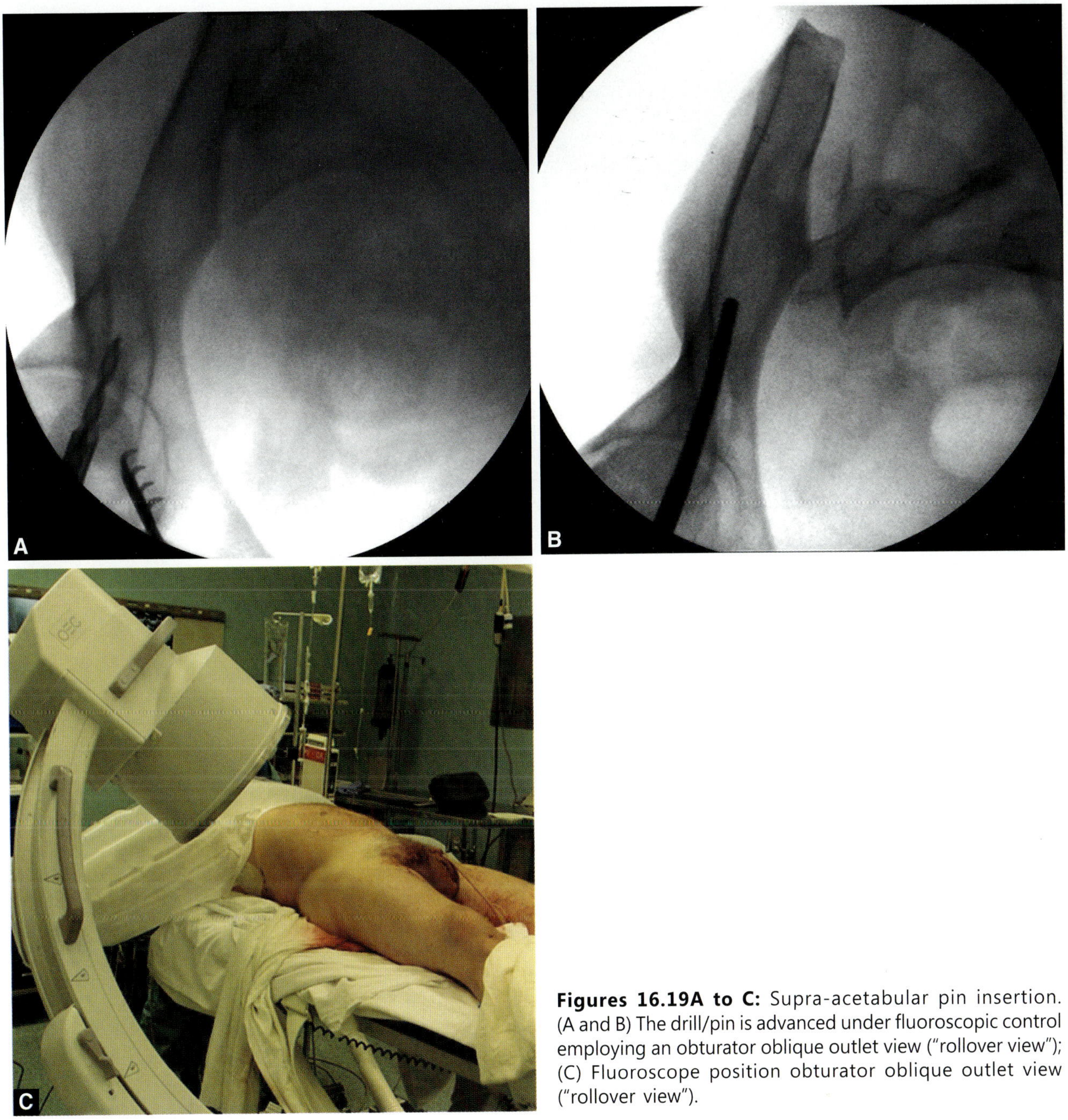

Figures 16.19A to C: Supra-acetabular pin insertion. (A and B) The drill/pin is advanced under fluoroscopic control employing an obturator oblique outlet view ("rollover view"); (C) Fluoroscope position obturator oblique outlet view ("rollover view").

parasymphyseal fractures to the extent of the iliopectineal eminence laterally. Fixation and exposure lateral to this may require formal dissection and control of the iliac vessels. Subcutaneous tissue dissection is carried down to the underlying fascia of the anterior rectus sheath. The robust interval of the linea alba identified vertically between the muscle bellies of the rectus abdominis is divided longitudinally. Blunt dissection continues to and through the posterior fascia of the rectus sheath which is of variable thickness. Accordingly, care is directed toward protection of the underling bladder while entering the potential space of Retzius. A malleable retractor enveloped in a well

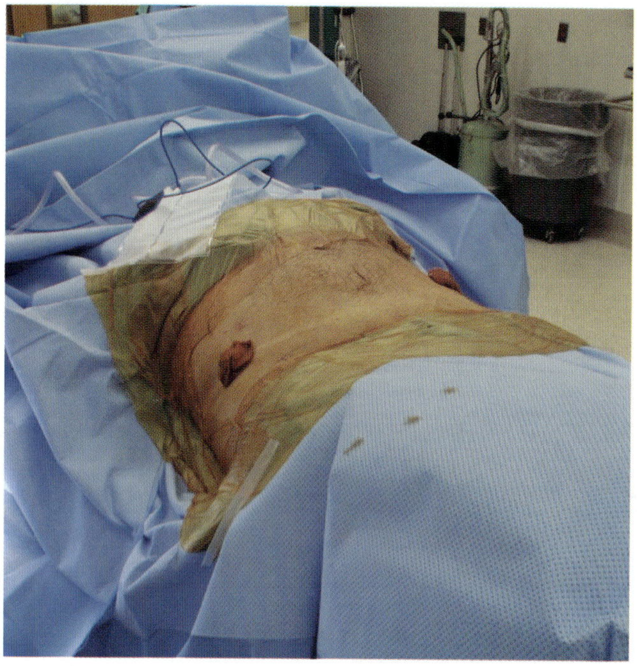

Figure 16.20: Anterior pelvic fixation. Draping should include both hemipelvic regions anteriorly to permit introduction of reduction devices in both. Retropelvic access may be required for insertion of posteriorly introduced percutaneous reduction devices and implants.

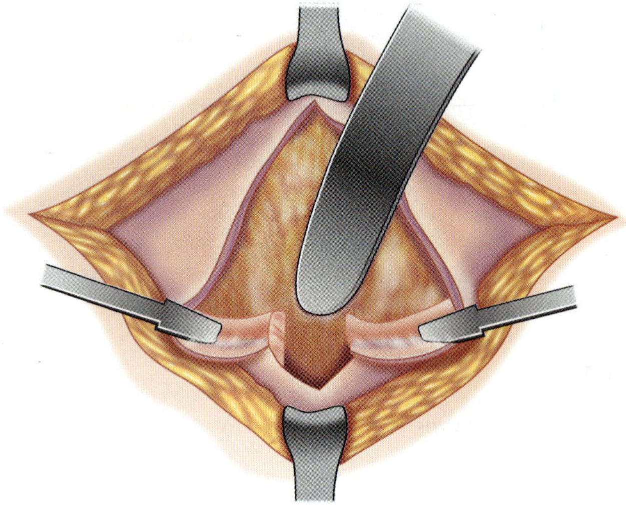

Figure 16.21: Anterior pelvic fixation (Pfannenstiel approach): 10–15 cm transverse incision superior to the pubis. A vertical incision is established in the rectus fascia (linea alba). Rectus insertions are preserved anteriorly. A malleable retractor serves to protect the bladder.

moistened laparotomy sponge is placed posterior to the symphysis to protect it. Any rents within the rectus fascia are appreciated and the integrity of the rectus insertion is established bilaterally. Commonly, traumatic detachment of the head of the rectus abdominis from the involved displaced hemipelvis is demonstrated.

The rectus abdominis is retracted laterally and its insertion subperiosteally elevated from the pubic body and superior ramus. Formal tenotomy is avoided and the anterior insertion is preserved as much as possible. Hohmann retractors are next placed lateral to each pubic tubercle and posterior to the elevated rectus insertion. As they are within close proximity to the iliac vessels, care is directed to both positioning and maneuvering of retractors. Symphyseal meniscus excision has been advocated by some to promote intentional surgical fusion of the symphysis. The exposure is carried sufficiently lateral to allow application of a 6-holed plate. Exposure of the superior rami is achieved on the inner pelvic brim as subperiosteal dissection continues beneath the iliac vessels. The presence of a corona mortis, an aberrant anastomosis of the obturator and external iliac arteries, is sought and controlled or ligated as needed (Fig. 16.22).[14]

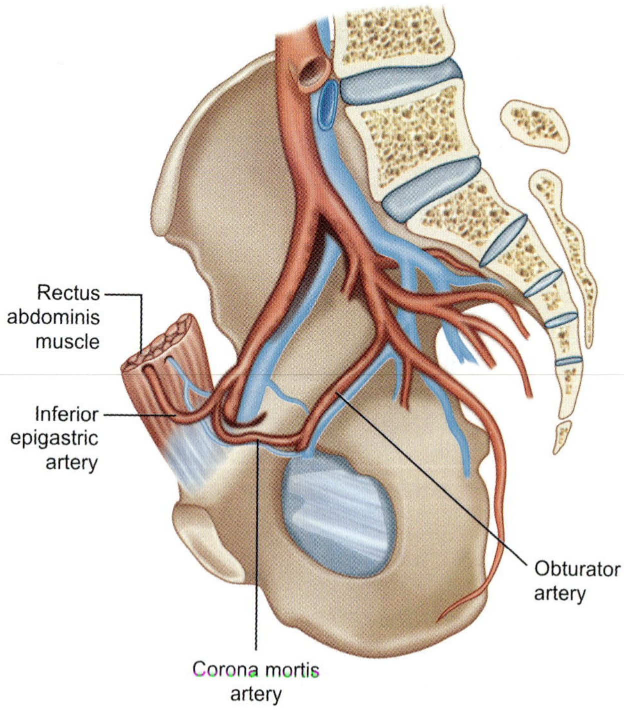

Figure 16.22: Corona mortis: Arterial connection between the obturator and external iliac systems.

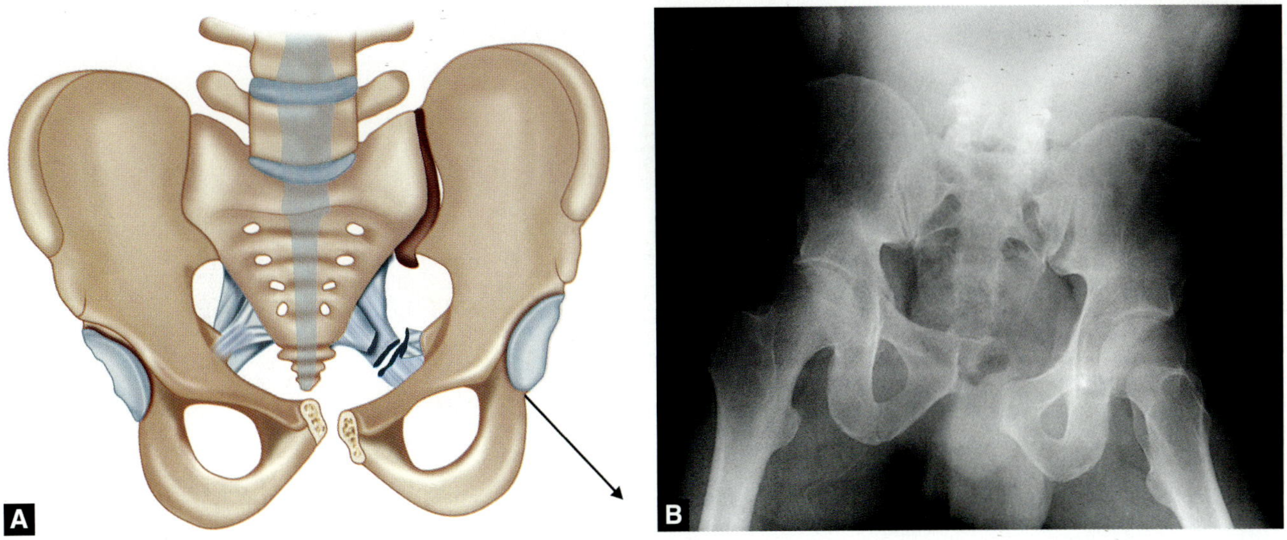

Figures 16.23A and B: Asymmetric pubic height may be apparent in the absence of vertical instability.

Occasionally, the Pfannenstiel exposure proves deficient with regard to fixation objectives. Such scenarios include fixation of lateral rami fractures which risk intra-articular implant penetration and injury to iliac vessels. This may require conversion to an ilioinguinal approach.[15]

A variety of techniques and instrumentation is available to affect reduction of anterior pelvic ring injuries. Schanz screws serving as joystick reduction aides can be placed in one or more pelvic sites. These include the iliac crest, anterior inferior iliac spine and proximal femur. Symphyseal disruption can present in company with pubic rami fractures due to lateral compression injury. The treating surgeon must recognize unstable lateral compression injury variants and the potential necessity for distraction techniques.

Subtle asymmetric pelvic height anteriorly does not necessarily denote posterior pelvic incompetence. Pure external rotation even in the presence of an intact posterior tension band will present with perceived inferior displacement anteriorly. This is owing to the obliquity of the SI joint in the coronal plane (Figs 16.23A and B).

A pointed weber reduction clamp conforms well to application on either side of each pubic tubercle (Figs 16.24A to D). It can be positioned anteriorly without violating the retained rectus insertion. Strategic placement of each tine of the tenaculum contributes to resolving the external rotational deformity. To a lesser degree, cephalad and posterior migration may be corrected. Asymmetric tine positioning may prove necessary to address multidirectional deformity. Reduction forces exerted by a weber reduction clamp are limited and adequate to address injuries of lesser magnitude. A Farabeuf or pelvic reduction clamp secured to screws (3.5 mm or 4.5 mm) within each pubic body offers enhanced multiplanar manipulation of the innominate bone (Figs 16.25A to E). This technique begins with a drill hole directed anterior to posterior within each pubic tubercle. A pelvic reduction or Farabeuf clamp captures the screw heads and properly directed vectors of force neutralize the deforming forces. Screw position and clamp orientation should not compete with the subsequent anticipated steps toward plate fixation (Fig. 16.26). Although this method of reduction may enable multiplanar mobilization, reduction within anatomic limits posteriorly, is unlikely. Prior to plate application, reduction anteriorly and posteriorly is confirmed on AP, inlet and outlet views.

Optimal plate length, gauge, as well as screw number and orientation remain controversial. A 2-holed 4.5 plate has been suggested to preserve physiologic motion diminishing risk of implant fatigue failure. It offers little control in the sagittal plane. This may contribute to construct failure, particularly when combined with vertically unstable patterns managed with insufficient posterior fixation. For most of the cases, a 6–8-holed plate with three bicortical screws on each side is satisfactory. This demands proper

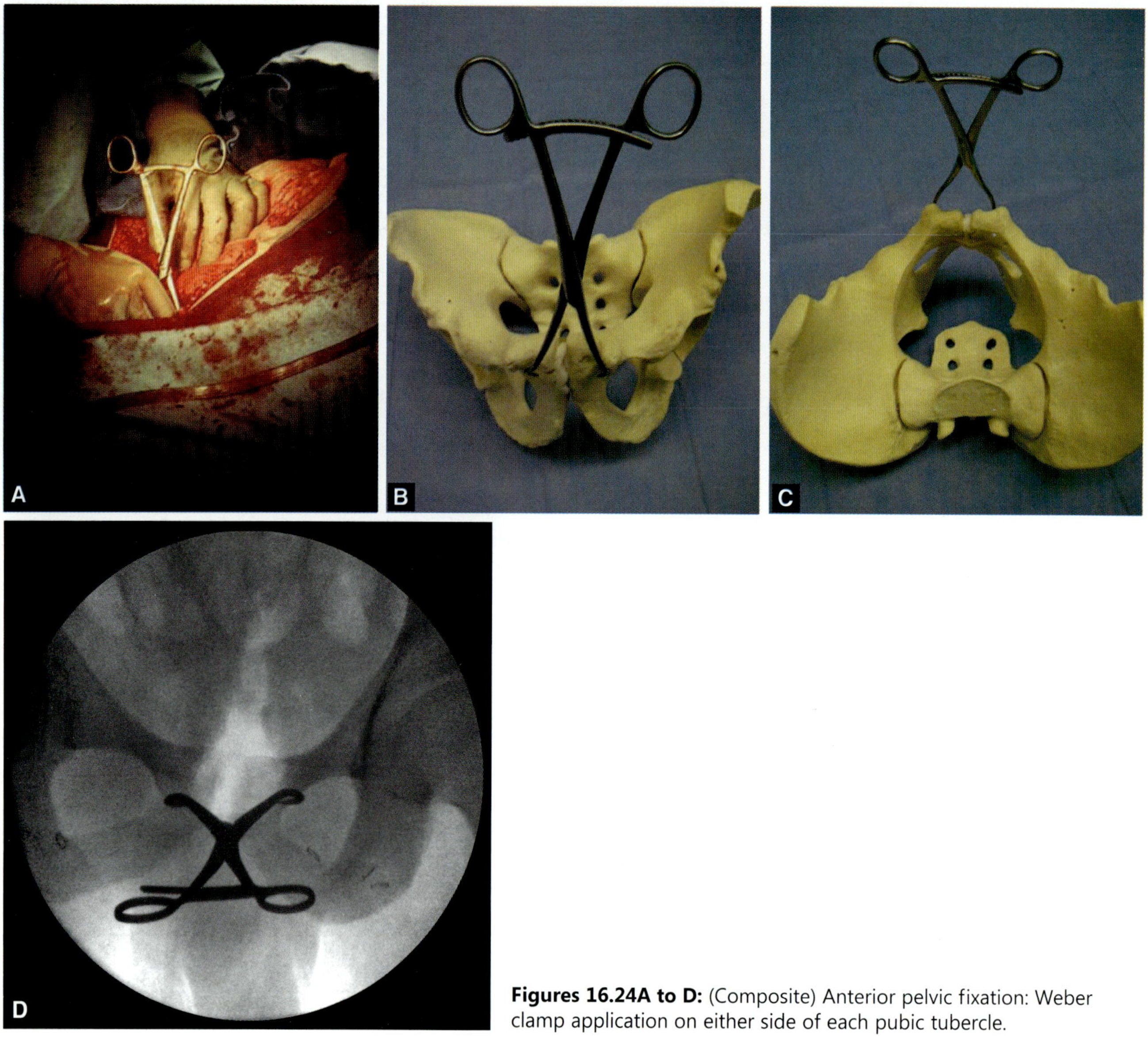

Figures 16.24A to D: (Composite) Anterior pelvic fixation: Weber clamp application on either side of each pubic tubercle.

indication and adequate posterior stabilization when required. Precontoured plates are often of thicker gauge and conform to many but not all cases applied. Any plate selected may require contouring to accommodate the pubic tubercle and curvature of the pelvis for which gender variations exist.

For anterior diastasis lesions, the plate is centered over the underlying reduced symphysis. Proper plate contour and desirable plate position at its lateral limits are confirmed. Next, it is provisionally secured with smooth wires within screw holes centrally and at its extremes laterally. Drilling is performed parallel to the posterior aspect of symphysis body to which the surgeon's digit is applied serving as a guide (Fig. 16.27A). Central screws are introduced first and are directed inferiorly toward the ischium (Fig. 16.27B). Eccentric drilling, tightening each in alternating fashion affords additional reduction and compression. The lateral aspects of the plate overlie the obturator foramen and hip joint. Accordingly, screws tend to be shorter and risk articular and obturator neurovascular jeopardy. A cephalad projection (outlet view) confirms screw length and pubic height symmetry (Fig. 16.27C). In addition to imaging studies, palpation on the inner surface of the pubis confirms reduction.

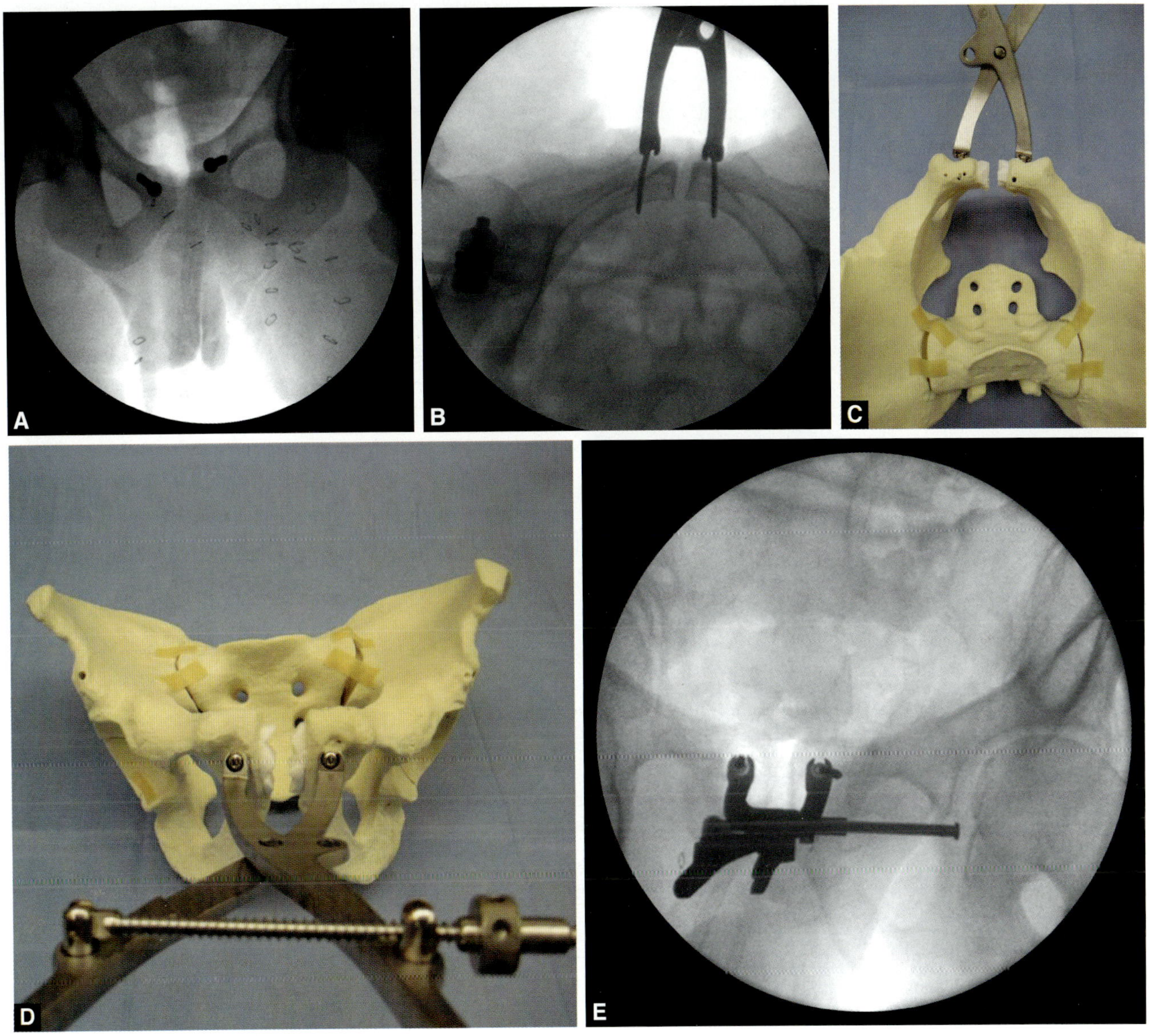

Figures 16.25A to E: (Composite) Anterior pelvic fixation: Pelvic reduction (or Farabeuf) clamp and screws. Screws are placed anteriorly in each pubic body. Deforming force vectors are neutralized and the clamp secured.

Modifications of symphyseal plating as described have been offered to enhance fixation rigidity. Pre-bending at the extremes of the plate bilaterally allows a crossing pattern screw configuration (Figs 16.28A and B). This method of screw "triangulation" permits insertion of longer screws and enhancing fixation. Trans-symphyseal plating may be considered in the presence of fracture comminution, inferior bone quality and with revision fixation (Fig. 16.29). The application of a second plate, anterior and accordingly orthogonal to the first, may enhance posterior stability. This may be applicable to vertically unstable patterns. It is however of transient benefit only and will not adequately or definitively address posterior concerns.

Medullary Ramus Screws

Plate fixation of anterior pelvic ring injuries as described is occasionally requirement of a wide surgical exposure. The dissection entailed may convey risk to regional vascular, urologic structures and a heightened risk of infection. Medullary screws inserted using percutaneous or minimally invasive techniques offer an attractive alternative.[16-18] Fixation attained offers comparable biomechanical stability to plating techniques.

These screws must be accurately positioned and maintained within the intramedullary cavity of the pubic rami. They can be inserted retrograde from the pubic tubercle directed superolaterally or inserted antegrade from the supra-acetabular region and directed inferomedially. Intramedullary diameter and anterior pelvic curvature may not accommodate screws in some individuals. Accordingly, variation in pelvic morphology may complicate and contraindicate medullary screw fixation. The rigidity of fixation is dependent on multiple covariables. Among these include bone quality, accuracy of reduction and fracture pattern comminution. Although the ambition with this technique is to minimize the complications of "surgical invasion" associated with more extensile exposures, it is not without potential peril. Extraosseous screw placement may prove hazardous. Despite adequate biplanar fluoroscopic imaging, undesirable extramedullary position cannot always be appreciated.

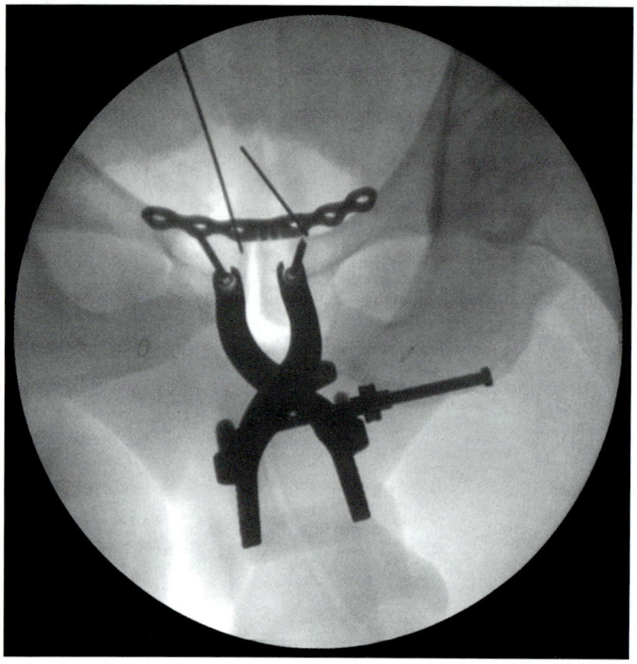

Figure 16.26: Anterior pelvic fixation: Provisional fixation of plate with wires. Anteriorly positioned pubic body screws and reduction clamp should not compete with subsequent plate fixation screws.

Retrograde medullary ramus screw: Retrograde pelvic rami medullary screw insertion is dependent upon adequate fluoroscopic imaging and tactile sensation (Figs 16.30A and B). This serves to assure intraosseous and non-articular screw position. It may be contraindicated in obese patients as thigh dimension may compromise proper targeting of implants. Another relative contraindication includes fractures lateral to the eminence which may be inadequately fixated due to insufficient distal screw purchase.

The fluoroscope, monitor and technician are situated on the involved side, the surgeon on the opposite. Patient positioning and draping should permit percutaneous posterior and contralateral pelvic access for open and closed reduction maneuvers. Low perineal access is required to enable sterile introduction of percutaneous

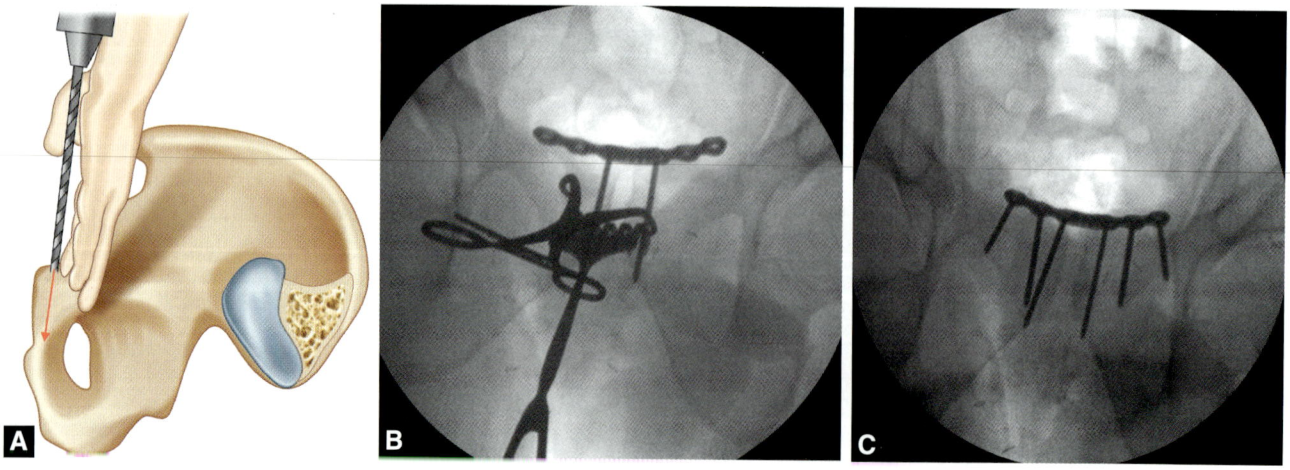

Figures 16.27A to C: Anterior pelvic fixation: Symphyseal plate fixation. (A) The surgeon's, digit serving as a guide is applied to the posterior aspect of the pubis; (B) Screws are first introduced within the central portion of the plate; (C) Screw length is assessed on a fluoroscopic outlet view.

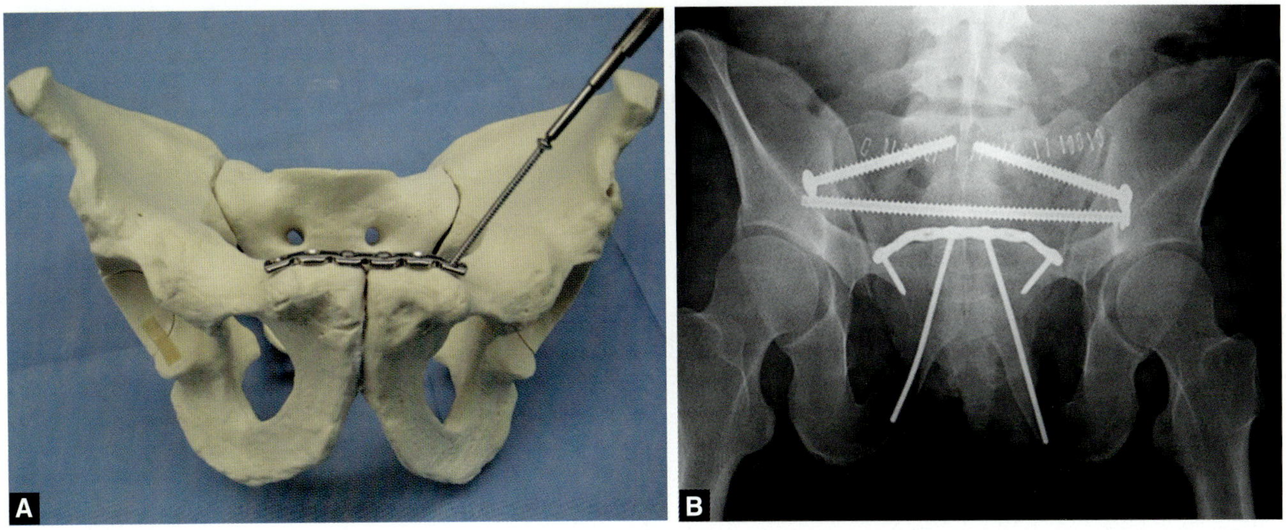

Figures 16.28A and B: Anterior pelvic fixation (Symphyseal plate fixation): Crossed screw fixation technique. (A) The plate is bent at both extremes prior to application. Screws are introduced in a crossing configuration; (B) Symphyseal plating "crossed screw fixation" technique (Postoperative radiograph).

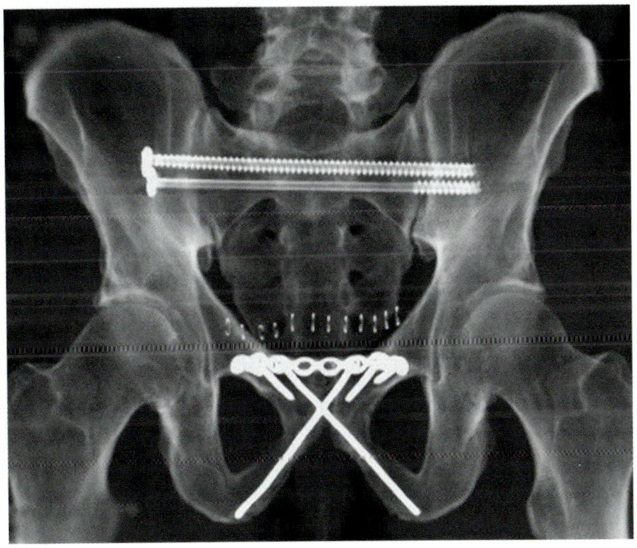

Figure 16.29: Anterior pelvic fixation: Trans-symphyseal fixation (optional; may include in anterior case revisions).

devices and implants. The inlet view determines the corridor for screw placement in the axial plane. Superimposition of superior and inferior rami on the inlet view is resolved by varying C-arm tilt. An obturator outlet view (combining outlet tilt with 20° of lateral C-arm rotation) demonstrates the safe zone for screw placement within the ramus, superior to the acetabulum.

Screws are inserted after successful closed reduction of the superior ramus. Fragment reduction and alignment should allow unimpeded intraosseous passage of drills and implants. Percutaneous joystick pins in the gluteus medius pillar, anterior inferior iliac spine and proximal femur as well distal femoral traction serve toward this goal. Lateral compression injury patterns with fracture impaction may demand distraction techniques. This is achieved with inclusion of the contralateral pelvis in an external fixator frame or with a femoral distractor. Failed closed reduction efforts are managed with open Pfannenstiel exposure. Fracture patterns lateral to the iliopectineal eminence may require a formal ilioinguinal dissection.

An ideal starting point just inferior to the pubic tubercle and lateral to the symphyseal meniscus is identified fluoroscopically. This is aided by a small caliber Kirschner (K)-wire on both pelvic inlet and obturator outlet views. The designated percutaneous portal is typically at the level of the contralateral pubic tubercle. Blunt dissection is next carried to the level of the injured pubic tubercle and a 3.5 mm drill sleeve introduced over the K-wire. A 3.5 mm drill is exchanged for the wire and a unicortical "pilot" gliding hole established. Next, a calibrated oscillating 2.5 mm drill bit is advanced retrograde within the pubis/rami under biplanar (inlet/obturator outlet) image control. It is advanced cephalad to the hip joint exiting the ilium laterally. Caudal and anterior misdirection risks intra-articular penetration. Screw length is determined and a 3.5 mm screw is advanced under image control. Although the cortical bone of the ilium laterally is a desirable target, fixation strength may be independent of screw length. Fixation stability next is assessed with a fluoroscopic manual stress view.

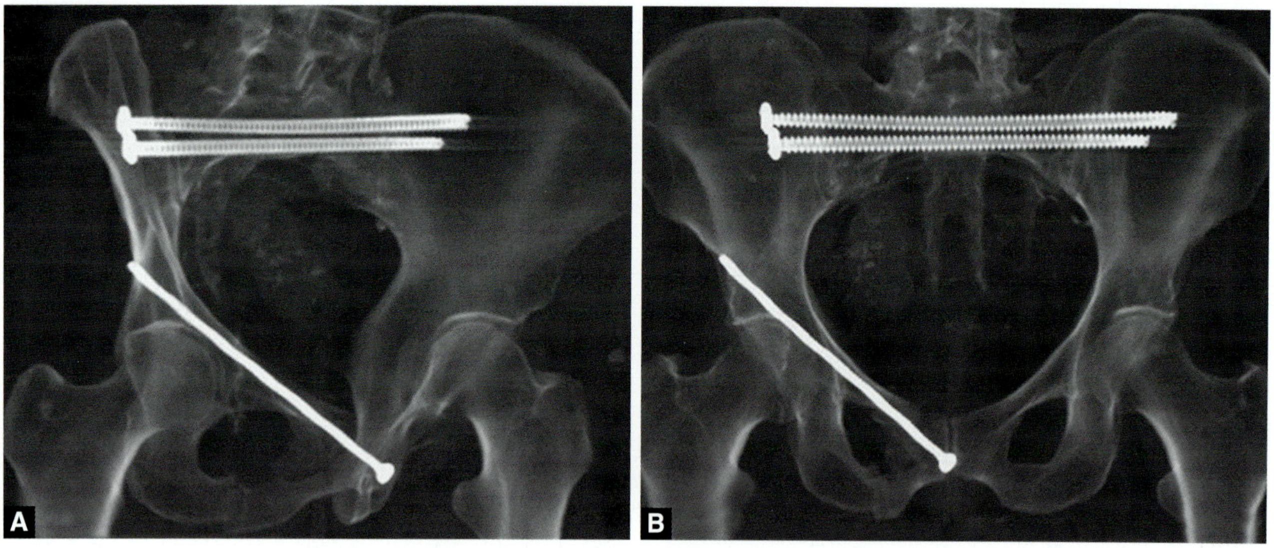

Figures 16.30A and B: Pubic rami medullary fixation (retrograde).

Retrograde medullary screw fixation may prove problematic in the presence of small or comminuted medial parasymphyseal fractures. In this scenario including those with impaired bone quality, medial screw purchase may prove deficient. An effective modification (trans-symphyseal fixation) in which the contralateral uninvolved pubic body is included in the fixation construct may be considered. The drill and subsequently screw are introduced in the adjacent uninvolved pubic tubercle traversing the symphysis, affording enhanced medial anchorage. Parasymphyseal fractures in combination with diastasis injuries of the symphysis pose an operative dilemma. Both lesions can be addressed with plate fixation alone. Retromedullary fixation of the rami fractures does not obviate plate fixation of the symphysis. Screw fixation of the ramus prior to symphyseal fixation facilitates manipulation and reduction of symphysis. Forceful symphyseal reduction efforts are unlikely to contribute to the displacement of rami fracture. The previously inserted retrograde medullary screw should not interfere with subsequent plate application.

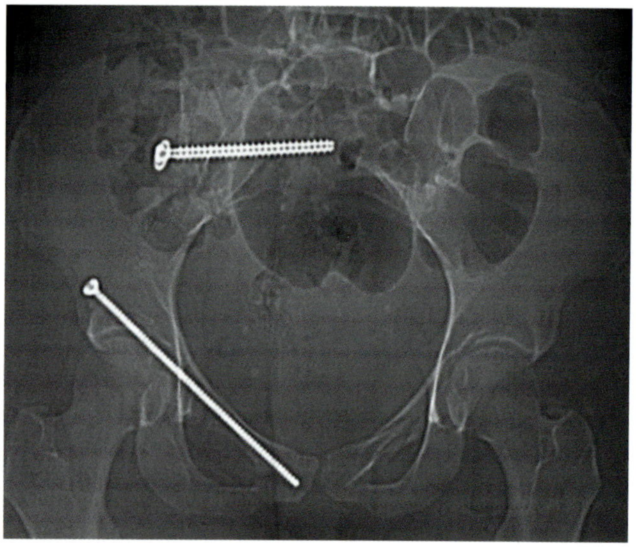

Figure 16.31: Pubic rami medullary fixation (antegrade).

Antegrade medullary ramus screw: Fractures lateral to the iliopectineal eminence require longer screw lengths to engage the lateral fragment adequately (Fig. 16.31). These screws in this setting risk intra-articular penetration and underperform biomechanically. Antegrade directed screws may be preferred particularly while managing fractures lateral to the obturator foramen. The sequence of steps is similar to retrograde screw insertion. The pelvic inlet view helps initiate a starting point along the gluteus medius pillar. Proper guidewire position is further confirmed on an obturator outlet view to direct cranial to caudal direction. Care is directed toward establishing a single soft tissue conduit through the tensor fascia lata. A 3.5 mm unicortical glide hole permits the entry of the blunt end of a guidewire. This helps to verify intramedullary passage. A 2.5 mm oscillating drill is directed within the intracortical path employing tactile and fluoroscopic guidance to diminish the risk of cortical penetration. Drilling continues until the far cortical limit is identified. A screw of determined length is inserted with the aid of image guidance.

ANTERIOR PELVIC FIXATION: Pearls and Pitfalls

- Screw "triangulation" with symphyseal plating allows longer crossing screws to enhance fixation
- Whereas, medullary screws provide minimally invasive anterior ring fixation, variation in pelvic morphology and poor imaging may complicate and contraindicate medullary screw fixation due to the potential for neurovascular injury
- Small or comminuted medial parasymphyseal fractures can be problematic for medullary screw fixation in which "trans-symphyseal fixation" may prove helpful

Technique 3: Iliosacral Screw Insertion

Iliosacral screw insertion is a well accepted method toward retropelvic fixation.[19,20] In their original description, Matta and Saucedo advocated open techniques of reduction in the prone position. Applicable described injury patterns include diastasis of the SI joint, as well as sacral fractures. Additional covariables that require consideration include severity of displacement, patient comorbidities, anterior pelvic traumatic lesions and anticipated required reduction maneuvers. This has significant impact on selection of open versus percutaneous techniques and patient positioning (supine vs open). Open reduction of SI diastasis can be managed in both the prone and supine positions. Sacral fractures requiring open methods of reduction demand prone positioning.

Percutaneous methods of fixation employing closed reduction maneuvers have been described to address SI joint and sacral fracture lesions in both prone and supine positions. These minimally invasive tactics are attractive as intrapelvic tamponade is maintained and surgical related hemorrhage minimized. Additionally, traumatically compromised retropelvic soft tissue integrity is not further violated. Supine positioning may be favored in the polytraumatized individual with respiratory impairment. Because many unstable hemipelvic injury patterns present with posterior displacement, supine positioning may favor reduction and facilitate closed reduction techniques. Prone positioning, despite proper bolstering techniques may however accentuate deformity. Another attribute of supine positioning includes anterior ring access. Simultaneous maneuvering of symphyseal and parasymphyseal (rami) structures is thus afforded (Figs 16.32A to C). This may contribute toward effective "combined" closed or open anterior and posterior pelvic reduction techniques.

Supine Considerations: Preparation, Approach and Reduction

The patient is suspended slightly on a longitudinally oriented folded sheet. This is placed directly beneath the sacrum or alternatively, the involved posteriorly displaced hemipelvis to aid in reduction. Its location should not compromise adequate sterile preparation of the region or instrument and implant insertion trajectory. The entire abdomen is included in the field to and including the suprapubic region (Fig. 16.33). The contralateral hemipelvis is included in the field to allow open and percutaneous insertion of implants and temporary reduction aids. In the event closed reduction efforts are unsuccessful, the preparation should allow open surgical access to the involved SI joint anteriorly (SI joint injuries), as well as the symphysis.

Lesions with an intact posterior tension band are often only requiring the correction of axial plane rotational deformity and anterior pelvic stabilization. These are most amenable to closed reduction maneuvers. In the absence of an intact posterior tension band, most diastasis lesions of the SI joint present with components of cephalad, flexion and external rotational ("triplanar") deformity. Ipsilateral distal femoral traction may resolve both cephalad and posterior hemipelvic migration (Fig. 16.34A). The traction pin may be placed preoperatively and isolated from the surgical field. Alternatively, it may be placed within the operative field employing sterile technique and traction rope. This latter technique permits intraoperative free and circumferential access to the lower extremity which may further aid in closed reduction maneuvers or prove necessary if conversion to open methods of reduction and fixation are pursued. Traction on the affected lower extremity may result in some undesired consequences that compromise its efficacy. These include deviation of the torso to the affected side which can be discouraged by placement of a thoracic bolster. Another concern is unintended caudal translation of the unaffected hemipelvis relative to the table. This may be resolved by either counter traction of the unaffected lower limb via a traction boot or by affixing the unaffected hemipelvis to the table via an external fixator apparatus (table assisted reduction) (Fig. 16.34B).

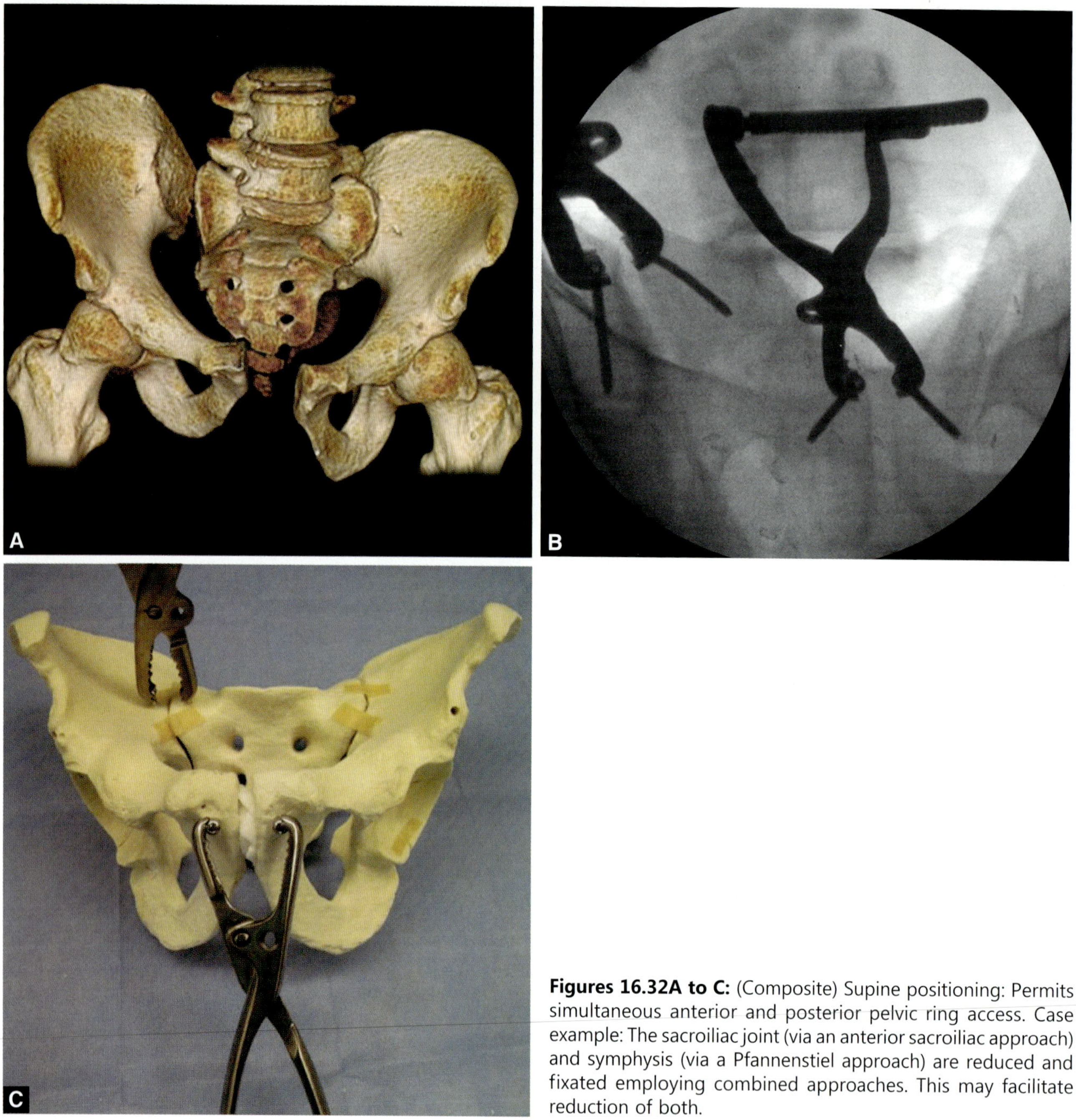

Figures 16.32A to C: (Composite) Supine positioning: Permits simultaneous anterior and posterior pelvic ring access. Case example: The sacroiliac joint (via an anterior sacroiliac approach) and symphysis (via a Pfannenstiel approach) are reduced and fixated employing combined approaches. This may facilitate reduction of both.

Several methods exist to address external rotational deformity whether in isolation or combined with other coexistent deformity patterns. Circumferential pelvic antishock sheeting is a commonly employed method for acute noninvasive mechanical pelvic stabilization may function as an operative reduction aid. Its application may offer accurate reduction of the posterior pelvis (sacral fracture and SI joint injuries). Working portals may then be established through which iliosacral screws, superior ramus screws or external fixator pins are introduced (Fig. 16.35).[21] Manual axial traction may be required with more unstable variants to enhance reduction. The sheet (approximately

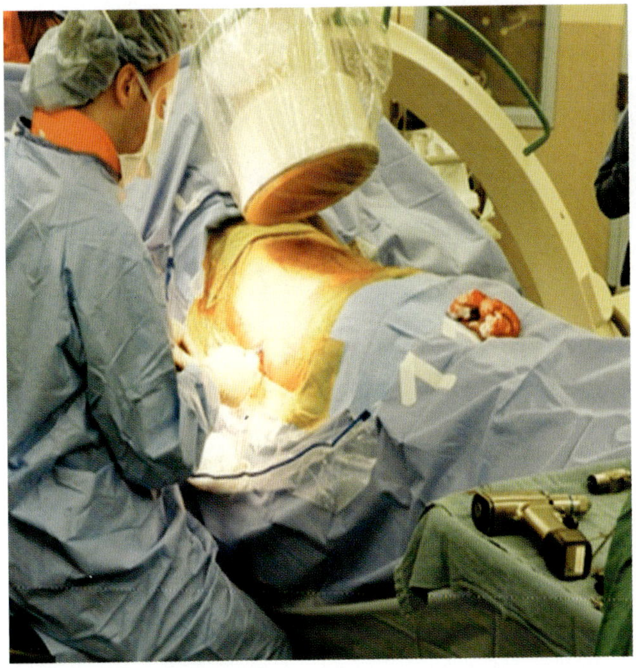

Figure 16.33: Iliosacral screw insertion (supine): Patient preparation (supine-percutaneous technique). The entire abdomen is included in the field including the contralateral hemipelvis.

3 feet wide) is circumferentially applied by spanning the iliac crests to the level of the greater trochanters. It may be shifted superiorly or inferiorly to afford abdominal access if necessary. Inclusion of the greater trochanters is crucial to affect the desired internal rotational and compression forces. To avoid soft tissue compromise, it is imperative that the sheet be applied smoothly and secured with clamps rather than a knot. Focal tissue pressure is thus minimized. A line is drawn from the anterior superior iliac spine perpendicular to the floor. This is then bisected by a line paralleling the femoral shaft. A 20 cm-diameter portal is established within the sheet centered upon this site of intersection. The skin within the portal is then sterilely prepped and draped. Additional portals can be established centered midline over the symphysis anteriorly or over the anterior superior and inferior iliac spines for purposes of Schanz pin insertion. Circumferential pelvic antishock sheeting is best suited for lesions requiring midline translation and internal rotation. It is not applicable for all variants particularly those of lateral compression type for which it may accentuate deformity and for those with sacral foraminal comminution at risk for sacral nerve root compression. Sagittal plane deformity (flexion) and vertical hemipelvic ascent require adjunctive methods of reduction.

For those cases in which circumferential antishock sheeting may be inappropriate (compromised peripelvic soft tissues, regional catheter insertion) internal rotational taping of the lower extremities may be of benefit (Fig. 16.36).[22] Much like

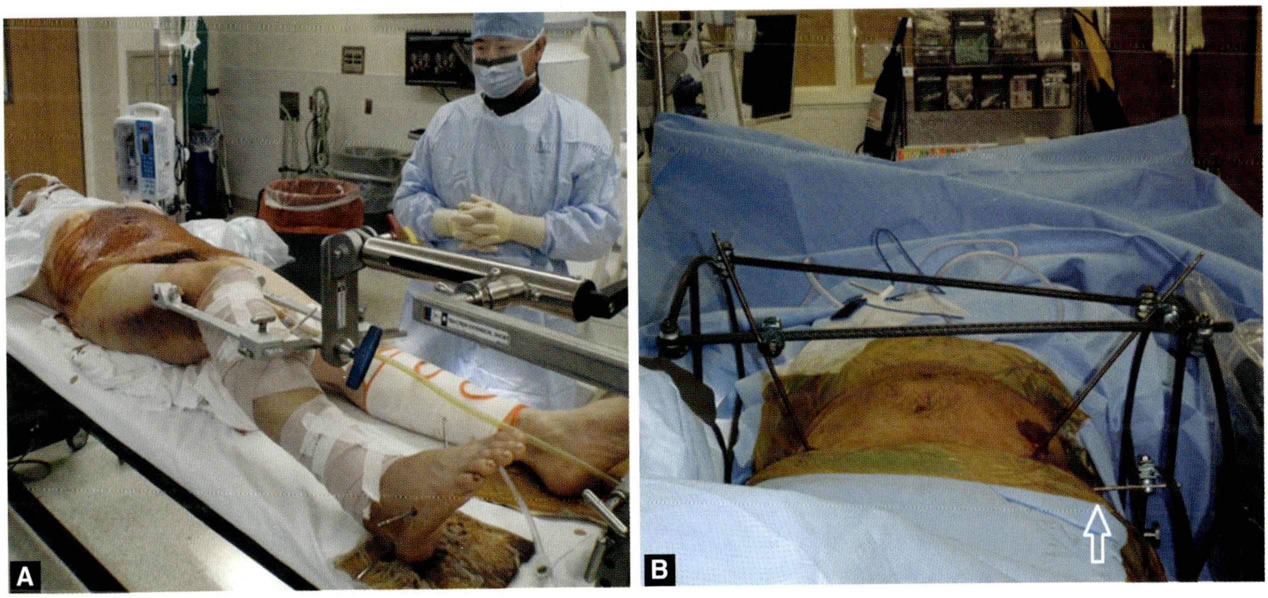

Figures 16.34A and B: Iliosacral screw insertion (supine). (A) Intraoperative skeletal traction serves to address vertical hemipelvic migration; (B) Skeletal traction can induce undesirable contralateral (uninvolved) hemipelvis migration. This can be resolved by affixing it to the table ("table assisted reduction") with an external fixation apparatus (white arrow).

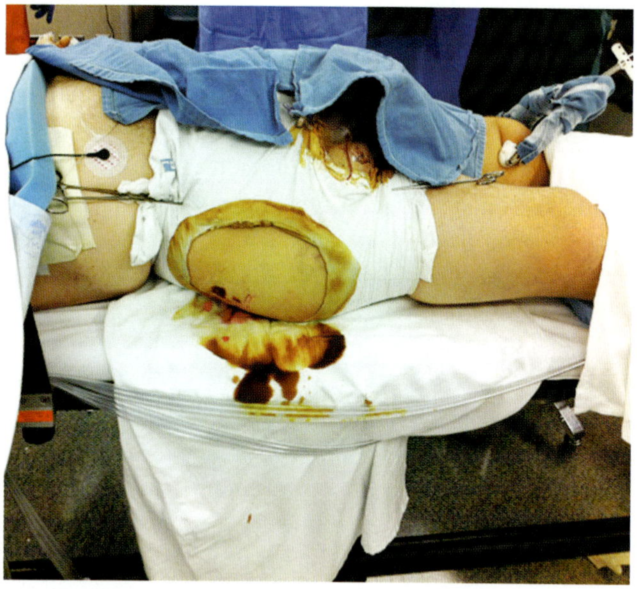

Figure 16.35: Iliosacral screw insertion (supine). Circumferential pelvic antishock sheeting working portals.

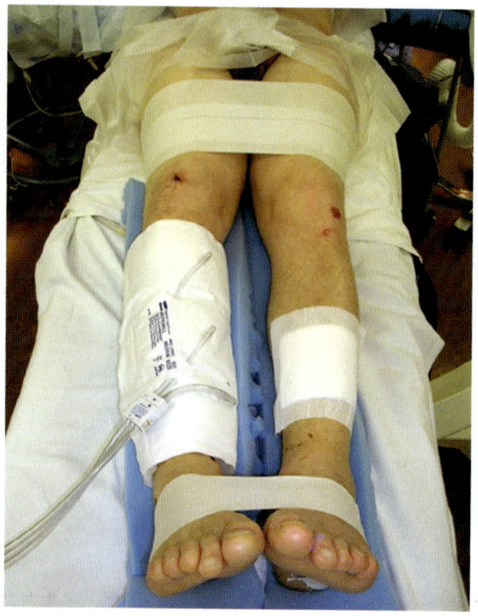

Figure 16.36: Iliosacral screw insertion (supine): Internal rotational taping lower extremities.

circumferential sheeting, it can serve both as a resuscitative and operative reduction aid. Typical application sites include the thighs and feet. Wide foam tape is applied to the already internally rotated lower extremities to limit soft tissue shear forces. Concomitant lower extremity fractures, ligamentous and soft tissue lesions must be identified prior to application. Circumferential and excessive forceful tape application should be avoided, particularly in regions of potential regional nerve compression or vulnerable subcutaneous osseous surfaces. This method of indirect reduction is most applicable in anterior compression type pattern cases, particularly in the presence of an intact posterior tension band. These techniques diminish or eliminate the need for intraoperative reduction instruments which can hinder intraoperative fluoroscopic imaging.

On occasion, multiple and more complicated vectors of force must be strategically oriented to counter multiplanar deformity. Fluoroscopic guided percutaneous insertion of Schanz pins serving as joysticks within the anterior superior and inferior iliac spines and pubic tubercle may serve these demands. Unlike pins within the crest, supra-acetabular pins (refer to external fixation section) offer purchase along the length of ilium to the depths of the posterior superior iliac spine (posterior to the SI joint) (Fig. 16.37A). A biomechanical study has suggested efficacy to be maintained with such pins introduced only as far as half this distance (approximately 70 mm).[23] Additionally these are advantageously within the plane of external rotational deformity. A femoral distractor in compression mode secured to these pins can exert a medially directed force imparting perpendicularly directed compression along the SI joint (Figs 16.37B to D).[24] Cephalad displacement may still be requiring longitudinal traction techniques. Unless specifically secured in distraction mode, external fixator application may exacerbate lateral compression injuries contributing to malreduction and deformity.

A more direct method of posterior reduction affording greater compressive force is the application of a pelvic C-clamp.[25-27] Various sites of application have described each with unique attributes and anatomic hazards. Indirectly, SI joint compression can be achieved by application at the greater trochanters comparable to a pelvic sheet or binder. This midsagittal site of application described as "coplanar" to the anterior and posterior pelvic ring elements affords compression to both. Alternatively, it can be positioned more posteriorly collinear with the SI joint.[28] Application at the S2 level is preferred as it offers satisfactory reduction efficiency without compromising access to S1 for purposes of iliosacral screw insertion.[29] This technique is discouraged in the presence of iliac wing fractures within proximity of the site of C-clamp application. The use of the pelvic C-clamp may

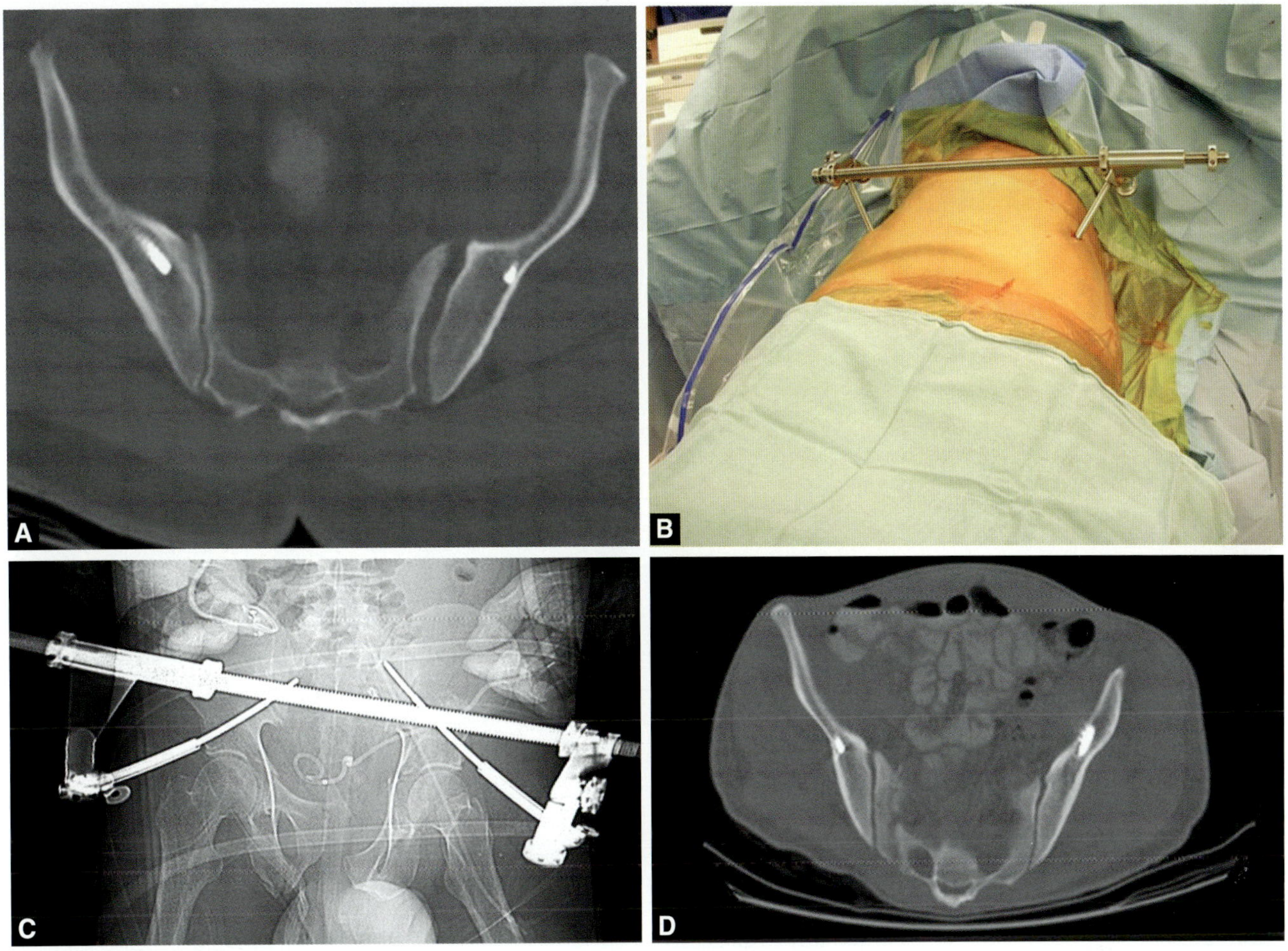

Figures 16.37A to D: Iliosacral screw insertion (supine). (A and B) Pelvic compressor: Pins are placed in the supra-acetabular region within the tables of the posterior hemipelvis to the level of the sacroiliac joint; (B) A femoral distractor in compression mode is applied; (C) An effective reduction force is applied; (D) Post reduction CT scan demonstrates improved posterior ring reduction.

aggravate nerve root compression in the presence of sacral foraminal comminution.

Described manipulation and reduction maneuvers are performed under fluoroscopic guidance. Adequacy of reduction of the SI joint is best appreciated on a tangential obturator-oblique inlet "rollover" view (Figs 16.38A and B). The quality of reduction of the anterior elements of the pelvic ring is assessed as well. Malreduction anteriorly is often accompanied by inaccurate posterior reduction. An accurate anterior reduction however does not ensure a satisfactory posterior reduction. The most common residual deformity after closed manipulation is posterior displacement of the ilium relative to the sacrum (Figs 16.39A and B). Pure lateral translation may persist despite otherwise successful reduction maneuvers. This can be addressed and final reduction accordingly achieved by accurate iliosacral screw placement (with proper insertion site and trajectory).

Inability to affect a satisfactory reduction may be secondary to entrapped debris within the SI joint. This may necessitate open techniques permitting anterior access to the joint (Fig. 16.40). Additional obstacles toward satisfactory reduction include delay in treatment and an excessively internally rotated contralateral hemipelvis disallowing satisfactory anterior reduction. Complete SI diastasis in which the posterior tension band is rendered incompetent may defy previously described less invasive methods of reduction. Ineffectual such efforts may require open methods of reduction.

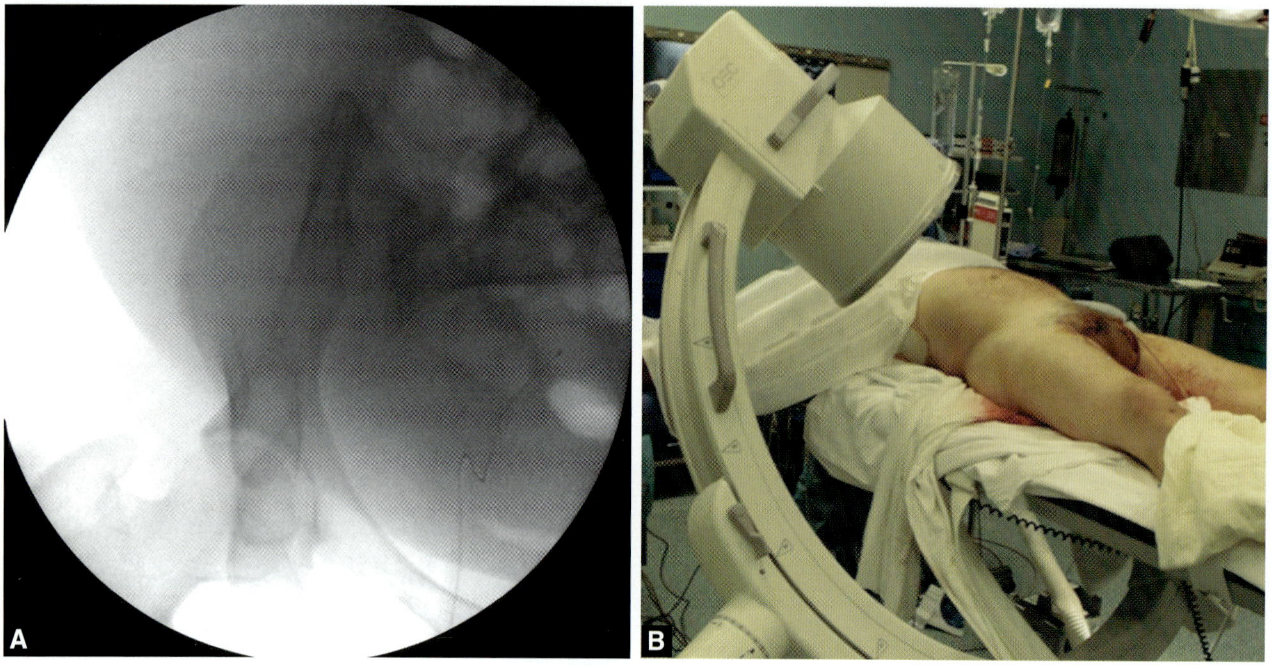

Figures 16.38A and B: Iliosacral screw insertion (supine). (A) Sacroiliac joint reduction is assessed on a fluoroscopic obturator-oblique inlet "rollover view"; (B) Fluoroscope position for obturator–oblique inlet "rollover" view.

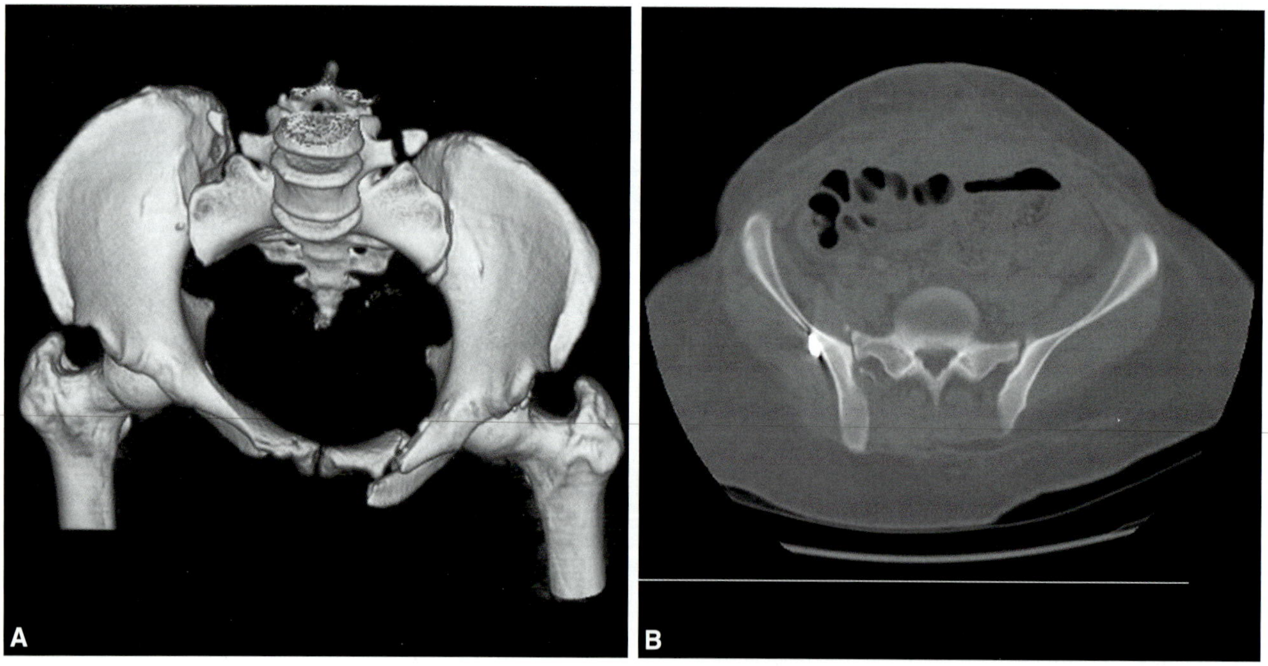

Figures 16.39A and B: Postfixation malreduction. Posterior displacement of the sacrum relative to the ilium is the most common residual deformity after fixation employing closed reduction and percutaneous fixation techniques. (A) Preoperative 3D reconstruction; (B) Postsurgical axial CT scan image.

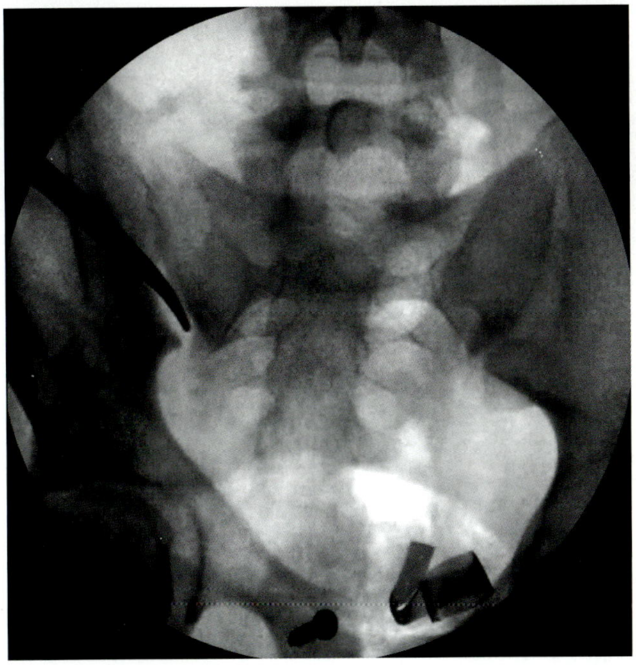

Figure 16.40: Retained osteochondral debris within the sacroiliac joint may complicate reduction. The sacroiliac joint was accessed anteriorly and a clamp introduced within it to remove interposed soft tissue and debris.

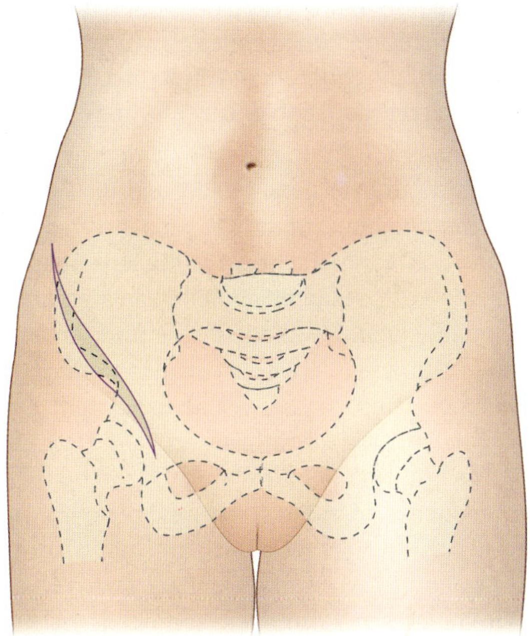

Figure 16.41: Iliosacral screw insertion (supine): Sacroiliac joint (anterior) approach. An incision is established laterally over the pelvic brim and carried as required, inferiorly to the level of the anterior superior iliac spine.

Open access to the SI joint anteriorly in the supine position may be of benefit in the event closed reduction maneuvers are unsuccessful. It offers more direct methods of reduction including visual assessment of the accuracy of reduction (superior limit of the joint). In contrast to prone positioning, retropelvic soft tissues are not threatened and simultaneous access to the anterior pelvic ring is permitted which may facilitate reduction efforts. Proximity to the lumbosacral plexus (L5 and S1 nerve roots) does demand an accurate presurgical assessment of the status of these structures, as well as care with regard to positioning of retractors and reduction device aids. This approach is inappropriate in the presence of sacral fractures as methods for reduction and assessment of are not afforded.

Surgical access to the SI joint anteriorly exploits the superior limit of the Smith-Peterson approach (equivalent to the lateral window of the ilioinguinal approach). The ipsilateral leg is draped free permitting flexion of both the hip and knee. This serves to facilitate both subperiosteal dissection and reduction maneuvers in addition to diminishing tension on the femoral nerve. An incision is established laterally over the pelvic rim and carried anteriorly to the level of the anterior superior iliac spine if required (Fig. 16.41). The lateral femoral cutaneous nerve is at risk and should be sought, identified and protected. Subcutaneous dissection is completed and the external oblique detached from the iliac crest. The iliacus is next elevated from the inner ilium and subperiosteal dissection carried posteriorly to the SI joint and the anterior portion of sacral promontory. Inspection within the SI joint is performed to extract any entrapped osteochondral debris and soft tissues. Blunt dissection and gentle soft tissue elevation on the sacral side follow with care to limit injury to the L5 nerve root. Hohmann retractors placed anterior and posterior to the sacral promontory serve to enhance visualization.

The majority of complete diastasis lesions of the SI joint present with combined deformity patterns of both external rotation and vertical hemipelvic migration. Indirect reduction methods previously described imparting longitudinal traction and internal rotation, are initially pursued under fluoroscopic guidance and direct visualization. Alternatively, owing to lesion severity, chronicity and considerable confounding muscular forces, more aggressive direct reduction efforts may prove necessary.

An asymmetric (offset) reduction clamp may effectively serve such a purpose (Figs 16.42A and B). The shorter tine is secured to the external iliac wing inserted through a small incision within the origin of the tensor fascia lata. The longer one is positioned upon the sacral ala anteriorly and superiorly lateral to the L5 nerve root. An alternate method of clamp assisted reduction incorporates the use of a Farabeuf clamp. A screw is inserted on either side of the SI joint into the sacral ala and ilium (Figs 16.43A and B). The drill path in both should be established prior to joint reduction to aid in screw path accuracy (parallel to the joint). The screw heads are maintained in a proud position to which the Farabeuf clamp is applied (Figs 16.43C and D). With either technique the surgeon must appreciate the site and vectors of force application as being beneficial or detrimental impact on joint reduction. Additionally, the location of clamp application and traction forces exerted on soft tissues should not compromise the L5 or S1 nerve roots.

When performing open reduction and fixation of the SI joint in the supine position, several caveats warrant consideration. Only the most superior and superoanterior aspect of the joint can be assessed with regards to reduction. Accordingly, a seemingly well reduced joint from this vantage point may exist in combination with an incompletely reduced posterior and inferior portion of the joint (Figs 16.44A and B). Additionally, although the surgeon is presented with the option toward simultaneous access of the anterior pelvic ring, definitive fixation anteriorly should be avoided prior to securing the SI joint. An incompletely reduced and surgically fixated anterior ring may impede posterior reduction. Temporary reduction of the symphysis or anterior ring elements with a clamp may facilitate posterior reduction without inherent rigidity sufficient to compromise posterior reduction efforts.

Prone Considerations: Preparation, Approach and Reduction

Iliosacral screw insertion imaging: Insertion of iliosacral screws by either open or closed techniques requires an accurate appreciation of regional soft tissue and osseous anatomy, anatomic variants and adequate imaging. This

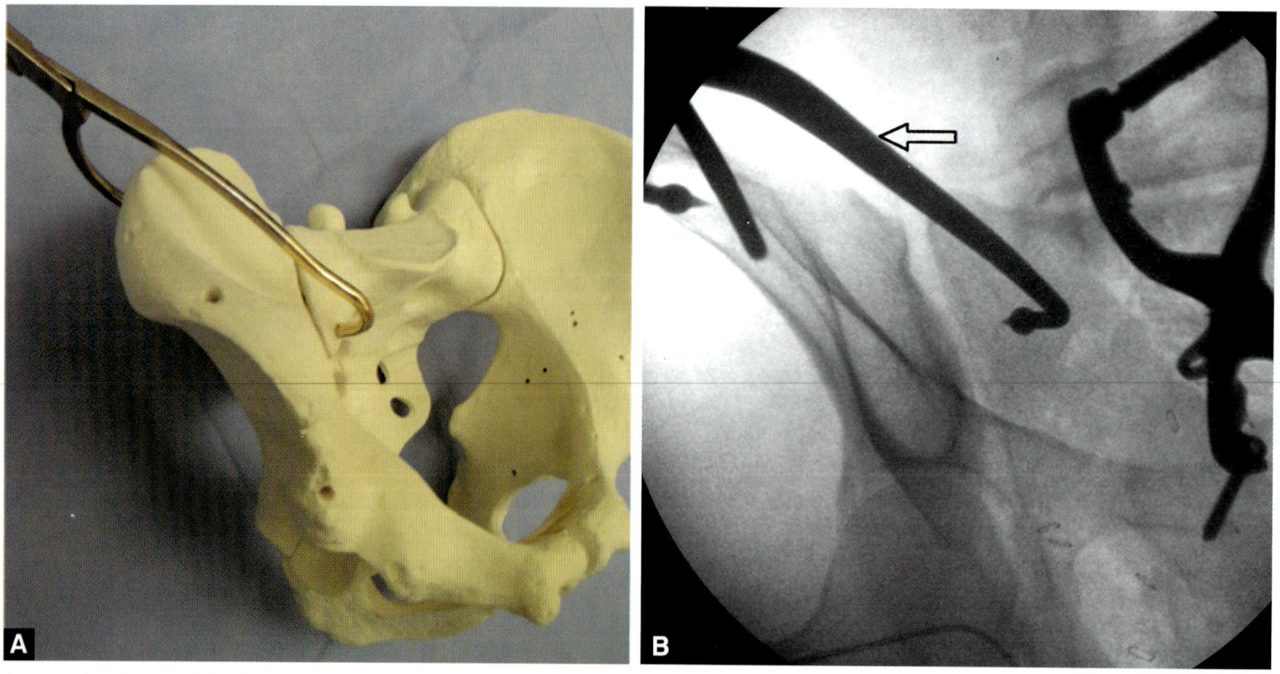

Figures 16.42A and B: Iliosacral screw insertion (supine): Sacroiliac joint reduction (anterior approach). An asymmetric "offset" clamp is applied with the shorter tine secured to the external iliac wing and the longer one (open arrow) upon the sacral ala. (A) Model depiction and (B) Intraoperative fluoroscopic image.

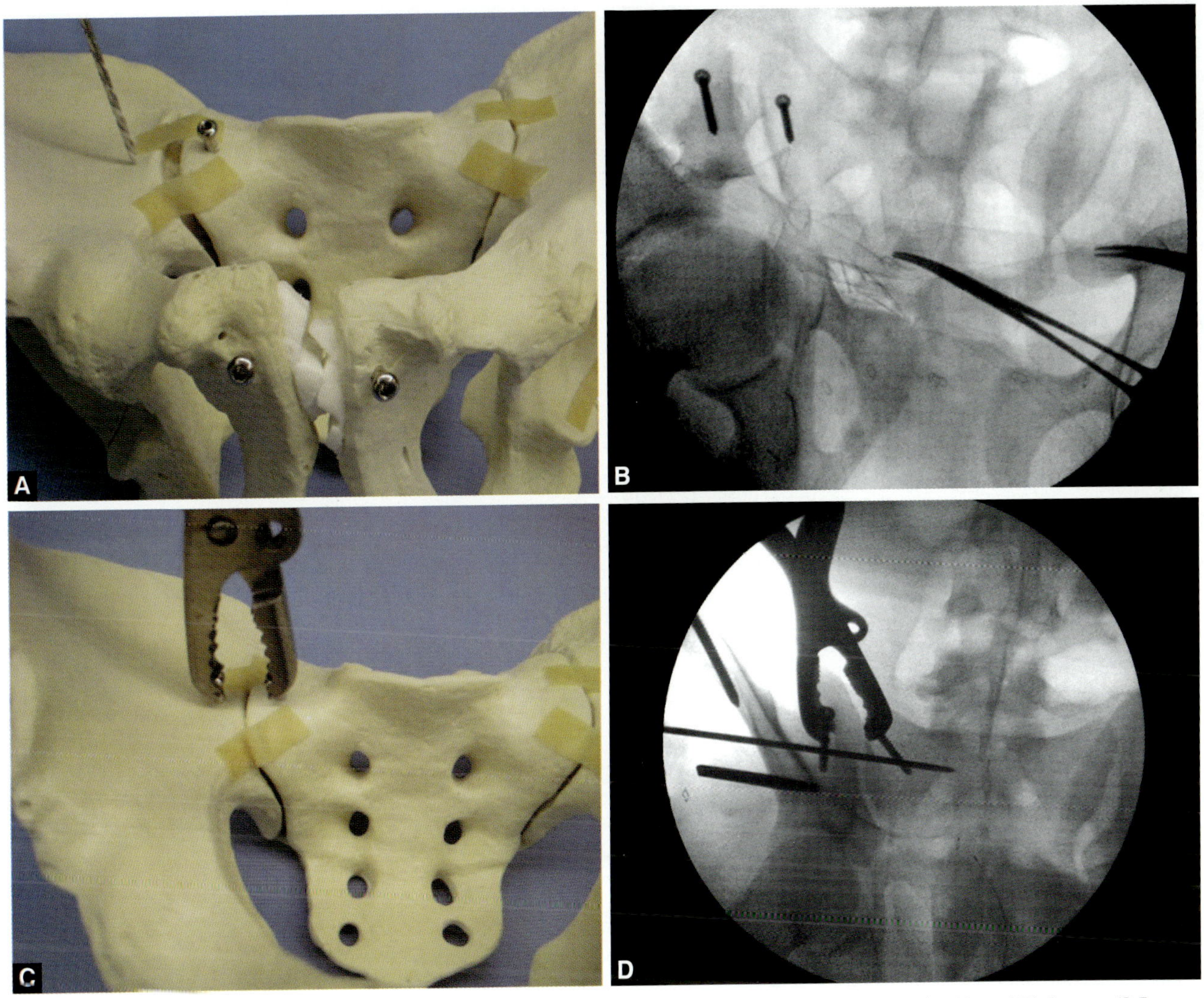

Figures 16.43A to D: Iliosacral screw insertion (supine): Sacroiliac joint reduction (anterior approach). (A and B) Screws (3.5 mm or 4.5 mm) are inserted on both sides of the sacroiliac joint in the nonreduced state. This offers an enhanced appreciation of joint inclination when introducing drills and screws; (C and D) A Farabeuf clamp is secured to the screw heads and reduction maneuvers performed.

demands a precise understanding of upper sacral morphology and pathoanatomy to determine whether the patient's unique sacral morphology possesses a "safe zone" which will accommodate screws. Both inadequate reduction of the posterior hemipelvis and inferior quality imaging preclude use of this technique.

Careful scrutiny of presurgically obtained radiographs and CT scans is performed. Conventional radiographic assessment begins with a review of orthogonally oriented inlet and outlet views in addition to a lateral sacral image. These should be correlated with subsequent fluoroscopic images obtained intraoperatively during the course of screw insertion. Any dysmorphic sacral characteristics either unilateral or bilateral must be recognized as they may have important impact on iliosacral screw indication and technique.[30] The following studies are pursued both with preoperative conventional radiographs to establish a treatment plan and fluoroscopically during the course of intraoperative fixation.

The pelvic inlet view is obtained by canting the imaging beam 45° caudally. An ideal inlet view will superimpose the upper sacral vertebral bodies depicting them as concentric circles (Fig. 16.45A). This however will be inapparent in the presence of sacral kyphosis or sagittal

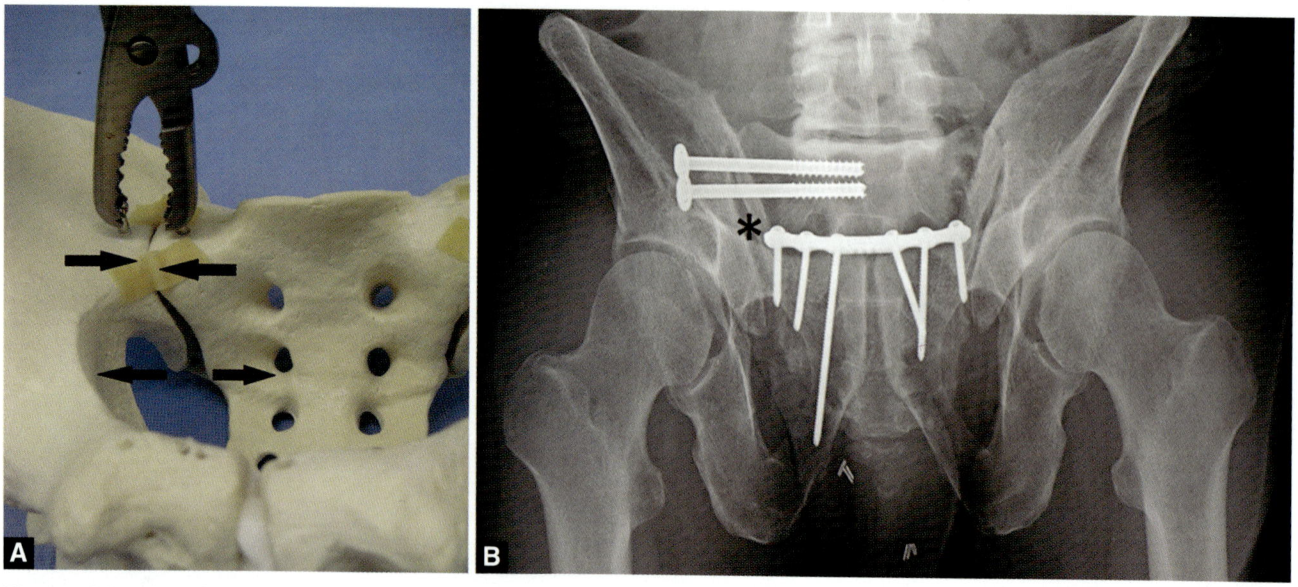

Figures 16.44A and B: Iliosacral screw insertion (supine): Sacroiliac joint reduction (anterior approach). The anterior approach to the sacroiliac joint permits reduction assessment only at its superior-anterior aspect. (A) Model, although reduction may appear adequate at the superior aspect reduction clamp techniques employing the anterior approach may render the inferior and posterior malreduction unappreciated intraoperatively; (B) Postoperative radiograph of a case in which an anterior approach with Farabeuf/screw reduction technique was employed. Diastasis of the inferior limit of the sacroiliac joint (*) remains unresolved.

plane fracture deformity. The sacral promontory is identified. Anterior osteophytes at the lumbosacral junction may render an inaccurate assessment of the anterior dimension of the upper sacral body. This may give an exaggerated impression of the safe zone for screw insertion. A review of the inlet view additionally serves to identify pelvic ring asymmetry and the impact sacral fracture or SI joint diastasis has on it.

To obtain a pelvic outlet view the imaging beam is directed 30–40° cephalad. It is most ideally demonstrated when the symphysis pubis is superimposed on the second sacral body (Fig. 16.45B). It may be, but is not necessarily truly orthogonal (90°) to the inlet view. This is dependent on unique upper sacral morphologic characteristics. Injury characteristics including vertical hemipelvic ascent and sagittal plane deformity may be observed on this view. The sacral foramen and cephalad limit of the sacral ala ("sacral slope") are inspected. From a radiographic perspective, the apparent superior limit of the sacrum actually represents its posterior aspect only (Figs 16.46A and B). It is the uppermost limit of an anteriorly descending slope upon which the L5 nerve root resides. Failure to appreciate this may result in errant extraosseous screw placement endangering both the L5 nerve root and iliac vessels. Although better discerned on CT axial imaging, subtleties regarding the sacral neural foramen can be ascertained from the pelvic outlet radiograph. These osseous tunnels begin superior/posteriorly originating centrally from the sacral spinal canal at the level of the lumbosacral disk space. They course inferior/anteriorly terminating as a ventral aperture. The pathway appreciated radiographically represents the corticated margin immediately superior and medial to the ventral aperture.

In addition to the aforementioned orthogonal inlet/outlet radiographs, a true lateral sacral image is obtained. Like the inlet view, anterior osteophytes at the lumbosacral articulation can and should be identified to establish a more accurate appreciation of the anterior limit of the sacral promontory. Superimposition of the greater sciatic notches facilitates accurate imaging (Fig. 16.46C). Limited magnification of the notch and hip joint nearer the beam will inhibit exact imaging overlap and should be accounted for. Any residual deformity or sustained malreduction will invalidate this view. The described technique in the presence of a well reduced pelvis will result in superimposition of the iliac cortical densities. These represent the cephalad surfaces of the sacral ala ("sacral slope") over which the L5 nerves

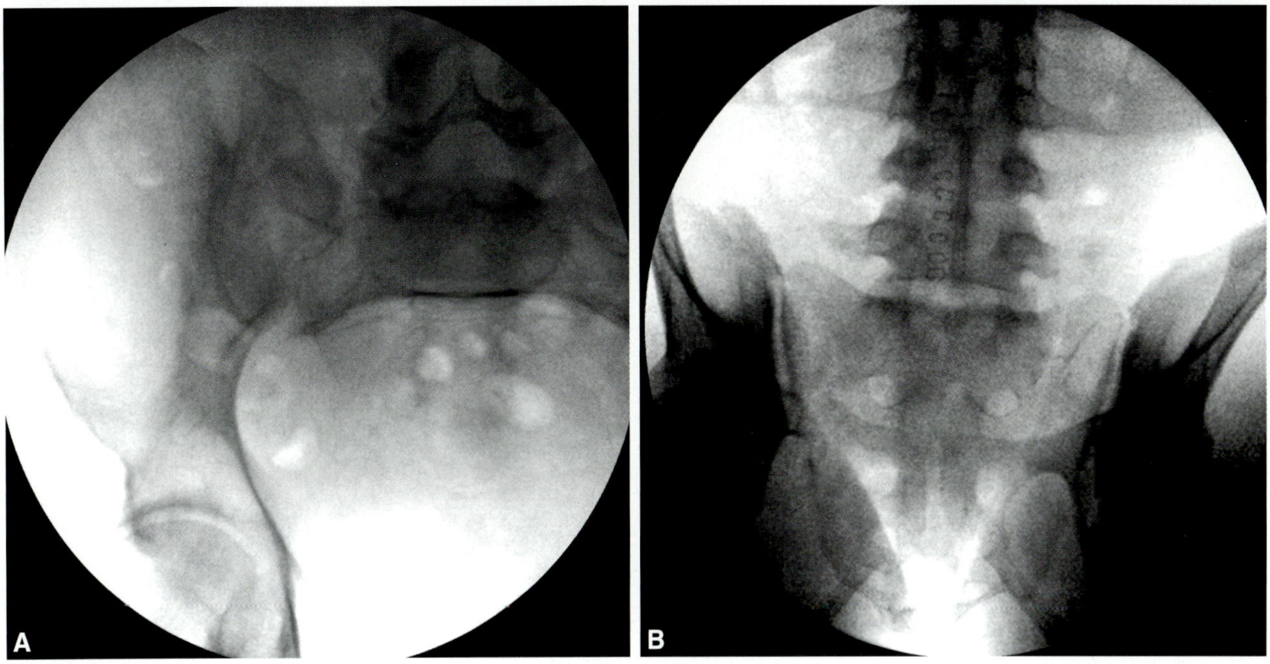

Figures 16.45A and B: Iliosacral screw insertion (supine). (A) Fluoroscopic inlet view; and (B) Fluoroscopic outlet view.

root traverses. Radiographically they present as oblique densities with varying inclination which help to define the safe zone for iliosacral screw accommodation.[31] Identification of this anatomic radiographic correlates is imperative to establish the course of the alar slope anteriorly. This serves to minimize neurologic and visceral injury during the course of screw insertion.

Iliosacral screw insertion technique: Adequate fluoroscopic imaging is an absolute prerequisite toward safe and effective iliosacral screw placement. Retained intraoperative bowel contrast agents, flatus, patient positioners and obesity may compromise required imaging of distinct anatomic landmarks rendering them ill-defined. Imaging adequacy should be confirmed prior to intubation and general anesthesia administration. Confirmation of reduction accuracy is equally important particularly when managing sacral fractures. Residual displacement as little as 10 mm may disallow safe intraosseous screw placement, jeopardizing adjacent neural and vascular structures.[32]

The fluoroscopic unit and technician are positioned opposite to the involved hemipelvis with the monitor placed within unobstructed view of both, the surgeon and the technician. Fluoroscopic tilt views (inlet and outlet) are obtained as described and magnitudes of tilt recorded for consistency and reproducibility. The arc of C-arm rotation is patient dependent and determined by individual sacral kyphosis. In addition to these an intraoperative fluoroscopic lateral image is scrutinized for accuracy and clarity.

During the course of defining optimum inlet and outlet views, lines are drawn on the operative field skin prep site (Fig. 16.47). These are perpendicular to the beam and serve as consistent references for imaging purposes. C-arm position referable to the table is recorded with floor landmarks in the form of pieces of tape.

Topographical landmarks aid in establishing a site to initiate percutaneous screw insertion (Fig. 16.48). A line is drawn on the operative site from the anterior superior iliac spine perpendicular to the floor. Next an intersecting line is drawn along the femoral shaft. This establishes four quadrants, the posterior/cranial of which serves as a cue to the skin starting position. A small caliber K-wire is directed through the abductor musculature within this quadrant under biplanar fluoroscopic control to the lateral surface of the ilium. Satisfactory starting point and trajectory are confirmed and a drill guide (2 mm) is directed over the wire. The guidewire is next exchanged for a terminally threaded 2 mm cannulated screw guide pin. The drill guide serves to protect soft tissues and aid

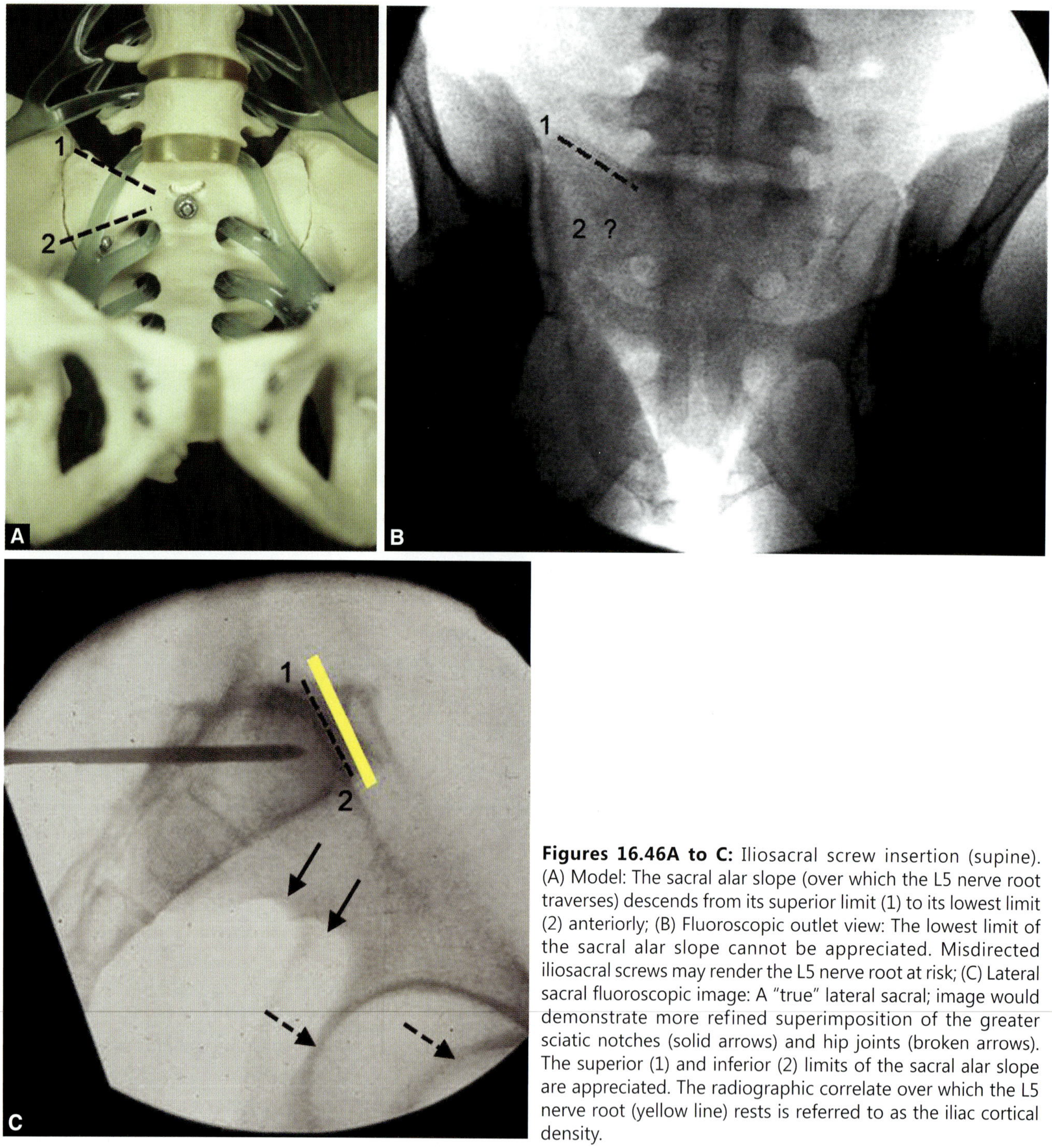

Figures 16.46A to C: Iliosacral screw insertion (supine). (A) Model: The sacral alar slope (over which the L5 nerve root traverses) descends from its superior limit (1) to its lowest limit (2) anteriorly; (B) Fluoroscopic outlet view: The lowest limit of the sacral alar slope cannot be appreciated. Misdirected iliosacral screws may render the L5 nerve root at risk; (C) Lateral sacral fluoroscopic image: A "true" lateral sacral; image would demonstrate more refined superimposition of the greater sciatic notches (solid arrows) and hip joints (broken arrows). The superior (1) and inferior (2) limits of the sacral alar slope are appreciated. The radiographic correlate over which the L5 nerve root (yellow line) rests is referred to as the iliac cortical density.

in maneuvering the terminally threaded pin while making minor directional changes as it enters the ilium. A single soft tissue path should be established and maintained during the course of these steps. It should be sufficiently dilated to allow unobstructed introduction of the screw and washer.

Guidewire starting point and its advancement are monitored with the three sacral fluoroscopic views described. The inlet view confirms pin position with respect to the sacral spinal canal and the anterior vertebral body limit, while the outlet view determines pin proximity to the S1 neural foramen (Figs 16.49A and B). Pin tip position

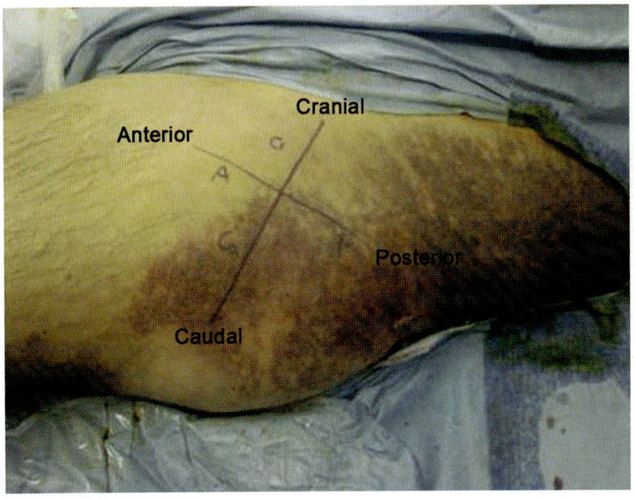

Figure 16.47: Iliosacral screw insertion (supine). Lines are drawn on the operative field to consistently reproduce preferential C-arm position. These are oriented perpendicular to the image beam (left hemipelvis depicted).

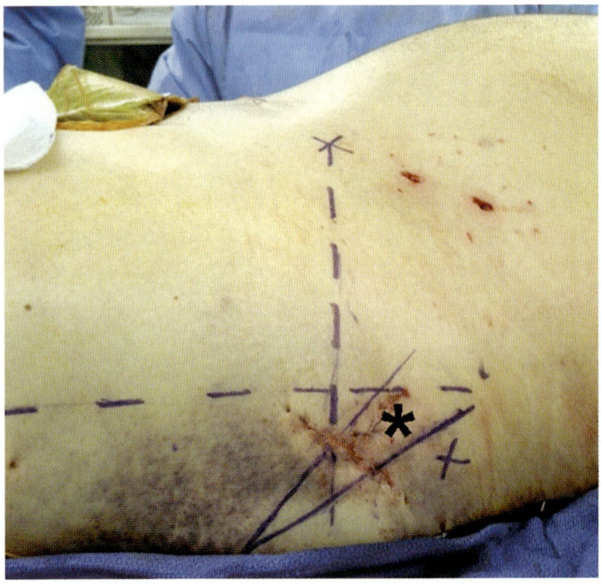

Figure 16.48: Iliosacral screw insertion (supine): Topographical landmarks. A line is drawn on the operative field from the anterior superior iliac spine descending inferiorly. A second line is drawn along the femoral shaft intersecting the first. Four quadrants are established, the posterior-superior one of which serves as a guide (*) to initiate iliosacral screw insertion (left hemipelvis depicted).

within the mid portion of sacral ala caudal to sacral slope is confirmed on the lateral sacral view (Fig. 16.49C).

At this time the guide pin is advanced until cephalad and just lateral to S1 neural foramen as appreciated on the outlet projection. This now identifies the tip relationship to iliac cortical density (ICD) which is verified on the lateral sacral view. On this view the guidewire tip should ideally be situated caudal and posterior to the ICD (Fig. 16.46C). This confirms safe position beneath sacral alar slope. It further assures that the wire tip is cranial to the neural tunnel (also visible on the true lateral sacral image), yet posterior to the anterior vertebral cortical limit. Properly executed insertion in a nondysmorphic proximal sacral segment will position the screw within the "safe zone". This is an elliptical shaped passageway bounded by the sloping sacral ala above and the upper sacral nerve root tunnel below.

The guide pin is advanced into the S1 body or contralateral alar depending on screw purpose and function. Guide pin depth is measured and the cannulated drill bit advanced over it. On occasion the guidewire may inadvertently advance ahead of the reamer if the guidewire becomes bent at its tip or incarcerated within the reamer. Accordingly in an effort to identify this and prevent intrapelvic penetration, reamer (and screw) insertion are performed under fluoroscopic control.

A 7 mm cannulated screw of appropriate length with washer is inserted over the guide pin. Excessive tightening may result in undesirable penetration of the lateral iliac cortex. To detect and prevent this, the final phase of screw insertion is performed with the benefit of a fluoroscopic "rollover" view (Figs 16.50A and B). To obtain this, the C-arm is rotated over the patient 20–30° with slight caudal inclination (obturator oblique-inlet view). This affords a tangential view of the posterior ilium to which the washer flattens out when full seated (Fig. 16.50C). Reduction and stability are next assessed with fluoroscopy and the wound is closed and dressed.

Sacroiliac versus sacral "style" screws: Iliosacral screws are ideally oriented perpendicular to the plane of disruption. Because SI joint injuries and sacral fractures occur in different planes (oblique and sagittal respectively), differing starting points and trajectories are required for each. Accordingly, screw orientation and length differ between SI and sacral fracture "style" screws. Several caveats exist common to both. First, screw pull out strength is superior within the sacral vertebral body relative to the alar region. Second, initial screw placement within the upper sacral

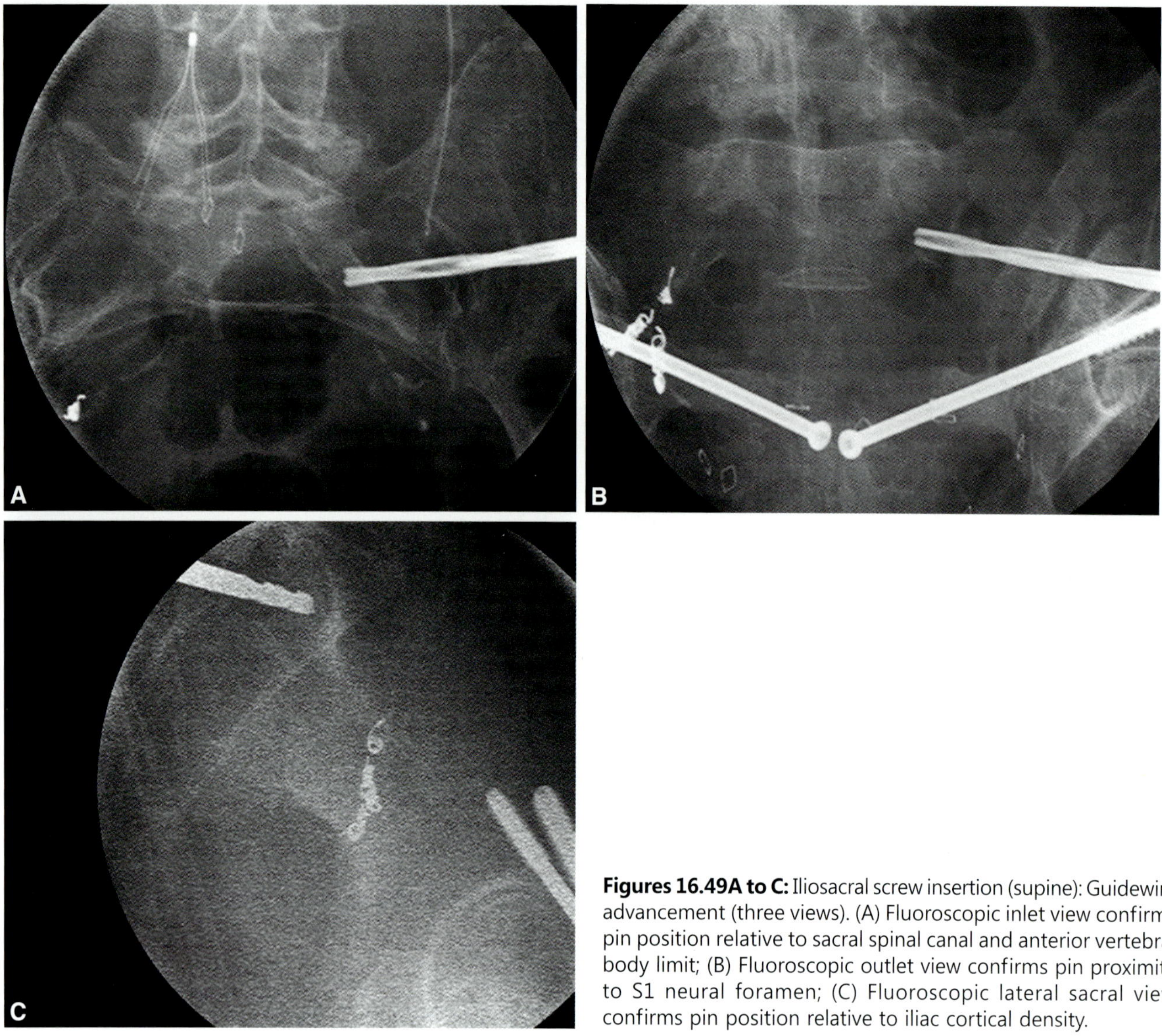

Figures 16.49A to C: Iliosacral screw insertion (supine): Guidewire advancement (three views). (A) Fluoroscopic inlet view confirms pin position relative to sacral spinal canal and anterior vertebral body limit; (B) Fluoroscopic outlet view confirms pin proximity to S1 neural foramen; (C) Fluoroscopic lateral sacral view confirms pin position relative to iliac cortical density.

segment should be low and anterior to accommodate additional screw insertion.

Sacroiliac style screws: To adopt a perpendicular relationship to the articulation, SI style screws are oriented obliquely in axial, sagittal and coronal planes. In contrast to sacral fracture style screws, they begin more posterior and caudal on the ilium and are directed cephalad and anterior (Figs 16.51A and B). They are posterior to, and uncompromising of the more anteriorly situated chondral surfaces of the sacroiliac joint. Desired final position is cephalad to the S1 neural foramen, caudal to L5–S1 disk space terminating within the body of S1. Because of its oblique orientation, these screws should not cross the midline anteriorly or risk extraosseous position. Selection of a 32 mm thread length partially threaded cancellous screw affords desired compression across the joint. If properly oriented, it may fine-tune the reduction as well. An additional fully-threaded noncompression screw serves to neutralize the construct.

Sacral fracture style screws: Sacral fractures, unlike the obliquely oriented SI joint, occur commonly in the sagittal plane. This favors a horizontally directed screw which mandates traversing the chondral component of the SI joint (Figs 16.51A to C). Longer screw lengths are thus

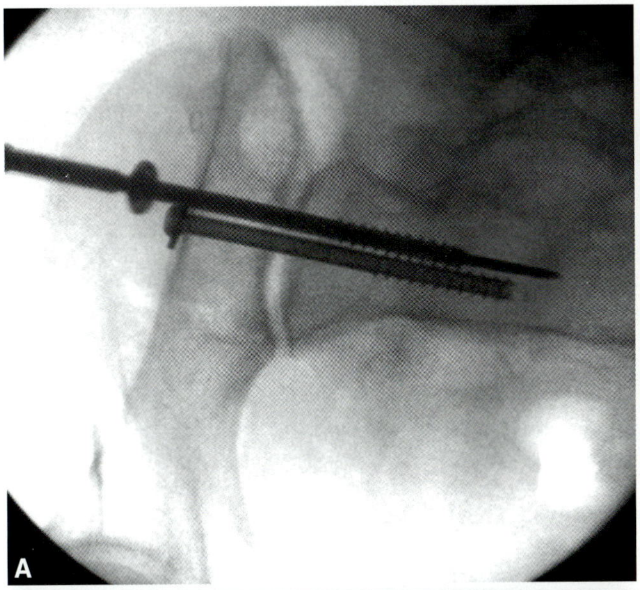

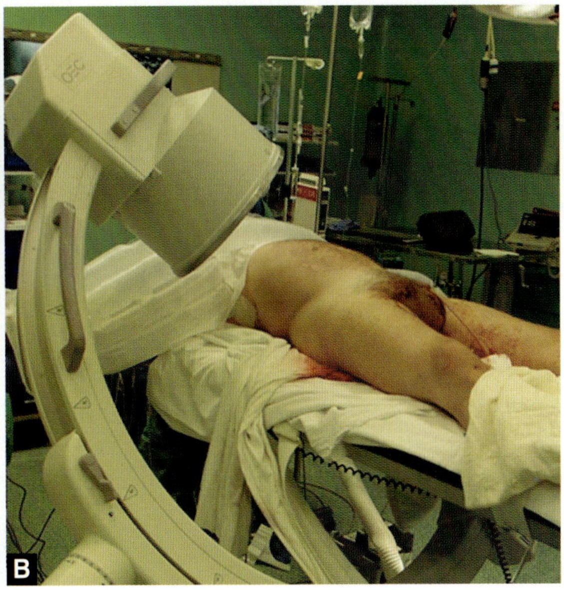

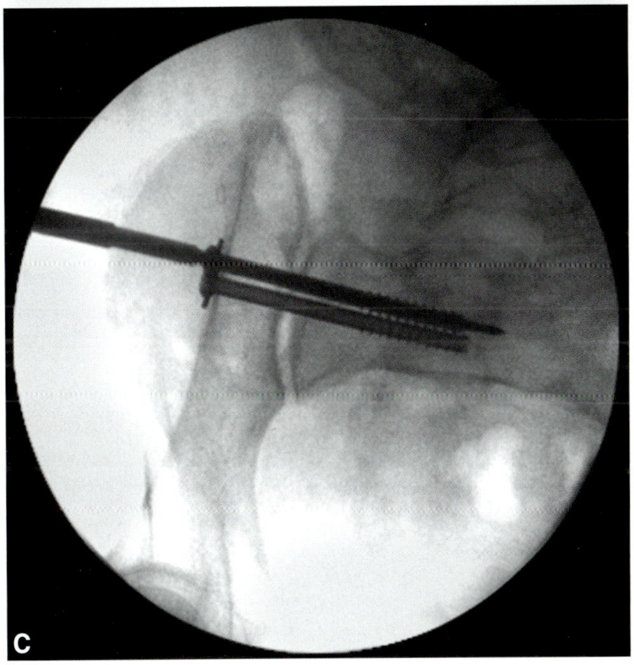

Figures 16.50A to C: Seating the screw: To avoid inadvertent penetration of the outer table of the ilium the screw is advanced under a fluoroscopic "rollover" view until fully "seated."

permitted. This is of considerable benefit owing to the more central location of sacral fractures compared to diastasis lesions of the SI joint. Fully threaded screws are well suited for transforaminal fractures at risk for neural compromise when compression is not desired.

Sacral dysmorphism: Variations in posterior pelvic ring osseous anatomy, referred to as "sacral dysmorphism" exist in as much as 30–40% of the population. Aberrant sacral morphology may complicate iliosacral screw insertion as safe zone sizes and angles for purposes of screw insertion are different and potentially less accommodating. These osseous anomalies although atypical, are fairly consistent (Fig. 16.52). Features that conform to dysmorphic criteria include (1) angulated and upsloping sacral ala, (2) colinearity of the iliac crest and the lumbosacral disc on an outlet view, (3) obliquely oriented atrophic residual transverse process ("mammillary bodies"), (4) sacral neural foramina whose anterior apertures are noncircular, (5) incomplete residual disk space between upper and second sacral segments.

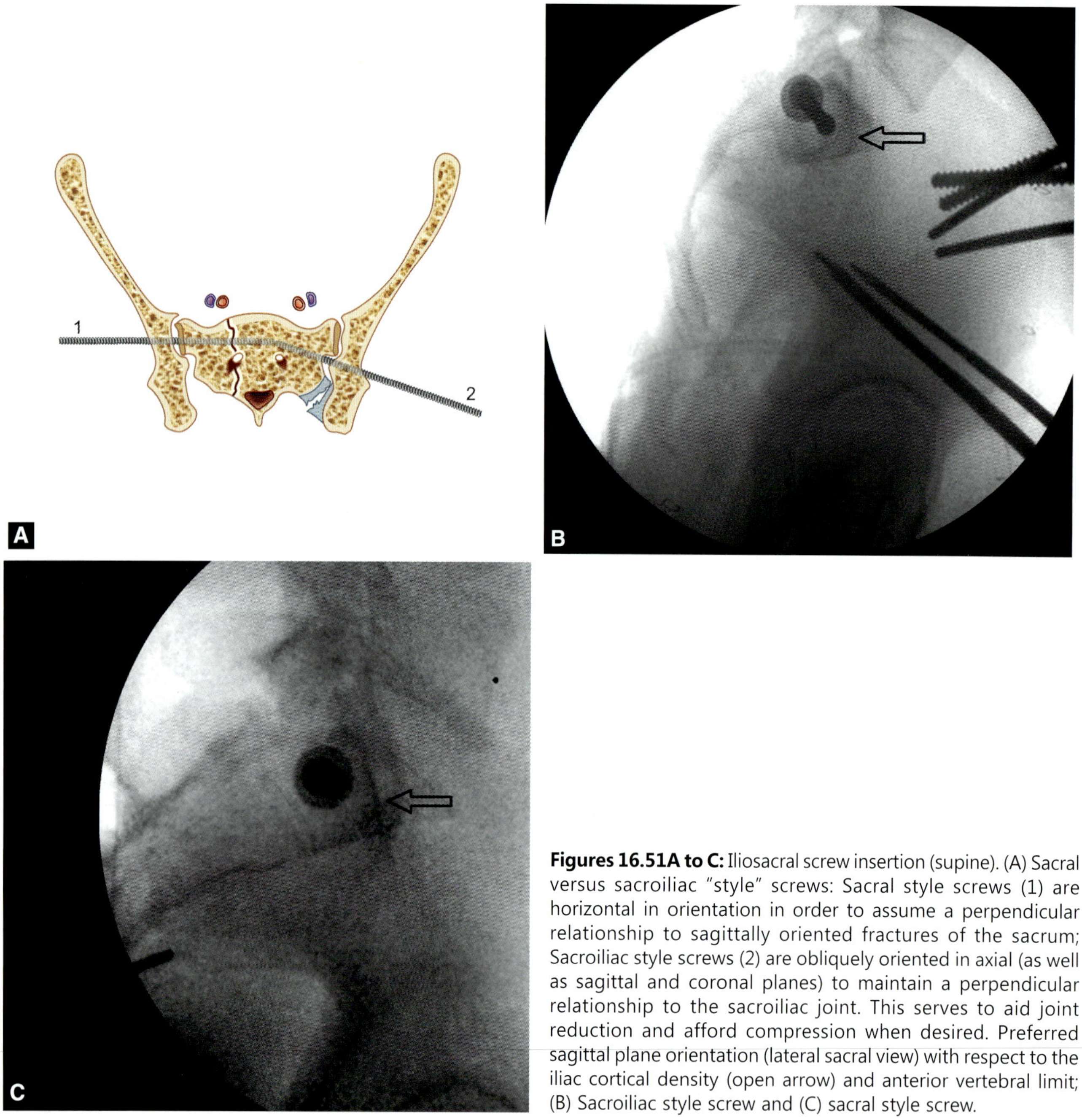

Figures 16.51A to C: Iliosacral screw insertion (supine). (A) Sacral versus sacroiliac "style" screws: Sacral style screws (1) are horizontal in orientation in order to assume a perpendicular relationship to sagittally oriented fractures of the sacrum; Sacroiliac style screws (2) are obliquely oriented in axial (as well as sagittal and coronal planes) to maintain a perpendicular relationship to the sacroiliac joint. This serves to aid joint reduction and afford compression when desired. Preferred sagittal plane orientation (lateral sacral view) with respect to the iliac cortical density (open arrow) and anterior vertebral limit; (B) Sacroiliac style screw and (C) sacral style screw.

Sacral dysmorphism may represent a continuum of sacral morphology and all criteria are therefore not required to meet this designation. Upper and second sacral safe zones are bordered by important neurovascular structures anteriorly/cranially (lumbar and sacral nerve roots) and posteriorly/caudally (spinal canal and sacral nerve roots). Errant screw placement in the presence of sacral dysmorphism may render these structures increasingly vulnerable. Screw insertion technique modifications are often accordingly required. Iliosacral screw starting points, trajectory and lengths differ between upper and second sacral segments and differ from normal variants. Required refined screw insertion techniques demand the surgeon to have a commanding understanding of these morphologic variations and radiographic correlates.

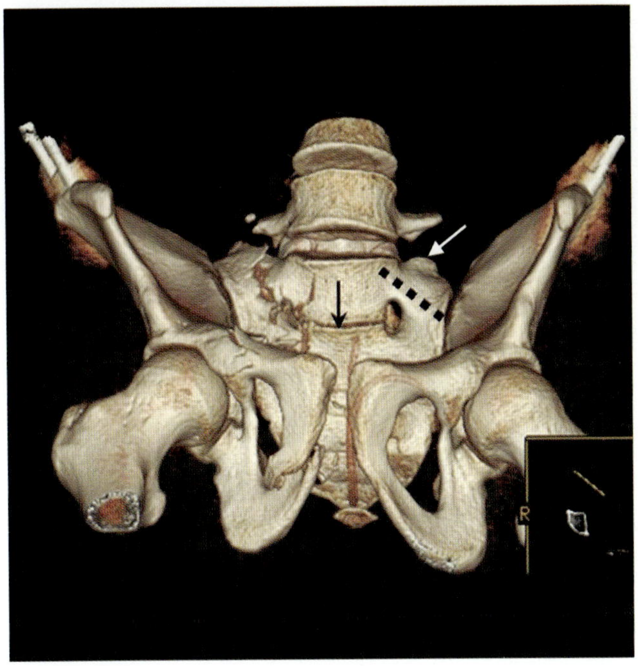

Figure 16.52: Sacral dysmorphism: (Criteria): Angulated and up-sloping sacral ala (dashed line)/colinearity of the iliac crest and lumbosacral disk on outlet view/"mammillary bodies"—obliquely oriented atrophic residual transverse processes (white arrow)/noncircular-elliptical sacral neural foramina/ incomplete residual disk—space between upper and second sacral segments (black arrow).

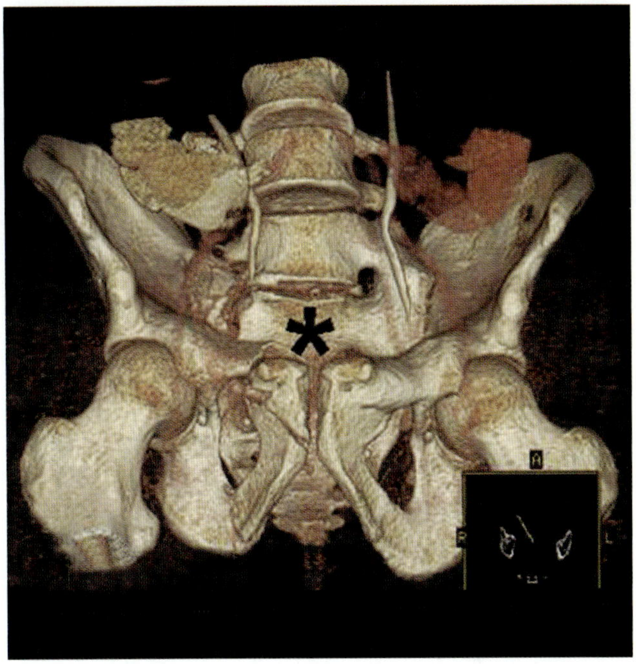

Figure 16.53: Sacral dysmorphism: The upper sacral segment is smaller and more obliquely oriented than normal variants. The second sacral segment (*) pathways in dysmorphic sacra are larger than the first sacral segment and more perpendicularly oriented. Second sacral segments in dysmorphic sacra are typically larger and more accommodating than second sacral segments in normal nondysmorphic variants.

The dysmorphic upper sacral segment zone is significantly smaller and more obliquely oriented than normal variants (Fig. 16.53). It has an increased caudal to cranial and posterior to anterior obliquity. Additionally, its safe zone cross-sectional area is over 30% smaller. This combination of variables precludes transverse screw insertion from either axial (inlet) or coronal (outlet) perspectives. Despite stenotic and obliquely oriented pathways, the dysmorphic upper sacral segment is often anatomically competent to contain a properly directed screw. This mandates a more posterior and caudally located lateral iliac cortical starting point and proper oblique trajectory (Figs 16.54 A and B). Screw length is limited by the required oblique screw orientation and the anterior sacral body cortical limit.

While the upper dysmorphic sacral segment anatomic screw pathways (axial and coronal) are obliquely oriented, the second sacral segment pathways in contrast are perpendicular. The second segment safe zone cross-sectional area is more than twice as large in dysmorphic sacral compared to normal.[33] Its capacious size and transverse orientation afford the opportunity for a screw of longer length. This second sacral potential screw pathway allows transiliac-transsacral screw placement into the contralateral lateral iliac cortical bone. The volume of bone within the dysmorphic second sacral segment permits safe passage through both neuroforaminal and alar zones. In summary, the dysmorphic sacrum has several unique and relevant morphologic features. An understanding of the unique dimensions and configurations of the dysmorphic posterior pelvis may allow multilevel iliosacral screw fixation.

S2 screws: Optimal iliosacral screw constructs with regard to screw length and number for specific injury patterns remain poorly defined. Multiplanar instability lesions have been associated with higher rate of fixation failure. Intuitively, the inclusion of more and longer screws should enhance construct stability (Fig. 16.55A). Size limitations in some patients may preclude the insertion of more than one screw into a normal S1 body. Screw order with regard to position is important to insure that both remain within the intraosseous safe zone beneath the sacral alar slope (Fig. 16.55B).

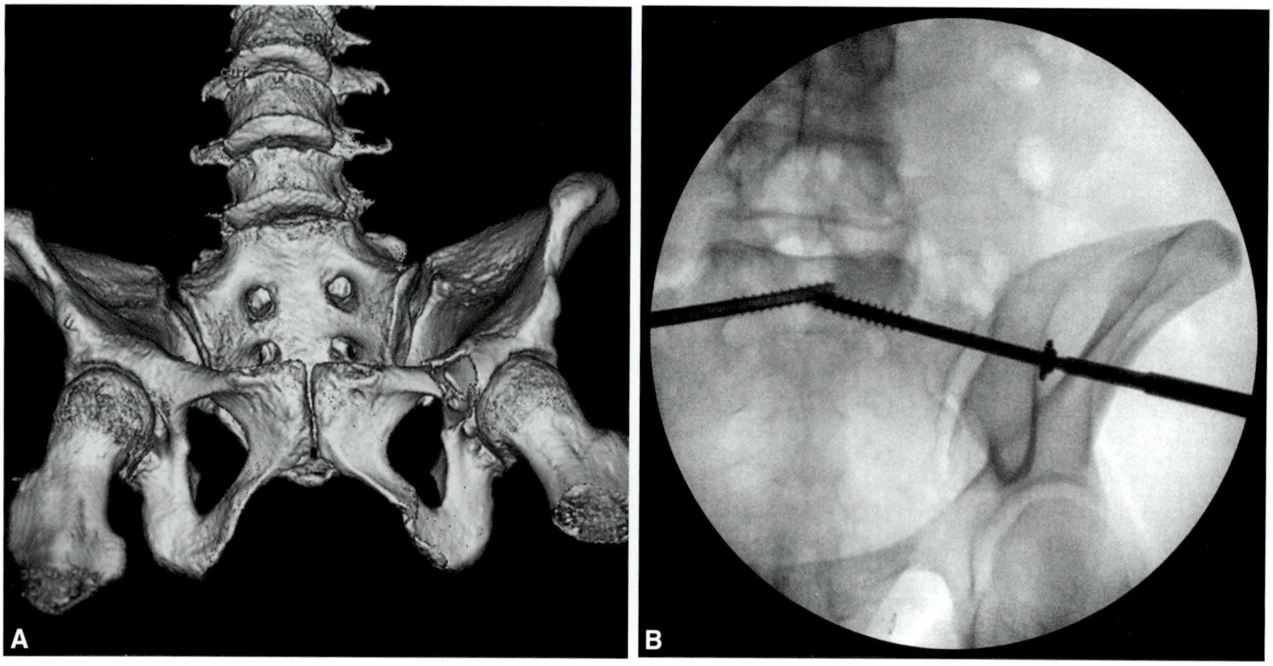

Figures 16.54A and B: (A) Dysmorphic sacral first segment screw insertion; Owing to the obliquely oriented safe zone in dysmorphic sacra transverse screw orientation is not afforded. (B) Dysmorphic sacral first segment screw insertion; transverse screw orientation is not afforded owing to the obliquely oriented safe zone. A more posterior and caudally located starting point is required in addition to an oblique screw trajectory.

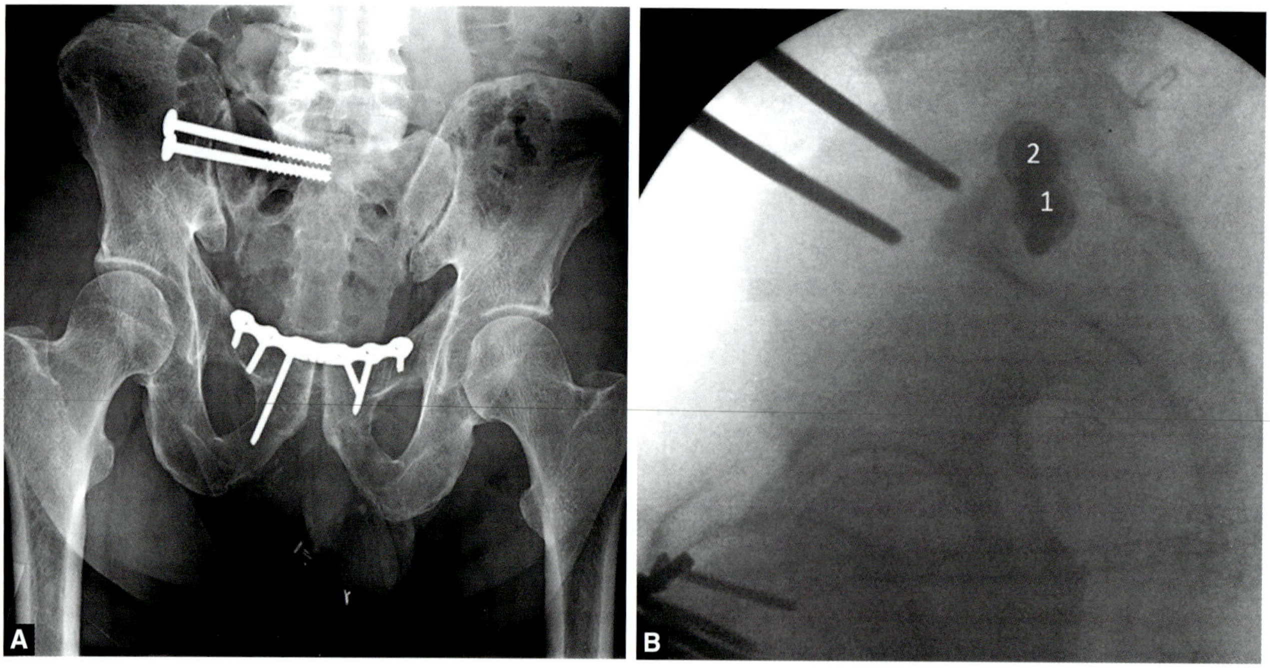

Figures 16.55A and B: (A) With the exception of small and dysmorphic sacra the upper sacral segment may accommodate two screws; (B) The initially inserted screw (1) should be caudal and anterior with respect to the iliac cortical density. The second (2) is more cranial and posterior. Both screws must remain within the intraosseous safe pathway beneath the sacral alar slope.

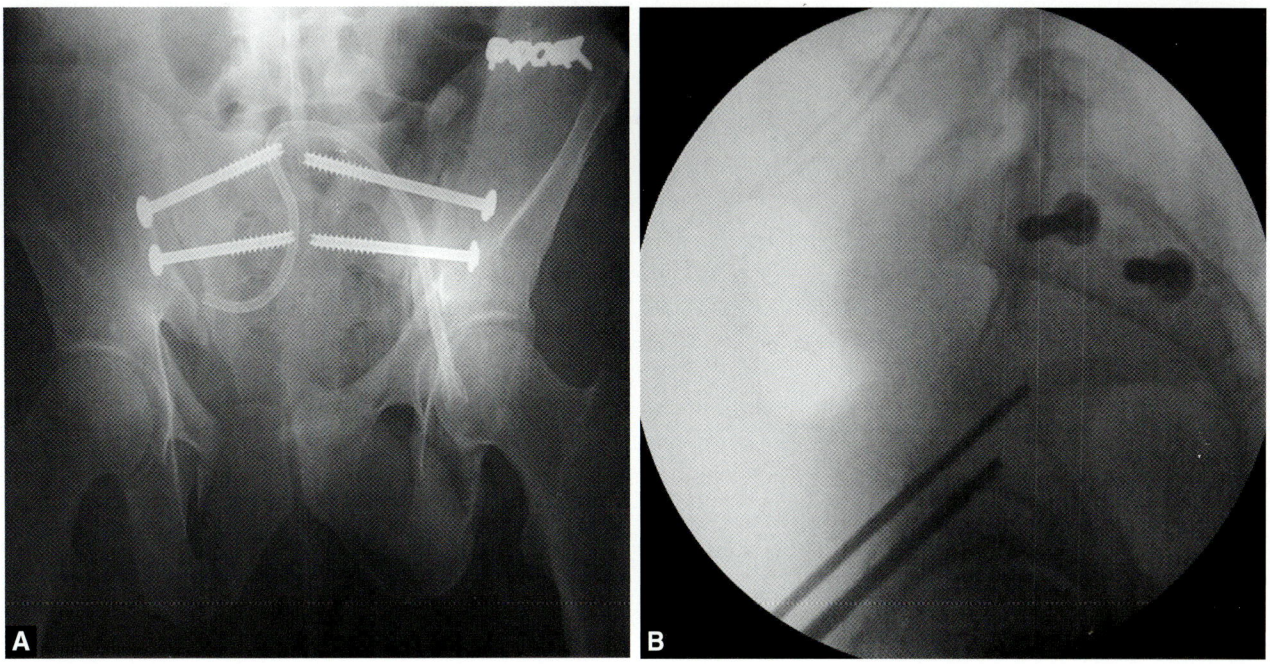

Figures 16.56A and B: Bilateral S1 and S2 screw insertion: (A) Outlet radiograph; (B) Lateral sacral fluoroscopic view.

The second sacral (S2) body despite its relatively small dimension and perceived increased risk for nerve root injury has been designated a safe and desirable site of screw fixation (Figs 16.56A and B).[34] Patient selection is predicated on a preoperative CT confirming adequate osseous volume. In a cadaveric biomechanical study, two screws outperformed single screw fixation when load to failure and rotational stiffness were studied.[35] This was independent of screw location (two in S1 vs one in both S1 and S2). The model design focused on a zone 1 extraforaminal noncomminuted otherwise stable pattern. Griffin et al. in a clinical study expressed concern when managing vertical sacral fractures with percutaneous iliosacral screws regardless of screw number, length and arrangement.[36]

Transiliac-transsacral screws: Iliosacral screws employed for sacral fracture fixation are typically inserted from the lateral iliac cortex into the safe upper sacral ala or body. Two or three cortices are engaged lateral to the injury and no or one cortical fixation point medial to the injury. Screws that terminate in the contralateral alar cancellous bone are at risk for fixation failure as osseous density is considerably less than that of the sacral body. This "unbalanced" construct with deforming forces acting perpendicular to the implant axis may prove insufficient in certain unstable injuries. In the presence of marked comminution or osteopenia, these screws may provide inadequate fixation and lead to reduction loss. Screw length is of particular importance in sacral fractures as short screw lengths may provide insufficient fixation strength when compared with longer and balanced screw constructs.

Longer iliosacral screws may offer superior fixation because they have a longer lever arm and accordingly greater resistance to toggle and vertical shear stress. A transsacral screw path, which courses from one ilium across the SI joint through the body of the sacrum and across the other SI joint exiting the contralateral iliac cortex may enhance fixation adequacy (Fig. 16.57A).[37-39] Engaging the cortical bone of the contralateral intact SI joint medial to the lesion may improve fixation and minimize reduction loss. This affords cortical fixation on the far side of the injury and permits the inclusion of a longer implant. Both the lever arm and distal screw purchase may be magnified. These "transiliac–transsacral screws" may be of benefit in the presence of osteoporosis, significant posterior pelvic instability, spinopelvic dissociation ("U" or "H" shaped sacral fractures) anticipated noncompliant behavior, bilateral posterior pelvic injuries and nonunion/revision fixation procedures.

Transiliac–transsacral screws are inserted from the injured hemipelvis' ilium through the sacral body and bilateral ala and exit from the contralateral iliac cortical bone. Safe passage requires careful preoperative planning and insertional precision as both sacral alar zones are traversed. To ensure that the patient's anatomy will accommodate full-length screws, the preoperative CT scan must be carefully scrutinized. The projected containment paths at both the S1 and S2 levels are studied. As described previously, in the dysmorphic sacrum the volume of bone available for a transiliac–transsacral screw is greater in the second compared with the upper sacral segment. The dysmorphic transverse safe zone size is also greater in the second sacral segment compared with S2 of a nondysmorphic sacrum. Accordingly, the S2 position is used exclusively for the transiliac–transsacral screw in patients with sacral dysmorphism (Fig. 16.57B).

Pelvic inlet and outlet fluoroscopic views are supplemented by a lateral sacral view used to target either the S1 or the S2 body. The starting trajectory for an upper sacral segment screw is perfectly transverse, cranial to the neural foramen on the outlet view and posterior to the ventral sacral cortex on the inlet view (Fig. 16.58A). In contrast to the oblique trajectory of an iliosacral screw, the starting point on the ilium is slightly more anterior and the projected screw trajectory parallel to the transverse axis and perpendicular to the long axis of the body. Owing to the anterior sacral alar slope, the screw should avoid a caudal and anterior position within the ala bilaterally. Trajectory is similar for both S1 and S2 targeting. The initial screw is positioned to permit the inclusion of a second and parallel transiliac-transsacral screw at the same or an adjacent level. This enhances sagittal plane rotational and overall construct stability.

Guide pin placement and wire insertion are monitored with sequential and progressive fluoroscopic pelvic inlet and outlet views. A true lateral sacral view is obtained prior to crossing both the near and far sacral nerve root tunnels to ensure safe placement. The guide pin is advanced until it exits the contralateral iliac cortex (Fig. 16.58B). This enables accurate length assessment with either the pin-based depth gauge or another guide pin of equal length (Fig. 16.58C). Fully threaded screws are preferred for comminuted transforaminal sacral fractures. Bilateral individual oblique fluoroscopic images with slight caudal inclination ("rollover" view) are obtained. These afford a perspective tangential to the posterior lateral iliac cortices confirming accurate screw length (uninvolved hemipelvis view) (Fig. 16.59A) and absence of screw head intrusion (involved hemipelvis view) (Fig. 16.59B). The fluoroscopic lateral view (Fig. 16.59C) confirms intraosseous "safe zone" containment of the screw throughout its course.

Transiliac–transsacral screw insertion if properly executed is a clinically effective technique without excessive hazard and is applicable in a variety of situations. The surgeon must confirm an inventory of screws of sufficient length prior to initiating the procedure. Disadvantages inherent to this technique include a smaller available bone volume (compared to conventional iliosacral screw insertion) and the technique accuracy accordingly required to maintain intraosseous screw placement (Figs 16.60A to C). An additional concern of indeterminate consequence is the violation of the otherwise uncompromised SI joint of the contralateral hemipelvis.

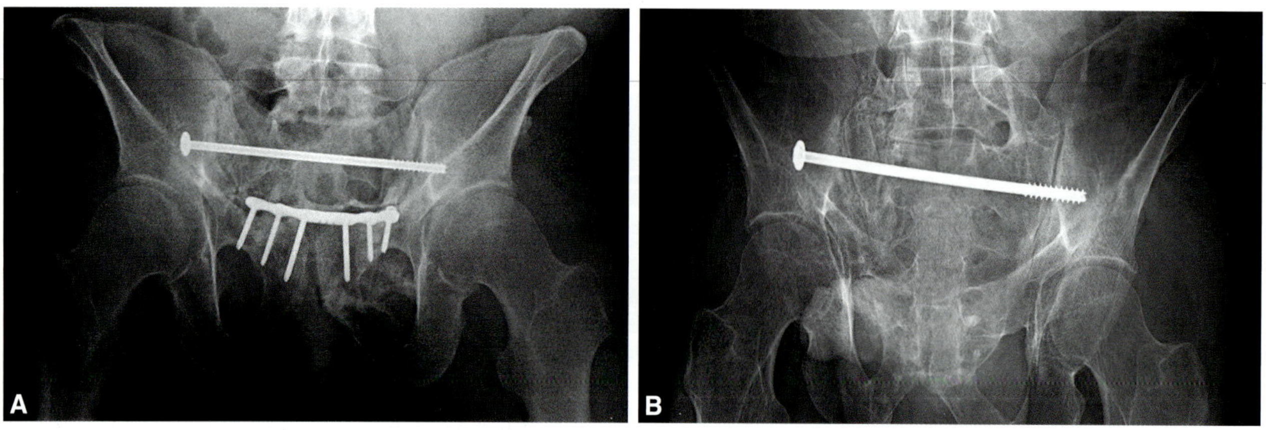

Figures 16.57A and B: (A) Transiliac-transsacral screw (upper sacral segment) nondysmorphic sacrum; (B) Transiliac-transsacral screw (second sacral segment) dysmorphic sacrum.

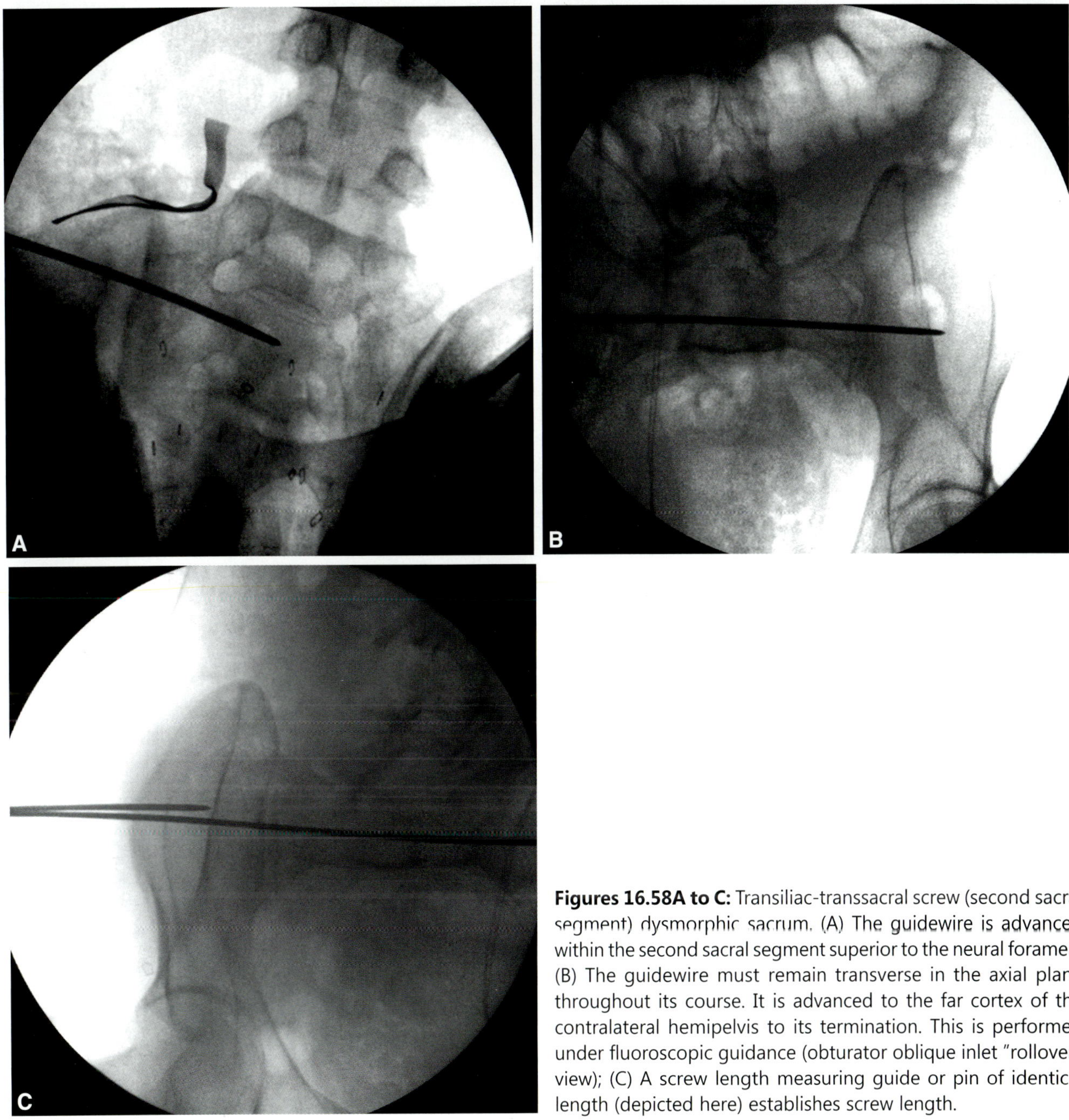

Figures 16.58A to C: Transiliac-transsacral screw (second sacral segment) dysmorphic sacrum. (A) The guidewire is advanced within the second sacral segment superior to the neural foramen; (B) The guidewire must remain transverse in the axial plane throughout its course. It is advanced to the far cortex of the contralateral hemipelvis to its termination. This is performed under fluoroscopic guidance (obturator oblique inlet "rollover" view); (C) A screw length measuring guide or pin of identical length (depicted here) establishes screw length.

ILIOSACRAL SCREW INSERTION: Pearls and Pitfalls

- Proper positioning and imaging is required to perform safe placement of iliosacral screws
- Ipsilateral femoral traction may be required to resolve cephalad and posterior hemipelvic migration
- Reduction of the pelvis can be achieved with external fixation, sheet application or taping the lower extremities together in internal rotation
- Special attention should be paid to anatomical variants, such as sacral dysmorphism, which can prevent certain screw trajectories such as the S1 transsacral screw

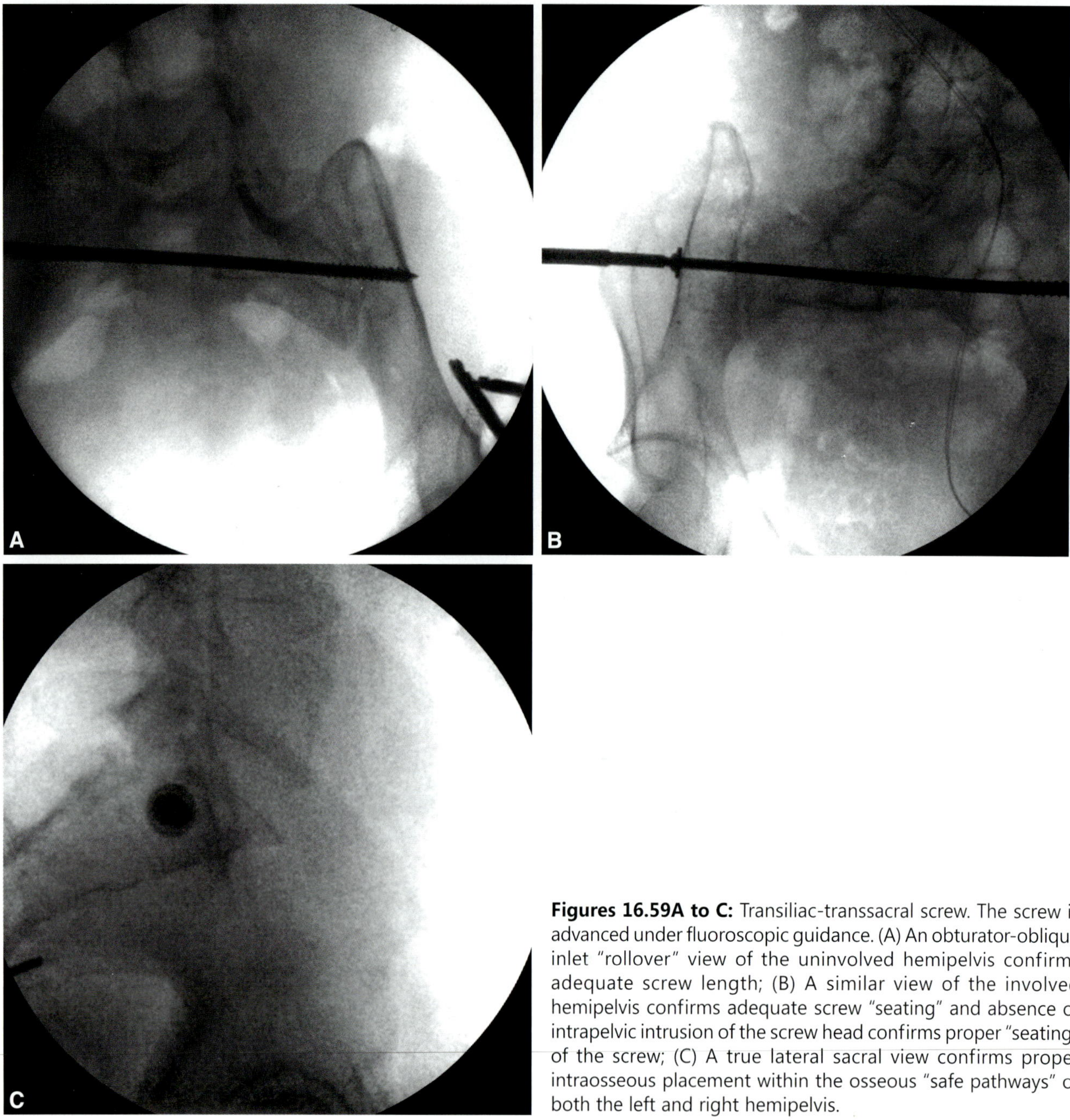

Figures 16.59A to C: Transiliac-transsacral screw. The screw is advanced under fluoroscopic guidance. (A) An obturator-oblique inlet "rollover" view of the uninvolved hemipelvis confirms adequate screw length; (B) A similar view of the involved hemipelvis confirms adequate screw "seating" and absence of intrapelvic intrusion of the screw head confirms proper "seating" of the screw; (C) A true lateral sacral view confirms proper intraosseous placement within the osseous "safe pathways" of both the left and right hemipelvis.

Authors' Preferred Management of Select Complications

Case 1: Malreduction of Sacroiliac Joint Fracture Dislocation with Iliosacral Screws

Iliosacral screw fixation of posterior ring injuries demands both reduction techniques and correct appreciation of the stability of the posterior tension band. Although satisfactory fixation can often be obtained with iliosacral screws, overcompression and internal rotation is a known phenomenon that the treating surgeon should be aware of.

In this case, a 26-year-old male was involved in a motor vehicle collision sustaining the pelvic injury shown in Figure 16.61A. The posterior tension band of the right

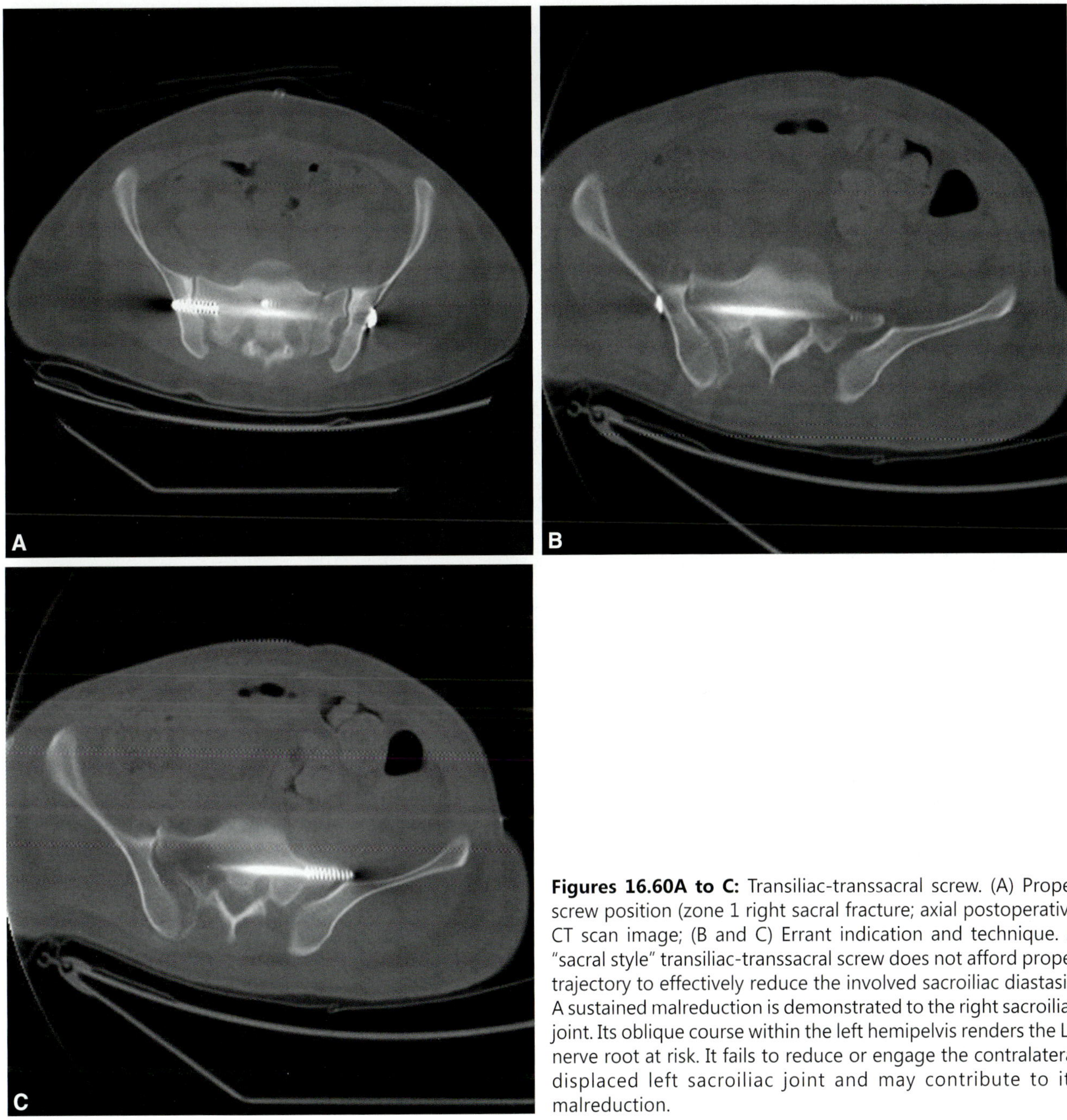

Figures 16.60A to C: Transiliac-transsacral screw. (A) Proper screw position (zone 1 right sacral fracture; axial postoperative CT scan image; (B and C) Errant indication and technique. A "sacral style" transiliac-transsacral screw does not afford proper trajectory to effectively reduce the involved sacroiliac diastasis. A sustained malreduction is demonstrated to the right sacroiliac joint. Its oblique course within the left hemipelvis renders the L5 nerve root at risk. It fails to reduce or engage the contralateral displaced left sacroiliac joint and may contribute to its malreduction.

hemipelvis was erroneously deemed intact and the significance of the left hemipelvic injury was underappreciated (Fig. 16.61B). The initial fixation effort included percutaneous iliosacral screw fixation of the right hemipelvis and symphyseal plating (Fig. 16.61C). During the course of the procedure diastasis of the contralateral SI joint (*) was revealed fluoroscopically. A left hemipelvis iliosacral "style" screw was introduced percutaneously in compression mode (Fig. 16.61D). Fixation of the right hemipelvis in a position of excessive internal rotation disallowed anatomic reduction of the left SI joint. The postoperative radiograph demonstrates internal "drift" of the right hemipelvis beyond the midsagittal line anteriorly (Fig. 16.61E). This forces the

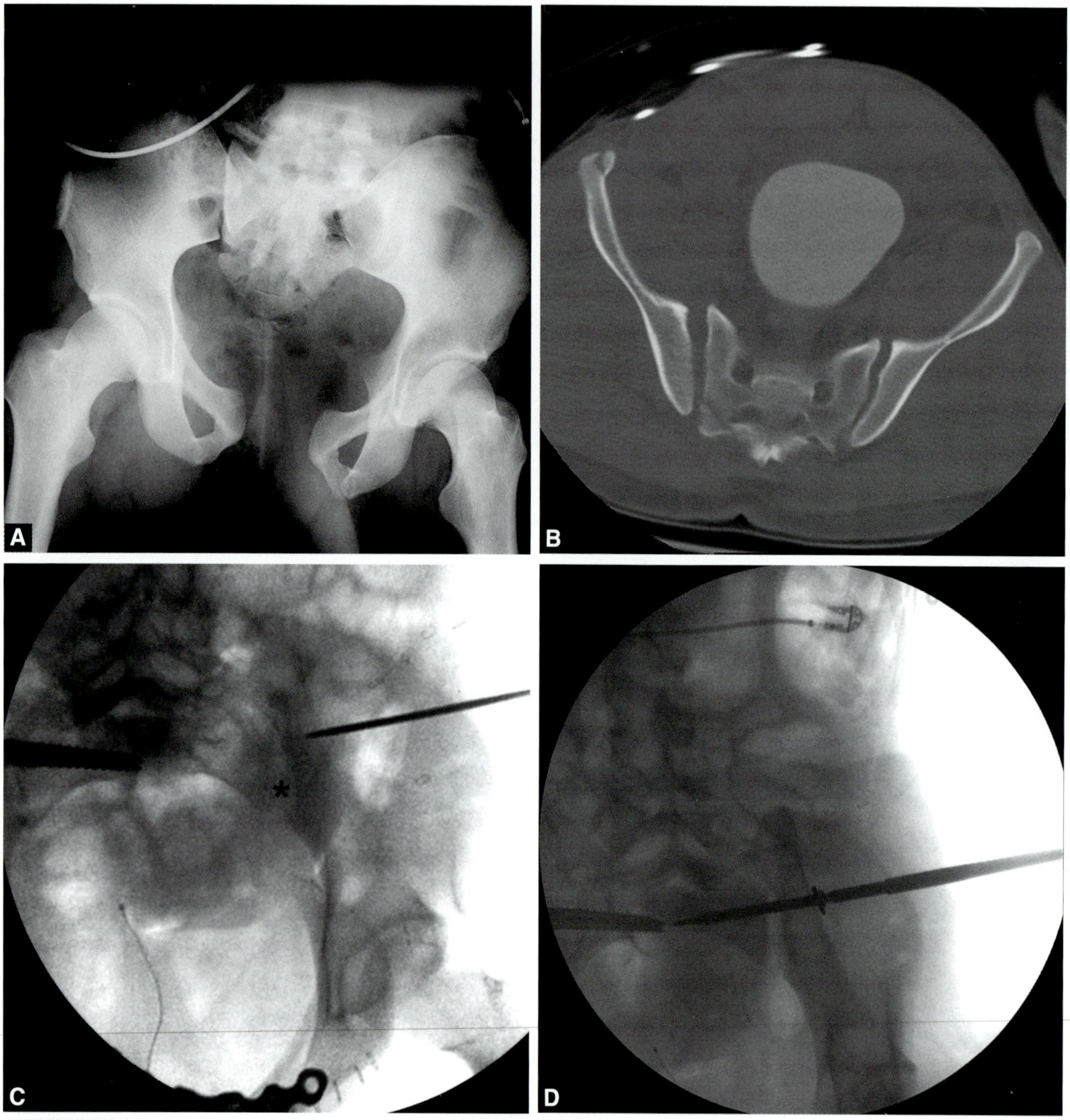

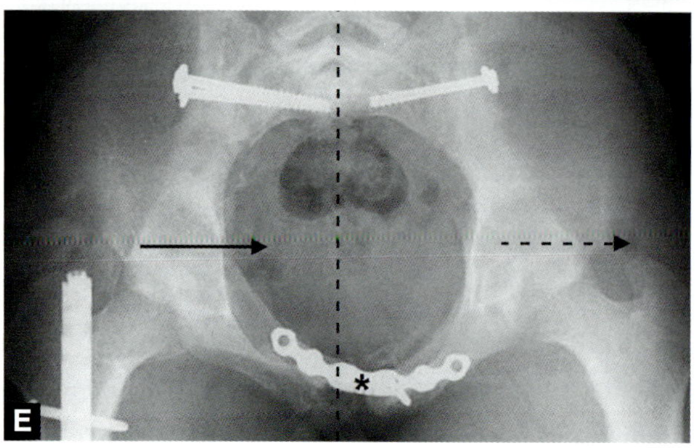

Figures 16.61A to E: Unstable pelvic ring injury with malreduction of posterior ring (see text for details). (A) Initial anteroposterior X-ray; (B) Initial CT scan demonstrating right sided sacral fracture with anterior sacroiliac widening and mild left sided anterior widening; (C) Intraoperative image after anterior plating, right sided iliosacral screw fixation and left sided guidewire placement. Anterior sacroiliac joint widening is noted with "*" in the figure; (D) Left sided anterior widening noted after compression iliosacral screw placement; (E) Postoperative radiograph demonstrating mild internal rotation "drift" on right (solid arrow) with persistent external rotation malreduction on left (dashed arrow). The center of the sacrum is shown with the vertical dashed line whereas the midsagittal line anteriorly [shown (as)*].

left hemipelvis into a state of sustained external rotation malreduction.

Fixation of the unstable pelvic ring demands an intact, stable contralateral hemipelvis or if unstable, the restoration of a stable one. The situation in the case outlined in Figures 16.61A to E could have been prevented in the following case, which demonstrates preferential treatment in a similar scenario. In this case, a 36-year-old woman involved in a motor vehicle collision sustained the pelvic ring injury demonstrated in Figure 16.62A. The CT scan in Figures 16.62B and C suggests a likely vertically unstable left hemipelvis with complete diastasis of the left SI joint. With the exception of a right L5 transverse process fracture, no obvious integrity compromise is suggested to the right hemipelvis. A supra-acetabular frame was applied during the initial effort toward pelvis stabilization. Diastasis of the right SI joint was appreciated fluoroscopically (Fig. 16.62D). The pin serving as a joystick facilitated reduction of the right SI joint to anatomic parameters (Fig. 16.62E). The left SI joint remained unreduced and the symphysis assumed a more midsagittal position. The right SI joint was then secured with a SI style screw in compression mode (Fig. 16.62F). Stability and reduction was accordingly restored to the right hemipelvis. This is then served as an adequate and accurate foundation upon which left hemipelvis reconstruction could be based. This was next pursued employing open techniques of reduction and SI fixation (left anterior SI plating and iliosacral screw insertion) (Fig. 16.62G).

Case 2: Errant Placement of Anterior External Fixation Pins

Common errors with placement of Schanz pins into the iliac crest include directing the pins through both inner and outer tables of the pelvis. This compromises pin fixation and subsequently pelvis stability. The following case illustrates this particular common error. In this case, a 55-year-old male involved in a high energy fall sustained an unstable fracture of the right hemipelvis. Clinical and radiographic exam were consistent with significant asymmetric internal rotation of the involved right hemipelvis. A distracting external pelvic fixator was applied employing iliac crest pin insertion technique. The postoperative radiograph and CT scan demonstrate resolution of the internal rotation deformity (Figs 16.63A and B). Findings additionally reveal errant extrapelvic pin

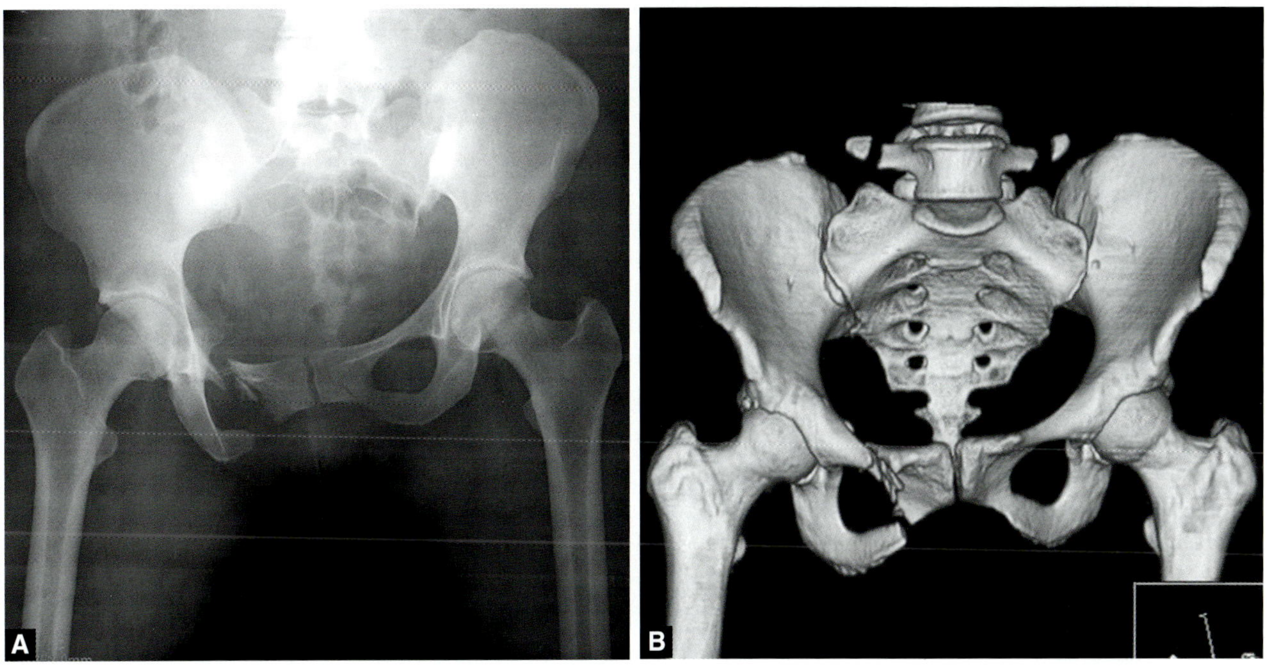

Figures 16.62A and B

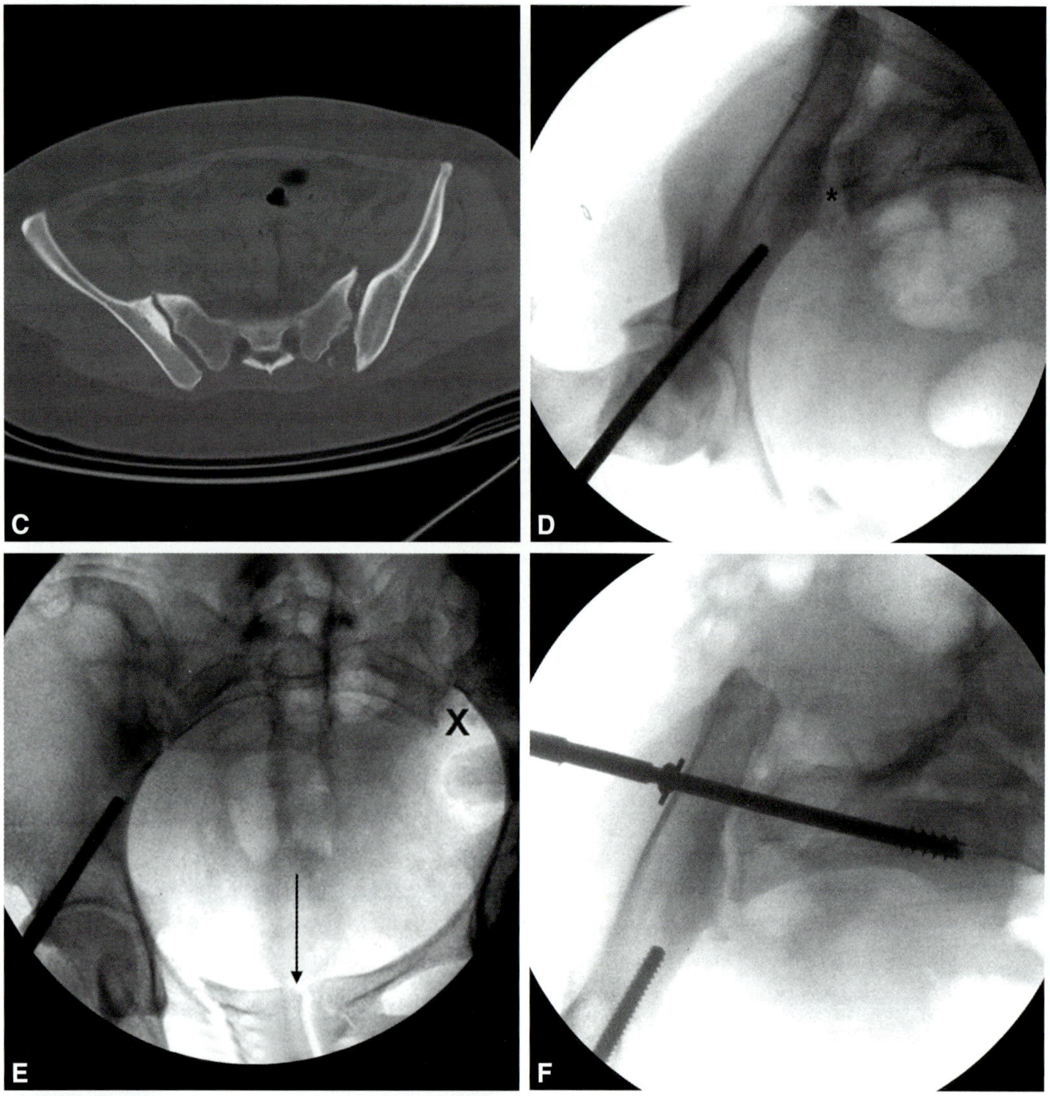

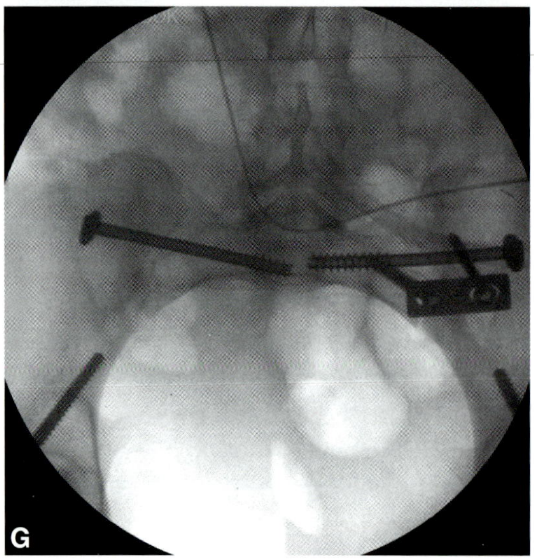

Figures 16.62A to G: Unstable pelvic ring injury with correction of initial malreduction of posterior ring (see text for details). (A) Initial anteroposterior pelvis radiograph; (B and C) CT images demonstrate left vertical instability but no obvious right sided hemipelvic posterior injury other than the L5 transverse process fracture; (D) After supra-acetabular external fixation was applied, anterior SI joint widening on the right is noted as(*); (E) The right sided external fixation pin was used as a joystick to reduce the right sacroiliac joint anatomically, although the left side remains unreduced (shown as "X"); (F) A sacroiliac style screw is used to compress the right sacroiliac joint. This stable right sacroiliac joint now provided a foundation for left sided reconstruction; (G) The left SI joint was treated with open reduction and anterior plating, as well as iliosacral screw fixation.

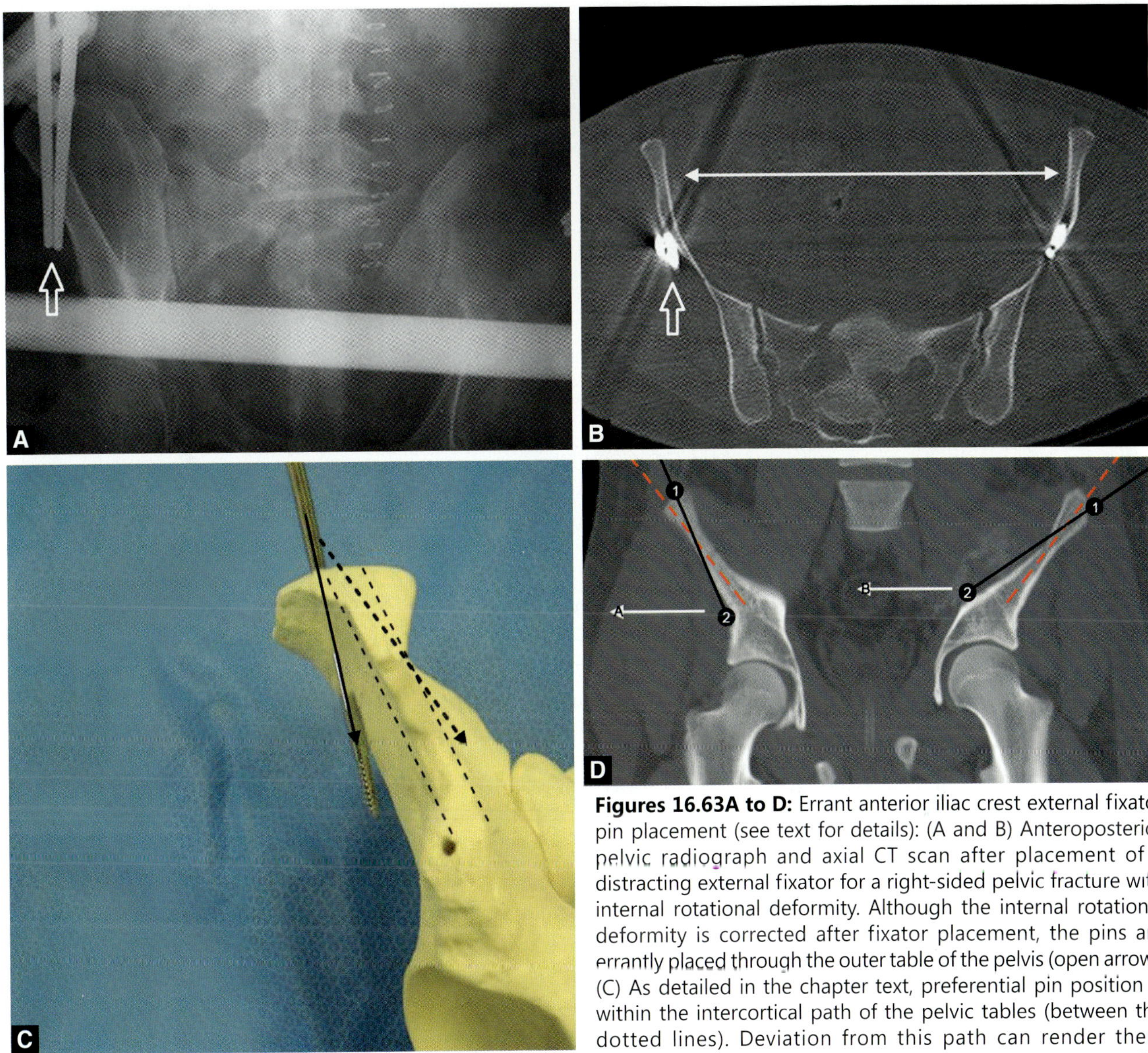

Figures 16.63A to D: Errant anterior iliac crest external fixator pin placement (see text for details): (A and B) Anteroposterior pelvic radiograph and axial CT scan after placement of a distracting external fixator for a right-sided pelvic fracture with internal rotational deformity. Although the internal rotational deformity is corrected after fixator placement, the pins are errantly placed through the outer table of the pelvis (open arrow); (C) As detailed in the chapter text, preferential pin position is within the intercortical path of the pelvic tables (between the dotted lines). Deviation from this path can render them extrapelvic (solid arrow) or intrapelvic (dashed arrow). In this model, the errant extrapelvic pin from this patient is replicated; (D) Within the depicted right hemipelvis, extrapelvic pin position would favor the application of distraction forces (arrow "A"). This may prove suitable when managing lateral compression injuries with sustained internal rotation deformity as depicted in this case. Conversely, intrapelvic pin position (as demonstrated in the left hemipelvis) favors the application of compression forces (arrow "B"). This would prove applicable when treating anteroposterior compression injury patterns and resolving external rotation deformity.

course inferiorly within the right hemipelvis. Correct pin placement trajectory is shown in Figure 16.63C. Whereas errant pin placement in either the extrapelvic or intrapelvic position is generally not desired, it may still prove satisfactory depending on the site of premature exit (intra vs extrapelvic) and intended purpose (Fig. 16.63D).

Case 3: Nonunion of Nondisplaced Pelvic Ring Fractures Treated with Percutaneous Compression Screws

A 46-year-old female had incidental trauma related to her equestrian activities. She noted some left groin pain but did not seek medical treatment initially. Several weeks later her left groin pain persisted and she consulted her local physician. She had a slight antalgic gait and mild tenderness to palpation of her pubis. She had no other relevant findings on physical examination. An AP pelvic plain radiograph revealed no fracture or other abnormality (Fig. 16.64A). Her pain worsened over the subsequent months and she was seen again and noted to have a more notable limp due to pain and persistent pubic tenderness. Another plain pelvic film identified left sided peripheral superior and mid-inferior pubic ramus fractures (Fig. 16.64B). Pelvic computed tomography confirmed the diagnosis and detailed the well-aligned hypertrophic nonunion sites. There were no other areas of fracture or instability seen on these imaging studies (Figs 16.64C to E). She was not able to work or participate in her routine activities due to her left inguinal-pubic pain. A complete medical evaluation ruled out any form of metabolic bone diseases. She was counseled regarding the variety of operative and nonoperative treatment options and she chose percutaneous stabilization of the symptomatic pubic ramus nonunion sites.

At surgery, medullary screws were inserted through small stab wounds under fluoroscopic guidance to stabilize the nonunion sites. First, the superior ramus site was fixed with an antegrade superior ramus medullary lag screw. The inferior ramus site was then secured using a large cortical lag screw (Figs 16.64F to I). Postoperative radiographs and CT scans demonstrate safe placement of the screws (Figs 16.64J to P).

Immediately after surgery, she noted good relief from her prior symptoms. She used crutches for 6 weeks thereafter limiting her weight bearing to light pressure only during the stance phase of gait. During weeks 7–12 after surgery, she progressed from partial weight bearing to full weight bearing along with light strengthening exercises. Four months after surgery, she had radiographic union at the nonunion sites, no pain complaints and had returned to her previous job and recreational impact activities (Fig. 16.64Q).

Case 4: Symptomatic Pelvic Nonunion after Routine External Fixation Treated with Anterior and Posterior Fixation

A 42-years-old healthy male cattle rancher was injured when he was bucked off of his horse. He had immediate low back and anterior pelvic pain. He was unable to stand to walk. He was transported by ambulance to a local medical center where an evaluation confirmed his pelvic pain complaints. He had ecchymosis in the pubic area. Pelvic instability was noted on manual compression over the iliac crests and this maneuver accentuated his pelvic pain significantly. There was not gross hematuria, but blood was identified on urinalysis. Pelvic plain radiographs and a CT scan identified a minimally displaced right-sided sacral alar fracture and a symphysis pubis disruption. A cystogram revealed an anterior extraperitoneal bladder disruption with contrast leak. He was treated operatively with an open reduction of the symphysis pubis using a Pfannenstiel exposure. The bladder injury was directly inspected by the consulting urologist during the surgery and partially involved the bladder neck area. On this reason, the planned repair was abandoned intraoperatively and a suprapubic tube was selected to treat the bladder injury. Concerned about potential contamination by the cystotomy tube, the orthopedic surgeon changed his planned symphyseal plating procedure and instead opted to use an anterior pelvic external fixator to treat the pelvic ring injuries (Fig. 16.65A). The patient was restricted to pivot transfers for bed to chair mobility only.

The suprapubic tube and pelvic frame were then removed 2 months after injury, and the patient was mobilized to crutch assisted activities for another 2 months. He had urinary incontinence after the suprapubic tube was removed, and used 8–10 adult diapers per day. Four months after injury, he was released to begin his regular activities but could not perform them due to continued pelvic pain, difficulty with ambulation and continuous urinary incontinence. His pelvic pain worsened over the next 6 months.

He was then referred to a tertiary center for evaluation. His symptoms were noted, as were his ongoing mobility and urological problems. He had no evidence of chronic pain behavior and was not addicted to analgesic medications. He had a cane assisted antalgic gait. His surgical wound and iliac pin sites were healed and his lower extremity neurological examination was without focal deficits. He had no perineal findings other than urinary incontinence. Pelvic plain films included alternating single leg standing (flamingo) images that demonstrated symphyseal widening and instability (Figs 16.65B and C). Pelvic CT demonstrated a nonunion of the sacral fracture (Figs 16.65D and E).

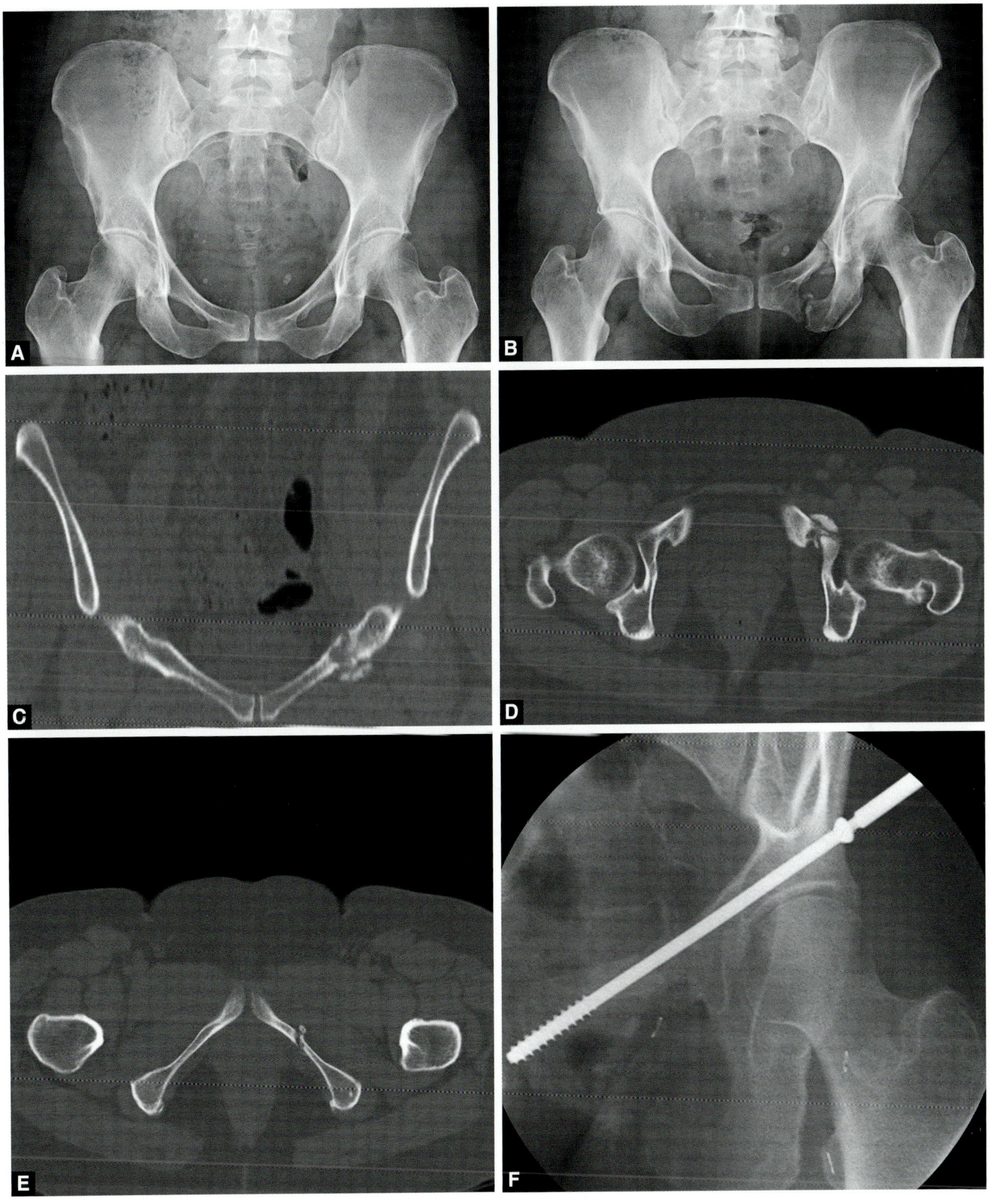

Figures 16.64A to F

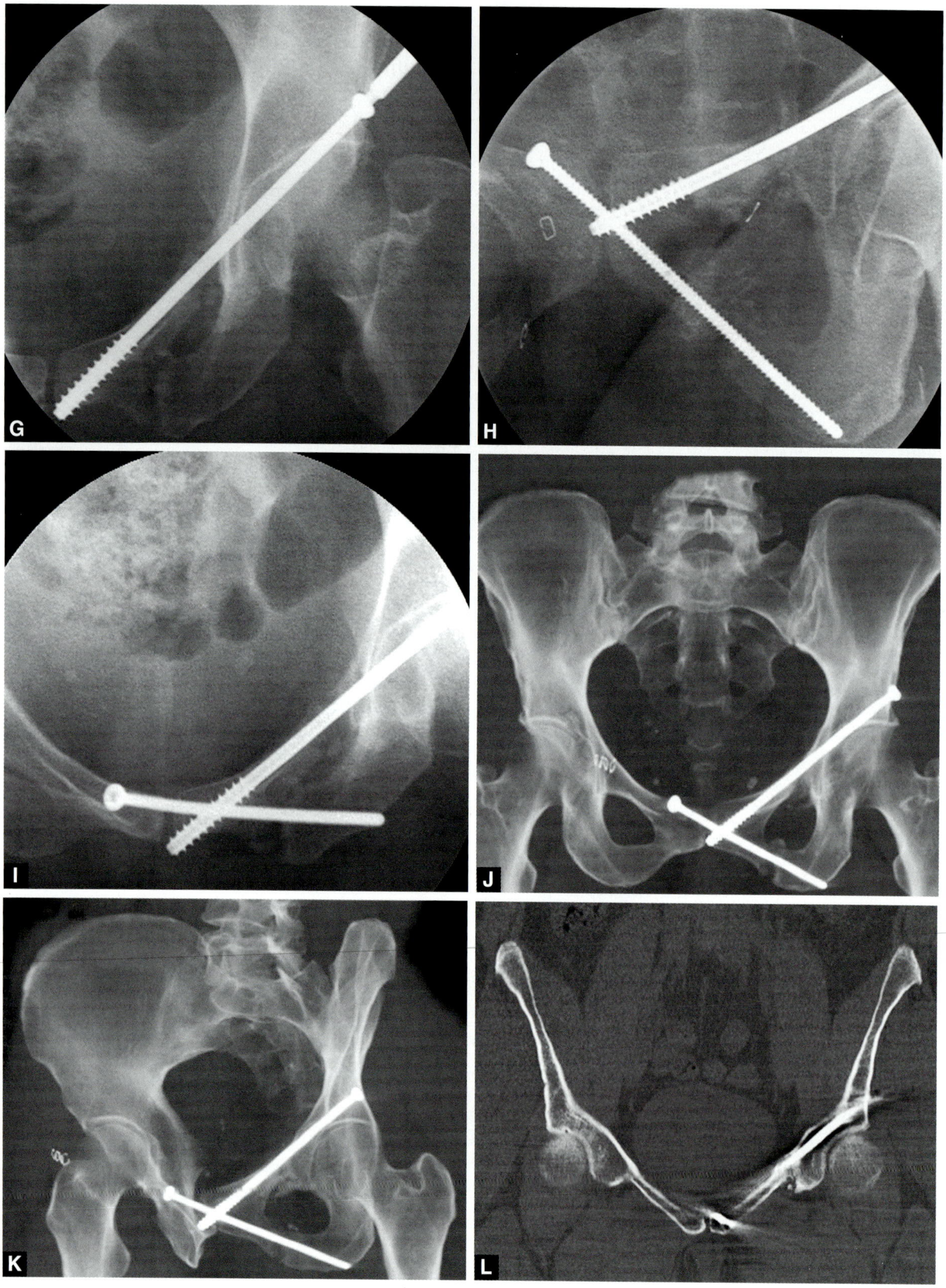

Figures 16.64G to L

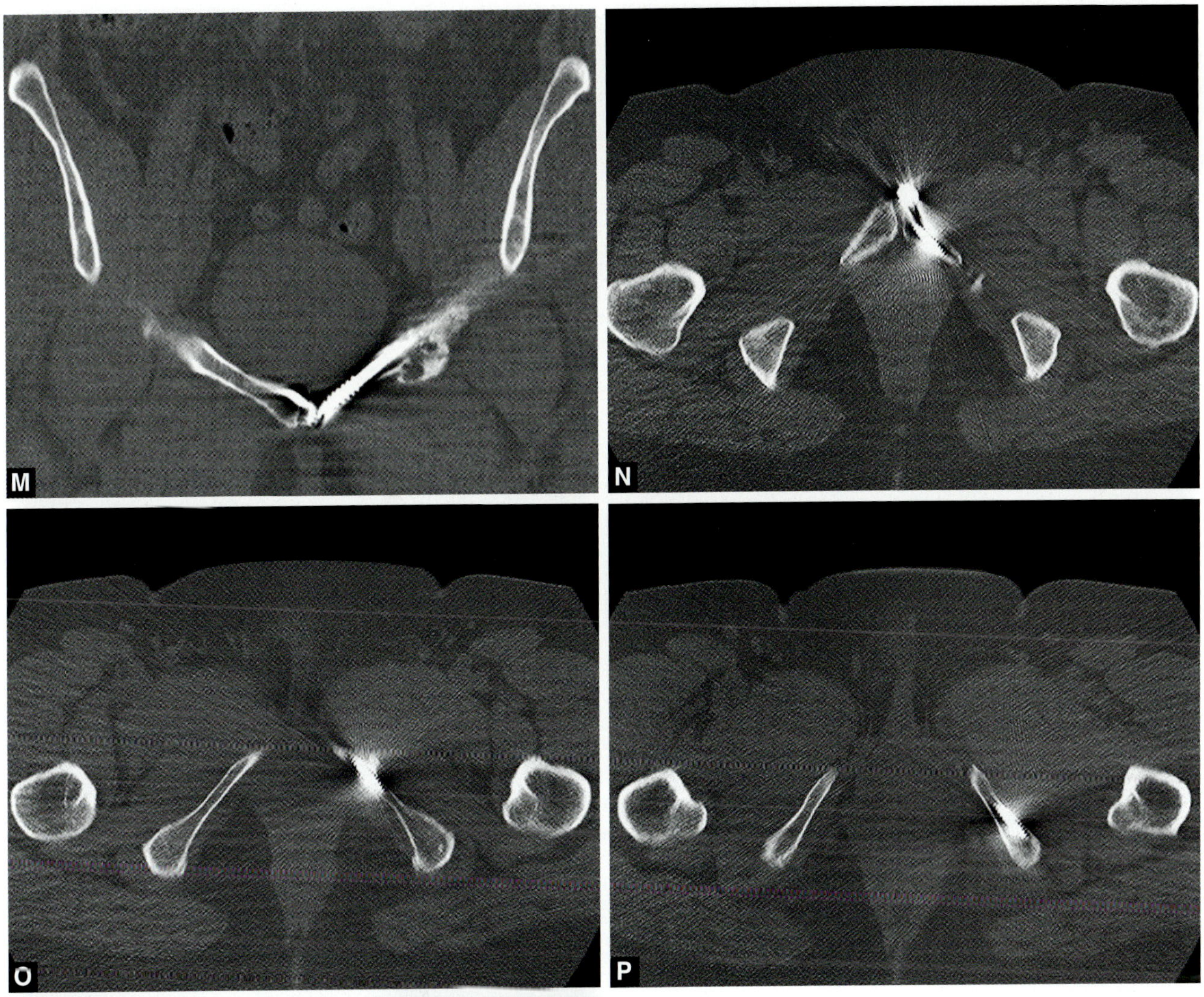

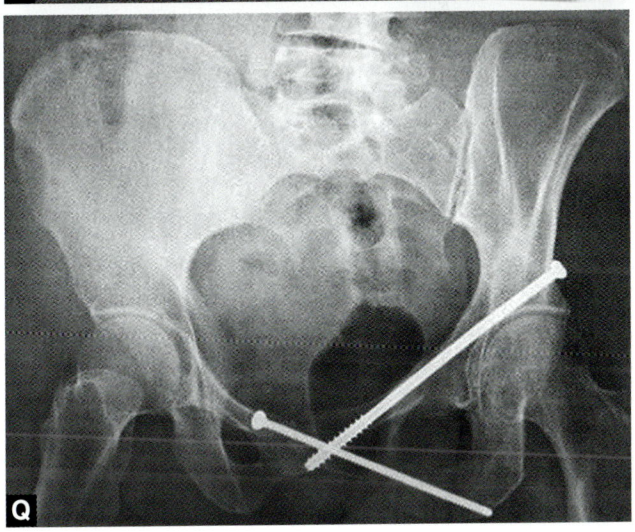

Figures 16.64A to Q: Percutaneous treatment of pelvic fracture nonunion (see text for details). (A) Initial anteroposterior pelvic radiograph of a 46-year-old female with groin pain after an equestrian injury does not demonstrate any obvious fracture; (B to E) Repeat radiograph and CT scan images after several months of persistent pain demonstrated unhealed left sided superior and inferior ramus fractures; (F to I) Intraoperative images demonstrate placement of medullary superior and inferior ramus screws; (J to P) Postoperative radiographs and CT scan images demonstrate safe placement of both screws; (Q) Follow-up radiograph at 4 months demonstrates healing of both fractures. The patient had resolution of pain and return to normal activities.

He opted for surgical management of his symptomatic unstable pelvic nonunion. An experienced urologist evaluated the patient before the nonunion surgery and recommended to follow exam several months after pelvic stabilization.

At surgery, the patient was positioned supine and his healed Pfannenstiel exposure was used again, and the anterior bladder was carefully peeled away from the posterior rectus abdominis sheath. No obvious bladder pathology was identified. The pubic symphysis scarring was excised and the pubis was then reduced using a clamp (Figs 16.65F and G). A contoured 3.5 mm pelvic reconstruction plate stabilized the symphyseal reduction (Fig. 16.65H). The wound was irrigated and closed. The patient was next positioned prone and a midline surgical exposure was centered over the lumbosacral area and used to debride and clamp the sacral nonunion site. Cancellous allograft and autograft were packed into the nonunion site. Transiliac- transsacral cannulated lag screws were inserted in the upper sacral segment and then unilateral lumbopelvic fixation was also used to stabilize the sacral nonunion (Fig. 16.65I). Postoperative CT scan images demonstrate reduction of the pelvis with safe placement of implants, particularly the transsacral screw posteriorly (Figs 16.65J).

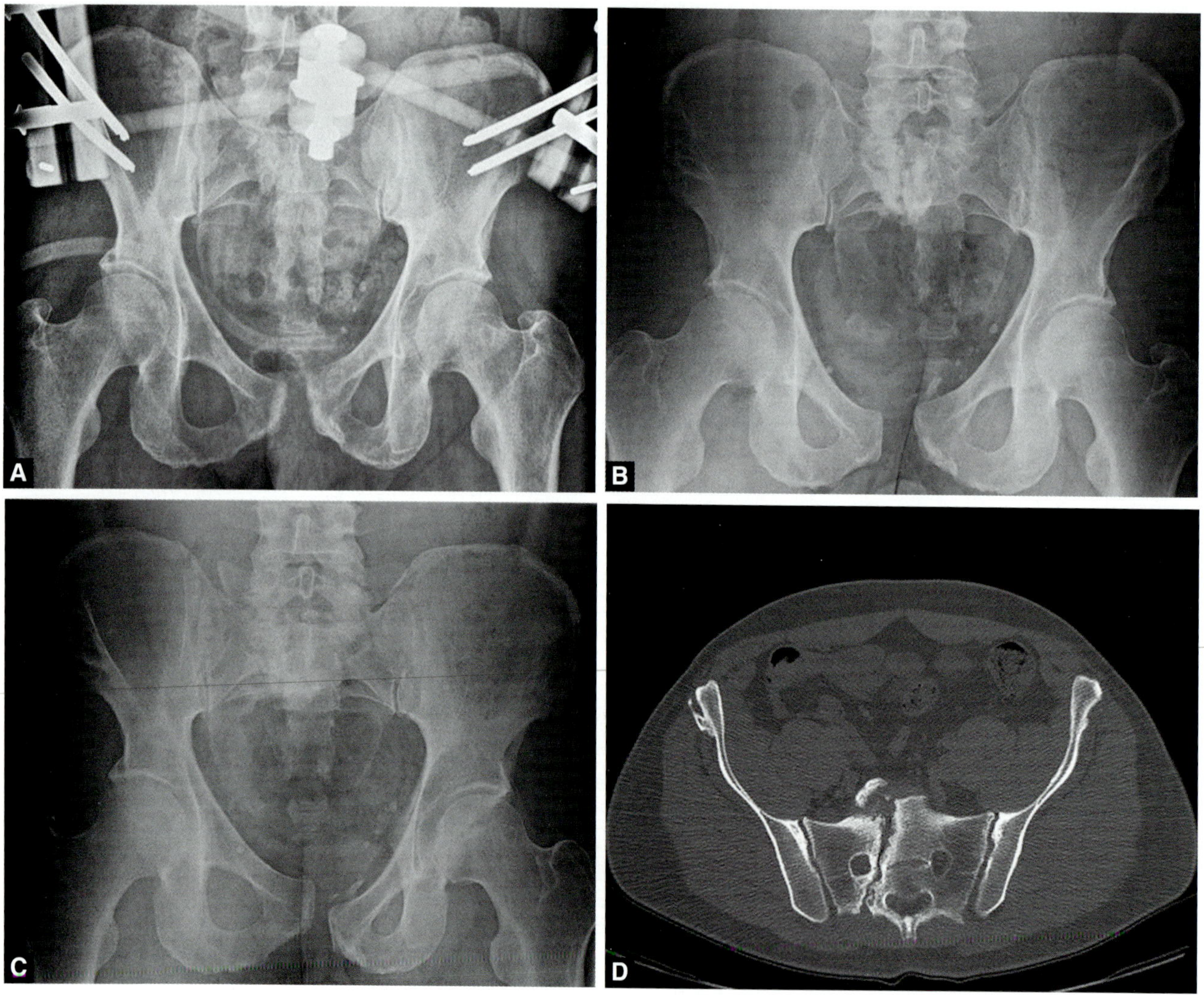

Figures 16.65A to D

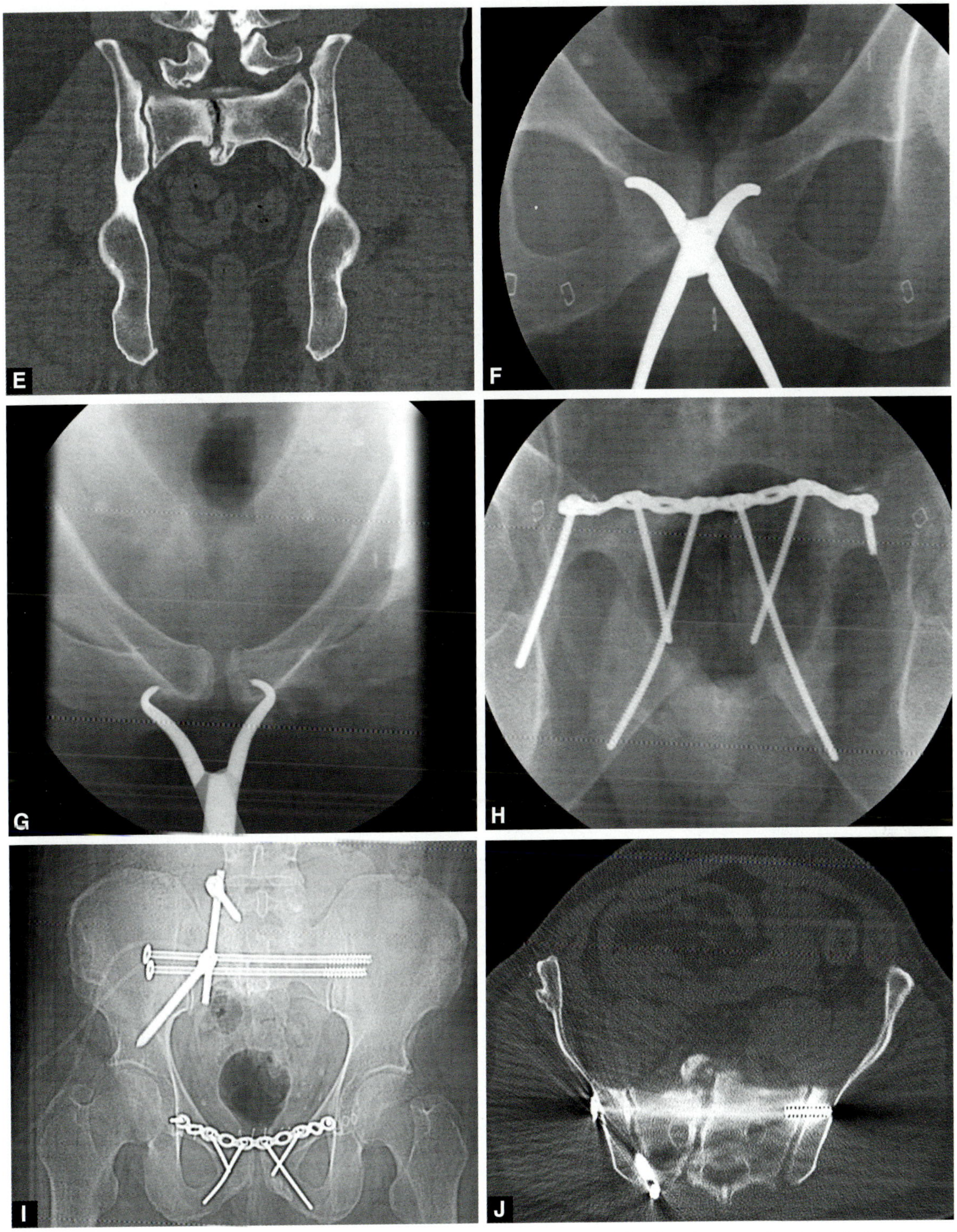

Figures 16.65A to J: Treatment of nonunion of the pelvis after anterior external fixation (see text for details). (A) Anteroposterior radiograph after external fixation for an unstable pelvic fracture in a 42-year-old male. Anterior symphyseal plating was planned but abandoned intraoperatively due to a bladder injury; (B to C) Single stance anteroposterior pelvic radiographs after eventual frame removal. The right leg is up in figure B, whereas the left leg is up in figure C; (D to E) CT scan images confirm a nonunion of the sacrum; (F to G) Intraoperative images demonstrating reduction of the anterior pelvis; (H) Intraoperative image demonstrating anterior 3.5 mm reconstruction plate fixation; (I to J) Postoperative radiograph and CT scan demonstrating excellent pelvic alignment and safe transsacral screw fixation. Iliolumbar fixation is also used to supplement fixation for the right posterior hemipelvis.

His immediate postoperative course was uncomplicated. His pain complaints and urinary incontinence were significantly improved immediately. He used crutches for 8 weeks after surgery to allow protected right-sided weight bearing. Progressive weight bearing and strengthening exercises were allowed for the next 6 weeks and he stopped using ambulatory aids 3 months after surgery.

Summary

Nonoperative treatment of unstable pelvic fractures may be associated with long-term complications including malunion, nonunion, chronic pain and neurologic dysfunction. Strategies toward treatment often distinguish between the anterior and posterior pelvic ring injury components. Because the pelvis is a ring, one injury may significantly impact the other. Posterior pelvic ring injuries result in a wide spectrum of severity, instability and functional deficits. Controversy exists regarding the importance of an anatomic reduction of various posterior pelvic fracture patterns. Several studies have related the quality of the reduction of the posterior pelvis to patient outcome.[40,41] Surgical reduction and fixation of pelvic fractures can be performed with external fixation, internal fixation and combinations of both. Fixation should offer sufficient stability to allow early mobilization of the patient, limiting complications associated with prolonged recumbency.

Displaced high-energy pelvic ring injuries have the potential for residual deformity and dysfunction if early reduction and maintenance of reduction until healing is not successful. Contemporary trends and techniques in pelvic fracture surgery continue to evolve in an attempt to resolve inadequacies of earlier efforts. These have focused on reduction of the pelvic ring and sustaining it once achieved. Obstacles have included the complex osseous anatomy of the pelvis and its variations, as well as seemingly difficult surgical access. In the broadest sense, the goal of surgery is to obtain "acceptable" reduction and introduce "adequate" fixation without generating serious complications. A proper understanding of the injury pattern and associated multiplanar displacement as well the required application of effective reduction force vectors initiate the fixation effort. Familiarity with the attributes and limitations of fixation constructs and surgical methods of introduction furthers the challenge. The pursuit of a percutaneous techniques attempts to address the concerns and complications of open treatment including wound breakdown and additional hemorrhage from decompression of the pelvic hematoma. These have proven applicable to both anterior and posterior lesions within the pelvic ring. As with any accepted paradigm, these methods will attempt to remedy what were previously considered "unsolvable problems". Some will be solved and new problems arising from the paradigm shift will be present and require resolution.

References

1. Blackmore CC, Cummings P, Jurkovich GJ, et al. Predicting major hemorrhage in patients with pelvic fracture. J Trauma. 2006;61(2):346-52.
2. Hak DJ, Smith WR, Suzuki T. Management of hemorrhage in life-threatening pelvic fracture. J Am Acad Orthop Surg. 2009;17(7):447-57.
3. Bottlang M, Krieg JC, Mohr M, et al. Emergent management of pelvic ring fractures with use of circumferential compression. J Bone Joint Surg Am. 2002;84-A Suppl 2:43-7.
4. Krieg JC, Mohr M, Ellis TJ, et al. Emergent stabilization of pelvic ring injuries by controlled circumferential compression: a clinical trial. J Trauma. 2005;59(3):659-64.
5. Kottmeier SA, Wilson SC, Born CT, et al. Surgical management of soft tissue lesions associated with pelvic ring injury. Clin Orthop Relat Res. 1996;(329):46-53.
6. Reilly MC, Zinar DM, Matta JM. Neurologic injuries in pelvic ring fractures. Clin Orthop Relat Res. 1996;(329):28-36.
7. Poka A, Libby EP. Indications and techniques for external fixation of the pelvis. Clin Orthop Relat Res. 1996;(329):54-9.
8. Kottmeier SA, Floyd JCP, Divaris N. External fixation of the pelvis. In: Wiesel SW (Ed). Operative Techniques in Orthopedic Surgery. Part 2 Section1 Chapter 1. Lippincott: Williams and Wilkins Publishers; 2011. pp. 462-75.
9. Kim WY, Hearn TC, Seleem O, et al. Effect of pin location on stability of pelvic external fixation. Clin Orthop Relat Res. 1999;(361):237-44.
10. de Ridder VA, de Lange S, Popta JV. Anatomical variations of the lateral femoral cutaneous nerve and the consequences for surgery. J Orthop Trauma. 1999;13(3):207-11.
11. Matta JM. Indications for anterior fixation of pelvic fractures. Clin Orthop Relat Res. 1996;(329):88-96.

12. Simonian PT, Schwappach JR, Routt ML Jr, et al. Evaluation of new plate designs for symphysis pubis internal fixation. J Trauma. 1996;41(3):498-502.
13. Webb LX, Gristina AG, Wilson JR, et al. Two-hole plate fixation for traumatic symphysis pubis diastasis. J Trauma. 1988;28(6):813-7.
14. Tornetta P 3rd, Hochwald N, Levine R. Corona mortis. Incidence and location. Clin Orthop Relat Res. 1996;(329):97-101.
15. Kottmeier SA, Farcy JP, Baruch HM. The ilioinguinal approach to acetabular fracture mangament.Op Techs in Orthop. 1993:60-70.
16. Routt ML Jr, Simonian PT, Grujic L. The retrograde medullary superior pubic ramus screw for the treatment of anterior pelvic ring disruptions: a new technique. J Orthop Trauma. 1995;9(1):35-44.
17. Simonian PT, Routt ML Jr, Harrington RM, et al. Internal fixation of the unstable anterior pelvic ring: a biomechanical comparison of standard plating techniques and the retrograde medullary superior pubic ramus screw. J Orthop Trauma. 1994;8(6):476-82.
18. Starr AJ, Nakatani T, Reinert CM, et al. Superior pubic ramus fractures fixed with percutaneous screws: what predicts fixation failure? J Orthop Trauma. 2008;22(2):81-7
19. Barei DP, Bellabarba C, Mills WJ, et al. Percutaneous management of unstable pelvic ring disruptions. Injury. 2001;32 Suppl 1:SA33-44.
20. Routt ML Jr, Simonian PT, Mills WJ. Iliosacral screw fixation: early complications of the percutaneous technique. J Orthop Trauma. 1997;11(8):584-9.
21. Gardner MJ, Osgood G, Molnar R, et al. Percutaneous pelvic fixation using working portals in a circumferential pelvic antishock sheet. J Orthop Trauma. 2009;23(9):668-74.
22. Gardner MJ, Parada S, Chip Routt ML Jr. Internal rotation and taping of the lower extremities for closed pelvic reduction. J Orthop Trauma. 2009;23(5):361-4.
23. Gardner MJ, Kendoff D, Ostermeier S, Citak M, Hüfner T, Krettek C, Nork SE.Sacroiliac joint compression using an anterior pelvic compressor: a mechanical study in synthetic bone. J Orthop Trauma. 2007;21(7):435-41.
24. Gardner MJ, Nork SE. Stabilization of unstable pelvic fractures with supraacetabular compression external fixation. J Orthop Trauma. 2007;21(4):269-73.
25. Archdeacon MT, Safian C, Le TT. A cadaver study of the trochanteric pelvic clamp for pelvic reduction. J Orthop Trauma. 2007;21(1):38-42.
26. Pohlemann T, Braune C, Gänsslen A, et al. A. Pelvic emergency clamps: anatomic landmarks for a safe primary application. J Orthop Trauma. 2004;18(2):102-5.
27. Richard MJ, Tornetta P 3rd. Emergent management of APC-2 pelvic ring injuries with an anteriorly placed C-clamp. J Orthop Trauma. 2009;23(5):322-6.
28. Schütz M, Stöckle U, Hoffmann R, et al. Clinical experience with two types of pelvic C-clamps for unstable pelvic ring injuries. Injury. 1996;27 Suppl 1:S-A46-50.
29. Wright RD, Glueck DA, Selby JB, et al. Intraoperative use of the pelvic c-clamp as an aid in reduction for posterior sacroiliac fixation. J OrthopTrauma. 2006;20(8):576-9.
30. Conflitti JM, Graves ML, Chip Routt ML Jr. Radiographic quantification andanalysis of dysmorphic upper sacral osseous anatomy and associated iliosacral screw insertions. J Orthop Trauma. 2010;24(10):630-6.
31. Routt ML Jr, Simonian PT, Agnew SG, et al. Radiographic recognition of the sacral alar slope for optimal placement of iliosacral screws: a cadaveric and clinical study. J Orthop Trauma. 1996;10(3):171-7.
32. Reilly MC, Bono CM, Litkouhi B, et al. The effect of sacral fracture malreduction on the safe placement of iliosacral screws. J Orthop Trauma. 2006;20(1 Suppl):S37-43.
33. Gardner MJ, Morshed S, Nork SE, et al. Quantification of the upper and second sacral segment safe zones in normal and dysmorphic sacra. J Orthop Trauma. 2010;24(10):622-9.
34. Moed BR, Geer BL. S2 iliosacral screw fixation for disruptions of the posterior pelvic ring: a report of 49 cases. J Orthop Trauma. 2006;20(6):378-83.
35. van Zwienen CM, van den Bosch EW, Snijders CJ, et al. Biomechanical comparison of sacroiliac screw techniques for unstable pelvic ring fractures. J Orthop Trauma. 2004;18(9):589-95.
36. Griffin DR, Starr AJ, Reinert CM, et al. Vertically unstable pelvic fractures fixed with percutaneous iliosacral screws: does posterior injury pattern predict fixation failure? J Orthop Trauma. 2006;20(1 Suppl):S30-6.
37. Gardner MJ, Routt ML Jr. Transiliac-transsacral screws for posterior pelvic stabilization. J Orthop Trauma. 2011;25(6):378-84.
38. Moed BR, Fissel BA, Jasey G. Percutaneous transiliac pelvic fracture fixation: cadaver feasibility study and preliminary clinical results. J Trauma. 2007;62(2):357-64.
39. Moed BR, Whiting DR. Locked transsacral screw fixation of bilateral injuries of the posterior pelvic ring: initial clinical series. J Orthop Trauma. 2010;24(10):616-21.
40. Tornetta P 3rd, Templeman DC. Expected outcomes after pelvic ring injury. Instr Course Lect. 2005;54:401-7.
41. Tornetta P 3rd, Matta JM. Outcome of operatively treated unstable posterior pelvic ring disruptions. Clin Orthop Relat Res. 1996;(329):186-93.

Chapter 17

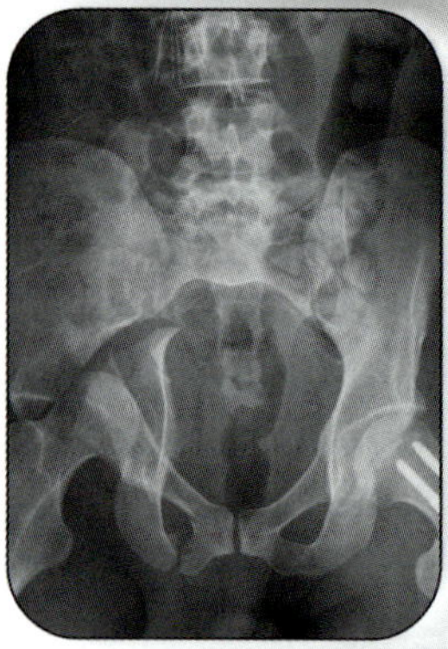

Acetabulum Fractures

Bruce Ziran, Stephen Becher

Chapter Outline

Introduction
- Historical Perspective
- Epidemiology and Outcome

Radiography and Classification
- Classification and Identification by Judet Views

Surgical Indications
- The Rationale for Operative and Nonoperative Treatment

Surgical Anatomy, Surgical Approaches and Techniques
- Approaches to the Acetabulum
- Posterior Wall and Column Injuries
- Anterior Column and Anterior Wall Fractures
- Transverse and Transverse Posterior Wall Fractures
- Both Column Fractures
- T-Type Fractures
- Anterior Column Posterior Hemitransverse Fractures
- Adjunct and Novel Methodologies

Complications
- Heterotopic Ossification
- Deep Vein Thrombosis and Pulmonary Embolism
- Nerve Palsy
- Malunion and Nonunion
- Late Stage Arthritis
- Late Instability after Open Reduction and Internal Fixation

Authors' Preferred Management of Select Complications
- Case 1: Management of Deep Infection
- Case 2: Surgical Management of Heterotopic Ossification of the Hip

Summary

Introduction

Historical Perspective

The acetabular fracture is a condition of the modern industrial era. The first detailed description of the fracture of acetabulum was made in 1820s.[1] Undoubtedly, injuries with the energy required to fracture an acetabulum before the modern era did occur, but were most likely fatal. Acetabular fractures began to be described more often in the 20th century, but the first half of the century was riddled with scattered terminologies and treatments. Nonoperative treatment was the rule until 1940s, when the World War II brought about a large increase in the number of these injuries.[2] Urist reported on 15 posterior wall fracture-dislocations treated with open reduction and internal fixation (ORIF) in soldiers injured during the war.[3] An early seminal work by Carter Rowe outlined the severity and problems of these injuries with a large portion of patients developing problems with pain, gait, function and post-traumatic arthritis.

Progress was made over the next 15 years, but a truly modern view did not arrive until 1960s, when Judet and Letournel published their classic work on acetabular fractures. They introduced the Judet views as well as an older version of the Letournel and Judet classification still used today. Since that time, ORIF of displaced acetabular fractures gradually became the standard of care. The origin of modern treatment can be seen in their infancy in the 1964 article, with approaches being dictated by the fracture pattern.[4] Their textbook translated into English in 1981 and allowed the modern Letournel classification to be disseminated widely in the United States.[5] The idea of weight-bearing dome was introduced by Matta in 1986,[6,7] and computed tomography (CT) scans were used to quantify the roof-arc previously defined by radiographs in 1993.[8] Throughout last 40 years, there have been modifications to the approaches described by Letournel, including the tri-radiate, Gibson, modified Rives-Stoppa, trochanteric osteotomy and numerous other "modifications". The synthesis of information has allowed the treatment of acetabular fractures to proceed in a more scientific manner, accounting for the involvement of weight-bearing dome, size of the posterior wall fracture and congruency of the joint space. This chapter focuses on the modern approach to acetabular fractures and their associated issues.

Epidemiology and Outcome

The original series presented by Judet had 159 patients, of which 77% received their injury due to a motor vehicle collision.[4] Patterns of injury have changed since the early 60s. The introduction of mandatory safety belts has been shown not only to reduce the incidence of acetabular fractures, but also to reduce associated injuries to the chest, abdominal cavity, head and other long bones.[9] A 16-year 2003 study from Edinburgh provides the most modern and applicable picture of acetabular fractures in the modern era,[10] showing an incidence of about 0.4% of all fractures treated. However, the associated injuries as measured by the Injury Severity Score declined in each 5-year period of the study, falling from 16 to 10. In addition, mortality was higher in earlier time periods of the study due to the increase in associated injuries to patients. Sixty two percent of all fractures were displaced and the distribution of displaced to nondisplaced fractures remained constant over time. The posterior wall fracture was the most common pattern in 23%. The mechanism of injury was substantially different from the days of Judet, with motor vehicle collisions accounting for 38% of injuries, falls from a height greater than 10 feet accounting for 27%, falls from a height less than 10 feet accounting for 12.8% and pedestrian accidents accounting for 8% of injuries.

Complications from acetabular fractures can occur from the injury itself or as a consequence of the treatment. The early complications from the result of injury are best dealt by a multidisciplinary team, which includes general trauma surgeons, intensivists and other specialists, as needed in addition to the orthopedic surgeon. The management of polytraumatized patients, retroperitoneal hematomas, hemorrhagic shock and Morel-Lavallee lesions are beyond the scope of this chapter, but the treating orthopedist should be comfortable with these situations. Perioperative complications occur frequently: sciatic nerve palsy (1–18%),[11] postoperative infection (4–6%),[2,5,10] deep vein thrombosis (DVT) (2–27%),[12-14] pulmonary embolism (PE) (0.6–2.2%),[12-14] postoperative arthritis (12–30%)[5,10,15] and heterotopic ossification (HO) (10–86%).[16-18]

Recently, two social trends have resulted in the need to examine the traditional "one size fits all" approach to these fractures. Specifically, the obese and active elderly populations are distinctly different than the young adults. Obese patients, defined as those with a basal metabolic index (BMI) greater than 30, are at greater risk for perioperative complications than those with a BMI less than 30. Morbidly obese patients (BMI > 40) are at much higher risk for postoperative infection (odds ratio: 5), blood loss of greater than 750 ml (odds ratio: 2.1) and symptomatic deep vein thrombosis (odds ratio: 2.6). Surprisingly, obesity did not affect the rate of pulmonary embolism, HO and sciatic nerve palsy.[19] Elderly patients have more medical comorbidities than younger patients do, but no study has shown particular increases with regards to complications in the elderly, though the sickest elderly patients simply do not undergo surgery. Recent series have shown that revision total hip arthroplasty occurs in 30% of elderly patients[15] contrasted with 12% overall in the Edinburgh review.[10] Letournel recommended an attempt at ORIF in medically stable patients and subsequent evidence has supported the conclusion he made from his series.[5] There is some recent work that proposes primary total hip arthroplasty in the elderly when there is gross comminution and extensive loss of articular cartilage.[20] With this approach, the acetabulum is still repaired to establish a stable foundation, within which a socket is secured, usually with supplemental fixation (screws or cement), with the understanding that these patients will be lower demand and with limited life spans.[21]

Radiography and Classification

The utility of the Letournel classification is both understanding the nature of the fracture as well as selecting the approach needed. Adjuncts found in recent years including the gull sign, roof-arc measurement, and percentage of posterior wall involvement, also guide the clinician towards or away from the operating room for selected fracture patterns. Before one can apply these tools, a thorough understanding of normal anatomy of the acetabulum and its radiographic landmarks must be understood.

The anteroposterior (AP) pelvis is the starting point for all radiographic evaluation of the pelvis. There are six major landmarks that should be seen on the AP view: iliopectineal line, ilioischial line, anterior rim of acetabulum, posterior rim of acetabulum, roof of acetabulum and teardrop (Fig. 17.1). The iliopectineal line best represents the anterior column of acetabulum. It runs from the superior border of the symphysis pubis, until it merges proximally with the ilioischial

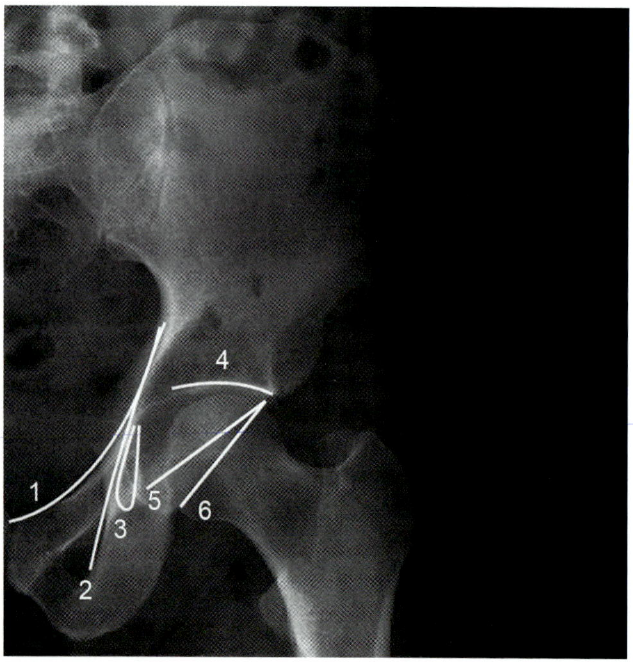

Figure 17.1: Anteroposterior (AP) pelvis radiograph with outline of six major radiographic landmarks (1) Iliopectineal line; (2) Ilioischial line; (3) Tear drop; (4) Dome; (5) Anterior wall; (6) Posterior wall.

line to form the true pelvic brim. The ilioischial line runs from the posterior or lateral aspect of obturator foramen up over the ischial spine, until it merges with the ilioischial line to form the pelvic brim. It represents the posterior column of acetabulum. The anterior and posterior lips of acetabulum themselves represent the anterior and posterior walls, respectively. The anterior rim line merges seamlessly into the superior border of obturator foramen, and the complete line is called the acetabulo-obturator line. The radiographic teardrop is not an actual structure, but rather a confluence of radiographic shadows. It represents the anterior and posterior aspects of the medial acetabulum and the quadrilateral surface at the same level, which is essentially the bone between the quadrilateral surface and cotyloid fossa. The sourcil (French for eyebrow) or roof of the acetabulum is just as it sounds, a radiographic density representing the subchondral bone supporting the weight bearing dome of the joint. It is important to evaluate roof-arc measurement on all views of the radiograph. Also, on the AP radiograph, impaction of the superiomedial dome of the acetabulum will produce a double lucency overlying the acetabulum—this is the "Gull Sign" as described first by Judet and Letournel,[5] and was noted to be a poor prognostic sign for ORIF of acetabular fractures in the elderly by Anglen.[22] It should be noted, but so should any obvious articular impaction that will need to be addressed at surgery.

The Judet views of pelvis enhance or remove these six landmarks from the radiograph so as to allow each one to be identified and evaluated separately. The obturator-oblique radiograph is taken with the patient's affected hip elevated at 45°, raising the injured hemipelvis (Fig. 17.2). This allows the obturator foramen to be in face and the iliac wing to be in profile (tangential) to the radiographic beam. The posterior rim or wall of the acetabulum is now much more clearly visible, and if fractured, will be the most obvious on this view. The iliopectineal line is now the only border on the medial pelvis seen and the anterior column can be evaluated without difficulty. Also of note is that the obturator foramen is well visualized and any fracture extending into it (such as a posterior column fracture or T-type fracture) will be best seen on this view. The teardrop is obliterated by the angle of the radiograph beam, and the ilioischial line and anterior wall landmarks are not clearly visible. The roof of acetabulum may still be seen and represents the posterior superior aspect of the acetabular dome.

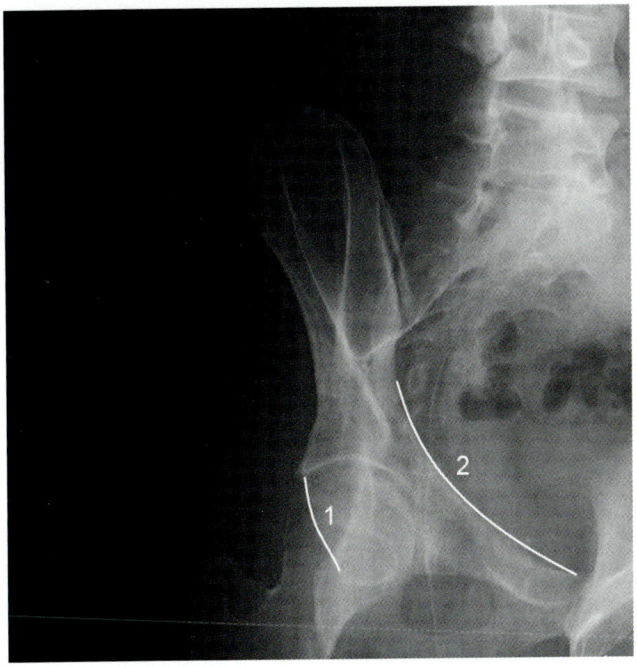

Figure 17.2: Obturator-oblique radiograph.
1. Posterior wall, 2. Anterior column.

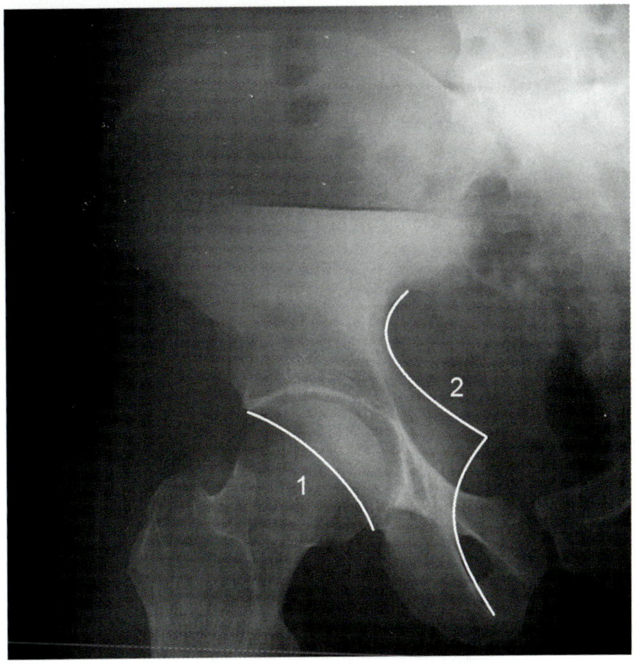

Figure 17.3: Iliac oblique radiograph.
1. Anterior wall, 2. Posterior column.

The iliac oblique view is taken with affected side down and the contralateral pelvis elevated 45° (Fig. 17.3). This will result in the affected iliac wing being seen in face and the obturator foramen (anterior rami) in profile (tangential). On this radiograph, the posterior column and ilioischial segment is seen well, and fractures of the posterior column are most easily diagnosed. Fractures of the iliac wing and upper anterior column are well visualized in this view. Finally, the anterior wall of acetabulum is easily evaluated. Of course, the roof of acetabulum is still seen and should be used to evaluate the roof-arc.

Classification and Identification by Judet Views

The five types are as follows:

1. *Isolated posterior wall*: Best seen on the obturator-oblique radiograph with a disruption of the posterior rim.
2. *Isolated posterior column*: Best seen on the iliac oblique radiograph with a disruption of the ilioischial line. By definition, it will extend through the obturator foramen and thus, have a fracture line through the ischium visible on the obturator-oblique radiograph.
3. *Isolated anterior wall*: Best seen on the iliac oblique radiograph with a disruption of the anterior rim line.
4. *Isolated anterior column*: Best seen on the obturator-oblique radiograph with a disruption of the iliopectineal line. It may have a fracture through the obturator foramen and thus, is visible on the iliac oblique radiograph.
5. *Transverse acetabular fractures*: Seen on all three views with a fracture line that disrupts both the ilioischial and iliopectineal lines on their respective radiographs. Transverse fractures can be further classified by the level of fracture in relation to the acetabular articular surface. Tectum is the level, where the superior edge of cotyloid fossa meets the acetabular weight-bearing dome. An infratectal fracture is low and does not involve the weight bearing fossa. A juxtatectal fracture shears through the junction of fossa and articular surface. A transtectal fracture involves the weight bearing surface. The higher up a fracture goes, worse is the prognosis and greater is a need for surgical intervention for anatomical reduction.

The five basic types of fractures can be combined to form five associated fracture patterns. When combined with five basic types, full ten types of acetabular fractures as classified by Letournel are obtained. The associated fracture patterns are as follows:

1. *T-shaped fractures:* A transverse fracture with an associated vertical fracture line that can occur in any plane. The transverse fracture component will have a fracture exiting through the obturator ring. The major difference between pure transverse and T-shaped fracture is that reduction of the transverse component will only stabilize one column, either anterior or posterior depending on the type of approach used. If both anterior and posterior limbs of the T-shaped fracture are displaced, a combined approach must be used.
2. *Posterior wall with posterior column:* A combination of two posterior injuries that may be addressed with a posterior approach alone.
3. *Posterior wall with a transverse fracture:* It is possible to reduce a transverse fracture through either an anterior or posterior approach. The posterior wall can only be addressed posteriorly, and in this associated type directs the surgeon to address the overall fracture posteriorly.
4. *Anterior column with a posterior hemitransverse pattern:* A variant of the T-shaped fracture, where the transverse component exits at different levels for the anterior and posterior columns.
5. *Both column fractures:* This fracture involves a complete separation of the articular surface of acetabulum from the remaining ilium still attached to the sacroiliac (SI) joint. A diagnostic aid radiographically is the "spur sign"—the image of intact ilium on the obturator-oblique view, while the two columns suffer medial displacement. The acetabulum is essentially floating in this fracture pattern. The femoral head can at times, produce secondary congruence, or the radiographic appearance of relatively circular and congruent acetabulum about the femoral head. Secondary congruence can be a rationale for nonoperative treatment in the elderly for both column fractures, where medical comorbidities can complicate the decision to proceed to surgery.

There is also the AO/OTA classification, which is based on increasing severity of pelvic and acetabular disruption. They modified the Letournel classification to match the overall AO classification. It is included for the sake of completeness in Table 17.1. While very useful for descriptive studies, the Judet-Letournel classification remains the mainstay amongst traumatologists.

Table 17.1: AO classification of acetabular fractures

Type A:	Partial articular fractures; one column
A1	Posterior wall fracture
A2	Posterior column fracture
A3	Anterior wall or column fracture
Type B:	Partial articular fractures; transverse
B1	Pure transverse
B2	T-shaped fracture
B3	Anterior column and posterior hemitransverse
Type C:	Complete articular fractures; both columns
C1	High
C2	Low
C3	With SI joint involvement

Prior to modern CT, radiographic interpretation was crucial for deciding treatment, surgical approach and tactic. With advances in CT scans, not only two-dimensional reconstructions are possible, but well-made three-dimensional (3D) reconstructions allow easy identification of the fracture pattern and greatly assist in decision making. In fact, due to modern CT scans, radiographic understanding of acetabular fractures is becoming a lost art form. In general, CT scans used to obtain 3D reconstructions need to be fine cut to allow adequate resolution in the reformatting. Computed tomography scans can also show nondisplaced fractures that are not seen on plain radiographs such as nondisplaced transverse fractures. Marginal impaction of the acetabular dome is best appreciated on CT scan and must be addressed at the time of surgery. Intra-articular fragments of varying size and injury to the femoral head can be seen on CT imaging. In addition, the size of the posterior wall fragment can be assessed as compared to the contralateral side. Some fractures that might be candidates for nonoperative treatment by plain radiography alone will need surgical intervention when analyzed with CT imaging, or vice versa, as in cases of elderly both column fractures with secondary congruence. Since, so many fracture and trauma patients are getting routine CT scans, the need for radiographs has been questioned with the use of CT radiographs. In these images, the CT scan is used to emulate a plain radiograph, without overlying soft tissues. Such modalities may in future obviate the need for routine plain radiographs, and avoid some pain associated with obtaining Judet views (rolling a patient on a fractured acetabulum is not well tolerated). It has been shown that CT scans have superior accuracy and interobserver reliability as compared to plain Judet films.[23,24]

Surgical Indications

The Rationale for Operative and Nonoperative Treatment

Letournel originally thought that any displaced fracture of the acetabulum should undergo operative intervention.[4] Casting such a large net would no doubt improve radiographic outcomes for all patients, but may cause unnecessary surgery. Many factors must be considered when the decision for surgery is weighed. The fracture involvement of the weight-bearing dome, hip stability, pattern, displacement and location, patient's age and functional status, and secondary congruence should all be weighed. The decision to undergo surgery is not a light one. An acetabular fracture that goes on to arthrosis after nonoperative treatment will no doubt be viewed with dismay by both patient and surgeon. Having an unnecessary surgery, or worse, unnecessary surgery causing a complication, is also not something any patient or surgeon would want. A careful balance must be struck, and unfortunately, there are no hard and fast rules in this area of orthopedics.

Involvement of the weight-bearing dome has long been known to be a poor prognostic factor for acetabular fractures. The incongruity of the weight-bearing area is thought to lead to elevated contact stresses and late arthrosis. However, what exactly "defines" the weight-bearing dome is not known at this time. The hip has a variety of weight-bearing surfaces as it moves through its wide range of motion. Initial classification of transverse fractures into infratectal, juxtatectal and transtectal shows a general understanding that the weight-bearing dome is important, although its exact parameters are poorly defined.[20]

Roof-arc measurements were first described by Matta in 1986 as a way of defining the weight-bearing dome of the acetabulum. The roof-arc is measured by taking the center of femoral head and drawing a vertical line through it (Fig. 17.4). A second line is then drawn between the

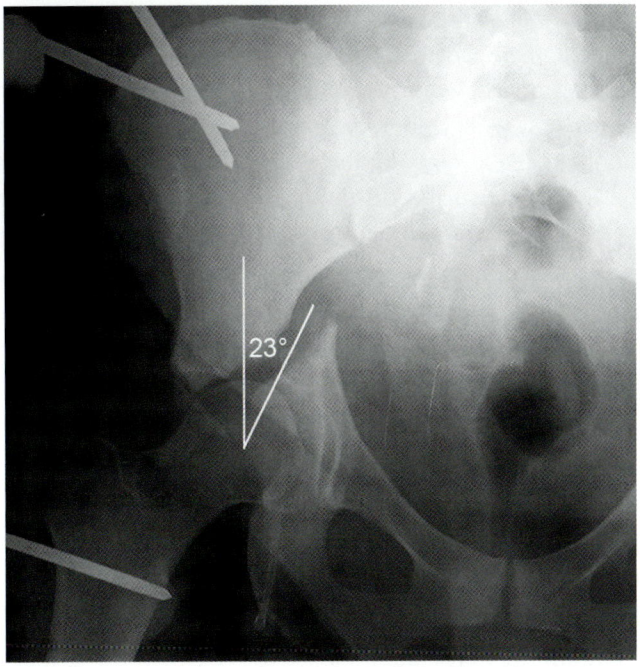

Figure 17.4: An example of roof-arc measured off the antero-posterior image. This medial roof-arc measures approximately 23° and thus involves the weight-bearing dome.

fracture fragment on the AP and Judet views through the center of femoral head. The angle subtended between the two lines is known as the roof-arc measurement. There are three angles to be measured. The medial roof-arc is measured off the AP film, the anterior roof-arc off the obturator-oblique and the posterior roof-arc off the iliac-oblique view. Initially, it was felt that if the angle was greater than 45° in all three views, the weight-bearing dome of the acetabulum was not involved.[6,7] Further investigation has altered the angle needed to preclude involvement of the weight-bearing dome. Multiple studies have differing angles, with the posterior roof-arc ranging from 60 to 70°, anterior roof-arc ranging from 25 to 50° and medial roof-arc ranging from 40 to 50°.[6,7,25,26]

Olson showed that a CT scan can be used to determine roof-arc measurement. If 2 mm cuts are used, five cuts from the subchondral arc of the weight-bearing dome on down are evaluated. If the fracture line does not involve 10 mm of superior acetabulum in this range, it is felt to be equivalent to roof-arc measurements of 45° using the method described first by Matta. Naturally, since the 45° arc measurement is a guide rather than a rule, the CT subchondral arc measurement is similarly only a guide. A fracture line that has a large roof-arc measurement and involvement well below the subchondral arc on CT scan, is very unlikely to involve the weight-bearing dome, and thus, may be considered for nonoperative treatment, but only in the overall context of the fracture. It would be unwise to use radiographic measurements alone to determine the treatment course.

In addition to weight-bearing involvement, hip stability is extremely important for long-term function of the hip. An unstable hip will lead to early arthritis and possibly dislocate recurrently. Posterior wall fractures often do not involve the weight-bearing dome, but may cause significant morbidity due to hip instability. There are several proposed methods to determine the stability of posterior wall segments. Recently, Moed expounded on the use of CT scan to evaluate size of the posterior wall fragment, and added the use of a fluoroscopic stress examination in order to determine which posterior wall segments are stable and require operative stabilization. Moed's method uses the CT axial cut with the greatest posterior wall involvement. A medial to lateral measurement of intact posterior wall and the uninjured side are taken. Involvement is then expressed as percentage. Moed's method has been shown to have the highest positive predictive value and should be the method of choice for measuring posterior wall fragment size. Only fragments with a size less than 20% were found to be stable. Fragments with a size greater than 50% were always unstable and those between 20% and 50% needed a fluoroscopic stress exam under anesthesia to determine stability. Patients found to have a stable hip either after stress exam of a CT fragment less than 20% or treated nonoperatively had a good clinical outcome. Stability is not, however, the only factor to consider in determining whether to proceed with surgery or not. Some surgeons have proposed that a nonosseous posterior lesion involving a labral tear is just as serious as a bony wall fracture. Again, the radiographic measurements must be taken as but one factor among many.[27,28] The pattern, location and displacement of the fracture must be taken into account. For example, low anterior column fractures, for instance, may be treated more as high rami fractures at times. Displacement of an articular surface greater than 2 mm is a cause for concern due to incongruity of the joint and should be addressed. Any marginal impaction or incarcerated fragments demand operative intervention as well.[2,5,20] Age alone is not a cause to change treatment course. However, as patients age, their medical comorbidities such as osteopenia and metabolic bone disease will make fixation difficult. Also, the stress of surgery in a patient with a number of medical comorbidities should be weighed. If the patient has secondary congruence of their acetabulum as well as advanced age and medical issues, nonoperative treatment should be considered. However, secondary congruence in a younger patient is not enough to warrant nonoperative management. Nonoperative treatment still consists of early motion, pain control, thromboembolic prophylaxis and serial radiographic imaging. It is recommended that weekly radiographs should be obtained during the first 6 weeks at a minimum to ensure that late fracture displacement does not occur. Progressive weight bearing may be begun after 8-12 weeks, if fracture healing is obvious on radiographs and clinically. Toe-touch weight bearing may be used initially as non-weight-bearing motion places greater stress on the hip joint due to contraction of the abductors. Any sign of displacement or instability should push the patient and surgeon towards operative intervention.

Surgical Anatomy, Surgical Approaches and Techniques

Approaches to the Acetabulum

Posterior Approach

Kocher-Langenbeck approach: The approach to the acetabulum will be dictated by fracture pattern. The workhorse of posterior pelvis is the Kocher-Langenbeck approach. It is usually familiar to most surgeons from hip arthroplasty. Posterior wall, posterior column and some transverse and certain T-fractures can be accessed by this approach. Rarely, a few both column fractures can be addressed via posterior approach. In certain fractures that involve the superior aspects of acetabulum, some transverse and T-fractures, and in obese patients, better visualization of the posterior pelvis can be achieved with a digastric trochanteric osteotomy.

Patient positioning may be either prone or lateral, but this aspect is hotly and passionately debated by both schools of thought. The proposed advantage of prone positioning is easier access through the notch, nullification of gravity and better imaging. The disadvantage is not having the leg freely mobile (e.g. femoral head fracture that needs anterior access) and an inability to perform a trochanteric osteotomy. The proposed advantage of lateral positioning is the ability to have the leg free, to perform a trochanteric osteotomy and familiarity with exposure. The authors are familiar with both prone and lateral positioning and believe that the lateral position offers the most advantage. The authors have not found an access to the notch to be problematic (if the surgeon's cephalad hand is used to palpate through the notch) and use of a perineal post or large pad as a fulcrum effectively to overcome the weight of the leg. Furthermore, if traction is desired, a setup similar to lateral femoral nailing provides an excellent luxation of the hip, when needed. Most importantly, in obese patients, the lateral position allows the tissues to fall away more than in the prone position and does not require constant assistance to hold the hindquarter. The lateral position also allows intraoperative decision to perform a digastric trochanteric osteotomy (as described by Siebenrock and Agudelo), so that concomitant femoral head fractures can be addressed with surgical hip dislocation. We have also found it suitable to place anterior column screws, if needed, using modified oblique views.

Three proximal incision lines can be used: (1) one in line with the femur while flexed, (2) one in line with the femur, while extended, and (3) one in between the two. The middle line is best suited for the skin incision. While there are several eponyms and modifications (modified Gibson, lateral, etc.), the end result Is fairly similar with little deep variations. In all approaches, the deep dissection is focused around the posterior column from superior acetabulum to ischium. We prefer an incision between the traditional Kocher and straight lateral, because it provides ample posterior access, while allowing the ability to obtain more anterior access (via an osteotomy described below), if needed. Superficially, sharp dissection should be made down to the gluteal fascia, cautery should be reserved until the gluteal and tensor fascia is incised, and a Charnley retractor is placed. The tension on the skin edges by Charnley retractor will often preclude the need for extensive electrocautery and shorten the operative time and thermal tissue damage from cautery. Excision of trochanteric bursal tissue will reveal the piriformis tendon as well as tendons of short external rotators. These should be tagged with a strong suture and released. Retraction of the piriformis should allow the sciatic nerve to come into view. A visual inspection of the nerve is in order to assess any variants of the piriformis/sciatic nerve relationship and ensure that no bone fragments are causing direct pressure on the nerve. Retraction of obturator internus will protect the nerve and a retractor may be placed along the tendon sheath into the lesser notch to allow visualization. Another retractor should be placed underneath the gluteus minimus and iliac wing periosteum to allow superior visualization. Care must be taken to place the retractor between minimus and periosteum and not in the plane between gluteus medius and minimus. Damaged minimus tissue should be debrided, as it is commonly the source of heterotopic ossification. The superior gluteal neurovascular bundle is at risk with excessive superior retraction of abductors and proximal extension of the incision through gluteus maximus. A stay suture in the proximal gluteal musculature may be used if the bundle is felt to be at risk. Inferior dissection with electrocautery of the ischial tuberosity will define the distal extent of the exposure and should be performed for inferior plate placement; at times, a portion of hamstrings may need to be partially detached. We prefer the use of Cobra retractors instead of sharp-tipped hohmans. One Cobra is placed superiorly towards the inferior spine, the second into the lesser notch and the third just anterior to the infra-acetabular groove near the ischium and into the obturator fossa (Fig. 17.5). We do not like to place retractors or clamps through greater sciatic notch for extended periods. The whole of the posterior column and posterior wall can be visualized with this approach. The major surgical risks are to the sciatic

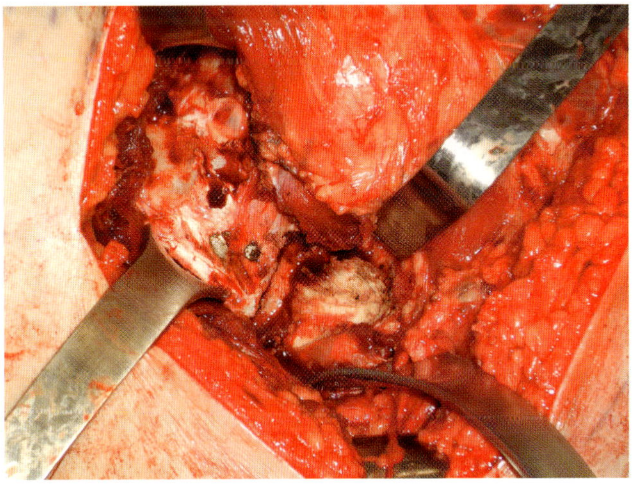

Figure 17.5: A clinical image showing proper placement of retractors during the Kocher approach.

nerve and superior gluteal neurovascular bundle. The sciatic nerve should be visualized in the traumatic situation (it is often not visualized during arthroplasty) and the hip should remain extended and the knee flexed.[2,5,20,29]

Trochanteric osteotomy: A trochanteric osteotomy is occasionally needed for very superior fractures, fractures of the femoral head requiring anterior access or dislocation and in obese individuals. This approach can also be used to facilitate reduction of anterior components of a fracture, as in certain transverse or T-type fractures treated from a posterior approach. A traditional osteotomy takes the top of the trochanter attached to the abductor mechanism (Fig. 17.6). It is reattached with screws, wires or special cleats.[30] The nonunion rate is variable, but has been reported as low as 0%[30,31] and is generally felt to be safe. If the repaired osteotomy fails to unite, gait can be affected, if migration exceeds 1.5–2.0 cm. We have adopted the digastric trochanteric osteotomy as described by Siebenrock.[30] This osteotomy maintains the vastus and medius attachments and separates the outer greater trochanter in a sagittal plane and along the lateral cortex of the femur. The advantage of this osteotomy is the counter opposing muscle forces of the gluteus and vastus, which serve to provide a small compressive force at the osteotomy surface, as well as prevent cephalad or caudad migration. The nonunion rate is exceeding low, and repair is with two or three small screws. We have found very little morbidity with the osteotomy that would not be incurred from the fracture itself. Since this osteotomy is used for fractures that involve anterior or superior aspects of the acetabulum, there is an inherent risk for heterotopic bone formation. The added effect of the osteotomy to such injuries predicates the consideration of prophylaxis against heterotopic bone. We do not use or advocate the use of indomethacin and have routinely used a single dose of therapeutic radiation as determined by the radiation oncologists. The dosimetry may vary with patient habitus, but they will provide ample prophylaxis. Historically, radiation was required within the first 24–48 hours, but some recent data suggest that even if unable to provide radiation in the early time frame, there is still a therapeutic benefit to prophylaxis, even if delayed up to 4 days.[32]

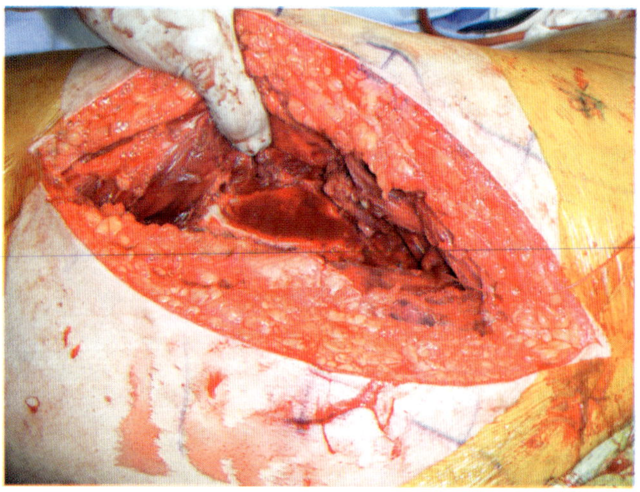

Figure 17.6: Clinical image of osteotomy showing maintained vastus and medius attachments to the osteotomized trochanter (underneath the surgeons thumb).

Other posterior approaches: There are a variety of other novel posterior approaches used including a chevron, a modified lateral and variations of the standard Kocher. Since the overwhelming majority of mainstream surgeons will use their own modification of the traditional Kocher, such novel, but marginally useful approaches are out of the scope of this report.

Anterior Approaches

If anterior exposure is necessary, the three approaches most used are the ilioinguinal, iliofemoral (Smith-Peterson) and modified stoppa. We have now used the modified stoppa for most anterior acetabular work, but will describe the ilioinguinal as well, since general familiarity with the less invasive stoppa approach is less prevalent, but is rising quickly. We feel that the modified stoppa combined with the lateral ilioinguinal window, is not only easier and allows for better reduction and fixation options, but is much safer than the traditional ilioinguinal approach, as it avoids dissection around the vascular bundle. It also allows access to the deep pelvis and posterior column from the front with an ability to directly access, reduce and fix such structures. With all anterior approaches, the patient should be placed supine on a radiolucent table with entire leg draped to allow flexion of the hip. Alternatively, a sloppy lateral position may be used, if a combined approach is going to be undertaken. However, we are not proponents of such a simultaneous tactics, since each approach (anterior and posterior) is compromised due to positioning limitations.

Iliofemoral (Smith-Peterson) approach: The iliofemoral approach is basically a modified Smith-Peterson approach. It is used primarily for pipkin lesions and has been utilized for periacetabular osteotomies. Centered over anterior superior iliac spine (ASIS), it provides access to the anterior column, anterior wall, can be extended to provide access to the iliac wing (both inner and outer tables) and can reach the SI joint. It provides limited access medial to the anterior wall, and if rami or symphyseal lesions need to be addressed, a separate Pfannenstiel incision may be necessary. This approach is well described in texts. The superficial dissection must manage the lateral femoral cutaneous nerve. If it is not seen or courses medial, without interfering with the surgical tactic, it is left alone. If it is in the way, we prefer surgical excision rather than excessive traction. Patients are told that they will have an anesthetic area on the lateral thigh. The surgeons have not seen any morbidity with such a cutaneous lesion, but traction lesions have resulted in cases of meralgia paresthetica, which is much more difficult to treat and is poorly tolerated by patients. The anesthetic area on the thigh often will decrease to a very small area due to local recruitment and adaptation. The deep dissection continues and the reflected head of the rectus is detached as needed. Cobra retractors can be placed strategically around the medial and lateral femoral neck and over the pelvic brim as needed. The hip can be dislocated anteriorly with gentle adduction/external rotation. We do not modify the approach as described in standard texts, except to suggest that for acetabular fractures, if the outer iliac fossa is dissected, consideration should be given to prophylaxis for heterotopic bone formation.

We have used few modifications including taking down some of the tensor fascia lata and placement of a blunt Cobra over the anterior rim and under the psoas to facilitate exposure. These exposures are more commonly used for femoral head fractures or more recently for anterior surgical dislocation of the hip.

Ilioinguinal approach: The ilioinguinal skin incision runs from the iliac crest in a curved fashion to include ASIS and course of the inguinal ligament. It ends at a point about two fingerbreadths above the symphysis. There will be three major windows to the ilioinguinal approach-medial, middle and lateral (Fig. 17.7). The lateral window begins by incising the fascial insertion of iliac crest and mobilizing the iliacus muscle off the iliac inner table. There is usually a nutrient vessel just anterior to the SI joint that requires bone wax. Blunt dissection can be used to palpate over the pelvic brim and allow visualization of the entire iliac wing. More medially, the surgeon will encounter the spermatic cord in males and round ligament in females exiting the superficial inguinal ring. The fascia of external oblique should be incised in the same direction as the skin incision from ASIS to inguinal ring. Once exposed, the contents of inguinal canal—the spermatic cord or round ligament, should be retracted medially using a flexible vessel loop. Retracting the external oblique fascia inferiorly and spermatic contents medially will allow visualization of the conjoint tendon medially and the floor of the inguinal canal consisting of fibers of the internal oblique and transversalis fascia (Fig. 17.8). Both should be incised in line with the skin incision leaving a cuff of tissue on each side to facilitate repair. Near the ASIS, care must be taken to avoid the lateral femoral cutaneous nerve, which is approximately 1 cm below the ASIS underneath the conjoint tendon. Traction injuries to this nerve can cause meralgia paresthetica. If at risk for traction injury, it may be preferable to excise the nerve, but the patient should be made aware of a small patch of numbness that will occur on the lateral thigh. We have not found this sensory deficit to be problematic and most patients report the size of the anesthetic area to decrease with time. Once the conjoint tendon is cut, the interval between the psoas muscle and external iliac neurovascular bundle should proceed. The iliopectineal fascia is a thin structure separating the muscle-nerve compartment from the

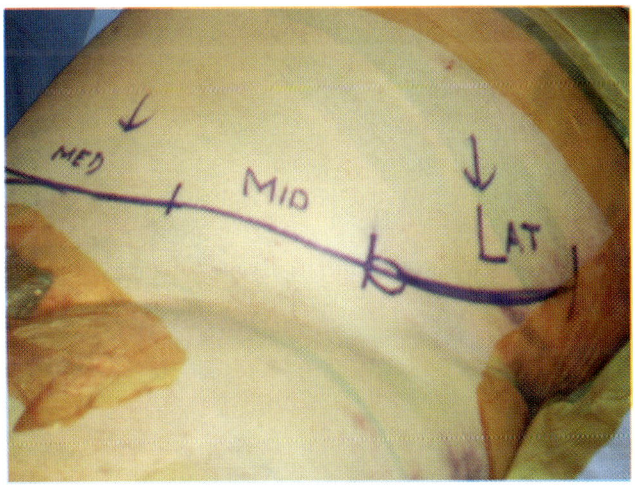

Figure 17.7: The three windows of ilioinguinal approach drawn on the skin.

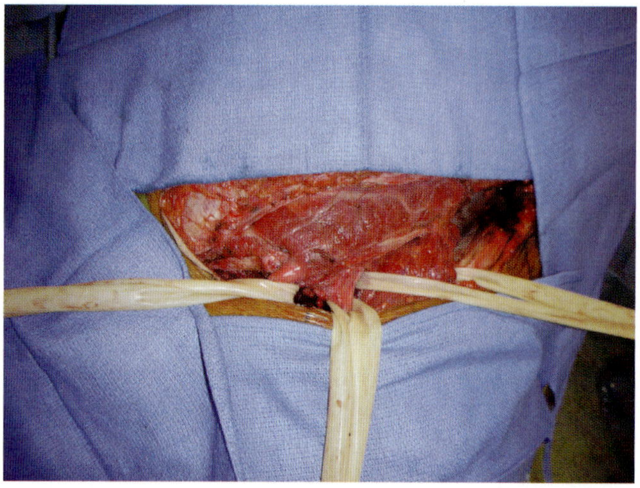

Figure 17.8: The ilioinguinal approach. The medial tagged structure is the vascular bundle, the middle one is the femoral nerve and the lateral one is the psoas muscle.

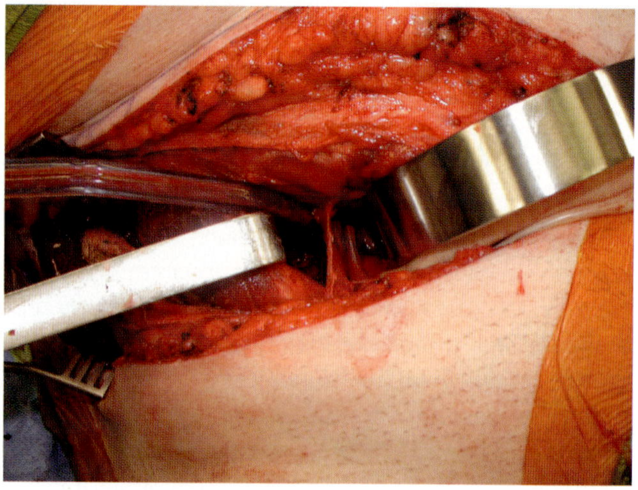

Figure 17.9: The iliopectineal fascia dividing the psoas/ femoral nerve (laterally) from the more medial structures.

vessel-lymph compartment (Fig. 17.9). It is the structure that Judet and Letournel described as providing access to the deep pelvis and its excision is a major reason the operative treatment of the acetabulum from the front is possible. The corona mortis, or connection between the external iliac and obturator vessels is at risk, when incising the iliopectineal fascia laterally and careful dissection must be performed in order to identify this structure, which is present in up to 30% of individuals (Fig. 17.10). It may be beneficial to develop the medial window first, as the corona mortis is easier to see on the medial side of the iliopectineal fascia than the lateral side. Take care not to retract the iliac vessels too vigorously, as it may predispose the patient to thrombosis or postoperative lymphedema. The femoral nerve lies on the iliopsoas muscle underneath the inguinal canal and vigorous retraction of this structure is to be avoided as well. The space of Retzius (between symphysis pubis and bladder) can be developed with a finger and the space is extended through the incised conjoint tendon laterally. The three windows are the medial (up to vessels), middle (between vessels and muscle) and lateral (between muscle and iliac crest). The lateral window allows visualization of the iliac wing, SI joint and pelvic brim with its medial border being defined by the iliopsoas muscle with the femoral nerve. The middle window between the iliopsoas and the iliac vessels can be used for anterior wall and upper anterior column. The medial window has the superior pubic ramus and symphysis medial to the iliac vessels.[2,5,14,27]

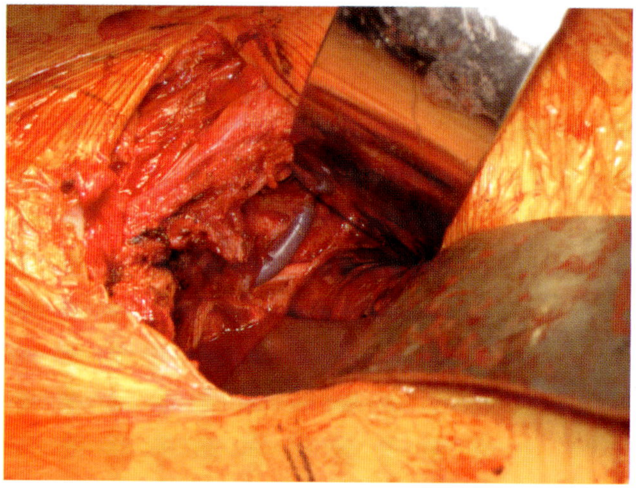

Figure 17.10: A large corona mortis seen through the medial window.

Modified Stoppa approach: The modified Stoppa is basically the ilioinguinal approach without the skin and deep dissection of the middle window. The surgeon however, works from the opposite side of the table and does most of their work "under" the inguinal contents (muscle, vessel and lymph). The main difference in deep exposure is a vertical split of the rectus abdominus muscle with the Stoppa versus a transverse split with the traditional ilioinguinal approach. The lateral window of the modified Stoppa is same as the lateral window of the ilioinguinal. The middle window is not developed and the iliopectineal fascia is taken down from the medial window and under

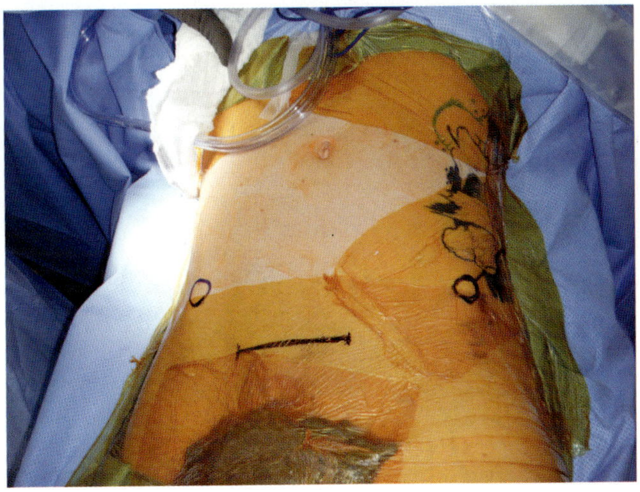

Figure 17.11: Skin incisions for the modified Stoppa approach.

the vessels (Fig. 17.11). We have found that this approach has avoided the following problems seen with the ilioinguinal approach: excessive retraction of the psoas and femoral nerve, manipulation of the vessels predisposing to thrombosis and lymphedema and lower abdominal hernias from pull off of the abdominal muscles. One minor disadvantage of the Stoppa, also present with traditional ilioinguinal is the obturator nerve, which must be retracted when working in the deep pelvis. From the medial window, and with the surgeon on the contralateral side of table, blunt dissection proceeds along pubic bone until the pelvic brim is reached and iliopectineal fascia is visualized "from below". It is easier and safer to release it from this aspect and it is retracted anteriorly along with the muscle vessel soft tissue envelope. The two windows in the Stoppa allow access to the entire anterior column and the quadrilateral surface. The iliac vessels may still be at some risk for thrombosis or injury during superior retraction of the abdominal musculature, but we have not seen this problem in over 300 cases.[2,33]

Both the modified Stoppa and ilioinguinal approach can be used for visualization of the anterior wall and column. There is no true intra-articular access, but we have been able to access the anterior wall and intra-articular acetabulum using two additional modifications. The first method is to flex the hip beyond the traditional 30° used for this approach by turning a triangular leg holder on end to flex the hip to about 60°. Then dissection over the iliopectineal eminence to the anterior hip capsule is performed bluntly with a wide Cobb elevator under the iliopsoas musculature. A blunt Cobra retractor can be placed over the hip capsule to allow access to the anterior-medial aspects of the hip via arthrotomy. The second method is to extend the incision of the lateral window from ASIS towards patella, thus allowing the iliofemoral approach (or Smith Peterson). Dissection distal to ASIS allows access to the hip joint via standard anterior approach.

One modification of the Stoppa used by the senior author is a version of "extended" ilioinguinal approach described by Mast. In this approach, the lateral window is further dissected on outer iliac fossa to provide limited access to the superior acetabulum and posterior ilium. An additional incision starting at ASIS and extending distally can be used for more access to the entire outer iliac fossa. This creates a "T" extension when using the ilioinguinal approach, but is a separate incision with the modified Stoppa. These additions are useful when there is a concomitant crescent fracture, or when a minimally displaced superior acetabular wall fracture needs a simple buttress plate.

Extensile Approaches (The Extended Iliofemoral, Texas T and Triradiate)

The extensile approaches are as their name implies, very extensile, and thus carry more morbidity than standard approaches. However, in certain fractures, they are the only way to adequately address the pathology and provide for an ample reduction. The most common extensile approach has traditionally been the extended iliofemoral (EIF) as described by Letournel. The patient is in the lateral position and the iliofemoral incision is used and extended more posteriorly along the iliac crest. The entire hindquarter is dissected off of the outer ilium. Historically, the abductor mechanism was detached using a tenotomy and was reattached with sutures. More recent modifications of this approach utilize a trochanteric osteotomy, either standard or digastric. The healing of bone to bone is theoretically less morbid than that of a tenotomy repair. With this approach, there is an excellent access to the outer ilium and posterior parts (Fig. 17.12). The access to the interior pelvis is possible, but potentially devascularizes some of the iliac bone.

The Texas T is similar to the EIF, but essentially uses distal extension of the ilioinguinal, with or without an

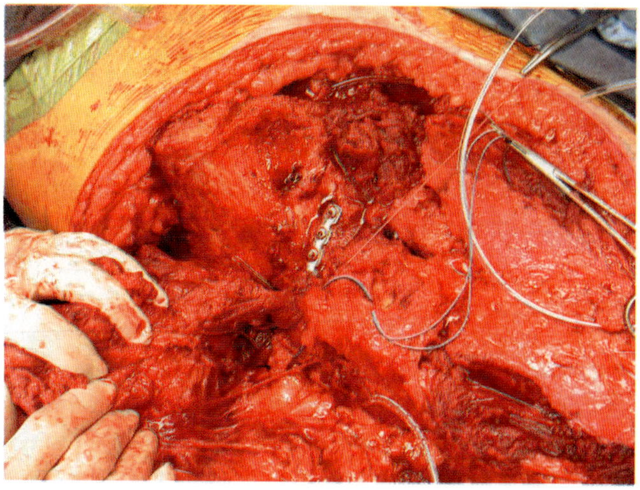

Figure 17.12: The extended iliofemoral with the gluteal mass retracted to the left exposes the outer table in its entirety—both anterior and posterior columns.

osteotomy of the anterior iliac spine to provide access to the outer ilium. With both these approaches, it is essential to consider the vascularity to the entire myocutaneous flap, which is primarily from the gluteal vessels. In cases, where vascularity is compromised, such as with gluteal embolization for bleeding, the flap may become ischemic and necrotic, which can lead to a devastating complication of flap loss or sloughing. The surgeon must consider the vascular status to the flap when undertaking such an extensile approach. The authors have found that with use of the modified stoppa, we have been able to address more complex fractures with one approach, and if an additional posterior approach is absolutely necessary, we prefer a sequential tactic, where a separate prep and drape surgery is performed, in order to optimize the access provided by each approach. The surgical tactic changes a bit, so that the surgeon is cognizant not to place fixation from one approach that might interfere with the subsequent approach. So, if an anterior approach is performed first, and there is a posterior column and wall fracture, fixation screws placed during the anterior approach should not be so long to interfere with reduction and fixation during the posterior approach.

The triradiate approach was popularized by Dana Mears and has a different focus. The patient is in a lateral position, as with the EIF, and a lateral incision is made over the femur up to the tip of trochanter. At that point, two incisions, one toward ASIS and one toward posterior superior iliac spine (PSIS), are made to create a "Y" or triradiate shape. The posterior leg of the approach is similar to the posterior Kocher-Langenbeck. The trochanter is osteotomized in the traditional fashion and the anterior leg of the approach is between the gluteus medius and anterior thigh, musculature.

Posterior Wall and Column Injuries

Posterior wall fractures are some of the most common types of acetabular fractures encountered. Posterior wall lesions that are very small and stable can be treated nonoperatively, although some surgeons feel that the disruption of joint mechanics with any lesion, including the soft tissue posterior wall (labral avulsion), makes these lesions worthy of operative treatment. Recently, Moed has advocated an intraoperative stress test to identify posterior wall fractures that are unstable and require fixation.[28] In our practice, we base treatment on two factors: (1) articular congruity and (2) joint stability. If the lesion is large enough or superiorly based (near weight-bearing area as described by Olson and Matta),[7,8] or if the joint is unstable as determined by Moed,[27] the operative reduction and fixation is warranted.

Superior wall lesions are inherently unstable and may require a trochanteric osteotomy. Very inferior wall lesions are generally irrelevant and not problematic, if not perfectly reduced. Extended posterior wall lesions that extend to or disrupt the posterior column are very difficult to address.

Marginal impaction is usually visualized on preoperative CT scan, but may be encountered intraoperatively. The impacted fracture fragments can be left alone, while the head is luxated to inspect the joint. Thereafter, the femoral head is relocated and is used as a template for impacted and loose osteochondral fragments. We then drill a non-weight-bearing aspect of the posterior femoral head to assess bleeding[34] and determine the risk of subsequent avascular necrosis.[35] The voids left after reduced impacted fragments behind should be bone grafted with either allograft cancellous bone chips, autogenous bone graft or a synthetic material. We have used a small trochanteric trap door to harvest local bone as needed without any issues. The posterior wall is then reduced and impacted in place using a ball spike pusher with a disk to prevent comminution. Kirschner (K) wires are then used to maintain the posterior wall and underlying fragments in place, while plates are applied. K-wires placed tangential to the joint,

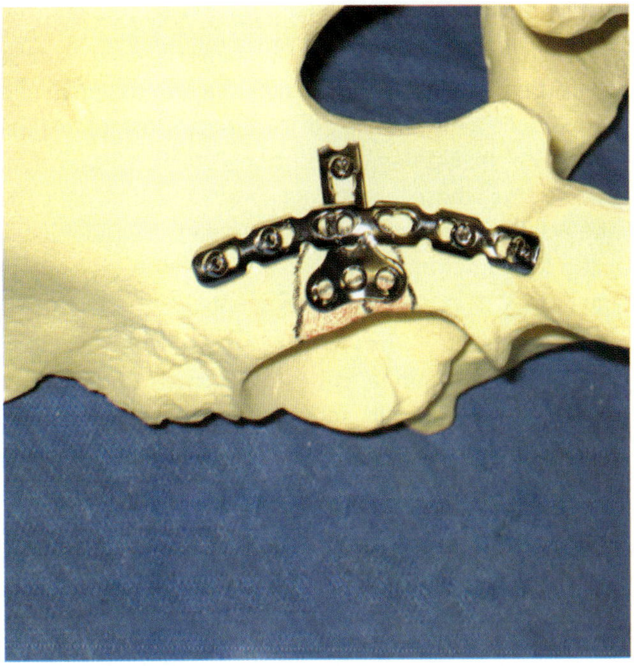

Figure 17.13: A T-plate used with a reconstruction plate for a posterior wall fracture.

can be a guide to screw placement later, since they provide a reference for aiming the drill to place the screws through the plate. Once reduced, a 6–8 hole curved 3.5 mm reconstruction plate is adequate for stabilization. Slightly undercontouring the plate will allow compression of the wall fragment. The two terminal screws are usually sufficient for fixation and minimize the risk of intra-articular screw placement through portions of the plate close to the articular rim. Highly comminuted fractures may at times need a one-third tubular or distal radius T-plate acting as a spring plate prior to the application of reconstruction buttress or neutralization plate (Fig. 17.13). These plates should have independent fixation in order to prevent plate migration. Cutting the end of the one-third tubular plate through last hole and bending the edges creates teeth and allows extra fixation into the comminuted fragment. Alternatively, commercially available "spring" plates are also available.

Posterior column fractures are relatively rare and usually present as part of a more complex lesion. They typically will have a more coronal orientation on the CT scan. When they present with a posterior wall lesion, the column needs to be addressed first, in order to provide a framework for the repair of posterior wall. Use of a Schanz pin in the ischium can help correct rotational deformities. A weber clamp or a farabeuf clamp around two small screws can reduce and compress the visualized fracture line posteriorly. Care should be taken to anticipate the placement of a small 4–6 hole 3.5 mm reconstruction plate, which is usually adequate for fixation. In other cases, if obliquity of the fracture permits, a single lag screw can be used to provide provisional fixation, while the clamps are removed to provide more room for plate fixation. It goes without saying that the sciatic nerve is at risk during all posterior column manipulations and whenever a clamp is placed through sciatic notch. Keeping hip extended and knee flexed will help reduce the chances of nerve injury.

Fluoroscopy is used to confirm reduction and screw placement. The use of drains after a Kocher-Langenbeck approach has not been shown to decrease the rate of infection or days of drainage in a small randomized trial.[36] Meta-analysis of thousands of orthopedic wounds does not support the use of routine drains in surgical wounds.[37] We have used a hemostatic agent (Arista, Medafor: Minneapolis, MN) to promote clot formation and prevent hematoma and seroma formation rather than drain usage. Obese patients are especially susceptible to postoperative infection. It is worth considering and has been shown in the literature that a wound vacuum dressing (KCI, San Antonio, TX) placed over a closed incision can decrease wound complications.[38,39] Placement of an incisional wound vacuum should be performed in obese patients (BMI > 30) in order to decrease postoperative infection. Postoperative CT scans have been shown to assess the accuracy of reduction better than plain radiographs.[40] The individual surgeon must decide, if the prognostic information gained from a postoperative CT scan is worth the extra irradiation to the patient. We do not currently perform routine postoperative CT scans at our institution.

Anterior Column and Anterior Wall Fractures

Isolated anterior wall fractures are rare and appear as a trapezoidal shaped fragment on obturator-oblique and AP radiographs. They are usually associated with more complex lesions. If they do present as isolated lesions, they are approached with one of the described anterior approaches, depending on the location and context. Small- and mini-fragment fixation may be needed. Because of the location, care should be taken to ensure that hardware is not intra-articular. While anterior wall fractures are generally not associated with instability; occasionally, a seemingly innocuous fracture will cause instability that requires fixation. Options include standard fixation with plates and screws or augmentation with bone blocks, either autogenous or bone bank.

Anterior column fractures are much more common than isolated anterior wall fractures. They also typically have a coronal orientation on the CT scan. The anterior column fractures occur in several varieties. The classic high anterior wall begins in the joint, usually superior, and exits the iliac crest somewhere posterior to ASIS. These fractures are amenable to reduction and fixation with screws placed just above the joint through ilium towards SI joint, and/or with plates along the crest. The middle anterior column fracture may be confused with an anterior wall and the surgeons have not really seen this variety. The low anterior column fracture is very common and often presents as a part of pelvic ring injury, and may be considered a "high ramus" fracture. In their isolated form, they probably do not warrant fixation, unless significantly displaced, or part of a more complex injury that requires fixation. We are not sure if the low anterior column fracture is better thought of as a part of a pelvic lesion or should remain an acetabular fracture. In either case, they are treated utilizing an ilioinguinal or stoppa approach. They are very amenable to retrograde ramus screws or standard supra-pectineal plating.

Transverse and Transverse Posterior Wall Fractures

Majority of transverse fractures are treated using a posterior approach, and those with a posterior wall fracture obligate the surgeon for posterior fixation. However, depending on location of the transverse fracture, presence of an anterior hinge and major part of displacement (anterior or posterior), an alternate approach may be needed. Transverse fractures are stratified by location of the transverse fracture line relative to the weight-bearing parts of the joint. The transtectal fracture is the most problematic as it occurs in the crucial weight-bearing aspects of the joint and requires a perfect reduction. In some cases, an extensile approach is required to allow access and visualization of the articular surface via luxation of the head. However, we have found that using appropriate traction set ups, a posterior approach can allow luxation of the head to visualize the intra-articular reduction as well. While ill-defined, most consider any fracture that involves the radiographic "dome" or "sourcil" to be transtectal. The juxtatectal fracture is below the crucial weight-bearing area down towards the cotyloid fossa, but still involving a major aspect of joint. These fractures require anatomical fixation as well, but imperfections are better tolerated than those through main weight-bearing area. The infratectal fractures involve the lower parts of acetabulum, and may sometimes be treated nonoperatively unless significantly displaced or part of a more complex lesion.

Transverse fractures will more often be displaced posteriorly with "hinge" on the symphysis pubis, which provides some help in achieving reduction. These are treated with a posterior approach, and use of Schanz pins in the ischium and angled "Matta" clamps placed through the sciatic notch facilitate reduction (Fig. 17.14). Fixation is with posterior 3.5 mm reconstruction plates. In these cases, the plates can be "overcontoured" to help provide an anterior closing force (similar to overcontouring plates in diaphyseal bone to achieve compression at the far cortex). If a posterior wall lesion occurs with a transverse fracture, the displaced transverse component is usually treated first along the most posterior aspect of the posterior column, to allow a second plate used for the posterior wall. In transverse/posterior wall fractures with minimally or

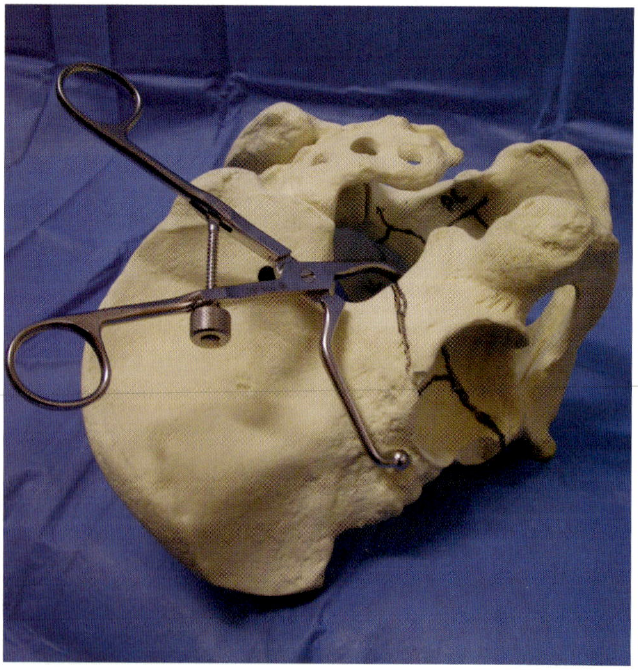

Figure 17.14: A Matta clamp placed through the sciatic notch can assist in reduction of a transverse fracture.

nondisplaced transverse components, a single plate addressing both the posterior wall and transverse lesion is generally sufficient. Some transverse fractures are displaced more along their anterior aspect. This characteristic makes use of the posterior approach more difficult. In these cases, an anterior approach is more suitable. Some surgeons feel that even with an anterior hinge, posterior fixation alone may be inadequate, so they place an anterior column screw. We have not found this to be the case, when there is no anterior instability in the form of a disrupted symphysis or ramus. In some isolated transverse fractures, we have used a modified stoppa approach to visualize the entire fracture and address both its anterior and posterior characteristics. The anterior fracture line can be reduced and treated with an anterior column screw, and the posterior fracture can be reduced and treated with a posterior column screw. Alternatively, a single plate along the pelvic brim is also sufficient.

Both Column Fractures

Both column fractures have an extreme range of fracture characteristics or "personality". The unifying factor is that there is no articular attachment to the intact posterior ilium. Most of these fractures can be accessed using either ilioinguinal or modified stoppa approach. In the case, where posterior access is needed, the authors recommend a sequential exposure instead of a simultaneous exposure for all the reasons previously mentioned. Extended approaches are occasionally used, but should be avoided, if possible, due to their morbidity.

One of the difficulties with these fractures is that there is no articular surface connected to the remaining ilium. Thus, the femoral head cannot be used as a template about which columns can be reconstructed, so that the surgeon must develop an appropriate surgical tactic. Most of the time, reconstruction is from posterior to anterior, but on occasion, the surgeon may work on the front before going to the back. The authors prefer a posterior to anterior reduction. The fixation begins with fixation of the anterior column to the posterior ilium, which is different from reconstructing the posterior column first. In many both column fractures, there is a triangular segment of the posterior aspect of the anterior column, which can be used as a keystone. In many cases, this fracture is incomplete, resulting in plastic deformation, which can make the crucial articular reduction more problematic. In these cases, the ilium should be osteotomized through the incomplete fracture to allow better reduction of the articular surface. Slight imperfections of the iliac crest are much better tolerated than those of the joint. Using the ilioinguinal or lateral stoppa window, the iliac wing can be reduced and held using small curved reconstruction plates or lag screws. Placement of plates on the inner cortex rather than on the edge of crest allows for optimal plate contouring and is least irritating to the patient postoperatively.

Small fragment reconstruction plates are adequate for most fractures and can be contoured for many surfaces, while being strong and stiff enough to help effect reductions when used as "push-pull" plates. The posterior column can be reduced through anterior exposures by use of a bone hook or co-linear clamp (Synthes, Paoli, PA) passing just medial to the quadrilateral surface of the medial acetabulum. If a fragment is large enough, lag or position screws from anterior to posterior may be enough to stabilize the fracture. Several screw locations have been previously identified and should be familiar to the surgeon including anterior column, posterior column, lateral compression-II (LC-II) screw and iliac crest screw. A sterile bag with sawbones pelvis that has fracture lines drawn can aid the surgeon in spatial orientation prior to screw placement. Medial wall comminution and protrusion can occur in both column fractures as in anterior column fractures and may need to have quadrilateral surface plates to address medial displacement. These plates have historically been called "spring" plates and are over-bent and placed over the pelvic brim. Some are now commercially manufactured. The authors have adopted a different approach and place a stronger 3.5 mm reconstruction plate directly over the quadrilateral surface, anchoring the plate to the posterior sciatic buttress. This plate can only be applied using the modified stoppa approach from the medial window. The undercontoured reconstruction plate functions as a buttress, or "push" plate that helps prevent protrusion and also become beneficial in the event of hip replacement as it defines the medial wall. The posterior column can be reduced with hooks or clamps, but we have adopted the use of co-linear clamp, which is analogous to some of the newer clamps found in hardware stores. This clamp is placed into the lesser notch and along the crest or brim. It then affects a reduction of the posterior column, and simultaneously provides a direction for placement of drill and screw for the posterior column. Posterior column screws are placed either independently or through a plate.

One technical point regarding drilling into complex anatomy such as the pelvis involves use of the drill as a guide to intraosseous placement. Resistance of the moving drill is due to a small "dynamic" coefficient of friction along the side wall of the drill and mostly due to resistance of the leading tip against the bone. Resistance of a stopped drill is due to both tip resistance of the bone and the static coefficient of friction, which is much larger than the dynamic coefficient. As such, if the drill remains spinning, and is gently advanced in a gentle oscillating manner (like an impact driver), a distinct proprioceptive sensation of the drill tip is felt. If the advance is performed gently, cancellous bone is easily drilled and felt, and when a "cortical" structure is reached by the drill point, the gentle oscillating force of the surgeon does not "advance" the drill point. This alerts the surgeon that a cortex has been reached and fluoroscopic verification is performed. If the surgeon increases the advancing force slightly, the drill point will have enough forward force to traverse the cortex. If the surgeon is able to continually "feel" gentle resistance while advancing, they are certainly in the cancellous bone. If there is no such sensation, they are most likely in soft tissues and should not advance the drill. A similar technique is advocated for placement of SI screws (Joel Matta MD, personal communication).

If the posterior column cannot be reduced through the ilioinguinal or stoppa approach, it is recommended to proceed with a Kocher-Langenbeck approach after the anterior exposure is closed and sterilely dressed (sequential approach). This does not have to be at the same operative setting and can be performed on a different day, if the patient requires further resuscitation. The authors feel that a sequential anterior-posterior exposure is preferred over the extensile approaches that would allow visualization in one incision.

T-Type Fractures

T-type fractures can be some of the most difficult fractures to treat. They are defined by a fracture that exits the inferior acetabulum and goes through the ischium. The femoral head pushes apart the anterior and posterior aspects of acetabulum like a trap door. Since it frequently results in loss of soft tissue attachments, ligamentotaxis alone is not enough to help with reduction. T-type fractures are classified by the location of "T" and that of stem. There is obviously overlap of many of the fracture patterns, e.g. a middle anterior column posterior transverse fracture will be very similar to a "T". Similarly, a both column fracture that has a high transverse fracture exiting the acetabulum with an inferior stem like a Y-shaped fracture, will also appear to be a "T". There are, however, several distinguishing features amongst these fractures as outlined eloquently by Judet and Letournel in their classic text. First, the T-type fracture has a distinctly transverse component, which is classified in the same manner as transverse fractures (transtectal, juxtatectal and infratectal). As a result, anterior column posterior hemitransverse and both column fractures, which both lack the relatively pure transverse fracture, can be differentiated based on the extension of one part of their fracture "up the column" along with its CT and radiographic features. The obliquity of the fracture lines in the both column and anterior hemi-transverse fractures is generally enough to differentiate them from T-type, even when there is a stem component present. There is a unique fracture, the extra-articular T, which has a "supratectal" fracture with an inferior stem that is technically a "both column" by Letournel's definition, but may have the personality of a T-type. Whatever it is called, the treatment is the same and requires assessing the best method of reduction, which is typically through an anterior approach.

The stem of the "T" is also classified based on whether it exits inferiorly, anteriorly or posteriorly. This feature may help the surgeon determine the best method of approach and fixation. A very anterior stem may be difficult to assess (and access) through a purely posterior approach, and vice versa. There is also a transischial stem that exits along the posterior column and can make its reduction problematic. One other fracture that has been grouped together with the T-type fracture is what would best be described as posterior column anterior hemitransverse pattern. Because of the more caudal location of the posterior column, a fracture traversing this aspect of the acetabulum and exiting anteriorly, will be very similar to a typical T-type fracture and thus, the surgeons grouped them together.

Treatment of T-type fractures should be based on several characteristics: location of the transverse component, location of the stem and presence of a posterior wall fracture. Any posterior wall fracture obligates at minimum a posterior approach. A complex transtectal fracture with a posterior wall may be one of the few true remaining indications for an extensile approach. If there is a wide displacement anteriorly and posteriorly in a transtectal fracture, the surgeon may consider an extensile approach in this situation also (Figs 17.15A to G). There is truly no well-defined rule book for T-type fractures, and in the authors' opinion, this particular fracture, when displaced, is one of the most difficult fractures to achieve a perfect reduction.

Anterior Column Posterior Hemitransverse Fractures

These fractures, along with both column and T-type fractures can be some of the most difficult fractures to treat, depending on the extent of posterior hemitransverse

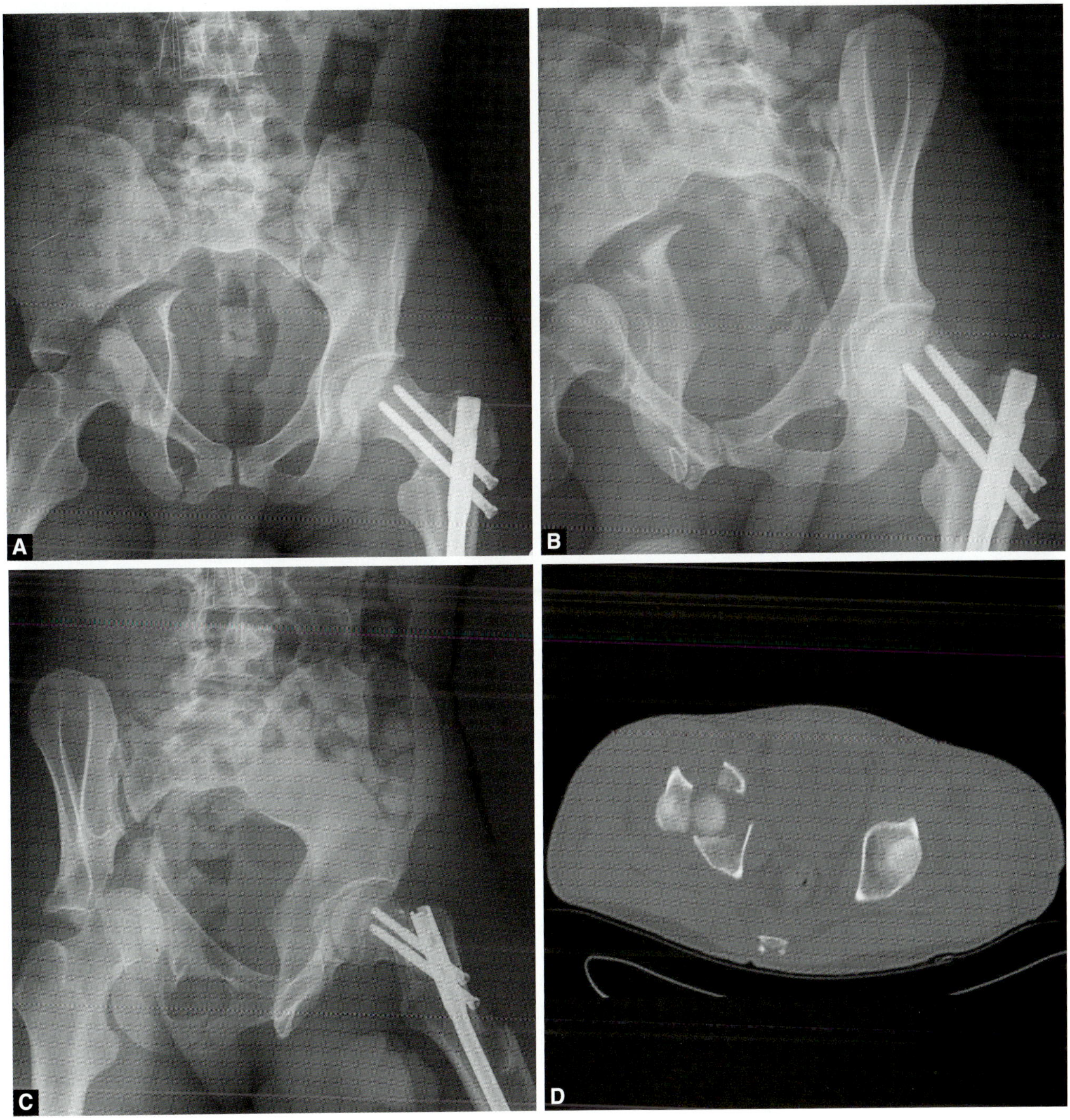

Figures 17.15A to D

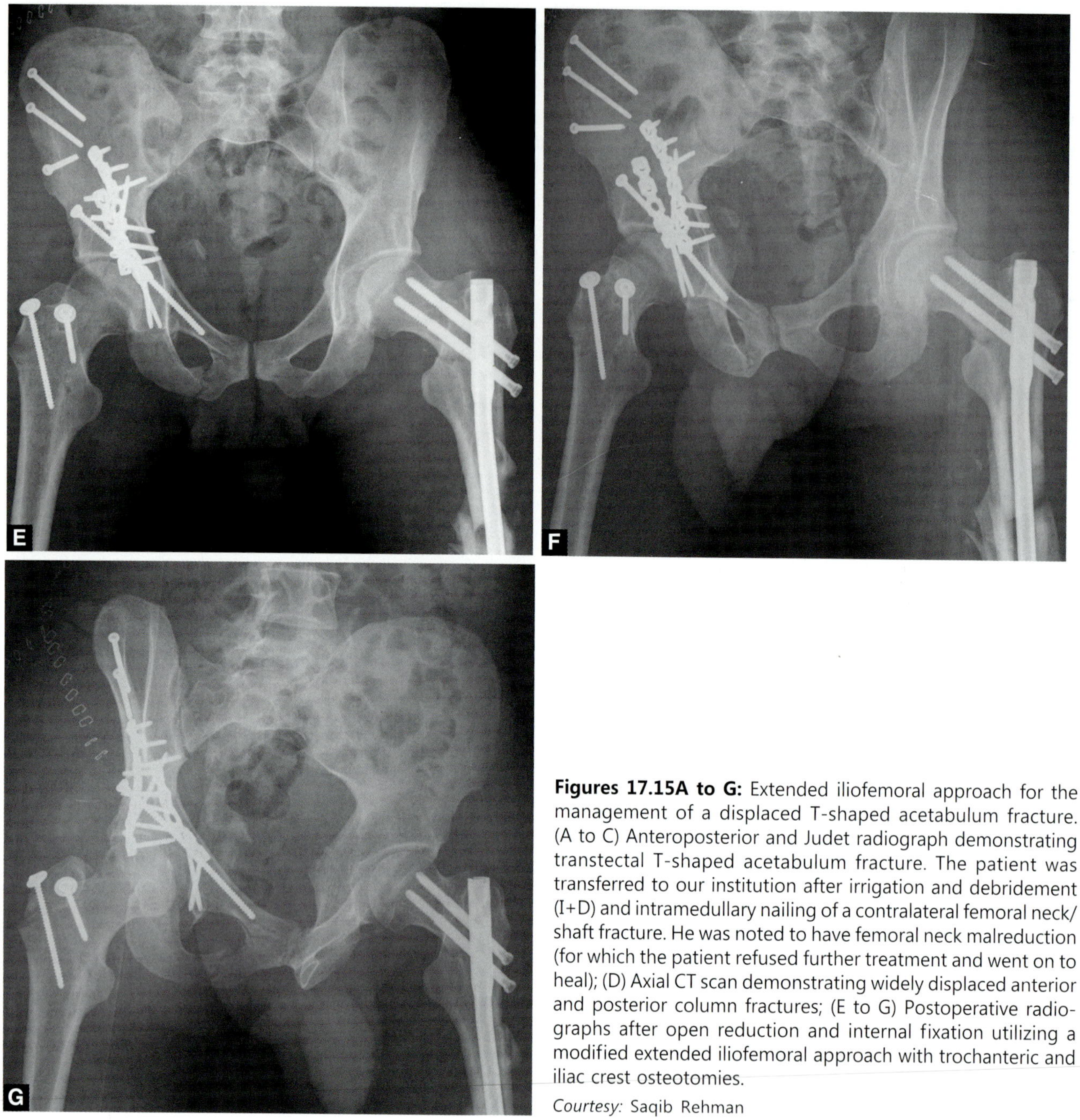

Figures 17.15A to G: Extended iliofemoral approach for the management of a displaced T-shaped acetabulum fracture. (A to C) Anteroposterior and Judet radiograph demonstrating transtectal T-shaped acetabulum fracture. The patient was transferred to our institution after irrigation and debridement (I+D) and intramedullary nailing of a contralateral femoral neck/shaft fracture. He was noted to have femoral neck malreduction (for which the patient refused further treatment and went on to heal); (D) Axial CT scan demonstrating widely displaced anterior and posterior column fractures; (E to G) Postoperative radiographs after open reduction and internal fixation utilizing a modified extended iliofemoral approach with trochanteric and iliac crest osteotomies.

Courtesy: Saqib Rehman

component. They are differentiated from both column fractures based on the presence of articular surface to the posterior ilium and by the presence of a columnar fracture pattern anteriorly (coronal on CT), with a transverse pattern posteriorly (sagittal). This fracture was also considered one of the more difficult patterns as per Letournel, and its treatment had both anterior and posterior approaches as well as extensile approaches utilized. We feel that this fracture can have various "personalities". The minimally displaced posterior hemitransverse component makes the fracture more of an anterior column fracture that just needs a little posterior work and fixation. When the fracture has a lot of protrusion from a middle anterior column fracture and quadrilateral surface comminution, it may have more of the "trap door" characteristics of the T-type fracture. When there is more extensive posterior displacement, depending on the level and obliquity of the fracture line, it may behave more like a both column fracture. In any case, the surgical approach and tactic should be based on the essential elements, and like any fracture crossing the tectum, this aspect is the most crucial. Also, the nature of the anterior column may facilitate reduction and actually changes the traditional posterior to anterior surgical tactic. The anterior column can usually be easily addressed with anterior approaches and then an intraoperative attempt at the posterior column fracture can be attempted with either a posterior column plate (via modified stoppa window) or posterior column screws. If successful, no further stabilization is needed, but if not, the surgeon should plan for a second posterior approach and ensure that none of the anterior column fixation will interfere with posterior hemitransverse reduction and fixation. From the authors' experience, this fracture typically behaves most like the both column fractures.

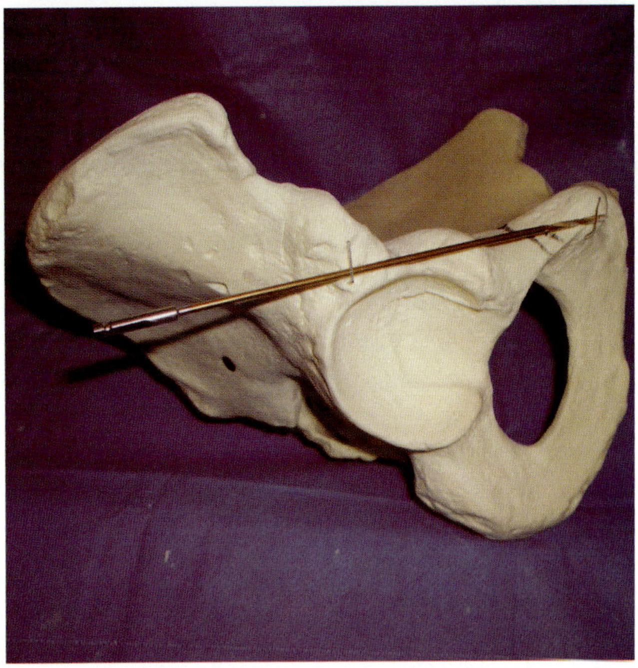

Figure 17.16: Path of an anterior column screw may be antegrade or retrograde.

Adjunct and Novel Methodologies

Two distinct technological advances have occurred since classic writings: (1) percutaneous fixation and (2) computer navigation. While out of the scope of this chapter, they are worth mentioning. Percutaneous fixation has been introduced and championed as less morbid. While hotly debated between the "purists" and the "progressives", the authors feel that it has a definite role in the acetabular surgeon's armamentarium. It requires an incredible 3D understanding of the pelvis, which is already non-cartesian. Certain osseous "windows" and percutaneous applications have been described, which we will review. However, the surgeons cannot understate that the percutaneous fixation is secondary to the surgical judgment regarding an appropriate reduction. It makes no sense to minimize surgery and accept imperfect reductions in a 20-year-old patient, but it makes complete sense to do so in an independent elderly patient with multiple medical problems. The screws discussed will be LC-II screw, antegrade anterior column screw, retrograde anterior column screw, posterior column screw and ischial posterior column screw.

The LC-II screw is typically used for isolated anterior column or LC-II fractures. It begins in the area of anterior inferior iliac spine (AIIS) and heads towards PSIS. It is best performed using an obturator outlet variant, where supra-acetabular corridor of the bone is visualized as a pear-shaped entity on the c-arm. The AIIS is a ridge-like structure, and the drill point often slips off the ideal starting point. We have found that a small rongeur allows creating of a concavity that facilitates placement.

The antegrade anterior column screw is one of the more difficult to place. It begins 3–4 cm superior to the acetabulum and traverses the narrow anterior column (Fig. 17.16). While multiple radiographic views are needed to verify screw placement, some authors (including present) advocate beginning with the obturator outlet and iliac inlet, which are roughly orthogonal to the anterior column's trajectory. Standard Judet views and AP are useful. The obturator-oblique and obturator-outlet verify that the screw is not in the joint, and the AP and iliac inlet provide some information regarding intrapelvic placement. The danger of this screw is very real as an error placing the screw too anterior places the vascular bundle at risk. As an alternative to this screw, a retrograde ramus screw can be placed through the anterior column. The authors typically place this screw through the anterior Pfannenstiel approach, where the "inner" table of the anterior column can be directly visualized and palpated. The same imaging is used for verification, but placement is easier and we believe it much safer, since there is an ability to visualize and triangulate the drill and screw relative to the dangers. The origin of this screw is typically just anterior, inferior and lateral to the pubic tubercle, and thus requires a more inferiorly placed skin incision, or a percutaneous stab wound to get the correct trajectory.

The posterior column screw begins anterior to the SI joint and just lateral to the pelvic brim. It should head down the posterior column behind the acetabulum and towards the ischial spine. Because of the convexity of posterior retroacetabular surface, it may exit just behind the posterior wall. It is best visualized using iliac oblique views to ensure that it is behind the acetabulum, and the obturator-oblique view to gauge its medial-lateral aspect. However, the authors will typically place this screw using only proprioceptive guidance of the drill in the cancellous bone and then verify with the iliac oblique image. The ischial posterior column screw, sometimes endearingly called the "up the butt" screw is a bit more difficult to place due to the need for patient positioning. The prep is perilously close to a visceral orifice (anus) and difficult to prep surgically. Also, the hip needs to be flexed and incurs weight of the leg. Once properly positioned, the obturator-oblique and AP views verify the starting point and initial trajectory in the medial to lateral plane, and the iliac-oblique view will verify the retroacetabular position of this screw.

All of these percutaneous screws can be placed using open technique and utilizing several different screw options. If cannulated screws are desirable, the 6.5 mm, 7.0 mm or 7.3 mm screw variety can be used. Alternatively, with more experience, a noncannulated version or smaller 4.5 mm or even 3.5 mm screw can be placed after predrilling. Considering the small corridors of bone involved, the authors are not big advocates of larger cannulated screws and prefer using only 4.5 mm or 3.5 mm columnar screws. We have not found them to be problematic for stability purposes and they function more like an intraosseous dowel. We do not feel that it is prudent to expect the screw to "lag" the fracture displacement into reduction. It is better to achieve reduction prior to screw placement.

Navigation may allow marriage of percutaneous fixation with closed or minimally open reduction, but currently the "line of sight" technology is not adequately efficient enough for more advanced acetabular surgeons, who can achieve nearly the same accuracy from their repetitive and extensive experience. Surgical navigation will undoubtedly be beneficial, once there is adequate innovation to make it an augment and not an impediment.

Table 17.2: Brooker's grading scale for heterotopic ossification after acetabular surgery

Brooker's Class	*Definition*
I	Islands of bone about the hip
II	Bone spurs from femur or acetabulum; space between surfaces is > 1 cm
III	Bone spurs from femur or acetabulum; space between surfaces is < 1 cm
IV	Apparent ankylosis of joint

Complications

Heterotopic Ossification

Heterotopic ossification is a common complication of acetabular surgery. The incidence ranges in the reported literature from 10% to 86%.[15-17] It is graded on the Booker's scale (Table 17.2), of which grade IV is associated with decreased hip scores in arthroplasty patients.[41] Obesity is not a risk factor for HO,[18] while use of extended iliofemoral, T-type fractures and injuries to the head and chest were found to be associated with HO formation.[42] Treatment of HO has long been a choice between indomethacin oral treatment or local irradiation of the operative site within 24–48 hours of surgery.

Multiple trials as well as a meta-analysis have proven the efficacy of irradiation in preventing the formation of Class III and IV HO in acetabular surgery.[15-17] Debridement of necrotic or damaged gluteal musculature is also associated with decreasing HO rates.[43] At this time, we recommend against using extensile approaches, local irradiation of 700 Gray within 48 hours of surgery and debridement of necrotic gluteal musculature for prevention of HO in acetabular surgery. The use of local irradiation is dependent on factors out of the surgeon's direct control, such as availability of radiology personnel and other hospital administrative issues. Thus, of the three recommendations we make, at least debridement and avoidance of extensile measures should be performed by the surgeon, with irradiation at the surgeon's discretion. Note that since fracture pattern may affect the incidence of HO, radiation is not best applied across all types of exposures and fractures. The decision to irradiate must be made in light of all risk factors the patient has.

Deep Vein Thrombosis and Pulmonary Embolism

The incidence of DVT with pelvic trauma is relatively high with reports ranging from 35% to 60%, symptomatic PE occurs in approximately 2–10% of patients with fatal PE occurring in a thankfully lower proportion of 0.5–2% of patients with pelvic and acetabular trauma.[12-14] Multiple studies have been performed on various interventions to prevent fatal PE, but they suffer from the fact that to detect significant differences in treatment, large numbers of patients need to be enrolled. Acetabular fractures are, statistically speaking, rare. Thus, recommendations specific to acetabular fractures with scientific evidence are not currently available. The American College of Chest Physicians (ACCP) guidelines for trauma patients has often been followed, though in recent years, recommendations for arthroplasty from the American Association of Orthopedic Surgeons (AAOS) have also been published. The AAOS guidelines do not deal with trauma patients and are not applicable to acetabular fracture patients, who often have multisystem injuries.

The ACCP guidelines for trauma patients recommend the use of a low molecular weight heparin (LMWH), if there are no contraindications and mechanical prophylaxis is able to be tolerated. The use of duplex ultrasound for screening should be reserved only for those patients, who have not had adequate prophylaxis for whatever reason. Inferior vena cava (IVC) filters are not recommended by the ACCP guidelines. All acetabular patients have impaired mobility by the nature of their injury; therefore, should have chemical prophylaxis beyond their inpatient stay. The exact length of time to continue the prophylaxis is left to the physician, although 35 days is recommended for patients with hip fractures. The patient should be ambulating prior to discontinuing prophylaxis.[44]

The treating physician must find which regimen he or she is most comfortable with. Certainly some forms of LMWH with mechanical prophylaxis should be used. The use of IVC filters is left for the treating physician. Despite the ACCP guidelines, we feel that IVC filters still have a role in patients with multiple fractures and organ trauma. We keep our patients on thromboprophylaxis until they are able to ambulate on their own with assistive devices or at least 6 weeks have passed and then reevaluate.

Nerve Palsy

Sciatic nerve palsy is a common sequelae of acetabular fractures. The Edinburgh series found a rate of 7.8%,[10] (of which 1% was iatrogenic and 6.8% was due to injury), while Letournel's older series had a rate of 12.2%.[4] Other published rates range between 1% and 18%.[11] The exact rate is not as important as realizing the high prevalence of sciatic nerve injury at the time of initial examination. The need for proper preoperative documentation cannot be underemphasized both for the patient and from a medicolegal stance. The most common fracture patterns to have sciatic nerve injury are displaced posterior column fractures and posterior wall fractures with an associated dislocation of femoral head. The difficult part of examining patients with acetabular fractures is their reticence to move the injured extremity due to pain, making a gross motor examination problematic. Sensory examination, preferably two-point discrimination using a tool as simple as an unwound paperclip, can be more effective at detecting sciatic nerve involvement.

Patterns of sciatic nerve involvement include peroneal division alone (mild or severe) and tibial division involvement (mild or severe) with severe peroneal involvement. Severe involvement of the peroneal division is more likely to have an unsatisfactory recovery, though mild isolated involvement of the peroneal division has a high likelihood of an excellent functional recovery. When both divisions are involved, tibial nerve returns quicker and to a greater degree than the peroneal. Majority of patients with sciatic nerve injury have no macroscopic lesions found during surgery suggesting that injury may occur at a higher level in the lumbar plexus as well. The importance of knowing patterns of involvement are primarily to provide prognosis to patients rather than attempt any secondary surgical intervention.[11]

Femoral nerve palsy is much rarer complication of acetabular fracture ranging in incidence from 0.2% to 0.4%. The likelihood of good recovery is very high. Iatrogenic injury as well as traumatic injury has been documented. The surgeon is most likely to injure the nerve during anterior exposure and should be careful in retraction of the iliopsoas muscle bundle during ilioinguinal and modified stoppa approaches.[45]

Malunion and Nonunion

Acetabular malunion is often not a complication of treatment at all. Indeed, when an elderly patient has secondary incongruence, a malunion is what is hoped for, albeit one that will have a functionally good result. Any surgically treated fracture would under ideal conditions have an exact anatomical reduction, but this is not always possible due to communition, impaction, visualization, fracture pattern or even surgical technique. Letournel himself noted that malunion and a poor radiographic outcome did not preclude a good or excellent clinical outcome. Which malunions will go on to symptomatic post-traumatic osteoarthrosis is difficult to predict, and even some fracture patterns with perfect unions may go on to late stage arthritis. The following malunited patterns are more likely to bring about a poor result leading to a painful hip.

1. Any union that causes an increased pressure on weight-bearing portion of the acetabulum. A decreased contact area will cause an increase in loading on remaining contact area leading to early wear and arthritis.
2. Malreduced fracture lines that cause increase in the wear on the femoral head.

A fracture treated either operatively or nonoperatively and found to have a malunion needs to have careful evaluation before embarking on a strategy for correction. To correct a malunion will require osteotomies in a region requiring a great deal of 3D thinking. Asymptomatic malunions are best left untreated. A patient can always undergo a total hip arthroplasty for pain relief, and if they are near an acceptable age treatment of symptomatic malunion. Even a younger patient may be treated with an arthroplasty, provided they understand the inevitable revision operation they will undergo at a later age. Any arthroplasty treatment for post-traumatic arthritis will fare poorer than one performed for primary degenerative osteoarthritis, likely due to scar tissue and heterotopic bone formation as well as atrophy and disrupted blood supply to the musculature of the hip girdle.

Nonunions of the acetabulum are rare. Any nonunion of an operatively treated fracture should make the physician concerned about deep infection. A laboratory workup with erythrocyte sedimentation rate (ESR), C-reactive protein (CRP) and white blood cell (WBC) count should be performed. The surgeon must decide in an infected setting whether to go for biopsy and treat the offending organism until union is achieved or removing all the hardware and cleaning the fracture site. Union of infected fractures can occur with suppression, and an unstable acetabular nonunion is a difficult problem for both patient and surgeon. For rare aseptic nonunion, the patient will have to undergo surgery for excision of the interposed fibrous tissue. Bone grafting and compression of the fracture line will be necessary to entice the bone to heal. The rich vascularity of this region makes most nonunions due to mechanical instability rather than atrophic biology.

Symptoms of malunion and nonunion are often the same—pain with motion, limp, limitation of hip motion and preclusion of weight bearing should all warrant evaluation.[46]

Late Stage Arthritis

Late stage arthritis is intimately linked to acetabular malunion. A malunited fracture has a higher chance of going on to arthritis. Other causes of arthritis include femoral head avascular necrosis (AVN) from hip dislocation and direct chondral injury to the acetabulum and femoral head from trauma. Late stage arthritis has a variable incidence and depends on the age of patient. Elderly patients, especially those with prior contralateral hip arthroplasty, malunion or poor reduction and head AVN, can have up to 31% rate of hip arthroplasty.[19] Letournel noted a rate of osteoarthritis of 19.7% in his original series.[4] His updated series found an overall rate of 17% with imperfect reductions having a rate of 35.7% and perfect reductions having a rate of 10.2%.[5] Modern studies show a rate around 14%.[10] Whatever the exact number, every acetabular surgeon will have several patients, who go on to have a painful and stiff hip that needs to be addressed with arthroplasty. The most effective way to reduce the number of posttraumatic arthritic hips is to become familiar and facile with reduction maneuvers. A perfect reduction reduces the chance that a hip will become arthritic.

As already mentioned, arthroplasty for traumatic arthritis of the hip has poorer outcomes than those for degenerative arthritis. This fact should not deter the trauma surgeon from offering his patients an arthroplasty option. The surgery will require careful preoperative planning and evaluation. Infection must be ruled out, if there is any suspicion. Often there will be significant deformity or bone loss associated with malunion or progressive wear that may need Judet and inlet/outlet views to appreciate. Three-dimensional reconstructions may help aid in planning the surgical tactic. Operative goals include a well-fixed acetabular and femoral component. The use of cementless acetabular cups has increased in recent decades. If possible, restoration of an anatomical hip center should be obtained.[21]

Late Instability after Open Reduction and Internal Fixation

Late instability from a fracture dislocation is due to an inadequate reduction of the fracture pattern associated with initial dislocation. A repeated reduction with fixation will be necessary, if the fracture has not yet united. If the fracture is united, either corrective osteotomies or a total hip with proper placement of acetabular version will be necessary to obtain stability. Thankfully this complication is exceedingly rare. Letournel does not even list it as a complication in his complete series.

Authors' Preferred Management of Select Complications

Case 1: Management of Deep Infection

The patient was a 42-year-old male, who was involved in an all-terrain vehicle accident and fell on his left hip sustaining both column acetabular fracture as well as left distal radius fracture with a scapholunate ligament tear. He underwent ORIF of both his left wrist and acetabulum during his Initial hospital stay (Figs 17.17A and B). A modified stoppa approach was used to access the fracture, and then, ORIF as performed. The patient was discharged home on fifth postoperative day.

On follow-up in the office 3 weeks later, he was noted to have purulent drainage from a percutaneous pin site on his left wrist being used for treatment of his scapholunate ligament repair. He was admitted to the hospital and underwent dorsal arthrotomy of his left wrist with removal of K-wires and irrigation and debridement of the infected left wrist. After being placed on antibiotics, he was discharged home. The patient over the next year went on to heal his acetabulum and wrist fracture, but developed posttraumatic arthritis of the wrist. He returned to clinic in year out from his injury with increasing hip pain and was noted to have eroded away much of his femoral head on radiograph and had beefy granulation tissue that now extruded from his former scar.

At this point, blood markers for infection were positive (CRP, ESR and WBC count) and the patient began with spiking fevers. With the clinical and laboratory picture, a diagnosis of advanced septic arthritis of the hip was made (Fig. 17.17C). He was admitted to the hospital and underwent a Girdlestone resection of the femoral head, removal of all accessible hardware in the pelvis and placement of an antibiotic coated nail in order to eradicate the infection (Fig. 17.17D). The plan is for total hip replacement, once infection is cleared. This case study demonstrates significant morbidity that can occur from infection due to open treatment of acetabular fractures, even if the infection is caused by seeding from another site at a time far from the index procedure.

Case 2: Surgical Management of Heterotopic Ossification of the Hip

This case involves a 41-year-old female, who was an unrestrained passenger in a motor vehicle crash and sustained multiple injuries including associated both column acetabulum fracture (Figs 17.18A to C). This was managed surgically with sequential Kocher Langenbeck and ilioinguinal approaches. Neither irradiation nor indomethacin prophylactic measures were taken after her surgery. Although, the fracture went on to heal, and she returned to work as a hair dresser, she could not stand comfortably for long periods of time due to painful lack of hip motion and associated low back pain, which the surgeons attributed to Brooker's III heterotopic ossification of the hip (Figs 17.18D to G). As noted on the CT imaging, most of the heterotopic bone was posterior and superior, corresponding with her physical examination findings of limited abduction and external rotation.

Surgical resection was discussed and nuclear imaging was noted to demonstrate significantly decreased bone metabolic activity at 2 years postoperatively. At this point, she was indicated for surgical resection of heterotopic ossification. It was felt that her symptoms were very likely due to the heterotopic bone itself and not arthritic pain or other factors. This was undertaken with a posterior surgical approach with the assistance of peripheral neurological monitoring (Fig. 17.18H). Although, blood loss was not overwhelming, a cell-saver system was utilized in anticipation of potentially significant blood loss. It is also important to identify the sciatic nerve early on. The sciatic nerve was completely encased in heterotopic bone, and

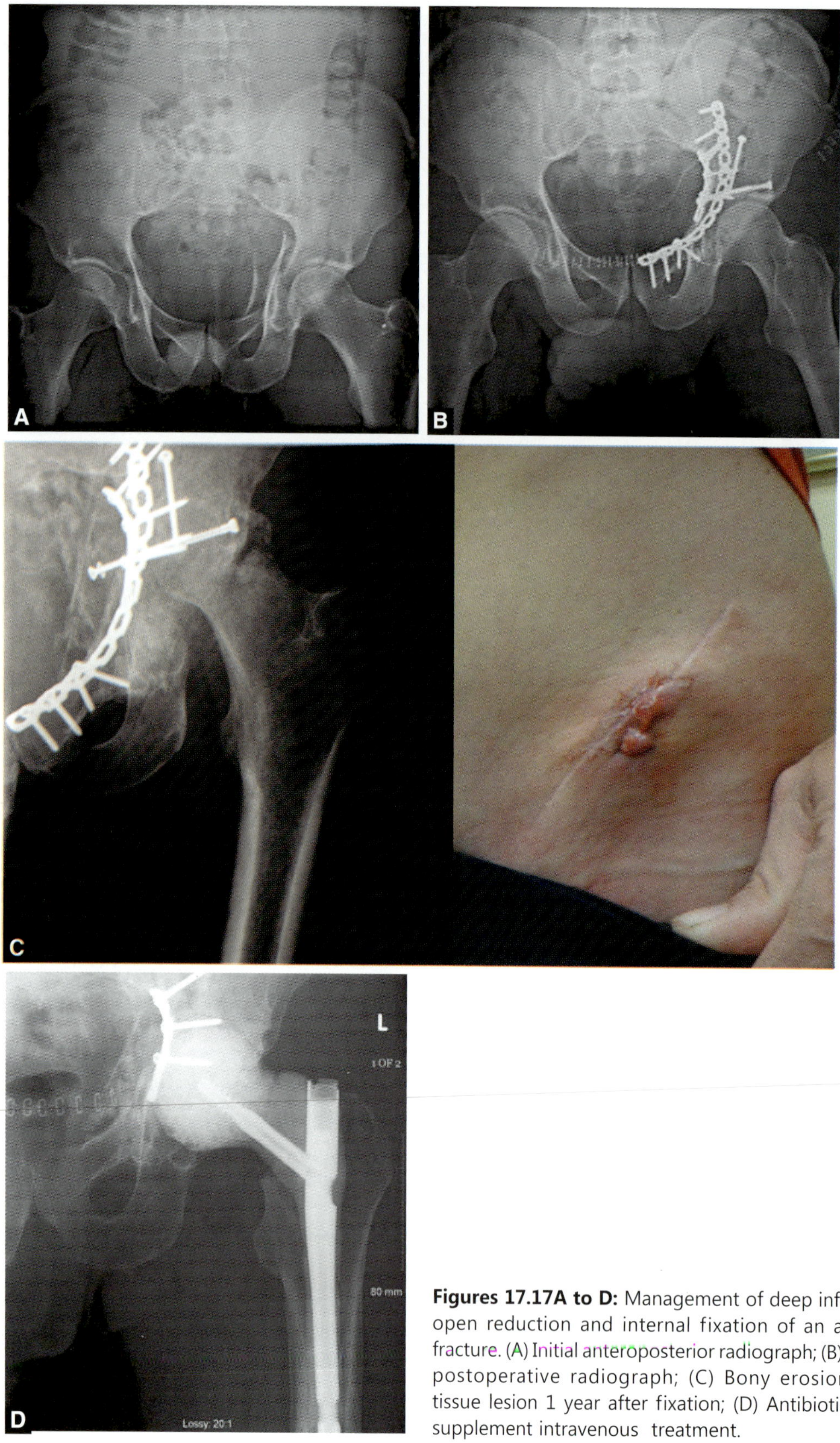

Figures 17.17A to D: Management of deep infection after open reduction and internal fixation of an acetabulum fracture. (A) Initial anteroposterior radiograph; (B) Immediate postoperative radiograph; (C) Bony erosion and soft tissue lesion 1 year after fixation; (D) Antibiotic spacer to supplement intravenous treatment.

spinal rongeurs (especially Kerrison rongeurs) are particularly helpful to avoid nerve injury. Both the sciatic nerve as well as native femoral neck are at risk for injury with indiscriminate removal of bone, particularly with osteotomes and Lexell rongeurs. Postoperatively, she received radiation therapy to the hip as a single dose. She did well during her recovery and returned to work without further complications.

The important principles of this case are as follows:

1. Heterotopic bone resection can incur significant blood loss, which should be prepared for.
2. Injury to both the sciatic nerve and femoral neck can be avoided with careful identification of these structures early on with the assistance of neurological monitoring and fluoroscopy, respectively. Kerrison rongeurs are particularly helpful to carefully remove bone in this area.

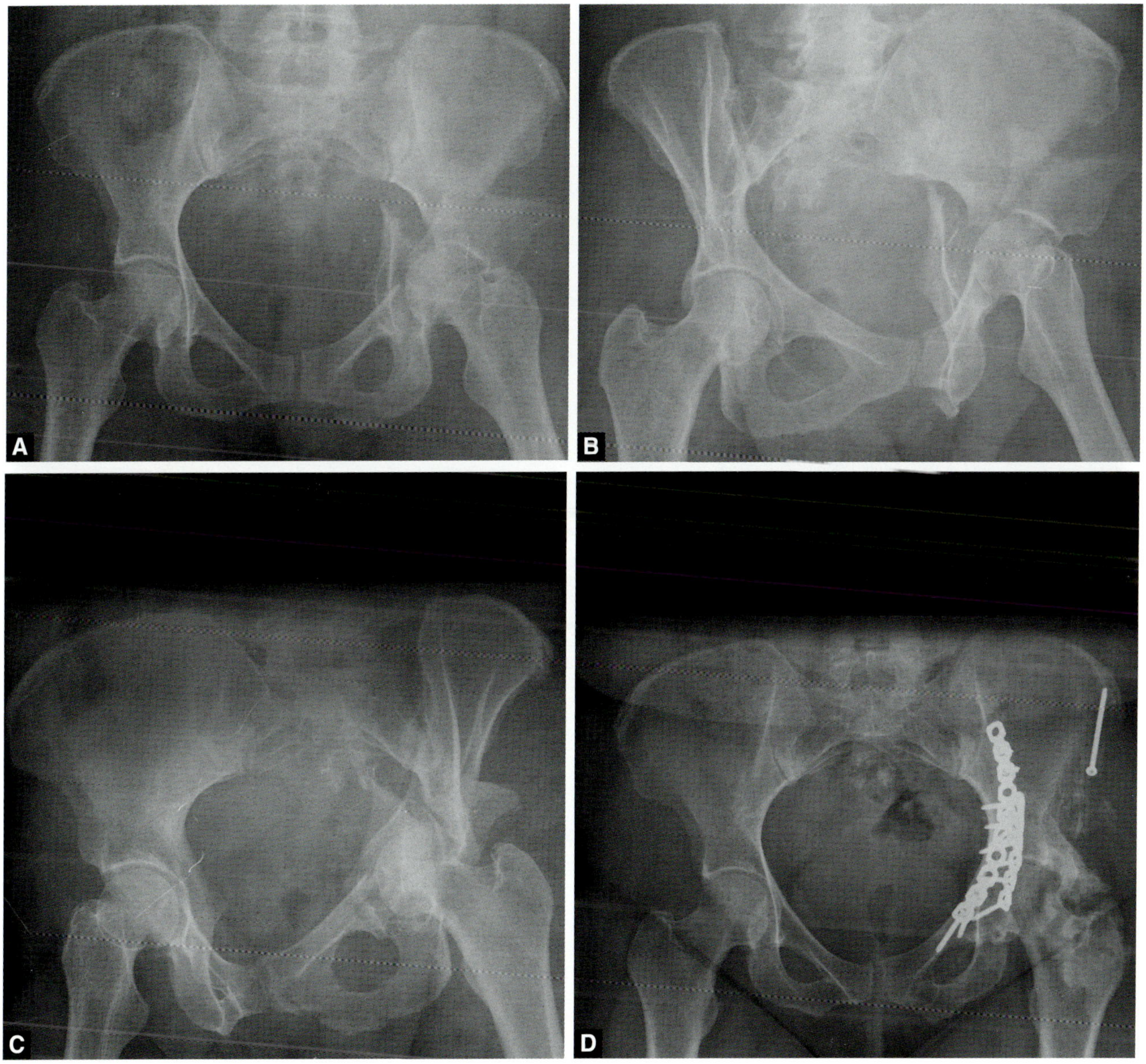

Figures 17.18A to D

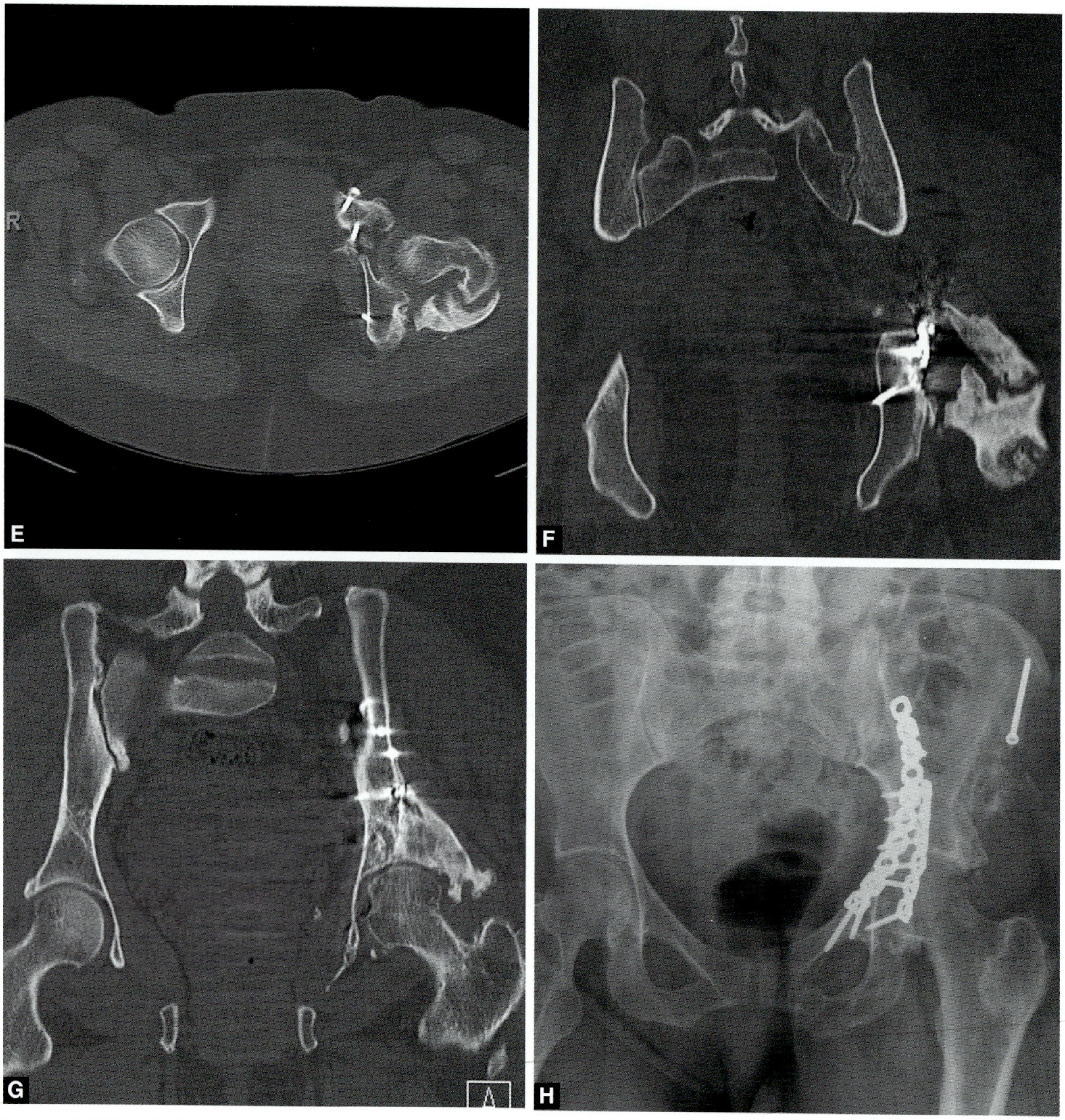

Figures 17.18A to H: Surgical management of heterotopic ossification after open reduction and internal fixation of an associated both column acetabulum fracture. (A to C) Anteroposterior and Judet radiographs demonstrating a displaced associated both column acetabulum fracture. Surgical management included ORIF via sequential Kocher-Langenbeck and ilioinguinal approaches; (D) Anteroposterior radiograph at 2-year follow up demonstrating healed fractures, but with significant Brooker's III heterotopic ossification and symptoms of painful lack of hip motion with associated back pain and hip flexion contracture; (E to G) CT imaging demonstrating primarily posterior and superior heterotopic bone corresponding to her complaints; (H) Follow-up radiograph after resection of heterotopic ossification demonstrating near-complete removal of posterior bone and near-complete removal of all impinging bone superiorly.

Courtesy: Saqib Rehman

3. In appropriate candidate with careful preoperative planning and execution, resection of heterotopic bone of the hip can be a rewarding procedure.
4. Due to the risks involved, significant surgical time should be reserved for this procedure in order to avoid surgical complications.

Summary

While this chapter is not nearly as thorough or seminal as the work of Letournel, and more recently Matta, it provides the reader with a firm foundation from which to pursue further study on acetabular fractures. There has been very little additional information regarding the description and etiology of these fractures, but there have been some advances in surgical treatment, at times hotly debated by the generational proteges of the great acetabular surgeons of the past. Most pelvic surgeons can trace their training back to one of the great surgeons, who began to develop their treatment tactics, and depending on their philosophy, their treatment will follow their surgical geneology. Still, we have noted that many of the opposing philosophies have begun to merge as our understanding and techniques have evolved. The resurrection of the modified stoppa approach may have been one of the most influential changes since it has provided surgeons the ability to address more complex fracture patterns without any violation of the neuro-vascular-lymphatic envelope, and to access fracture lines that would previously require either an extensile or dual approaches. Also, the understanding of fractures and advanced imaging methods allow surgeons to reduce and visualize these very complex problems. It is not unforeseeable that sometime in the future, an endoscopic or minimally invasive technique may become available.

References

1. Cooper SA. Surgical essays 1818; Part I (Second Ed.):51.
2. Ziran B, Morgan S, Smith W (eds). Fractures of the Pelvis and Acetabulum. New York, NY: Informa Healthcare Publishers; 2007.
3. Urist MR. Fracture-dislocation of the hip joint; the nature of the traumatic lesion, treatment, late complications and end results. J Bone Joint Surg. 1948;30A(3):699-727.
4. Judet R, Judet J, Letournel E. Fractures of the acetabulum: classification and surgical approaches for open reduction. Preliminary report. J Bone Joint Surg. 1964;46:1615-46.
5. Letournel E, Judet, R. Fractures of the Acetabulum, 2nd Edition. New York: Springer-Verlag; 1993.
6. Matta JM, Anderson LM, Epstein HC, et al. Fractures of the acetabulum. A retrospective analysis. Clin Orthop Relat Res. 1986;(205):230-40.
7. Matta JM, Mehne DK, Roffi R. Fractures of the acetabulum. Early results of a prospective study. Clin Orthop Relat Res. 1986;(205):241-50.
8. Olson SA, Matta JM. The computerized tomography subchondral arc: a new method of assessing acetabular articular continuity after fracture. J Orthop Trauma. 1993;7(5):402-13.
9. al-Qahtani S, O'Connor G. Acetabular fractures before and after the introduction of seatbelt legislation. Can J Surg. 1996;39(4):317-20.
10. Laird A, Keating JF. Acetabular fractures: a 16-year prospective epidemiological study. J Bone Joint Surg Br. 2005; 87(7):969-73.
11. Fassler PR, Swiontkowski MF, Kilroy AW, et al. Injury of the sciatic nerve associated with acetabular fracture. J Bone Joint Surg Am. 1993;75(8):1157-66.
12. Montgomery KD, Geerts WH, Potter HG, et al. Thromboembolic complications in patients with pelvic trauma. Clin Orthop Relat Res. 1996;(329):68-87.
13. Borer DS, Starr AJ, Reinert CM, et al. The effect of screening for deep vein thrombosis on the prevalence of pulmonary embolism in patients with fractures of the pelvis or acetabulum: a review of 973 patients. J Orthop Trauma 2005;19(2):92-5.
14. Slobogean GP, Lefaivre KA, Nicolaou S, et al. A systematic review of thromboprophylaxis for pelvic and acetabular fractures. J Orthop Trauma. 2009;23(5):379-84.
15. Carroll EA, Huber FG, Goldman AT. Treatment of acetabular fractures in an older population. J Orthop Trauma. 2010;24(10):637-44
16. Bosse MJ, Poka A, Reinart CM, et al. Heterotopic ossification as a complication of acetabular fracture. Prophylaxis with low-dose irradiation. J Bone Joint Surg Am. 1988;70(8): 1231-7.
17. Blokhuis T, Frolke JP. Is radiation superior to indomethacin to prevent heterotopic ossification in acetabular fractures? Clin Orthop Relat Res. 2009;467(2):526-30.
18. Burd TA, Lowry KJ, Anglen JO. Indomethacin compared with localized irradiation for the prevention of heterotopic ossification following surgical treatment of acetabular fractures. J Bone Joint Surg Am. 2001;83-A(12):1783-8.
19. Karunakar MA, Shah SN, Jerabek S. Body mass index as a predictor of complications after operative treatment of acetabular fractures. J Bone Joint Surg Am. 2005;87(7):1498-1502.

20. Tile M, Helfet DL, Kellam JF (eds). Fractures of the Pelvis and Acetabulum 3rd Edition. Philadelphia, PA: Lippincott Williams & Wilkins; 2003. pp 61-79.
21. Mears DC, Velyvis JH. Primary total hip arthroplasty after acetabular fracture. Instr Course Lect. 2001;50:335-54.
22. Anglen JO, Burd TA, Hendricks KJ, et al. The "Gull Sign": A harbinger of failure for internal fixation of geriatric acetabular fractures. J Orthop Trauma. 2003;17(9):625-34.
23. O'Toole RV, Cox G, Shanmuganathan K, et al. Evaluation of computed tomography for determining the diagnosis of acetabular fractures. J Orthop Trauma. 2010;24(5):284-90.
24. Ohashi K, El-Khoury GY, Abu-Zahra KW, et al. Interobserver agreement for Letournel acetabular fracture classification with multidetector CT: are standard Judet radiographs necessary? Radiology. 2006;241(2):386-91. Epub 2006 Sep 27.
25. Chuckpaiwong B, Suwanwong P, Harnroongroj T. Roof-arc angle and weight-bearing area of the acetabulum. Injury. 2009;40(10):1064-6.
26. Vrahas MS, Widding KK, Thomas KA. The effects of simulated transverse, anterior column, and posterior column fractures of the acetabulum on the stability of the hip joint. J Bone Joint Surg Am. 1999;81(7):966-74.
27. Moed BR, Ajibade DA, Israel H. Computed tomography as a predictor of hip stability status in posterior wall fractures of the acetabulum. J Orthop Trauma. 2009;23(1):7-15.
28. Moed BR, Grimshaw CS. Outcomes of posterior wall fractures of the acetabulum treated nonoperatively after diagnostic screening with dynamic stress examination under anesthesia. J Bone Joint Surg Am. 2010;92(17):2792-2800.
29. Hoppenfeld S, deBoer P. Surgical Exposures in Orthopaedics. The Anatomic Approach. 3rd ed. Philadelphia, PA: Lippincott Williams & Wilkins; 2003.
30. Siebenrock KA, Gautier E, Ziran BH, et al. Trochanteric flip osteotomy for cranial extension and muscle protection in acetabular fracture fixation using a Kocher-Langenbeck approach. J Orthop Trauma. 2006;20(1 Suppl):S52-6.
31. Hadjicostas PT, Thielemann FW. The use of trochanteric slide osteotomy in the treatment of displaced acetabular fractures. Injury. 2008;39(8):907-13. Epub 2008 Jul 2.
32. Childs HA, Cole T, Falkenberg E, et al. A prospective evaluation of the timing of postoperative radiotherapy for preventing heterotopic ossification following traumatic acetabular fractures. Int J Radiat Oncol Biol Phys. 2000; 47(5):1347-52.
33. Sagi HC, Afsari A, Dziadosz D. The anterior intra-pelvic (modified rives-stoppa) approach for fixation of acetabular fractures. J Orthop Trauma. 2010;24(5):263-70.
34. Gill TJ, Sledge JB, Ekkernkamp A, et al. Intraoperative assessment of femoral head vascularity after femoral neck fracture. J Orthop Trauma. 1998;12(7):474-8.
35. Reddix RN, Russell G, Woodall J, et al. Relationship between intraoperative femoral head bleeding and development of avascular necrosis after acetabular fracture surgery. J Surg Orthop Adv. 2009;18(3):129-33.
36. Hsu JR, Stinner DJ, Rosenzweig SD, et al. Is there a benefit to drains with a Kocher-Langenbeck approach? A prospective randomized pilot study. J Trauma. 2010;69(5):1222-5.
37. Parker MJ, Livingstone V, Clifton R, et al. Closed suction surgical wound drainage after orthopaedic surgery. Cochrane Database Syst Rev. 2007;18(3):CD001825.
38. Reddix RN, Tyler HK, Kulp B, et al. Incisional vacuum-assisted wound closure in morbidly obese patients undergoing acetabular fracture surgery. Am J Orthop (Belle Mead NJ). 2009;38(9):446-9.
39. Reddix RN Leng, Woodall J, et al. The effect of incisional negative pressure therapy on wound complications after acetabular fracture surgery. J Surg Orthop Adv. 2010; 19(2):91-7.
40. Moed BR, Carr SE, Gruson KI, et al. Computed tomographic assessment of fractures of the posterior wall of the acetabulum after operative treatment. J Bone Joint Surg Am. 2003;85-A(3):512-22.
41. Brooker AF, Bowerman JW, Robinson RA, et al. Ectopic ossification following total hip replacement: incidence and a method of classification. J Bone Joint Surg Am. 1973; 55(8):1629-32.
42. Ghalambor N, Matta JM, Bernstein L. Heterotopic ossification following operative treatment of acetabular fracture. An analysis of risk factors. Clin Orthop Relat Res. 1994;(305):96-105.
43. Rath EM, Russell GV, Washington WJ, et al. Gluteus minimus necrotic muscle debridement diminishes heterotopic ossification after acetabular fracture fixation. Injury. 2002; 33(9):751-6.
44. Geerts WH, Bergqvist D, Pineo GF, et al. Prevention of venous thromboembolism: American College of Chest Physicians evidence-based clinical practice guidelines (8th Edition). Chest. 2008;133(6 Suppl):381S-453S.
45. Gruson KI, Moed BR. Injury of the femoral nerve associated with acetabular fracture. J Bone Joint Surg Am. 2003;85-A(3):428-31.
46. Letournel E. Diagnosis and treatment of nonunions and malunions of acetabular fractures. Orthop Clin North Am. 1990;21(4):769-88.

Chapter 18

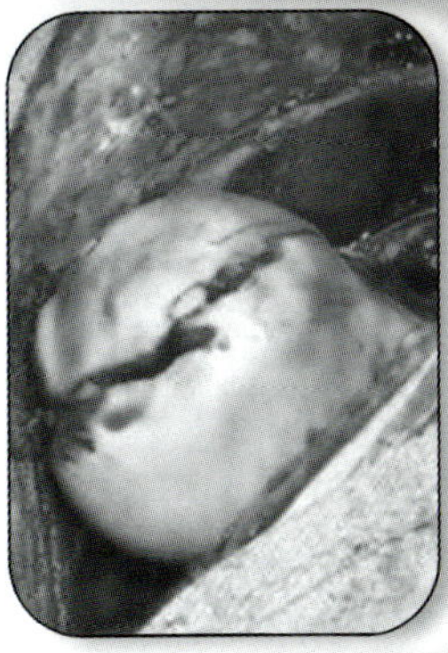

Femoral Head Fractures and Hip Dislocations

Kaan Irgit, Zhiyong Hou, Wade Smith

Chapter Outline

Introduction
Diagnosis
Classification
Surgical Indications
Surgical Anatomy, Positioning and Approaches
- Applied Anatomy
- Positioning
- Approaches

Surgical Techniques
- Technique 1: Anterior Dislocation of the Femoral Head with a Smith-Peterson Approach
- Technique 2: ORIF of Femoral Head with a Kocher-Langenbeck Posterior Approach
- Technique 3: Trochanteric Flip Osteotomy

Rehabilitation
Outcomes
Complications
- Post-traumatic Arthritis
- Osteonecrosis
- Heterotopic Ossification
- Sciatic Nerve Injury
- Retained Loose Bodies
- Residual Instability

Authors' Preferred Management of Select Complications
- Case 1: Management of Osteonecrosis of the Femoral Head
- Case 2: Management of Nonunion and Osteonecrosis after Femoral Head Fracture

Summary

Introduction

The hip is a diarthrodial joint which is inherently stable due to osseous and soft-tissue restraints. A force which exceeds the durability of the surrounding soft tissues causes hip dislocation. Arvidsson demonstrated that a traction force of 400 N (90 lbs) was needed in order to cause separation of the hip joint.[1] Traumatic dislocation of the hip accounts for 2–5% of all joint dislocations.[2] Due to its inherent stability, a high energy mechanism is needed to dislocate the hip joint. The incidence of hip dislocation and fracture-dislocation is increasing due to increasing survival from motor vehicle accidents.[3]

Femoral head fractures occur with a relative infrequency, with a reported incidence of 6–16% after hip dislocation.[4] The most common mechanism of injury for hip dislocation is a dashboard injury in a motor vehicle accident. Falls from heights, automobile-pedestrian accidents and athletic injuries are other common causes of hip fracture-dislocations. The amount and direction of the force applied combined with the position of the hip at the time of load, determines the type of hip dislocation. Hip dislocations are classified as central, anterior and posterior (approximately 90%, the most common type) dislocations. If a direct force is applied through the knee in line with femur with hip flexed, internally rotated and adducted, a posterior hip dislocation occurs. An anterior dislocation occurs when the hip is forcibly loaded in an abducted and externally rotated position. Anterior dislocations are subdivided into the superior type (10%) and the inferior type (90%). When the hip is in flexion the femoral head dislocates into the obturator foramen (inferior type). Dislocating in extension causes a pubis dislocation. If a fracture of the femoral head occurs during posterior dislocation, a shear type injury results. Anterior dislocations cause an impaction injury of osteochondral surface of the femoral head. Associated musculoskeletal injuries are common, particularly of the knee. As many as 26% of patients may have a significant associated knee injury with patellar fractures present in 4%.[2] Traumatic dislocation is a true orthopedic emergency and failure to recognize and treat the injury promptly is associated with a significantly poorer prognosis.[5] Despite timely management, osteonecrosis of the head and post-traumatic arthrosis are major concerns after treatment of hip dislocations and femoral head fractures. Heterotopic ossification (HO), postreduction instability and neurological injury are other common complications. These high-energy injuries occur in a younger population than other hip fracture entities. The severity of the injury and the potential for lifetime disability in this population emphasizes the need for prompt diagnosis and appropriate treatment.

Diagnosis

High-energy injury patterns from motor vehicle accidents or falls from height are the most common mechanisms of these injuries. Posterior dislocation frequently results from a dashboard injury in which the flexed hip is pushed posteriorly by an impact of the knee on the car dashboard. As with all high-energy trauma, Advanced Trauma Life Support (ATLS) protocols should be followed when assessing these patients. Awake patients will present with severe hip pain with palpation or motion of the lower extremity. The lower limb is slightly shortened and held typically in internal rotation, flexion and adduction with posterior hip dislocations. With anterior dislocations, the leg appears shortened with extreme external rotation, less pronounced abduction and flexion. Femoral head, neck or shaft fractures and obtunded patients may present with nonclassical posturing. A slight but fixed flexion in immobile neutral rotation and obvious leg length discrepancy on the physical examination should alert the surgeon for a possible irreducible dislocation without posterior wall fracture.[6] Motor and sensory examination of the affected extremity is mandatory because of the frequent association of sciatic nerve injuries (4–13%).[3] Motor function of the nerve and sensation of the peroneal and tibial nerve distribution should be documented in the initial examination and after reduction attempts.

Following history taking and a thorough physical examination, imaging is needed to confirm the diagnosis. Imaging permits assessment of the dislocation pattern and identification of associated injuries particularly of the femoral neck and acetabulum. Post-reduction imaging assists in assessment of the adequacy of reduction and with planning for surgical intervention. An anteroposterior (AP) pelvis radiograph as part of the initial ATLS trauma series is adequate for the initial diagnosis of hip fracture dislocations. On the AP radiograph in posterior dislocations, the femoral head appears to be displaced proximally and is smaller in diameter than the contralateral head. The femoral head will lie superior to the acetabulum with the femur in adduction and internal rotation, so that the lesser trochanter will be less visible than normal (Figs 18.1A and B). If there is a suspicion for associated injuries such as femoral neck fractures, acetabular fractures, or pelvic fractures, additional imaging including lateral X-rays of the hip, Judet views, or pelvic inlet and outlet radiographs should be obtained but not at the expense of any significant further delay in reduction of the femoral head (Figs 18.2A to D). Sixty percent of posterior dislocations are associated with a fracture of the acetabulum and these fractures potentially may prevent the reduction or produce residual instability after reduction. Anterior dislocations may occur in different locations. In obturator dislocations the femoral head overlies the obturator foramen. Iliac or pubic dislocations may be difficult to distinguish from posterior dislocations because both may come to overlie the iliac wing.

A 2–3 mm cut computerized tomography (CT) scan of the pelvis and femoral neck with coronal and sagittal reconstructions should be routinely obtained after hip reduction. CT scan is rarely required before reduction and

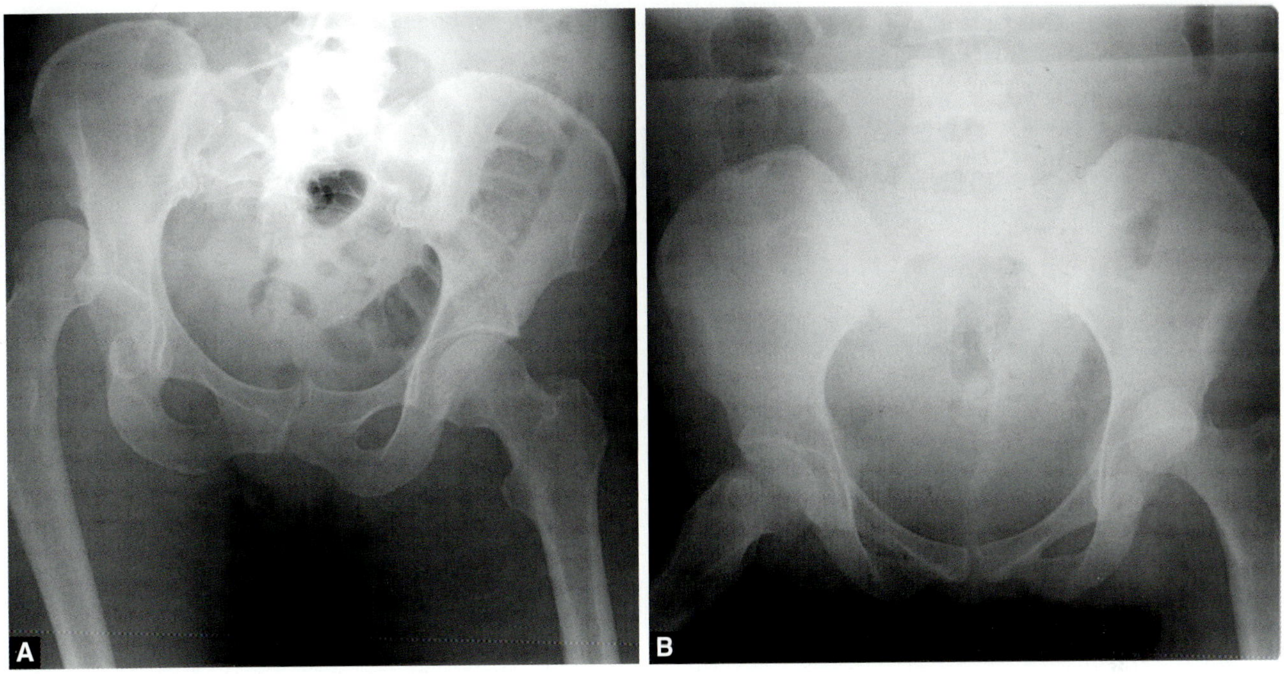

Figures 18.1A and B: Anteroposterior radiography of two pure posterior dislocations. Note that the lesser trochanters are not visible due to excessive internal rotation. In both films, dislocated head appears smaller than the contralateral side.

should not be routinely ordered. CT scan can reveal a nondisplaced neck or head fracture, the congruity of reduction, small intra-articular fragments and size of bony fragments (Fig. 18.3). Occult impactions or the severity of displacement of a femoral head fracture can accurately be assessed by CT. When an open reduction is planned after unsuccessful closed reduction attempts, CT should be ordered in a timely fashion that will not delay the initial closed reduction attempt. The period between presentation and reduction should be as short as possible. There is some evidence that dislocations of greater than 6 hours may have an increased risk of osteonecrosis. Several methods using fine cut CT scan images have been proposed to calculate hip stability after reduction, however the reliability of these calculations is low. Examination under fluoroscopy provides the most reliable assessment of hip stability after reduction.

Magnetic resonance imaging (MRI) in the acute setting is not indicated although it is superior in visualizing labral tears, femoral head contusions and microfractures, sciatic nerve injury, intra-articular fragments and pelvic vein thrombosis. Some surgeons advocate the use of MRI to evaluate possible damage to the obturator externus muscle that protects the medial femoral circumflex artery (MFCA) which is the main blood supply to the femoral head.[2,7] Additionally, MRI can be used to evaluate and monitor femoral head osteonecrosis in the follow-up period. However, the role of MRI is not clearly defined in the management of hip dislocations. Currently, the most valuable way to utilize MRI in the acute setting would be to evaluate the widened hip joint for any interposed soft tissues in the presence of a normal CT after a nonconcentric closed reduction.

FEMORAL HEAD FRACTURES AND HIP DISLOCATIONS DIAGNOSIS: Pearls and Pitfalls

- The initial trauma AP radiograph should be carefully scrutinized as most hip fractures or dislocations can be seen without the need for more extensive imaging
- CT of the involved hip should be routinely obtained following successful closed reduction as well as before open reduction of an irreducible femoral head
- Associated injuries to the knee (e.g. patella fracture, ligamentous injury, meniscal tears) are common
- When possible, prereduction documentation of lower extremity neurological function is important. The

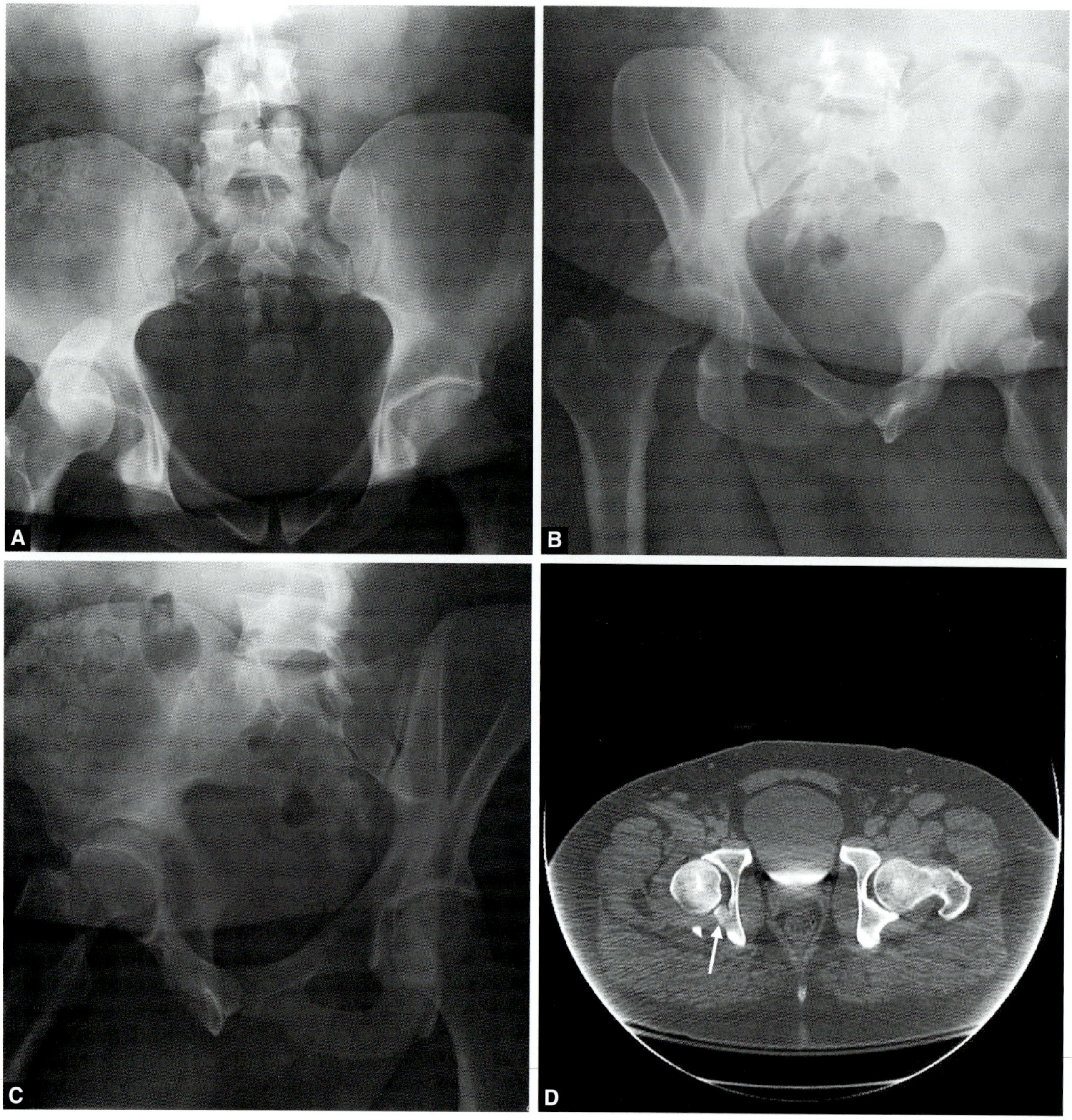

Figures 18.2A to D: Radiographic evaluation of hip dislocations with acetabular fractures. (A) Right hip posterior fracture dislocation on an anteroposterior pelvic X-ray; (B) Obturator oblique view; (C) Iliac oblique view. Judet or inlet/outlet views should only be done prior to femoral head reduction if they can be performed immediately in order to prevent any significant delay in reduction of the femoral head. Otherwise, they can be performed as a postreduction study; (D) Axial CT image after reduction is done to confirm a concentric reduction and rule out intra-articular loose bodies as well as assess acetabular fracture patterns. In this case, a posterior wall fragment is identified and is determined to be large enough to be a risk for instability and is therefore indicated for open reduction and internal fixation.

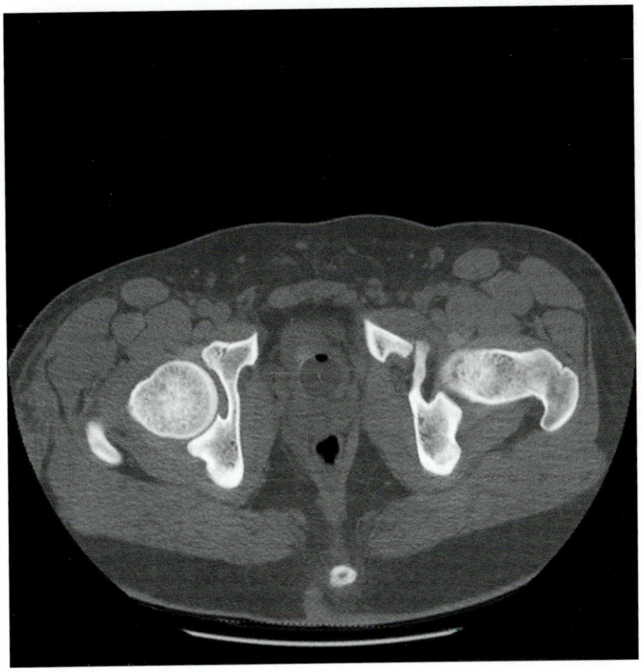

Figure 18.3: Occult anterior wall acetabular fracture detected with CT after an anterior hip dislocation of the right hip. An otherwise congruent reduction with no loose bodies is confirmed with this CT scan.

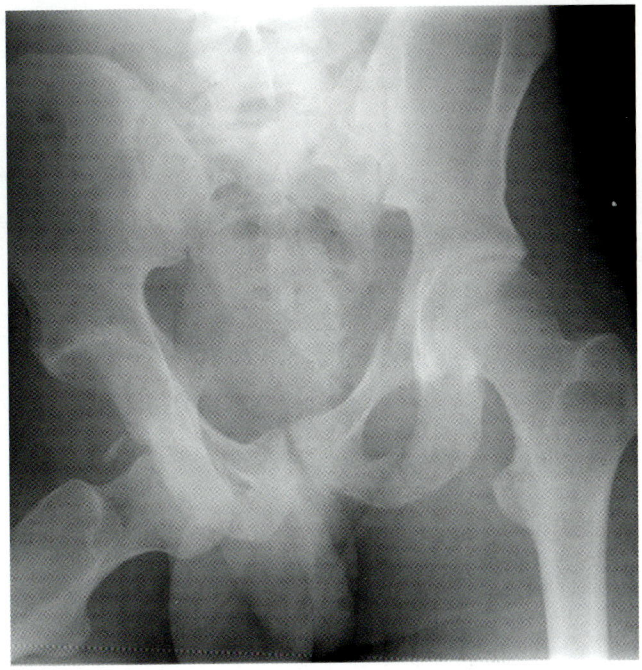

Figure 18.4: Right anterior obturator hip dislocation.

peroneal nerve is most affected thus toe and ankle dorsiflexion with first dorsal web space sensory function assessment should be assessed routinely

- Even with thin cut CT imaging some osteochondral or chondral loose bodies can be missed

Classification

Various classification schemes are proposed for both hip dislocations and femoral head fractures. Hip dislocations are classified as anterior, central and posterior types. Ninety percent of all hip dislocations are anterior and further subdivided by anatomic locations into inferior (obturator or perineal) and superior (pubic or subspinous) types (Fig. 18.4). One percent of the dislocations may occur bilaterally (Figs 18.5A to D).

The Levin classification can be used for both anterior fracture-dislocations and posterior fracture-dislocations. The Thomas and Epstein classification is commonly used for hip dislocations and includes associated fractures from Types II to V[8] (Table 18.1). Type V fractures include femoral head fractures. Stewart and Milford proposed a commonly used classification scheme which addresses postreduction stability in case of an acetabular fracture and has prognostic value.[9] Since the publication of Garret Pipkin in 1957, the Pipkin classification scheme remains the most widely used to describe femoral head fractures[10] (Figs 18.6A to D). Pipkin published his treatment results on 25 hips of 24 patients.[11] Reviewing 29 articles for femoral head fractures, Giannoudis et al. found that Pipkin classification is the most commonly used classification scheme (Table 18.2). Among 301 eligible femoral head fractures included in the study, there were 79 type 1 (26.2%), 100 type 2 (33.2%), 26 type 3 (8.6%), 88 type 4 (29.2%) and 8 were unclassified (2.7%) fractures of the femoral head.[10]

Surgical Indications

Fracture-dislocation of the hip is a relative orthopedic emergency. When a hip dislocation without a fracture of the neck is diagnosed a closed reduction attempt should be performed as soon as possible, preferably within 6 hours, in order to decrease the risk of osteonecrosis of the femoral head. Early reduction may assist in returning

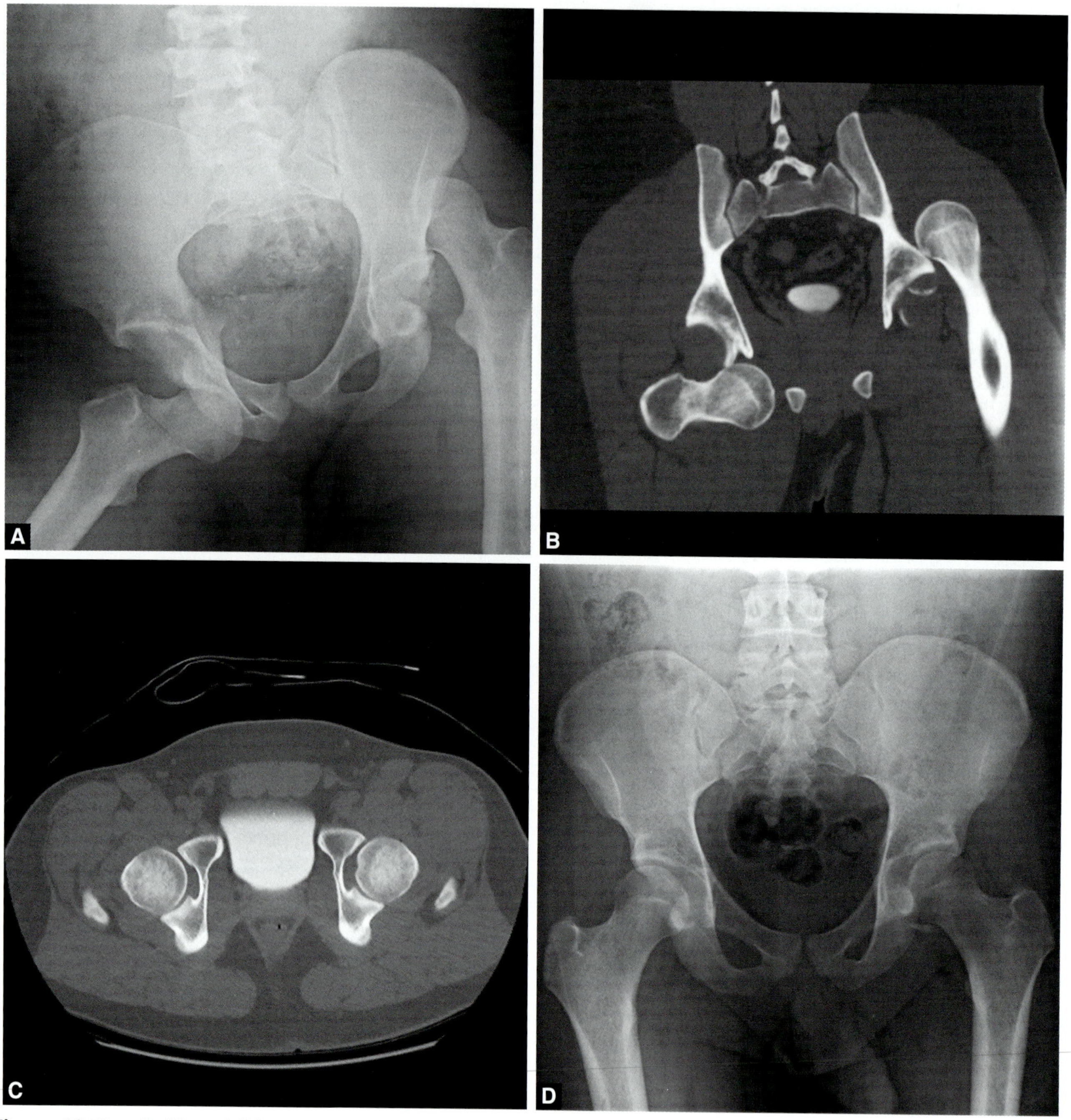

Figures 18.5A to D: Bilateral dislocation, right anterior obturator and left posterior hip dislocations. (A) Pelvic X-ray anteroposterior (AP); (B) Coronal CT scan before reduction. (Note the bony fragments in the left hip joint); (C) Postreduction CT shows concentric reduction without incarcerated bony fragments in the joint; (D) Six months postreduction AP pelvic X-ray demonstrates no obvious sign of osteonecrosis or arthritic changes.

normal blood flow to the hip, thus reducing the duration of ischemia to the femoral head. Ideally closed reduction should be performed under general anesthesia with complete muscle relaxation but some surgeons prefer to perform reduction under deep sedation. Optimal conditions such as an experienced surgeon, anesthesia, operating room adequate AP pelvic imaging should be established before any reduction attempt. Multiple closed

Table 18.1: Thomas and Epstein classification

1. Dislocation with or without minor fracture
2. Posterior fracture-dislocation with a single, significant fragment
3. Dislocation in which the posterior wall contains comminuted fragments with or without a major fragment
4. Dislocation with a large segment of posterior wall that extends into the acetabular floor
5. Dislocation with fracture of the femoral head

Table 18.2: Pipkin classification

1. Hip dislocation with fracture of the femoral head caudal to the fovea
2. Hip dislocation with fracture of the femoral head cephalad to the fovea
3. Type I or II injury with associated fracture of the femoral neck
4. Type I or II injury with associated fracture of the acetabular rim

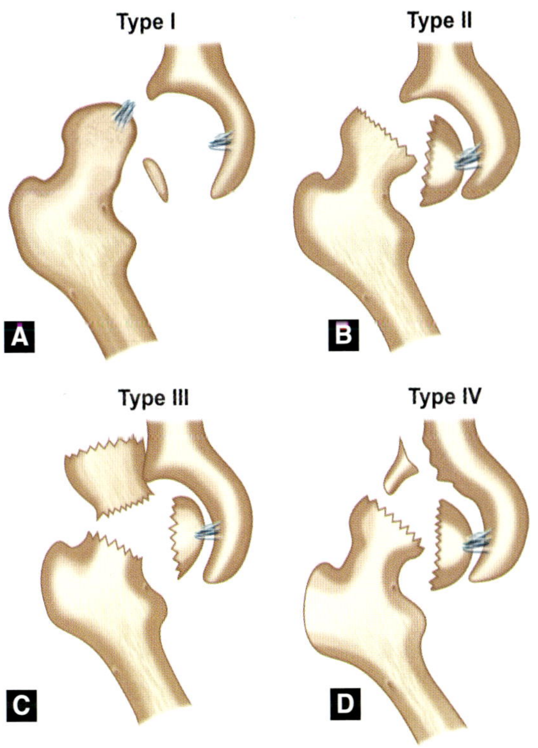

Figures 18.6A to D: Pipkin classification of femoral head fractures. (A) Type I: Fracture inferior to foveal depression; (B) Type II: Fracture superior to foveal depression; (C) Type III: Concomitant fractures of femoral head and neck; (D) Type IV: Concomitant fractures of femoral head and acetabulum.

reduction attempts should be avoided to prevent further damage to the femoral head cartilage.[5] For dislocations without associated fractures that result in congruent reduction by closed means, nonoperative management is usually definitive. However, irreducible dislocations, those with incongruent reductions and those with associated fractures may require subsequent operative management.

Closed reduction is usually accomplished via traction in line with the deformity. There are various reduction techniques described for posterior hip dislocations and our recommendation is to become familiar with at least two different techniques. The Allis maneuver, Stimson gravity technique and East Baltimore lift are the most commonly used techniques to reduce hip dislocations.

In the Allis maneuver, the patient is positioned supine on the table. While an assistant is holding the pelvis stable on the table, traction is applied in the direction of the deformity. The hip is then slightly flexed and is internally and then externally rotated with a slight adduction until an audible and a palpable clunk may be noted. The patient is prone in the Stimson gravity technique, which may not be possible in multiply injured patients. Within this technique, the affected extremity hangs off the stretcher with the hip and knee flexed to 90°. Downward pressure is then applied on the flexed knee. The East Baltimore lift reduction technique can be effective but necessitates two assistants. While the patient's knee and hip are placed in 90° of flexion, the surgeon rests one arm under the calf of the patient, with the surgeon's hand positioned on the shoulder of the assistant across the table. The surgeon uses the other hand to control rotation of the dislocated extremity. The assistant also positions his arm in a similar fashion as that of the surgeon. A second assistant counterpressures the pelvis. Both the surgeon and the first assistant apply an anteriorly directed traction. The lateral decubitus reduction technique (which is a modification of Allis technique) and the "piggy back" method are other simple and widely used techniques. There is a high risk of iatrogenic femoral neck fracture with the Bigelow forceful rotational technique, so this technique should be avoided. In fact, for all types of reduction, sudden forceful movements can cause fractures of the neck and damage the cartilage surface of the femoral head.

An AP pelvic radiograph and a 2 mm CT should be ordered to confirm the reduction. In order to control the stability after verification of reduction, a strong posteriorly directed force is applied to the flexed hip between 90° and 95° in neutral abduction or adduction and neutral rotation. In the presence of an associated wall fracture, stability should be fluoroscopically evaluated in the surgical suite by placing the hip in 90° of flexion, 20° of adduction and slight internal rotation and then applying a posteriorly-directed force. The presence, location and size of a posterior wall fracture should be assessed radiographically after a posterior dislocation.[2] Although there are available CT evaluations to estimate stability, clinical evaluation under fluoroscopy appears to be the most reliable method. After reduction, if the joint is congruent and stable without large fragments in the joint, nonoperative management is generally definitive. Small fragments making no contact with the articular surface of the head during movement and fragments which are not in the joint, do not require wash-out and debridement.

Pipkin type I fractures that anatomically reduce with a closed attempt can be treated with early weight-bearing and mobilization. Fixation or excision of a Pipkin type I or II fracture are indicated when the reduction of the hip is not congruent.

About 2–15% of hip dislocations are irreducible by closed means and they require immediate open reduction (Table 18.3). The reasons for irreducible dislocation include inadequate sedation, buttonholing through the joint capsule and interposition of muscle or bone fragments.

A dislocated hip can be irreducible due to soft tissue interposition (e.g. capsular, tendinous, labral or muscular) or osteochondral or purely cartilaginous fragments. The interposed soft tissue can be diagnosed with MRI or during the open reduction. Iliopsoas or piriformis tendons (for anterior dislocations) and more commonly the displaced posterior wall fragment caught between the femoral head and acetabulum may prevent reduction. If the irreducible hip dislocation is associated with a femoral head or acetabular fracture, the fracture pattern must be fully understood prior to performing open reduction. A thin cut CT image through acetabulum will demonstrate the location, size and the number of the bony fragments and it will be helpful in planning the surgical approach. The femoral head injury associated with posterior hip dislocation is almost always in the anterior portion of the head. In this situation, direct lateral or anterior approaches are more convenient for direct exposure and appropriate management.

Table 18.3: Surgical indication for open reduction

- Irreducible hip dislocation
- Incarcerated fragment
- Incongruent reduction
- Associated femoral neck fracture
- Sciatic nerve injury caused by reduction

Incarcerated fragments are the most common cause of instability after reduction. All the free fragments located between the femoral head and acetabular articular cartilage must be removed. The source of the bony fragments may be the femoral head avulsions, inferior femoral head fractures, loose fragments from the posterior wall or cartilage fragments detached from the femoral head. Small foveal avulsion fragments associated with a symmetric reduction can be left in place.

Posterior wall fractures that cause instability and incarceration, femoral head fractures that cause incongruence or are in the weight-bearing dome and all femoral neck fractures associated with hip dislocation require open reduction. If there is a femoral neck fracture preventing reduction by closed manipulation, open reduction and internal fixation (ORIF) of the femoral neck fracture is indicated. In case of a nondisplaced neck fracture, ORIF can follow the closed reduction attempt for the hip dislocation. In young patients with neck fracture and hip dislocation, immediate ORIF should be considered whereas for elderly patients with associated neck fractures hemiarthroplasty or total hip arthroplasty may be a better option (Figs 18.7A to D). When there is an associated neck fracture, the direct lateral of the hip or anterolateral approach should be performed with the assistance of fluoroscopic control.

In the presence of a femoral head fracture, surgical management depends upon size, location and stability of the fragments. The treatment goal for these injuries should be to preserve the joint and prevent post-traumatic arthrosis if at all possible. Indications for surgical management include nonanatomic reduction of the femoral head fragment, an unstable hip joint and the presence of intra-articular incarcerated fragments that are

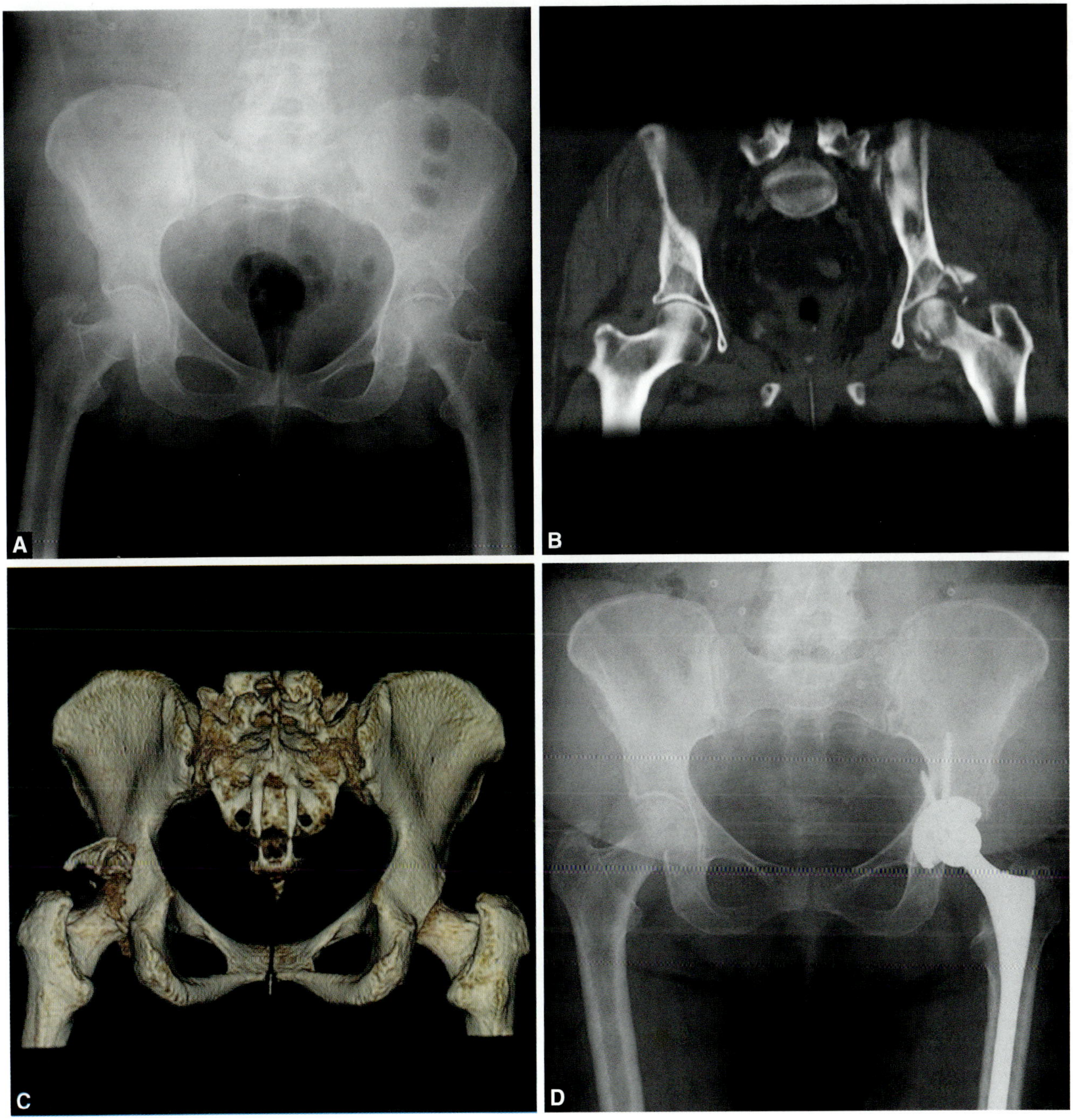

Figures 18.7A to D: Radiographic evaluation of an 80-year-old male who sustained left hip posterior dislocation after a motor vehicle accident. Due to the extensive comminution and cartilage damage the patient was managed with total hip arthroplasty. (A) Anteroposterior pelvic radiograph demonstrates a reduced femoral head but a displaced acetabulum fracture; (B) Coronal reformatted CT scan image demonstrates comminution of the weight-bearing dome of the acetabulum; (C) 3-D rendered CT image demonstrates a comminuted acetabulum fracture from a posterior perspective; (D) Anteroposterior pelvic radiograph after definitive treatment with total hip arthroplasty.

preventing congruent hip relocation. There is controversy whether to fix or excise the fractured head fragments. After a closed reduction of a Pipkin type I fracture, if an anatomic or near anatomic (< 2 mm) reduction is achieved and the hip is considered stable with no interposed fragments, nonsurgical management can be chosen. Pipkin type II fragments often extend into the weight-bearing portion of the femoral head and they may constitute a relatively large amount of the femoral head, so surgical management should be attempted if the fragments are large enough for screw fixation (Figs 18.8A to E). However, if the criteria for the type I fractures are met, nonsurgical management also may be considered for a Pipkin type II fractures. Following the emergent closed reduction and assessment of joint stability of a Pipkin type I or II fracture, if the hip is deemed to be unstable such that concern exists for redislocation while the patient is in bed, skeletal traction can be applied. Traction is also beneficial in the setting of joint incongruity with a large fracture fragment lying incarcerated within the joint space. Without application of traction and restriction of motion, such a fragment has the potential to further damage the articular surface. Surgical treatment to internally fix or excise such fragments should be considered relatively urgent. However, the anterior approach to the hip joint and fixation of femoral head fragments is potentially difficult. If the surgical team is unsure of their experience or technique, delaying operative intervention may be appropriate. If a large portion of the weight-bearing surface of the femoral head is involved and cannot be reduced and fixed, a more definitive procedure such as arthroplasty should be performed. Elderly patients with osteoarthritis (OA) who sustain a femoral head fracture of any type with unsatisfactory closed reduction alignment may benefit from primary hemiarthroplasty or total hip arthroplasty. Osteosynthesis should be the first choice in younger patients.

Nonsurgical treatment of femoral head fractures is possible in the presence of anatomic or near-anatomic reduction, a stable hip joint and no incarcerated fragments. However, Pipkin type III fractures must be treated surgically whereas all other types have a nonsurgical treatment option if meeting the above described criteria (Fig. 18.9). Pipkin III fractures are treated with emergent ORIF of the femoral neck. Pipkin type IV fractures generally are treated with emergent closed reduction, and management may require temporary skeletal traction. The type of associated acetabular fracture, instability and size of the posterior wall fragment on the posterior wall dictate the surgical approach, generally.

Surgical Anatomy, Positioning and Approaches

Applied Anatomy

Hip stability is directly related to the bony anatomy of the acetabulum and femoral head. The bony stability is achieved through the size and relationship of the femoral head and neck to the acetabular socket, which is deepened by osteocartilaginous labrum. The acetabulum is formed by 3 bones: ischium, ilium and pubis by converging as triradiate cartilage. Anterior, superior and posterior portions of acetabulum are covered with articular cartilage. The labrum is a horseshoe-shaped structure attached to the perimeter of the portion of the acetabulum covered by articular cartilage. The acetabular labrum increases the articular surface area by 22% and acetabular volume by 33%,[12] thus increasing the stability of the joint. One role of the labrum is a sealing function that is to resist distraction of the femoral head from the socket by acting like a suction cup and maintaining the negative pressure within the joint. The transverse acetabular ligament connects the anteroinferior and posteroinferior edges of the labrum in the most inferior portion of the acetabulum. The ligamentum teres lies in the acetabular notch in the mid-inferior portion of the acetabulum.

A thick capsule, which consists of iliofemoral, pubofemoral and ischiofemoral ligaments, run in a spiral and circular fashion and surrounds the hip joint. The iliofemoral ligament, the strongest of the three, courses inferiorly from the iliac body and anterior iliac spine in two distinctions. The pubofemoral ligament serves as a restraint for excessive extension of the hip joint. The ischiofemoral ligament lies posteriorly to the hip in an oblique and horizontal fashion.

Osteonecrosis of the femoral head after a traumatic posterior hip dislocation is a well known and devastating complication so the vascular structures around the hip and their anatomical, histological and angiographic features during dislocations are widely studied.

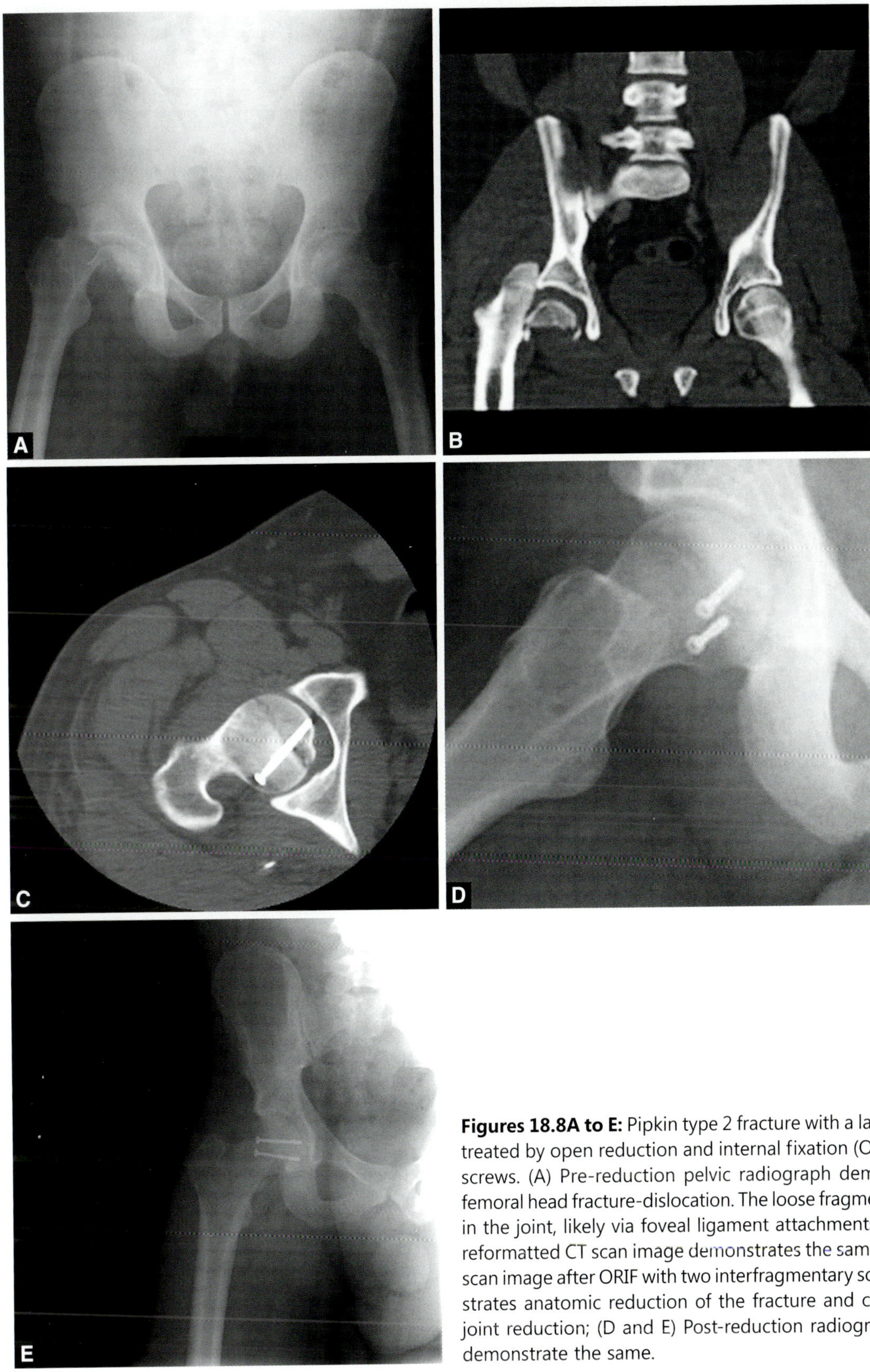

Figures 18.8A to E: Pipkin type 2 fracture with a large fragment treated by open reduction and internal fixation (ORIF) with two screws. (A) Pre-reduction pelvic radiograph demonstrating a femoral head fracture-dislocation. The loose fragment is retained in the joint, likely via foveal ligament attachments; (B) Coronal reformatted CT scan image demonstrates the same; (C) Axial CT scan image after ORIF with two interfragmentary screws demonstrates anatomic reduction of the fracture and concentric hip joint reduction; (D and E) Post-reduction radiographic images demonstrate the same.

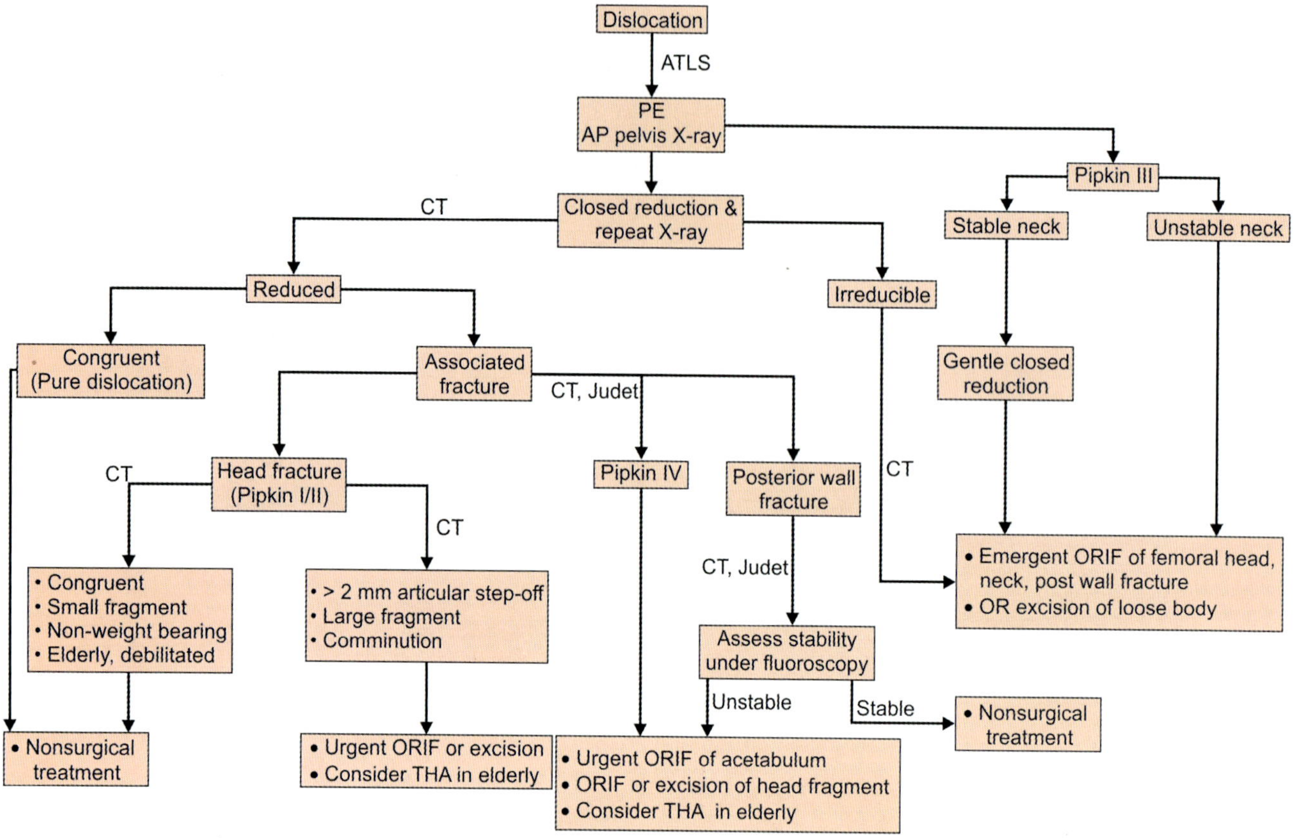

Figure 18.9: Algorithm for management of hip dislocations and femoral head fractures.

Abbreviations: AP, Anteroposterior; ATLS, Advanced Trauma Life Support; ORIF, Open reduction and internal fixation; THA, total hip arthroplasty

The intraosseous vascular anatomy of the head of the femur has been well described. The blood supply to the weight-bearing portion is derived from the MFCA.[4,13]

The MFCA commonly originates from the profunda femoris artery and occasionally from the common femoral artery. The MFCA has five branches: trochanteric, posterior, anterior, transverse and deep. The deep branch runs toward the intertrochanteric crest between pectineus medially and the iliopsoas tendon laterally along inferior border of obturator externus. Crossing posterior to obturator externus and anterior to the superior gemellus, obturator internus and inferior gemellus, the main division of the deep branch perforates the capsule superior to the insertion of superior gemellus and distal to the piriformis. In their comprehensive anatomical cadaver study, Gautier et al. clarified the relationship between the consistent branches of the MFCA and external rotatory muscles.[14] While using a Kocher-Langenbeck approach, they suggested dividing the conjoint tendon from distal to proximal about 1.5 cm or more from the trochanteric crest preserving the tendon of the obturator externus muscle. Their findings demonstrated that the deep branch of the MFCA courses along the inferior border of the tendon of the obturator externus and is at risk during a posterior approach.

Positioning

Positioning of the patient for surgery depends upon the direction of the dislocation, associated injuries (femoral head, neck, lung, abdominal, pelvic, knee, etc.), surgical approach chosen and experience of the surgeon. Anterior approaches (Smith-Peterson and Watson-Jones) can be performed supine. The Kocher-Langenbeck approach can be performed in a lateral decubitus or prone position with or without traction. Trochanteric osteotomy and surgical dislocation of the hip, as described by Ganz et al. require a lateral decubitus position.[15]

Approaches

Historically, surgeons were instructed to perform open reductions of a hip dislocation from the direction of the dislocation. The direction of the dislocation alone should not be a factor in determining postreduction management. Approaching the hip from a posterior direction may be more familiar to most surgeons and may also provide easy access to fractures of the posterior wall. A relative indication for an anterior approach may be associated femoral head and neck fracture. Due to the multitude of posterior dislocations the majority of the femoral head fractures occur on the anterior portion of the head. Regardless of the approach chosen, every attempt should be made to anatomically fix the osteochondral fragments and repair the avulsed soft tissue and labral tears. The joint should be irrigated to clear out the debris before reduction. Following reduction, one should be certain about the stability, especially in the presence of a posterior wall fracture. Our preference is to perform a direct anterior approach for posterior dislocations with associated femoral head fractures. The incidence of osteonecrosis with this strategy does not increase according to several recent studies and the exposure permits anatomic reduction and fixation of the femoral head fragments.

Anterior and Anterolateral Approach

A Smith-Peterson (between the sartorius and tensor fascia lata) or a Watson-Jones incision (between tensor fascia lata and gluteus medius) can be used for an anterior approach. A Watson-Jones incision may be better if there is a combined femoral neck and head fracture or an irreducible dislocation. The Smith-Peterson incision gives the advantage of more direct visualization of the anterior femoral head so that reduction and screw insertion are easier. The anterior approach can be used for ORIF of anterior head fractures, anteriorly located impaction head injuries, ORIF of combined neck fractures and arthrotomy and excision of loose bodies. Manual distraction by an assistant or a femoral distractor is helpful to visualize the joint. One advantage of the anterior approaches is that the vascular supply of the femoral head is not compromised although extensive stripping of the abductors from the lateral ilium may increase the risk of HO.

Posterior Approach

The Kocher-Langenbeck approach is a commonly used posterior approach for the treatment of posterior wall fractures and posterior hip dislocations. Other indications for the posterior approach are irreducible posterior dislocation and nonconcentric reductions with posterior interpositions of soft tissue or bone fragments. Complications after posterior approach include iatrogenic nerve palsies (3–18%), wound infections (3–12%), deep vein thrombosis or pulmonary embolism (8%), osteonecrosis of the femoral head (2–10%), HO (4–30%) and post-traumatic OA of the hip (4–35%).[16,17] A major limitation of the Kocher-Langenbeck approach is the limited access to the entire acetabulum and the femoral head but it allows direct visualization of the sciatic nerve. Identification of the sciatic nerve is the first step of the procedure. Gluteus muscle insertion can be released at its distal insertion to identify the sciatic nerve. The sciatic nerve itself or piriformis tendon, capsular attachments, labrum, ligamentum teres, gluteus maximus muscle and osteochondral or bony fragments may prevent the reduction and they should all be removed from the joint for a successful reduction. Care should be taken not to damage the MFCA which passes below the obturator externus muscle and is often intact despite the dislocation.

Transtrochanteric Approach

The trochanteric flip osteotomy (digastric osteotomy) and surgical dislocation of the hip, as described by Ganz et al. require a lateral decubitus position.[15] Gautier et al. presented a technique of surgical dislocation of the hip through a trochanteric osteotomy for preservation of the remaining blood supply to both the quadratus femoris and obturator externus muscles. In order to locate these muscles accurately, the trochanteric branch of the deep portion of the MFCA should be identified [14] (Fig. 18.10). After a Z-shaped capsulotomy staying anterior to the lesser trochanter to avoid the MFCA, the femoral head can be dislocated without further damage to the main vascular supply of the head. Excision of fragments or fixation of femoral head and acetabular fractures can be accomplished through this exposure. This approach provides surgical dislocation of the femoral head with minimal risk of osteonecrosis of the femoral head when

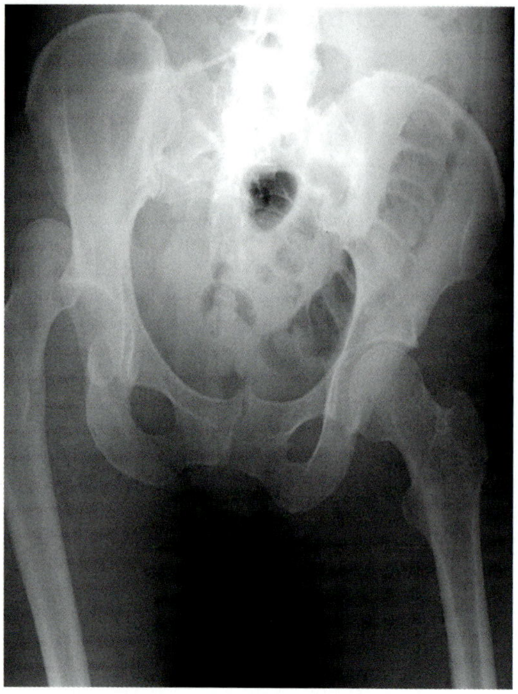

Figure 18.10: Step-cut and straight trochanteric osteotomy.

performed correctly. This allows a full view of the acetabulum to be obtained so that the adequacy of the reduction can be judged. It also avoids further devascularization of the fragments of the acetabular wall which remains attached to the capsule. This approach can be used for all four types of Pipkin fractures and has the advantage of exposing the entire hip joint, facilitating labral repair and improving the ability to ensure the implants are not intra-articular. Solberg et al. published their results with trochanteric flip osteotomy in Pipkin IV fractures. Eleven out of twelve of their patients achieved healing of the femoral head with only one patient with the osteonecrosis of the femoral head.[18] Eighty percent of the patients in their series had good or excellent outcomes at an average 4-year follow-up.

Arthroscopic Excision of Loose Bodies

Over the last two decades, hip arthroscopy has become an increasingly popular and a more frequently performed procedure. Generally as a technique, arthroscopy is a safe alternative to arthrotomy for addressing intra-articular pathology, particularly for removal of loose bodies. In the case of hip trauma, arthroscopy can be useful in cases of retained loose bodies which do not otherwise require open reduction and internal fixation of any fractures. There are several advantages over arthrotomy, including less disruption of the capsuloligamentous structures of the joints, less blood loss, reduced potential for neurovascular injury and decreased recovery time. However, hip arthroscopy is not harmless. Complications include broken intra-articular instruments, traction neurapraxia (sciatic and femoral), direct injury of nearby neurovascular structures (e.g. lateral femoral cutaneous nerve), portal hematoma or bleeding, osteonecrosis, retroperitoneal fluid extravasation and iatrogenic articular cartilage injuries.

Loose bodies represent a clear indication for hip arthroscopy. If an attempt is made to extract the loose bodies by arthroscopy, care must be taken to explore the peripheral compartment and even the iliopsoas tendon sheath, because loose bodies will often reside there. Arthroscopy also has been shown to be useful in diagnosing and treating labral tears.

Hip arthroscopy can be performed in two positions: supine and lateral. One of the primary goals of patient positioning for hip arthroscopy should be to allow for adequate distraction of the hip joint. Supine positioning is technically easier than the lateral position and they both require a traction table. In the supine position, the perineal post is placed more laterally than one placed for a hip fracture because a certain amount of abduction combined with the lateralizing force of a perineal post are both required to create the appropriate resultant force in line with the femoral neck. Another reason for the lateralization of the post is to protect the pudendal nerve and its perineal branch, which passes just medial to the ischial tuberosity. Lateral position can be advantageous for the obese patients and because it allows the use of 30° scope, visualization may be superior in the lateral position.

During hip arthroscopy 8–10 mm of joint distraction is necessary for adequate visualization. The recommended time for traction is typically less than 2 hours and a complete motor blockade is required with the anesthesia. The three most commonly used portals in hip arthroscopy are the anterior, anterolateral and posterolateral portals. Together, these give excellent visualization to the central compartment of the hip. The anterior portal is made at the intersection of a transverse line tangential to the tip of the greater trochanter and a longitudinal line made distal to the anterior superior iliac spine. The anterolateral and posterolateral portals are made on their respective sides at the tip of the greater trochanter. A posterior portal has been described when the patient is placed in the lateral position. Hypotensive anesthesia and higher pump pressures may be needed to overcome the excessive bleeding from fracture surfaces which impairs visualization. However, higher pressures also increase the risk for retroperitoneal fluid extravasation. For this reason, some surgeons advocate waiting until the capsule is healed, if possible.

Even after a concentric reduction of a simple dislocation, some but not all loose bodies are detectable by standard imaging, although chondral loose bodies can be missed. Although there is basic science evidence to suggest that hip arthroscopy may be beneficial for patients because it enables detection of loose bodies, no clinical evidence yet supports this.

Surgical Techniques

Technique 1: Anterior Dislocation of the Femoral Head with a Smith-Peterson Approach

After being medically cleared for surgical intervention, the patient is taken to the operating room, administered general anesthesia with muscle relaxation, and positioned supine on the operating table (See Fig. 19.11 in chapter 19). A folded blanket (or a sandbag) is placed posterior to the lumbosacral region to elevate the pelvic area from the table. The hair of the perineum and surgical site should be shaved. The entire injured lower extremity, hip, region and ipsilateral flank are next prepared with iodine. Skin preparation and draping were completed especially for the inguinal and posterior thigh region. After IV antibiotic administration and patient specific identification, the skin incision is made. A long incision is made following the anterior half of the iliac crest to the anterior superior iliac spine. From there, the incision is curved down so that it runs vertically for 8–10 cm, pointing toward the lateral side of patella. The gap between the tensor fascia lata and the sartorius is palpated and the intermuscular interval is dissected down with a scissor. Iatrogenic injury to the lateral femoral cutaneous nerve should be avoided. The sartorius is retracted medially and upward and tensor fascia lata downward and laterally. At this point the large ascending branch of the lateral femoral circumflex artery below the anterior superior iliac spine should be ligated or coagulated. Deep to these muscles, the rectus femoris and gluteus medius muscles are exposed. Both heads of the rectus femoris, including the direct head that originates from the anterior inferior iliac spine and the reflected head that originates from superior lip of the acetabulum should be detached and retracted medially. After retracting the gluteus medius laterally, the anterior hip joint capsule can be exposed. Next an obliquely oriented Z-shaped capsulotomy is made with the upper limb paralleling and sparing the anterior acetabular labrum parallel to the femoral neck. At this point the joint is irrigated and the hematoma and debris is washed out. The femoral head and the acetabulum are evaluated for occult or evident fractures. Titanium screws, Herbert screws, or alternatively, bioabsorbable pins can be used for fixation of the femoral head fractures (Figs 18.11 and 18.12A to D). Irreducible femoral head fracture fragments within the acetabulum and the residual osteochondral debris are removed. The joint can be relocated with the aid of a bone hook while assuring skeletal muscle relaxation and the hip in flexion, adduction, internal rotation and anterior translation. Femoral neck fractures can be easily assessed and reduced by this exposure. In such cases, femoral head fractures should be fixed to allow screw fixation for femoral neck fractures. After the fixation and reduction of the hip joint passive full extension

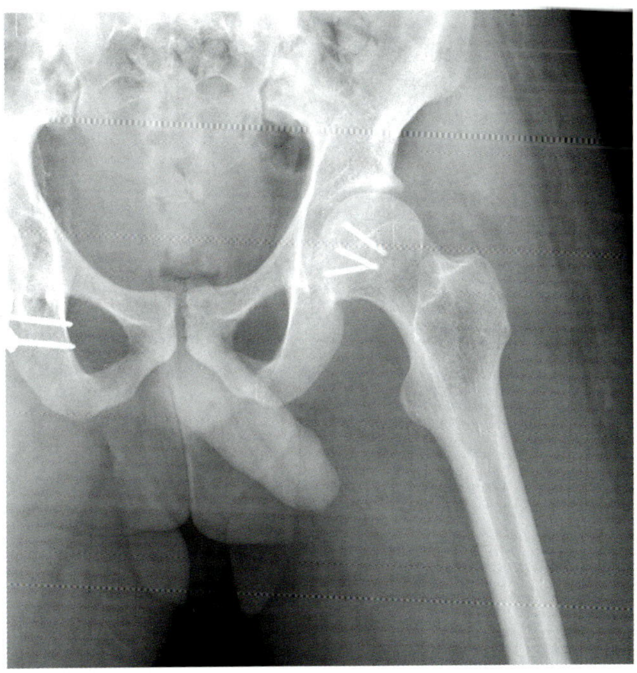

Figure 18.11: An example of Herbert-Whipple headless screw fixation for a femoral head fracture.

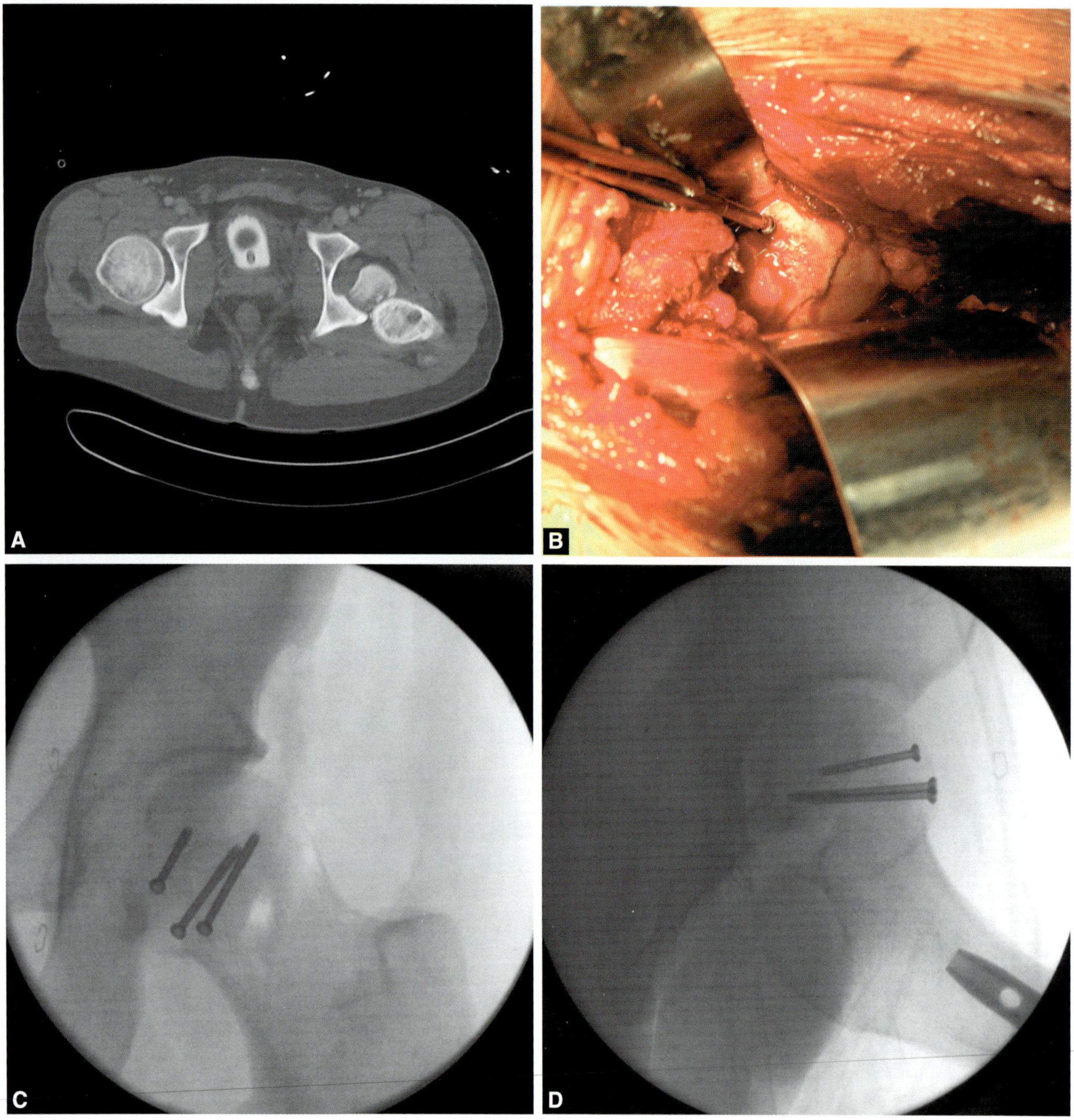

Figures 18.12A to D: Fixation of a Pipkin type 2 femoral head fracture through an anterior Smith-Peterson exposure without dislocation of the head fragments: (A) Axial CT image demonstrates the fracture dislocation. Due to an ipsilateral open femoral shaft fracture, closed reduction in the emergency department was unsuccessful; (B) Operative exposure: the patient's feet are to the right, the rectus is shown retracted medially (to top of photo), gluteus medius and tensor fascia muscle are retracted laterally (to bottom of photo and fixation with 3.5 mm countersunk AO partially threaded cancellous screws is shown. With the femoral head reduced in the acetabulum, proper screw trajectory (typically directed from anteromedial to posterolateral) is dependent on both external rotation of the hip and satisfactory retraction of the rectus and sartorius and can be difficult in obese patients; (C and D) Anteroposterior and lateral fluoroscopic images demonstrating anatomic reduction and fixation.

Courtesy: Saqib Rehman

and flexion of the hip joint is assessed and confirmed for hip congruency, reduction accuracy and implant safety before closure. The anterior surgical capsulotomy and the rectus femoris tenotomy is repaired directly and the fascia and dermal layers and skin are closed primarily.

ANTERIOR DISLOCATION OF THE FEMORAL HEAD WITH A SMITH-PETERSON APPROACH: Pearls and Pitfalls

- This approach preserves the blood supply to the head by sparing the external rotators and MFCA passing through them
- There is a relatively high risk of HO
- Most of the femoral head fractures are on the anterior portion of the head thus this approach is advantageous for young patients with hip dislocations associated with femoral head fracture
- One cannot fix posterior wall fractures via this approach
- Beware not to damage lateral cutaneous femoral nerve during the fascial dissection

Technique 2: ORIF of Femoral Head with a Kocher-Langenbeck Posterior Approach

After the patient is taken into the operating room, general anesthesia with muscle relaxation is applied and an intravenous antibiotic is given prior to the start of the procedure. The hip is sterilely prepped and draped. Before the incision the bony landmarks, (1) posterior superior iliac spine, (2) greater trochanter and (3) shaft of femur can be outlined by a sterile marking pen. A 10–15 cm incision is made beginning a few centimeters distal and lateral to the posterior superior iliac spine (Figs 18.13 and 19.13 in chapter 19). The incision can be extended in obese patients. The incision is carried anteriorly over the greater trochanter and curved distally along the tip of the greater trochanter towards the lateral aspect of the femoral shaft. The incision ends approximately to the distal insertion of the gluteus maximus tendon. After dividing the subcutaneous tissue over the fascia, the gluteus maximus muscle and the tractus iliotibialis is incised by a scalpel or scissors in line with the skin incision. The anterior part of the split muscle belly includes muscle of the tensor fasciae latae. After freeing the fat and bursae now the external rotators (piriformis tendon, the gemelli superior and inferior, external and the

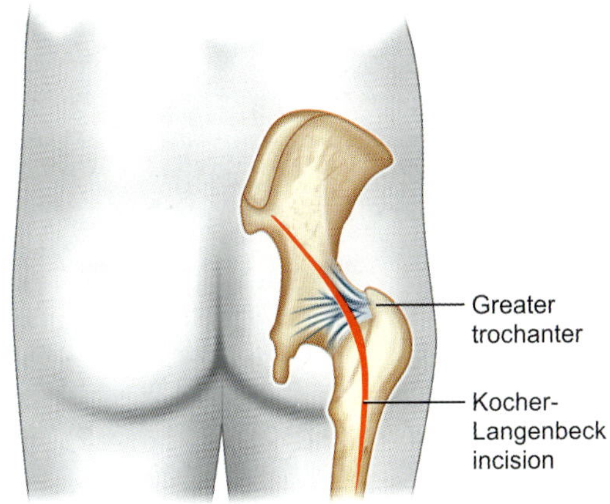

Figure 18.13: Kocher-Langenbeck incision.

internal obturator muscle and the quadratus femoris) are exposed. The sciatic nerve is identified over the quadratus femoris muscle and is traced proximally toward the greater sciatic notch where it emerges at the inferior border of the piriformis muscle. The sciatic nerve lies posterior to the gemelli and internal obturator muscles and anterior to the piriformis muscle, between the greater trochanter and the ischial tuberosity (Fig. 18.14). Care should be taken not to exert pressure or stretch the nerve during the surgery. The nerve can be protected by a free hand or gently by a retractor all through the operation. The hip should also be kept in an extended position while the knee is kept flexed throughout the procedure to reduce tension on the sciatic nerve. External rotators are partly or totally torn by the force generated by dislocation. Excessive soft tissue stripping should be avoided from the bony fragments. At this stage, the femoral head and acetabulum should be inspected to detect if there is any marginal impaction or damage to the cartilage of the acetabulum and femoral head. Any free intra-articular fracture fragment(s) should be localized, removed and/or cleaned and reinserted. Acetabular posterior wall fractures should be reduced and fixed properly. A meticulous debridement of all soft tissues should be performed before wound closure. Labral defects should be recorded. If possible a labral abrasion is repaired by bone anchors or they should be resected. Any necrotic tissue (especially in gluteus minimus muscle) should be removed and the entire wound should be irrigated promptly to decrease the risk of HO. Before closure all tendons should be repaired. The short external rotators should be repaired through bone tunnels through the greater trochanter. The

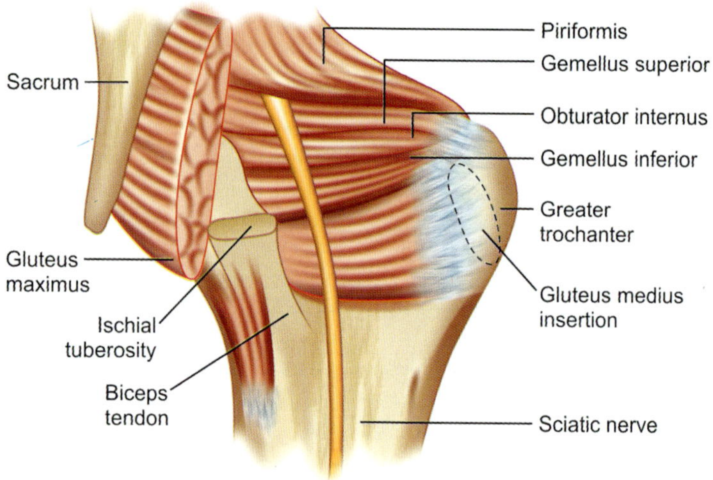

Figure 18.14: The sciatic nerve and its relationship with the short external rotator muscles.

iliotibial tract, subcutaneous tissue and skin are closed after insertion of suction drain.

ORIF OF FEMORAL HEAD WITH KOCHER-LANGENBECK POSTERIOR APPROACH: Pearls and Pitfalls

- Creates suboptimal access for the anteriorly located fractures of femoral head
- Pipkin type IV fractures are best treated through this approach
- The sciatic nerve should be protected throughout the operation. Any direct pressure with a retractor may cause neuropraxia. Keeping the knee flexed and hip extended help to relieve tension on the sciatic nerve and must be employed throughout the procedure

Technique 3: Trochanteric Flip Osteotomy

The preferred position of the patient is lateral decubitus for this approach. Draping should be performed in a manner to allow free movement of the injured leg. A sterile bag should be fixed in the ventral side of the patient for positioning of the leg during hip dislocation. After a longitudinal skin incision, fascia lata is incised in the line with the skin incision. Trochanteric bursa is than dissected. Internally rotate the leg to facilitate identification of the gluteus medius muscle. An osteotomy is made from the posterosuperior edge of the greater trochanter extending distally to the posterior border of the ridge of vastus lateralis with an oscillating saw as shown in Figure 18.10. The thickness of the osteotomised fragment should not exceed 1.5 cm. The osteotomy should stay lateral to the insertion of the short external rotators, which remain attached to the proximal femur. Alternatively the osteotomy can be done as a step-cut osteotomy. After completion of the osteotomy, the fragment is rotated 90° and retracted anteriorly including the digastric attachment of vastus lateralis and gluteus medius muscles. The vastus lateralis is then released from the femoral shaft about 5 cm distal to the origin of the vastus lateralis at the trochanteric ridge. Proximally the most posterior fibers of the gluteus medius tendon are released from the stable trochanter. The piriformis tendon should remain with the stable portion. By gently flexing and externally rotating the leg, the vastus lateralis and intermedius are dissected sharply from the femur. By gently retracting the posterior border of the gluteus medius anterosuperiorly, the tendon of the piriformis is visualized. The interval between the gluteus minimus and the piriformis is then developed to expose the superior capsule. By additional external rotation and flexion of the hip the anterior, superior and posterosuperior capsule can be exposed. A Z-type capsulotomy is now made starting anterolaterally along the long axis of the femoral neck. The capsulotomy is then extended distally along an anteroinferior line ending anterior to the lesser trochanter. This will prevent damage to the main branch of MCFA, which is located just superior and posterior to the lesser trochanter. The posterior extension of the capsulotomy runs parallel to the labrum. The capsulotomy can be modified according to the fracture pattern in order to preserve capsular attachments to acetabular rim fragments when present. In order to dislocate the hip, the leg is brought into further flexion and external rotation. The leg is then placed into a sterile bag placed on the opposite side of the operating table. By manipulating the leg, 360° views of the acetabulum and the femoral head are possible. After dislocation of the head, the acetabular cartilage and the labrum should be carefully inspected for traumatic damage. Small labral tears are debrided and the larger tears can be fixed with suture anchors. Most of the time ligamentum teres would be found torn and the stump should be removed from the head to allow reduction. Loose fragments of the femoral head without any capsular attachment should be removed and placed on a back table for potential later reassembly. Any soft tissue attachments to bony fragments are preserved in order to avoid further devascularization of these fragments. The vascularity of the fragment and the main head after fixation can be confirmed by 2 mm drillings or intraoperative Doppler flow. Fixation of the head fragments can be performed with mini or small fragment cortical screws (2.0–2.7 mm), Herbert screws, titanium cannulated

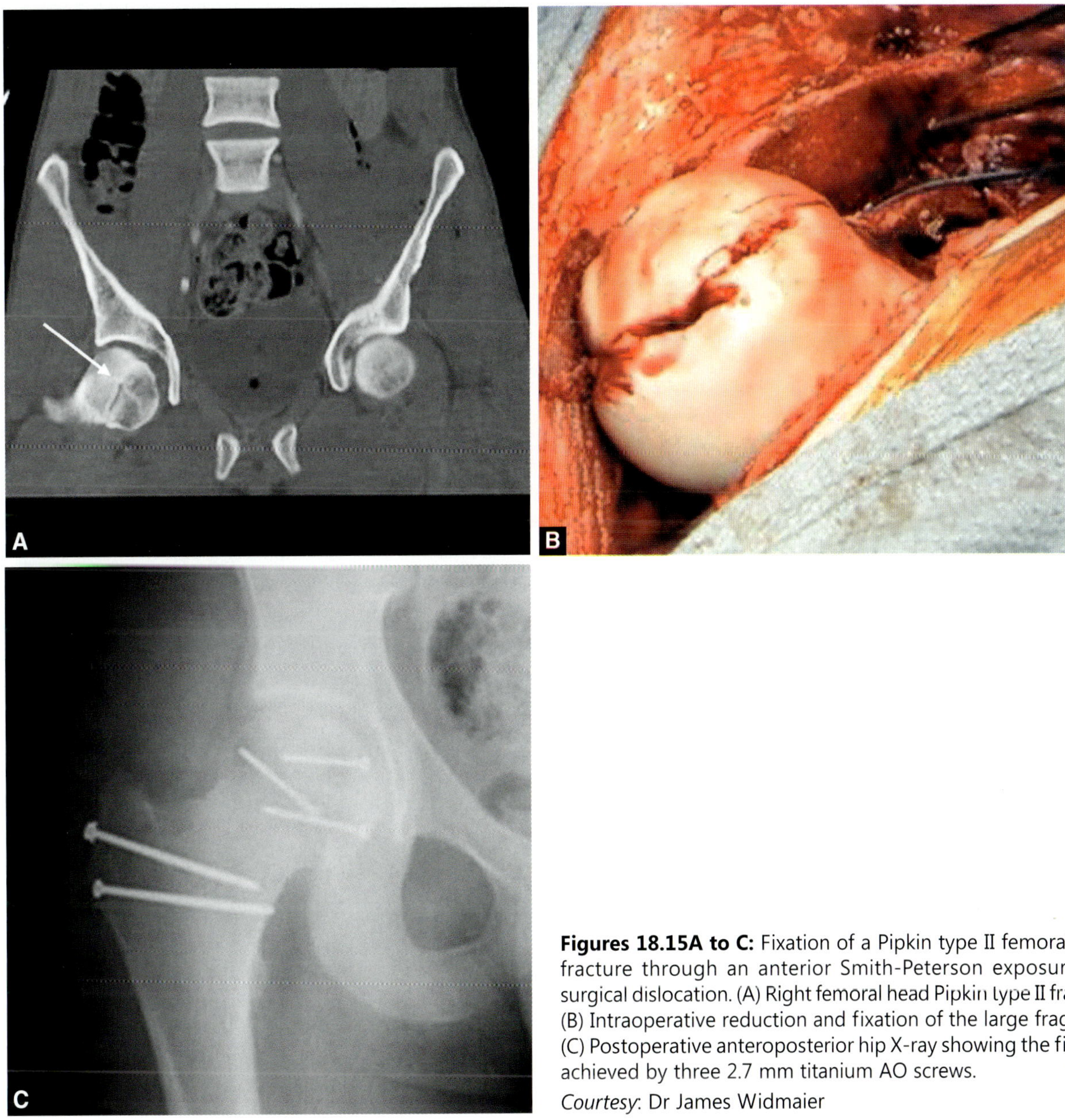

Figures 18.15A to C: Fixation of a Pipkin type II femoral head fracture through an anterior Smith-Peterson exposure and surgical dislocation. (A) Right femoral head Pipkin type II fracture; (B) Intraoperative reduction and fixation of the large fragment; (C) Postoperative anteroposterior hip X-ray showing the fixation achieved by three 2.7 mm titanium AO screws.
Courtesy: Dr James Widmaier

screws or bioabsorbable screw (Figs 18.15A to C). If there is a femoral neck fracture (Pipkin type III) it should be addressed initially. ORIF of the femoral neck component can be performed through the same approach. Depending on the type of fracture and visibility, the short external rotators may have to be released off the proximal femur with a safety distance of about 2 cm from the greater trochanter to prevent damage to the main blood supply of the femoral head. After fracture fixation the hip can be reduced by manual traction on the flexed knee and internal rotation. The capsule should be re-approximated without too much tightening in order to prevent tension on the retinacular vessels with potential drop in femoral head perfusion. Finally, the trochanteric osteotomy is reduced and fixation is achieved with two 3.5 mm screws or 6.5 mm cancellous screws. The wound is closed in layers after placement of a drain.

TROCHANTERIC FLIP OSTEOTOMY:
Pearls and Pitfalls

- There is a high risk of HO
- Use of the step osteotomy could reduce the degree and length of the postoperative reduced weight-bearing period
- There is limited access for reduction of the anterior column with visual control of the extra-articular placement of long column screws

Rehabilitation

Rehabilitation after reduction and/or surgical intervention of a hip dislocation is controversial. Some surgeons suggest a short period of skeletal traction until pain is improved. Bucks traction and/or traction pin can be applied for unstable patients, and the surgical treatment must be delayed such as in multiple injured patients.

After closed reduction or surgical reduction, early gentle range of motion and patient mobilization should be initiated as soon as possible. Sahin et al. showed bed rest does not improve outcomes.[5] Eight weeks of toe-touch weight-bearing can be encouraged after posterior wall fractures or femoral head fractures. Immediate and full weight-bearing can be advised after pure dislocations.

When there is a femoral head fracture associated in patients for whom fracture-healing is a goal, weight-bearing generally is restricted to toe-touch weight-bearing for 3 months. This allows fracture fragments to heal and is believed to diminish loads that could result in sub-chondral collapse in a patient who goes on developing osteonecrosis. Some surgeons advocate prolonged delay to weight-bearing in cases whose reduction is delayed beyond 6 hours (thus increasing their risk for osteone-crosis). If fracture fragments have been excised and a congruent joint remains, however, weight-bearing may be initiated as tolerated by the patient. Physical therapy focusing on hip abductor, flexor and quadriceps streng-thening, is instituted after weight-bearing is allowed. Hip flexion beyond 90° must be restricted during the next 8 weeks after the reduction.

Outcomes

Outcomes following simple hip dislocation vary from a functionally normal hip to a severely painful, arthritic hip joint. Factors which influence the outcome include the extent of other severe injuries, the time to reduction, the direction of the dislocation, the overall condition of the patient prior to dislocation and postreduction management and rehabilitation.[5,19] In general, anterior dislocations do better than posterior ones and patients with multiple injuries do worse than those without additional injuries.[19,20] Good to excellent long-term outcomes are reported in half to nearly all patients with simple hip dislocations managed with rapid reduction.[21] In general, anterior dislocations have better prognosis than posterior dislocations whereas fracture dislocations have a better prognosis than pure dislocations. Associated femoral head fractures adversely affect the outcome by causing osteonecrosis or OA. Timing of treatment is another crucial factor affecting the outcome, as the longer delay between injury and reduction the worse is the outcome. In this sense, it is likely to expect poor prognosis with the multiple injured patients who have a delay in reduction due to other vital organ injuries.

The most commonly used functional assessment tool is established by Thompson and Epstein.[8] Giannoudis et al. reviewed the literature to investigate data regarding femoral head fractures, particularly focusing on their management, complications and clinical results.[10] Thompson-Epstein criteria were used in 18 out of 29 articles available. The overall results according to Thompson-Epstein criteria and regardless of fracture type or treatment, were excellent in 40 (14.3%) cases, good in

111 (39.8%), fair in 54 (19.3%) and poor in 74 (26.5%). The authors also reviewed 16 articles (256 cases) including definite nonoperative or surgical treatment. For the conservative group (54 cases-21%), the results were excellent in 7 (13%), good in 16 (29.6%), fair in 15 (27.8%) and poor in 16 (26.9%) patients. Among surgical fractures (202 cases-79%), the outcomes were excellent in 31 (15.3%), good in 92 (45.5%), fair in 32 (15.8%) and poor in 47 (23.3%). They extracted 155 femoral head fractures from 11 articles and found no difference in outcome among Pipkin subtypes.

The decision of intraoperative surgical approaches may also affect the outcomes. Brian recently reported 12 patients with Pipkin IV fracture treated with trochanteric flip osteotomy. Out of 12, ten had good or excellent outcomes, one had a fair outcome and one had a poor outcome. Eleven achieved healing of the femoral head fracture and osteonecrosis developed in one patient.[18] Development of OA of the hip joint or osteonecrosis of the femoral head also contributes to bad outcomes.

The natural history of symptomatic osteonecrosis has been documented to lead to collapse and subsequent OA. The rate of both post-traumatic coxarthrosis and osteonecrosis is much higher for posterior fracture-dislocation, with an incidence of up to 70%. There are various factors to predict poorer outcomes: delay in reduction (more than 6 hours), direction of dislocation (posterior dislocations show more late complications than anterior), the severity of injuries (acetabular fractures, other associated fractures, closed head injuries, thoracic injuries, peripheral nerve injuries, labral or other soft tissue injuries) and the surgical approach (posterior approach intervention show more osteonecrosis than an anterior or trochanteric-flip osteotomy approach).[19,22,23]

Complications

Simple hip dislocations and/or femoral head dislocations have significant long-term complications: as reported in the literature, 0–24% osteonecrosis of the femoral head, 0–72% post-traumatic arthritis, 7–27% peripheral nerve injury and 2–64% formation of HO.[13,24] Information concerning complications was also extracted by Giannoudis et al. who reviewed 26 articles describing 405 femoral head fractures. Within their systematic review the overall incidence of major late complications (mean follow-up 59.7 months) included osteonecrosis 11.8% (48/405), post-traumatic arthritis 20% (81/405) and HO 16.8% (68/405).[10] As a general rule, the choice of the surgical approach mainly influences osteonecrosis and HO; time to reduction of the femoral head mainly influences osteonecrosis and OA.

Post-traumatic Arthritis

Post-traumatic arthritis is the most common long-term complication after hip dislocation. It is thought to result from articular cartilage injury during the initial dislocation because small amounts of strain may have deleterious effects on the articular cartilage. Upadhyay et al. reported a 16% incidence of post-traumatic arthritis.[21] Arthritis is more likely to develop after an acetabular fracture or associated femoral head fracture. It is more common after posterior approaches than anterior approaches. A higher incidence was found in case of an anterior or posterior approach respectively versus a trochanteric-flip osteotomy in a review done by Giannoudis et al.[10] If a patient continues to perform heavy labor after hip dislocation, it is more likely for that patient to have OA. Additionally, a higher rate of arthritis is found in patients who continue heavy labor after hip dislocation.[3]

Osteonecrosis

The rate of osteonecrosis following hip dislocation varies widely, which is reported up to 40% in some series.[3] This is seen more after posterior dislocation and correlates with the time to reduction. Osteonecrosis rates are close to 0% when the reduction is done in the first 6 hours of the trauma. Yue et al. and other researchers showed that dislocation causes a kinking effect and spasm on the vascular supply to the femoral head, which is relieved by early reduction.[25] Generally, radiographic appearance of osteonecrosis occurs within 2 years after hip dislocation.[26] However, osteonecrosis may appear 8 years after a simple dislocation in a hip without previous evidence of radiographic changes.[27] Thus, longer-term follow-up for the hip dislocation is needed.

Osteonecrosis of the femoral head has been reported after both surgical and nonsurgical treatment and the choice of surgical approach may also affect the risk of osteonecrosis. There is a tendency to develop osteonecrosis after a posterior approach more than after an anterior or trochanteric-flip osteotomy approach.

Osteonecrosis in young patients is a difficult problem to treat because these patients are usually active and total hip arthroplasty may not be an appropriate solution. Other treatment options for osteonecrosis of the femoral head include vascularized fibular grafting and femoral osteotomy.

Heterotopic Ossification

There is a high incidence of HO following hip dislocation and acetabular surgery. It is particularly related to the approach and common after open reduction of a posterior dislocation. Stripping and trauma to the gluteal muscles predispose to HO formation (Figs 18.16A to C). It occurs with a higher incidence in cases of patients who undergo an anterior surgical approach.[4]

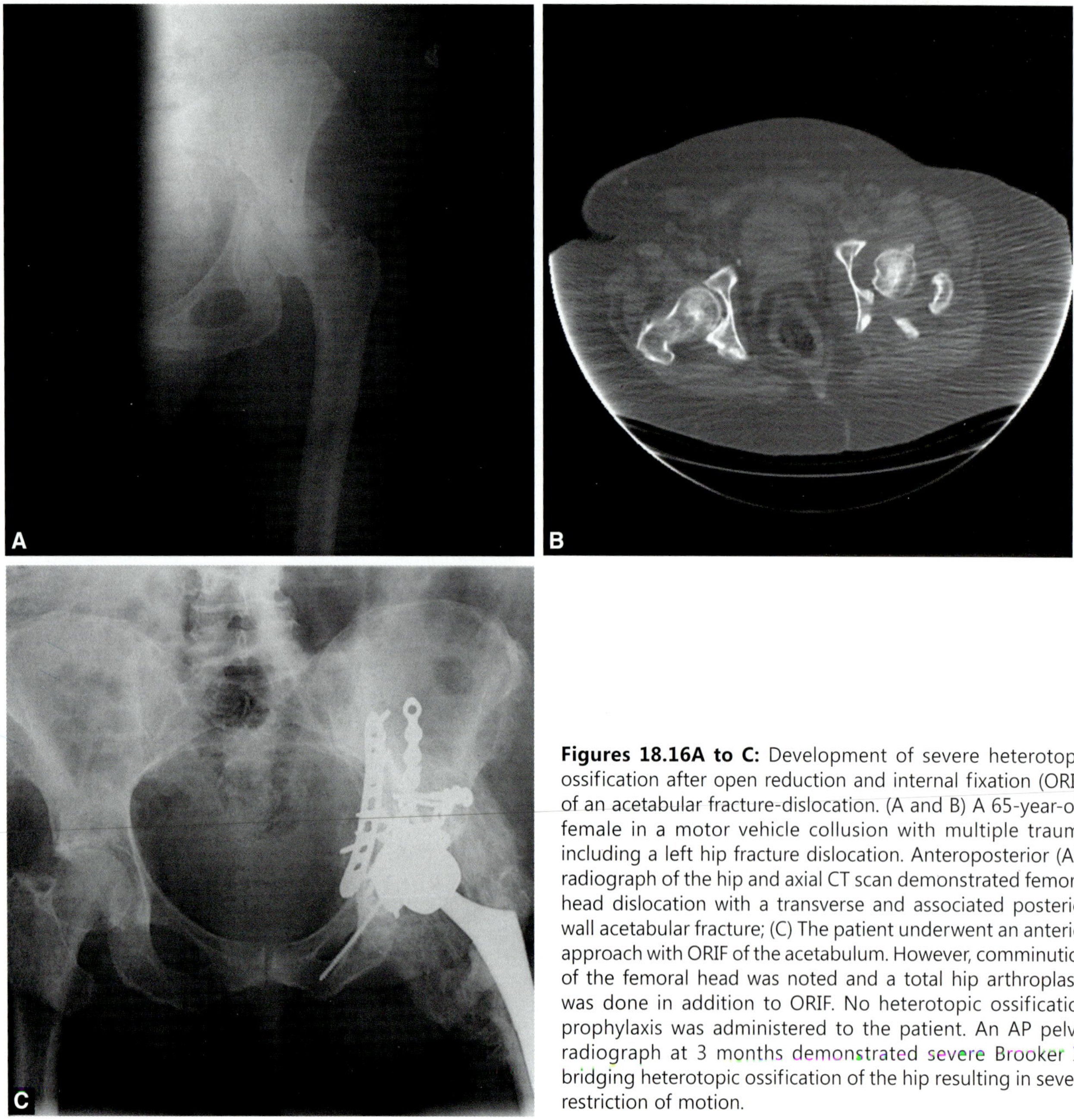

Figures 18.16A to C: Development of severe heterotopic ossification after open reduction and internal fixation (ORIF) of an acetabular fracture-dislocation. (A and B) A 65-year-old female in a motor vehicle collusion with multiple trauma including a left hip fracture dislocation. Anteroposterior (AP) radiograph of the hip and axial CT scan demonstrated femoral head dislocation with a transverse and associated posterior wall acetabular fracture; (C) The patient underwent an anterior approach with ORIF of the acetabulum. However, comminution of the femoral head was noted and a total hip arthroplasty was done in addition to ORIF. No heterotopic ossification prophylaxis was administered to the patient. An AP pelvic radiograph at 3 months demonstrated severe Brooker IV bridging heterotopic ossification of the hip resulting in severe restriction of motion.

Swiontkowski reported 3 of 12 patients who underwent a posterior Kocher-Langenbeck approach developed HO whereas 7 of 12 patients who underwent an anterior Smith-Petersen approach developed HO; these were cases with femoral head fractures.[28] Risk of HO is partly related to the degree of stripping of gluteal muscles from the ilium and can be minimized by appropriate surgical technique. The influence of the trochanteric-flip osteotomy on the development of HO is controversial. Giannoudis et al. demonstrated a trend to a higher incidence of HO after a trochanteric-flip osteotomy exposure in comparison to the posterior one, even there was no compromise to the final functional outcome.[10] Ganz et al. thought it seems to be very unlikely related with the trochanteric-flip osteotomy because there is minimal heterotopic bone formation with the same approach in a nontraumatic setting.[15]

Brain or spinal cord injury is known to systemically induce osteogenesis, therefore being an important risk factor for the development of HO.[24] Systemic factors such as hormones, cytokines and bone morphogenetic proteins have been shown to be involved in regulation of fracture healing as well as the physiological process of bone formation but their role in the development of HO is not clear.[24] Prophylaxis should be considered in patients with an extensile approach, significant muscle trauma, brain or spinal cord injury, a history of HO and delayed treatment. Strategies for prophylaxis include nonsteroidal anti-inflammatory drugs and irradiation. Either indomethacin can be administered in a dosage of 25 mg three times daily or as a single dose of 75 mg per day for 3 weeks. Alternatively, 700 Gy radiation in one dose can be used as prophylaxis. Both methods may be effective in prophylaxis against heterotopic bone formation but might also negatively affect fracture healing. Excision may be a treatment option for symptomatic HO (Figs 18.17A to C). Complications due to excessive blood loss (e.g. hypotension, myocardial infarction, death) are not uncommon after an excision surgery.

Sciatic Nerve Injury

Sciatic nerve palsy occurs in approximately 10–15% of persons with hip dislocation.[3] The peroneal division of the sciatic nerve is most commonly affected because of the anatomy and composition of the peroneal division, as a result of the nerve being stretched over the displaced femoral head. Other less common causes of sciatic injury include acute laceration, compression or encasement in HO.[19] Sciatic nerve injuries are more common with fracture dislocations than after pure dislocations.

Delayed reduction of the dislocation also increases or worses the nerve injury. Hillyard and Fox looked at the incidence of sciatic nerve injury in patients with dislocated hips who were transferred from one facility to another prior to closed reduction.[29] They found that a major nerve injury was much more common (16%) in patients transferred prior to reduction of hip dislocation versus those reduced prior to transfer (4%).

Partial nerve recovery can be expected in more than half of patients, with complete palsies having worse prognosis than partial palsies. Exploration of the nerve is not generally recommended. A longer period of observation may be needed with recalcitrant cases.

Rehabilitation for the nerve injury is important to prevent skin complications and contractures.[3] The mainstays are protective skin barriers and dorsiflexion splints (ankle foot orthosis), with the latter used to maintain the foot in neutral position for a plantigrade foot. If the recovery does not occur, posterior tibial tendon transfers can be performed.

Late sciatic nerve injuries after reduction are due to HO either compressing the nerve or causing it to be stretched.

Retained Loose Bodies

About 2–15% of hip dislocations are irreducible by closed means.[19] The reasons for irreducible dislocation include inadequate sedation, buttonholing through the joint capsule and interposition of muscle or bone fragments. In these patients, an emergent open reduction should be performed. Absolute indications for surgery include irreducible dislocations and nonconcentric reductions. A preoperative CT scan can be extremely beneficial to the surgeon if it can be performed in a timely manner.

Residual Instability

Recurrent hip dislocation following a simple hip dislocation is rare and is reported to occur only 1% of the time.[19]

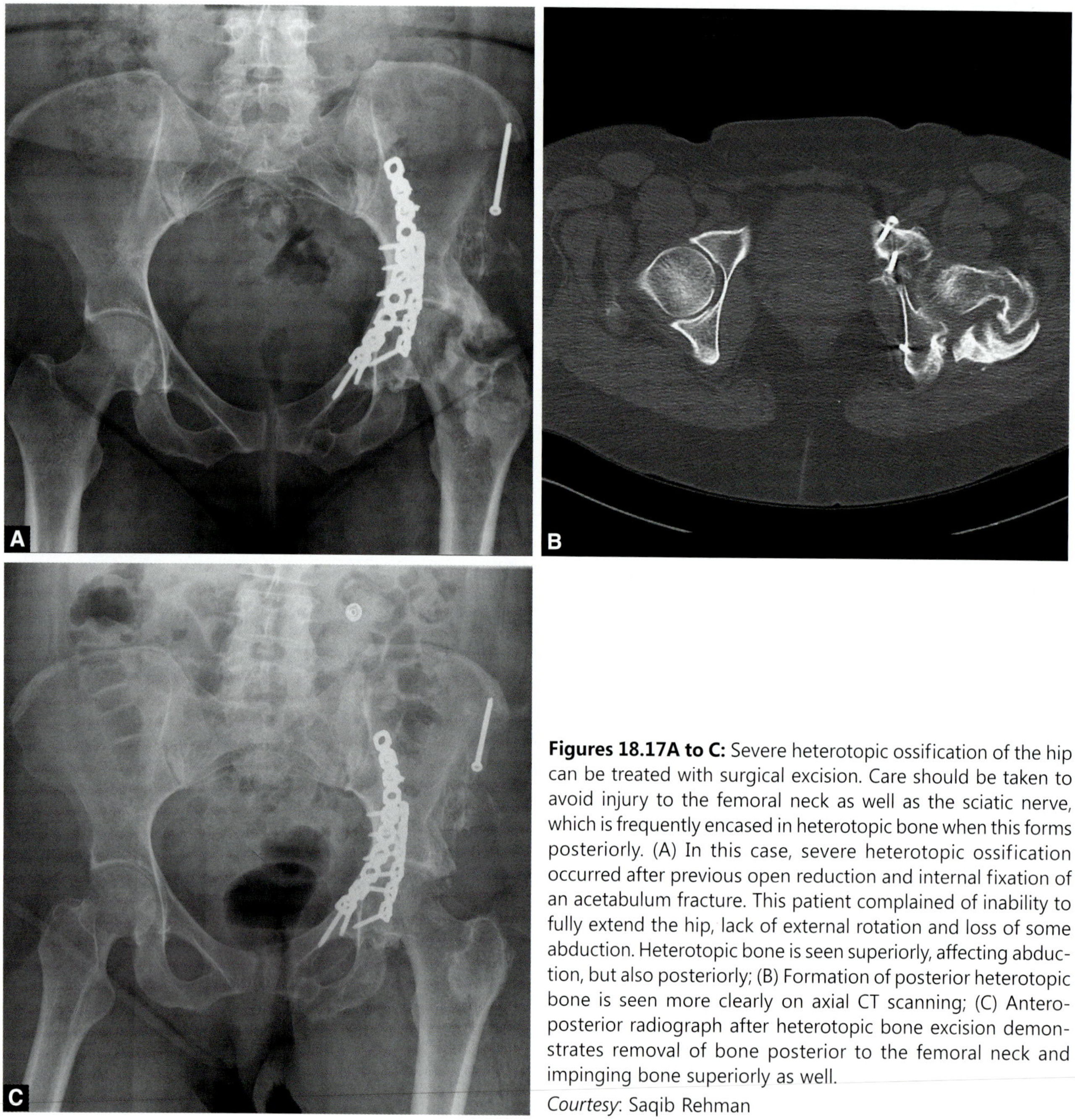

Figures 18.17A to C: Severe heterotopic ossification of the hip can be treated with surgical excision. Care should be taken to avoid injury to the femoral neck as well as the sciatic nerve, which is frequently encased in heterotopic bone when this forms posteriorly. (A) In this case, severe heterotopic ossification occurred after previous open reduction and internal fixation of an acetabulum fracture. This patient complained of inability to fully extend the hip, lack of external rotation and loss of some abduction. Heterotopic bone is seen superiorly, affecting abduction, but also posteriorly; (B) Formation of posterior heterotopic bone is seen more clearly on axial CT scanning; (C) Anteroposterior radiograph after heterotopic bone excision demonstrates removal of bone posterior to the femoral neck and impinging bone superiorly as well.

Courtesy: Saqib Rehman

COMPLICATIONS: Pearls and Pitfalls

- Recognizing these injuries in time, and immediate and anatomic reduction is the key to successful outcome
- Many trauma centers have routine AP pelvis radiography to help recognize potentially missed injuries in the multiply injured patient
- Peroneal and anterior tibialis tendon functions should be tested and monitored for recognition of sciatic nerve injuries

After reduction, Judet views and thin-sliced cut CT should be obtained if acetabular fractures are suspected.

Authors' Preferred Management of Select Complications

Case 1: Management of Osteonecrosis of the Femoral Head

A 49-year-old female sustained motor vehicle collusion (MVC) as an unrestrained driver. She had a left posterior wall fracture dislocation with a Pipkin IV femoral head fracture, a right comminuted proximal femur fracture, multiple rib fractures, a pulmonary contusion and an abdominal injury (Figs 18.18A and B). On the examination, a splenic rupture was diagnosed and emergent splenectomy was performed. The vitals were in normal range so the left hip was reduced in the emergency room under sedation within the next 12 hours after the initial injury. After the reduction the hip appeared unstable under examination so a temporary traction pin was performed during the abdominal surgery (Figs 18.18C and D). On the 5th day of the injury the patient was operated for the left posterior wall fracture or dislocation and the femoral head fracture. Operation was performed through a lateral incision over the greater trochanter with a trochanteric flip osteotomy. Three large cartilaginous femoral head fragments were removed during the surgery and the posterior wall fragment was reduced and fixed by a two hole plate (Fig. 18.18E). She also had an ORIF for the right

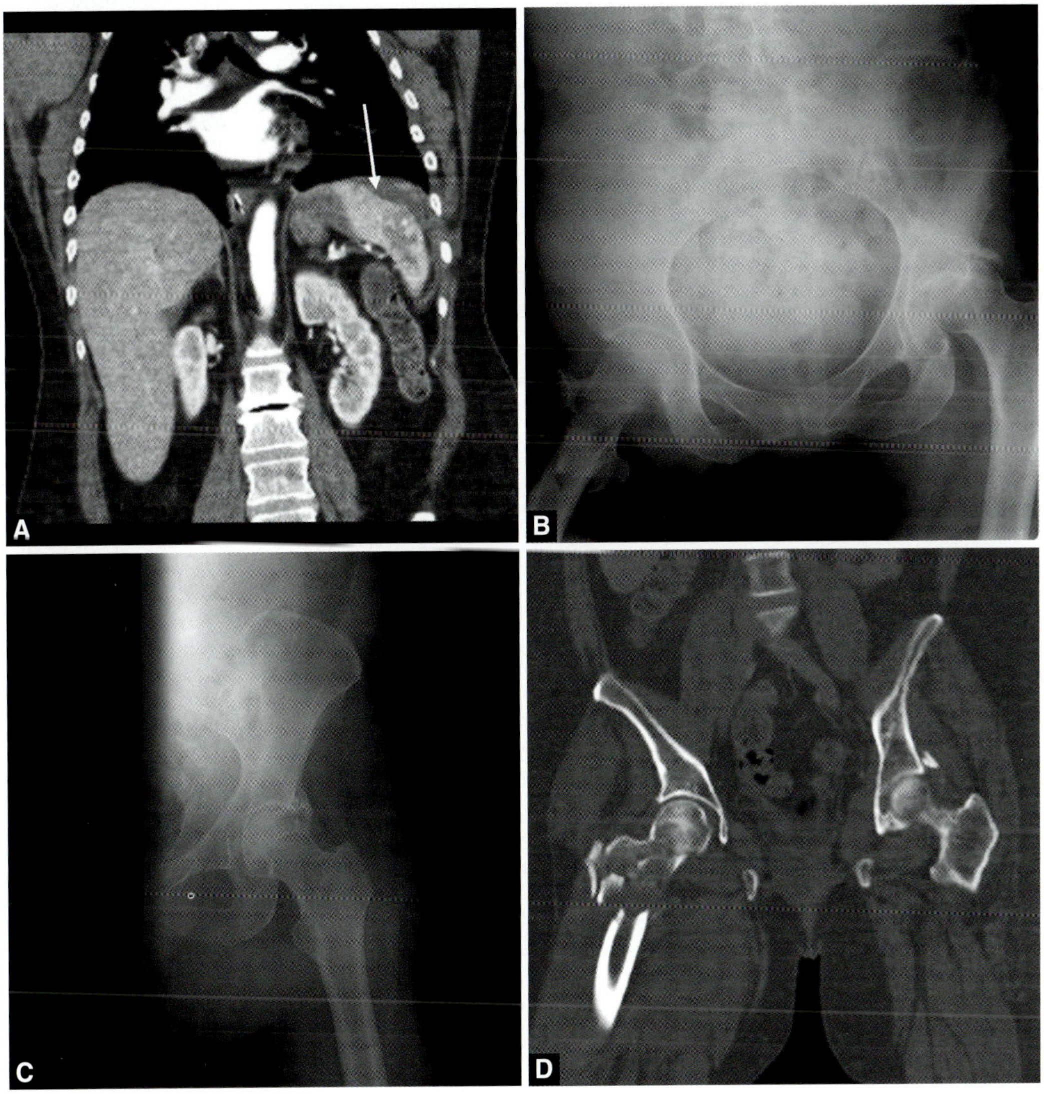

Figures 18.18A to D

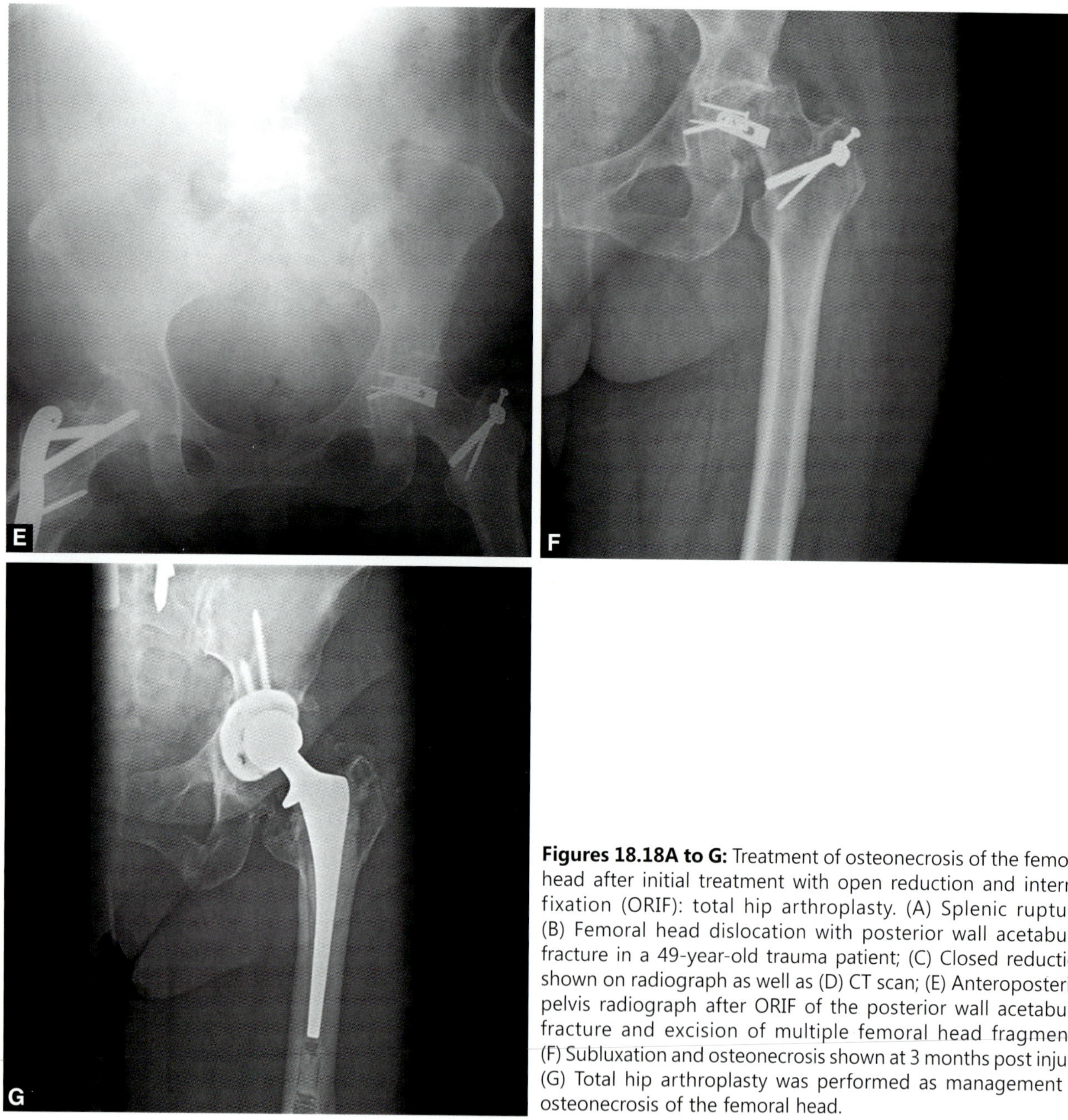

Figures 18.18A to G: Treatment of osteonecrosis of the femoral head after initial treatment with open reduction and internal fixation (ORIF): total hip arthroplasty. (A) Splenic rupture; (B) Femoral head dislocation with posterior wall acetabular fracture in a 49-year-old trauma patient; (C) Closed reduction shown on radiograph as well as (D) CT scan; (E) Anteroposterior pelvis radiograph after ORIF of the posterior wall acetabular fracture and excision of multiple femoral head fragments; (F) Subluxation and osteonecrosis shown at 3 months post injury; (G) Total hip arthroplasty was performed as management of osteonecrosis of the femoral head.

intertrochanteric femur fracture. The patient was ordered to be non weight-bearing for the following 8 weeks. After gradual onset of weight-bearing the patient started having pain on the left hip. Anteroposterior pelvic X-rays were obtained on the third month follow-up and demonstrated osteonecrosis on the left femoral head. A total hip arthroplasty was the choice of management for treating the osteonecrosis with severe arthritic changes (Fig. 18.18F). After 3 years she developed mild HO on the left hip and severe HO on the right hip (Fig. 18.18G).

Case 2: Management of Nonunion and Osteonecrosis after Femoral Head Fracture

A 38-year-old male sustained a fall resulting in a displaced femoral head fracture dislocation of the right hip (Figs 18.19A to C). He was treated with emergent ORIF from a posterior approach. Herbert-Whipple headless screws were used to fix the fragment with a posterior to anterior trajectory as shown in Figures 18.19D and E. A residual gap was noted on the CT scan as shown. The patient was made non-weight-bearing on the hip, however, lost fixation of the femoral head fragment and redislocated 3 weeks later, which was treated with closed reduction only (Figs 18.19F and G). Although his reduction remained stable, progressive loss of fracture reduction as well as subchondral collapse of the remaining femoral head indicated nonunion of the fracture fragment as well as osteonecrosis of the intact portion of the femoral head (Fig. 18.19H). By 15 months after his initial injury, a ceramic-on-ceramic total hip arthroplasty was done for painful osteonecrosis and nonunion of the femoral head (Fig. 18.19I). Despite hesitations due to his relatively young age, nonarthroplasty reconstruction options were deemed unsatisfactory to properly address the pathology. The nonunion in this case was likely due to inadequate compression of the fracture initially and no attempt at refixation after the incident where fixation was lost. The etiology for the osteonecrosis could be due to devascularization of the femoral head during the emergent posterior approach to the hip rather than any sort of delay in the initial reduction (which was done emergently). (Case courtesy of Bruce Vanett, MD)

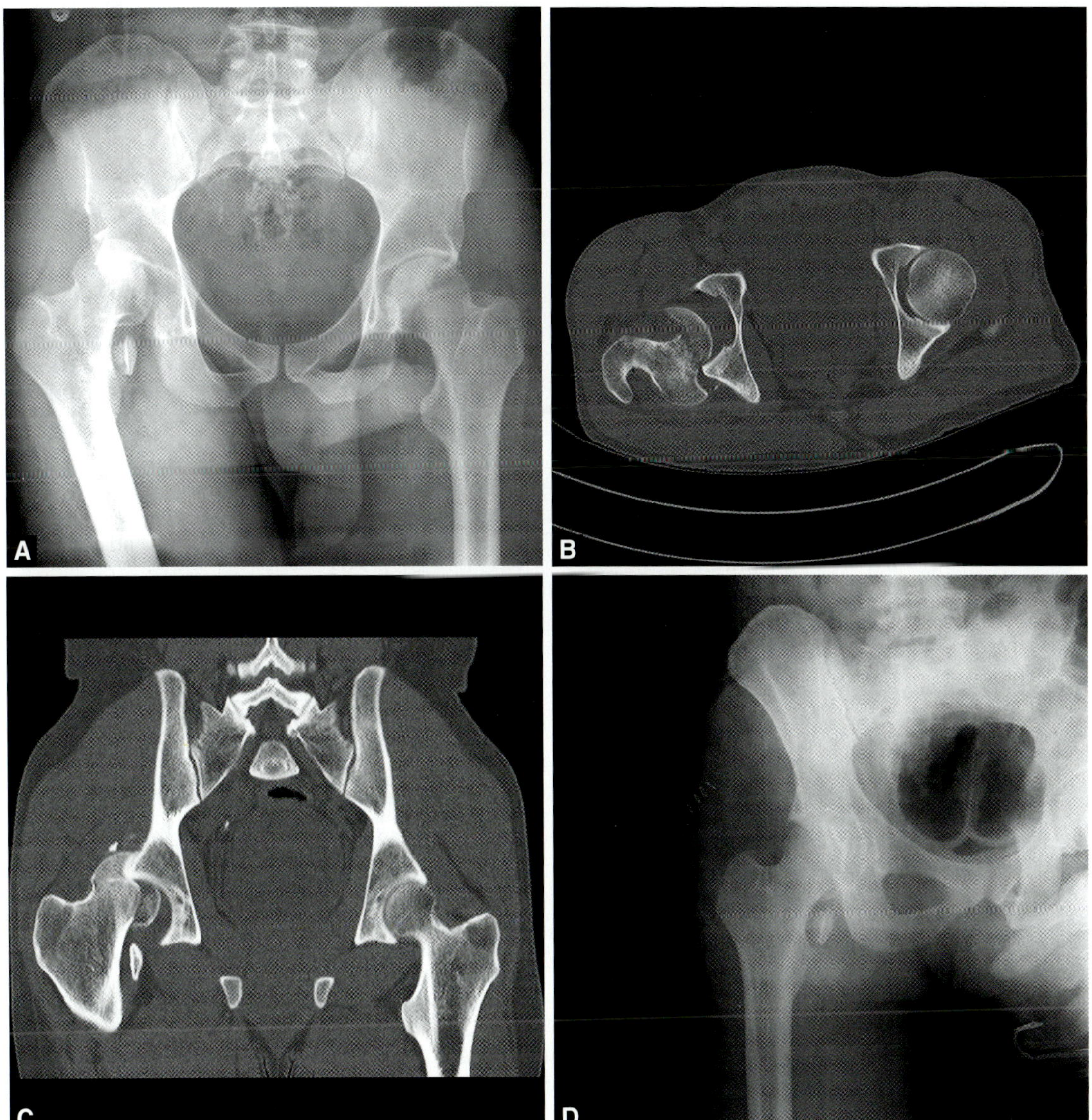

Figures 18.19A to D

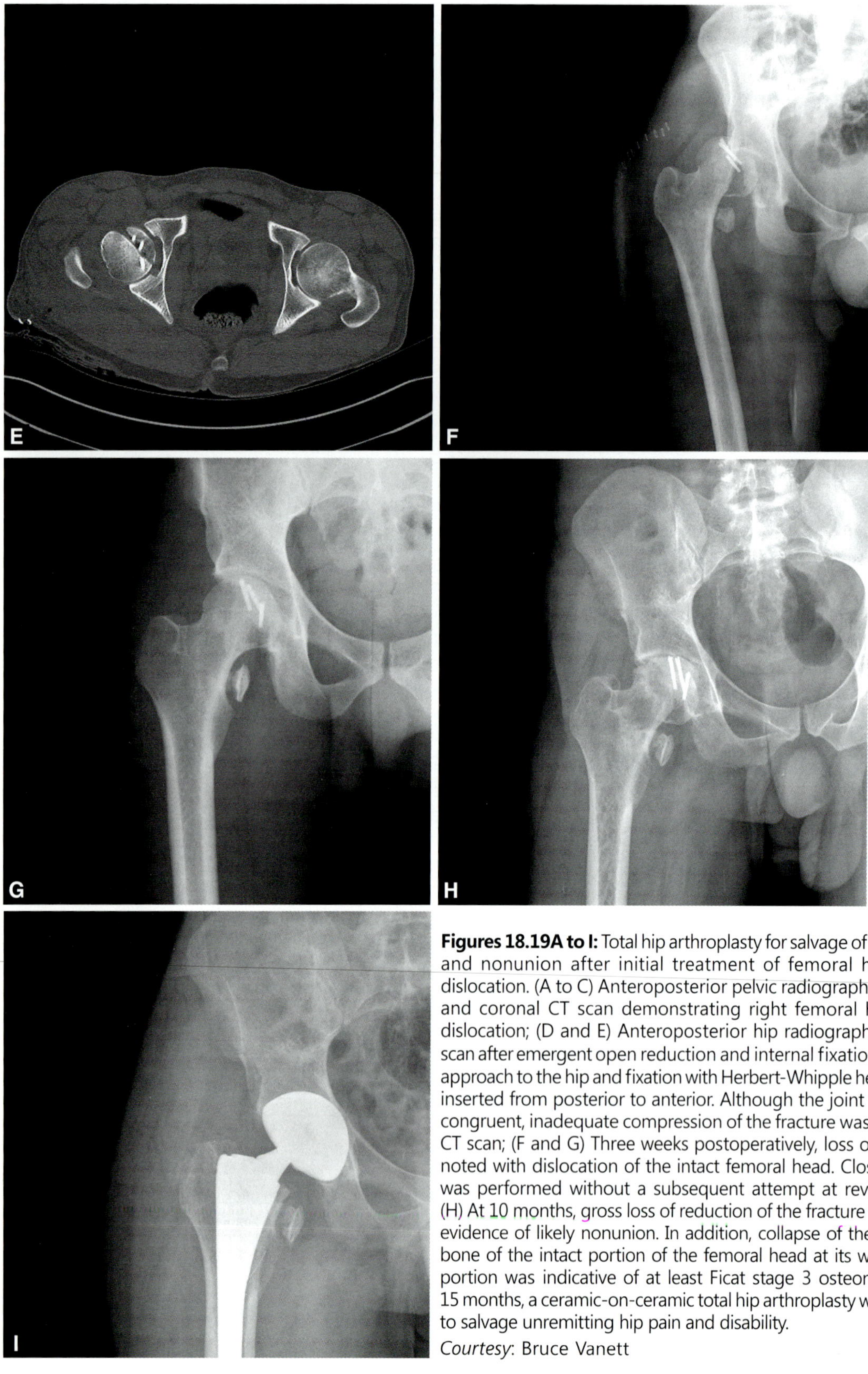

Figures 18.19A to I: Total hip arthroplasty for salvage of osteonecrosis and nonunion after initial treatment of femoral head fracture dislocation. (A to C) Anteroposterior pelvic radiograph, axial CT scan and coronal CT scan demonstrating right femoral head fracture dislocation; (D and E) Anteroposterior hip radiograph and axial CT scan after emergent open reduction and internal fixation via posterior approach to the hip and fixation with Herbert-Whipple headless screws inserted from posterior to anterior. Although the joint was relatively congruent, inadequate compression of the fracture was noted on the CT scan; (F and G) Three weeks postoperatively, loss of fixation was noted with dislocation of the intact femoral head. Closed reduction was performed without a subsequent attempt at revision fixation; (H) At 10 months, gross loss of reduction of the fracture fragment was evidence of likely nonunion. In addition, collapse of the subchondral bone of the intact portion of the femoral head at its weight-bearing portion was indicative of at least Ficat stage 3 osteonecrosis; (I) At 15 months, a ceramic-on-ceramic total hip arthroplasty was performed to salvage unremitting hip pain and disability.

Courtesy: Bruce Vanett

The important principles of this case are the following:

- Adequate compression of the femoral head fracture is important for maintaining stability. In most cases, this can be difficult to achieve from a posterior approach when the fragment is anterior. In this particular case, it did not appear that optimal compression was achieved, perhaps contributing to the loss of fixation, hip instability and eventual nonunion. Consideration for revision ORIF after the redislocation or loss of fixation could have been undertaken given that his eventual outcome was a total hip arthroplasty.
- Osteonecrosis of the femoral head with collapse of the weight-bearing portion of the femoral head in addition to gross incongruity due to nonunion of the anterior femoral head fragment is extremely difficult to salvage without arthroplasty. Arguably, other arthroplasty options can be offered, but a total hip arthroplasty provides a reliable method of achieving painless functional use of the hip. Due to the patient's age, there were clearly concerns for early wear and need for revision surgery.

Summary

Because of the various treatment protocols and approaches used in the literature it is difficult to establish the best approach for a particular hip dislocation. The treating surgeon should be a master in the comprehensive anatomy of the hip and the extraosseous and intraosseous blood supply for the femoral head and all surgical approaches for the hip. A decision to make the right approach should not be based on the direction of the dislocation, solely. In fact, associated femoral neck or head fracture, acetabular wall fracture should help determine the surgical approach chosen. Timely recognition of the injury, reduction of the hip in less than 6 hours, knowledge of the mechanism of injury, precise planning for irreducible dislocations, meticulous surgical technique and preserving the blood supply to the femoral head by not harming the MFCA are mandatory for better results. A recent improvement in arthroscopic techniques has given a tremendous advantage on diagnosis and management of loose bodies in the hip joint. No matter the most convenient management is applied in a timely manner, hip dislocations and femoral head fractures are caused by high energy mechanisms and excellent or good results do not exceed 50%. Therefore, surgeons should warn the patients for possible complications and bad results. Total hip arthroplasty should be kept as an alternative for elderly patients with a comminuted head fracture who have had a delayed reduction or who already have cartilage degeneration on the hip joint.

References

1. Arvidsson I. The hip joint: forces needed for distraction and appearance of the vacuum phenomenon. Scand J Rehabil Med. 1990;22(3):157-61.
2. Brooks RA, Ribbans WJ. Diagnosis and imaging studies of traumatic hip dislocations in the adult. Clin Orthop Relat Res. 2000;377:15-23.
3. Foulk DM, Mullis BH. Hip dislocation: evaluation and management. J Am Acad Orthop Surg. 2010;18(4):199-209.
4. Asghar FA, Karunakar MA. Femoral head fractures: diagnosis, management, and complications. Orthop Clin North Am. 2004;35(4):463-72.
5. Sahin V, Karakas ES, Aksu S, et al. Traumatic dislocation and fracture-dislocation of the hip: a long-term follow-up study. J Trauma. 2003;54(3):520-9.
6. Mehta S, Routt ML. Irreducible fracture-dislocations of the femoral head without posterior wall acetabular fractures. J Orthop Trauma. 2008;22(10):686-92.
7. Kloen P, Siebenrock KA, Raaymakers E, et al. Femoral head fractures revisited. Euro J Trauma. 2002;28(4):221-33.
8. Thompson VP, Epstein HC. Traumatic dislocation of the hip: a survey of two hundred and four cases covering a period of twenty-one year. J Bone Joint Surg Am. 1951;33(3): 746-78.
9. Stewart MJ, Milford LW. Fracture-dislocation of the hip; an end-result study. J Bone Joint Surg Am. 1954;36(2):315-42.
10. Giannoudis P, Kontakis G, Christoforakis Z, et al. Management, complications and clinical results of femoral head fractures. Injury. 2009;40(12):1245-51.
11. Pipkin G. Treatment of grade IV fracture-dislocation of the hip. J Bone Joint Surg Am. 1957;39(11):1027-42.
12. Seldes RM, Tan V, Hunt J, et al. Anatomy, histologic features, and vascularity of the adult acetabular labrum. Clin Orthop Relat Res. 2001;382:232-40.
13. Droll KP, Broekhuyse H, O'Brien P. Fracture of the femoral head. J Am Acad Orthop Surg. 2007;15(12):716-27.
14. Gautier E, Ganz K, Krugel N, et al. Anatomy of the medial femoral circumflex artery and its surgical implications. J Bone Joint Surg Br. 2000;82(5):679-83.
15. Ganz R, Gill T, Gautier E, et al. Surgical dislocation of the adult hip: a technique with full access to the femoral head

and acetabulum without the risk of avascular necrosis. J Bone Joint Surg Br. 2001;83(8):1119-24.

16. Petsatodis G, Antonarakos P, Chalidis B, et al. Surgically treated acetabular fractures via a single posterior approach with a follow-up of 2-10 years. Injury. 2007;38(3):334-43.
17. Giannoudis P, Grotz M, Papakostidis C, et al. Operative treatment of displaced fractures of the acetabulum: A meta-analysis. J Bone Joint Surg Br. 2005;87(1):2-9.
18. Solberg BD, Moon CN, Franco DP. Use of a trochanteric flip osteotomy improves outcomes in pipkin IV fractures. Clinical Orthop Relat Res. 2009;467(4):929-33.
19. Clegg TE, Roberts CS, Greene JW, et al. Hip dislocations—epidemiology, treatment, and outcomes. Injury. 2010; 41(4):329-34.
20. Dreinhofer K, Schwarzkopf SR, Haas N, et al. Isolated traumatic dislocation of the hip. Long-term results in 50 patients. J Bone Joint Surg Br. 1994;76(1):6-12.
21. Upadhyay S, Moulton A. The long-term results of traumatic posterior dislocation of the hip. J Bone Joint Surg Br. 1981;63(4):548-51.
22. Upadhyay S, Moulton A, Srikrishnamurthy K. An analysis of the late effects of traumatic posterior dislocation of the hip without fractures. J Bone Joint Surg Br. 1983;65(2): 150-2.
23. Hougaard K, Thomsen PB. Coxarthrosis following traumatic posterior dislocation of the hip. J Bone Joint Surg Br. 1987;69(5):679-83.
24. Henle P, Kloen P, Siebenrock KA. Femoral head injuries: which treatment strategy can be recommended? Injury. 2007;38(4):478-88.
25. Yue JJ, Wilber JH, Lipuma JP, et al. Posterior hip dislocations: a cadaveric angiographic study. J Orthop Trauma. 1996; 10(7):447-54.
26. Brav EA. Traumatic dislocation of the hip: army experience and results over a twelve-year period. J Bone Joint Surg Br. 1962;44(6):1115.
27. Cash DJ, Nolan JF. Avascular necrosis of the femoral head 8 years after posterior hip dislocation. Injury. 2007;38(7): 865-7.
28. Swiontkowski MF, Thorpe M, Seiler JG, et al. Operative management of displaced femoral head fractures: case-matched comparison of anterior versus posterior approaches for pipkin I and pipkin II fractures. J Orthop Trauma. 1992;6(4):437-42.
29. Hillyard RF, Fox J. Sciatic nerve injuries associated with traumatic posterior hip dislocations. Am J Emerg Med. 2003;21(7):545-8.

Chapter **19**

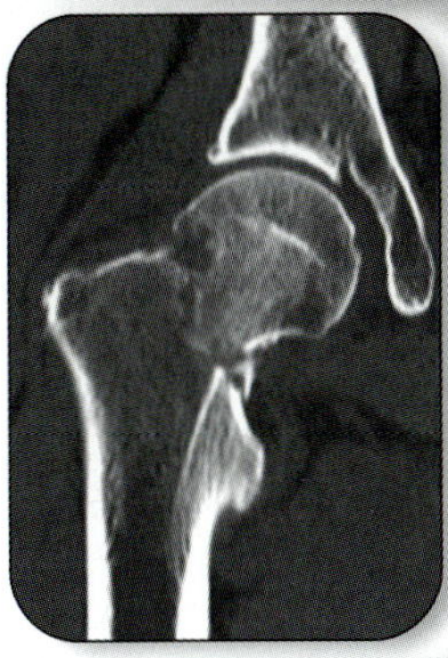

Femoral Neck Fractures

Christopher Haydel, Saqib Rehman

Chapter Outline

Introduction
Diagnosis
Classification
Surgical Indications
Surgical Anatomy, Positioning and Approaches
Surgical Techniques
- Technique 1: Closed Reduction and Cannulated Screw Fixation of Femoral Neck Fractures
- Technique 2: ORIF of Displaced Femoral Neck Fracture
- Technique 3: Hemiarthroplasty of Femoral Neck Fracture

Outcomes
Complications
Authors' Preferred Management of Select Complications
- Case 1: Displaced Femoral Neck Fracture with Nonunion Treated with Total Hip Arthroplasty
- Cases 2 and 3: Treatment of Femoral Neck Nonunion with Valgus Osteotomy and Angled Blade Plate Fixation
- Case 4: Treatment of a Subtrochanteric Femur Fracture as a Complication of Femoral Neck Pinning
- Case 5: Loss of Fixation of Femoral Neck Fracture Treated with Screws, Revised with Sliding Hip Screw

Summary

Introduction

Femoral neck fractures continue to challenge the US health care system. The number of displaced femoral neck fractures in the US annually is 250,000 and the annual health care expenditures are expected to exceed $15 billion.[1] The distribution of femoral neck fractures has a bimodal age distribution. In younger patients, these fractures, which only account for 2–3%,[2] are the result of high-energy trauma such as motor vehicle collisions. Young patients have great bone quality, high levels of activity and minimal, if any, comorbidities. In contrast, the elderly sustain femoral neck fractures after a simple fall from standing height because of poor bone quality, multiple medical problems and gait disturbances. Fractures in this age group carry a 1-year mortality rate of 36%[2] and are most common in Caucasian women.[3]

Documentation of femoral neck fractures dates back to the 14th century.[4] Upon examination of the remains of Charles IV, the King of Bohemia and Roman Emperor, he was noted to have a left transcervical femoral neck fracture with posterior cortical comminution and a near vertical fracture line. The first classification system of femoral neck fractures was published in 1819 by Sir Astley Paton Cooper, which grouped the fractures into intracapsular or extracapsular.[5] This was shortly after the publication of the first study on femoral neck fractures in 1818 by Abraham Colles, which described a peritrochanteric fracture line and a nonunion of the femoral neck.[5] A few years later, in the 1850s, Bernhard Rudolf Konrad von Langenbeck was the first to attempt percutaneous internal fixation of an extra-articular femoral neck fracture nonunion.[5] Unfortunately, the patient developed an infection and died. However in 1875, Franz König was the first to successfully treat a young patient with a femoral neck fracture with a percutaneous gimlet under aseptic conditions.[5] Also during this time period, while working with cadavers, Friedrich Trendelenburg developed a technique of internal fixation of intracapsular neck fractures with an ivory peg, ivory screw or silver screw.[5] Finally in 1925, Marius Nygaard Smith-Petersen, Cave and Van Gordor used a flanged nail that gained worldwide acceptance and marked the beginning of a new era.[5]

Despite the diligent efforts of orthopedic surgeons, the complications of femoral neck fractures continue to arise. The most notable are nonunion of the fracture and osteonecrosis of the femoral head.[6] These complications can be devastating, especially in a young active patient. Salvage procedures that preserve the femoral head are technically demanding and sometimes carry a high failure rate, and arthroplasty is not ideal in chronologically young patients with high activity levels.[6] Surgical treatment of femoral neck fractures is usually performed with closed or open reduction and internal fixation with cannulated screws or a sliding hip screw device in the chronologically and physiologically young or arthroplasty in the less active and elderly patients. Although the complications are multifactorial, when performing internal fixation of these fractures, the surgeon must scrutinize the fracture reduction and position of hardware to ensure a biomechanically stable construct to improve union rates and hopefully avoid avascular necrosis (AVN).

Diagnosis

A thorough history is necessary in all patients with a suspected femoral neck fracture. Often, young and elderly patients present in the emergency department after a specific traumatic event that has resulted in groin pain and the inability to ambulate. Elderly patients may report hearing a crack just before falling.[6] Remember that young patients sustain femoral neck fractures as the result of a high-energy impact and may present unconscious or with concomitant injuries that act as pain distractors. Also it is very important to remember that patients with very active lifestyles, such as runners or soldiers in basic training, may present without history of trauma, ambulating without pain and report pain only during physically strenuous activity. These findings raise a high level of suspicion for a stress fracture.

Physical exam findings include a shortened, flexed and externally rotated lower extremity. This position usually is the most comfortable for the patient because the capsule is relaxed and the intracapsular pressure is the lowest.[6] This position is also the result of the displacement of the fracture as the distal fragment is pulled cranially causing varus and apex anterior angulation. In the conscious patient, log rolling the extremity and placing an axial load on the heel or knee will cause discomfort. This skin must be inspected for ecchymosis, abrasions or lacerations. Motor function, sensation and distal pulses also must be documented. In the polytrauma patient, a full secondary survey must be performed because of the high rate of associated injuries.[6]

Diagnostic imaging begins with plain radiographs that include an anteroposterior (AP) view of the pelvis, AP and lateral films of the affected hip as well as the entire femur (Figs 19.1A to C). It is important to internally rotate the affected hip approximately 15° to accurately view the femoral neck on the AP film. This will allow the observer to describe the location, inclination and coronal displacement of the fracture. A cross-table lateral will reveal posterior cortical comminution and sagittal plane displacement. Frog leg lateral films are avoided because they cause discomfort and more importantly can displace the fracture fragments. Computed tomography (CT) will better define bony pathology that is not easily seen on plain film (Figs 19.2A to C). This has proven to be very helpful in revealing nondisplaced femoral neck fractures in polytrauma patients with ipsilateral femur fractures. Tornetta et al. found that nondisplaced femoral neck fractures are present in 1–9% and missed in 20–50% of patients with an ipsilateral femoral shaft fracture.[7] Using a protocol including an internal rotation AP plain film, 2 mm fine cut CT scan, intraoperative fluoroscopy and postoperative AP and lateral films, before the patient was awakened, significantly improved the detection of femoral neck fractures (Figs 19.3A to C). Magnetic resonance imaging (MRI) is especially useful in detecting stress fractures with increased signal intensity representing edema from a fracture in the femoral neck (Fig. 19.4).

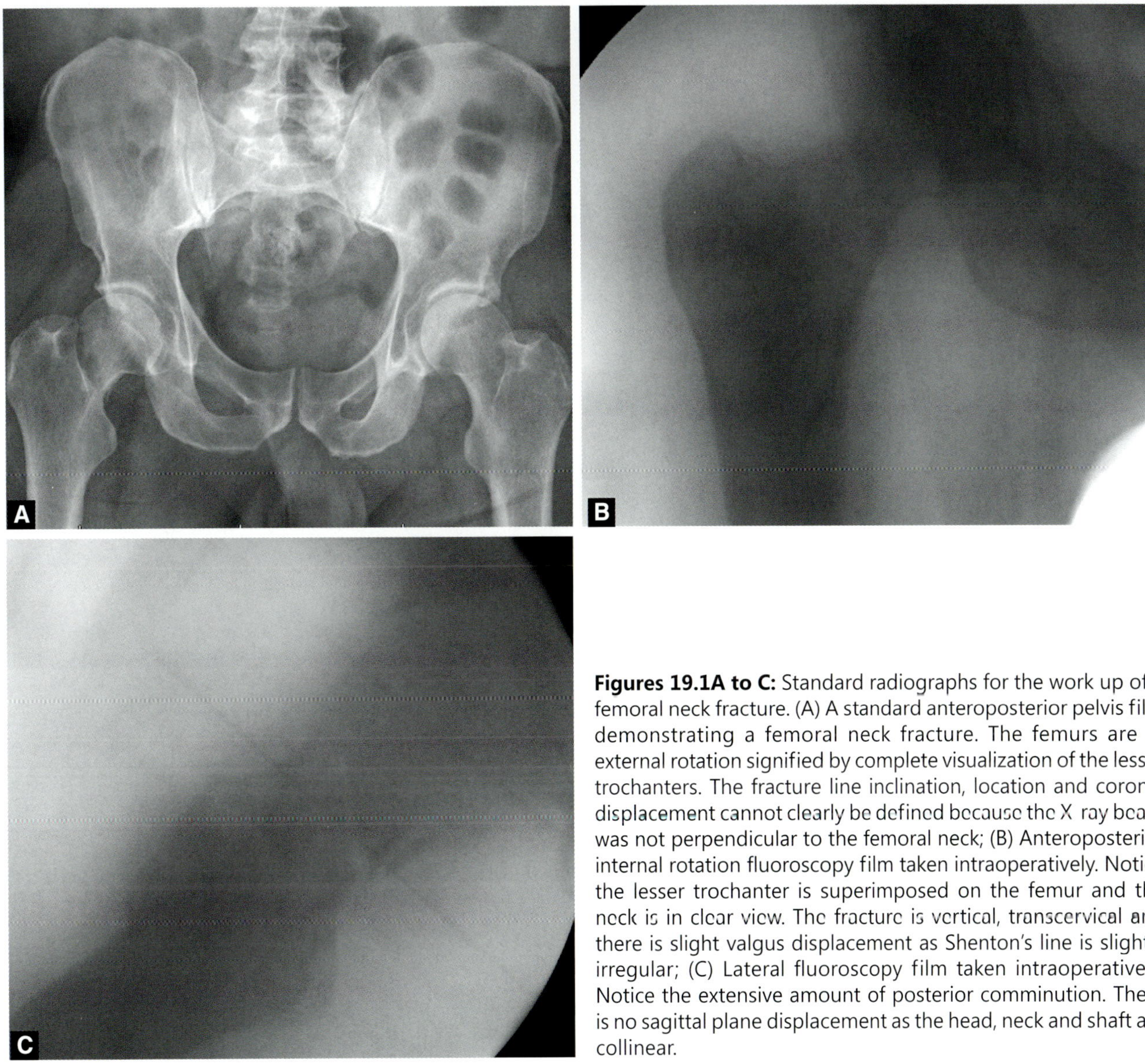

Figures 19.1A to C: Standard radiographs for the work up of a femoral neck fracture. (A) A standard anteroposterior pelvis film demonstrating a femoral neck fracture. The femurs are in external rotation signified by complete visualization of the lesser trochanters. The fracture line inclination, location and coronal displacement cannot clearly be defined because the X ray beam was not perpendicular to the femoral neck; (B) Anteroposterior internal rotation fluoroscopy film taken intraoperatively. Notice the lesser trochanter is superimposed on the femur and the neck is in clear view. The fracture is vertical, transcervical and there is slight valgus displacement as Shenton's line is slightly irregular; (C) Lateral fluoroscopy film taken intraoperatively. Notice the extensive amount of posterior comminution. There is no sagittal plane displacement as the head, neck and shaft are collinear.

FEMORAL NECK FRACTURES DIAGNOSIS:
Pearls and Pitfalls

- In polytrauma patients, be suspicious of a non-displaced femoral neck fracture with ipsilateral femoral shaft fracture
- 2 mm fine cut CT scan can identify nondisplaced femoral neck fractures
- Obtain an MRI when a stress fracture is suspected

Classification

The most comprehensive classification for fractures of the femoral neck was designed by the Orthopaedic Trauma Association (OTA) and the Swiss Association for the Study of Internal Fixation (AO/ASIF) (Fig. 19.5). This classification is based on the fracture fragment configuration on AP and lateral plain radiographs.[8] These fractures are denoted as 31B. The number 3 identifies the femur, the number 1

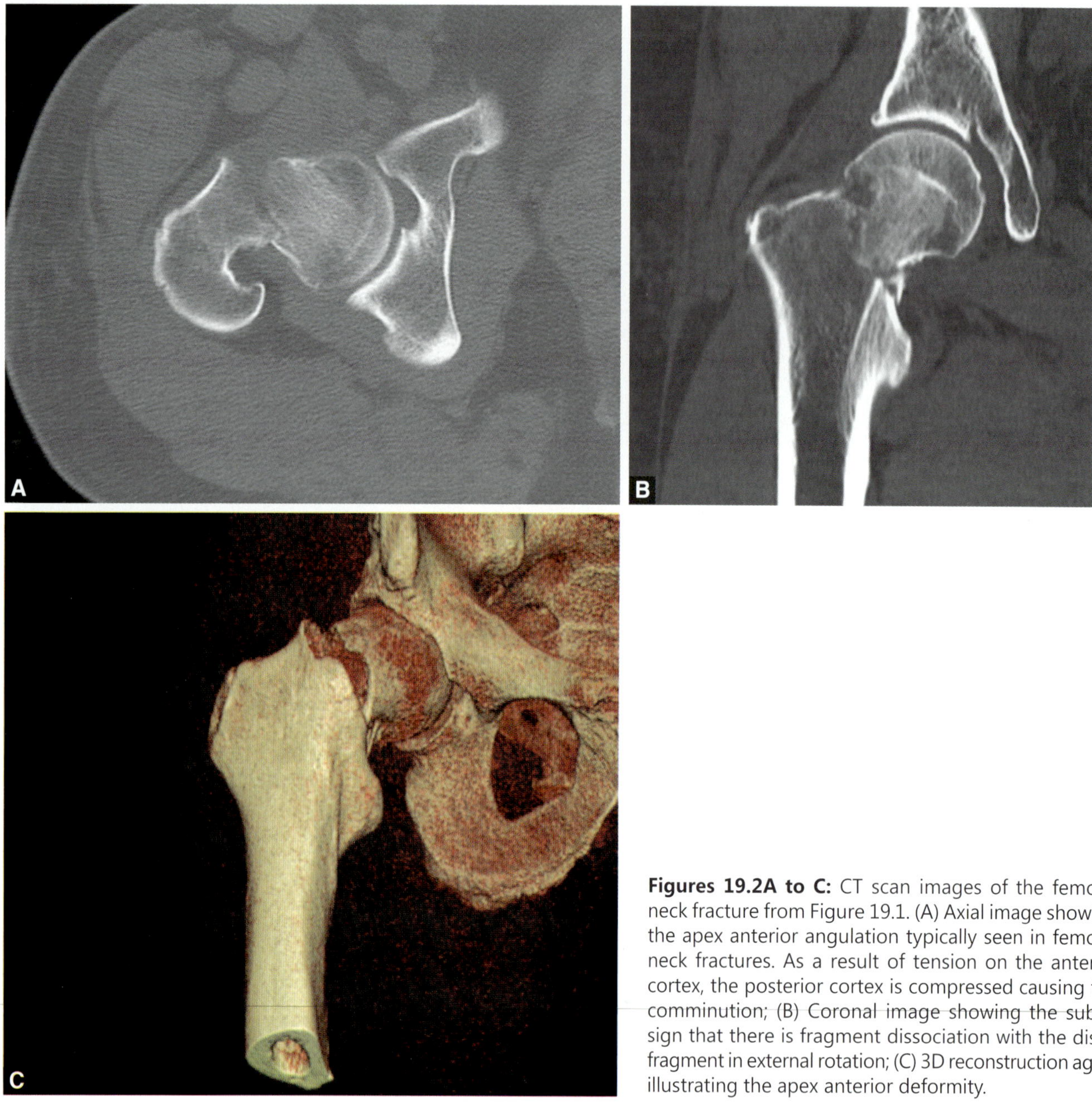

Figures 19.2A to C: CT scan images of the femoral neck fracture from Figure 19.1. (A) Axial image showing the apex anterior angulation typically seen in femoral neck fractures. As a result of tension on the anterior cortex, the posterior cortex is compressed causing the comminution; (B) Coronal image showing the subtle sign that there is fragment dissociation with the distal fragment in external rotation; (C) 3D reconstruction again illustrating the apex anterior deformity.

identifies the proximal end, and letter B identifies the neck. The fractures are further divided into subgroups by adding a 1, 2 or 3. Subgroup 1 includes minimally displaced subcapital fractures, subgroup 2 includes basicervical and transcervical fractures, and subgroup 3 includes displaced subcapital fractures. The subgroups are further divided adding a 1, 2 or 3, which define the amount or type of displacement. This fracture classification has low intraobserver and interobserver reliability using all of the subgroups, but reliability significantly improves when the fractures are grouped into nondisplaced and displaced.[9]

The Garden Classification (Fig. 19.6) is more commonly used to describe femoral neck fractures in elderly population.[6] This fracture classification includes four types.[8] Type I is an incomplete fracture in which the distal fragment is externally rotated and the proximal fragment is in valgus and impacted. Type II is a complete fracture without displacement. Type III is a complete fracture that is

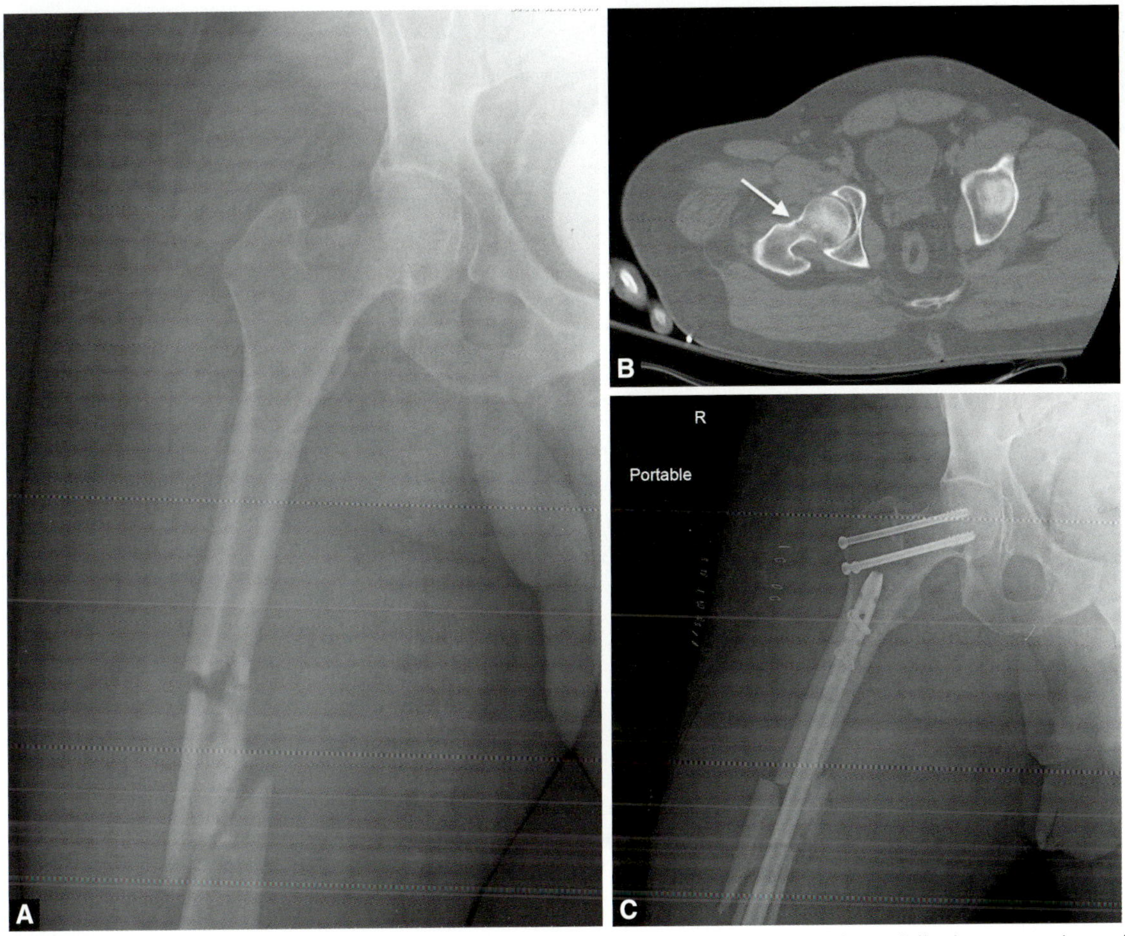

Figures 19.3A to C: Treatment of femoral neck/shaft fractures. (A) Anteroposterior radiograph partially demonstrating a displaced femoral shaft fracture in a 45-year-old man in a motorcycle crash. There is no obvious fracture of the femoral neck noted; (B) CT scan of the abdomen and pelvis demonstrates a nondisplaced femoral neck fracture as shown with the arrow; (C) This was treated with cannulated screw fixation of the femoral neck followed by retrograde intramedullary nailing of the femoral shaft.

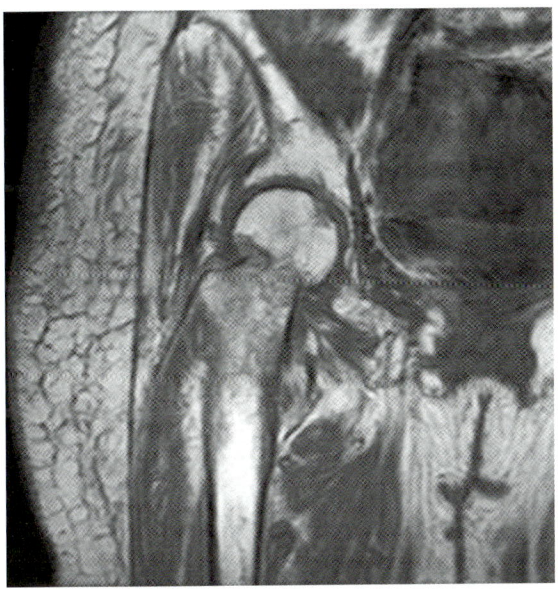

Figure 19.4: T1-weighted MRI image demonstrating a minimally displaced femoral neck fracture.

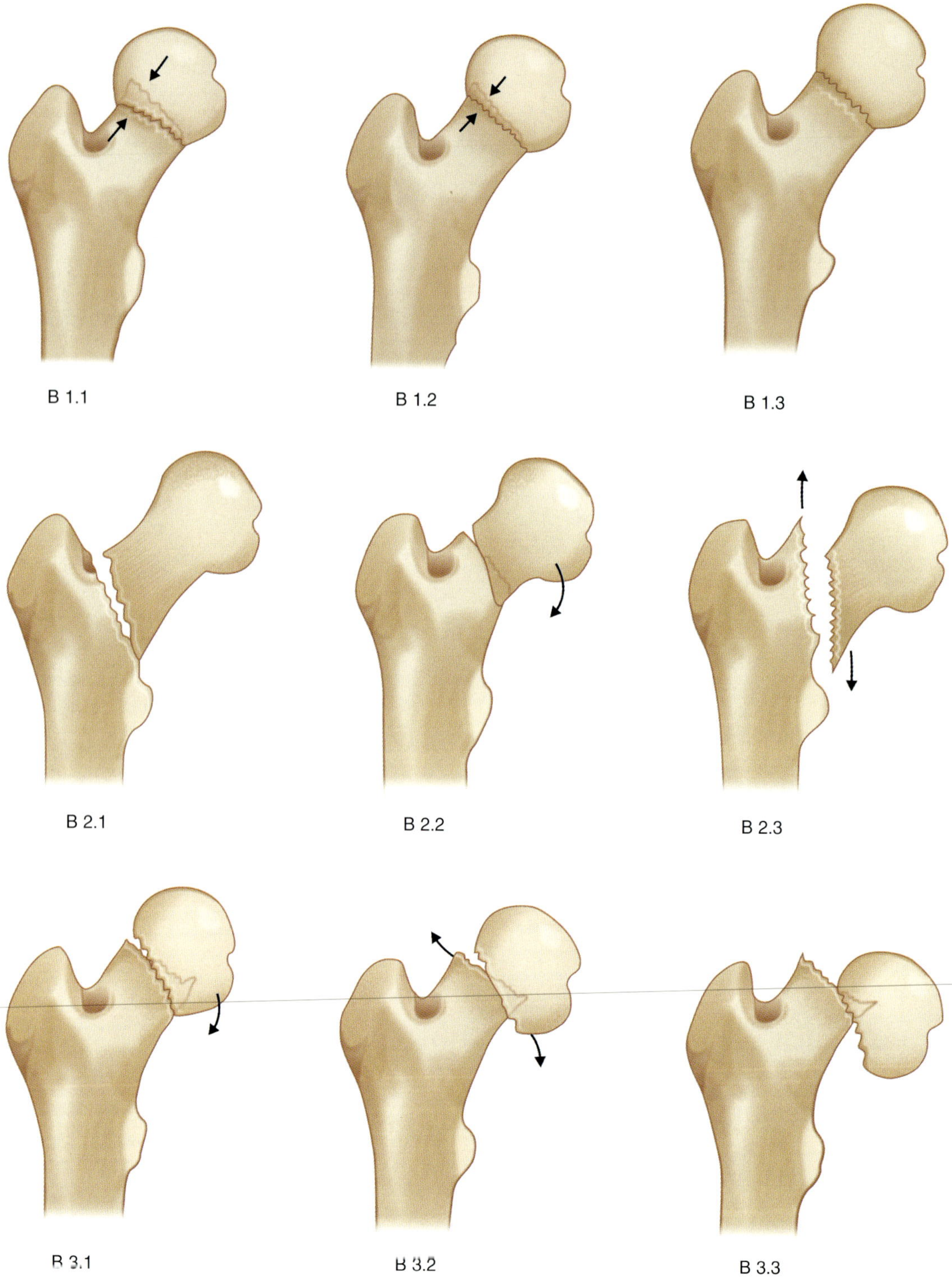

Figure 19.5: The AO/OTA classification of femoral neck fractures.

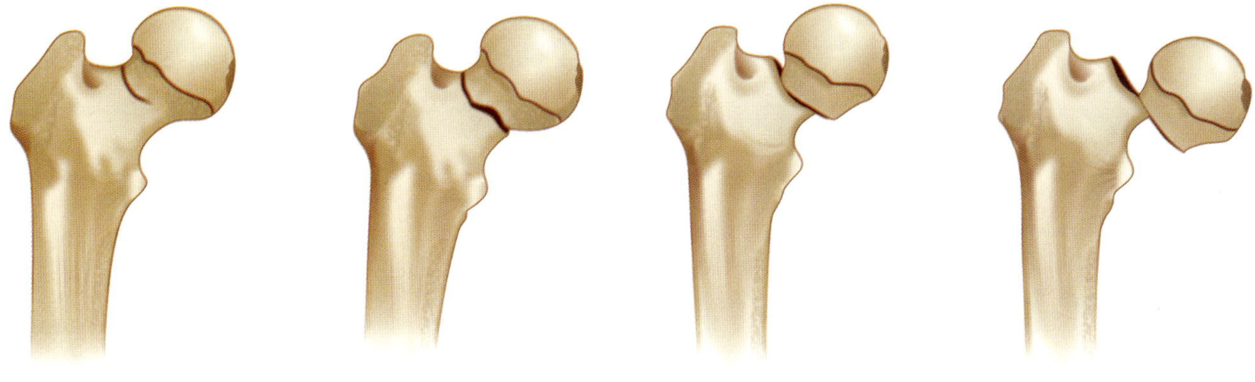

Figure 19.6: The Garden Classification for femoral neck fractures. Type I fractures are incomplete and valgus impacted. Type II fractures are complete and nondisplaced. Type III fractures are complete, less than 50% displaced, and in varus. Type IV fractures are complete, greater than 50% displaced, and complete dissociation between fracture fragments.

displaced less than 50% in which the distal fragment is in external rotation and the proximal fragment is in varus and rotated medially. The trabecular lines in the femoral head are not in line with the trabecular lines in the pelvis signifying that the fracture fragments are still moving as a unit. Type IV is a complete fracture with greater than 50% displacement. The trabecular lines in the femoral head are in line with trabecular lines in the pelvis signifying complete dissociation of the fragments. Despite being used quite frequently,[10] numerous studies have shown that there is low interobserver reliability when using all four types.[10-15] These studies have consistently shown that the interobserver reliability significantly increases when the fractures are classified as nondisplaced (types I and II) and displaced (types III and IV).

In the younger population, the Pauwels classification (Fig. 19.7) is used to quantify the degree of inclination of the fracture line.[8] Type I fractures have a fracture line that is oriented less than 30° from the horizontal. Type II is between 30° and 70°. Type III is greater than 70°. The premise behind this classification is that as the fracture line inclination increases, the forces across the fracture line are converted from compressive to shearing. Unfortunately there is also low interobserver reliability between the fracture types mainly because inclination of the fracture line changes with rotation of femur.[16] There is also evidence that the Pauwels classification does not correlate with union rates, but can be a predictor of future displacement with nonoperative treatment.[17]

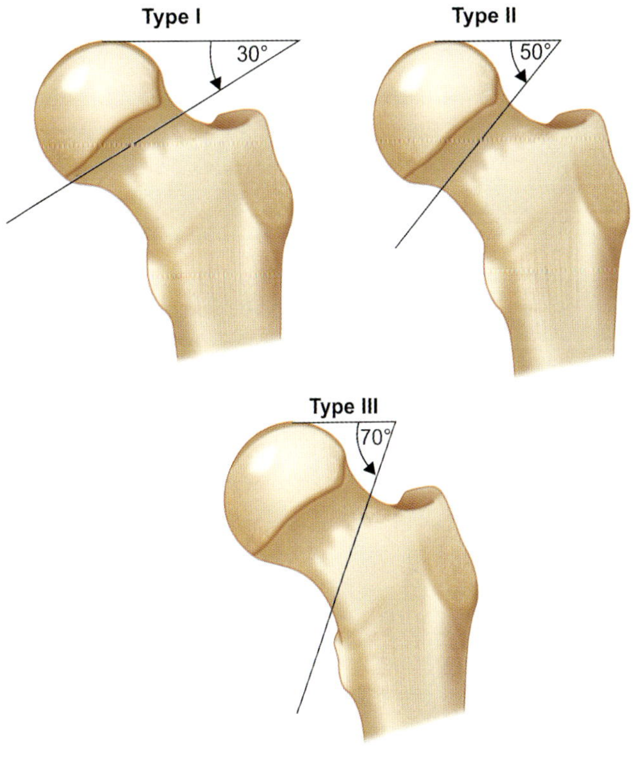

Figure 19.7: The Pauwels classification for femoral neck fractures. The fracture line inclination increases as the classification progresses from I to III. The forces across the fracture site are converted from compressive in Type I to shearing in Type III.

Surgical Indications

The surgical procedures to treat femoral neck fractures vary widely because of the bimodal age distribution. In general, young patients are less than 60-year-old and elderly patients are greater than 60-year-old. However, there is a group of patients that may be chronologically characterized as elderly because they are between the ages of 60 years and 80 years, but can also be physiologically characterized as young because they are active, have minimal comorbidities, and have good bone quality. We will call this group the "physiologically young" elderly population. For this particular group of patients, the indications for specific procedures may become ambiguous as reflected in a survey of 442 orthopedic surgeons in 2005 concerning patients in the age range of 60–80 years old in which there was no consensus on type of treatment or implant used.[18]

All femoral neck fractures should be considered for operative fixation. Please note that basicervical femoral neck fractures are treated like intertrochanteric femur fractures as described in chapter 20. The indications for nonoperative treatment of femoral neck fractures are limited to patients who are medically unfit for any type of anesthesia and patients who are nonambulators and have adequate pain control. Studies have shown that nonoperative management of nondisplaced femoral neck fractures has led to a 41–46% operation rate for secondary displacement.[19,20] The goals in young patients are to achieve union and preserve the femoral head, avoiding osteonecrosis, thus internal fixation is the procedure of choice for displaced as well as nondisplaced fractures. Anatomic reduction and stable fixation are the most important surgeon controlled factors.[6] This typically requires an open reduction in order to ascertain that an anatomic reduction has been achieved. In the "physiologically young" elderly patients, the goals are to restore the preoperative level of function and avoid complications associated with prolonged bed rest, such as deep vein thrombosis, pressure ulcers and pneumonia. For nondisplaced fractures, internal fixation is the best choice. For displaced fractures, arthroplasty is the best choice. Studies have shown that patients over the age of 60–70 years have reoperation rates between 22.6% and 47% for those who underwent internal fixation compared with 2.9–9% who underwent arthroplasty.[21-23] To further divide the arthroplasty group, it is generally accepted that the "physiologically young" elderly patients and patients with rheumatoid arthritis will undergo total hip arthroplasty, and those who are elderly or have cognitive impairment or neurological disorders will undergo hemiarthroplasty. It is very important to remember that medical optimization before surgery is critical to reduce complication rate and lower hospital costs.[24,25]

Surgical Anatomy, Positioning and Approaches

Understanding the skeletal and soft tissue anatomy is vital for treating femoral neck fractures (Figs 19.8A and B). Normally the neck-shaft angle is 130±7° and the femoral neck anteversion is 10.4±6.7°.[3] The intertrochanteric line separates the anterior surface of the neck from the femoral shaft, and intertrochanteric crest traverses the two trochanters posteriorly.[3] The greater trochanter is approximately 2 mm below the femoral head, and a horizontal line drawn between the superior border of the greater trochanters should pass through the center of the femoral head.[3]

The blood supply to the femoral head (Figs 19.9A and B) comes from three arteries: the medial and lateral femoral circumflex arteries and the obturator artery.[6] The obturator artery contributes to the vascularity of femoral head via the artery of ligamentum teres. The lateral femoral circumflex artery gives rise to the inferior metaphyseal artery via the ascending branch, which supplies the majority of anteroinferior femoral head.[6] The medial femoral circumflex artery is the major contributor to the femoral head supply, especially the superolateral portion.[6] The medial femoral circumflex artery gives rise to the lateral epiphyseal artery, which travels along the posterosuperior femoral neck and dives into the capsule to form the retinacular branches. Distortion or disruption of these branches with fracture displacement plays a critical role in the development of osteonecrosis of the femoral head.[6]

The ligaments of the hip joint (Figs 19.10A and B) travel from the upper portion of the acetabulum and transverse acetabular ligament to the intertrochanteric ridge anteroinferiorly and the intertrochanteric crest postero-inferiorly.[3] There are two types of capsular reinforcements:

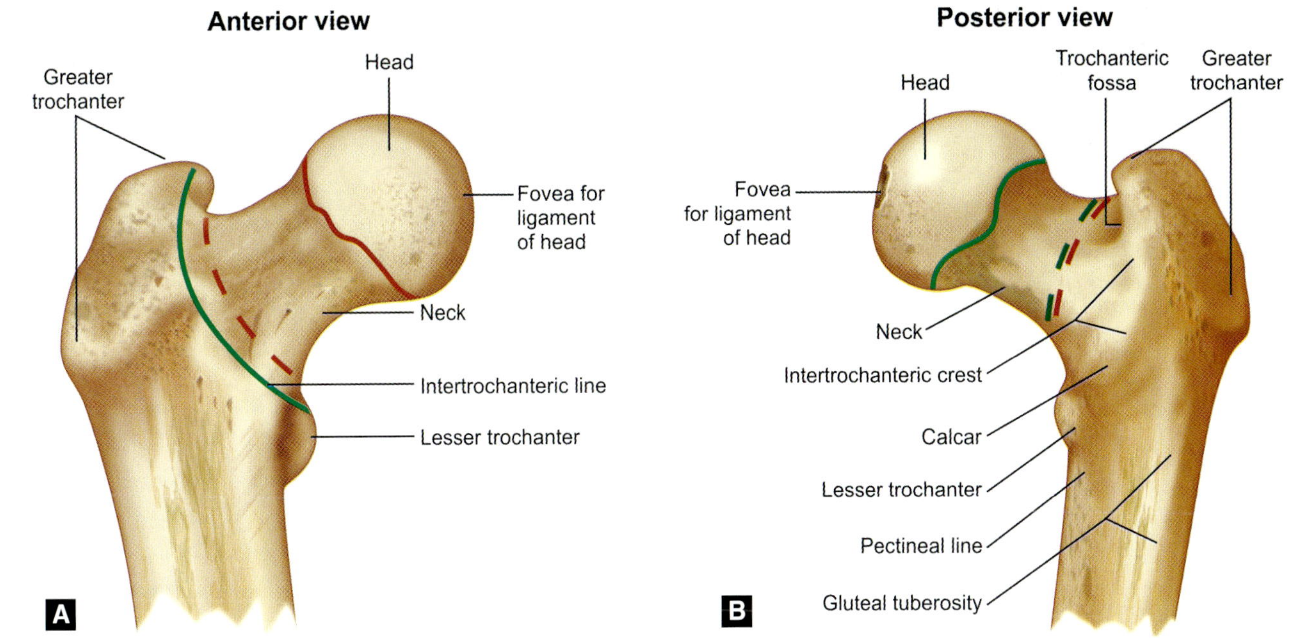

Figures 19.8A and B: The skeletal anatomy of the proximal femur. (A) Anterior view; (B) Posterior view.

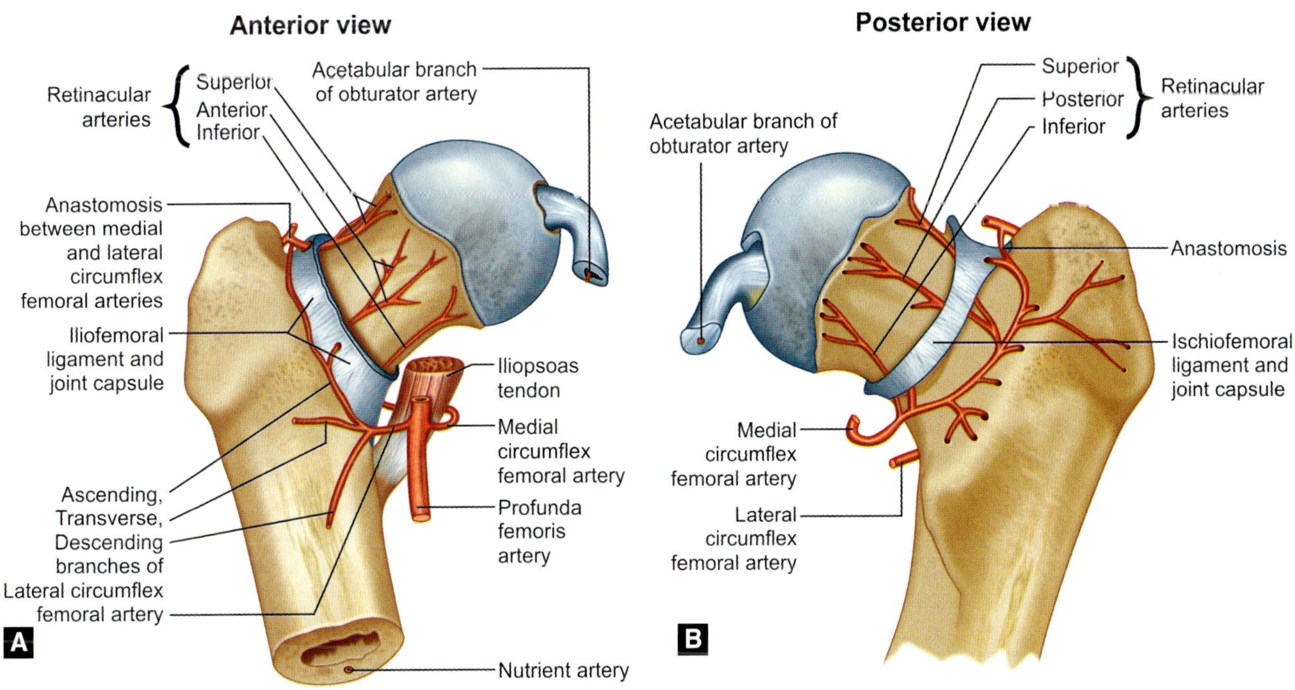

Figures 19.9A and B: The blood supply to the femoral head. (A) Anterior view; (B) Posterior view. The three blood vessels that supply the femoral head are the medial and lateral femoral circumflex arteries and the obturator artery. The medial femoral circumflex artery is the main blood supply as it becomes the lateral epiphyseal artery which then divides into the retinacular arteries.

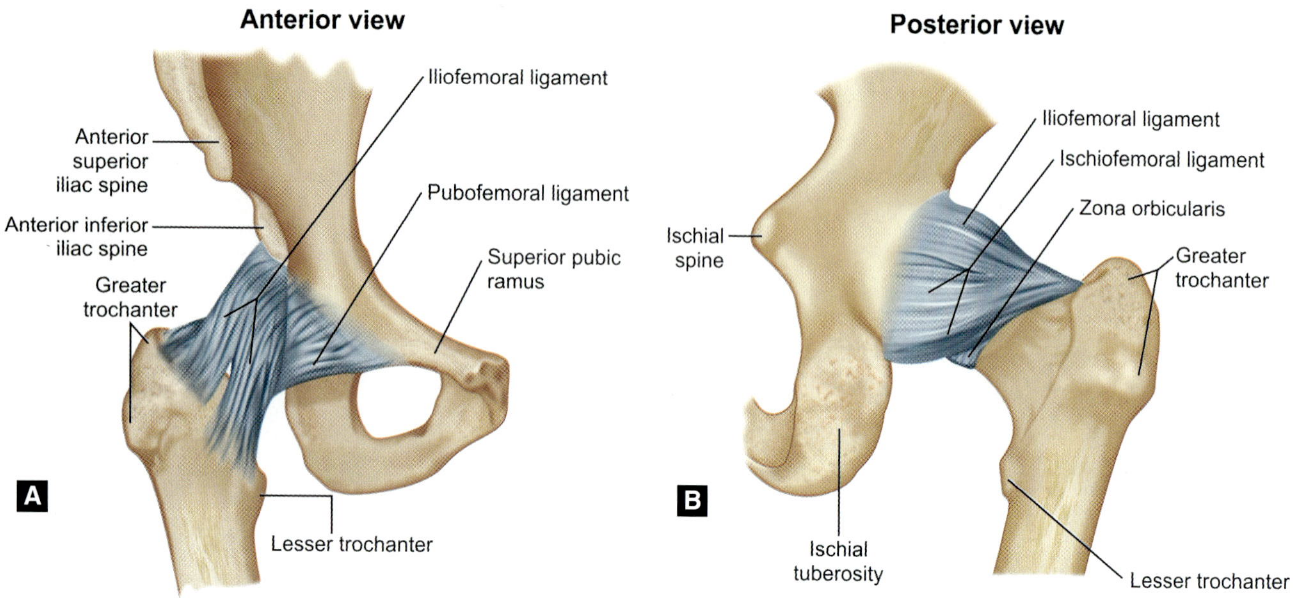

Figures 19.10A and B: The ligaments of the hip joint. (A) Anterior view; (B) Posterior view. The most important is the iliofemoral ligament, also known as the Y ligament of Bigelow.

(1) the circular fibers or zona orbicularis and; (2) the longitudinal fibers.[3] The zona orbicularis forms a sling at the inferior and posterior portions of the neck. The longitudinal fibers are more superior and anterior and are comprised of three distinct ligaments: the iliofemoral, ischiofemoral and pubofemoral ligaments.[3] The iliofemoral ligament or Y ligament of Bigelow is important in resisting hyperextension. It travels from the anterior inferior iliac spine and the acetabular rim to the intertrochanteric ridge. The ischiofemoral ligament travels from the ischial portion of acetabular rim to the femoral neck just medial to the base of greater trochanter. It blends with the zona orbicularis and provides posterior support. The pubofemoral ligament travels from the pubic portion of the acetabulum and iliopectineal eminence to the inferior aspect of the anterior neck and provides inferior support.[3]

Patient positioning is dependent on what approach will be used. For open reduction and internal fixation using an anterior approach, the patient is placed supine on a traction table or radiolucent table. If the patient is placed on a traction table, the foot of the injured limb is placed into a boot mounted on the traction table. If there are injuries in the ipsilateral knee or tibia, a traction pin can be placed in the femur. The unaffected lower extremity is placed in the hemilithotomy position and secured to a well-leg holder with a gel pad or can be secured in a traction boot in the "scissor" position (see Chapter 21). (It should be noted that the hemilithotomy position is a risk for well-leg compartment syndrome and should only be used for relatively short cases unless the leg is "let down" periodically). Pads or blankets are placed on the patient's chest and the upper extremity on the same side as the injured hip is draped over the chest and secured with tape. The upper extremity on the side of the uninjured hip is abducted and secured to a well-padded arm board. The C-arm is then placed in between the lower extremities at an angle when the well-leg is in the hemilithotomy position or on the contralateral side perpendicular to the table when the legs are "scissored." Anteroposterior and lateral views are taken to ensure that proper imaging can be obtained.

Alternatively, for anterior exposures, the patient can be placed supine on a radiolucent table with bumps made of towels along the back and buttock to elevate the injured hip approximately 20°. This will ensure that the hip joints will not be overlapped on the lateral view. Towels are placed on the patient's chest and the upper extremity on the same side as the injured hip is draped over the chest and secured with tape. The contralateral upper extremity is abducted and secured to a well-padded arm board.

The contralateral lower extremity is placed on a gel pad and secured to the table with tape. The C-arm is positioned on the contralateral side and is perpendicular to the table. Anteroposterior and lateral views are taken to ensure that proper imaging can be obtained. Traction can be executed from an assistant or a traction pin placed through the tibia or femur after the leg is prepped. A sterile traction bow is placed on the pin and rope is positioned over an IV pole with a sterile Mayo stand cover and weights are placed on the end of the rope.

Positioning for the posterior approach for arthroplasty is in the lateral decubitus position with the injured hip in the air. A bean bag is used to secure the body of the patient. An axillary role is placed just distal to the axilla to prevent brachial plexopathy. The proximal fibula of the well-leg is off loaded by placing "egg crate" foam padding proximally and distally. This will help prevent peroneal nerve palsy. The upper extremity on the well-leg side is secured to a well-padded arm board. The upper extremity on the side of the injured hip is secured to an elevated well-padded arm board. A padded sterile draped Mayo stand will aid in positioning of the injured lower extremity.

Once the patient is positioned, a closed reduction can be attempted by gently flexing the hip to 45° while slightly abducted, and then extending and internally rotating the hip while pulling traction.[6] The reduction maneuver should not involve excessive manipulation and should only be attempted once. If closed reduction is unsuccessful, open reduction should commence through one of the two approaches: the Smith-Petersen or Watson-Jones.

The Smith-Petersen or iliofemoral approach (Figs 19.11A to D) is the direct anterior approach to the hip that utilizes a true internervous plane between the superior gluteal nerve and the femoral nerve.[26] The incision begins over the lateral iliac crest and travels anterior to the anterior superior iliac spine (ASIS) and is taken distally over the anterior thigh aiming for the lateral edge of the patella. The subcutaneous tissue is dissected carefully as to avoid damage to the lateral femoral cutaneous nerve. Once the fascia over the tensor fascia lata is exposed, it is incised and then split with Mayo scissors proximally and distally. Blunt dissection is used to separate the tensor fasciae lata from the sartorious. The ascending branch of the lateral femoral circumflex artery must be identified and ligated. The fascia over the rectus femoris is identified and incised and the rectus femoris is retracted medially and the gluteus medius is retracted laterally. The rectus femoris had two heads: (1) the direct head attached to the anterior inferior iliac spine and; (2) the reflected head to the superior lip of the acetabulum and anterior hip capsule. For increased exposure, the heads of the rectus femoris can be released from their respective origins and the abductor muscles can be released from the lateral iliac crest. The pericapsular fat is swept away with a Cobb elevator and a vertical incision is made in the capsule from the labrum superiorly to the intertrochanteric ridge inferiorly. The capsulotomy is completed by making a horizontal limb that is parallel to the anterior labrum. Avoid placing retractors that lever on the posterior neck to prevent further damage to the blood supply to the femoral head. Place suture tags in the capsule for retraction. This approach provides excellent exposure of the femoral neck and head, but can only be used for reduction. A separate incision must be made for implant placement.

The Watson-Jones or anterolateral approach to the hip (Figs 19.12A to F) does not have a true internervous plane of dissection because the muscles that form the interval are both innervated by the superior gluteal nerve.[26] The incision is made over the lateral femur with a curve slightly anterior in the proximal limb of the incision aiming for the tubercle of the iliac crest. Use sharp dissection down to the fascia over the tensor facia lata and incise it. Take the fascial incision proximally following the posterior border of the tensor facia lata. Retract the tensor fascia lata anteriorly and develop the plane between it and the gluteus medius with blunt dissection. Identify the group of vessels that cross the interval proximally and ligate them. A right angle retractor is then placed under the gluteus medius and minimus to reveal the fat over the joint capsule. The hip is externally rotated and the origin of vastus lateralis is released from vastus ridge. The pericapsular fat is swept away to reveal the joint capsule and the reflected head of the rectus femoris is released. A T-shaped capsulotomy is made as described with the Smith-Petersen approach. The visualization can be improved with a greater trochanteric osteotomy. This approach allows reduction of the fracture and implant placement through the same incision, but the anterior musculature may limit visualization. It can also be used for arthroplasty.

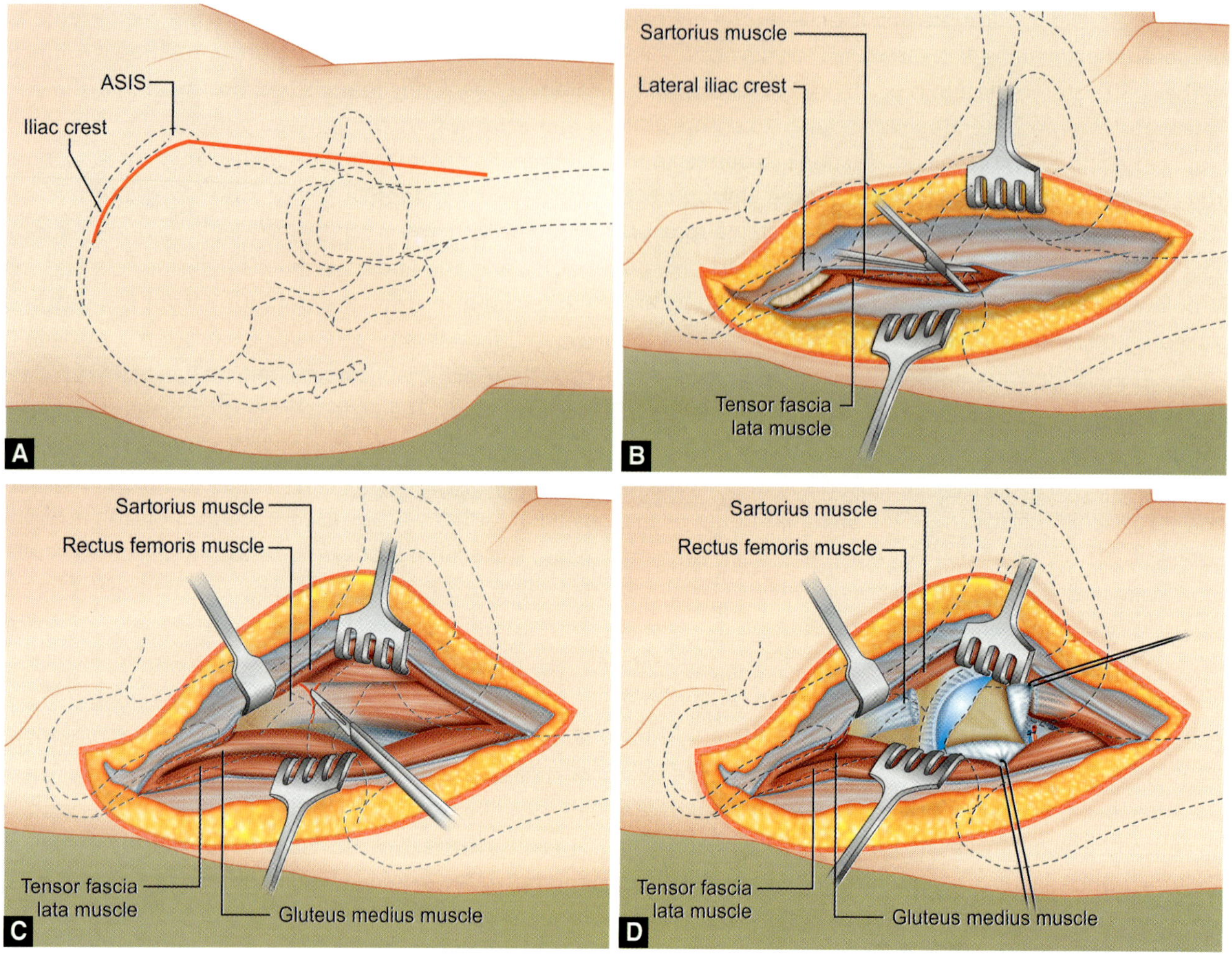

Figures 19.11A to D: The Smith-Petersen approach. (A) The skin incision parallels the iliac crest and is curved distally on the anterior thigh aiming for the lateral edge of the patella; (B) The superficial interval between the sartorius and the tensor facia lata is developed; (C) The deep interval between the rectus femoris and the gluteus medius is developed by releasing the two heads of the rectus femoris; (D) The approach is complete when a T-shaped capsulotomy is performed to expose the femoral neck and head.

The posterior or Southern approach (Figs 19.13A to F) was popularized by Moore and does not have a true internervous plane.[26] The incision is placed over the posterior aspect of the femoral shaft and greater trochanter and is curved proximally toward the posterior superior iliac spine. Sharp dissection is taken down to the tensor fascia and then it is incised proximally and distally in line with the incision. The gluteus maximus is split bluntly revealing the fat over the short external rotators. A sharp retractor is placed in between the gluteus minimus and the piriformis. The piriformis and obturator internus tendons are tagged with sutures and released from their femoral insertions and retracted posteriorly. Note that only the obturator internus tendon protects the sciatic nerve. The piriformis tendon is normally posterior to the sciatic nerve and will not protect it when retracted posteriorly. A T-shaped incision is made in the capsule exposing the femoral neck and acetabulum. The quadratus femoris can be released to the level of lesser trochanter where the ilipsoas tendon inserts. For more visualization, the tendinous insertion of the gluteus maximus can be partially released from the gluteal ridge of the femur. This exposure offers excellent visualization of the acetabulum for arthroplasty, but is not routinely used for open reduction due to the potential danger to the vessels that supply the femoral head.

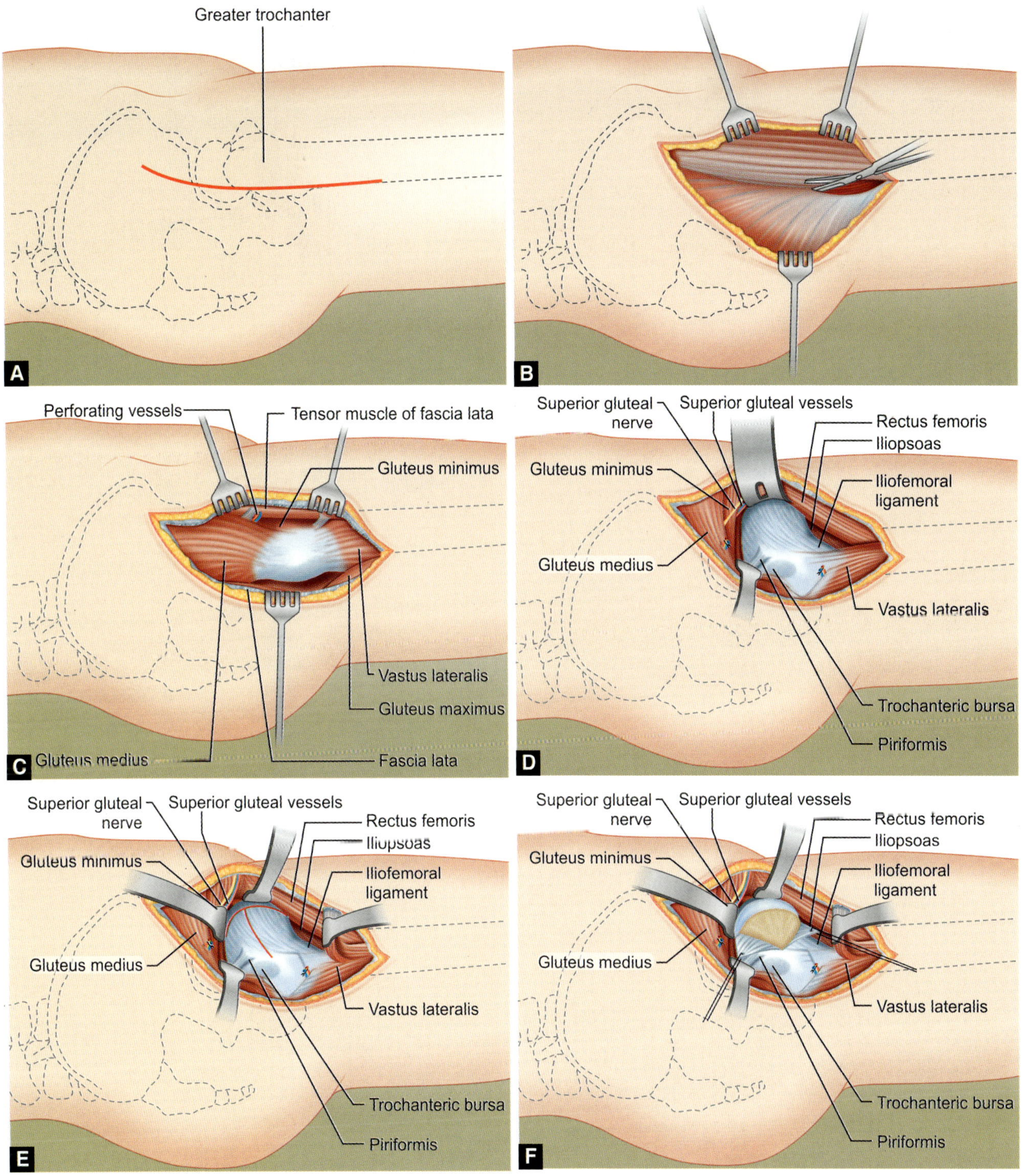

Figures 19.12A to F: The Watson-Jones approach. (A) The skin incision is taken over the lateral femur and curved anteriorly above the greater trochanter; (B) The tensor facia is incised and the interval between the tensor fasciae lata and the gluteus medius is developed; (C) Extend the interval proximally; (D) The vessels that cross the interval are ligated and retractors are placed deep to the rectus femoris and the gluteus medius. The origin of the vastus lateralis and insertion of the gluteus medius are partially released from the vastus ridge and anterior greater trochanter; (E and F) A T-shaped capsulotomy exposes the femoral neck and completes the exposure.

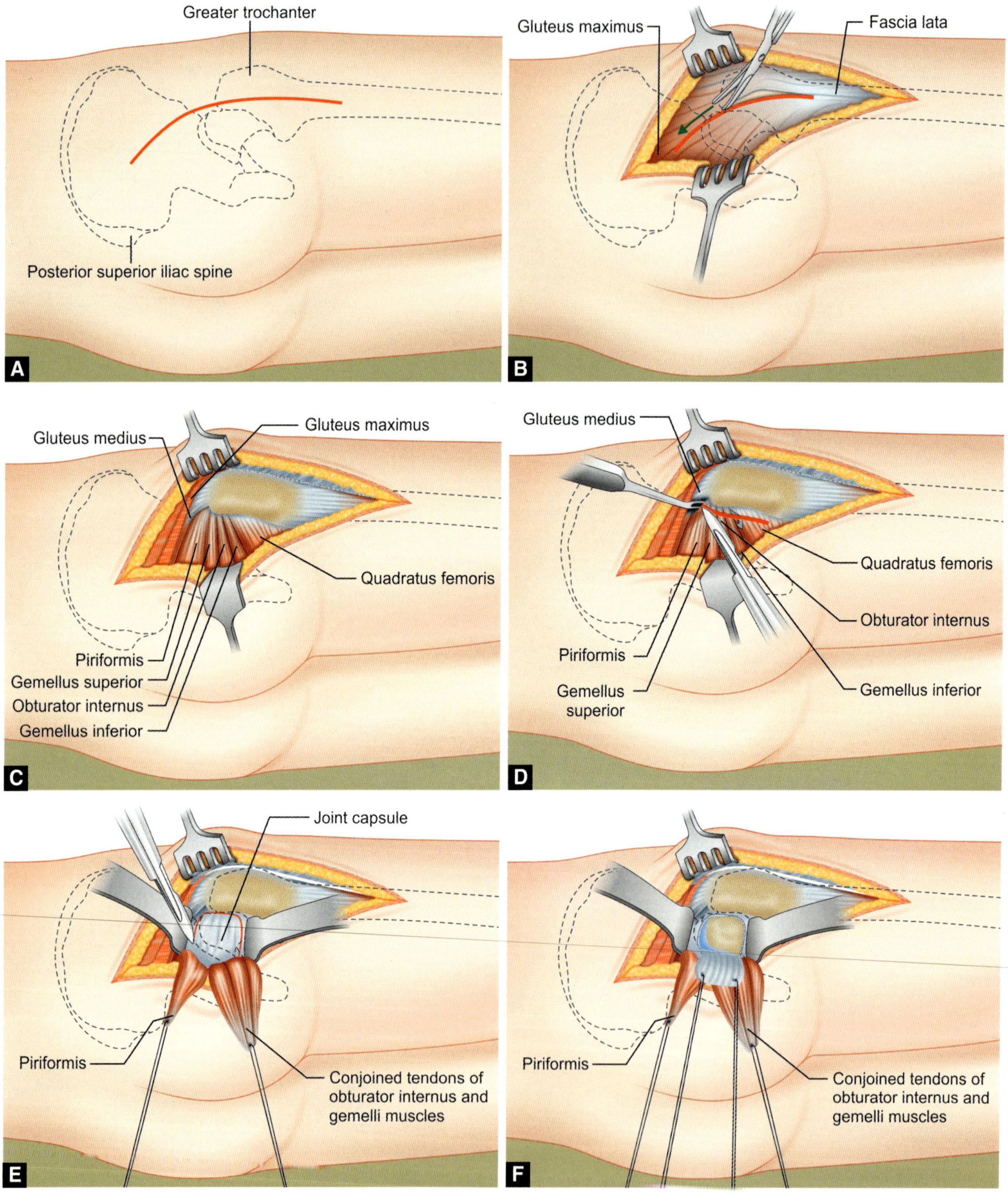

Figures 19.13A to F: The posterior approach. (A) The incision is carried over the posterior shaft and greater trochanter and curved posteriorly to the posterior superior iliac spine; (B) The tensor fascia is split along with the fibers of the gluteus maximus; (C) The external rotators are identified. The piriformis and the obturator internus are tagged with heavy suture; (D) The external rotators are sharply released from the proximal femur; (E) The external rotators are then retracted posteriorly to expose the capsule. The obturator internus protects the sciatic nerve; (F) A capsulotomy is performed exposing the femoral head and neck.

Surgical Techniques

Technique 1: Closed Reduction and Cannulated Screw Fixation of Femoral Neck Fractures

Preoperative Planning and Anatomic Considerations

Closed reduction and cannulated screw fixation is typically performed for patients who have nondisplaced or minimally displaced subcapital or transcervical fractures of the femoral neck. It is important not to allow these fractures to go to displace. Therefore, bed rest is typically prescribed except in cases of stress fractures. Since the majority of these cases are in elderly patients, a thorough medical evaluation for preoperative cardiac risk stratification should be performed prior to surgery. This workup should be done in an expeditious manner in order to get the patient to the operating room as soon as possible (within the first 24 hours, preferably) in an effort to mobilize the patient out of bed.

Anatomic considerations should be taken into account when preoperatively planning cannulated screw fixation. However, most adult proximal femurs will allow placement of cannulated screws between 6 mm and 8 mm in diameter (Figs 19.14A and B). Proper imaging should be done to rule out posterior comminution, previous implants or deformity. However, screws can even be placed in the setting of previous femoral nail; although this can create difficulties (Figs 19.15A to F). Templating can be done to determine the screw lengths needed and the ability for the threads to cross the fracture for the given implants chosen for fixation.

Instrumentation, Implant and Patient Positioning Considerations

A large cannulated screw set (typically anywhere from 6 to 8 mm in diameter) is utilized. Varying screw lengths should be available up to 110 mm unless careful preoperative planning with templating has been done. A power drill, preferably with a wire driver attachment should be available.

A radiolucent table is mandatory, typically with traction attachments, but can be done without traction attachments in nondisplaced and minimally displaced fractures. C-arm fluoroscopy is mandatory for these procedures as well. If traction attachments are used, either the well-leg holder can be used in the hemilithotomy position or the well leg can be placed in the "scissor" position (see Fig. 21.4). It is important to note that although lateral imaging is more straightforward with the hemilithotomy position, this is a risk for "well-leg" compartment syndrome. For this reason, the scissor position is preferable in most cases in which the traction table is utilized. In either case, the perineal post should be well-padded and traction should not even be necessary in cases of nondisplaced or minimally

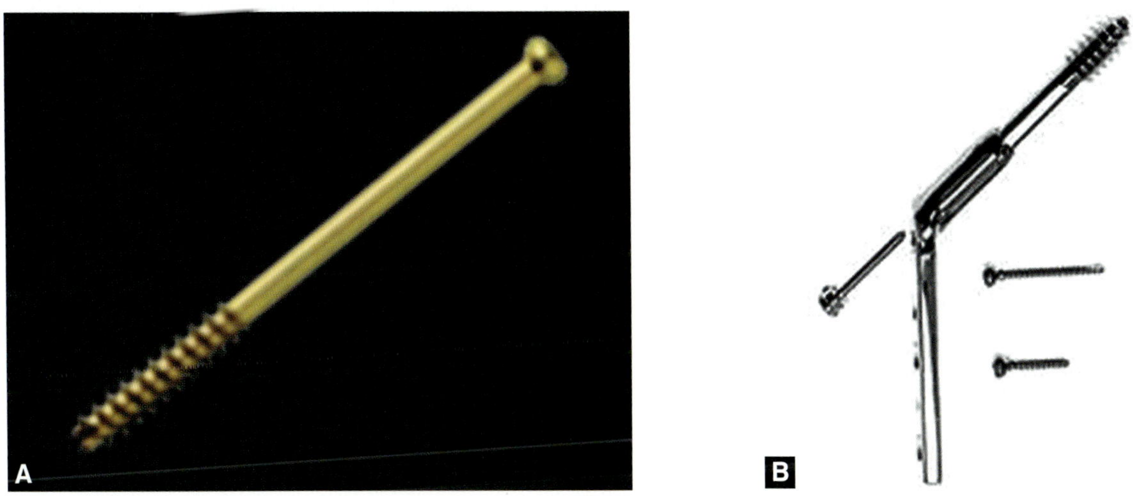

Figures 19.14A and B: Commonly used implants for the internal fixation of femoral neck fractures. (A) A 7.3 mm cannulated screw with 16 mm and 32 mm threads; (B) Sliding hip screw device with side plate.

displaced fractures. Supine positioning is used routinely for these cases. Navigation systems, if available, can help to reduce fluoroscopic radiation during the procedure.

Technique

After positioning as described above, fluoroscopic images are taken before prepping to make sure that imaging will be optimal when the procedure starts. After prepping and draping, images are taken with the guidewire overlying the skin in the proposed trajectory of the screw. A short incision can then be made just distal to the greater trochanter on the lateral proximal thigh. Alternatively, the wire can be placed percutaneously. Care should be taken not to place the wires distal to the lesser trochanter as drill holes here in the lateral femur are particular risks for late iatrogenic subtrochanteric femur fracture. Furthermore, multiple lateral cortical perforations with the drill at and below the level of the lesser trochanter can also present a risk for late fracture (Figs 19.16A to F).

Typically, three wires are placed across the fracture in parallel fashion, into the femoral head. Multiple acceptable configurations exist although the "inverted triangle" method is fairly popular (See Figs 19.3A to C). The main principle of screw fixation in osteoporotic bone is to place the screws peripherally in the femoral neck so that the screws are not sitting in the middle of the femoral neck where there is minimal bone to counter potential migration of the screw (Fig. 19.17).

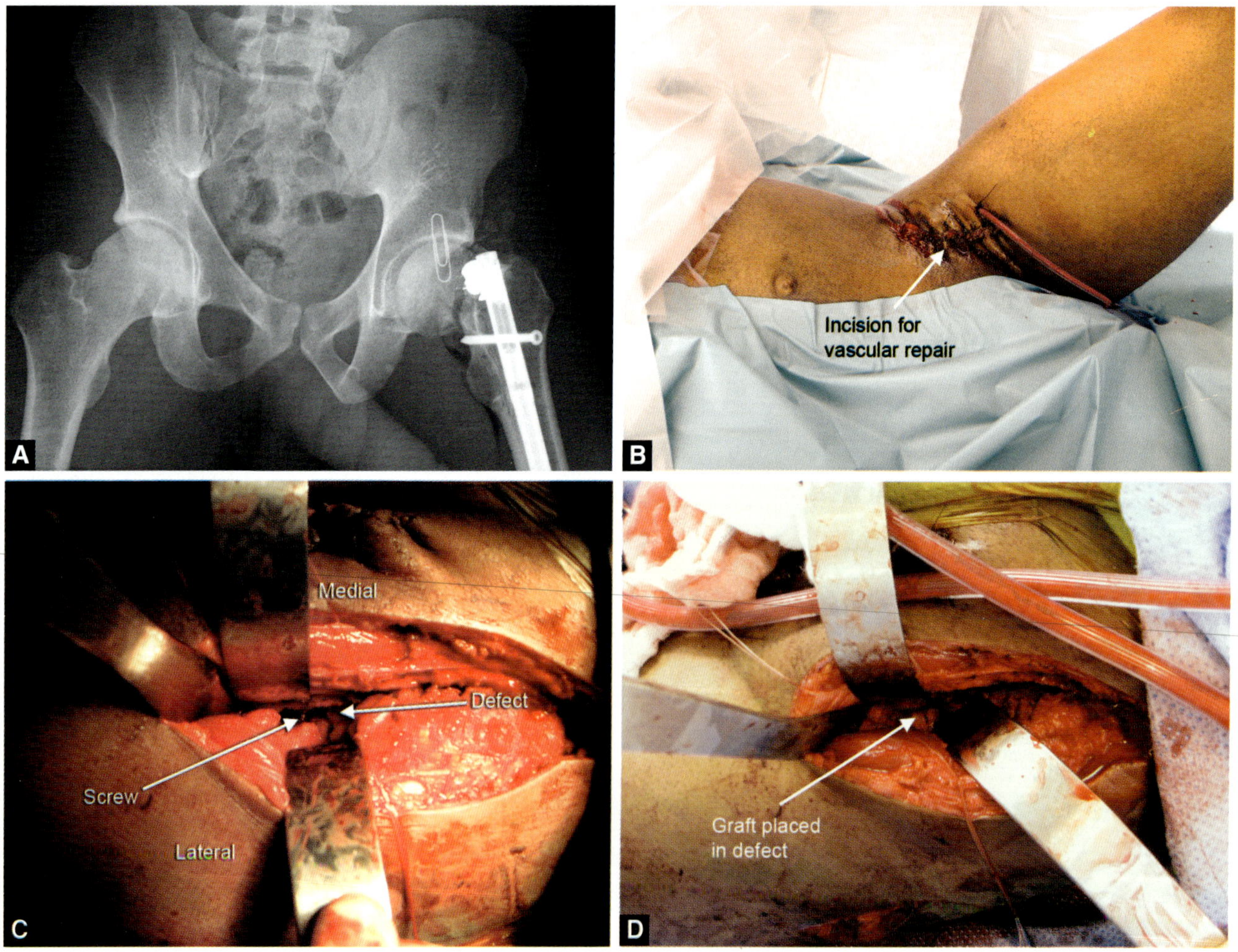

Figures 19.15A to D

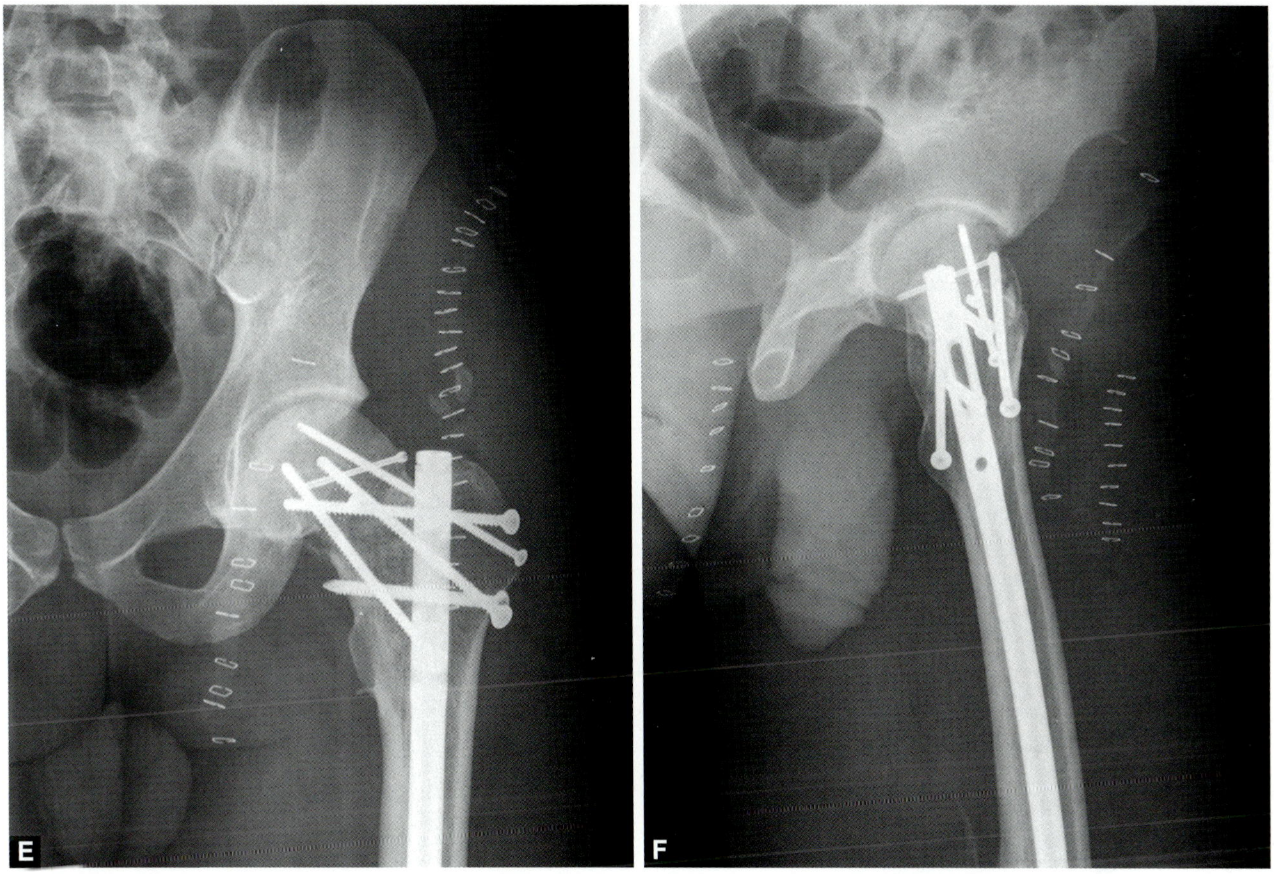

Figures 19.15A to F: Open reduction and internal fixation of a displaced femoral neck fracture from a gunshot injury. (A) Anteroposterior radiograph of a displaced femoral neck fracture from a low-velocity gunshot injury. The patient also had a vascular injury and a previous history of an antegrade femoral nail as seen. Given the emergent need to go to surgery and unknown femoral nail implant, a decision was made to fix the femoral neck while leaving the previous femoral nail in place; (B) The patient underwent a vascular repair through an anteromedial proximal thigh exposure. After this was completed, the patient was kept supine but with a slight bump placed under the buttock and was reprepped and draped, (C) A Smith-Petersen approach was performed and the fracture was exposed and reduced directly. This was highly comminuted with bone loss of the anterior femoral neck. Multiple 3.5 mm and 4.5 mm screws were placed through a separate lateral incision. As shown here with the arrow, an anterior femoral neck defect is seen with a screw passing through this space; (D) Through the same incision, an iliac crest graft was obtained, shaped and gently impacted into the defect as shown here; (E and F) Postoperative radiographs demonstrate good overall reduction with multiple screws as well as retention of the previous intramedullary nail and interlocking screw.

Anteroposterior, lateral and intermediate images are taken to make sure that the wires are safely placed and are not penetrating the articular surface (Figs 19.18A to H). After all the three wires are placed, measurements are taken, and the screws are placed sequentially after overdrilling with the cannulated drill. Washers are frequently used to prevent lateral wall fracture of the proximal femur when the screws are used to compress the fracture. Final images are taken and the wound is irrigated and closed. A capsulotomy can be performed in order to decompress the intracapsular hematoma, although the evidence to support this technique is lacking.

Postoperatively, weight bearing can usually be allowed. Follow-up radiographs should be taken after the procedure and 1 week afterwards. Staples are removed 2 weeks postoperatively.

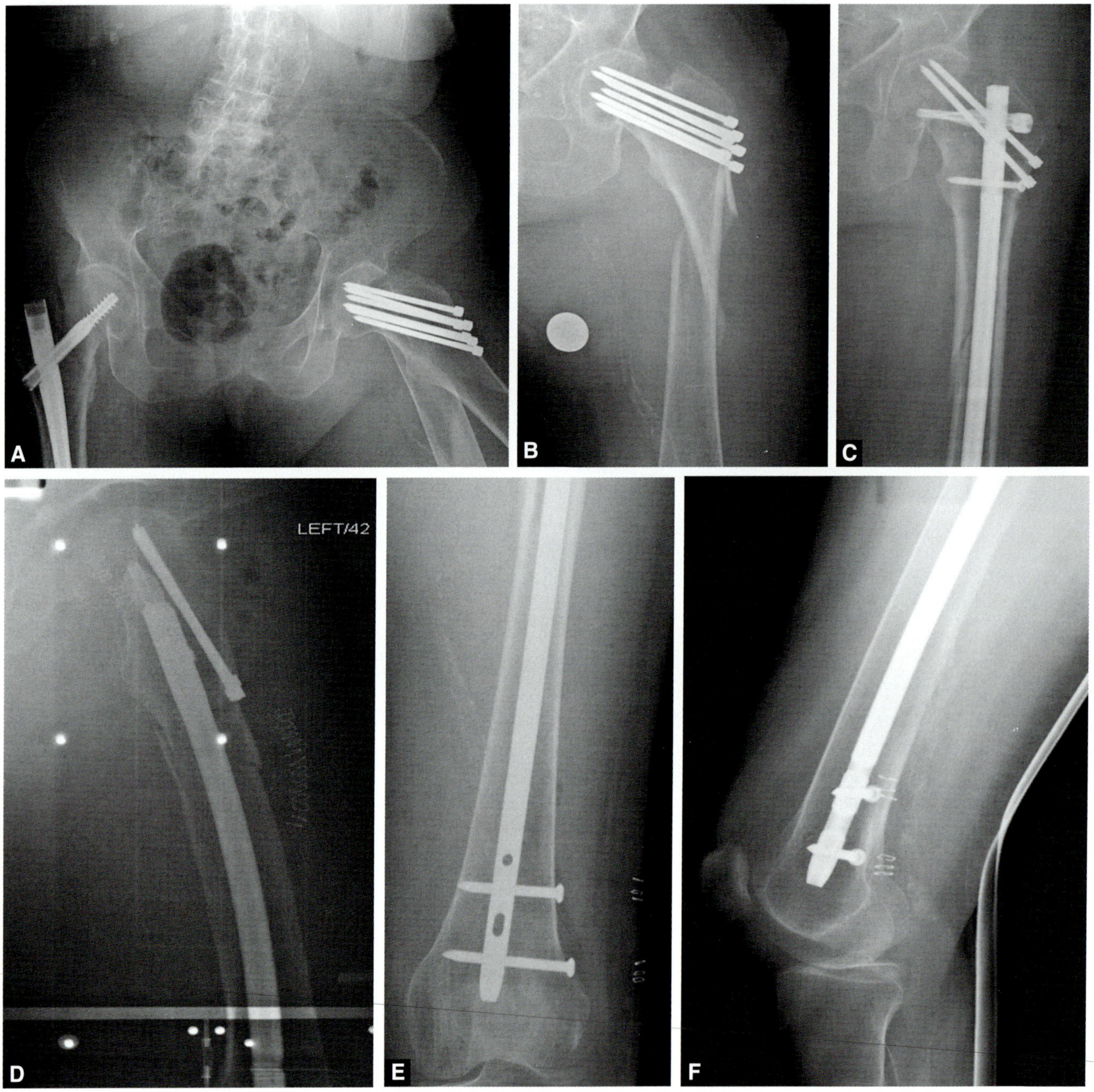

Figures 19.16A to F: Treatment of late subtrochanteric femur fracture after prior femoral neck pinning. (A and B) An 86-year-old female with prior Knowles pinning procedure of left femoral neck fracture with a fall and new subtrochanteric femur fracture; (C to F) Multiple postoperative radiographs demonstrating removal of four of the six Knowles pins, reduction of the subtrochanteric femur fracture, and placement of a cephalomedullary nail with a spiral blade and interlocking screws proximally and distally.

Courtesy: Jaimo Ahn

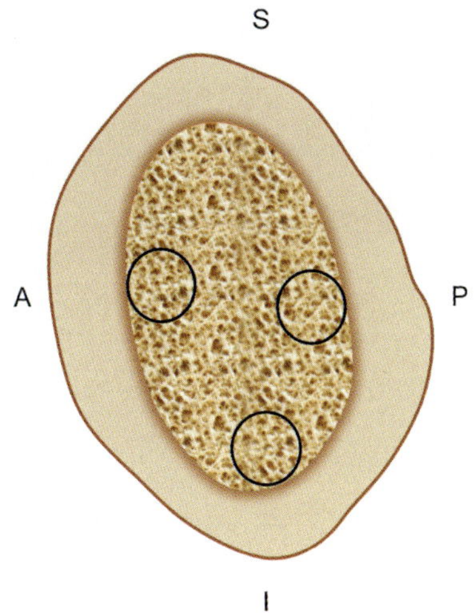

Figure 19.17: Strategy of screw placement for femoral neck fractures as shown in cross section. (S, superior; I, inferior; A, anterior; P, posterior)

CLOSED REDUCTION AND CONNULATED SCREW FIXATION OF FEMORAL NECK FRACTURES: Pearls and Pitfalls

- Peripheral placement of the screws is important, particularly in osteoporotic bone, typically in an "inverted triangle" configuration
- Avoid multiple lateral cortical perforations, and avoid screw placement inferior to the lesser trochanter in order to avoid a late subtrochanteric femur fracture
- Parallel placement of the screws will allow the most efficient compression

Technique 2: ORIF of Displaced Femoral Neck Fracture

Preoperative Planning and Anatomic Considerations

Displaced femoral neck fractures have 30% risk of nonunion and osteonecrosis. In many cases, these complications are unavoidable. Whereas fracture nonunion can be due to technical issues related to fracture reduction and fixation, osteonecrosis is due to disruption of the blood supply to the femoral head at the time of injury. It is generally agreed upon that surgical reduction and fixation within 6–8 hours from the time of injury should improve outcomes with regard to avoiding osteonecrosis. Therefore, displaced femoral neck fractures in young patients (younger than 65 years of age) should be considered surgical emergencies. The preoperative process should be expedited because a priority should be placed on the time to get into the operating room.

Since fracture reduction is also paramount, in order to prevent nonunion, open reduction methods are usually preferred to closed reduction. Whereas closed reduction can be successful, it is often hard to accurately judge the reduction with only fluoroscopic images. Furthermore, the surgeon will have a tendency to overestimate the quality of reduction when done through closed methods. We feel that in all cases preparations should be made to perform an open reduction.

From a templating standpoint, careful attention should be paid to the location of the primary fracture line, and the degree of comminution. The Pauwels angle should be measured if a proper AP radiograph of the hip has been obtained. Attention should also be made to determine if a patient has a basicervical femoral neck fracture versus a transcervical or basicervical fracture. As described earlier, basicervical femoral neck fractures can be treated like intertrochanteric femur fractures with regard to timing and fixation methods (see Chapter 20).

Instrumentation, Implant and Patient Positioning Considerations

As described above, preparations should be made for open reduction. This can be done via one of the multiple surgical approaches, but the authors feel that the anterior Smith Petersen approach offers the most direct access to the femoral neck and allows convenient supine positioning which can be done either with a traction table or a flat radiolucent table. An additional lateral surgical approach can then be performed for placement of internal fixation. With the patient in the supine position, either the traction table can be set up as shown in "Technique 1" previously, or the flat radiolucent table can be used and a tibial traction pin placed with weights placed over the end of the table.

Closed reduction can be attempted with simple traction either from the traction pin or with the traction table, and fluoroscopic images can be taken before draping to determine the quality of the imaging and of the reduction. In many cases, a proper AP radiograph of the hip with 15° of internal rotation is not available at the time of surgery due to emergent nature of the preoperative process. If it is not available preoperatively, then appropriate imaging

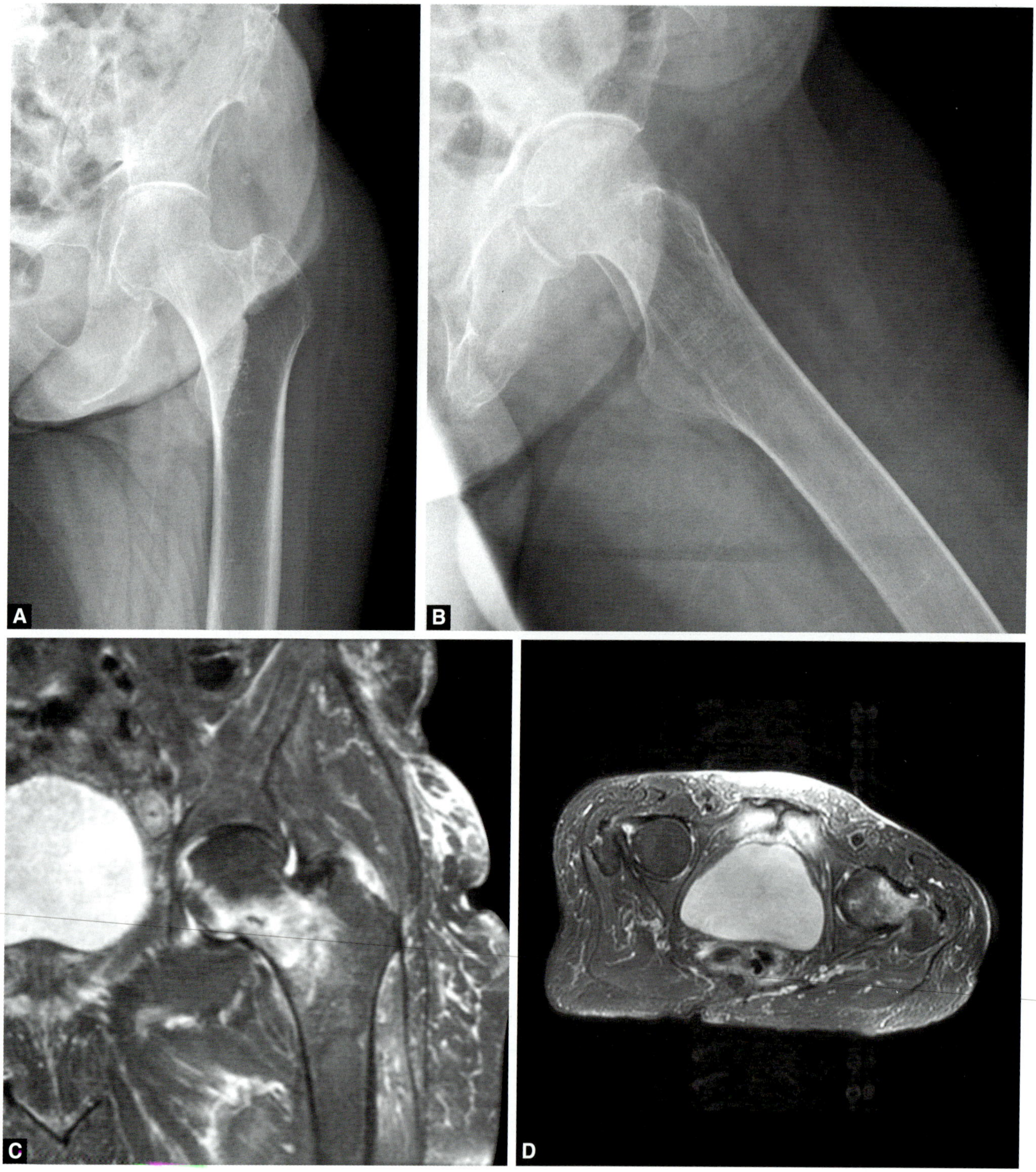

Figures 19.18A to D

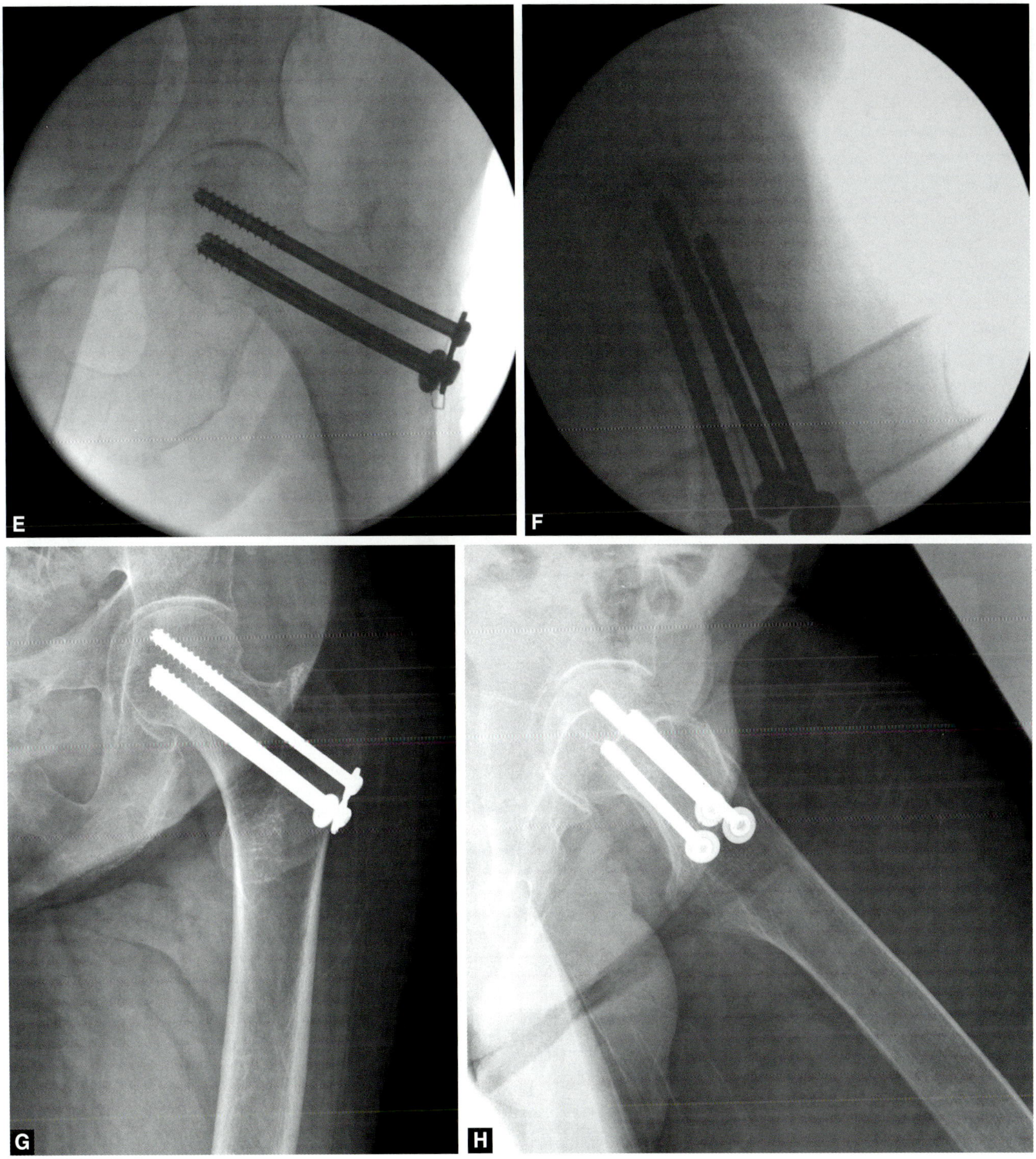

Figures 19.18A to H: Cannulated screw fixation of a nondisplaced femoral neck fracture. (A and B) Anteroposterior and lateral images of an 80-year-old female with groin and hip pain after a fall. No obvious fracture is seen although it is suspected clinically; (C and D) MRI images demonstrating bone edema and a fracture line of the femoral neck; (E and F) Anteroposterior and lateral fluoroscopic images demonstrating parallel placement of three cannulated screws in a triangular configuration; (G and H) Follow-up radiographs demonstrating a healed fracture of the femoral neck.

should be taken at this point, particularly to properly assess the Pauwels angle. Prepping and draping should be done in such a manner that full access to the hip is available from both the operative side as well as contralateral side of the table so that the surgical assistant can provide appropriate retraction. A C-arm cover should be used rather than the "shower curtain."

Instrumentation and implants are similar to those used for closed reduction and cannulated screw fixation as described in "Technique 1." However, a sliding hip screw device can also be utilized, and is arguably biomechanically superior to parallel cannulated screws. In certain cases, 3.5 mm or 4.5 mm solid cortical screws of appropriate length might be needed, particularly in more comminuted cases. With severe comminution, bone grafting might be necessary. With lateral wall and greater trochanteric fracture involvement, cannulated screw fixation alone may not have sufficient near cortical fixation, and treatment with a sliding hip screw with trochanteric stabilization plate fixation might be needed (Figs 19.19A to K). Minifragment fixation has been advocated by some to augment traditional compression screw fixation. However, locked fixation either with locked plates or fixed angled nail devices is a risk for nonunion and should not be done for femoral neck fractures. Appropriate retractors and instruments for an open anterior approach to the hip should be available (Figs 19.20A to G).

Technique

Patient positioning, prepping and draping is done as described. Traction is applied either through the traction boot/table below the drapes, or through the traction pin and bow. If a "free leg" draping is done with skeletal traction and a bow, then the entire limb is prepped, and an impervious stockinette for the lower leg and foot can be used. Sterile rope will also be necessary. The C-arm should be placed at the contralateral side of the table. An anterior Smith-Petersen approach is performed (See Figs 19.11A to D).

`The fracture should be exposed at this time. Kirschner wires are placed as "joysticks" into the medial fragment, and an anatomic reduction is achieved with this along with appropriate use of traction and manipulation. Once this is achieved, a guidewire from the cannulated screw set is placed as described in "Technique 1". Additional guidewires are placed in parallel fashion, and after drilling, screws are placed as shown in "Technique 1."

As mentioned previously, Pauwels three type fractures can often benefit from an additional transverse screw placed perpendicular to the fracture line. In cases of having to "work around" other implants, such as an antegrade femoral nail, sometimes smaller caliber screws such as 3.5 mm and 4.5 mm screws, might be needed instead of 6.5 mm or 7.3 mm screws (See Figs 19.15A to F).

At the conclusion of the procedure, the capsule can be loosely approximated and the tissues are closed in layers over a drain, if necessary. Final images with the C-arm are done to ensure that there is no articular penetration and that the reduction is anatomic.

Postoperatively, weight bearing should be restricted in contradistinction to postoperative weight bearing for nondisplaced or minimally displaced fractures in the elderly. Hip precautions, however, are not needed.

ORIF OF DISPLACED FEMORAL NECK FRACTURE: Pearls and Pitfalls

- Anatomic reduction is more important in the femoral neck for bony healing than it is in most other locations. Therefore, displaced femoral neck fractures, if being treated with fixation, typically require an open reduction through an anterior or anterolateral approach. If closed reduction is done, an anatomic reduction cannot always be assured
- If a Smith-Petersen approach is used, fixation can still be placed through a separate, lateral incision
- Fixation can be performed with either cannulated screws or a sliding hip screw. If a sliding hip screw is used, the surgeon must be careful not to allow "spinning" of the head with reaming and screw placement. A "derotational" additional pin can help prevent this
- Currently, locked plates do not have a place in the treatment of femoral neck fractures due to their unacceptable failure rate

Technique 3: Hemiarthroplasty of Femoral Neck Fracture

Preoperative Planning

Planning from a medical perspective is similar to that for closed reduction and cannulated screw fixation (Technique 1). Timing of the surgery is similar (preferably

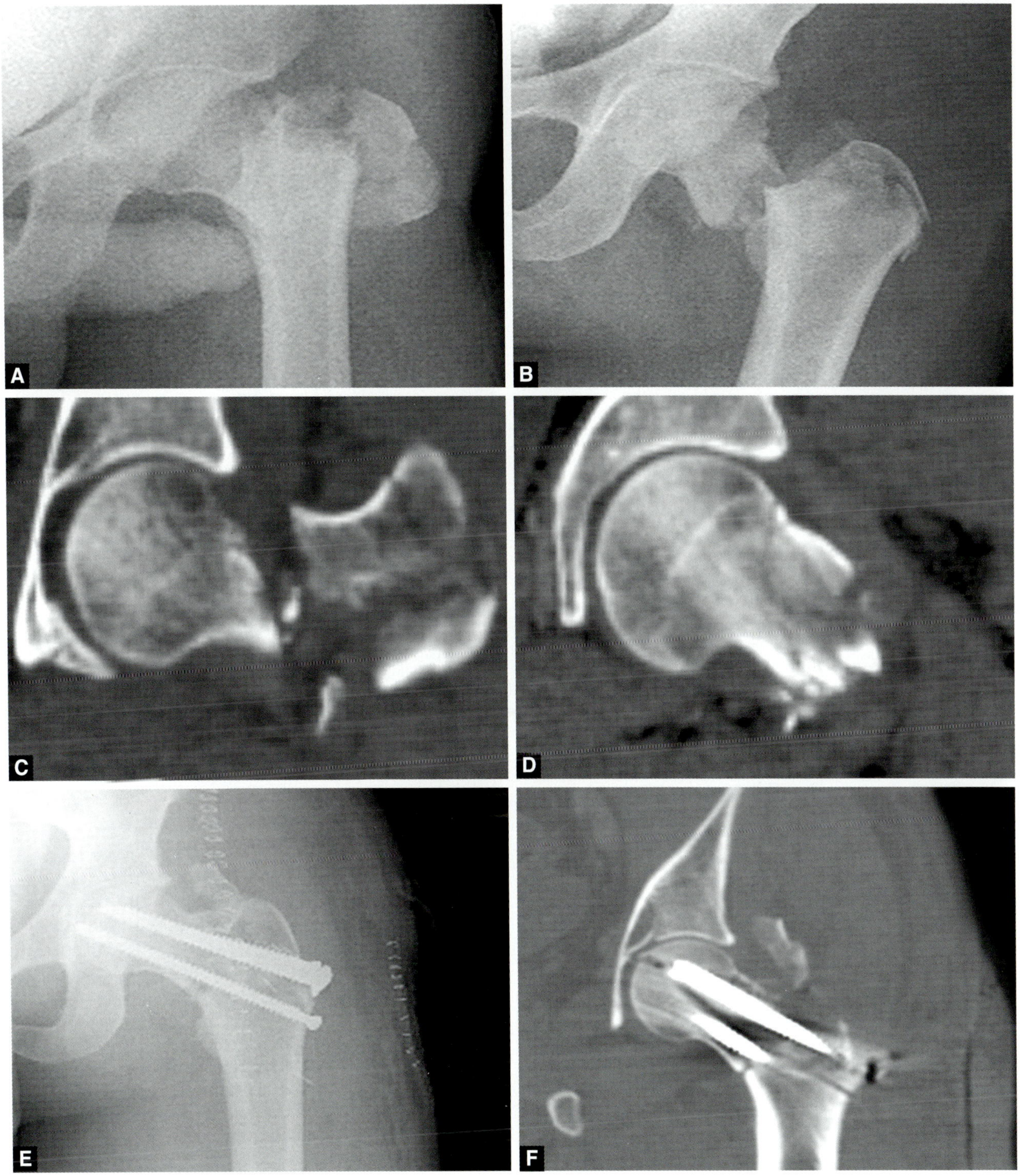

Figures 19.19A to F

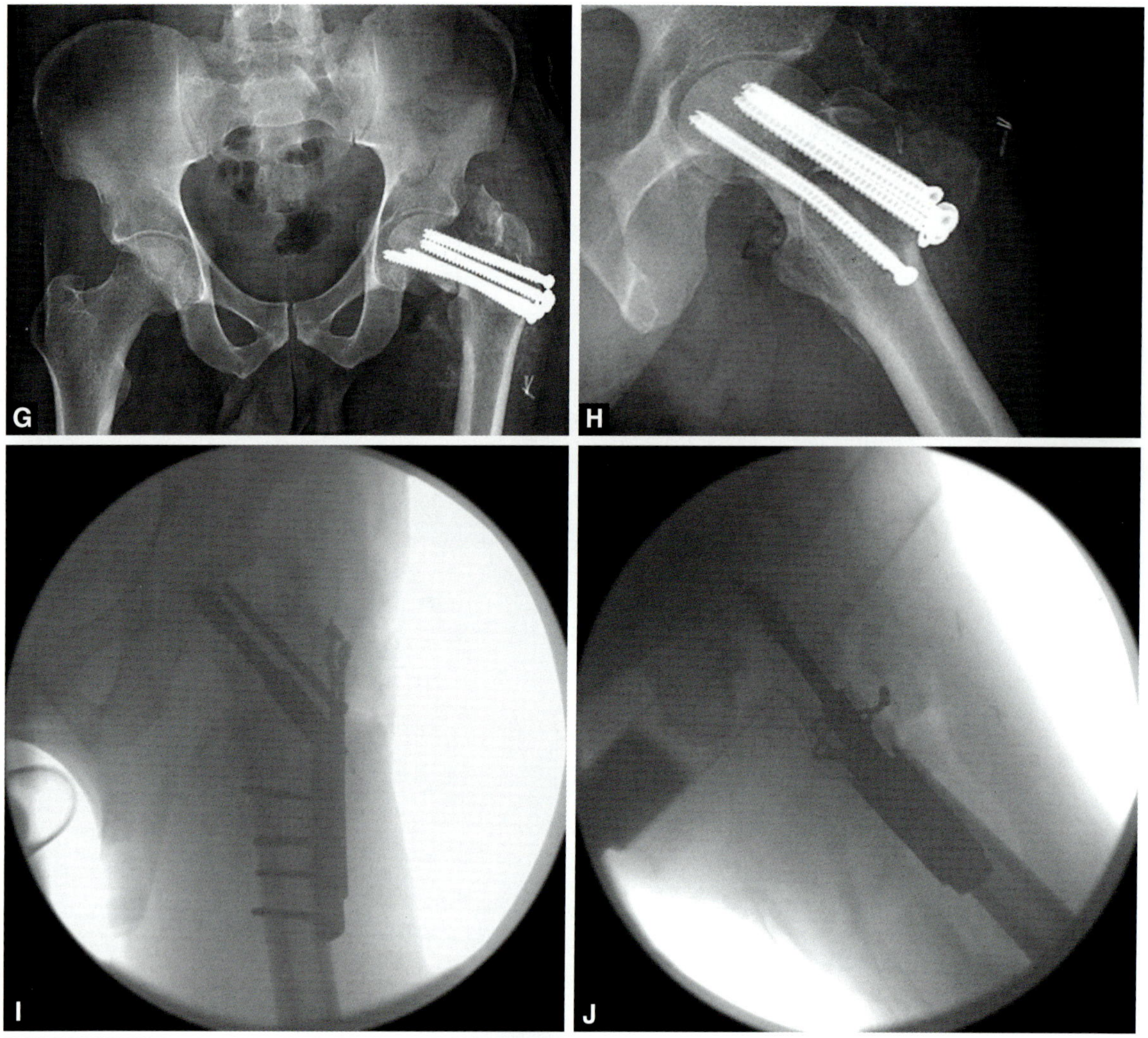

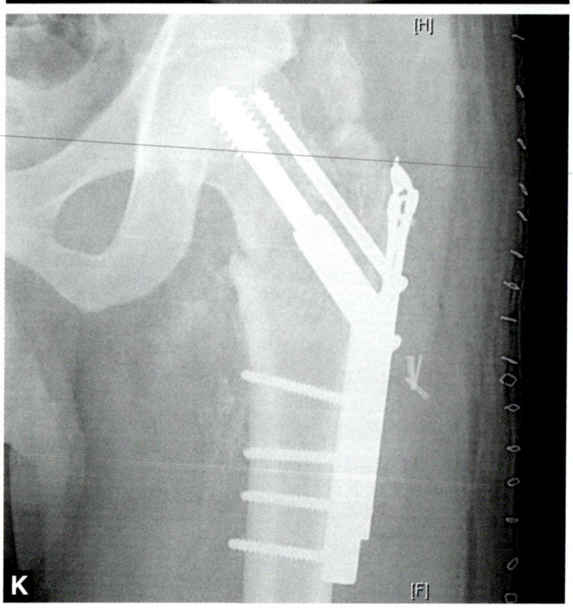

Figures 19.19A to K: Failure of fixation after cannulated screw fixation of a displaced femoral neck fracture. (A to D) Radiographs and CT scan images of a displaced, comminuted Pauwels 3 type vertical femoral neck fracture with lateral wall and greater trochanteric involvement in a 37-year-old male; (E and F) Postoperative radiograph and CT scan demonstrating slight varus reduction of the fracture. Fixation of the near cortex with the cannulated screws was noted to be compromised by the lateral wall fracture; (G and H) Radiograph at 4 weeks postoperatively demonstrating further collapse and screw migration as well as early heterotopic ossification; (I to K) Anteroposterior and lateral, intraoperative and anteroposterior postoperative images after revision ORIF. After removal of the screws (including one bent screw inferiorly), a 135° sliding hip screw with side plate was utilized. Due to the lateral wall fracture, a trochanteric stabilization plate was used to prevent uncontrolled sliding. A slight valgus reduction was intentionally done to improve the biomechanics for healing, and a "derotational" screw was also placed through the plate.
Courtesy: Chinenye Nwachuku

within 24 hours) as well, but there are anatomical considerations that need to be accounted for and do not pertain to screw fixation. Firstly, the need for good-quality imaging is arguably more important. A proper AP pelvis image, lateral image of the affected hip, and full length images of the involved femur are important for several reasons. The AP pelvis image allows the surgeon to determine what the "normal" side looks like. The full length femur imaging is done to rule out any separate fracture lines or possibly lytic lesions or deformity in the femoral canal. Femoral canal diameter can also be measured. These are important for hemiarthroplasty because a femoral stem has to be placed down into the femoral canal, and the risk of periprosthetic fracture (early or late) can be minimized with an appreciation of femoral anatomy before hand.

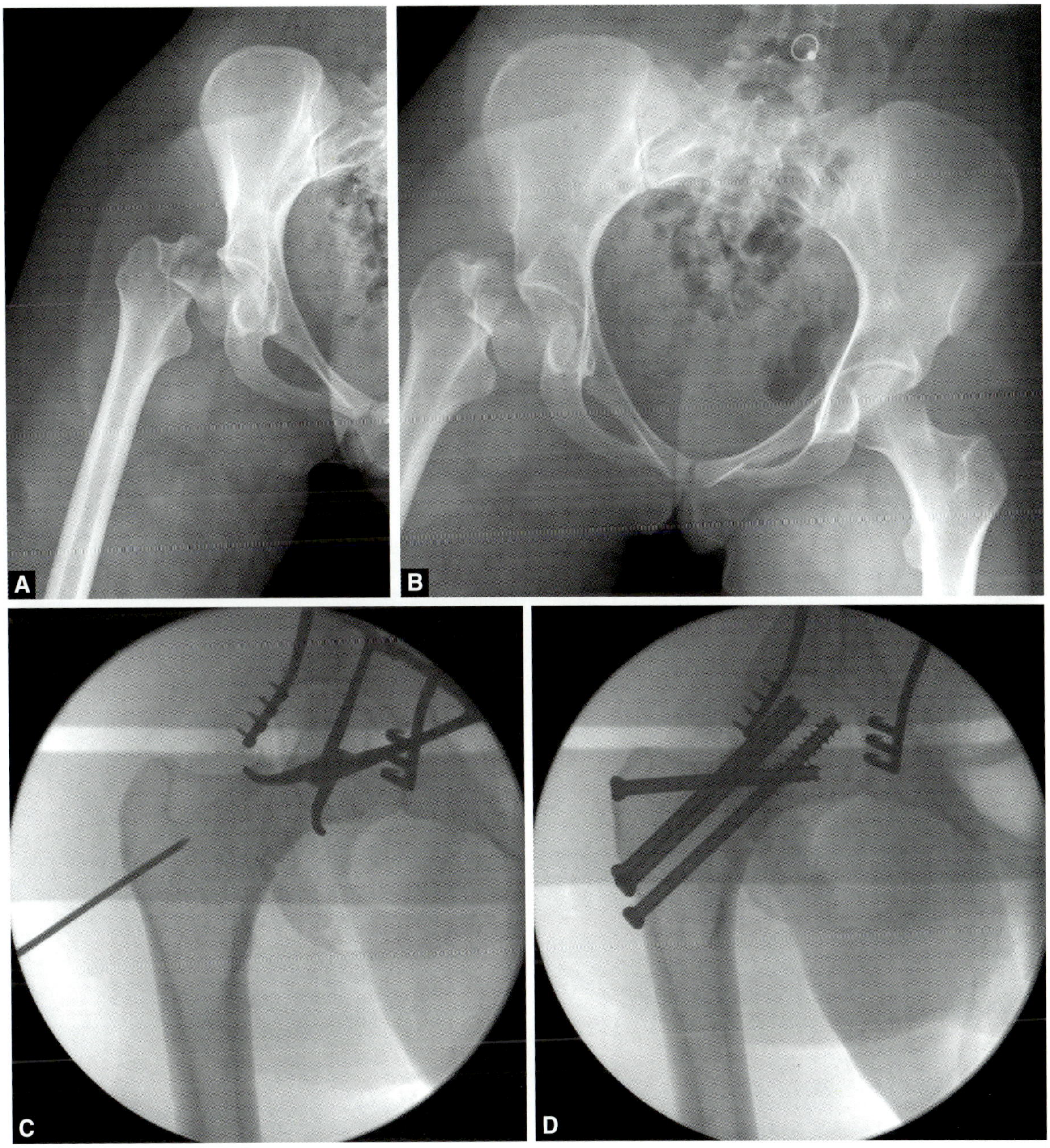

Figures 19.20A to D

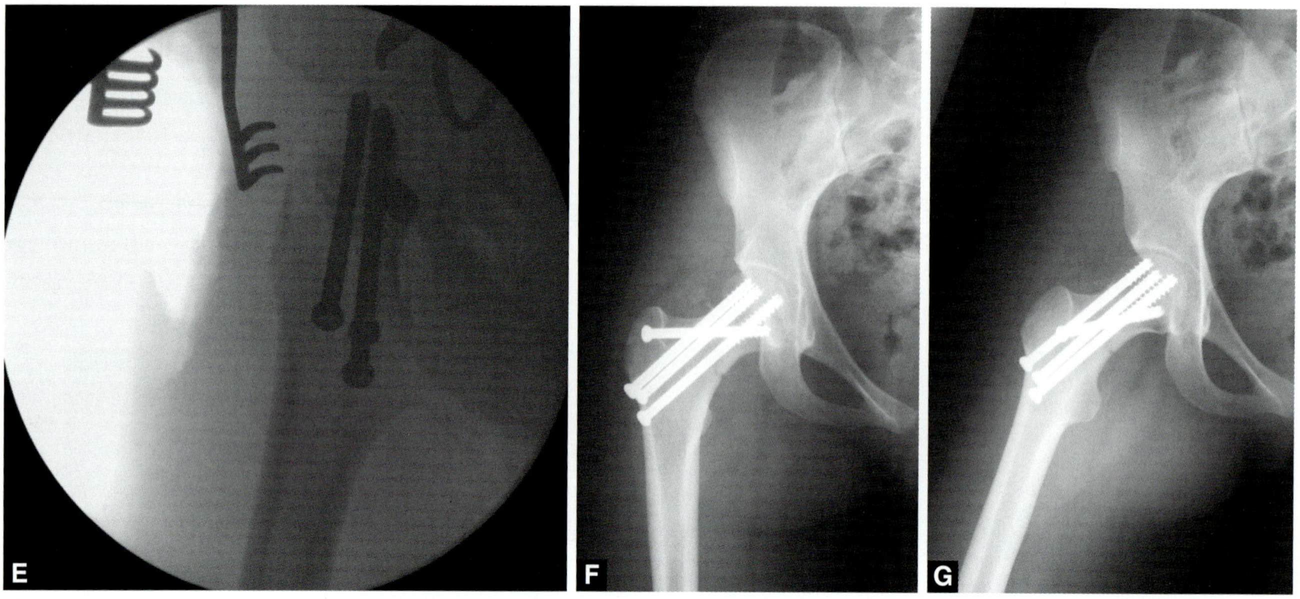

Figures 19.20A to G: Open reduction and internal fixation of a displaced femoral neck fracture. (A and B) Anteroposterior hip and anteroposterior pelvic radiographs in a 19-year-old female after a motor vehicle crash with a displaced femoral neck fracture; (C to E) A Smith-Petersen approach was done on a radiolucent table with skeletal traction applied through a tibial traction pin with the entire limb prepped into the field. After an open approach was done, the fracture was exposed and an open reduction of the fracture was performed as shown. Fluoroscopic images show the fracture well reduced with placement of multiple cannulated screws; (F and G) Postoperative radiographs demonstrate final fixation. One of the screws appears to be violating the superior cortex of the femoral neck although this was not apparent on intraoperative views. A more critical evaluation of multiple views of the femoral neck intraoperatively might have prevented this. Also, the three parallel screws could have ideally been placed at a slightly more horizontal angle in order to have a more proximal starting point on the lateral femur (to lessen the risk of late development of a subtrochanteric fracture).

Templating should be done in order to determine the location of the neck cut as well as the size of the proposed implants that will be utilized.

Instrumentation, Implants and Patient Positioning Considerations

Appropriate retractors for hip arthroplasty should be available. Instrumentation should include broaches, reamer and trial components and related instruments whichever are necessary for the particular hip implants. A power saw should also be available for making a neck cut. This same instrument should ideally be able to operate the calcar planer as well.

The surgical approach (anterior, anterolateral or posterior) as well as the patient positioning can be chosen based on surgeon preference. Patient positioning is either supine (for anterior approach) or lateral (for anterolateral or posterior approaches). For lateral positioning, either a beanbag or lateral positioning device is utilized.

Technique

Surgical approaches for arthroplasty of the hip are well described elsewhere. In this section, the authors will discuss only the posterior approach to the hip (See Figs 19.13A to F). The femoral head fragment is removed at this point and its diameter is sized for trial implant purposes. Based on preoperative templating, the neck cut is made accordingly with the sagittal saw. The following steps will vary depending on the implant manufacturer. But essentially, the canal finder is placed followed by curettage or the use of a "lateralizer" reamer or broach. At this point, calcar planning can be done followed by reaming, if needed. This is followed by broaching. Care is taken to maintain anatomic version during broaching. It is important for the assistant to maintain the rotation of the hip during broaching, which is best accomplished with having the lower leg perpendicular to the floor. After broaching is completed to the appropriate size, a trial stem and head is placed and the joint is reduced. Soft tissue tension is checked for either joint instability or excessive "tightness" by taking the hip through a range of motion including full hip extension with knee flexion and with gentle provocative maneuvers with internal rotation and adduction. Although leg lengths can be checked with the contralateral limb through the drapes, this method is somewhat inaccurate. Other than accurate preoperative templating with an accurate neck cut, there are other methods to ensure proper leg length equality when the case is over. This is a bit more difficult in cases of arthroplasty for femoral neck fracture than that for arthritic conditions. A portable radiograph can be taken with the trials in place if there is doubt regarding the implant position and neck cut. If necessary, the neck cut can be revised or trials can be changed as needed for sizing or soft tissue "balancing" purposes.

Once the appropriate trials are chosen, the joint is irrigated and preparations are made for implant insertion and assembly. If cement fixation has been chosen then a cement restrictor is placed to the appropriate depth, the canal is brushed, irrigated with a canal irrigator, and then dried with sponges. Cement is prepared with a vacuum method and inserted with a pressurized cement "gun." The authors generally use cement with tobramycin premixed. If uncemented fixation is chosen, then an implant with porous coating is inserted with a press-fit technique. With either method, care is taken to ensure proper placement with regard to depth, version (rotation) and varus/valgus alignment. Once femoral stem placement is completed (and cement is dried for cemented implants) then the head component is placed. This can be either a unipolar head or a bipolar head, which is assembled in two steps.

After the components are placed and assembled, the hip joint is reduced and soft tissue balancing is again assessed. The capsule and short external rotators are then repaired to the greater trochanter. A drain is placed at the discretion of the surgeon, and then the fascia lata is repaired followed by approximation of the subcutaneous tissues and skin closure. A low AP pelvic and lateral hip radiograph is then taken on the patient bed in the operating room to confirm joint reduction, proper implant placement, and lack of any periprosthetic fracture (Figs 19.21A to D and 19.22A to C). Leg lengths are checked clinically, and the patient is then awakened and taken to the post anesthesia recovery unit. Postoperatively, posterior hip precautions are employed (no hip adduction past midline, no internal rotation past neutral, no hip flexion beyond 90°). Weight bearing as tolerated with an assist device and supervision by a physical therapist is allowed.

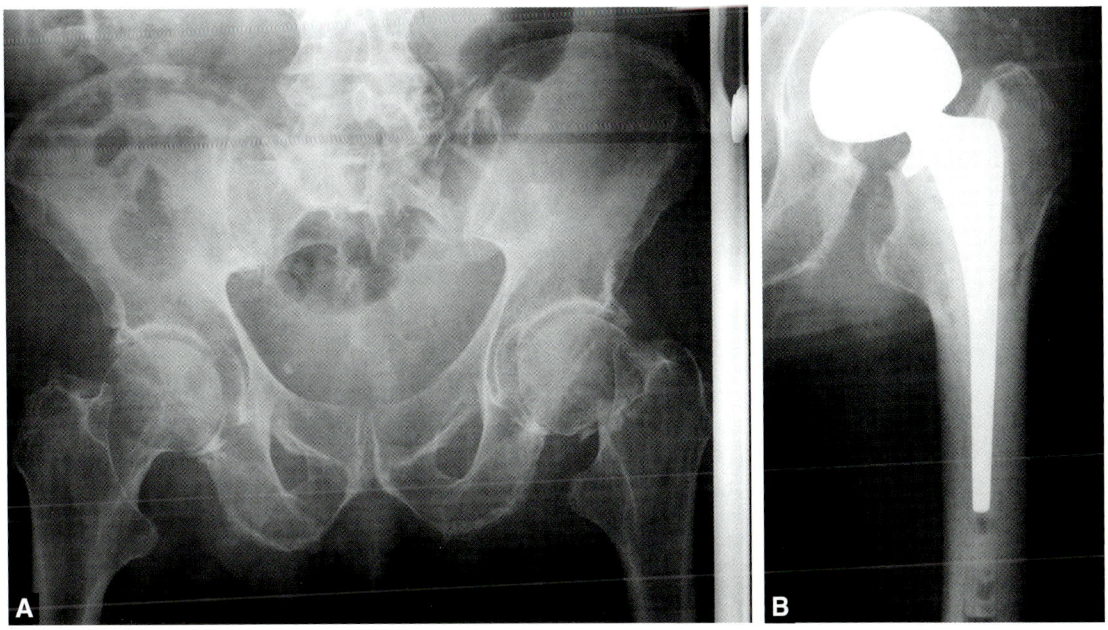

Figures 19.21A and B

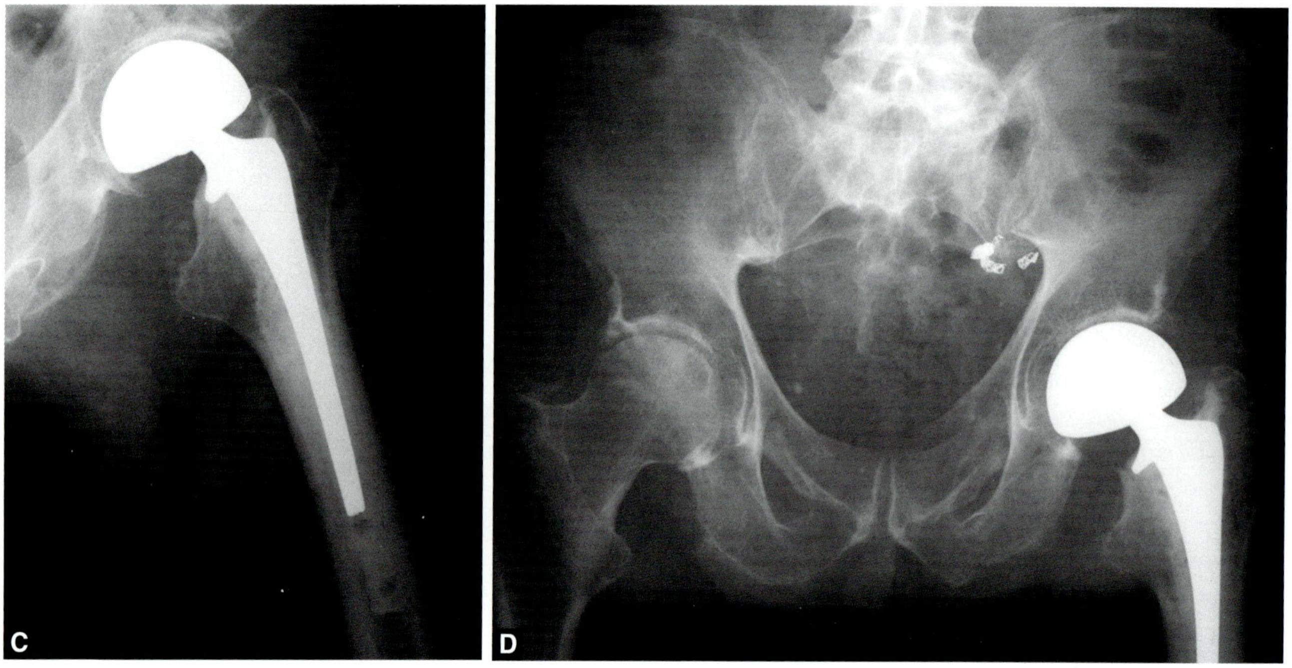

Figures 19.21A to D: Cemented hemiarthroplasty for treatment of a displaced femoral neck fracture in an elderly patient. (A) Anteroposterior pelvic radiograph demonstrating a displaced left femoral neck fracture in an elderly patient with osteoporosis after a low energy fall; (B to D) A cemented bipolar hemiarthroplasty was performed through a posterior approach. Postoperative radiographs demonstrate the implants in relatively good position with restoration of appropriate limb length.

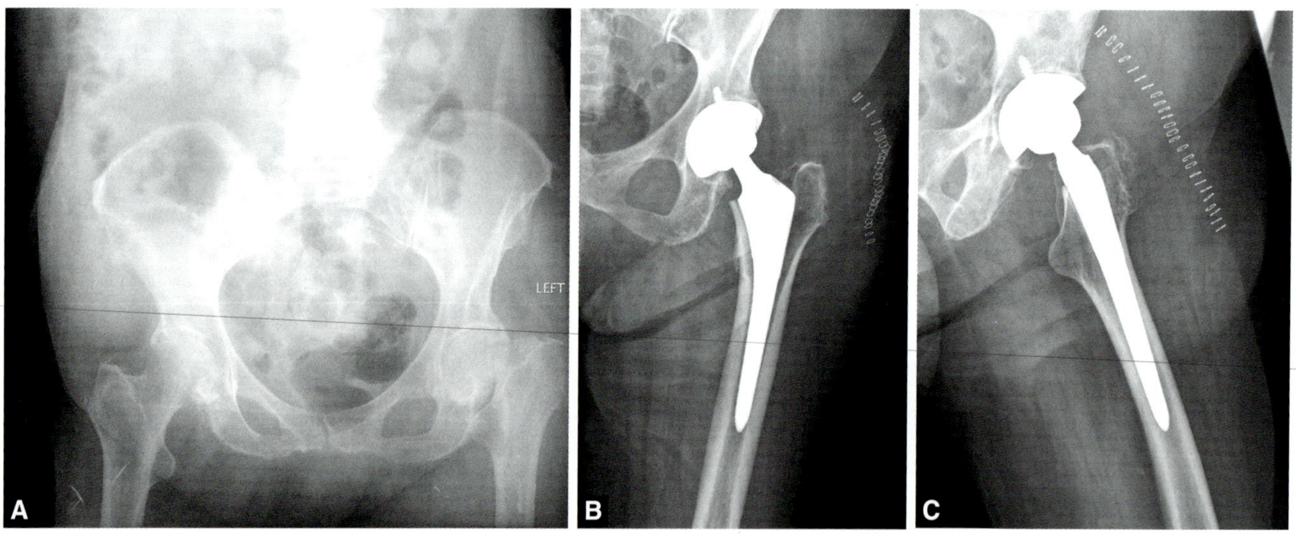

Figures 19.22A to C: Treatment of a displaced femoral neck fracture with total hip arthroplasty. (A) Anteroposterior pelvic radiograph demonstrating a displaced left femoral neck fracture in a relatively active 70-year-old female. A decision was made to do a total hip arthroplasty rather than hemiarthroplasty in order to avoid the risks of acetabular wear and subsequent protrusion of the component; (B and C) Postoperative radiographs of the hip demonstrating a noncemented total hip arthroplasty done through a posterior approach with components in good position.

HEMIARTHROPLASTY OF FEMORAL NECK FRACTURES: Pearls and Pitfalls

- Do not perform hemiarthroplasty in the "physiologically young" and active elderly patients or in young patients. If arthroplasty must be performed in these groups, total hip arthroplasty is preferable in order to prevent acetabular wear
- If a cementing technique is chosen for fixation of the stem, antibiotic cement (usually with tobramycin) is preferable
- Care must be taken to avoid periprosthetic femoral fractures particularly if a press fit technique is chosen for the femoral stem fixation. These are typically osteoporotic fractures, and iatrogenic fractures are possible if excessive force is used during instrumentation

Outcomes

Treatment of femoral neck fractures with reduction and internal fixation is well documented in the literature.[27-37] Union rates range from 61% to 100%. Quality of reduction is the most important factor influencing union rates.[33] A varus reduction of greater than 10° created a nonunion rate of 90% and initial displacement significantly decreases the union rates.[37]

Different types of implants used for fixation have also been compared. There is no apparent biomechanical advantage of using three cannulated screws versus a sliding hip screw with a side plate in certain models, although the sliding hip screw has shown an advantage in other models.[31] The sliding hip screw did have a higher blood loss and operative time, but some prefer this implant in osteoporotic bone.[38] Unfortunately, there is no evidence supporting the use of a fourth screw, but theoretically it may help in fractures with extensive posterior comminution. The use of a posterolateral femoral locking plate for femoral neck fractures was shown to have 7/18 catastrophic results.[35] Femoral neck fractures require compression for healing. The locked plate was excessively rigid, prevented compression and resulted in implant failure.

The position of the screws in the femoral neck can influence nonunion rates. One study showed that a larger distance between screws on the lateral view and placement of the middle screw more anterior increased union rates.[34] Navigational systems may help with accurate screw placement, but the clinical benefit has not been established.[28,29]

Internal fixation has been compared with arthroplasty for displaced femoral neck fractures in patients that were older than 60–70 years.[21-23] In patients who were independent and did not have cognitive impairment, total hip arthroplasty provided the best functional outcomes and highest satisfaction with their surgery. In patients with cognitive impairment, significantly greater benefit was gained from hemiarthroplasty over internal fixation.

Multiple outcome studies have been done to compare hemiarthroplasty with total hip arthroplasty.[1,39-42] The dislocation rate for total hip arthroplasty is significantly higher than hemiarthroplasty. Despite this, total hip arthroplasty is clearly superior in the independent, active patient. The Harris Hip Scores continue to increase past the 1st year after surgery in total hip arthroplasty groups while the Harris Hip Scores tend to level off at 1 year for hemiarthroplasty. Pain continued to be an issue in the hemiarthroplasty group, most likely due to acetabular erosion. The reoperation rate for hemiarthroplasty was significantly higher with conversion to total hip arthroplasty as the most common corrective procedure.

Complications

The major complications that result from the treatment of femoral neck fractures are nonunion and AVN of the femoral head. Infection is a risk with any surgical procedure. The infection rate for internal fixation is about 5% including superficial and deep infections.[43] For prosthetic replacement, the rate varies from 2–20%.[43] To avoid infections, sterile technique must be utilized at all times. Perioperative antibiotics must be used as well.

Nonunion rates are between 0–39%.[28-34,37] The cause of nonunion is multifactorial and infection must always be eliminated from the differential. The most important factor is the quality of reduction. In a study by Estrada et al. the nonunion rate was 70% with malreduction and 18% with adequate reduction.[44] To avoid malreduction, it is crucial to be aware of posterior comminution, avoid excessive reduction maneuvers and never accept a varus fragment configuration. If there is an ipsilateral femoral shaft fracture, there are two options. One can consider using two separate implants and fix the neck fracture first or a cephalomedullary nail can be used to fix both fractures simultaneously (Figs 19.23A to I). Inadequate fixation is another cause of nonunion.[44] A parallel configuration of screws and screw thread placement completely past the fracture site will allow for maximum compression. Starting the screw path at or above the lesser trochanter will help avoid creating a subtrochanteric fracture. If an intramedullary nail is used to treat an ipsilateral shaft fracture, a reconstruction screw configuration is ideal. Two screws will be in the head and neck, and earlier weight bearing is allowed because there is a shorter lever arm. Initial displacement is the last factor, but unfortunately it cannot be influenced by surgical intervention.

Avascular necrosis is a devastating complication, especially in the young patient. Disruption or distortion of the main blood supply of femoral head is the main cause and there are many factors that compromise this blood supply.[45] The most important is the initial displacement of the fracture. Avascular necrosis rates for nondisplaced fractures are between 5–8.5% and increase significantly to 29–35% with displacement.[43,45] Another factor is tamponade by hematoma. The role of capsulotomy is controversial, but experimental and clinical data suggest that increased blood flow occurs with hematoma evacuation.[45] Impaired venous outflow is also a proposed cause that may be alleviated with postoperative anticoagulants used in the prevention of deep vein thrombosis.[45] Reduction quality affects the AVN rates as well, increasing from 29–58% when the fracture is malreduced.[44] Time to surgery has implications in the development of AVN. Because initial displacement may "kink" the vessels, reducing the fracture in a timely manner may improve AVN rates.[43,45] Lastly, technical skill of the surgeon can decrease AVN rates. As with nonunion, reduction maneuvers must be executed in a controlled and cautious manner.[45]

Authors' Preferred Management of Select Complications

Case 1: Displaced Femoral Neck Fracture with Nonunion Treated with Total Hip Arthroplasty

When a femoral neck fracture goes onto a nonunion, multiple questions must be considered and answered: Is there an infection? Was the reduction and fixation poorly done? Does the patient have an endocrine disorder which needs to be addressed (such as diabetes or vitamin D deficiency)? Is the patient a smoker and

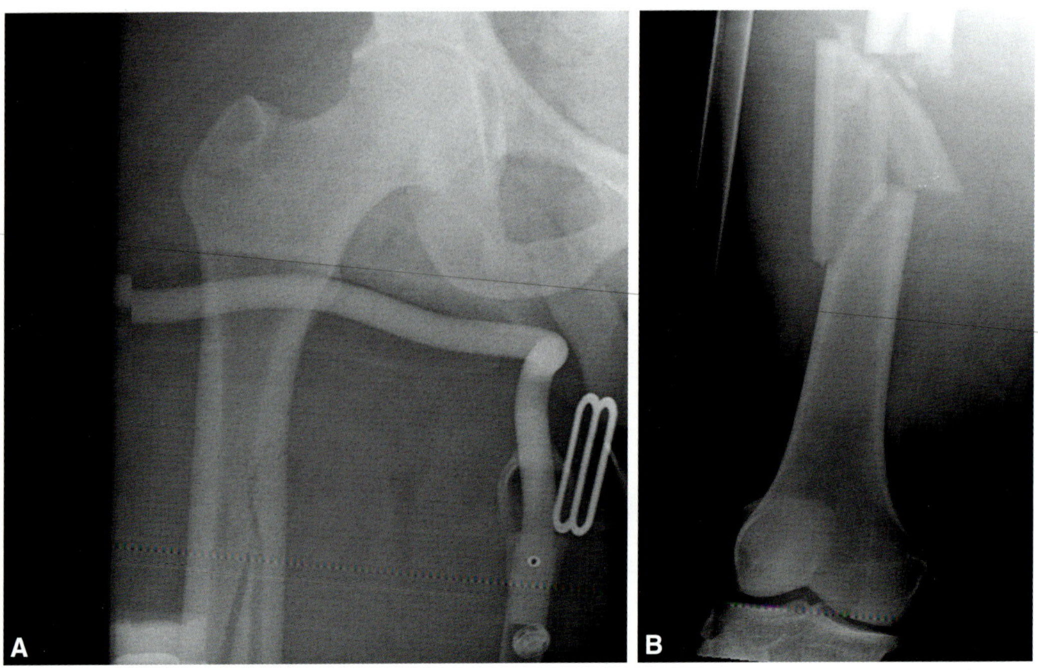

Figures 19.23A and B

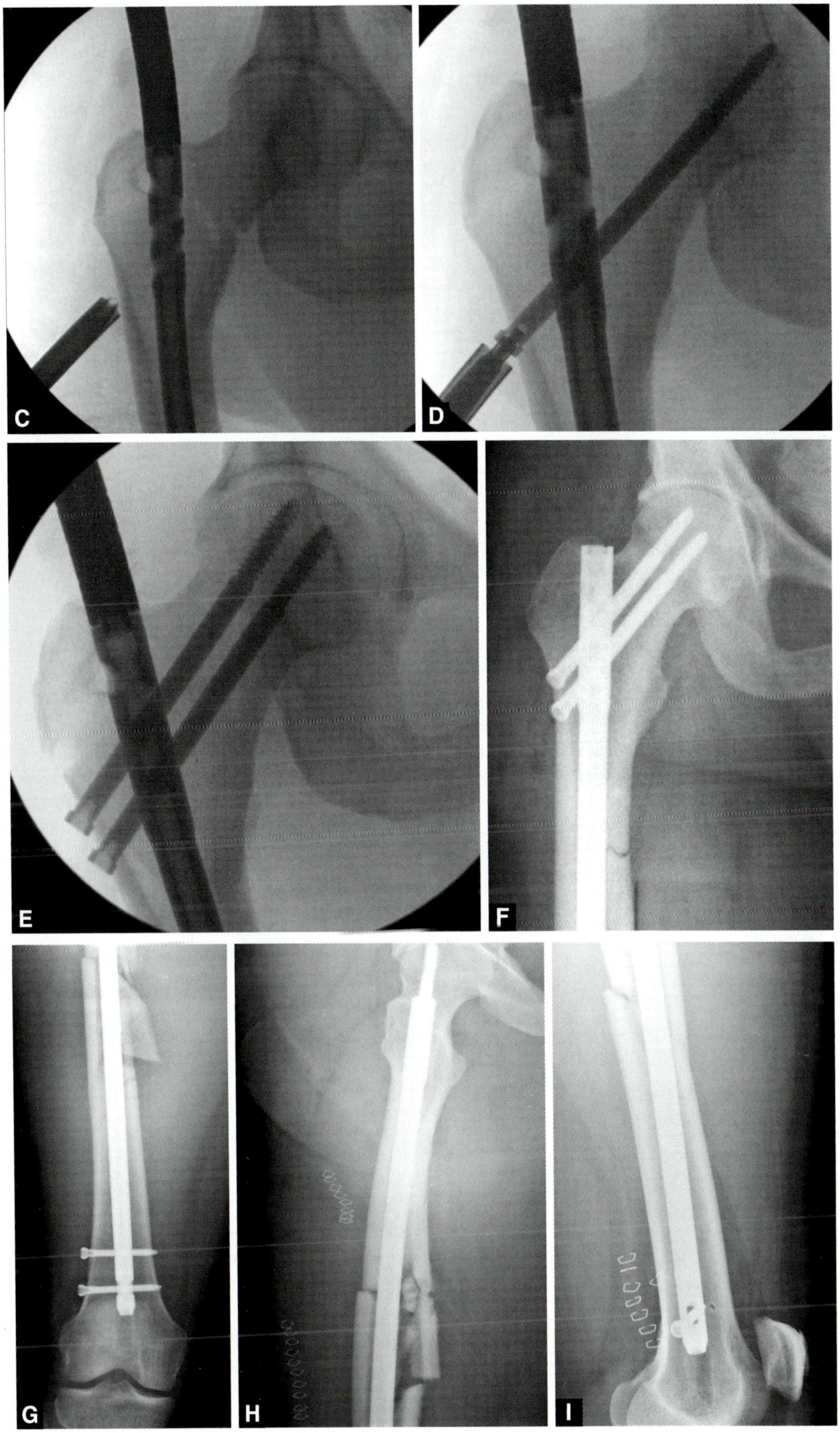

Figures 19.23A to I: Treatment of a missed or iatrogenic femoral neck fracture discovered during intramedullary nailing of a femoral shaft fracture. (A and B) Preoperative radiographs of a 42-year-old male with a right femoral shaft fracture and multiple trauma from a motor vehicle crash. There is no obvious femoral neck fracture; (C) During insertion of the femoral nail, a femoral neck fracture is clearly apparent and preparations for "reconstruction" locking screws into the femoral head are done. This particular implant fortunately allowed this option; (D and E) Sequential placement and tightening of two partially threaded screws demonstrated anatomic compression of the fracture; (F to I) Postoperative radiographs demonstrate excellent reduction of the femoral neck and shaft fractures. Open reduction of the femoral neck was therefore not necessary.

Courtesy: Jaimo Ahn

needs help to quit? These are similar questions one must answer when dealing with almost any nonunion. Once these are considered and addressed, the surgeon must now answer other questions to further narrow down the course of action. How old is the patient, and what are their functional demands? Is the patient going to tolerate additional future surgeries if your revision fails? The surgeon must also ask himself/herself: What are my capabilities with regard to either nonunion repair or arthroplasty, and should this patient be referred to a colleague? Essentially, the age and activity level of the patient is the dominant factor in determining one of the two broad courses of action: either total hip arthroplasty or intertrochanteric valgus osteotomy and revision fixation. In this case, the former option was pursued after considering all of these questions.

A 58-year-old gentleman sustained a displaced left femoral neck fracture after a fall (Figs 19.24A and B). He underwent emergent ORIF through an anterolateral Watson-Jones approach (Figs 19.24C to F). Screw fixation was performed, and reduction appeared to be satisfactory, but perhaps not perfectly anatomic due to posterior comminution. There appeared to be clustering of the screws posteriorly possibly causing asymmetric compression with gapping of the fracture anteriorly. He was initially not weight bearing for 3 months and then was allowed to progress weight bearing at that point.

Unfortunately, he continued to have hip pain and was unable to wean from crutches or a cane at 11 months. Radiographs suggested a possible nonunion although there were no broken screws and only slight collapse (Figs 19.24G and H). CT scanning was done to confirm this and a nonunion was confirmed (Figs 19.24I and J). An infection workup was done including blood work (erythrocyte sedimentation rate and C-reactive protein) and a nuclear medicine scan. All tests were negative for infection. He was a nonsmoker and an endocrine workup was negative. An operative biopsy or joint aspiration was not done although these could have been considered as well to rule out an occult infection.

At this point, treatment options for either nonunion repair versus total hip arthroplasty were discussed with the patient. Nonunion repair with a valgus osteotomy was considered as a treatment option. However, the authors felt that at age 58 with a relatively sedentary lifestyle, total hip arthroplasty was a good definitive treatment option. He had a previous Watson-Jones anterolateral approach, but the authors felt that satisfactory exposure could be achieved with a posterior approach and the abductors could be spared. Therefore, he agreed to go ahead with the total hip arthroplasty.

Surgery was performed in the lateral position and a posterior approach to the hip. The screws were removed without difficulty. An extensive capsular release was necessary in order to dislocate the hip which was perhaps the most tedious part of the case. After this, the usual steps of total hip arthroplasty with noncemented components and highly crosslinked polyethylene were performed (Figs 19.24K and L). He was doing well at 3 years postoperatively thus far.

Total hip arthroplasty would not have been considered if he was much younger. One could certainly make the case that he could have also benefited from an osteotomy at his age of 58. Nevertheless, the authors believe that this was a good choice for him and would be for similar cases.

The key points of this case are as follows:

- Although timely treatment of a displaced femoral neck fracture might help to prevent osteonecrosis, fracture healing is more dependent on anatomic fracture reduction. Even slight posterior comminution, as in this case, can be a cause for concern and potentially lead to nonunion.
- Total hip arthroplasty is a viable treatment option in the 50–60 year old age group, though intertrochanteric osteotomy is also a good option.
- Be prepared for an extensive capsulotomy and releases when converting a previous ORIF to a total hip arthroplasty.

Cases 2 and 3: Treatment of Femoral Neck Nonunion with Valgus Osteotomy and Angled Blade Plate Fixation

Courtesy: Stephen Kottmeier

Femoral neck nonunions in young patients are classically treated with valgus osteotomy and angled blade plate fixation. The essential problem with most of these nonunions is the vertical nature of the fracture, particularly the Pauwels type 3. The crux of the procedure is to convert this shearing into compression by creating wedge, valgus osteotomy. Although elegant in its concept, this is a technically demanding procedure which requires careful preoperative templating and planning.

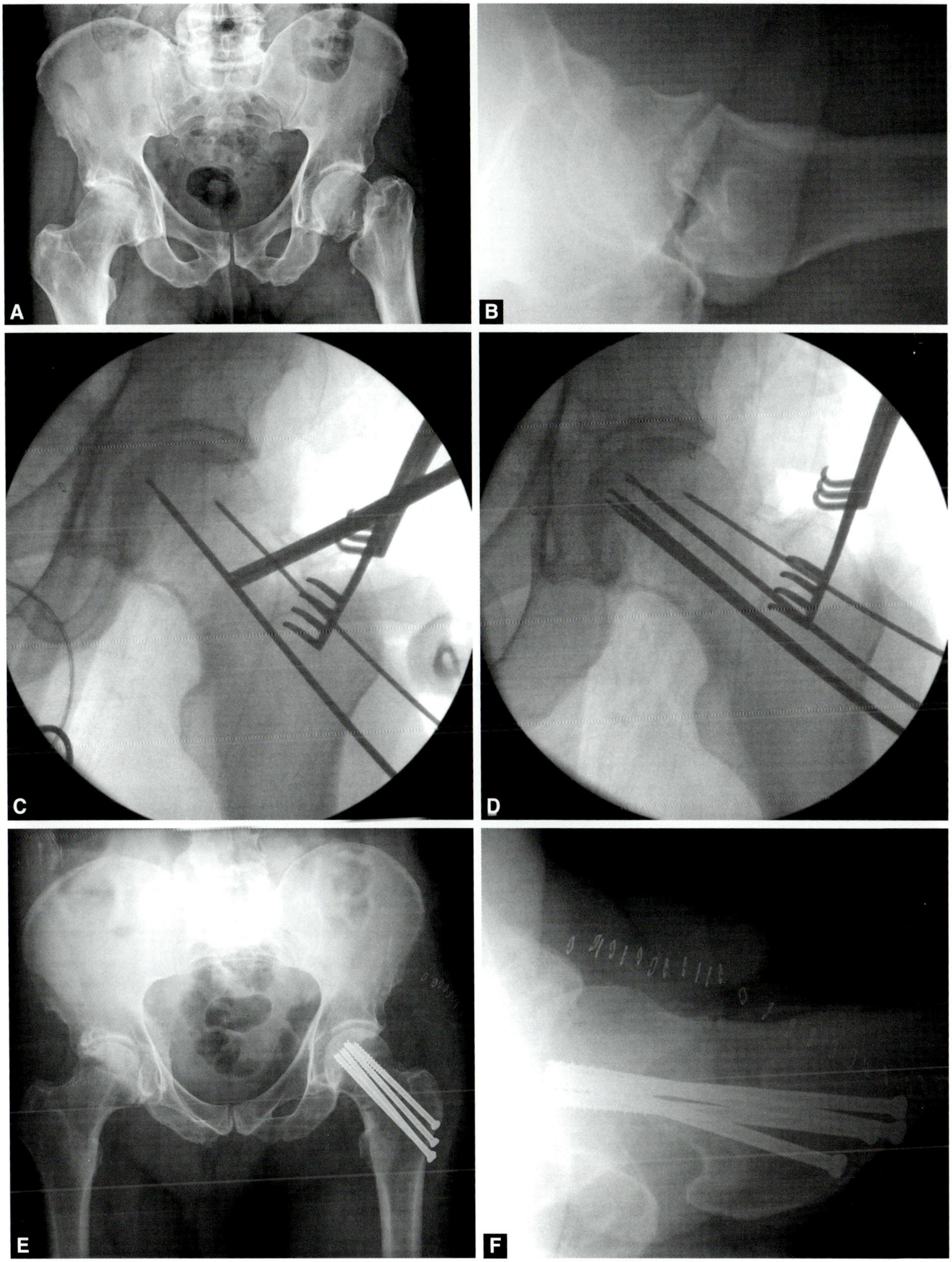

Figures 19.24A to F

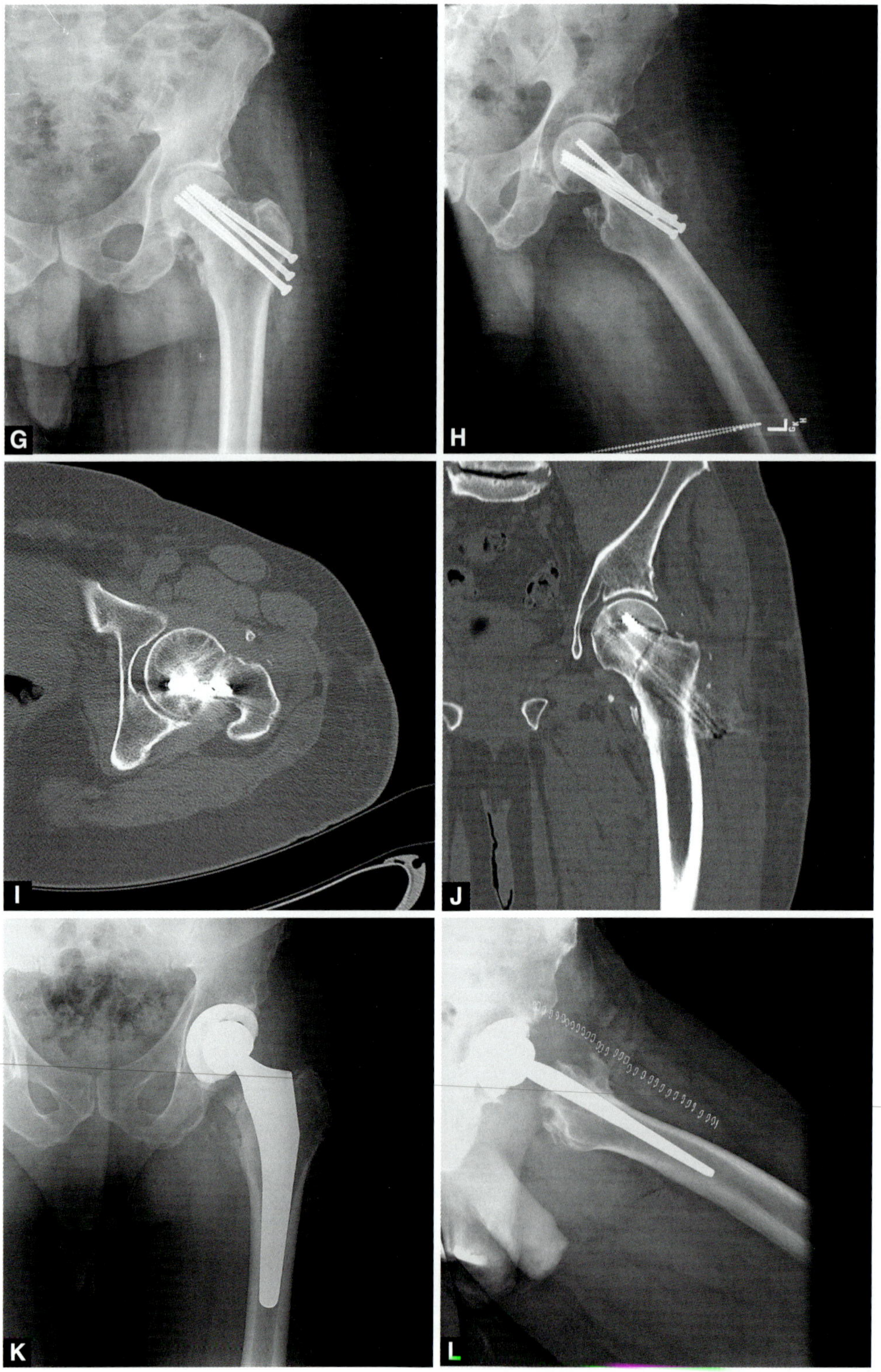

Figures 19.24A to L: Treatment of a femoral neck nonunion with total hip arthroplasty (see text for details). (A and B) Radiographs of a 58-year-old man with a displaced femoral neck fracture; (C and D) Intraoperative images of an emergent open reduction and internal fixation with a Watson-Jones approach and cannulated screws; (E and F) Postoperative radiographs after ORIF; (G and H) Nonunion at 11 months as seen on radiographs; (I and J) CT scan images; (K and L) Radiographs after noncemented total hip arthroplasty done through a posterior approach.

Case 2 involves a 59-year-old male with a femoral shaft fracture who was treated with antegrade intramedullary nailing (Fig. 19.25A). A preoperative CT scan did not demonstrate any evidence of a femoral neck fracture. Nevertheless, a vertical femoral neck fracture was noted postoperatively (Figs 19.25B to D). It is unclear whether or not the fracture was missed by the CT scan (a known phenomenon) or was a complication of femoral nailing procedure itself. This was treated with cannulated screw fixation with retention of the antegrade femoral nail (Figs 19.25E to G). Unfortunately, this did not heal and resulted in a nonunion of the femoral neck although the femoral shaft healed (Fig. 19.25H). A decision was made to proceed with femoral nail removal and a valgus intertrochanteric osteotomy with angled blade plate fixation (Figs 19.25I to L). With the more favorable biomechanics with the valgus alignment, the fracture went on to heal (Figs 19.25M and N). The patient subsequently did well with excellent return to function.

In case 3, a 56-year-old female equestrian sustained a displaced femoral neck fracture which was initially treated with cannulated screw fixation. This went on to nonunion and was mistakenly treated by the referring surgeon with removal of the implants because it was assumed that the symptoms were due to painful implants (Fig. 19.26A). However, it became quite clear at this point that there was a nonunion and the patient was referred for treatment. At this point, an MRI scan was done in an attempt to determine the viability of the femoral head (Figs 19.26B and C). The imaging was, in fact, interpreted as demonstrative of viability of the femoral head, and a decision was made to move forward with valgus intertrochanteric osteotomy with blade plate fixation (Fig. 19.26D). This was done in a similar manner to that in case 2, although an additional cortical screw was used as well. Both the femoral neck nonunion as well as the osteotomy went on to heal (Figs 19.26E and F).

The key points of these cases are as follows:

- Careful preoperative planning is necessary to properly execute a valgus intertrochanteric osteotomy for nonunion of the femoral neck. The procedure's success lies in the concept of converting the shearing forces at the femoral neck into compressive forces.
- Even with preoperative CT scanning, nondisplaced femoral neck fractures can be missed. Therefore, proper radiographs of the hip postoperatively should be done after femoral nailing to rule this out.

Case 4: Treatment of a Subtrochanteric Femur Fracture as a Complication of Femoral Neck Pinning

Courtesy: Jaimo Ahn

Careful placement of cannulated screws for fixation of femoral neck fractures is important both to achieve satisfactory fixation and also to avoid iatrogenic fractures. Triangular placement of the screws in a periphery of the femoral neck improves fixation and prevents inferior translation of the head. Multiple cortical perforations, particularly below the level of the lesser trochanter, are risks for late subtrochanteric femur fracture. If a fracture occurs, surgical management often requires removal of previous implants, and either antegrade femoral nailing or plate fixation of the proximal femur. In this particular case, the pins were not placed too inferior, but a multiplicity of pins might have been a risk for a fracture to occur at the subtrochanteric level. Regardless, this case does make the point that subtrochanteric fractures can occur in the setting of previous pinning for a femoral neck fracture.

An 86-year-old female with a previous history of left femoral neck pinning, right hip nailing and multiple medical problems was referred from another hospital after a low-energy fall resulting in a left subtrochanteric femur fracture (See Figs 19.16A and B). The original pinning procedure involved the use of six Knowles pins as shown and was done in the 1980s. It is presumed that this fracture most likely occurred due to the multiplicity of pins and possibly additional drill holes along the lateral cortex approaching the subtrochanteric region. In this particular case, the patient had done fine for approximately 30 years so it may be unfair to call this iatrogenic and the fracture could be coincidentally adjacent to the pins. But it nevertheless brings up the teaching point as described in "Technique 1" above: screws should not enter the lateral cortex distal to the lesser trochanter, and multiple perforations into the lateral cortex at and below the level of the lesser trochanter is also a risk for late fracture. The subtrochanteric femur fracture can be treated with intramedullary nailing or plate fixation. In this particular case, cephalomedullary nail fixation was performed with retention of two of the original Knowles pins (See Figs 19.16C to F). The posterior and central pins had to be removed to allow passage of

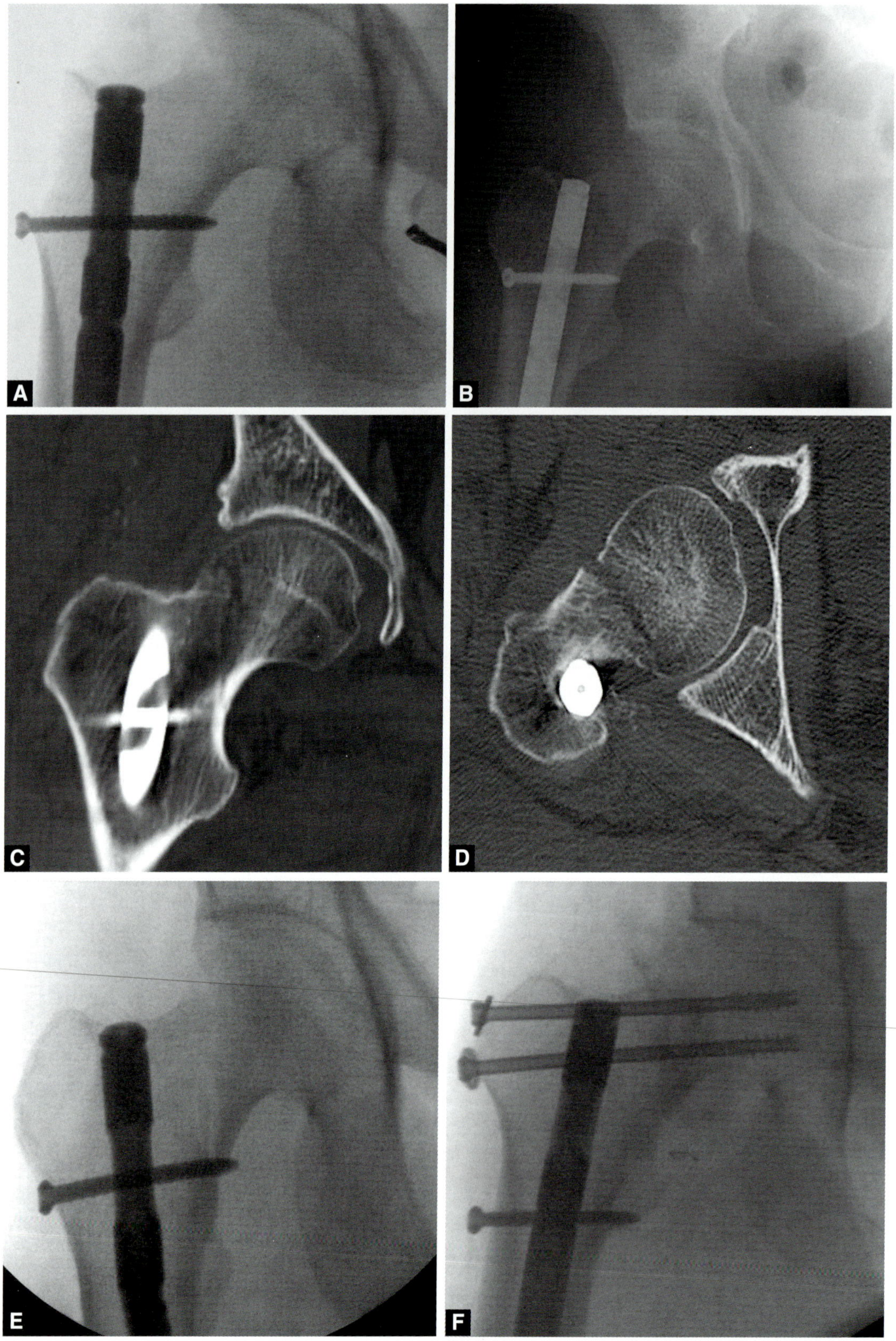

Figures 19.25A to F

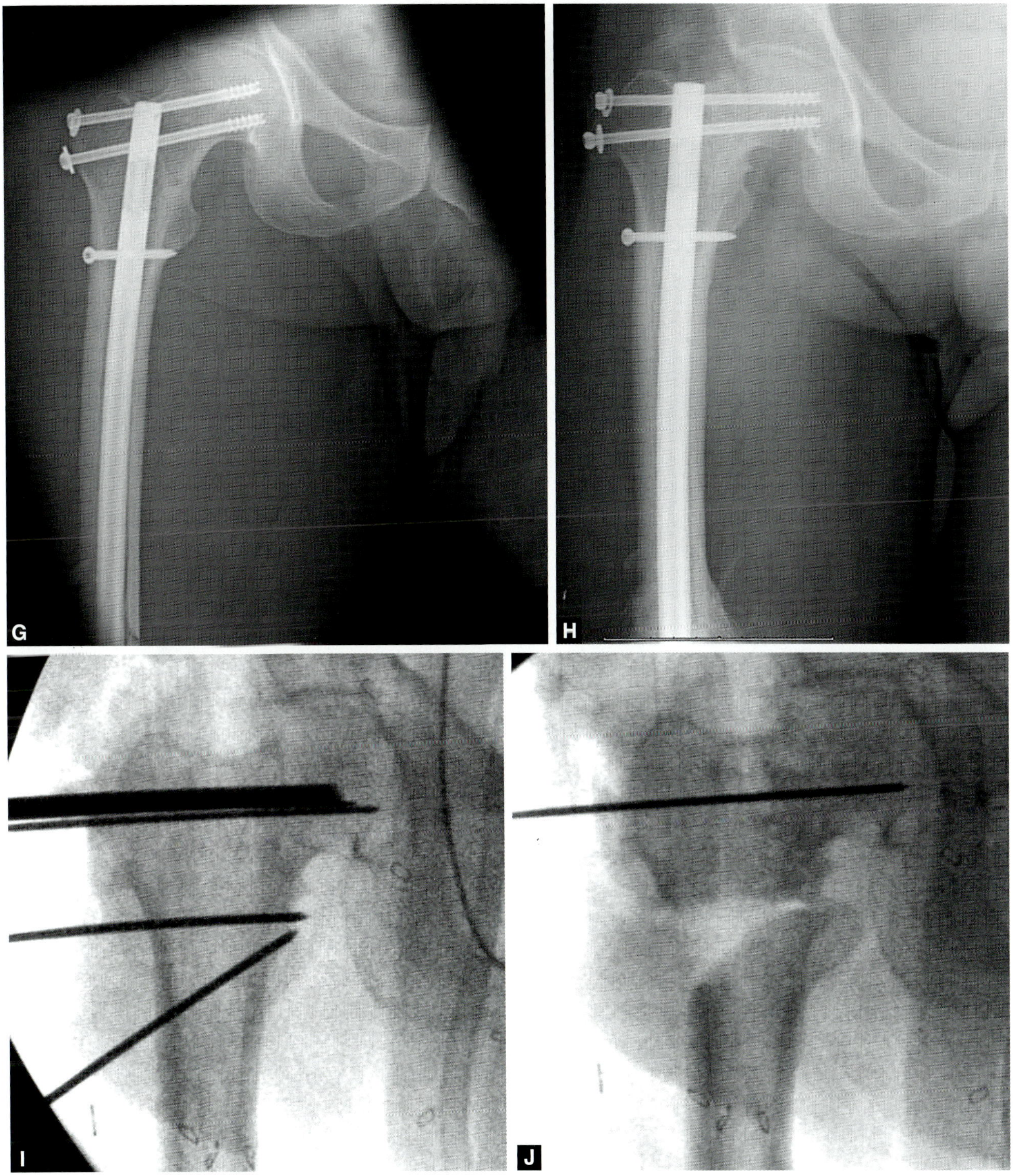

Figures 19.25G to J

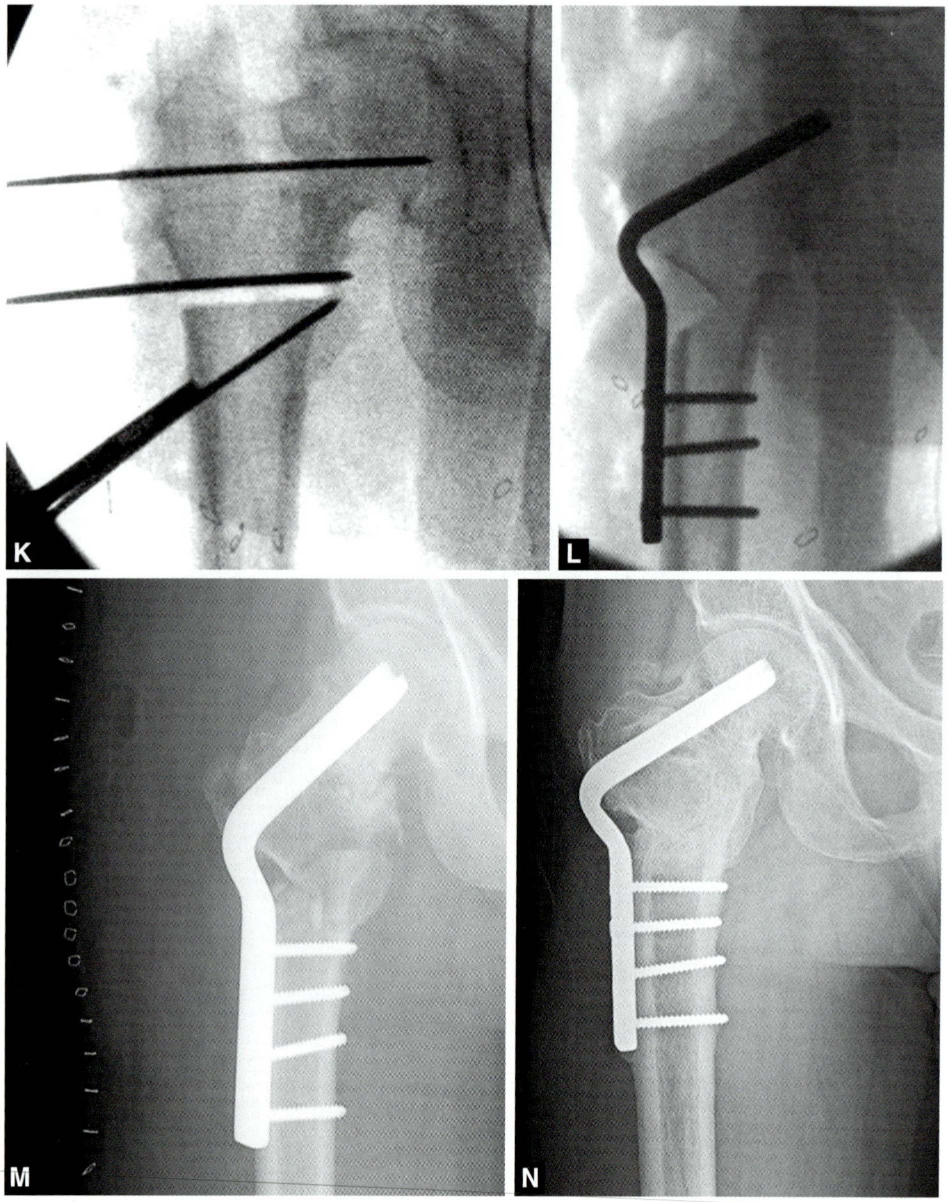

Figures 19.25A to N: Treatment of a femoral neck nonunion with valgus intertrochanteric osteotomy and angled blade plate fixation. (A) Intraoperative fluoroscopic image of the hip after antegrade intramedullary nailing in a 59-year-old male; (B) A postoperative radiograph shows a nondisplaced vertical femoral neck fracture. Note that preoperative CT scan images did not show evidence of a fracture; (C and D) Postoperative CT images demonstrate a minimally displaced vertical (Pauwels type 3) femoral neck fracture; (E and F) The patient was taken to surgery for cannulated screw fixation around the existing antegrade femoral nail. An intraoperative image now more clearly shows the fracture followed by demonstration of parallel screw fixation perpendicular to the fracture line; (G and H) Although a postoperative radiograph demonstrates satisfactory alignment, the fracture did go on to collapse in varus. The femoral neck fracture eventually went on to nonunion although the femoral shaft fracture healed. At this point, the femoral neck nonunion was treated with valgus intertochanteric osteotomy. The femoral nail was also removed; (I) Wires are placed in accordance to preoperative templating measurements. Here, the chisel for the blade is demonstrated as well; (J) The proximal cut of the osteotomy is complete and the osteotome for the inferior cut is shown here; (K) The osteotomy is complete and ready for correction with valgus and translation; (L) The angled blade is inserted first, followed by angular correction and slight translation. Cortical screws are then placed with dynamic compression across the osteotomy; (M and N) Postoperative and final follow-up radiographs demonstrate excellent alignment and eventual healing of the osteotomy as well as the femoral neck nonunion.

Courtesy: Stephen Kottmeier

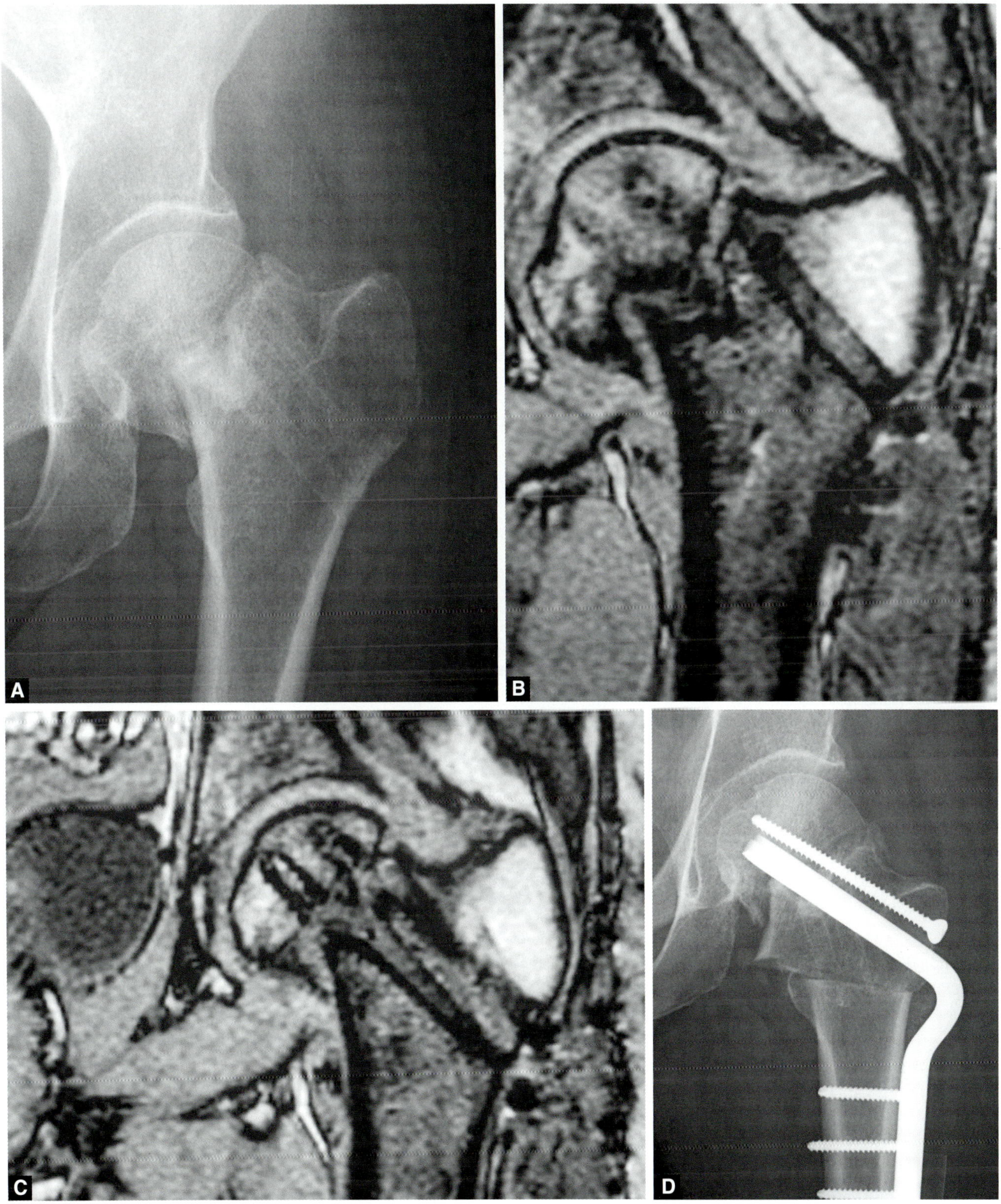

Figures 19.26A to D

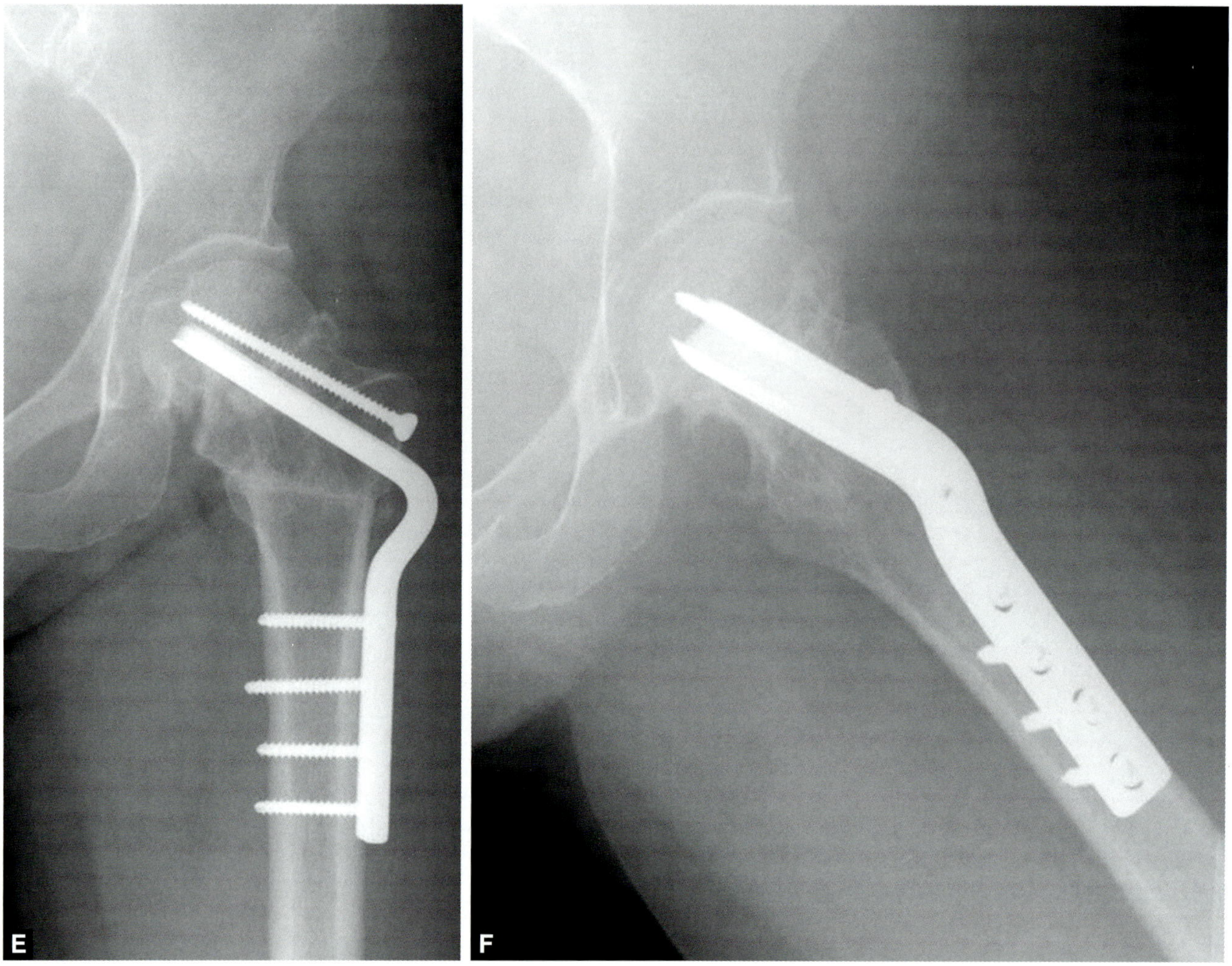

Figures 19.26A to F: Treatment of a femoral neck nonunion with valgus intertrochanteric osteotomy and angled blade plate fixation. (A) A 56-year-old female with a displaced femoral neck fracture initially treated with cannulated screws. Implants had been removed by referring surgeon. A nonunion is demonstrated; (B and C) MRI images are interpreted to demonstrate viability of the femoral head; (D) Intertrochanteric valgus osteotomy and blade plate fixation is performed as in Figure 19.25; (E and F) At final follow-up, the osteotomy and femoral neck nonunion have both healed.
Courtesy: Stephen Kottmeier

the nail, and the anterior pins were kept in place for protecting against further intraoperative iatrogenic fracture comminution. The 90° blade here was chosen in order to provide fixation into the inferior part of the femoral head and avoid multiple screw tracks proximally in the head.

The key points of this case are as follows:

- Subtrochanteric fractures after femoral neck pinning are often iatrogenic. They are preventable in most cases by avoiding multiple cortical perforations laterally and not allowing pins to be placed distal to the lesser trochanter.
- When treating the subtrochanteric femur fracture, fixation into the femoral head might be compromised by the previous screws. Therefore, injectable bone-cement materials (such as hydroxyapatite or tricalcium phosphate materials) in the old screw tracks or a completely different screw/blade trajectory might be needed.

Case 5: Loss of Fixation of Femoral Neck Fracture Treated with Screws, Revised with Sliding Hip Screw

Courtesy: Chinenye Nwachuku

Fixation of femoral neck fractures can be difficult to achieve in cases of osteoporosis or comminution.

Although cannulated screws alone work in many cases, sliding hip screw devices are potentially biomechanically superior and can be helpful in more challenging cases. Fixation is also compromised by even subtle varus alignment after ORIF. Early loss of fixation requires the surgeon to take a detached, critical look at the initial reduction and fixation to determine if either the reduction or the fixation was suboptimal and can be improved. Whereas a total hip arthroplasty is a good salvage option in an older patient, a younger patient would require revision ORIF. In this particular case, extreme comminution, including lateral wall comminution, compromised fixation along with slight varus malalignment, allowed for early loss of reduction and fixation.

A 37-year-old male involved in a motor vehicle crash sustained multiple trauma including a displaced, comminuted Pauwels type 3 femoral neck fracture with lateral wall and greater trochanteric involvement as well (See Figs 19.19A to D). Unfortunately, he was unable to undergo surgery initially due to persistent hemodynamic instability from a liver laceration. On hospital day 5, he underwent open reduction and internal fixation through an anterior Smith-Petersen approach (See Figs 19.19E and F). Fixation was performed with multiple cannulated screws placed through a separate short lateral incision. Screw purchase laterally was felt to be somewhat compromised due to lateral cortical fractures as seen on the imaging. Critical evaluation of the reduction and fixation shows that there is slight varus malalignment. The patient recovered well, then was seen at 4 weeks postoperatively with complaints of a limb length discrepancy. Unfortunately, radiographs at this point demonstrated loss of reduction with migration of one screw through the articular surface of the femoral head (See Figs 19.19G and H). Heterotopic ossification was also noted as seen in this image.

At this point, treatment options were discussed and it was determined that revision ORIF would be necessary. A sliding hip screw construct was planned preoperatively. In addition, a trochanteric stabilization plate was planned in order to prevent uncontrolled collapse due to fracture of the lateral wall. An intramedullary nail is also an option, particularly because of the lateral wall fracture, but reaming and placement of a nail essentially through the fracture site can be fraught with difficulties including lateralization of the distal fragments. Locked plate fixation was considered, but the current evidence is not in favor of locked plate fixation for the treatment of femoral neck fractures. Unacceptable rates of failure have been reported and it was felt that a sliding hip screw would provide fixed angle stability with controlled compression.

At revision surgery, one of the inferior screws was noted to be bent. This also raised the suspicion of early (noncompliant) weight bearing by the patient as another contributor to failure. The patient was positioned supine on a fracture table with traction attachments. The surgical approach utilized the previous lateral incision (but not the anterior incision) and extended this into a Watson-Jones anterolateral approach. Reduction was achieved both with traction and with the plate itself. The guide pin was placed centrally in the femoral head, followed by a "derotational" pin to prevent spinning of the head with reaming. After the lag screw was placed centrally in the head using the 135° angled guide, valgus reduction was created with bringing the plate to the shaft with the clamp and then screw fixation. A trochanteric stabilization plate was then added and an additional "derotational" screw was added through the plate (See Figs 19.19I to K). Satisfactory alignment and improved fixation was noted at this point.

The key points of this case are the following:

- Comminuted femoral neck fractures, particularly with lateral wall involvement, cannot be reliably fixed with cannulated screws alone. A sliding hip screw device should be strongly considered.
- In cases of lateral wall involvement, a trochanteric stabilization plate must be used in conjunction with the sliding hip screw device. In intertrochanteric fractures (including basicervical femoral neck fractures), cases involving lateral wall fractures can also be treated with an intramedullary device.
- Varus alignment is not only poorly tolerated by most patients but also is a risk for nonunion and should therefore be avoided.

Summary

Femoral neck fractures continue to be a surgical challenge. Patient factors, such as chronological and physiologic age, activity level and medical comorbidities, will influence the type of surgical intervention. Fracture classification and fragment configuration will also aid in the surgical planning process. There are multiple surgical approaches so a thorough understanding of hip joint anatomy is vital for successful outcomes. A number of implants are available for internal fixation, but cannulated screws or a sliding hip screw are most commonly used. Anatomic or slightly valgus fracture reduction is vital for decreasing nonunion and AVN rates. In the physiologically young or elderly patients, arthroplasty should be considered in displaced femoral neck fractures because of the high reoperation rates with internal fixation in these age groups. If nonunion should occur, an infection workup must be done. Chronologically young patients should undergo a femoral head sparing procedure such as a valgus osteotomy to decrease the fracture line inclination and convert shearing to compressive forces. Arthroplasty is the treatment of choice for nonunion in the physiological young and elderly population. Avascular necrosis in the chronologically young can also be treated with an osteotomy to off load the necrotic portion of the femoral head. In the physiologically young and elderly patient population, arthroplasty is again the treatment of choice. Hemiarthroplasty should be reserved for the low demand elderly patient or a patient with a cognitive impairment or neurological disorder.

References

1. Liao L, Zhao JM, Su W, et al. A meta-analysis of total hip arthroplasty and hemiarthroplasty outcomes for displaced femoral neck fractures. Arch Orthop Trauma Surg. 2012:1-9.
2. Macaulay W, Pagnotto MR, Iorio R, et al. Displaced femoral neck fractures in the elderly: hemiarthroplasty versus total hip arthroplasty. J Am Acad Orthop Surg. 2006;14(5):287-93.
3. DeLaMora SN, Gilbert M. Introduction of intracapsular hip fractures: anatomy and pathologic features. Clin Orthop Relat Res. 2002;399:9-16.
4. Bartonícek J, Vlcek E. Femoral neck fracture–the cause of death of Emperor Charles IV. Arch Orthop Trauma Surg. 2001;121(6):353-4.
5. Bartonícek J. Proximal femur fractures: the pioneer era of 1818 to 1925. Clin Orthop Relat Res. 2004;419:306-10.
6. Ly TV, Swiontkowski MF. Treatment of femoral neck fractures in young adults. J Bone Joint Surg Am. 2008;90(10):2254-66.
7. Tornetta III P, Kain MS, Creevy WR. Diagnosis of femoral neck fractures in patients with a femoral shaft fracture improvement with a standard protocol. J Bone Joint Surg Am. 2007;89(1):39-43.
8. Caviglia HA, Osorio PQ, Comando D. Classification and diagnosis of intracapsular fractures of the proximal femur. Clin Orthop Relat Res. 2002;399:17-27.
9. Blundell CM, Parker MJ, Pryor GA, et al. Assessment of the AO classification of intracapsular fractures of the proximal femur. J Bone Joint Surg Br. 1998;80:679-83.
10. Zlowodzki M, Bhandari M, Keel M, et al. Perception of Garden's classification for femoral neck fractures: an international survey of 298 orthopaedic trauma surgeons. Arch Orthop Trauma Surg. 2005;125(7):503-5.
11. Frandsen PA, Andersen E, Madsen F, et al. Garden's classification of femoral neck fractures. An assessment of inter-observer variation. J Bone Joint Surgy Br. 1988;70(4):588-90.
12. Oakes DA, Jackson KR, Davies MR, et al. The impact of the garden classification on proposed operative treatment. Clin Orthop Relat Res. 2003;409:232-40.
13. Thomsen NO, Jensen CM, Skovgaard N, et al. Observer variation in the radiographic classification of fractures of the neck of the femur using Garden's system. Int Orthop. 1996;20(5):326-9.
14. Van Embden D, Rhemrev SJ, Genelin F, et al. The reliability of a simplified Garden classification for intracapsular hip fractures. Orthop Traumay Surg Res. 2012;98(4):405-8
15. Beimers L, Kreder HJ, Berry GK, et al. Subcapital hip fractures: the Garden classification should be replaced, not collapsed. Can J Surg. 2002;45(6):411-4.
16. van Embden D, Roukema G, Rhemrev S, et al. The Pauwels classification for intracapsular hip fractures: is it reliable? Injury. 2011;42(11):1238-40.
17. Parker MJ, Dynan Y. Is Pauwels classification still valid? Injury. 1998;29(7):521-3.
18. Bhandari M, Devereaux PJ, Tornetta P, et al. Operative Management of Displaced Femoral Neck Fractures in Elderly Patients. An International Survey. J Bone Joint Surg Am. 2005;87(9):2122-30.
19. Shuqiang M, Kunzheng W, Zhichao T, et al. Outcome of non-operative management in Garden I femoral neck fractures. Injury. 2006;37(10):974-8.
20. Verheyen CC, Smulders TC, van Walsum AD. High secondary displacement rate in the conservative treatment of impacted femoral neck fractures in 105 patients. Arch Orthop Trauma Surg. 2005;125(3):166-8.
21. Blomfeldt R, Törnkvist H, Ponzer S, et al. Comparison of internal fixation with total hip replacement for displaced femoral neck fractures. Randomized, controlled trial performed at four years. J Bone Joint Surg Am. 2005;87 (8):1680-8.

22. Keating JF, Grant A, Masson M, et al. Randomized comparison of reduction and fixation, bipolar hemiarthroplasty, and total hip arthroplasty. Treatment of displaced intracapsular hip fractures in healthy older patients. J Bone Joint Surg Am. 2006;88(2):249-60.
23. Gjertsen JE, Vinje T, Engesaeter LB. Internal screw fixation compared with bipolar hemiarthroplasty for treatment of displaced femoral neck fractures in elderly patients. J Bone Joint Surg Am. 2010;92(3):619-28.
24. Macfie D, Zadeh RA, Andrews M, et al. Perioperative multimodal optimisation in patients undergoing surgery for fractured neck of femur. Surgeon. 2012;10(2):90-4.
25. Nikkel LE, Fox EJ, Black KP, et al. Impact of comorbidities on hospitalization costs following hip fracture. J Bone Joint Surg Am. 2012;4;94(1):9-17.
26. Hoppenfeld S, DeBoer P, Buckley R, et al. Surgical exposures in orthopaedics: the anatomic approach. Philadelphia: Lippincott, Williams & Wilkins; 2009. pp. 683-6.
27. Lee YS, Chen SH, Tsuang YH, et al. Internal fixation of undisplaced femoral neck fractures in the elderly: a retrospective comparison of fixation methods. J Trauma. 2008;64(1):155-62.
28. Liebergall M, Ben-David D, Weil Y, et al. Computerized navigation for the internal fixation of femoral neck fractures. J Bone Joint Surg Am. 2006;88(8):1748-54.
29. Weil YA, Khoury A, Zuaiter I, et al. Femoral neck shortening and varus collapse after navigated fixation of intracapsular femoral neck fractures. J Orthop Trauma. 2012;26(1): 19-23.
30. Lu-Yao GL, Keller RB, Littenberg B, et al. Outcomes after displaced fractures of the femoral neck. A meta-analysis of one hundred and six published reports. J Bone Joint Surg Am. 1994;76(1):15-25.
31. Parker MJ, Blundell C. Choice of implant for internal fixation of femoral neck fractures. Meta-analysis of 25 randomised trials including 4,925 patients. Acta Orthop Scand. 1998;69(2):138-43.
32. Parker MJ. Prediction of fracture union after internal fixation of intracapsular femoral neck fractures. Injury. 1994;25: B3-6.
33. Saito N, Miyasaka T, Toriumi H. Radiographic factors predicting non-union of displaced intracapsular femoral neck fractures. Arch Orthop Trauma Surg. 1995;114(4):183-7.
34. Gurusamy K, Parker MJ, Rowlands TK. The complications of displaced intracapsular fractures of the hip: the effect of screw positioning and angulation on fracture healing. J Bone Joint Surg Br. 2005;87(5):632-4.
35. Berkes MB, Little M, Lazaro LE, et al. Catastrophic Failure After Open Reduction Internal Fixation of Femoral Neck Fractures With a Novel Locking Plate Implant. J Orthop Trauma 2012.
36. Swiontkowski MF, Winquist RA, Hansen ST. Fractures of the femoral neck in patients between the ages of twelve and. J Bone Joint Surg Am. 1984;66:837-46.
37. Haidukewych GJ, Rothwell WS, Jacofsky DJ, et al. Operative treatment of femoral neck fractures in patients between the ages of fifteen and fifty years. J Bone Joint Surg Am. 2004;86(8):1711-6.
38. Rodríguez-Merchán EC. In situ fixation of nondisplaced intracapsular fractures of the proximal femur. Clin Orthop Relat Res. 2002;399:42-51.
39. Hedbeck CJ, Enocson A, Lapidus G, et al. Comparison of bipolar hemiarthroplasty with total hip arthroplasty for displaced femoral neck fractures: a concise four-year follow-up of a randomized trial. J Bone Joint Surg Am. 2011;93:445-50.
40. Rodríguez-Merchán EC. Displaced intracapsular hip fractures: hemiarthroplasty or total arthroplasty? Clin Orthop Relat Res. 2002;399:72.
41. Yu L, Wang Y, Chen J. Total Hip Arthroplasty Versus Hemiarthroplasty for Displaced Femoral Neck Fractures: Meta-analysis of Randomized Trials. Clin Orthopa Relat Res. 2012:1-9.
42. Mabry TM, Prpa B, Haidukewych GJ, et al. Long-term results of total hip arthroplasty for femoral neck fracture nonunion. J Bone Joint Surg Am. 2004;86(10):2263-7.
43. Koval KJ, Zuckerman JD. Hip fractures: I. Overview and Evaluation and Treatment of Femoral-Neck Fractures. J Am Acad Orthop Surg. 1994;2(3):141-9.
44. Estrada LS, Volgas DA, Stannard JP, et al. Fixation failure in femoral neck fractures. Clin Orthop Relat Res. 2002; 399:110-8.
45. Bachiller FG, Caballer AP, Portal LF. Avascular necrosis of the femoral head after femoral neck fracture. Clin Orthop Relat Res. 2002;399:87-109.

Chapter 20

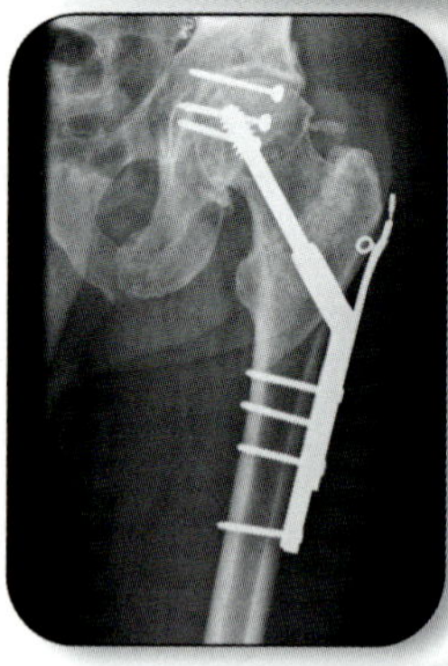

Intertrochanteric Femur Fractures

Stephen Kayiaros, Christopher Born

Chapter Outline

Introduction
Diagnosis
Classification
Surgical Indications
Surgical Anatomy, Positioning and Approaches
- Applied Anatomy
- Positioning
- Approaches

Surgical Techniques
- Fracture Reduction
- Technique 1: Open Reduction and Internal Fixation of Intertrochanteric Hip Fracture
- Technique 2: Intramedullary Nailing of Intertrochanteric Hip Fracture

Outcomes
Complications
Authors' Preferred Management of Select Complications
- Case 1: Lag Screw Cut-out
- Case 2: Nonunion of Intertrochanteric Fracture

Summary

Introduction

Intertrochanteric hip fractures are one of the most common fractures treated by orthopedic surgeons. In the United States alone, the incidence approaches 250,000 per year, with numbers expected to increase dramatically as the population ages and the prevalence of osteopenia grows. The management of intertrochanteric hip fractures is almost always universally surgical. This allows for immediate mobilization of the elderly patient, thus avoiding complications of prolonged bed rest. Pitfalls of varus malunion and leg shortening, which are typically expected with nonoperative treatment, are avoided with operative intervention. With the advent of the modern sliding hip screw and cephalomedullary nail implants, complications related to fixation failure have dropped significantly.[1]

Diagnosis

Intertrochanteric hip fractures most commonly occur as a result of a fall in elderly patients. In younger patients, a high-energy mechanism is required to produce this fracture pattern. The affected extremity is usually shortened and externally rotated. The skin overlying the trochanter can exhibit ecchymosis. Careful inspection of the patient's skin to look for evidence of breakdown should be included in the evaluation. The remaining three extremities, pelvis, and the spine should all be examined to look for occult injury. Range of motion of the contralateral hip should be assessed, as restriction can affect patient positioning in the operating room.

Radiographic assessment should include anteroposterior pelvis and hip views, cross table lateral of the hip, as well as films of the entire femur. Further delineation of the fracture with computed tomography (CT) is usually not required. Magnetic resonance imaging is a useful diagnostic tool in cases of suspected occult fracture, or isolated greater and/or lesser trochanteric fractures to evaluate for extension into the intertrochanteric region.[2]

INTERTROCHANTERIC FEMUR FRACTURES DIAGNOSIS: Pearls and Pitfalls

- Occasionally, a traction radiograph may be needed to better delineate the fracture pattern
- Clinically significant hemorrhage is possible with these injuries which can be problematic in elderly patients with medical comorbidities. Hemoglobin levels should be checked serially after admission to the hospital
- Magnetic resonance imaging can be useful to diagnose suspected occult fractures

Classification

Although many classifications have been proposed for intertrochanteric hip fractures, what is more important is recognizing and distinguishing between specific fracture patterns that will guide treatment and choice of implant fixation.[3,4] The AO/OTA comprehensive fracture classification categorizes intertrochanteric hip fractures into three main types: (1) Type A1 (simple pertrochanteric), (2) Type A2 (multi-fragmentary pertrochanteric), and (3) Type A3 (intertrochanteric or reverse obliquity patterns) (Fig. 20.1).[5]

It is useful to be able to divide intertrochanteric fractures into stable and unstable injury patterns. In general, an intertrochanteric hip fracture is said to be unstable when the fracture line extends into the region of the lesser trochanter causing displacement, or when the integrity of the posteromedial buttress is compromised. Of equal importance is recognition of the reverse obliquity fracture pattern that can sometimes occur with subtrochanteric extension. The major fracture parallels the axis of the femoral neck, making the sliding hip screw fixation construct predestined for failure. The failure rates of using the sliding hip screw to stabilize this fracture pattern have been well documented. It has been shown that posteromedial comminution, failure to obtain medial cortical apposition, and the reverse obliquity fracture pattern are all components that constitute instability.[4,6] A study of over 600 intertrochanteric hip fractures demonstrated the degree of collapse of the sliding hip screw correlated directly with instability of the posteromedial buttress.[4] The surgeon should be able to recognize three distinct types of intertrochanteric hip fractures: (1) stable fractures with medial cortical apposition and intact posteromedial buttress, (2) unstable fractures with loss of integrity of the posteromedial buttress, and (3) reverse obliquity fractures.

Surgical Indications

Nearly all intertrochanteric hip fractures are treated surgically. Surgical management offers the patient the best chance for safe mobilization and early rehabilitation. The goal is to return patients to their preinjury functional status.[1] The timing of when to operate on patients with intertrochanteric hip fractures continues to be a source of debate. Some studies have shown increased mortality when surgery is performed on the day of admission, while others have demonstrated a ten fold increase in mortality when surgery is delayed past 48 hours for nonmedical issues.[7,8] While these injuries are not considered emergent, it is of paramount importance, so that any unneeded delays in surgery can be avoided to stabilize these fractures in a semi-urgent manner.

Nonoperative management is rarely indicated and is reserved for special circumstances. Nonambulatory patients and those who are medically unfit to withstand surgery can generally be treated nonoperatively. Nondisplaced and/or occult fractures can undergo a trial of nonoperative treatment as long as the patient can be made comfortable and safely mobilized to a chair.[9] Close follow-up with X-ray evaluation is mandatory in these latter cases. A certain degree of varus and shortening may be accepted in lieu of the risks of surgery.

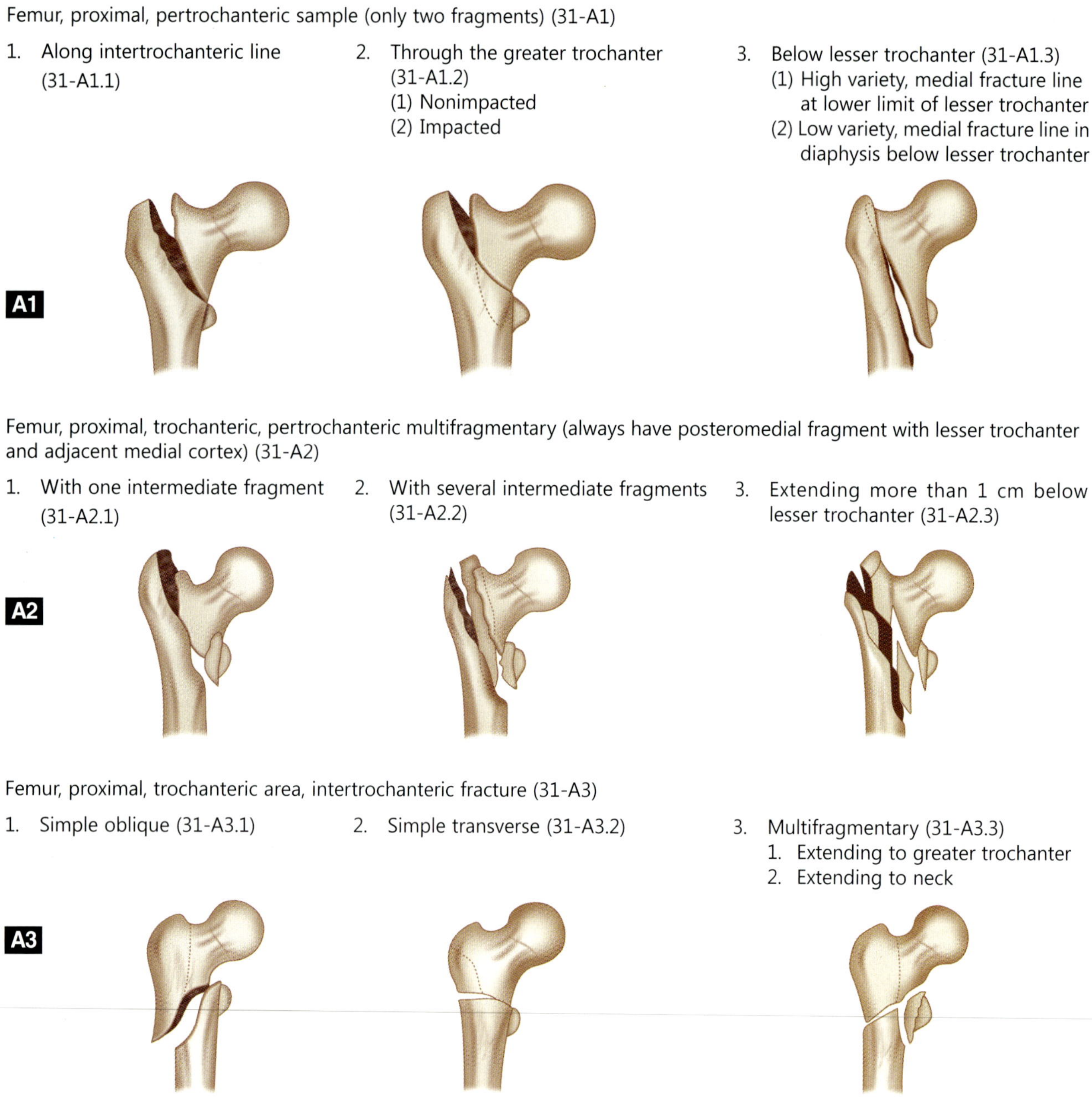

Figure 20.1: AO/OTA classification of proximal femur fractures.

Surgical Anatomy, Positioning and Approaches

Applied Anatomy

An understanding of the bony anatomy of the proximal femur and its deforming forces is critical to be able to obtain a satisfactory reduction.[1] The femoral neck and head, greater trochanter, lesser trochanter, and the subtrochanteric region or femoral shaft are all involved in the spectrum of intertrochanteric hip fractures. The femoral neck and head are usually not involved by virtue of their intracapsular location, although the extracapsular region of the femoral neck can occasionally comprise the fracture. The gluteus medius exerts a strong abducting force through its insertion on the greater trochanter, while the gluteus minimus and the short external rotators will externally rotate the proximal femur away from the femoral neck and head. The hip adductors exert a strong medial deforming force through their insertion on the femoral shaft. The iliopsoas pulls the fragment containing the lesser trochanter into flexion and adduction. The quadriceps and hamstring muscles will contribute to overall axial shortening of the limb and must also be considered during fracture reduction. Elementary fractures typically exhibit predictable displacement patterns that reduce easily, while more complex fracture patterns with severe displacement can make reduction more challenging for the surgeon.

Positioning

The most efficient way to obtain satisfactory reduction and fixation of intertrochanteric hip fractures is through the use of a fracture table. The patient is positioned supine on the fracture table with traction applied to the injured leg through the foot or a traction pin. The contralateral leg is flexed, abducted, and externally rotated in a well-padded leg holder and the ipsilateral arm is draped across the torso. Alternatively, in cases of limited contralateral hip motion, the uninvolved leg can be "scissored" in extension and neutral abduction/adduction. Once the patient is safely secured to the fracture table, fluoroscopic views are obtained to accurately assess the fracture and quality of the reduction. The three essential views are an anteroposterior (AP) of the hip, lateral, and the true lateral of the femoral neck, which can be obtained by angling the c-arm beam approximately 15° from horizontal (Figs 20.2 to 20.4). The latter view helps to evaluate femoral anteversion and helps guide accurate pin or screw placement into the femoral neck and head.[1]

Approaches

The surgical approach for intertrochanteric hip fractures will depend on the type of implant used. For a sliding hip screw and side plate construct, the incision is placed on the lateral aspect of the thigh, starting at the level of the vastus ridge, extending distally approximately 15–20 cm in length. The incision should be made in line with the femoral shaft or just slightly posterior, with the inferior pole directed slightly anterior to account for the femoral bow. Dissection is carried down through the subcutaneous

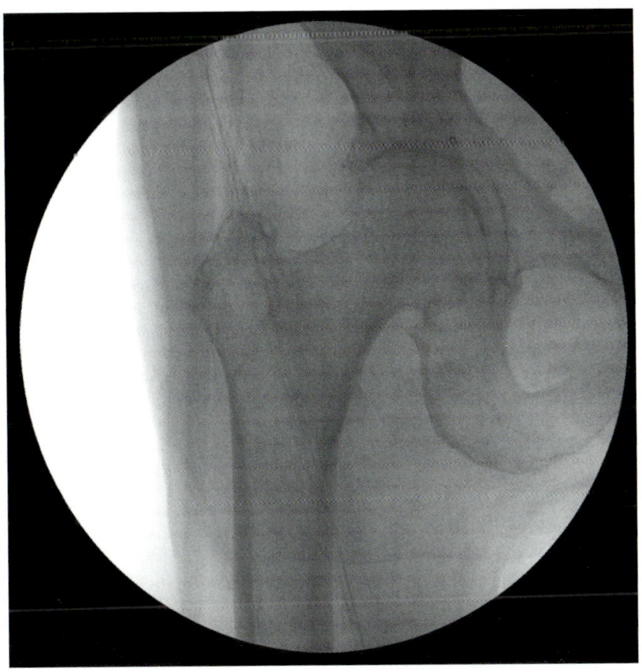

Figure 20.2: Anteroposterior (AP) fluoroscopic image of the right hip with slight internal rotation.

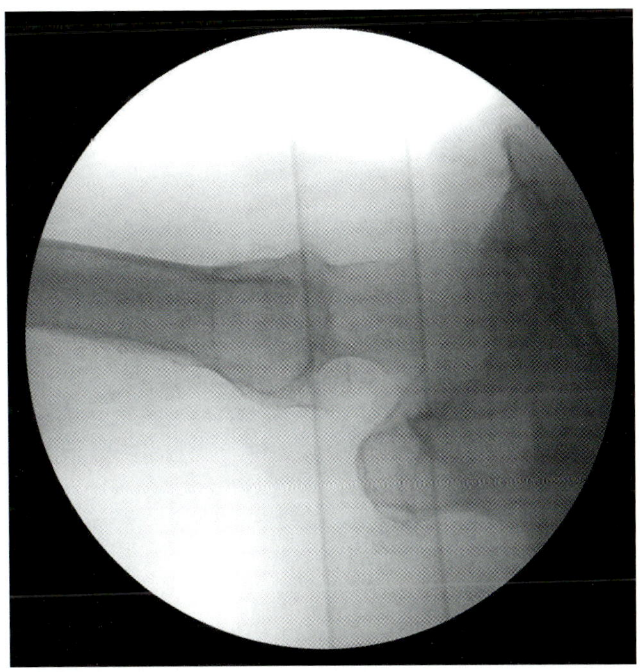

Figure 20.3: Lateral fluoroscopic image of the right hip. The normal anteversion of the femoral neck is noted.

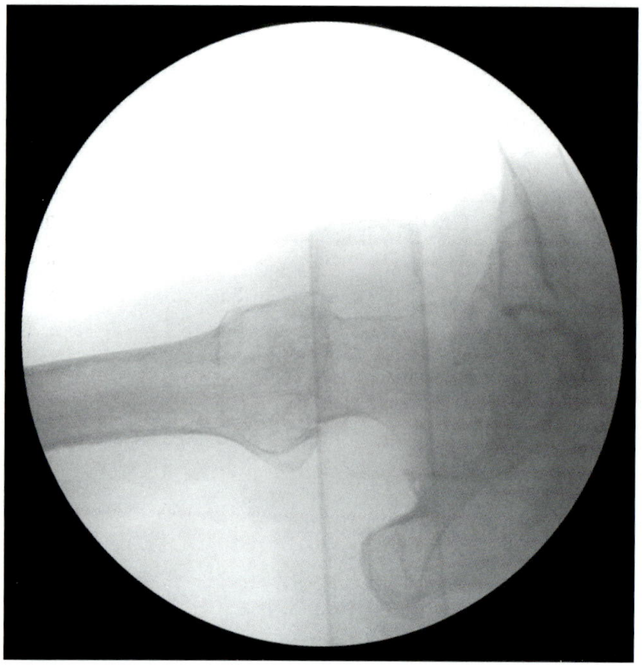

Figure 20.4: Lateral fluoroscopic image of the same hip as shown in Figure 20.3 but with 15° of rotation of the c-arm to show a true lateral image.

tissues with electrocautery and down to the level of the fascia lata, which is incised in line with the skin incision. At this point, the vastus lateralis muscle can be split bluntly in line with the femur to gain access to the fracture site. Alternatively, the vastus can be elevated off the lateral intermuscular septum. Hohman or Bennet retractors are used to maintain adequate visualization of the femur during instrumentation. Perforating vessels should be identified and clamped before they are allowed to retract behind the femur.

For a cephalomedullary nail construct, the incision is placed approximately two finger breadths proximal to the tip of the greater trochanter, which can be palpated manually or marked out with fluoroscopy. The incision made is generally about 3 cm in length, but can vary depending on the patient's soft tissues. In obese patients, the incision should be extended even more proximally to facilitate guide pin placement in the proximal femur and to avoid eccentric and lateral reaming of the greater trochanter. Adduction of the patient's torso on the fracture table can also assist the surgeon in obtaining a proper starting point for the nail when soft tissues are impeding or if the patient has a prominent iliac wing. Once the skin incision is made, dissection is carried down to the fascia lata with electrocautery, which is incised in line with the skin incision. The tip of the greater trochanter should be manually palpable and the guide pin can be placed.

If a closed reduction cannot be obtained, the surgeon must be prepared to perform an open reduction. An extensile lateral incision should be utilized in these instances, starting proximal to the greater trochanter and extending distally in line with the proximal femoral shaft. The iliotibial band and fascia lata are incised in line with skin incision, allowing excellent exposure to the entire proximal femur. The fracture fragments can be directly manipulated to obtain a direct reduction. Meticulous care should be applied when handling the fracture fragments to avoid periosteal stripping, especially in osteoporotic bone, as iatrogenic fractures can be created if the surgeon is not careful. Once the reduction is obtained and maintained, fixation and instrumentation is carried out.

Surgical Techniques

Fracture Reduction

Reduction of the fracture is first obtained by applying traction to the leg. The external rotation deformity must be corrected by aligning the leg with the patella pointing directly anterior. Confirmation of the reduction is checked with fluoroscopy, paying close attention to the alignment of the femoral neck and inferomedial calcar on the AP view.[1] The lateral view will determine if the leg needs to be flexed or extended in order to properly align the femoral shaft. This view will also show if there is excessive posterior sagging of the fracture. If present, posterior sag must be corrected and maintained during the entire operation before final implant instrumentation. This can be done by placing a Cobb elevator posterior to the proximal femur and exerting upward pressure (Fig. 20.5). Alternatively, a Steinmann pin can be placed from the lateral cortex into the femoral neck anteriorly to maintain the reduction. Infrequently, fracture fragments may have significant impaction, and in younger patients involving high-energy trauma, incarcerated soft tissue with significant displacement will prevent reduction. In these cases, the fracture table is used to determine proper leg

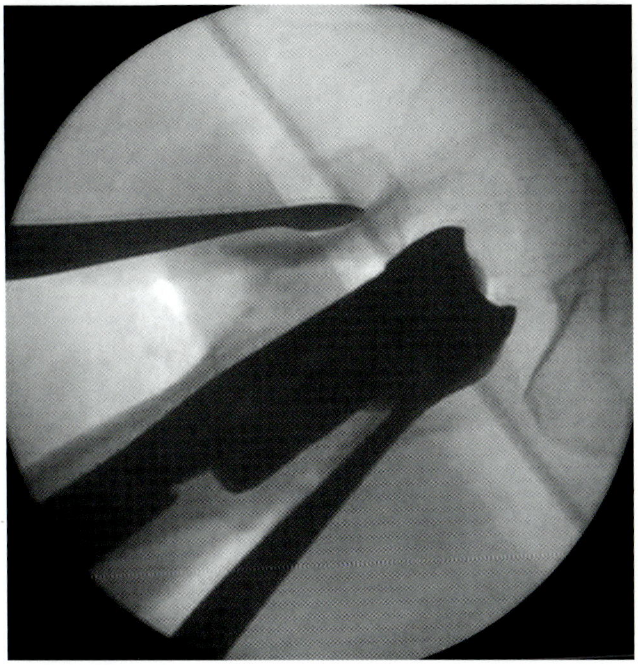

Figure 20.5: The use of a Cobb elevator posteriorly can help with reduction of posterior "sag" which frequently occurs.

length, alignment and rotation, and the surgeon should then proceed to formal open reduction employing reduction techniques with clamps, Schanz pins, a ball-spike pusher, cerclage wire, etc. (Figs 20.6A to C). It is critical to point out that in all cases, the reduction must be obtained prior to and maintained during fixation because the implant will not reduce the fracture.

Technique 1: Open Reduction and Internal Fixation of Intertrochanteric Hip Fracture

Preoperative Planning

For fractures with an intact posteromedial buttress and minimal to no comminution, the sliding hip screw and side plate construct are excellent implant choices. Preoperative planning should include obtaining an AP pelvic radiograph to template from the contralateral hip. When possible, internally rotated views of both hips should be obtained to best determine the true neck-shaft angle. This will allow the surgeon to select the ideal implant angle needed to obtain compression at the fracture site, taking advantage of the biomechanics of sliding hip screws.[1]

Technique

After the reduction and exposure have been performed, fluoroscopy is used to determine the starting point for the hip screw guide pin. The starting point will vary on the implant angle chosen; for more valgus-angled implants, the starting point will be more distal on the femur.[1] Once the appropriate starting point is determined, the pin is inserted from the posterolateral aspect of the femur, aiming toward the center of the femoral neck and head. The trajectory is aimed slightly anterior to account for femoral anteversion. Fluoroscopy is used on all three views to confirm appropriate pin placement. This is the critical point of the case as pin placement will determine final hip screw position. Adjustments should be made prior to fully advancing the pin, avoiding multiple passes in the femoral neck, which may already be osteopenic in nature.

Pitfalls include starting too anterior on the femoral cortex or starting too proximal and preventing pin placement at the apex of the femoral head. A proximal starting point will place the pin too superior in the femoral head, risking implant failure and lag screw cut-out. The premise of the tip-apex distance (TAD) has been well described by Baumgaertner et al.[10,11] Tip-apex distance is the sum of the distances from the apex of the femoral head to the tip of the hip screw as measured on the AP and lateral radiographic views. Tip-apex distance of greater than 25 mm greatly increases the risk of screw cut-out and eventual implant failure.[10]

Once the pin has been inserted properly, the screw length and reaming depth are determined. The surgeon should be aware of the particular implant manufacturer's measurement requirements. The chosen screw length should be sufficiently long to engage the barrel of the plate, but not so long as to disallow active compression with the compression screw. The reamer is then slowly advanced over the guide pin. Reaming should be performed with periodic fluoroscopy to monitor potential advancement of the guide pin into the pelvis, as serious complications can occur from this. If the guide pin comes out with the reamer, it should be reinserted in the proper position for final screw placement and checked by X-ray. The screw hole is then tapped by hand to appropriate depth. The cannulated hip screw is then advanced over the guide pin and down to the subchondral bone of the femoral head. The guide pin

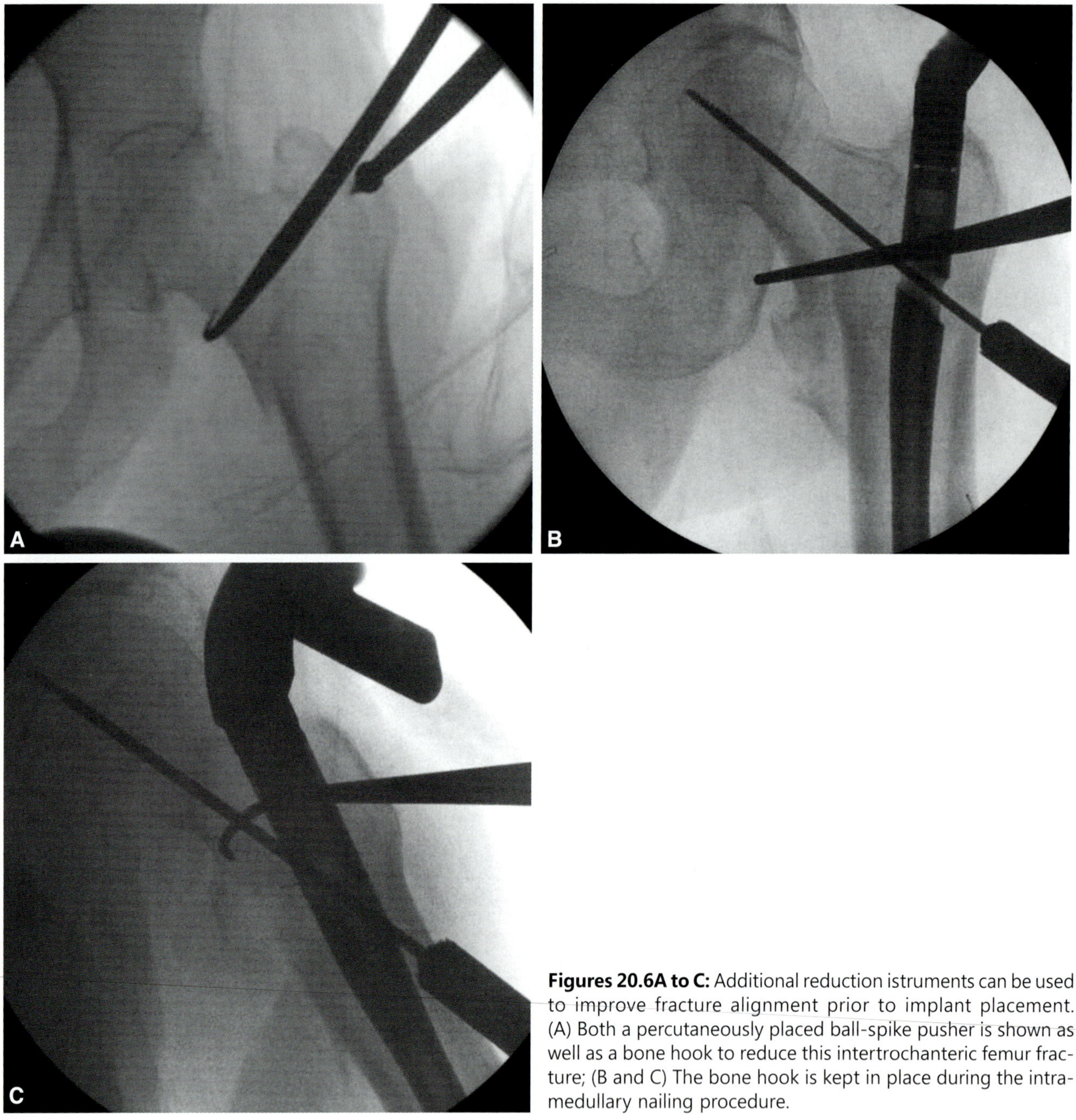

Figures 20.6A to C: Additional reduction istruments can be used to improve fracture alignment prior to implant placement. (A) Both a percutaneously placed ball-spike pusher is shown as well as a bone hook to reduce this intertrochanteric femur fracture; (B and C) The bone hook is kept in place during the intramedullary nailing procedure.

is then removed and attention is turned toward application of the side plate.

The side plate is then advanced over the screw and impacted until it sits flush with the femoral cortex. Some systems are designed to have the plate "key" into the screw to reduce rotation. Proper rotational orientation of the screw will be necessary to allow the plate to align appropriately on the femoral shaft. The plate is then secured to the femoral shaft with 2–6 bicortical screws in standard fashion. Most stable fractures require only two screws. Additional screws may be used for more unstable fractures or in patients with poor bone stock (Figs 20.7A and B and 20.8).

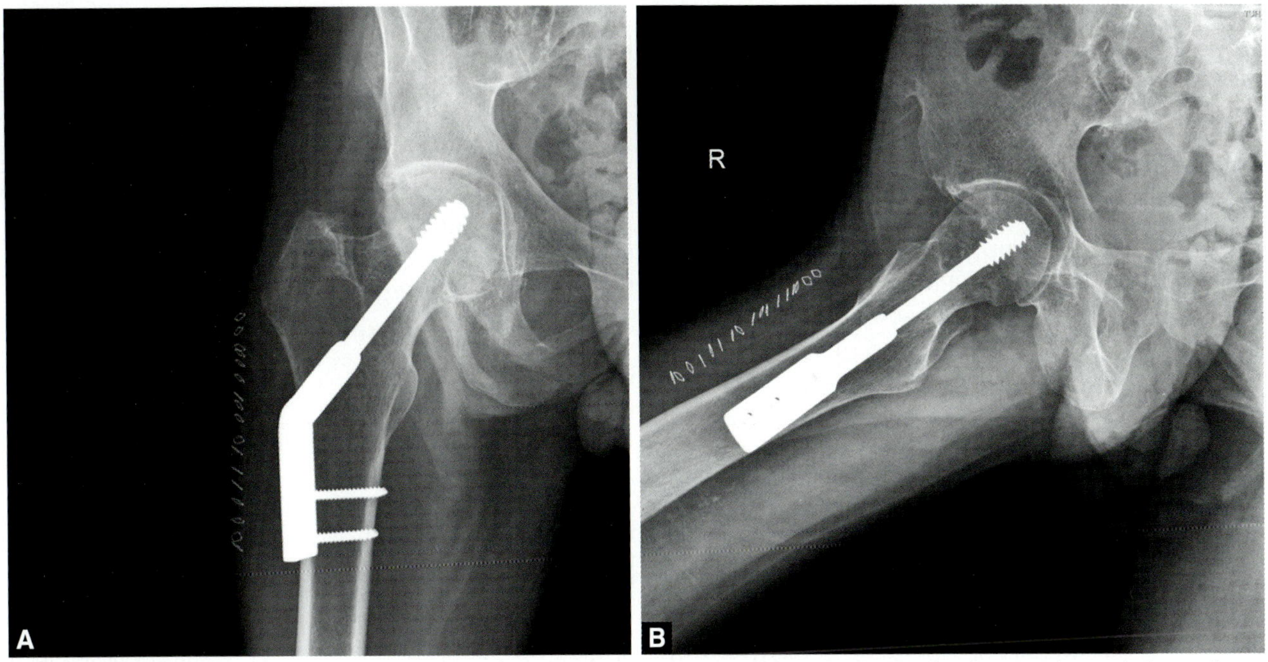

Figures 20.7A and B: Radiographic images after open reduction and internal fixaton (ORIF) of an intertrochanteric femur fracture with a sliding hip screw and side plate device. (A and B) Anteroposterior (AP) and lateral images. Central and deep placement of the lag screw is essential to prevent complications of cut-out from the femoral head. In this case, the lag screw is in acceptable position, but ideally could be slightly more inferior and deeper to lower the tip-apex distance (TAD).

Courtesy: Saqib Rehman

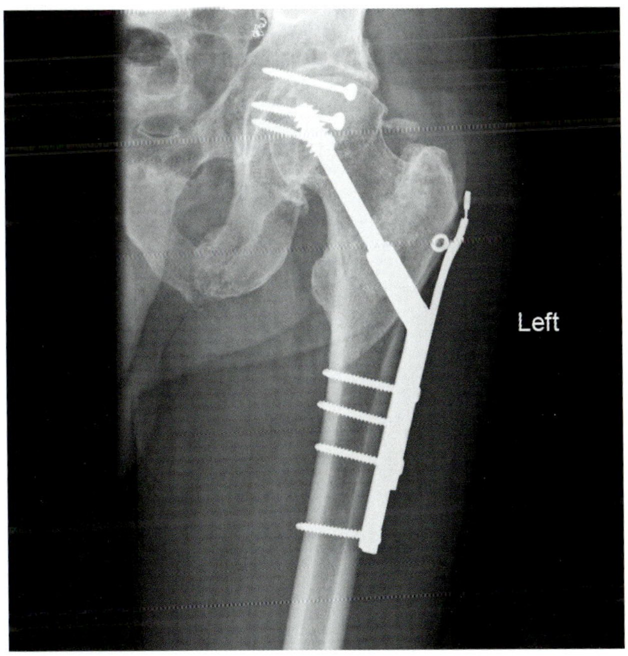

Figure 20.8: If the greater trochanter requires lateral buttressing and a sliding hip screw is being used for intertrochanteric fracture fixation, a trochanteric stabilization plate as shown here can be helpful. Screws can also be placed into the proximal portion of this plate if needed. Incidentally, this patient also had previous fixation of an acetabular fracture.

Courtesy: Saqib Rehman

ORIF OF INTERTROCHANTERIC HIP FRACTURE: Pearls and Pitfalls

- A 15° internally-rotated view of bilateral hips will help demonstrate the neck-shaft angle most accurately
- Central placement of the guidewire deeply in the femoral head will minimize the TAD, which should be less than 25 mm to minimize the chance of lag screw cut-out

Technique 2: Intramedullary Nailing of Intertrochanteric Hip Fracture

Preoperative Planning

Although the sliding hip screw has an excellent track record for stabilizing intertrochanteric hip fractures, more unstable fractures, especially those with disruption and comminution of the posteromedial buttress, may be better suited for fixation with a cephalomedullary nail.[1] The reverse obliquity fracture pattern should be considered a contraindication to use the sliding hip screw, evidenced by failure rates. This fracture type should be stabilized with an intramedullary nail.[12] Antegrade femoral nails for intertrochanteric fractures are designed to be inserted through the greater trochanter. Studies by Lindsey et al. and Davis et al. demonstrated multiple benefits of a cephalomedullary nail including: (1) providing stable head and neck fixation, (2) allowing for controlled collapse and impaction of the fracture site, (3) decreasing the lever arm on the proximal fragment compared to the side plate by virtue of its intramedullary location, (4) providing bone graft from intramedullary reaming, (5) providing excellent axial and rotational control, (6) allowing for early weight bearing, (7) allowing minimal dissection and "percutaneous" insertion, and (8) serving as a load-sharing implant device.[13,14]

Trochanteric nails come in many varieties; most come in short and long lengths; some have one single femoral neck screw, while others utilize two screws. There is some concern for periprosthetic fractures with the use of short nails, and there has been a trend in stabilizing intertrochanteric hip fractures with long nails to protect the entire femur. Compression across the fracture is obtained in a similar manner to the sliding hip screw; however, several implants are designed with devices that allow for immediate fracture compression intraoperatively.

Technique

After the reduction and exposure have been performed, fluoroscopy is used to determine the starting point of the guide pin for nail insertion. The starting point is critical for proper nail insertion. It should be at or on the downslope of the tip of the trochanter on the AP view, and just anterior to the midline of the greater trochanter-femoral shaft axis on the lateral view (Figs 20.9A and B). This is critical in order to ensure central lag screw placement in the anterior/posterior (coronal) plane. Once the correct starting point has been established, the guide pin is advanced toward the lesser trochanter on the AP view and in line with the femoral shaft on the lateral view. The pin is then overreamed with a starting reamer.

The ball-tipped guidewire is then advanced through the starting hole, across the fracture site and into the distal femur. When using a long nail, the surgeon must try to place the guidewire in the center of the distal femur on both the AP and the lateral view. In osteoporotic bone, it may be difficult to achieve this, as the ball-tipped guidewire will tend to "swim" in the distal femur and drift anterior. Placing a small bend on the end of the guidewire

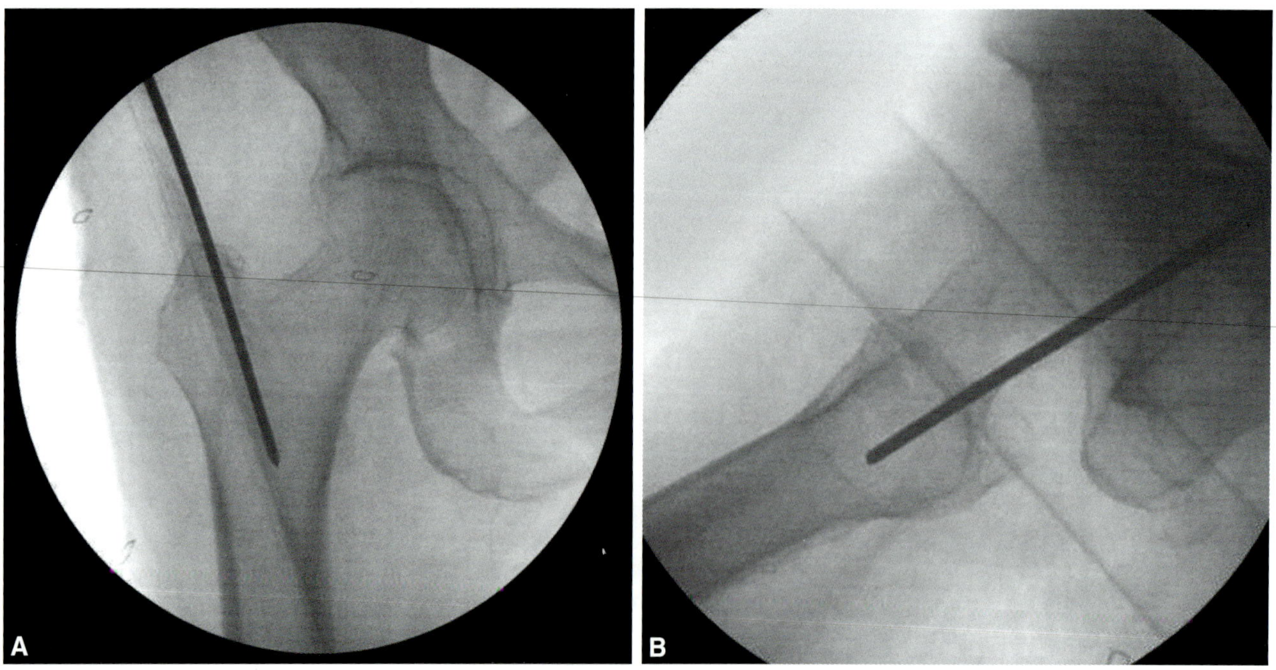

Figures 20.9A and B: (A) Anteroposterior (AP) and (B) lateral fluoroscopic images demonstrating proper placement of the opening guidewire.

and gentle tapping as it is passed through the distal metaphysis may facilitate proper placement rather than forcefully pushing it. By rotating the guidewire, the bend may act as a "skid" to help steer the tip into a proper, final position. A more anterior starting point for the nail on the lateral view of the hip may also be helpful. Once satisfactory placement of the guidewire has been established, the proximal femur is prepared for nail insertion with differential proximal and distal reaming (Figs 20.10A to L). Most implant systems are designed with standard proximal and distal reaming for proper nail placement. Reaming should be performed over the guidewire in standard fashion. A mallet or small Richardson retractor can be placed on the lateral aspect of the reamer with a medial directed force to avoid eccentric reaming of the trochanter, and loss of the lateral cortex.

The nail is assembled with its outrigger targeting device and is advanced manually into the femur over the guidewire. The nail should be advanced gently and carefully to avoid iatrogenic fracture or loss of reduction. Proper nail depth is confirmed with fluoroscopy on the AP view and the final resting position of the nail should be so that the lag screw will end up in the center of the femoral neck and head or just slightly inferior on the AP view. Seating of a cephalomedullary nail with a mallet should be avoided except to fine tune the last few millimeters of placement. If the force of a mallet is required, the nail should be removed and the canal should be reamed to a larger diameter. Careful review of the X-rays may reveal that the proximal metaphysis will not accommodate the proximal shoulder of the nail. In that case, the reamers should be used to bore out this area even further. The guidewire can now be removed.

The guide pin for the lag screw is now inserted via outrigger and advanced into the femoral head. Proper placement of the pin requires fluoroscopy on AP, lateral, and true femoral neck lateral views. The outrigger can be rotated accordingly to account for femoral anteversion. Adjustments in pin placement should be made prior to fully advancing it, because it needs to be removed entirely before changing the trajectory. As in the sliding hip screw construct, the pin should be aimed for the apex of the femoral head, utilizing the same TAD criteria described previously. Screw length is determined, the guide pin is overreamed, and the screw is advanced manually to the proper end position. Specific system designs allow for immediate fracture compression and can be performed at this point. In unstable fracture patterns, the nail should be locked distally to provide rotational control. If a long nail is used, we recommend a single dynamic screw as there will be some perceptible axial compression migration with weight bearing that takes place after locking screw placement. Releasing the traction on the leg prior to distal locking screw deployment is particularly important in cases of reverse obliquity fractures so as to allow cortical impaction of the proximal and distal segments.

INTERMEDULLARY NAILING OF INTERTROCHANTERIC HIP FRACTURES:
Pearls and Pitfalls

- More unstable intertrochanteric femur fracture patterns, including reverse obliquity patterns, are more appropriately treated with an intramedullary nail rather than a sliding hip screw
- Starting guidewire placement should be just medial to the tip of the greater trochanter on the AP image and just anterior to the midline of the greater trochanter-femoral shaft axis on the lateral image
- The long ball-tipped guidewire should be placed into the central part of the distal femur on both AP and lateral images. Excessive anterior placement can lead to anterior cortical perforation of a long nail
- Minimization of the TAD is critical, similar to what is done for the sliding hip screw, in order to prevent lag screw cut-out

Outcomes

The primary goal of surgical treatment of intertrochanteric hip fractures is early mobilization and rehabilitation for the patient to restore preinjury level of function.[1] Until recently, outcomes after intertrochanteric hip fractures were deemed successful if the patient survived and the fracture united. General health assessment tools and hip function scores are now being employed to better characterize patient outcomes. Cornwall et al. showed that the strongest predictor of outcome was the patient's preinjury level of function.[15] Interestingly, they found that those with unstable fracture patterns demonstrated the worst outcomes, but there were also the patients that were the most frail and debilitated preoperatively.

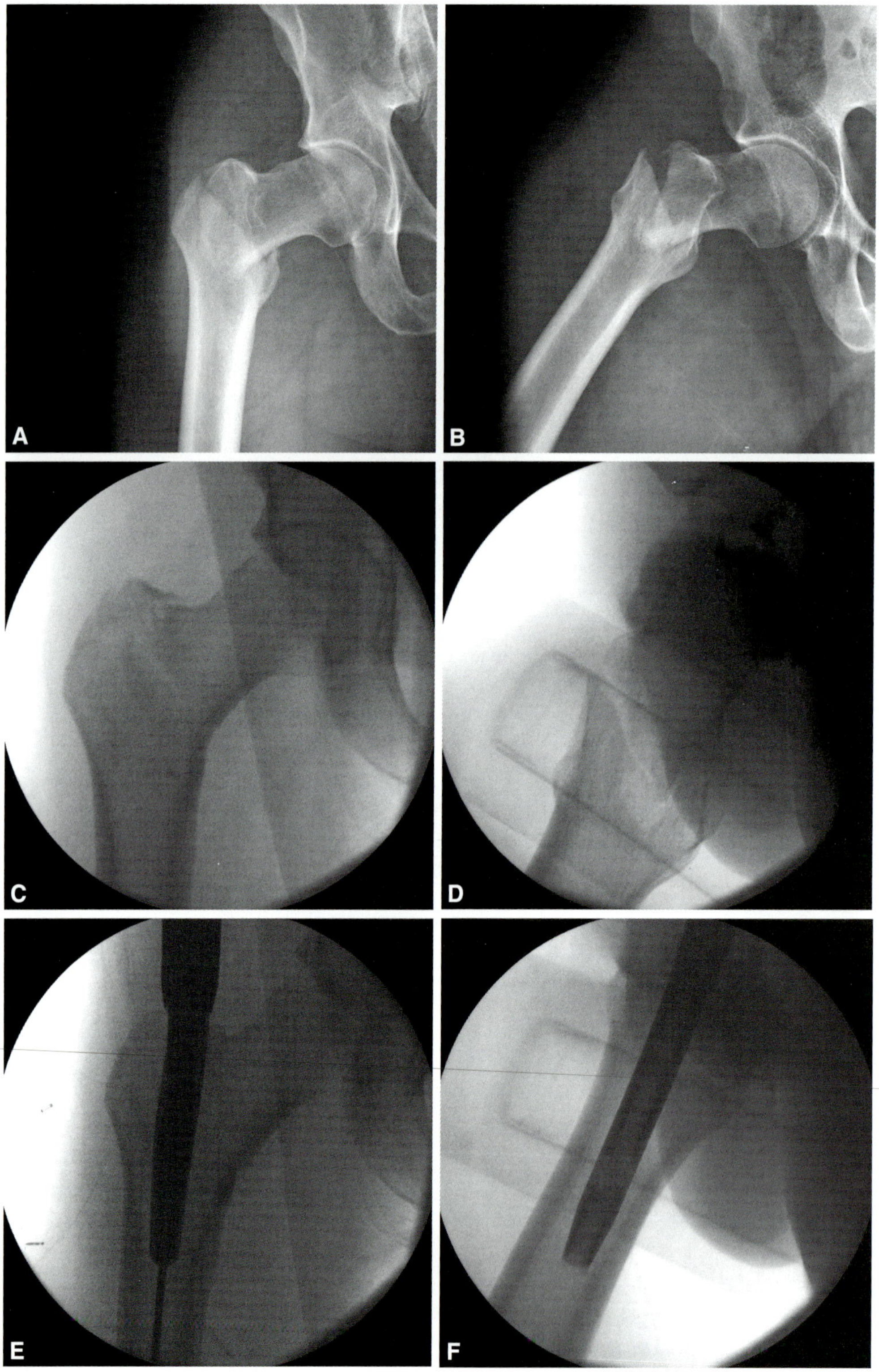

Figures 20.10A to F: Intramedullary nailing of an intertrochanteric femur fracture. (A and B) Anteroposterior (AP) and lateral radiographs demonstrating a displaced intertrochanteric femur fracture; (C and D) The fracture is satisfactorily reduced with simple distraction using the traction table as shown on these intraoperative fluoroscopic images; (E) After guidewire placement as shown in Figure 20.9, the opening reamer is inserted with care not to damage either the lateral wall or the medial cortex; (F) Lateral image demonstrating insertion of the short intramedullary nail after reaming.

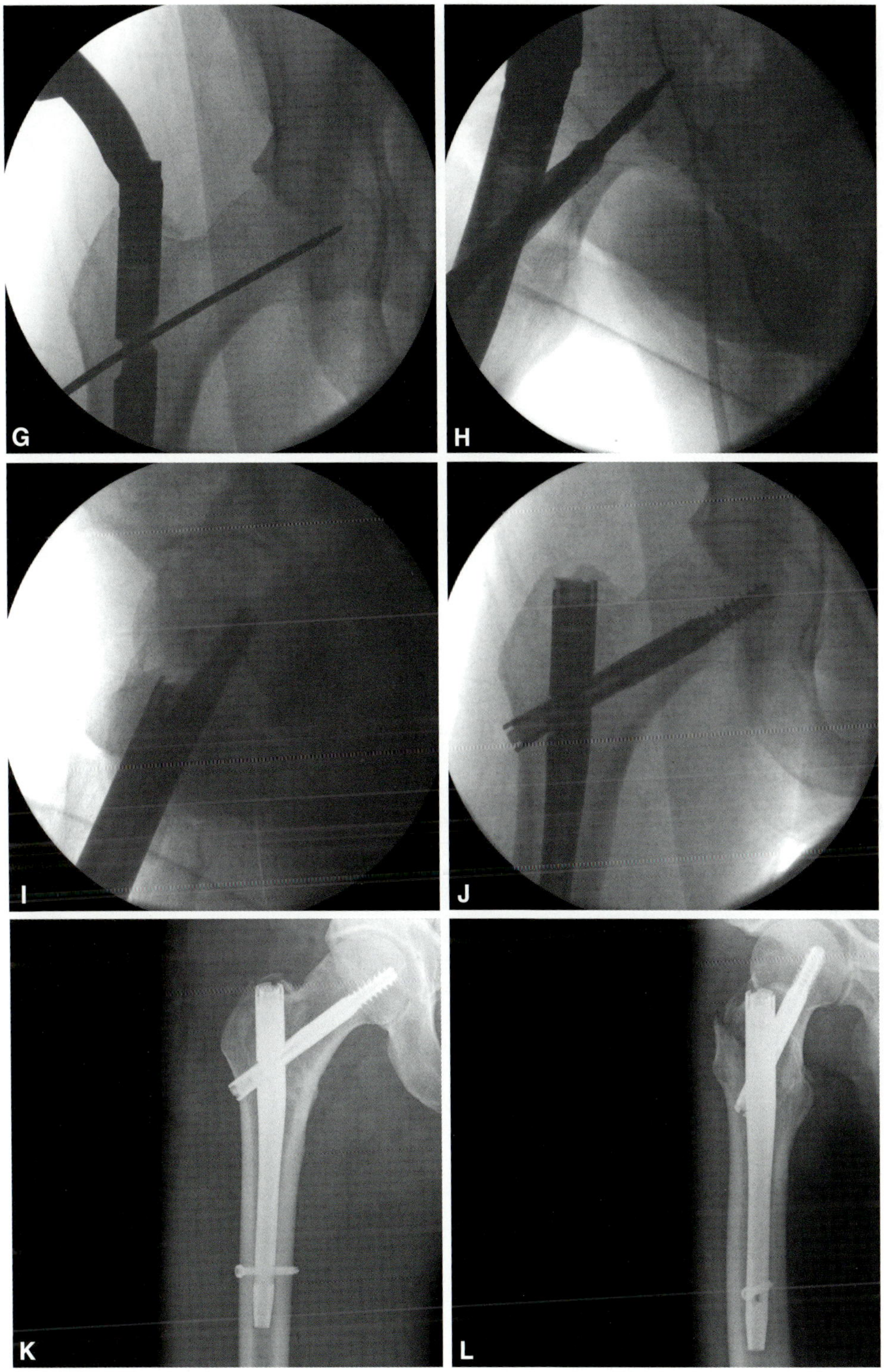

Figures 20.10G to L: (G) After placement of the nail to appropriate depth, the guidewire for the lag screw is placed such that it is central or just inferior to the central position in the head; (H) Reaming for the lag screw should be done under fluoroscopic control to avoid inadvertent intra-articular penetration of the reamer. Reaming can also bind the guidewire potentially sending it intra-articular or even intrapelvic if not checked under image control; (I and J) Lateral and AP images demonstrating final placement of the nail and lg screw; (K and L) Postoperative AP and lateral images demonstrating final reduction and fixation with the intramedullary nail, lag screw, and distal locking screw.

Courtesy: Saqib Rehman

Accurate fracture reduction, appropriate implant selection, and proper implant instrumentation and fixation will all directly affect and optimize outcomes.[1] In a recent randomized clinical trial, Barton et al. showed no significant difference in reoperation rates, outcomes scores, mortality rates, and secondary outcomes measures between a long cephalomedullary nail and a sliding hip screw.[16] They found that the rate of cut-out for both implants correlated directly to the TAD. The authors concluded that the sliding hip screw should remain the gold standard for treatment of these fractures because of similar outcomes and less expense.[16] Another comparative study by Utrilla et al. demonstrated better walking ability in patients with unstable fractures treated with a cephalomedullary nail.[17] This may be due to the intramedullary position of the implant, allowing for fracture union with less deformity, better femoral offset, less leg lengthening, and potentially better abductor function. Parker and Handoll recently published a series of meta-analyses of 32 randomized clinical trials as part of the Cochrane Library of Systematic Reviews.[18] Twenty of these studies compared the cephalomedullary nail to the sliding hip screw. Their conclusions were that patients treated with a cephalomedullary nail had an increased risk of intra- and postoperative periprosthetic fracture and a higher rate of reoperation. Other studies in the report looked at the intramedullary hip screw and the sliding hip screw, again noting more fracture related complications in the former group. Two studies examined reverse obliquity or transverse fractures at the level of the lesser trochanter specifically. These studies showed that the cephalomedullary nails were associated with better results and fewer fracture fixation complications as compared to a 95° blade plate or dynamic condylar plate. Overall, the report by Parker and Handoll in the Cochrane review concluded that the sliding hip screw is superior for most intertrochanteric hip fractures, but that intramedullary nails have advantages in select fracture patterns, such as the reverse obliquity and subtrochanteric types.[18] One might speculate that the studies used by the Cochrane group were older and that current technology and usage expertise might mitigate problems with cephalomedullary nails vis-à-vis any intertrochanteric fracture pattern. There is no question as to the cost differential between sliding hip screws and intramedullary nails, with the plates being less expensive.[16]

Complications

Complications in the management of intertrochanteric hip fractures include systemic complications, such as mortality, myocardial infarction, other medical complications, thromboembolism, and pressure sores; and fracture-related complications, such as nonunion, malunion, loss of fixation/cut-out and/or hardware failure, iatrogenic fracture, and infections.

- Patients who have developed a nonunion are faced with two surgical options: (1) total hip arthroplasty usually with a calcar-replacing femoral component, or (2) revision ORIF, with or without a valgus osteotomy. Bartonicek et al. showed 93% healing rate (14 out of 15 patients), improved Harris hip scores and no osteoarthritis or avascular necrosis of the femoral head in patients treated with a valgus osteotomy for intertrochanteric nonunion or malunion, and concluded that it is an effective procedure.[19]
- Loss of fixation is a common complication, especially in patients with osteopenia and severely comminuted fractures. Bone quality, fracture stability, reduction accuracy, and implant position will all affect final outcomes. Proper instrumentation of the implant with close attention to minimize the TAD, continues to a critical factor in reducing failure rates. It has been shown that in unstable fracture patterns, intramedullary devices perform better than sliding hip screws, evidenced by lower rates of failure of fixation. If loss of fixation is associated with cut-out and intra-articular protrusion of the femoral head screw, an arthroplasty is mandated. Haidukewych and Berry reported on a series of 60 patients that underwent arthroplasty for failed intertrochanteric hip fractures.[20] Thirty-two patients underwent total hip arthroplasty, while 28 underwent hemiarthroplasty. Forty-four out of 60 patients were followed for a mean of 5 years. Forty patients were ambulatory, 39 had mild or no pain, while 5 had moderate to severe pain. Survivorship analysis of the implants using revision for any reason demonstrated 100% survival at 7 years and 87.5%

survival at 10 years. The authors concluded that arthroplasty is an effective salvage procedure in older patients with failed intertrochanteric hip fractures.[20]

- Iatrogenic fractures are common when utilizing intramedullary implants. It is crucial for the surgeon to exercise caution when inserting these devices, and be critical at maintaining the reduction throughout the operation, as the nail will not reduce the fracture. The implant should always be inserted manually and periodically using fluoroscopy to visualize the nail bypassing the fracture site and assuring that no additional fractures are inadvertently created.

Authors' Preferred Management of Select Complications

Case 1: Lag Screw Cut-out

A 77-year-old relatively healthy female community ambulator presented to the emergency room with left-sided hip pain following a fall. She was diagnosed with an intertrochanteric hip fracture (Fig. 20.11A). She was operated on the next day; fixation was achieved with a cephalomedullary nail (Figs 20.11B and C). The patient was allowed immediate weight bearing postoperatively and was seen in the office on two occasions following her surgery. At her 6-week visit, she complained of pain in the hip. Radiographs revealed that the lag screw had failed catastrophically (Figs 20.11D and E). All markers for infection were negative or normal. The option to revise the reduction and fixation with either a blade plate or a proximal femoral locking plate was discussed. Ultimately the patient opted for a total hip replacement because this would allow her to bear weight immediately after surgery, an important consideration for this age group. She underwent successful total hip replacement (Fig. 20.11F). Intraoperative Gram stain and frozen sections were not suggestive of infection. The remainder of her course of recovery and rehabilitation was unremarkable. When arthroplasty is chosen following lag screw cut-out, a calcar replacement prosthesis will frequently be needed. In this particular case, the final resting position of the lag screw in the femoral head led to premature failure of the hardware and eventual lag screw cut-out. Note that the TAD exceeds 25 mm.

Case 2: Nonunion of Intertrochanteric Fracture

An 84-year-old female community ambulator sustained a left intertrochanteric fracture following a low-energy fall (Fig. 20.12A). She was managed with a cephalomedullary nail. Her immediate postoperative X-rays showed what appeared to be satisfactory placement of the nail and the lag screw (Fig. 20.12B). She was started on immediate weight bearing after surgery. At her 2-month follow-up visit, she complained of modest continued groin pain (Figs 20.12C and D). She was continued in physical therapy. The groin pain persisted through subsequent follow-up visits. Infection markers of white blood count, sedimentation rate and C-reactive protein were all normal. At 6 months, her aching and discomfort in the groin region persisted. Radiographs showed maintenance of the reduction and intact hardware (Fig. 20.12E). A CT scan was obtained showing lucency at the fracture site consistent with a nonunion (Figs 20.12F to I). Options were discussed with the patient. These included removal of the hardware and a valgus osteotomy versus arthroplasty. The patient elected to undergo arthroplasty to facilitate her postoperative mobility. A hemiarthroplasty was selected because of her age and absence of any arthritis on her X-rays (Fig. 20.12J). In younger patients, valgus osteotomy is the preferred management for intertrochanteric nonunions to preserve the native hip.

Summary

Intertrochanteric hip fractures continue to be one of the most common fractures that are treated by orthopedic surgeons. Surgical treatment is almost always indicated as there is almost never any role for nonoperative management. Loss of the posteromedial buttress and the reverse obliquity fracture pattern constitute unstable injuries and should be recognized. The hallmark of surgical technique is that the reduction must be obtained prior to implant instrumentation, and needs to be maintained throughout to avoid malreduction. Majority of these fractures, with the exception of the reverse obliquity pattern, can be stabilized with a sliding hip screw and side plate construct. Cephalomedullary devices can be inserted percutaneously and offer biomechanical

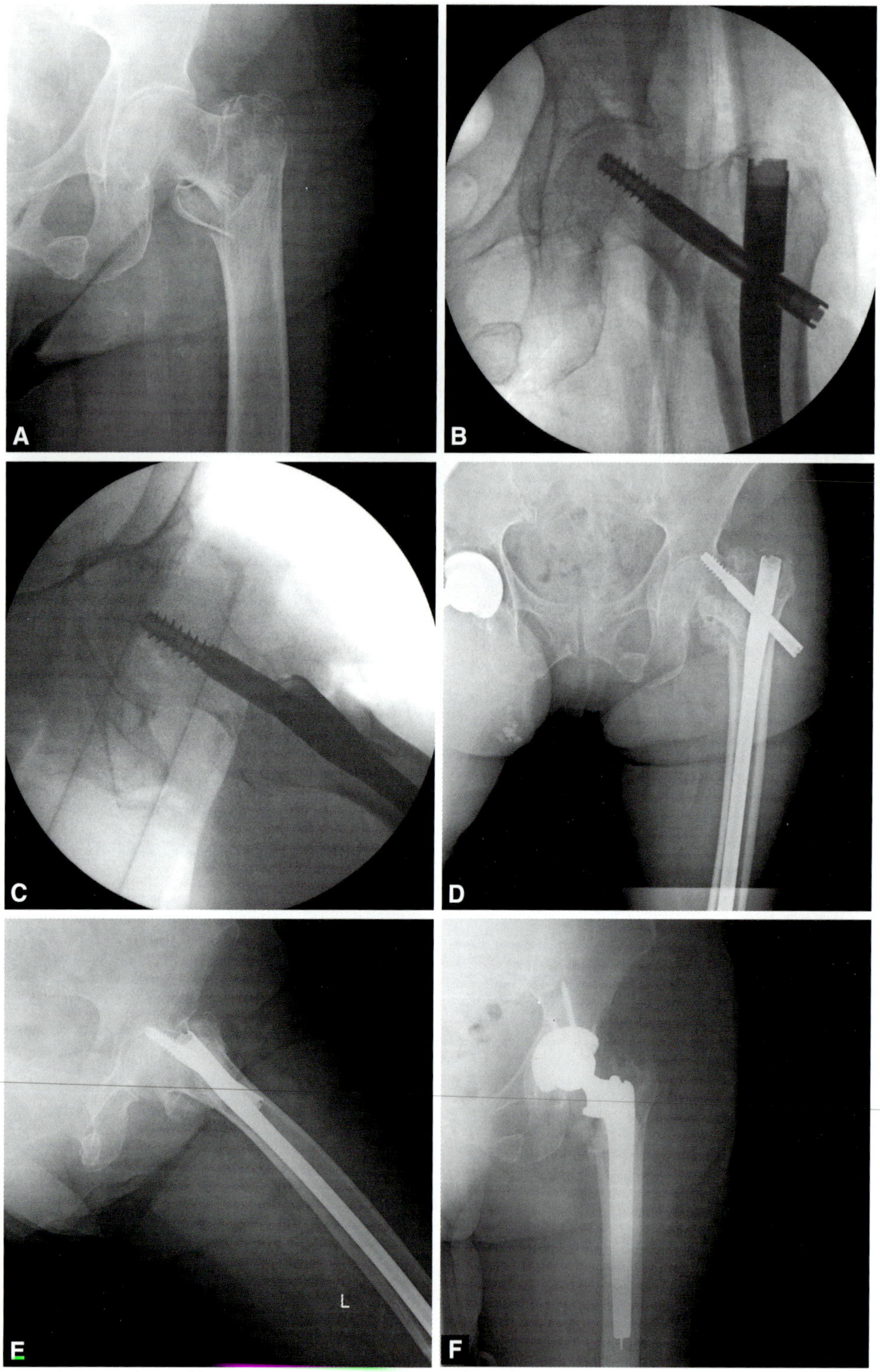

Figures 20.11A to F: Management of lag screw cut-out in an elderly patient after fixation of an intertrochanteric femur fracture. (A to C) Preoperative anteroposterior (AP) and intraoperative AP and lateral images demonstrating an intertrochanteric femur fracture treated with intramedullary nailing. Critical evaluation reveals that the lag screw position is somewhat superior in the femoral head; (D and E) Cut-out of the lag screw from the femoral head is noted at 6 weeks postoperatively on AP and lateral images; (F) Due to her age and articular injury at the weight-bearing surface of the femoral head, this was managed with total hip arthroplasty with a calcar-replacing stem.

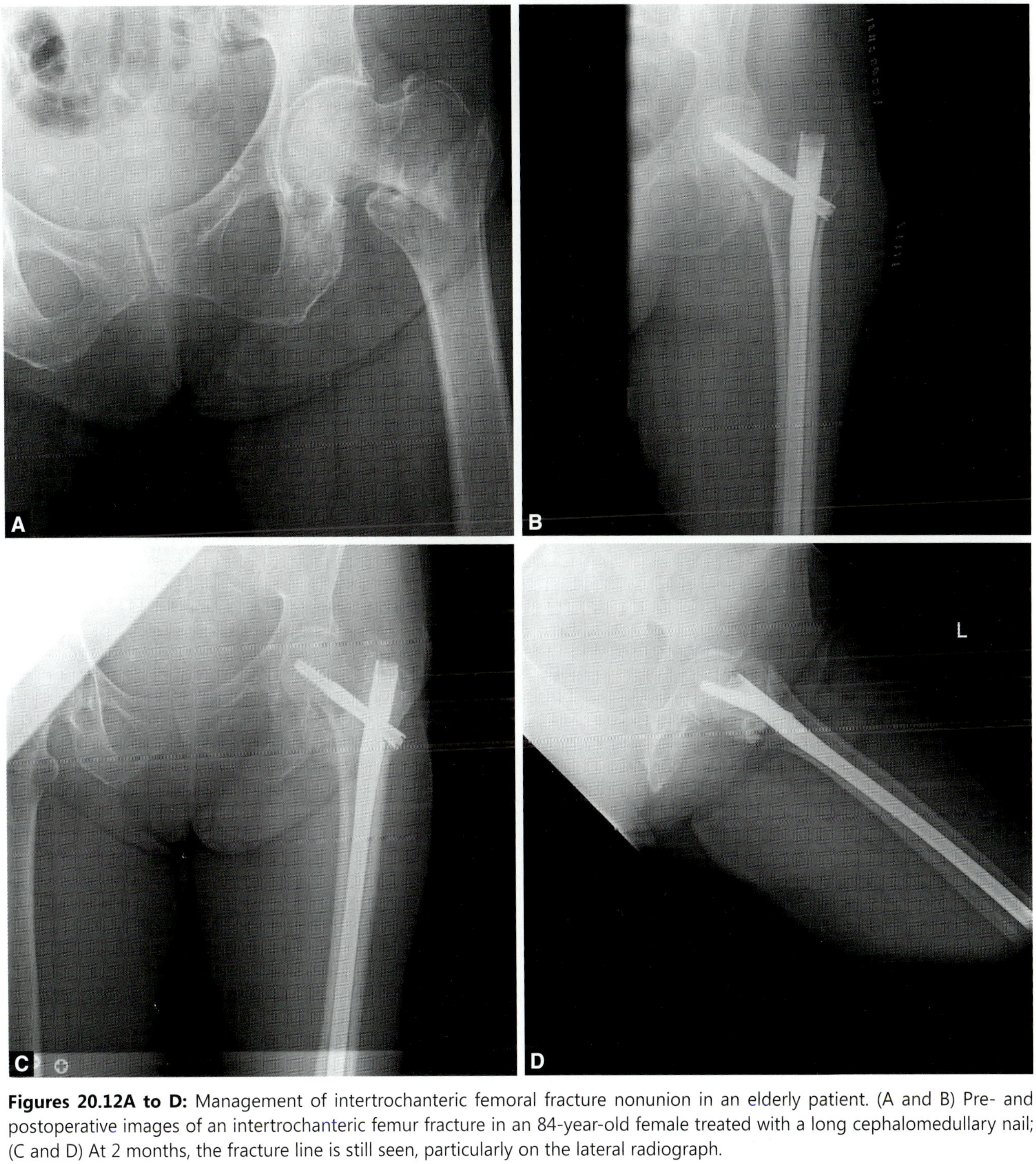

Figures 20.12A to D: Management of intertrochanteric femoral fracture nonunion in an elderly patient. (A and B) Pre- and postoperative images of an intertrochanteric femur fracture in an 84-year-old female treated with a long cephalomedullary nail; (C and D) At 2 months, the fracture line is still seen, particularly on the lateral radiograph.

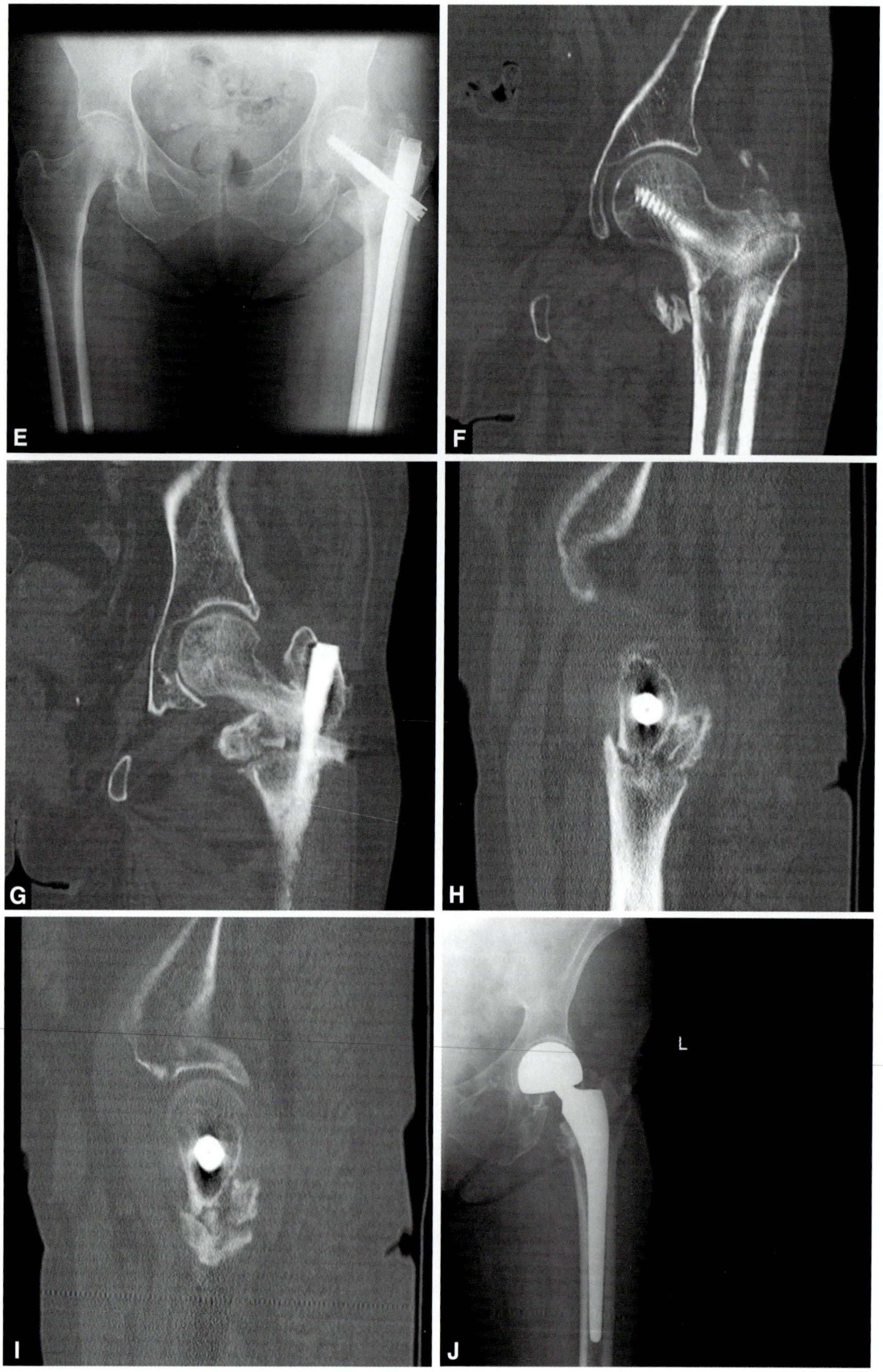

Figures 20.12E to J: (E to I) At 6 months, radiographs and CT scan demonstrate that the implants are intact, alignment is maintained, but the lucent fracture line is still visible; (J) Her persistently painful aseptic nonunion was treated with hemiarthroplasty due to her age and lack of any obvious arthritic changes.

advantages. Regardless of the implant utilized, the TAD should be minimized to avoid complications and ensure bony healing. Complications such as nonunion and loss of fixation with hardware failure can occur, and these will be frequently managed with joint arthroplasty in this age-group patient.

References

1. Stannard JP, Schmidt AH, Kregor PJ. Surgical treatment of orthopaedic trauma. New York, NY: Thieme; 2007. p. 940.
2. Lubovsky O, Liebergall M, Mattan Y, et al. Early diagnosis of occult hip fractures MRI versus CT scan. Injury. 2005; 36(6):788-92.
3. Evans EM. The treatment of trochanteric fractures of the femur. J Bone Joint Surg Br. 1949;31B(2):190-203.
4. Kyle RF, Gustilo RB, Premer RF. Analysis of six hundred and twenty two intertrochanteric hip fractures. J Bone Joint Surg Am. 1979;61(2):216-21.
5. Marsh JL, Slongo TF, Agel J, et al. Fracture and dislocation classification compendium-2007: Orthopaedic Trauma Association classification, database and outcomes committee. J Orthop Trauma, 2007;21(10 Suppl):S1-133.
6. Kyle RF, Ellis TJ, Templeman DC. Surgical treatment of intertrochanteric hip fractures with associated femoral neck fractures using a sliding hip screw. J Orthop Trauma. 2005; 19(1):1-4.
7. Kenzora JE, McCarthy RE, Lowell JD, et al. Hip fracture mortality. Relation to age, treatment, preoperative illness, time of surgery, and complications. Clin Orthop Relat Res. 1984;(186):45-56.
8. McNeill DH. Hip fractures. Influence of delay in surgery on mortality. Wis Med J. 1975;74(12):129-8.
9. Lyon LJ, Nevins MA. Management of hip fractures in nursing home patients: to treat or not to treat? J Am Geriatr Soc. 1984;32(5):391-5.
10. Baumgaertner MR, Curtin SL, Lindskog DM, et al. The value of the tip-apex distance in predicting failure of fixation of peritrochanteric fractures of the hip. J Bone Joint Surg Am. 1995;77(7):1058-64.
11. Baumgaertner MR, Solberg BD. Awareness of tip-apex distance reduces failure of fixation of trochanteric fractures of the hip. J Bone Joint Surg Br. 1997;79(6):969-71.
12. Bridle SH, Patel AD, Bircher M, et al. Fixation of intertrochanteric fractures of the femur. A randomised prospective comparison of the gamma nail and the dynamic hip screw. J Bone Joint Surg Br. 1991;73(2):330-4.
13. Davis J, Harris MB, Duval M, et al. Pertrochanteric fractures treated with the Gamma nail: technique and report of early results. Orthopedics. 1991;14(9):939-42.
14. Lindsey RW, Teal P, Probe RA, et al. Early experience with the gamma interlocking nail for peritrochanteric fractures of the proximal femur. J Trauma. 1991;31(12):1649-58.
15. Cornwall R, Gilbert MS, Koval KJ, et al. Functional outcomes and mortality vary among different types of hip fractures: a function of patient characteristics. Clin Orthop Relat Res. 2004;(425):64-71.
16. Barton TM, Gleeson R, Topliss C, et al. A comparison of the long gamma nail with the sliding hip screw for the treatment of AO/OTA 31-A2 fractures of the proximal part of the femur: a prospective randomized trial. J Bone Joint Surg Am. 2010;92(4):792-8.
17. Utrilla AL, Reig JS, Munoz FM, et al. Trochanteric gamma nail and compression hip screw for trochanteric fractures: a randomized, prospective, comparative study in 210 elderly patients with a new design of the gamma nail. J Orthop Trauma. 2005;19(4):229-33.
18. Parker MJ, Handoll HH. Gamma and other cephalocondylic intramedullary nails versus extramedullary implants for extracapsular hip fractures in adults. Cochrane Database Syst Rev. 2005;(4):CD000093.
19. Bartonicek J, Skala-Rosenbaum J, Dousa P. Valgus intertrochanteric osteotomy for malunion and nonunion of trochanteric fractures. J Orthop Trauma. 2003;17(9): 606-12.
20. Haidukewych GJ, Berry DJ. Salvage of failed internal fixation of intertrochanteric hip fractures. Clin Orthop Relat Res. 2003;(412):184-8.

Chapter 21

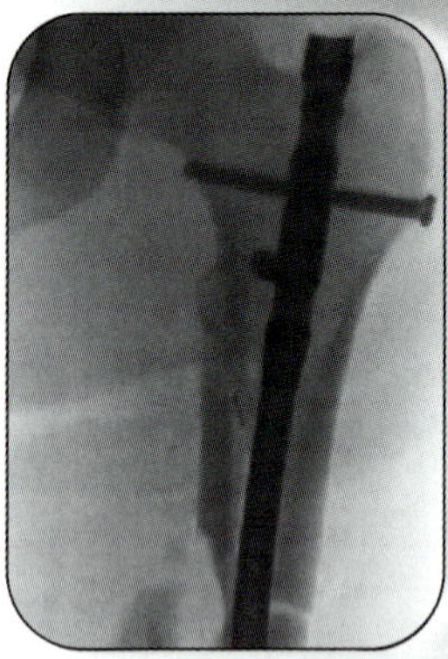

Subtrochanteric Femur Fractures

Paul Lafferty, Emily Keener, Peter Cole

Chapter Outline

Introduction
Diagnosis
- Physical Examination
- Diagnostic Imaging

Classification
- Seinsheimer's Classification
- Russell-Taylor Classification
- AO/OTA Classification

Surgical Indications
- Temporizing Measures
- Definitive Fixation

Surgical Anatomy and Positioning
- Anatomy
- Positioning

Surgical Techniques: General Concepts
- Intramedullary Nails
- Reconstruction Nails
- Trochanteric Nails
- 95° Angled Plates
- Proximal Femoral Locking Plates
- Preoperative Planning
- Reduction
- Length, Alignment and Rotation

Surgical Techniques: Specific Procedures
- Technique 1: Cephalomedullary Nailing
- Technique 2: Proximal Femoral Locking Plate
- Technique 3: Blade Plate

Outcomes
Complications and Management
- Deep Vein Thrombosis
- Loss of Fixation and Malunion
- Nonunion
- Malrotation

Authors' Preferred Management of Select Complications
- Case 1: Nonunion Repair of an Intertrochanteric Femur Fracture with a Blade Plate
- Case 2: Nonunion Repair of a Pertrochanteric Femur Fracture with Blade Plate Fixation
- Case 3: Nonunion Repair of a Pertrochanteric Femur Fracture with Proximal Femur Locking Plate

Summary

Introduction

Subtrochanteric femur fractures involve the region of proximal femur with primary fracture line existing between the lesser trochanter and 5 cm below the lesser trochanter.[1] Wiss and Brien described subtrochanteric femur fractures as fractures extending from the lesser trochanter to the junction of the proximal and middle third of the femur.[2] These types of fractures are difficult for the orthopedic surgeons to treat secondary to the high-stress loads in this portion of the femur along with deforming muscle forces present in this region. Subtrochanteric femur fractures occur in a bimodal age distribution resulting from high-energy injuries, including motor vehicle accidents and motorcycle crashes in young individuals, and from lower-energy mechanisms, such as falls from standing heights in elderly individuals.[3] Suspicion should be raised for pathological fractures in young individuals that sustain these types of fractures from low-energy mechanisms. There has also been a growing number of subtrochanteric insufficiency fractures in the elderly population resulting from long-term bisphosphonate therapy.[4]

Diagnosis

Physical Examination

Patients with subtrochanteric femur fractures can have other associated life-threatening injuries and conditions that need to be addressed acutely including hypovolemic shock. Patients with subtrochanteric femur fractures present with proximal thigh pain and swelling. The affected extremity is shortened and externally rotated. A careful neurological and vascular examination should be performed on the affected extremity. The skin should be examined for any open injuries as well as any lacerations or abrasions that may affect future surgical incision sites. The ipsilateral knee should also be evaluated for ligamentous injury.[3]

Diagnostic Imaging

The X-rays of the entire femur are required to adequately image the fracture. An axial traction view of the affected femur can help elucidate the fracture pattern. The hip and knee should also be imaged. An anteroposterior (AP) view of the pelvis is also required to look for any associated injuries including ipsilateral femoral neck fractures and acetabular fractures especially in high-energy mechanisms. A computerized tomography (CT) scan can be helpful in detecting complex fracture patterns with extension into the intertrochanteric region and femoral neck and/or distal extension into the femoral diaphysis. Computerized tomography scans are also helpful in identifying any nondisplaced fracture lines that may not be appreciated on X-rays of the femur.[4] A bone scan or magnetic resonance imaging may be used to identify stress fractures of the subtrochanteric region of the femur that are not appreciated on X-ray or CT scan of the femur.[5]

SUBTROCHANTERIC FEMUR FRACTURES DIAGNOSIS: Pearls and Pitfalls

- Patients with subtrochanteric femur fractures present with proximal thigh swelling and pain. It is important to appreciate and not to overlook any associated injuries including ipsilateral knee injuries
- Patients must have a neurovascular examination of the affected extremity. The skin should be examined carefully for any open injuries associated with the subtrochanteric femur fracture
- The X-rays of the entire femur as well as the hip and knee in both the AP and lateral views are necessary for diagnosis. Axial traction views of the femur help characterize the fracture pattern
- Computerized tomography scan of the proximal femur can elucidate the subtrochanteric femur fracture patterns and any extension of the fracture lines proximally into the intertrochanteric and/or femoral neck region or distally into the diaphysis of the femur

Classification

Seinsheimer's Classification

Seinsheimer created a classification system in 1978 for subtrochanteric femur fractures based on major fracture fragments and the fracture lines and their extensions (Fig. 21.1). The fracture fragment must measure 1 cm or greater in its largest diameter to be considered a major fragment. The classification includes Types I–V. Type I fractures are nondisplaced fractures that have less than 2 mm displacement of any fracture piece. Type II fractures are two-part fractures that are subdivided into A, B and C. Type IIA is a two-part transverse fracture. Types IIB and IIC are spiral fractures with the lesser trochanter attached to the proximal fragment in IIB and to the distal fragment in IIC. Type III subtrochanteric femur fractures are three-part fractures. Type IIIA is a spiral fracture of the proximal femur with the lesser trochanter attached to the third fragment, which also includes an inferior spike of cortex. Type IIIB is a spiral fracture in which the third part is a butterfly fracture fragment. Type IV fractures are

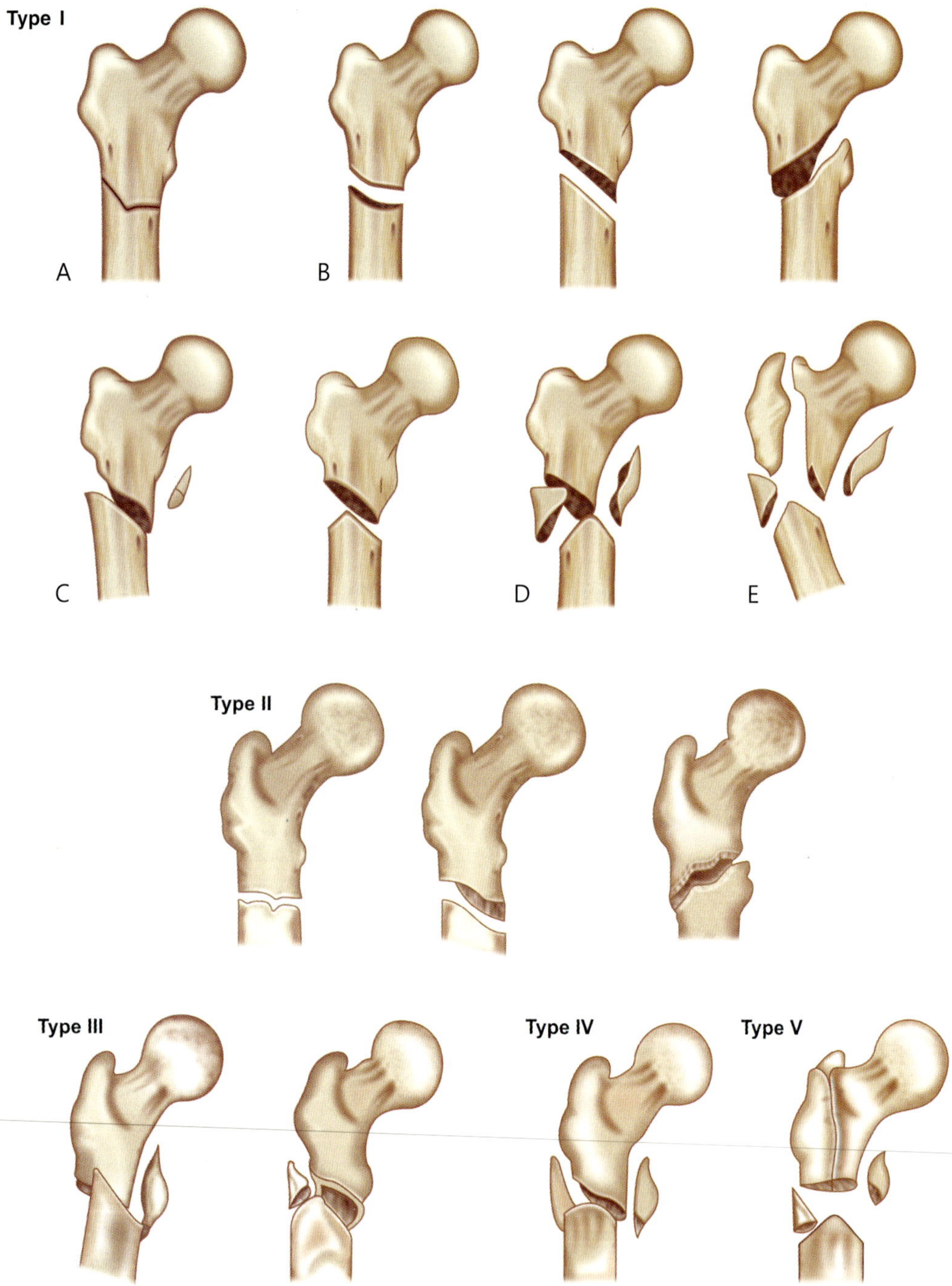

Figure 21.1: Seinsheimer's classification of subtrochanteric femur fractures.

comminuted subtrochanteric femur fractures with four parts. Type V fractures are subtrochanteric femur fractures with extension into the intertrochanteric region and also into the greater trochanter. In Seinsheimer's study, Type IIIA fractures had the highest failure rates when treated with internal fixation secondary to the large bending forces at the implant at the level of the fracture sites.[1]

Russell-Taylor Classification

The Russell-Taylor classification of subtrochanteric femur fractures examines the extension of the fracture into the piriformis fossa as well as involvement of the lesser trochanter (Fig. 21.2). Type I fractures do not involve the piriformis fossa. Type IA does not have comminution of the

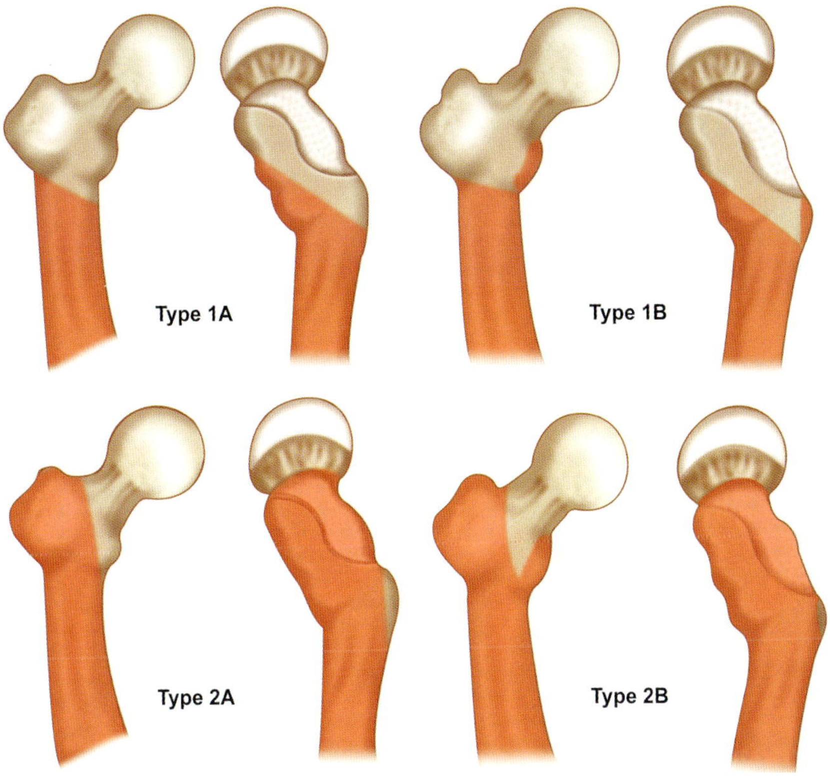

Figure 21.2: Russell-Taylor classification of subtrochanteric femur fractures.

lesser trochanter, while Type IB has comminution present in this region. Type II fractures have fracture lines that extend into the piriformis fossa. Type IIA fractures again do not involve comminution of the lesser trochanter and Type IIB fracture patterns have comminution in the lesser trochanter region. Comminution of the lesser trochanter indicates a lack of intact medial proximal femoral cortex. This leads to increased varus stress loads after internal fixation of the proximal femur. Extension into the piriformis fossa is important to note when using a piriformis starting point for intramedullary (IM) nail fixation. The fracture line into the fossa can affect this starting point.[6]

AO/OTA Classification

The AO/OTA also classified subtrochanteric femur fractures. The femur is named 3 and the proximal femur 31. The trochanteric portion of the femur is 31-A which is then divided into three subtypes: (1) reverse obliquity intertrochanteric fractures are 31-A3.1, (2) transverse subtrochanteric fractures are 31-A3.2, and (3) comminuted subtrochanteric fractures are 31-A3.3 (Fig. 21.3).[7]

Surgical Indications

Surgical stabilization is recommended in almost all subtrochanteric femur fractures. Nonoperative therapy is only employed for patients that cannot survive a surgical procedure secondary to concomitant medical or severe trauma issues. Even for nonambulatory patients, surgical fixation of subtrochanteric femur fractures helps with nursing care. Operative therapy for subtrochanteric femur fractures aids in mobilizing the patient and thus, decreases the risk of pneumonia, decubitus ulcers and deep venous thrombosis.[3]

Temporizing Measures

Open subtrochanteric femur fractures should undergo an emergent irrigation and debridement and either temporary or definitive fixation. Skeletal traction should be applied if the patient does not undergo immediate fixation. Traction helps with pain control and also decreases the potential third space caused by the injury, thus, decreasing blood loss into the thigh. External fixation is a temporizing measure

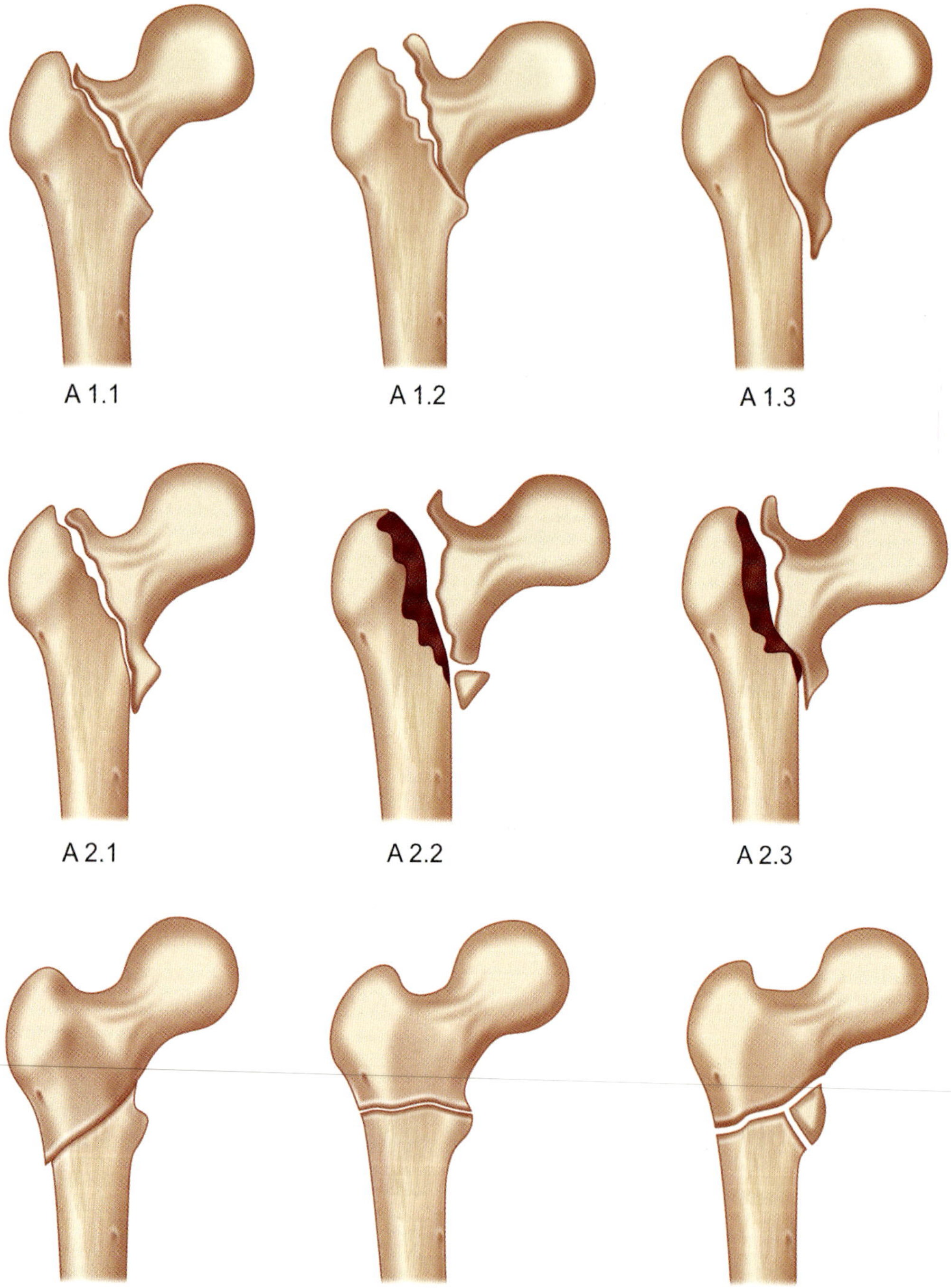

Figure 21.3: AO/OTA classification of subtrochanteric femur fractures.

of subtrochanteric femur fractures used on severely injured trauma patients.[3] However, external fixation of proximal femur fractures can be technically difficult due to the small proximal fragment. Furthermore, there tends to be more drainage from proximal thigh and pelvic pins, potentially compromising future internal fixation, particularly with hospital acquired organisms frequently found in intensive care units. Therefore, this is not an ideal temporizing measure as it is for the knee or ankle, by comparison.

Definitive Fixation

Operative fixation of subtrochanteric femur fractures with IM nail fixation or plate and screw techniques is preferred over nonoperative therapy, skeletal traction and external fixation, when the patient is stable to undergo a surgical procedure. Definitive operative therapy helps with mobilization postoperatively and thus, decreases many risks which are incurred by remaining on bed rest.[8]

Surgical Anatomy and Positioning

Anatomy

Subtrochanteric femur fractures are difficult to treat operatively because of the bony anatomy of this region of the femur as well as the strong muscular attachments in this region. The femoral shaft has an anterior bow with an average curvature between 109° and 120°. The neck-shaft angle averages 129° in males and 133° in females. Koch's biomechanical study in 1917 showed that axial loads of 100 pounds in the subtrochanteric region led to compression forces greater than 1,000 pounds per square inch most pronounced on the medial side. These forces on the medial side of the subtrochanteric femur are greatest at 1–3 cm distal to the lesser trochanter. This leads to dense cortical bone in this region.[9] The linea aspera is an area of cortical thickening on the posterior femoral shaft, in which the adductor group inserts and the vastus intermedialis and short head of the biceps femoris attaches.

The greater trochanter has several muscular attachments including the abductor muscles: the gluteus medius and minimus; and the external rotators: the piriformis, gemelli muscles and quadratus femoris. These muscular attachments cause the proximal fracture fragment of subtrochanteric femur fractures to externally rotate and abduct. The iliopsoas is a powerful hip flexor attached to the lesser trochanter. This causes flexion of the proximal or distal fracture fragment depending on which fragment the lesser trochanter is attached. The adductor muscles attach to the distal femur and thus, pull the distal fragment of subtrochanteric femur fractures into adduction.

The blood supply to the femur is from the nutrient artery that arises from the area of linea aspera. There are also contributions from multiple periosteal arteries. The medial femoral circumflex artery is the main supply to the femoral head and neck (Fig. 21.4).[10]

Positioning

Traditionally, the traction table has been the operating table of choice for subtrochanteric femoral fractures; however, many surgeons use the radiolucent operating table without traction devices. The patient usually is positioned either in the supine or in the lateral position, although some surgeons prefer a so-called sloppy lateral position, that is, supine position with a large bump under the affected hip.

There has been a significant amount written about the advantages and disadvantages of the above mentioned techniques for antegrade femoral nailing. The focus of most studies has been comparisons between positioning on a fracture table versus supine positioning on a flat radiolucent table with the affected limb draped free. Advantages of the fracture table include sustained longitudinal traction without the need for an additional assistant as well as circumferential access to the injured extremity for manipulation, exposure and imaging. Disadvantages include difficulty in accommodating an obese patient, establishing the correct starting point and limited access to the polytraumatized patient. Additionally, there are also several complications associated with the use of fracture table, including pudendal nerve injury, skin slough associated with the peroneal post, compartment syndrome of the well leg and internal malrotation deformity. Advantages of supine positioning on a flat radiolucent table are decreased operative time and increased versatility for multiple-injured patients. Disadvantages have been cited as difficulty in obtaining lateral imaging of the proximal femur and in obtaining and holding alignment throughout the procedure.

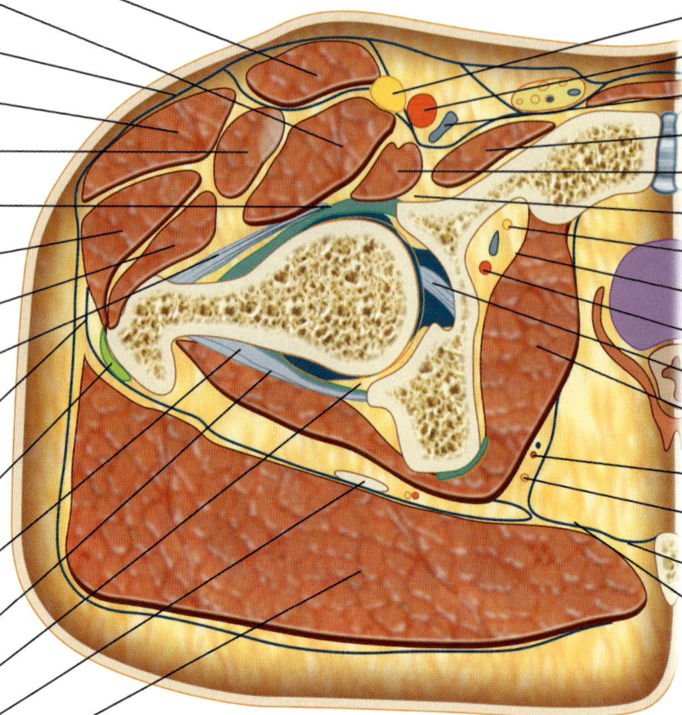

Figure 21.4: Surgical anatomy of the hip as viewed anteriorly and posteriorly.

Lateral positioning has several advantages. As with supine femoral nailing on the radiolucent table, the potential complications and inconveniences unique to the fracture table are avoided. Lateral positioning allows improved access to both piriformis fossa and trochanteric entry points, particularly in obese patients. The larger incisions typically required in obese patients are also much more accessible in the lateral position. The lateral position is also versatile in allowing for conversion to an open procedure, if the need arises. Additionally, the operative limb is accessible from both sides of the operating room table. High quality AP and lateral imaging of the proximal femur is performed without difficulty, as the C-arm does not have to be positioned at extremes of its arc range or in an oblique angle to the femur, as is necessary with traction table positioning.

Open reduction and internal fixation with plate and screws can be performed through a lateral approach. The incision is made over middle of the greater trochanter and extended distally along the axis of the femoral shaft. The tensor fasciae latae is split and the vastus lateralis is then exposed and elevated anteriorly. Perforating branches of the profunda femoris artery lie along the vastus lateralis and must be coagulated. The lateral femur is then exposed. Intramedullary nail fixation of subtrochanteric femur fractures is often performed percutaneously and thus, an open surgical approach is often unnecessary, but may be required if a closed or percutaneous reduction cannot be achieved.[10]

Surgical Techniques: General Concepts

Implants used for fixation of subtrochanteric femur fractures can be divided into two broad categories: (1) plate and screw devices inserted with either standard or minimally invasive techniques, or (2) IM nails inserted via open or minimally invasive techniques. Antegrade IM femoral nails are further divided into either centromedullary (standard interlocked femoral nails) or cephalomedullary (reconstruction and trochanteric femoral nails).

Intramedullary Nails

A subtrochanteric femoral fracture can be stabilized with standard piriformis-entry first-generation interlocking nail if it has an intact proximal fragment large enough to accommodate the nail and proximal interlocking screws. Failure to stabilize the proximal fragment can adequately result in malreduction, which typically consists of a combined procurvatum and varus deformity. Standard locking techniques may not adequately secure the proximal fragment, and the nail may toggle in the wide canal of the proximal fragment.

Reconstruction Nails

Reconstruction nails are typically inserted via piriformis fossa and utilize screws that engage the bone in the femoral neck and head. This allows the implant to better secure the proximal fragment because of an increased contact with the bone in the femoral neck and head. Reconstruction nails can be used to stabilize all patterns of subtrochanteric femur fractures, including those with comminution of the lesser trochanter, extension into the piriformis fossa and intertrochanteric or femoral neck involvement.

Trochanteric Nails

Trochanteric entry nails are frequently employed in subtrochanteric fractures. These devices have an apex-medial bend in the proximal aspect of the nail to allow the nail to easily traverse the IM canal. Similar to reconstruction nails, trochanteric nails feature screws or a spiral blade that engage the bone in the femoral head and neck, making them suitable for treating subtrochanteric fractures. Many surgeons find that these trochanteric nails are easier to insert than the nails with an entry point at the piriformis fossa. Like reconstruction nails, trochanteric entry nails can be used to stabilize all patterns of subtrochanteric femur fractures.

95° Angled Plates

Many of the early advances in stabilizing difficult proximal femoral fractures were in large part of the result of the successful deployment of the 95° condylar blade plate. Nevertheless, the surgical technique is very challenging; the plate must be inserted precisely in all three planes: (1) axial, (2) sagittal, and (3) coronal. Many surgeons found that using this device was a difficult experience.

The 95° compression screw plate has also been used successfully for many years in treating subtrochanteric fractures. The technique is familiar to orthopedic surgeons, who use 135° compression hip screws in treating intertrochanteric femoral fractures. An advantage of the 95° compression hip screw as compared to the 95° condylar blade plate is that the construct can be adjusted in the sagittal plane after the compression screw has been placed. As a result, this device has less potential for error in placement, particularly in the sagittal plane.

Proximal Femoral Locking Plates

Precontoured proximal femoral locking plates can be inserted using both open and minimally invasive techniques. They are useful in the treatment of comminuted and unstable subtrochanteric fractures, fractures with extension into the piriformis fossa, and combined intracapsular and extracapsular fractures.

Preoperative Planning

Treatment of these fractures is technically demanding. The surgeon requires flexibility in the choice of implant and approach. When proximal comminution requires the use of a fixed angle device, detailed templating is required to ensure that an implant with the proper blade or compression screw length, as well as plate length, is available. When an IM device is chosen, templating for length, as well as canal diameter and bow, is necessary for proper planning. In addition, because significant comminution could make limb length determination difficult, it can be helpful to obtain radiographs of the unaffected femur with a ruler to ascertain the normal femur length. High-quality standard AP and lateral X-rays of the hip, femur and knee should be obtained. Cross-table lateral and films in traction are useful if the fracture pattern is complex. Full-length radiographs including the joints above and below are required before surgery to evaluate the full extent of damage to the femur, to estimate the length and diameter of implant selections and to assess the femoral bow.

Computerized tomography scans are also useful in complex fracture patterns. The radius of curvature of some commercially available nails may be greater than the average femoral curvature of 109–120 cm. Excessive bow, which may be found in elderly patients and patients of short stature, may make passage of long IM nail difficult and results in perforation of the anterior distal cortex with long nail insertion.

Reduction

The reduction technique depends on the "personality" of the fracture. In case of subtrochanteric fracture, care must be taken to correct the typical deformities of flexion, abduction and external rotation of the proximal fragment. Alternatively, the distal fragment can be externally rotated to match the proximal fragment. These deformities are due to forces exerted on the proximal fragment by the iliopsoas, hip abductors and short external rotators. The distal fragment is typically displaced medially and shortened due to the deforming forces of the adductor, quadriceps and hamstring complexes. The fracture can be reduced using any number of described techniques, including traction applied either manually or via traction table, femoral distractor, closed manipulation of the limb (utilizing well-padded mallet or "F" tool), percutaneous Steinmann pin manipulation of fracture fragments (Figs 21.5A to D), a fracture reducer (preloaded with a reaming guidewire) introduced through the proximal entry portal, or a limited open approach to the fracture.

Examples of limited open approaches include the use of a ball-spike pusher with or without a spike disk (Figs 21.6A and B) via percutaneous incisions to correct flexion and/or abduction of the proximal fragment and placement of a bone hook percutaneously around the medial cortex of the distal fragment. Small incisions can also be made to facilitate placement of a large point-to-point clamp, when the fracture pattern is amenable.

When closed reduction is inadequate, the fracture should undergo formal open reduction to ensure that adequate alignment is achieved. Open reduction techniques should be employed that minimize soft tissue dissection and subsequent devascularization of the fracture site. The viability of the medial femoral fragments is very important; these pieces should be handled carefully to avoid iatrogenic injury.

Blocking screws can be utilized to assist in attaining reduction in subtrochanteric femur fractures. As in other locations, the concave side of the short segment is the appropriate location for the screws. A screw placed medially in the proximal segment will assist in correcting a varus deformity (Fig. 21.7A) and a screw placed posteriorly in the proximal segment will help correct a recurvatum deformity. These screws can be placed temporarily or left in place following nail placement. Blocking screws can also be placed in the distal fragment when necessary (Fig. 21.7B).

Length, Alignment and Rotation

When assessing the adequacy of the reduction, the surgeon should strive for anatomical alignment; however, 10° of angulation or 1 cm of shortening is common in difficult subtrochanteric fractures, such as those with extensive comminution. Restoration of femoral length should be assessed by judging the alignment of the reduced fragments or by comparison with the contralateral femur. Rotational alignment can be assessed by a variety of methods.

Fluoroscopic Measurement of Anteversion

The uninjured extremity is assessed prior to surgery. With the patient supine, a true lateral view of the proximal femur is obtained, and the position of the C-arm is noted. The true lateral view is delineated by the overlap of the medial and lateral cortices of the femoral neck. The leg is held still, while fluoroscopy is used to obtain a perfect lateral view of the ipsilateral knee. The perfect lateral view demonstrates overlap of the posterior cortices of medial and lateral condyles. The difference in angles of the intensifier determines the femoral version. This same technique is used on the injured leg following placement of the proximal interlocks in the nail. The femoral version is matched to that on the contralateral side, and the distal interlocks are placed.

Lesser Trochanteric Profile

This technique utilizes assessment of the profile of the lesser trochanter on an AP fluoroscopic image. This method can be performed at any time with the patient supine, with or without a fracture table and can be performed intraoperatively. The profile of the lesser trochanter on an

AP image serves as the basis for comparing the lower limbs. First, a true lateral image of the femoral condyles is obtained. The C-arm is then rotated 90° from that point, without moving the limb. This AP view of the proximal femur is used to assess the profile of the lesser trochanter. The double screen of the image intensifier can be used to compare the sides. This method is not appropriate for lesser trochanteric fractures or bilateral femur fractures and should not be used in patients with preexisting hip disease.

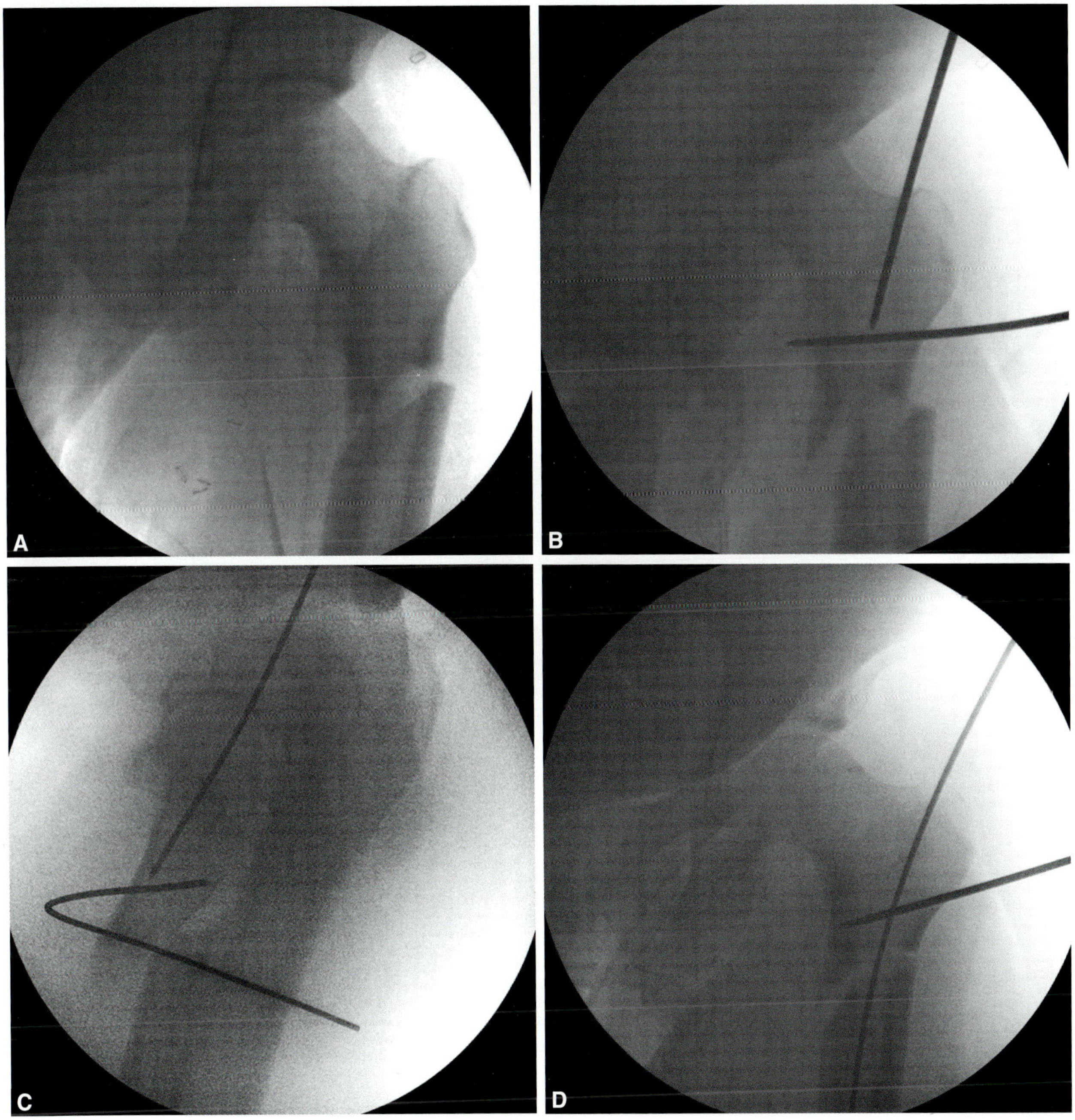

Figures 21.5A to D: Use of percutaneous Steinmann pin as a reduction tool. (A) Intraoperative image in a 23-year-old male with a left subtrochanteric femur fracture as a result of a motor vehicle crash; (B and C) A guidewire is placed through the greater trochanteric starting point. A Steinmann pin is placed percutaneously transversely into the proximal fragment as a reduction tool; (D) The guidewire is passed from the proximal fragment into the distal fragment after reduction of the fracture.

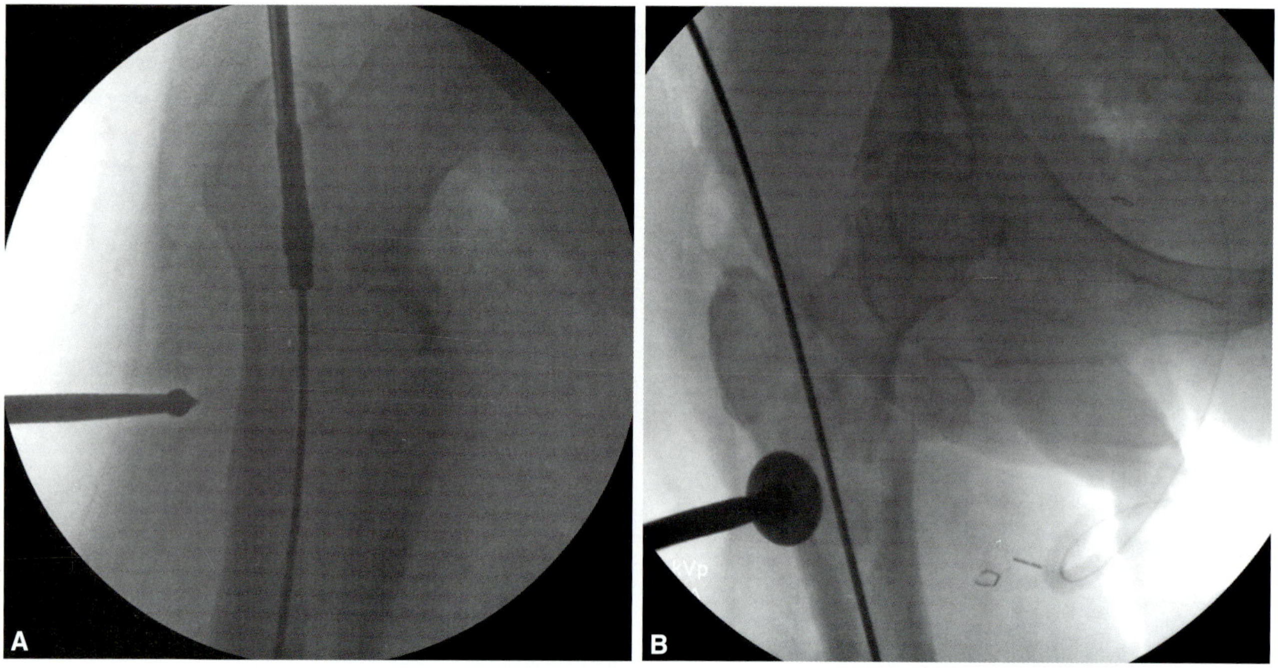

Figures 21.6A and B: Use of a percutaneous ball-spike pusher with and without a disk as a reduction tool. (A) A ball-spike pusher without and (B) with a spiked disk being used to correct varus and procurvatum deformities.

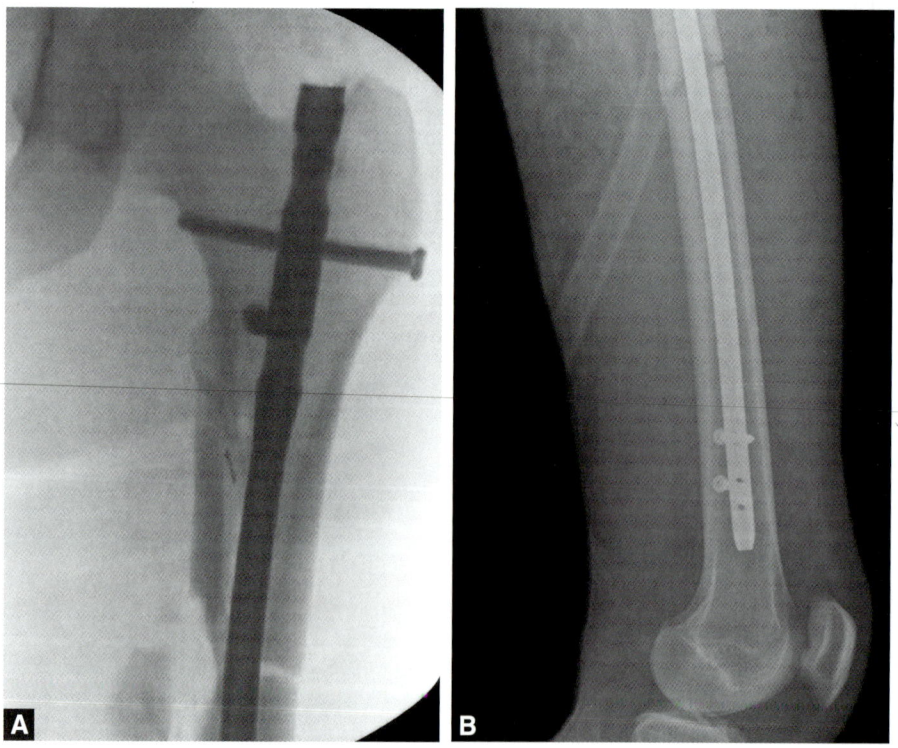

Figures 21.7A and B: Placement of blocking screws to prevent malalignment. (A) Anterior to posterior blocking screw placed on the medial side of the proximal fragment helps to correct varus deformity; (B) A blocking screw can also be placed in the distal fragment if necessary.

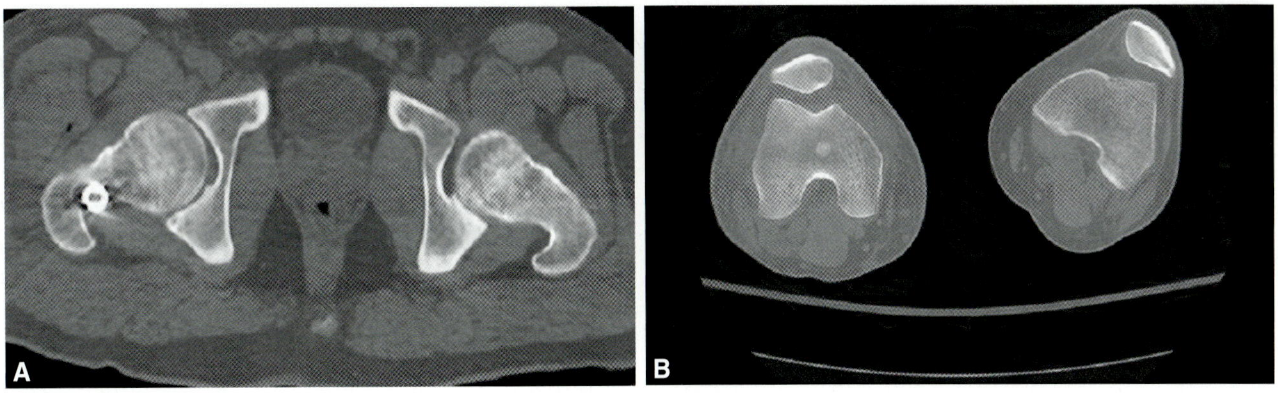

Figures 21.8A and B: Use of CT scanning to assess rotational alignment. (A and B) Internal malrotation of the right femur after antegrade intramedullary nailing of a comminuted midshaft femur fracture is shown on axial CT scanning proximally and (B) distally.

Computerized Tomography Scan

Computerized tomography can be used for preoperative and postoperative assessment of femoral rotation. Femoral anteversion is measured based on the angle between a line drawn through the center of femoral neck and a tangent drawn across the posterior aspect of distal femoral condyles (Figs 21.8A and B).[11] A prior limitation of this technique is that it cannot be used intraoperatively. The use of CT scan intraoperatively as a way to prevent malrotation has been investigated.[12] However, concerns exist regarding patient's exposure to radiation as well as the availability and cost of equipment. The biggest challenge in determining anteversion is accurate and reliable identification of the axis of femoral neck.

Computer Assisted Surgery

Computer assisted surgery (CAS) is being used more frequently in arthroplasty and realignment osteotomy procedures. The use of CAS in orthopedic trauma has also been investigated.[13] Computer assisted surgery has been shown to significantly decrease the amount of malrotation. However, CAS has been found to add to surgical time in arthroplasty surgery, and equipment costs may be significant. The future of CAS in fracture care remains uncertain.

Clinical Assessment

Clinical assessment of rotation is often used in surgical and office settings. Comparison of the orientation of greater trochanter to that of distal lateral femoral epicondyle through palpation of these structures and comparison of their positions has been described. Rotation can also be clinically measured by flexing the hip and knee of each lower limb with the patient supine or prone. Prone positioning has been described as offering more accurate result, but many surgeons prefer the supine position for ease of use.[14] Each hip is fully rotated internally and externally. If each hip is free of pathology and has a similar amount of total rotation, side-to-side difference can be attributed to malrotation through the fracture site. For example, 20° of external malrotation alters the profile of the hip so that it has 20° more external rotation from neutral and 20° less internal rotation as compared with the other side.

Despite widespread use, clinical assessment of the rotational profile has been shown to be inaccurate.[15] However, other studies have demonstrated accuracy to within 5° using clinical examination.[16] The accuracy of clinical examination alone must be questioned in patients with symptomatic complaints consistent with malrotation and in those, in whom preexisting hip disease is suspected.

Intraoperative Assessment

Regardless of the technique chosen to assess rotation, each patient must be examined thoroughly following static locking of the IM nail before leaving the operating room. If there are adjustments to be made, these are the best made while the patient is still under anesthesia. This systematic examination must assess rotation and limb length and the knee should be evaluated for ligamentous stability.

Radiographic assessment of the femoral neck is required to ensure the absence of femoral neck fracture following fixation.

Surgical Techniques: Specific Procedures

Technique 1: Cephalomedullary Nailing

Successful cephalomedullary nailing depends on three fundamental concepts to ensure maximal bone and soft tissue conservation during instrumentation and to minimize the potential for malreduction: (1) precise portal placement, (2) trajectory control, and (3) portal preservation (Figs 21.9A to S).[17]

A precise starting point is crucial to ensure accurate reduction of subtrochanteric femur fractures to avoid common malalignments of varus and procurvatum. Correct portal placement is predicated on the selected implant. Three options for portal placement have been described:[18] (1) lateral trochanteric for nails with a proximal lateral angulation of more than 5°, (2) medial trochanteric portal for nails with a proximal lateral angulation of 4–5°, and (3) piriformis portal for straight proximal segment nails. Regardless of the implant chosen, starting farther lateral than the implant is designed to be inserted will lead to a varus malreduction. In placing the nail, it is also important to establish the correct anterior-to-posterior position on the greater trochanter to avoid procurvatum and to ensure that the screws will be in line with the axis of the femoral neck.

Trajectory control is the development of a precise path for the nail through the proximal fragment, which is crucial in restoring the appropriate proximal alignment in coronal and sagittal planes. The correct trajectory parallels the anterior lateral cortex of the proximal femur and allows nail juxtaposition against a solid cortical structure. An incorrect trajectory is very difficult to recover from, and will result in malalignment with nail insertion. Once the correct trajectory is established, the portal must be protected from erosion and fragmentation by subsequent instrumentation during reduction, canal preparation and fixation.

First, a 3.2 cm guidewire is precisely placed in an appropriate starting position on the AP view depending on the implant chosen. Regardless of implant choice, all portals should be centered in the femoral neck on the lateral view to allow safe screw passage into the femoral head. The guidewire is inserted 15–20 mm into the bone. In the event of errant pin placement, the original pin may be left in place and a honeycomb-type targeter can be adjusted to precisely place a second pin. The definitive guidewire should be inserted 15–20 mm and does not have to be in correct canal alignment, as the definitive trajectory will be established with passage of the starting reamer. Insertion of the guidewire too deep may force the reamer to cut a varus path through the proximal fragment, which can be difficult to compensate for.

Next, a cannulated rigid starting reamer approximating the proximal nail diameter is introduced over the guidewire through a protective sleeve to prevent excessive damage to the abductor tendons. The reamer is advanced to a central position in the proximal fragment on the AP view. After the appropriate trajectory has been established on the AP view and the reamer has been inserted 15–20 mm, its trajectory is confirmed with a lateral C-arm view. The reamer should be directed along the anterior cortex of the proximal femur on the lateral view. The insertion of the reamer can be adjusted during reaming to approximate the position described and is most helpful in avoiding a varus position of the proximal femur. The reamer is inserted until it reaches the medullary canal just below the region of lesser trochanter.

A long ball-tip guidewire is then inserted into the physeal scar distally. It is important to confirm that the wire does not impinge on the anterior cortex distally, as cortical perforation can result. Insertion of the guidewire into the lateral femoral condyle should also be avoided, as this may lead to varus malreduction of the fracture in patients with wide-diameter canals. Length is checked with an appropriate ruler, allowing for fracture distraction and desired final nail position.

The diaphyseal region is reamed in 0.5 mm increments beginning with an end-cutting reamer. The canal should be reamed up to 1–1.5 mm over the desired nail diameter and up to 2 mm when excessive anterior bow is present. Reaming should always be performed with a high speed and slow advancement to prevent excessive heat generation, incarceration of the reamer tip and pressurization of the IM canal, which can cause embolization of fat. Reaming is typically continued until chatter is encountered.

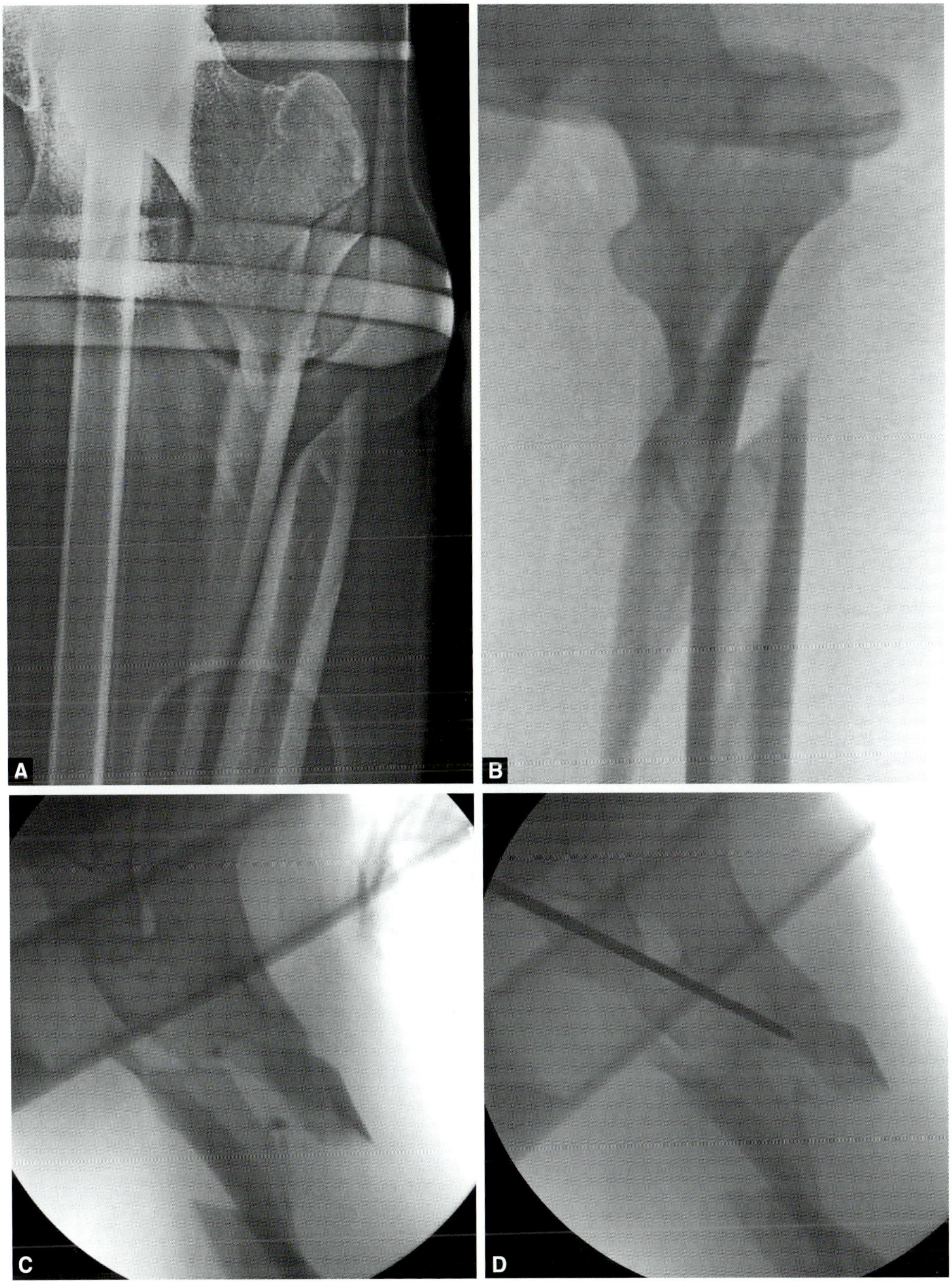

Figures 21.9A to D

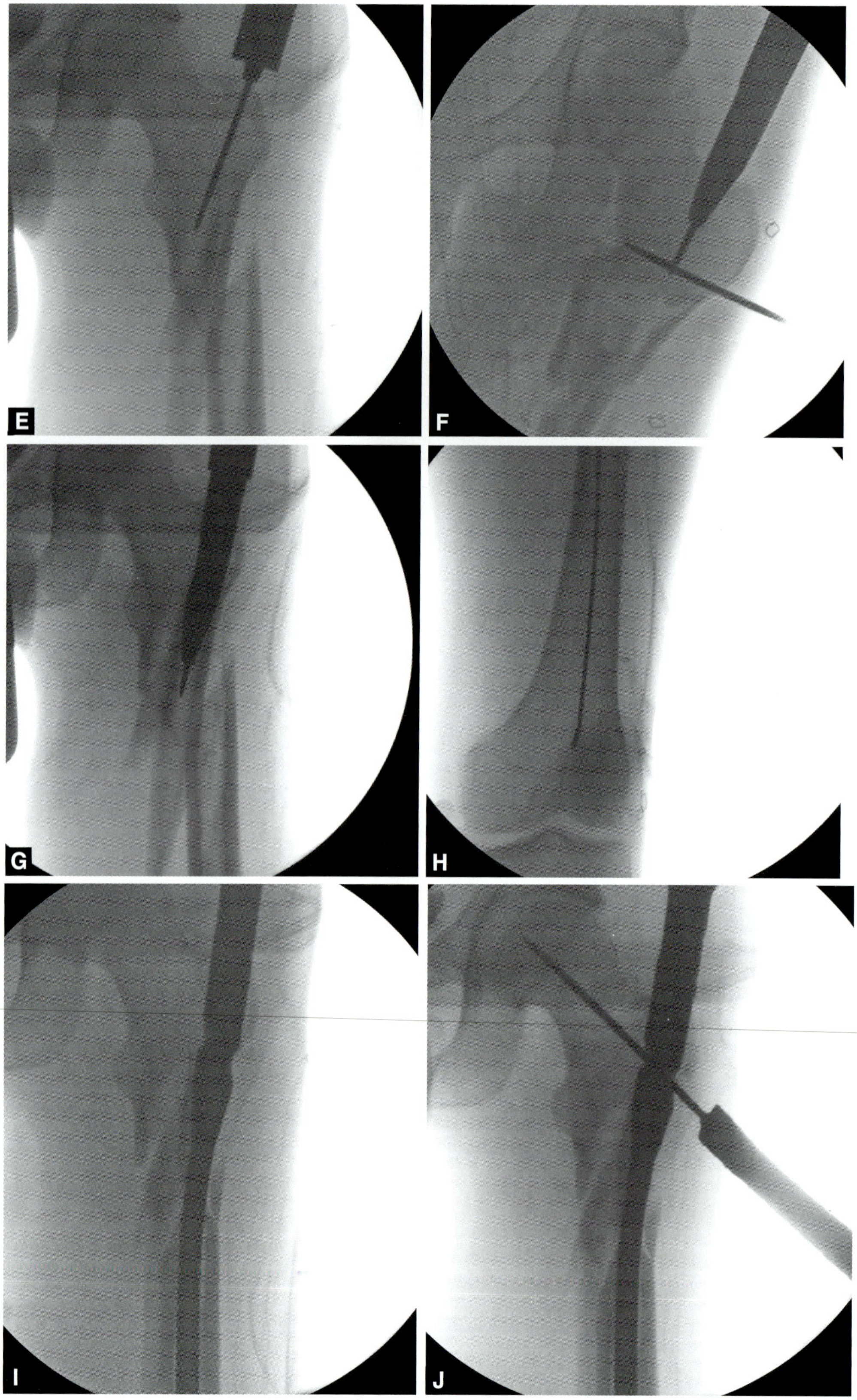

Figures 21.9E to J

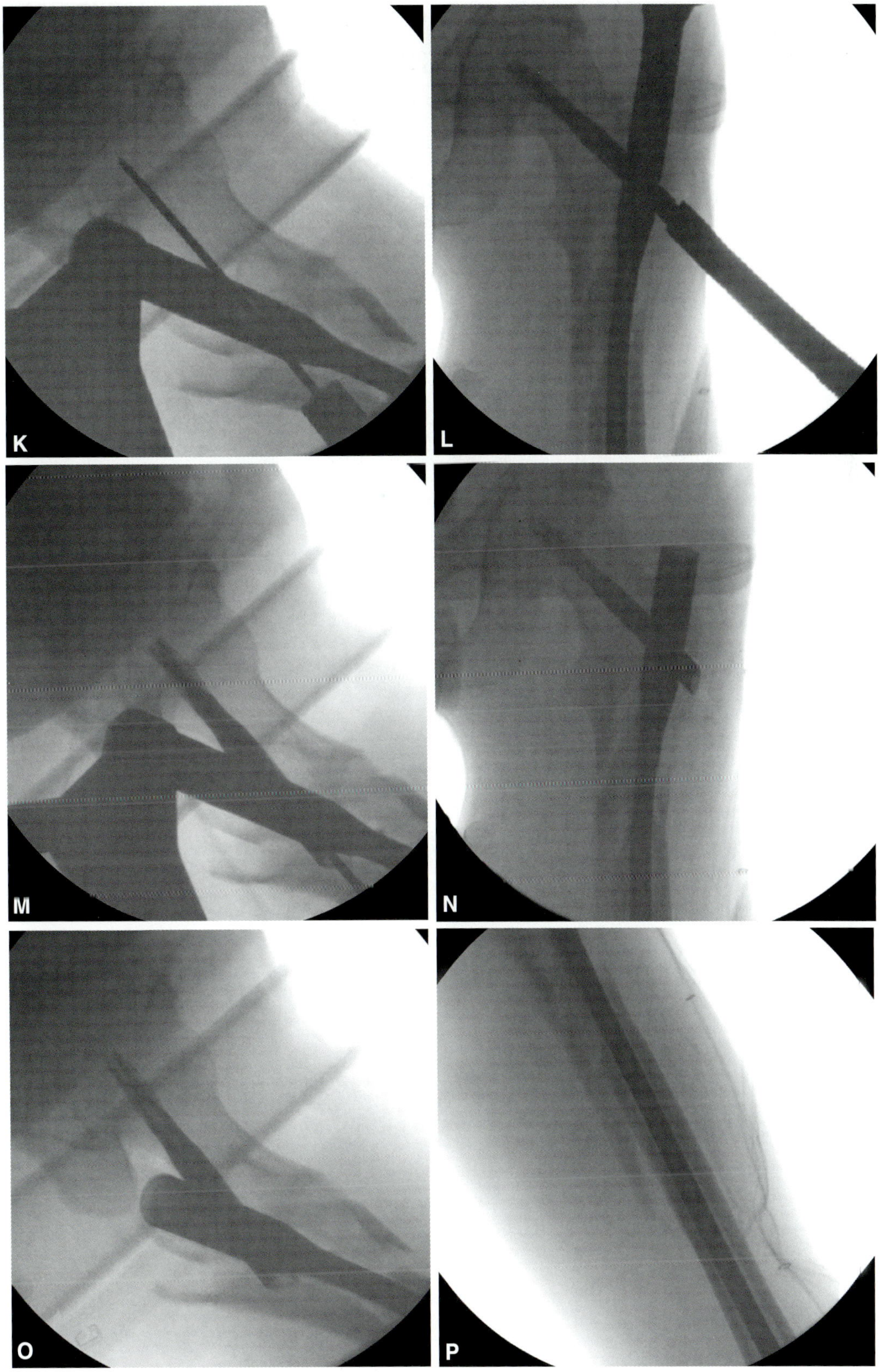

Figures 21.9K to P

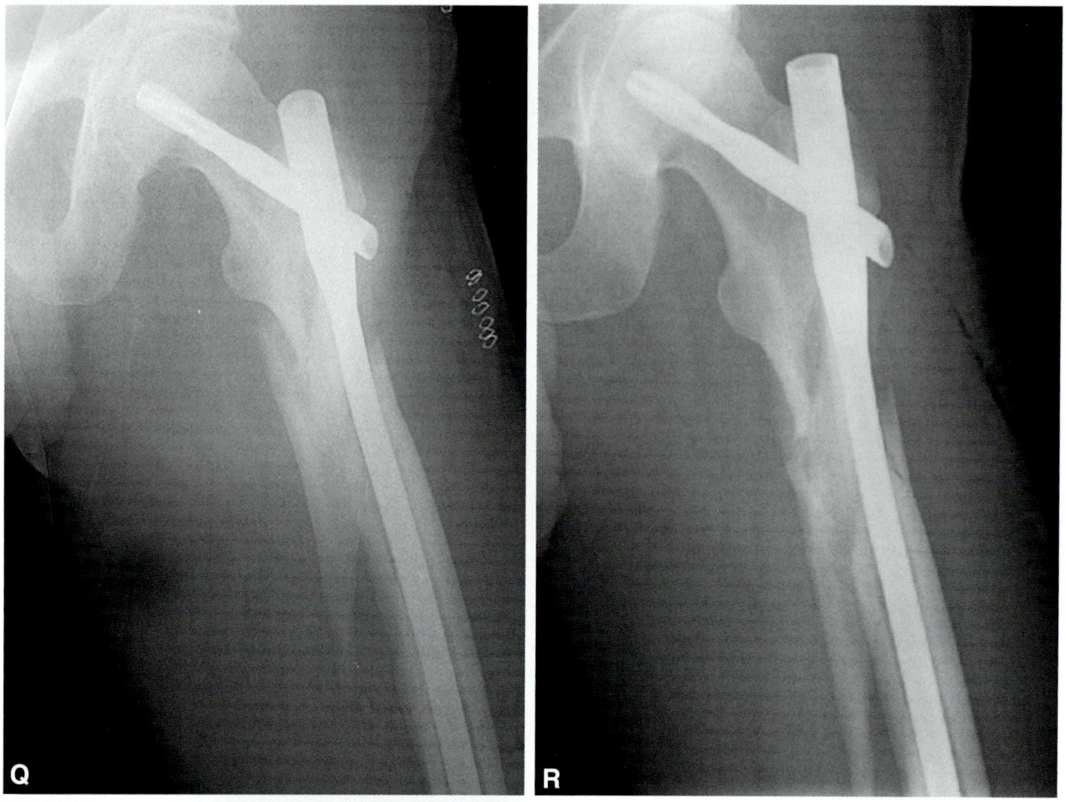

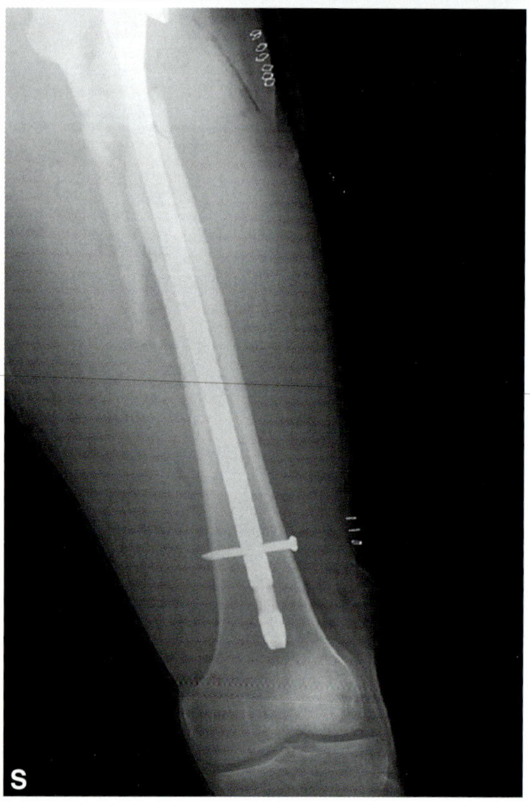

Figures 21.9A to S: Cephalomedullary nailing of a subtrochanteric femur fracture. A 39-year-old male, presented with an injury from an all-terrain vehicle. (A) Preoperative radiograph; (B) Intraoperative anteroposterior and (C) lateral fluoroscopic images on the traction table. (D) Placement of the starting portal guidewire shown on lateral image; (E to G) The opening portal reamer is introduced into the greater trochanter; (H) The ball-tipped guidewire is centrally placed in the distal femur; (I) The cannulated cephalomedullary nail is placed into the left femur over the guidewire; (J and K) The Kirschner (K) wire is inserted into the proximal femur through nail; (L and M) The spiral blade is inserted into the femoral neck and head; (N to P) Cephalomedullary nail is in place as shown on intraoperative images and (Q to S) on postoperative radiographic images.

During trochanteric nail insertion, it is helpful to rotate the nail 90° anteriorly during the first half of the nail advancement to minimize hoop stresses in the proximal femur. After partial insertion, the nail is rotated simultaneously, while it is advanced with gentle mallet taps to the anticipated anteversion required for insertion of the screw or blade into the femoral head.

The guidewire is removed to allow interlocking. Proximal interlocking technique varies depending on the chosen implant. Many implants have a radiolucent targeting device, which indicates the projected position of the guidewire in femoral head and neck. This is useful in avoiding multiple passes of the guidewire and potential perforation of the head and neck. Most designs recommend the screw or blade be placed in a center-center position. If a second screw is included in the nail design, there is usually a sufficient room for the second screw inferiorly; however, care should be exercised in small patients, in whom the initial screw may need to be placed slightly superior.

Trochanteric nails have distal locking capability with either static holes or a combination of static and dynamic. For length-stable fractures, one bicortical screw is sufficient in a dynamic mode. Conversely, for segmental fractures or extensive comminution, two screws are preferred. Distal interlocking is most commonly done using freehand "perfect-circles" technique, although long radiolucent targeting devices have recently become available. Additionally, a three-dimensional imaging system has recently become available, which obviates the need for fluoroscopy during distal interlocking, thereby decreasing radiation exposure to the surgical team.

With attention to detail and judicious use of soft tissue protectors, minimal damage to soft tissues is incurred with cephalomedullary nail insertion. Wound irrigation and standard layered closure are performed. Drains are not typically required.

CEPHALOMEDULLARY NAILING: Pearls and Pitfalls

- The key to reduction is rotation of the distal fragment to the externally rotated proximal fragment and apposition of the anterior cortex of proximal and distal fragments
- These two maneuvers will allow the correction of flexion and malrotation deformities
- After nail insertion, the length and rotational alignment of the proximal femur may change; therefore, before distal interlocking, the surgeon should recheck length and alignment
- Appropriate trajectory control will place the nail in apposition to the anterolateral cortex, minimizing varus and procurvatum deformities at the fracture site. Rotation of the trochanteric nail during the first half of insertion minimizes hoop stresses on the greater trochanter and medial cortex of the femur below the lesser trochanteric region in long nail designs
- Guidewire insertion and reaming should always be performed with a high speed and slow advancement. Guidewires and reamers can bend and be misdirected with excessive axial force during drilling
- For single-device and integrated screw femoral head fixation, the surgeon should use a center-center position for the large lag screw or spiral blade. For two-device femoral head fixation (reconstruction), the inferior screw is placed first along the medial calcar of the femoral neck. This will ensure adequate room for the proximal screw

Technique 2: Proximal Femoral Locking Plate

The following technique is modified from Hasenboehler et al.[19] Surgery is performed with the patient supine either on a radiolucent operating table or on a fracture table. For the latter option, closed fracture reduction is obtained before surgery under fluoroscopic guidance in AP and lateral planes. Care must be taken to achieve adequate rotation of the femur with patella in a horizontal position. In highly comminuted and unstable fractures that cannot be adequately reduced by traction on a fracture table, free draping of the lower extremity in the supine position on a radiolucent operating table is performed (Figs 21.10A to E).

A standard lateral approach is performed utilizing a longitudinal incision extending from the greater trochanter, approximately 10 cm distally in the direction of the lateral epicondyle. The iliotibial band is incised in line with the skin incision and the fascia of the vastus lateralis is incised in an L shape at its proximal insertion and the muscle is retracted anteriorly to visualize the lateral aspect of the proximal femur. Care should be taken to preserve soft

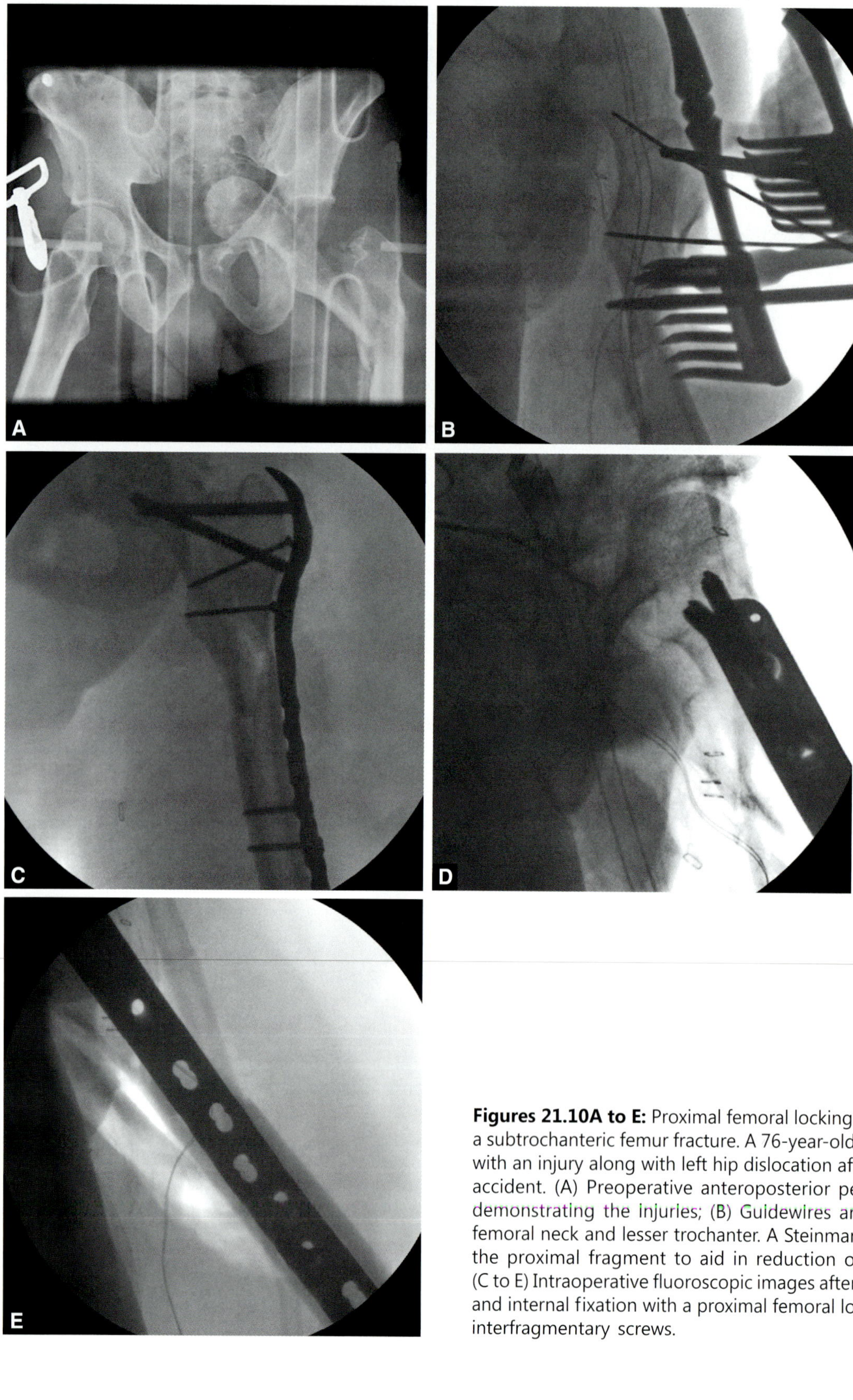

Figures 21.10A to E: Proximal femoral locking plate fixation of a subtrochanteric femur fracture. A 76-year-old male presented with an injury along with left hip dislocation after a motorcycle accident. (A) Preoperative anteroposterior pelvis radiograph demonstrating the injuries; (B) Guidewires are placed in the femoral neck and lesser trochanter. A Steinmann pin is used in the proximal fragment to aid in reduction of the fragment; (C to E) Intraoperative fluoroscopic images after open reduction and internal fixation with a proximal femoral locking plate with interfragmentary screws.

tissue attachments to comminuted fragments to preserve vascularity of the fracture zone.

In cases where a closed reduction is successful, a minimally invasive plating technique may be feasible. The plate is slid distally in the submuscular plane by the use of a distal counter incision at the level of the tip of the plate. The distal most hole of the plate can be used to attach a suture that is pulled through the distal counter incision to facilitate correct distal alignment of the plate to the bone, which must be visualized under fluoroscopy.

For more complex and comminuted fractures, the plate can be used as a reduction tool. In this case, the proximal fragment is first fixed to the plate and the plate is reduced to the femoral shaft. This maneuver is possible due to the angular-stable interface between the plate and the locking head screws in the proximal fragment. To facilitate reduction, a strong Kirschner (K) wire or Schanz pin can be temporarily fixed to the greater trochanter as a joystick to reduce the proximal segment.

In order to simplify reconstruction, the proximal fragment may be temporarily transfixed to the acetabulum with a smooth Steinmann pin to hold the alignment and allow proximal plate fixation. After ensuring appropriate placement of the plate on the proximal fragment, the plate is provisionally fixed to the head and neck. Depending on which currently available plate is selected, either 3 or 6 points of fixation into the head and neck are available. The plate is provisionally fixed to the proximal fragment with appropriately sized guidewires. The guidewires are advanced to the subchondral bone and their correct placement is confirmed by fluoroscopy in AP and lateral views. At this point, before the placement of proximal locking screws, it is crucial to recheck the alignment of the distal part of the plate to the femoral shaft. Appropriate screw length is determined by a measuring device placed over the guidewires. Depending on fracture configuration, one may choose to place a nonlocking screw initially to achieve interfragmentary compression prior to length-stable fixation with locking screws. This conical screw can later be replaced with a locking screw to augment fixation. Correct placement and screw length is ensured under fluoroscopy in two planes and the guidewires are removed.

The plate fixed to the proximal segment may now be used for anatomical reduction to the shaft in cases, where the initial closed reduction was unsuccessful. The plate can be held provisionally to the shaft via guidewires placed through locking trocars or via reduction clamp. Appropriate reduction must be ensured again under fluoroscopy. Once acceptable alignment is ensured, the plate may be fixed to the shaft utilizing either conventional or locking screws, depending on the fracture configuration.

In cases with extensive metaphyseal comminution, at least 3–4 holes of the plate should be left empty at the level of the fracture. This allows a larger area of stress distribution on the plate and reduces strain at the fracture. Filling all screw holes may lead to stress concentration and high strain, which can lead to implant failure after cyclic loading. One should ideally aim for 50% screw density and 6–8 cortices of fixation distally. The wound is closed in layers over a drain.

PROXIMAL FEMORAL LOCKING PLATE:
Pearls and Pitfalls

- After the approach to the proximal femur has been performed, the plate should be placed using minimally invasive techniques submuscularly from proximal to distal to minimize devascularization of fracture fragments
- Check the reduction again with respect to the axial alignment, length, and rotation following provisional fixation of the plate to the proximal fragment. This is done prior to proximal fragment screw insertion
- In complex fractures, the clinical judgment of the rotation becomes more important, while the radiological findings in that respect is challenging to interpret
- In the lateral position, prior to the placement of second screw in the shaft, ensure that sagittal plane reduction is appropriate. Reduction can be adjusted with use of sterile bolsters using the initial screw as a pivot
- In osteoporotic bone and comminuted fractures, the use of all locking screws is advantageous

Technique 3: Blade Plate

Meticulous preoperative planning is essential in order to insert the 95° angled blade plate correctly. The implant is unforgiving. Four crucial degrees of freedom must be controlled: (1) point of entry of the blade into the bone, (2) parallelism to the anteversion of the femoral neck, (3) angle between the blade and the femoral shaft axis, and (4) rotation of the seating chisel about its long axis (Figs 21.11A to H).

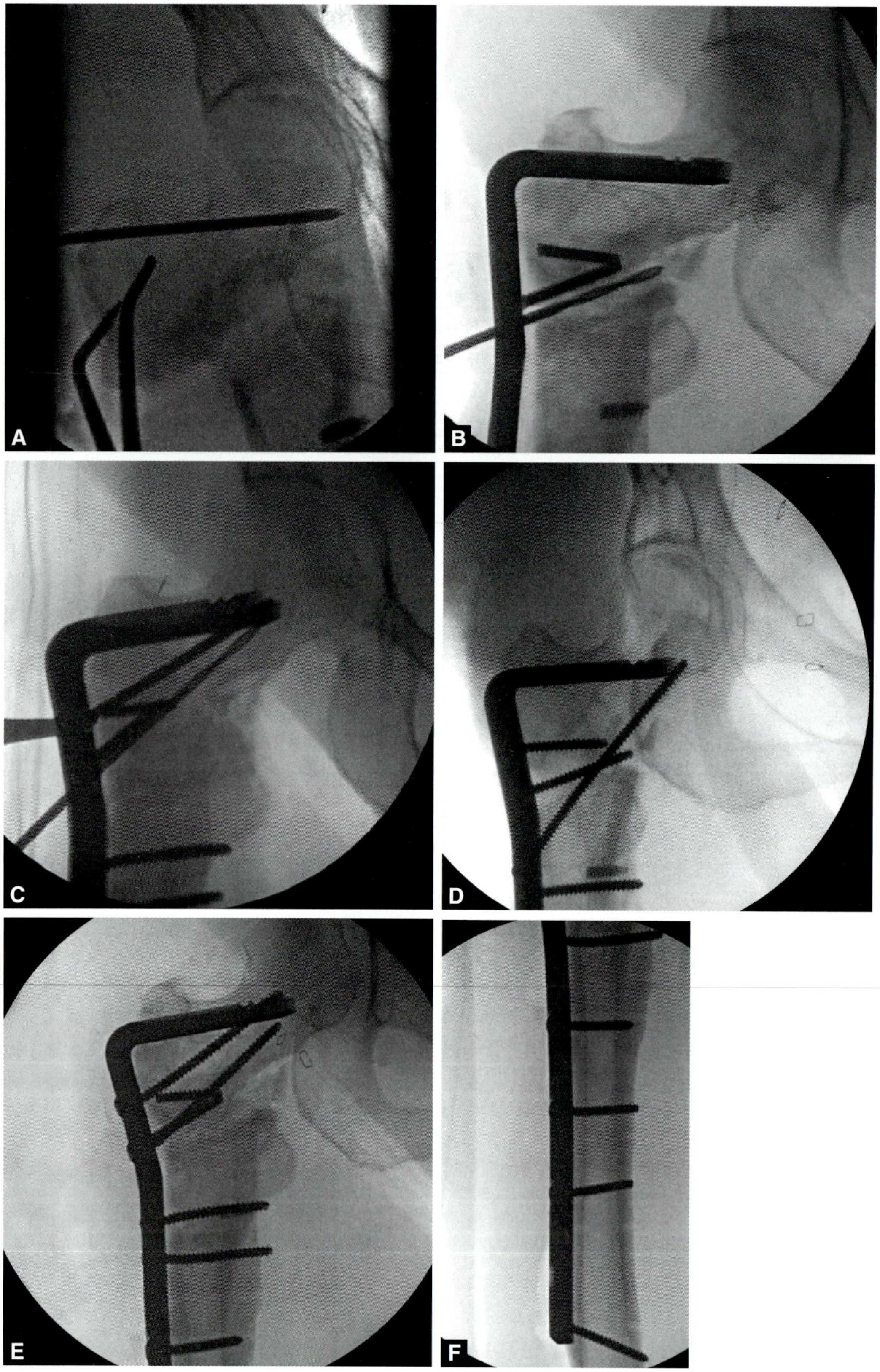

Figures 21.11A to F

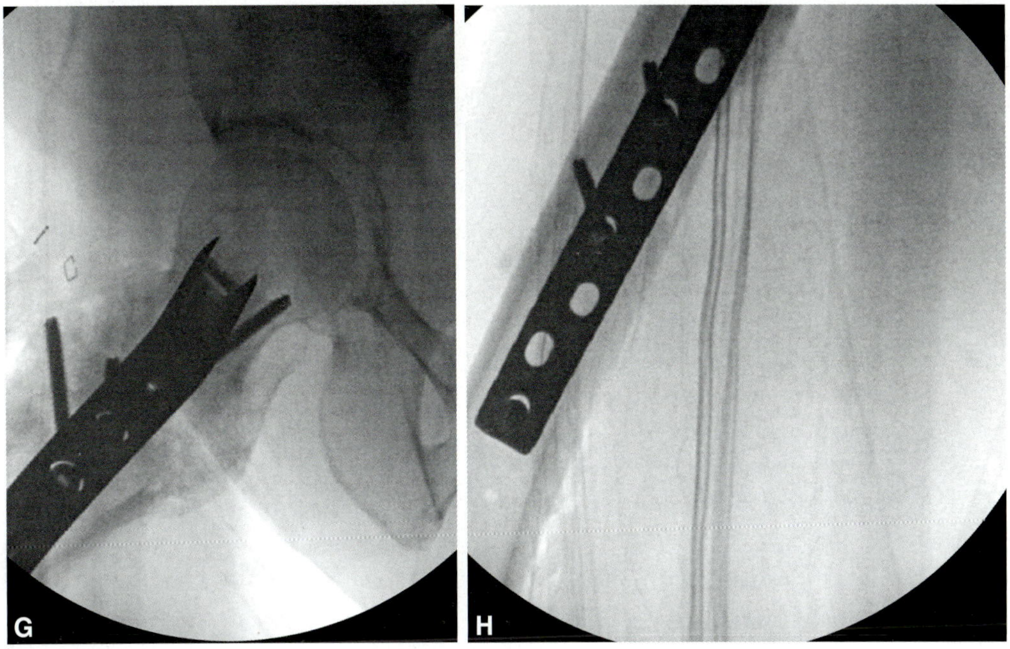

Figures 21.11A to H: Blade plate fixation of a subtrochanteric femur fracture. (A) Guidewire in place for the blade in the proximal femur as shown on this intraoperative image; (B) Blade plate in place in the proximal femur; (C) A drill is entered into the femoral neck; (D to H) Blade plate in place with final fixation construct.

The initial step during insertion of a 95° angled blade plate is creating a channel for the blade. Parallelism to the anteversion of the femoral neck and the angle between the blade and the femoral shaft axis must be correctly identified prior to proceeding with channel creation. Guidewires are used to mark the plane of anteversion of the femoral neck and also to mark the appropriate inclination of the seating chisel in relation to the long axis of femur. The surgeon will be guided in the chisel insertion by a definitive guidewire.

First, a guidewire is passed along the anterior aspect of the femoral neck. This guidewire indicates the axis of the neck in axial plane. This wire must pass distal to the anterior intertrochanteric ridge, or may be deflected anteriorly. Second, the 95° plate guide is placed along the lateral cortex and a definitive guidewire is inserted, parallel in the axial view to the first guidewire and parallel with the upper edge of the condylar plate guide in the AP view. Guided by the measurement made on the preoperative plan, the point of entry on the outer face of the greater trochanter is determined. It is important to remember that, at this level, the posterior edge of the greater trochanter overhangs more than the anterior edge and the center of the point of insertion is at the junction of anterior one third and middle one third of the outer face of the greater trochanter. The guidewire is drilled into the greater trochanter just above the planned point of entry. The track for the seating chisel will be parallel to this wire. The wire's position should be checked radiologically in both planes and adjusted accordingly as necessary.

Three 4.5 mm drill holes are made. These holes are enlarged with a router to produce a horizontal slot matching the width and height of the seating chisel. The lower edge of the entry hole should be beveled, using a chisel, to accommodate the curve of shoulder of the angled blade plate. The seating chisel can now be inserted through the prepared entry slot parallel in both axial and AP views to the definitive guidewire. This parallelism is judged by frequent visual reference in both planes, to the advancing seating chisel, and to the guidewire. The use of the slotted hammer over the seating chisel aids the control of this track. Throughout the insertion of the seating chisel, the parallelism of the tongue of the seating chisel guide to the femoral shaft axis is also carefully maintained. This is the most demanding step of the procedure, and the grip on the slotted hammer and the seating chisel guide is crucial.

Once the seating chisel has been inserted, its position should be checked with fluoroscopy. This also determines whether the planned blade length is appropriate. The seating chisel bears markings that indicate the depth of its insertion. The seating chisel is then removed by back strokes with the slotted hammer.

The 95° angled blade plate is then mounted into the plate holder and the blade is advanced by hand into the prechiseled track. The blade should pass easily into the precut track and light taps with a mallet should be all that is required to insert it into the femoral neck. When the plate is about 5 mm from the bone, remove the plate holder and fully seat the plate.

The blade should be stabilized with a proximal screw. After the angled blade plate has been inserted into the proximal femur, it is secured with a fully threaded 6.5 mm cancellous screw through the most proximal of the holes of the plate. The use of a cortical screw at this site would require drilling of the calcar of the femur, which results in weakening of this important bony buttress. A unicortical locking screw can also be used, if the situation dictates.

Once the angled blade plate is firmly anchored in the proximal fragment, the distal femur is aligned onto the plate and held, if necessary, with a clamp. In single plane transverse or short oblique fractures, the first screw in the distal fragment should be a compression screw in order to compress the fracture and to achieve primary bone healing. An articulating tension device can also be used when adequate compression can be challenging to achieve. The remaining, neutral screws are then inserted. At least 6–8 cortices of fixation are necessary in the shaft fragment. Again, a 50% screw density is recommended to distribute stress across the implant.

Customized blade plates fashioned from standard plates can be applied to a number of challenging situations involving acute or ununited subtrochanteric femur fractures. By placing a long screw across the long and short axes of the custom blade plate after it is inserted, the implant is effectively locked into the metaphyseal fragment with excellent fixation.[20] The wound is closed in layers over a drain.

BLADE PLATE: Pearls and Pitfalls

- In order to insert the 95° angled blade plate correctly into bone, four degrees of freedom must be controlled: (1) point of entry of the blade into the bone, (2) parallelism to the anteversion of the femoral neck, (3) angle between the blade and the femoral shaft axis, and (4) rotation of the seating chisel about its long axis
- The first guidewire passed in close contact with the front of femoral neck will indicate the axis of the neck in axial plane
- Place the 95° condylar plate guide along the lateral cortex and insert the definitive guidewire parallel in the axial view to the first guidewire and parallel with the upper edge of the condylar plate guide in the AP view
- Sufficient compression may only be achieved by the use of an external compression device

Postoperative Protocol

Regardless of fixation method, drains are removed when the output is less than 20 cc per shift or after 48 hours. Antibiotic prophylaxis is given for 24 hours in closed fractures and 48 hours in open fractures. Deep vein thrombosis (DVT) prophylaxis is utilized unless contraindicated. Patients are mobilized to a chair in upright position on the first day postoperatively. Ambulation with supervision is allowed with weight bearing as tolerated in length-stable patterns and toe-touch weight bearing in unstable patterns. Multiple trauma or patients with other complications may have delayed ambulation, but it should begin as soon as possible to minimize secondary complications. Patients are re-evaluated with an examination and radiographs at 2, 6, 12, 24 and 52 weeks. Fracture healing is documented and the patients usually have maximized ambulatory capabilities by 6 months after the injury.

Outcomes

Kuzyk et al.[21] performed a meta-analysis of intramedullary versus extramedullary internal fixation of subtrochanteric femur fractures to determine if clinical evidence exists to recommend one method of internal fixation over the other. Three level I and nine level IV studies were identified. They concluded that there is grade B evidence that operative time is reduced and that fixation failure is reduced with the use of IM implants for subtrochanteric fractures.

Starr et al.[22] performed a prospective, randomized clinical trial comparing nails placed through the greater trochanter versus piriformis fossa in high-energy proximal femoral fractures. They found no difference with respect to the blood loss, rate of nonunion, complications or duration of surgery between the two techniques. Robinson et al.[23] reported a 7.1% incidence of nail revision because of fracture or implant complications in their series of patients with subtrochanteric fractures treated with a trochanteric IM nail.

Multiple authors have found that with indirect reduction techniques and maintenance of the biology of the fracture environment, high rates of union can be achieved with 95° condylar plate, with reported rates of union of 93.7–100%.[24–26]

Sadowski et al.[27] compared results of using trochanteric IM femoral nail with 95° condylar plate in 39 elderly patients, who had either transverse or reverse obliquity proximal femoral fractures. They found that the nail group had shorter surgical times and hospital stays and that the patients required fewer blood transfusions. These authors also noted seven nonunions or hardware failures in 19 patients treated with the blade-plate; by contrast, only 1 of the 20 patients treated with the femoral nail developed a nonunion. They recommended that this fracture pattern could be treated with a trochanteric femoral nail.

Yoo et al.[28] reported an average of 19 weeks to union in 38 patients with subtrochanteric or reverse obliquity type fractures treated with 95° angled blade plate. Only one patient developed nonunion and hardware failure.

Glassner and Tejwani[29] reported a series of seven failures of the proximal femoral locking compression plate. Of seven cases, two were acute peritrochanteric fractures, one was a periprosthetic fracture at the site of a prior hip fusion, one was an early failure of compression hip screw, and three were nonunions. The failure mode was implant fracture in four cases and loss of fixation in three cases resulting from varus collapse and implant cutout. Five of seven failures were within first 3 weeks (average 12.4 days). The average time to failure for all cases was 37.9 days (range, 5–175 days). The average patient age was 56.7 years (range, 36–72 years).

Modern indirect reduction techniques have allowed most subtrochanteric fractures to be treated successfully without the use of bone grafts. Kinast et al.[30] demonstrated that indirect reduction techniques resulted in good outcomes and dramatically reduced the need for bone grafts. When the vascularity of comminuted bone on the medial side of the proximal fragment is maintained and when the fracture is stabilized sufficiently to reduce substantial stresses in this area, the fracture has a good chance of healing.

Complications and Management

Deep Vein Thrombosis

In treating patients with subtrochanteric femoral fractures, the relatively high incidence of DVT should be kept in mind. Both mechanical and chemical prophylaxis should be considered, based on the clinical situation. Pneumatic compression devices on lower extremities should be applied before surgery, and the surgeon should add chemical prophylaxis postoperatively when the clinical situation allows. The treating surgeon should be sensitive to the signs and symptoms associated with DVT as well as pulmonary embolism and should thoroughly evaluate any patient with suspected thromboembolic phenomena with Doppler ultrasound or chest CT scans.

Loss of Fixation and Malunion

The limited proximal bone available for fixation, poor bone quality in the proximal femur in elderly patients and tremendous forces acting on the proximal femur all contribute to the loss of fixation seen in subtrochanteric femur fractures. Careful attention in choosing an appropriate implant and obtaining optimal fixation in well-aligned fracture provides the most consistent results.

Ensuring anatomical alignment of the fracture decreases the possibility of fixation failure. The surgeon must be aware of deforming muscle forces that affect the fracture fragments. The proximal fragment often remains flexed, resulting in apex anterior malreduction (Figs 21.12A to D). The distal fragment should be flexed to match the

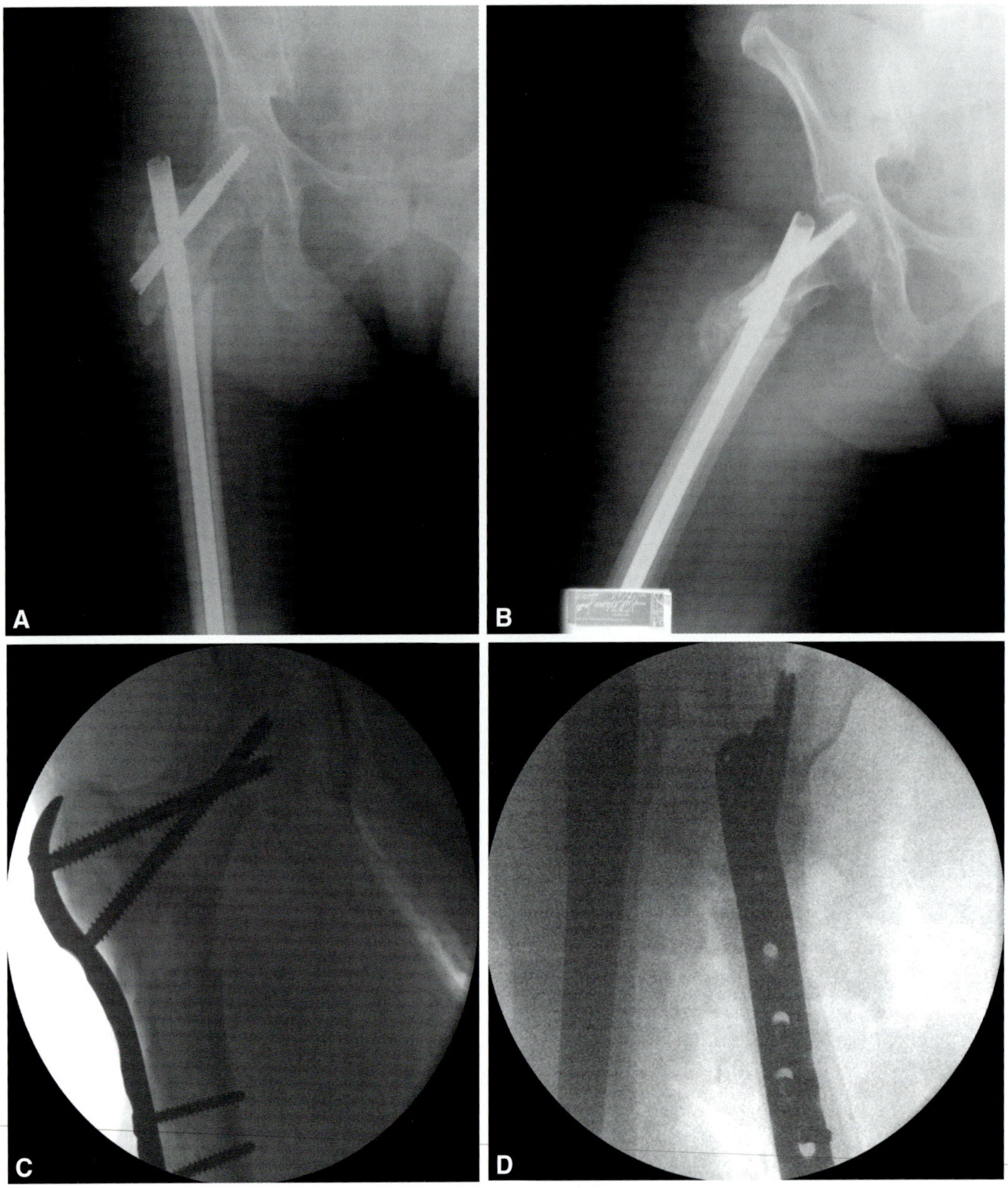

Figures 21.12A to D: Malreduction of proximal femur fracture resulting in nonunion requiring repair. (A and B) Anteroposterior (AP) and lateral radiographs of a painful subtrochanteric nonunion with previous intramedullary nailing, nail dynamization and in situ autogenous iliac crest bone grafting; (C and D) AP and lateral images after nonunion repair with removal of implants, grafting of lag screw hole, compression locked plating and repeated autogenous bone grafting of the subtrochanteric nonunion.
Courtesy: Saqib Rehman

alignment of the proximal fragment and should be rotated appropriately. Understanding that the reamers and nail will not reduce a subtrochanteric fracture is a key in determining appropriate preliminary steps to achieve anatomical reduction. When reduction cannot be achieved, the fracture should be opened with a careful attention paid to minimize soft tissue stripping.

Nonunion

Before operating on a nonunion, the surgeon must first understand the etiology. Brinker et al.[31] stressed on the importance of appropriate referral to endocrinology for patients who had unexplained nonunions. These patients included those who failed to heal their fractures despite adequate reduction and stabilization, and had a history of multiple low-energy fractures with at least one progressing to nonunion, or a nondisplaced pubic ramus or sacral alar fracture that progressed to nonunion. In their study, 31 of 37 patients (83.8%), who met the above screening criteria, had one or more new diagnoses of metabolic or endocrinal abnormalities. The most common newly diagnosed abnormality was vitamin D deficiency (25 of 37 patients; 68%). Other newly diagnosed abnormalities included calcium imbalances, central hypogonadism, thyroid disorders and parathyroid hormone disorders. All newly diagnosed abnormalities were treated medically. Eight patients, who underwent no operative intervention following the diagnosis and treatment of a new metabolic or endocrine abnormality, achieved bony union in an average of 7.6 months (range, 3–12 months) following their first visit to the endocrinologist.

Wiss and Brien reported a nonunion rate of 1% (1 of 95).[2] Their sole nonunion was in a fracture that was initially open and healed after bone grafting. Kang et al.[32] reported a union rate of 92%, and French and Tornetta[33] reported 100% union at an average of 13.5 weeks. These reports indicate that nonunion is unusual in the management of subtrochanteric femoral fractures; however, nonunion can be problematic, when it does occur. Excessive soft tissue stripping and reckless handling of the medial fragments may contribute to nonunion.

Haidukewych and Berry[34] reported on 21 patients with subtrochanteric nonunions that underwent revision surgery and were stabilized with a variety of methods. Eight patients were treated with a cephalomedullary nail, seven patients were treated with a standard antegrade femoral nail, five patients were treated with a 95° angled blade plate, one patient was treated with a sliding hip screw, one patient was treated with a 95° dynamic condylar screw, and one patient was treated with dual large fragment plates. They bone-grafted 78% of the nonunions with either autograft or allograft. They had only one recalcitrant nonunion in their series, indicating that subtrochanteric nonunions can be successfully managed with revision fixation and bone grafting using a variety of fixation methods.

Brinker and O'Connor[35] reviewed the literature on exchange nailing and concluded that exchange nailing is an excellent choice for aseptic nonunions of noncomminuted diaphyseal femoral fractures, with union rates reported to range from 72% to 100%. Exchange nailing is most appropriate for nonunion without substantial bone loss. The exchange nail should be at least 1 mm larger in diameter than the nail being removed, and it has been recommended that it should be up to 4 mm larger when the nail being removed is greatly undersized. Canal reaming should progress until osseous tissue is observed in the reaming flutes.

de Vriesa et al.[36] treated 33 subtrochanteric nonunions with blade plates. Union was achieved in 32 of 33 hips after an average of 5 months. Complications were seen in nine patients; five complications required intervention and four minor complications were treated conservatively. This study shows that treatment of a subtrochanteric nonunion with a blade plate is a viable option that can consistently lead to bony union.

Subtrochanteric nonunions may involve considerable shortening. A method of concomitantly treating both issues was reported by Wu.[37] He reported on 23 consecutive patients who were treated by femoral condylar skeletal traction, one-stage lengthening to 4 cm maximum, static locked nail stabilization and corticocancellous bone grafting. Indications for this technique included aseptic nonunions, patient younger than 60 years, and 2–5 cm shortening. Postoperatively, protected weight bearing ambulation was encouraged. All nonunions healed with a median period of 4 months.

Malrotation

No universally accepted guidelines exist for defining the degree at which malrotation becomes significant. The key to early identification of malrotation is to listen to the patient's concerns regarding rotation. Typically, the patient will make it known that the functional or cosmetic aspects of a malrotated femur are unacceptable. The surgeon should perform an appropriate examination. A CT rotational profile will help in quantifying the degree of malrotation and in determining whether a corrective procedure is indicated. Despite its limitations, the CT rotational profile offers the best means of quantifying rotational asymmetry. Correction is easier to perform before fracture union and this should be discussed with the patient. Following diagnosis of significant malrotation, the corrective procedure can be planned.

A high potential for drill-hole cutout exists in patients with less than 20° of malrotation, in whom the previous distal locking site is to be used. This is due to the proximity of the new interlock site to the previous interlock site.[38] This may be an issue when correction is performed early in the postoperative period before the bone has healed. Depending on the nail used, this risk can be overcome by using alternative locking holes or a dynamic locking slot. Alternatively, the nail could be advanced or retracted to avoid the previous site of locking.

Derotational osteotomy is used to correct malrotation after the fracture has healed. A CT rotational profile must be obtained to determine the degree of malrotation. Before performing the correction, two stout (3.8 mm) Steinmann pins are placed. One pin is placed in the trochanteric region, either in front of or behind the nail; the other is inserted into the distal femoral condylar region. The pins may be placed at an angle to each other, so that the two pins will be parallel, once the correction is made. Alternatively, the pins may be placed parallel and used as a goniometer to measure the correction as it occurs. Stout Steinmann pins must be used because soft tissues will bend smaller Kirschner wires, thereby preventing an accurate guide to the needed correction.

The nail is removed and a transverse osteotomy is performed with an IM saw or an open technique with multiple drill perforations and an osteotome. Transverse osteotomy with an IM saw reduces the disruption of the periosteal blood supply and aids in bone healing. Following removal of the nail, the IM canal is reamed an additional 1.5 mm greater than the diameter of the saw.

On completion of osteotomy, the correction is made, as measured using the Steinmann pins and a goniometer. A new IM nail is placed and statically locked, with attention paid to the proximity of the new distal interlocks to the previously placed screws.

Authors' Preferred Management of Select Complications

Case 1: Nonunion Repair of an Intertrochanteric Femur Fracture with a Blade Plate

The patient is a 53-year-old woman, who was shoveling her sidewalk when she slipped on the ice and fell on her left buttock. She could not stand or mobilize her left hip due to pain. The AP view of the left hip revealed an intertrochanteric hip fracture with osteopenia (Fig. 21.13A). Though there was some comminution evident, the medial calcar and lesser trochanter was intact. The femur was externally rotated as one could tell from the prominent profile of the lesser trochanter.

The lateral X-ray of the left hip as shown in Figure 21.13B corroborated the finding of an intertrochanteric hip fracture. Due to the patient's obesity, the soft tissue shadows made it difficult to appreciate the detail of proximal femur.

The fracture was fixed with a cephalomedullary nail as shown in the postoperative AP view of the patient's hip (Fig. 21.13C). Note that the lesser trochanter is now fractured; something that is likely better appreciated on this properly rotated view, or perhaps an occult fracture became complete and displaced. Also referred to as a reconstruction nail, this implant was presumably chosen by the surgeon for a number of reasons. First of all, it prevents excessive medialization common to dynamic hip screw and side plate. With the nail, the femur can only medialize to a point at which the nail impacts the medial calcar inside the canal proximally. Secondly, this device may be superior biomechanically, because the IM position of the implant puts it closer to the center of rotation of the femoral head, thus providing a shorter moment arm than a plate. Lastly, the nail can be placed through a small incision proximally, accomplishing the procedure less invasively perhaps. The implant seems to be well-placed, as the screws are nicely centralized in the head. The lateral postoperative view reveals that the screws are nicely centralized in the head as well, in addition to the anterior cortex being nicely lined up implying no rotational displacement (Fig. 21.13D). Immediate weight bearing as tolerated would be an appropriate way to mobilize this patient. The advantage of obtaining an AP view of the pelvis (Fig. 21.13E) is to verify that the neck-shaft angle is symmetrical, as it is in this patient. There is some shortening already appreciated, but this should be okay because medialization can be expected with this device, since the proximal screws traverse the nail but do not lock into it. Medialization is considered to be good, because it means that the fracture can impact or compress. This fracture should heal!

The AP X-ray view taken 8 months after the original surgery revealed that there had been substantial shortening by virtue of the proud screws at the lateral cortex (Fig. 21.13F). These prominent screws can sometimes be painful and

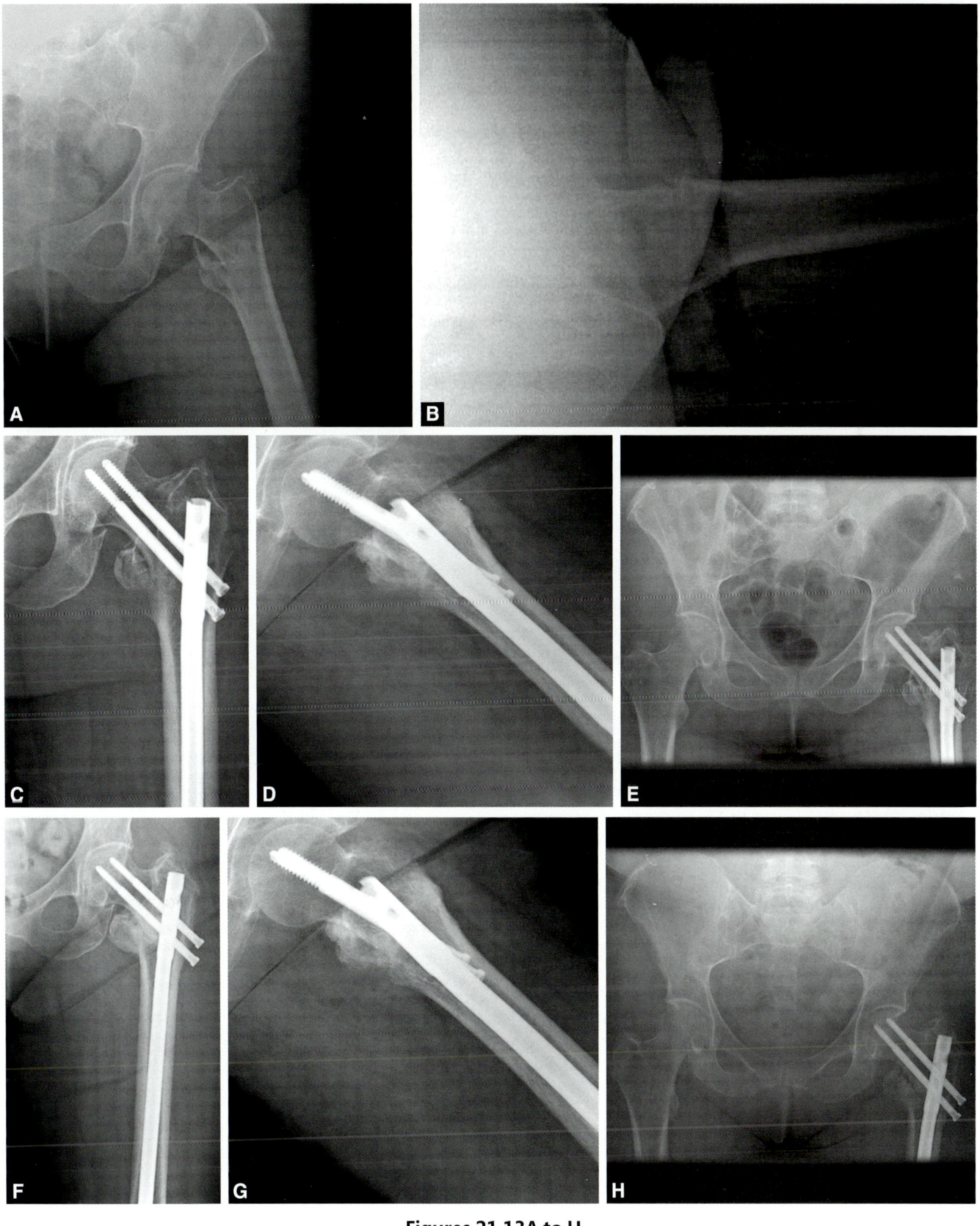

Figures 21.13A to H

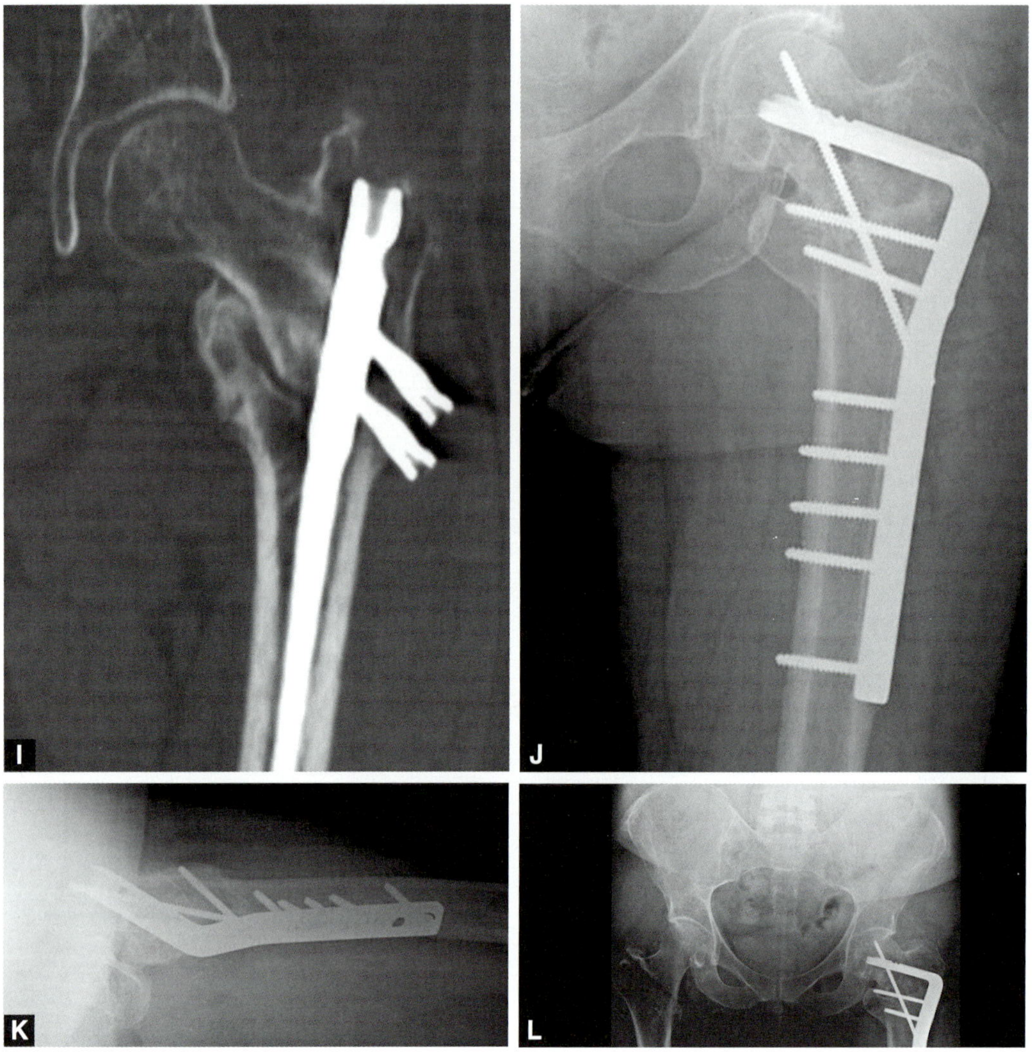

Figures 21.13A to L: Repair of an intertrochanteric fracture nonunion with blade plate fixation after initial cephalomedullary nailing. (A and B) Anteroposterior (AP) and lateral radiographic images of an intertrochanteric femur fracture; (C to E) AP and lateral hip and AP pelvis radiographs after cephalomedullary nailing with note of improved alignment and a minimally displaced fracture of the lesser trochanter; (F and G) AP and lateral hip radiographs 8 months after fixation. The fracture line is still evident with lack of cortical bridging at the medial margin; (H) AP pelvis radiograph demonstrates that fracture reduction has been maintained; (I) CT scan with coronal reconstruction confirms nonunion as well as the need for operative reconstruction; (J to L) AP and lateral hip and AP pelvis radiographs at 4 months after nonunion repair revision surgery. Alignment is adequate and fracture lines are no longer visible.

need to be removed, but since the neck-shaft angle had also fallen (possibly healed) into slight varus, and the patient complained of deep pain in the hip, a CT scan was obtained to investigate the possibility of nonunion. The lateral view of the hip taken at the same time revealed that the version of the femoral neck had been nicely maintained, and there was no displacement (Fig. 21.13G). Hypertrophic callus consistent with healing was evident on both anterior and posterior to the proximal neck. The AP view of the pelvis is good to appreciate both the relative medialization which has occurred in the left hip, as well as the varus deformity relative to the right hip (Fig. 21.13H).

A coronal CT cut through the proximal femur revealed a nonunion as suspected (Fig. 21.13I). The surgeon at this juncture decided to perform a nonunion repair with a blade plate, which was a good device to correct malalignment as well as to create a compression across the nonunion site to ensure healing (Fig. 21.13J). Compression should be achieved with an articulating tension device at the distal end of the plate, a tool available in large fragment fracture fixation sets. After compression, the patient would be allowed to bear weight immediately. A lateral view of the proximal femur showed the blade plate contained in the neck and head, and though this view was not a perfect lateral, the perfect lateral view demonstrated that it was well-placed into the head (Fig. 21.13K). The most vertically oriented screw traversed both the side plate and the blade itself which made the proximal fixation more stable. Note that the goal of surgery is not to address the medialization, a deformity which is generally accepted in a reconstruction, because otherwise, to get the patient back out to original neck length, would leave an unstable bone defect at the base of the neck, so the medialization is accepted.

A final AP view of the pelvis showed a healed proximal femur approximately 1 year post reconstruction (Fig. 21.13L). Generally, the blade plate can be left in place, but if the side plate is symptomatic due to impingement of the iliotibial band, there is no problem in removing it, though the senior surgeon's preference is to wait at least for 12 months, if not 18 months in the scenario of a proximal femur nonunion in a patient with osteoporosis. The patient had a good result and resumed life as a community, ambulatory with minimal symptoms.

Case 2: Nonunion Repair of a Pertrochanteric Femur Fracture with Blade Plate Fixation

This case involves a 48-year-old garbage man, who was swinging a 50 pound trash bag into the garbage truck, when he lifted off the ground to fall onto his left hip. This resulted in an unstable pertrochanteric femur fracture with a transverse fracture line extending from the lesser trochanter and exiting laterally (Fig. 21.14A). There was another fracture line extending distal and lateral to this transverse fracture line, which made it a reverse intertrochanteric fracture pattern. The lateral X-ray of the proximal femur and hip clearly showed that the cortex was broken laterally, underscoring that this was a very unstable fracture pattern (Fig. 21.14B). Furthermore, there was a coronal plane fracture extending through the greater trochanter.

Peritrochanteric fractures are considered unstable if they have a fractured posteromedial calcar, a fragmented lateral wall, or if they have a reverse intertrochanteric pattern as shown here. The treatment implication of these unstable variants is that they should not be treated with a dynamic hip screw and side plate unless the side plate has a trochanteric extension plate, which would prevent excessive medialization. Otherwise, a length stable proximal femur fixed angle device such as a proximal femoral locking plate or a blade plate should be used.

A decision was made to treat this fracture with a proximal femoral locking plate (Figs 21.14C to E). What is shown is an AP view of the proximal femur. There is a proximal femoral locking plate in place. This demonstrates three screws which extend into the head at different angles and are fixed to the side plate making this a locking plate. The neck-shaft angle of the proximal femur has been restored to a near normal angle of 135°. There are four conventional 4.5 mm screws and two thicker 5 mm locking screws in the shaft. Some surgeons prefer to add locking screws after conventional screws are placed to enhance the fixation, which is appropriate in patients with osteoporosis. Note that there is no hole in the bone distal to the locking plate, proving that the surgeon did not use the articulating tension device to compress the proximal fracture. Not applying the principles of primary rigid fixation for direct fracture healing can lead to complications. The lateral X-ray view of the proximal femur showed good central contained screw placement in the neck and head, as well as good reduction (Fig. 21.14D). The greater trochanter was left unfixed, which is fine when it is minimally displaced as it is in this situation.

Five months after surgery, the patient had persistent pain as well as a persistent fracture line on radiographs. Therefore, a CT scan was ordered which confirmed a nonunion (Fig. 21.14F). The surgeon decided to use a blade plate to fix this problem. This was done because the patient had acceptable alignment, but a simple incompletely healed cleft of proximal femur was never compressed adequately. Therefore, the proximal femoral locking plate was removed, a 95° angled blade plate was inserted and the proximal fragment was compressed to the distal fragment before placing screws into the diaphysis. This was done with an articulating tension device for which there was evidence due to the holes below side plate in the femur shaft. Because the patient had a nonunion, autogenous bone graft was used, as well as local decortication around the nonunion was done with a sharp gouge to stimulate bone healing and incorporation of the graft. The nonunion healed and the bone graft consolidated by 9 months after the nonunion repair (Figs 21.14G and H).

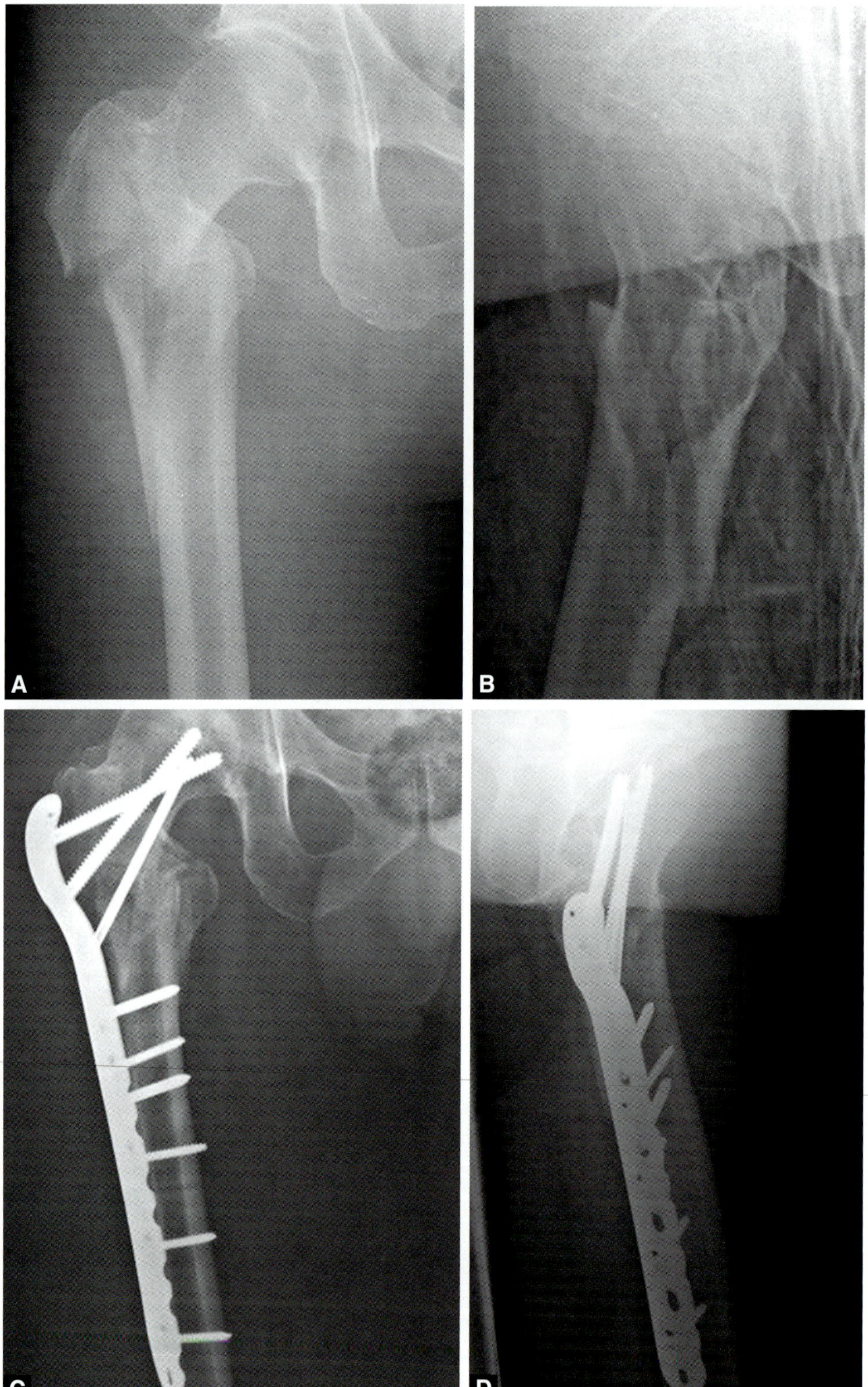

Figures 21.14A to D

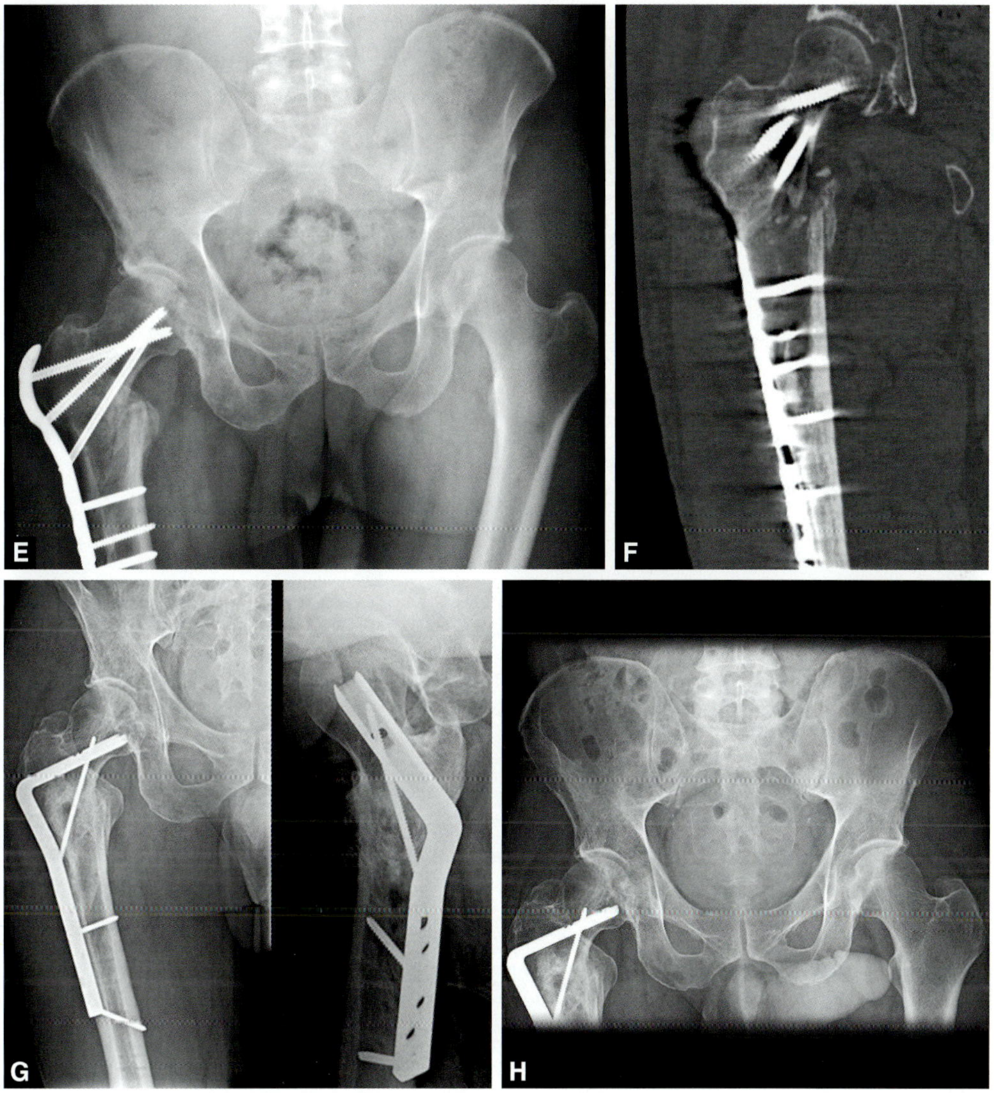

Figures 21.14A to H: Repair of an intertrochanteric proximal femur fracture with subtrochanteric involvement with a proximal femoral locking plate. (A and B) Anteroposterior (AP) and lateral hip radiographs of a 48-year-old male with a comminuted reverse obliquity right proximal femur fracture, which includes intertrochanteric and subtrochanteric involvement; (C to E) AP hip, lateral hip and AP pelvis radiographs 3 months after open reduction and internal fixation with a proximal femoral locking plate. Alignment is satisfactory, but fracture is still evident and patient cannot bear weight; (F) CT scan image with coronal reformat taken 6 months postoperatively demonstrates no evidence of solid osseous union across majority of the fracture; (G and H) AP hip, lateral hip and AP pelvic radiographs 9 months after reconstruction with a 95° angled blade plate demonstrating that the subtrochanteric nonunion has gone on to heal.

Case 3: Nonunion Repair of a Pertrochanteric Femur Fracture with Proximal Femur Locking Plate

This case involves the repair of a failed fixation with a compression hip screw device. As shown in Figure 21.15A, compression hip screw with side plate has failed, indeed, has ripped out of the femur. The screws placed through the side plate are loose, and there is bone loss around the lag screw as evidenced by lucency and sclerosis around the barrel of the side plate which slides over the lag screw. The lateral radiograph confirms the diagnosis and shows complete displacement in the sagittal plane of the distal fragment relative to the proximal fragment (Fig. 21.15B). An AP view of the pelvis should be obtained for preoperative planning, specifically to measure the right to left neck-shaft angles (Fig. 21.15C).

A decision was made to repair this nonunion with a blade plate device. An AP view of the right hip revealed postoperative reconstruction of the proximal femur with a 95° angled blade plate (Figs 21.15D and E). The neck-shaft angle was nicely restored, and there was a large fragment screw running up the base of the femoral neck to help augment fixation in the proximal fragment as well as to prevent varus collapse. Blade plates are ideal for this salvage situation, because of the bone loss in the neck and head from the previous lag screw. Because this was a case of nonunion, which was quite atrophic, based on the lack of evidence for bone healing and callus in the original failure films, autogenous bone graft harvested from the iliac crest was used to supplement the reconstruction, thus providing osteoinductive elements to the milieu to enhance the healing process (Fig. 21.15E).

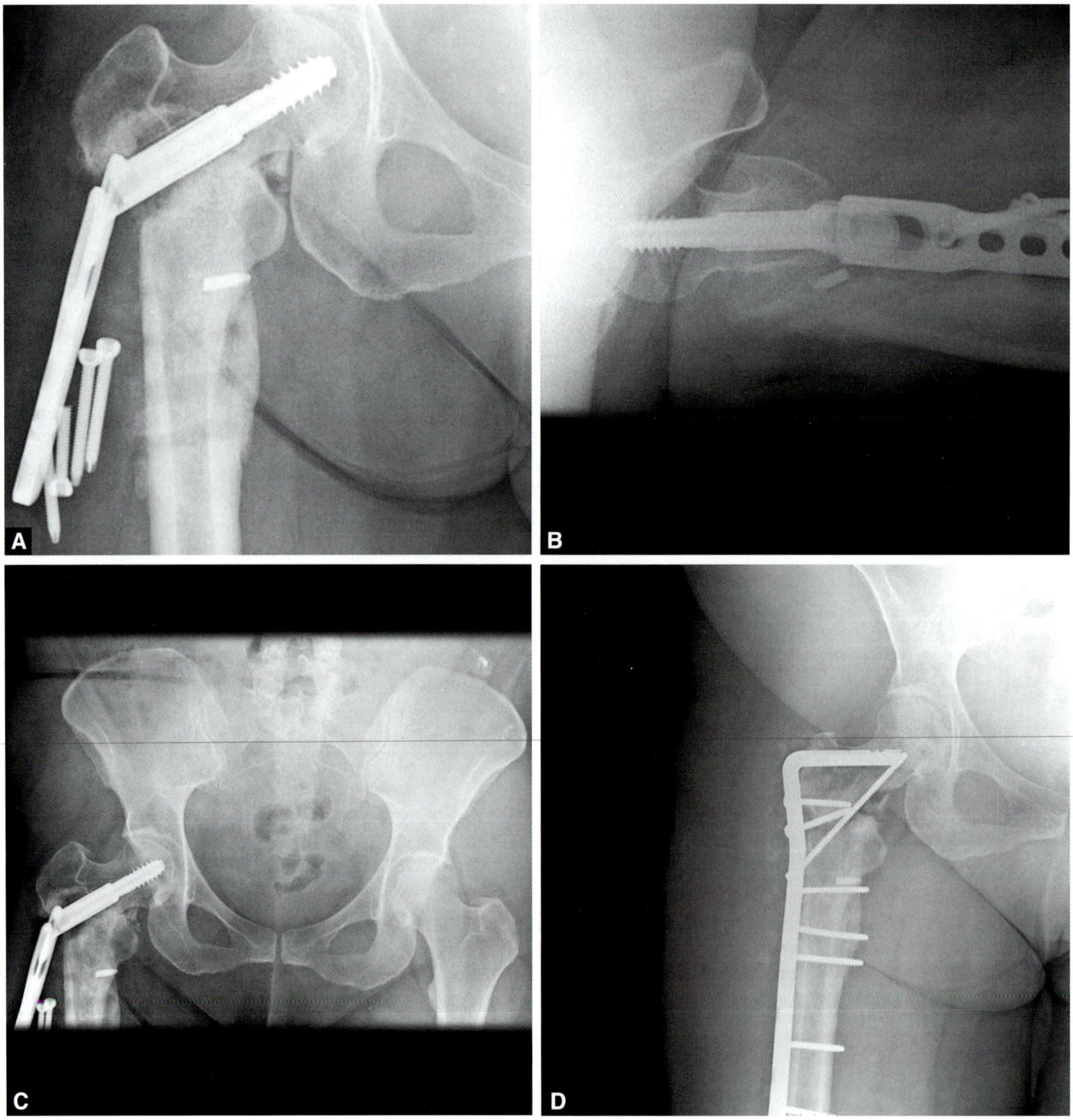

Figures 21.15A to D

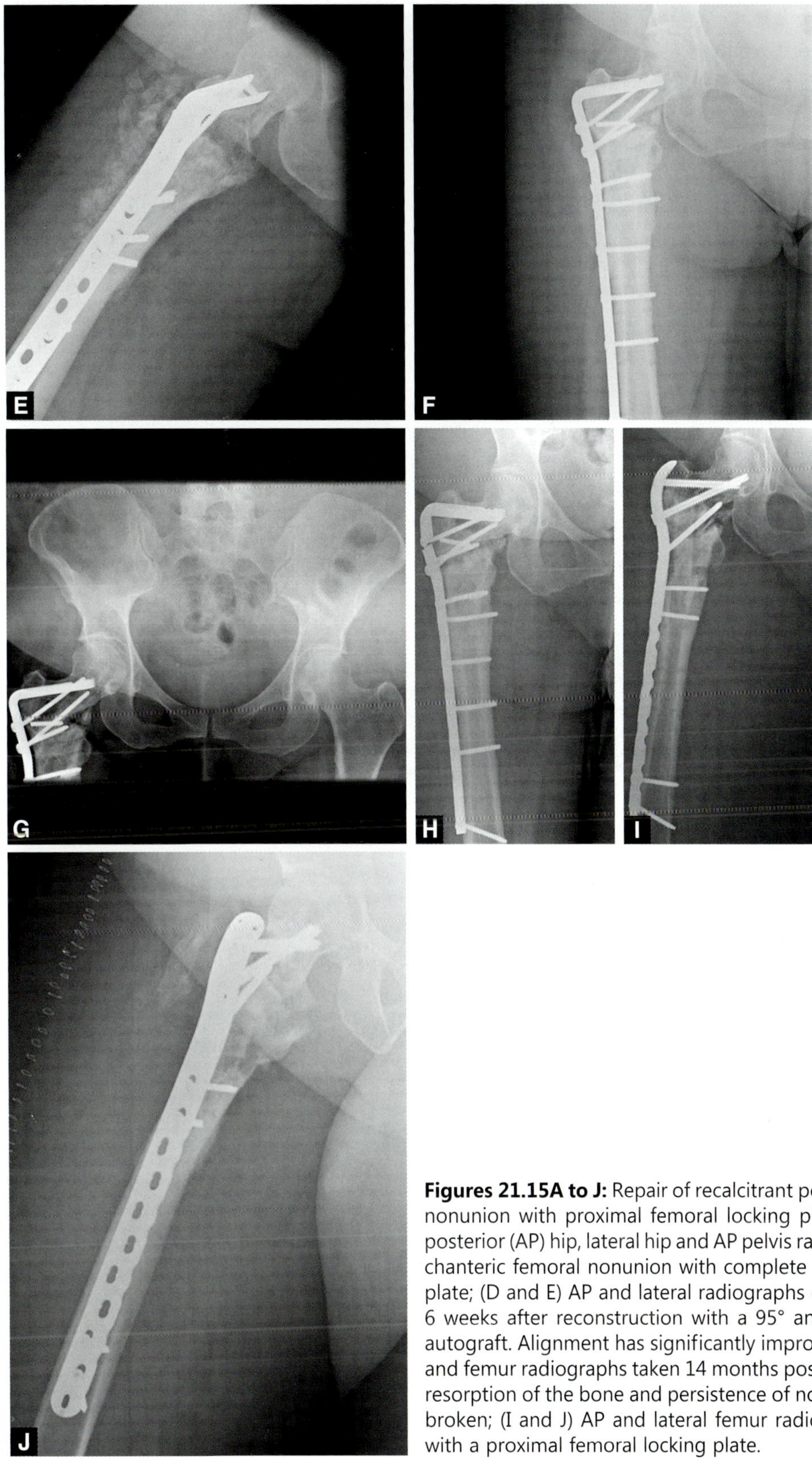

Figures 21.15A to J: Repair of recalcitrant pertrochanteric femoral nonunion with proximal femoral locking plate. (A to C) Anteroposterior (AP) hip, lateral hip and AP pelvis radiographs of a pertrochanteric femoral nonunion with complete loss of fixation of the plate; (D and E) AP and lateral radiographs of the proximal femur 6 weeks after reconstruction with a 95° angled blade plate and autograft. Alignment has significantly improved; (F to H) AP pelvis and femur radiographs taken 14 months post reconstruction show resorption of the bone and persistence of nonunion with the plate broken; (I and J) AP and lateral femur radiographs after revision with a proximal femoral locking plate.

Fourteen months after the original injury and 10 months after reconstruction, the patient had persistent pain with weight bearing. Radiographs showed a lack of healing and consolidation in the intertrochanteric region (Figs 21.15F and G). Furthermore, this clinical scenario prompted a CT scan. Figures 21.15G and H show AP X-ray views of the patient depicting a lucent zone in the intertrochanteric region at 10 months post reconstruction, associated with a broken blade plate.

The surgeon in this case chose to use a proximal femoral locking plate to resolve this nonunion. The reason was that with previous blade plate placement and lag screw placement up into the head, there was a significant bone loss, and the proximal femoral locking plate was allowed for three large locking screws all at different vectors to be placed to enhance fixation (Figs 21.15H and I). This reconstruction was augmented with two types of bone grafts. One was a fibular allograft placed intramedullary in the proximal femur to provide a medial cortex and enough bone stock for mechanical stability and screw purchase. The third screw from the proximal end of the plate can be seen traversing this allograft strut. The second was an autogenous bone graft obtained with the reamer irrigator aspirator (RIA) system (Synthes USA, Paoli, PA), from the opposite femur. This bone graft was packed up into prior bone defects, as well as intramedullary in the proximal and distal femoral fragment to provide osteoinductive capacity. Figure 21.15J shows the corresponding lateral view of the proximal femur demonstrating fixation with the proximal femoral locking plate for definitive reconstruction.

Summary

Subtrochanteric femur fractures demand special consideration, giving high rate of complications associated with their management. The intense concentration of compressive, tensile and torsional stresses in the subtrochanteric region along with decreased vascularity of this area has challenged orthopedic surgeons with problems of malunion, delayed union and nonunion resulting from loss of fixation, implant failure and iatrogenic devascularization due to operative exposure. Only recently, a better understanding of fracture biology, reduction techniques, minimally invasive surgical techniques and biomechanically improved implants has allowed for subtrochanteric fractures to be addressed with consistent success.

References

1. Seinsheimer F. Subtrochanteric fractures of the femur. J Bone Joint Surg Am. 1978;60(3):300-6.
2. Wiss DA, Brien WW. Subtrochanteric fractures of the femur. Results of treatment by interlocking nailing. Clin Orthop Relat Res. 1992;(283):231-6.
3. Lundy DW. Subtrochanteric femoral fractures. J Am Acad Orthop Surg. 2007;15(11):663-71.
4. Goh SK, Yang KY, Koh JS, et al. Subtrochanteric insufficiency fractures in patients on alendronate therapy: a caution. J Bone Joint Surg. 2007;89(3):349-53.
5. Ivkovic A, Bojanic I, Pecina M. Stress fractures of the femoral shaft in athletes: a new treatment algorithm. Br J Sports Med. 2006;40(6):518-20.
6. Russell TA. Subtrochanteric fractures of the femur. In: Browner BD, Jupiter JB, Levine AM, Trafton PG, Krettek C (Eds). Skeletal Trauma: Basic Science, Management, Reconstruction. Philadelphia: Saunders; 2009. pp. 1977-2034.
7. Mueller ME. Mueller AO classification of fractures-long bones. Pamphlet. Switzerland: AO Publishing; 2007. pp 1-10.
8. Rahme DM, Harris IA. Intramedullary nailing versus fixed angle blade plating for subtrochanteric femoral fractures: a prospective randomized controlled trial. J Orthop Surg. 2007;15(3):278-81.
9. Koch JC. The laws of bone architecture. Am J Anatomy. 1917;21:177.
10. Hoppenfeld S, deBoer P, Buckley R. Surgical exposures in orthopaedics: the anatomic approach. Philadelphia: Lippincott Williams & Wilkins; 2007. pp 463-67.
11. Jeanmart L, Baert A, Wackenheim A. Computer tomography of neck, chest, spine and limbs. New York, NY: Springer; 1983(3):171-7.
12. Khoury A, Whyne CM, Daly M, et al. Intraoperative cone-beam CT for correction of periaxial malrotation of the femoral shaft: a surface-matching approach. Med Phys. 2007;34(4):1380-7.
13. Mosheiff R, Weil Y, Peleg E, et al. Computerized navigation for closed reduction during femoral intramedullary nailing. Injury. 2005;36(7):866-70.
14. Jaarsma RL, Pakvis DF, Verdonschot N, et al. Rotational malalignment after intramedullary nailing of femoral fractures. J Orthop Trauma. 2004;18(7):403-9.
15. Bråten M, Terjesen T, Rossvoll I. Torsional deformity after intramedullary nailing of femoral shaft fractures: Measurement of anteversion angles in 110 patients. J Bone Joint Surg Br. 1993; 75(5):799-803.

16. Ruwe PA, Gage JR, Ozonoff MB, et al. Clinical determination of femoral anteversion. A comparison with established techniques. J Bone Joint Surg Am. 1992;74(6):820-30.
17. Russell TA, Mir HR, Stoneback J, et al. Avoidance of malreduction of proximal femoral shaft fractures with the use of a minimally invasive nail insertion technique (MINIT). J Orthop Trauma. 2008;22(6):391-8.
18. Perez EA, Jahangir AA, Mashru RP, et al. Is there a gluteus medius tendon injury during reaming through a modified medial trochanteric portal? A cadaver study. J Orthop Trauma. 2007;21(9):617-20.
19. Hasenboehler EA, Agudelo JF, Morgan SJ, et al. Treatment of complex proximal femoral fractures with the proximal femur locking compression plate. Orthop. 2007;30(8):618-23.
20. Schmidt AH, Templeman DC. Custom locking blade plate for periarticular fractures and nonunions. Tech Orthop. 2003;18(4):329-33.
21. Kuzyk PR, Bhandari M, McKee MD, et al. Intramedullary versus extramedullary fixation for subtrochanteric femur fractures. J Orthop Trauma. 2009;23(6):465-70.
22. Starr AJ, Hay MT, Reinert CM, et al. Cephalomedullary nails in the treatment of high-energy proximal femur fractures in young patients: a prospective, randomized comparison of trochanteric versus piriformis fossa entry portal. J Orthop Trauma. 2006;20(4):240-6.
23. Robinson CM, Houshian S, Khan LA. Trochanteric-entry long cephalomedullary nailing of subtrochanteric fractures caused by low-energy trauma. J Bone Joint Surg Am. 2005;87(10):2217-26.
24. Vaidya SV, Dholakia DB, Chatterjee A. The use of a dynamic condylar screw and biological reduction techniques for subtrochanteric femur fracture. Injury. 2003;34(2):123-8.
25. Blatter G, Janssen M. Treatment of subtrochanteric fractures of the femur: reduction on the traction table and fixation with dynamic condylar screw. Arch Orthop Trauma Surg. 1994;113(3):138-41.
26. Pai CH. Dynamic condylar screw for subtrochanteric femur fractures with greater trochanteric extension. J Orthop Trauma. 1996;10(5):317-22.
27. Sadowski C, Lübbeke A, Saudan M, et al. Treatment of reverse oblique and transverse intertrochanteric fractures with use of an intramedullary nail or a 95 degrees screw-plate: a prospective, randomized study. J Bone Joint Surg Am. 2002;84-A(3):372-81
28. Yoo MC, Cho YJ, Kim KI, et al. Treatment of unstable peritrochanteric femoral fractures using a 95 degrees angled blade plate. J Orthop Trauma. 2005;19(10):687-92.
29. Glassner PJ, Tejwani NC. Failure of proximal femoral locking compression plate: a case series. J Orthop Trauma. 2011;25(2);76-83.
30. Kinast C, Bolhofner BR, Mast JW, et al. Subtrochanteric fractures of the femur. Results of treatment with the 95 degrees condylar blade-plate. Clin Orthop Relat Res. 1989; (238):122-30.
31. Brinker MR, O'Connor DP, Monla YT, et al. Metabolic and endocrine abnormalities in patients with nonunions. J Orthop Trauma. 2007;21(8):557-70.
32. Kang S, McAndrew MP, Johnson KD. The reconstruction locked nail for complex fractures of the proximal femur. J Orthop Trauma. 1995;9(6):453-63.
33. French BG, Tornetta P 3rd. Use of an interlocked cephalomedullary nail for subtrochanteric fracture stabilization. Clin Orthop Relat Res. 1998;(348):95-100.
34. Haidukewych GJ, Berry DJ. Nonunion of fractures of the subtrochanteric region of the femur. Clin Orthop Relat Res. 2004;(419):185-8.
35. Brinker MR, O'Connor DP. Exchange nailing of ununited fractures. J Bone Joint Surg Am. 2007;89(1):177-88.
36. de Vries JS, Kloenab P, Borens O, et al. Treatment of subtrochanteric nonunions. Injury. 2006;37(2):203-11.
37. Wu CC. Locked nailing for shortened subtrochanteric nonunions: a one-stage treatment. Clin Orthop Relat Res. 2009;467(1):254-9.
38. Piper K, Chia M, Graham E. Correcting rotational deformity following femoral nailing. Injury. 2009;40(6):660-2.

Chapter 22

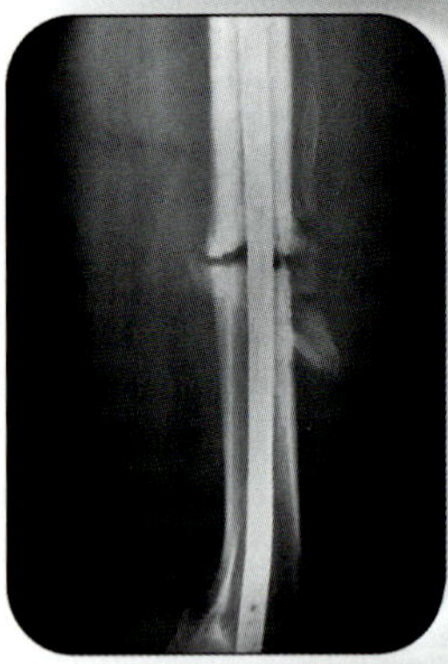

Femoral Shaft Fractures

Matthew Mendez-Zfass, Ryan Ficco, Fernando Vilella-Hernandez

Chapter Outline

Introduction

Diagnosis
- History and Physical Examination
- Imaging

Classification

Surgical Indications
- Plate Fixation
- Intramedullary Nailing

Surgical Anatomy, Positioning and Approaches

Surgical Techniques
- Technique 1: Antegrade Nailing
- Technique 2: Retrograde Intramedullary Nailing
- Postoperative Management for Antegrade and Retrograde Nailing
- Technique 3: Traction Pin Placement
- Technique 4: Placement of Antibiotic Cement-Coated Nails

Outcomes

Specific Situations
- Open Fractures
- Fractures from Gunshot Wounds
- Damage Control Orthopedics
- Floating Knee
- Associated Femoral Neck Fractures
- Vascular Injury

Complications
- Nonunion
- Malunion
- Leg Length Discrepancy
- Infection
- Heterotopic Ossification
- Traction Related

Authors' Preferred Management of Select Complications
- Case 1: Femur Nonunion
- Case 2: Femur Fracture Infection

Summary

Introduction

Diaphyseal femur fractures are common injuries treated by orthopedic surgeons and their treatment has undergone rapid evolution in the 20th century. In the time of Hippocrates the treatment of such fractures consisted of manual isometric traction and splinting the extremity in extension. This was felt by Hippocrates to be an overriding principle of fracture management and of femur fractures in particular. "When the thigh-bone is broken, particular pains should be taken with regard to the extension that it may not be insufficient, for when excessive, no great harm results from it."[1] This dictum of diaphyseal femur fracture treatment progressed relatively unchallenged until Sir Percival Pott, after suffering an open femur fracture, recognized that contraction of soft tissue attachments provided the deforming forces in diaphyseal femur fractures and the goal of treatment should be to minimize these forces.[2] He advocated splinting with the hip and knee in flexion in order to relax the soft tissue envelope.[3]

It was not until the 19th century that the idea of isotonic traction written about by Galen, but first described in the management of femur fractures by Guy de Chauliac some 500 years earlier, began to take hold.[4] Continuous isotonic traction via skin traction (Buck's traction) or traction splints (Thomas Splint) became the popular method of treating such injuries during the time of the American Civil War and World War I respectively.[5] The Thomas splint consists of a long leg splint with the proximal end secured to the proximal femur and pelvis, and the distal end with continuous traction applied through the foot. Its wide use in World War I has been the source of controversy regarding its reported dramatic success in morbidity reduction.[6] Yet an analysis of two battles in World War I by Sir Henry Gray demonstrated a death rate of 80% from gunshot femur fractures without the use of the splint versus 15.6% with the splint accompanied by an organized method for evacuation and treatment.[7] The Thomas splint is still widely employed today in emergency situations, but the shortcomings of skin traction in terms of wound complications led Fritz Steinmann to develop skeletal traction through the insertion of a metal pin through the distal femur or proximal tibia. The advantages of such skeletal traction over skin traction include the ability to apply a greater force, less wound complications and the ability to monitor the soft tissue envelope. Unfortunately, treatment of femoral shaft fractures by immobilization led to poor outcomes.

The gold standard for surgical treatment of these injuries has long been considered intramedullary fixation. Its ability to provide correct alignment and early mobilization was postulated to significantly minimize complications resulting from these injuries. Despite early attempts in the late 19th century at providing such fixation in long bone fractures, it was not until 1939 when after much experimentation and research Gerhard Küntscher performed the first marrow nail or "Marknagelung" on a femoral shaft fracture.[8] Küntscher's ideas in developing the marrow nail stemmed from his use of the Smith Peterson stainless steel nail for the treatment of femoral neck fractures. He believed that diaphyseal femoral shaft fractures could be treated using the same basic principles.[9] His principles included: (1) closed nailing to reduce the risk of infection, (2) stable fixation with rotational control and (3) early weight bearing.[10] In November 1939, he inserted a stainless steel V-shaped nail that was said to be "elastic" and inserted antegrade without the use of reaming. This marked the first use of intramedullary fixation for a femoral shaft fracture.

Küntscher continued to refine his technique, and the start of World War II provided him with a surge in casualties. During World War II Küntscher was drafted as a surgeon and sent to the eastern front in Finland. It is rumored that the German medical establishment's displeasure with his new surgical technique led to his exile from Germany.[11] He became close with the Finnish surgeons and instructed them on his technique. The Finnish collaboration allowed for the first English language paper of the Küntscher technique to be published in 1947. After the war, word of his technique spread throughout Europe and the United States, both in the medical literature and in the long bones of prisoners of war whom he treated with marrow nails. In the late 1940s, Küntscher began to redesign his marrow nail shape from his original V-shape to a cloverleaf shape that he hoped would improve fixation by increasing elastic expansion of the nail. Troubled by a high rate of nonunion, Küntscher also began to experiment with the use of flexible intramedullary reaming to expand the canal diameter and surface area for nail-canal contact and ultimately nail stability.

The majority of diaphyseal fractures of the femur occurs as a result of high-energy trauma. Salminen found that the incidence in males' ages 15–24 years was the highest with over four times the baseline population.[12] The trend for higher femur fracture incidences in males persists until the age of 75 years when females suffer a dramatic increase in injuries secondary to osteopenia, which allows minor or moderate trauma to provide injuries to appear as from a higher energy mechanism.[13] Middle one-third diaphyseal injuries accounted for approximately 80% of the fracture patterns. Arneson demonstrated an overall incidence 19 per 100,000 patient years, with men 15–24 years demonstrating and an overall "severe" traumatic etiology of 70%. These included motor vehicle collisions, pedestrians hit by vehicles and falls from heights and sports related injuries.[14]

Diagnosis

History and Physical Examination

The diagnosis of femoral shaft fractures is not subtle. Owing to the deforming soft tissue forces there is usually an obvious deformity in the extremity with the proximal fragment flexed, externally rotated and abducted, while the distal fragment is shortened and adducted. Patients commonly present with significant pain, swelling and ecchymosis in the affected extremity. The thigh muscle can hold approximately 3 units of blood and significant blood loss is not uncommon.[14] Vital signs and other signs of shock should be carefully evaluated for in these patients. The challenge in these injuries is not to allow the obvious deformity of the femur to act as a distraction for other serious or life-threatening injuries. All trauma patients with associated femur fractures should be first evaluated and treated according to advanced trauma life support protocols. Due to the blunt, high-energy mechanism of trauma, particular attention should be paid to head, chest and visceral trauma. During physical examination all four extremities should be carefully palpated to check for tenderness and range of motion. A careful vascular exam should be performed on the affected leg to assess pulses and capillary refill, particularly in those injuries caused by penetrating trauma. Determination of neurologic status should include an examination of motor strength and sensation in the involved extremity. Additionally, the knee should be carefully examined for an effusion, ligamentous injury or fracture as a coincident knee injury may modify the planned operative technique.

Imaging

Radiographic diagnosis of femoral shaft fractures can easily be made with anteroposterior (AP) and lateral radiographs of the affected extremity. Because of the reported incidence of up to 9% of ipsilateral femoral neck fractures, a protocol for evaluating for these injuries should be institutionally established. Two millimeter thin cut computed tomography (CT) through the femoral neck, or internal rotation AP view radiograph of the femoral neck may be used to carefully assess for an associated femoral neck fracture.[15] Additionally, fractures in the pelvis and acetabulum can also occur in association with shaft fractures and an AP pelvis radiograph or dedicated CT of the pelvis should be obtained.

FEMORAL SHAFT FRACTURES DIAGNOSIS: Pearls and Pitfalls

- Massive hemorrhage up to 3 liters can occur in a closed femoral shaft fracture, so vital signs and signs of shock should be carefully evaluated
- Examine the knee as well to help determine the potential for bone or ligamentous injury which could affect the planned surgical technique and approach
- Be careful not to miss occult femoral neck fractures. CT scans are increasingly being done to rule this out

Classification

The two main classification systems in use for femoral shaft fractures are the Winquist-Hansen and the AO/OTA classification systems. The Winquist-Hansen system classifies femoral shaft fractures from Type I to Type IV based on the amount of comminution present (Fig. 22.1).[16] Type I fractures are transverse with no or minimal comminution. Type II fractures have a small amount of comminution and a small butterfly fragment, but at least 50% of the bone at the fracture site is intact which allows for rotation and length control. Type III fractures have a large butterfly fragment which prevents control of length or rotation, or both. Type IV fractures are segmental with severe comminution and no abutment of the cortices at the fracture level to prevent shortening.

The AO/OTA classification is based on the Müller system. The diaphyseal femur is coded as 32 (Figs 22.2A to C). Type 32-A fractures are simple fractures with A1 demonstrating a spiral pattern, A2 demonstrating an oblique—greater than 30° from a line orthogonal to the long axis of the femur—and A3 demonstrating a transverse pattern—less than 30° from the orthogonal. Type 32-B fractures are wedge fractures and these are classified as B1 or spiral wedge, B2 or bending wedge and B3 or fragmented wedge. Type 32-C fractures are complex fracture patterns. C1 fractures are complex spiral, C2 fractures are complex segmental and C3 fractures are complex irregular and highly comminuted.

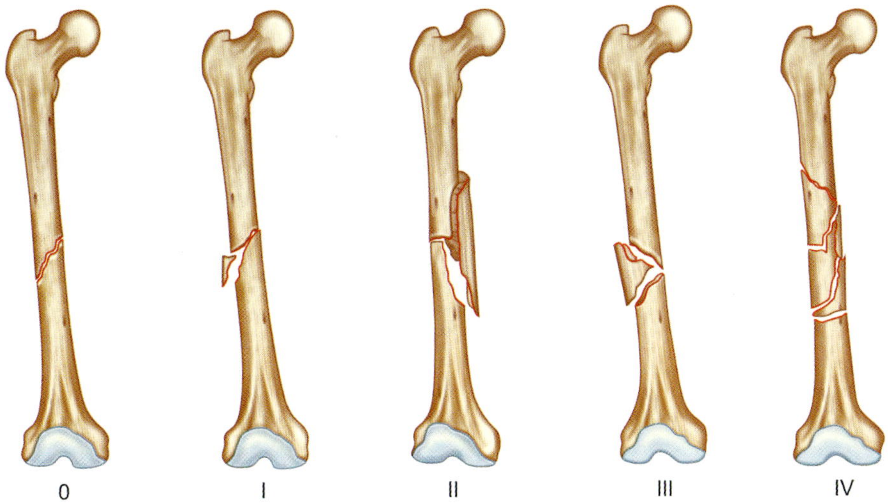

Figure 22.1: Winquist-Hansen classification of diaphyseal comminution.

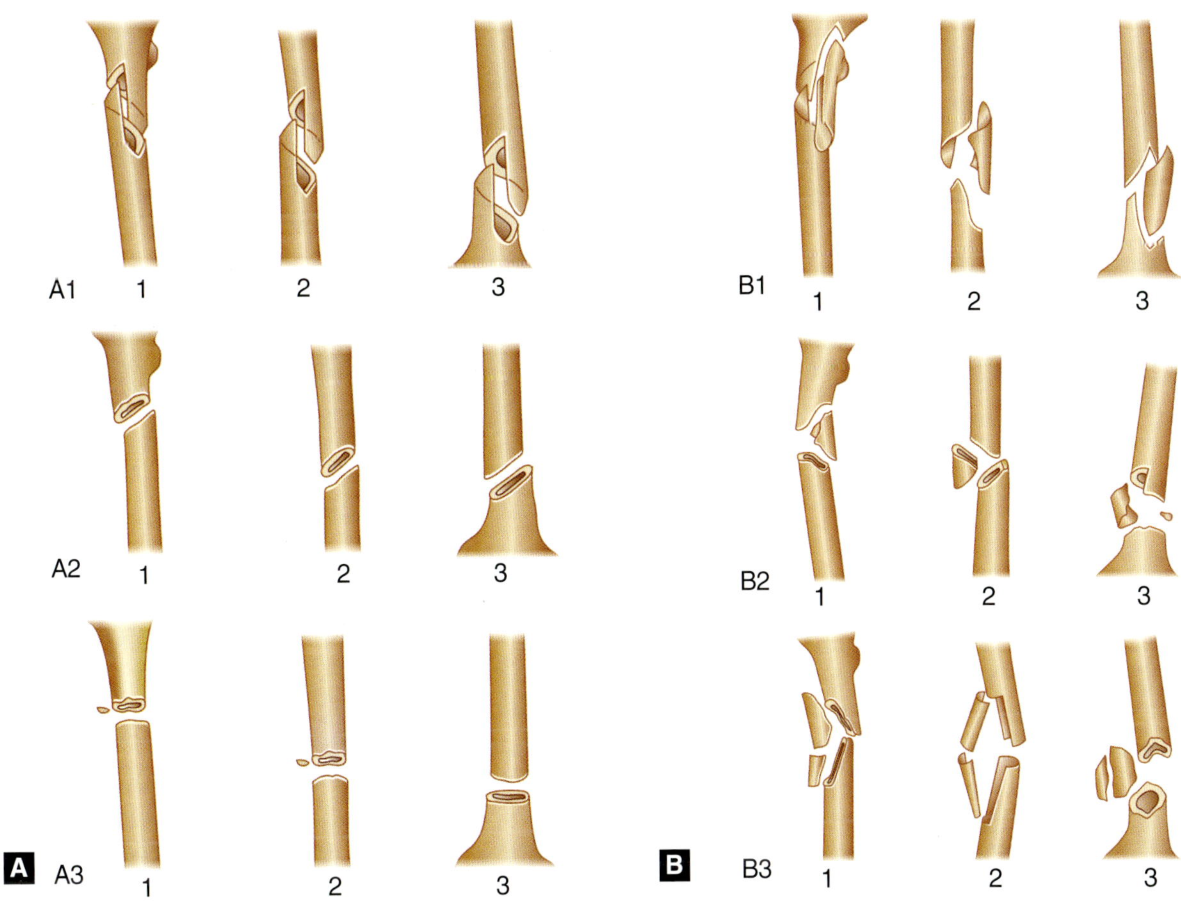

Figures 22.2A and B

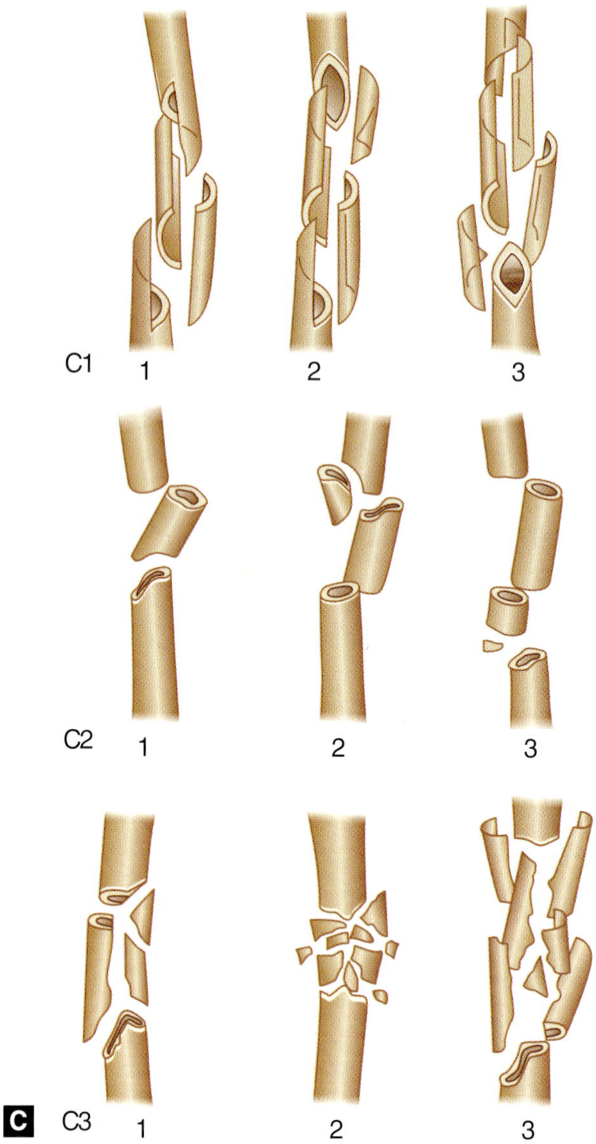

Figures 22.2A to C: AO/OTA classification of diaphyseal fractures.

Surgical Indications

Surgical fixation of femoral shaft fractures is nearly universally indicated in order to optimize fracture reduction, union rates, time to healing and avoid the morbidities of prolonged immobilization. Reamed, interlocked intramedullary nailing is considered the standard by most surgeons. Skeletal traction is an effective temporary stabilization method but should not be used for definitive treatment except perhaps in situations where no other options are available. External fixation is indicated when large open wounds or contamination is present at the fracture site or entry point for nailing. External fixation is also used when surgical time must be limited due to hemodynamic instability or concomitant head, chest, abdominal, or extremity trauma. The external fixator can later be converted to an intramedullary nail albeit with potentially increased infection risk. Occasionally, external fixation can be used as definitive treatment in patients who remain too unstable to return to the operating room (OR) for nailing, patients with severe soft tissue compromise over their femur that precludes internal fixation, or those who have a poor functional prognosis.

Plate Fixation

Plating of femoral shaft fractures is an effective treatment method, particularly in patients with extremely narrow medullary canals, or a femoral deformity that precludes nailing (Figs 22.3A and B).[17] Traditional compression plating with emphasis on anatomic fracture reduction and rigid internal fixation has been associated with suboptimal rates of nonunion, implant failure and infection.[18] Techniques, such as bridge plating with indirect fracture reduction and "minimally invasive" percutaneous plate insertion that avoids subperiosteal dissection have led to improved results.[19-21] Locked plating techniques can improve fixation in osteopenic bone.[17,22] Since the fixation construct does not rely on friction of the plate against bone for fixation, damage to the periosteal blood supply may be limited. Similarly, wave plates with a mid-portion contour away from the fracture site minimize plate to bone contact in the area where blood supply is most critical.

Intramedullary Nailing

Intramedullary nailing has become the standard for the treatment of diaphyseal femur fractures. It is easily reproducible with high union rate and low rate of complications. However, there is a myriad of decisions that must be made with regard to positioning, entry point, reaming, type of nail and locking. All these decisions must be made within the context of the patient, associated traumatic injuries, technical expertise of the surgeon, institutional capabilities and the fracture pattern itself.

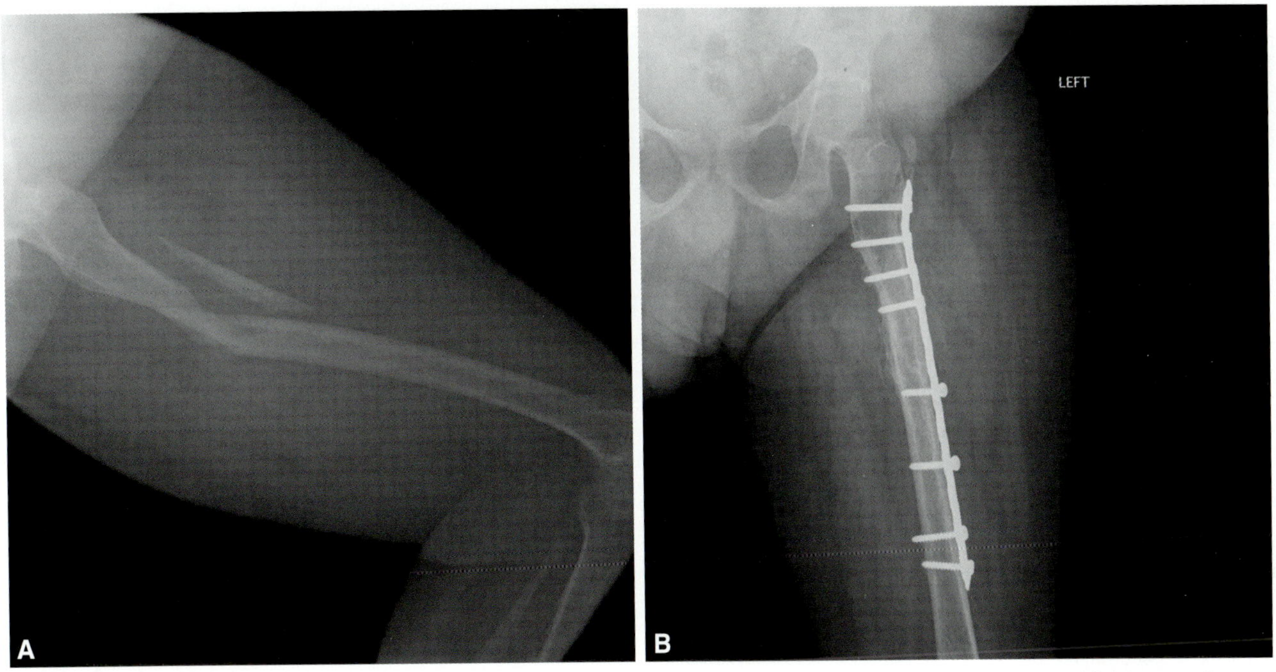

Figures 22.3A and B: (A) Injury radiograph of a left femur fracture in a 30-year-old nonambulatory male with history of mental retardation. Note the small diameter of the canal and the excessive bow; (B) Follow-up radiographs of a left femur fracture treated with compression plating through an open subvastus approach.

Surgical Anatomy, Positioning and Approaches

Antegrade nailing is done through a percutaneous approach and retrograde nailing is done through either a percutaneous or open arthrotomy of the knee. Open reduction during intramedullary nailing or open reduction as part of a plate fixation procedure is typically done through a lateral incision with either a split of the vastus lateralis or elevation of the vastus lateralis from the lateral intermuscular septum and the femur from a posterolateral to anterior direction. A true open reduction with direct visualization of the fragments and application of bone clamps can rarely be done through short incisions and the surgeon should be prepared to have the appropriate retractors (such as Bennett retractors, large self-retaining retractors) for this portion of the case.

Details about the particular positioning and approaches for each procedure are discussed in the following section.

Surgical Techniques

Technique 1: Antegrade Nailing

Positioning

Antegrade femoral nailing can be performed with the patient on a fracture table, lateral decubitus or a "sloppy lateral" position. The use of a fracture table may be limited in patients with unstable spine or pelvic fractures. Patients should first be given adequate anesthesia on their hospital bed then the patient should carefully be transferred over to the fracture table with an assistant ensuring that traction is maintained on the injured extremity. After the patient is placed on the fracture table, a post is placed in between the patient's legs to provide countertraction (Fig. 22.4). Traction boots with extensive padding can be used for both extremities or a traction pin and bow may be used for the affected limb. To optimize fluoroscopic access, the legs can be positioned in a scissor position with the affected extremity elevated slightly higher. To obtain views

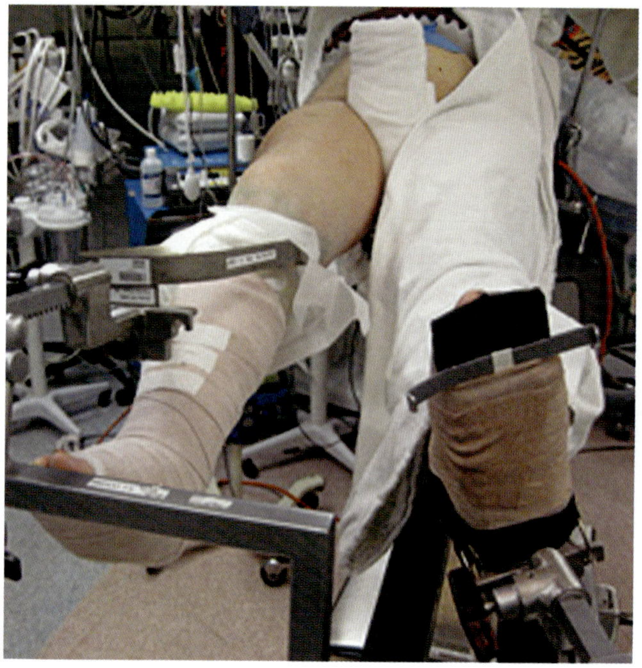

Figure 22.4: Patient set-up on a fracture table in a scissor position. A well padded post is placed at the perineum. The contralateral extremity is placed in a well padded boot, lowered as much as possible and covered. The patient's injured extremity is placed in traction that is first set at the bottom rail and fine adjustments in traction are made with the dial on the lower right hand corner. This particular patient also sustained an ipsilateral ankle fracture that is immobilized in a splint.

in the area of the hip the fluoroscopy machine may have to be angled in caudally by approximately 45° (Fig. 22.5). This permits lateral visualization of the hip without interference of the other extremity. Alternatively, to avoid interference from the uninvolved extremity, it can be abducted and placed in a hemilithotomy position for fluoroscopic access, but this should only be done for short cases (i.e. under 2 hours). It has been reported that the hemilithotomy position has been associated with increased risk of compartment syndrome and nerve injury.[23,24]

Prior to prepping the extremity, fluoroscopic images in all views of the hip and of the fracture site should be obtained. This allows visualization of fracture alignment, length and rotation. The appropriate corrections can now be made without having the added difficulty of a prepped leg. A crutch can be placed to assist with maintenance of fracture reduction but must be left out of the field when prepping (Fig. 22.6). Traction can be increased or decreased to establish length. Abduction and adduction of the extremity can establish alignment. The patient should be prepped and draped from just proximal to the iliac crest down to the knee allow for placement of distal locking screws (Fig. 22.7). The lateral decubitus position on a radiolucent table is an alternative for antegrade

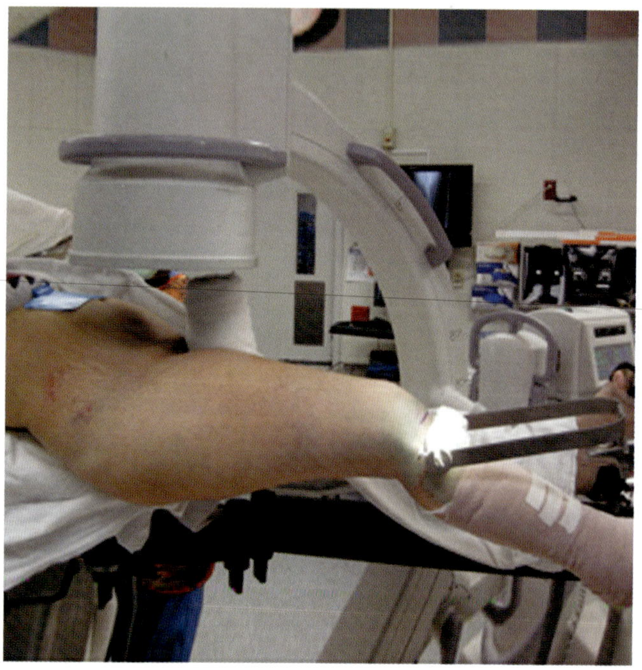

Figure 22.5: The C-arm is brought in from the opposite side of the injury at 45°. This will allow better visualization of the proximal femur on the lateral view without interference from the contralateral extremity.

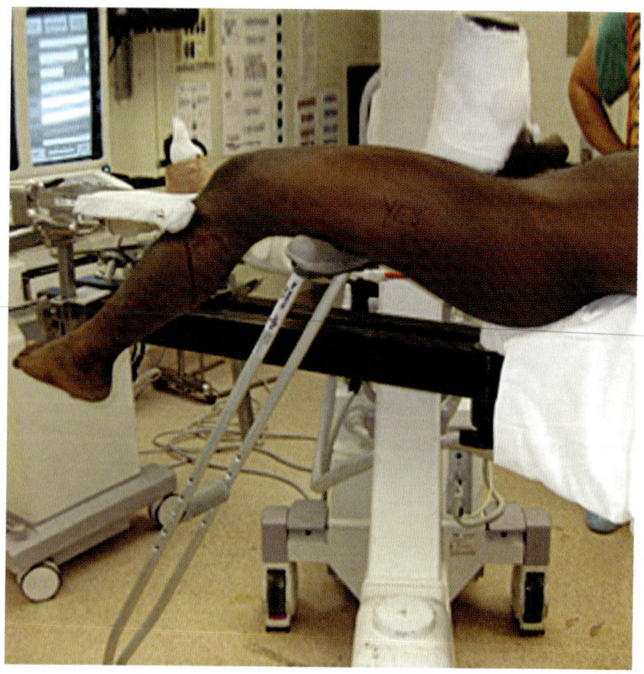

Figure 22.6: Patient placed on a fracture table. Initial images are being taken before prepping. A crutch is place underneath the distal fragment as a reduction tool. The crutch is removed and then placed back after the leg is prepped.

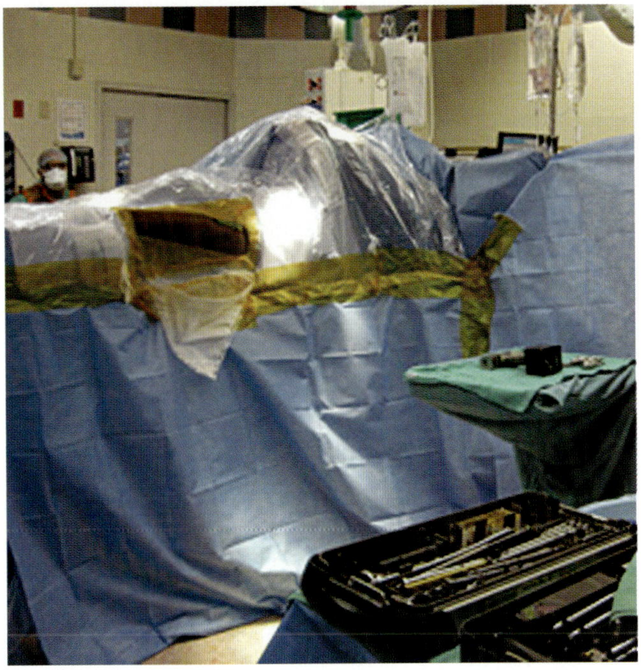

Figure 22.7: The extremity has been fully prepped. Ideally, the leg should be prepped from just above the iliac wing to provide space for entry point to just past the knee and to provide space for distal locking. Notice the blue drape on the right providing sterile space that provides protection proximally during the process of reaming.

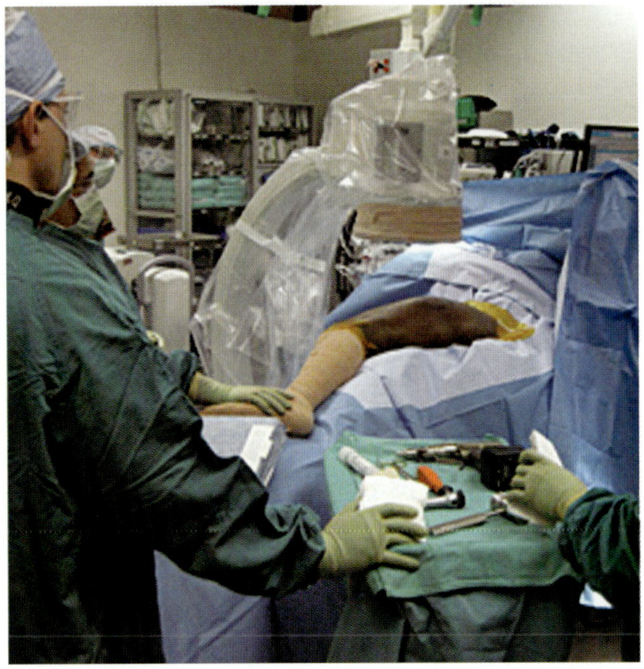

Figure 22.8: Lateral decubitus position. The patient is held in lateral position by a radiolucent bean bag. The C-arm is brought in from the opposite side and an anteroposterior image will provide visualization of the lateral hip. A lateral image will provide an anteroposterior visualization of the hip.

nailing of femoral shaft fractures. After anesthesia is given, the patient is transferred onto a radiolucent table and then placed in lateral decubitus position and held with a radiolucent bean bag. Adequate padding is applied at all pressure points (Fig. 22.8). Prior to prepping, ensure that adequate AP and lateral fluoroscopy views of the hip, femoral shaft and knee can be obtained. An assistant is required to apply traction, control rotation and maintain fracture reduction for the procedure (Fig. 22.9). A "sloppy lateral" is a variation in which bean bag or large bump is placed under the involved hip/torso approximately 30°. Ensure that appropriate fluoroscopy views can be obtained of the hip prior to prepping if this position is chosen, particularly lateral views where the C-arm must be brought over the operative field.

A retrospective study of 988 patients has shown that utilizing the lateral position was not a significant predictor of mortality or ICU admission when compared to the supine position.[25] This position will allow for easier reduction of some proximal fractures as it allows the leg to be flexed and adducted to a larger extent than a fracture

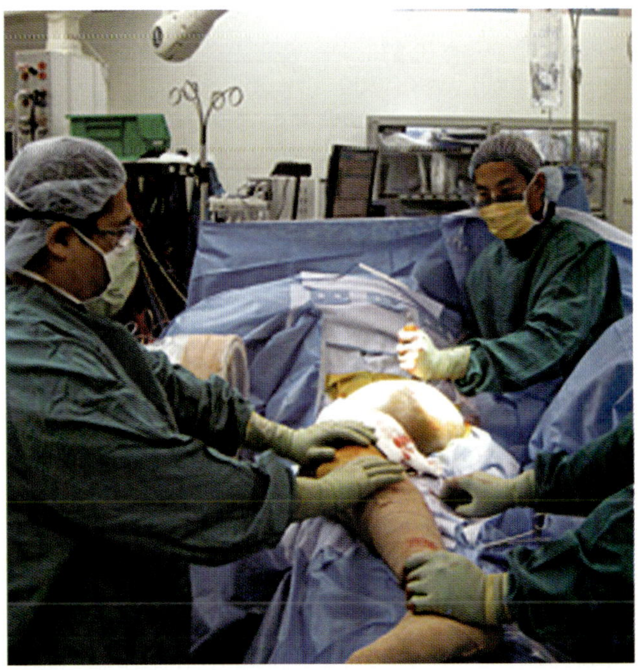

Figure 22.9: Entry point in the lateral position. The assistant on the opposite side of the bed is critical in providing traction and reduction maneuvers that must be held during the procedure.

table, but it requires intense labor from an assistant. Risk of injury to the superior gluteal nerve and gluteus medius may be lower with the increased hip flexion and adduction enabled by the lateral position.[26] The increased ability to adduct the hip also can improve access to the entry point, especially for obese patients. A prospective study of 87 patients showed that using manual traction compared to a fracture table significantly diminished overall operative time and improved rotational alignment.[27,28] Comparison with the other leg intraoperatively can help with clinical assessment of leg length. Rotational evaluation can be enhanced by matching the relationship between an AP of the hip and knee with that of the opposite site, which can be checked prior to draping. Bishop and Rodriguez noted that external rotation errors were more common in their series of patients due to the tendency of gravity to internally rotate the proximal fragment in this position.[29]

Traction-related complications should be avoided. Traction should only be applied when absolutely needed and should be relaxed when it is no longer needed. This will diminish the risk for traction-related complications, such as pudendal nerve palsy and perineal soft tissue necrosis. Generous padding of the perineal post is also required. As discussed earlier, the hemilithotomy position and the use of the well-leg holder is discouraged, particularly for longer cases due to the risk of well-leg compartment syndrome. If it must be utilized, it is recommended that the well-leg be brought down from the elevated position after 2 hours, and if necessary, once an hour afterwards.

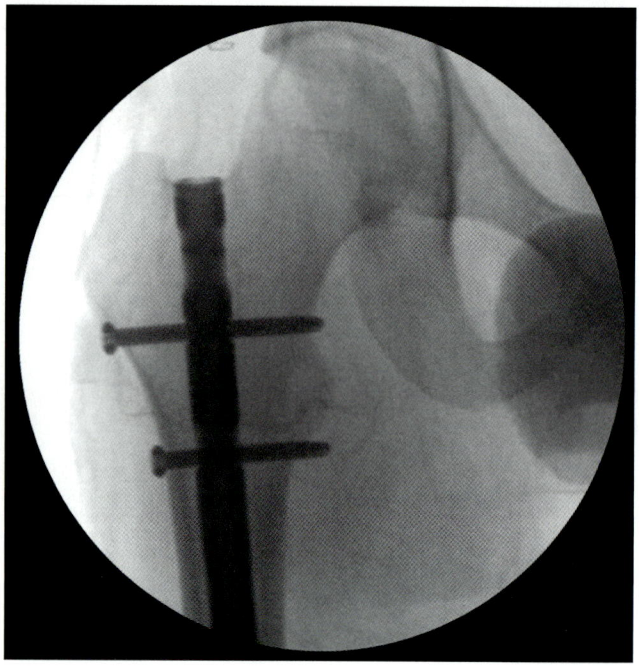

Figure 22.10: Fluoroscopic view of a piriformis type femoral nail. The entry point is in line with the femoral canal.

Entry Point

A piriformis entry point offers the advantage that the piriformis fossa is in line with the center of the femoral canal in both planes (Fig. 22.10). In patients with unusual anatomy, such as an overhanging greater trochanter, the appropriate entry point can be determined by centering the start down the femoral canal on AP and lateral fluoroscopic views. The guide pin can then be advanced down the center of the canal to the level of the lesser trochanter, checking appropriate position and depth on fluoroscopy. Since this entry point is more medial than a trochanteric entry, it can be somewhat more difficult to access, especially in obese patients.[30] An excessively medial or anterior starting point has the potential to cause a femoral neck fracture.[31] This entry point has potential to injure the piriformis and obturator internus tendons, as well as the deep branch of the medial circumflex femoral artery.[32] In younger adolescent patients, the piriformis entry should be avoided due to potential avascular necrosis of the femoral head.[33] Damage to the superior gluteal nerve has also been reported.[34] A trochanteric entry point can be used with appropriately designed nails incorporating a proximal lateral bend into their design (Fig. 22.11). Union rate, low complication rate and functional results have been shown to be similar to piriformis entry nailing with significantly lower fluoroscopy time.[35] On the AP view, the starting point is generally based on the tip of the trochanter, although an optimal starting point may be slightly medial or lateral to the tip depending on the implant and patient anatomy.[36] Excessively lateral entry points may cause difficulty passing the nail past the medial cortex and predispose more proximal fractures to go into varus malalignment.[37] On the lateral view, the starting point should be centered with the femoral canal. If cephalomedullary screws are going to be used, ensure that the starting point is also well-aligned with the femoral neck which is usually slightly anterior to the canal.

Antegrade entry points have been associated with trochanteric pain, limp, diminished abduction strength and

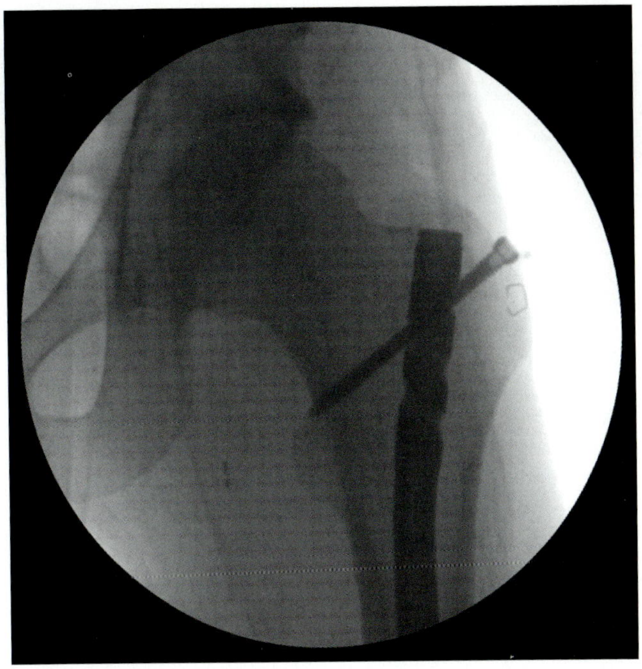

Figure 22.11: Fluoroscopic view of a trochanteric entry femoral nail. Notice that the entry point is slightly medial to the greater trochanter, but lateral to the piriformis fossa. The bend on these nails is usually between 4° and 6°.

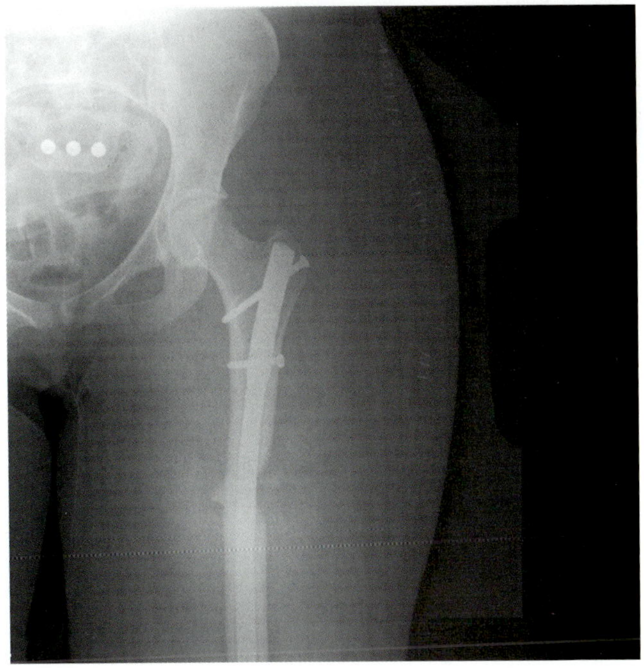

Figure 22.12: Postoperative radiograph of an obese patient with a proximal femoral shaft fracture treated with a lateral entry nail. The entry point is slightly lateral the greater trochanter, at the level of the piriformis fossa. The proximal bend of this nail is 10°.

altered hip kinematics.[38,39] A lateral entry point on the greater trochanter may minimize these effects (Fig. 22.12). A cadaver study has shown that there is a "bald spot" where injury to tendons and neurovascular structures can be minimized. This point was centered 11 mm distal to the tip on the lateral aspect of the greater trochanter and 5 mm anterior to the midline on the lateral view.[40] Another cadaveric study utilizing nails with approximately 10° of lateral bend in the frontal plane proximally showed that bone strain was comparable during insertion of lateral, piriformis and trochanteric nails. Fluoroscopy assists with obtaining an appropriate lateral entry point as anatomic landmarks may be variable. The entry point is 10° lateral to the center of the femoral canal on the AP view and in line with the center of the canal laterally.[41] Anterior third starting points on the lateral view are associated with increased valgus malalignment and iatrogenic fracture compared with middle-third entry.[42] Nails have been designed for lateral entry use with a 10° lateral bend in the AP plane. As with trochanteric entry nails, internally rotating the nail 90° during advancement through the proximal segment facilitates passage.

Technique

Regardless of position and entry point chosen, the skin incision is made in line with the femoral shaft approximately four fingerbreadths above the lesser trochanter. Deep dissection is angled toward the greater trochanter which can be palpated during dissection for guidance. Alternatively the starting point can be located percutaneously and the approach can be guided by the position of the pin. After locating the starting point as above and advancing the guide pin down the center of the canal, an entry reamer or an awl is used to create the entry hole. This should be done through a soft tissue protector in order to protect the abductor musculature. Fluoroscopy can be used to check the position of the reamer and pin during reaming because their position can shift during reaming, especially in osteopenic bone. The entry reamer is advanced to the level of the lesser trochanter. A ball tipped guide wire is then advanced into the canal after removal of entry components. A gentle bend can be made in the tip of the guidewire to aid with guidance down the canal and across the fracture site, after it has been reduced to the superior pole of the patella. Biplanar fluoroscopy is used to verify that fracture reduction and depth of insertion.

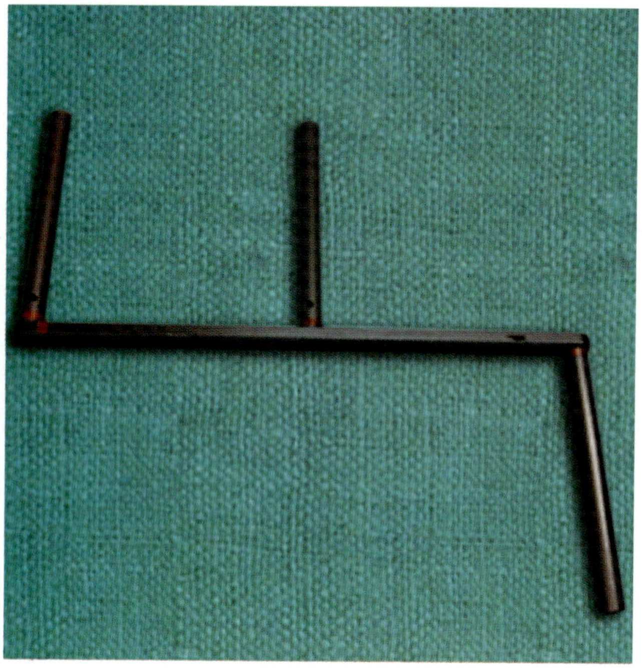

Figure 22.13: "F-tool" for manipulative closed reduction maneuvers. This is useful to correct displacement in the anteroposterior or medial-lateral planes.

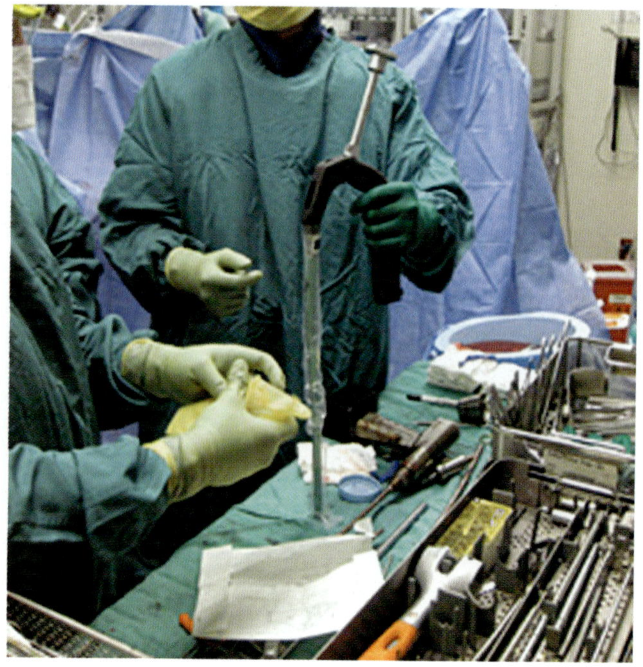

Figure 22.14: Back table assembly of the femoral nail. At this point, it is critical that the external jig be assembled in order to assure proper alignment for locking.

Fracture reduction maneuvers vary depending on patient position. Traction is applied with a fracture table or manually with assistance of a skeletal traction pin for other positions. Strategically placed bumps, towels, mallets, F-tool or a crutch can be used for further adjustment (Fig. 22.13). Percutaneous insertion of a ball spike pusher, a bone hook, clamp or a Schanz pin can provide additional control of the reduction. When closed techniques are not effective, opening the fracture for reduction may be necessary and fracture clamps can be used.[43] The length of the nail can be measured off of the guidewire, but the fracture must be out to length and have adequate alignment for an accurate measurement, making sure that the ruler is properly placed on the hip.

Flexible reaming begins below the expected canal size and advances 1 mm increments until good "chatter" is felt along the canal, then it advances at 0.5 mm increments. The reamer should be advanced slowly and steadily, avoiding forceful and eccentric reaming. Extra caution should be used in patients with dense bone and thin canal diameters to minimize thermal complications. Generally, a nail is selected with a diameter 1.5–2 mm less than the largest flexible reamer used in order to accommodate the bow of the femur. Reaming should occur with the fracture held in a reduced position, especially in osteopenic bone and proximal or distal nonisthmal fractures. If reaming is performed malreduced then chances are that the final reduction after nail insertion will also end up malreduced. The nail is not a reduction tool.

The nail is assembled on the back table with the insertion handle, ensuring that all drills guides and bits enter the locking holes appropriately (Fig. 22.14). The nail is advanced carefully into the femur with the apex of the bow facing anteriorly. Alternatively, the nail can be temporarily internally rotated 90° to facilitate entry proximally. This is particularly true in trochanteric or lateral entry nails. Manual pressure and/or gentle strikes by the mallet can be used to advance the nail. When crossing the fracture site, fluoroscopy is used to verify fracture reduction and confirm that the nail is advancing easily across the fracture site and it is not impinging on the cortical bone of the distal segment. After the nail has crossed the fracture site, the guidewire is removed. Ensuring that there is adequate room for advancement on a lateral view of the knee, the nail is seated in the greater trochanter or piriformis fossa. Rotation of the limb should be verified by clinical examination, fluoroscopic evaluation of the fracture site, the hip and the knee, ensuring that the nail is facing anteriorly in accordance with native femoral anatomy.

Proximally, locking screws can be inserted through small incisions using the aiming arm attached to the nail insertion handle. Recon and cephalomedullary screws can be used if indicated, but the nail must be inserted to the appropriate depth and rotation in order for the proximal locking screws to engage to femoral head in a proper direction. Axially stable fracture patterns can be impacted after proximal locking and after the traction has been released. The perfect circles technique can be used for insertion of the distal locking screws. Less stable fracture patterns or those where the contact between the nail and isthmus is limited, require more than one distal locking screw.

ANTEGRADE NAILING: Pearls and Pitfalls

- Patient positioning is surgeon's choice. Lateral decubitus positioning provides easier access to the entry point but requires an assistant to provide traction and manipulation for reduction. The fracture table takes longer time to set up, and the entry point might be more difficult to obtain. However, the reduction and manipulation does not require an assistant, it is held relatively constant and the fracture table does not complain or get tired
- Entry point is also surgeon's choice. Femoral shaft fractures in adolescents should never be treated with piriformis entry nails due to the risk of osteonecrosis. A piriformis entry point is in line with the femoral shaft in both AP and lateral fluoroscopic views. A trochanteric entry point is slight medial to the trochanter, aiming towards the distal shaft on the AP view and in line with the shaft on the lateral view
- Lateral entry point nails can be used on obese patients with femoral shaft fractures that are not amenable to retrograde nailing
- Monitor the initial reamer as it enters the femur on both fluoroscopic views to prevent eccentric reaming or canal penetration
- Small bends with shallow angles on the distal ball tipped guidewires are preferable
- Pass the ball tipped guidewire through the fracture after reduction maneuvers have been established. Verify reduction and guidewire placement on both views before reaming
- Gently impact the ball tip distally on the femur at the level of the superior pole of the patella. This will create a collar of bone around the ball tip that will hold the guidewire in place during reaming
- Start with a cutting reamer that correlated with canal size on the initial X-ray of the fractured femur
- Reaming should be performed with the fracture reduced. As the reaming progresses and the intervening soft tissue is removed from the fracture site, maintaining an acceptable reduction should become easier
- If you ream malreduced, the fracture will end up malreduced
- Reaming should progress at 1 mm intervals until the initial chatter is felt, then it should progress at 0.5 mm intervals. The reamer size of the first significant chatter will usually correlate with final nail diameter
- Ream to 1.5–2.0 mm above the final nail diameter
- Length measurement should be done after final reaming because of the easier reduction after reaming. Make sure the guidewire is well placed distally, the fracture is adequately reduced and the depth gauge is well seated on the proximal femur before the final length is determined
- Assemble the nail on the back table, making sure the proximal jig lines up with the proximal locking holes
- Nail insertion should be done by hand or gentle malleting. The nail can be rotated so that its bow is pointed laterally to facilitate insertion. The nail can then slowly be rotated while it is inserted
- Monitor the nail as it passes the fracture to maintain reduction and ensure that the nail is not hitting the cortex of the distal fragment. Small, rapid taps at this point may facilitate nail passage through the fracture site
- Remove the guidewire after the nail has passed the fracture site. This distance will help generate enough momentum for the guidewire to pass freely through the nail
- Monitor the nail distally above the knee, keeping in mind the distance to the knee and make sure this correlates with the distance left proximally as the nail is inserted into the hip

- After nail placement, verify its distal and proximal positions, as well as fracture reduction before the locking process begins
- Consider distal locking first to provide for fracture impaction in stable patterns
- Lock proximally and distally
- Evaluate length and rotation of the injured extremity before the instruments are contaminated and before leaving the room so that correction can be undertaken
- Avoid pudendal nerve palsy by generously padding the perineal post and using traction only when needed (i.e. relax the traction when the reduction is obtained and instruments are in place)
- Avoid well-leg compartment syndrome by not using the well-leg holder

Technique 2: Retrograde Intramedullary Nailing

Indications for retrograde femoral nailing include multisystem injury, trauma involving multiple extremity fractures and isolated fracture in the morbidly obese patient, bilateral femur fractures. Pregnancy is a relative indication. Contraindications include skeletal immaturity and a history of knee joint sepsis. Relative contraindications are limitation of knee flexion to less than 45°, fractures within 5 cm of the lesser trochanter, and severe soft tissue injury about the knee.[44] Excellent results can reliably be obtained in distal femoral fractures, though technical challenges exist.[45]

The patient is given anesthesia on the hospital bed. The patient is then transferred and positioned supine on a radiolucent table or a regular table with an extension. When prepping and draping the involved limb, adequate access must be left proximally for insertion of locking screws, therefore draping should be proximal to the level of the iliac crest. A radiolucent triangle is placed beneath the femur to keep the knee flexed to 30-40° (Fig. 22.15). A longitudinal incision is made through the skin over the patellar tendon. Depending on surgeon preference, the patellar tendon can be split longitudinally in the midline or dissection can proceed under the paratenon medially around the tendon. A guide pin is inserted into the center of the femoral notch on a fluoroscopic AP view of the knee and just anterior to Blumensaat's line on the lateral view (Fig. 22.16). Exact position on the lateral is dependent

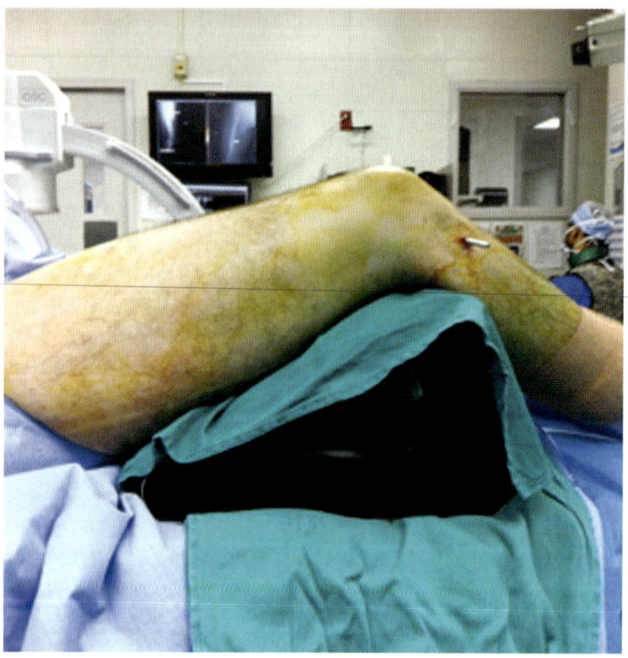

Figure 22.15: Positioning of the involved femur for retrograde nailing. The leg has been prepped as proximally as possible to provide ample space for proximal locking. The triangle is placed underneath the thigh with the longer side aiming proximally.

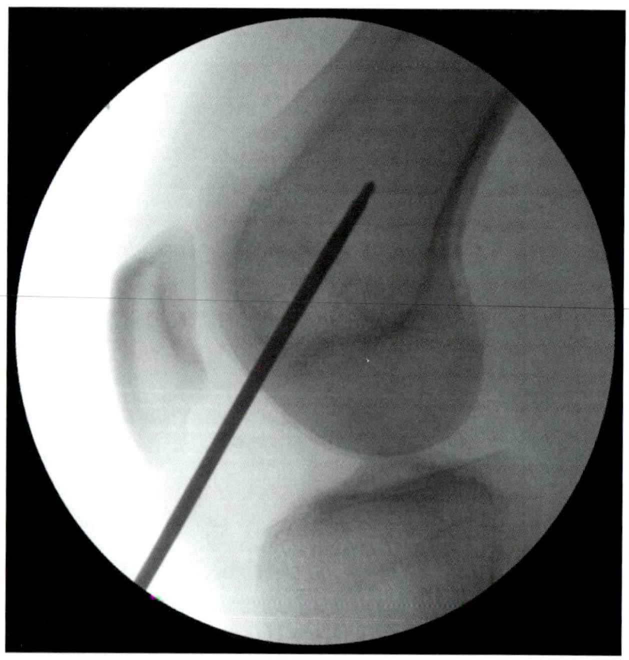

Figure 22.16: Lateral view of retrograde entry point just above Blumensaat's line. Notice that the femoral condyles are perfectly in profile for this view. Inaccurate lateral imaging can lead to misplacement of the starting portal.

on nail design and ability to match the femoral bow. The pin is advanced several centimeters in line with the center of the canal. After the entry hole is then established with an entry reamer, the ball-tapped guidewire is advanced into the canal across the fracture site after reduction, and up to the level of the lesser trochanter. Fracture reduction can also be accomplished with the tools previously mentioned. Usually a towel bump under the fracture to correct to the posterior angulation of the fracture with an appropriately placed F-tool to correct varus/valgus alignment, and traction are all that is necessary (Fig. 22.17). Once the fracture is reduced, the length of the nail to be utilized can be measured off of the guidewire, with fluoroscopic confirmation that the ruler is appropriately seated on a lateral fluoroscopic view of the knee. Reduction must be held throughout the reaming process until the nail has been locked proximally and distally. As is the case with antegrade nails, if reaming is done malreduced then chances are final reduction after nail placement will end up malreduced. After reaming with same technique as mentioned above, and determining appropriate nail size, the nail is assembled on the back table with the insertion handle, ensuring that all drill guides and drill bits line up appropriately with the nail. The nail is advanced carefully into the femur with the apex of the bow facing anteriorly. Manual pressure and/or gentle strikes with the mallet can be used to advance the nail. When crossing the fracture site, fluoroscopy is used to verify fracture reduction and confirm that the nail is advancing easily across the fracture site, without impinging on proximal fragment cortical bone. Once the nail has crossed the fracture site, the guidewire is removed. Ensuring that there is adequate room for advancement proximally, the nail is seated just below the subchondral bone on a lateral view of the knee (Fig. 22.18).

Rotation of the limb should be verified by clinical examination, comparison to the contralateral extremity, fluoroscopic evaluation of the fracture site, of the hip and knee and verifying that the nail is pointing anteriorly. Especially in more distal fractures, blocking pins or screws can be utilized to correct malalignment in the AP and/or lateral planes. They act as an "artificial cortex" to guide the nail to an appropriate position. If malalignment is noted, the nail is removed leaving the guidewire in place. Most commonly, blocking screws are inserted in the short segment on the concave aspect of the deformity though other patterns may be required for particular fractures. If a blocking screw is used, it can be left in place to prevent

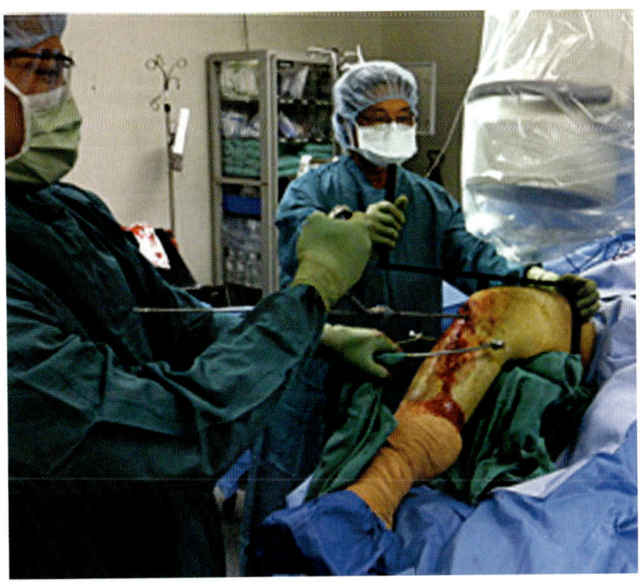

Figure 22.17: Reduction maneuvers for retrograde nailing are demonstrated here. Skeletal traction, a bump underneath the distal segment of the fracture, a cannulated reduction tool for manipulation of the distal segment and an F-tool to correct for medial-lateral displacement are all shown.

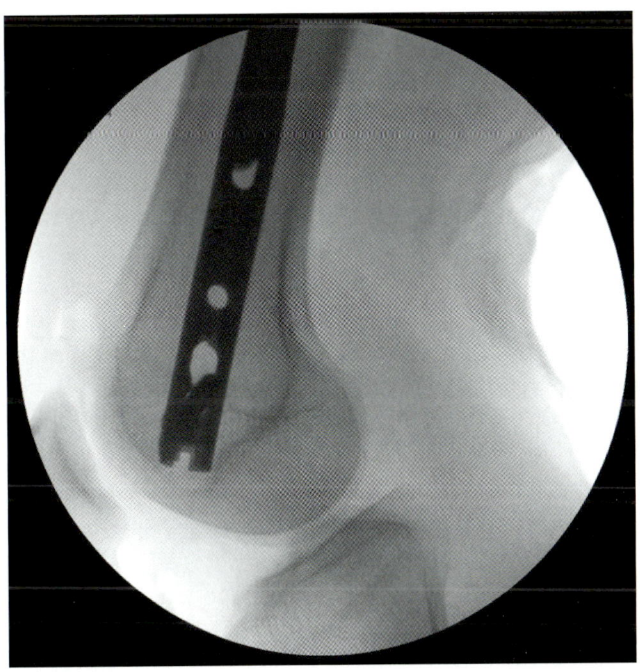

Figure 22.18: Final placement of the retrograde nail just deep to Blumensaat's line.

later displacement of the fracture.[46] Distally, locking screws can be inserted through small incisions using the aiming arm attached to the nail insertion handle. At least two locking screws are inserted distally to prevent the nail from subsiding into the knee joint. Screw heads should be buried within metaphyseal bone to prevent later symptomatic hardware. The number of screws used proximally and distally depends on factors, such as fracture pattern, the isthmal contact of the nail, bone quality, bone contact and axial stability at the fracture site. For fractures with good bone contact and axial stability, such as transverse fractures, the fracture should be impacted prior to proximal locking. Proximal locking screws can be inserted using the perfect circles technique. The presence of a fracture can alter the position of nerves and vessels during proximal locking, especially with acetabular fractures.[47] Careful dissection and use of tissue protectors can help minimize the risk of injury to neurovascular structures. Some authors have suggested that lateral to medial locking screws may be less injurious than those placed anteroposteriorly.[48]

Reaming

There has been considerable debate regarding using reamed or unreamed nails for femur fractures. Reaming has become more acceptable over time due to its enhancement of fracture healing, but there continue to be concerns with its use.

Reamed intramedullary nails have been shown to improve healing time and union rate with a lower rate of reoperation.[49,50] Larger implants can be inserted which add strength and stability to the fixation construct. Reaming debris has the potential to enhance fracture healing as well. However, reaming does temporarily cause damage to the endosteal blood supply. However, the effect of this phenomenon on fracture healing has not been clearly shown to be detrimental. Potential thermal damage to bone can be minimized by utilizing appropriately sharp reamers, reaming in small increments when appropriate and avoiding excessive reaming of small diameter canals. Reamer designs that include a narrower shaft, sharp cutting edges, deep flutes and a conical shape can help minimize increases in marrow pressures.[51,52] The Reamer Irrigator Aspirators (RIA), Synthes, Paoli, PA, have been introduced as a way to minimize pressure increases during reaming as well. Studies have not shown clinically significant changes in pulmonary complications though they may have an effect on some serum inflammatory markers.[53-55]

Consideration of the systemic effects of reaming is important to maximize patient outcomes. Reaming does increase intramedullary pressure, which can force fat droplets into the blood stream with potential adverse effects on other organ systems.[56] However, introducing unreamed nails into the canal can have this effect as well.[57] Several clinical studies have not shown different rates of adult respiratory distress syndrome, pulmonary complications or mortality with reamed nailing when compared to unreamed nailing or plating.[58-60] The effects of additional mediators of systemic effects with reaming, such as interleukin-6, continue to be studied.

RETROGRADE INTRAMEDULLARY NAILING: Pearls and Pitfalls

- Patient should be supine on a radiolucent table with a triangle inserted with its longer side proximally below the thigh
- Entry point is in line with the shaft on the AP view and just above Blumensaat's on the lateral view
- Fracture reduction can be achieved with towel bumps directly underneath the fracture to counter act deforming force, traction and an F-tool to correct for varus/valgus
- A cannulated reduction tool can be used to manipulate the distal fragment to provide for adequate guidewire placement into the proximal segment
- Reaming and nail placement should proceed as in antegrade nails
- The distal nail should be buried under Blumensaat's on the lateral view
- Two distal locking screws should be used, preferably those with the most distance in between them
- The more metaphyseal locking screw should be shorter than usual so it is buried enough within the bone so that it is not bothersome postoperatively
- Lock proximally
- Verify length and rotation postoperatively

Postoperative Management for Antegrade and Retrograde Nailing

The postoperative management of femoral shaft fractures includes adequate pain management, wound care and prophylaxis for deep vein thrombosis. The weight bearing status is dependent on the location and pattern of the fracture, the implant, the level of comminution and the amount and location of locking screws.

Midshaft transverse femur fractures, short oblique fractures or those with adequate cortical contact treated with large diameter intramedullary nails can be weight bearing as tolerated. This does not always mean that the patient will be walking on it right away, rather they will slowly put more pressure on the extremity as their pain level and confidence improves. Usually, the bigger the diameter of the nail, the better the isthmal contact of the nail, then the prospect for immediate weight bearing improves. In the case of significant comminution, more locking screws should be used. If the comminution is distal or proximal to the isthmus, then two locking screws should be used distally or proximally, respectively. However, intramedullary nails should always have at least one proximal and one distal locking screw to prevent rotation of the nail. In the case of retrograde nails, two distal locking screws should be used to prevent nail penetration into the knee joint. Particular attention should be paid to those systems where smaller nails have smaller diameter locking screws. In this case, consideration should be given to have a greater number of locking screws.

Technique 3: Traction Pin Placement

Skeletal pin traction for femoral shaft fractures is used in the context of temporary stabilization and fracture reduction before definitive surgical management. The applied traction will align the fracture and provide fracture immobilization which helps with patient comfort, patient transport and pain management. The pin can be placed either through the distal femur or the proximal tibia. The proximal tibia is preferred because of its ease of insertion. Traction through the distal femur may provide more longitudinal force. Contraindications to skeletal traction include an ipsilateral ligamentous knee injury and an ipsilateral fracture about the knee.

TRACTION PIN PLACEMENT: Pearls and Pitfalls

- Do not place traction pin until AP and lateral knee X-rays are available to rule out an ipsilateral fracture about the knee
- Ideally, the patient should be in a minor procedures room with intravenous sedation and cardiac monitoring
- The area should be prepped and draped sterile
- Local anesthetic should be injected into the skin, soft tissues and into the periosteum in a sequential manner
- The largest diameter Schanz pin should be chosen
- Make a stab incision at the insertion site on the skin
- Proximal tibia traction pins should be inserted at the level of the tibial tubercle or two fingerbreadths below the inferior pole of the patella in a lateral to medial direction
- Distal femur traction pins should be inserted at the level of the superior pole of the patella in a medial to lateral direction
- The leg should be held with the patella pointing straight upward and the pin should be inserted parallel to the floor and parallel to the joint line
- If the pin is not inserted parallel to the joint line, traction during the definitive intramedullary nailing may not result in an adequate reduction
- Make a stab incision on the far side as the pin starts to protrude under the skin
- The traction bow should be applied after sterile dressings
- Traction should be built around a pulley system with 20–25 lbs of traction. Make sure that the foot is off the foot plate of the bed and the ropes are not impinging on any portion of the lower extremity. Also, make sure the weights are not touching the floor
- Post-traction AP and lateral X-rays of the femur and knee should be taken to confirm fracture reduction and pin placement

Technique 4: Placement of Antibiotic Cement-Coated Nails

The indications for placement of antibiotic cement-coated nails are medullary infection with or without the presence of fracture healing in the femur. In the case of acute or chronic osteomyelitis, an antibiotic cement-coated nail helps to reduce dead space in the medullary canal in the event of medullary infection. It also helps to deliver high doses of antibiotics to control the infection but should not be relied upon to "cure" an infection. Furthermore, it should be kept in mind that depending on the type and concentration of antibiotics used, drug elution drops off typically after several weeks. After this, the nail continues to be a foreign body in the face of possible persistent infection and should be removed. Reaming and irrigation is important to perform prior to placement of antibiotic cement-coated nails. Details about and images of antibiotic cement nail preparation are also discussed in chapter 26 (Tibial Shaft Fractures).

PLACEMENT OF ANTIBIOTIC CEMENT-COATED NAILS: Pearls and Pitfalls

- Utilize a full dose of 40 grams of cement mixed in with 2 grams of Vancomycin and 4.8 grams of Tobramycin
- Make sure the antibiotic powder is properly crushed before mixing it in with the antibiotic powder
- Add the monomer from the full dose and another from a half dose of cement in order to provide a more liquid mixture that is easier to manage
- After mixing, pour the cement into a large 60 cc syringe with predrilled holes around the 60 cc level. These holes will let the air out as the syringe's pusher is inserted without forcing cement out the other side
- Use a 40 French chest tube. This size is equivalent to a 10 mm diameter nail. Length of the chest tube should be equal to the length of the removed, infected nail or slightly smaller
- The ball tipped guidewire should be bent onto itself, opposite the ball tip, at a length slightly longer than the chest tube. The bent proximal hook of the guidewire will facilitate its later removal. Also, bend the guidewire so that it correlates with the nail bow
- Lubricate the chest tube with 5 cc of sterile mineral oil before insertion of the cement mixture. The oil will help prevent the cement from curing and melting onto the chest tube. Remove the extra oil before cement insertion
- Hold the chest tube vertically with the bottom sealed off and insert the cement under pressure with the syringe. If necessary, make holes on the upward side of the chest tube to allow air to escape and not force the cement out the other side
- After the chest tube is full of the still liquid cement, insert the ball tipped guidewire down the center removing any excess cement that pours out of the chest tube
- Insert the guidewire to a level where the ball tip is slightly past the cement at one end of the chest tube, and where the bent hook is also slightly short of the chest tube on the other end. A collar of cement should be molded around the ball tip so that it will help with nail removal. The nail's hook should be left free of cement so that it provides something with which to hold the nail during removal and insertion
- As the cement starts to cure and heat up, start by cutting open the ends of the chest tube with a sharp knife until wet, uncured cement is reached. Leave this area unopened so that it can cure within the tube. Work your way towards the center of the tube as it cures
- Cutting open the chest tube too early will cause the cement to spill and lose its form. Cutting the chest tube too late will cause the cement to adhere to the tube and will make its removal extremely hard
- After the nail has been taken out of the chest tube, remove any excess melted plastic from the chest tube with a knife
- Make sure the nail is totally cooled down before insertion
- The smoother and rounder the periphery of the nail, the easier is its insertion and removal
- Remove and/or exchange the nail at 4–6 weeks

Outcomes

Management of femoral shaft fractures with intramedullary nailing continues to be the standard for treatment. Outcomes include high union rate between 95% and 99%, low complication rate and high return to function.[61] Similar rates of healing, delayed union and malunions have been demonstrated between antegrade and retrograde nailing when appropriately sized nails are utilized.[45] However, there are some conflicting studies that suggest longer time to union and slightly lower rate of union with retrograde nails.[62,63] Even though intramedullary nailing of femoral shaft fractures is highly successful, it does not mean that it is not without its problems.

Hip function, hip strength, as well as gait alterations, continue to be a common sequelae of antegrade nailing with the persistent need for early therapy and strengthening exercises.[39] Hip and thigh pain are also more commonly reported when using antegrade nails.[64] Alterations in knee function and knee pain are more related to retrograde nailing, however knee stiffness and septic complications have not shown to be a significant complication.[64,65]

More patients with retrograde nails require removal of hardware for symptomatic distal locking screws.[62] At 1 year postoperative, knee flexion, Lysholm scores and isokinetic evaluation did not show a significant difference after retrograde nailing with comparison to the contralateral limb.[65] Knee sepsis is also a potential concern with open fractures treated with retrograde nailing, though the incidence was shown to be 1.1% in a retrospective study of 90 patients.[66]

Specific Situations

Open Fractures

The soft tissue envelope that surrounds the femur makes open injuries not as common as in the tibia. On the other hand, small wounds about an open femur fracture may be indicative of severe soft tissue trauma and periosteal stripping of bone. Upon initial presentation, the location of the size of the wound must be correlated with the location and pattern of the fracture. A small puncture wound around a transverse femur fracture represents less trauma than the same wound over a highly comminuted injury.

The timing of the initial debridement is dependent on the patient's condition and the availability of hospital resources. A thorough debridement starts with a systematic approach. The superficial tissues must be examined first, with the removal of any contaminated or nonviable tissue. Then the deeper layer of the wound is examined in a sequential fashion down to bone. Any nonviable bone should also be removed. It is the severity of the injury and not the timing of the debridement that affects infection risk.[67]

After the initial debridement, an initial irrigation should be done with normal saline with a low pressure, high volume system. Once the initial irrigation is done, a second look debridement should be performed in order to re-examine the tissues. Once satisfied with the debridement, bony stabilization can be performed. Antibiotics-impregnated cement beads should be considered in a setting of highly contaminated tissues and/or bone loss. Wound closure should be performed in order to prevent hospital acquired infection. Seventy-two hours of intravenous antibiotics should be administered after each debridement.

The majority of open femur fractures can be stabilized initially with intramedullary nailing. External fixation is reserved for cases where the soft tissue injury and the contamination are so severe that it requires aggressive management with multiple trips to the OR, in which case the patient should be kept on intravenous antibiotics until after definitive stabilization and management have been undertaken.

Fractures from Gunshot Wounds

Gunshot wounds are penetrating injuries therefore patient evaluation requires special attention to neurovascular status. Examination of the wound should document location and extent. The wounding capability of the bullet is dependent on the kinetic energy imparted on the tissues which in turn depends on the velocity of the projectile and its mass.[68] High-velocity injuries are secondary to projectiles traveling at greater than 2,000 fps (feet per second) and these therefore are associated with more significant tissue damage. Shotgun injuries at close range because of their associated blast effect also cause significant tissue damage.

High-velocity and shotgun wounds, because of the severity of their soft tissue injury, should be treated like severe open injury, with consideration given to temporary

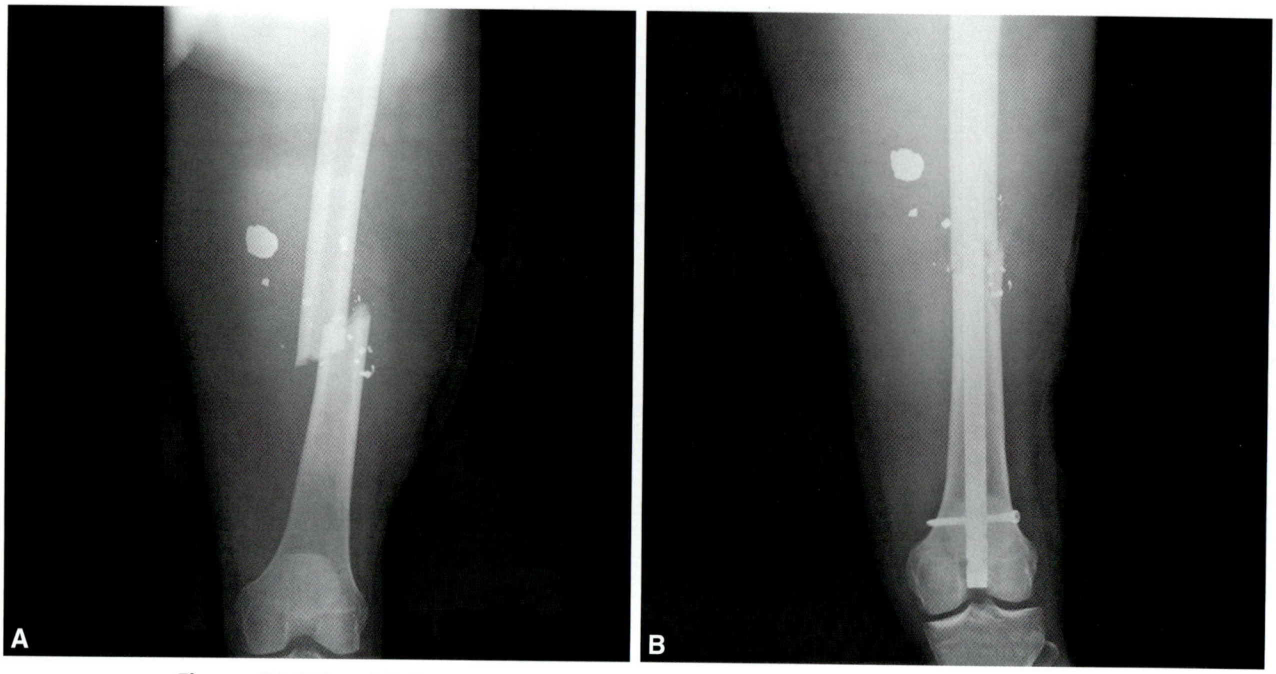

Figures 22.19A and B: Preoperative and postoperative radiographs of a distal femoral shaft fracture from a low-velocity gunshot wound treated with a retrograde nail.

external fixation with serial debridement and aggressive soft tissue management. Low-velocity injuries are caused by bullets with muzzle velocities below 2,000 fps. These femur fractures are generally treated like closed injuries with irrigation and debridement of superficial tissues only, and stabilization with an intramedullary nail (Figs 22.19A and B). However, a low-velocity gunshot wound at close range releasing all of its kinetic energy, might cause severe soft tissue damage; therefore, the treating surgeon should always remember to treat the wound, not the weapon.[68,69]

Damage Control Orthopedics

Damage control orthopedics is a management approach that emphasizes fracture management in the context of overall patient physiology. The rapid stabilization of fractures controls hemorrhage, helps soft tissue management and delays the physiologic insult of major orthopedic procedures until the patient's condition is optimized. Early intramedullary nailing of femur fractures in patients who are borderline, unstable or in extremis can cause the release of inflammatory mediators, blood loss and hypothermia. Additionally, the systemic effects of reaming, especially in patients with head and pulmonary injury, are associated with worsening of a patient's overall physiology.[70,71]

External fixation of femur fractures in polytrauma patients is the workhorse of damage control orthopedics

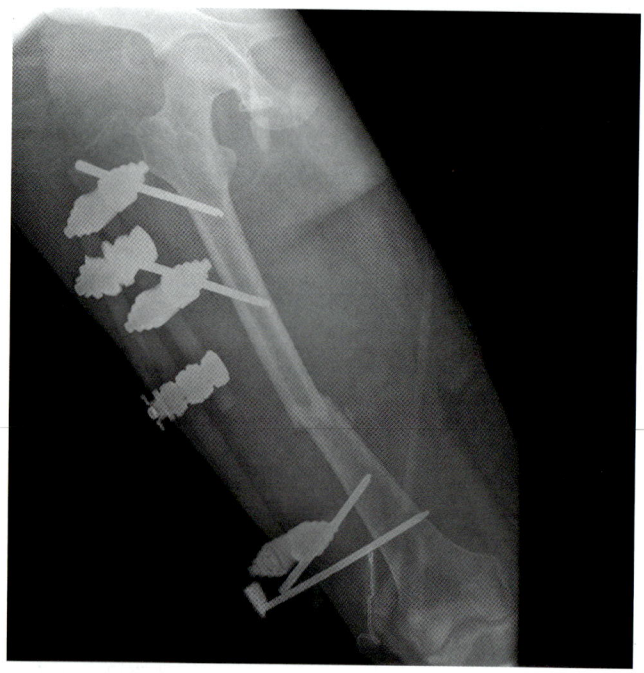

Figure 22.20: Damage control orthopedics. Postoperative radiograph of a right femur fracture stabilized with an anterolateral external fixator in a hemodynamically unstable patient.

(Fig. 22.20). It provides fracture stability that promotes patient mobility, easier bedside management of the patient and associated soft tissue injuries, as well as preventing further damage to surrounding tissues that may be detrimental to patient physiology. Conversion of the external fixator to an intramedullary nail within 2 weeks can be performed safely and effectively in polytrauma patients in the absence of a pin site infection.[72]

Placement of the external fixator should be performed with Schanz pins placed anterolaterally between the quadriceps and vastus lateralis. They should be placed bicortically after predrilling to prevent heat injury to the bone and the surrounding tissues. Two stable bases should be created, one proximally and one distally with a connecting rod to provide greater modularity for ease of alignment and reduction of the fracture.

In more recent literature, the concept of damage control nailing has been introduced. This is when a multiple trauma patient is undergoing other surgical procedures, and the associated femur fracture is stabilized through a rapidly placed unreamed small diameter retrograde intramedullary nail with or without static locking. This provides the same benefits of early stabilization from external fixation with the added decrease in risk of pin site infection. It also does not burn any bridges in terms of definitive stabilization. The nail can be locked, exchanged, and any other potential problems, such as malrotation or leg length discrepancy, can be corrected when the patient is optimized. The disadvantage of this procedure is potential deleterious pulmonary effects associated with intramedullary nailing.[73]

Floating Knee

The term floating knee denotes ipsilateral fracture of the femur and tibia in a single patient. These usually are secondary to high-energy trauma, such as motor vehicle and motorcycle accidents. They are associated with a high rate of multiple extremity trauma, visceral injury, head injury, ligamentous knee injuries and vascular injuries. Preoperative workup and documentation is paramount in patients with vascular injury, as is a ligamentous knee exam and/or reconstruction after bony stabilization. Open injuries are commonly located on the tibial side due to its poor soft tissue coverage, and its severity is a prognostic factor in the outcome of floating knee injuries.

The most accepted treatment for floating knee injuries are retrograde intramedullary nailing of the femoral shaft and intramedullary nailing of the tibial shaft through the same approach.[74] This is performed during a single surgery with the patient supine on a radiolucent OR table. Both intramedullary nailings can be performed through patellar splitting or medial parapatellar approaches with the femur being addressed first. This is due to the more serious implication of the femur fracture with regard to the overall patient physiology, the ease of transport without the need for traction, the ability to gain better knee flexion for access to the tibial starting point and greater control of the lower extremity during management of the associated soft tissue defect.

Associated Femoral Neck Fractures

Femoral neck fractures can occur in up to 10% of femoral shaft fractures and they are missed up to 50% of the time. Because of the prognostic implications of femoral neck fracture of osteonecrosis and nonunion, they should ideally be recognized and managed early. As discussed previously, a protocol has been described that significantly improves the ability to diagnose these early. This includes a dedicated AP internal rotation views of the involved hip providing a profile view of the neck, a fine cut CT scan of the femoral neck as part of the initial abdominal pelvic CT scan, intraoperative fluoroscopy of the hip and immediate postoperative films.[13]

The majority of femoral neck fractures associated with shaft injuries are unstable, vertically oriented and located at the base or the mid portion of the neck (Fig. 22.21). These injuries should be managed first with a dynamic hip screw type implant and derotational screw proximally—with open reduction of the neck if necessary, with subsequent retrograde nailing of the shaft component.[75] Antegrade intramedullary nailing of these injuries is dangerous because it can cause displacement of the neck component, especially with piriformis entry nails.

Vascular Injury

Vascular injuries associated with femur fractures are rare and are usually associated with penetrating injury. The hallmark of treatment of these injuries is initial stabilization of the bone injury to establish proper length and rotation, then vascular repair. Stabilization can be accomplished either through placement of a temporary external fixator, rapid intramedullary nailing or sequential treatment with a vascular shunt, bony stabilization and then definitive vascular repair.[76]

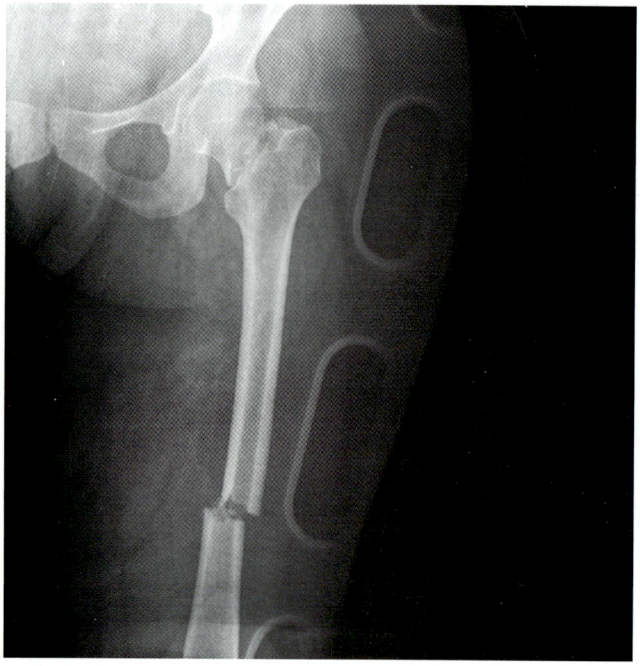

Figure 22.21: Initial radiograph of a left femoral shaft fracture sustained during a high-energy motor vehicle collision with an ipsilateral, vertically-oriented femoral neck fracture.

Complications

Nonunion

The diagnosis of a femoral nonunion is dependent on three criteria. The first is time. Femoral shaft fractures should heal within 3 months. A nonunion should be suspected when there is no evidence of union by 9 months. Second, serial radiographs show continued presence of fracture lines, no callus maturation, absence of bridging callus and no serial progression of healing. Clinically, the patient continues to have pain at above or below the fracture with disturbances in gait and function, with pain and tenderness on palpation and manipulation of the fracture site.

Nonunions of the femur can be classified as hypertrophic or atrophic. Hypertrophic nonunions demonstrate exuberant callus formation radiographically with a typical "elephant's foot" appearance without progression to healing. These usually occur in the presence of good vascularity with an adequate healing response but inadequate stability. Atrophic nonunions do not have an adequate healing response and therefore they radiographically demonstrate no evidence of callus formation with osteopenic bone and sclerosis at persistent fracture lines.

Diagnosis of a nonunion includes a thorough history and physical exam with evaluation of the extremity, associated wounds and drainage as well its neurovascular status. Careful attention should be paid to the possibility of metabolic or endocrine issues with the patient. Adequate radiographs and/or a CT scan should be carefully examined to determine the type of nonunion, its pattern and its extent. It is imperative that infection be ruled out as the cause of the nonunion. Workup should include complete blood count (CBC) with differential, sedimentation rate and quantitative C-reactive protein with a radionuclide leukocyte scan if the diagnosis of infection is equivocal.

Management of femoral nonunions can be discussed in increasing order of complexity. First, in the cases of femoral nonunions associated with distraction, nail dynamization may be performed, and by allowing early weight bearing, the compressive forces across the fracture site promote bony healing. This has met with a moderate success of about 50% rate of union.[77] Complications include shortening and loss of rotational control of the fracture.

Closed, exchange nailing of hypertrophic femoral nonunions has a reported success rate of 86%.[78] The process of removing the old nail, reaming and inserting a larger implant provides biology with the reamings that can locally act as bone graft, and stability with a more stable implant. An increase of at least 2 mm in nail diameter has had a positive correlation with union rate after nonunion.[78] In the case of atrophic nonunions, exchange nailing should be accompanied with debridement of the fibrous tissue at the nonunion site and bone grafting with a bone substitute, autograft harvested through the RIA system, and/or a combination of both.[79] Recalcitrant femoral nonunions, as well as those more metaphyseal in nature, can be treated with open debridement, plate fixation and autogenous bone grafting.[80]

Malunion

Malalignment in the treatment of femur fractures can be discussed in two separate aspects. One is angular malalignment and the other is rotational malalignment. Angular malalignment is mostly associated to nonisthmal proximal (30%) and distal (10%) shaft fractures with a wide canal where there is no less contact between cortical bone and the nail. This can be avoided intraoperatively with proper reduction and alignment of the fragments during the process of reaming, as well as the use of blocking screws on the concave side of the short deformity. The use of antegrade nails in proximal shaft fractures and retrograde nails in distal shaft fractures has also been associated with a decrease in the incidence of angular malalignment.[81]

Rotational malalignment of 15° can occur in approximately 28% of patients with femur fractures, and malalignment of 10° or less can occur in up to half of patients when compared to the contralateral extremity. Deformities of external rotation have the most serious implications on patient function.[82]

There are several ways to establish proper rotation intraoperatively. First, the proper alignment of the anterior superior iliac spine with the patella and the second metatarsal should be evaluated. Fluoroscopically, a proper AP view of the hip, with enough visualization of the lesser trochanter should be in concordance with an AP view of the knee where the patella is central on the condyles of the femur. Intraoperatively, there should be good fit among the fracture fragments and proper congruency of the cortical widths. Finally, after the procedure is over, a clinical assessment rotation should take place, and any differences can be corrected by redraping, removing a locking screw, changing the reduction to proper rotation and reinserting a new locking screw. A chronic rotational malunion should have a CT performed in order to determine the degree of malrotation and provide a preoperative plan.

Leg Length Discrepancy

Leg length discrepancy can also be a significant complication of intramedullary nailing of femoral shaft fractures.[83] However, the degree of leg length discrepancy that can cause clinically relevant problems remains controversial. It has been shown that discrepancies as small as 5 mm can be associated with hip and back pain. Increasing the amount of leg length discrepancy can lead to changes in gait energy expenditure, hip and knee degeneration, equinus contracture of the short leg and compensatory scoliosis.[84]

Prevention of leg length discrepancy in femur fractures starts with a preoperative radiographic examination of the nonfractured femur in order to determine proper length, especially in more comminuted fractures—Winquist III and higher. Intraoperatively, a modified scanogram can be performed with the use of a sterile electrocautery cord. Immediately postoperatively, leg length should be assessed along with potential malalignment. Measurement can performed from the anterior superior iliac spine to the medial malleolus and any correction can be undertaken while still in the OR. Late presentation of leg length discrepancy after intramedullary nailing of femur fractures can be evaluated through clinical examination, a block test, a scanogram or a CT scanogram.[85] Treatment should include shoe lifts or surgical lengthening if the discrepancy is more than 2 cm. Surgical lengthening is best achieved with removal of the distal locking screw, transport over a rail type external fixator and relocking once the proper length is achieved.

Infection

Infection after intramedullary nailing of femoral shaft fractures has been reported as high as 4–5%, with open fractures and the degree of openness significantly associated with the development of deep infection and subsequent nonunion.[67] Acute infections within the early postoperative period can be treated with irrigation and debridement, nail retention and organism specific antibiotics with or without oral antibiotic suppression to healing and eventual hardware removal of hardware in more recalcitrant cases.

In cases of chronic infection, the recommended treatment includes nail removal, thorough irrigation and debridement of the canal and removal of any nonviable bone. More recently, the effectiveness of the RIA has been reported as an important tool in the debridement of the intramedullary canal.[86] The placement of an antibiotic coated cement nail within the canal offers some mechanical stability and at the same time delivers local concentrations of antibiotic to treat the infection.[87] Treatment should also involve at least 6 weeks of culture specific intravenous antibiotics with weekly CBC and differentials, sedimentation rate and quantitative C-reactive protein to monitor response. Once treatment is complete, the antibiotic nail should be removed and/or exchanged.

Heterotopic Ossification

The incidence of heterotopic ossification after intramedullary nailing of femoral shaft fractures has been reported to be as high as 55–68%. It usually occurs within the abductor musculature after antegrade nailing. Risk factors include prolonged intubation, CT evidence of brain injury, male gender and long delay for surgery. From a technique standpoint, the dissection of abductors should be as sharp as possible, a soft tissue protector should always be used and any leftover reamings within the abductor musculature should be irrigated out. Excision of the heterotopic bone should be considered when there is significant pain and/or loss of hip range of motion.[88]

Traction Related

Pudendal nerve palsy is a common complication due to pressure against the perineal post. Higher traction forces induced by hip adduction and fracture reduction maneuvers are associated with the risk of nerve injury.[89] Rate of erectile dysfunction in young males up to 40.5% after femoral fracture fixation on a fracture table has been reported although symptoms of numbness and dysfunction are typically self-limited and usually resolve over time. Appropriate muscle relaxation intraoperatively may help minimize this issue.[90,91] Occlusion of a low-flow artery by the perineal post requiring a revascularization procedure has been described.

Authors' Preferred Management of Select Complications

Case 1: Femur Nonunion

This is the case of a 23-year-old male involved in a motor cycle collision, 1 year prior to evaluation. In the accident, he sustained an isolated left femur fracture that was treated with a size 9 mm diameter retrograde nail. Upon initial evaluation, the patient complained of persistent left thigh and left knee pain 1 year post injury. The patient had been placed on an ultrasound bone stimulator at 6 months post injury.

Anteroposterior and lateral radiographs of the involved area demonstrated an atrophic nonunion of the fracture (Figs 22.22A and B). Infection workup, including sedimentation rate, quantitative C-reactive protein and CBC with differential were all negative.

After consent from the patient, he was taken to the OR, for exchange nailing with open debridement of the fracture site, and reaming with the RIA system. The

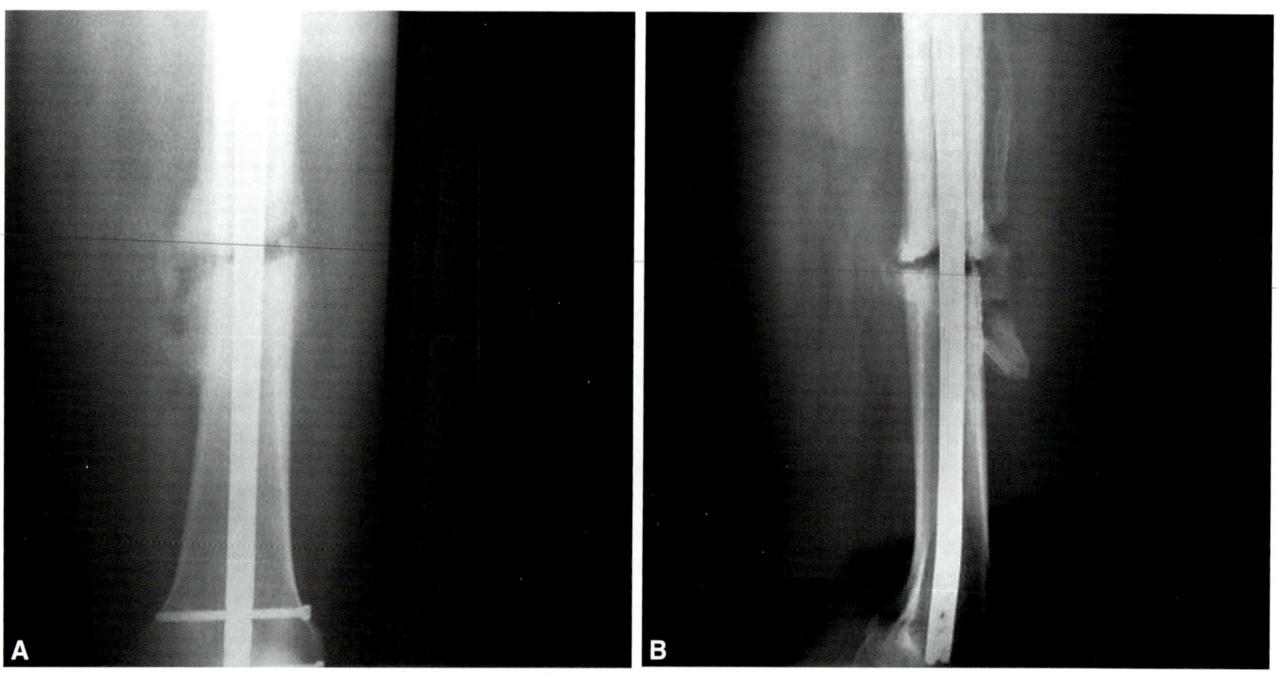

Figures 22.22A and B: Anteroposterior and lateral radiographs of an atrophic femoral nonunion 1 year post injury.

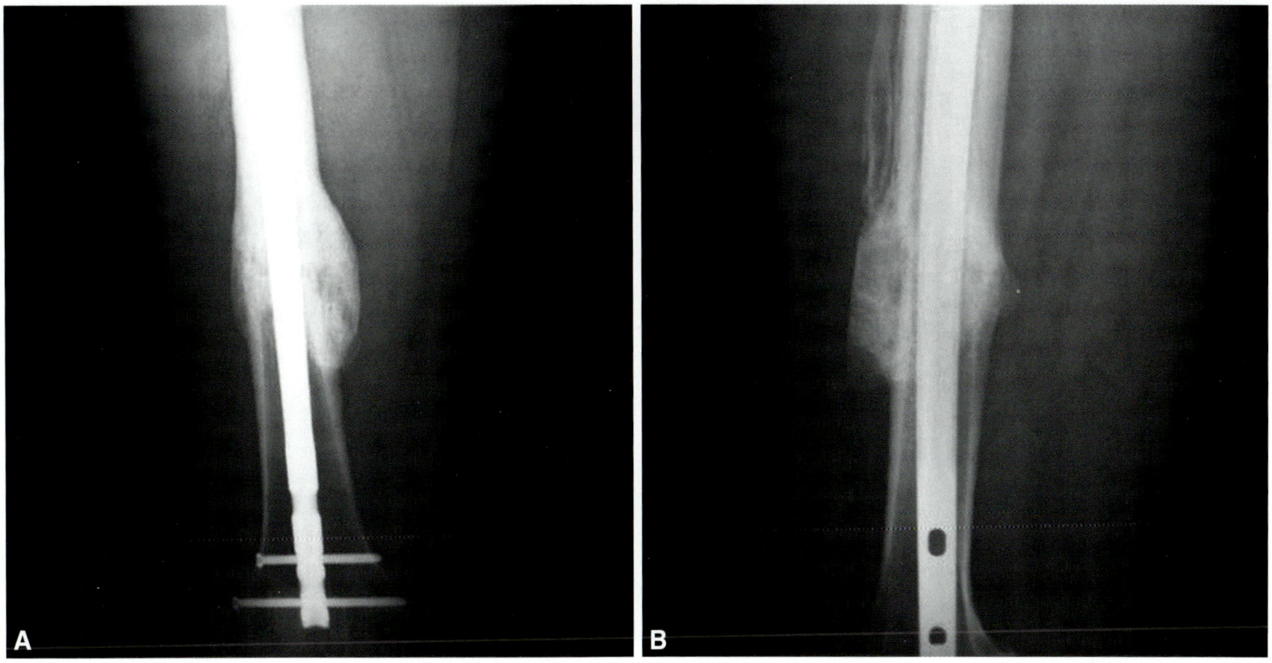

Figures 22.23A and B: Anteroposterior and lateral radiographs of the same femoral nonunion 1 year after exchange nailing with take down of the nonunion and bone grafting utilizing the Reamer Irrigator Aspirator system.

harvested bone graft was then placed around the debrided nonunion and a size 11 mm retrograde nail was placed. One year post injury, the fracture demonstrated signs of union and he remained pain free (Figs 22.23A and B).

Case 2: Femur Fracture Infection

This is the case of a 47-year-old female involved in a motor vehicle collision in Colombia 15 years ago, sustaining a right open femur fracture. The fracture was originally treated with multiple debridement procedures and eventual plating. The fracture progressed to nonunion and was revised to an intramedullary nail after debridement of the nonunion. Patient presented to our clinic with a chief complaint of persistent pain of the lateral thigh associated with a draining sinus.

Initial workup included AP and lateral radiographs of the femur (Fig. 22.24), sedimentation rate and quantitative C-reactive protein. A CT of the affected limb revealed a sequestrum associated with a posterior defect of bone at the level of the broken drill bit (Fig. 22.25). After informed

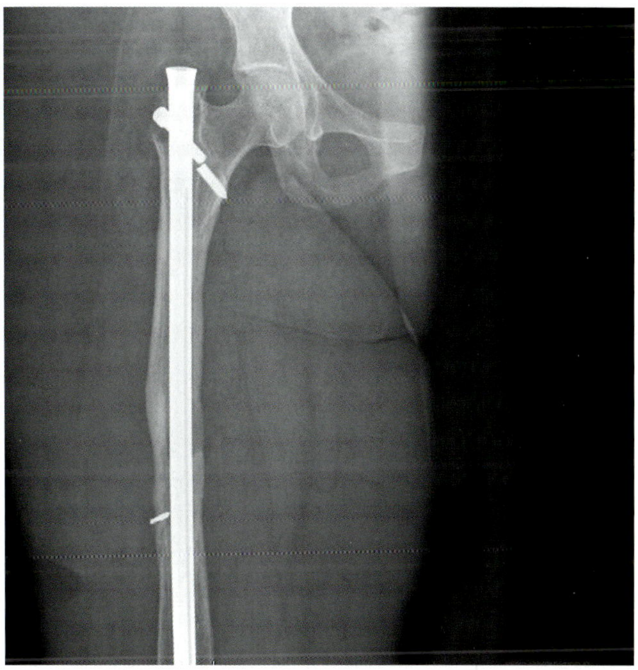

Figure 22.24: Anteroposterior radiograph of a chronically infected femoral fracture. Note the soft tissue silhouette of the draining sinus laterally.

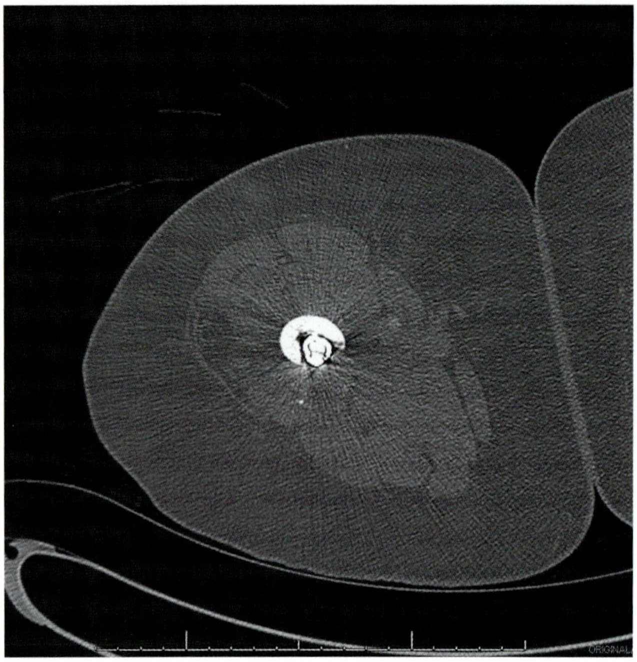

Figure 22.25: Preoperative computed tomography of an infected femoral nail. Note the missing posterior aspect of bone that is in direct communication with the infected nail.

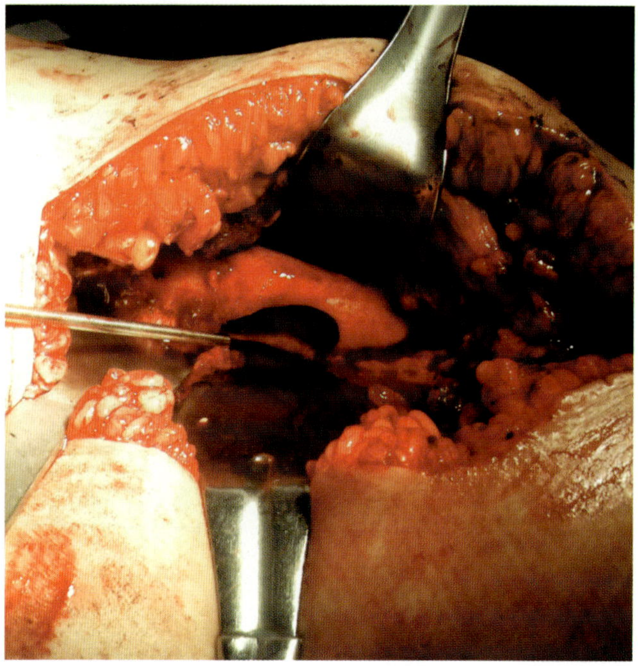

Figure 22.26: Intraoperative radiograph of the debrided sequestrum.

consent, the patient was taken to the OR for exploration and removal of the draining sinus, removal of the nail, over-reaming and irrigation with the RIA system, with placement of an antibiotic nail. The posterior defect in the bone involved approximately one third of diaphyseal diameter (Figs 22.26 and 22.27). A small flat disk of antibiotic cement was placed over the defect to create pseudoperiosteum with osteogenic potential.

The patient completed 6 weeks of culture specific intravenous antibiotics and after normalization of sedimentation rate and C-reactive protein. The antibiotic nail was removed at 8 weeks and the canal was again reamed. A standard piriformis intramedullary rod was then placed for stabilization of concern for the weakened bone and the large area of bony defect posteriorly.

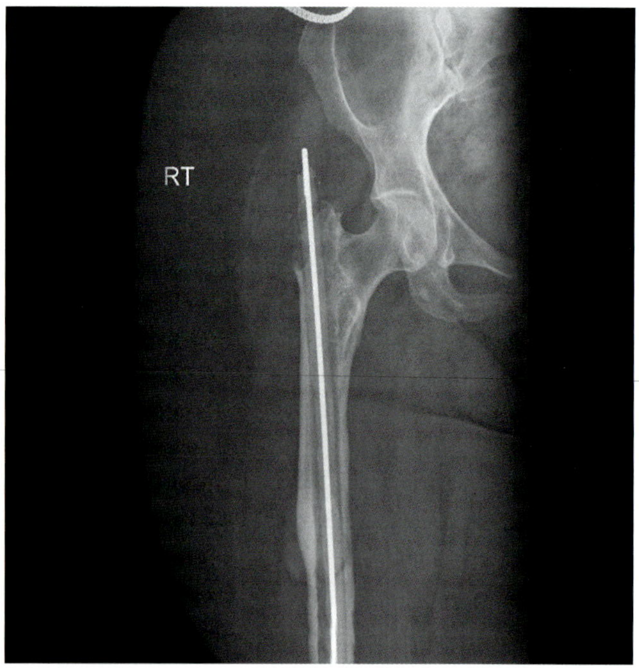

Figure 22.27: Postoperative radiograph of the antibiotic coated cement nail.

Summary

In just over 70 years, intramedullary nailing has become the gold standard of treatment for diaphyseal femoral fractures. It is associated with good functional outcomes, high rate of healing and low rate of complications. These are mostly associated to high-energy trauma in the young and low-energy trauma in the elderly. The technical considerations and principles of surgery apply for both populations. The decision for the type of nail, the positioning of the patient, entry point of the nail, it's locking and the postoperative management is dependent on multiple variables. Ultimately, these decisions should be individualized to the patient. They should be based on the type of patient and their physiology. These decisions should also be based on surgeon expertise and level of comfort. Technically, the two most important aspects of surgery are entry point and reduction. A misplaced entry point can not only make the rest of the procedure a serious challenge but also cause severe damage to the patient. As far as reduction, it is imperative that the reduction be maintained during the reaming process, especially in nonisthmal, metaphyseal fractures. A fracture that is malreduced during reaming will end up malreduced after nail placement. The nail is not a reduction tool.

References

1. Hippocrates. On Fractures, Part 19, Mobile Reference, 2009.
2. Peltier LF. Percival Pott and Pott's Fracture. Surgery. 1962; 51:280-6.
3. Percival Pott. Some Few General Remarks on Fractures and Dislocations, 2nd edition. London; 1773.
4. Malgaigne JF. Recherches historiques et practiques sur les appareils employes dans le traitement des fractures en general depuis hippocrate jusqu'a nos jours. Paris: H. Cousin. 1841.
5. Peltier LF. A brief history of traction. J Bone Joint Surg Am. 1968;50:1603-17.
6. Henry BJ, Vrahas MS. The Thomas splint. Questionable boast of an indispensable tool. Am J Orthop. 1996;25(9): 602-4.
7. Robinson PM, O'Meara MJ. The Thomas splint: its origins and use in trauma. J Bone Joint Surg Br. 2009;91;540-3.
8. Fischer. Gerhard Kuntscher 1900-1972. J Bone Joint Surg Am. 1974;56:208-9.
9. Bong MR, Koval KJ, Egol KA. The history of intramedullary nailing. Bull NYU Hosp Jt Dis. 2006;64(3-4):94-7.
10. Kuntscher G. Intramedullar Surgical Technique and Its Place in Ortthopaedic Surgery: My Present Concept. J Bone Joint Surg Am. 1965;47:808-18.
11. Cross AT. Gerhard Kuntscher: A Surgical Giant. AO Dialogue Volume 15, Issue 11. December. 2001.
12. Salminen ST, Pihlajamäki HK, Avikainen VJ, et al. Population based epidemiologic and morphologic study of femoral shaft fractures. Clin Orthop Relat Res. 2000;372:241-9.
13. Arneson TJ, Melton LJ 3rd, Lewallen DG, et al. Epidemiology of diaphyseal and distal femoral fractures in Rochester, Minnesota, 1965-1984. Clin Orthop Relat Res. 1988; 9234):188-94.
14. Lieurance R, Benjamin JB, Rappaport WD. Blood loss and transfusion in patients with isolated femur fractures. J Orthop Trauma. 1992;6(2):175-9.
15. Tornetta P 3rd, Kain MS, Creevy WR. Diagnosis of a femoral neck fracture in patients with a femoral shaft fracture. Improvement with a standard protocol. J Bone Joint Surg Am. 2007;89:39-43.
16. Winquist RA, Hansen ST, Clawson DK. Closed intramedullary nailing of femoral fractures. A report on five hundred and twenty cases. J Bone Joint Surg Am. 1984;66:529-39.
17. El-Sayed Khalil A. Locked plating for femoral fractures in polio patients. Arch Orthop Trauma Surg. 2010;130:1299-1304.
18. Loomer RL, Meek R, De Sommer F. Plating of femoral shaft fractures: the Vancouver experience. J Trauma. 1980;20(12): 1038-42.
19. Apivatthakakul T, Chiewcharntanakit S. Minimally invasive plate osteosynthesis in the treatment of the femoral shaft fracture where intramedullary nailing is not indicated. Int Orthop. 2009;33:1119-26.
20. Angelini AJ, Livani B, Flierl MA, et al. Less invasive percutaneous wave plating of simple femur shaft fractures: a prospective series. Injury. 2010;41:624-8.
21. Zlowodzki M, Vogt D, Cole PA, et al. Plating of femoral shaft fractures: open reduction and internal fixation versus submuscular fixation. J Trauma. 2007;63:1061-5.
22. Abdel-Aa MA, Farouk OA, Elsayed A, et al. The use of a locked plate in the treatment of ununited femoral shaft fractures. J Trauma. 2004;57:832-6
23. Dugdale TW, Schutzer SF, Deafenbaugh MK, et al. Compartment syndrome complicating use of the hemi-lithotomy position during femoral nailing. A report of two cases. J Bone Joint Surg Am. 1989;71(10):1556-7.
24. Tait GR, Danton M. Contralateral sciatic nerve palsy following femoral nailing. J Bone Joint Surg Br. 1991; 73(4):689-90.
25. Apostle KL, Lefaivre KA, Guy P, et al. The effects of intraoperative positioning on patients undergoing early definitive care for femoral shaft fractures. J Orthop Trauma. 2009;23(9):615-20.
26. Ozsoy MH, Basarir K, Byramoglu A, et al. Risk of superior gluteal nerve and gluteus medius muscle injury during femoral nail insertion. J Bone and Joint Surg Am. 2007; 89(4):829-34.
27. Wolinsky PR, McCarty EC, Shyr Y, et al. Length of operative procedures: reamed femoral intramedullary nailing performed with and without a fracture table. J Orthop Trauma. 1998;12(7):485-95.

28. Stephen DJ, Kreder HJ, Schemitsch EH, et al. Femoral intramedullary nailing: comparison of fracture-table and manual traction. A prospective, randomized study. J Bone Joint Surg Am. 2002;84-A(9):1514-21.
29. Bishop JA, Rodriguez EK. Closed intramedullary nailing of the femur in the lateral decubitus position. J Trauma. 2010;68(1):231-5.
30. Starr A, Hay M, Reinert CM, et al. Cephallomedullary nails in the treatment of high-energy proximal femur fractures in young patients: a prospective, randomized comparison of trochanteric versus piriformis fossa entry portal. J Ortho Trauma. 2006;20(4):240-6.
31. Khan FA, Ikram MA, Badr AA, et al. Femoral neck fracture: a complication of femoral nailing. Injury. 1995;26:319-21.
32. Dora C, Leunig M, Beck M, et al. Entry point soft tissue damage in antegrade femoral nailing: a cadaver study. J Orthop Trauma. 2001;15:488-93.
33. Mileski RA, Garvin KL, Crosby LA. Avascular Necrosis of the femoral head in an adolescent following intramedullary nailing of the femur. A case report. J Bone Joint Surg Am. 1994;76:1706-8.
34. Moein CA, Duis H, Oey L, et al. Functional outcome after antegrade femoral nailing: a comparison of trochanteric fossa versus tip of greater trochanter entry point. J Orthop Trauma. 2011;24(4):196-201
35. Ricci WM, Schwappach J, Tucker M, et al. Trochanteric verus piriformis entry portal for the treatment of femoral shaft fractures. J Orthop Trauma. 2006;20:663-7.
36. Streubel P, Wong AHW, Ricci W, et al. Is there a standard trochanteric entry site for nailing of subtrochanteric femur fractures? J Orthop Trauma. 2011;25(4):202-7.
37. Ostrum RF, Marcantonio A, Marburger R. A critical analysis of the eccentric starting point for trochanteric intra-medullary femoral nailing. J Orthop Trauma. 2005;19(10):681-6.
38. Bain GI, Zacest AC, Paterson DC, et al. Abduction strength following intramedullary nailing of the femur. J Orthop Trauma. 1997;11(2):93-7.
39. Archdeacon M, Ford KR, Wyrick J, et al. A prospective functional outcome and motion analysis evaluation of the hip abductors after femur fracture antegrade nailing. J Orthop Trauma. 2008;22(1):3-9.
40. Gardner M, Robertson WJ, Boraiah S, et al. Anatomy of the greater trochanteric 'bald spot': a potential portal for abductor sparing femoral nailing? Clin Orthop Relat Res. 2008;466:2196-2200.
41. Linke B, Moein CA, Bosl O, et al. Lateral insertion points in antegrade femoral nailing and their influence on femoral bone strains. J Orthop Trauma. 2008:22(10):716-22.
42. Prasarn ML, Cattaneo MD, Achor T, et al. The effect of entry point on malalignment and iatrogenic fracture with the Synthes lateral entry femoral nail. J Orthop Trauma. 2010;24(4):224-9.
43. Pape HC, Tarkin IS. Intraoperative reduction techniques for difficult femoral fractures. J Orthop Trauma. 2009;23(Suppl 5):S6-11.
44. Moed BR, Watson JT. Retrograde nailing of the femoral shaft. J Am Acad Orthop Surg. 1999;7(4):209-16.
45. Handolin L, Pjarinen J, Lindahl J, et al. Retrograde intra-medullary nailing in distal femoral fractures: results in a series of 46 conseceutive operations. Injury. 2003;35:517-22.
46. Ostrum RF, Maurer JP. Distal third femur fractures treated with retrograde femoral nailing and blocking screws. J Orthop Trauma. 2009;23(9):681-4.
47. Brown GA, Firoozbaksh K, Summa CD. Potential of increased risk of neurovascular injury using proximal interlocking screws of retrograde femoral nails in patients with acetabular fractures. J Orthop Trauma. 2001;15(6):433-7.
48. Shuler FD, Busam M, Beimesch CF, et al. Retrograde femoral nailing: computed tomography angiogram demonstrates no relative safe zone for prevention of small diameter arterial vascular injury during proximal anteroposterior interlocking. J Trauma. 2010;69(5):E42-5
49. Forster MC, Aster AS, Ahmed S. Reaming during antero-grade femoral nailing: is it worth it? Injury. 2005; 36:445-9.
50. Chapman MW. The effect of reamed and nonreamed intramedullary nailing on fracture healing. Clin Orthop Relat Res. 1998;355:S230-8.
51. Muller C, Mciff T, Rahn BA, et al. Intramedullary pressure, strain on the diaphysis, and increase in cortical temperature when reaming the femoral medullary cavity: a comparison of blunt and sharp reamers. Injury. 1993;24:S22-30.
52. Bong MR, Kummer FJ, Koval KJ, et al. Intramedullary nailing of the lower extremity: biomechanics and biology. J Am Acad Orthop Surg. 2007;15(2):97-106.
53. Steubel PN, Desai P, Suk M. Comparison of RIA and conventional reamed nailing for treatment of femur shaft fractures. Injury. 2010;41(S2):S51-6.
54. Giannoudis PV, Tan HB, Tzioupis C, et al. The systemic inflammatory response following femoral canal reaming using the reamer-irrigator-aspirator device. Injury. 2010; 41(S2):S57-61.
55. Hartsock LA, Barfield WR, Kokko KP, et al. Randomized prospective clinical trial comparing reamer irrigator aspirator to standard reaming in both minimally injured and multiply injured patients with closed femoral shaft fractures treated with reamed intramedullary nailing. Injury. 2010;41(S2):S94-8.
56. Rudloff MI, Smith WR. Intramedullary nailing of the femur: current concepts concerning reaming. J Orthop Trauma. 2009;(23)5:S12-7.

57. Hogel F, Gerlach UV, Sudkamp NP, et al. Pulmonary fat embolism after reamed and undreamed nailing of femoral fractures. Injury. 2010;(41):1317-22.

58. Bosse MJ, Mackenzie EJ, Riemer BL, et al. Adult respiratory distress syndrome, pneumonia, and mortality following thoracic injury and a femoral fracture treated with with intramedullary nailing with reaming or with a plate. A comparative study. J Bone Joint Surg Am. 1997;79A(6):799-809.

59. Canadian Orthopaedic Trauma Society. Reamed versus undreamed nailing of the femur: comparison of the rate of ARDS in multiple injured patients. J Orthop Trauma. 2006;20(6):384-7.

60. Anwar IA, Battistella FD, Neiman R, et al. Femur fractures and lung complications. Clin Orthop Relat Res. 2004;422: 71-6.

61. Wolinsky, P, Tejwani, N, Richmond, JH, et al. Controversies in intramedullary nailing of femoral shaft fractures. Instr Course Lect. 2002;51:291-303.

62. Ostrum RF, Agarwal A, Lakatos R, et al. Prospective comparison of retrograde and antegrade femoral intramedullary nailing. J Orthop Trauma. 2000;14(7):496-501.

63. Papadokostakis G, Papakostidis C, Dimitriou R, et al. The role and efficacy of retrograding nailing for the treatment of diaphyseal and distal femoral fractures: a systematic review of the literature. Injury. 2005;36:813-22.

64. Ricci WM, Bellabarba C, Evanoff B, et al. Retrograde versus antegrade nailing of femoral shaft fractures. J Orthop Trauma. 2001;15(3):161-9.

65. Daglar B, Gungor E, Delialioglu O. Comparison of knee function after antegrade and retrograde intramedullary nailing for diaphyseal femoral fractures: results of isokinetic evaluation. J Orthop Trauma. 2009;23(9):640-4.

66. O'Toole RV, Riche K, Cannada LK, et al. Analysis of postoperative knee sepsis after retrograde nail insertion of open femoral shaft fractures. J Orthop Trauma. 2010; 24(11): 677-82.

67. Noumi T, Yokoyama K, Ohtsuka H, et al. Intramedullary nailing of open fractures of the femoral shaft: Evaluation of contributing factors on deep infection and nonunion using multivariate analysis. Injury. 2005;36(9):1085-93.

68. Bartlett CS, Helfet DL, Hausmann MR, et al. Ballistics and Gunshot Wounds: Effects on Musculoskeletal Tissues. J Am Acad Orthop Surg. 2000;8(1):21-36.

69. Cooper GJ, Ryan JM. Interaction of penetrating missiles with tissues: Some common misapprehensions and implications for wound management. Br J Surg. 1990;77:606-10.

70. Roberts CS, Pape HC, Jones AL, et al. Damage Control Orthopaedics: Evolving concepts in the treatment of patients who have sustained orthopaedic trauma. Instr Course Lect. 2005;54:447-62.

71. Pape HC, Tornetta P, Tarkin I, et al. Timing of fracture fixation in multitrauma patients: the role of early total care and damage control surgery. J Am Acad Orthop Surg. 2009; 17(9):541-9.

72. Nowotarski PJ, Turen CH, Brumback RJ, et al. Conversion of external fixation to intramedullary nailing for fractures of the shaft of the femur in multiply injured patients. J Bone Joint Surg. 2000;82A(6):781-8.

73. Higgins TF, Horwitz DS. Damage control nailing. J Orthop Trauma. 2007;21(7):477-83.

74. Ostrum RF. Treatment of floating knee injuries through a single percutaneous approach. Clin Orthop Relat Res. 2000; 375:43-50.

75. Watson JT, Moed BR. Ipsilateral femoral neck and shaft fractures: complications and their treatment. Clin Orthop Rel Res. 2002;399:78-86.

76. McHenry TP, Holcomb JB, Aoki N, et al. Fractures with major vascular injuries from gunshot wounds: Implications and surgical sequence. J Trauma. 2002;53(4):717-21.

77. Wu CC. The effect of dynamization on slowing the healing of femur shaft fractures after interlocking nail. J Trauma. 1997;43:263-7.

78. Shroeder JE, Mosheiff R, Khoury A, et al. The outcome of closed, intramedullary exhange nailing with reamed insertion in the treatment of femoral shaft nonunions. J Orthop Trauma. 2009;23(9):653-7.

79. Giannoudis PV, Tzioupis C, Green J. Surgical techniques: how do I do it? The Reamer/Irrigator/Aspirator (RIA) System. Injury. 2009;40:1231-6.

80. Bellarba C, Ricci WM, Bolhofner BR. Results of indirect reduction and plating of femoral shaft nonunions after intramedullary nailing. J Orthop Trauma. 2001;15:254-63.

81. Ricci WM, Bellarba C, Lewis R. Angular malalignment after intramedullary nailing of femoral shaft fractures. J Orthop Trauma. 2001;15:90-5.

82. Jaarsma RL, Pakvis DF, Verdonschot N, et al. Rotational malalignment after intramedullary nailing of femoral shaft fractures. J Orthop Trauma. 2004;18(7):403-9.

83. Reina R, Vilella FE, Ramirez N, et al. Knee pain and leg length discrepancy after retrograde femoral nailing. Am J Orthop (Belle Mead NJ). 2007;36:325-6.

84. Karapinar L, Kaya A, Ozturk H, et al. Leg length discrepancies in adult femoral shaft fractures treated with intramedullary nailing. Ulus Travma Acil Cerrahi Derg. 2009;15(3)256-61.

85. Harris I, Hatfield A, Walton J. Assessing leg length discrepancy after femoral fracture: Clinical examination or computerized tomography? ANZ J. Surg. 2005;75: 319-21.
86. Zalavras CG, Sirkin M. Treatment of long bone intramedullary infection using the RIA for removal of infected tissue: indications, method and clinical results. Injury. 2010;41: S43-7.
87. Thonse R, Conway J. Antibiotic cement coated interlocking nail for the treatment of infected nonunions and segmental bone defects. J Orthop Trauma. 2007;21(4):258-68.
88. Steinberg GG, Hubbard C. Heterotopic ossification after femoral intramedullary rodding. J Orthop Trauma. 1993; 7(6):536-42.
89. Brumback RJ, Ellison TS, Molligan H, et al. Pudendal nerve palsy complicating intramedullary nailing of the femur. J Bone Joint Surg Am. 1992;74(10):1450-5.
90. Mallet R, Tricoire JL, Rischmann P, et al. High prevalence of erectile dysfunction in young male patients after intramedullary femoral nailing. Urology. 2005;65(3):559-63.
91. Kadzielski J, Vrahas M. A vascular complication of trochanteric entry femoral nailing on a fracture table. Am J Orthop. 2010;39(7):E64-6.

Chapter 23

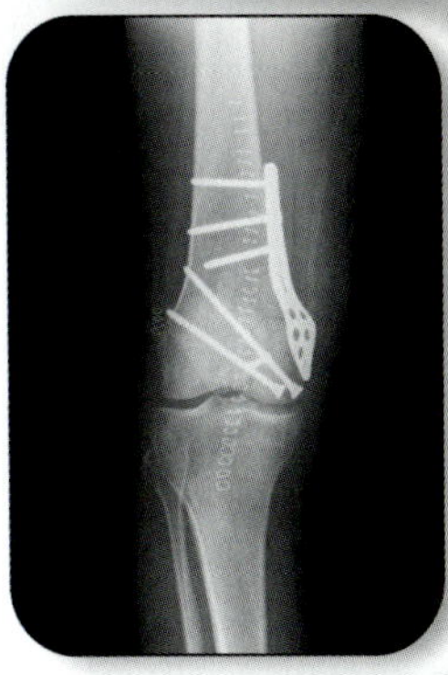

Distal Femur Fractures

Matthew Mellon, William DeLong, Saqib Rehman

Chapter Outline

Introduction
Diagnosis
Classification
Surgical Indications
- Open Reduction and Internal Fixation
- Intramedullary Fixation
- External Fixation
- Acute Knee Arthroplasty

Surgical Anatomy, Positioning and Approaches
- Anatomy
- Positioning
- Approaches

Surgical Techniques
- Technique 1: Minimally Invasive Plate Osteosynthesis Plating of Type A (Extra-articular) Fracture
- Technique 2: Retrograde Intramedullary Nail of Type A Fracture
- Technique 3: ORIF of Type C Fracture
- Technique 4: ORIF of Type B (Unicondylar) Fracture
- Technique 5: ORIF of Type B3 (Hoffa) Fracture

Outcomes
Complications
- Knee Stiffness
- Nonunion
- Malunion

Authors' Preferred Management of Select Complications
- Case 1: Nonunion with Implant Failure
- Case 2: Atrophic Nonunion with a Stable Implant
- Case 3: Chronic Deep Infection and Loss of Extensor Mechanism Treated with Knee Arthrodesis

Summary

Introduction

Distal femur fractures make up about 0.4% of all fractures with an estimated rate of 4.5 fractures per 1,00,000 population per year.[1] They are 10–30 times less common than proximal femur fractures.[1,2] Martinet and coauthors reviewed over 2,100 distal femur fractures and identified a bimodal age distribution of these fractures. The first peak involved patients in the second and third decades; these patients were primarily male with high-energy trauma as the cause of injury. The second peak consisted of osteoporotic injuries with most patients being women in the seventh through ninth decades, who had sustained low-energy trauma.[2]

Prior to 1970, most supracondylar femur fractures were treated nonoperatively with resulting complications of angular deformity, joint incongruity and loss of motion.[3] In more recent decades, most surgeons have favored

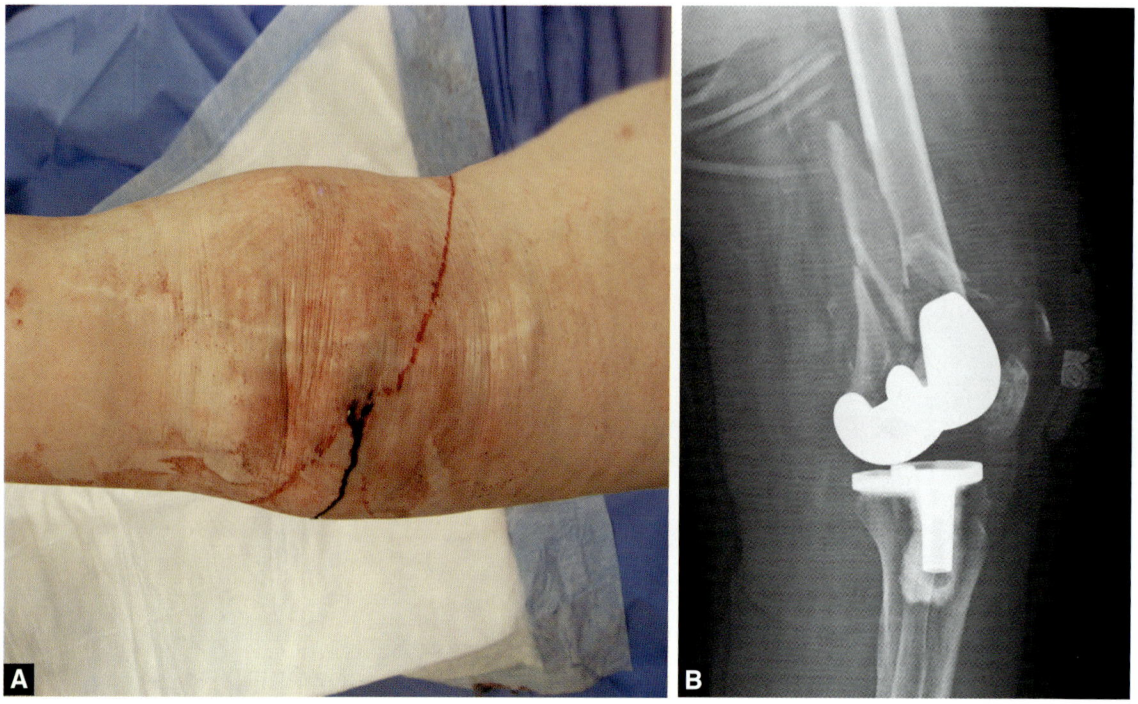

Figures 23.1A and B: Grade 1 open distal femoral fracture. (A) Clinical photograph; (B) X-ray of an open periprosthetic distal femur fracture in an 82-year-old woman after ground level fall. Note the small anterior laceration from distal translation of the proximal segment.

operative fixation of distal femur fractures. Operative treatment has been shown to reduce the risk of poor results as compared to nonoperative treatment in a randomized controlled trial.[4] Fixation of these injuries can be challenging due to fracture comminution, thin cortices and a wide medullary canal. Several factors are important for successful management of these injuries including avoidance of angular or rotational malalignment, stable fixation to allow early motion and avoidance of complications such as nonunion, mechanical malalignment or arthrofibrosis.

Diagnosis

Distal femoral fractures resulting from high-energy trauma are often only one of several injuries sustained by the individual. The entire patient must be evaluated in a multidisciplinary team approach. The orthopedic surgeon should be alert especially for associated injuries including hip dislocation, acetabular fractures and fractures of the hip, femoral diaphysis, patella and tibia.

Evaluation of distal femoral injuries should include evaluation of the soft tissues and neurovascular status. Overlying injuries associated with open fractures are often anterior and distal due to distal translation of the sharp proximal diaphyseal fragment at the time of injury (Figs 23.1A and B). Due to the proximity of the joint capsule, an open fracture may include a traumatic arthrotomy.

Associated ligamentous knee injuries have been reported in 20% of patients.[5] Evaluation of these injuries is difficult on clinical examination, until the fracture has been stabilized. The popliteal artery is in relative proximity to the medial femoral cortex as it exits the adductor hiatus 10 cm above the joint line and is at risk of injury with higher energy or gunshot fractures. While the overall rate of vascular injury has been reported as low as 0.2%,[6] it may rise up to 40% with associated ligamentous injuries (especially posterior dislocation).[5] If concern for a vascular injury exists, an ankle-brachial index should be obtained and patients with values less than 0.9 should proceed to angiography.[7]

Imaging of these injuries should include anteroposterior (AP) and lateral X-rays of the knee and entire femur. If significant shortening is noted, a traction view X-ray can improve characterization of the fracture. Due

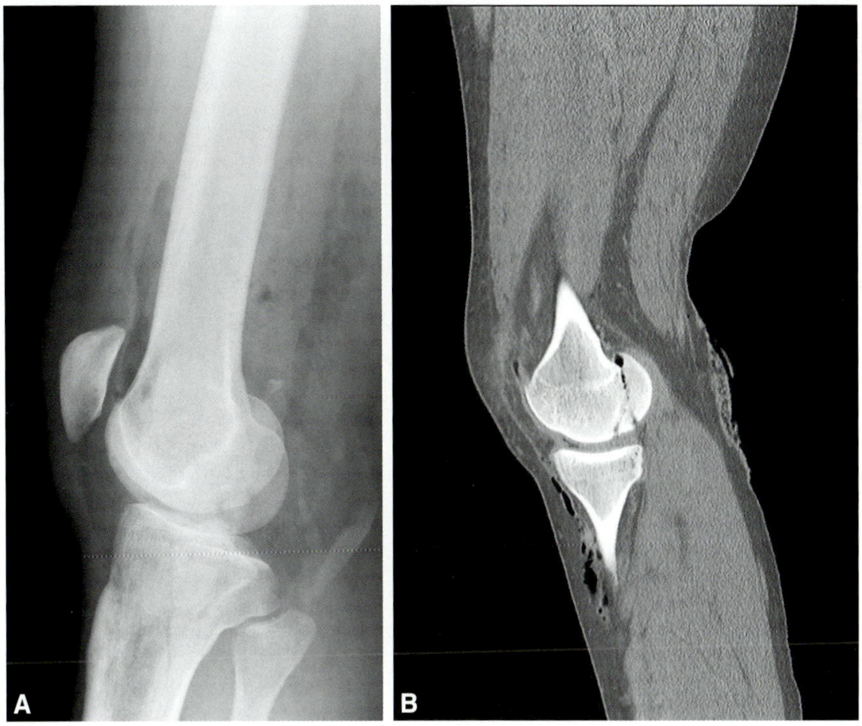

Figures 23.2A and B: Imaging of the distal femoral fracture. (A) Lateral knee X-ray; (B) Sagittal reformatted CT scan showing a B3 type (Hoffa) fracture. These coronal plane fractures are frequently missed on standard radiographs. CT scanning should include axial, coronal and sagittal imaging, and three-dimensional reconstructions can also be helpful.

to the inability of standard radiographs to adequately characterize intra-articular distal femoral fracture patterns and with the increasing availability of advanced imaging modalities, we recommend routine use of computed tomography (CT) if there is any concern for intra-articular involvement. Three-dimensional reconstructions are necessary to avoid missing a coronal plane (Hoffa) fracture (Figs 23.2A and B). Magnetic resonance imaging (MRI) may also be obtained, if there is a suspicion of ligamentous injury requiring repair. This should be ideally obtained preoperatively as metallic implants and postsurgical changes may degrade image quality.

DISTAL FEMUR FRACTURES DIAGNOSIS:
Pearls and Pitfalls

- Open fractures, vascular injury and ligamentous injury are all common with high-energy distal femur fractures and should be rigorously evaluated
- Traction X-rays may improve fracture characterization in the case of significant comminution or shortening
- Computed tomography imaging is useful to visualize intra-articular comminution and evaluate for a coronal plane (Hoffa) fracture
- Consider preoperative MRI if suspicion exists for an associated ligamentous injury

Classification

Classification systems for distal femur fractures typically divide the fractures into extra-articular, unicondylar and bicondylar groups. Neer, Egund and Kolmert, and Seinsheimer have all described classification systems. The most widely used classification system today is the AO/OTA Müeller's classification.[6] This fracture classification is categorized into three main types: (1) Type A (extra-articular), (2) Type B (partial articular), and (3) Type C (complete articular) with subtypes given for further fracture characteristics (Fig. 23.3).[8] A B3 subtype is also known as a Hoffa fracture and the posterior piece is referred to as the Hoffa fragment.

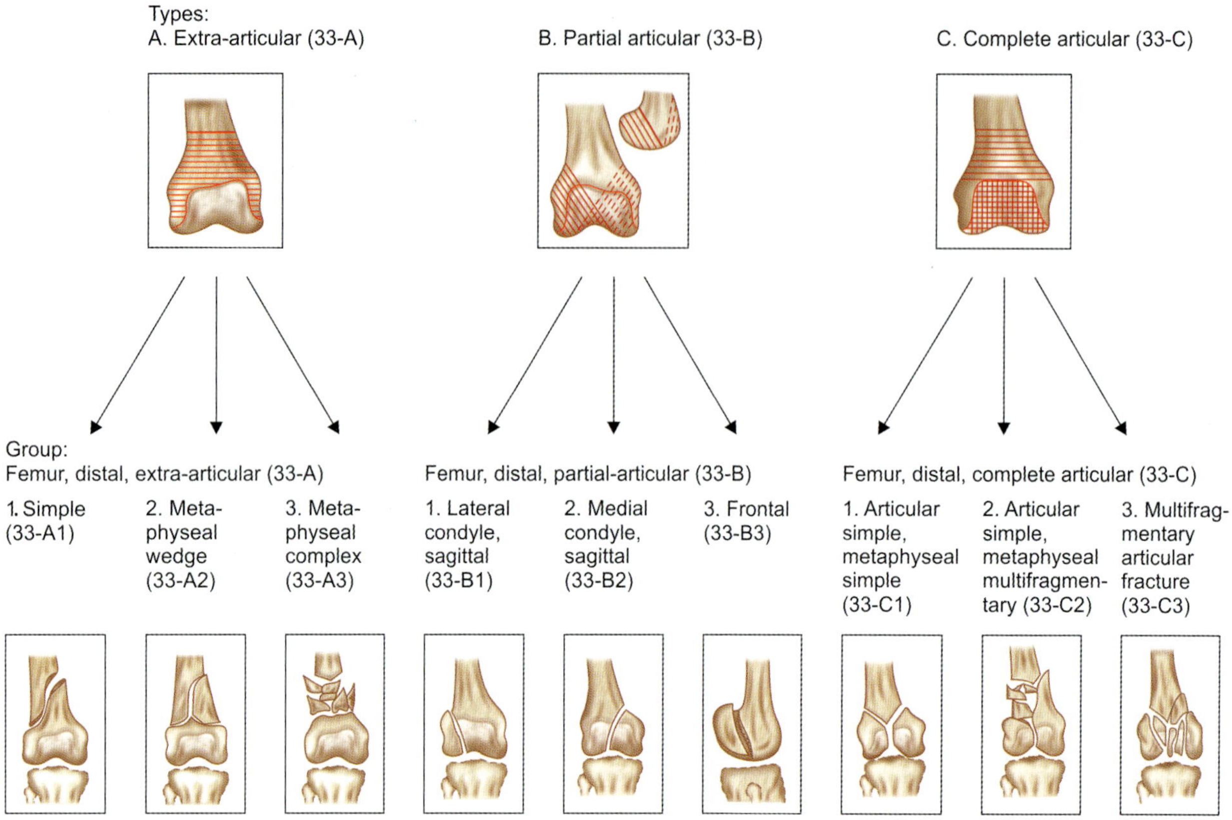

Figure 23.3: AO/OTA fracture classification of distal femur fractures.

Surgical Indications

Fractures of the distal femur are routinely treated operatively. It is rare for fractures of this region to be inherently stable. Due to the multiple deforming forces and a short fracture segment, a reduction of the distal femur is difficult to maintain with casting alone. Traction followed by cast bracing was previously the mainstay of therapy. However, this resulted in complications due to prolonged recumbency, loss of motion and poor articular reduction.[9] Contemporary indications for nonoperative treatment include incomplete fractures, stable, impacted fracture in elderly patients and advanced medical comorbidities.

Operative treatment has been shown to reduce the risk of poor results as compared to nonoperative treatment in a randomized controlled trial.[4]

Indications for operative management include most distal femur fractures, but especially open injuries, injuries with vascular compromise, and injuries with articular involvement. Operative management may include open reduction and internal fixation (ORIF), intramedullary (IM) fixation and external fixation. A review of operative treatment of distal femur fractures did not show any difference between implants in nonunions, infections, fixation failures and revision surgeries. There is evidence that surgeons with increased experience may reduce the rate of revision surgery.[10] Acute knee arthroplasty may be an option for the treatment of highly comminuted distal femur fractures in elderly patients.

Open Reduction and Internal Fixation

Open reduction and internal fixation is the most versatile method of surgical fixation for distal femur fractures. It can be employed to restore anatomical relationships in Type A, B and C fractures including the restoration of articular congruity in Type B and C fractures. Newer implants such as locking condylar plates can act as a fixed angle device, when applied in locking mode and restore appropriate distal femoral valgus, when applied properly.

Intramedullary Fixation

Intramedullary fixation is utilized for spanning diaphyseal and metaphyseal fractures. It can function as a load-sharing device and can often be inserted with smaller incisions and less soft tissue mobilization than with ORIF. It is primarily indicated for Type A fractures, especially A2 and A3 fractures, though the indications may be expanded to include simple articular involvement after limited ORIF. Intramedullary fixation may allow for early weight bearing. As the distal fragment is metaphyseal, there is a limited capacity for the nail to reduce the fracture and care must be taken to avoid an angular malreduction.

External Fixation

Joint-spanning external fixation is occasionally indicated when skeletal stability is required, but other treatments are not indicated. Examples include severe open fractures requiring repeated debridement, severe soft tissue swelling, or to protect a vascular repair. External fixation may also be used to augment internal fixation in the setting of severe comminution or osteoporosis. If motion is desired, a hinged external fixator may be employed.

Acute Knee Arthroplasty

Surgical fixation can be challenging in the setting of osteoporosis and severe comminution. Total knee arthroplasty has been recommended as an option for acute treatment of comminuted distal femur fractures in elderly patients[11] or for the revision of a distal femur nonunion.[12] Arthroplasty in these patients can allow for immediate weight bearing and range of motion as well as the elimination of fracture healing issues. In most cases, the femoral prosthesis must replace the distal fractured bone. This usually results in the loss of collateral ligaments, requiring a hinged prosthesis.

Surgical Anatomy, Positioning and Approaches

Anatomy

Understanding the applied anatomy of the distal femur is critical to successful treatment fractures of the distal femur.

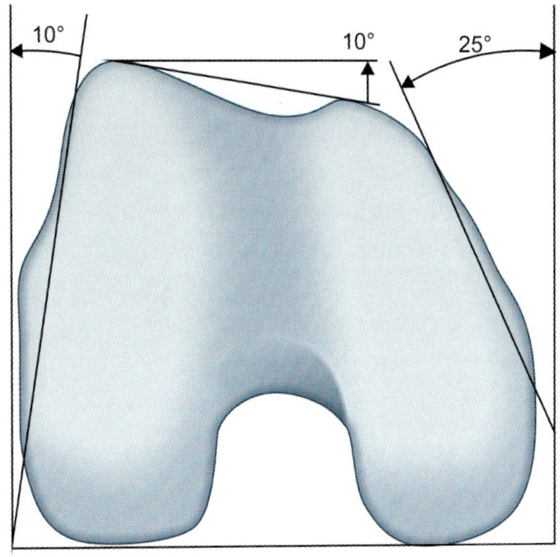

Figure 23.4: Anatomy of the distal femur. Note the trapezoidal shape as viewed distally.

The distal femur is trapezoidal in shape and is narrower anteriorly, when viewed from its distal end. The lateral metaphyseal surface is angulated approximately 10° with respect to the sagittal plane, while the medial metaphyseal surface is angulated approximately 25° (Fig. 23.4). When viewed from the lateral side, the medullary canal is in line with the anterior half of the medial and lateral condyles. The medial femoral condyle is larger and projects further distally than the lateral femoral condyle. This produces the normal 9° of anatomic valgus of the distal femur (range 7–11°).

While knowledge of osteology of the distal femur is important to all techniques of surgical stabilization, it is especially critical in the positioning of precontoured plates. These plates should be placed on the anterior aspect of the lateral metaphysis to ensure proper screw placement. The longer precontoured plates are designed to accommodate the anterior bow of the femur; a lateral image is critical to ensure that the proximal aspect of the plate is properly positioned on the femur. Due to the trapezoidal shape of the distal femur, distal screws may be quite long and still appear short on AP imaging. Screw lengths can be checked by rotating the image intensifier from the AP position approximately 25° toward the lateral to obtain an image orthogonal to the plane of medial metaphysis of the distal femur.

The pull of local musculature produces characteristic deformities of distal femur fractures. The gastrocnemius muscle takes its origin from the posterior aspect of the distal femur. Contraction of this muscle produces an apex posterior deformity that may be reduced by flexing the knee. Contraction of the quadriceps and hamstrings will produce shortening, while the pull of adductors on medially located adductor tubercle will produce a varus deformity. In the event of an intracondylar fracture, the soft tissue attachments will tend to produce rotational malalignment of the respective condyles.

Positioning

These injuries may be addressed with the patient positioned supine or in the lateral decubitus position. The supine position is generally preferred and will allow both medial and lateral approaches to be performed if needed. However, the lateral position may facilitate dissection from a lateral approach in an obese patient, or maybe beneficial in a patient being positioned lateral for other surgical procedures.

For supine positioning, a bump placed under the ipsilateral buttock may be utilized to internally rotate the femur allowing greater distance between the table and lateral femur. The knee should be flexed over a bump or a radiolucent triangle (Fig. 23.5A). This serves to relax the gastrocnemius muscle and facilitates fracture reduction. For the same reason, the knee should be flexed if a lateral approach is utilized. A pneumatic tourniquet is routinely utilized.

Approaches

Lateral

The standard lateral approach is performed with an incision directly lateral over the thigh. The incision is carried distally over the lateral femoral condyle staying anterior to the lateral collateral ligament (Fig. 23.5B). Depending on the articular involvement, the distal limb of the incision may be brought anteriorly toward the lateral aspect of the tibial tubercle. The iliotibial (IT) band is identified and incised in line with the skin incision. The distal fibers may need to be incised anteriorly to allow for adequate exposure (Figs 23.5C and D). The synovium and capsule can then be incised. The superior lateral geniculate artery must generally be ligated at this stage. The vastus lateralis is then elevated anteriorly from the intramuscular septum. Perforating vessels must be identified and coagulated. A blunt Hohmann retractor can then be placed across the anterior femur to allow for visualization of the joint surface (Fig. 23.5E). While lateral condyle visualization is generally adequate, it is difficult to visualize the medial condyle or patellofemoral groove from this approach.

Lateral Parapatellar

A lateral parapatellar approach will allow for improved joint visualization in Type C fractures, especially if extensive comminution is present in the patellofemoral groove. An incision is made over the anterior aspect of the knee from the tibial tubercle to a point 10–15 cm proximal to the superior pole of the patella (Fig. 23.6A). A lateral parapatellar arthrotomy is then performed with the incision brought proximally through the quadriceps tendon between the rectus femoris and vastus lateralis (Fig. 23.6B). The superior and inferior lateral geniculate arteries must be ligated in this approach, which can compromise the vascular supply to the patella, if the patient has had a recent medial parapatellar arthrotomy.

Subluxation of the patella medially provides for excellent visualization of the articular surface. Lateral plate application is more challenging through this approach than the standard lateral approach (Fig. 23.6C). A small lateral incision may be required proximally to ensure appropriate proximal implant placement and fixation.

Medial Parapatellar

A medial parapatellar approach may be utilized for a medial condyle fracture, acute arthroplasty or for the placement of an IM nail utilizing the inferior aspect of this approach. As this incision is also used for total knee arthroplasty, it will be familiar to most surgeons. It is not possible to place a laterally-based plate through this incision. In this approach, an incision is made over the anterior aspect of the knee from the medial side of the tibial tubercle to a point 3–5 cm proximal to the superior pole of the patella (Fig. 23.7A). A medial parapatellar arthrotomy is then performed, and the medial geniculate arteries are ligated. The patella is inverted or subluxed laterally allowing excellent joint visualization (Fig. 23.7B). The inferior aspect of this approach is used in isolation for the placement of a retrograde IM nail.

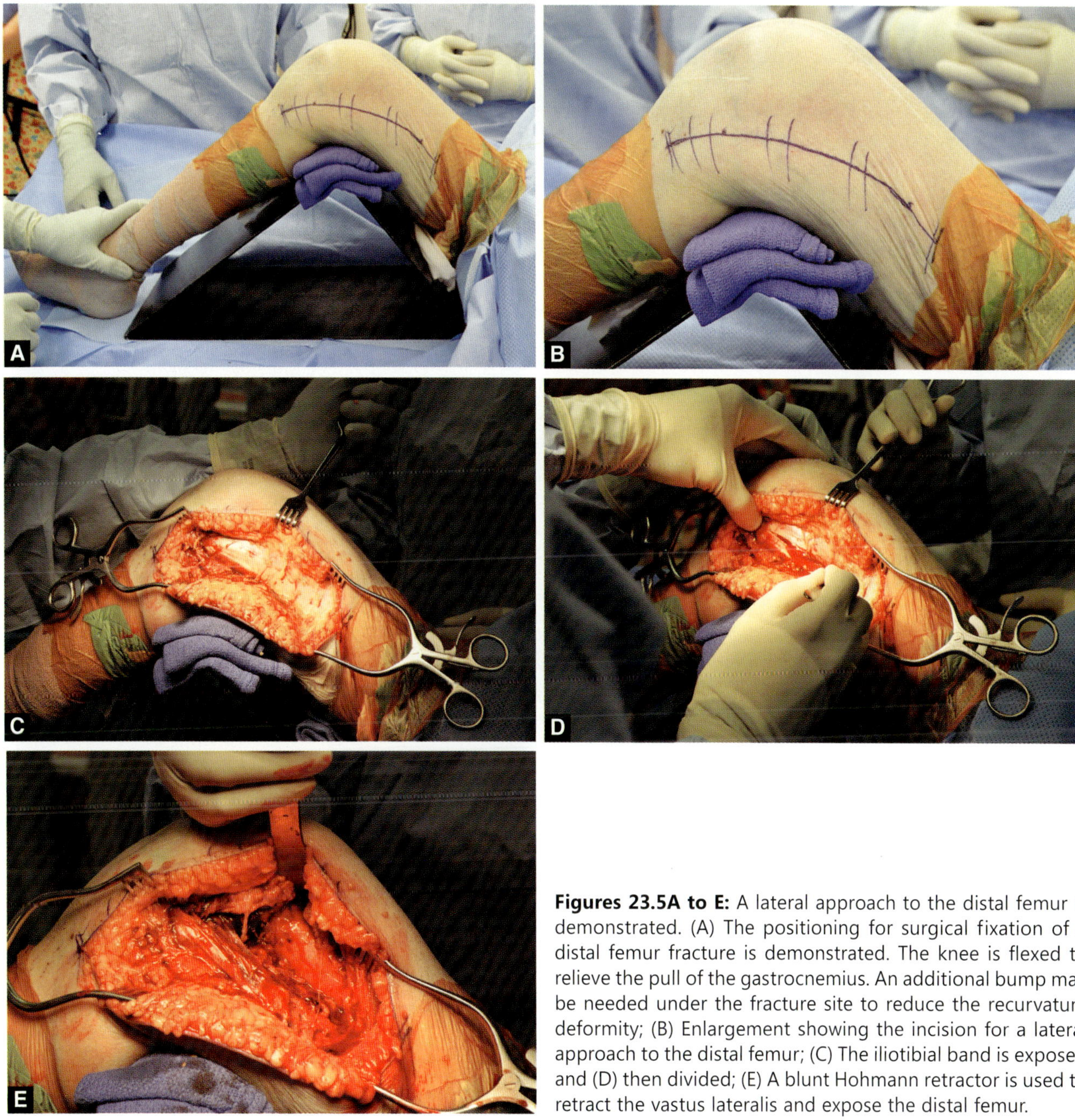

Figures 23.5A to E: A lateral approach to the distal femur is demonstrated. (A) The positioning for surgical fixation of a distal femur fracture is demonstrated. The knee is flexed to relieve the pull of the gastrocnemius. An additional bump may be needed under the fracture site to reduce the recurvatum deformity; (B) Enlargement showing the incision for a lateral approach to the distal femur; (C) The iliotibial band is exposed and (D) then divided; (E) A blunt Hohmann retractor is used to retract the vastus lateralis and expose the distal femur.

Medial Subvastus

This approach may be utilized to address a medial condyle fracture. Compared to a medial parapatellar approach, a medial subvastus approach will offer an improved position for implant placement, but with less visualization of the patellofemoral grove and intracondylar notch.

A medial plate may be required for an isolated medial condyle fracture (B2), or when double-plating of the distal femur is indicated for severe supracondylar comminution or bone defects requiring additional stabilization. In this approach, a straight medial incision is made just anterior to the adductor tubercle. The deep fascia is incised in line

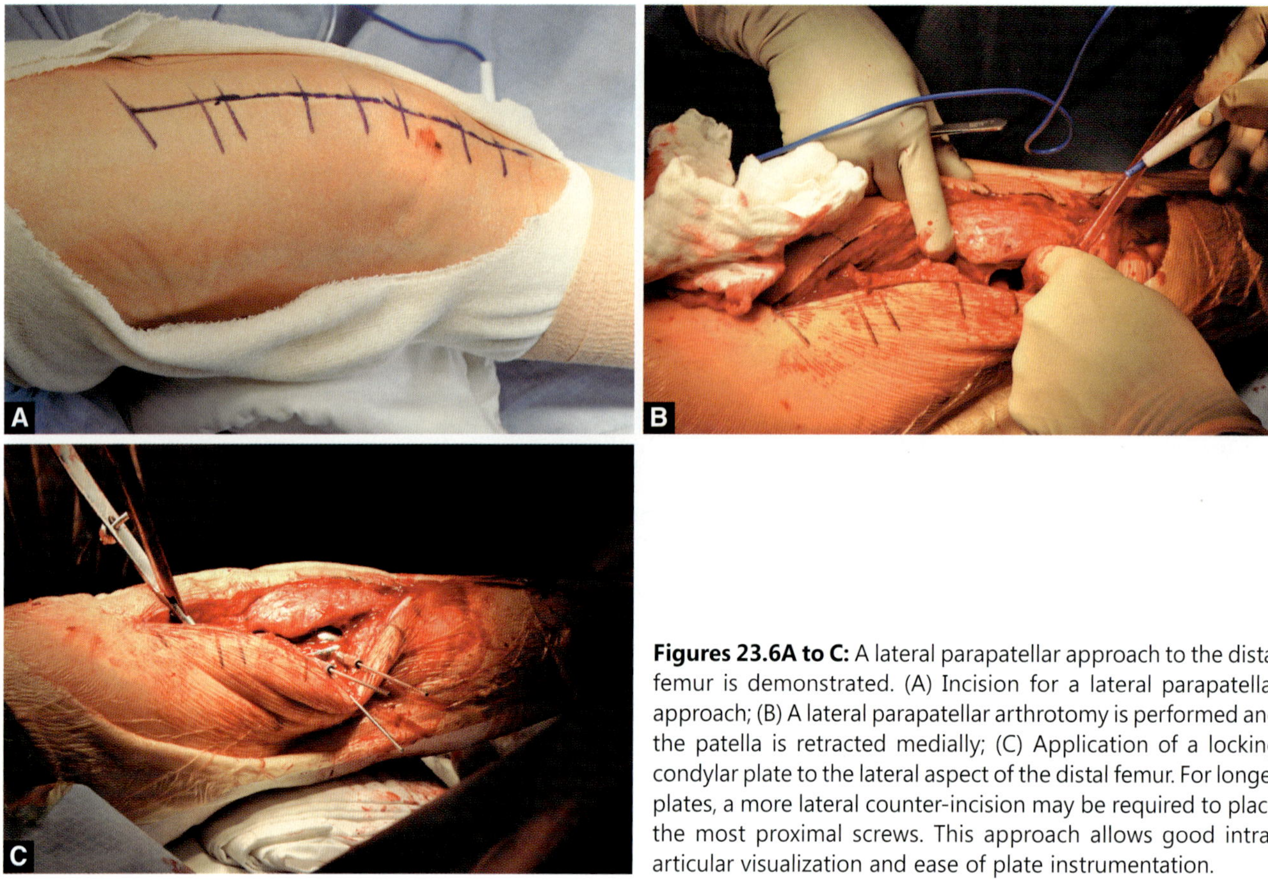

Figures 23.6A to C: A lateral parapatellar approach to the distal femur is demonstrated. (A) Incision for a lateral parapatellar approach; (B) A lateral parapatellar arthrotomy is performed and the patella is retracted medially; (C) Application of a locking condylar plate to the lateral aspect of the distal femur. For longer plates, a more lateral counter-incision may be required to place the most proximal screws. This approach allows good intra-articular visualization and ease of plate instrumentation.

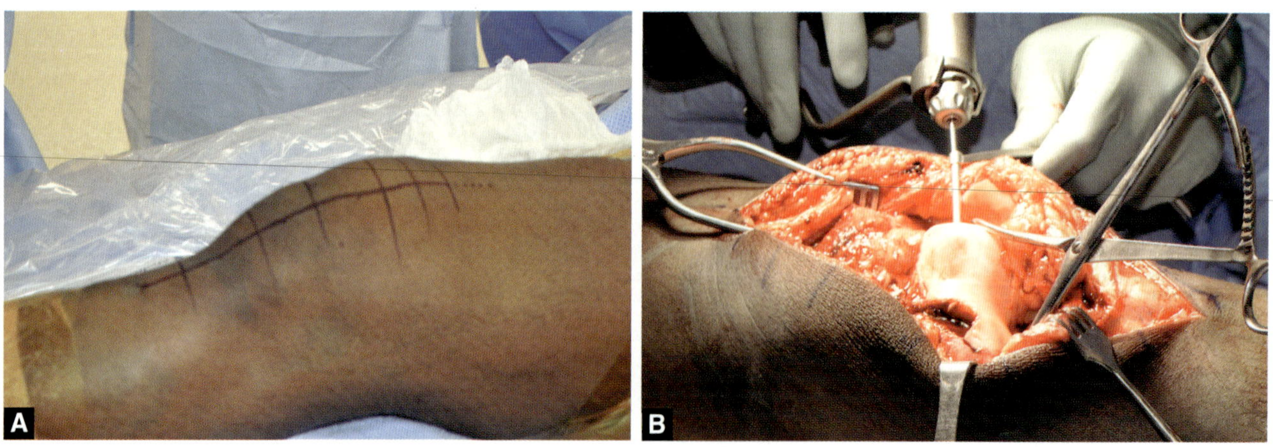

Figures 23.7A and B: Medial parapatellar approach to the distal femur. (A) Incision for a medial parapatellar approach; (B) Retraction of the patella laterally during a medial parapatellar approach provides for excellent visualization of the articular surface, especially the medial condyle and patellofemoral groove. Application of a tenaculum clamp to reduce the fracture is also demonstrated. Excellent articular visualization is provided, but plate instrumentation is difficult.

with the skin and the vastus medialis is elevated off the adductor magnus, exposing the distal femur. The superior medial geniculate artery is identified and ligated. The retinaculum can then be incised exposing the joint surface. A Hohmann retractor may be placed under the extensor mechanism to improve visualization of the joint surface. Care must be taken to avoid damage to the femoral artery, which pierces the adductor hiatus 10 cm proximal to the joint line.

Surgical Techniques

Technique 1: Minimally Invasive Plate Osteosynthesis Plating of Type A (Extra-articular) Fracture

In cases, where an articular reduction is not required, plating may be achieved in a biologically friendly, minimally invasive manner. This may include periprosthetic fractures (Figs 23.8A to F). Instrumentation and equipment to be available for these surgeries include a lateral periarticular plate, radiolucent triangle and bolster, fluoroscopy, and large fragment instrumentation. In minimally invasive plate osteosynthesis (MIPO) plating, the fracture site and reduction are not directly visualized; therefore, it is critical to scrutinize both the limb and fluoroscopic images to avoid malreduction.

The patient is positioned with the knee over a radiolucent triangle; this serves to remove the pull of the gastrocnemius and aids in fracture reduction. An additional bolster, such as a roll of sterile towels directly under the fracture site may be required to reduce the expected recurvatum deformity (Fig. 23.5A). A valgus stress at the fracture site may be required to complete the reduction.

An incision is then made over the lateral femoral epicondyle. The IT band is then incised in line with the skin incision. Fibers of the IT band may need to be elevated at the distal and anterior insertion of the IT band to allow the plate to be placed. The joint is not opened in the MIPO approach. A Cobb elevator can then be passed proximally along the femur to clear sufficient vastus lateralis to allow for passage of the plate.

Once an adequate reduction is obtained, the plate is placed submuscularly along the lateral femur. A second small lateral incision at the proximal end of the plate may be necessary to move the proximal aspect of the plate and ensure that it is on the bone. Especially with longer plates, small malalignments at the distal end of the plate may result in the proximal aspect of the plate not being on the femur. If the reduction and plate placement appear adequate at this time, the plate can then be affixed to the bone proximally and distally with screws or Kirschner (K) wires placed through guide towers (Fig. 23.8C). If residual malalignment remains before the plate is affixed, the plate can be used as a reduction device. For sagittal plane malalignment, the plate can be affixed to the bone distally and then rotated until the proximal portion of the plate is overlying the bone. For coronal plane malalignment (usually varus), the plate can be affixed to the bone distally, and a long cortical screw is used to bring the proximal portion of the plate down to the diaphysis.

Once proximal and distal provisional fixation is obtained and the fracture is reduced, the remaining number of desired screws can be placed. Distally, they are placed through the incision. Proximal screw placement is carried out through small incisions that are guided by fluoroscopy or a targeting guide attached to the plate (Fig. 23.8D).

The reduction and implant position are then checked on fluoroscopy. Distal screw lengths can be checked by rotating the image intensifier from AP position approximately 25° toward lateral to obtain an image orthogonal to the plane of the medial metaphysis of the distal femur. The wounds are then irrigated and closed in layers (Figs 23.8E and F).

MINIMALLY INVASIVE PLATE OSTEOSYNTHESIS PLATING OF TYPE A FRACTURE: Pearls and Pitfalls

- Flex the knee to reduce the pull of the gastrocnemius muscle and to improve the recurvatum deformity. A bump under the fracture site may also be required
- Small distal sagittal plane malalignments can result in the proximal aspect of the plate being well anterior or posterior to the femur. Check alignment on the lateral view
- Rotate the C-arm laterally to check screw lengths on the medial femoral condyle. Palpate the medial condyle to assure that no screws are prominent
- A longer plate with lower screw density and the use of unlocked screws proximally will decrease the construct rigidity and may improve healing

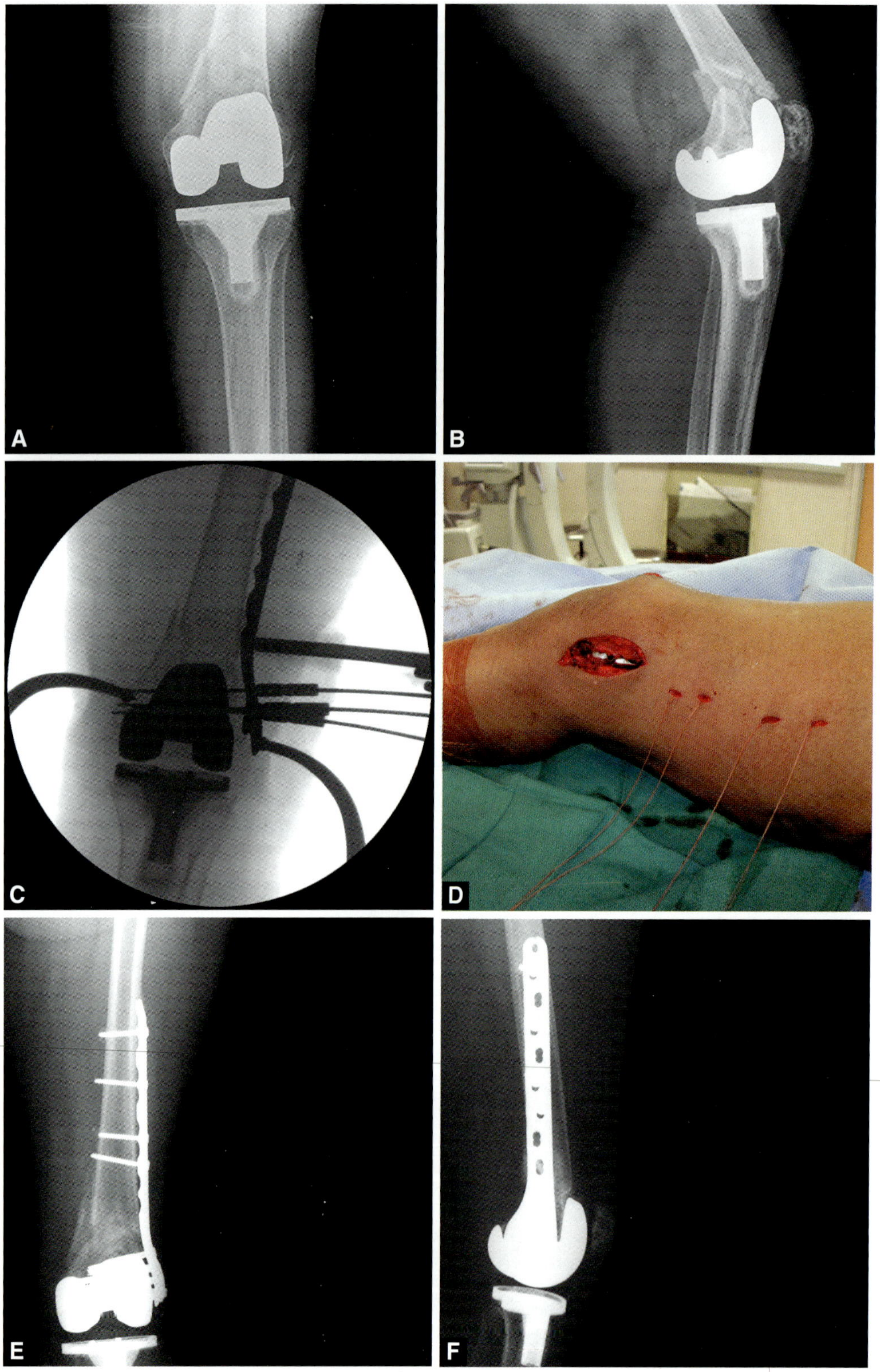

Figures 23.8A to F: Minimally invasive plate osteosynthesis of a periprosthetic supracondylar femur fracture. (A and B) Anteroposterior and lateral X-rays of a 74-year-old woman with a periprosthetic distal femur fracture; (C) Fluoroscopic images of another patient showing provisional plate application intraoperatively; (D) Proximal screws are placed through small incisions as is customary for MIPO technique; (E and F) Anteroposterior and lateral X-rays of the woman 5 months after surgery.

Technique 2: Retrograde Intramedullary Nail of Type A Fracture

In cases where an articular reduction is not required, surgical fixation with an IM nail allows for biologically friendly fixation and may allow for early weight bearing (Figs 23.9A to E). Instrumentation and equipment to be available include a retrograde femoral nail or supracondylar nail, radiolucent triangle and bolster, fluoroscopy

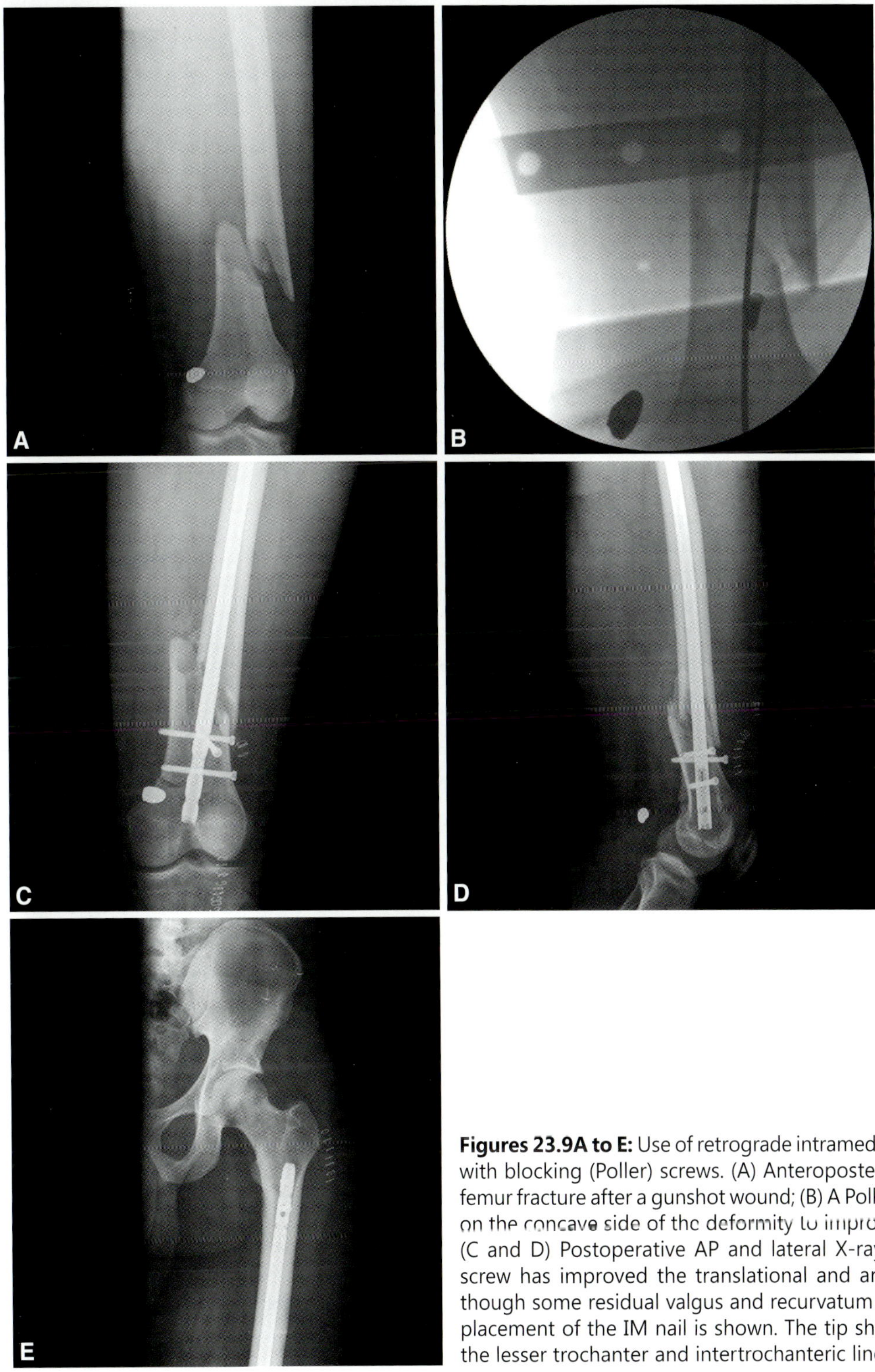

Figures 23.9A to E: Use of retrograde intramedullary (IM) nailing with blocking (Poller) screws. (A) Anteroposterior (AP) X-ray of femur fracture after a gunshot wound; (B) A Poller screw is placed on the concave side of the deformity to improve the reduction; (C and D) Postoperative AP and lateral X-rays; (E) The Poller screw has improved the translational and angular deformity, though some residual valgus and recurvatum remain. Proximal placement of the IM nail is shown. The tip should be between the lesser trochanter and intertrochanteric line.

and large fragment instrumentation. In IM nailing, the fracture site and reduction are not directly visualized; therefore, it is critical to scrutinize both the limb and fluoroscopic images to avoid malreduction.

The patient is positioned with the knee over a radiolucent triangle; this serves to remove the pull of the gastrocnemius and aids in fracture reduction. Chemical paralysis may aid in achieving fracture reduction. An additional bolster such as a roll of sterile towels directly under the fracture site may be required to reduce the expected recurvatum deformity. A valgus stress at the fracture site may be required to complete the reduction. This may require an F-tool or mallet held by a scrubbed assistant. It is critical to remember that the distal femoral condyles should be in 7–9° of anatomic valgus with respect to the diaphysis. If the condyles are orthogonal to the diaphysis, a varus malreduction is present. As these are not diaphyseal fractures, there is minimal potential to use the nail to reduce the fracture. The fracture must be reduced prior to reaming.

If there is an intra-articular component to the fracture, it must be reduced prior to reaming and placement of the IM device. Once the intra-articular component of the fracture is reduced, it can be held with screws placed outside of the nail trajectory or held with a clamp. Newer implants may have condylar screw interlocking options available which incorporate flared washers into the medial and lateral aspect of the screw and may improve fixation of the intra-articular fracture.

With the knee flexed over a radiolucent triangle or bolster, an incision is made over the medial aspect of the patellar tendon. A small medial parapatellar arthrotomy is then made just medial to the patellar tendon. The incision and arthrotomy may need to be extended proximally depending on the patient's laxity and ability to sublux the patella laterally to allow access to the intracondylar notch. Under fluoroscopic guidance, a starting point is obtained with an awl or threaded guide pin. The starting point is at the tip of Blumensaat's line on the lateral view and at the center of the intracondylar notch on the AP view. If a threaded guide pin is used to obtain the starting point, it is overreamed with a cannulated opening reamer. A ball-tipped guidewire is then advanced through the length of the IM canal from the starting point. The length is then measured. For a full-length retrograde femoral nail, the distal end of the nail should be 3–5 mm deep to the articular surface and the proximal end of the nail should rest between the lesser trochanter and intertrochanteric ridge. The canal is then reamed with flexible IM reamers 1.5 mm above initial cortical chatter. A nail 1.5 mm smaller than the final reamer is then advanced with blows from the mallet. The guidewire is then removed. Distal interlocking screws are then placed with the attached targeting guide and proximal interlocking screws are placed under fluoroscopic guidance utilizing perfect circle technique. If compression of the fracture site is desired, the nail may be counter-sunk and the proximal interlocking screws are placed first. The nail can then be back-slapped with a slap hammer to generate compression and then distal interlocking screws are placed.

Blocking screws may be required to aid in the reduction due to large metaphyseal volume of the distal fragment. Blocking screws, also known as Poller screws, act as a fulcrum to redirect the nail and aid in fracture reduction (Fig. 23.9B). They are placed on the concave side of the deformity. An anterior to posterior directed screw is placed in the proximal and medial aspect of the distal fragment. This screw will serve to redirect the reamer and nail path further lateral, thereby correct a varus deformity. Likewise, a lateral to medial directed screw placed in the anterior-proximal aspect of the distal fragment will help to correct a recurvatum deformity. Poller screws should be placed before reaming. If an inadequate reduction is noted after nail placement, when Poller screws are lacking or poorly positioned, the nail can be removed and appropriate Poller screws can be placed. Reaming should then be repeated prior to reinsert the nail. Large fragment screws are recommended, as small fragment screws may bend significantly upon nail insertion.

After the nail is inserted and the interlocking screws are placed, it is critical to assess the limb alignment and rotation prior to leaving the operating room. Rotation can be assessed radiographically by scrutinizing the relative cortical widths around the fracture site and assessing the position of the lesser trochanter, when the knee is properly positioned for AP imaging. Clinically, the internal and external rotation of the limb can be checked and compared to the contralateral limb. The incisions are then irrigated; the arthrotomy incision should be closed in layers, while single layer closure alone may suffice for incisions for the interlocking screws.

RETROGRADE INTRAMEDULLARY NAIL OF TYPE A FRACTURE : Pearls and Pitfalls

- Flex the knee over a bump and radiolucent triangle to reduce the recurvatum deformity
- An F-tool or padded mallet may be utilized to reduce the varus deformity
- Poller screws placed on the concave side of the deformity may be required to obtain and hold the reduction
- Proximal interlocking screws should be secured with a suture or a screwdriver that screws into the screw head to avoid losing the screw in the thigh during insertion

Technique 3: ORIF of Type C Fracture

Operative treatment of a type C fracture requires an articular reduction. The goals of the surgery are anatomical reconstruction of the articular surface followed by reduction of the reconstructed condyles to the femoral diaphysis. Implants to be available include K-wires, headless compression screws which can be advanced deep to the articular surface, long (60–70 mm) cortical screws, and a laterally-based periarticular locking plate. If severe supracondylar comminution or bone loss is present, a small fragment or reconstruction plate should be available for medial-sided plating. Alternatively, a medially-based distal femur osteotomy plate can also be used.

The choice of approach and implants will depend on the extent and location of the comminution. If there is comminution within the patellofemoral groove, a lateral parapatellar approach will provide the best access and visualization. Distally, a laterally-based distal femur locking plate can be applied through this incision, though a more lateral counter-incision may be required proximally to place proximal screws into the femoral diaphysis. If there is no comminution within the patellofemoral groove, a lateral approach brought slightly anterior at its distal aspect will provide sufficient visualization and allow for improved access to the femoral diaphysis (Fig. 23.10A). In addition, a medial subvastus approach will allow access for medial plating and improved visualization of the medial aspect of the medial femoral condyle.

The patient is positioned supine with the knee over a sterile radiolucent triangle; this serves to remove the pull of the gastrocnemius and aids in fracture reduction. Chemical paralysis may aid in achieving fracture reduction. An additional bolster such as a roll of sterile towels directly under the fracture site may be required to reduce the expected recurvatum deformity. A pneumatic tourniquet is routinely used to improve visualization of the articular fragments. The patient should be draped to allow for free manipulation of the knee during the procedure. Hyperflexion of the knee will improve visualization of the more posterior articular fractures. If the fracture is severely comminuted or the fracture has shortened, a femoral distractor will be useful in fracture reduction.

After the surgical approach, the articular surface is visualized. Whether a lateral, lateral parapatellar or medial subvastus approach is utilized, a Hohmann retractor placed under the quadriceps tendon may improve visualization of the articular surface. The articular fragments are then visualized. K-wires are inserted into the fragments to act as joysticks. Small fragment reduction clamps may aid in the reduction of smaller fragments, while a larger periarticular reduction forceps can be used to reduce the larger medial and lateral condyle pieces, providing compression across the intercondylar notch (Fig. 23.10B). Disimpaction of the fragments with a Freer may be required. Fracture hematoma is removed to allow for anatomical reduction under direct visualization. Once reduction is achieved, the previously placed K wires can be driven across the fracture lines to provide provisional fixation (Fig. 23.10C).

Definitive fixation is begun with screws. This may require headless compression screws, which can be inserted deep to the articular surface (Fig. 23.10D). If the fracture fragment is sufficiently large or posterior, fixation may be achieved with a long cortical screw directed into the fragment from a location just proximal to the articular surface on the anterior femur. Lag screws are then placed across the sagittal plane fracture lines. A distal plate template is generally included in the locking condylar plate set and should be used to make sure that the lag screws are outside of the footprint of the plate.

Once an articular reduction is achieved, the articular surface is reduced to the femoral diaphysis. The plate may be used as an aid in reduction. A laterally-based condylar plate becomes a fixed angle device, when it is applied in locking mode. If the anatomically designed plate is applied correctly to the distal femur as a fixed angle device, it will restore the appropriate distal femur valgus alignment. The plate can be fixed provisionally to the distal femur with K-wires through guide towers (Fig. 23.10E). A trial reduction can then be performed to assure that the proximal aspect of the plate will position appropriately on the diaphysis with the fracture reduced. A small positioning error on the distal fragment may result in the proximal aspect of the plate being well anterior or posterior to the femoral diaphysis. This problem is exacerbated with longer plates. Once the plate is positioned appropriately, definitive fixation is placed in the distal femur. Any compression screw required to compress sagittal plane fractures should be placed before locking screws are placed. Once sufficient distal fixation is placed, the proximal aspect of the plate is fixed to the diaphysis. If at all possible, the plate should be loaded with either the AO tensioning device or by drilling the first cortical screw eccentrically in compression mode. Standard cortical screws

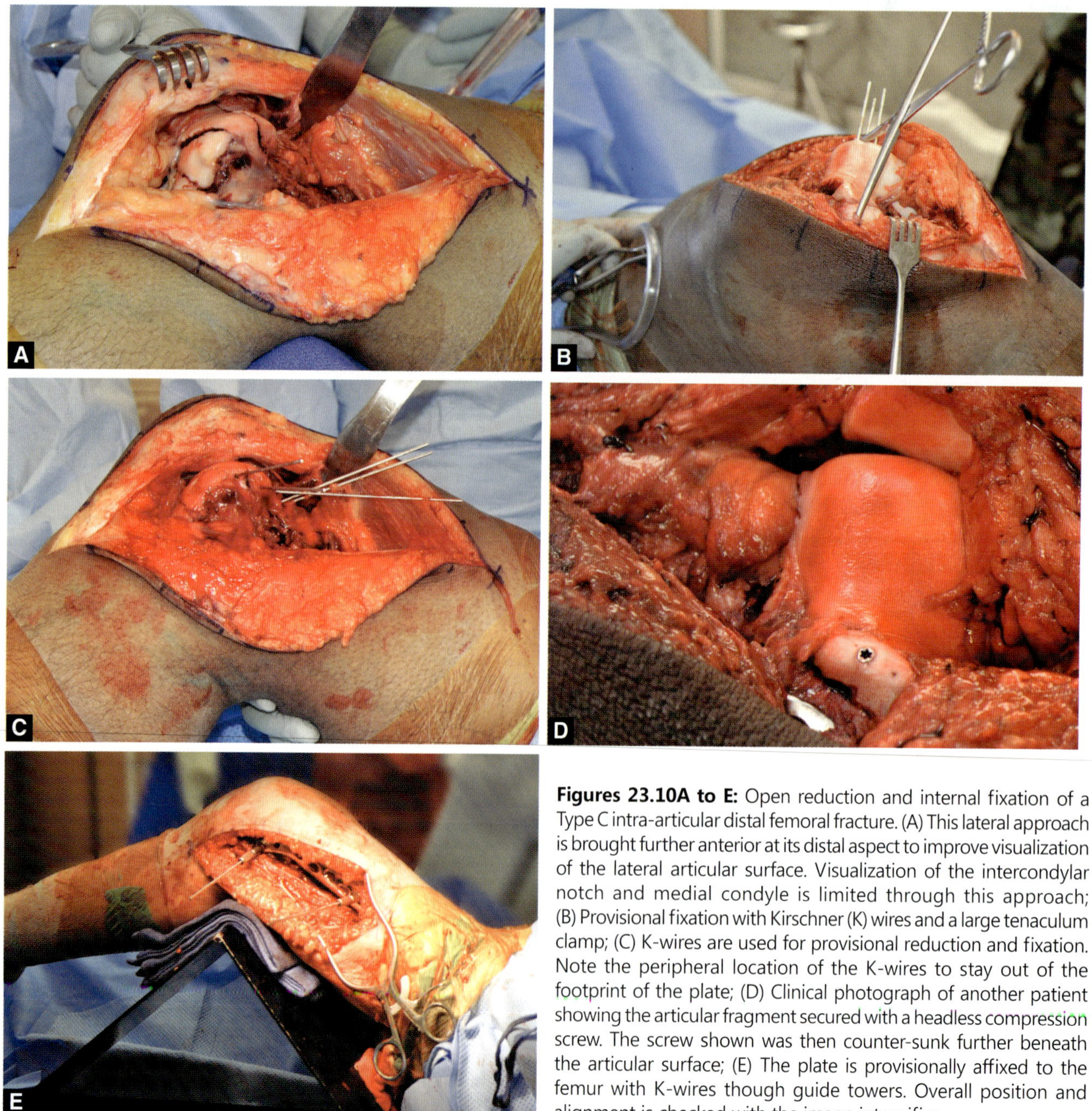

A B C D E

Figures 23.10A to E: Open reduction and internal fixation of a Type C intra-articular distal femoral fracture. (A) This lateral approach is brought further anterior at its distal aspect to improve visualization of the lateral articular surface. Visualization of the intercondylar notch and medial condyle is limited through this approach; (B) Provisional fixation with Kirschner (K) wires and a large tenaculum clamp; (C) K-wires are used for provisional reduction and fixation. Note the peripheral location of the K-wires to stay out of the footprint of the plate; (D) Clinical photograph of another patient showing the articular fragment secured with a headless compression screw. The screw shown was then counter-sunk further beneath the articular surface; (E) The plate is provisionally affixed to the femur with K-wires though guide towers. Overall position and alignment is checked with the image intensifier.

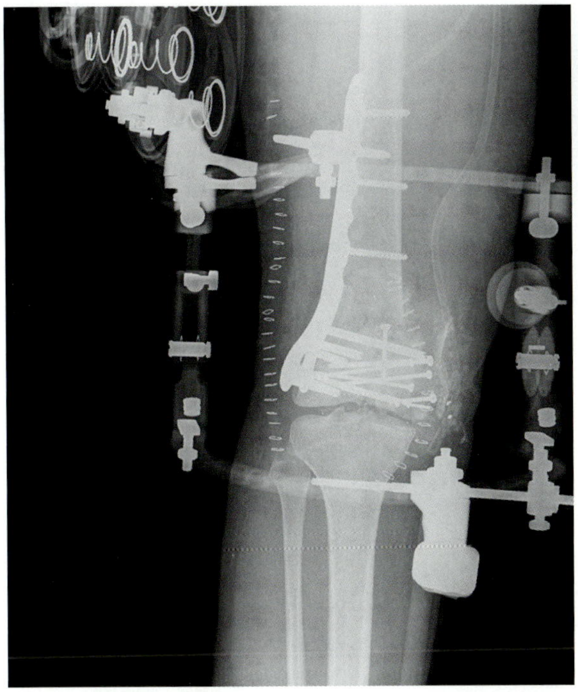

Figure 23.11: This patient had a C3 type fracture with severe medial condylar comminution due a gunshot injury. A hinged external fixator was used as neutralization due to the extensive comminution.

may be used, if there is good bone quality. If necessary, a medial plate can then be placed through a medial subvastus approach. Three to four screws proximal to the fracture are utilized. It is preferable to utilize a longer plate with a lower screw density. In the setting of severe comminution, an external fixator (static or preferably hinged) may be necessary as an adjunct to fixation to prevent collapse of the construct (Fig. 23.11).

Implant position, limb alignment and rotation are critically assessed prior to leaving the operating room. The articular reduction can be assessed both on fluoroscopy and direct visualization. It is critical to restore the mechanical alignment of the limb by restoring appropriate valgus alignment of the distal femoral condyles. Metaphyseal comminution may lead to a varus or valgus malreduction even in the setting of an anatomical articular reduction. Clinically, the internal and external rotation of the limb can be checked and compared to the contralateral limb. The tourniquet is deflated and any major bleeding is controlled. A drain is placed, if necessary, and the wound is closed in layers taking care to achieve a water-tight closure of the IT band and arthrotomy.

The patient is kept non-weight bearing on the knee for 10–12 weeks. Early range of motion is allowed, generally in a hinged knee brace.

ORIF OF TYPE C FRACTURE: Pearls and Pitfalls

- Plan incisions appropriately. Extensive notch comminution can be best visualized through a parapatellar arthrotomy. Additional incisions may be needed for the proximal aspect of a lateral plate or to add a medial plate
- Extensive comminution can lead to an angular malreduction. Scrutinize images
- Double-ended K-wires can be utilized to provisionally fix multiple fragments
- In the setting of severe comminution, an external fixator may be utilized to augment fixation

Technique 4: ORIF of Type B (Unicondylar) Fracture

A unicondylar type fracture may involve either the lateral (B1) or medial (B2). The fracture may consist of a single sagittal plane fracture separating the condyle from the femoral metaphysic, or there may be substantial comminution. A CT is usually required to characterize the displacement and comminution (if any) of this fragment. As these fractures require an anatomical articular reduction, ORIF is generally the treatment of choice. A buttress plate is generally added to prevent vertical displacement of the fracture. However, in a nondisplaced or minimally displaced fracture with a minimal shear component, screw fixation alone may suffice (Figs 23.12A to E). Percutaneous fixation may also be considered in a nondisplaced fracture with a minimal shear component.

The choice of implants and approach will be determined by the nature of the fracture. A lateral unicondylar fracture may be approached via a lateral or lateral parapatellar approach, while a medial unicondylar fracture may be addressed through a medial parapatellar or medial subvastus approach. Hohmann retractors may be inserted to improve visualization. Implants to be available include K-wires, headless compression screws which can be advanced deep to the articular surface, long (40–70 mm) cortical screws and reduction clamps.

The patient is positioned supine with the knee over a sterile radiolucent triangle; this serves to remove the pull of the gastrocnemius and aids in fracture reduction. Chemical paralysis may aid in achieving fracture reduction.

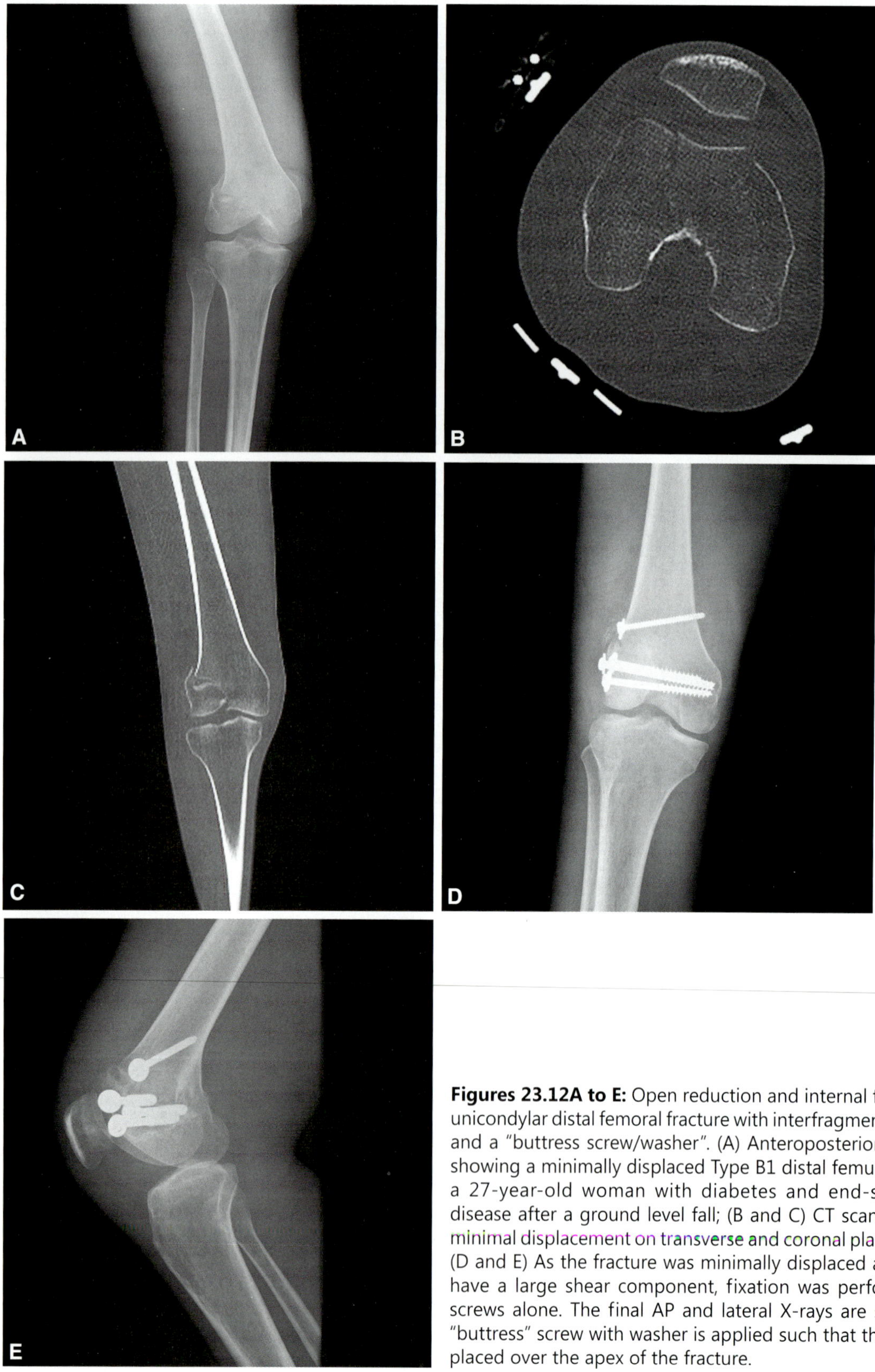

Figures 23.12A to E: Open reduction and internal fixation of a unicondylar distal femoral fracture with interfragmentary screws and a "buttress screw/washer". (A) Anteroposterior (AP) X-ray showing a minimally displaced Type B1 distal femur fracture in a 27-year-old woman with diabetes and end-stage renal disease after a ground level fall; (B and C) CT scan confirmed minimal displacement on transverse and coronal plane imaging; (D and E) As the fracture was minimally displaced and did not have a large shear component, fixation was performed with screws alone. The final AP and lateral X-rays are shown. The "buttress" screw with washer is applied such that the washer is placed over the apex of the fracture.

An additional bolster such as a roll of sterile towels directly under the fracture site may be required to reduce the expected recurvatum deformity. A pneumatic tourniquet is routinely used to improve visualization of the articular fragments. The patient should be draped to allow for free manipulation of the knee during the procedure. Hyperflexion of the knee will improve visualization of the more posterior articular fractures. If the fracture is severely comminuted or the fracture has shortened, a femoral distractor will be useful in fracture reduction.

The general strategy in a Type B fracture is to begin with the intact portion of the distal femur and sequentially reduce the fragments working from "known to unknown." Once the fracture site is visualized, the fracture(s) are disimpacted and fracture hematoma is removed. Kirschner wires may be inserted to use as joysticks in fracture reduction. A large periarticular reduction forceps is used to reduce the fractured condyle to the intact portion of the femur (Fig. 23.10B). Small fragment clamps may be used to reduce smaller comminuted pieces within the fractured condyle. When a provisional reduction is obtained, it is held with the clamps or K-wires driven across the fracture line(s). The pieces are then lagged together using either extra-articular screws or headless compression screws depending on the orientation of the fracture line. A buttress plate is then applied to prevent proximal subluxation of the fractured condyle (Figs 23.13A to C).

Implant position, limb alignment and rotation are critically assessed prior to leaving the operating room. The articular reduction can be assessed both on fluoroscopy and direct visualization. It is critical to restore the mechanical alignment of the limb by restoring appropriate valgus alignment of the distal femoral condyles. Metaphyseal comminution may lead to a varus or valgus malreduction even in the setting of an anatomical articular reduction. Clinically, the internal and external rotation of the limb can be checked and compared to the contralateral limb. The tourniquet is deflated and any major bleeding is controlled. A drain is placed, if necessary, and the wound is closed in layers taking care to achieve a water-tight closure.

The patient is kept non-weight bearing on the knee for 10–12 weeks. Early range of motion is allowed, generally in a hinged knee brace.

ORIF OF TYPE B FRACTURE: Pearls and Pitfalls

- Sequentially reduce the fracture fragments to the intact condyle. Double-ended K-wires may be utilized to affix multiple fragments to one wire
- A plate template can be used to prevent extra-articular screws from interfering with plate position
- Utilize additional K-wires to stabilize the fracture fragments when advancing screw to prevent rotation

Technique 5: ORIF of a Type B3 (Hoffa) Fracture

Type B3 (Hoffa) fracture is a coronal plane fracture separating the posterior aspect of femoral condyle from the femur. This is difficult to fully characterize on plain-film X-ray and a CT scan is usually required to characterize the displacement and comminution (if any) of this fragment (Figs 23.14A and B). Hoffa fractures are most common in the lateral condyle, though medial condyle and bicondylar injuries are also reported.[13] The choice of implants and approach will be determined by the nature of the fracture. A lateral B3 fracture may be approached via lateral or lateral parapatellar approach, while a medial B3 fracture may be addressed through medial parapatellar or medial subvastus approach. Hohmann retractors may be inserted to improve visualization. Implants to be available include K-wires, headless compression screw, which can be advanced deep to the articular surface, long (60–70 mm) cortical screws and reduction clamps.

The patient is positioned supine with the knee over a sterile radiolucent triangle or bolster. The patient should be draped to allow for free manipulation of the knee during the procedure. After the joint is exposed, the knee is brought into additional flexion until the fracture line of the Hoffa fragment is visible. The more posterior the fracture, the greater flexion will be required.

Once the fracture is visualized, the fragments are disimpacted. Fracture hematoma is removed to allow for anatomical reduction under direct visualization. Fragments are then reduced. Small fragment reduction clamps, tenaculum clamps and K-wires used as joysticks may aid in fracture reduction. The reduction is checked under direct

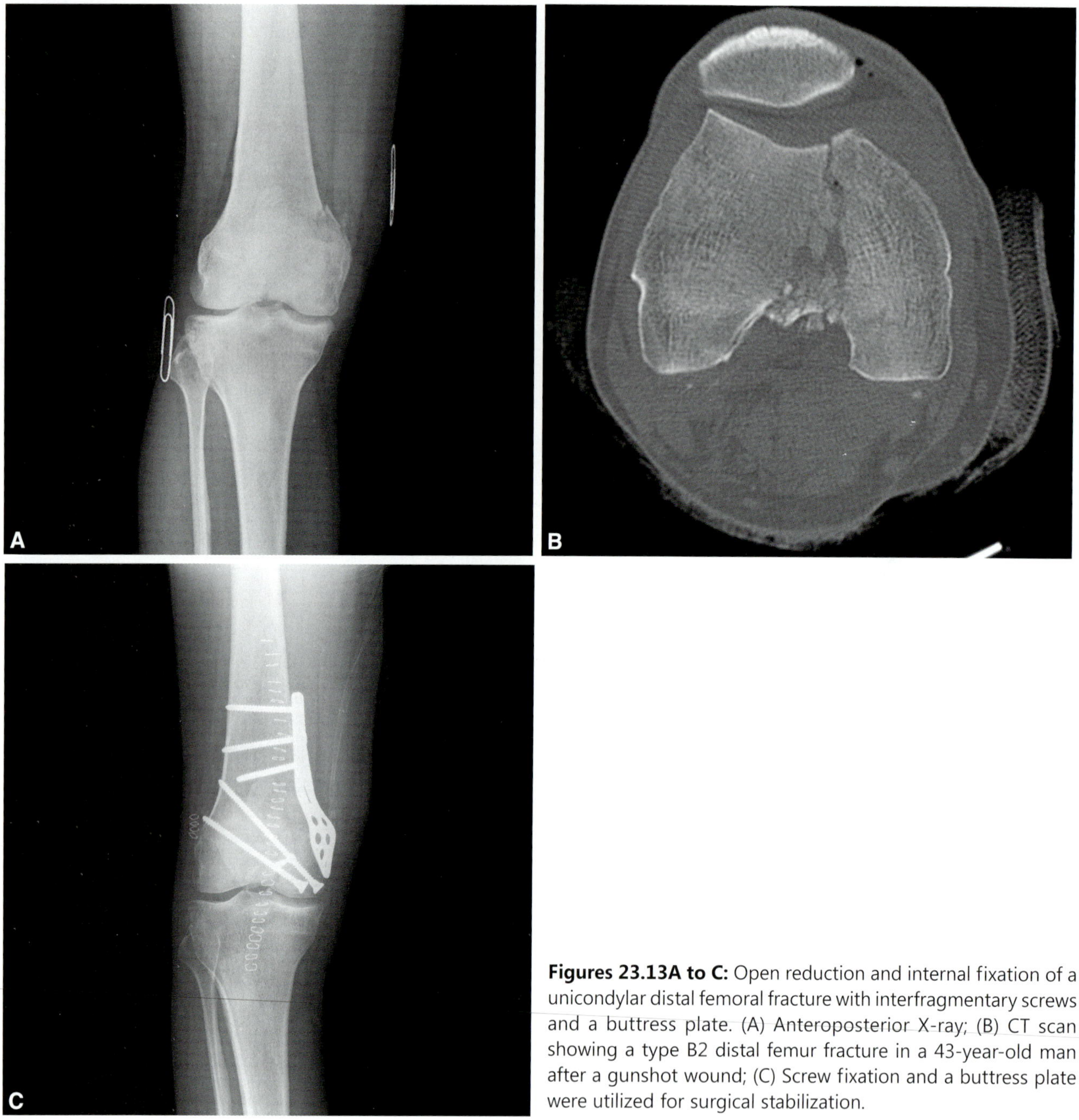

Figures 23.13A to C: Open reduction and internal fixation of a unicondylar distal femoral fracture with interfragmentary screws and a buttress plate. (A) Anteroposterior X-ray; (B) CT scan showing a type B2 distal femur fracture in a 43-year-old man after a gunshot wound; (C) Screw fixation and a buttress plate were utilized for surgical stabilization.

visualization with a goal of achieving an anatomical reduction. It is important to visualize the entire articular aspect of the fracture line to assure that the fragment is not rotated. Definitive fixation should be performed with headless compression screws, which can be inserted deep to the articular surface. If the fracture fragment is sufficiently large or posterior, fixation may be achieved with an extra-articular screw. This is a long (60–70 mm) cortical screw directed into the posterior fragment from a location just proximal to the articular surface on the anterior femur. Two screws are utilized to prevent the fragment from rotating around a single point of fixation (Figs 23.14C and D). Fluoroscopy is utilized to guide screw trajectory. After implants are placed, the reduction is again visualized and

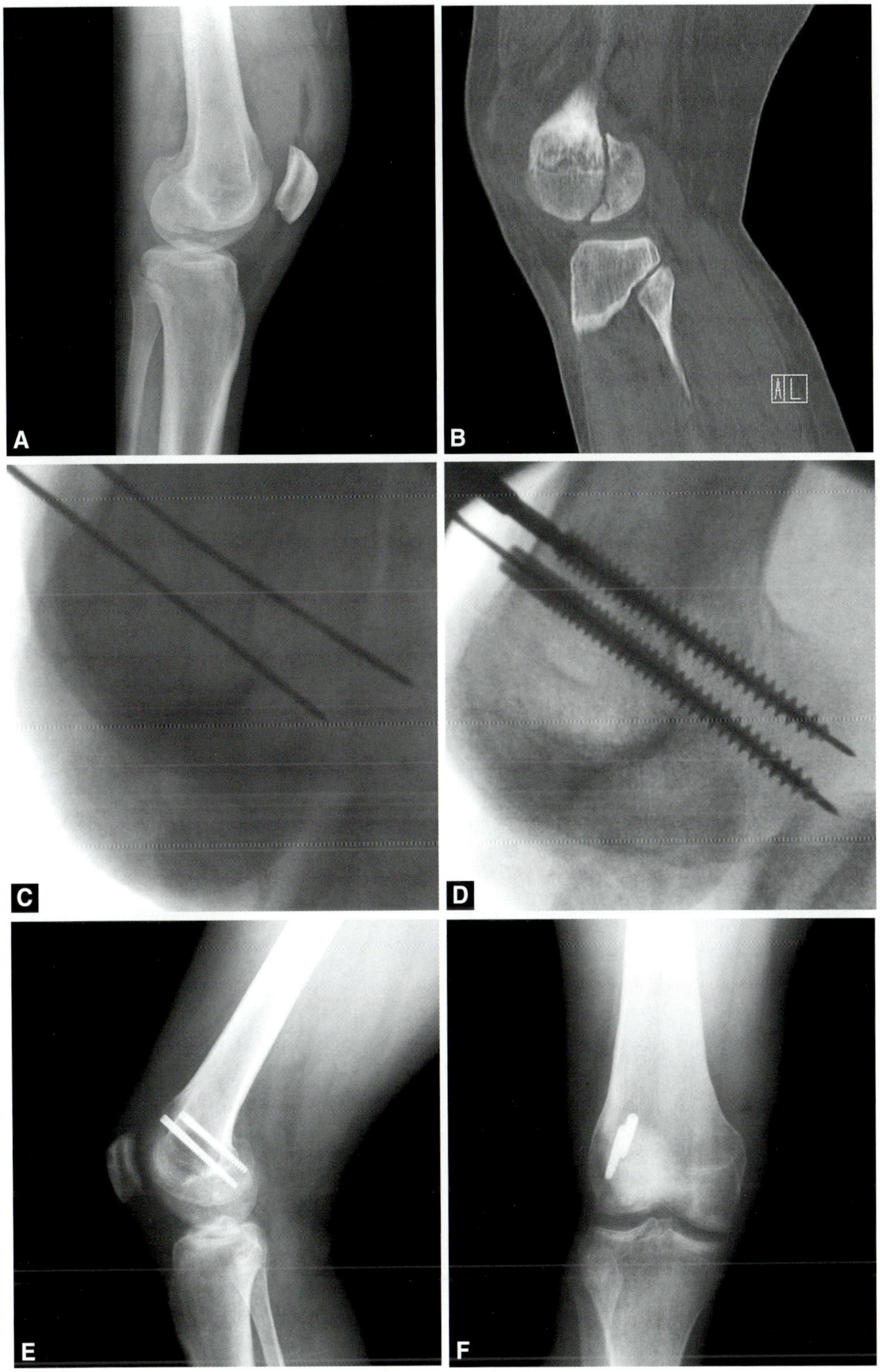

Figures 23.14A to F: Open reduction and internal fixation of a coronal plane type B3 (Hoffa) posterior condylar distal femoral fracture. (A) Lateral knee X-ray; (B) CT scan of a 20-year-old man struck by an automobile with a B3 type (Hoffa fragment) distal femur fracture; (C) The fracture was provisionally stabilized with Kirschner (K) wires; (D) Headless compression screws were advanced over the K-wires; (E and F) Final lateral and anteroposterior X-rays. Note that in this example, the screws were started just proximal to the articular surface.

reduction and implant position are visualized on fluoroscopy. The screws are again checked by visualization to assure that they are either extra-articular or are buried deep to the articular surface (Figs 23.14E and F).

The tourniquet is then deflated and the incision is closed in layers. A drain may be placed. A dressing is applied and the patient is kept non-weight bearing for 8–12 weeks, but an early range of motion is allowed in a hinged knee brace.

ORIF OF TYPE B3 FRACTURE: Pearls and Pitfalls

- Hoffa fracture is easy to miss on X-ray. A CT scan should be ordered if clinical suspicion exists
- Flexion of the knee is often required to visualize the fracture. Greater flexion will be required for a more posterior fracture
- Fixation may be achieved with an extra-articular screw started just proximal to the articular surface. Alternatively, headless compression screws may be utilized

Outcomes

Prior to 1970, most supracondylar femur fractures were treated nonoperatively with resulting complications of angular deformity, joint incongruity and loss of motion.[3] During more recent decades, operative fixation has become the standard treatment. Operative treatment has been shown to reduce the risk of poor results as compared to nonoperative treatment in a randomized controlled trial of elderly patients.[4] In this series, good to excellent results by Schatzker's criteria were noted in 52% of operatively treated patients and 31% of nonoperatively treated patients. The nonoperative group had longer hospital stays and a higher complication rates including urinary tract infection, deep venous thrombosis, pressure sores and respiratory infections.

Zlowodzki and coauthors reviewed the English language literature with the goal of comparing results and complications of different surgical management techniques of 33A and 33C distal femur fractures. Included in the review were one randomized control trial (noted above), one prospective cohort study and 45 case series. The prospective cohort study did not show any difference between locked internal fixation with a less invasive stabilization system (LISS) plate and retrograde IM nail with regard to nonunion, fixation failure, infection or secondary surgical procedure at 1 year. With regard to the case series reviewed, there were no statistically significant differences among compression plating, locked internal fixation, antegrade IM nailing, retrograde IM nailing, or external fixation with regard to nonunion, fixation failure, infection, or secondary surgical procedure. Average follow-up was 2.5 years. The noted complication rates were nonunion 6%, fixation failure 3.3%, deep infection 2.7% and secondary surgical procedure 16.8%. When locked internal fixation was compared to compression plate, there were non-significant trends toward decreased infection, increased fixation failure and increased rates of secondary procedures in the locked internal fixation group.[10]

Long-term follow-up from distal femur fractures was published by Rademakers and coauthors. In this study, 32 patients were available for long-term (5–25 years, mean 14 years) follow-up from an initial cohort of 68 patients with 33B or 33C distal femur fractures treated by ORIF. Mean range of motion was 118°. By the Neer scoring system, 84% of patients had good or excellent results, while 75% of patients had good or excellent results by the hospital for special surgery scoring system. By the Ahlback score, 36% of patients had moderate to severe osteoarthritis; however, 72% of these patients still had good to excellent functional results. There were no differences noted between the 33B and 33C groups. Patients with isolated injuries had better outcome scores than those with multiple injuries.[14]

Complications

Common complications of distal femur fractures include nonunion, malunion and limited knee motion.

Knee Stiffness

Moore and coauthors reported that limitation of knee motion was the most common complication of a distal femur fracture requiring referral. Furthermore, they found that patients with decreased motion were often young patients who had sustained high-energy trauma. In many of these patients, the extent of their soft tissue injuries and severity of the fracture necessitated immobilization even after surgical fixation. Early motion may be beneficial in restoring range of motion in these patients.[15]

Posttraumatic knee stiffness can result from a variety of sources including articular malreduction, intra-articular implants, arthrofibrosis, ligamentous contractures, quadriceps or hamstring scarring and posttraumatic arthritis.[5] Addressing the limitation in motion will require identifying and addressing the underlying cause. If articular malreduction or intra-articular implants are identified, this should be addressed surgically to allow improvement of knee motion. Posttraumatic arthritis may respond to anti-inflammatory medication, physical therapy, viscosupplementation, intra-articular corticosteroids or arthroplasty. Arthrofibrosis, ligament or muscle contractures or scarring may require surgical release.

Patients with quadriceps scarring or adhesions may benefit from quadricepsplasty. Quadricepsplasty for extension contracture of the knee was first described by Thompson in 1944 and Judet in 1956. The Thompson quadricepsplasty is a release of the vastus medialis, vastus lateralis and vastus intermedius near the patellar insertion. The rectus femoris is left intact. Residual extensor lag has been reported. The Thompson quadricepsplasty is a stepwise procedure. Step 1 is release of the retinaculi, medial and lateral gutter adhesions and pin tract adhesions all through a parapatellar approach. If this does not provide sufficient flexion, then step 2 is release of the vastus intermedius from the femur and vastus lateralis from the linea aspera through a long posterolateral incision. If flexion is still limited, the final step is release of the rectus femoris origin from the anterior inferior iliac spine.[16]

Masse and coauthors reported on the 2-year outcomes of 21 patients treated with Judet quadricepsplasty for extension contracture after an extra-articular femur fracture. They reported an average flexion gain of 72° from 23° to 95°. There were five complications including two cases of deep sepsis, one fracture of the lateral femoral condyle, one case of skin necrosis and one intraoperative rupture of the quadriceps tendon.[16]

Wang and coauthors reported on 2-year outcomes of 21 patients treated with quadricepsplasty for extension contracture after a variety of lower extremity trauma. The technique was performed in a stepwise manner through a 2–4 cm incision 3 cm proximal to the superior lateral corner of the patella. The stages were as follows: (1) release of the lateral retinaculum, (2) release of intra-articular adhesions and separation of the vastus intermedius from the rectus femoris, (3) release of medial retinaculum, (4) transaction of the vastus intermedius near its musculotendinous junction, (5) lengthening of the rectus femoris by transecting it near the patellar insertion and suturing to the cut vastus intermedius insertion. Following this, knee arthroscopy was performed to remove remaining intra-articular adhesions and scar tissue. They reported a mean gain of 88° of flexion, from 27° preoperatively to 115° at final follow-up. There was one superficial infection, 15 patients with transient extensor lag and one permanent extensor lag.[17]

Nonunion

Nonunion is not an uncommon complication of distal femur fractures. Risk factors for nonunion include open fracture, comminution, bone loss, poor surgical fixation and patient systemic disease or endocrine abnormality. Zlowodzki and coauthors noted a 6% nonunion rate among all fixation methods.[10]

A more recent review by Henderson and coauthors of studies on locking plates for distal femur fractures since 2000 showed a high rate of late implant failure and other healing difficulties. The studies reported a 0–19% rate of nonunion, 0–15% rate of delayed union and a 0–20% rate of implant failure. In the implant failure group, it was noted that 50% occurred after 6 months and 16% occurred more than 1 year after surgery. An overly rigid construct may increase the rate of nonunion. Preliminary studies included in the review described a statistically significant higher nonunion rate in stainless steel versus titanium plates (23% vs 7%) as well as a statistically significant increase in the number of empty screw holes near the fracture in those fractures that went on to union.[18]

Treatment options for nonunion include revision fixation, addition of bone graft or bone graft substitute, or conversion to a total knee arthroplasty. Haidukewych and coauthors reported on 17 patients with distal femur nonunions treated with total knee arthroplasty. They reported a 91% 5-year prosthesis survival rate. There were large improvements in the Knee Society Pain Score from 2–89 and Knee Society Functional Score from 2–45 from before surgery to 2 years after surgery.[12]

Studies have reported good results with surgical repair of distal femur nonunions. Gardner and coauthors reported on 31 patients with distal femur nonunions treated with debridement of the nonunion site, revision

ORIF, and augmentation with iliac crest autograft or demineralized bone matrix. They reported a 97% union rate with large increase in the patients' Knee Society Rating Scale Score. Nearly half of the patients experienced some shortening of the limb, which averaged 1.6 cm.[19] Bellabarba and coauthors similarly reported on 20 patients treated with debridement of the nonunion site and revision ORIF. Iliac crest autograft was utilized for those patients who deemed to have atrophic or oligotrophic nonunions. They reported a 100% union rate with substantial increase in the patients' Böstman and Hospital for Special Surgery knee scores.[20] Other authors have reported good results with the addition of allograft struts,[21] vascularized bone graft[22] and distraction osteogenesis.[23]

Malunion

Malunion may occur from axial malalignment or intra-articular step-off from malreduction or loss of fixation. It is more common in nonoperatively treated distal femur fractures, and avoidance of malunion is a primary indication for operative treatment of these fractures.[9,10] Even with operative fixation, there is a tendency toward varus malunion in the setting of severe comminution.[24]

Proper preoperative planning and careful attention to anatomy can help reduce surgical malunions. After reduction and fixation, the distal femoral condyles should be restored to 7–9° of anatomic valgus with respect to the diaphysis. If the condyles are orthogonal to the diaphysis, a varus malreduction is present.

The reported incidence of malunion varies in the literature. In a review of different fixation methods for distal femur fractures, Forster and coauthors found published malunion rates from 0–19%.[6] A prospective study of distal femur fractures fixed with LISS plate found a malunion rate of 26% with malunion defined at axial malalignment of 5 or more degrees from anatomic valgus. However, only one patient underwent a secondary procedure for correction of axial malalignment. The authors did not find any statistically significant correlation between fracture types, reduction method, or implant length and occurrence of a malreduction.[25]

Symptomatic malalignment is an indication for corrective osteotomy. Prior to this, conservative measures such as bracing and pain medication should be attempted. A shoe lift may be beneficial, if there is a leg-length discrepancy. Preoperative planning should include full length, weight bearing AP and lateral radiographs of both lower extremities with woodblocks in place to level the pelvis. If a rotational deformity is present, this can be confirmed and measured with the use of a CT scanner.

Options for osteotomies include acute correction with an opening wedge, closing wedge or dome osteotomies. Advantage of acute correction is that it can be achieved in a single operative procedure and can allow for earlier return of function. Alternatively, these deformities can be corrected gradually with the use of an external fixator. This can allow for concomitant lengthening with distraction osteogenesis and allow for correction of complex deformities. However, this must be weighed against the patient's ability to tolerate such a device.

There are few published reports dealing specifically with supracondylar malunion treatment.[26] Good results have been reported with a variety of techniques including dome osteotomy fixed over an IM nail,[27] closing wedge osteotomy with the far cortex left intact,[28] internal fixation after intraoperative use of a Taylor Spatial Frame,[29] and antegrade nailing.[26] Preoperative planning is essential in deformity correction and has been described elsewhere in detail. Poorly placed osteotomies can result in additional iatrogenic deformities.[30]

Authors' Preferred Management of Select Complications

Case 1: Nonunion with Implant Failure

A 56-year-old woman presented with increased leg pain after feeling a "pop" in her leg while performing activities of daily living. She had undergone ORIF for a distal femur fracture 7 months prior to presentation at our facility. She had multiple medical comorbidities including Type II diabetes, hypertension and congestive heart failure. At the time of her presentation, she had been treated with a bone stimulator for the past 3 months.

The patient had previously undergone ORIF with a locked condylar plate. She was noted to have a persistent fracture with failure of implants (Fig. 23.15A). Her inflammatory markers were moderately elevated; therefore, a bone biopsy was first obtained to rule out infection. At this procedure, an additional cortical screw was placed proximally to prevent further displacement of the implant (Fig. 23.15B).

The patient was returned to the operating room 7 days later. All cultures were negative at this time. Through small, lateral stab incisions, new cortical screws were placed through the combi holes of the plate adjacent to the broken locking screws. No attempt was made to remove the broken portions of screws that were buried within the bone. An anterior incision was then made with a medial parapatellar arthrotomy. This allowed for an access to the nonunion site and provided an access to place a medial plate. The nonunion site was debrided sharply. A high-speed burr with irrigation was then used to debride the bone ends until appearing healthy. Bleeding bone ends were noted. The nonunion site was then packed with an allograft, bone morphogenetic protein (BMP)-2 and allograft bone. She had extensive skin irritation at her iliac crests due to an overlying panus, which made her a poor candidate for iliac crest autograft (Fig. 23.15C). A medial plate was placed to provide additional stability and prevent varus collapse (Fig. 23.15D).

Postoperatively, the patient regained good motion with good control of pain. Her weight bearing was advanced slowly as radiographic evidence of healing was delayed. Due to the delayed union, she was prescribed an ultrasonic bone stimulator 6 months after the nonunion repair. This was a different mechanism of action than the bone stimulator that she had used prior to the nonunion repair. Fourteen months after the nonunion repair, X-rays showed some evidence of healing and she was able to ambulate with a cane. At the time of final follow-up 21 months after surgery, the nonunion site was healed (Figs 23.15E and F). She was ambulatory with good range of motion at the knee and minimal pain. She was quite happy with the results.

Case 2: Atrophic Nonunion with a Stable Implant

A 40-year-old man had pain with attempted weight bearing and a nonunion of his distal femur 2 years after sustaining an open distal femur fracture. He was initially treated with surgical debridement, irrigation and fixation with a retrograde IM nail. His radiographs taken 2 years after the initial injury revealed an atrophic nonunion with an intact and functional implant (Figs 23.16A and B).

Since the nonunion was atrophic with a stable and intact implant, the surgical goal was to provide biologic stimulus to the nonunion. At surgery, fibrinous tissue was sharply removed from the nonunion site, and the bone ends were trimmed to viable, bleeding bone (Fig. 23.16C). The defect was grafted with allograft bone mixed with concentrated autologous bone marrow aspirate from the patient's iliac crest (Fig. 23.16D).

The patient continued to have pain with weight bearing and no radiographic evidence of healing. Fourteen months later, he underwent a second surgical repair of his femur nonunion. At this procedure, the fibrinous tissue was again resected and the bone ends were trimmed to reveal viable, bleeding bone. The gap was again filled with allograft bone mixed with concentrated autologous bone marrow aspirate. Bone morphogenetic protein-2 was also added to the nonunion site (Fig. 23.16E).

At nearly 5 years postoperatively, the patient was able to bear full weight on his leg and ambulate with a normal gait. Final radiographs are shown in the Figures 23.16F and G. He had full extension and nearly 120° range of motion and had been able to resume riding his motorcycle.

Case 3: Chronic Deep Infection and Loss of Extensor Mechanism Treated with Knee Arthrodesis

This case describes a 39-year-old man who sustained gunshot injuries resulting in an open left distal femoral intra-articular fracture with comminution of the inferior pole of the patella as well. In addition, there was also substantial injury to the patellar tendon itself. He was treated with urgent irrigation, debridement, and open reduction and internal fixation of the fractures as well as patellar tendon repair. Unfortunately, he developed a deep infection requiring serial irrigation, debridement, and antibiotic bead placement over the course of several weeks until the infection was resolved. With the infection under control, the fractures eventually healed at 11 months post-injury although the patient demonstrated minimal extensor function (Figs 23.17A to C).

At this point, he was treated with removal of the implants and partial resection of the lateral heterotopic ossification. Due to the extensive articular surface injury, transarticular heterotopic ossification, and loss of extensor mechanism function, salvage treatment options were considered. The patient could not ambulate comfortably due to his relatively fixed position of flexion and development of more extensive heterotopic ossification (Figs 23.17D and E). At this point,

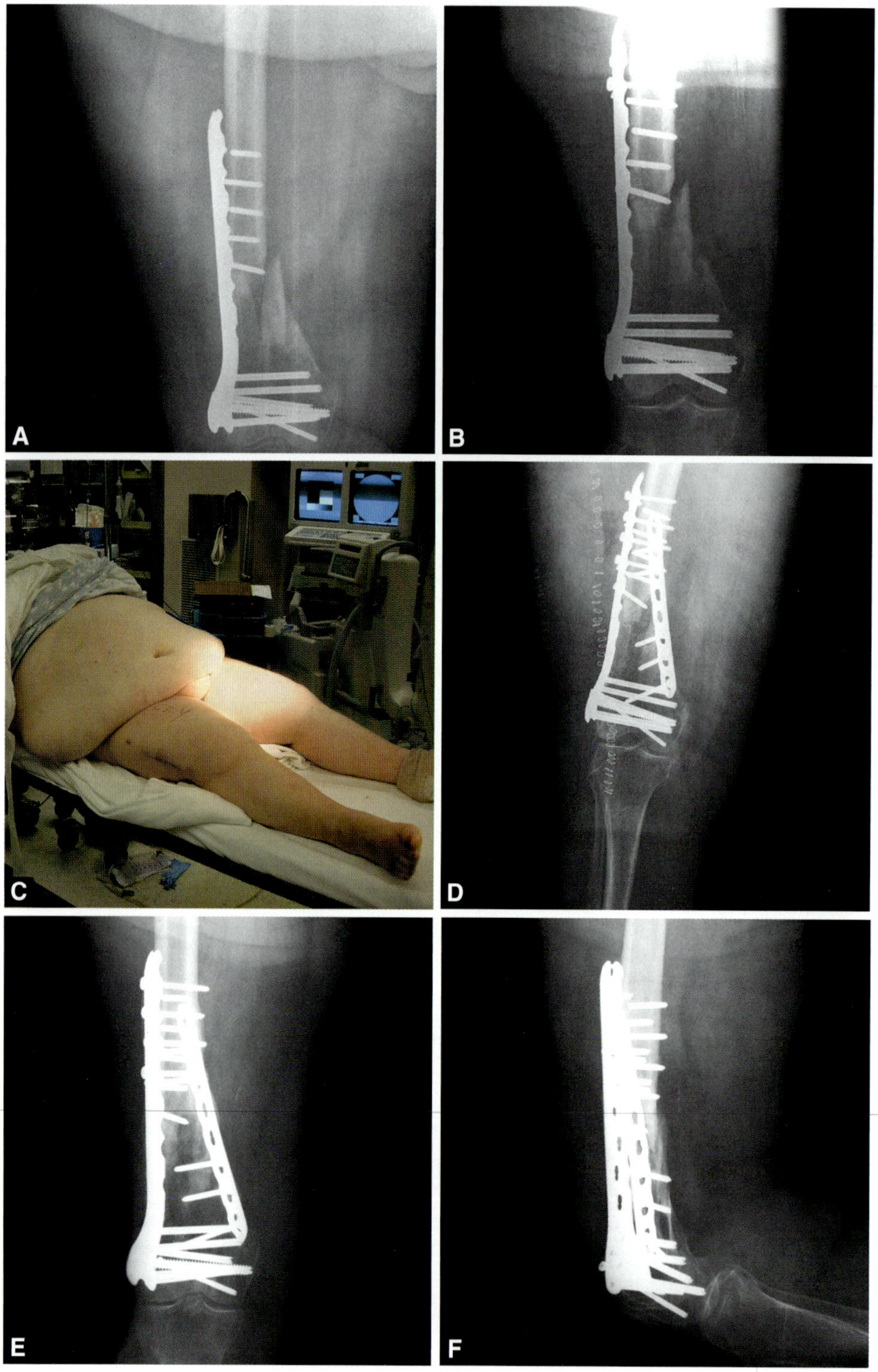

Figures 23.15A to F: A 56-year-old woman with a distal femur nonunion. (A) Anteroposterior X-ray of the distal femur showing a persistent nonunion with loss of fixation at the proximal aspect of the plate due to screw breakage; (B) This X-ray shows addition of a single cortical screw proximally to prevent further pull-off of the plate. Note that the broken screws were not removed from the femur; (C) Clinical photograph at the time of the nonunion repair. Bone morphogenetic protein -2 was utilized instead of iliac crest bone graft due to the large pannus overlying the iliac crest. The incision from the biopsy and single screw insertion can be seen laterally; (D) Anteroposterior X-ray taken postoperatively after the nonunion repair. Note the addition of proximal cortical screws and a medial plate; (E and F) Anteroposterior and lateral knee X-rays showing healing of the nonunion. These X-rays were 21 months after nonunion repair.

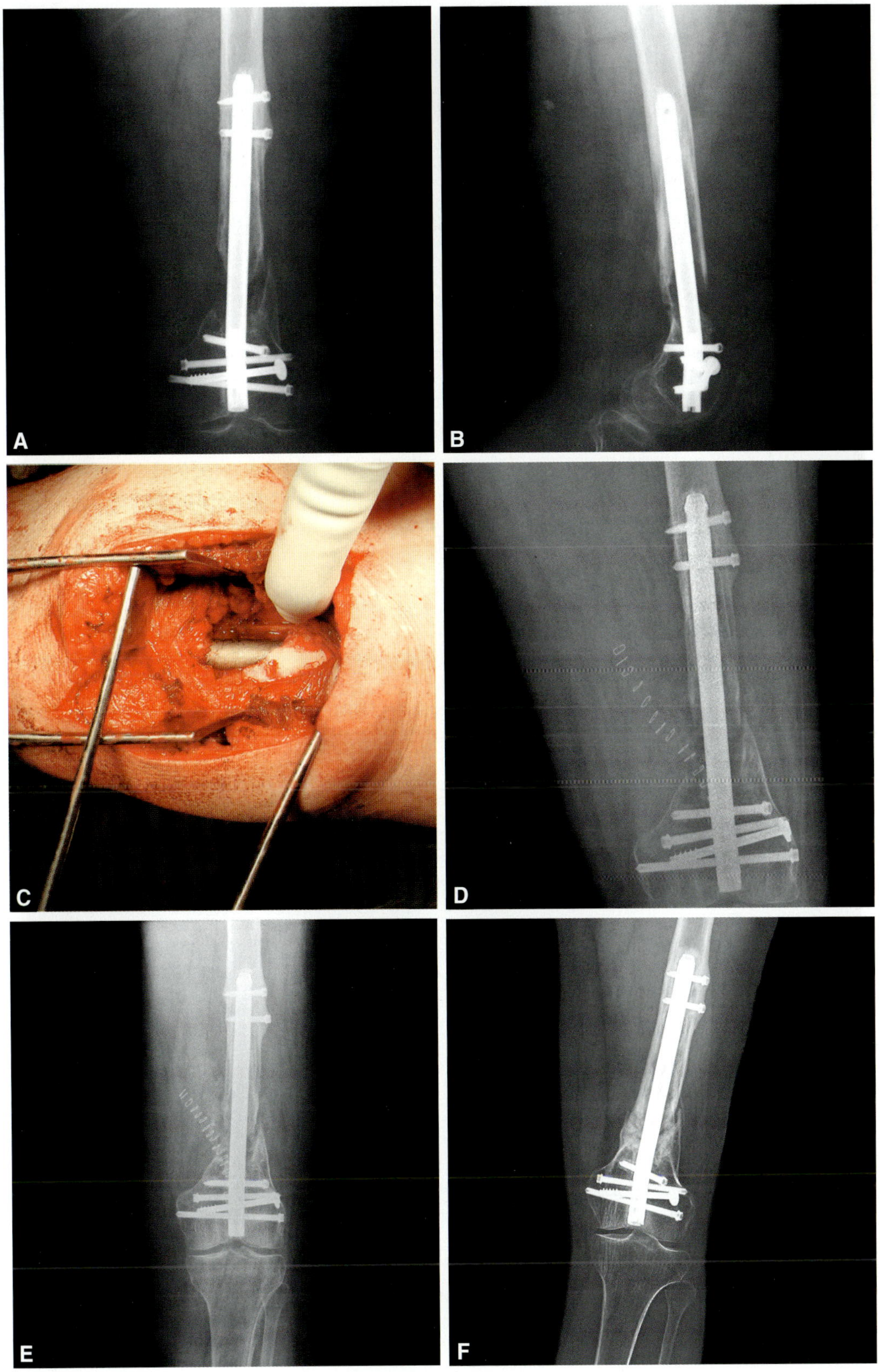

Figures 23.16A to F

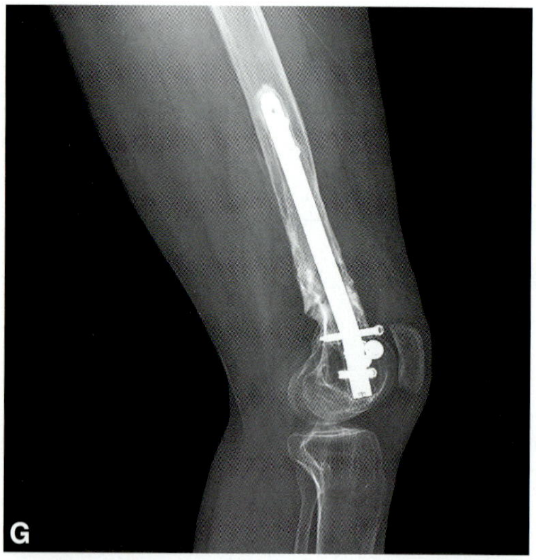

Figures 23.16A to G: A 40-year-old man with a distal femur nonunion. (A and B) Anteroposterior and lateral X-ray showing a stable supracondylar nail and presence of an atrophic nonunion; (C) The bone defect as visualized at the time of the first nonunion repair; (D) Anteroposterior X-ray of the distal femur after nonunion repair with allograft bone and concentrated autograft bone marrow aspirate; (E) Anteroposterior X-ray of the distal femur after repeat nonunion repair with allograft bone, concentrated autograft bone marrow aspirate and bone morphogenetic protein -2. The second nonunion repair was 14 months after the initial nonunion repair; (F and G) Anteroposterior and lateral X-rays of the distal femur showing healing of the nonunion.

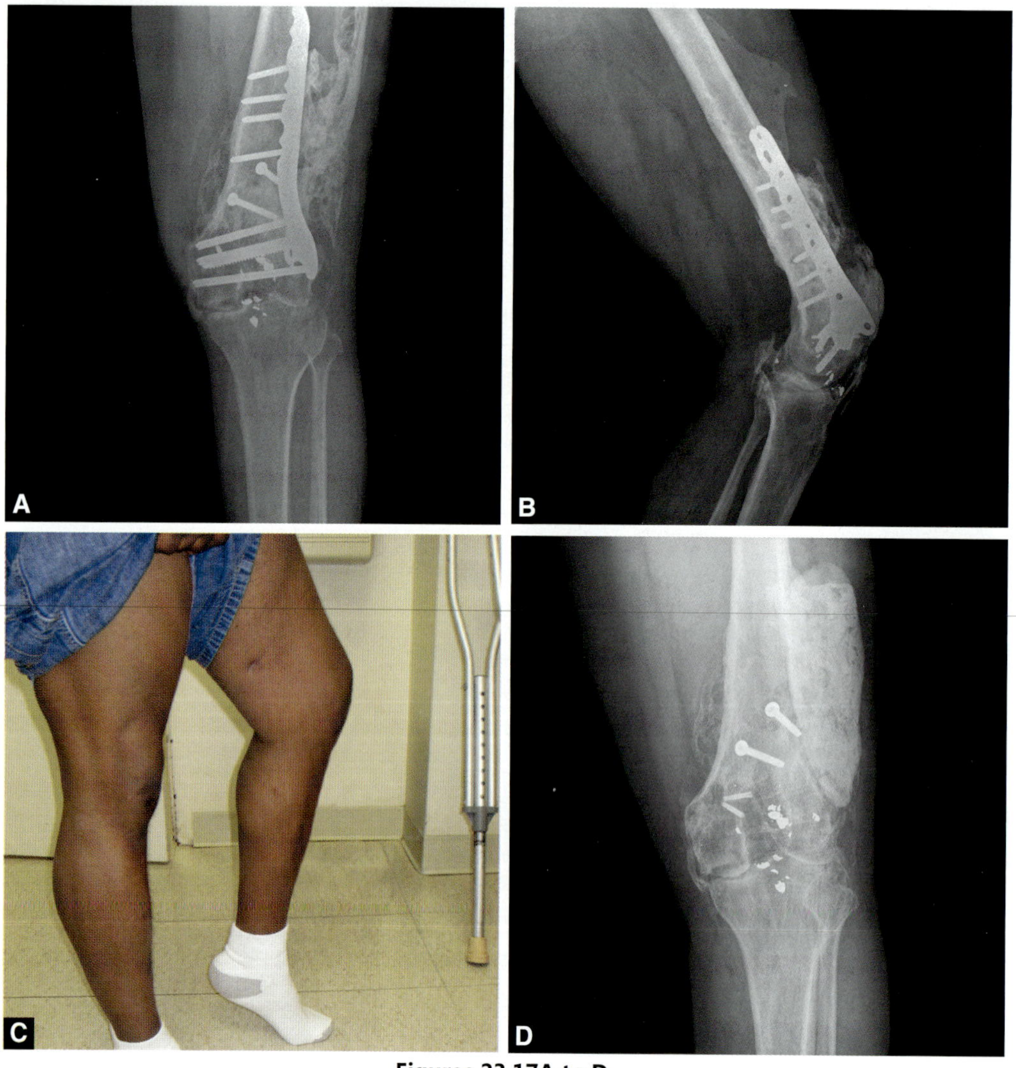

Figures 23.17A to D

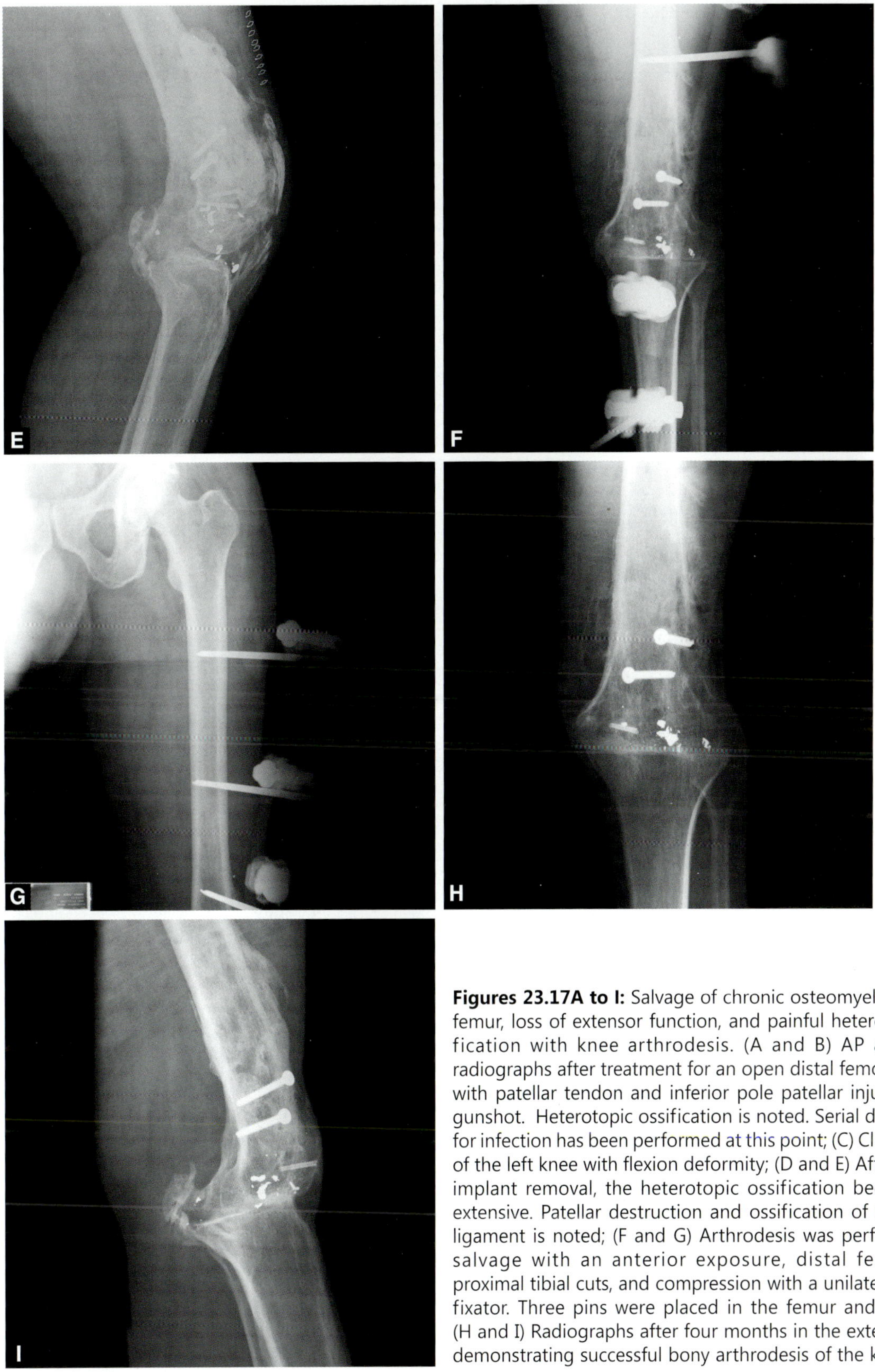

Figures 23.17A to I: Salvage of chronic osteomyelitis of distal femur, loss of extensor function, and painful heterotopic ossification with knee arthrodesis. (A and B) AP and lateral radiographs after treatment for an open distal femoral fracture with patellar tendon and inferior pole patellar injury from an gunshot. Heterotopic ossification is noted. Serial debridement for infection has been performed at this point; (C) Clinical image of the left knee with flexion deformity; (D and E) After eventual implant removal, the heterotopic ossification became more extensive. Patellar destruction and ossification of the patellar ligament is noted; (F and G) Arthrodesis was performed as a salvage with an anterior exposure, distal femoral and proximal tibial cuts, and compression with a unilateral external fixator. Three pins were placed in the femur and tibia each; (H and I) Radiographs after four months in the external fixator demonstrating successful bony arthrodesis of the knee.

he did not have any recurrence of his infection. But with his history of infection and age, total knee arthroplasty was not considered the optimal treatment for him although it was discussed with the patient. We felt that although not performed often, his case was an indication for knee arthrodesis. This would allow him to ambulate with his foot flat on the ground, provide pain relief, and would provide a more durable result with less chance of infection recurrence than total knee arthroplasty. Given his history of infection, arthrodesis with external fixation rather than internal fixation was chosen. Simple transverse distal femoral and proximal tibial cuts were made through an anterior incision, bony apposition was achieved, and external fixation was performed (Figs 23.17F and G). External fixation was maintained for four months and then removed. At this point, bony fusion was achieved and he was able to ambulate with minimal discomfort (Figs 23.17H and I).

The key points of this case are the following:

- Preservation of extensor mechanism function is extremely critical to knee function. Although extensor function loss in this case was one of many factors leading to a decision for fusion, it was a main factor.
- Although knee fusion in most cases is not an acceptable treatment option for the vast majority of cases, it should be considered for the treatment of chronic infection of a non-functioning, painful stiff knee with loss of extensor function.
- External fixation is an excellent option for arthrodesis in the setting of chronic osteomyelitis. This avoids potentiating an infection recurrence which would be more likely with the use of internal fixation devices.

Summary

Distal femur fractures are generally treated surgically to prevent complications of malunion and prolonged recumbency. Surgical fixation has been shown to lead to good long-term results. Many of these patients develop radiographic signs of moderate to severe osteoarthritis, though they may still have good to excellent clinical results. Common complications include nonunion, malunion, loss of range of motion and posttraumatic arthritis. While the incidence of complications can be reduced by proper surgical planning and technique, these remain challenging fractures for the surgeons. Surgeons should be prepared to deal with the complications of these injuries, if they arise and strive for durable long-term results.

References

1. Court-Brown CM, Caesar B. Epidemiology of adult fractures: a review. Injury. 2006;37(8):691-7.
2. Martinet O, Cordey J, Harder Y, et al. The epidemiology of fractures of the distal femur. Injury. 2000;31(Suppl 3): C62-3.
3. Schmidt AH, Teague DC. Orthopaedic Knowledge Update: Trauma 4, 1st edition. Rosemont, Illinois: American Academy of Orthopaedic Surgeons; 2010.
4. Butt MS, Krikler SJ, Ali MS. Displaced fractures of the distal femur in elderly patients. Operative versus non-operative treatment. J Bone Joint Surg Br. 1996;78(1):110-4.
5. Browner BD, Jupiter JB, Levine AM, et al. Skeletal Trauma; 4th edition. Philadelphia, PA: Saunders Elsevier; 2009.
6. Forster MC, Komarsamy B, Davison JN. Distal femoral fractures: a review of fixation methods. Injury. 2006; 37(2):97-108.
7. Mills WJ, Barei DP, McNair P. The value of the ankle-brachial index for diagnosing arterial injury after knee dislocation: a prospective study. J Trauma. 2004;56(6):1261-5.
8. Marsh JL, Slongo TF, Agel J, et al. Fracture and dislocation classification compendium—2007: Orthopaedic Trauma Association classification, database and outcomes committee. J Orthop Trauma. 2007;21(10 Suppl):S1-133.
9. Stover M. Distal femoral fractures: current treatment, results and problems. Injury. 2001;32(Suppl 3):SC3-13.
10. Zlowodzki M, Bhandari M, Marek DJ, et al. Operative treatment of acute distal femur fractures: systematic review of 2 comparative studies and 45 case series (1989 to 2005). J Orthop Trauma. 2006;20(5):366-71.
11. Rosen AL, Strauss E. Primary total knee arthroplasty for complex distal femur fractures in elderly patients. Clin Orthop Relat Res. 2004;(425):101-5.
12. Haidukewych GJ, Springer BD, Jacofsky DJ, et al. Total knee arthroplasty for salvage of failed internal fixation or nonunion of the distal femur. J Arthroplasty. 2005;20(3): 344-9.
13. Holmes SM, Bomback D, Baumgaertner MR. Coronal fractures of the femoral condyle: a brief report of five cases. J Orthop Trauma. 2004;18(5):316-9.
14. Rademakers MV, Kerkhoffs GM, Sierevelt IN, et al. Intra-articular fractures of the distal femur: a long-term follow-up study of surgically treated patients. J Orthop Trauma. 2004;18(4):213-9.

15. Moore TJ, Watson T, Green SA, et al. Complications of surgically treated supracondylar fractures of the femur. J Trauma. 1987;27(4):402-6.
16. Masse A, Biasibetti A, Demangos J, et al. The judet quadricepsplasty: Long-term outcome of 21 cases. J Trauma. 2006;61(2):358-62.
17. Wang JH, Zhao JZ, He YH. A new treatment strategy for severe arthrofibrosis of the knee. A review of twenty-two cases. J Bone Joint Surg Am. 2006;88(6):1245-50.
18. Henderson CE, Kuhl LL, Fitzpatrick DC, et al. Locking plates for distal femur fractures: is there a problem with fracture healing? J Orthop Trauma. 2011;25(Suppl 1):S8-14.
19. Gardner MJ, Toro-Arbelaez JB, Harrison M, et al. Open reduction and internal fixation of distal femoral nonunions: long-term functional outcomes following a treatment protocol. J Trauma. 2008;64(2):434-8.
20. Bellabarba C, Ricci WM, Bolhofner BR. Indirect reduction and plating of distal femoral nonunions. J Orthop Trauma. 2002;16(5):287-96.
21. Wang JW, Weng LH. Treatment of distal femoral nonunion with internal fixation, cortical allograft struts, and autogenous bone-grafting. J Bone Joint Surg Am. 2003; 85-A(3):436-40.
22. Yoshida A, Yajima H, Murata K, et al. Pedicled vascularized bone graft from the medial supracondylar region of the femur for treatment of femur nonunion. J Reconstr Microsurg. 2009;25(3):165-70.
23. Kabata T, Tsuchiya H, Sakurakichi K, et al. Reconstruction with distraction osteogenesis for juxta-articular nonunions with bone loss. J Trauma. 2005;58(6):1213-22.
24. Sanders R, Swiontkowski M, Rosen H, et al. Double-plating of comminuted, unstable fractures of the distal part of the femur. J Bone Joint Surg Am. 1991;73(3):341-6.
25. Schutz M, Muller M, Regazzoni P, et al. Use of the less invasive stabilization system (LISS) in patients with distal femoral (AO33) fractures: a prospective multicenter study. Arch Orthop Trauma Surg. 2005;125(2):102-8.
26. Wu CC. Femoral supracondylar malunions with varus medial condyle and shortening. Clin Orthop Relat Res. 2007;456:226-32.
27. Gugenheim JJ Jr, Brinker MR. Bone realignment with use of temporary external fixation for distal femoral valgus and varus deformities. J Bone Joint Surg Am. 2003;85-A(7): 1229-37.
28. Stahelin T, Hardegger F, Ward JC. Supracondylar osteotomy of the femur with use of compression. Osteosynthesis with a malleable implant. J Bone Joint Surg Am. 2000;82(5): 712-22.
29. Rogers MJ, McFadyen I, Livingstone JA, et al. Computer hexapod assisted orthopaedic surgery (CHAOS) in the correction of long bone fracture and deformity. J Orthop Trauma. 2007;21(5):337-42.
30. Paley D, Tetsworth K. Mechanical axis deviation of the lower limbs. Preoperative planning of uniapical angular deformities of the tibia or femur. Clin Orthop Relat Res. 1992;(280):48-64.

Chapter 24

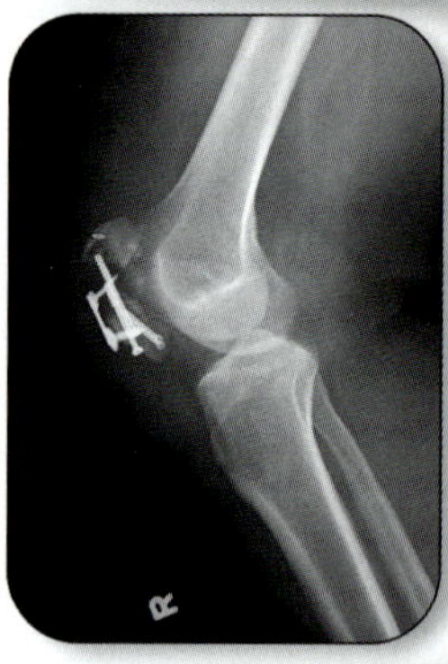

Patellar Fractures

Peter Krause, Melissa Gorman, Barton Wax

Chapter Outline

Introduction
Diagnosis
Classification
Surgical Indications
Surgical Anatomy, Positioning and Approaches
Surgical Techniques
- Tension Band Technique
- Partial Patellectomy

Outcomes
Complications
- Infection
- Loss of Reduction
- Hardware Irritation
- Nonunion
- Knee Stiffness
- Arthritis

Authors' Preferred Management of Select Complications
- Case 1: Hardware Failure–Revision Fixation
- Case 2: Hardware Failure–Partial or Total Patellectomy
- Case 3: Knee Stiffness

Summary

Introduction

Patella fractures, in isolation, make up a very small proportion of lower extremity fractures, occurring most commonly as a consequence of a direct blow to the knee. These injuries often occur in older patients with osteoporosis and medical comorbidities. Less often, patella fractures may occur in the setting of a high-energy collision injury such as a motor vehicle accident. These high-energy patella fractures are often open and frequently associated with other injuries, such as ipsilateral femur or acetabular fractures.[1,2] Displaced transverse or comminuted fractures of the patella imply a disruption of the extensor mechanism, and are usually treated operatively.

With our aging population, patella fractures may also occur as periprosthetic fractures after knee arthroplasty and may pose a challenge to reconstruction due to implants and loss of bone stock. Rarely, patella fractures may occur after anterior cruciate ligament graft harvest,[3] as osteochondral fractures after patellar dislocation, and as stress fractures.

Diagnosis

A thorough history and physical examination are always necessary for the evaluation of a patella fracture. Patients will often complain of an inability to extend the knee along with pain, swelling, and loss of strength. Injury mechanisms

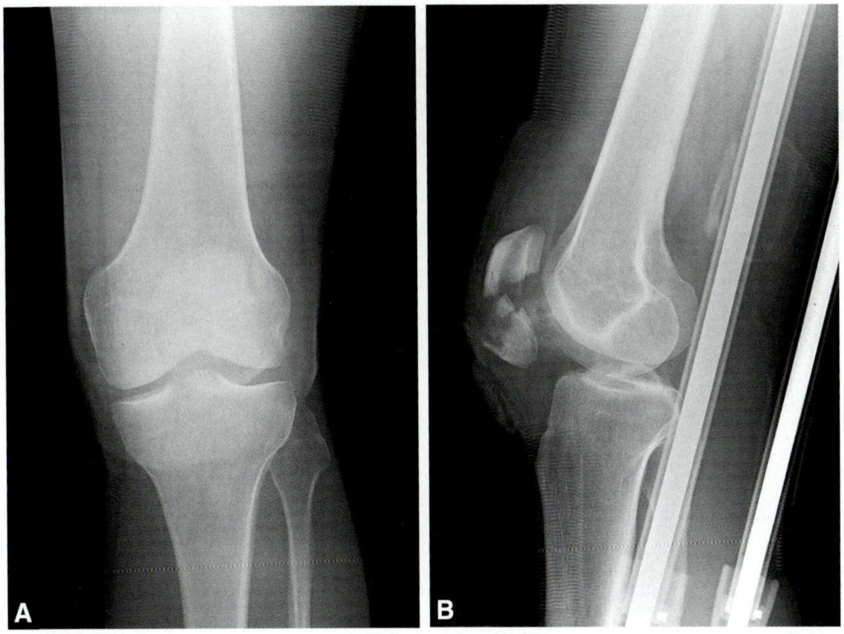

Figures 24.1A and B: Anteroposterior and lateral radiographs of a patella fracture.

can be either direct or indirect trauma. Direct trauma will most often result from a fall, while indirect trauma often takes the form of an eccentric quadriceps contraction.

Physical examination findings include tenderness over the patella or extensor mechanism, a palpable defect, or frank separation of fracture fragments. Extensor mechanism weakness is often present, but is not necessary for the diagnosis of a patellar fracture. Skin should be examined to ensure that no open fracture is present. A saline load test may be performed to rule out an open knee joint. This test can be combined with an arthrocentesis for pain relief. Lack of extensor mechanism function implies rupture of both the medial and lateral retinaculum. The ability to extend against gravity signifies continuity of the extensor mechanism, but does not necessarily preclude patellar fracture.

Radiographic evaluation should include anteroposterior (AP) and lateral views, but a sunrise view can be helpful if the diagnosis is not apparent. Figures 24.1A and B show a typical moderately comminuted mid-distal patella fracture. Comparison views of the unaffected limb can be obtained in the face of severe loss of native anatomy, which can aid in preoperative planning to restore appropriate patellar height. Computed tomography or magnetic resonance imaging is rarely necessary. A bipartite patella can be mistaken for an acute fracture, but careful history taking will often help to separate this entity from acute traumatic injuries. A bipartite patella is often bilateral and the fragment is usually superior lateral and well corticated. Figures 24.2A to H show a typical bipartite patella which also has a transverse patella fracture.

PATELLAR FRACTURES DIAGNOSIS: Pearls and Pitfalls

- Usually, the history and physical examination and anteroposterior and lateral X-ray are sufficient for diagnosis
- Be vigilant for patellar fractures in association with ipsilateral acetabular, femur and tibia fractures
- A congenital bipartite patella may be mistaken for a fracture. Look for smooth as opposed to sharp edges

Classification

Classification of patellar fractures is mainly descriptive in nature. Fractures are described as either displaced or nondisplaced and characterized by location and pattern. Patella fractures have been classified in the Orthopaedic Trauma Association's alpha-numeric compendium of fractures, but this classification has no prognostic significance.

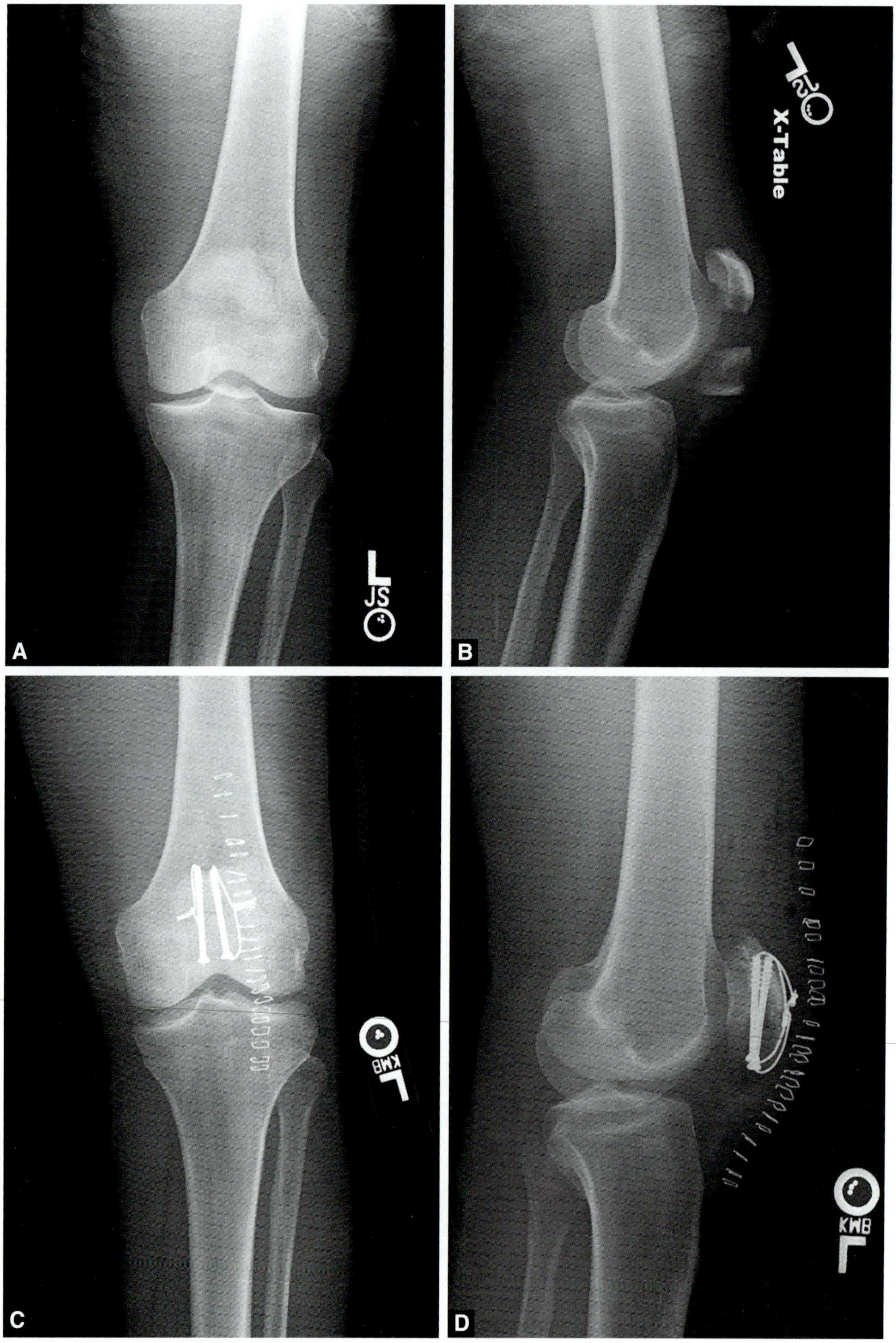

Figures 24.2A to D

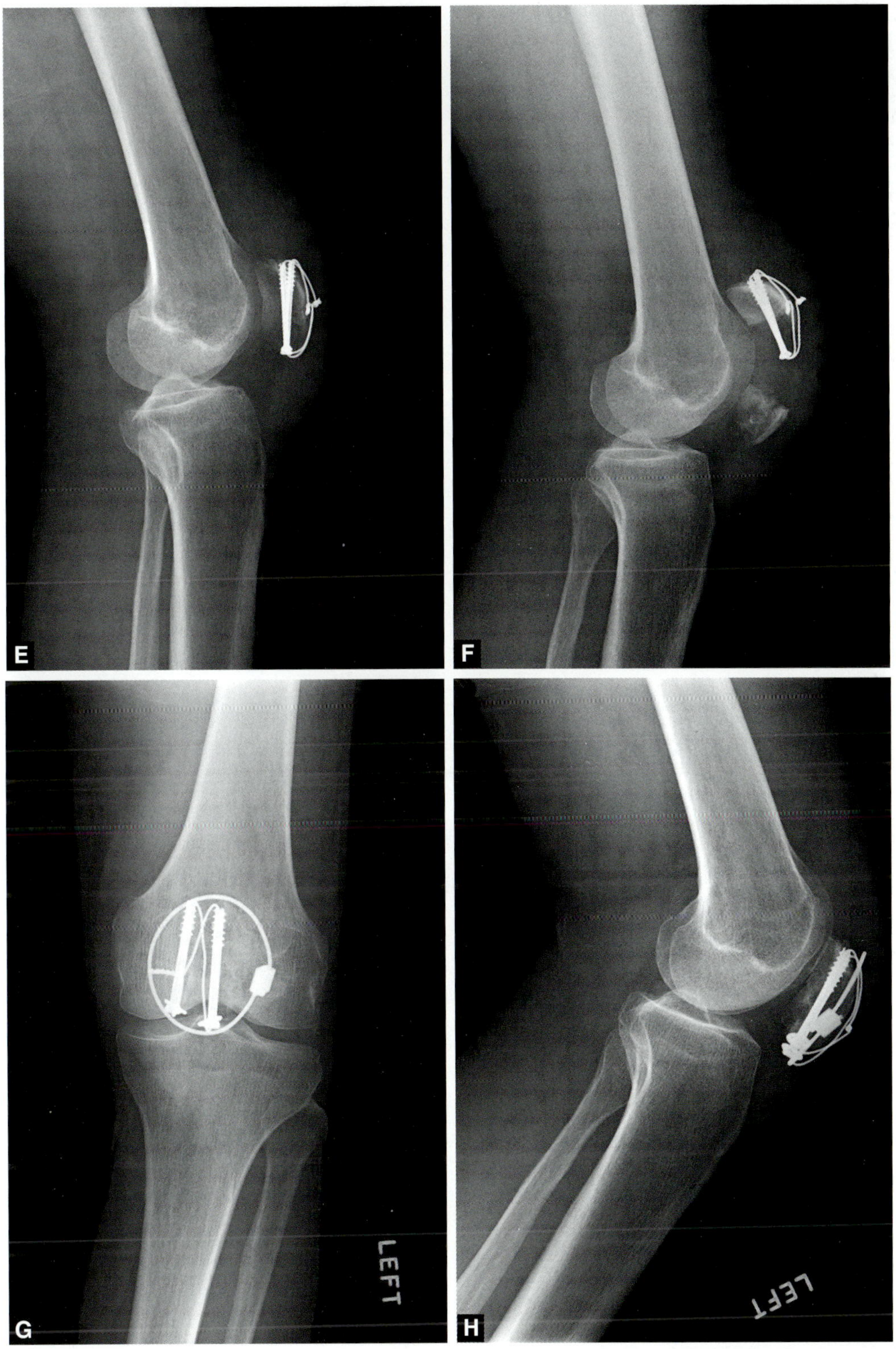

Figures 24.2A to H: Salvage of hardware failure with revision fixation. (A and B) Injury radiographs show a typical fracture with incidental bipartite patella; (C and D) Immediate postoperative radiographs show satisfactory reduction and fixation although two single loops of wire instead of a figure-of-eight were used. This construct may be more prone to failure; (E) Fracture appears to have healed uneventfully at 2 months follow-up; (F) A second fall at 5 months lead to dramatic failure; (G and H) Revision fixation with larger cannulated screws, figure-of-eight wire and supplemental cerclage cable goes on to complete healing.

Commonly used fracture pattern descriptors include transverse, vertical, stellate or comminuted. Location may be described as proximal, distal or osteochondral. Patellar fractures in the setting of knee arthroplasty are described as periprosthetic.

Surgical Indications

Indications for nonoperative management of patella fractures include vertical nondisplaced fractures and nondisplaced transverse fractures. Typically, patella fractures can be treated nonoperatively in a knee immobilizer or long leg cast, as long as the extensor mechanism remains intact. The patient must be able to perform a straight leg raise (maintain active extension against gravity). This can sometimes be difficult to determine secondary to the pain that occurs with the injury. Consideration may be given to inject local anesthetic intra-articularly in order to alleviate the pain to allow patients to demonstrate their ability to perform the straight leg raise.

It is important to remember that displaced transverse patella fractures are far more likely to involve the extensor mechanism than non- or minimally displaced vertical fractures. As with other intra-articular fractures, articular congruity must also be intact with less than 2 mm of articular step off. The primary complication of nonoperative treatment of patella fractures is knee stiffness.

Nonoperative treatment typically consists of bracing or casting for a period of 4–6 weeks. The patient is allowed to weight bear as tolerated on the extended extremity. At that time, if radiographs demonstrate healing and clinical exam is improved, the patient may then begin progressive range of motion exercises. Typically, this is gradual, beginning at 30° of flexion and advancing to 20–30° a week until full motion is obtained while protecting the knee in a hinged knee brace.

Indications for surgical treatment of displaced patella fractures are similar to the treatment of all other displaced articular fractures. The patella has a large chondral surface, and fractures that are displaced greater than 2 mm should be reduced operatively. All patellar fractures that disrupt the extensor mechanism also require operative intervention, regardless of the amount of displacement. Surgical intervention for patella fractures should also be considered when associated with other fractures about the knee (tibial plateau fractures, supracondylar femur fractures) in order to allow earlier knee motion and rehabilitation. Open fractures also warrant surgical debridement as is the case with most of the open fractures.

There are primarily two operative approaches to patella fractures: open reduction and internal fixation (ORIF) versus a partial or total patellectomy. Open reduction is most appropriate when the fracture fragments are large with minimal comminution. Partial patellectomy is typically considered when a portion of the patella is so comminuted or a fragment is so small that a more secure repair can be obtained by reattaching either the patellar or quadriceps tendon to the remaining patella rather than repairing the fracture. This often allows the patient to rehab more rapidly as there is less concern for loss of fixation. Finally, as a salvage procedure, a total patellectomy can be considered, but should be a surgery of last resort.

Surgical Anatomy, Positioning and Approaches

The patella is the largest sesamoid bone in the body, lying encased in the quadriceps tendon. It is the central portion of the extensor mechanism which consists of the four quadriceps muscles; the patella, the patella tendon, the retinaculum and the tibial tuberosity. The skin overlying the knee is extensively mobile, allowing the knee to flex to greater than 120° without putting undo stress on the skin. The superior three quarters of the surface of the patella consist of articular cartilage with the inferior one quarter being extra-articular. The medial and lateral facets can be divided into superior, middle and inferior portions, with the odd facet located on the most medial edge.[4] The patella articulates in the groove on the anterior aspect of the femur throughout the entirety of the knee range of motion. Contact stresses are the greatest in the patellofemoral joint at 90° of flexion[5] and mechanically, the moment arm of extension of the quadriceps is increased by as much as 50% by the patella.[6]

The blood supply to the patella is very complex. A vascular plexus surrounds the patella receiving contributions from 6 different arteries. These include the supreme geniculate artery that branches from the superficial femoral artery, the four geniculate arteries from the popliteal artery and the recurrent anterior tibial artery.[7] Typically, this increased vascularity ensures adequate blood supply to all fragments, even in significantly comminuted fractures.

Positioning for operative intervention is the same regardless of the treatment chosen. The patient is placed supine on a radiolucent operative table. Care must be taken to assure that appropriate AP and lateral fluoroscopic views can be attained. A small bump is then placed underneath the hip of the operative side, allowing the patella to point directly toward the ceiling. A well-padded tourniquet may be used if the surgeon prefers, although the tourniquet should be placed high on the thigh to ensure that it remains outside the operative field. If a tourniquet is used, the limb is exsanguinated after the limb has been appropriately prepped and draped. The knee is then flexed to advance the patella, although this may be ineffective and the tourniquet is inflated. A vertical incision is then made centered over the patella from slightly above the proximal pole of the patella to the tibial tubercle. In open fractures, the traumatic wound should be incorporated into this wound. As the patella lies subcutaneously, the fractured patella is then easily exposed as dissection is taken down sharply with a scalpel. Proximally, the incision is carried down to the quadriceps tendon and distally to the patellar tendon. The entire expanse of the quadriceps tendon, patellar tendon and patella should be visualized. The medial and lateral retinaculum should then be exposed to determine the extent that they are disrupted. The traumatic disruption of the retinaculum can be extended in order to expose the fracture on either or both sides. This can be done with a vertical incision in the retinaculum, creating a T-type wound. This allows the greatest visibility of the articular surface of the patella. Then the surgeon can proceed with the definitive approach for fixation.

Surgical Techniques

Tension Band Technique

Instrumentation and Implant Consideration

Patella fractures are typically repaired with some combination of a tension band construct, interfragmentary screws and cerclage wire. The construct depends on the fracture pattern. Transverse fractures are most successfully treated with a tension band construct, while more comminuted fractures may be the best treated by leaving the 'bag of bones' intact and using a cerclage wire. All of these options should be available when treating a patella fracture operatively. Typically, small and mini-fragment sets, 4.0 mm and 4.5 mm cannulated screw sets, Kirschner wires (K-wires), 18 gauge wire and cables should be available. Reduction instruments should include small and large bone clamps. Intraoperative C-arm should be available.

Surgical Approach

Surgical approach is as listed above, with a midline incision extending from above the proximal pole of the patella to the tibial tuberosity. Once the medial and lateral retinaculum have been exposed, the fracture fragments are then identified. Care must be taken to fully clean the surfaces of all debris and hematoma. The knee joint should also be thoroughly irrigated to ensure removal of any loose fracture fragments and loose articular cartilage. The articular surface of the fragments should be inspected by gently displacing the fracture fragments. The articular surface of the distal femur should also be examined, as any disruption here may also be treated through this approach if necessary. If any free osteochondral fragments are found on the undersurface of the patella, these should be either excised or stabilized.

Fracture Reduction Techniques

Next, attention is directed to reduction of the articular surface. Larger osteochondral fragments should be maintained, while very small fragments can be excised and discarded. Rigid stabilization of all free osteochondral fragments is imperative to prevent displacement during postoperative knee motion. Small or mini-fragment screws can be used if necessary. Once the joint has been adequately irrigated, the larger articular surface pieces should be reduced. This is typically accomplished with the use of either one or two pointed reduction clamps. A finger can be placed through the retinacular incision to feel the articular reduction. The anterior cortical reduction is important but the articular reduction is critical for a good outcome. At this time fluoroscopy should be used to verify reduction prior to fixation.

Using guidewires from the 4.0 mm cannulated screw system, two guidewires are then placed parallel to each

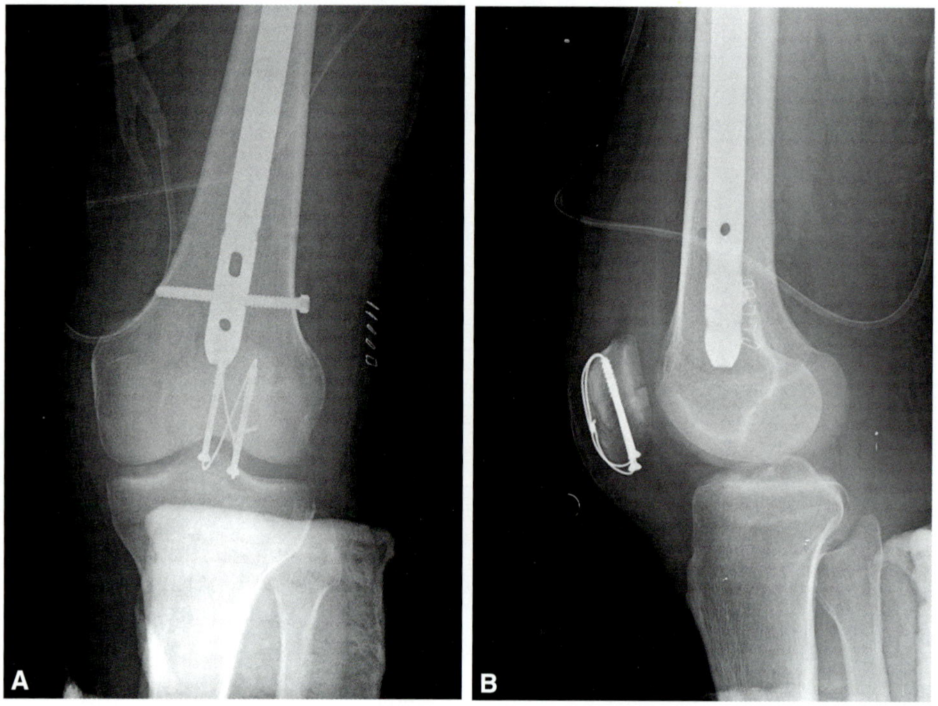

Figures 24.3A and B: Typical figure-of-eight fixation through cannulated screws.

other (one at the junction of the medial and middle one-third of the patella and the second at the junction of the lateral and middle one-third of the patella), parallel to the joint surface and as close to it as possible to engage harder bone. Typically, these are placed from inferior to superior, but they can also be placed from superior to inferior. The guidewires are left short of the second cortex and measurements are taken. It is important to measure short of the far cortex, as the screws should not penetrate out of the far cortex of the patella. The wires are then driven out of the patella and brought up out of the quadriceps tendon. The patella is then drilled, and the appropriate length 4.0 mm partially threaded cancellous screws are then placed. Figures 24.3A and B show a typical construct.

The screws are left short for placement of the tension band wire. If they are allowed to penetrate the far cortex, they run the risk of cutting the tension band wire. Figure 24.4 shows screws placed too long. The best way to determine exact length of the screws is by directly visualizing the tip of the guidewire to ensure that it is the right length and then subtracting several millimeters. Fluoroscopy is not a reliable way to make this measurement. An 18 gauge wire is then placed through the cannulated screws in a figure-of-eight fashion and tensioned. Two separate wires can be placed in

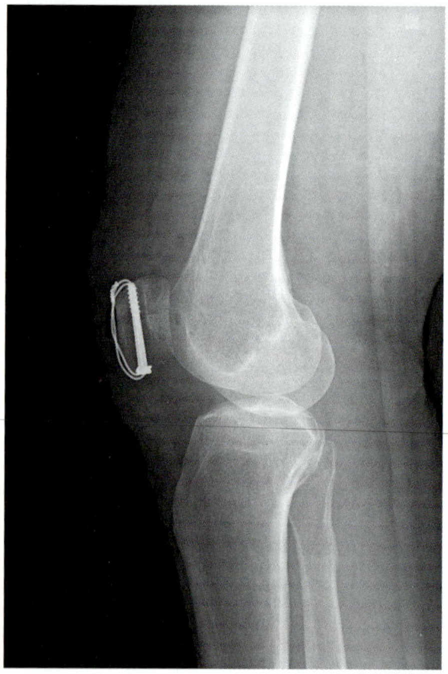

Figure 24.4: Proximal pole fractures pose a dilemma. Screws that are too short may leave threads across the fracture site preventing compression. Screws that are too long may cause the wire to be tensioned against the sharp cutting edge of the screw. In this case the screws were left slightly too long which was felt to be the best compromise with the equipment available. Healing was uneventful.

a parallel fashion; however, the surgeons prefer a single wire because a wire in-line with a screw appears more likely to fail by cutting through the patella (Figs 24.2A to H). The wire is then cut and bent laterally and impacted into the bony surface of the patella. The wire should not be impacted inferiorly secondary to a risk of irritating or lacerating the patellar tendon. Fluoroscopy is then brought in to confirm reduction and hardware placement. The knee should be taken through a gentle range of motion to determine at what degree of flexion stress is placed on the repair.

Although in our practice this is seldom done, K-wires can be used in place of the cannulated screws. Two 2.0 mm K-wires are positioned in the same place as the guidewires from the cannulated screw technique above. The ends must be left long in order to accommodate a tension band wire. The 18 gauge wire is then passed along the anterior surface of that patella in a figure-of-eight and then passed behind the K-wires. Care should be taken to assure that no soft tissue intervenes between the wire and the patella. Once the wire is tensioned, the K-wires should be bent and impacted onto the superior surface of the patella, making sure that the cerclage does not slip anterior to the K-wires (Figs 24.5A to D).

In cases of delayed presentation, additional reduction measures may be required and additional fixation measures should be considered to prevent loss of reduction. With a delayed presentation, the quadriceps may require release from the femur and intraoperative traction of the proximal fragment may be utilized to slowly stretch the quadriceps contracture to permit the patellar fragments to reduce (Figs 24.6A to F). Again, the knee should be taken through a gentle range of motion prior to closure.

Closure

Once final fluoroscopic images are taken to ensure reduction and placement of the hardware, the knee should be copiously irrigated with normal saline. The medial and lateral retinaculum is then closed with #1 Vicryl or 0 Vicryl suture. The extensor retinaculum should then be repaired over the hardware. The skin is closed in an interrupted fashion with a subcutaneous suture, followed by staples. Sterile dressings are then placed and the patient is placed into a hinged knee brace locked in full extension.

Rehabilitation

The patient may weight bear as tolerated with the knee in full extension. At the 2-week mark, the patient may begin range of motion exercises in a hinged knee brace. Typically, the patient is initially limited to 45° of flexion and advances range of motion 10–15° every week until full range of motion is accomplished. In reliable patients with a good soft tissue envelope, the surgeons begin short arc range of motion within the first week and advance 10–15° per week. The surgeons' goal is to be at 90° by 4 weeks, although this program may be modified based on the degree of stability obtained intraoperatively. Typically, resistive exercises and gentle weight lifting can begin at 12 weeks postoperatively. The patient is followed in clinic until the fracture heals, the patient has good extension strength and the patient is walking without an assistive device.

TENSION BAND TECHNIQUE: Pearls and Pitfalls

- The retinacular tears can be extended to allow further exposure. One must visualize or palpate the articular surface through the retinacular tear to ensure adequate reduction
- When using cannulated screws, it is imperative to ensure that the screw tips do not extend beyond the patella to avoid cutting of the tension band wire by the sharp screw threads
- Cannulated screws should be directed parallel to and as close to the articular surface as possible to engage harder bone.

Partial Patellectomy

Instrumentation and Implant Considerations

One should be prepared to perform a partial patellectomy whenever approaching a patella fracture. Often the articular surface is much more comminuted than appreciated on initial X-rays. Equipment needed for a partial patellectomy includes a small fragment drill bit (2.5 mm or 2.0 mm), a suture passer and some large sized suture. The surgeons prefer #2 Ethibond suture but equivalents can be used.

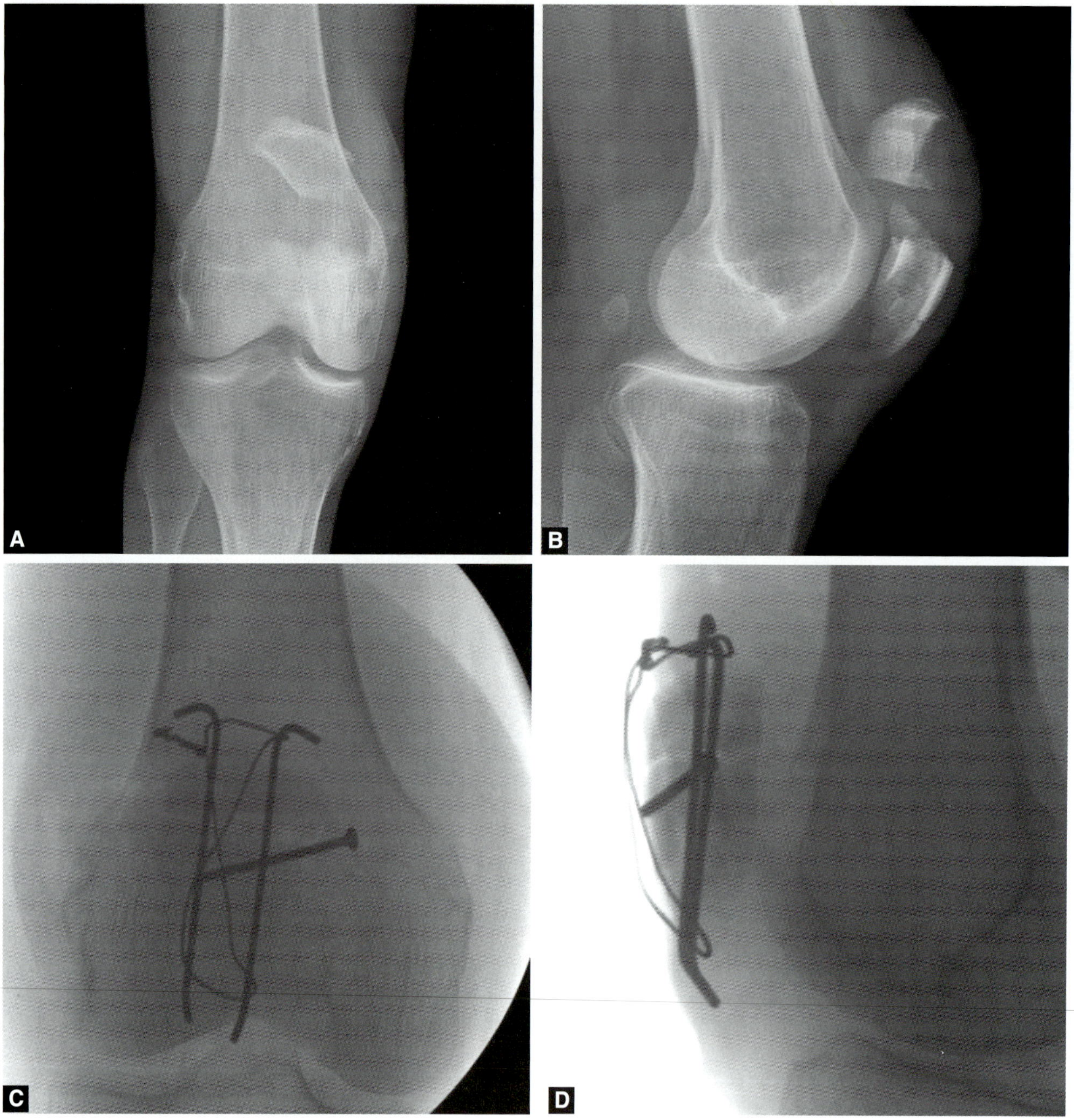

Figures 24.5A to D: Fixation with tension band wiring. (A and B) AP and lateral images of a transverse patella fracture with slight comminution; (C and D) This was treated with open reduction, lag screw fixation of the smaller fragment, then compression with a tension band wire technique.

Surgical Approach

The surgical approach is unchanged from that listed above.

Fracture Reduction Techniques

Once the patella is adequately exposed, the fracture fragments should be identified. Although it is typically the

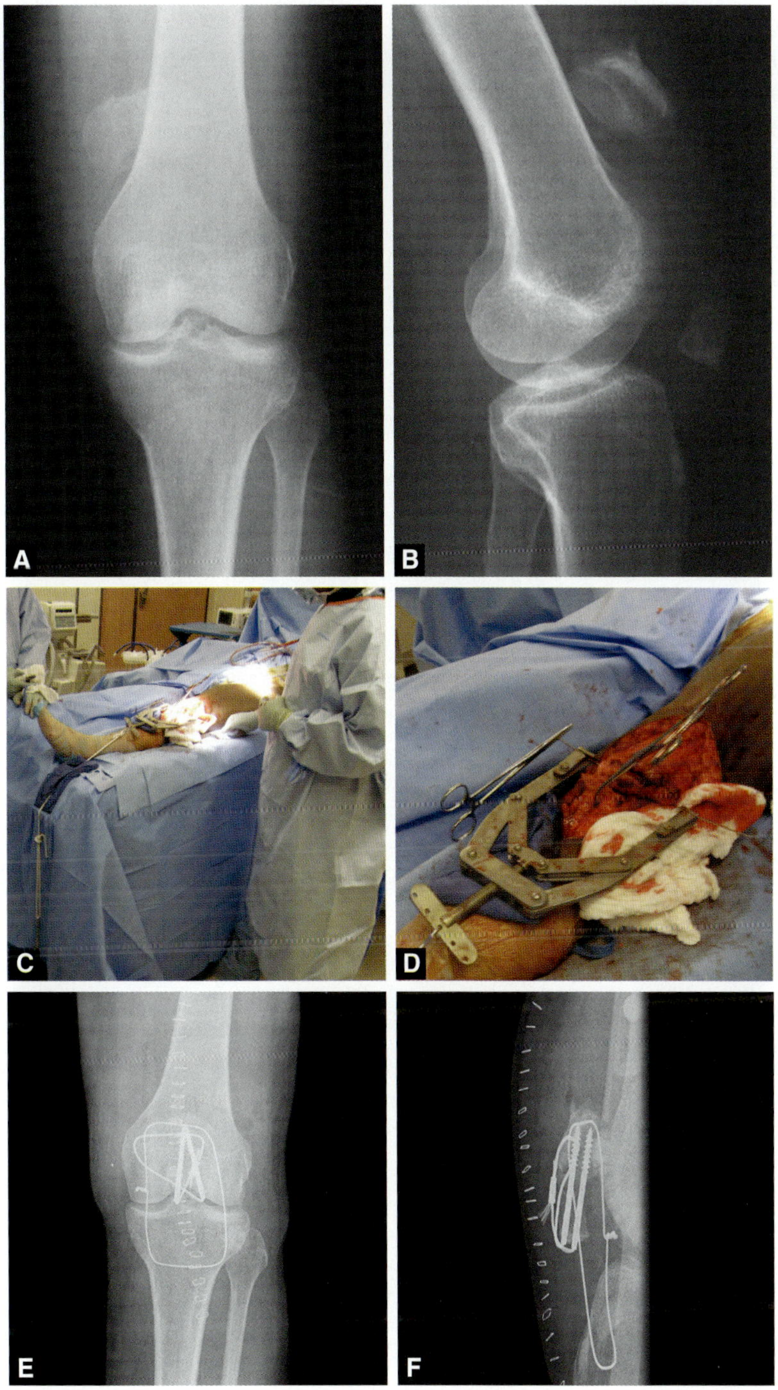

Figures 24.6A to F: Use of intraoperative traction for reduction in fractures with delayed presentation. (A and B) Anteroposterior and lateral radiographs demonstrate a widely displaced patellar fracture presenting 3 months after initial injury. This was treated with wide exposure, removal of intervening scar tissues, elevation of the quadriceps muscle from the distal femur and open reduction and internal fixation; (C and D) Due to the development of contracture of the quadriceps, standard reduction forceps were insufficient to reduce the fragments. Quadriceps lengthening could be performed but can lead to an extensor lag. In this case, intraoperative traction is demonstrated in these photos. A Kirschner pin is placed transversely in the proximal fragment and tensioned with a Kirschner bow attached to traction as shown; (E and F) Intraoperative images demonstrate reduction and fixation with a partially threaded cable-pin device (Zimmer, Warsaw, IN, USA) and protected with a wire from the superior patella to the proximal tibia. Anatomic reduction could not be achieved, although there was satisfactory bony contact. The wire was removed by 3 months with the patient having achieved 90° of flexion by this point and the fracture apparently healing.

Courtesy: Saqib Rehman

inferior pole that is comminuted and excised, the superior pole can be resected as well depending on the presenting injury pattern. The injured pole of the patella is then excised from the adjacent tendon, as well as any other comminuted fragments of the patella. Saltzman et al. have demonstrated that there does not seem to be any correlation between outcome and the size of the remaining patella.[8]

Therefore, the largest fragment of the patella should be retained for repair. When enucleating the damaged pole, care should be taken to preserve the tendon as much as possible.

Next, the borders of the tendon (either patellar or quadriceps) are identified, and anchoring sutures are placed in a Krakow-type suture technique. One suture should be run up either side of the tendon providing four strands for attachment to the retained portion of the patella. A 2.0 mm or 2.5 mm drill bit is then used to drill three holes through the long axis of the patella in a parallel fashion. These should avoid penetrating the articular surface and should be placed in the midcoronal plane. It is essential to avoid placing the drill holes too anteriorly, as such positioning will result in malalignment of the patella. A suture passer is then passed through the drill holes beginning at the intact portion of the patella. The medial and lateral most sutures should be passed through the more medial and lateral drill holes respectively. The midline sutures are passed through the middle drill hole together. The suture is then tied over the superior (or inferior) pole of the patella, tying the medial two sutures together and the lateral two sutures together. Care should be taken at this time to appropriately tension these sutures in order to maintain the appropriate length of the extensor mechanism. The knee is then taken through a gentle range of motion, noting the degree of flexion which begins to put tension on the repair.

Total patellectomy can be considered for unsalvageable patella fractures. The patient will be functional after this, however they will be left with a significant extensor lag and decreased quadriceps power.[9] To repair the tendons following excision of all of the fragments of the patella, multiple sutures are placed above and below the defect. The key to avoiding a significant extensor lag is to attempt restoration of the appropriate tension of the entire extensor mechanism. Soft tissue imbrication procedures should be considered in order to accomplish this goal. The sutures are then tied with care to place some tension in the extensor mechanism with the knee in full extension. It is however equally important to assure that the knee can flex at least 90° without failure of the repair.

Closure

It is imperative to repair the retinacular tears following partial patellectomy in order to further reconstruct the extensor mechanism. Also, a cerclage wire or cable can be passed from above the patella through the tibial tubercle to augment the repair if necessary. This cable or wire will have to be removed, and this removal is typically scheduled at 6–8 weeks following the index procedure. The skin is then closed in standard fashion.

Rehabilitation

Generally, gentle active range of motion is allowed immediately to the degree that the repair is stable. The condition of the soft tissues and surgical incision should also be considered, and the patient may be held at full extension for a period of days in order to allow these to calm down appropriately. Typically the range of motion is allowed in an over the counter type of hinged knee brace, and the patient is allowed to weight bear as tolerated. The surgeons' goal is to have the patient attaining at least 90° of flexion by 4–6 weeks postoperatively. Resistive exercises are typically allowed at the 12 weeks point, and the patient should be followed until the patient has good strength and is ambulating well without an assistive device.

PARTIAL PATELLECTOMY: Pearls and Pitfalls

- Either the superior or inferior portion of the patella can be excised and the surgeon should retain the largest portion of the patella possible
- Avoid repairing the tendon too anterior on the patella. This will cause a malalignment and improper tilting of the patella
- Be sure to repair the retinacular tears in order to support the patellar/quadriceps tendon repair to the patella
- Following a total patellectomy, the appropriate tension of the extensor mechanism must be reconstructed in order to avoid an extensor lag

Outcomes

Overall outcomes of patellar fractures are good, although most studies attempt to combine heterogeneous treatment methods, fracture patterns and outcome measurements. Complication rate including loss of fixation, stiffness, infection, arthritis and especially the need for hardware removal appears to be high.

Describing tension band results, Hung et al. showed 81% excellent or good results with operative fixation, although only 73% of the fractures in that study were transverse in nature.[10] Reporting on open fractures treated with immediate fixation, Catalano et al. found 73% with excellent or good results at an average follow-up of 21 months, but a large number was lost to follow-up.[11] Berg reported his results at 2 years to be particularly encouraging with the use of wires through cannulated screws and continuous passive motion (CPM) in the immediate postoperative period. All fractures united at an average of 8 weeks. There were no losses of reduction, no cases of implant migration and no implant failures.[12]

Hardware removal is a common occurrence after internal fixation and should be discussed with the patient preoperatively. Most of the above studies listed high rate of reoperation for hardware removal ranging up to 60%. One approach to decrease this rate has been to use suture instead of wire. Several authors have reported on using suture or bioabsorbable implants.[13,14]

Partial patellectomy, as an alternative to fixation, can have satisfactory results with several authors reporting similar rate of functional recovery to primary internal fixation.[15,16] Total patellectomy, however, appears to have inferior results primarily due to loss of quadriceps function.[17,18] As a special group, elderly patients with displaced fractures can do well, possibly better when treated surgically.[19]

Complications

The surgical fixation of patella fractures has a high rate of early complications, reported in some series to be greater than 20%.[20] The most common early complications are infection and loss of reduction. The most common late complications are knee pain and stiffness. Late knee pain and stiffness may be caused by hardware irritation, arthrofibrosis, nonunion or arthritis.

Infection

Infection in the setting of closed patella fracture surgery is relatively uncommon with a reported incidence similar to other closed fractures. Open fractures may have extensive soft tissue injuries that predispose to infection, especially if grossly contaminated and not adequately debrided. In closed fractures, causes for infection should be sought. These may include fracture-specific factors, such as failed fracture fixation or host factors, such as an immunocompromised state (Figs 24.7A to E).

Loss of Reduction

Loss of reduction, which is the most common early complication, can occur because of poorly executed fracture fixation, severe fracture comminution or patient noncompliance. In general, avoidance is the best remedy for this problem. Fixation should be manually tested in the operating room and ideally, fixation should be stable with 90° of flexion. The arc of stability in the operating room should be documented and the postoperative protocol should restrict motion to this safe arc until healing occurs. Additionally, one should never hesitate to use redundant fixation and never leave questionable fixation in place (Figs 24.2 and 24.6).

Hardware Irritation

The subcutaneous position of the patella almost guarantees some degree of soft tissue irritation and pain. Wire knots are sometimes difficult to bend over fully without damaging them. Fixation with K-wires often leaves proud wires either at the patella tendon or at the quadriceps insertions. These can cause pain and limit knee flexion.

Nonunion

Nonunion appears to be relatively rare although good data is hard to find. Presumably these cases are treated at tertiary referral centers and no large series have been reported. One small case series suggests that patellar nonunions may be asymptomatic and should only be treated, if they cause symptoms[21] (Figs 24.8A to F).

Knee Stiffness

Stiffness in the absence of arthritis is often a consequence of inadequate early range of motion, which in turn can be due to inadequate fixation, patient non-compliance or pain. Arthrofibrosis can occur (Figs 24.9A to I).

Arthritis

Arthritis may occur due to damage to the patellar articular cartilage at the time of injury due to a malreduction of the joint surface or due to altered joint mechanics as a consequence of patella baja or alta. A careful reduction of the joint and restoration of mechanics similar to the contralateral side may reduce this incidence.

Authors' Preferred Management of Select Complications

Case 1: Hardware Failure—Revision Fixation

A 45-year-old man tripped over a curb landing on his flexed knee sustaining a direct blow to the patella. The patient was diagnosed with an isolated displaced patella fracture in the emergency department, placed in a compressive dressing and a knee immobilizer, and sent to clinic for follow-up (Figs 24.2A and B). He underwent elective outpatient surgery 8 days later using two 4.0 mm cannulated screws and two loops of 18 gauge cerclage wire, one placed through each screw (Figs 24.2C and D). He was started on early range of motion within 2 weeks of surgery without the use of CPM and he appeared to heal uneventfully (Fig. 24.2E). A subsequent fall 5 months after his initial injury resulted in hardware failure with the screws and wire pulling out of the distal pole (Fig. 24.2F). The fracture was re-reduced and fixed using two 5.0 mm cannulated screws with a figure-of-eight 18 gauge cerclage wire placed through the screws supplemented with a circumferential cerclage cable (Figs 24.2G and H). Healing was then uneventful.

Hardware failure after ORIF of the patella is an uncommon but potentially disastrous complication. Fixation, which can be difficult due to the small space available for fixation and the need for early motion, can be further compromised by fracture factors, such as a high degree of comminution or osteoporosis. The best remedy is prevention with redundant stable fixation that is able to tolerate motion.

The best treatment for hardware failure is revision fixation with either repeat ORIF or partial or total patellectomy. The surgeons' preference is to attempt revision fixation in the active patient if the bone quality appears sufficiently good to hold new fixation. However, if the bone quality appears poor, the surgeons have a low threshold to proceed to partial or even total patellectomy (see Case #2 below). Revision fixation should be performed with a larger diameter cannulated screw often with washers and additional cerclage wires, or cables should be added to supplement fixation.

Case 2: Hardware Failure—Partial or Total Patellectomy

A 65-year-old man fell from a ladder sustaining a closed, comminuted patella fracture (Fig. 24.7A), and ORIF was performed on an outpatient basis one week later. Fixation was apparently difficult requiring the unconventional use of a locking plate (Fig. 24.7B). Early fixation failure occurred through the proximal screws (Fig. 24.7C). The distal pole was too comminuted to salvage and therefore a partial patellectomy was performed (Fig. 24.7D). That surgery failed due to infection and therefore a total patellectomy was performed (Fig. 24.7E), which resulted in a satisfactory result. Final outcome was a minimally symptomatic knee with range of motion of 5–95°, an intact extensor mechanism and a healed soft tissue envelope.

In this case, salvage was attempted with a partial patellectomy in order to preserve quadriceps strength, but a deep infection necessitated a debridement and a total patellectomy. Total patellectomy is usually the only option in deep infections. Although a total patellectomy does not predictably provide as satisfactory a result as a partial patellectomy, results can be quite good especially in thinner low demand patients.

Case 3: Knee Stiffness

A 73-year-old woman tripped and fell while dancing and sustained a highly comminuted patella fracture (Figs 24.9A and B). She underwent ORIF the next day (Figs 24.9C and D). Despite routine early mobilization and satisfactory radiographs, the patient developed severe knee stiffness limiting flexion to about 45° Physical therapy failed to make significant progress and therefore around 3 months postoperatively the patient underwent

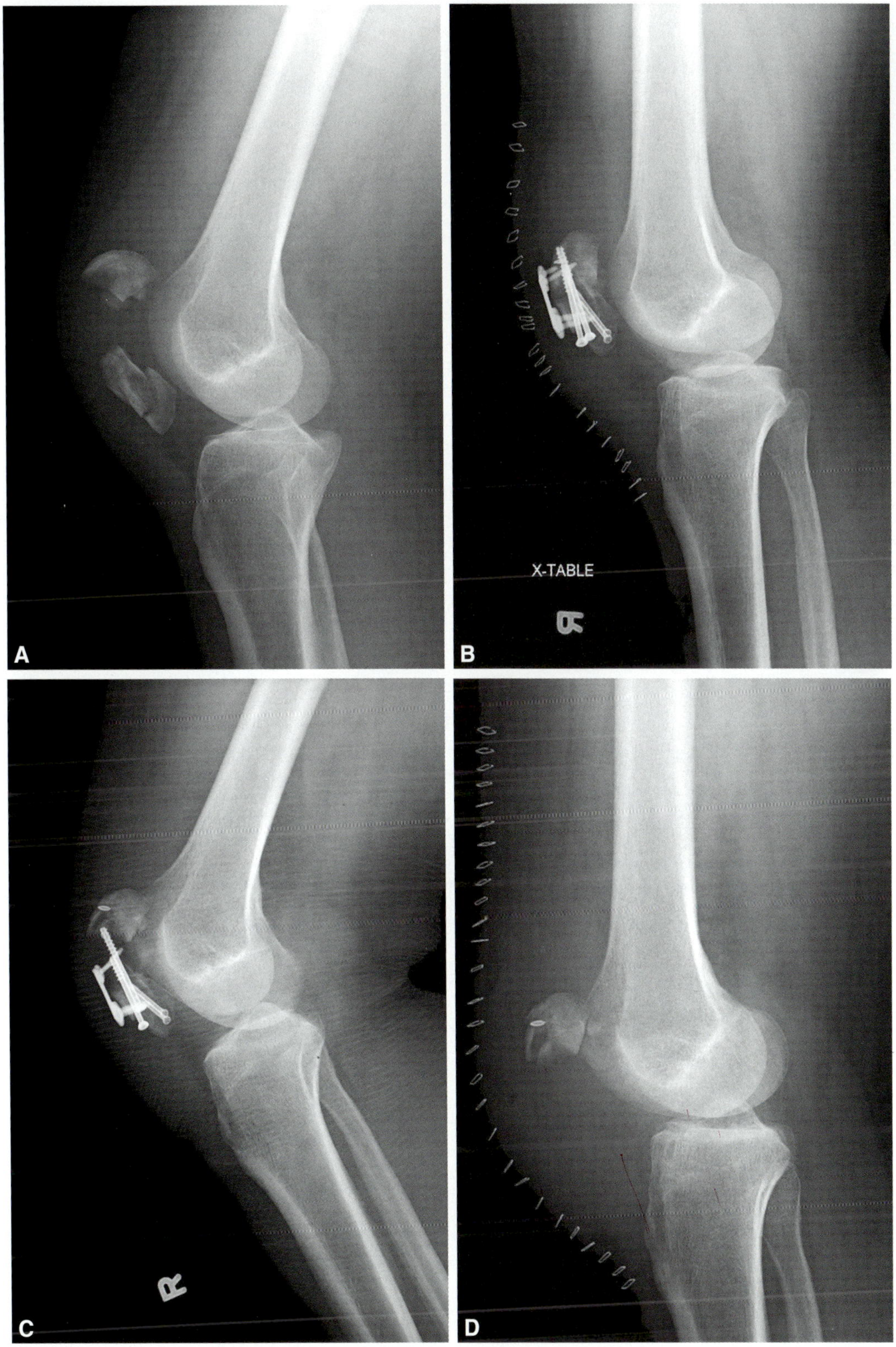

Figures 24.7A to D

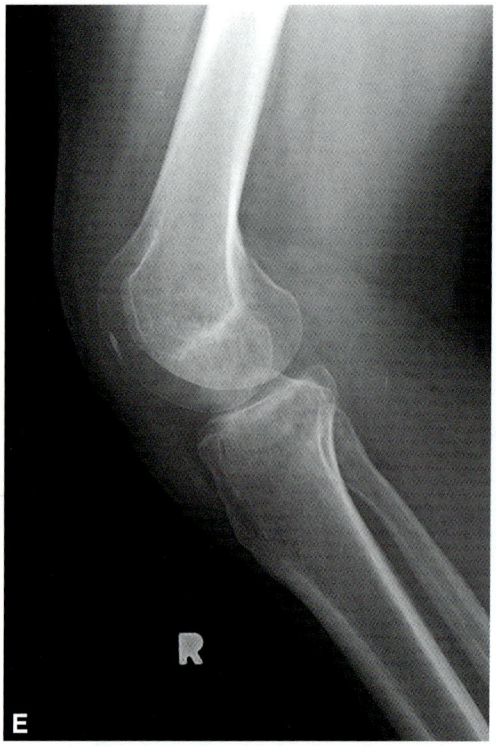

Figures 24.7A to E: Salvage of hardware failure with patellectomy. (A) Injury lateral radiograph shows a highly comminuted fracture; (B) Immediate postoperative lateral radiograph shows an unusual plate and screw construct suggesting difficulty was encountered with fixation. Angulation at the fracture has caused a malreduction at the articular surface and also decreased bone available for fixation; (C) Early fixation failure has occurred through the proximal screws; (D) Salvage was attempted by excision of the distal pole and advancement of the patellar tendon; (E) Subsequent persistent wound drainage and deep infection necessitated a complete patellectomy which yielded a satisfactory result. Final outcome was a minimally symptomatic knee with range of motion of 5–95°, an intact extensor mechanism and a healed soft tissue envelope.

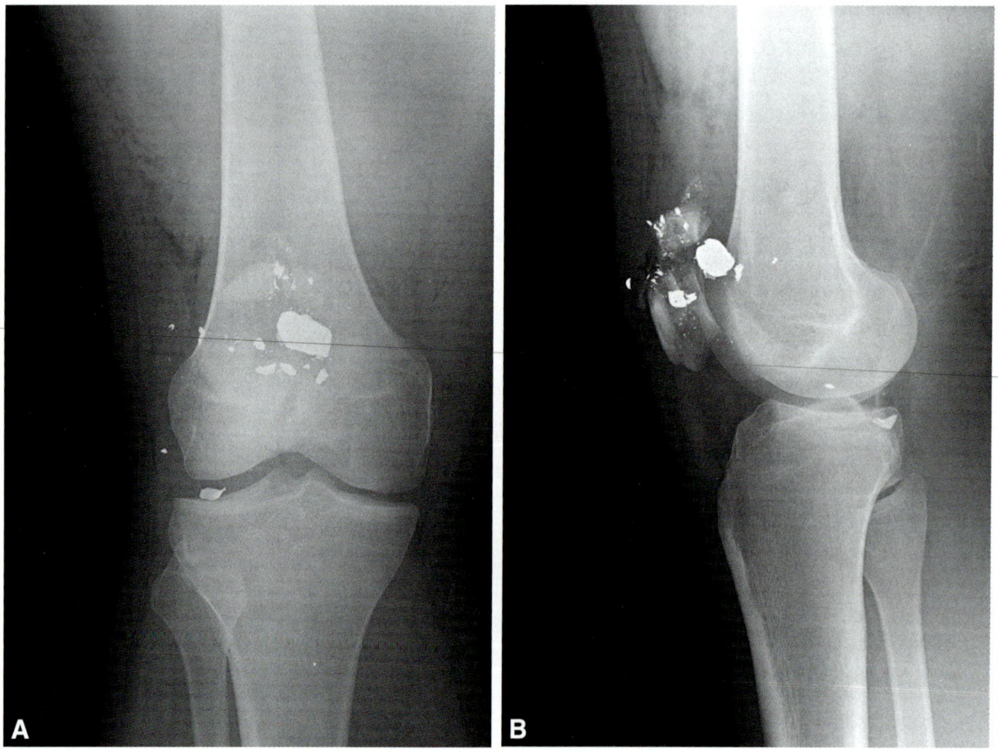

Figures 24.8A and B

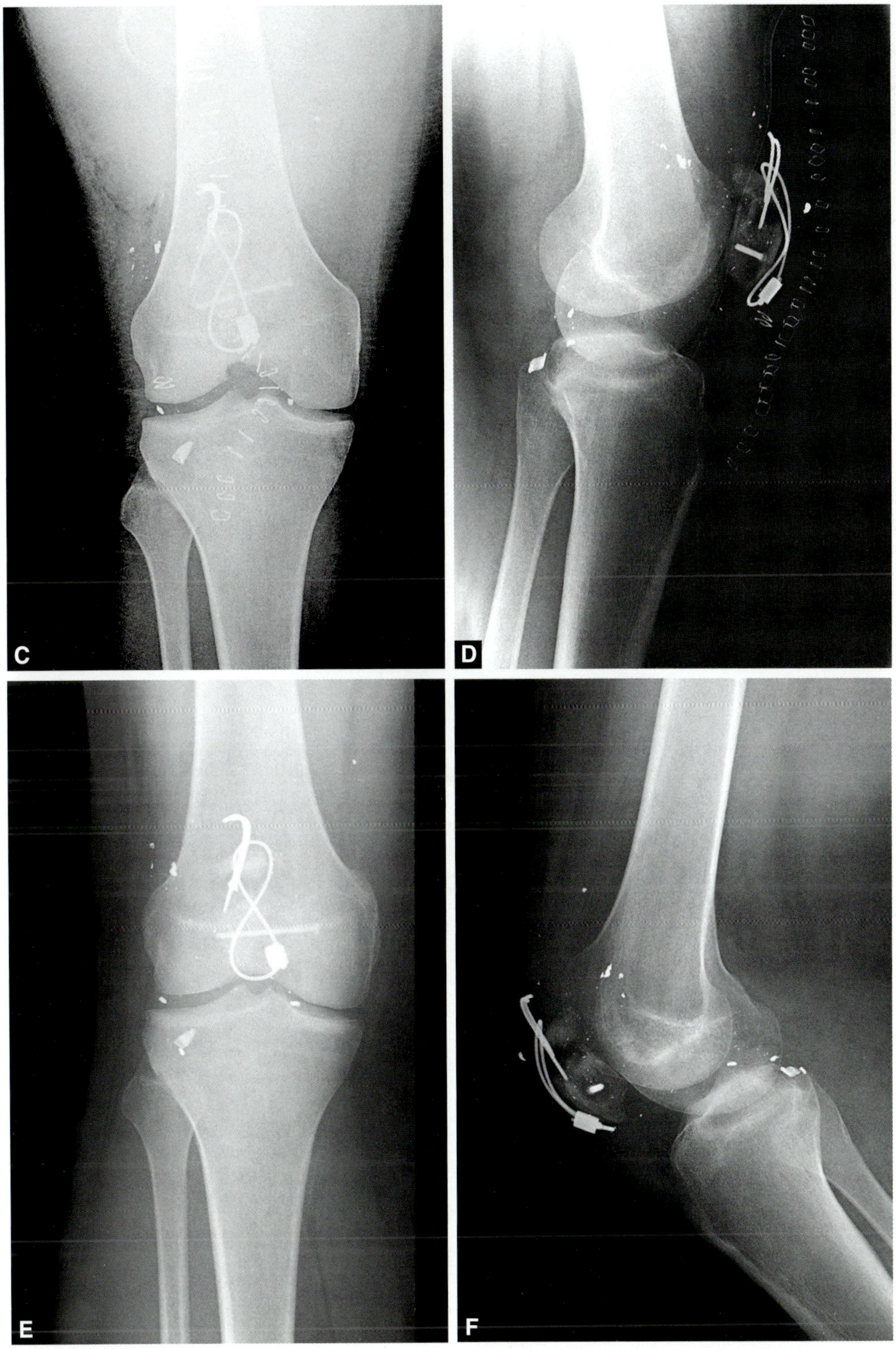

Figures 24.8A to F: Patellar nonunion. (A and B) Injury radiographs show a comminuted patellar fracture due to a low-velocity gunshot wound; (C and D) Postoperative radiographs after arthroscopic exam of the knee and open reduction and internal fixation of the fracture using a cable anchored on two Kirschner wires due to extensive comminution. Fixation appears suboptimal; (E and F) Although a nonunion is apparent at 4 months follow-up, the patient's knee is asymptomatic and therefore no additional treatment is needed at this time.

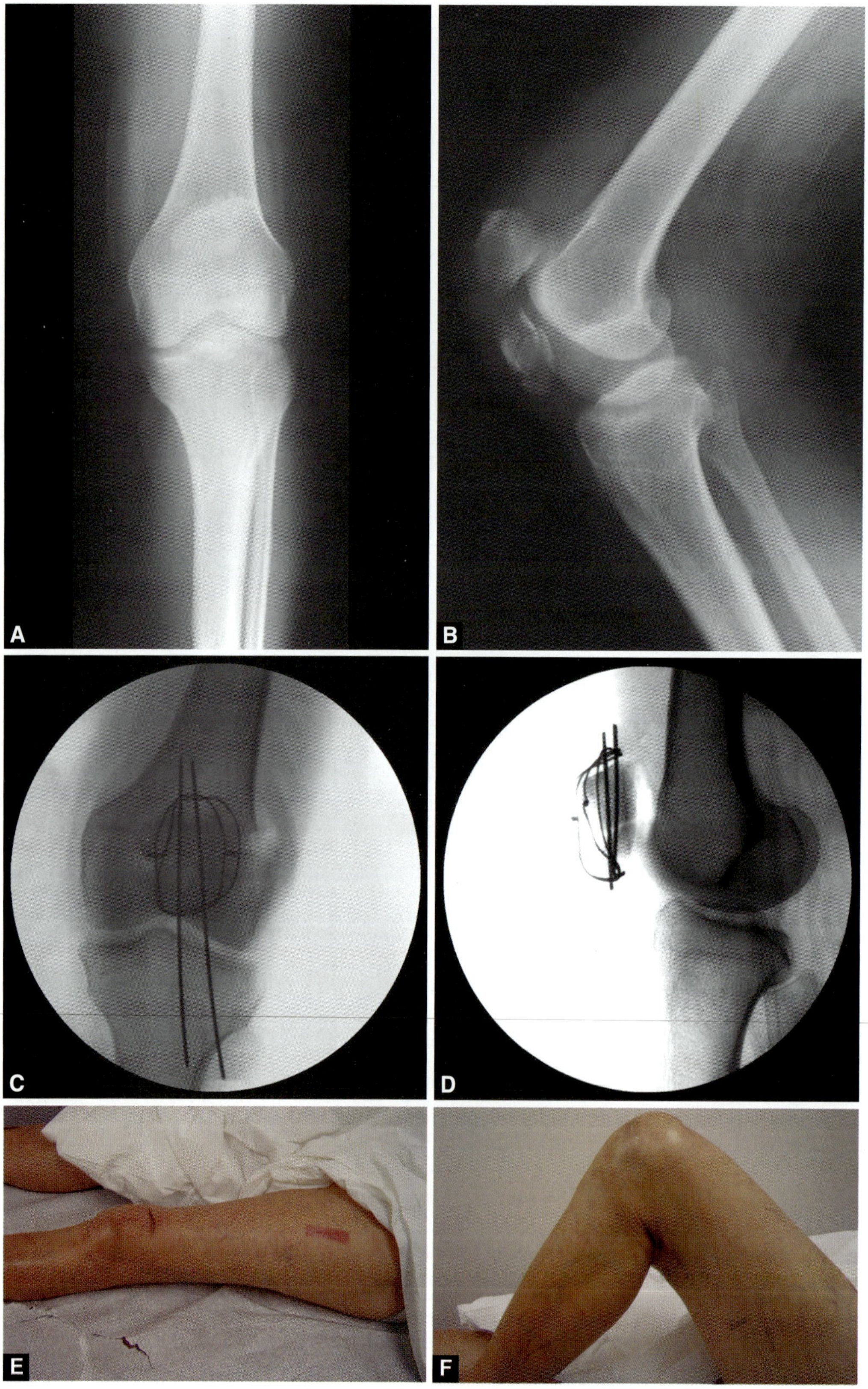

Figures 24.9A to F

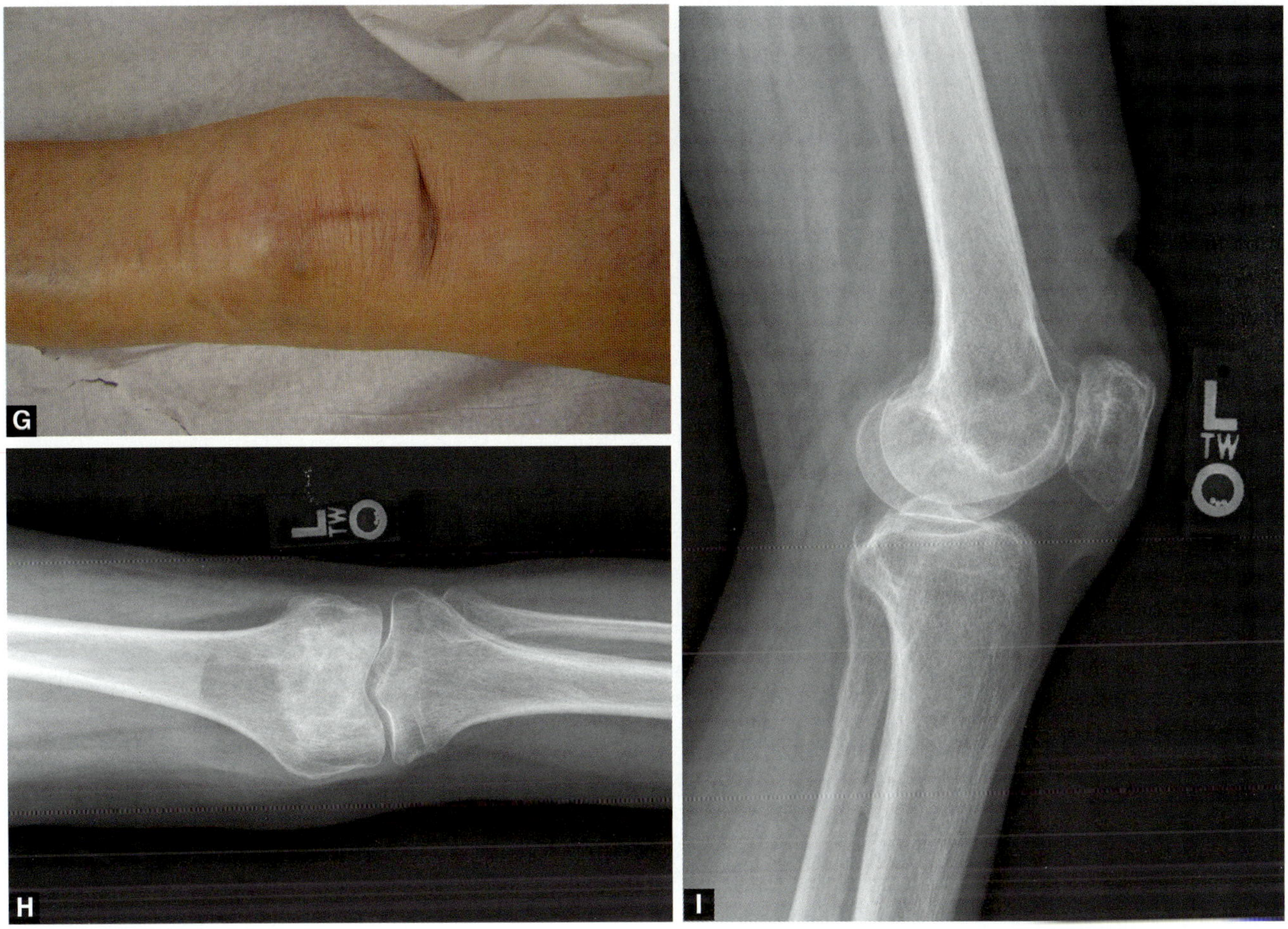

Figures 24.9A to I: Stiffness after patellar open reduction and internal fixation. (A and B) Comminuted patellar fracture in an elderly patient; (C and D) Intraoperative fixation with Kirschner wires and cerclage due to the comminution; (E and F) Patient developed knee stiffness but had healed her fracture 3 months postoperatively. She underwent manipulation under anesthesia and achieved excellent range of motion, but tore her skin requiring split-thickness skin grafting; (G to I) Hardware was removed after 1 year. Late outcome was fair due to the development of patellofemoral arthritis. Patient is considering arthroplasty but has not undergone it at 5 years follow-up.

arthroscopy and gentle manipulation under anesthesia. The manipulation resulted in a superficial transverse skin tear above the patella. In order to preserve motion this wound was skin grafted a few days later and the patient was placed on a CPM. The skin graft was held in placed with a negative pressure wound dressing. Excellent motion was regained and wound healing was uneventful (Figs 24.9E to G). At 3 years follow-up the patient had developed some patellofemoral arthritis but motion remained good (Figs 24.9H and I).

Knee stiffness is relatively common after patella fracture fixation and is best avoided by anatomic fixation and early range of motion. Despite optimal low-profile fixation and early encouragement, some patients will develop knee stiffness. This may be due to hardware irritation or due to articular damage at the time of injury (either of which may have been the case here).

Early range of motion should begin as early as possible, and always within the first 1–2 weeks. If there is concern about patient compliance with the surgeon's instructions, physical therapy should be involved to supervise their activity. The patients are allowed active and active assisted range of motion in a hinged knee brace starting usually at 45° and advancing 10–15° per week. Usually, the goal is to be at 90° by 4 weeks, although this program may be modified based on the degree of stability obtained intraoperatively. Weight bearing as tolerated is allowed with the knee brace locked in extension and therefore a brace with drop locks is preferred.

If patients are not making adequate progress with range of motion early on but their fixation constructs appear stable and satisfactory, the author would initially simply provide reassurance and encouragement. At 2–3 months, if range of motion is not satisfactory, the author would consider a gentle manipulation under anesthesia in the operating room. Risks of manipulation include hardware failure, patellar tendon rupture, femur fracture and exceptionally, as in this case, a skin tear. At the same time as manipulation, consideration can also be given to arthroscopy of the knee to verify that there is no treatable intra-articular etiology for the stiffness. A lysis of intra-articular adhesions, if there are any, is then performed. In the older patient with recalcitrant knee stiffness, especially with patellofemoral arthritis, consideration can be given after fracture healing to knee arthroplasty.

Summary

The surgical treatment of patella fractures has a high rate of complications due to the relative difficulty of stable internal fixation, the subcutaneous position of the bone and the high mechanical loads placed across the fracture during ordinary knee motion. Despite this, the best outcomes are achieved by an anatomically reduced fracture fixed with low-profile secure and redundant internal fixation followed by early postoperative protected range of motion. Attention to detail and careful monitoring after surgery can help reduce the incidence of complications and ameliorate their consequences.

References

1. Anand S, Hahnel JC, Giannoudis PV. Open patellar fractures: high energy injuries with a poor outcome? Injury. 2008; 39(4):480-4.
2. Torchia ME, Lewallen DG. Open fractures of the patella. J Orthop Trauma. 1996;10(6):403-9.
3. Viola R, Vianello R. Three cases of patella fracture in 1,320 anterior cruciate ligament reconstructions with bone-patellar tendon-bone autograft. Arthroscopy. 1999;15(1): 93-7.
4. Wilberg G. Roentgenographic and anatomic studies on the patellofemoral joint. Acta Orthop Scand. 1941;12: 319-29.
5. Hueberti HH, Hays WC. Patellofemoral contact pressures. The influence of Q-angle and tendofemoral contact. J Bone Joint Surg Am. 1984;66:715-24.
6. Kaufer H. Patellar biomechanics. Clin Orthop Relat Res. 1979;144:51-4.
7. Scapinelli, R. Blood supply of the human patella. J Bone Joint Surg Br. 1967;49:563-70.
8. Saltzman CI, Goulet JA, McClellan RT, et al. Results of treatment of displaced patellar fractures by partial patellectomy. J Bone Joint Surg Am. 1990;72:1279-85.
9. Lennox IA, Cobb AG, Knowles J, et al. Knee function after patellectomy: a 12- to 48-year follow-up. J Bone Joint Surg Br. 1994;76: 485-7.
10. Hung LK, Chan KM, Chow YN, et al. Fractured patella: operative treatment using the tension band principle. Injury. 1985;16:343-7.
11. Catalano JB, Iannacone WM, Marczyk S, et al. Open fracture of the patella: long-term functional outcome. J Trauma. 1995;39:439-44.
12. Berg EE. Open reduction internal fixation of displaced transverse patella fractures with figure-eight wiring through parallel cannulated compression screws. J Orthop Trauma. 1997;11:573-6.
13. Gosal HS, Singh P, Field RE. Clinical experience of patellar fracture fixation using metal wire or non-absorbable polyester: a study of 37 cases. Injury. 2001;32:129-35.
14. Qi L, Chang C, Xin T, et al. Double fixation of displaced patella fractures using bioabsorbable cannulated lag screws and braided polyester suture tension bands. Injury. 2011; 42(10):1116-20.
15. Saltzman CL, Goulet JA, McClellan RT, et al. Results of treatment of displaced patellar fractures by partial patellectomy. J Bone Joint Surg Am. 1990;72:1279-85.
16. Hung LK, Lee SY, Leung KS, et al. Partial patellectomy for patellar fracture: tension band wiring and early mobilization. J Orthop Trauma. 1993, 7:252-60.
17. Einola S, Aho AJ, Kallio P. Patellectomy after fracture. Long-term follow-up results with special reference to functional disability. Acta Orthop Scand. 1976;47:441-7.
18. Sutton FS, Thompson CH, Lipke J, et al. The effect of patellectomy on knee function. J Bone Joint Surg Am. 1976; 58:537-40.
19. Shabat S, Mann G, Kish B, et al. Functional results after patellar fractures in elderly patients. Arch Gerontol Geriatr. 2003;37:93-8.
20. Smith ST, Cramer KE, Karges DE, et al. Early complications in the operative treatment of patella fractures. J Orthop Trauma. 1997;11:183-7.
21. Klassen JF, Trousdale RT. Treatment of delayed and nonunion of the patella. J Orthop Trauma. 1997;11:188-94.

Chapter 25

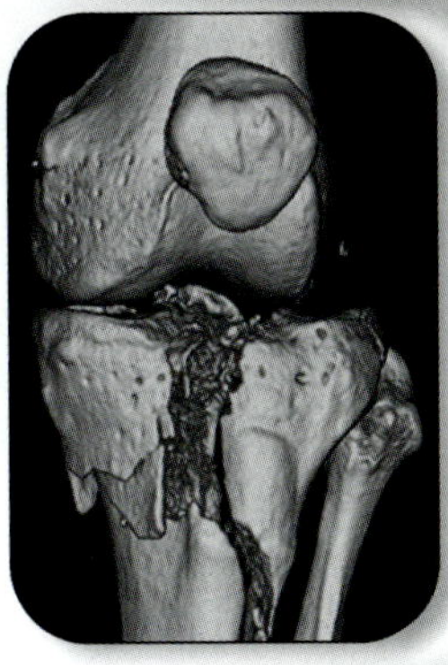

Proximal Tibia Fractures

J Spence Reid

Chapter Outline

Introduction

Diagnosis
- Patient Evaluation
- Mechanism of Injury
- Associated Injuries

Classification
- The Schatzker Classification
- AO/OTA Classification
- The Moore Classification of Fracture-Dislocations

Surgical Indications
- Overview and Guiding Principles of Fracture Repair

Surgical Anatomy, Positioning and Approaches
- Relevant Anatomical Features
- Approaches

Surgical Techniques
- Emergent Treatment
- Surgical Technique and Rationale by Classification
  - Lateral Tibial Plateau Fractures
  - Medial Tibial Plateau Fractures
  - Bicondylar Tibial Plateau Fractures
- High-Energy Tibial Plateau Fracture—Approach to Treatment
- Postoperative Care

Complications and Author's Preferred Management of Select Cases
- Loss of Fixation
- Infection
- Malunion and Nonunion
- Post-traumatic Arthritis

Summary

Introduction

Tibial plateau fractures encompass an extremely broad group of injuries from both an osseous and soft tissue perspective. Optimal treatment must give equal attention to both elements of the injury. A complete understanding of the fracture pattern, aided by modern imaging techniques and coupled with a careful, experienced evaluation of the nonosseous injuries is critical to achieve the best possible reduction of the articular surface, restoration of axial alignment and initiation of early joint range of motion (ROM), while minimizing complications. There have been significant advances in the last several years in our understanding of the role of calcium ceramics in void filling, and the appropriate role and limitations of locked plating and hybrid fixation techniques in these injuries. The optimal method and timing to stabilize a severe bicondylar fracture remains controversial and continues to undergo refinement. The importance of reduction and stability of the posteromedial fragment has been investigated. There are several new surgical approaches for the exposure and treatment of the posterolateral fracture fragment.

Diagnosis

Patient Evaluation

Physical Examination

Fractures of the tibial plateau can occur either with indirect trauma such as a valgus loading injury or as a result of direct trauma such as "bumper" injury from a motor vehicle. Careful examination of the extremity at presentation and during hospital admission is important for assessing and documenting skin, soft tissues and neurovascular injury. Compartment syndrome, seen most frequently in fracture dislocations, higher grade fractures and "bumper" injuries, is a particularly devastating complication that requires careful and repeated physical examination. Splints and braces can limit direct evaluation of the soft tissues. Compartment syndrome or cases that are at higher risk for blistering often require a period of spanning external fixation, which stabilizes the limb, while allowing direct access to the soft tissues. This is described in the section on surgical techniques.

Imaging

Orthogonal radiographs are usually made in the emergency room or trauma bay. These are sufficient to identify the injury, but are inadequate for classification and preoperative planning. A patient with a high-energy tibial plateau fracture should have radiographs of the adjacent femur, entire tibia or ankle to identify associated injuries. In cases, where a spanning external frame is planned to regain length and improve reduction, further imaging should be delayed until after frame placement. When obtaining radiographs and intraoperative fluoroscopic images of the tibial plateau, it is useful to angle the beam in the anteroposterior (AP) plane to match the posterior slope of the concave medial condyle. This is achieved when the medial articular surface appears as a single line indicating that the beam is tangent to the subchondral bone of the anterior and posterior edge of the joint. This defines the "plateau view" of the proximal tibia and should be used, whenever screws are being inserted to avoid intra-articular penetration (Figs 25.1A to C).

Axial computed tomography (CT) with sagittal and coronal reconstructions has become the standard for evaluating tibial plateau fractures. Chan et al.[1] noted that the addition of CT scanning improved intra and inter-observer agreement for both fracture classification and surgical planning as compared to plain films alone. The treatment plan was changed 26% of the time with the addition of CT to plain films. The more recent advent of three-dimensional (3D) CT reconstruction to evaluate tibial plateau fractures has been shown to further improve intraobserver and interobserver reliability in both classification and surgical planning as compared to axial CT and two-dimensional (2D) reconstructions.[2] Three-dimensional reconstructions, particularly of complex fractures, are also very valuable in a teaching environment, in which an inexperienced medical student or resident can rapidly visualize a fracture pattern (Figs 25.2A to D). As the cost and time involved in obtaining 3D reconstructions has decreased, the surgeons now routinely obtain them for all medial and bicondylar fractures.[3] With the high incidence of associated injuries of the knee in tibial plateau fractures, it is not surprising that magnetic resonance imaging (MRI) is playing an increasing role in the preoperative assessment of these injuries. Combining CT with MRI[4] allows surgeons to visualize the fracture, the status of cruciate and collateral ligaments, the meniscus and the involved soft tissue envelope. Mui et al.[5] compared the results of CT and MRI findings in 41 plateau fractures and found that CT yielded 80% sensitivity and 98% specificity for the detection of ligament tears. Magnetic resonance imaging was still needed for the detection of meniscal injury. The relative utility of the addition of CT or MRI in both fracture classification and surgical planning was investigated by Yacobian et al. For fracture classification, radiographs alone yielded a mean kappa coefficient of 0.68, which increased to 0.73 for radiographs with CT scan and 0.85 for radiographs with MRI. Fracture classification (Schatzker) was changed on an average of 6% with the addition of CT scan and 21% based on radiographs with MRI. For the fracture management plan, the mean interobserver kappa coefficient for radiographs alone was 0.72, which increased to 0.77 for radiographs with CT scan and 0.86 for radiographs with MRI. Magnetic resonance imaging changed treatment plan in 23% of cases. The high sensitivity of MRI can lead to false positive findings with respect to meniscal tears. Mustonen et al.[6] noted in a study of 78 menisci in 39 patients that 42% had an abnormal meniscal signal, but in 52% of these, there was contusion only with no tear, and this subgroup would not benefit from surgical treatment.

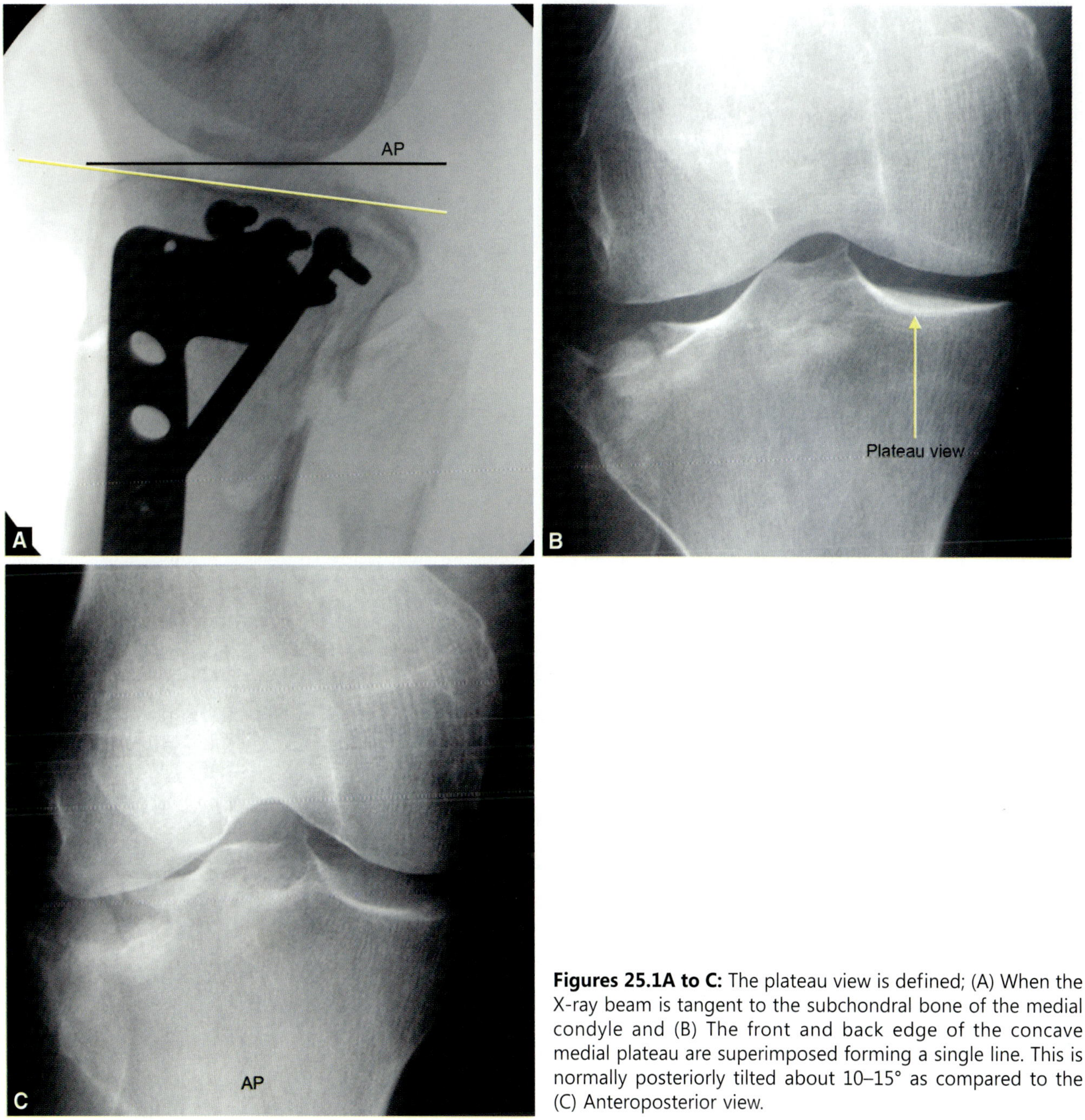

Figures 25.1A to C: The plateau view is defined; (A) When the X-ray beam is tangent to the subchondral bone of the medial condyle and (B) The front and back edge of the concave medial plateau are superimposed forming a single line. This is normally posteriorly tilted about 10–15° as compared to the (C) Anteroposterior view.

The purpose of imaging is to characterize and classify the fracture and associated injuries, so that an optimal plan of treatment can be formulated. It appears that after plain radiographs, CT scanning with 2D or 3D reformatting remains the standard of care for all plateau fractures with the addition of MRI or as needed basis in high-energy or fracture-dislocation patterns. If a spanning external fixator is being placed, both repeat plain radiographs and CT scanning should be performed after the length is re-established with the fixator. If the routine use of preoperative MRI scans is being contemplated, an MRI compatible external fixation system should be utilized.

Mechanism of Injury

Injuries to the tibial plateau and associated structures occur as a result of both translationally and axially directed forces.

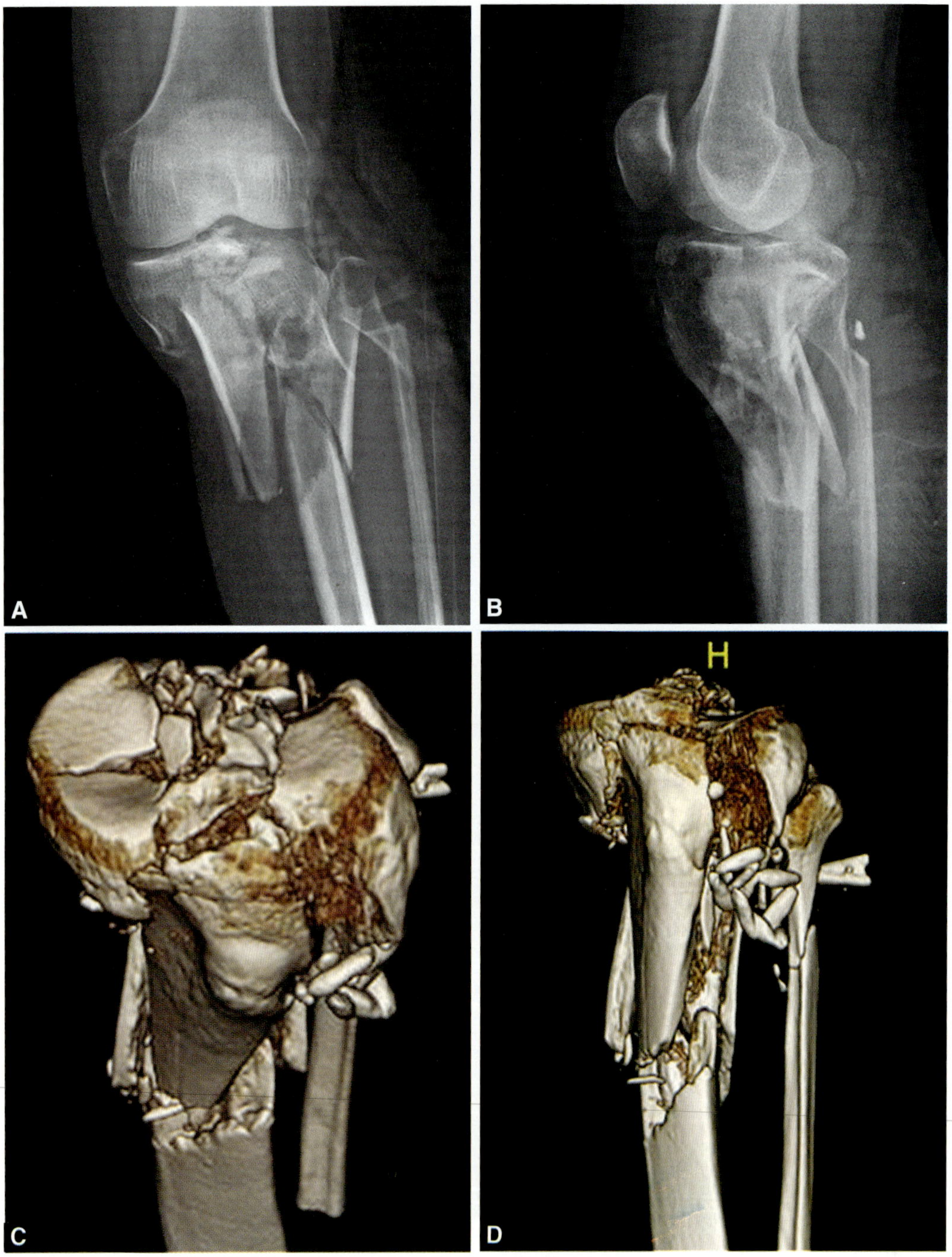

Figures 25.2A to D: A complex bicondylar fracture. (A and B) Anteroposterior and lateral radiographs are difficult to interpret; (C and D) CT with three-dimensional (3D) reconstructions allow better fracture classification and preoperative planning than plain radiographs or axial CT or two-dimensional (2D) reconstructions.

The interplay of the force vector and bone and ligament strength yields the wide spectrum of observed injury patterns—both fractures and fracture-dislocations. In most cases, the opposing femoral condyle exerts compressive and shearing forces on the underlying tibial condyle, while the joint capsule and ligament structures can exert tensile forces causing avulsion fractures. The relative strength of the cortical bone to the cancellous bone is a function of age and bone health and determines how the condyle responds to a compressive load. In young patients, the cancellous bone is very strong and allows the overlying compressive force from the femoral condyle to be transmitted as shear to the cortex, which then fails. The bone trabeculae are not crushed. This results in pure split fractures rarely seen in patients older than early twenties. In older bone, the ratio of the strength of cancellous bone to cortical bone is much closer. The applied compressive force is still transmitted to the metaphyseal cortex resulting in a split, but cancellous trabeculae fail as well, yielding a region of depression adjacent to the split. As overall bone density continues to fall in elderly patients, the cancellous bone is much weaker than the adjacent cortical bone and compressive forces are absorbed almost entirely via crush of cancellous trabeculae with little energy extending to the cortex to yield a split fracture.

The magnitude of forces involved also play a role in the observed fracture patterns. Kennedy and Bailey[7] created many of the commonly observed tibial plateau fracture patterns by combining varus and valgus forces with axial loads applied to cadaver knees. Valgus moments in the range of 2,250–3,750 inch-pounds produced a classical lateral plateau fracture with joint impaction and condylar separation. Pure axial loading greater than 8,000 pounds resulted in a severely comminuted bicondylar fracture akin to that observed clinically after a fall from a height or loading an extended knee in a motor vehicle accident. Early investigators felt that a varus or valgus moment could not be generated, unless the collateral ligaments were intact to act as a fulcrum. More recent studies using MRI and arthroscopy reveal that collateral ligament injuries can occur in conjunction with a pure varus or valgus applied load.[8,9] Gardner et al.[10] reported that a complete medial collateral ligament (MCL) injury was noted in 36% of lateral split depression fractures. A varus producing force creates an analogous situation with the lateral collateral ligament (LCL). A medial plateau fracture often occurs with an associated tear of the LCL complex and posterior cruciate ligament (PCL). The peroneal nerve can sustain a traction injury and the displacement can extend sufficiently to injure the popliteal vessels.

Associated Injuries

Soft tissue injury in the presence of a tibial plateau fracture is common. Gardner et al. performed MRI scans on a consecutive series of 103 preoperative tibial plateau fracture patients and noted a 91% incidence of lateral meniscal injury, 44% incidence of medical meniscal injury, 61% incidence of posterolateral corner tear and 77% incidence of avulsion or tear of one or more cruciate or collateral ligaments. Sixty percent of these fractures were Schatzker II.[10] Plain radiographs are usually not critiqued to ascertain the likelihood of meniscus and ligament injuries. Nonetheless, several studies report a strong association between amount of joint line depression and condylar widening as well as the incidence of meniscal injuries. A study comparing plain radiographs with MRI scans in split-depression fractures[11] demonstrated that when depression was greater than 6 mm and condylar widening was greater than 5 mm on plain radiographs, lateral meniscal injury was present in 83% of fractures. Ringus et al.[12] compared operative findings with preoperative CT and noted that patients with greater than 10 mm of plateau depression had an 8X greater likelihood of a lateral meniscal tear as compared to patients with less than 10 mm of depression. This correlation between the amount of joint depression and the presence of a meniscal tear was not found by Mustonen et al.[6]

Several authors have reported the spectrum of soft tissue injury using arthroscopy at the time of operative repair of the fracture and noted a 50% incidence of meniscal tear that was usually on the side of the plateau fracture and in the peripheral vascular zone. No significant association was noted between the fracture type and the presence of a meniscal tear.[13] The incidence of all ligament injuries except the anterior cruciate ligament (ACL) was noted to be less than 6%. Anterior cruciate ligament tears were noted in 25% of patients, usually associated with Schatzker type IV and VI fractures.[9]

When the findings from the published studies are coalesced, it appears that meniscal injuries in tibial plateau fractures are very common findings by MRI scan, but up to 50% may be contusions[6] that do not require surgical treatment. Nonetheless, it is incumbent upon the surgeon to ascertain the status of the meniscus at the time of open or arthroscopic repair of the plateau fracture. When present, meniscal tears are usually in the vascular zone and are amenable to repair. Anterior cruciate ligament injuries either in the form of bone avulsions or mid-substance tears are also common in bicondylar fractures and fracture-dislocations. The bone avulsions should be

Overview and Guiding Principles of Fracture Repair

The principles of articular fracture treatment are well-established and grounded in the basic science of articular cartilage repair. Reduction and stability of the articular surface is paramount and is strongly correlated to outcome.[21] The tolerance of articular cartilage to residual step-off is a matter of some debate, but studies suggest that a step-off greater than the local cartilage thickness will not remodel with hyaline cartilage.[23] This concept has been reinforced by detailed fracture follow-up studies—both CT[24] and arthroscopy. Cetik et al.[25] performed second look arthroscopy in 12 patients at an average of 19 months after repair of a plateau fracture. Anatomically reduced fractures healed with hyaline cartilage, while residual step-offs showed grade I–II chondral defect at the fracture line and adjacent femoral condyle. After articular congruity, restoration of axial alignment, particularly in bicondylar fractures, is paramount and is also closely associated with long-term outcome. Residual varus is not well-tolerated. In a long-term follow-up study of tibial plateau fractures, Rasmussen noted that patients with normal axial alignment as an independent variable had a 13% incidence of post-traumatic arthritis at 7 years, while patients with 5–10° of varus had a 70% incidence of arthritis, and that rose to 100% in cases of greater than 10° of residual varus.[26] The importance of recognition and repair of meniscal injuries is crucial for the long-term outcome after plateau fracture repair.[21,27] The incidence of post-traumatic arthritis is doubled, if the meniscus is removed.[22]

Role of Locking Plates in Tibial Plateau Fractures

There exists a considerable confusion regarding when and how locking plates versus nonlocking periarticular plates should be used to stabilize tibial plateau fractures. This has resulted in the overuse of locking plates and in some situations, making it more difficult to create a stable construct, particularly when a depressed segment requiring elevation and grafting is present. In general, locking proximal tibial plates are unnecessary in the treatment of unicondylar fractures (Schatzker I–IV or OTA B). The locking plates are not needed in unicondylar fractures, as they actually have a downside—mainly the difficulty they create in placing "rafting" screws very close to the subchondral bone of the reconstructed articular surface to support elevated segments. The use of locking screws also limits the ability to independently direct these screws around other implants, such as small threaded wires or AP directed lag screws. The locking implants are not necessary in unicondylar fractures because of the engineering concept that with the far cortex intact (the definition of a unicondylar fracture), the end of the screw essentially rests in intact bone that cannot be "shorten" and is in effect "locked". The plate itself fixes the position of the near side of the screw and the intact bone fixes the distal end of the screw, placing the screw in 4-point bending. The use of a locking screw in this situation will essentially add no additional stability to the construct, since rotation of the screw in the plate is already constrained. In most situations, Schatzker I, II and III fractures can be stabilized with a laterally-based nonlocked periarticular plate, and Schatzker IV fractures with a medially-based nonlocked periarticular plate. Exceptions are the very osteopenic patient or certain fracture-dislocation patterns, in which the fracture extends well into the far condyle leaving a narrow fragment of bone for anchoring the end of the nonlocked screw.

Surgical Anatomy, Positioning and Approaches

Relevant Anatomical Features

The proximal tibial articular surface is not symmetric with respect to the medial and lateral condyles. Compared to the lateral condyle, the medial condyle is 50% larger, has thinner cartilage (also matched by thinner cartilage on the femoral side) (Fig. 25.7A) and substantially, less of its articular surface is covered by meniscus. All these factors in combination render the medial plateau less tolerant of articular incongruity as compared to the lateral condyle. The lateral plateau is higher (2–3 mm) and convex, and the medial plateau is lower and concave. This allows the respective condyles to be recognized on the lateral radiograph. In the sagittal plane, both condyles slope posteriorly about 10°. The two plateaus are separated by the nonarticular intercondylar eminence with medial and lateral tubercles. The tibial attachment of the ACL is just anterior to the medial intercondylar tubercle. The PCL attaches in the posterior intercondylar area and extends onto the posterior metaphysis.

The bony landmarks of tibial plateau serve as sites of attachment for the tendinous structures that stabilize and move the knee. They are also important landmarks for surgical approaches to the tibial plateau. The tibial tubercle is located on the anterior tibial crest about 2–3 cm distal to the anterior joint line and functions as the insertion site for the patellar tendon. On occasion, this tubercle can be contained as a separate fracture fragment in a complex injury and mechanical restoration is important to restore active knee extension. The iliotibial (IT) band inserts into an almond-sized prominence on the lateral metaphysis known as Gerdy's tubercle. The fibular head is more posterior and slightly more proximal than Gerdy's tubercle and serves as the site of attachment of the LCL and biceps tendon. The proximal tibiofibular joint is a true synovial joint, and in about 10% of the population, it communicates with the knee joint (Fig. 25.7B).[28] Mechanically, the lateral condyle is buttressed by the fibular head and this can be exploited during surgical stabilization.

Approaches

Exposure of the Lateral Plateau

The lateral exposure is standard for both treatment of an isolated lateral condyle fracture as well as the lateral portion of a bicondylar fracture. The skin incision is lateral parapatellar along the lateral side of the tibial tubercle extending proximal to the joint line by 4–5 cm (Figs 25.8A and B). Alternatively, the proximal portion of the incision can turn laterally just above the joint line into a "hockey stick" incision. In either case, the deep dissection remains the same. The deep exposure detaches fibers of the tibialis anterior from the tibial crest and extends along the lateral border of the patella tendon insertion to a point about 5 mm distal to the joint line and extends laterally parallel to the joint line as needed. The location of the joint line in a displaced fracture can be difficult to determine by palpation, and we routinely place an 18-gauge needle in the joint line and verify its position by C-arm prior to making the horizontal limb of the deep incision. A scalpel is then used to remove Sharpy's fibers from the most proximal 5 mm of subchondral bone of the plateau, until the joint is entered in a submeniscal position. The vertical portion of the deep incision can be extended across the joint line to the level of the meniscus to improve anterior exposure. Exposure of the lateral condyle for plate placement reflects the cut portion of the IT band inferiorly exposing Gerdy's tubercle. Care is taken to expose just enough to allow plate placement, but not to devascularize the split fragment. The tibialis anterior is reflected off of the lateral side of the tibia as needed to accommodate the distal extension of the lateral plate. In the situation, in which a very long lateral plate is needed as in a bicondylar fracture, the distal extent can be managed using percutaneous screw placement and obviate the need for a long distal skin incision. Visualization of the lateral articular surface can be improved with flexion and varus loading or with use of a femoral distractor.

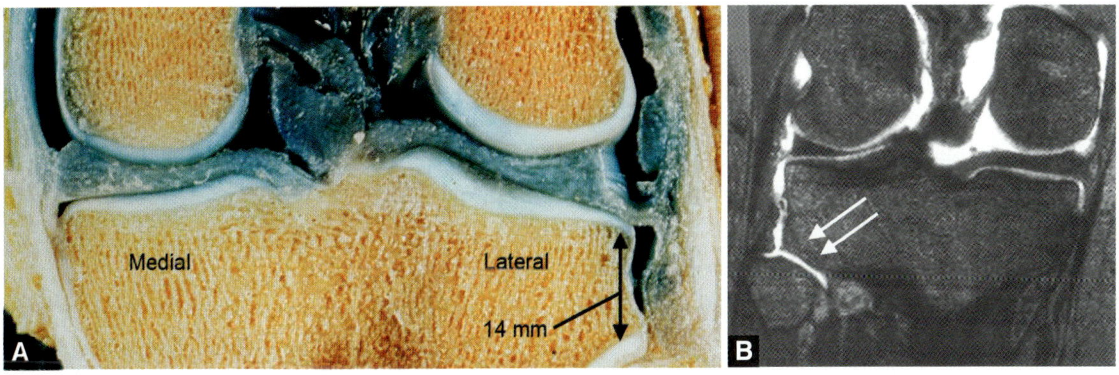

Figures 25.7A and B: (A) Coronal section through the knee just anterior to the tibiofibular joint. The lateral plateau is higher and has thicker cartilage than the medial plateau. Also note the medial and lateral reflections of the joint capsule (in blue). The lateral joint capsule extends up to 14 mm from the subchondral bone; (B) Coronal MRI arthrogram through the proximal posterior tibia showing contrast extending into the proximal tibiofibular joint (white arrows), indicating communication between this joint on the synovial cavity of knee joint. This is present in about 10% of the population.

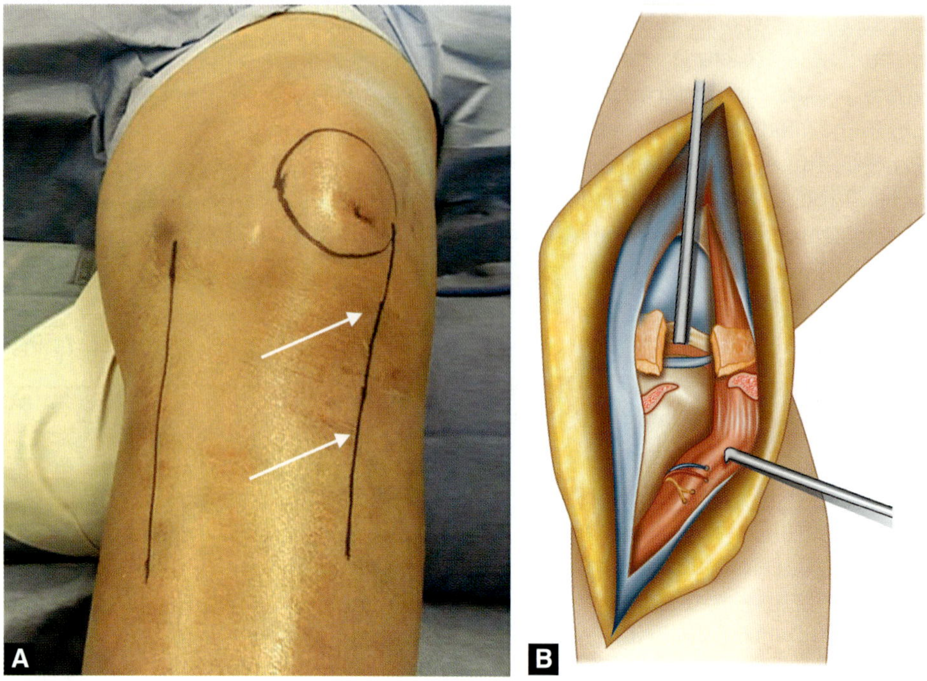

Figures 25.8A and B: (A) The approach to the lateral side of a tibial plateau fracture is lateral parapatellar superficially (white arrows); (B) and then the deep exposure includes a horizontal limb of the deep incision about 5 mm distal to the subchondral bone of the lateral plateau, which is then entered under the meniscus by elevating the meniscotibial ligaments with a scalpel. Sharpey's fibers are elevated off of Gerdy's tubercle and proximal fibers of the tibialis anterior are reflected laterally, as far as needed, to accommodate the length of plate required.

Additional Exposures: Posterolateral, Medial and Posteromedial

Whereas the anterolateral exposure is used commonly, fractures involving the posterolateral, medial and posteromedial portions of the tibial plateau frequently require separate direct exposures either from the supine or prone position. These are described in the following section on "Surgical Techniques".

Surgical Techniques

Emergent Treatment

Since tibial plateau fractures encompass such a broad spectrum of pathology, emergent care must be individualized. Low-energy compression or split-depression fractures in osteopenic patients rarely result in compartment syndrome or significant swelling. The distal neurovascular examination is usually intact, and the patients can be placed in a well-padded splint and imaged as needed. On the other end of the spectrum, an open bicondylar fracture from a motorcycle accident may require all the skill and decision points of limb salvage. These fractures may be opened with concominant bone loss, a substantial and evolving zone of injury, significant contamination, risk of compartment syndrome and neurovascular compromise, if the fracture pattern incorporates wide displacement or a dislocation pattern. Early treatment of these high-energy patterns must rule out vascular injury by use of the ankle-brachial index, and include a detailed examination of the status of tibial and superficial and deep peroneal nerves. In some cases, an emergent operative treatment is indicated to debride an open wound, release a compartment syndrome, or place a spanning external fixator across an unstable fracture pattern. Which patterns benefit from temporary spanning external fixation is based on two features of the injury. The first is axial stability and/or translational stability. Most lateral unicondylar patterns (Schatzker I–III) are length stable, when kept out of varus and can be splinted or braced prior to surgery. The bicondylar injuries (Schatzker V and VI) are, by definition, axially unstable and external fixation is beneficial to relieve pain, restore length and stabilize tissues to allow functional recovery. The Schatzker IV and the Moore patterns of fracture dislocation benefit from external fixation to effectively maintain reduction of the knee joint in addition to restoring length. These fracture-dislocation patterns do not shorten in the same sense as the bicondylar injuries. Rather, they translate and shorten along the obliquity of the major fracture line. In this situation, external fixation controls both translation and shortening and helps protect neurovascular structures prior to definitive fixation. The other injury feature that is an independent indication for external fixation is the status of the soft tissues. An open wound that will require delayed closure or an obvious compartment syndrome requiring fasciotomy is an excellent indication for a spanning frame. A leg that is at risk for compartment syndrome over subsequent 24–48 hours also benefits from an external frame, as it is difficult to monitor the status of an extremity concealed in a padded splint. The threshold for placing a spanning frame should be low, as there is often little downside, if the injury severity is less than originally expected. Soft tissue is stabilized, length is restored and appropriate imaging studies and preoperative planning can be performed with minimal discomfort to the patient.

Technique of Spanning Frame

The key concept in placing a spanning frame across a plateau fracture is to keep the tibial pins outside both the zone of injury and the zone of future hardware placement, if possible. There are fracture patterns and zones of injury that extend very distally in the tibia, but these are rare. In general, two 5 mm bicortical half pins in the anteromedial face of the tibia and two 5 mm half pins in the distal third of the femur along the rectus femoris/vastus lateralis interval is sufficient (Figs 25.9A to C).[29] We prefer to use an MRI compatible frame to allow both the axial skeleton as well as the knee joint to be studied, if needed. We prefer to predrill and place these pins by hand to prevent thermal bone necrosis. C-arm imaging of the pin placement and the fracture reduction should be performed. Although the intent of the frame is usually temporary, care should be taken to reduce the fracture as well as possible, and allow unimpeded joint visualization. Sepsis or acute respiratory distress syndrome in a critically ill patient may prevent a timely return to the open reduction for definitive reconstruction, and a good initial reduction may become the final reduction.

Compartment Syndrome in Tibial Plateau Fractures

Compartment syndrome is not uncommon in the setting of bicondylar plateau fractures or fracture-dislocations. In a retrospective case series, Stark et al. found an incidence of compartment syndrome following external fixation of a Schatzker type IV fracture of 53% as compared to 18% in a Schatzker type VI fracture. They noted that the onset of compartment syndrome can be delayed up to 24–48 hours after injury and recommended careful monitoring of the patients at risk.[30] This delayed presentation of compartment syndrome may be secondary to slow bleeding into the involved compartments following injury. Placing the foot at neutral at the time of compartment release may increase the risk of compartment syndrome in these patients due to increased pressure in the posterior compartments. It is better to allow the foot to rest in "gravity equinus", which is the position the foot naturally assumes following compartment release—usually 15–20° of equinus. The technique of fasciotomy with a plateau fracture is controversial. Both one-and two-incision techniques are supported.[31,32] The single-incision technique is a laterally-based incision, in which the superficial and deep posterior compartments are released along the posterior border of fibula. A separate more anterior incision is then used for the placement of internal fixation. The most challenging scenario is the need for a two-incision fasciotomy in the presence of a bicondylar plateau fracture requiring both medial and lateral plating. This can be handled in one of two ways. Some surgeons suggest that the incision for the lateral fasciotomy should be placed very anterior. The lateral fascial release and internal fixation are then performed via this single lateral incision. On the medial side, the medial fasciotomy incision can be extended proximally to allow placement of medial or posteromedial fixation as needed. The downside of this approach is that often, the lateral fasciotomy wound cannot be closed primarily, and must be skin grafted, leading to a nonimmunocompetent coverage over the lateral hardware. We prefer a staged, three-incision technique, in which the skin incision for the lateral fasciotomy incision is brought very laterally, almost in line with the fibula. The medial incision to release the deep and superficial posterior compartments is placed distal to, but in line with the proposed incision for the medial plate placement (Figs 25.10A to K). At the time of definitive

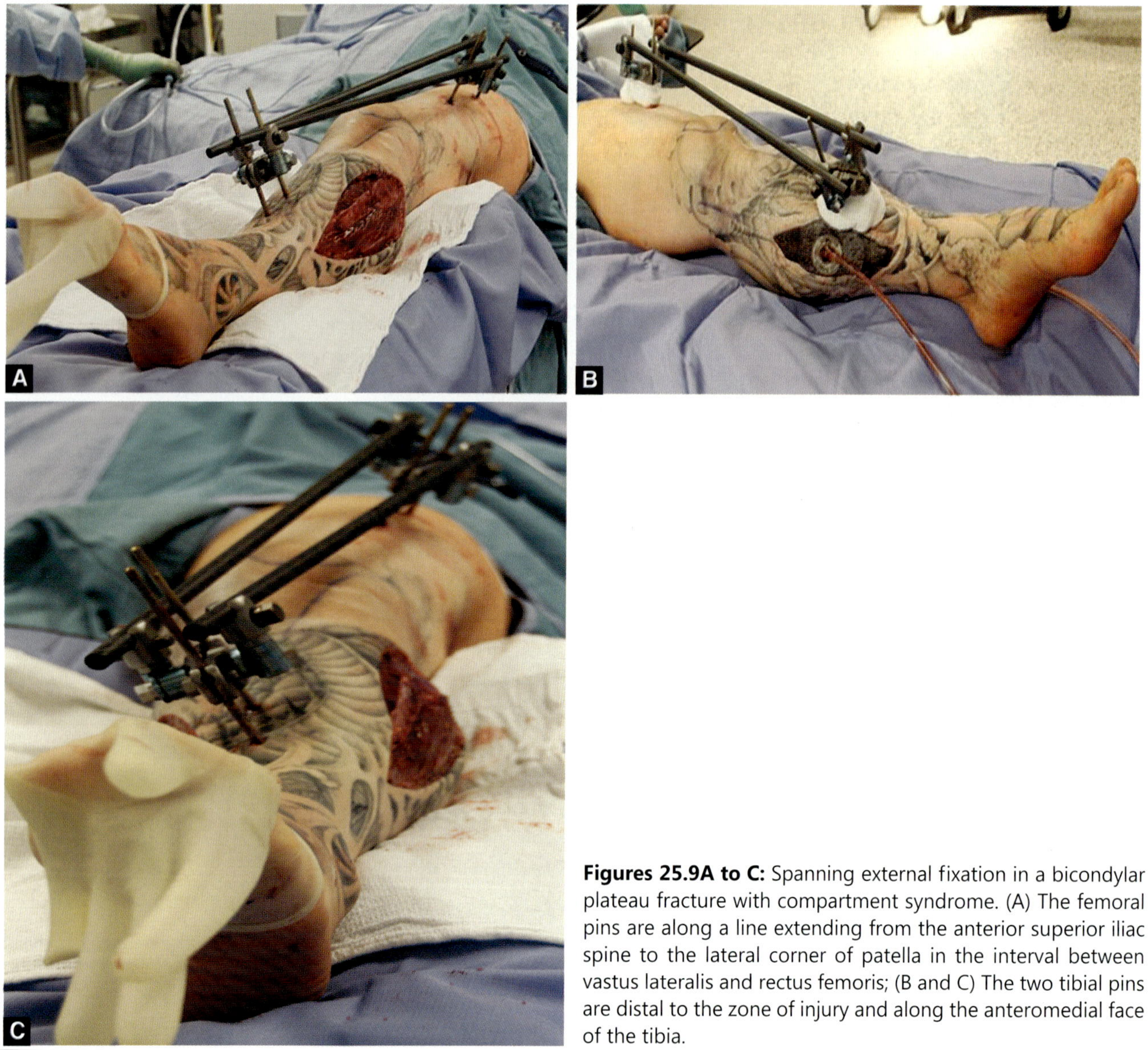

Figures 25.9A to C: Spanning external fixation in a bicondylar plateau fracture with compartment syndrome. (A) The femoral pins are along a line extending from the anterior superior iliac spine to the lateral corner of patella in the interval between vastus lateralis and rectus femoris; (B and C) The two tibial pins are distal to the zone of injury and along the anteromedial face of the tibia.

reconstruction (5–15 days), incision for the lateral fixation is separate from the lateral fasciotomy incision and is placed in an anterolateral (almost midline) parapatellar position. A full-thickness bridge between the anterolateral and lateral incision is maintained (Fig. 25.10D). In general, plate placement is delayed, until swelling has resolved and the fasciotomy wounds are ready for closure or grafting. The medial and anterolateral incisions can generally be closed at the conclusion of open reduction and internal fixation (ORIF). The lateral fasciotomy incision will often require a split thickness skin graft at the same operative setting. The incisions over the hardware are closed primarily with this approach. We feel that this technique allows primary closure over all hardware at the conclusion of the internal fixation.

EMERGENT TREATMENT: Pearls and Pitfalls

- Fractures with shortening such as bicondylar fractures or displaced Schatzker type IV fractures benefit from spanning external fixation
- When performing external fixation, pins are kept out of the zone of injury in the tibia

- Allow the foot to assume a position of gravity equinus after performing fasciotomy for compartment syndrome
- Be mindful of incision placement with fasciotomies with regard to future reconstruction particularly with bicondylar injuries

Surgical Technique and Rationale by Classification

Split Fracture (Schatzker I)

The Schatzker I fracture can be treated either percutaneously or via an open or arthroscopic technique depending on

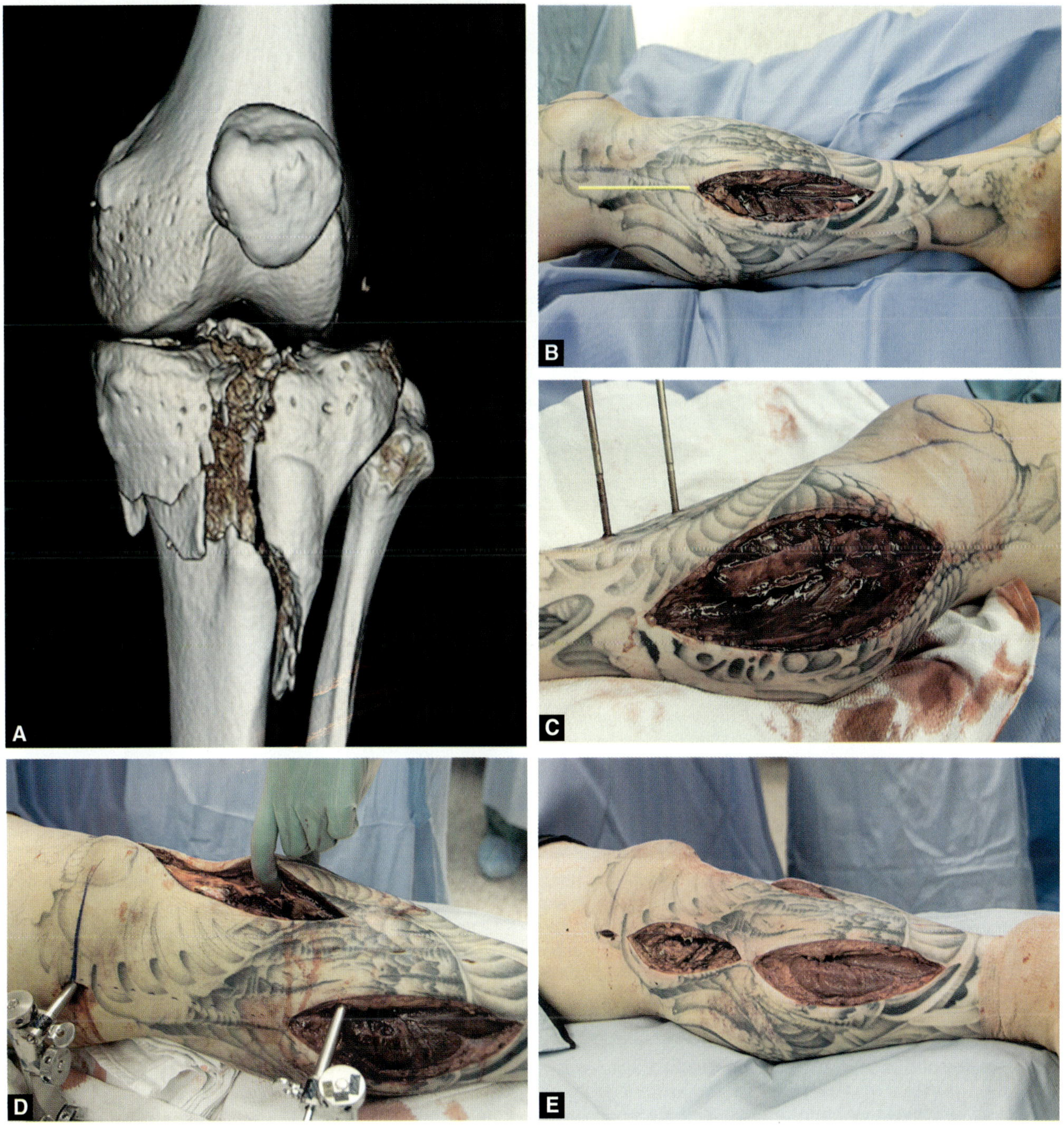

Figures 25.10A to E

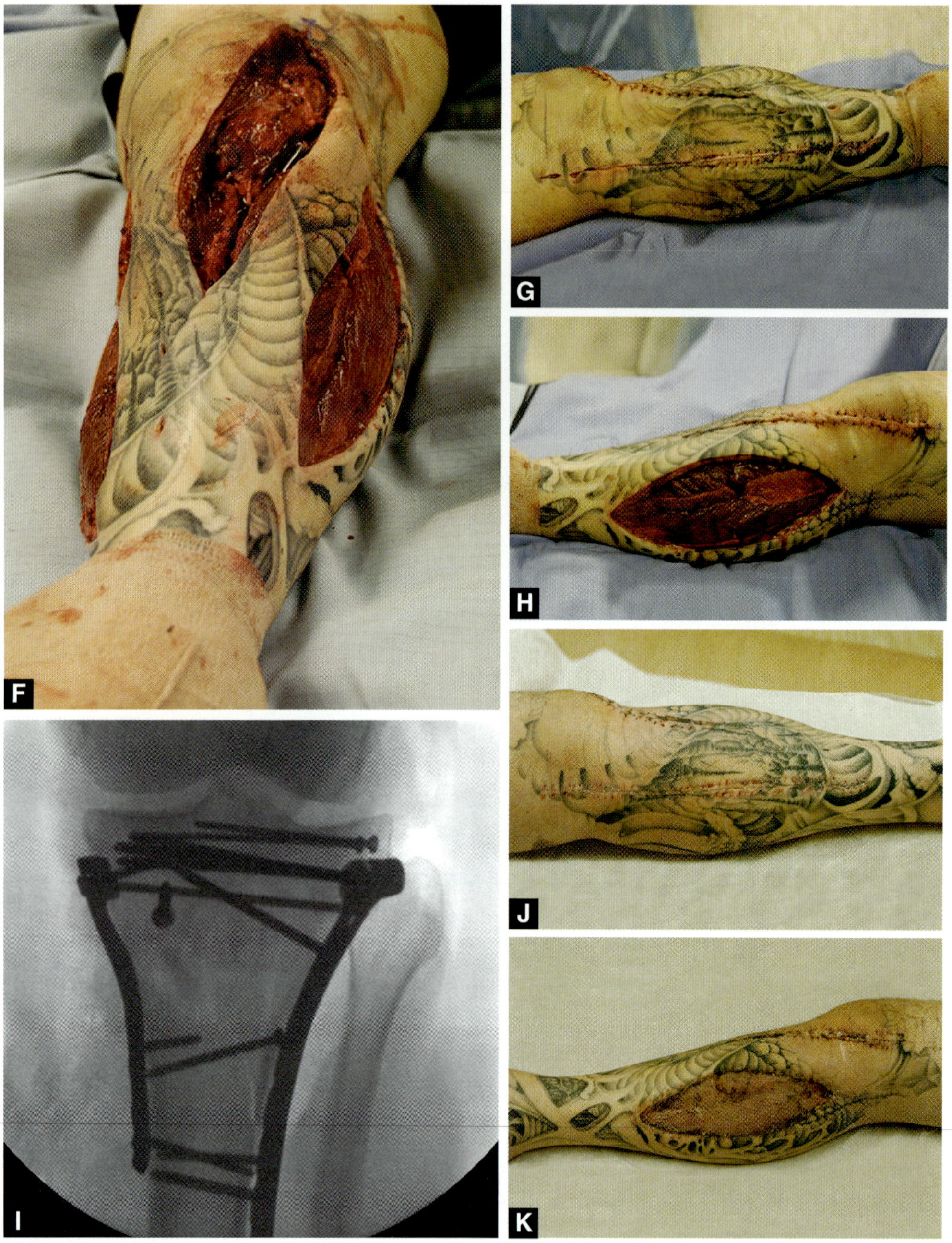

Figures 25.10A to K: Three incision technique of four compartment fasciotomy and staged dual plating of bicondylar tibial plateau fractures with compartment syndrome. (A) Bicondylar high energy tibial plateau fracture as seen on 3D CT image; (B) The medial fasciotomy is along the posterior border of the tibia and distal to and in line with the proposed posteromedial incision that will be used for plate placement; (C) The lateral fasciotomy is along the anterior border of the fibula; (D) At the time of definitive internal fixation (5–10 days), the spanning external fixator is removed. A medial view of the leg shows a separate anterior lateral parapatellar incision for fracture exposure and a medially placed distractor. The skin bridge is maintained by keeping it completely attached to the underlying fascia and muscle; (E and F) Medial and anterior views showing another medial incision for posteromedial fixation. This is in line with, and can be incorporated into the medial fasciotomy incision. The anterior incision is well seen here as well; (G and H) At the completion of internal fixation, the medial and anterior incisions are generally closable. Furthermore, priority is given to closing the incisions over the implants, so they were closed. Although attempts are made to close the lateral fasciotomy wound, there was excessive tension in this case and the wound was left open. Therefore, split thickness skin grafting was performed laterally. (I) Final intraoperative fluoroscopic image demonstrating excellent articular reduction and restoration of tibial alignment; (J & K) (Follow-up) views of the leg with healing of the incisions and skin graft.

the status of the lateral meniscus. If the split is significant (>5 mm),[11] or preoperative studies (MRI) indicate a meniscal tear, then the meniscus should be visualized for extraction and repair. If a percutaneous technique is selected, but the split is unable to be anatomically reduced with a clamp with C-arm confirmation, the surgeon should be prepared to alter the technique to ensure that the meniscus is not entrapped in the split and responsible for the inability to close the fracture gap. Since the bone is of good quality, two lag screws are usually sufficient for stabilization. A third percutaneous lag screw at the inferior apex of the split fragment in the antiglide position has not been shown to provide any biomechanical advantage over two lag screws alone.[33] Alternatively, if an open approach has been made, a small low profile nonlocked periarticular plate will also suffice.[34,35]

Split Depression Fracture (Schatzker II)

This is the most common pattern of the lateral condyle fractures and has great variability of presentation both in location within the condyle and degree of comminution and depression. We prefer a formal open exposure for majority of these fractures, although some can be successfully reduced using arthroscopic techniques.[36] Following exposure, the meniscus should be elevated and completely inspected to determine if a tear exists and if it is repairable. In general, sutures to repair the meniscus are easier to place prior to reduction of the condyle. The depressed segment is approached by exploiting the split and rotating the cortex posteriorly (Figs 25.11A to F). This can be aided by use of a lamina spreader. With the split fragment rotated, the meniscus elevated and a varus moment on the knee, the depressed articular fragments can be disimpacted from the underlying cancellous bone maintaining as much cancellous bone on the fragments as possible. It is often useful to place a kirschner (K) wire into the depressed fragment to maintain orientation and act as a handle. This is particularly useful in situations of multiple depressed fragments. The depressed fragment(s) are then anatomically reduced to either the intact segment of the articular surface or occasionally to the split fragment, whichever provides a more accurate "read" of the reduction. Multiple small diameter k-wires are then placed across the reduced articular surface. The defect can be filled with impacted allograft[37] followed by closing and clamping the split fragment. Alternatively, the split fragment can be closed first and clamped, followed by use of one of the injectable calcium ceramic products. Finally, a nonlocked small fragment[34] buttress plate is applied, preferably with a construct that allows multiple screws parallel and close to the depressed articular segment. A construct of four 3.5 mm subchondral screws ("rafting screws") either through the buttress plate or superior to it has been shown to be significantly better in supporting the depressed segment as compared to a large fragment plate.[38] The meniscotibial ligaments are then repaired. This portion of the closure can be aided by using the most superior k-wire holes in the lateral limb of modern periarticular plates to anchor sutures holding the lateral edge of the meniscus.[39]

Pure Depression Fracture (Schatzker III)

This group represents the lowest-energy fractures in the most osteopenic patients of lateral condyle group. As alluded to by Gardner et al.,[10] this pattern may be very rare as more detailed imaging generally reveals a cortical split not visible on plain radiographs. This fracture can be reconstructed using an open technique and exploiting the small split fracture as described above, or via a closed technique using arthroscopy[36] or C-arm imaging to judge reduction. While not as common in this group, meniscal injuries do occur with significant depression and need to be addressed. The surgeon will face three problems in the surgical treatment of this fracture. The first is the judgment of reduction, if the articular surface is not directly visualized. Due to variability in intraoperative fluoroscopy, arthroscopic assessment of reduction has been shown to be more accurate than C-arm.[40] The second issue is the choice of material to fill the void following reduction of the articular segment. This is a situation, which particularly lends itself to the use of injectable calcium ceramics. As will be discussed in a separate section, the calcium ceramics are an evolving class of materials with excellent immediate compressive strength, exhibiting less subsidence in this setting than cancellous bone.[41–47] After reduction and stabilization of the depressed segment, a closed cavity is created, which is ideal for the injection of the calcium ceramics. The final problem is the fracture stabilization complicated by significant osteopenia that is the hallmark of this injury. As discussed above, rafting screws are ideal for supporting the reduced joint segment. If the lateral cortex is very thin, a small nonlocked buttress plate incorporating rafting screws should be used (Figs 25.12A to E).

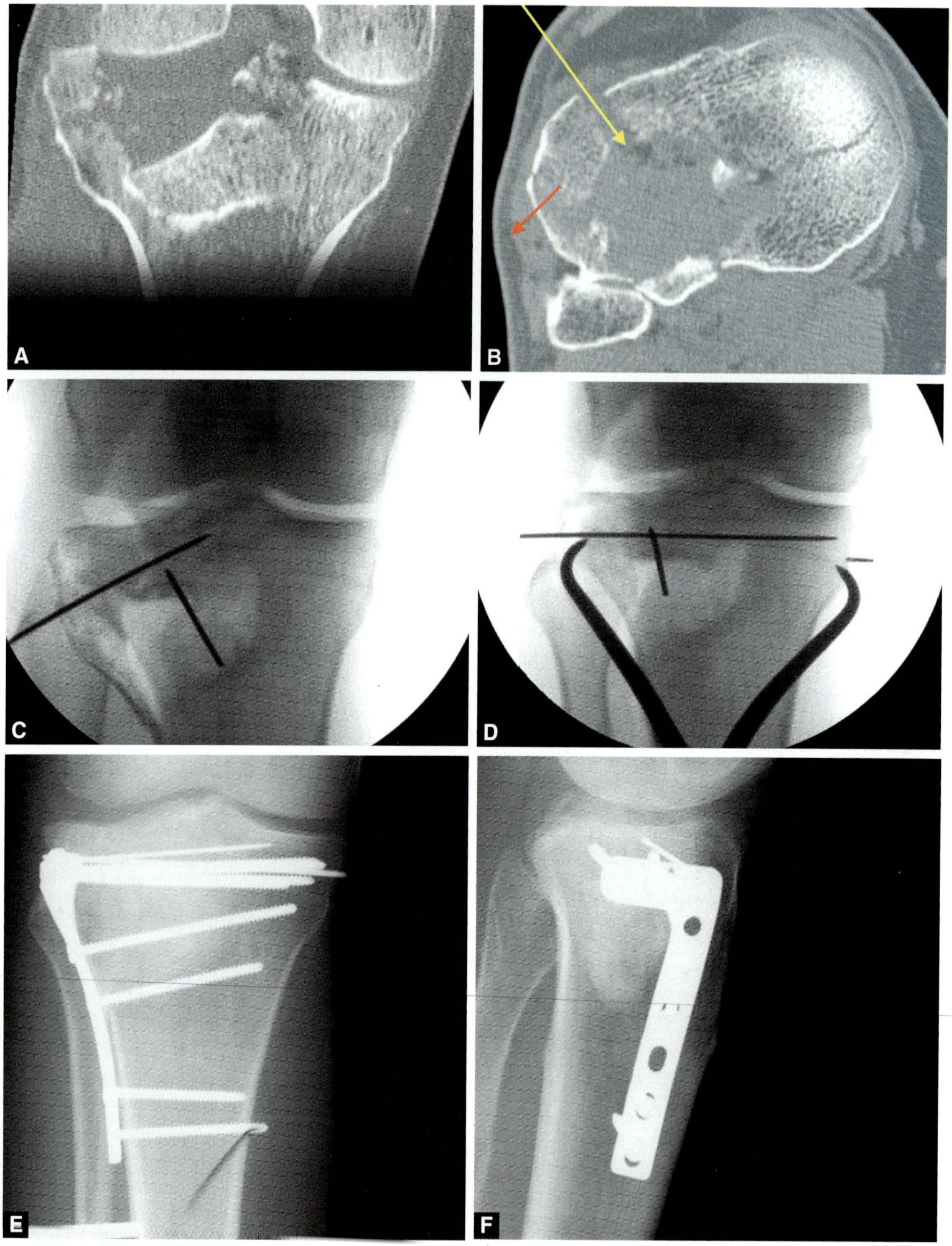

Figures 25.11A to F: (A) Split depression fracture; (B) The split fragment is rotated externally (red arrow) and the depressed segment is entered via the split (yellow arrow); (C and D) The depressed segment is freed at the zone of compressed cancellous bone and is anatomically reduced under direct vision and is fixed with a smooth wire. The split fragment is compressed with a percutaneous tenaculum after filling the void with cancellous allograft; (E and F) Finally, a nonlocked lateral small fragment buttress plate is applied with rafting screws close to the articular surface. Alternatively, the void can be filled with a calcium phosphate ceramic.

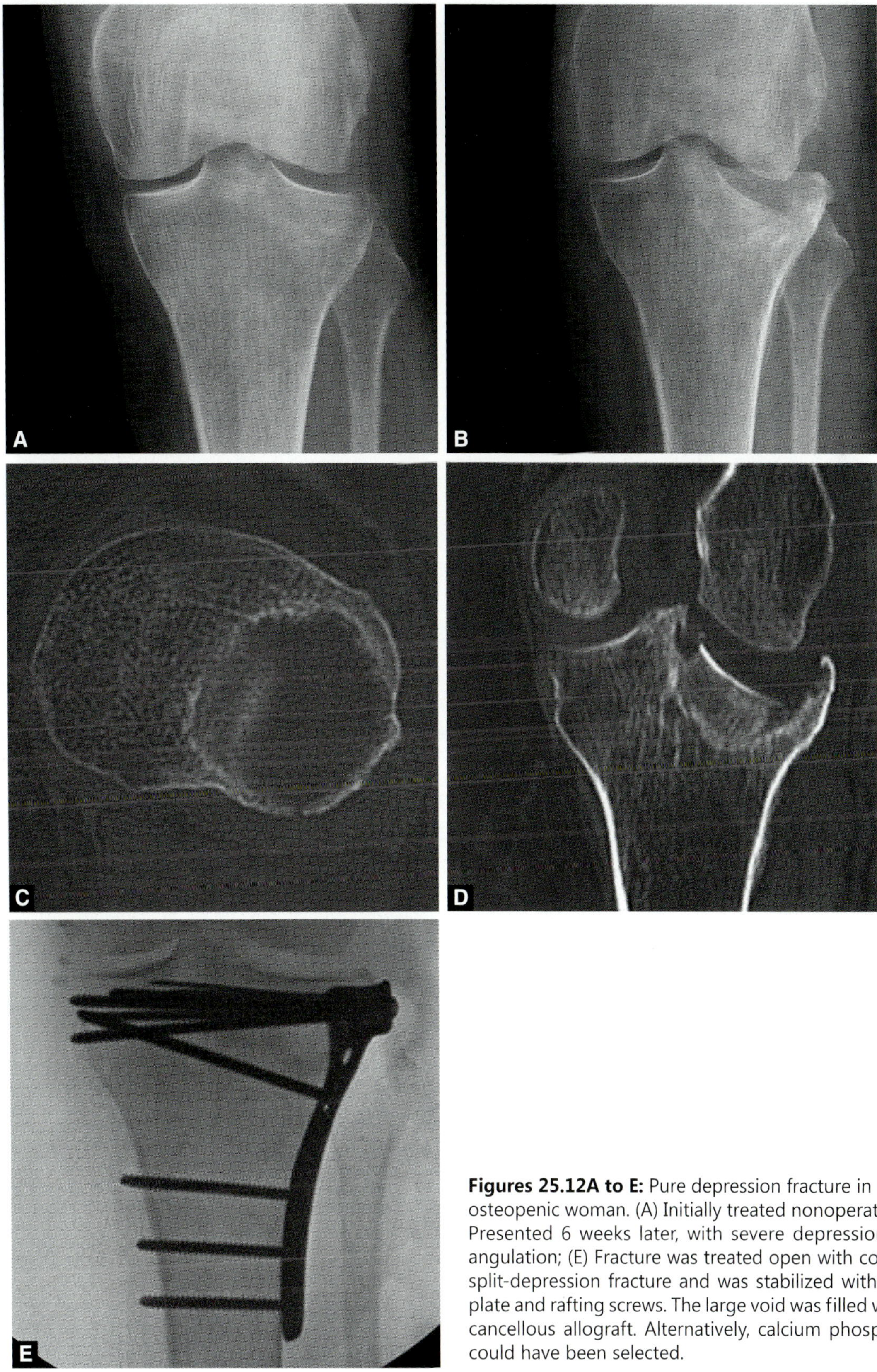

Figures 25.12A to E: Pure depression fracture in a 63-year-old osteopenic woman. (A) Initially treated nonoperatively; (B to D) Presented 6 weeks later, with severe depression and valgus angulation; (E) Fracture was treated open with conversion to a split-depression fracture and was stabilized with a nonlocked plate and rafting screws. The large void was filled with impacted cancellous allograft. Alternatively, calcium phosphate cement could have been selected.

Lateral Fracture Dislocations

This group of injuries is not described in the Schatzker classification and includes those, in which the fracture line exiting out the lateral cortex crosses the midline to enter the medial plateau (Fig. 25.13). This will render the cruciate ligaments incompetent from avulsion. There is often a fracture or avulsion of the fibular head including the LCL insertion. Consideration should be given to MRI scanning of these injuries to fully characterize the soft tissue component. Foremost, these injuries need to be recognized as highly unstable variants with attendant risks to the peroneal nerve and posterior vasculature associated with a knee dislocation. Meniscal injuries are likely to be present due to the significant translation that can occur during the injury. As in their medial counterparts, there is in some cases, the need to plate the fracture on the lateral side, but visualize the reduction, where the fracture exists in the medial plateau. This can be accomplished via C-arm arthroscopy or a small anteromedial arthrotomy. If the median eminence is separate from the main lateral fragment, the cruciate origins need to be reduced and stabilized to restore functional tension. If the attached bone fragment is small, this can be accomplished with heavy suture or FiberWire (Arthrex Inc.–Naples Fla) placed through the base of the ligament at the time of fracture reduction and then brought out through the anterior cortex through drill holes and tied. If the attached bone fragment is larger, it can be anatomically reduced and stabilized to the intact medial subchondral bone via long subchondral horizontal screws. Finally, the avulsed LCL should be repaired to the proximal fibula via a lag screw or tension band construct. In some cases, a formal repair of the posterolateral corner is indicated based on the MRI scan and intraoperative examination of the knee.

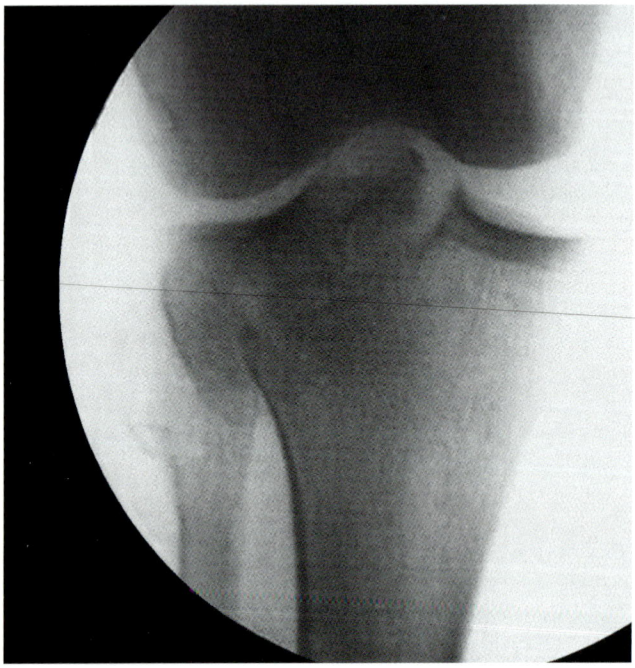

Figure 25.13: Lateral fracture dislocation (Moore type 2). This was fixed with a lag screw across the lateral condyle and a nonlocked lateral buttress plate.

The Posterolateral Fracture

Fractures of the posterolateral corner of the tibial plateau are uncommon but problematic. They occur in about 10% of operatively treated plateau fractures.[48,49] The fragments are usually covered by the fibular head and ligamentous structures in the corner region of the popliteus muscle. These fractures are very difficult to treat using a standard anterior or anterolateral approach. Osteotomy of the intact anterior tibial cortex is an option for exposure. However, this is inefficient and biomechanically unsound in that despite its aggressiveness, this osteotomy does not provide adequate exposure for anatomical reduction, or the ability to properly buttress the reduced fragment. Carlson[50] described a posterolateral approach, in which the posterior tibia was exposed between the fibula and medially retracted lateral head of the gastrocnemius. This approach was used in combination with a posteromedial approach to treat posterior bicondylar fractures in five patients. Bhattacharyya et al.[49] described an extensile posterior approach, in which the medial head of the gastrocnemius was released exposing the entire posterior aspect of the proximal tibia. Both of these exposures require prone patient positioning making it difficult to address other elements of a complex fracture pattern. To address the difficulties associated with this fracture pattern, alternative approaches have been proposed. In 1979, Gossling and Peterson[51] described an extensile approach exposing the entire lateral aspect of the proximal tibia—anterior, lateral and posterior. Anteriorly, tibialis anterior was detached and reflected distally. Posteriorly, biceps femoris and LCL were detached from the fibular head. In 1997, Lobenhoffer et al.[52] described an extensile approach utilizing fibular neck osteotomy with good results in 12 patients. Solomon et al.[48] described a transfibular approach with the patient in supine position allowing direct reduction and buttressing of a posterolateral fragment, while preserving the proximal tibial soft tissue envelope and blood supply. Good results were described in eight patients, with uneventful healing of the fibular neck osteotomy and no injury to the peroneal nerve. A modified posterolateral approach without the use of fibular osteotomy was proposed by Frosch et al.[53] In this technique, patient is placed in a lateral position and a 15 cm posterolateral incision is made beginning 3 cm above the joint line. A lateral submeniscal arthrotomy is made after detaching the IT band from Gerdy's tubercle. This window allows visualization of the articular surface. Manipulation of the fragment and buttress plate placement are performed via a separate posterolateral window created through the same skin incision exploiting the interval between lateral gastrocnemius and biceps femoris. The peroneal nerve is mobilized with the biceps muscle. The authors successfully treated seven patients via this approach and noted that a major disadvantage was restriction imposed by the lateral position.

LATERAL TIBIAL PLATEAU FRACTURES:
Pearls and Pitfalls

- Whereas pure split fractures can be treated with percutaneous reduction and fixation, split depression injuries often require open reduction, articular elevation with grafting and rafting screws and traditional plate fixation. Meniscal injuries are common and should be repaired
- Pure depression (Type 3) fracture patterns are suited for injectable bone graft substitutes
- Magnetic resonance imaging can be helpful to identify ligamentous injury in lateral fracture dislocations
- Posterolateral fracture patterns often require alternative lateral and posterolateral approaches rather than standard anterolateral exposures

Medial Plateau Fractures (Schatzker IV) and Fracture Dislocations

The medial plateau fractures as per the Schatzker classification overlaps with the Moore[15] type 2 fracture-dislocation classification. The spectrum of stability observed in this group depends largely on which side of the median eminence, fracture exits the articular surface. A subclassification of medial fractures based on this concept was proposed by Wahlquist et al.[54] in which a fracture line medial to the intercondylar spine was ascribed as type A, within the intercondylar spine as type B and lateral to the intercondylar spine as type C. Peroneal nerve and arterial injuries were seen only in the subtype C, which also had 67% incidence of compartment syndrome as compared to 33% in type B and 14% in type A. The predilection for compartment syndrome (53%) in the fracture-dislocation group was also reported by Stark et al.[30] Isolated, medial plateau fractures should be stabilized with a medial buttress plate. In a biomechanical study, Ratcliff et al.[55] compared the use of a medial buttress plate (nonlocked) with a lateral locked plate to stabilize a vertically oriented medial fracture and found that the medial buttress plate provided significantly greater stability in static loading and a trend towards improved stability with cyclic loading. The placement of the buttress plate can be directly medial, in which the plate can be slid under the pes tendons or posteromedially (see section on posteromedial approaches) depending on the orientation of the fracture line and location of the spike of the medial fragment. Sometimes, a plate is required both medially and posteromedially (Figs 25.14A to E) because of extensive medial comminution. If the fracture disrupts the lateral articular surface, a separate lateral arthrotomy or arthroscopy may be needed to verify the reduction of the articular surface. Alternatively, an isolated medial plateau fracture can be approached via a midline anterior incision employing a full-thickness skin flap and medial parapatellar arthrotomy.[56]

Medial fracture dislocation patterns can be subtle. Figures 25.15A to D show a medial fracture that does not cross the midline, yet displays a tension failure of the medial plateau with rotation. Intraoperatively, this fracture was found to be very unstable with an avulsion of the LCL from the femoral origin. This was classified as a Moore type 4.

The Posteromedial Fracture

First described by Hohl in 1967,[57] the posteromedial fragment can present in isolation often as the osseous element of a fracture-dislocation (Moore type I).[15] It is very commonly seen as a part of a bicondylar fracture (30–60%). It is usually displaced (>5 mm) and contains about

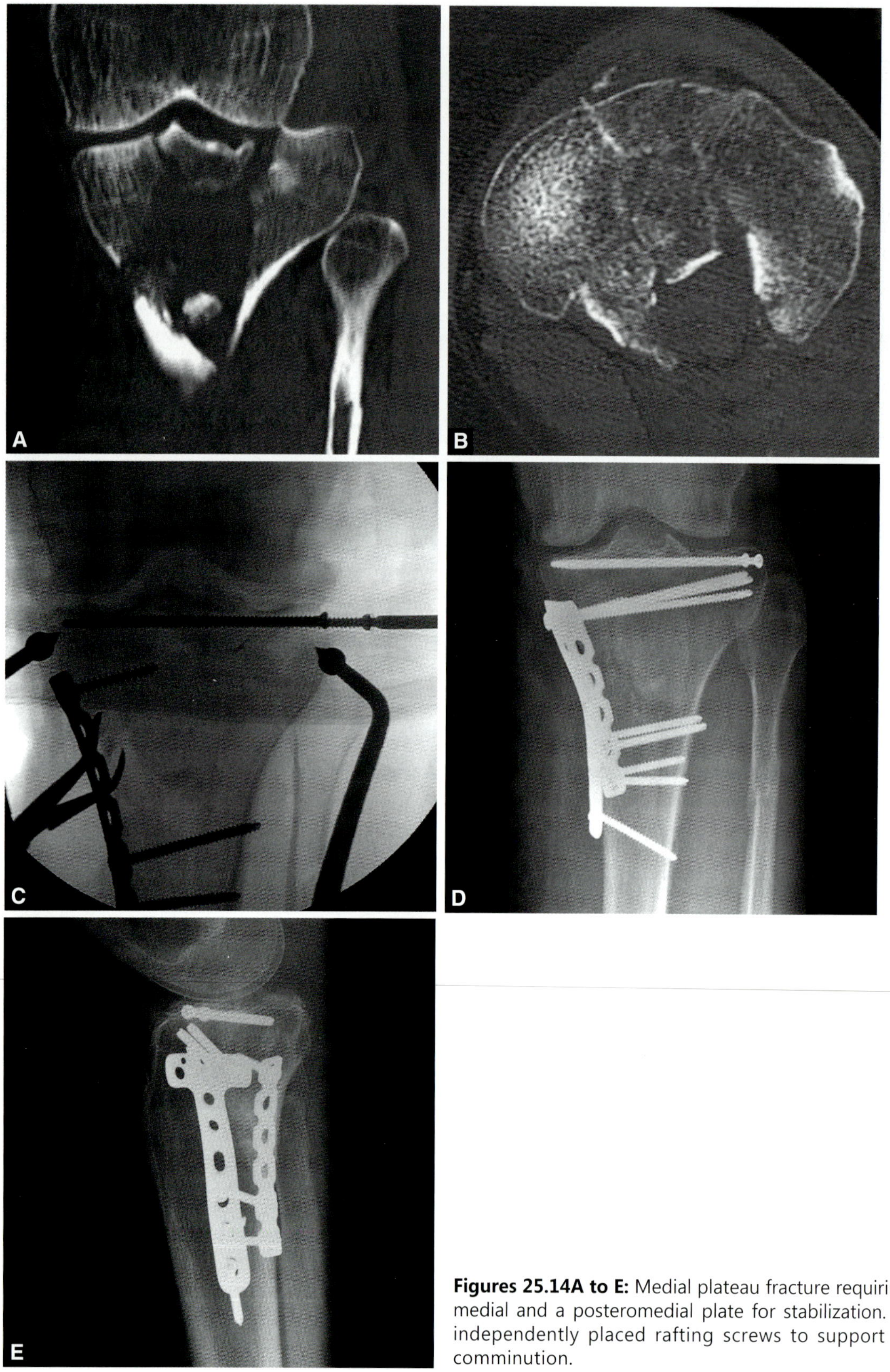

Figures 25.14A to E: Medial plateau fracture requiring both a medial and a posteromedial plate for stabilization. Note the independently placed rafting screws to support the joint comminution.

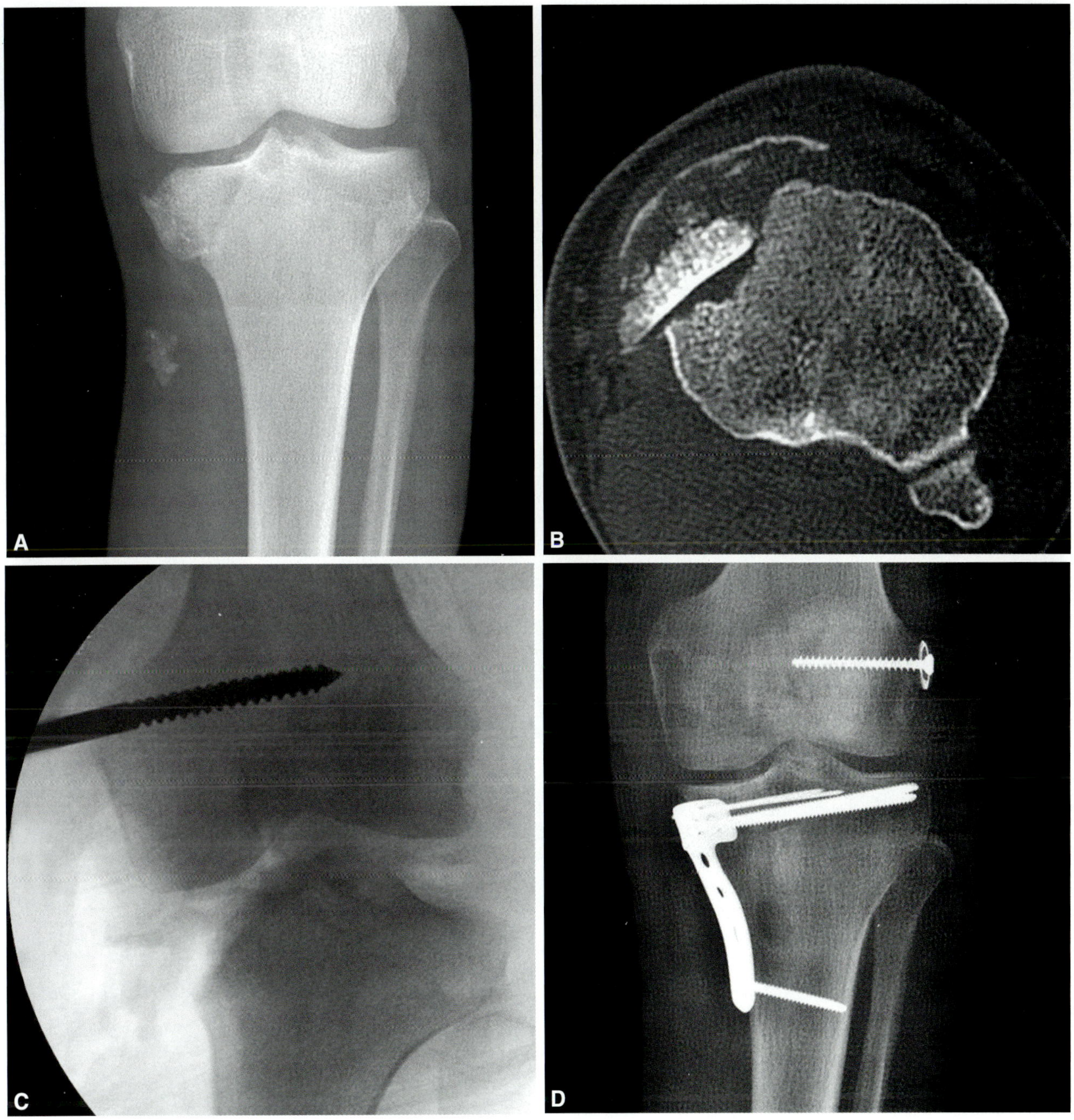

Figures 25.15A to D: (A and B) A medial plateau fracture-dislocation with avulsion of lateral collateral ligament (LCL) from the femoral condyle (Moore Type 4) creating a very unstable pattern; (C) Repair was done by a medial buttress plate; (D) Reattachment of the bone avulsion of LCL from the femur.

25% of the plateau area. Due to the size and location, it is often associated with subtle posterior rotatory subluxation of the femur. The fracture pattern is generally quite vertical and unstable with a high shearing angle[58,59] creating a fragment that may be quite difficult to control without the use of an antiglide plate (Figs 25.16A to C). Failure to stabilize this fragment can result in persistent subluxation of the femoral condyle and poor long-term outcome. In general, this fragment is not fixed well from any lateral plating technique[60–62] and usually requires a direct approach.

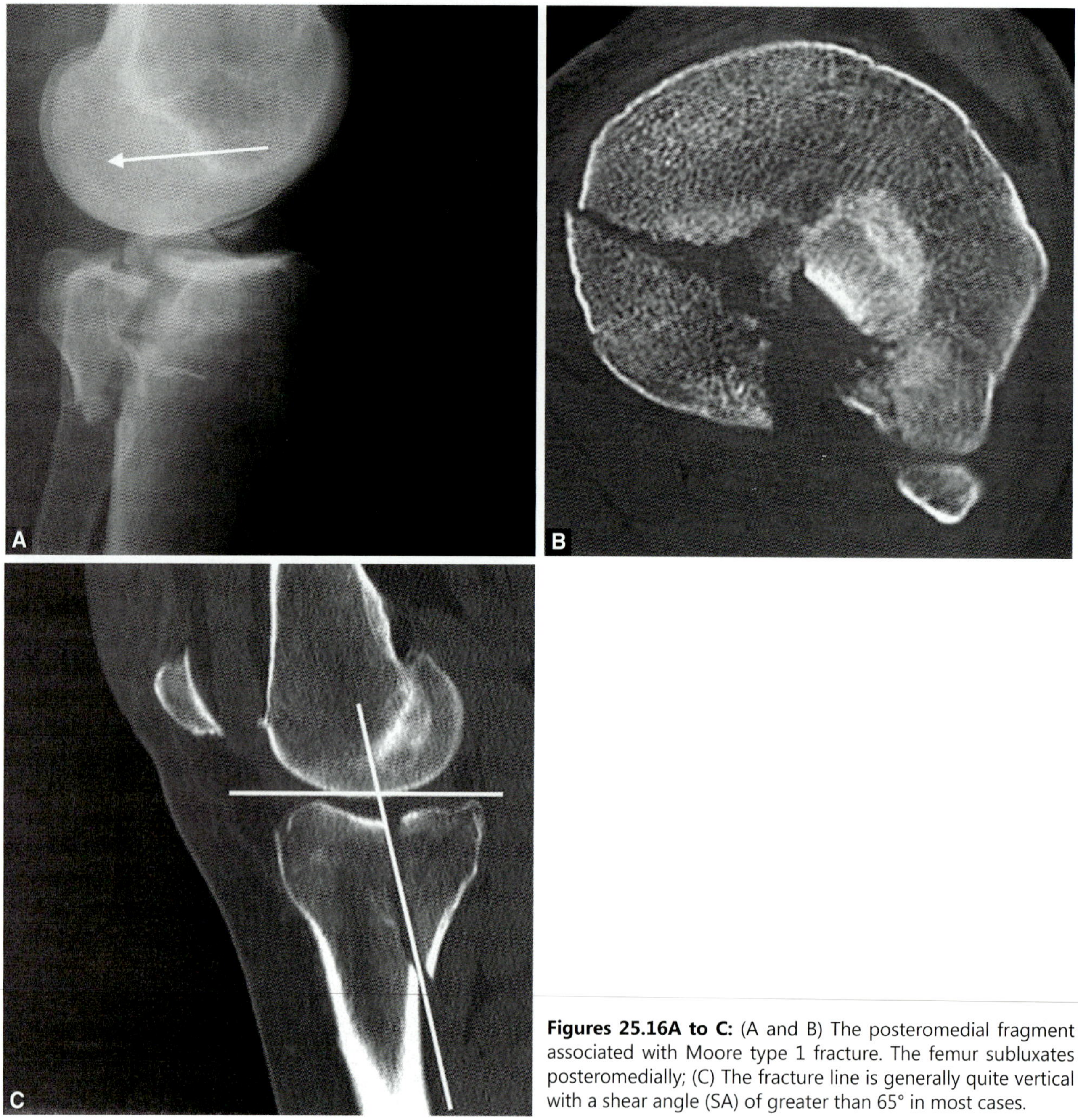

Figures 25.16A to C: (A and B) The posteromedial fragment associated with Moore type 1 fracture. The femur subluxates posteromedially; (C) The fracture line is generally quite vertical with a shear angle (SA) of greater than 65° in most cases.

Both extensile and modified Lobenhoffer[52,63] approaches have been described to gain access. The approach can be done prone in case of an isolated posteromedial fragment. More commonly, it is done supine as a part of combined medial and lateral reconstruction for a bicondylar fracture.[64–67] The skin incision is made along the medial head of gastrocnemius muscle extending from medial femoral epicondyle proximally to the posterior border of tibia 6–8 cm beyond the tip of posteromedial fragment distally (Figs 25.17A to L). The deep dissection is between the medial border of gastrocnemius and pes anserinus. There is no true internervous plane. The MCL remains intact anteriorly. If needed, the semimembranosus insertion can be released off of the bone using an elevator. The pes tendons are

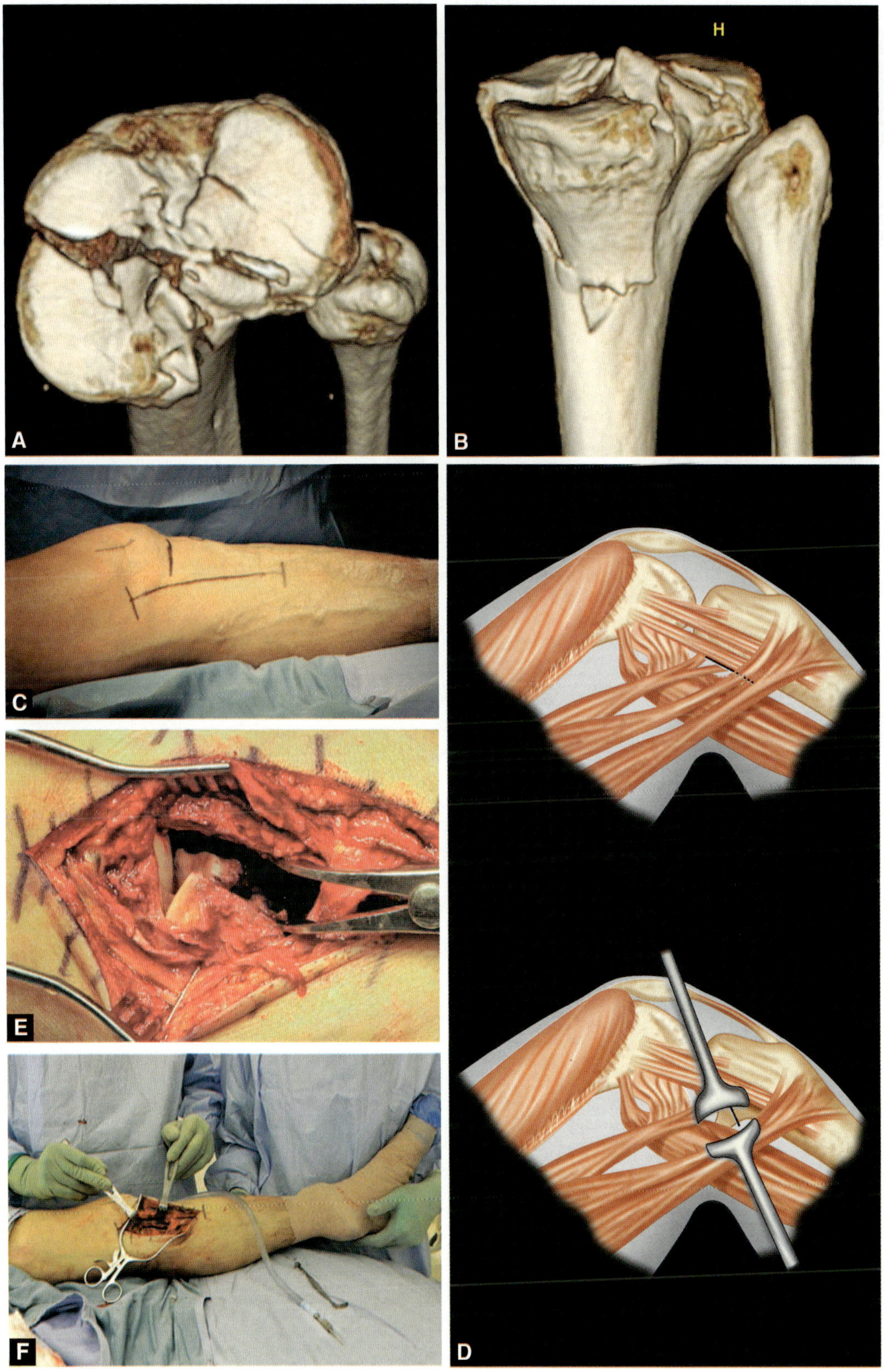

Figures 25.17A to F

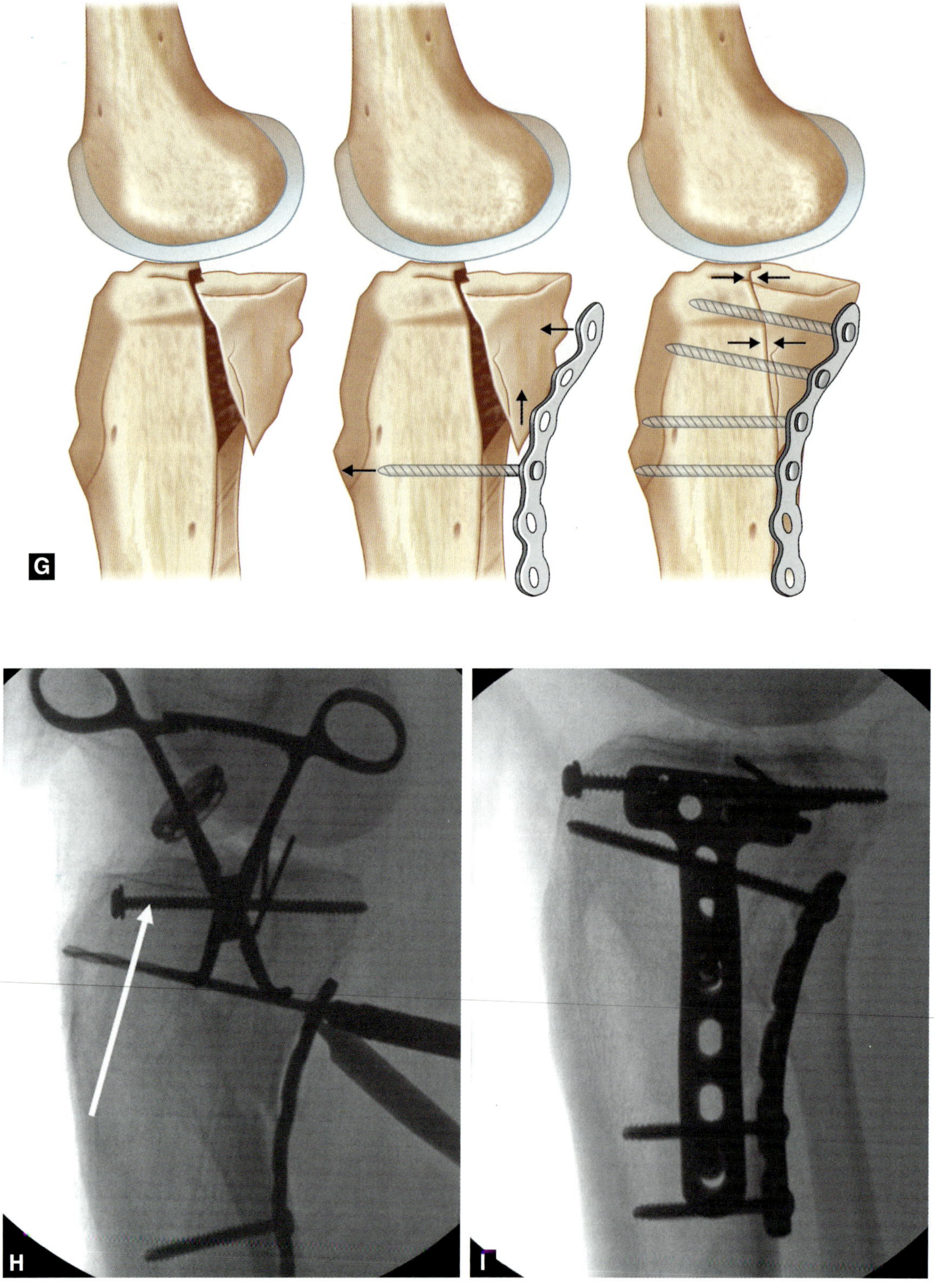

Figures 25.17G to I

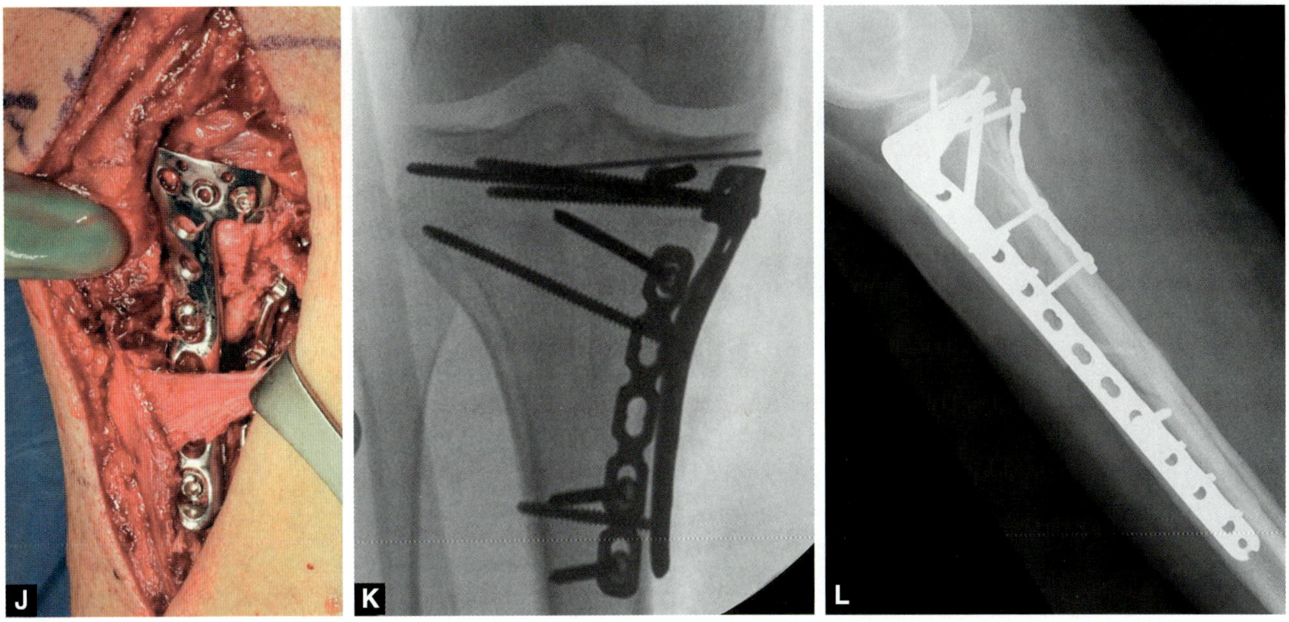

Figures 25.17A to L: (A and B) Three-dimensional reconstruction of a large posteromedial fragment; (C) The Lobenhoffer approach can be utilized in supine position, in which the skin incision is along the posterior border of the tibia; (D) The deep interval is between the medial collateral ligament and the posterior oblique ligament; (E) The joint can be exposed by a submeniscal arthrotomy; (F) Reduction is achieved by knee extension, traction and valgus and is confirmed at both the joint line and metaphysis; (G and H) An antiglide plate is placed with the first screw just distal to the apex of the fragment. A front to back lag screw just distal to the joint line can be useful (white arrow 17H); (I to K) Due to the size of the posteromedial fragment, a second direct medial plate was placed in this case; (L) The position of posteromedial plate in conjunction with lateral locking plate in the treatment of a bicondylar fracture.

mobilized anteriorly keeping their insertion intact. In case of supine positioning, the surgeon stands on the opposite side of the table. In this approach, the articular surface can be visualized via submeniscal arthrotomy, if needed. When the fragment is large and noncomminuted, reduction can be achieved at the level of the metaphysis and can be verified at the joint line via fluoroscopy, without opening the joint. The reduction maneuver is traction on the tibia and extension of the knee. Anterior translation of the femur is often needed. A medially placed femoral distractor may be useful to regain length. After reduction is achieved, it can be held with a k-wire and a pointed reduction clamp. An antiglide buttress plate consisting of a small fragment third tubular or reconstruction plate is sufficient. There are also newer, site specific precontoured plates available. The key is to place first screw just distal to the apex of the fragment on the intact tibial cortex and let the slightly undercontoured plate aid the reduction as the screw is tightened.[65]

MEDIAL TIBIAL PLATEAU FRACTURES:
Pearls and Pitfalls

- Medial and particularly posteromedial fracture patterns should not be fixed with lateral locked plates. Direct medial or posteromedial plate fixation is required
- Medial fracture dislocation patterns can be subtle and ligamentous stability should be evaluated properly to rule this out
- Posteromedial fracture reduction can be assisted with traction and extension of the knee, for which a femoral distractor can be utilized
- Medial fractures and fracture-dislocation have a high incidence of compartment syndrome, which may present late following the injury

Bicondylar Fractures (Schatzker V and VI, AO/OTA Type C and Moore 5)

The bicondylar fractures present special problems in timing, surgical approach and fracture stabilization that can render them a significant surgical challenge. These fractures are generally high energy, may be open, and often occur with associated injuries. They may be functional knees dislocations (Moore 5). Arterial injuries, meniscus and ligament injuries are common and must be addressed. Compartment syndrome both immediate and delayed is common. From a reconstruction standpoint, reduction and stability of both sides of the joint must be achieved and maintained. Early studies proposed medial and lateral plating through a single midline skin incision with poor results secondary to incision breakdown and wound infection.[68–70] This was probably a result of both poor surgical timing as well as excessive bone fragment devascularization. The current treatment of bicondylar fractures has resulted in significantly improved outcomes largely through understanding and respect of the soft tissue envelope. Staged and individualized treatment of these injuries often with initial use of spanning external fixation allows soft tissue recovery, analogous to pilon fracture treatment, and has become the standard of care in most trauma centers.[29,71,72] Definitive treatment must address the need for articular congruity of both condyles and stability sufficient to allow joint motion. Contemporary methods of fixation of bicondylar plateau fractures include appropriately timed medial (or posteromedial) plating combined with lateral plating through two separate skin incisions, circular frame fixation and single-sided fixation (medial or lateral) only with locked plates.

Plating Options in Bicondylar fractures—Dual Plating

Since the fracture of the lateral condyle is usually stabilized by a standard plating technique, the decision making in the treatment strategy of a bicondylar tibial plateau fracture usually centers on the morphology of fracture of the medial condyle. The medial fracture is generally addressed first and may be aided with use of a femoral distractor (Figs 25.18A to D). Typically, the medial condyle has a coronal fracture line creating a posteromedial and anteromedial fragment of varying size (Figs 25.19A to H). A coronal fracture line that is relatively midline or anterior, creates two medial segments that can often be compressed with a lag screw, and then stabilized by a direct medially applied plate. The exposure is directly medial; the articular surface is exposed by elevating the meniscotibial ligament analogous to the lateral side, and a small fragment plate can be placed under the pes tendons. When the coronal fracture line is relatively posterior, the classic posteromedial fragment is present. This fragment is usually displaced,[58,59] has a high shear angle (SA) and is often undertreated by inexperienced surgeons. Reduction and fixation generally requires a direct posteromedial approach and placement of an antiglide plate. The problems associated with this fragment and its treatment are discussed in a separate section. The lateral condyle is usually reduced after the medial side through a standard lateral approach and is stabilized by a locked or nonlocked plate. Again, a femoral distractor can be quite helpful to regain length or visualize the articular surface. The key to prevent soft tissue complications in dual plating is to time the surgery after soft tissue recovery and perform no interval stripping between two incisions. Barei et al.[72] reported on 83 patients with high-energy tibial plateau fractures treated with this approach and found only 11% incidence of nonseptic and 8% incidence of septic complications.

Plating Options in Bicondylar fractures—Locked Plating

Prior to the development of locked proximal tibial plates, bicondylar fractures required dual plating to achieve stability. The introduction of proximal tibial locking plates has raised the clinical question of which (if any) bicondylar fracture patterns can be stabilized with a locked plate from one side only, potentially eliminating the need to make another incision and place a second implant. This is analogous to the situation in the distal femur, in which dual plating is rarely required. The available biomechanical studies that compare dual plating to single locked plating in the stabilization of a bicondylar fracture show a trend toward more movement of the opposite fragment under load with a locked plate than when an antiglide plate is present.[61,62,73,74] The clinical question becomes how much motion is too much, how large of a condylar fragment is needed and of what bone quality to permit the elimination of the second plate? What appears to be clear from the available studies is that the common

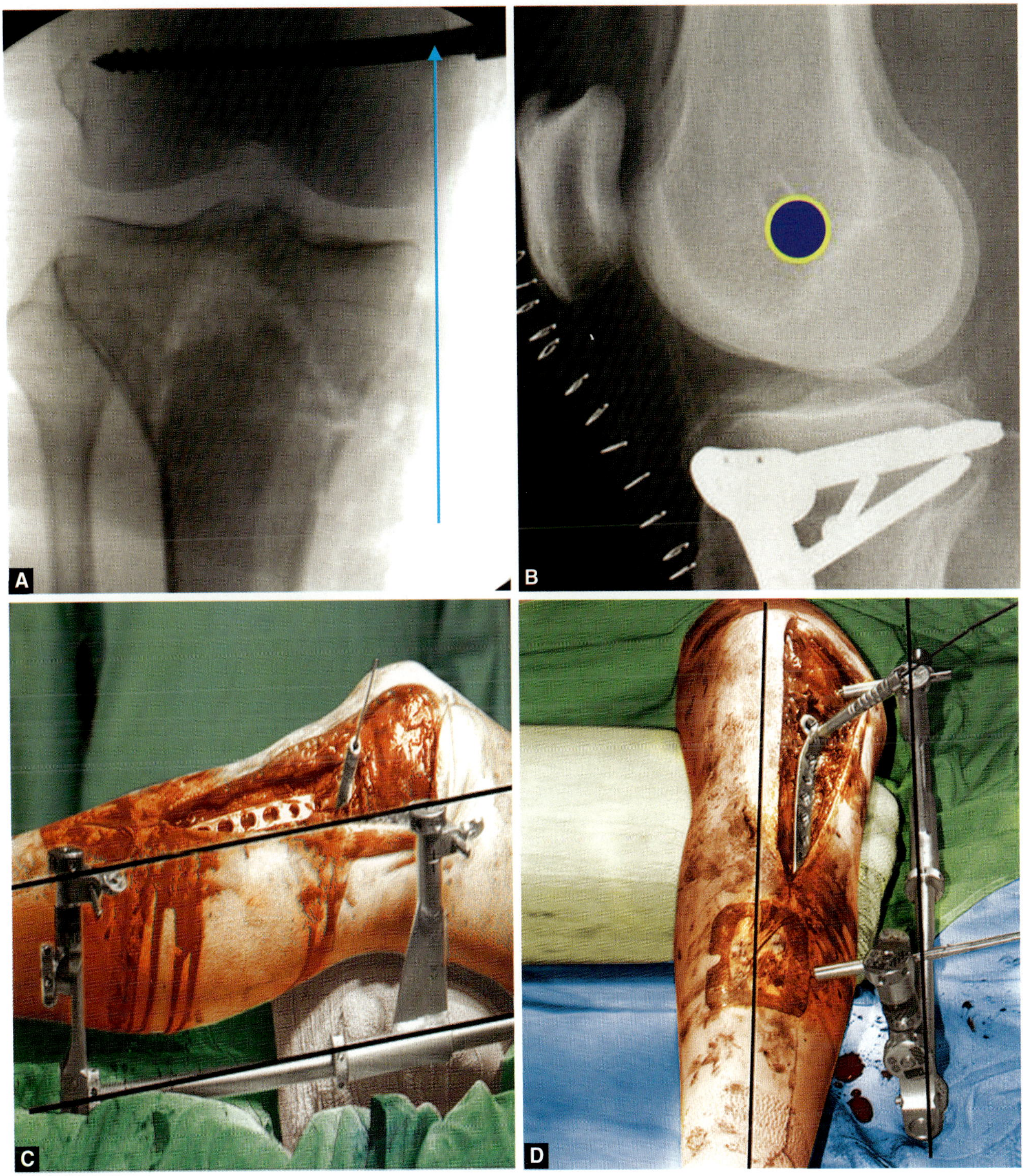

Figures 25.18A to D: Use of the femoral distractor as an aid to reduction in a bicondylar plateau fracture. Since the fibula is intact, the distractor is placed from the medial side in this case. (A) The femoral pin is placed parallel to the joint line; (B) At the intersection of the posterior cortex of the femur and Blumensatt's line, which is the instant center of rotation of the femur. The tibial pin is placed perpendicular to the long axis of the tibia and parallel to the femur pin; (C and D) The axis of the distractor bar is parallel to the tibial shaft in both anteroposterior and lateral projections. This avoids translation during distraction.

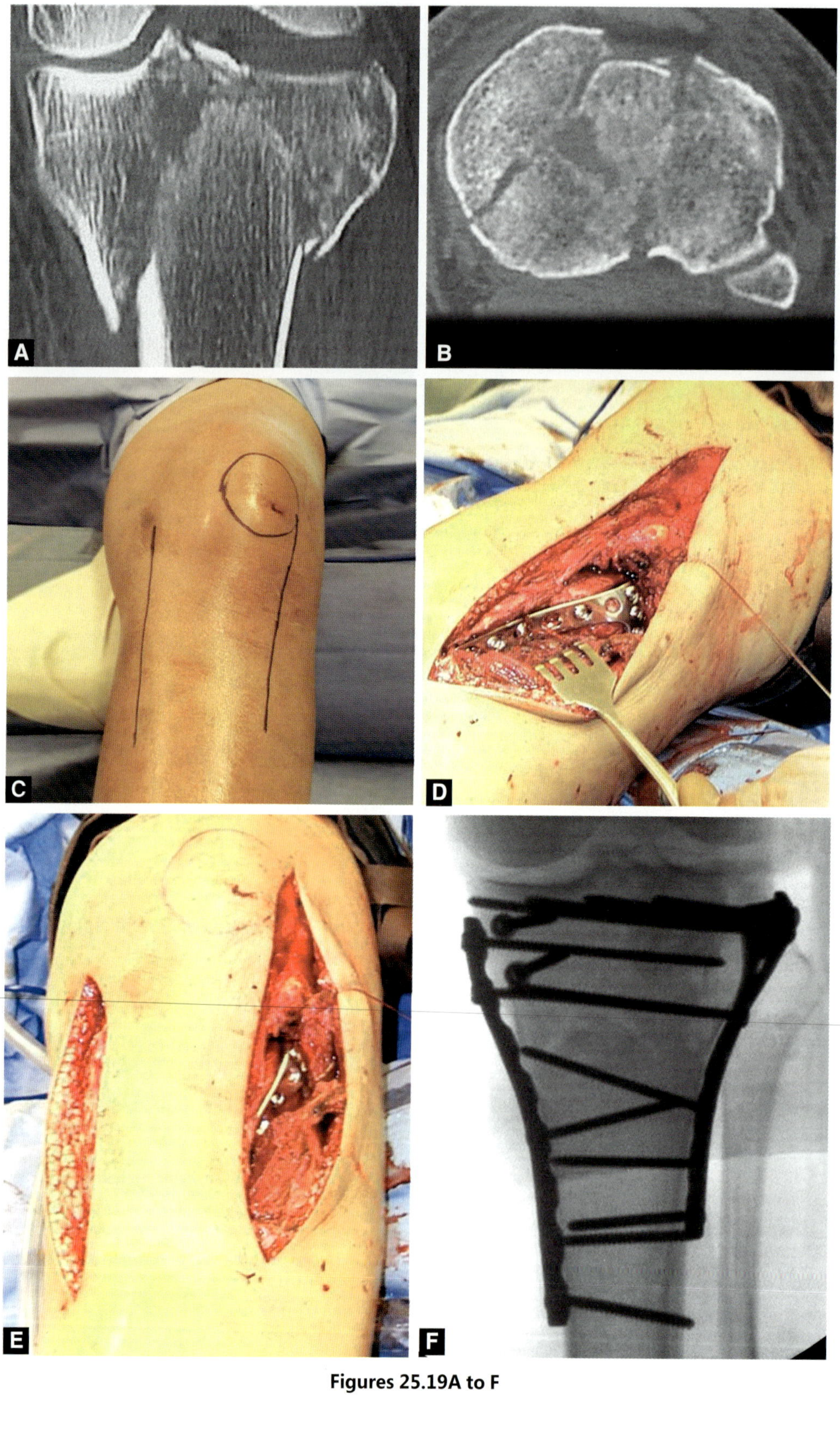

Figures 25.19A to F

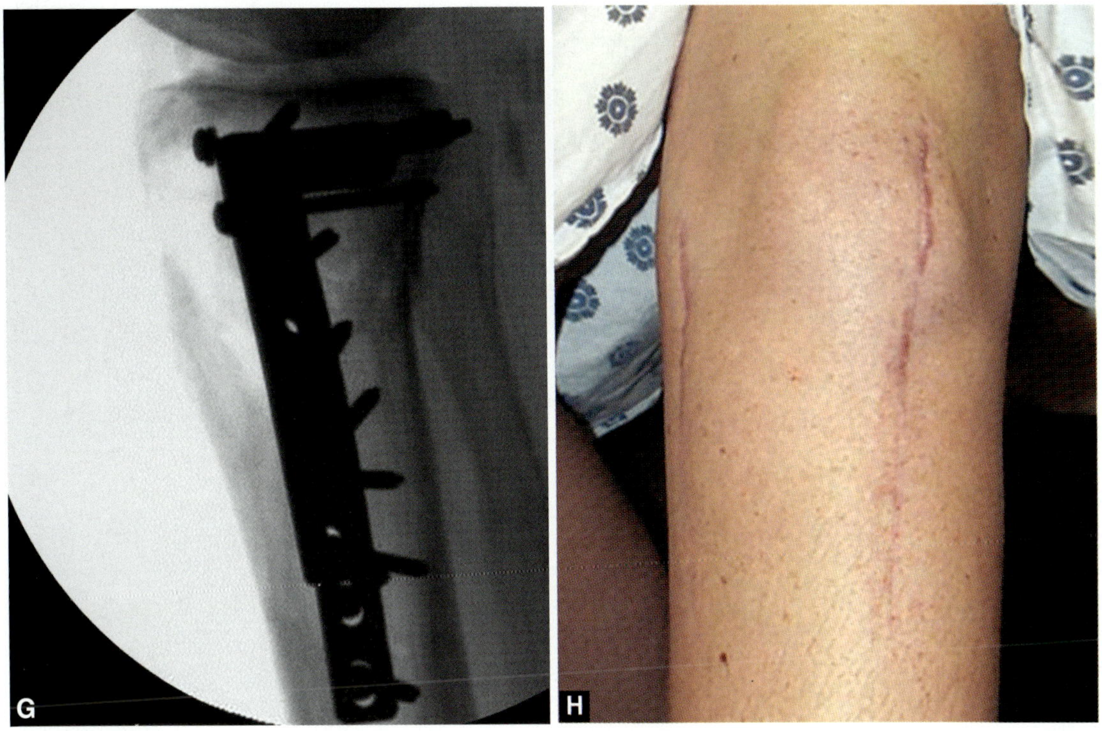

Figures 25.19A to H: (A and B) Bicondylar fracture in a 32-year-old woman; (C to H) She was treated at 8 days post injury with medial and lateral plating via two incisions without intervening stripping.

posteromedial shear fracture discussed earlier cannot be adequately stabilized from the lateral side with a locked plate and needs to be addressed via a separate posteromedial incision (Fig. 25.17L).

Currently, locked plates are available specifically made for both the medial and lateral sides of the proximal tibia. This gives surgeons great flexibility in creating a stable construct from one side of the joint only in selected fracture patterns. Figures 25.20A to H display a bicondylar fracture with medial comminution stabilized with a lateral locked plate without loss of reduction at healing. In some fracture patterns, there exists significant articular depression in addition to condyle displacement. Following elevation of the joint depression, it is advantageous to place rafting screws as described earlier to support the reduction. Usually, these must be placed proximal to the locking plate as either free 2.7 mm or 3.5 mm screws (Figs 25.20G and H). A horizontally oriented three-hole third tubular plate directly proximal to the locking plate can also be an effective rafting construct. A bicondylar fracture with medial displacement and minimal lateral displacement may be stabilized from the medial side only with a locked plate. An intact fibula is a marker that the lateral side of the joint is usually fairly stable and amenable to this technique.

The plating options discussed above, both locking and nonlocking, coupled with staged fracture management have given surgeons increased flexibility and options for stabilizing a bicondylar fracture. Small wire circular external fixation is an alternative technique that allows surgeons to create stability of a complex proximal tibia fracture with minimal additional soft tissue insult. This technique can be extended to incorporate a diaphyseal shaft fracture and can also be extended across the knee to maintain ligamentotaxis in severe fractures. There is a learning curve associated with these circular frame techniques and the occasional user will find them difficult to master.

Hybrid Circular External Fixation for Bicondylar Plateau Fractures

Reduction and stabilization of bicondylar plateau fractures (Schatzker V and VI) demand that both condyles of the joint should be addressed. This technique is usually coupled with percutaneous or open reduction of the joint surface as needed. Circular external fixation involves minimal additional soft tissue injury, and is extremely adaptable to specific fracture patterns. It can be employed in various configurations both in joint sparing, in which

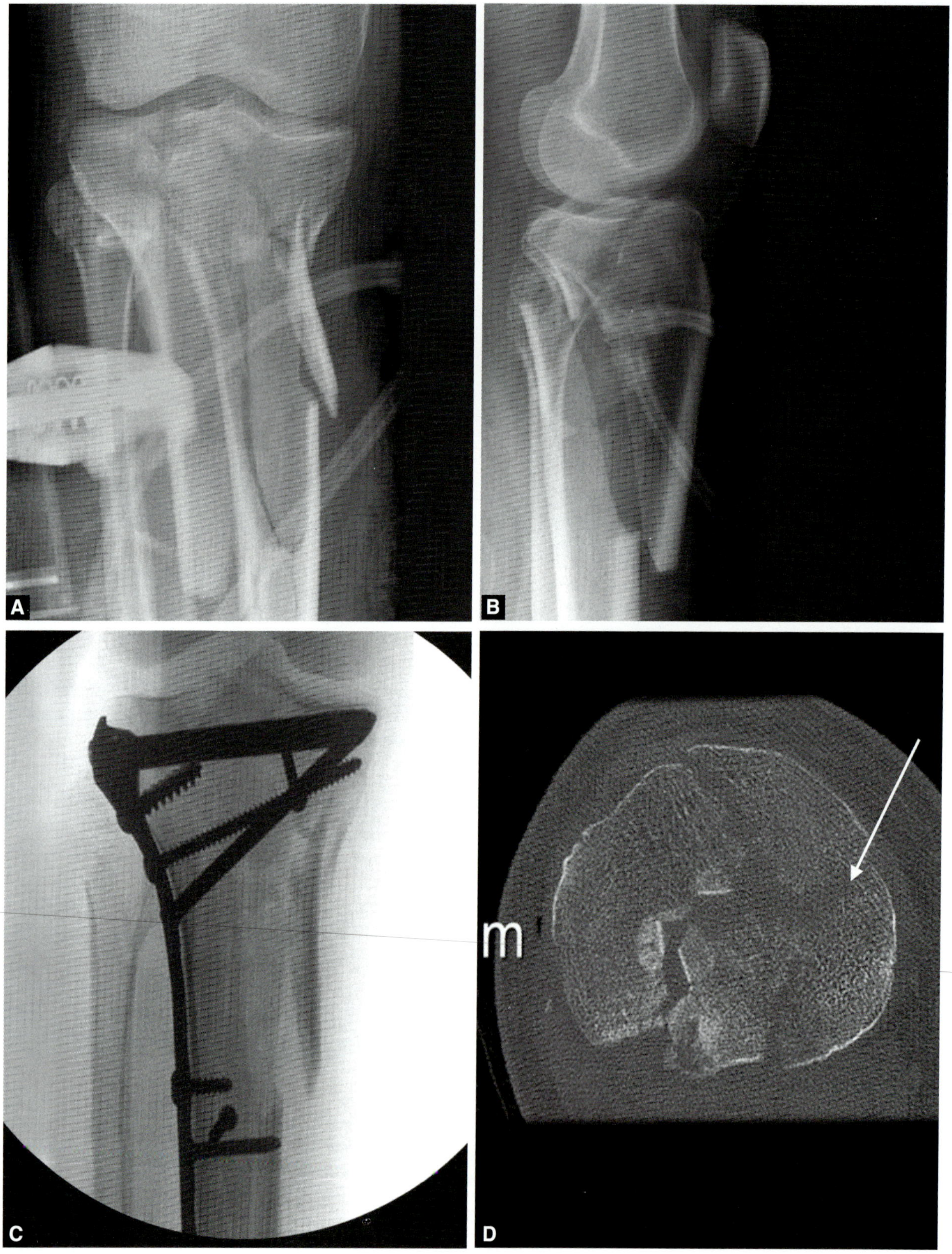

Figures 25.20A to D

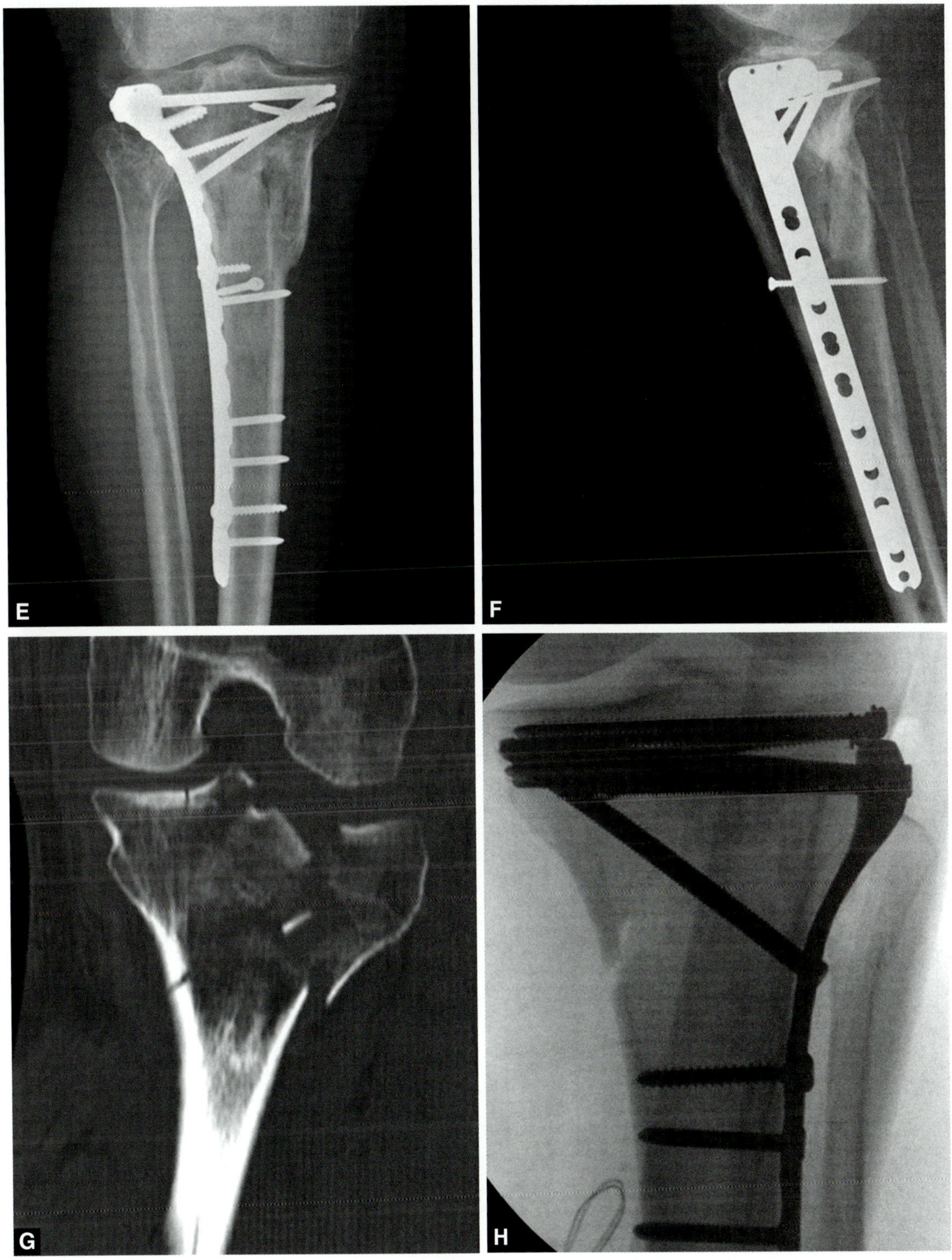

Figures 25.20A to H: (A and B) Bicondylar plateau fracture; (C) fixed from the lateral side only with a locked plate; (D) Note that the coronal split in the medial condyle (arrow) is first anatomically reduced and is fixed with a front to back lag screw; (E and F) The medial comminution heals with callus; (G and H) A bicondylar fracture with extensive joint depression stabilized with a locked lateral plate with rafting screws placed in a subchondral position proximal to the locked plate.

the frame is within the tibia, or in a joint spanning mode, in which the frame is extended to the femur either statically or hinged at the center of knee rotation.[75,76] Indications for joint spanning include severe comminution, knee instability, vascular injury/repair, extensor mechanism disruption severe soft tissue injury.[77] Joint spanning configurations are useful in highly comminuted injuries, as it allows for joint distraction during the early phases of healing. Biomechanically, ring fixator constructs at the level of the tibial plateau exhibits axial stiffness that is very similar to dual buttress plating,[78] and may be less sensitive to bone quality than plate fixation as a result of the nature of tensioned fine wire purchase[79] in the metaphysis. The term "hybrid" fixator refers to the use of both fine wire (1.5–2.0 mm) and half pins (5–6 mm) within the same frame. Half pins are generally restricted to metadiaphysis and diaphysis. Use of a monolateral rail on the diaphysis attached to a ring in the metaphysis should be discouraged, as this creates tremendous cantilever bending forces on the ring/bar junction.[80]

The treatment strategy for fine-wire fixation of a bicondylar plateau fracture begins with injury assessment and reduction strategy. A preoperative CT scan preferably after placement of the spanning external fixator is invaluable in preoperative planning. The accuracy of joint reduction should not be different, when circular frame fixation is chosen as compared to plate fixation. The technique relies heavily on ligamentotaxis to achieve a metaphyseal reduction. This "traction" can be applied via external fixator that is often placed initially. Alternatively, femoral distractors (one or two), or use of a fracture table with distal tibia or calcaneal pin traction may be used. Following distraction and restoration of length, joint reduction can be performed under fluoroscopy with percutaneous "joy sticks" and externally applied clamps. If successful, lag screws or olive wires can be placed to maintain reduction and provide interfragmentary compression. In many cases, the articular surface will require an appropriately timed surgical approach to key areas of the joint to directly control reduction and elevate/graft depressed segments. Since less dissection is required with circular frame techniques, surgical treatment can often be undertaken earlier following injury, which makes percutaneous techniques more efficacious (Figs 25.21A to H).

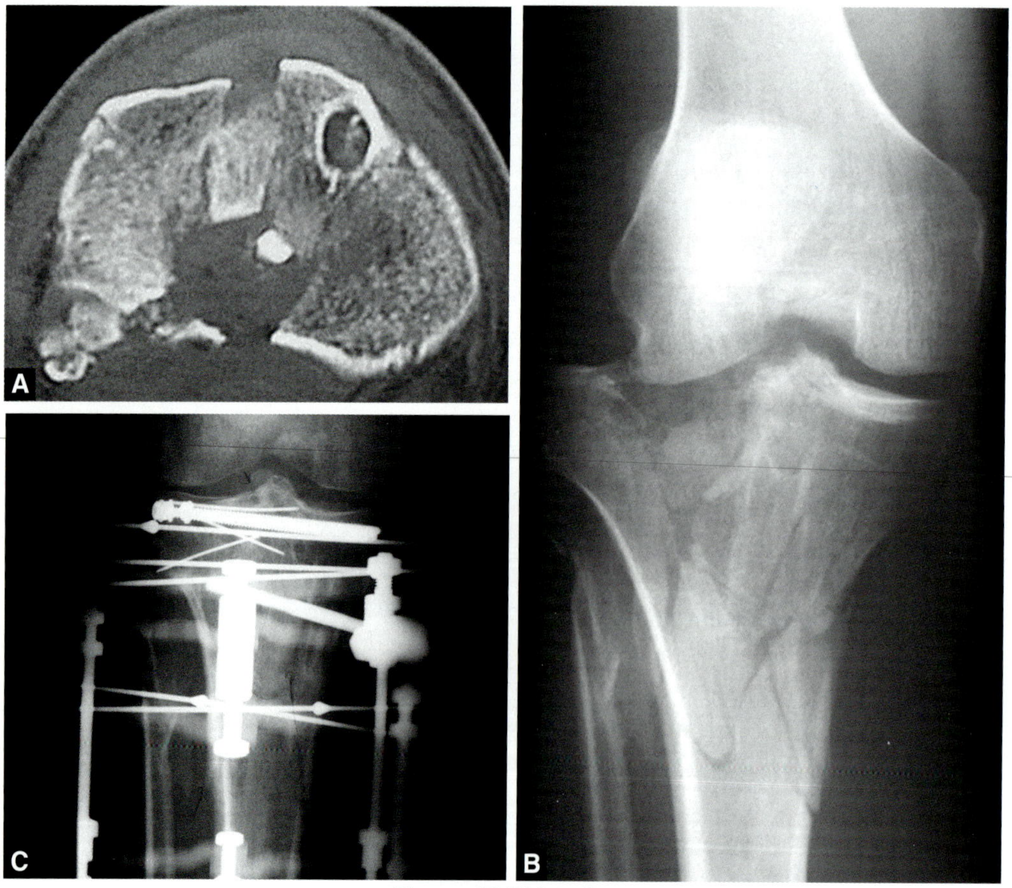

Figures 25.21A to C

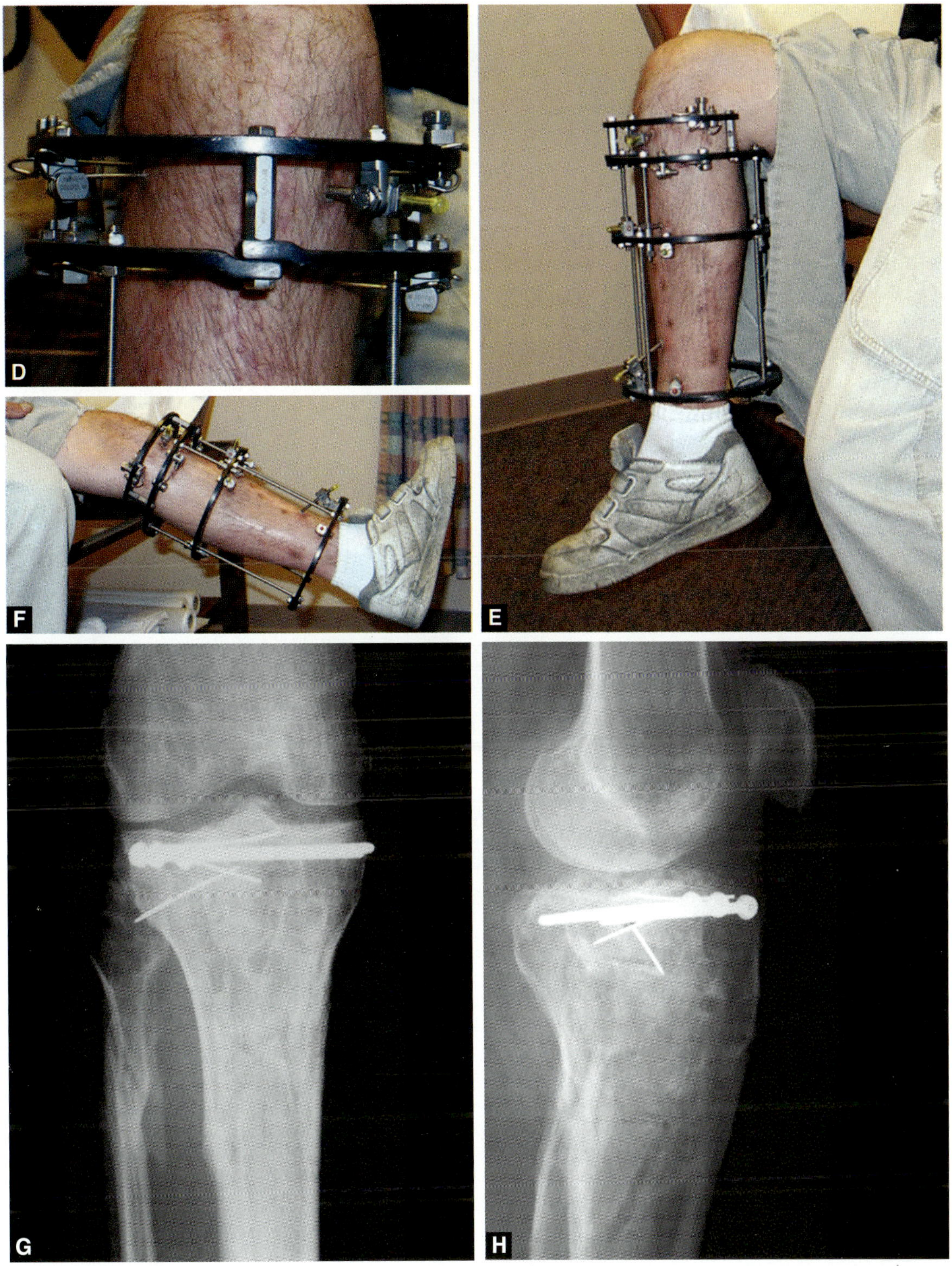

Figures 25.21A to H: (A to C) A 49-year-old male s/p closed bicondylar plateau fracture with significant soft tissue injury; (D to F) A formal open reduction and internal fixation (ORIF) of the articular surface was performed via lateral submeniscal approach and a stable small-wire frame was applied at day 7 post injury. Knee range of motion was maintained in the frame and the patient was allowed full weight bearing on week 10; (G and H) Excellent final reduction and outcome was achieved. The frame was removed on week 20.

Application of circular fixation in the proximal tibia requires knowledge of, and respect for, the interplay of biomechanics and anatomy. The metaphyseal segment must be stable to protect reduction of the articular surface and to allow bone healing. Particularly challenging is control of the flexion/extension moment on the metaphyseal segment due to rotational forces from the patella tendon. The ability to maintain condylar reduction depends on the creation of compressive forces across the fracture lines. If the cross-sectional anatomy permits, this can be achieved by counter-opposed olive wires coming from opposite sides of major fracture lines. Ideally, the wires should be applied such that they cross perpendicular to the major fracture lines to maximize compression. Coronal fracture lines are difficult to control in this way, because they require anterior to posterior fixation, which is outside the anatomic safe zone in the proximal tibia. This is the ideal place for a percutaneous lag screw. Another difficult fragment to control is the posteromedial fragment discussed earlier, this usually presents as a coronal fracture with a high SA and can be controlled with a combination of front to back lag screw and posteromedial to anterolateral olive wire. This wire can be a source of patient discomfort as a result of pes anserinus irritation and may need to be removed prior to overall frame removal to enhance knee motion. Each fragment needs to have at least two points of fixation to provide compression and control rotation. Care must be taken when placing wires near the articular surface of the proximal tibia to avoid capsular reflection. Wires should be kept at least 14 mm from the subchondral bone to remain extra-articular (Fig. 25.7A). Wires placed through the fibular head are even at more risk, since 10% of the population exhibits a communication between the proximal tibiofibular joint and knee joint.[28] Wires that violate the articular reflection may seed the knee joint and result in septic arthritis (Fig. 25.7B).[81] The stability of various wire configurations in the proximal tibia was investigated in a biomechanical study by Watson et al.[80] They compared two or four counter-opposed olive wires with or without a 6.5 mm cannulated screw to dual plating. The most stable construct was the four olive wires and the cannulated screw followed by the dual plating construct. Two opposed olive wires with or without screw fixation were inadequate (Fig. 25.22). The four olive wires were placed with two opposed wires proximally and two more inferiorly near the apex of the condyle. This configuration also improves flexion/extension rotational control of the proximal segment by the creation of a force couple in the short segment.

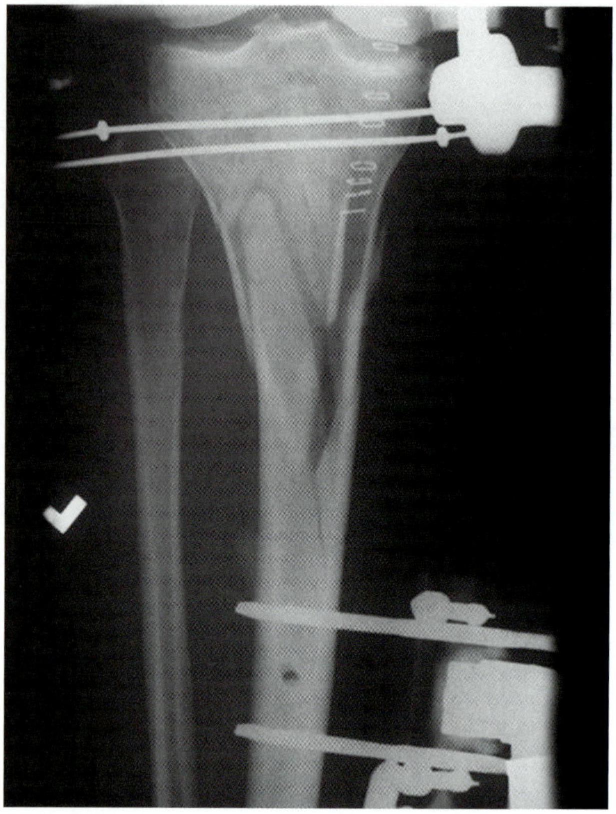

Figure 25.22: Bicondylar plateau fracture fixed with a hybrid frame. This is an example of unstable fixation with only two closely placed wires in the proximal segment. Four divergent wires, or three wires and an anteroposterior half pin are required for sufficient stability.

The purchase of tibial diaphysis is generally with two rings widely spaced with orthogonal half pin or wire fixation at each level. When the fracture pattern allows, compression between the reconstructed articular segment and metadiaphysis should be obtained. This requires a fibular fracture to be present that can be slightly shortened. Compression will result in improved load transmission through the bone with lower stress on pins and wires. The frame will have greater stability and will be more comfortable for the patient. Bone healing will be enhanced in the metaphysis. Achieving compression may result in limb shortening of up to a centimeter (or more in severe cases) and should be discussed with the patient preoperatively. Postoperatively, joint ROM is encouraged with attention to avoid a flexion contracture. Weight bearing can be advanced when the articular portion of the fracture is healed, generally 6–10 weeks. Full unassisted weight bearing in the frame is preferred prior to frame removal, which is usually at 16–20 weeks. If osseous union is uncertain, CT scan may be helpful.

The studies available in the literature documenting the outcome of treatment of bicondylar tibial plateau fractures with hybrid fixation are generally small, retrospective, single-surgeon series.[75,82–90] These reports have demonstrated the efficacy of this technique and generally encouraging results. Watson[83] reported one of the earliest series of 31 high-energy plateau fractures fixed with circular external fixation and noted articular healing at an average of 15 weeks. Average knee ROM was 106° and average hospital for special surgery (HSS) knee score was 82. Reductions were judged as good or excellent in 27 of 31 fractures. There was one shaft nonunion and no serious pin tract infections. Katsenis et al.[77] retrospectively reported on 129 patients with a minimum of 5 years of follow-up. This was a high-energy population with 32% AO/OTA C3 fractures and 36% open fractures. They noted that 82% had a good or excellent score at 3 years and 78% at 5 years. In their series, 14% of patients had a residual step-off of 4–6 mm and 3 patients had a step-off of greater than 6 mm. All of these patients had early arthritic changes at 4 years ($p = 0.004$), again verifying that the quality of the articular reduction drives the long-term outcome. The Canadian Orthopaedic Trauma Society[91] published one of the few studies directly comparing conventional (nonlocked) plating with hybrid fixation techniques in this population. This level I study was a multicenter, prospective, randomized clinical trial with 40 patients in the internal fixation group and 43 in the circular frame group. Sixteen different surgeons were involved in surgical care of these patients. The circular frames were applied using the technique of Watson et al.[83,92] with a minimum of four points of fixation in the proximal segment (i.e. olive three wires and a half pin). Bilateral plates were used in all cases for internal fixation. A single anterior, or combined medial and lateral incisions were used at the discretion of the treating surgeon. There were no significant differences between the groups in terms of demographics, mechanism of injury or fracture severity. The patients in the circular fixator group had less intraoperative blood loss and spent less time in the hospital (9.9 days versus 23 days). The quality of osseous reduction was similar in the two groups. There was a trend for patients in the circular fixator group to have superior early outcomes in terms of HSS knee scores and the ability to return to preinjury activity at 6 months and 1 year. These outcomes were not different at 2 years. There was no difference in total arc of motion. The short form (SF)-36 scores at 2 years were significantly decreased as compared to controls for both groups, although there was less impairment in the circular fixator group in the bodily pain category (score of 46) as compared to the ORIF group (score of 35). The incidence of deep infection in the ORIF group was 18%. The number of unplanned repeat surgical interventions and their severity was greater in the ORIF (37 procedures) as compared to the circular fixator group (16 procedures, $p = 0.001$). Average time to frame removal was 16 weeks. Overall, circular frame fixation was felt to provide a good quality of fracture reduction, shorter hospital stay, marginally faster return to function and fewer and less severe complications as compared to conventional ORIF.

This multicenter study was critiqued by Mahadeva et al.[93] who noted that the hybrid fixator group tended to have better results overall, but were frequently outside statistical significance. Due to inadequate power of the study, this may be a beta type error, accepting no difference when a real difference is present. Unfortunately, this high-quality study was performed before the widespread use of locking plates and employed an unknown number of single anterior incisions to place both the lateral and medial plates. This single-incision technique has been historically associated with a high rate of soft tissue complication.[68–70] Hopefully, another study of this caliber consistently using a two-incision technique as described by Barei et al.[72] and/or employing locked plating in the internal fixation arm will be forthcoming.

BICONDYLAR TIBIAL PLATEAU FRACTURES: Pearls and Pitfalls

- Dual plate fixation for bicondylar fractures should be done directly with two incisions rather than a single midline incision to lessen the chances of infection and wound breakdown
- Rafting screws for articular fragment support should be placed prior to plate fixation

- If tensioned wire external fixation is chosen (often in cases of severe soft tissue injury), diaphyseal rings rather than monolateral bars should be utilized for biomechanical superiority
- Success with ring fixators depends on proper extra-articular pin spread in the metaphysis, compression of the metaphysis to the articular segment, early ROM and weight bearing well before eventual frame removal

High-Energy Tibial Plateau Fracture—Approach to Treatment

The high-energy tibial plateau fracture generally occurs in younger patients as a result of blunt injury or gunshot wounds. A common prototype for this injury is a pedestrian struck by the bumper of a motor vehicle. These patients are often multiply injured, and these fractures are often bicondylar, open, contaminated and highly displaced, precluding nonoperative management. The fractures often defy easy classification and incorporate elements of both bicondylar and fracture dislocation patterns. The soft tissue envelope will also absorb an extensive amount of energy resulting in internal shearing at the skin, muscle and bone interface. Neurovascular injury, bone loss, compartment syndrome (immediate or delayed), and massive degloving are not uncommon. A surgeon not experienced in treating these injuries can be overwhelmed by complexity of the decision-making involved.[94]

Staged Management

Care of this injury begins with care of the patient. Life-threatening injuries must be identified and treated in parallel with care of the injured limb. Radiographs should include the pelvis, femur, knee, tibia and foot, as associated lower extremity injuries are common. Neurovascular status of the limb at knee and foot level should be documented. If injury is open, surgical treatment should commence as soon as the general condition of the patient allows. Staged treatment to allow full injury evaluation and recovery of soft tissue is recommended by many authors.[29,71,72,83] Spanning external fixation as discussed previously, is extremely useful in these situations, as it restores length, provides a preliminary reduction via ligamentotaxis and stabilizes the soft tissue envelope. In addition, spanning external fixation will allow both the physician and the nursing staff to perform dressing changes and wound evaluation in absence of a splint and minimal additional pain to the patient. If the limb is at risk for compartment syndrome, a spanning frame also allows the extremity to be suspended off the bed at heart level, minimizing external pressure and permitting easy measurement of compartment pressure at the bedside. The frame can be extended to ankle and foot, as needed, to incorporate associated fractures and create a stable "working unit". In addition to the placement of a spanning frame, the first operative intervention will include wound debridement and careful check of compartment pressures. If wound coverage is anticipated, the plastic surgical service should be consulted early. In majority of open fractures, a negative pressure wound dressing can be placed over polymethylmethacrylate (PMMA) antibiotic beads for temporary management of the dead space. On occasion, large well-debrided fracture fragments can be definitively reduced and fixed with lag screws at this operative setting, particularly if this closes dead space and stabilizes soft tissues.

Complete imaging, as discussed previously, should be performed following debridement and external fixation. It is at this point that a comprehensive plan of care can be developed. The most difficult decisions surround the technique, approach and timing of the definitive fracture reduction and stabilization. The plan must be individualized based on the fracture pattern and available soft tissue corridors. If fracture is closed, the timing is based on soft tissue recovery. In open fractures, we prefer to couple definitive internal fixation with wound closure or coverage, as this may minimize the chance of infection. This is not always possible and a reapplication of a negative pressure dressing with or without PMMA antibiotic beads over the internal fixation awaiting soft tissue coverage is appropriate. This is a clinical scenario, in which circular frame techniques may have a theoretical advantage over standard plating. However, modern minimally invasive locked plating techniques may negate much of this advantage. The technique employed will usually be surgeon dependent, but it must be remembered that outcomes are correlated to reduction of the articular surface and restoration of axial alignment. A metaphyseal nonunion or malunion is a relatively easy problem to deal with, if the articular surface is well-reduced. Metaphyseal bone loss can be managed with bone grafting (or substitute) at the time of wound closure, or in a delayed fashion depending on the perceived degree of contamination and surgeon preference. If the defect is large and metadiaphyseal, we prefer to treat in a delayed fashion and manage the dead space in the interim with PMMA antibiotic beads. Graft material is either iliac crest autograft, or bone from the ipsilateral femur harvested with the reamer aspirator irrigator (RIA) (Synthes, West Chester, PA, USA).

At the conclusion of definitive reconstruction and soft tissue coverage, consideration should be given in selected severe cases to maintain the spanning external fixator for 2–6 weeks. Mild knee joint distraction should be created in these cases. The ongoing ligamentotaxis can protect the reduction of a comminuted articular surface. Holding the joint in full extension will protect against the common and difficult to treat flexion contracture. Finally, tenuous skin closures and flap coverage will be protected from the shearing effects of early motion and promote immunocompetent primary wound healing. These frames are routinely removed in the operating room and are coupled with careful knee manipulation to maximize the return of knee flexion. Obviously, delay in the initiation of joint motion may have a negative impact on the final degree of knee flexion. Figures 25.23A to I show a very complex high-energy fracture treated with dual plates, in which the spanning frame was maintained for 4 weeks after the internal fixation was performed. The frame was removed in the operating room and a gentle knee manipulation was performed. Figure 25.28 shows a similar high-energy fracture treated with a circular frame technique.

HIGH-ENERGY TIBIAL PLATEAU FRACTURES: Pearls and Pitfalls

- Complications such as compartment syndrome, neurovascular injury and infection are common with these injuries, necessitating careful staged soft tissue and fracture management
- Spanning external fixation is used commonly as a preliminary treatment and can extend to the ankle and foot to incorporate associated fractures

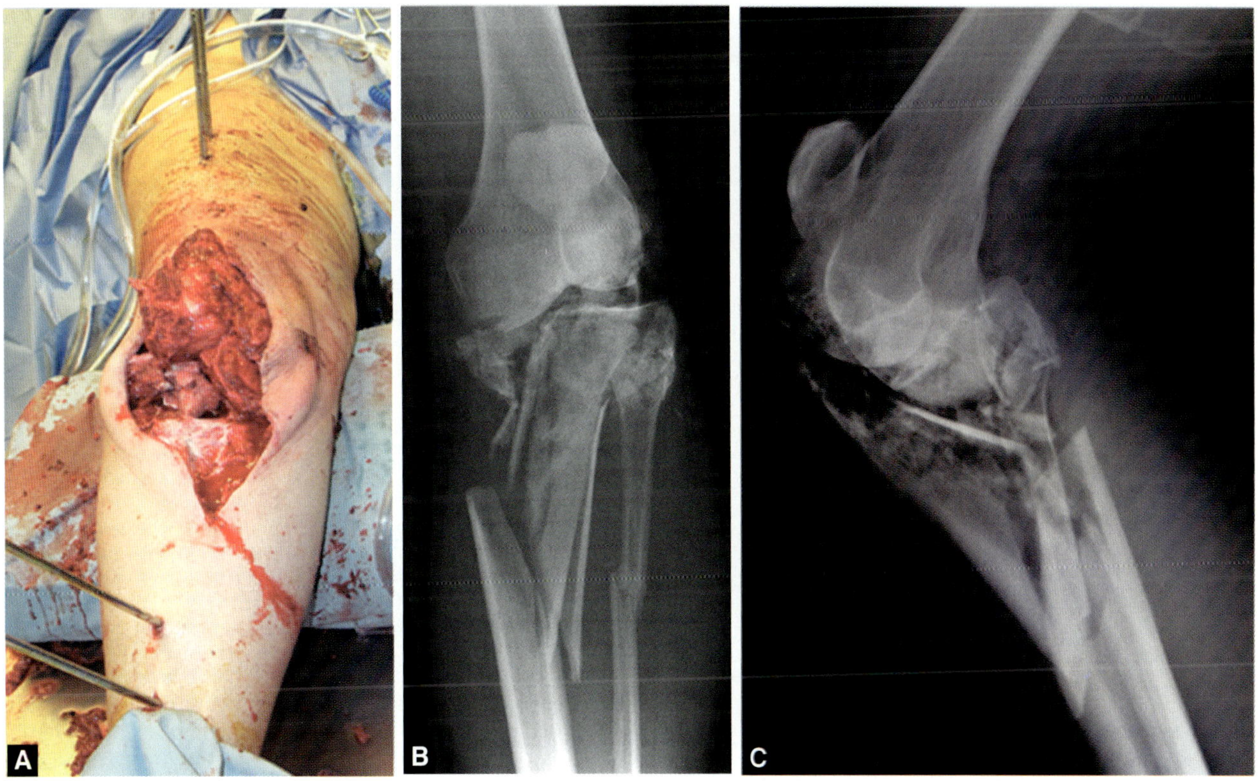

Figures 25.23A to C

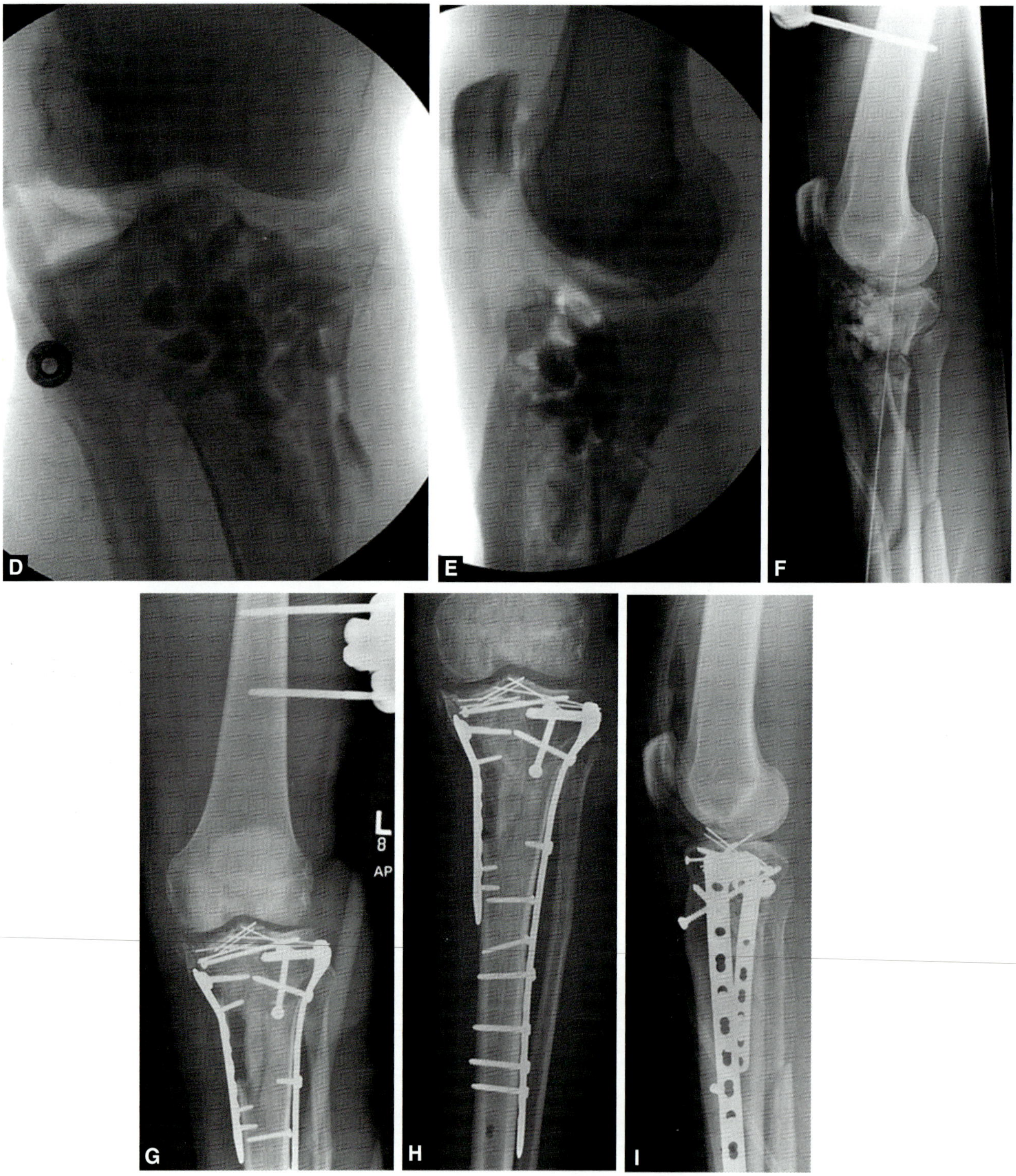

Figures 25.23A to I: (A-F) This grade IIIb open tibial plateau fracture was treated in a staged fashion with initial debridement and placement of a spanning frame. The dead space was managed with antibiotic beads and a negative pressure dressing. Internal fixation was performed via extension of the open wound and was followed by flap coverage on day 8 post injury; (G) The spanning frame was continued for 2 weeks after flap coverage to maintain terminal extension and provide soft tissue stability; (H and I) Delayed (4 weeks) iliac crest bone grafting was performed to the metaphyseal defect. Final range of motion was 3–115°.

- In selective cases of severe comminution, spanning external fixation can be kept in place for 2–6 weeks after ORIF. In most cases; however, stable fixation should allow early motion to be initiated as soon as the soft tissues permit this to be done safely

Filling the Void—Bone Graft and Calcium Ceramics

Historically, autogenous bone was the material of choice for backfilling the defect after reducing depressed segment of a tibial plateau fracture.[95] Since the need for bone induction is rarely an issue in this anatomical location, and to eliminate donor site morbidity, impacted allograft has become widely used in this situation with good success.[37] The introduction of the spectrum of calcium ceramic products has provided surgeons with a variety of injectable bioabsorbable products that offer immediate resistance to compressive forces. Majority of published studies have focused on calcium phosphate products. These substrates exhibit a crystalline-dependent rate of incorporation, meaning that the nature of the crystalline structure will dictate the rate of osteointegration.[96] These are "true ceramics" in that they will not dissolve if they enter a joint. The immediate and significant improvement in compressive strength with calcium phosphate cement as compared to cancellous bone was noted in several biomechanical studies.[41,47] In one of the few animal studies, Welch et al.[42] noted significantly decreased fracture subsidence over time in the calcium phosphate group as compared to autograft in a tibial plateau fracture model. Calcium phosphate was observed to be rapidly resorbed with the volume fraction of cement reduced to 4% at 6 months. The trabecular bone volume in the defect was restored to that of controls by 6 months. In clinical studies, calcium phosphate cement was well-tolerated in the tibial plateau and yielded good results.[43–45] Russell and Leighton and the Tibial Plateau Fracture Study Group[46] reported level I evidence in a multicenter, randomized, prospective study comparing calcium phosphate cement to iliac autograft in tibial plateau fractures. They found a significantly higher rate of fracture subsidence ($p = 0.009$) in the autograft group at 1 year.

Calcium sulfate substrates[97] behave as a true salt in a fluid dynamic sense and will dissolve, if they enter a synovial cavity. They exhibit a crystalline-independent rate of incorporation. Dissolution is associated with a significant increase in osmotic load at the site of implantation and can lead to increased sterile wound drainage.[96] It is available in a self-setting cement, (e.g. Osteoset, Wright Medical Technology, Arlington TN, USA) that will harden quickly and can be instrumented with hardware.

The Use of Bone Morphogenic Proteins in Tibial Plateau Fractures

Bone morphogenic proteins (BMPs) are potent osteoinductive agents. Commercially available BMP products have been approved by the Food and Drug Administration (FDA) for use in both long bone nonunions (Infuse, Medtronic, Minneapolis) and open tibia fractures (Osteogenic protein-1, Stryker Biotech, Hopkinton, Mass). The off-label use of BMP in tibial plateau fractures with bone loss in an effort to decrease healing time has been investigated. Scheafer et al.[98] used a canine tibial plateau model with a subchondral defect to determine if the addition of recombinant human bone morphogenic protein-2 (rhBMP-2) to a calcium phosphate matrix was superior to the use of calcium phosphate alone or autogenous bone graft. At 6 weeks, the BMP group showed significantly increased trabecular bone volume as compared with the other two groups. In clinical studies, the use of BMP as an adjunct to fill the subchondral defect in tibial plateau fractures has been associated with a significant risk of the development of heterotopic bone formation. Boraiah et al.[99] reported that 10 of 17 patients treated with BMP developed heterotopic bone versus 1 of 23 not receiving BMP. Resection of symptomatic heterotopic bone was required in 4 of 17 (24%) of patients, who received BMP as compared to 0 of 23 not receiving BMP. It appears that the applied BMP may not stay contained in the defect and may communicate with the intra-articular and extracapsular space during healing. Figures 25.24A to C show such a case, in which BMP was placed into a large post-traumatic open tibial plateau fracture defect prior to closure with the development of severe heterotopic bone formation about the knee and joint ankylosis.

USE OF BONE GRAFT SUBSTITUTES: Pearls and Pitfalls

- Structural support may be needed for support of previously depressed fragments, although osteoinductive and osteogenic grafts (such as autograft, concentrated stem cells, and BMPs) are typically not needed

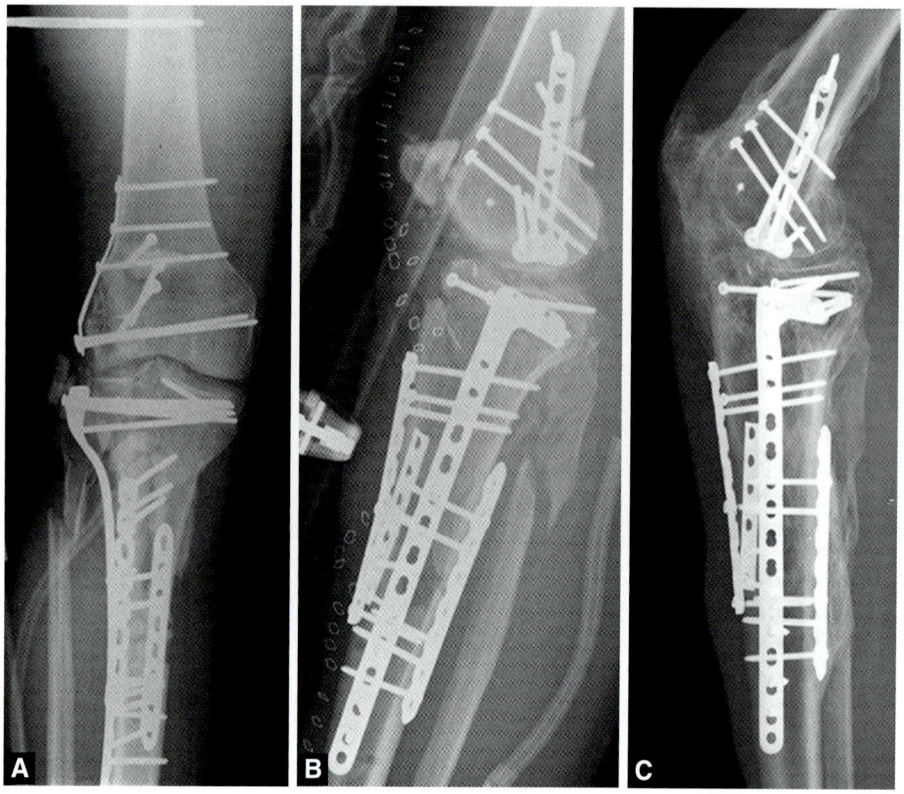

Figures 25.24A to C: (A and B) A 43-year-old male s/p open bicondylar fracture treated in a staged fashion with multiple plates; (C) At the time of wound closure, a bone morphogenic protein sponge was placed into a large metaphyseal defect. Severe heterotopic bone formed around the entire zone of injury essentially rendering the knee joint ankylosed 5 months later.

- Structural osteoconductive grafts that are useful for tibial plateau fractures include allograft cancellous bone, calcium phosphate and sulfate cements and similar "ceramics"
- The rate of resorption varies for bone graft substitutes with hydroxyapatite being the longest and calcium sulfate being the shortest
- Pitfalls include intra-articular leakage (with resulting sequelae) with improper technique of application by the surgeon and postoperative sterile wound drainage with calcium sulfate, in particular

Postoperative Care

Patient care following surgical treatment of a tibial plateau fracture centers on restoration of the joint function and protection of the surgical correction. Joint motion should not be initiated until surgical incisions are dry, which may range from 24 hours to several days in a patient with an injured soft tissue envelope after a long operation. Systemic factors such as low serum protein levels or immune suppression can prolong the wound drainage. In these types of patients, consideration can be given to a short duration wound vaccum assisted closure-KCI over the incision for 72 hours as suggested by Stannard et al.[100] Immunologically competent primary wound healing is the goal at this point. Shearing forces created at the incision edges by joint motion hinder this primary healing and should be avoided. When the wound is dry, initiation of ROM either by a physical therapist or continuous passive motion machine is appropriate. There is no study that supports one technique over the other. Two points regarding joint ROM postoperatively, are important. First, if the fracture configuration split the tibial tubercle from the tibial diaphysis (usually Schatzker IV, VI and selected V's), active extension should be avoided for the first 4–6 weeks. Passive extension and quadriceps sets (attempted straight leg raising) are appropriate. This is to protect fixation of the tubercle fragment. Second, attention must be paid to the avoidance of a flexion contracture. This is common following surgical treatment of a tibial plateau fracture and can occur in up to 20% of patients.[101] We never allow a pillow under the knee and use a terminal extension period of 1 hour three times a day with a pillow under the heel to promote terminal extension. Patients need to be instructed on avoidance of flexion contracture in the postoperative phase of care and needs to be carefully monitored at postoperative visits. If a surgical incision that was dry at the initiation of joint motion begins to drain during therapy, motion is halted and the limb is placed straight and elevated until the incision is again dry. Weight bearing is usually restricted for 8–12 weeks depending on the presence of joint depression and the quality of fixation. While "toe-touch" weight bearing is widely prescribed, this position of the leg promotes knee flexion contractures and ankle equinus. Instead, "foot flat" is much preferred, in which the therapist teaches the patient to rest weight of their leg on the floor with heel contact to promote terminal extension of the knee and an ankle neutral position. Supervised physiotherapy is continued for 12 weeks. Recovery of quadriceps strength generally lags behind hamstrings recovery. At 1 year, most patients have recovered only about 80% of their quadriceps strength,[101] highlighting the need to continue self-directed therapy after discharge from supervised physiotherapy.

Patients without risk factors for deep vein thrombosis are discharged on once a day prophylactic low molecular weight heparin (LMWH) for 3 weeks. If the patient is mobilizing well by the third week, this is converted to 325 mg acetylsalicylic acid until weight bearing is initiated. Patients at higher risk or very slow to ambulate are either continued on LMWH or converted to prophylactic warfarin until weight bearing.

The progression of knee flexion in the postoperative period should be closely monitored. Most patients will achieve greater than 100° by 3 months.[101] In a severe fracture, the recovery of 90° of flexion by 4 weeks is a good prognostic indicator. Failure to achieve 90° by 8–10 weeks is an indication, in our practice, for a knee manipulation under anesthesia, followed by 3 days of regional block and intensive physiotherapy. After 10 weeks, knee manipulation can be considered, but often, the collagen cross-linking is too extensive for success. Arthroscopic and/or open lysis of adhesions and quadricepsplasty may be required after this point.[102] If the patient was placed in a spanning external fixator for an extended period of time either preoperatively, or as an adjunct postoperatively, adhesions can develop between the femoral pin sites and overlying muscle groups. This can be an independent source of restricted knee motion and may require a separate surgical approach (direct lateral) for release.

POSTOPERATIVE CARE: Pearls and Pitfalls

- Joint motion should be initiated as soon as wounds are dry
- Avoid allowing a flexion contracture to develop
- Avoid active extension for 4–6 weeks in fracture types involving a split of the tibial tubercle
- Failure to achieve 90° of flexion by 8–10 weeks is an indication to proceed to a knee manipulation under anesthesia followed by 3 days of regional block and intensive physiotherapy

Complications and Author's Preferred Management of Select Cases

Loss of Fixation

Loss of fixation following reconstruction of a tibial plateau fracture can take two forms. In the first type, implants have remained essentially stable, but articular fragments have moved during the period of healing resulting in a residual deformity in the form of articular step-off, condylar widening or varus/valgus deformity not present in the immediate postoperative radiographs. It is important to note that these are not nonunions. This type of loss of fixation can be subtle and not recognized unless specifically searched for by comparing radiographs at healing with immediate postoperative radiographs. The second, more familiar type of loss of fixation occurs during the period of fracture healing and consists of gross failure of hardware, with screw pullout and screw or plate breakage associated with visible loss of reduction.

The first type of loss of fixation was specifically addressed in a rather unique paper by Ali et al.[103] The authors of the 12 leading articles on tibial plateau fractures were contacted to find a consensus on the definition of "failure of fixation". Remarkably, the responses were fairly consistent and were summarized as articular step-off greater than 3 mm or a malalignment of greater than 5°. Interestingly, these criteria were essentially the same as the indications for surgical treatment outlined earlier in this chapter.[22] Ali et al. retrospectively reviewed 43 of their own fractures using these failure criteria, and found that bone quality (age) and fracture complexity strongly correlated to failure of fixation. The fractures that failed were in patients with a mean age of 70 years as compared to 38 years for the fractures that did not fail ($p < 0.001$). All patients with osteoporosis failed. The incidence of failure in AO/OTA B3 and C3 fractures was 40% as compared to 0% and 20% in AO/OTA B1 and C1 fractures respectively. Noncompliance with weight bearing instructions was also statistically correlated with loss of fixation. Overall rate of loss of fixation was 31% in this study. Figures 25.25A to G show a bicondylar fracture in a severely osteopenic patient treated with dual plates. There was substantial loss of fixation of the medial plateau resulting in varus collapse and an eventual need for knee arthroplasty. Note that the position of the hardware did not change during the loss of fixation, rather the medial plateau "settled" secondary to osteopenia.

The second type of failure of fixation (implant failure) presents at a variable time during the period of healing. Although, not specifically studied, it is our experience that noncompliance with weight bearing restrictions is also highly correlated. Painless presentation of gross hardware failure should alert surgeons to a possible Charcot joint or other neuropathic process. This clinical scenario usually requires a revision surgery, if the loss of reduction is significant and the joint is to be salvaged. The principles employed in the treatment of this problem are in many ways identical to those of nonunion surgery. Occult infection should always be considered and multiple intraoperative cultures should be obtained in all cases. Staging these reconstructions to allow culture results to manifest is appropriate. Hardware can be removed, cultures are obtained, and antibiotic beads and simple spanning external fixation are placed. If cultures are negative, the definitive reconstruction can be performed often in the same hospitalization. If cultures are positive, the patient can be discharged on appropriate antibiotics and can be scheduled for delayed reconstruction. These surgical cases are usually quite demanding and much more

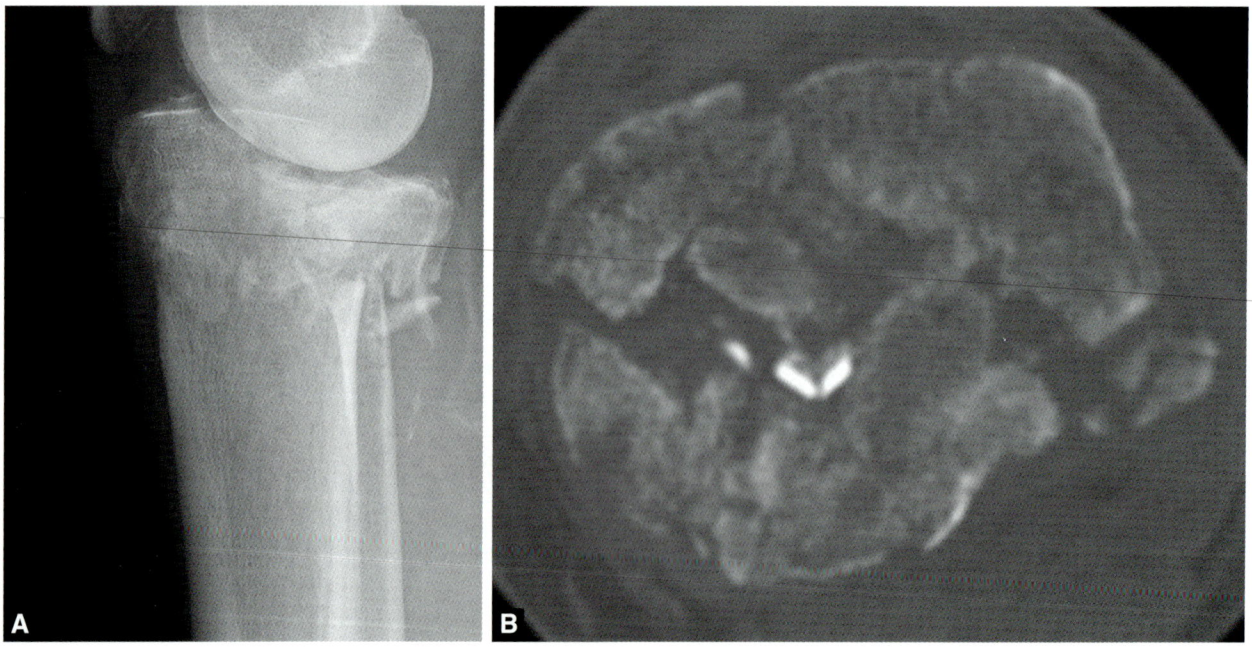

Figures 25.25A and B

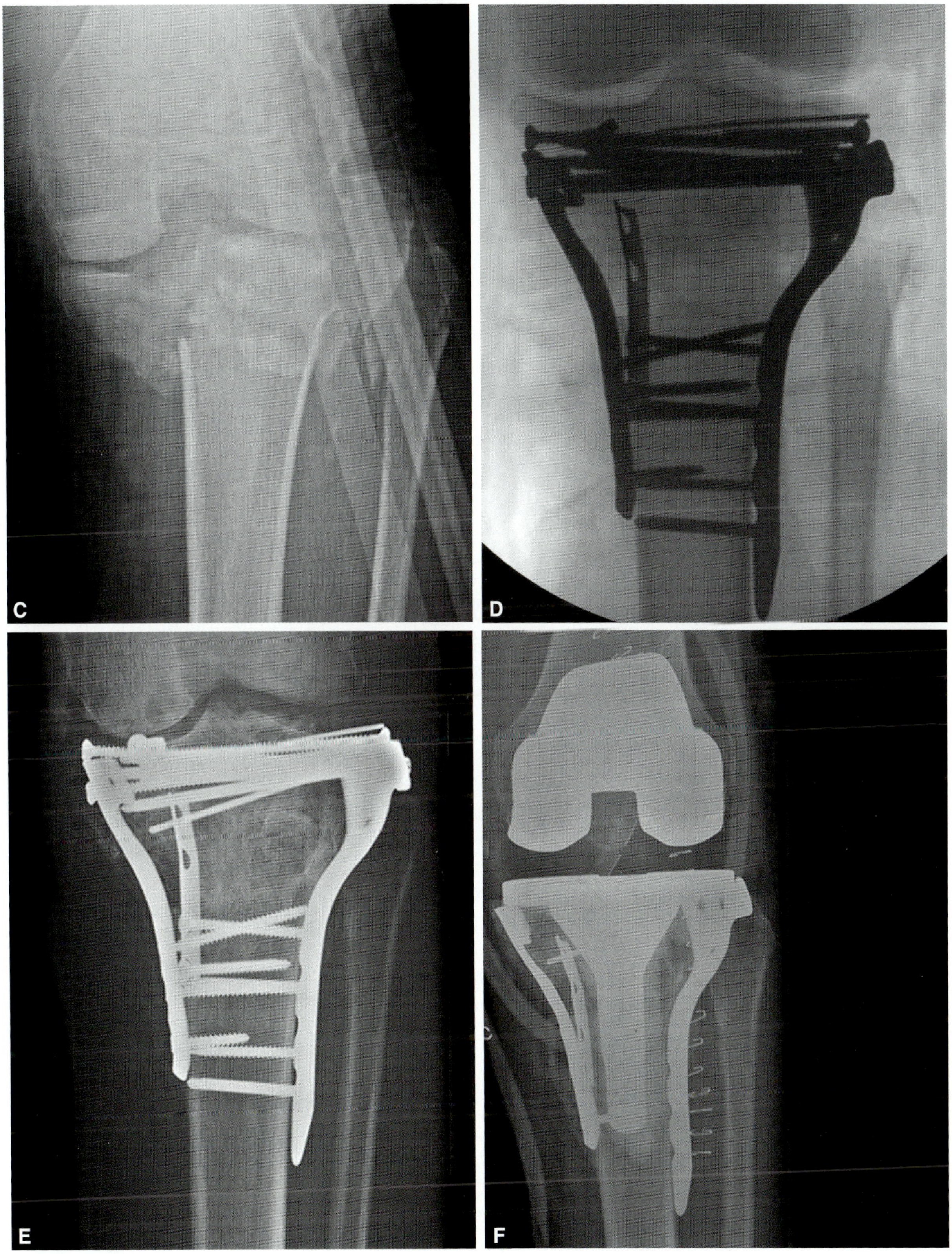

Figures 25.25C to F

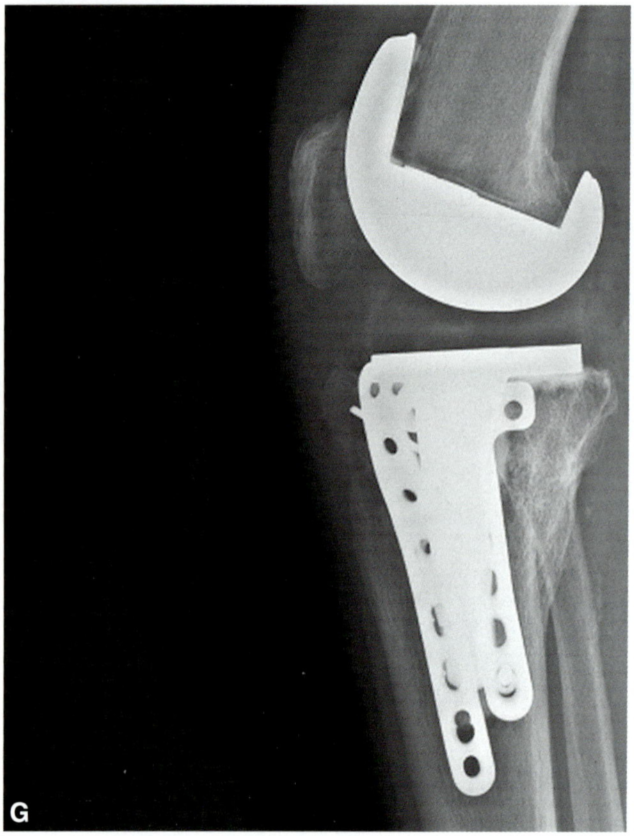

Figures 25.25A to G: (A to C) A 68-year-old osteopenic female with an impacted bicondylar fracture fixed with dual plating; (D and E) During healing, the fracture settled into varus; (F and G) The post-traumatic arthritis was treated with a one-stage total knee replacement with partial removal of hardware.

difficult than the index case. Consideration should be given to referral to a center with experience in their management. The previous incisions must be reopened and the failed hardware must be removed. Anatomical re-reduction of the articular surface and restoration of the joint axis in both coronal and sagittal planes is necessary. The biomechanical stability of original construct should be critiqued to determine if a conceptual change in reconstruction is needed, and longer plates with better load sharing are often indicated. We have successfully utilized circular fixation in the scenario of an infected bicondylar fracture with failure of fixation.

Infection

Infection after operative treatment of a tibial plateau fracture can occur from failure of primary wound healing or as a result of inadequate debridement following an open fracture. Wound healing complications can be secondary to underestimation of the damage to the soft tissue leading to inappropriate surgical timing or extensive dissection and secondary surgical trauma with subsequent wound breakdown. Patient factors such as smoking, malnutrition and diabetes will often be associated cofactors. The incidence of deep infection following internal fixation of tibial plateau fractures varies widely. Older studies reported infection rates up to 32% in unicondylar fractures and even higher in medial and bicondylar fractures.[70] As methods of soft tissue management have evolved including use of low-profile implants with better timed, less traumatic insertion techniques, infection rates have fallen significantly in more recent series. Egol et al.[29] reported a 5% deep infection rate in 57 high-energy tibial plateau fractures treated with a staged management. In a similar high-energy patient series treated with dual plating via two incisions, Barei et al. reported an 8.4% deep infection rate and 3.6% incidence of septic arthritis in 83 patients.[72] As a result of less injury to the tissue envelope and no deep implanted hardware, circular external fixation is reported to have a lower infection rate than internal fixation. This has been borne out in several studies.[77,87,91,104] Small-wire external fixation for tibial plateau fractures is associated with an incidence of pin/wire infections that may require removal/exchange and an incidence of septic arthritis, for which the surgeon must be vigilant.[81]

Infection following treatment for a tibial plateau fracture can present in multiple clinical settings. Following internal fixation, infection can develop early, prior to fracture union, in which the decision to retain or remove infected hardware becomes critical. Hardware retention can be attempted, if the infection has been present for less than 2 weeks (implying minimal biofilm formation), the implants are stable, the cultures are unambiguous, the bacteria is suppressible with an oral agent, the patient is a nonsmoker, and the patient has normal immune function. In this clinical setting, a thorough debridement is performed with or without the use of castile soap solution to breakdown the biofilm. Viable soft tissue coverage must be present with a meticulous closure. This may involve local flap coverage, usually in the form of a medial or lateral gastrocnemius flap, if the existing soft tissue envelope will not permit an immunocompetent closure.[105] Intravenous antibiotics are given for 4–6 weeks guided by laboratory assessment of infection parameters[102] like erythrocyte sedimentation rate (ESR), C-reactive protein (CRP) and white blood cell (WBC) count followed by oral suppression until fracture union. This technique may be successful in up to 68% of selected cases as reported by Rightmire et al.[106] In their series, 40% of patients required hardware removal after fracture union. Debridement coupled with hardware removal should be considered in patients not meeting the aforementioned criteria. If hardware removal is selected, then external fixation, either knee spanning or knee sparing, will usually be required to provide stability to permit fracture union. Less frequently, infection can present late following fracture union, in which hardware removal, thorough debridement of the hardware and adjacent bone and soft tissue and culture specific antibiotics will often be curative. The presence of septic arthritis in conjunction with hardware and bone infection should always be considered, as the findings can be subtle and symptoms can be masked by the pain of the fracture and/or nonunion. The knee joint should always be opened, formal cultures should be obtained and thoroughly irrigated. Following debridement, metaphyseal bone defects may be present particularly in cases of infected nonunions. This dead space can be managed with a negative pressure wound dressing prior to closure and antibiotic beads at closure. Bead removal and bone grafting can be performed, when the signs of infection have resolved (2–4 weeks). Figures 25.26A to J show a 58-year-old male s/p dual plating via two incisions for a bicondylar plateau fracture with recurrent infection and hardware failure.

Malunion and Nonunion

Malunion of a tibial plateau fracture can occur in the metaphysis and can lead to a varus or valgus deformity (or flexion/extension in the sagittal plane). As shown by Rasmussen,[19] significant varus or to a lesser extent valgus deformity is an independent risk factor for the development of post-traumatic arthritis. Failure to adequately buttress the medial side of a bicondylar plateau fracture or failure of a laterally-based locked plate to control the medial side, is a common etiology of a varus malunion in our experience (Figs 25.27A to E). If the articular surface is congruent, these can be salvaged with a medial opening wedge osteotomy to re-establish axial alignment and can be stabilized with a medial buttress plate.[102] The space can be filled with a tricortical iliac crest autograft or calcium ceramics.

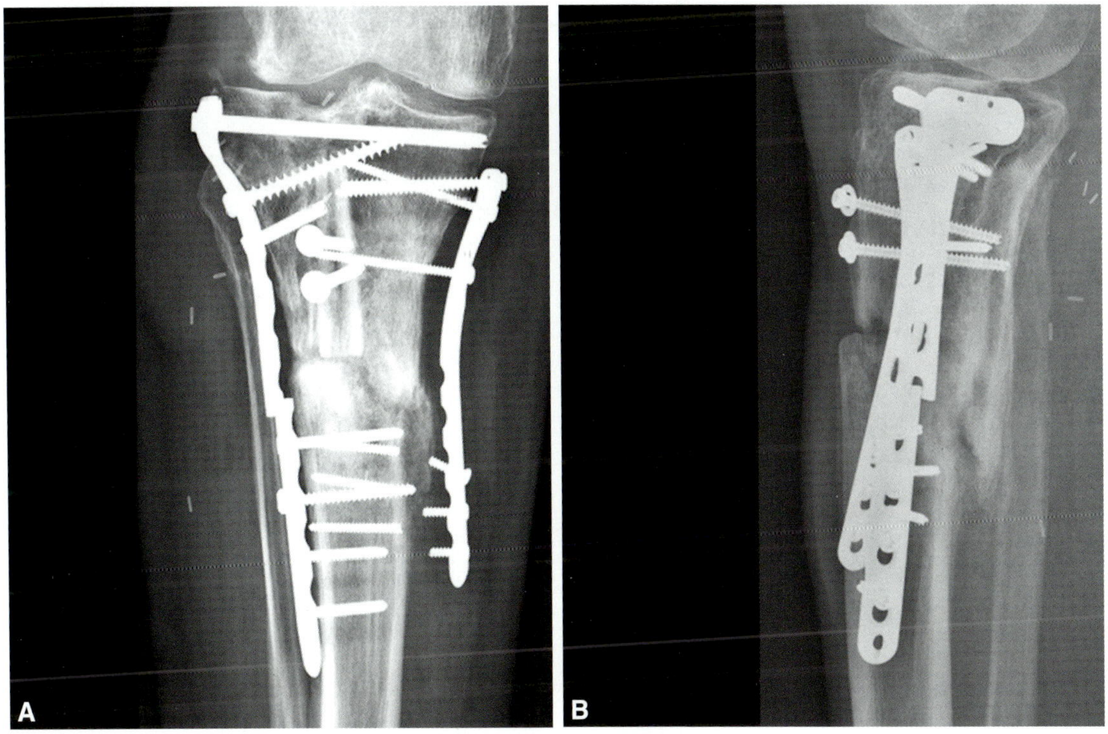

Figures 25.26A and B

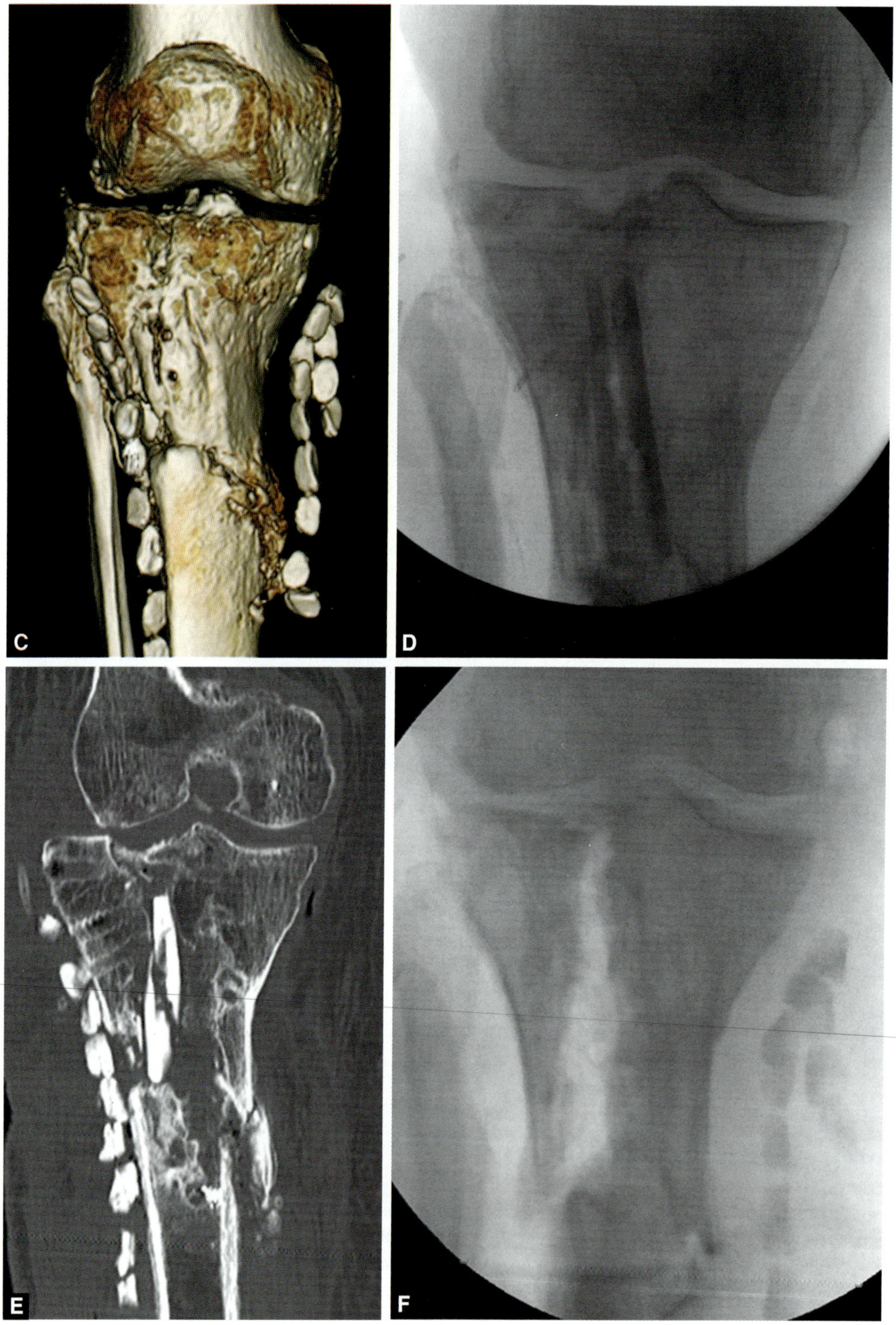

Figures 25.26C to F

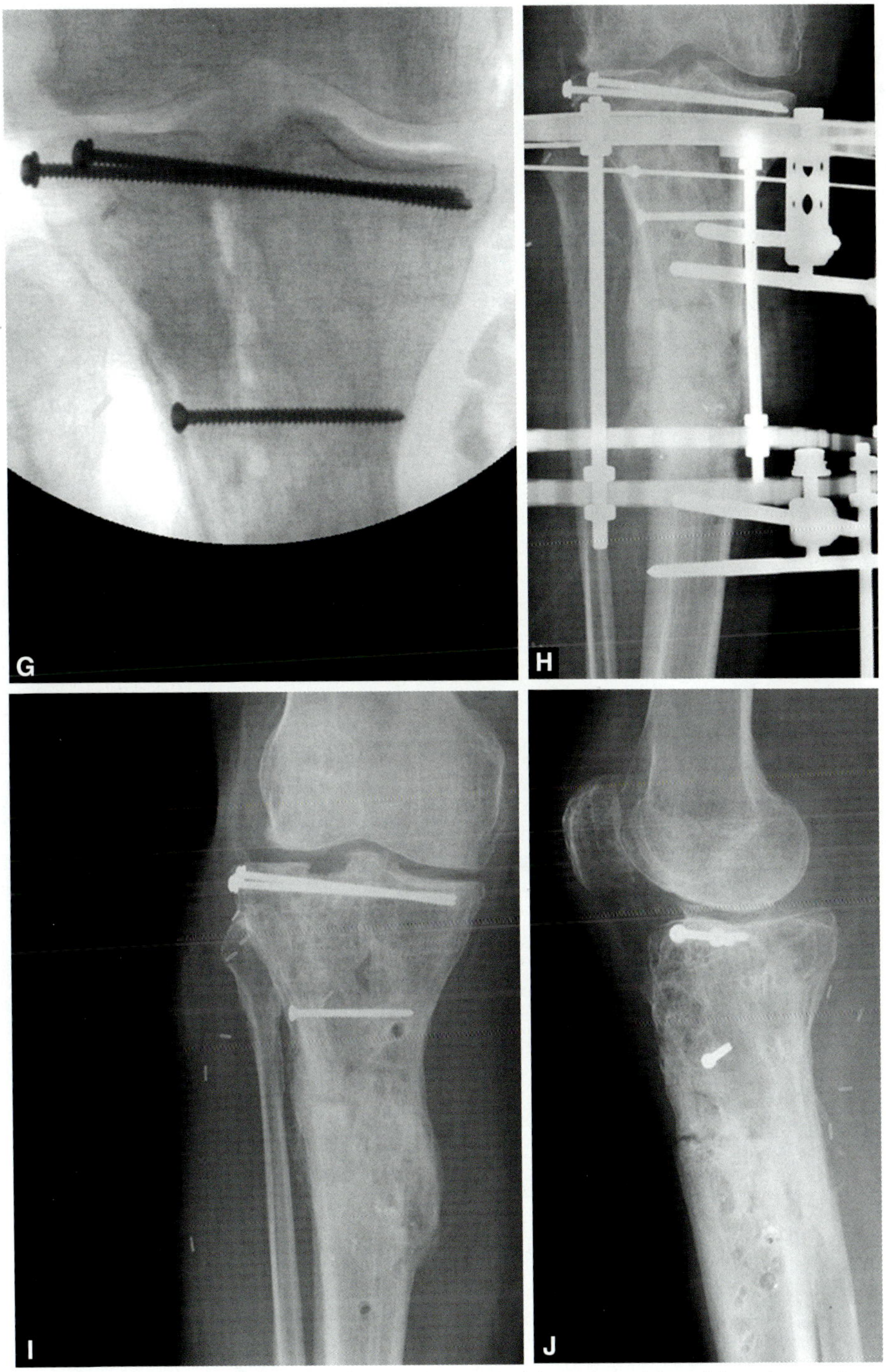

Figures 25.26A to J: A 58-year-old male s/p dual plating via two incisions for a bicondylar plateau fracture with a recurrent infection and hardware failure. (A and B) The patient presented at six weeks with wound erythema and elevated infection markers and was treated for 4 weeks with intravenous vancomycin with resolution of symptoms. He then presented again at 4 months with recurrence of the infection with drainage and complete failure of hardware. The patient was referred to our institution at this point. All hardware were removed, underlying bone was debrided, and the knee joint was opened and irrigated. Cultures were methicillin resistant *Staphylococcus aureus* (MRSA) positive; (C) Temporary spanning fixation was placed; (D to F) There was a fibular allograft present in the metaphysis that required osteotomizing of the lateral condyle for removal; (G) A revision internal fixation of the articular surface was performed followed by placement of antibiotic impregnated autograft, wound closure and (H) Application of an Ilizarov frame for definitive fixation; (I and J) Frame was removed at 20 weeks.

Intra-articular malunions are more difficult to correct as they will require an intra-articular osteotomy. However, in physiologically young patients with a viable joint surface, this may be an appropriate and gratifying procedure. Careful preoperative planning is required to completely restore congruency, condylar width, posterior slope and preserve the meniscus. Figures 25.27A to E show a 26-year-old male with malunion of a bicondylar plateau fracture poorly treated initially, and salvaged with an intra-articular osteotomy and stable fixation. The patient had an excellent long-term outcome.

Tibial plateau nonunions are uncommon due to large opposed cancellous bone surfaces and robust blood supply of the proximal tibia.[107] Blokker et al.[108] reported two cases

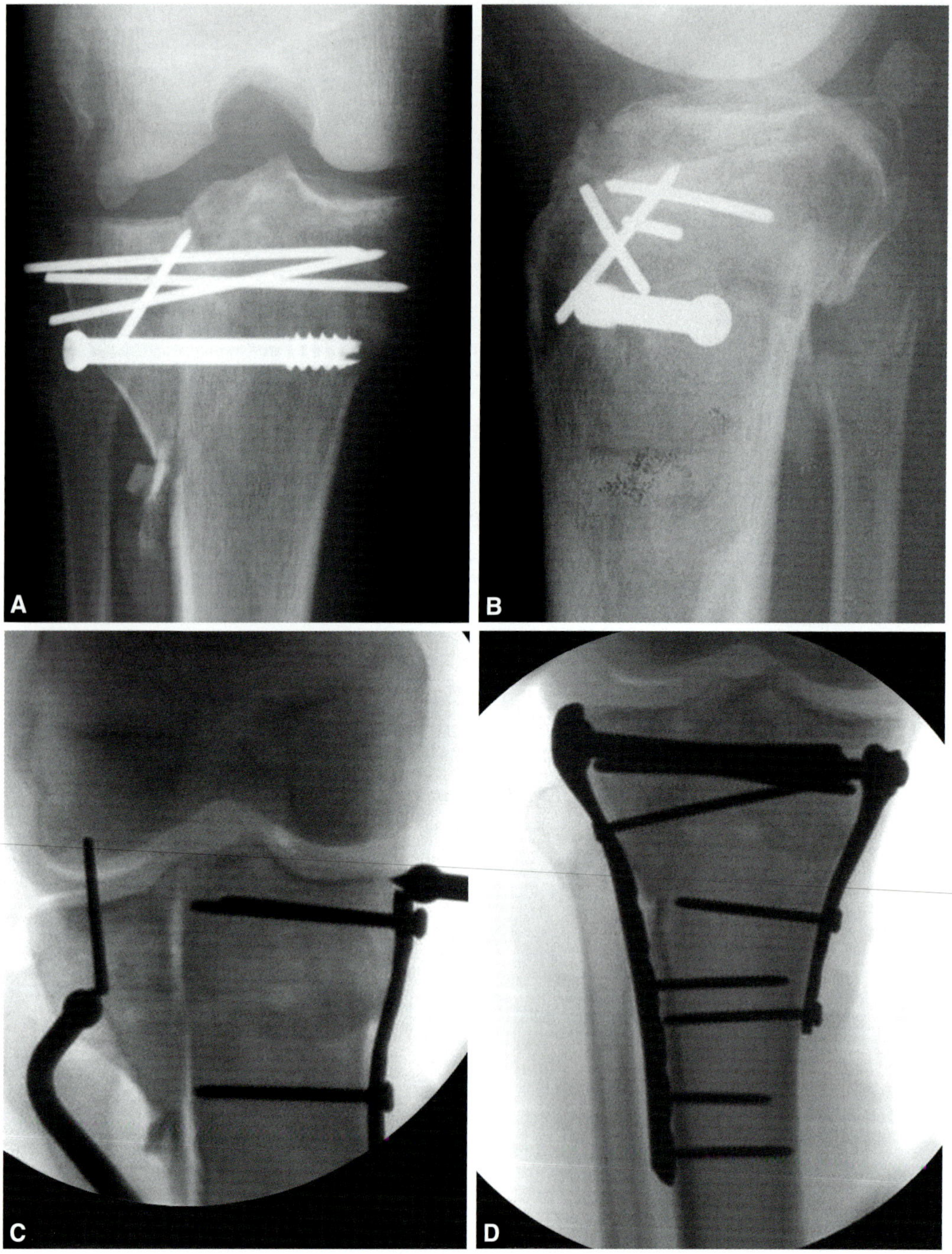

Figures 25.27A to D

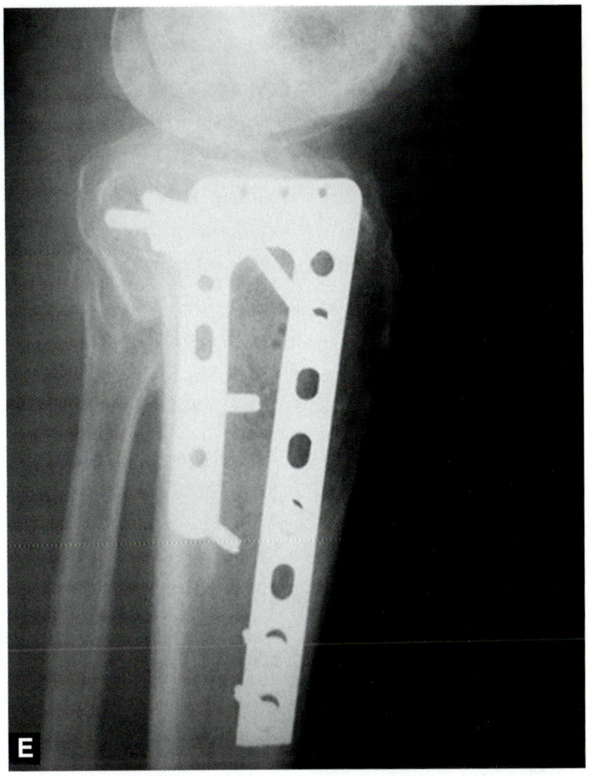

Figures 25.27A to E: A 26-year-old male with malunion of a bicondylar plateau fracture fixed with percutaneous pins/screws. This required an intra-articular osteotomy and fixation with dual plates via two incisions with an excellent long-term outcome.

of nonunion in a series of 60 fractures (3%). Moore et al.[68] reported one metaphyseal nonunion in 988 tibial plateau fractures (0.1%). Barei et al. reported one (1.5%) metadiaphyseal nonunion in 83 high-energy bicondylar fractures.[72] Many series report no nonunions.[109,110] Metadiaphyseal nonunions may occur in the context of a high-energy fracture,[83,111,112] particularly if open and with bone loss, but intra-articular nonunions are quite rare.[113]

The accepted principles of treatment of nonunions are applicable in this setting. Since these are unusual nonunions, systemic etiologies must be considered and treated. Vigorous attempts at smoking cessation, often with use of oral Varencline (Chantix) are indicated. Patients often present using substantial amounts of nonsteroidal anti-inflammatory drugs (NSAIDs) and these must be stopped preoperatively. Endocrine workup as outlined by Brinker et al.[114] should be considered, if clinical presentation is suspicious. Vitamin D deficiencies are much more common than previously recognized and may play a role in the development of nonunions. Vitamin D levels should be checked and supplemented as needed.

The presence of infection must always be considered. Preoperative WBC count, ESR and CRP are useful, but not always diagnostic of deep infection. Multiple intraoperative cultures, off of antibiotics, remain the gold standard for the presence of infection. If deep infection is suspected preoperatively, or encountered intraoperatively, the staged treatment with placement of a temporary spanning external fixator as discussed in the preceding section is appropriate. In the absence of infection, reconstruction can proceed in a single stage. Computed tomography scanning with 2D and 3D reconstructions is very useful to confirm the nonunion in questionable cases, as well as to determine the plane of orientation of the nonunion. Often, the original fracture might have presented with a wide zone of comminution in the metaphysis and was treated with a bridge plate construct without an opportunity for interfragmentary compression. During healing, the comminuted region will often coalesce into two major fragments with only a single nonunited fracture line. This should be searched for at every opportunity, as it provides the ability to generate interfragmentary compression after axial realignment, with either lag screws or compression plate techniques or external fixation. It must be remembered that the use of a locking plate to gain proximal purchase of an articular segment does not preclude compression of the nonunion along the bone axis either with combination holes in plate or with use of compression device at the end of the plate. Compression of a nonunion may result in limb shortening. The benefit of, and the tolerance for, limb shortening should be discussed with the patient preoperatively. Shortening of 10–15 mm in a young patient is usually very well-tolerated, and can result in a much more stable construct and substantially shortened healing time. Larger amounts of shortening can be tolerated in the elderly, as use of a postoperative shoe lift is usually a lesser cosmetic problem. Autogenous bone graft should be strongly considered in the setting of bone defects following axial relalignment and compression due to the need for bone induction. Infected nonunions can also be treated with autogenous bone graft in a staged fashion after debridement and with appropriate course of antibiotics. Consideration can be given to adding culture-specific antibiotics to the autogenous graft. This may decrease the rate of infection recurrence and still permit bone healing.

Toro-Arbelaez et al.[113] retrospectively reported on intra-articular nonunions treated by a single surgeon. Five patients averaging 50 years of age were referred from 4–8 months to the author's institution. According to the Schatzker classification, there were two type IV, one type V and two type VI. All cases were originally treated with ORIF. The major complaint preoperatively was pain (4 of 5) and deformity (4 of 5). Flexion contracture from 10° to 30° was present in 3 of 5 patients. Three patients had significant meniscal pathology. All patients were treated with revision ORIF with debridement of the nonunion, correction of deformity in both sagittal and coronal planes, arthrolysis, and internal fixation with bone grafting. A strict postoperative rehabilitation protocol was followed. All patients achieved union by an average of 12.8 weeks. At an average follow-up of 44 months, the coronal plane deformity was corrected in all patients. The final knee arc of motion averaged 120° with one patient having a persistent 10° flexion contracture. In two patients, the nonunion healed, but due to persistent pain, successful knee arthroplasty was performed at 5th and 16th months following healing of the nonunion. Both patients, who underwent knee arthroplasty, had significant meniscal pathology. On the Knee Society Rating Scale (KSRS), the knee function subscore improved from 45 to 87 ($p < 0.05$) and the pain subscale improved from 28 to 70 ($p < 0.05$).

Treatment of metadiaphyseal nonunions are simplified as compared to intra-articular nonunions in that the articular segment behaves as a single unit. Nonetheless, attention must be paid to restoration of both coronal and sagittal plane alignment. Axial realignment is often aided with use of the femoral distractor placed on the shorter side. If soft tissue envelope is favorable, one or more plates can be reapplied as indicated by the fracture pattern. Stable small-wire fixation may be indicated, if the soft tissue envelope is compromised, or in situations of significant osteopenia (Figs 25.21A to H and 25.28A to N).

Post-traumatic Arthritis

Despite optimal treatment, a certain number of patients with tibial plateau fractures will develop debilitating post-traumatic arthrosis.[115] This may be the result of cartilage apoptosis originating from the time of original injury.[102,116] Other factors, such as residual deviations in axial alignment, articular incongruity, residual instability or significant meniscal damage can exacerbate the effects of initial cartilage injury. Since the population sustaining tibial plateau fractures is considerably younger than those undergoing total knee replacement for primary osteoarthritis, this creates a significant dilemma for the treating surgeons. If the cartilage remains viable, and significant axial malalignment or intra-articular incongruity exists, consideration can be given to an extra or intra-articular osteotomy to restore normal joint mechanics. If this is not indicated, or the status of the cartilage precludes corrective osteotomy, the options for surgical treatment include total knee arthroplasty or knee fusion.

Knee fusion for post-traumatic arthritis following tibial plateau fractures without a history of infection, is best performed using a long intramedullary nail after hardware removal and preparation of the joint surfaces. Arthroplasty alignment and cutting jigs are very useful to achieve congruent opposing bone surfaces. The type of knee fusion nail that enters via piriformis fossa and has provisions for locking screws in both the proximal femur and distal tibia is preferable. These types of nails can be removed intact via piriformis fossa in the event a complication ensues such as nonunion or infection. If the plateau fracture has been complicated by significant infection, there is considerable risk in extending the infection into medullary canal of both the tibia and femur if an intramedullary nail is chosen as the fusion technique in that situation.[117] Circular or biplanar unilateral external fixation should be considered when fusing a knee after a tibial plateau with a history of significant infection.[118,119]

The problems and results of total knee arthroplasty following tibial plateau fracture have been addressed by multiple authors. In the largest series, Weiss et al.[120] reviewed 62 patients with total knee replacements after 62 plateau fractures. The mean age was 63 years, and 23 patients were originally treated nonoperatively for their plateau fractures. Knee society scores improved significantly for both pain and function following total knee arthroplasty. Complications; however, were significant. There were 13 reoperations, including five knee manipulations, five component revisions and three wound revisions. Postoperative complications occurred in 16 knees (26%). There were two deep infections, both treated successfully. Partial detachment of the patella tendon from the tubercle occurred in five patients, which were repaired

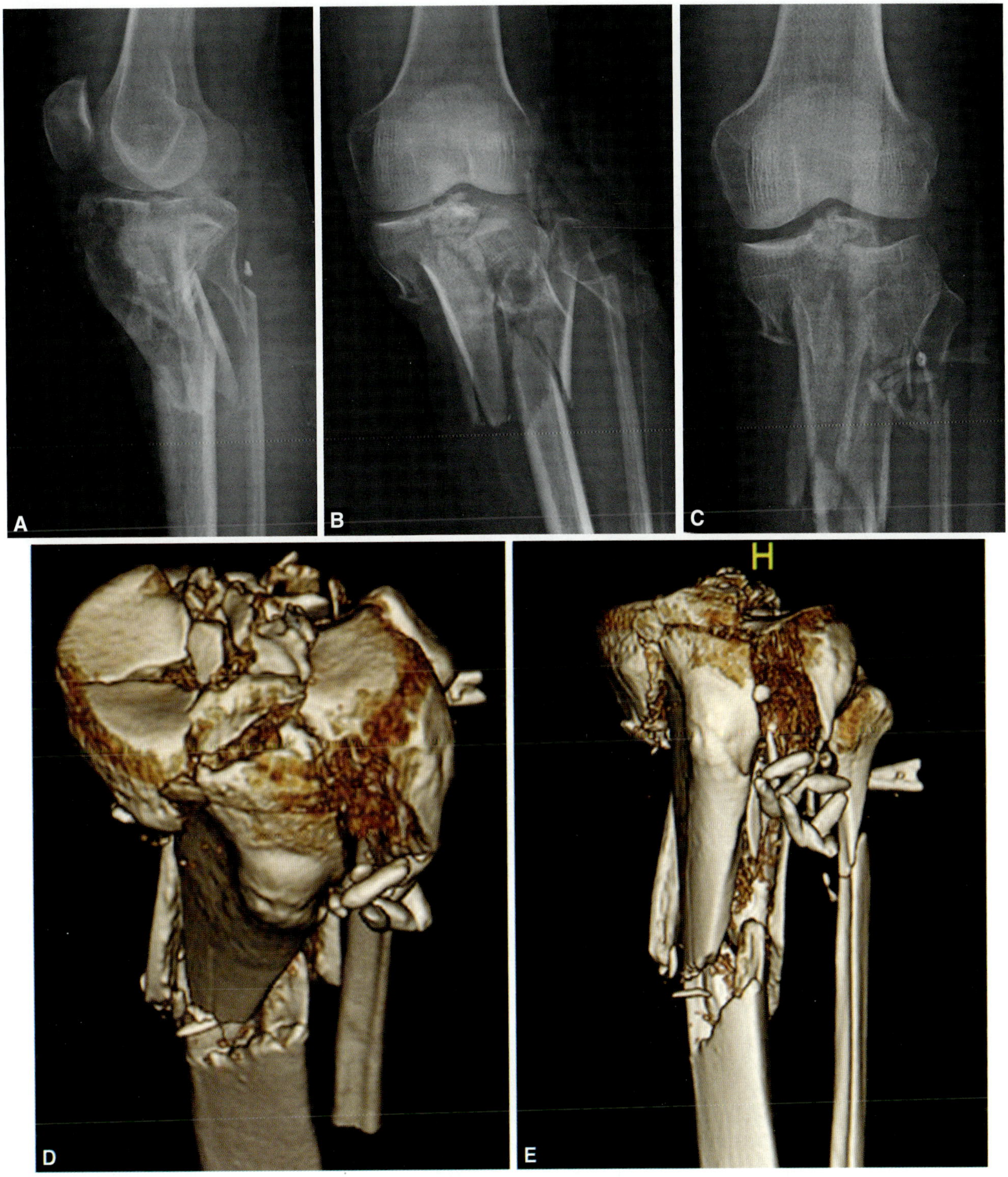

Figures 25.28A to E

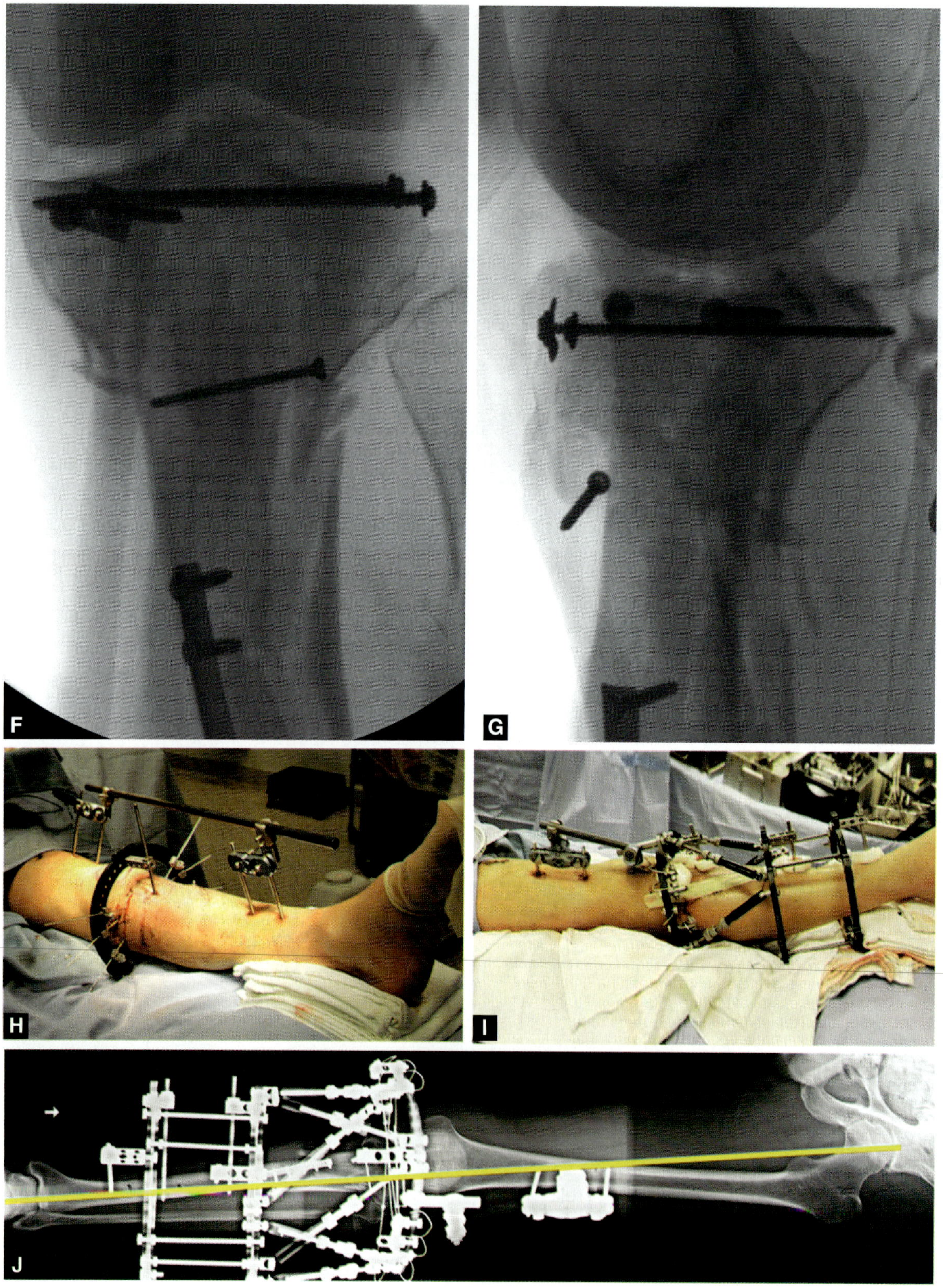

Figures 25.28F to J

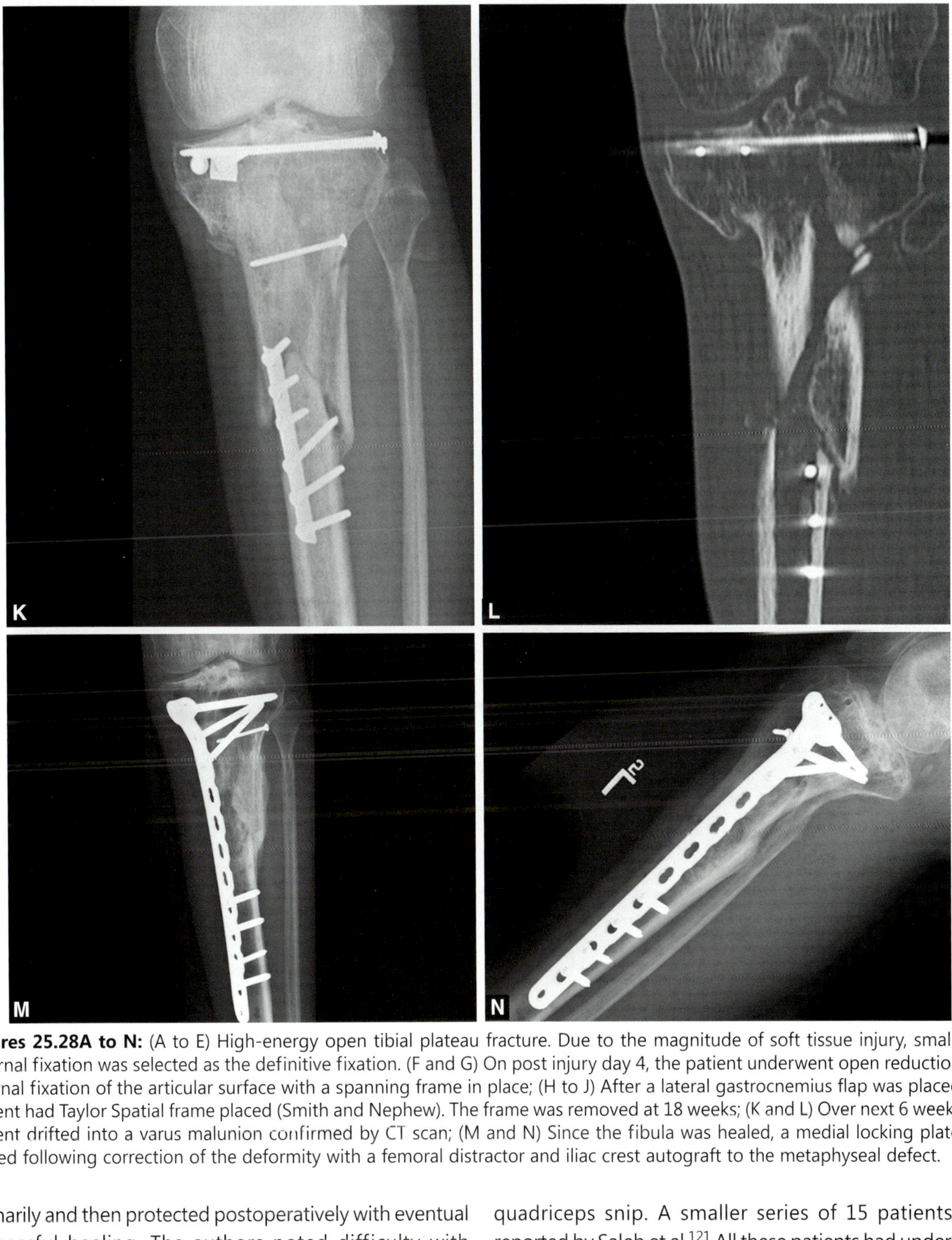

Figures 25.28A to N: (A to E) High-energy open tibial plateau fracture. Due to the magnitude of soft tissue injury, small-wire external fixation was selected as the definitive fixation. (F and G) On post injury day 4, the patient underwent open reduction and internal fixation of the articular surface with a spanning frame in place; (H to J) After a lateral gastrocnemius flap was placed, the patient had Taylor Spatial frame placed (Smith and Nephew). The frame was removed at 18 weeks; (K and L) Over next 6 weeks, the patient drifted into a varus malunion confirmed by CT scan; (M and N) Since the fibula was healed, a medial locking plate was placed following correction of the deformity with a femoral distractor and iliac crest autograft to the metaphyseal defect.

primarily and then protected postoperatively with eventual successful healing. The authors noted difficulty with exposure, particularly with respect to the extensor mechanism and recommended consideration of a quadriceps snip. A smaller series of 15 patients was reported by Saleh et al.[121] All these patients had undergone ORIF for their plateau fractures between 8 months and 11 years prior to their total knee replacement. The average follow-up after total knee replacement was 6.2 years. The HSS knee score improved on average from 51 to 80. A high rate of postoperative complications was also noted by these authors. Two patients sustained a patellar tendon disruption. Three patients developed deep infection (20%), two requiring arthrodesis and one resolving after two-stage treatment.

A very difficult clinical scenario is the patient with post-traumatic arthritis of the knee following a tibial plateau fracture, which was complicated by infection. In a unique study, Larson et al.[122] attempted to address this question in a matched case-control series comparing 19 patients undergoing primary total knee replacement following an infected tibial plateau fracture with 19 patients undergoing total knee replacement following a tibial plateau fracture with no history of infection. The mean time from infection to arthroplasty was 5.6 years, and the minimal follow-up after arthroplasty was 2 years. All fracture fixation hardware was removed during a separate procedure prior to total knee arthroplasty. In the infection group, recurrent infections occurred in five patients (26%) at a mean of 1.1 years. The 5-year infection free survival in the control group was 100% versus 73% in the case group. As compared with matched control subjects, patients with a previously infected tibial plateau fracture were four times more likely to have a complication requiring additional surgery. Knee Society pain score improvement was greater in the control group ($p = 0.002$), but the change in functional score was similar between the two groups. Given the high rate of recurrent infection in a patient with a history of infection, the authors suggested a protocol of careful preoperative screening including knee aspiration, measurement of inflammatory markers (CRP and ESR) and selected indium-labeled leukocyte scans. If any study is positive, the two-stage primary total knee arthroplasty is selected. They further recommended that antibiotic-impregnated cement should be used in all total knee arthroplasties following a tibial plateau fracture.

Total knee arthroplasty following a tibial plateau fracture internal fixation can be quite demanding. The challenges encountered often rival those of complex revision arthroplasty. Extensive preoperative planning is required to evaluate the need for augmentation of osseous defects, the need for long-stem components and the correction of limb malalignment.[120] Protection of the extensor mechanism is important. A history of previous infection demands careful evaluation and patient education as to the risks of arthroplasty. Despite the challenges, successful total knee arthroplasty following tibial plateau fracture can be quite gratifying for both patient and surgeon. Figures 25.25A to G show a bicondylar plateau fracture in a severely osteopenic patient treated with dual plating. There was loss of fixation, varus malunion and eventual conversion to a knee arthroplasty. In this type of case of severe osteopenia in an age-appropriate patient, consideration can be given to primary knee arthroplasty rather than an attempt at internal fixation.[123]

Summary

The entire spectrum of absorbed energy and bone quality is represented in tibial plateau fractures. The goals of axial alignment and a congruent articular surface correlate directly to long-term outcome. Thorough imaging to allow a complete understanding of the bone and soft tissue injuries is critical for planning specific treatment. In high-energy fractures, a staged approach using initial spanning external fixation followed by internal or circular external fixation is very useful. Posteromedial fractures generally require an antiglide plate via a separate approach. Consideration should be given to the use of calcium ceramics as void fillers following reduction of depressed segments. Finally, avoidance of a flexion contracture in addition to early motion as the soft tissue allows is important.

References

1. Chan PS, Klimkiewicz JJ, Luchetti WT, et al. Impact of CT scan on treatment plan and fracture classification of tibial plateau fractures. J Orthop Trauma. 1997;11(7):484-9.
2. Hu YL, Ye FG, Ji AY, et al. Three-dimensional computed tomography imaging increases the reliability of classification systems for tibial plateau fractures. Injury. 2009; 40(12):1282-5.
3. Suero EM, Hufner T, Stubig T, et al. Use of a virtual 3D software for planning of tibial plateau fracture reconstruction. Injury. 2010;41(6):589-91.
4. Markhardt BK, Gross JM, Monu JU. Schatzker classification of tibial plateau fractures: use of CT and MR imaging improves assessment. Radiographics. 2009;29(2):585-97.
5. Mui LW, Engelsohn E, Umans H. Comparison of CT and MRI in patients with tibial plateau fracture: can CT findings predict ligament tear or meniscal injury? Skeletal Radiol. 2007;36(2):145-51.

6. Mustonen AO, Koivikko MP, Lindahl J, et al. MRI of acute meniscal injury associated with tibial plateau fractures: prevalence, type, and location. AJR Am J Roentgenol. 2008;191(4):1002-9.
7. Kennedy JC, Bailey WH. Experimental tibial-plateau fractures. Studies of the mechanism and a classification. J Bone Joint Surg Am. 1968;50(8):1522-34.
8. Bennett WF, Browner B. Tibial Plateau Fractures: a study of associated soft tissue injuries. J Orthop Trauma. 1994; 8(3):183-8.
9. Abdel-Hamid MZ, Chang CH, Chan YS, et al. Arthroscopic evaluation of soft tissue injuries in tibial plateau fractures: retrospective analysis of 98 cases. Arthroscopy. 2006; 22(6):669-75.
10. Gardner MJ, Yacoubian S, Geller D, et al. The incidence of soft tissue injury in operative tibial plateau fractures: a magnetic resonance imaging analysis of 103 patients. J Orthop Trauma. 2005;19(2):79-84.
11. Gardner MJ, Yacoubian S, Geller D, et al. Prediction of soft-tissue injuries in Schatzker II tibial plateau fractures based on measurements of plain radiographs. J Trauma. 2006;60(2):319-23; discussion 324.
12. Ringus VM, Lemley FR, Hubbard DF, et al. Lateral tibial plateau fracture depression as a predictor of lateral meniscus pathology. Orthopedics. 2010;33(2):80-4.
13. Vangsness CT Jr., Ghaderi B, Hohl M, et al. Arthroscopy of meniscal injuries with tibial plateau fractures. J Bone Joint Surg Br. 1994;76(3):488-90.
14. Schatzker J, McBroom R, Bruce D. The tibial plateau fracture. The Toronto experience 1968–1975. Clin Orthop Relat Res. 1979;(138):94-104.
15. Moore TM. Fracture-dislocation of the knee. Clin Orthop Relat Res. 1981,(156).128-40.
16. Marsh JL, Slongo TF, Agel J, et al. Fracture and dislocation classification compendium - 2007: Orthopaedic Trauma Association classification, database and outcomes committee. J Orthop Trauma. 2007;21(10 Suppl):S1-133.
17. Swiontkowski MF, Agel J, McAndrew MP, et al. Outcome validation of the AO/OTA fracture classification system. J Orthop Trauma. 2000;14(8):534-41.
18. Lansinger O, Bergman B, Korner L, et al. Tibial condylar fractures. A twenty-year follow-up. J Bone Joint Surg Am. 1986;68(1):13-9.
19. Rasmussen PS. Tibial condylar fractures. Impairment of knee joint stability as an indication for surgical treatment. J Bone Joint Surg Am. 1973;55(7):1331-50.
20. Brown TD, Anderson DD, Nepola JV, et al. Contact stress aberrations following imprecise reduction of simple tibial plateau fractures. J Orthop Res. 1988;6(6):851-62.
21. Bai B, Kummer FJ, Sala DA, et al. Effect of articular step-off and meniscectomy on joint alignment and contact pressures for fractures of the lateral tibial plateau. J Orthop Trauma. 2001;15(2):101-6.
22. Honkonen SE. Indications for surgical treatment of tibial condyle fractures. Clin Orthop Relat Res. 1994;(302): 199-205.
23. Llinas A, McKellop HA, Marshall GJ, et al. Healing and remodeling of articular incongruities in a rabbit fracture model. J Bone Joint Surg Am. 1993;75(10):1508-23.
24. Mustonen AO, Koivikko MP, Kiuru MJ, et al. Postoperative MDCT of tibial plateau fractures. AJR. Am J Roentgenol. 2009;193(5):1354-1360.
25. Cetik O, Cift H, Asik M. Second-look arthroscopy after arthroscopy-assisted treatment of tibial plateau fractures. Knee Surg Sports Traumatol Arthrosc. 2007;15(6):747-52.
26. Rasmussen P. Tibial condylar fractures as a cause of degenerative arthritis. Acta Orthop Scand. 1972;43(6): 566-75.
27. LeRoux MA, Arokoski J, Vail TP, et al. Simultaneous changes in the mechanical properties, quantitative collagen organization, and proteoglycan concentration of articular cartilage following canine meniscectomy. J Orthop Res. 2000;18(3):383-92.
28. Reid JS, Van Slyke MA, Moulton MJ, et al. Safe placement of proximal tibial transfixation wires with respect to intra-capsular penetration. J Orthop Trauma. 2001;15(1):10-7.
29. Egol KA, Tejwani NC, Capla EL, et al. Staged management of high-energy proximal tibia fractures (OTA types 41): the results of a prospective, standardized protocol. J Orthop Trauma. 2005;19(7):448-55; discussion 456.
30. Stark E, Stucken C, Trainer G, et al. Compartment syndrome in Schatzker type VI plateau fractures and medial condylar fracture-dislocations treated with temporary external fixation. J Orthop Trauma. 2009;23(7):502-6.
31. Crist BD, Della Rocca GJ, Stannard JP. Compartment syndrome surgical management techniques associated with tibial plateau fractures. J Knee Surg. 2010;23(1):3-7.
32. Weinlein J, Schmidt A. Acute compartment syndrome in tibial plateau fractures—beware! J Knee Surg. 2010;23(1): 9-16.
33. Parker PJ, Tepper KB, Brumback RJ, et al. Biomechanical comparison of fixation of type-I fractures of the lateral tibial plateau. Is the antiglide screw effective? J Bone Joint Surg Br. 1999;81(3):478-80.
34. Ballmer FT, Hertel R, Notzli HP. Treatment of tibial plateau fractures with small fragment internal fixation: a preliminary report. J Orthop Trauma. 2000;14(7):467-74.
35. Westmoreland GL, McLaurin TM, Hutton WC. Screw pullout strength: a biomechanical comparison of large-fragment and small-fragment fixation in the tibial plateau. J Orthop Trauma. 2002;16(3):178-81.
36. Hung SS, Chao EK, Chan YS, et al. Arthroscopically assisted osteosynthesis for tibial plateau fractures. J Trauma. 2003;54(2):356-63.

37. Veitch SW, Stroud RM, Toms AD. Compaction bone grafting in tibial plateau fracture fixation. J Trauma. 2010;68(4): 980-3.
38. Karunakar MA, Egol KA, Peindl R, et al. Split depression tibial plateau fractures: a biomechanical study. J Orthop Trauma. 2002;16(3):172-7.
39. Barrett MO, Kazmier P, Anglen JO. Repair or reattachment of the meniscus after fixation of a tibial plateau fracture. J Orthop Trauma. 2005;19(3):198-200.
40. Lobenhoffer P, Schulze M, Gerich T, et al. Closed reduction/ percutaneous fixation of tibial plateau fractures: arthroscopic versus fluoroscopic control of reduction. J Orthop Trauma. 1999;13(6):426-31.
41. Trenholm A, Landry S, McLaughlin K, et al. Comparative fixation of tibial plateau fractures using alpha-BSM, a calcium phosphate cement, versus cancellous bone graft. J Orthop Trauma. 2005;19(10):698-702.
42. Welch RD, Zhang H, Bronson DG. Experimental tibial plateau fractures augmented with calcium phosphate cement or autologous bone graft. J Bone Joint Surg Am. 2003;85-A(2):222-31.
43. Shen C, Ma J, Chen XD, et al. The use of beta-TCP in the surgical treatment of tibial plateau fractures. Knee Surg Sports Traumatol Arthrosc. 2009;17(12):1406-11.
44. Simpson D, Keating JF. Outcome of tibial plateau fractures managed with calcium phosphate cement. Injury. 2004;35(9):913-8.
45. Lobenhoffer P, Gerich T, Witte F, et al. Use of an injectable calcium phosphate bone cement in the treatment of tibial plateau fractures: a prospective study of twenty-six cases with twenty-month mean follow-up. J Orthop Trauma. 2002;16(3):143-9.
46. Russell TA, Leighton RK, Alpha BSMTPFSG. Comparison of autogenous bone graft and endothermic calcium phosphate cement for defect augmentation in tibial plateau fractures. A multicenter, prospective, randomized study. J Bone Joint Surg Am. 2008;90(10):2057-61.
47. Yetkinler DN, McClellan RT, Reindel ES, et al. Biomechanical comparison of conventional open reduction and internal fixation versus calcium phosphate cement fixation of a central depressed tibial plateau fracture. J Orthop Trauma. 2001;15(3):197-206.
48. Solomon LB, Stevenson AW, Baird RP, et al. Posterolateral transfibular approach to tibial plateau fractures: technique, results, and rationale. J Orthop Trauma. 2010;24(8):505-14.
49. Bhattacharyya T, McCarty LP 3rd, Harris MB, et al. The posterior shearing tibial plateau fracture: treatment and results via a posterior approach. J Orthop Trauma. 2005; 19(5):305-10.
50. Carlson DA. Posterior bicondylar tibial plateau fractures. J Orthop Trauma. 2005;19(2):73-8.
51. Gossling HR, Peterson CA. A new surgical approach in the treatment of depressed lateral condylar fractures of the tibia. Clin Orthop Relat Res. 1979;(140):96-102.
52. Lobenhoffer P, Gerich T, Bertram T, et al. Particular posteromedial and posterolateral approaches for the treatment of tibial head fractures (German). Unfallchirurg. 1997;100(12):957-67.
53. Frosch KH, Balcarek P, Walde T, et al. A new posterolateral approach without fibula osteotomy for the treatment of tibial plateau fractures. J Orthop Trauma. 2010;24(8): 515-20.
54. Wahlquist M, Iaguilli N, Ebraheim N, et al. Medial tibial plateau fractures: a new classification system. J Trauma. 2007;63(6):1418-21.
55. Ratcliff JR, Werner FW, Green JK, et al. Medial buttress versus lateral locked plating in a cadaver medial tibial plateau fracture model. J Orthop Trauma. 2007;21(7):444-8.
56. Espinoza-Ervin CZ, Starr AJ, Reinert CM, et al. Use of a midline anterior incision for isolated medial tibial plateau fractures. J Orthop Trauma. 2009;23(2):148-53.
57. Hohl M. Tibial Condylar Fractures. J Bone Joint Surg Am. 1967;49(7):1455-67.
58. Higgins TF, Kemper D, Klatt J. Incidence and morphology of the posteromedial fragment in bicondylar tibial plateau fractures. J Orthop Trauma. 2009;23(1):45-51.
59. Barei DP, O'Mara TJ, Taitsman LA, et al. Frequency and fracture morphology of the posteromedial fragment in bicondylar tibial plateau fracture patterns. J Orthop Trauma. 2008;22(3):176-82.
60. Gosling T, Schandelmaier P, Marti A, et al. Less invasive stabilization of complex tibial plateau fractures: a biomechanical evaluation of a unilateral locked screw plate and double plating. J Orthop Trauma. 2004;18(8):546-51.
61. Mueller KL, Karunakar MA, Frankenburg EP, et al. Bicondylar tibial plateau fractures: a biomechanical study. Clin Orthop Relat Res. 2003(412):189-95.
62. Higgins TF, Klatt J, Bachus KN. Biomechanical analysis of bicondylar tibial plateau fixation: how does lateral locking plate fixation compare to dual plate fixation? J Orthop Trauma. 2007;21(5):301-6.
63. Galla M, Riemer C, Lobenhoffer P. Direct posterior approach for the treatment of posteromedial tibial head fractures. Oper Orthop Traumatol. 2009;21(1):51-64.
64. Georgiadis GM. Combined anterior and posterior approaches for complex tibial plateau fractures. J Bone Joint Surg Br. 1994;76(2):285-9.
65. Weil YA, Gardner MJ, Boraiah S, et al. Posteromedial supine approach for reduction and fixation of medial and bicondylar tibial plateau fractures. J Orthop Trauma. 2008;22(5):357-62.
66. Fakler JK, Ryzewicz M, Hartshorn C, et al. Optimizing the management of Moore type I postero-medial split fracture dislocations of the tibial head: description of the Lobenhoffer approach. J Orthop Trauma. 2007;21(5):330-6.

67. Oznur A, Aksoy C, Tokgozoglu AM. Posteromedial approach and posterior plating of the tibia. J Trauma. 2002; 53(4): 722-4.
68. Moore TM, Patzakis MJ, Harvey JP. Tibial plateau fractures: definition, demographics, treatment rationale, and long-term results of closed traction management or operative reduction. J Orthop Trauma. 1987;1(2):97-119.
69. Mallik AR, Covall DJ, Whitelaw GP. Internal versus external fixation of bicondylar tibial plateau fractures. Orthop Rev. 1992;21(12):1433-6.
70. Young MJ, Barrack RL. Complications of internal fixation of tibial plateau fractures. Orthop Rev. 1994;23(2):149-54.
71. Dirschl DR, Del Gaizo D. Staged management of tibial plateau fractures. Am J Orthop. 2007;36(4 Suppl):12-7.
72. Barei DP, Nork SE, Mills WJ, et al. Complications associated with internal fixation of high-energy bicondylar tibial plateau fractures utilizing a two-incision technique. J Orthop Trauma. 2004;18(10):649-57.
73. Jiang R, Luo CF, Wang MC, et al. A comparative study of less invasive stabilization system (LISS) fixation and two-incision double plating for the treatment of bicondylar tibial plateau fractures. Knee. 2008;15(2):139-43.
74. Lindeque B, Baldini T. A biomechanical comparison of three different lateral tibia locking plates. Orthopedics. 2010;33 (1):18-21.
75. Catagni MA, Ottaviani G, Maggioni M. Treatment strategies for complex fractures of the tibial plateau with external circular fixation and limited internal fixation. J Trauma. 2007;63(5):1043-53.
76. Katsenis DL, Dendrinos GK, Kontos SJ. High energy tibial plateau fractures treated with hybrid fixation: is knee bridging necessary? Orthopedics. 2006;29(4):355-61.
77. Katsenis D, Dendrinos G, Kouris A, et al. Combination of fine wire fixation and limited internal fixation for high-energy tibial plateau fractures: functional results at minimum 5-year follow-up. J Orthop Trauma. 2009;23 (7):493-501.
78. Ali AM, Saleh M, Bolongaro S, et al. The strength of different fixation techniques for bicondylar tibial plateau fractures—a biomechanical study. Clin Biomech. 2003; 18(9):864-70.
79. Ali AM, Saleh M, Eastell R, et al. Influence of bone quality on the strength of internal and external fixation of tibial plateau fractures. J Orthop Res. 2006;24(11):2080-6.
80. Watson JT, Ripple S, Hoshaw SJ, et al. Hybrid external fixation for tibial plateau fractures: clinical and biomechanical correlation. Orthop Clin North Am. 2002 2002;33 (1):199-209.
81. Hutson JJ Jr, Zych GA. Infections in periarticular fractures of the lower extremity treated with tensioned wire hybrid fixators. J Orthop Trauma. 1998;12(3):214-8.
82. Stamer DT, Schenk R, Staggers B, et al. Bicondylar tibial plateau fractures treated with a hybrid ring external fixator: a preliminary study. J Orthop Trauma. 1994;8(6):455-61.
83. Watson JT. High energy fractures of the tibial plateau. Orthop Clin North Am. 1994;25(4):723-52.
84. Weiner LS, Kelley M, Yang E, et al. The use of combination internal fixation and hybrid external fixation in severe proximal tibia fractures. J Orthop Trauma. 1995;9(3): 244-50.
85. Gaudinez RF, Mallik AR, Szporn M. Hybrid external fixation of comminuted tibial plateau fractures. Clin Orthop Relat Res. 1996(328):203-10.
86. Mikulak SA, Gold SM, Zinar DM. Small wire external fixation of high energy tibial plateau fractures. Clin Orthop Relat Res. 1998(356):230-8.
87. Dendrinos GK, Kontos S, Katsenis D, et al. Treatment of high-energy tibial plateau fractures by the Ilizarov circular fixator. J Bone Joint Surg Br. 1996;78(5):710-7.
88. Katsenis D, Athanasiou V, Megas P, et al. Minimal internal fixation augmented by small wire transfixion frames for high-energy tibial plateau fractures. Erratum appears in J Orthop Trauma. 2006;20(1):69. Note: Vasilis, Athanasiou [corrected to Athanasiou, Vasilis]; Panayiotis, Megas [corrected to Megas, Panayiotis]; Minos, Tillianakis [corrected to Tyllianakis, Minos]. J Orthop Trauma. 2005;19(4):241-8.
89. Kataria H, Sharma N, Kanojia RK. Small wire external fixation for high-energy tibial plateau fractures. J Orthop Surg. 2007;15(2):137-43.
90. Chin TY, Bardana D, Bailey M, et al. Functional outcome of tibial plateau fractures treated with the fine-wire fixator. Injury. 2005;36(12):1467-75.
91. Canadian Orthopaedic Trauma Society. Open reduction and internal fixation compared with circular fixator application for bicondylar tibial plateau fractures. Results of a multicenter, prospective, randomized clinical trial. J Bone Joint Surg Am. 2006;88(12):2613-23.
92. Hall JA, Beuerlein MJ, McKee MD; Canadian Orthopaedic Trauma Society. Open reduction and internal fixation compared with circular fixator application for bicondylar tibial plateau fractures. Surgical technique. J Bone Joint Surg Am. 2009;91 Suppl 2 Pt 1:74-88.
93. Mahadeva D, Costa ML, Gaffey A. Open reduction and internal fixation versus hybrid fixation for bicondylar/severe tibial plateau fractures: a systematic review of the literature. Arch Orthop Trauma Surg. 2008;128(10):1169-75.
94. Berkson EM, Virkus WW. High-energy tibial plateau fractures. J Am Acad Orthop Surg. 2006;14(1):20-31.
95. Segal D, Franchi AV, Campanile J. Iliac autograft for reconstruction of severely depressed fracture of a lateral tibial plateau. Brief note. J Bone Joint Surg Am. 1985; 67(8):1270-2.
96. Watson JT. Overview of biologics. J Orthop Trauma. 2005;19(10 Suppl):S14-6.
97. Beuerlein MJ, McKee MD. Calcium sulfates: what is the evidence? J Orthop Trauma. 2010;24 (Suppl 1):S46-51.

98. Schaefer SL, Lu Y, Seeherman H, et al. Effect of rhBMP-2 on tibial plateau fractures in a canine model. J Orthop Res. 2009;27(4):466-71.
99. Boraiah S, Paul O, Hawkes D, et al. Complications of recombinant human BMP-2 for treating complex tibial plateau fractures: a preliminary report. Clin Orthop Relat Res. 2009;467(12):3257-62.
100. Stannard JP, Robinson JT, Anderson ER, et al. Negative pressure wound therapy to treat hematomas and surgical incisions following high-energy trauma. J Trauma. 2006; 60(6):1301-6.
101. Gaston P, Will EM, Keating JF. Recovery of knee function following fracture of the tibial plateau. J Bone Joint Surg Br. 2005;87(9):1233-6.
102. Papagelopoulos PJ, Partsinevelos AA, Themistocleous GS, et al. Complications after tibia plateau fracture surgery. Injury. 2006;37(6):475-84.
103. Ali AM, El-Shafie M, Willett KM. Failure of fixation of tibial plateau fractures. J Orthop Trauma. 2002;16(5):323-9.
104. Watson JT, Coufal C. Treatment of complex lateral plateau fractures using Ilizarov techniques. Clin Orthop Relat Res. 1998;(353):97-106.
105. Chou YC, Wu CC, Chan YS, et al. Medial gastrocnemius muscle flap for treating wound complications after double-plate fixation via two-incision approach for complex tibial plateau fractures. J Trauma. 2010;68(1):138-45.
106. Rightmire E, Zurakowski D, Vrahas M. Acute infections after fracture repair: management with hardware in place. Clin Orthop Relat Res. 2008;466(2):466-72.
107. Borrelli J Jr., Prickett W, Song E, et al. Extraosseous blood supply of the tibia and the effects of different plating techniques: a human cadaveric study. J Orthop Trauma. 2002;16(10):691-5.
108. Blokker CP, Rorabeck CH, Bourne RB. Tibial plateau fractures. An analysis of the reslults of treatment in 60 patients. Clin Orthop Relat Res. 1984;(182):193-9.
109. Burri C, Bartzke G, Coldewey J, et al. Fractures of the tibial plateau. Clin Orthop Relat Res. 1979;(138):84-93.
110. Tscherne H, Lobenhoffer P. Tibial plateau fractures. Management and expected results. [Review]. Clin Orthop Relat Res. 1993;(292):87-100.
111. King GJ, Schatzker J. Nonunion of a complex tibial plateau fracture. J Orthop Trauma. 1991;5(2):209-12.
112. Wu CC. Salvage of proximal tibial malunion or nonunion with the use of angled blade plate. Arch Orthop Trauma Surg. 2006;126(2):82-7.
113. Toro-Arbelaez JB, Gardner MJ, Shindle MK, et al. Open reduction and internal fixation of intraarticular tibial plateau nonunions. Injury. 2007;38(3):378-83.
114. Brinker MR, O'Connor DP, Monla YT, et al. Metabolic and endocrine abnormalities in patients with nonunions. J Orthop Trauma. 2007;21(8):557-70.
115. Manidakis N, Dosani A, Dimitriou R, et al. Tibial plateau fractures: functional outcome and incidence of osteoarthritis in 125 cases. Int Orthop. 2010;34(4):565-70.
116. Borrelli J Jr. Chondrocyte apoptosis and posttraumatic arthrosis. J Orthop Trauma. 2006;20(10):726-31.
117. Mabry TM, Jacofsky DJ, Haidukewych GJ, et al. Comparison of intramedullary nailing and external fixation knee arthrodesis for the infected knee replacement. Clin Orthop Relat Res. 2007;464:11-5.
118. Garberina MJ, Fitch RD, Hoffmann ED, et al. Knee arthrodesis with circular external fixation. Clin Orthop Relat Res. 2001(382):168-78.
119. Salem KH, Kinzl L, Schmelz A. Circular external fixation in knee arthrodesis following septic trauma sequelae: preliminary report. J Knee Surg. 2006;19(2):99-104.
120. Weiss NG, Parvizi J, Trousdale RT, et al. Total knee arthroplasty in patients with a prior fracture of the tibial plateau. J Bone Joint Surg Am. 2003;85-A(2):218-21.
121. Saleh KJ, Sherman P, Katkin P, et al. Total knee arthroplasty after open reduction and internal fixation of fractures of the tibial plateau: a minimum five-year follow-up study. J Bone Joint Surg Am. 2001;83-A(8):1144-8.
122. Larson AN, Hanssen AD, Cass JR. Does prior infection alter the outcome of TKA after tibial plateau fracture? Clin Orthop Relat Res. 2009;467(7):1793-9.
123. Vermeire J, Scheerlinck T. Early primary total knee replacement for complex proximal tibia fractures in elderly and osteoarthritic patients. Acta Orthop Belg. 2010;76(6): 785-93.

Chapter 26

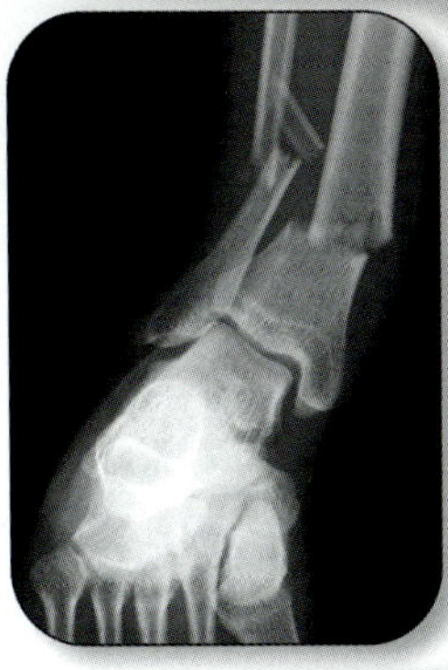

Tibial Shaft Fractures

Saqib Rehman, Katharine Criner

Chapter Outline

Introduction
Diagnosis
Classification
Surgical Indications
Surgical Anatomy, Positioning and Approaches
Surgical Techniques
- Technique 1: Reamed, Locked Intramedullary Nailing of Tibial Shaft Fracture
- Technique 2: Intramedullary Nailing of a Proximal Tibial Shaft or Metadiaphyseal Fracture
- Technique 3: Intramedullary Nailing of a Distal Tibial Metadiaphyseal Fracture
- Technique 4: ORIF of a Tibial Diaphyseal Fracture

Outcomes
Complications
Authors' Preferred Management of Select Complications
- Case 1: Treatment of an Acute Infection of the Tibia after Intramedullary Nailing
- Case 2: Treatment of an Established Infected Nonunion of the Tibia
- Case 3: Treatment of an Aseptic, Atrophic Nonunion of the Tibia
- Case 4: Treatment of Hypertrophic Nonunion of the Tibia
- Case 5: Treatment of Acute Tibial Bone Loss with Massive Autogenous Bone Grafting
- Case 6: Treatment of Compartment Syndrome of the Leg

Summary

Introduction

The tibia (Latin) is named after the aulos, an ancient Greek wind instrument. It is the second largest bone in the body and a major weight-bearing structure. The fibula is responsible for 6–17% of the weight-bearing load.[1] Tibia fractures are the most common long bone fractures and there are about 26 tibial shaft fractures per 100,000 population per year.[2] Tibia shaft fractures occur most commonly in young men and the average age of the patient is 37 years.[2] The tibia sustains the highest percentage of open long bone fractures and approximately 24% of tibial diaphysis fractures are open.[2]

The first evidence of tibial shaft treatment dates back to the ancient Egyptian era. The Egyptians used bandages and wooden splints to immobilize and stabilize tibia fractures. Since then several operative techniques for tibial shaft fractures have been established. Intramedullary (IM) nailing was introduced in the early 20th century. Küntscher invented the interlocking nail and pioneered reamed IM nailing.[3] Intramedullary nailing is currently the standard of treatment for most tibial shaft fractures.

Complications from infection, nonunion and compartment syndrome are relatively more common than are seen in other fractures encountered by orthopedic surgeons. Treatment, therefore remains a challenge even at experienced trauma centers. Surgical management of the fracture itself is frequently accomplished by IM nailing although external fixation and plating methods are more advantageous in certain situations. Successful management of tibial shaft fractures requires careful attention to detail in order to achieve bony union while avoiding these complications.

Diagnosis

Physical examination findings for a tibia fracture in the conscious patient are pain, deformity, and soft tissue swelling at the fracture site. Unconscious patients require a thorough skeletal survey and findings include skeletal instability, deformity and soft tissue swelling. Neurovascular status must be assessed to determine if there are distal pulses and intact motor and sensation of the posterior tibial nerve, deep peroneal nerve and superficial peroneal nerve. Sensation from the sural and saphenous nerves should also be checked. The patient's severity of pain is important since compartment syndrome can occur with tibial fractures.

Compartment syndrome is defined as microvascular compromise from interstitial pressure elevation in a closed fascial compartment. Myoneural function is compromised and soft tissue necrosis occurs as interstitial pressure increases and is prolonged. Significant physical examination findings are extreme pain out of proportion to the injury and pain on passive range of motion of the toes. The examiner should passively dorsiflex and plantarflex the toes to stretch the involved compartments. Other findings include pallor of the extremity, paralysis and paresthesia with early loss of vibratory sensation. Loss of pulses from the dorsalis pedis and posterior tibial arteries can occur in the late stage of compartment syndrome.

The skin of the lower extremity needs to be thoroughly assessed. Any superficial abrasions, skin avulsions or open wounds need to be noted. The size of the open wound and degree of contamination should be recorded. Photographs of the skin are helpful for documentation and legal issues. Crush injury to the soft tissues are suspected in patients found lying on the ground for a prolonged time, alcoholics, the elderly, drug addicts and in motor vehicle accidents. Crush injury can cause myonecrosis and myoglobinuria. Myoglobinuria can produce acute renal failure.

The tibial fracture can be associated with other injuries, especially in the setting of high-energy trauma. Templeman et al. found a high incidence of knee ligament injuries.[4] Keating et al. have shown that 5% of tibial fractures involve two distinctly separate fractures in the tibia.[5]

Diagnostic imaging modalities of importance are anteroposterior (AP) and lateral radiographs. The knee and ankle must be imaged as well, since the fracture line could be intra-articular or there could be other associated injuries. Magnetic resonance imaging (MRI) scans and technetium bone scans are only used in the diagnosis of stress fractures. Information from the radiographs include the fracture location, secondary fracture lines, presence and degree of comminution, fracture displacement, bone defects and intra-articular extension. The condition of the bone, such as osteopenia, osteoarthritis, cysts, tumor or previous fracture can be determined. Gas in the tissues can be seen—an indicator of an open fracture or anaerobic infection of the soft tissues.

TIBIAL SHAFT FRACTURES DIAGNOSIS: Pearls and Pitfalls

- Be sure to perform a careful neurovascular examination and always be vigilant for compartment syndrome, particularly in obtunded patients in which examination is unreliable
- Perform a careful examination of the skin and soft tissues to evaluate for open wounds and skin tenting
- Radiographic evaluation should include AP and lateral radiographs of entire tibia, knee and ankle. Computed tomography (CT) scanning can help in cases of suspected intra-articular extension

Classification

The Orthopedic Trauma Association (OTA) classification described by the Swiss AO/ASIF is the most comprehensive classification system for tibial shaft fractures (i.e. AO-OTA classification) (Fig. 26.1). The AO-OTA classification is based on the morphology of the fracture as it presents on the initial AP and lateral radiographs.[6] There are three

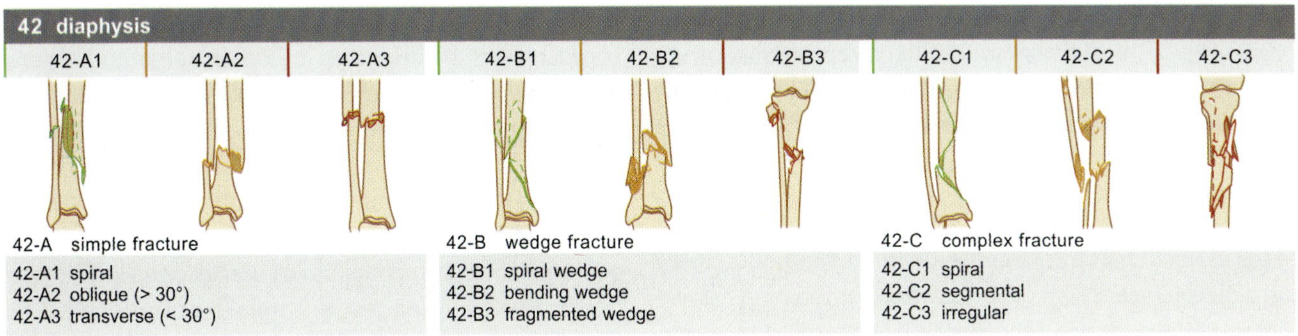

Figure 26.1: AO/OTA classification of tibial diaphyseal fractures.

fracture groups based on the amount of comminution as shown in Figure 26.1.

Group A includes all simple fractures with no comminution. Group B includes wedge fractures or butterfly fragments, in which one cortex is fractured once and the other cortex has several fractures. Group C involves the highest level of comminution and complex fractures. The three groups are further divided into three subgroups 1, 2 and 3 based on the mechanism of injury and nature of the fracture. Subgroup 1 includes all spiral fractures, which mainly occur by torsion and indirect impact. Subgroup 2 involves all oblique fractures (fracture line greater than 30°) which are caused by uneven bending and direct impact. Subgroup 3 is all transverse fractures (fracture line less than 30°), which are caused by pure bending and direct impact.

Group A1 are unifocal spiral fractures. Group A2 are simple oblique fractures. Group A3 are simple transverse fractures. Group B1 are intact spiral wedge fractures. Group B2 are oblique bending wedge fractures with one butterfly fragment. Group B3 are wedge fractures with more than one butterfly fragments. Group C1 are comminuted spiral fractures. Group C2 involves segmental fractures. Group C3 includes all severely comminuted fractures.

The nine morphologic groups are further divided based on the presence and location of a fibula fracture. The suffix 1 is used when no fibula fracture is present. The suffix 2 is for fibula fractures that occur at a different level than the tibia fracture. The suffix 3 is when the fibula and tibia fractures are at the same level.

The Gustilo and Anderson classification and the Tscherne classification are both based on the extent of soft tissue damage. The Tscherne classification is for closed fractures with soft tissue damage and the Gustilo and Anderson classification is used for open fractures. Open fractures are those that communicate with an open wound which implies that the fracture has been exposed to the environment.

The Gustilo and Anderson classification divides open fractures into three types. Type I involves fractures with a clean soft tissue defect of less than 1 cm in length. Type II fractures have a wound larger than 1 cm in length without periosteal stripping. Type III open fractures have a wound larger than 10 cm in length or a wound with extensive soft tissue damage. Other factors that characterize a Type III open fracture are open segmental fractures, traumatic amputation, gunshot injuries, farmyard injuries, fractures more than 8 hours old and fractures associated with a vascular repair. Type III open fractures are further subdivided into three groups of A, B and C. Subtype IIIA is open fracture with adequate periosteal covering and adequate skin coverage. Subtype IIIB has extensive periosteal stripping and the soft tissue coverage of the bone is poor and will likely require soft tissue reconstructive surgery. Subtype IIIC involves a vascular injury that requires repair and revascularization.[1]

The Tscherne classification of closed fractures has four different grades. Grade C0 is a simple fracture with minimal soft tissue injury. Grade CI fractures are from low to moderate energy mechanisms with superficial abrasions or contusions of the soft tissue. Grade CII fractures are from moderate to severe energy mechanisms with significant muscle contusions and skin abrasions that could be deeply contaminated. This group is at a high risk for compartment syndrome. Grade CIII fractures involve a high-energy mechanism with extensive crushing of the soft tissues, subcutaneous degloving or avulsion, arterial disruption or compartment syndrome.[1]

Surgical Indications

Closed tibial shaft fractures can be treated nonoperatively in a long leg cast with progressive weightbearing if there is acceptable fracture reduction with minimal comminution. Close observation while in the cast must be maintained, since there is a risk of varus malunion, especially in patients older than 20 years. A tibial shaft fracture with less than 5° of varus or valgus angulation is acceptable in the coronal plane. Less than 10° of anterior or posterior angulation is acceptable in the sagittal plane, however, less than 5° is preferred. There should be less than 10° of rotational deformity. External rotation is tolerated better than internal rotation. There should be less than 1 cm of shortening and less than 5 mm of distraction. More than 5 mm of distraction could delay healing. Acceptable rotational reduction allows the anterior superior iliac spine, center of the patella and base of the second proximal phalanx to be collinear.[1]

Operative treatment is indicated when the fracture does not meet the acceptable fracture reduction guidelines and when the fracture is highly comminuted or open. Intramedullary nailing of tibial shaft fractures is currently the standard operative technique. Intramedullary nailing preserves the periosteal blood supply and causes minimal soft tissue damage. Furthermore, it controls alignment, rotation and translation.

The operative technique of external fixation is indicated in severe open fractures or closed fractures with simultaneous soft tissue burns or compartment syndrome treated with fasciotomies.

Surgical Anatomy, Positioning and Approaches

The leg is comprised of four compartments—anterior, lateral, superficial posterior and deep posterior. The compartments are enveloped by nondistensible fascia. The anterior compartment contains the tibialis anterior, extensor hallucis longus, extensor digitorum longus and peroneus tertius muscles. Neurovascular structures of the anterior compartment are the deep peroneal nerve and anterior tibial artery. The lateral compartment includes the peroneus longus and peroneus brevis muscles, as well as the superficial peroneal nerve. The superficial posterior compartment holds the medial and lateral heads of the gastrocnemius, soleus and plantaris muscles. The deep posterior compartment contains the flexor hallucis longus, flexor digitorum longus and tibialis posterior muscles. Neurovascular structures in the deep posterior compartment are the posterior tibial artery, nerve and vein.

The two nerves located superficial to the fascia are the sural and saphenous nerves. They are entirely sensory nerves. The sural nerve is a branch off the common peroneal nerve. The sural nerve is located on the posterolateral side of the leg and courses to the dorsal lateral foot. It provides sensation to the lateral and posterior third of the leg and lateral aspect of ankle and foot. The saphenous nerve is a branch off the femoral nerve and it supplies sensation to the medial aspect of the leg.

The anteromedial aspect of the tibia has a thin subcutaneous border, which makes it susceptible to open fractures. The main arterial blood supply to the tibia is the nutrient artery, which is a large branch of the posterior tibial artery. The periosteal vessels stem from the anterior tibial artery and also provide blood supply.[7]

The patient should be positioned supine on a radiolucent table for tibia diaphyseal fracture fixation. Intramedullary nailing of the proximal tibia requires knee flexion to at least 90°. The leg can be placed in such a manner with either padding of blankets and/or towels under the popliteal fossa or with a radiolucent triangle. The leg can also be positioned in the arthroscopic figure of four positions with the hip and knee flexed over the opposite leg. The authors prefer to position the leg on a radiolucent triangle covered with padding under the popliteal fossa. Prior to prepping and draping, the fracture should be imaged with C-arm fluoroscopy to check for adequate positioning and reduction.

Traction can be applied to the foot manually from an assistant or through a calcaneal pin. Calcaneal pin traction on a fracture table has a greater risk of neurologic injury versus no traction. The third traction option is to hold the reduction with an external fixator or an AO universal distractor. The proximal pin should be placed posteriorly to allow room for the nail entry site. The common peroneal nerve is at risk during proximal pin placement. The distal pin can be placed in the distal tibia or calcaneus. If placed in the distal tibia, it should be distal to the insertion site of distal locking screws.

The surgical approach for IM nailing from the proximal tibia begins with locating the starting point. The optimal entry site for the IM nail is extra-articular and 1–1.5 cm distal to the joint line. Tornetta et al. defined the intra-articular safe zone to be a starting point 3 mm lateral to the center of the tibial tubercle.[8] On the AP radiographic view, the entry site is medial to the lateral tibial spine. The entry site on the lateral radiographic view is on the anterior edge of the tibial plateau along the long axis of the tibia.[9] Once the entry site is found with C-arm fluoroscopy, the skin incision can be made either longitudinally or transverse. A transverse incision 2–3 cm long that is parallel to Langer lines is made halfway between the joint line and tibial tuberosity. A longitudinal incision crosses Langer lines and is made midline from the inferior pole of the patella to tibial tuberosity. A postoperative scar that crosses Langer lines can have more issues with a painful scar.

The approach continues with an incision either medial paratendinous or transtendinous. The most common complication of tibial IM nailing is chronic anterior knee pain. It is controversial whether the transtendinous approach has a higher incidence of chronic anterior knee pain. Keating found anterior knee pain in 77% of transtendinous patients.[10] However, Jarmo did not find a clinically significant difference between the two approaches.[11] They had chronic anterior knee pain in 67% of their transtendinous patients and 71% of their paratendinous patients.

Pros of the transtendinous approach are it allows easy access to the nail entry point. Cons of the transtendinous approach are patellar tendon and sheath dessication with weakening of the tendon. Pros of the paratendinous approach are it preserves the tendon. Cons of the paratendinous approach are it can make access to the optimal starting point more difficult, since the tendon can push the bone awl medial to the safe zone.

The proximal aspect of the incision is down to deep fascia and the fat pad prevents entry into the joint. The distal incision is down to bone and the anterior surface of the proximal tibia is exposed once the infrapatellar fat pad is pushed proximally and posteriorly.

Open surgical approaches for plate osteosynthesis of the tibial shaft include the anterolateral approach and the anteromedial approach. The anterolateral approach is generally preferred for improved soft tissue coverage of the implant. A skin incision is made just lateral to the crest of the tibia which is extensile to the ankle and the knee. The anterior compartment fascia is opened and the anterior compartment muscles are elevated from the lateral aspect of the tibial shaft. The anteromedial approach also involves an anterior skin incision with elevation of the subcutaneous tissues from the medial tibia. This can also be extended to the very proximal and distal tibia but the plate has a thinner soft tissue coverage and the pes anserinus tendons obstruct visualization in the very proximal portion of the tibia.

Surgical Techniques

Technique 1: Reamed, Locked Intramedullary Nailing of Tibial Shaft Fracture

Preoperative Planning

Anatomical considerations: The tibial diaphysis has a triangular morphology with a relatively cylindrical medullary canal with muscle coverage posteriorly and laterally. Therefore, the medial surface of the tibia has minimal soft tissue coverage and implants placed through the medial cortex should not be left prominent as they may cause discomfort long after the fracture has healed. Intramedullary nailing by nature requires the implant to fit properly in the medullary canal and commercially available IM nails exist in a finite number of diameters. Preoperative planning should include both the measurement of length (from radiographs of the injured tibia and even the contralateral tibial imaging if necessary) and IM canal diameter. In certain cases, a tibial canal could be 8 mm or less, which is the smallest size tibial nail typically available. Intramedullary nailing of tibia, which has a smaller diameter than this, is contraindicated for risk of iatrogenic fracture or potential inability to pass the nail at all across the fracture site.

Instrumentation and implant considerations: After making the appropriate radiographic measurements, the surgeon should be sure that the appropriately sized implants including the nail, interlocking screws and endcaps (if desired) are readily available. Instrumentation required for reamed locked IM nailing includes a pneumatic or battery-powered reamer and drill, ball-tipped guidewires, and an "exchange tube" and smooth guidewire for a certain implant systems. A radiolucent table and fluoroscopic C-arm for intraoperative imaging is also required except in rare instances [e.g. Surgical Implant Generation Network (SIGN) nail]. A "triangle" knee positioner is the authors' preferred method although positioning can be achieved by alternative methods. Reduction of the fracture can require the use of free-hand Steinman pins, an AO large distractor or external fixator, or large bone clamps, such as a Weber bone forcep, serrated bone holding forceps, or ball-point pelvic forceps.

Patient considerations (local and systemic): Finally, systemic and local patient factors should be assessed before performing IM nailing. A multiply-injured patient who is either hemodynamically unstable or "borderline" and therefore, not adequately resuscitated could be at considerable risk for acute respiratory distress syndrome or multiple organ system failure if IM nailing is performed.[12] Although controversial and more often applied in the treatment of femoral fractures, this "damage control" concept should be considered when making the decision to perform IM nailing of the tibia. The presence of uncontrolled systemic sepsis is also a contraindication for performing IM nailing although the mere presence of fevers is more controversial and not an absolute contraindication. The condition of the limb itself should also be considered before performing nailing. Excessive swelling preoperatively can potentially be a risk for compartment syndrome with nailing although this is a subjective finding and clinical experience is necessary to recognize patients at risk. Local infection in the leg is also a contraindication for IM nailing. Furthermore, converting treatment from an external fixator to an IM nail even without obvious pin tract sepsis is a potential risk for deep infection via contamination of the IM canal. Therefore, conversion should be done within about 14 days and if this is delayed further or if pin tract infections have developed, the fixator should be removed, a splint should be placed, and a "pin holiday" should be given to the limb and pin tract infections treated appropriately until nailing can be safely performed.

Technique

The patient is given a general or spinal anesthetic. The placement of an indwelling epidural catheter for postoperative pain control is not advised in order to allow a reliable postoperative neurologic examination in the event that a compartment syndrome or related ischemic event has occurred. Intravenous antibiotics for skin flora bacterial prophylaxis should be given within 1 hour of skin incision. The patient is placed supine on the radiolucent operating table. A tourniquet can be placed, but the surgeon should exercise caution not to leave the tourniquet inflated during the reaming process in order to provide the venous circulation to help prevent thermal necrosis of the bone. A rolled sheet or blanket "bump" placed under the ipsilateral buttock can help in cases of excessive external rotation of the hips. However, the surgeon should be mindful of the contralateral limb external rotation this can create and should therefore not use the contralateral limb for intraoperative comparison for rotational alignment if the "bump" is used. The limb should be scrubbed and prepped with care not to allow excessive deformity to prevail during this process.

The surgeon utilizes a triangular knee positioner to place the knee at three different degrees of flexion. He must first ensure that a reduction of the fracture can be achieved. This is preferably done with closed manipulation and gentle traction, but percutaneous and open methods may be required as well. In long oblique and spiral fracture patterns, a percutaneously placed Weber large pointed bone forcep can be utilized to achieve a reduction (Figs 26.2A to E). Be careful not to crush the skin particularly on the medial face of the tibia with the use of blunt instruments.

After it is demonstrated that a reduction can be achieved, the procedure for nail placement is started. A midline skin incision is made from the inferior pole of the patella extending inferiorly, but just short of the tibial tubercle. After skin incision, the surgeon makes a medial parapatellar incision and retracts the patellar tendon laterally (Figs 26.3A to E). Alternatively, a midline split in the patellar tendon can be performed. Although both techniques work well, the medial parapatellar incision is potentially extensile in case the semiextended approach is required for more proximal metadiaphyseal fractures (Figs 26.4A to D). Depending on the instrumentation system utilized, either a guidewire or curved awl is placed at the "rollover" position of the proximal tibia as seen on

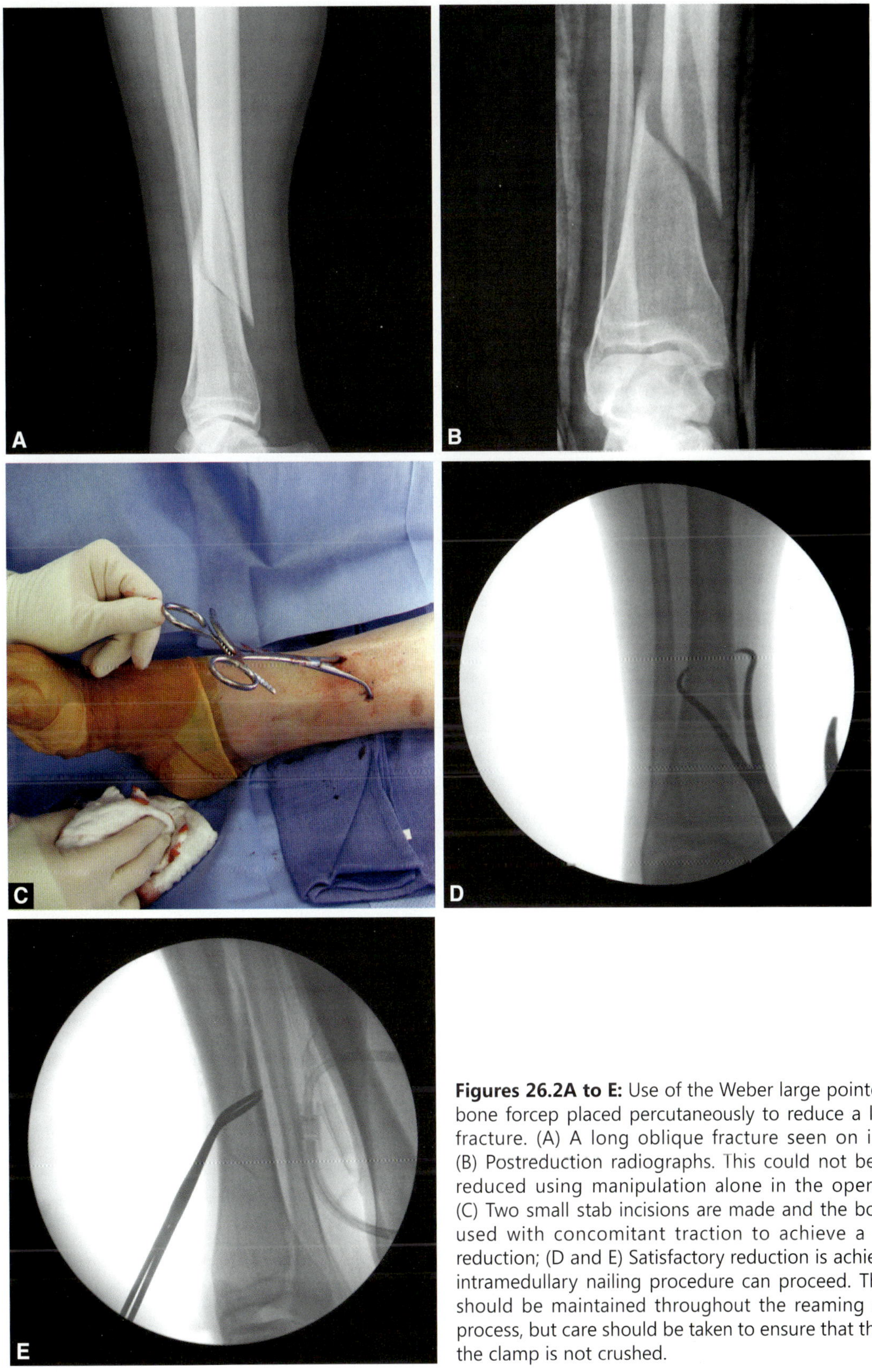

Figures 26.2A to E: Use of the Weber large pointed reduction bone forcep placed percutaneously to reduce a long oblique fracture. (A) A long oblique fracture seen on initial injury; (B) Postreduction radiographs. This could not be adequately reduced using manipulation alone in the operating room; (C) Two small stab incisions are made and the bone forcep is used with concomitant traction to achieve a satisfactory reduction; (D and E) Satisfactory reduction is achieved and the intramedullary nailing procedure can proceed. The reduction should be maintained throughout the reaming and fixation process, but care should be taken to ensure that the skin under the clamp is not crushed.

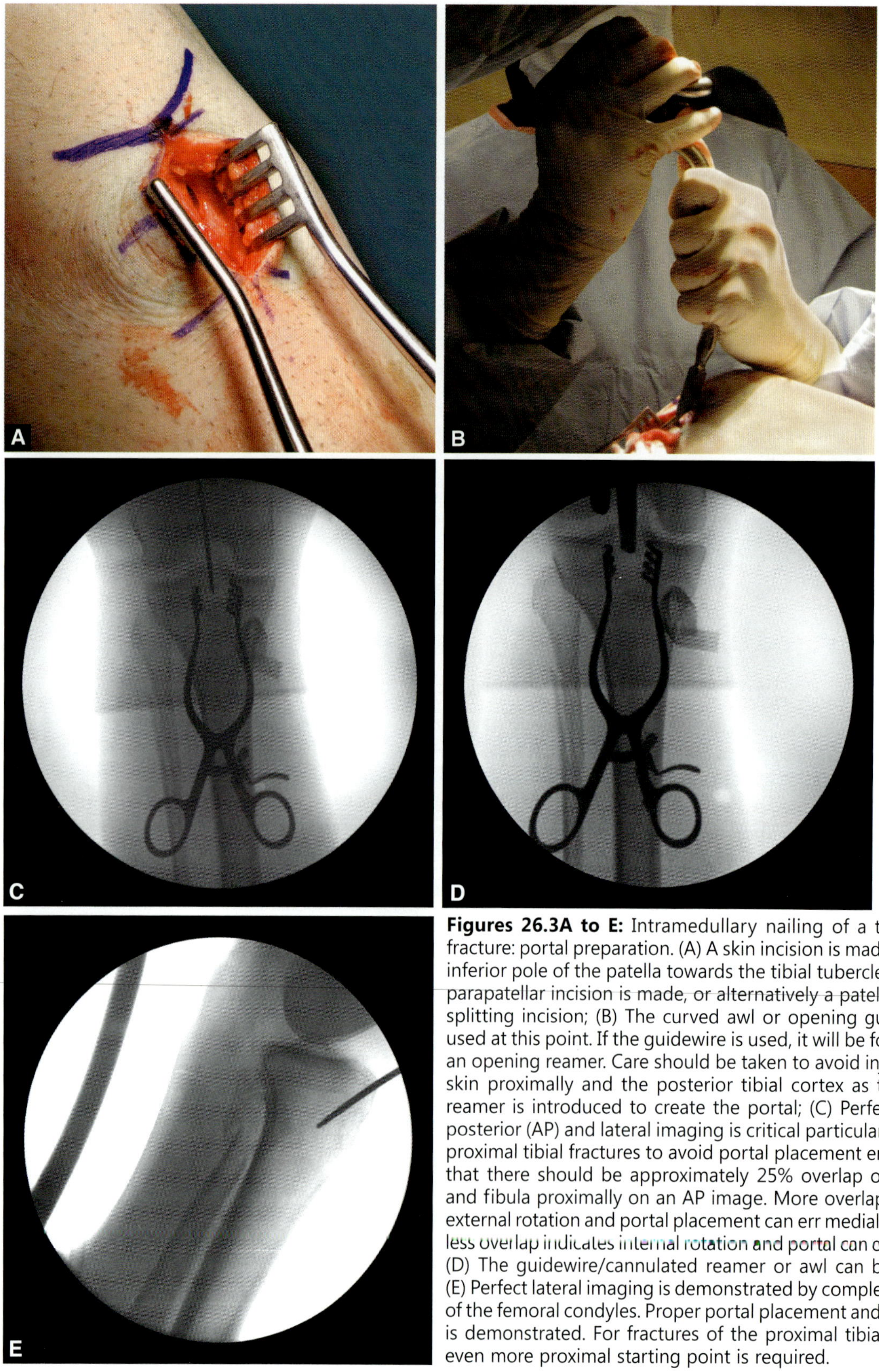

Figures 26.3A to E: Intramedullary nailing of a tibial shaft fracture: portal preparation. (A) A skin incision is made from the inferior pole of the patella towards the tibial tubercle. A medial parapatellar incision is made, or alternatively a patellar tendon splitting incision; (B) The curved awl or opening guidewire is used at this point. If the guidewire is used, it will be followed by an opening reamer. Care should be taken to avoid injury to the skin proximally and the posterior tibial cortex as the awl or reamer is introduced to create the portal; (C) Perfect antero-posterior (AP) and lateral imaging is critical particularly in more proximal tibial fractures to avoid portal placement errors. Note that there should be approximately 25% overlap of the tibia and fibula proximally on an AP image. More overlap indicates external rotation and portal placement can err medially whereas less overlap indicates internal rotation and portal can err laterally; (D) The guidewire/cannulated reamer or awl can be utilized; (E) Perfect lateral imaging is demonstrated by complete overlap of the femoral condyles. Proper portal placement and trajectory is demonstrated. For fractures of the proximal tibial shaft, an even more proximal starting point is required.

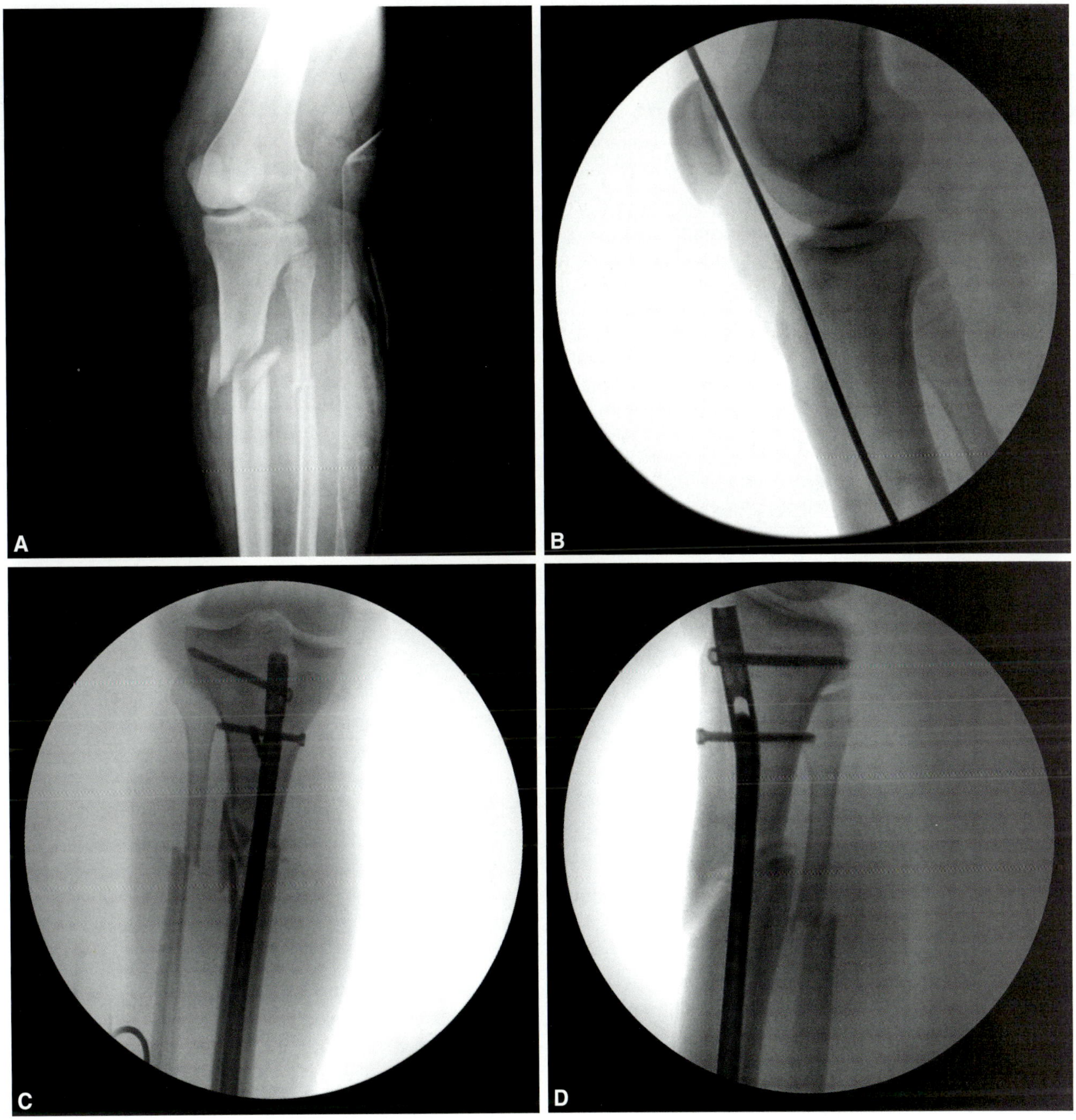

Figures 26.4A to D: Preventing malalignment when nailing a proximal tibial fracture: the semiextended arthrotomy approach. (A) Preoperative image of a proximal third tibial fracture; (B) The semiextended arthrotomy approach allows lateral subluxation of the patella which in turn permits a more proximal placement and anterior trajectory of the portal and guidewire. Furthermore, the added relaxation of the extensor mechanism reduces the tendency for the proximal fragment to extend; (C) A blocking screw is also placed in an anterior to posterior direction to prevent valgus malalignment; (D) Acceptable alignment is seen on the lateral image with slight residual translation of the fragments.

the lateral fluoroscopic image and at the medial border of the lateral tibial spine on an AP image (Figs 26.3A to E). It is critical to make sure that the imaging is performed with perfect AP and lateral imaging to avoid errors in portal placement due to image rotation. Whereas the lateral image can often be perfected by demonstrating perfect overlap of the femoral condyles, AP imaging is a bit more difficult. The tibia-fibular overlap is a good radiographic relationship to pay close attention to. In general, there should be approximately 25% overlap of the fibular head with the tibia on the AP image. Whereas this absolute perfection of the portal position is not always critical in the treatment of the mid-shaft tibial fracture, it is often critical when nailing proximal tibial fractures as described later.

The guidewire is then reamed or the awl is appropriately inserted to the depth required by the instrumentation system being utilized. Care is taken to avoid penetrating the posterior tibial cortex. The fracture is reduced by whatever means necessary (closed manipulation, percutaneous instruments, open reduction, etc.) and a ball-tipped guidewire is passed through the portal and across the fracture site (Figs 26.5A to L). The surgeon attempts to place the tip of the wire into the central portion of the distal tibial metaphysis on both AP and lateral images. A measurement of nail length is then taken using a second guidewire of equal length (subtraction method) or a radiographic ruler. Reaming is performed typically starting with a 9 mm end-cutting reamer. The surgeon must be careful not to allow the guidewire to come out or for the fracture to lose reduction during the reaming process. Care should also be taken to avoid progressively reaming anteriorly at the portal "reaming out anteriorly". To avoid this, the power reaming can be stopped well before exiting because the opening reamer creates space for the smaller reamer to be removed the last few centimeters by hand. Reaming is increased in either 0.5 or 1.0 mm increments. Furthermore, adequate flexion of the knee is necessary to allow a more direct trajectory of the reamer with the tibial shaft. If the knee is allowed to assume a position of more extension, the reamer is blocked by the patella which can allow for reaming out anteriorly. The surgeon typically places a loose-fitting nail and do not attempt to ream up to "chatter". Although in the femoral shaft, the surgeon does ream up to "chatter" in an attempt to place an isthmus-fitting nail and avoid a hypertrophic nonunion, there is evidence to suggest that over-reaming in the tibia can further compromise the endosteal blood supply without any purported mechanical advantage. Therefore, most adult tibias in his patient population are fixed with a 10 mm nail.

The tibial nail implant with chosen length and diameter is then inserted with gentle taps of the mallet. If the fracture is gapped at this point, distal interlocking is performed and then a back-tapping technique is performed to compress the fracture. After drilling and placing the distal interlocking screws using a freehand "perfect circle" technique with fluoroscopy, the extraction rod is placed on the insertion handle and gentle back tapping is performed. This will allow compression of the fracture which is desirable for predictable healing. Proximal interlocking can then be done after it is clear that rotational alignment is satisfactory. This should be checked with both radiographic and clinical examination findings. Proximal interlocking is generally done using a targeting device on the insertion handle depending on the instrumentation system being utilized. If there is no fracture gap after the nail is inserted, then proximal interlocking can be performed before distal interlocking.

The surgeon typically places at least two interlocking screws proximally and distally for a tibial shaft fracture. If a smaller diameter nail with smaller diameter screws is utilized (likely due to a small canal size), one should consider a third screw since the incidence of screw breakage is higher with these smaller implants.

The fibular diaphyseal fracture generally does not require reduction and fixation, although this can be considered in cases of wide displacement that do not reduce with tibial reduction and fixation, but these cases are rare. Distal fibular diaphyseal or lateral malleolar fractures seen concomitantly with a distal tibial shaft or metadiaphyseal fracture, however, may benefit from open reduction internal fixation (ORIF) (Figs 26.6A to E). Retrograde IM fixation can be performed with Kirschner wires or Rush pins particularly in transverse or simple fracture patterns. But if the soft tissues permit ORIF, plating methods are more versatile and work well. In a simple fracture pattern, the fibula can be fixed anatomically before tibial fixation as long as varus malalignment of the tibia can be avoided. However, if there is a comminuted fibular fracture, the fibula should not be fixed before the tibia because a nonanatomic reduction of the fibula is more likely and this can lead to inability to properly reduce the tibia fracture. The authors generally prefer to reduce

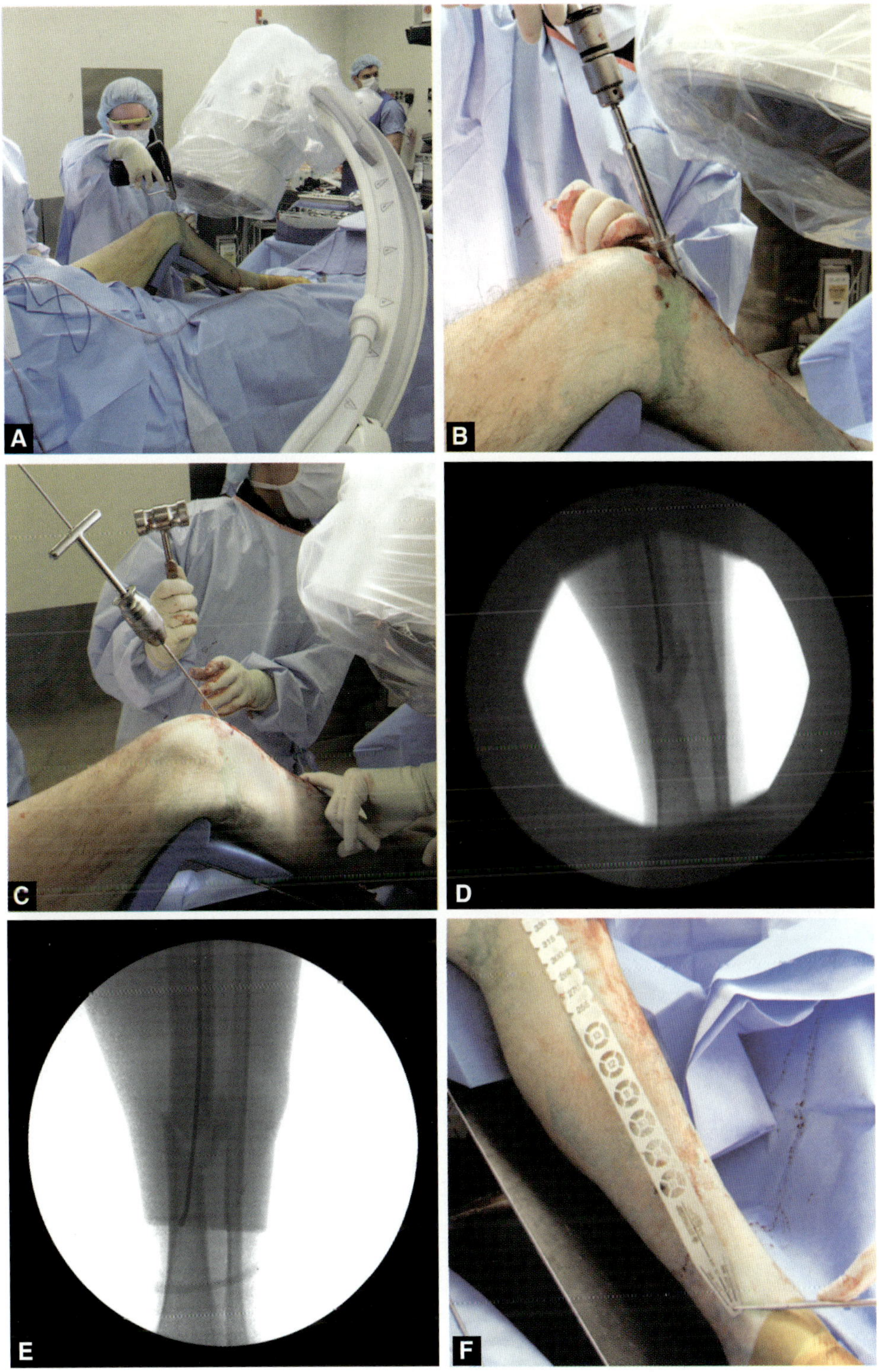

Figures 26.5A to F: Intramedullary nailing of a tibial shaft fracture: guidewire placement, reaming, and implant placement. (A) The fluoroscopic C-arm is positioned as shown from the opposite side of the table while the starting portal is instrumented; (B) Once the opening guidewire is confirmed to be properly placed on perfect anteroposterior and lateral images, it is reamed as shown; (C) The ball-tipped guide rod is placed into the portal and a closed or open reduction of the fracture is performed to allow passage of the guide rod across the fracture; (D and E) Passage of the guidewire across the fracture site. The wire is rotated and the bent tip can be navigated across the fracture site; (F) A length measurement is taken.

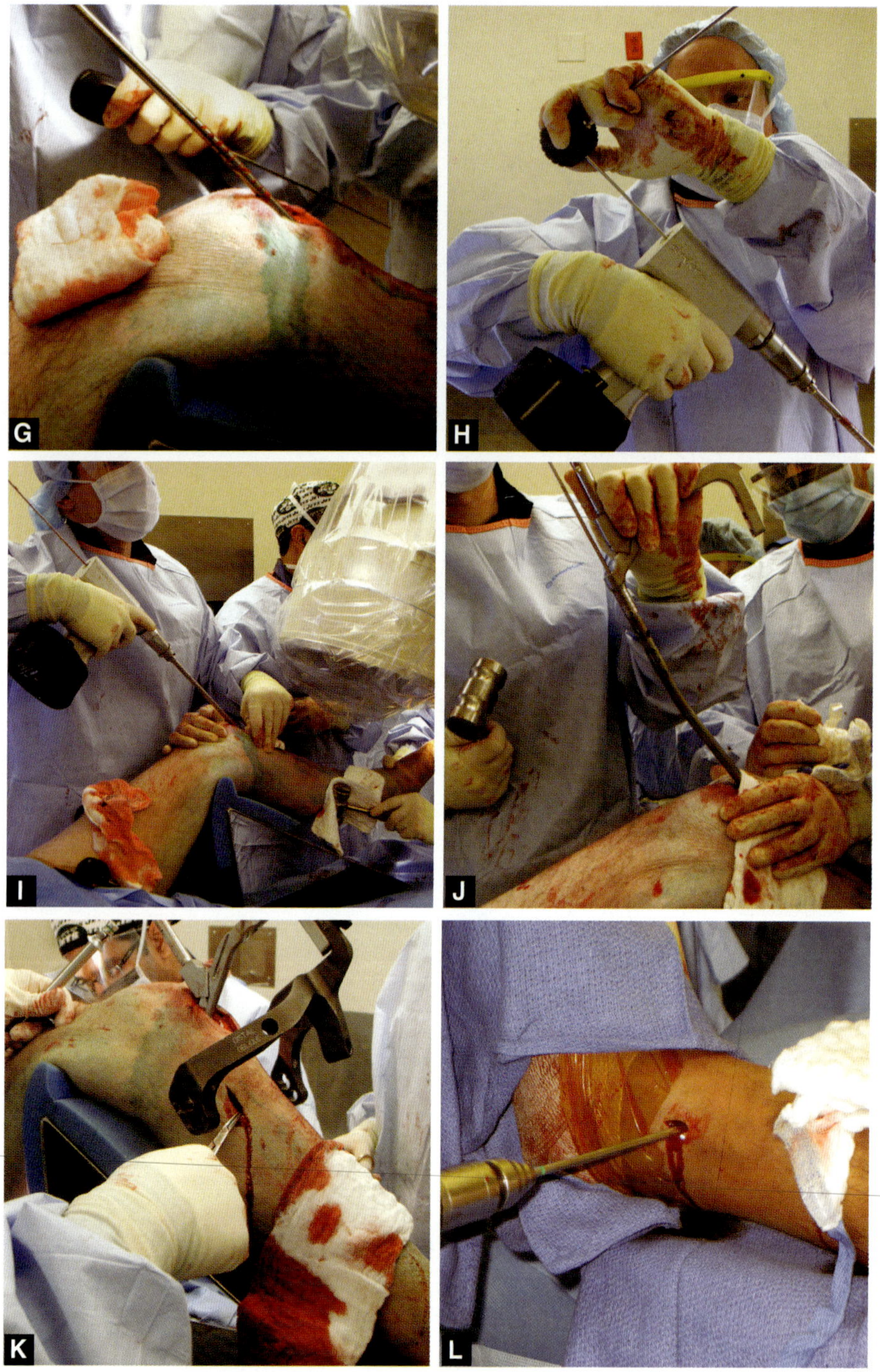

Figures 26.5G to L: (G) Reaming is performed. Reaming typically starts with a 9 mm reamer and increases in 0.5 mm or 1.0 mm increments depending on how difficult it is to pass the reamer. Care is taken to avoid using excessive force which can cause mechanical or thermal bone injury as well as pressurize the canal causing marrow embolization; (H) Care should be taken to prevent "backing out" of the guide rod during the reaming process; (I) Fracture reduction should be maintained throughout the procedure; (J) The nail is then inserted by hand and then with gentle mallet blows; (K) A targeting device is used to lock proximally. Distal locking followed by "back-tapping" can be done before proximal locking if the fracture is gapped and requires compression; (L) Distal locking is done with a freehand method. "Perfect circles" are visualized using the C-arm and drill holes are placed from medial to lateral followed by interlocking screws. The surgeon must ensure that rotational alignment and length is correct before the final locking screws are placed.

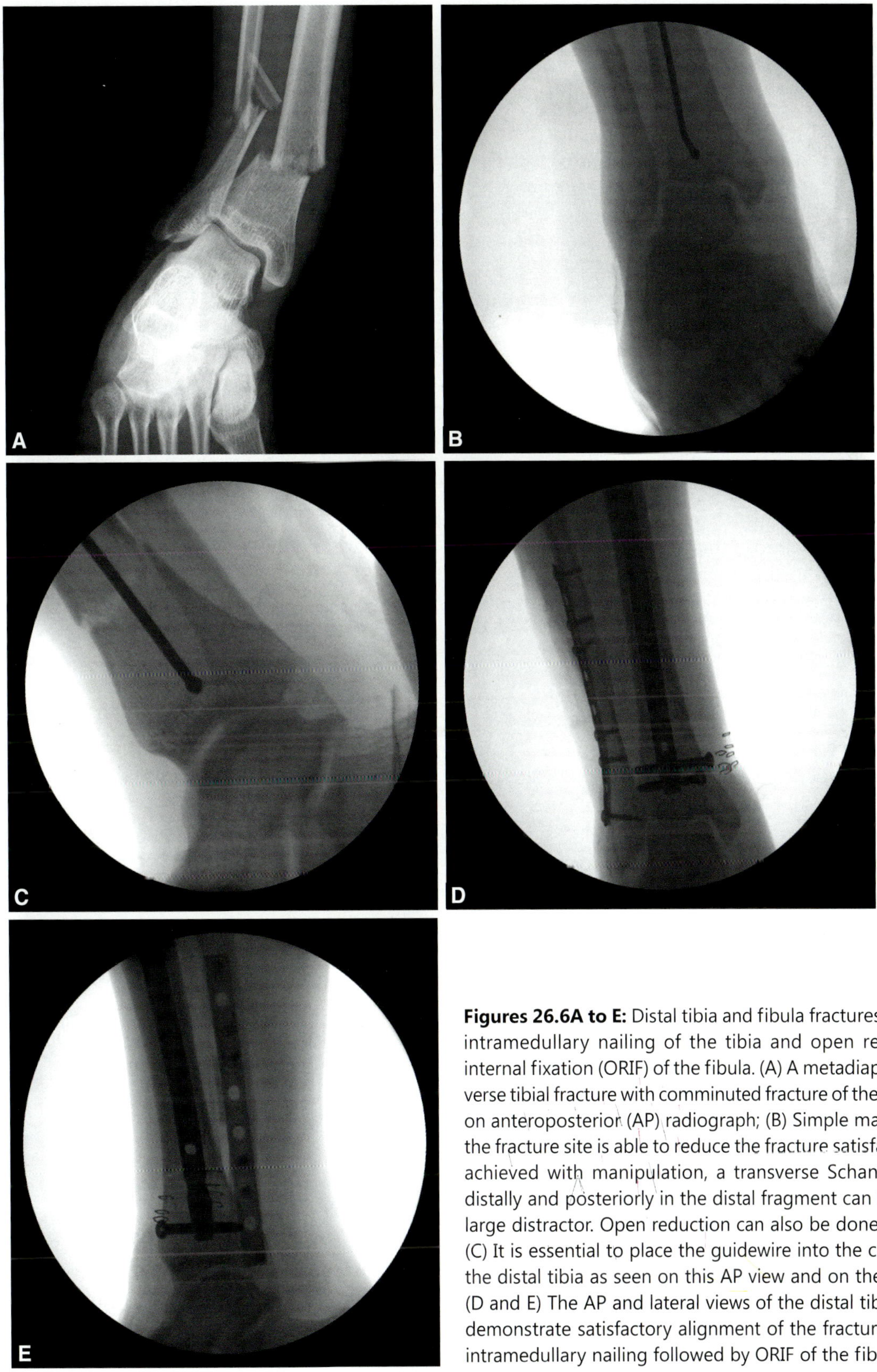

Figures 26.6A to E: Distal tibia and fibula fractures treated with intramedullary nailing of the tibia and open reduction and internal fixation (ORIF) of the fibula. (A) A metadiaphyseal transverse tibial fracture with comminuted fracture of the fibula shown on anteroposterior (AP) radiograph; (B) Simple manipulation of the fracture site is able to reduce the fracture satisfactorily. If not achieved with manipulation, a transverse Schanz pin placed distally and posteriorly in the distal fragment can help as can a large distractor. Open reduction can also be done if necessary; (C) It is essential to place the guidewire into the central part of the distal tibia as seen on this AP view and on the lateral view; (D and E) The AP and lateral views of the distal tibia and fibula demonstrate satisfactory alignment of the fractures after tibial intramedullary nailing followed by ORIF of the fibula.

and fix the tibia first since its reduction is more critical than that of the fibula. Manipulation of the tibial fracture is easier when the fibula fracture is mobile and not yet stabilized.

After fixation is completed, be sure to check fluoroscopic images in multiple planes to ensure that the implants are not intra-articular, the locking screws are properly seated and not excessively long, and that the locking screws are actually passing through the nail and not outside of it. Rotation of the leg should also be checked critically using both clinical examination and radiographic parameters. Radiographically, try to minimize magnification and check that the appropriate tibiofibular relationships are seen on the AP image of the knee and ankle without repositioning the limb. A proper lateral image of the knee and ankle with excellent joint space visualization should be able to be seen similarly without repositioning the limb. After the drapes are removed at the conclusion of the case, the pelvis should be made perfectly level and rotational alignment should be examined and compared to the contralateral limb. If there is a significant malalignment (particularly in internal rotation), consideration should be made for immediate removal of the necessary locking screws, correction of the malrotation, and revision of the locking screws.

Wounds should be irrigated and bony debris particularly from the proximal wound should be removed. The proximal incision is closed in layers and the smaller incisions for screw placement usually are short and only in need of skin closure. Loosely applied dressings should be placed to avoid constriction since swelling is likely to occur postoperatively. Distal pulses should be checked before waking the patient and a neurologic examination should be performed as soon as the patient is able to follow commands. Later postoperative examinations will focus mainly on the neurovascular status of the limb, so a good baseline examination is critical. Weight bearing is generally allowed postoperatively as tolerated with an assist device such as crutches except in cases of bone loss or intra-articular extension. Range of motion exercises are encouraged of the knee, hip, and ankle.

REAMED, LOCKED INTRAMEDULLARY NAILING OF TIBIAL SHAFT FRACTURE: Pearls and Pitfalls

- Make sure that a fracture reduction can be achieved before inserting the implants
- Do not rely on the implant to achieve the reduction for you, particularly in metadiaphyseal fracture patterns
- Do not "ream out" the anterior cortex
- Be sure to check rotational alignment before leaving the operating room

Technique 2: Intramedullary Nailing of a Proximal Tibial Shaft or Metadiaphyseal Fracture

Intramedullary nailing of proximal tibial shaft fractures is technically demanding with regard to maintaining the fracture reduced throughout the procedure. There are several special reduction techniques which have been described in this section to avoid malreduction. Otherwise, most of the methods utilized in technique 1 above are also used when performing IM nailing of the proximal tibial shaft fracture. Preoperative planning is also similar. The main issue is to simply identify the fact that the fracture, particularly where the posterior cortex is involved, is proximal enough to potentially cause problems with malreduction during this procedure. Options for surgical treatment of this injury also include locked anterolateral plating and ring external fixation. Preoperative radiographs, and if necessary, CT scanning is checked to rule out intra-articular involvement. Although this is not a strict contraindication for IM nailing, it is preferred that intra-articular fractures be nondisplaced or minimally displaced and that these are fixed before any reaming and nail insertion is performed. It is also important to choose an IM nail which does not have a very distal Herzog bend as this may create difficulties with maintaining the reduction once the nail is inserted.

The extensor mechanism can create either anterior displacement of the proximal fragment or this combined with an apex anterior deformity. Flexion of the knee which is typically performed during IM nailing can accentuate this deformity (Figs 26.7A to D). If the guidewire and reaming is not kept anterior in the proximal fragment and is allowed to be directed towards the posterior cortex, reduction of the fracture will likely be lost as the nail is inserted, recreating the initial deformity or even making it worse. Furthermore, errant placement of the guidewire will also easily produce varus or valgus deformities of the fracture seen on AP imaging (Fig. 26.7C). Particular attention to both the starting position and trajectory of the guidewire or awl is extremely important when performing IM nailing of a proximal tibial fracture. Even a slightly errant placement or trajectory can cause a deformity of the fracture. Making sure that proper

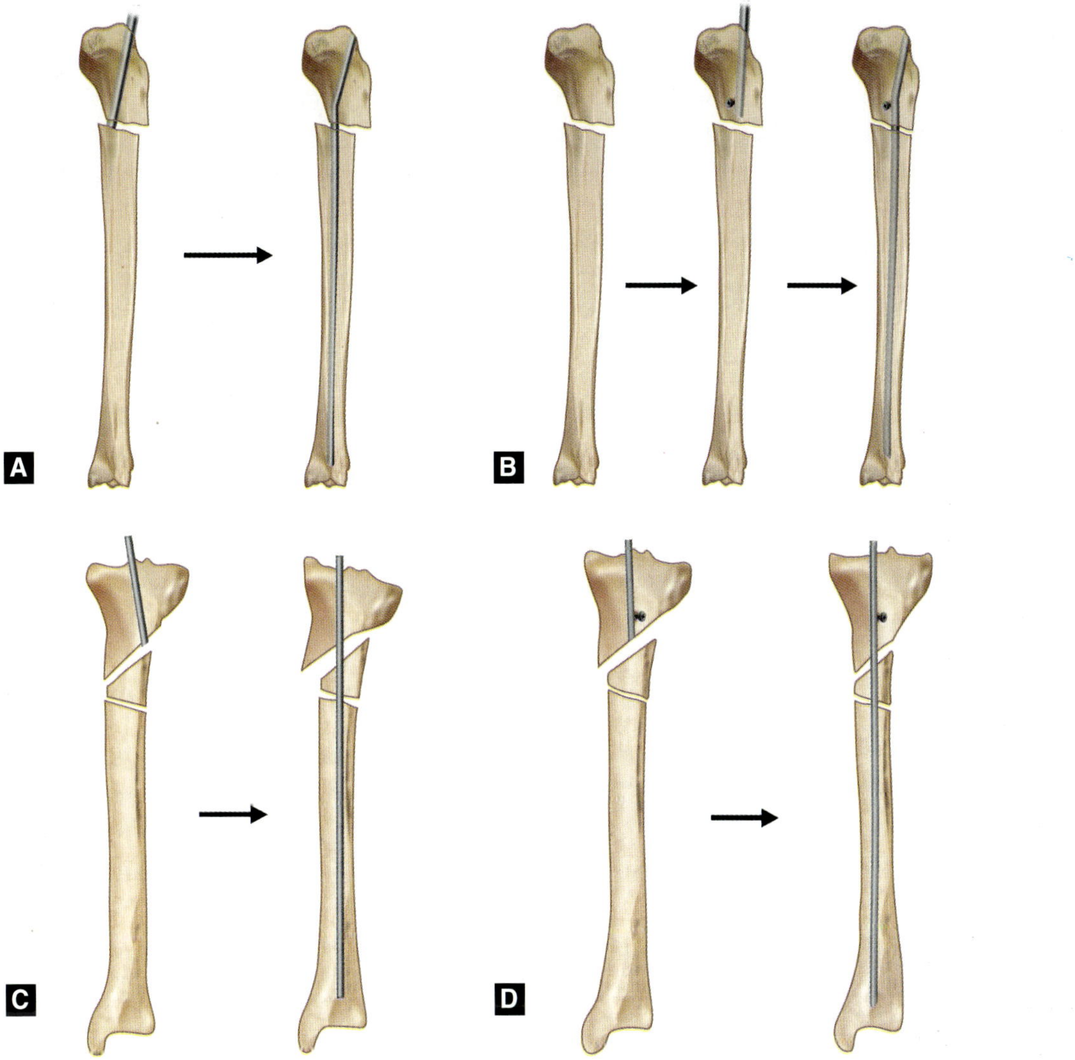

Figures 26.7A to D: Preventing malalignment when nailing a proximal tibial fracture: blocking screws. (A) Apex anterior deformity with anterior translation of the proximal fragment can be exaggerated by increased flexion of the knee. If the nail portal is directed too posteriorly as shown here, this deformity will persist or even become worse when the nail is inserted. A more proximal and anteriorly directed portal could have prevented this; (B) This can be corrected with the placement of a medial to lateral blocking screw to effectively create a new posterior "cortex" and keep the nail anterior. As the nail centers itself in the canal, the deformity seen in 26.7A is prevented; (C) Valgus deformity seen due to lateral comminution. An excessively medial starting point will cause the nail to be directed from medial to lateral. As the nail centers itself, the valgus deformity is made even worse. A more laterally placed portal could have prevented this; (D) This can be corrected with the placement of a blocking screw to effectively create a new lateral cortex and keep the nail medial. As the nail centers itself in the canal, the deformity seen in Figure 26.7C is prevented. An example of this is shown in Figure 26.4.

AP and lateral imaging is obtained, and that the AP images are not rotated, is critical to actually knowing if portal placement is correct.

To achieve and maintain appropriate fracture alignment, several methods can be performed that are not typically needed for IM nailing of the mid-diaphyseal fracture. These methods include the semiextended approach, blocking (Poller) screws, open reduction and temporary unicortical plating, and temporary external fixation or distractor placement. If necessary, a combination of these techniques can be utilized in order to prevent deformity during IM nailing.

The semiextended approach essentially negates the deformity caused by the extensor mechanism by moving the patella out of the way and allowing the nailing procedure to occur with the knee in a much more extended position.[13] The initial knee incision as described in technique 1 above is made extensile into a full parapatellar arthrotomy as is used in total knee arthroplasty. The patella is then everted or subluxed laterally and the knee is kept on a bump roll in slight flexion of approximately 30° at most. This is far less flexion than is typically possible with the standard positioning and approach described in technique 1. The initial guidewire or awl is placed at the proximal "rollover" position and directed as anteriorly as possible (Figs 26.3A to E). The key is to prevent the initial guidewire or awl to be directed from anteriorly to posteriorly which will create a subsequent extension deformity particularly when the implant is inserted (Figs 26.7A to D). If the reduction can be maintained during guide wire or awl placement, reaming is performed in the same position and IM nailing proceeds as described in technique 1. Care is taken to ensure that all reamings are carefully irrigated and removed from the joint and the authors prefer to place an intra-articular suction drain at the end of the procedure. Weight bearing is allowed depending on the degree of cortical contact. It should be noted that manufacturers have now introduced instrumentation that allows for the semiextended approach to be performed through a miniarthrotomy without subluxation of the patella. This "retropatellar" approach is performed through long cannulas that are placed between the patella and femur.

Blocking "Poller" screws are another effective method to avoid not only an extension deformity (apex anterior angulation) of the proximal tibia but also varus and valgus deformities (Figs 26.4A to D and 26.7A to D). The key concept of blocking screws is that they essentially try to narrow the canal of the tibia in order to channel the guidewire and implant in a straight path. They are used mainly in the proximal tibial metaphysis or metadiaphyseal region but can also be used in the distal tibia. A blocking screw is meant to block the path of the guidewire and implant from taking an errant path, which is typically a path into either a posterior, medial, or lateral area of comminution. The most common error is to place the portal slightly medial, which allows the implant to be directed from medial to lateral, creating a valgus deformity (Figs 26.7A to D). In order to prevent this, many surgeons prefer to use a lateral parapatellar starting point for nailing the proximal tibia fracture. The authors have found that this is not usually necessary and this does not allow the approach to be easily converted to the medial parapatellar semiextended approach as described above, if necessary.

Blocking screws are placed either pre-emptively or if initial guidewire placement is not taking a central trajectory in the tibial canal despite efforts to do so. The interlocking screws from the locked IM nailing set can be utilized. These must be placed under image guidance to ensure that they are placed exactly where needed to help direct the guidewire in the correct direction. If the screw is placed too conservatively, the expected result may not be achieved and errant guidewire or nail placement may still occur. On the other hand, if the screw is placed too close to the center of the medullary canal, the nail will be completely blocked altogether from being passed distally. Understand that if the blocking screw is properly placed, the flexible reamers will indeed hit against the screw as they are passed which can lead to dulling of the reamer tip and obvious damage to the screw. If the screw is placed too close to the center of the medullary canal, it may not allow the reamer to be passed at all and aggressive reaming attempts can lead to dislodgement of the screw and subsequent fracture propagation. After the nail and interlocking screws are placed, the blocking screws can be removed but there is usually no advantage of doing so and the authors generally leave them in place.

Open reduction and temporary unicortical plating is yet another method which can prevent proximal tibial deformity with IM nailing. A small anterolateral approach to the tibia is performed, the anterior compartment muscles are carefully elevated, and standard AO fracture reduction methods are performed to achieve fracture reduction. A unicortical 3.5 mm plate is plated, typically with 6 screws (Figs 26.8A to J). Although bicortical screws can be utilized if strategically placed to avoid the path of the nail and reamers, this can be difficult to achieve. Ideally, unicortical plating is performed with locked plate and screws to prevent loosening during the nailing procedure although this is a very expensive option to use as a temporary measure. Open fractures can offer the opportunity for this technique after formal debridement is done if IM nailing is chosen as definitive management rather than plating. Care should be taken to avoid excessive manipulation of the fracture site during the nailing procedure to avoid screw loosening, particularly if nonlocked implants are used or if fixation is not adequate. The authors generally remove this implant at the conclusion of the IM

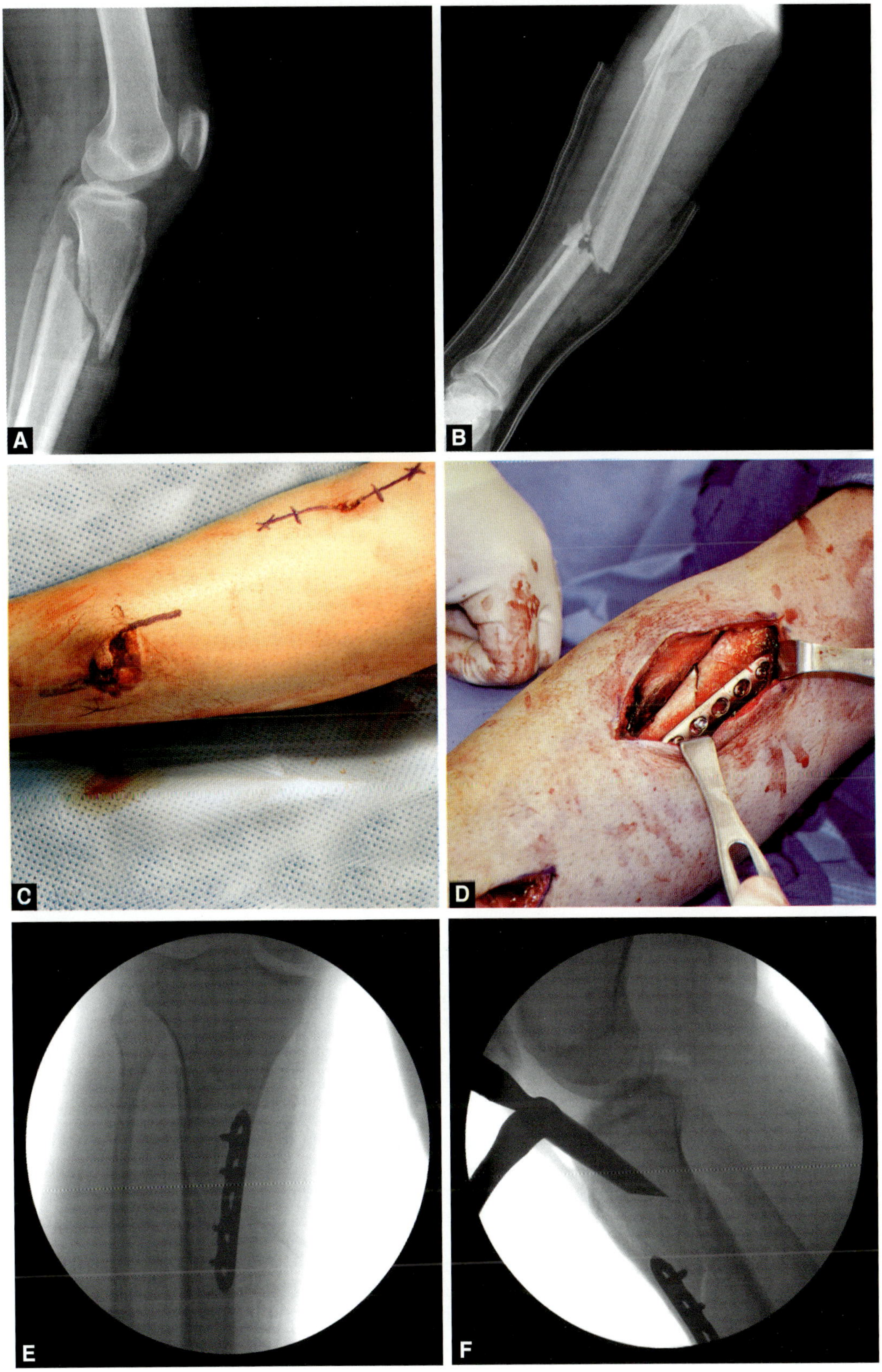

Figures 26.8A to F

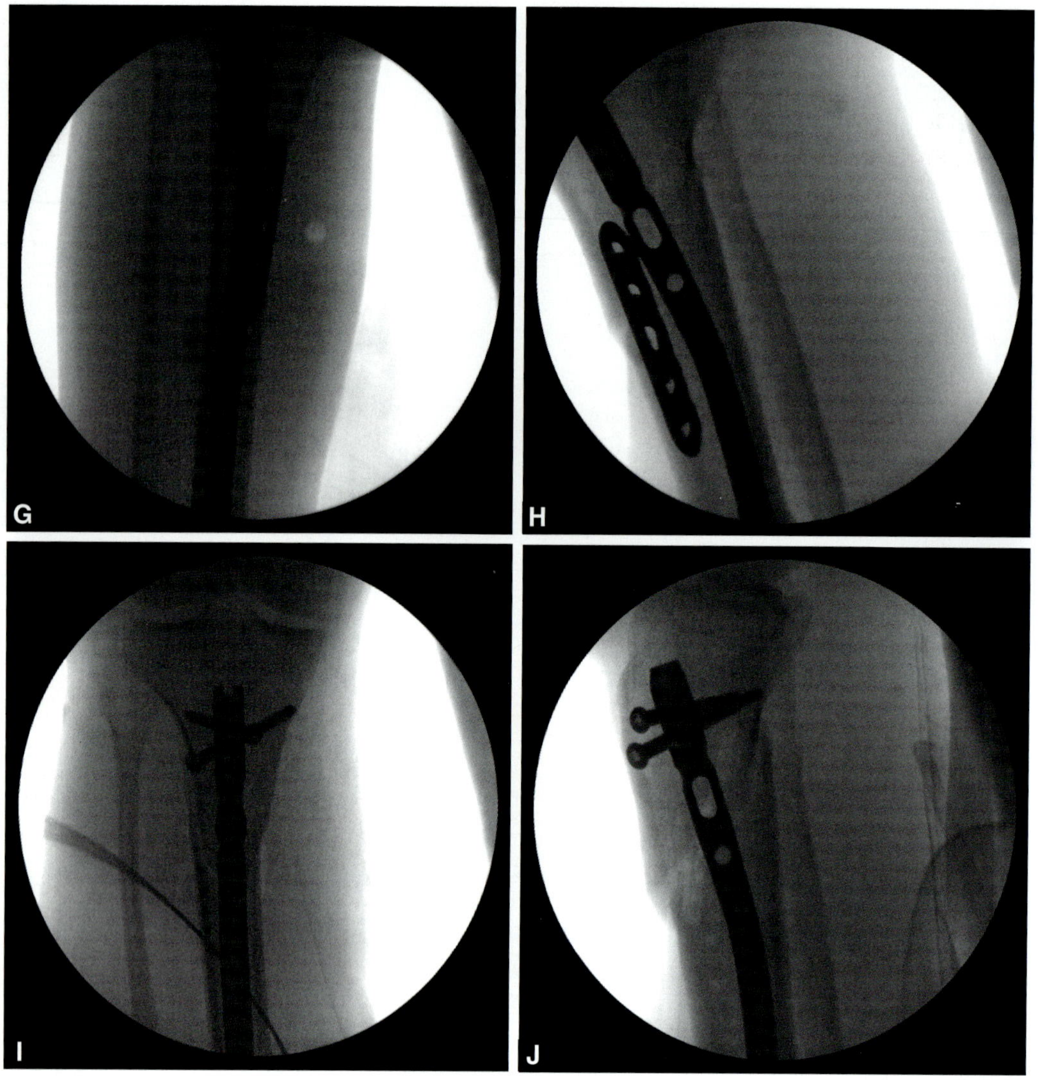

Figures 26.8A to J: Preventing malalignment when nailing a proximal tibial fracture: temporary unicortical plating. (A) Anteroposterior (AP) and (B) lateral radiographs of an open segmental tibial shaft fracture; (C) For debridement, both wounds are to be extended and the fracture ends and wounds debrided; (D) Open reduction and temporary unicortical plating is performed to maintain alignment throughout the intramedullary nailing procedure; (E) AP and (F) lateral images after plating. Care is taken to make the nail portal proximal and directed as anterior as possible; (G and H) Reduction is maintained after nail placement although the nail is countersunk more than is required; (I and J) Since this was an open fracture which was well-stabilized with the nail, the plate was removed but slight loss of reduction is seen on the lateral image although overall alignment is quite acceptable.

nailing procedure. If unacceptable displacement occurs after the plate is removed, it can be re-reduced and placed back on the tibia. This is probably the most costly method in terms of implant price of these four techniques, particularly if a locked plate and locked screws are utilized.

Temporary external fixation can be performed with either large external fixator components or the large distractor. A Schanz pin is placed transversely in the proximal tibia posteriorly, and into the distal tibia also transversely and posteriorly in order to avoid the path of the guidewire and nail. After placement of the pins, a closed reduction of the fracture is attempted and the frame is locked into position when reduction is achieved. The fixator is then removed at the conclusion of the IM nailing procedure. Care should be taken to avoid injury to the common peroneal nerve proximally and the posterior tibial artery distally. The authors have generally found this method to be the more useful for correcting varus and valgus deformities rather than extension deformities or translational deformities.

INTRAMEDULLARY NAILING OF A PROXIMAL TIBIAL SHAFT OR METADIAPHYSEAL FRACTURE: Pearls and Pitfalls

- It is critical to achieve the perfect starting portal and trajectory of the awl or guidewire. A proximal starting point at the "roll-over" position best allows a more anterior trajectory. Perfect AP and lateral imaging is necessary to achieve a perfect position and trajectory
- Do not be afraid to use one of the methods described above in order to achieve and maintain a reduction. If the fracture is not reduced, the nail will not achieve the reduction for you like it can in the mid-diaphyseal fracture. In fact, even if the fracture is reduced during reaming, reduction can be lost with nail insertion if the reaming trajectory is not ideal and the implant has a distal Herzog bend
- Be sure to have the appropriate implants available (such as a small fragment set and distractor or external fixator) when planning for an IM nailing of a proximal tibia fracture in case they are needed as described above
- Blocking screw placement must be precise. If a blocking screw is too close to the center of the canal and the reamer will not go past it, insert a more conservatively-placed screw and remove the prior screw. Over-aggressive attempts to get past this initial screw can lead to excessive damage to the reamer or even dislodgement of the screw and fracture propagation

Technique 3: Intramedullary Nailing of a Distal Tibial Metadiaphyseal Fracture

As tibial nails manufacturers have allowed more distal placement of locking screws recently, tibial nailing can be performed for distal metadiaphyseal fractures of the tibia as well. With better understanding of minimally invasive techniques and the popularity of locked plates, plating methods are also an attractive technique for treating these injuries. Open fractures, patients with a poor soft tissue envelope or very thin patients are in the authors' opinion better suited for IM nailing rather than plating for risk of infection or wound complications. Plating, however, avoids the common complaints of anterior knee pain and may be preferable particularly in patients who kneel frequently such as carpenters, plumbers, and other laborers. If nailing is chosen, similar preoperative considerations as described in technique 1 should be followed. In addition, it is important to make preoperative measurements to ensure that at least two distal locking screws will be able to be placed in the nail safely distal to the fracture site. Furthermore, imaging should ideally include CT scanning to rule out a posterior malleolar fracture or intra-articular extension. Although intra-articular extension is not a contraindication for nailing if nondisplaced, it cannot be missed preoperatively.

In distal tibial fracture cases, achieving reduction is generally easier than in the proximal tibia. The distal tibia is easier to manipulate manually although excessive pressure to the skin around the ankle should be avoided. When necessary, a Steinman pin can be placed in the posterior distal tibia transversely as described in the previous section in order to manipulate the fragment in order to achieve a reduction (Fig. 26.9). Be sure not to

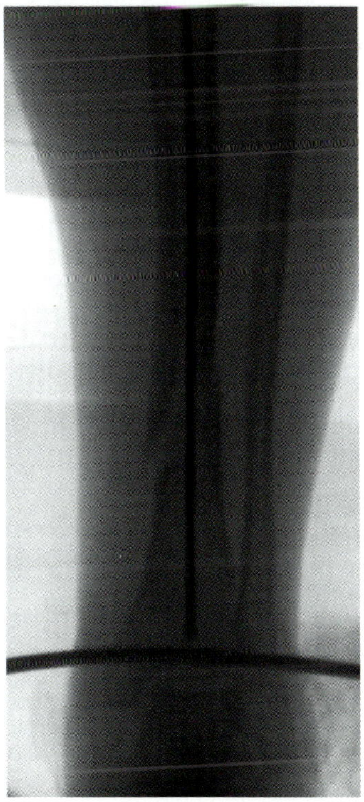

Figure 26.9: Preventing malalignment in distal tibial fractures: Steinman pin reduction maneuver. A Steinman pin is placed posteriorly and distally through the tibia and manipulated in order to obtain a reduction.

place this if there is a posterior malleolar fracture or intra-articular fracture extension that has not yet been stabilized, as this may lead to late migration of the nail by widening this gap. Also, a pointed reduction forcep can be used in more oblique or spiral type fracture patterns as described in technique 1 above. Regardless of the method chosen, once reduction is achieved, the reaming ball-tipped guidewire must be placed into the central position of the distal tibia on both AP and lateral images before reaming is done (Figs 26.6A to E).

A distal fibula or lateral malleolus fracture and occasionally a posterior malleolar fracture can occur concomitantly with the distal tibia fracture. Posterior malleolar fractures are generally nondisplaced but can be missed if not looked for with proper ankle radiographs and/or a CT scan. If seen, these should be fixed at the start of the procedure. One or two lag screws can be placed in a distal position avoiding the central portion of eventual tibial nail path and avoiding potential interlocking screw paths. After this is fixed, IM nailing can proceed. A true lateral malleolar ankle fracture is typically treated with ORIF using standard methods followed by external stress of the syndesmotic ligaments and fixation of that if necessary. But the distal fibular fracture that usually accompanies the distal tibia fracture often spares the lateral malleolus and its treatment is more controversial. Generally, the surgeon will treat this with ORIF with a third tubular plate after IM nailing is completed as long as the soft tissues permit this to be done safely (Figs 26.6A to E). It can be done before IM nailing as a tibial reduction method. That is, it can help to achieve length, angular alignment, and rotation if reduced correctly. This should only be attempted if the fracture is a simple, noncomminuted fracture which can be reliably anatomically reduced. If comminuted, it is less likely that anatomic reduction will be achieved and this can actually lead to difficulty in subsequently reducing the tibia properly. Even if fixed anatomically, it can sometimes allow for tibial varus to occur if the tibia is comminuted. This can be hard to overcome during the nailing procedure (as is the case with the tibia fracture without fibula fracture) and therefore, the authors tend to fix the fibula after tibial fixation.

After wound closure, the authors usually immobilize these injuries with a below knee plaster splint for 2 weeks, most particularly if there has also been a concomitant distal fibular or lateral malleolar fracture. The authors treat these non-weight-bearing (as opposed to weight-bearing as tolerated in tibial diaphyseal fractures without bone loss) for 6 weeks.

INTRAMEDULLARY NAILING OF A DISTAL TIBIAL METADIAPHYSEAL FRACTURE: Pearls and Pitfalls

- Preoperative planning should ensure that at least two interlocking screws will be able to be safely placed distal to the fracture with the implant used and that nondisplaced intra-articular fractures are not missed
- The ball-tipped guidewire should be placed in the central position of the tibia on both AP and lateral intraoperative fluoroscopic images
- Nondisplaced intra-articular fractures are not a contraindication but should be fixed prior to the IM nailing portion of the procedure
- If fixing a concomitant distal fibula fracture before the tibial nailing procedure, be sure to achieve anatomic reduction otherwise tibial reduction will not be satisfactory. If it does not appear that an anatomic reduction can be guaranteed, then tibial nailing should be done first followed by fibular ORIF if needed

Technique 4: ORIF of a Tibial Diaphyseal Fracture

Intramedullary nailing has essentially become the standard of care for the treatment of displaced diaphyseal fractures of the adult tibia. Fracture union, return to function, early weight bearing, and the familiarity of this technique have made this the treatment of choice for most orthopedic surgeons. External fixation (either uniplanar or circular) has problems with pin tract infections, malunion, nonunion, and poor patient tolerance. Its use is invaluable in treatment of complex soft tissue injury and in cases of deformity correction, but its advantages for the closed or low grade open tibial diaphyseal fractures are limited. The ORIF of the tibial diaphyseal fracture unfortunately has a higher incidence of infection and does not allow immediate weight bearing, which is often allowed for patients treated with tibial nailing. The orthopedic surgeon should be familiar with standard AO methods of ORIF of the tibial shaft, however, for cases in which it is needed.

Indications for ORIF with plate and screw implants of the tibial diaphysis include patients with an exceedingly narrow IM canal (which will not permit IM nailing), tibial diaphyseal deformity (either congenital or acquired), and pre-existing total knee arthroplasty or similar implant of the proximal tibia. It can also be considered in patients who need to avoid any chance of acquiring anterior knee pain often seen with tibial nailing. Also, surgeons not comfortable with or without the resources to perform locked IM nailing can obtain excellent results with ORIF of the tibia, although the infection risks are not diminished. The ORIF methods can also be employed in proximal or distal tibial fractures which have significant extension into the tibial shaft. In these cases, IM nailing methods can be challenging and ORIF can provide a technically easier and more predictable surgical result. Finally, ORIF techniques are frequently employed in the case of nonunion repair.

Preoperative planning methods should follow AO principles and ensure that the fracture pattern is thoroughly understood through radiographic imaging. The soft tissue status should also be carefully evaluated. Patients with severe soft tissue injury without adequate skin coverage are contraindicated, as are active infection or impending compartment syndrome. Standard 4.5 AO plates are typically used although 3.5 plates can work well in certain patients and fracture patterns. Locking instrumentation and implants are helpful in metadiaphyseal fracture patterns and in osteoporotic patients, but are otherwise not needed. The surgeon should be sure that the proper implants and instruments are available. Intraoperative imaging is preferable, although not as essential as it is for closed locked IM nailing.

Technique

Preoperative IV antibiotics are given within 1 hour of skin incision. A pneumatic tourniquet placed on the thigh may be utilized for upto 120 minutes if desired by the surgeon, but should not be utilized in cases of vascular injury or disease. Reperfusion with release of the tourniquet can also lead to excessive swelling in certain cases and may be dangerous in cases of significant preoperative swelling. A radiolucent table is utilized in order to allow intraoperative fluoroscopic imaging. Either blankets or foam positioners can be utilized under the leg in order to help facilitate lateral imaging and also raise the operative field away from the contralateral limb as shown in Figures 26.10A to P. The limb is prepped and draped in the usual manner.

An anterolateral approach is usually an excellent method to facilitate exposure of the tibial diaphyseal fracture. This also avoids the pes anserinus insertion proximally and provides better soft tissue coverage for the implant. The anterior compartment muscles are carefully elevated from the tibia and the periosteum is stripped only from the area of the fracture site (Fig. 26.10G).

Standard AO methods and strategies are employed in order to achieve reduction and fixation. Simple fracture patterns should be reduced and compressed anatomically and fixed with rigid absolute stability as shown in Figures 26.10A to P. Although soft tissue attachments to bone should be preserved whenever possible to maintain bone vascularity, standard bone clamps are utilized for direct reduction. These may include both pointed reduction or serrated jaw large bone forceps. In these cases lag screws should be used when possible and 6–8 cortices of fixation should be achieved both proximally and distally.

Comminuted fractures may be fixed with a bridge plating method in which longer plates are utilized and anatomic reduction of the fracture fragments is not attempted and relative stability is achieved in a similar fashion to IM nailing (Figs 26.11A to K). Reduction is achieved with indirect methods, such as distraction with the large distractor or simple traction. Anatomically contoured plates can also allow the fragments to reduce to the plate with cortical screws. Six to eight cortices of fixation should also be achieved in these cases although much longer plates are generally used than in cases of rigid fixation and absolute stability. As described earlier, 4.5 mm plates with cortical screws are generally sufficient. Locking screws are helpful in the metaphysis and in osteoporotic bone. Minimally invasive submuscular reduction and fixation techniques can be utilized in the diaphysis in a similar fashion as is shown in Figures 26.11A to K for the tibial metaphysis.

Wound closure should be done with careful skin and soft tissue handling. Suction drains are used at the discretion of the surgeon. Joint mobilization should be allowed as soon as possible. In cases in which wound healing is of a concern either due to local or systemic risk factors, joint mobilization can be delayed upto 2 weeks. Weight bearing is allowed at 6 weeks, although this may be variable depending on the degree of bone contact and reliability of the fixation and bone.

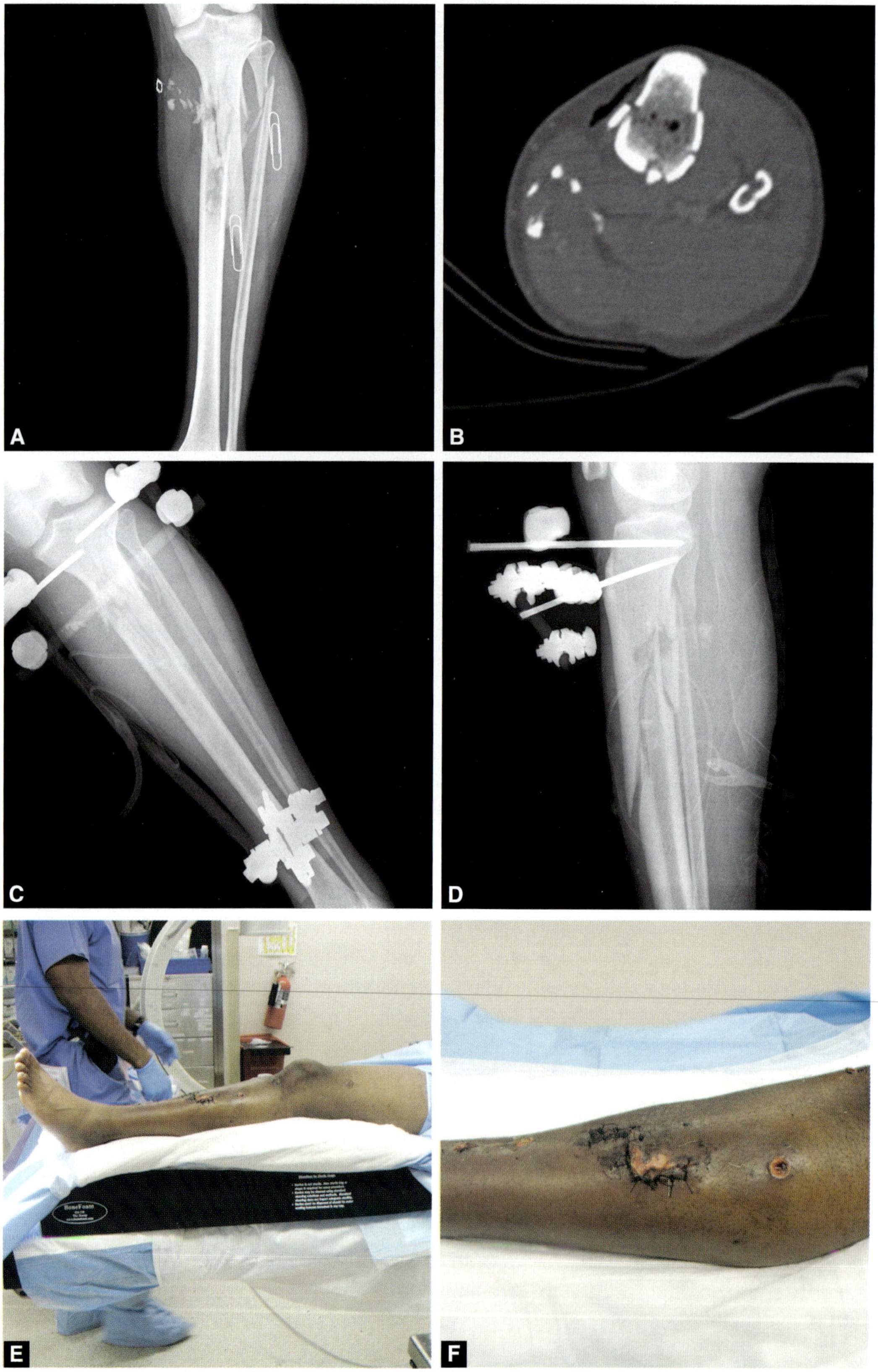

Figures 26.10A to F

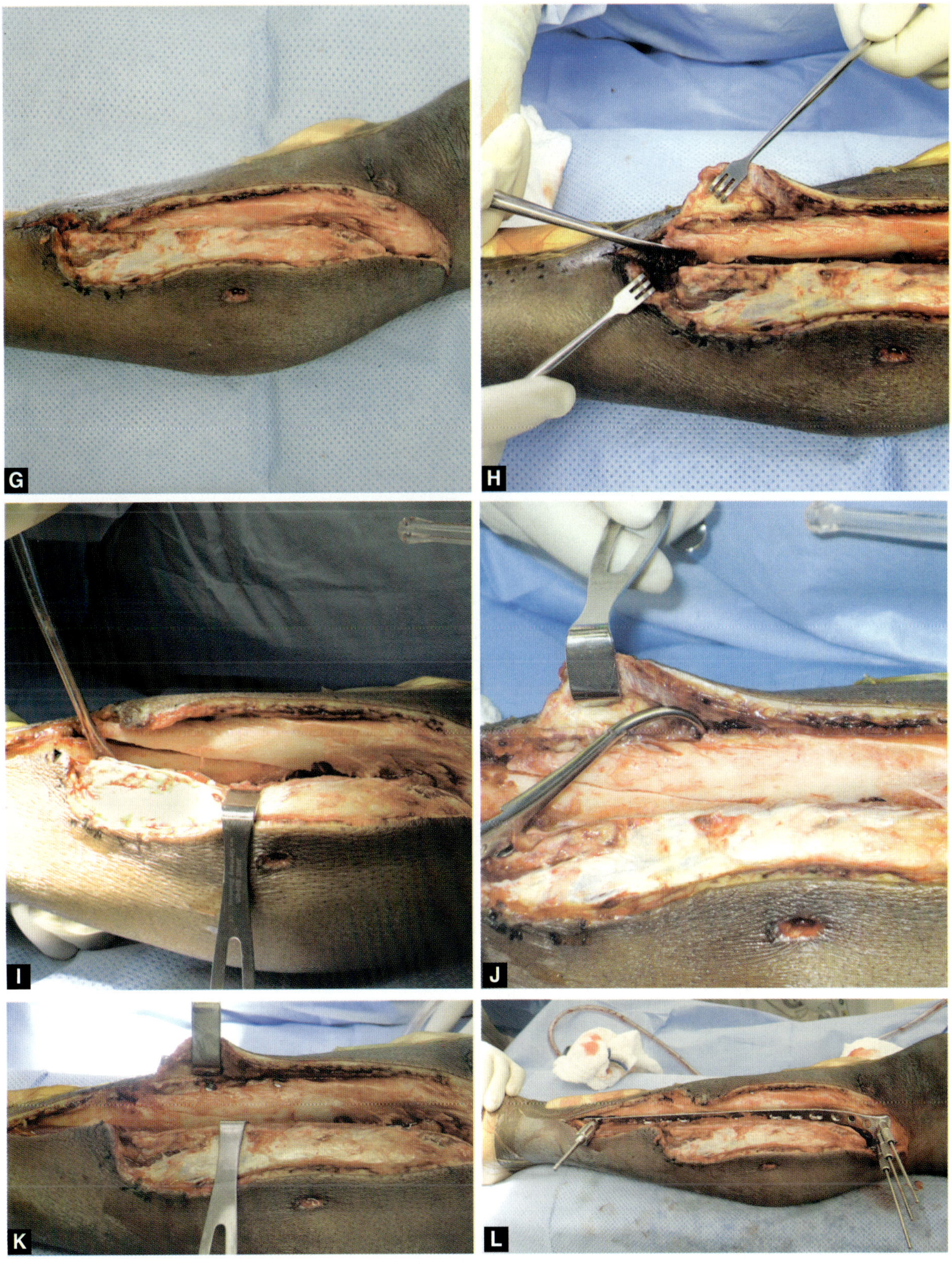

Figures 26.10G to L

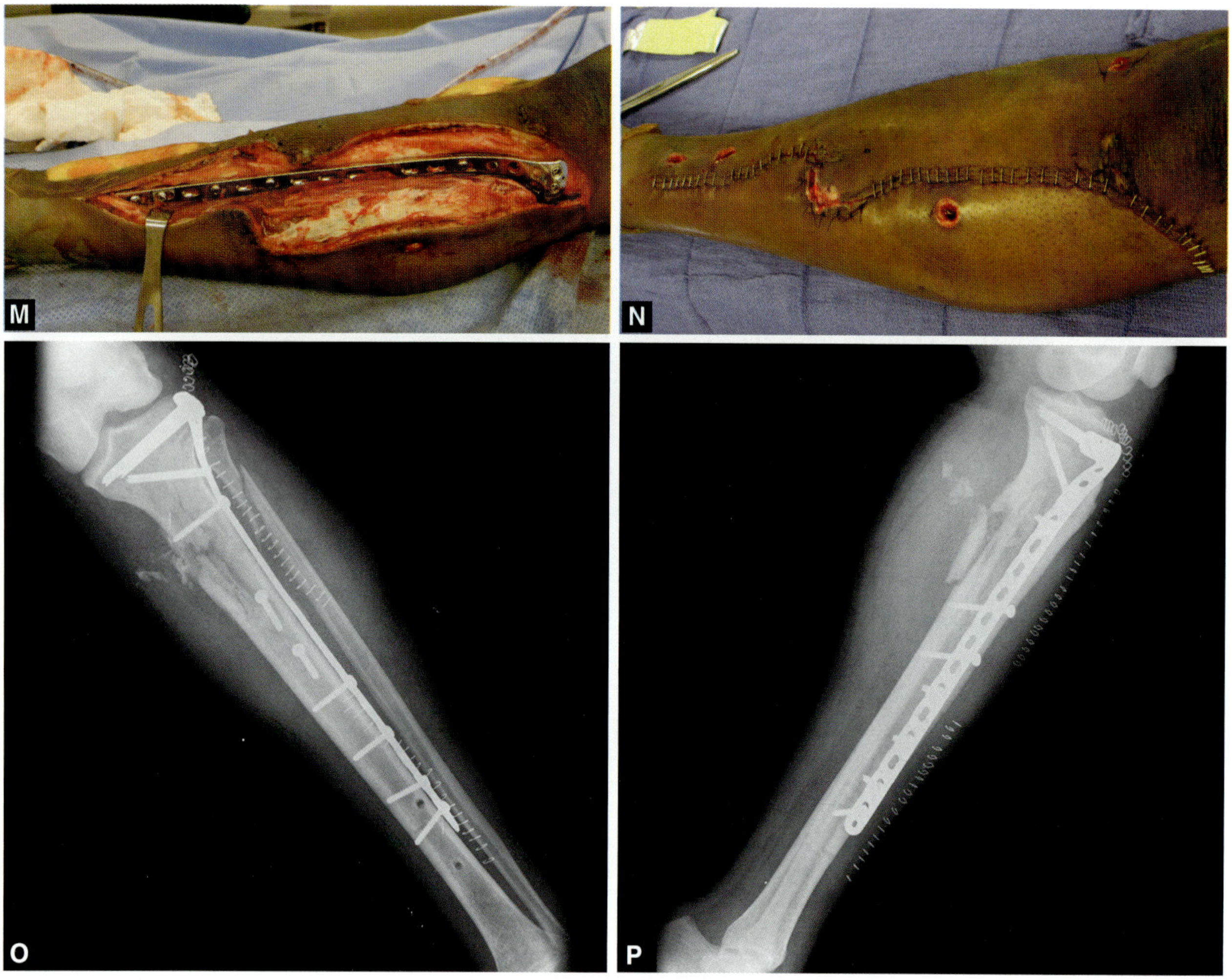

Figures 26.10A to P: Open reduction and internal fixation (ORIF) of a tibial shaft fracture with proximal intra-articular extension. (A) Preoperative anteroposterior radiograph as well as (B) CT scanning after a low velocity gunshot injury demonstrate an oblique tibial shaft fracture with proximal extension and comminution just posterior to the tibial tubercle. The patient was treated by irrigation and debridement of the fracture followed by (C and D) external fixation. After 1 week, the wounds were improved, swelling was improved, and consideration for definitive fixation was given. Intramedullary nailing was also an option here, but it was felt that this could lead to displacement of the fracture while instrumenting the portal essentially right into the proximal fracture site. Therefore, ORIF was chosen; (E) The operative leg is elevated on a foam positioner to facilitate lateral imaging and to get the contralateral limb out of the way. A radiolucent table is utilized and the fluoroscopic C-arm is brought from the opposite side of the table; (F) A missile entry wound is seen proximally and a separate open wound from the open fracture has been now closed in the mid-portion of the leg; (G) Anterolateral exposure with muscle elevation is performed from the proximal tibia to the fracture site. Periosteum is strictly preserved except along the fracture site; (H) Fracture hematoma is cleared from the fracture site; (I) The long oblique tibial fracture is now fully exposed with the missile injury to soft tissue and bone seen proximally. The diaphyseal fracture is essentially a simple fracture pattern and should be reduced anatomically and fixed with rigid plate and screw fixation (absolute stability); (J) A simple pointed bone reduction forcep is utilized in order to achieve an anatomic reduction of the fracture; (K) Two 4.5 mm countersunk AO screws are placed using AO lag technique of overdrilling the near cortex; (L) A neutralization plate is placed along the tibia. Care is taken to ensure that this plate is perfectly contoured. Otherwise, cortical screws placed through it can cause displacement of the previously anatomically reduced fracture. Since this fracture has significant proximal extension, a long proximal tibial periarticular plate is chosen. Locked screws will be placed in the proximal fragment and cortical screws placed along the shaft. In this photo, guidewires for the locking screws are placed proximally to ensure that the screws will not be intra-articular and a temporary fixation device is used distally to ensure that the plate is properly contoured and placed on the bone; (M) Final fixation before wound closure; (N) Wound closure. The open fracture wound is incorporated into the extensile anterolateral surgical approach; (O) Postoperative AP and (P) lateral radiographs demonstrate good overall alignment and stable fixation.

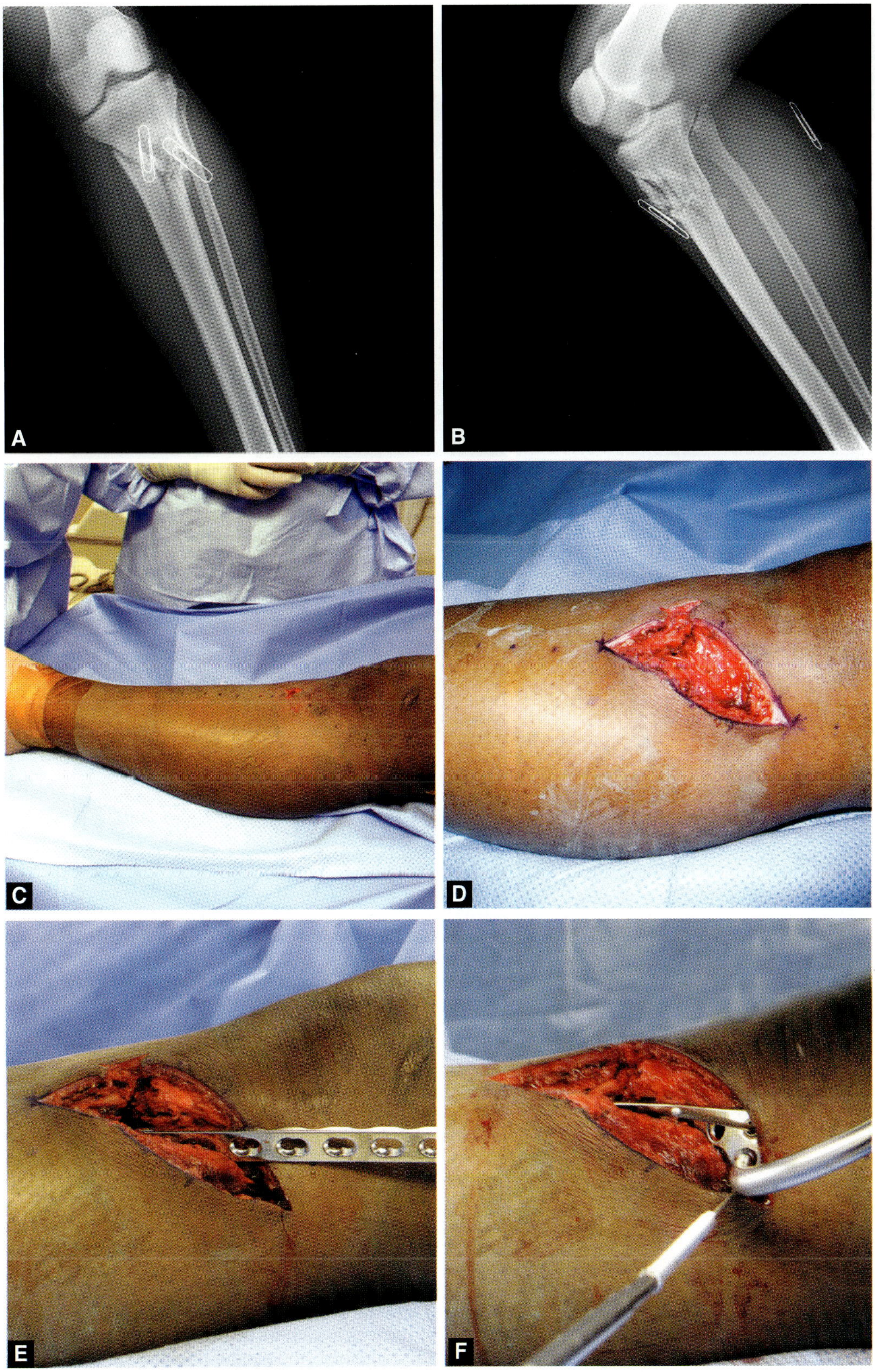

Figures 26.11A to F

after tibial nailing, although not all are clinically significant to the patient. Malalignments tend to be more common after any procedures involving indirect reduction, such as closed nailing or minimally invasive plate osteosynthesis (MIPO) of the tibia and are less common after direct reduction and plating. Malalignment has been discussed in the following section as well. Particular attention should be paid by the surgeon to angular and rotational alignment during and immediately postoperatively. Both clinical evaluation of the appearance of the limb as well as fluoroscopic and radiographic bony relationships should be used to avoid malalignment during surgery. At the end of the procedure, it should be checked again and compared with the contralateral limb while the patient is on the flat OR table under anesthesia. If malalignment is still missed at this point and diagnosed later, it is always better to correct a significant malalignment before the patient leaves the hospital rather than convincing oneself that it is okay only to end up dealing with it later. If a malunion occurs which is clinically significant, this may need to be treated surgically with osteotomy and fixation depending on the location and characteristics of the malunion.

Compartment syndrome is a devastating condition if missed and can lead to irreversible muscle death if emergent fasciotomy surgery is not performed. It can be difficult to prevent compartment syndrome as this condition usually occurs as part of the natural history of the injury sustained by the patient. Sustained hypotension, excessive elevation, and very tightly wrapped dressings should all be avoided as they may potentially precipitate a compartment syndrome in certain patients. The key is early diagnosis as described in the following section. Clinical examination should evaluate for this carefully and pressure measurements should be taken if necessary.

Authors' Preferred Management of Select Complications

Case 1: Treatment of an Acute Infection of the Tibia after Intramedullary Nailing

Acute or semiacute deep infection of the tibial diaphysis after IM nailing of the tibia is an unfortunate situation because the tibia has not yet healed and some form of stabilization is required in order to achieve union. The surgeon basically has to make a decision between removing the implants and going with external fixation or exchanging the nail. In both cases, the initial implants must be removed and debridement of the medullary canal must be performed. In addition, any obvious sequestrum from the fracture site must be debrided. If substantial bone is removed in this process, the entire situation may change and a new plan may have to be drawn up in order to account for the infection with bone loss (which in the authors' hands often means using a circular fixator with an antibiotic spacer and staged bone grafting or transport).

In this particular case, a 16-year-old male sustained a shotgun injury to the leg resulting in an open tibial fracture with vascular injury as shown in Figures 26.12A to N. He had been treated with vascular repair, external fixation and serial debridement, and eventual conversion to IM nailing with rotational flap coverage within 2 weeks of the initial injury. He developed a severe deep infection with gross purulence from the medial and lateral sides of the leg. The nail was not obviously visible from either wound. The tibia was accessible through the medial wound, but there was adequate muscle coverage over the tibia although there was a deep lateral wound as shown in Figures 26.12D and E. According to Cierney-Mader classification of osteomyelitis, this is a 1A (medullary infection in a normal host). This was treated by serial debridement, partial fibular resection, IV antibiotics, and negative pressure wound therapy before being transferred to the authors' institution. Debridement was repeated and no gross purulence or necrotic tissue was then seen. At this point, the patient had undergone five debridements over a 2-week period and the gross infection appeared under control. Cultures grew methicillin-resistant *Staphylococcus aureus* (MRSA). The authors typically exchange the initial implants for an antibiotic-impregnated cement nail spacer once gross purulence is under control. After 1–2 weeks, he exchanges this for a new locked IM nail as long as the infection still appears to be under control. Therefore, he planned for removal of this patient's IM nail with exchange for an antibiotic-impregnated cement nail spacer as shown in Figures 26.12F to J.

The locked nail is removed using standard techniques. The IM canal is then reamed 1–2 mm greater than the size of the removed IM nail. Bone cultures are taken. The canal is then irrigated clear and all debris is removed from the IM canal by either suction tubing in the canal or venting from a wound distally in the leg. If there is

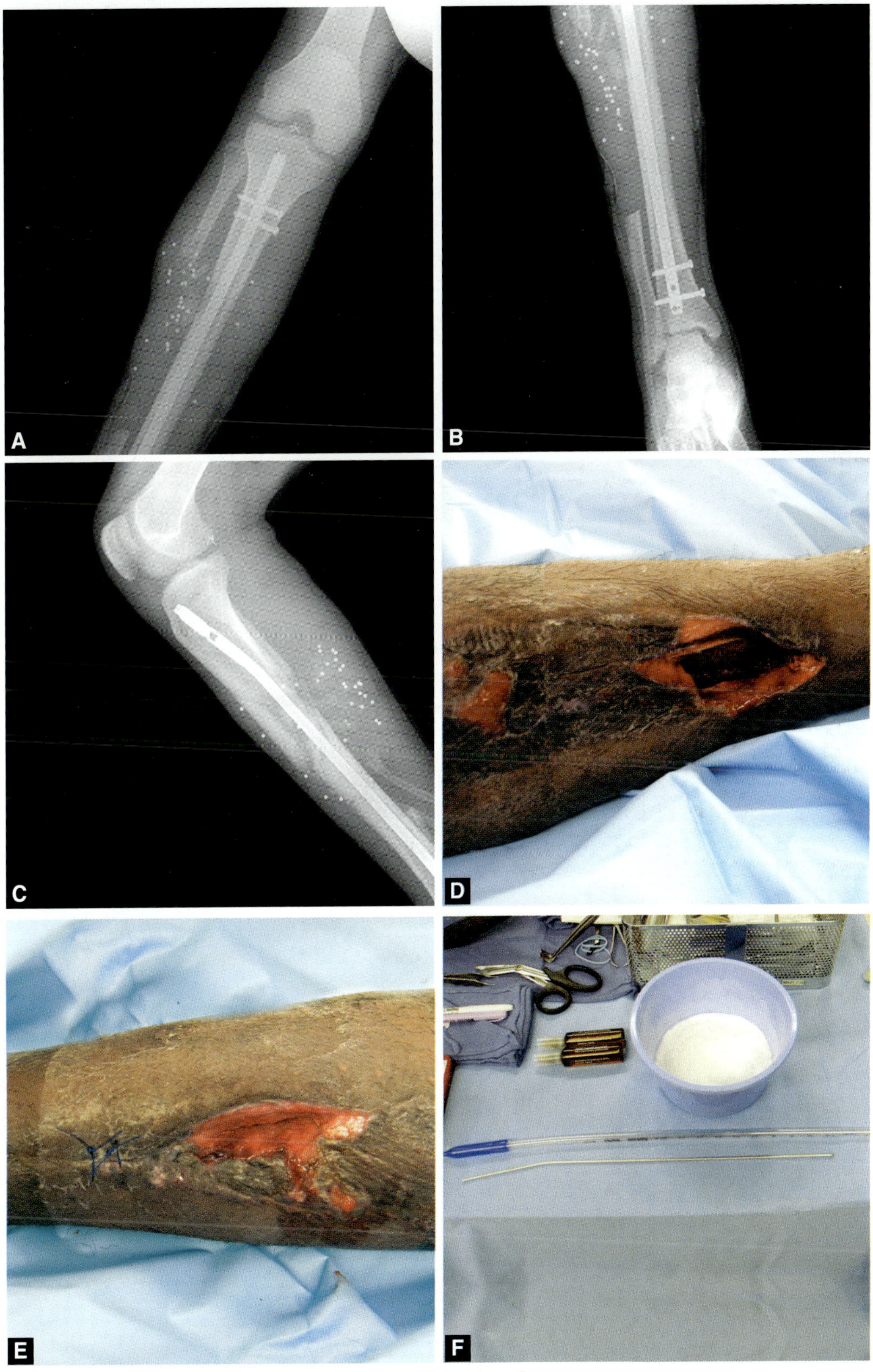

Figures 26.12A to F

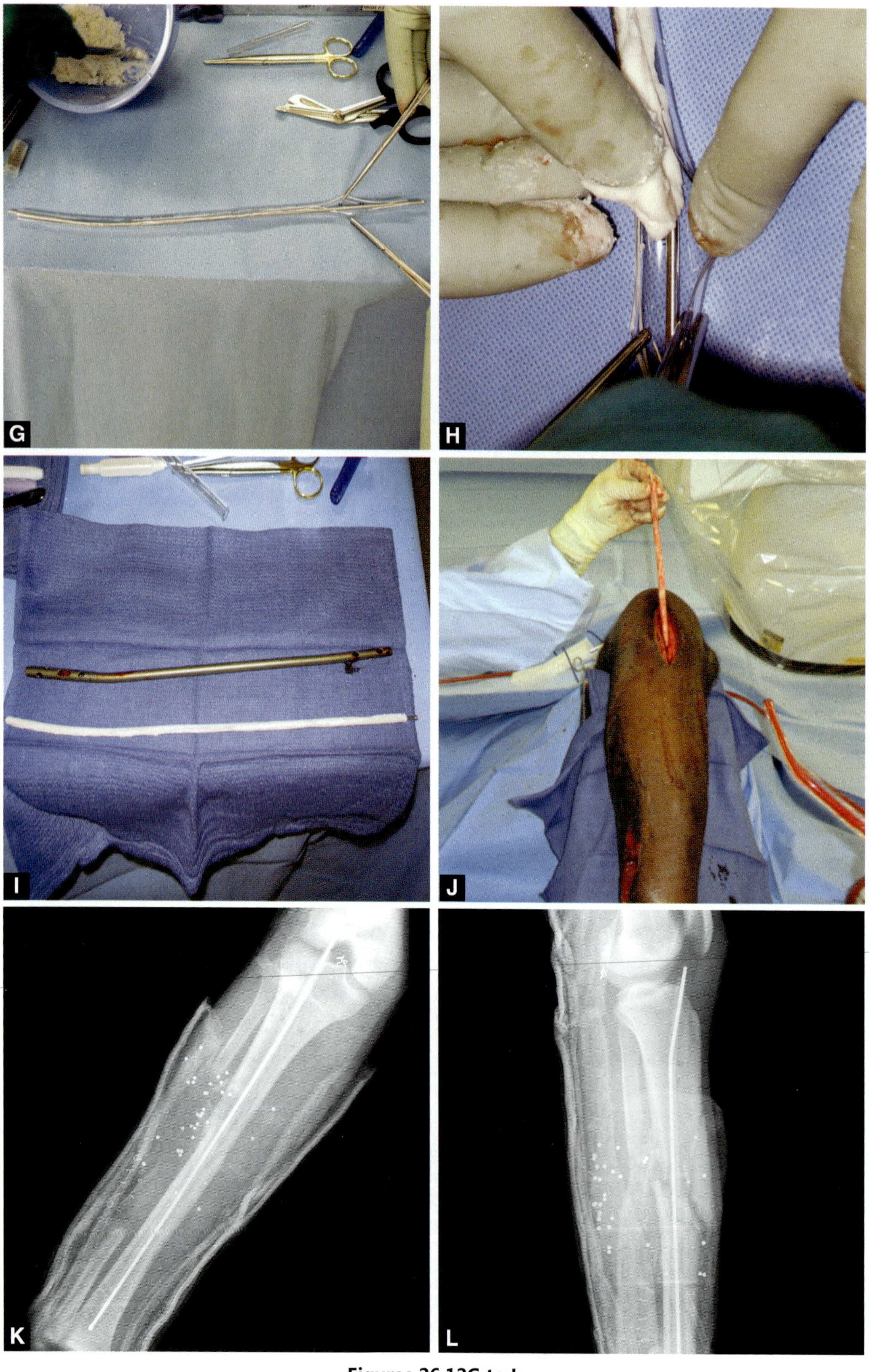

Figures 26.12G to L

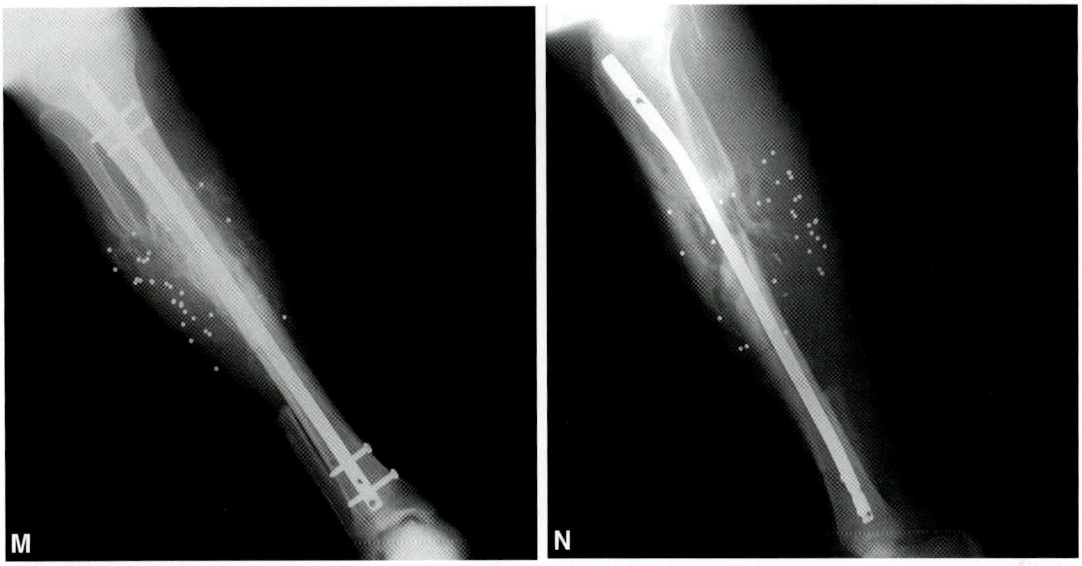

Figures 26.12A to N: Treatment of an acute infection of the tibia after intramedullary nailing. (A and B) Anteroposterior (AP) and (C) lateral images of the tibia after shotgun injury leading to vascular injury and open tibia fracture. See text for details; (D) Lateral and (E) medial wounds after serial debridement and negative pressure wound therapy; (F) The implants were removed, the canal was reamed and irrigated, and an antibiotic cement spacer nail was inserted. Two packets of PMMA cement and antibiotic powder are mixed. A ball-tipped guide rod is cut slightly longer than the explanted nail and the thoracostomy tube is cut slightly shorter than the guide rod. A slight proximal Herzog bend is also created in the guide rod; (G) The guide rod is placed inside the thoracostomy tube and the activator is added and mixed with the PMMA/antibiotic mixture. A longitudinal slit is cut in the thoracostomy tube as shown; (H) The antibiotic cement mixture is then finger packed into the tube over the guide rod. After the cement has cured, the tube is peeled away; (I) The final antibiotic cement spacer rod is shown next to the implanted rod; (J) The antibiotic cement spacer rod is then inserted gently into the tibia. If significant resistance is encountered, it should be removed and a burr can be used to narrow the diameter where needed to facilitate smooth passage; (K) AP and (L) lateral radiographs postoperatively with the antibiotic cement spacer nail in place. The tip of the guide rod is intentionally left slightly proud in order to facilitate later removal. A long leg splint is used for rotational control of the fracture and negative pressure wound therapy was resumed. After 1 week, exchange nailing for a new locked nail is performed; (M) AP and (N) lateral radiographs demonstrate interval fracture healing as well as abundant reactive bone formation. Although there has been no sign of recurrence of infection, the implants will require removal once the fracture has fully healed.

suspected sequestrum at the fracture site, this may need to be exposed and debrided as well. The reason for the antibiotic-impregnated cement nail spacer is two fold. It functions as a spacer to eliminate the dead space of the medullary canal. If the nail is removed and external fixation or casting is immediately performed, this dead space of the reamed canal can essentially fill with hematoma and is at high risk for redeveloping the deep infection. The second reason is that the spacer nail can deliver high doses of antibiotics directly to the site of the infection (the tibial medullary canal).

A 24 or 32 F-sized thoracostomy tube is used along with a ball-tipped IM guide rod and two 40 g packets of polymethylmethacrylate (PMMA) bone cement are utilized. It is important that the guidewire is ball tipped and a washer can also be placed at the distal end in order to prevent inadvertent retention of the cement upon attempted removal of the cement rod at a later date. 4.0 g of powdered vancomycin and 4.8 g of powdered tobramycin are added to the powdered PMMA and thoroughly mixed. The activator liquid is then added and the cement is hand-mixed. Because this mixture is typically much more viscous than bone cement without the antibiotics, the authors have found it difficult to inject this mixture and perform this by hand packing instead. The guide rod is given a slight proximal Herzog bend and cut slightly longer than the explanted nail. The chest tube is chosen which has an inner diameter at least 1 mm smaller than the explanted nail in order to prevent difficulty with later removal of the antibiotic cement spacer nail. The chest tube is cut slightly shorter than the guide rod and is placed over the guide rod. A longitudinal slit is made in the chest tube and the mixed cement is finger packed into the chest tube with care not to overstuff this (Figs 26.12H and I).

Once the cement has cured, the chest tube is removed and the nail is ready for insertion into the tibial canal (Figs 26.12J to L). The authors always make sure that there is minimal to no resistance to insertion of the nail. If significant resistance is encountered, this could signify a tight fit and could hamper later efforts to remove this nail. If the nail is tight upon later removal, the cement is at risk for dislodging from the guidewire. Since this nail is slightly longer than the explanted nail, it will sit proud as shown in Figures 26.12K and L which helps facilitate later removal of the nail. Since there is poor rotational control of the fracture, a long leg splint is still needed and negative pressure wound therapy is continued.

One week later, the patient was taken back to surgery for removal of the antibiotic cement spacer nail and reimplantation of a new locked tibial nail and the patient was discharged home 2 days later with per os antibiotics and negative pressure wound therapy by a visiting nurse. Repeat reaming was not performed and there was no sign of gross infection. Cultures were repeated and were found to be negative for infection at this time. At 2 months, his medial wound had closed and the lateral wound was nearly closed with no sign of infection. Antibiotics were taken per os for 6 weeks as per consultation with an infectious diseases specialist and radiographs showed some interval healing and reactive bone formation was as shown in Figures 26.12M and N. Once a patient has confirmed osteomyelitis, the authors will remove their implants once the fracture has healed, which is the plan for this patient.

The important principles of this case were as follows:

- The infection was classified according to Cierney-Mader. This was a 1A (medullary infection in a normal host) infection of the tibia. The authors believe that this helps the surgeon determine the course of action. A medullary infection unfortunately means that the entire canal will require debridement. But it also means that there are no localized areas of sequestrum requiring cortical debridement. Because the patient is a normal host, resolution of the infection is achievable with proper treatment.
- Recognize that simple serial debridements of the wounds and fibula helped to control the infection. Revision nailing was not performed in a grossly infected tibia or tissue bed.
- Although conversion to external fixation could have been done instead of nail exchange, excellent alignment and stability had been achieved with the IM nail initially. Therefore, it was desirable to continue with this method of fixation if possible. However, a temporary antibiotic cement nail was required both for stabilization as well as for dead space management and high-dose local antibiotic delivery.
- Do not think that the infection is completely eradicated even though there is no obvious sign of infection. Once the fracture is healed and satisfactorily remodeled, the implants should be removed before waiting for infection to recur.

Alternative treatments could have involved retention of the implants from the beginning, conversion to external fixation instead of exchange nailing, or one stage exchange nailing instead of using the interim antibiotic cement nail. In the authors' opinion, IM nailing had provided excellent alignment and stability and he felt that the infection in this case could be well controlled. In the absence of significant bone loss, it did not seem that external fixation would be necessary. Retention of the implants without any exchange could have been attempted but would not allow for proper debridement of the medullary osteomyelitis. One step exchange nailing is a good option and would allow improved rotational stability over the antibiotic cement nail, but does have the additional risk of infection recurrence and does not provide the high doses of local antibiotic delivery afforded by the antibiotic cement nail.

Case 2: Treatment of an Established Infected Nonunion of the Tibia

An infected nonunion of the tibia with established chronic osteomyelitis involves surgical debridement of all infected and dead bone and either bone grafting or distraction osteogenesis (Ilizarov method) to reconstitute the defect. The difference between these cases and the acute infection as shown in Case 1 is that in the acute case, the bone is usually not necrotic and sclerotic unless completely devitalized fragments in an open fracture were left in place after attempted debridement. In the chronic case, the authors generally use imaging to help identify the most likely extent of infection and the sequestrum itself. In most instances, the sequestrum is quite difficult to identify with imaging. The CT scanning is helpful in identifying sinus tracts and seeing what part of the fracture is healed versus nonunion. The MRI is helpful in identifying fluid collections, such as IM extension. Nuclear scanning can help identify infection in equivocal cases and can help in determining the general extent of the infection. However, biopsy and bone cultures are required to establish the diagnosis. Furthermore, despite all the imaging studies, direct intraoperative visualization of the bone to look for punctate bleeding and absence of sclerosis and obviously necrotic bone is the only way to truly identify the extent of bone infection.

Once the authors have made a diagnosis of chronic osteomyelitis and nonunion of the tibia (infected nonunion), it usually means that surgical treatment will be indicated. Whereas waiting and seeing if callus will form sometimes works out, this method cannot be relied upon. Furthermore, in cases in which there is gross purulence and substantial drainage, surgical debridement is clearly indicated. The only way to cure a patient of chronic osteomyelitis is through aggressive resection. The problem is that this can lead to a critical sized defect that may not heal without bone grafting. As mentioned above, this may also require other methods of bone reconstruction, such as distraction osteogenesis or free vascularized bone transfer. The authors' preference in smaller defects is to perform bone grafting once the infection is under control and to perform resection and distraction osteogenesis (bone transport) in larger defects greater than 3 cm.

Two cases will be briefly described here. In the first case, only a small defect resulted from debridement and exchange nailing with delayed bone grafting was performed. In the second case, substantial debridement was required resulting in a large defect, which was treated with Ilizarov method of distraction osteogenesis by bone transport.

The first case involved a 45-year-old male who had sustained a closed tibial shaft fracture, which was treated with IM nailing (Figs 26.13A to L). Four months after tibial nailing, partial union was noted posteriorly but a moderate gap anteriorly did not heal (Figs 26.13A and B). Furthermore, purulent drainage occurred from the fracture site at this point confirming infection. At this point, incision and drainage of the infection was performed, cultures were taken, and antibiotics were administered as per the recommendation of an infectious diseases consultant. The IM nail and screws were removed, the canal was reamed, and the fracture site was debrided. Careful bone debridement was performed in order to remove all sclerotic bone down to healthy bone with punctate bleeding. After a second debridement 3 days later, an antibiotic cement spacer was placed as shown in Figures 26.12K to M in the previous case and shown in Figures 26.13C and D. At this point, the acute infection was under control and the

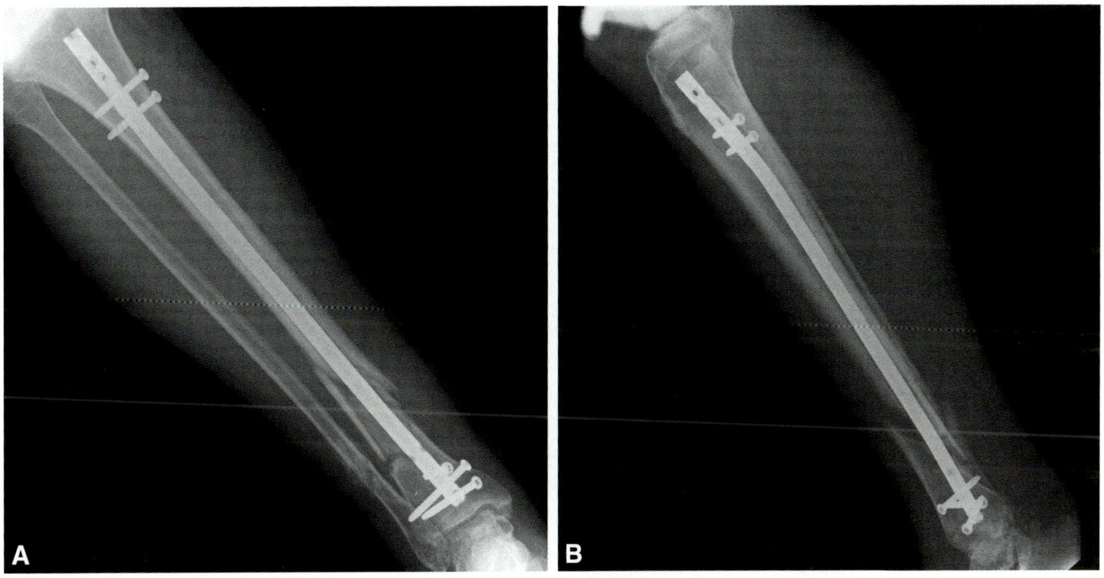

Figures 26.13A and B

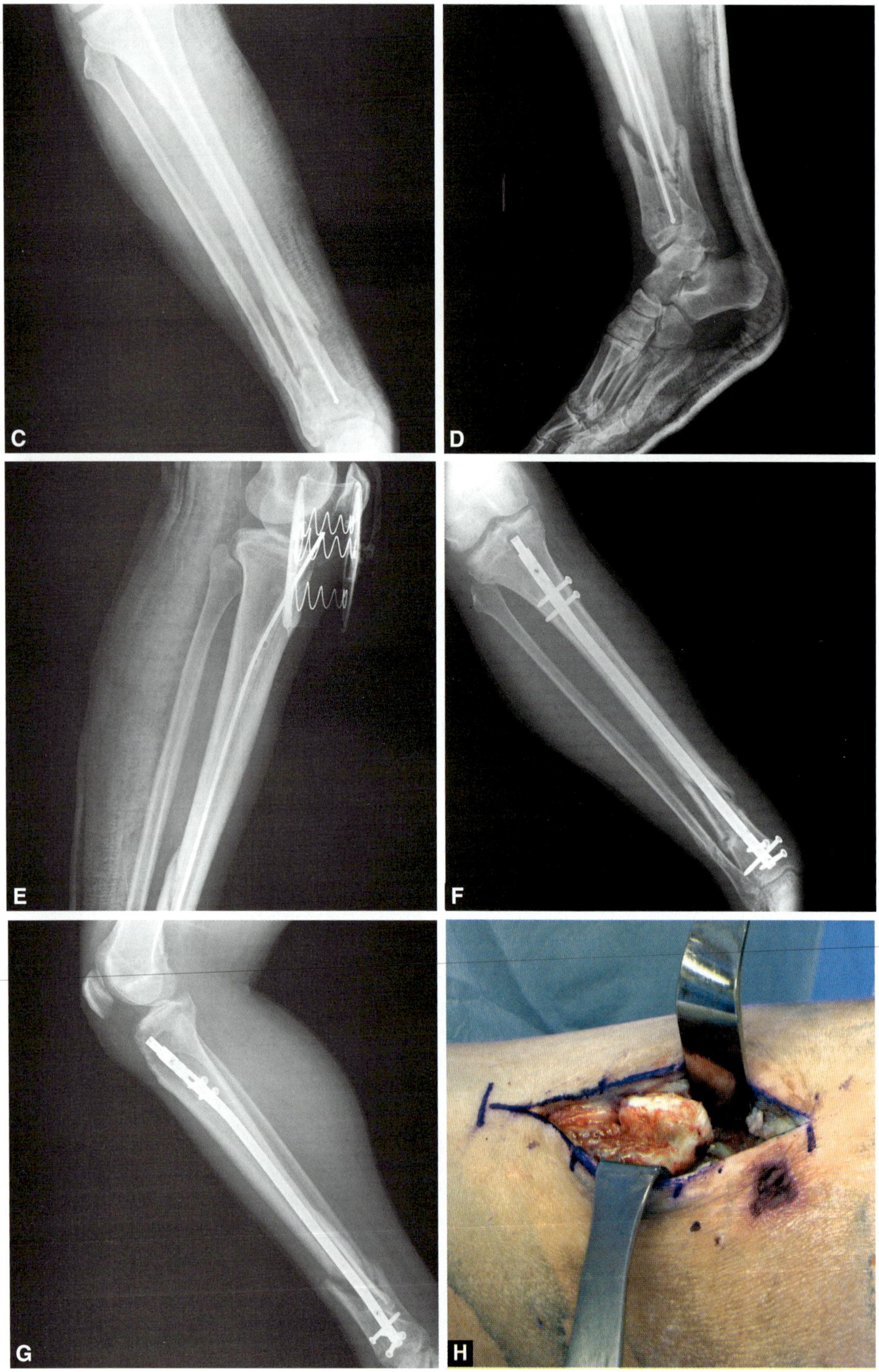

Figures 26.13C to H

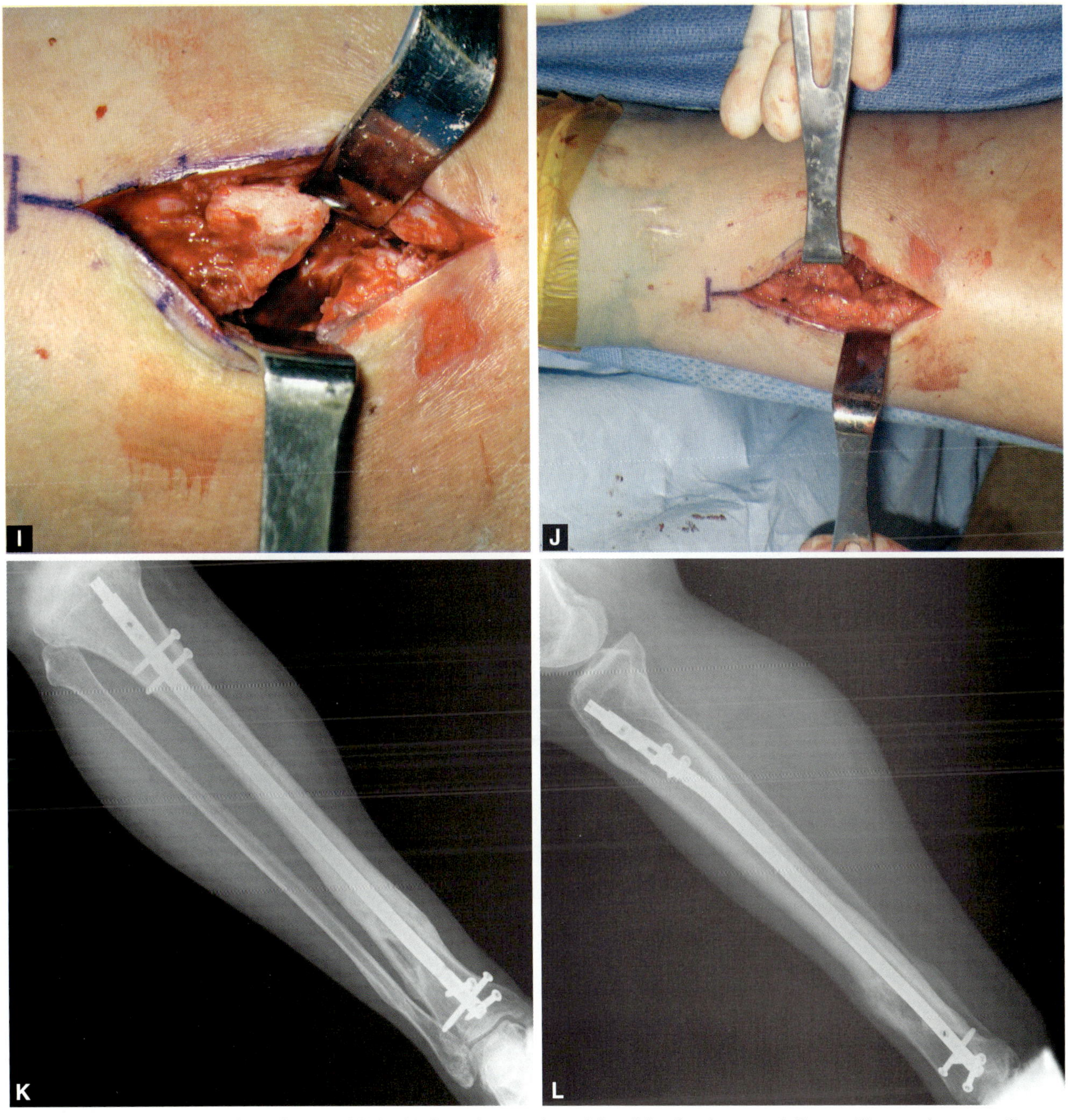

Figures 26.13A to L: Treatment of an established infected nonunion of the tibia after intramedullary nailing: exchange nailing and delayed bone grafting. (A) anteroposterior (AP) and (B) lateral radiographs taken 4 months after intramedullary nailing of a closed tibia fracture in a highway construction worker. A persistent gap anteriorly was noted and there was no obvious fracture bridging at the other cortices. Onset of purulent drainage and cellulitis at the fracture site indicated osteomyelitis. See text for details. After drainage was performed and antibiotics were given, the patient was brought back to the operation room for implant removal and reaming with irrigation of the canal followed by; (C to E) implantation of an antibiotic cement spacer nail with a suction drain at the fracture site. After continued administration of oral antibiotics, the spacer nail was exchanged for a locked nail after 2 weeks as shown on; (F) AP and (G) lateral images. Cultures remained negative at this time. Despite the lack of recurrence of infection, nonunion persisted anteriorly; (H) An anterior approach is made with careful debridement of all fibrous tissue until (I) punctate bleeding bone is seen; (J) Autogenous iliac crest bone graft is then placed in addition to bone morphogenetic protein (BMP)-2; (K and L) AP and lateral images with healing of the nonunion. The patient has returned to full time work duties.

patient was discharged with oral antibiotics. After 2 weeks, the antibiotic cement nail was removed and exchanged for another locked IM nail as shown in Figures 26.13E to G.

An antibiotic spacer block could have been placed, but the defect was relatively small and the tibia was healing posteriorly. Therefore, the spacer block was not placed. Antibiotics were administered per os for a total of 6 weeks and radiographic and clinical follow-up was performed. There was no evidence of bone healing anteriorly at 8 weeks, at which time the authors decided to proceed with bone grafting. The patient delayed this procedure until 20 weeks due to personal reasons during which time an electric bone stimulator device was used. This, however, did not lead to union of the fracture and he agreed to proceed with bone grafting.

The fracture site was exposed anteriorly and all fibrous tissue was sharply debrided as shown in Figures 26.13H to J. Punctate bleeding at the fracture ends was noted and autogenous iliac crest bone graft was harvested and packed at the nonunion site. Recombinant human bone morphogenetic protein-2 (rH BMP-2) (Infuse) was also used as a bone graft at the nonunion site. There was no sign of infection at the time of surgery. A surgical drain was placed at the iliac crest harvest site and weight bearing was allowed at 3 weeks postoperatively. His pain eventually improved and he returned to work full time as a highway repair laborer (Figs 26.13K and L). His radiographs at most recent follow-up demonstrate near complete union of the fracture. Once his fracture is fully healed and remodeled satisfactorily, his implants will be removed.

In the second case, a 28-year-old man with an open tibial fracture and multiple other injuries from a motorcycle crash was treated with irrigation and debridement and external fixation. This was converted to IM nailing after 1 week. He went on to heal his other injuries including an associated both column acetabulum fracture but his tibia fracture went on to develop a chronic infected nonunion with a draining sinus (Figs 26.14A to H). This was initially treated unsuccessfully with removal of the IM nail and exchange nailing. Therefore, the implants were removed and weight bearing in a custom-fitted fracture brace was allowed which also failed. Therefore, radical resection of all the necrotic bone and all marginal appearing bone was performed as shown in Figure 26.14D along with reaming of the tibial canal. An Ilizarov circular frame was applied and a proximal corticotomy was performed after the infection was controlled and purulent drainage had stopped. An antibiotic spacer block was placed at the defect and after a latency period of 7 days, bone transport was commenced at the rate of 1 mm per day in 0.25 mm increments as is typically done for the adult tibia. Once the defect became smaller, the spacer block was removed and bone transport was continued. Once docking was performed, autogenous bone grafting was performed at the docking site. Regenerate bone formed proximally and the docking site eventually healed at 8 months. The external fixator was eventually removed at 18 months as shown in Figure 26.14H. Over the course of his treatment, multiple procedures were required in all which include the above procedures in addition to treatment of pin tract infections, superficial wound infections and loose pins.

The important principles of these cases are as follows:

- Chronic osteomyelitis cannot be effectively treated without resection of all of the infected bone. In cases in which there has been no bone healing and a significant amount of infected or dead sclerotic bone appears to be present, radical resection may be required to effectively remove this. If a nail is present, this may need to be removed and Ilizarov methods can be employed in order to reconsitute the bone defect.
- Cases in which the sequestrum is very small and the infection is mostly a medullary type (by Cierney-Mader classification) can be treated with medullary reaming, local debridement of the fracture site and bone grafting. If an IM nail is in place, this can be exchanged for an antibiotic spacer nail and then exchange nailing with subsequent bone grafting.
- A prolonged treatment course can be expected in order to eradicate the infection and achieve bony union. The patient should be prepared for this and understand what is involved. Ilizarov methods of bone transport cannot be done in patients who cannot tolerate external fixation pins. They must be able to advance the distractor four times a day and be able to care for pin sites successfully. Most of all, you need a

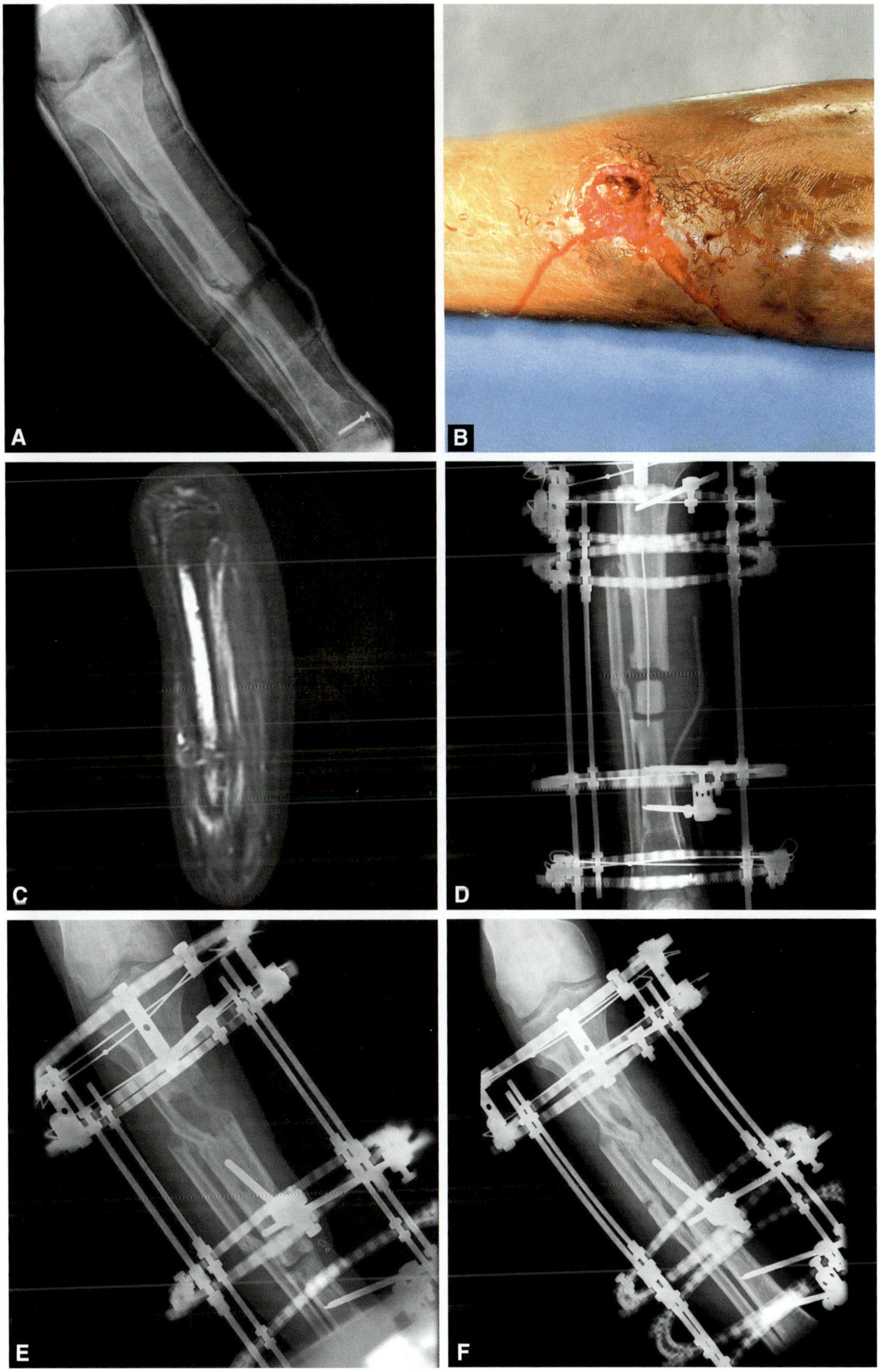

Figures 26.14A to F

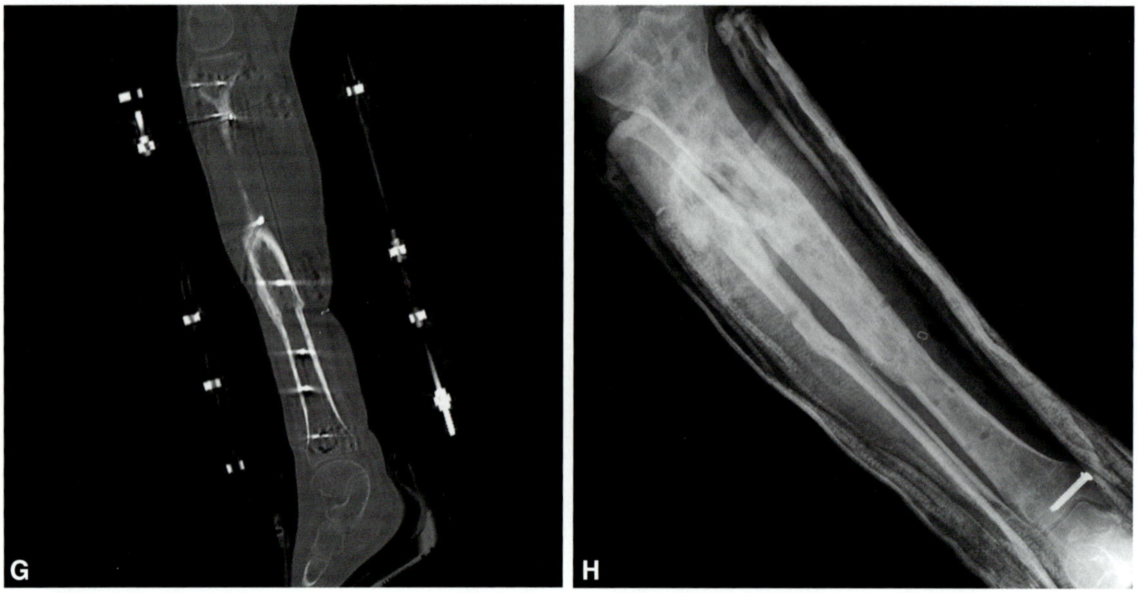

Figures 26.14A to H: Treatment of an established infected nonunion of the tibia after intramedullary nailing and failed exchange nailing: radical resection and Ilizarov bone transport. (A) Anteroposterior (AP) radiograph of infected nonunion of the tibia. Initially an open tibial fracture treated with external fixation staged to an intramedullary nail, this developed a recalcitrant chronic infection. Exchange nailing was unsuccessful. Removal of implants, casting and local wound care and antibiotic cement bead treatment failed; (B) Purulent drainage persisted from the nonunion site; (C) MRI imaging demonstrated a fluid collection throughout the intramedullary canal; (D) After radical debridement and control of the infection as described in the text, a Ilizarov bone transport frame and a new antibiotic spacer block was placed as shown. A proximal corticotomy was then performed and bone transport was performed as described in the text for this 6 cm defect; (E) The transport segment is shown docked but without union at 6 months after initial placement of the frame. Some early regenerate bone is seen proximally. Bone grafting is performed at the docking site; (F) Union is achieved at the docking site with regenerate bone proximally at 14 months after initial fixator placement as shown on radiograph and; (G) CT scan image; (H) The frame is removed at 18 months after initial placement with union without sign of infection.

patient with the patience to tolerate being in a frame for up to an year or longer. Unfortunately, many patients do not fit these criteria and this treatment should not be performed on them.

In patients who are type C hosts (e.g. severe peripheral vascular disease, uncontrolled diabetes mellitus, etc.) recalcitrant infection in which acute flare-ups with cellulitis and fevers occur might need to be treated with amputation and prosthetic fitting in select cases. As opposed to chronic osteomyelitis without fracture or in a healed fracture, the chronic infected nonunion is difficult to treat with antibiotic suppression alone in the type C host. The mechanical instability usually does not allow functional use of the limb despite the fact that the draining sinus may be tolerated by the patient.

Case 3: Treatment of an Aseptic, Atrophic Nonunion of the Tibia

Open fractures, lack of cortical contact and fracture gapping and avascularity are implicated as risk factors for aseptic nonunion of the tibia. Diagnosing the nonunion is typically easy. The patient has persistent pain at the fracture site along with tenderness and radiographs show the fracture line to still be visible without callus formation. The atrophic nonunion has smooth fracture ends due to resorption but without any presence of fracture healing. If in doubt, a CT scan can help demonstrate the nonunion. What is more difficult is determining if there is an infection when there are no obvious local signs of infection such as drainage, redness, swelling or fevers. In these cases, the surgeon typically initiates a workup consisting of blood tests and imaging studies. Blood tests include a C-reactive protein (CRP) and a complete blood count with differential. If there is any reason to suspect an endocrinologic etiology of the nonunion, then vitamin D levels and other serologic workup can help to reveal treatable risk factors for nonunion that have been recently described.[16] Imaging studies include white blood cell-labeled nuclear scanning and possibly MRI imaging if implants are compatible with the scanner. Unfortunately, these tests even in combination are often not helpful in clearly ruling out the presence of a chronic indolent osteomyelitis. Therefore, in equivocal cases, a bone biopsy and culture (or polymerase chain reaction analysis if available) is performed before performing definitive nonunion repair.

In this particular case, a 35-year-old male construction worker sustained a fall from a height on the job, sustaining a closed tibial diaphyseal fracture which was treated with IM nailing. He went on to develop an atrophic painful nonunion and was referred to us for definitive management (Figs 26.15A to H). Laboratory workup demonstrated an elevated CRP but his complete blood count was normal and nuclear imaging did not suggest an obvious osteomyelitis. The authors interpreted these studies as being overall equivocal, so he proceeded with biopsy and culture of the tibia. Since he was going to need a nonunion repair in either case (although the method of repair could differ whether or not infection is present), he decided to proceed with implant removal and biopsy and culture of the tibia. Since the patient's CRP was elevated, he did not rely on an intraoperative gram stain or a pathologist's microscopic count of nucleated cells per high power field but rather relied on formal microbiological cultures. This would take 5 days to have a final result, so the patient was informed that this would be a staged procedure with return to the OR after 2 weeks. He would return to the office after 1 week for culture results and an operative plan would be made at that time and he was scheduled for nonunion repair the following week.

The patient was taken to the OR, the implants were removed and there was no sign of gross infection. A small incision was made over the fracture site and bone trephines were used to retrieve small bone plugs for culture. The canal was also reamed 1 mm over the size of the nail and reamings were also sent for cultures. Rather than risk hematoma formation in the canal (particularly in this patient who was being treated with anticoagulation for a venous thrombosis) with subsequent risk for colonization and infection of the hematoma, an antibiotic spacer nail was placed (Figs 26.15C and D). Cultures were negative for bacterial growth and he was brought back to the OR after 2 weeks for removal of the nail and nonunion repair with compression plating and autogenous iliac crest bone grafting. Cultures taken at this time were also negative for bacterial growth. An anterolateral approach was utilized and the fracture nonunion was exposed and fibrous tissue was carefully excised. Periosteum was preserved except along the fracture lines. Curettes were used and a high speed burr was used only when needed with frequent saline cooling to prevent thermal osteonecrosis. Bone grafting was then packed at the nonunion site as well. This went onto uneventful healing and the patient returned to work although not in heavy labor.

The important principles of this case are as follows:

- Infection needs to be ruled out in any case of atrophic nonunion.
- Compression should be performed with adjunctive bone graft whenever possible rather than relying only on bone graft to heal defects. In atrophic nonunions, the authors always perform either autogenous grafting or an equivalent osteoinductive graft material, such as concentrated stem cells or BMP-2. Allograft cancellous bone or osteoconductive bone graft substitutes alone should not be used in atrophic nonunions except as graft "extenders". Compression is best achieved with plate fixation but can be performed in a limited fashion with certain IM nails.
- Care should be taken not to excessively strip periosteum or cause bone necrosis (e.g. by indiscriminate use of the high speed burr) in the course of a nonunion repair.

Case 4: Treatment of Hypertrophic Nonunion of the Tibia

A hypertrophic nonunion of the tibia indicates that excessive motion at the fracture site is not allowing callus to properly bridge the gap. Callus is seen and an "elephant foot" appearance on radiographs is diagnostic

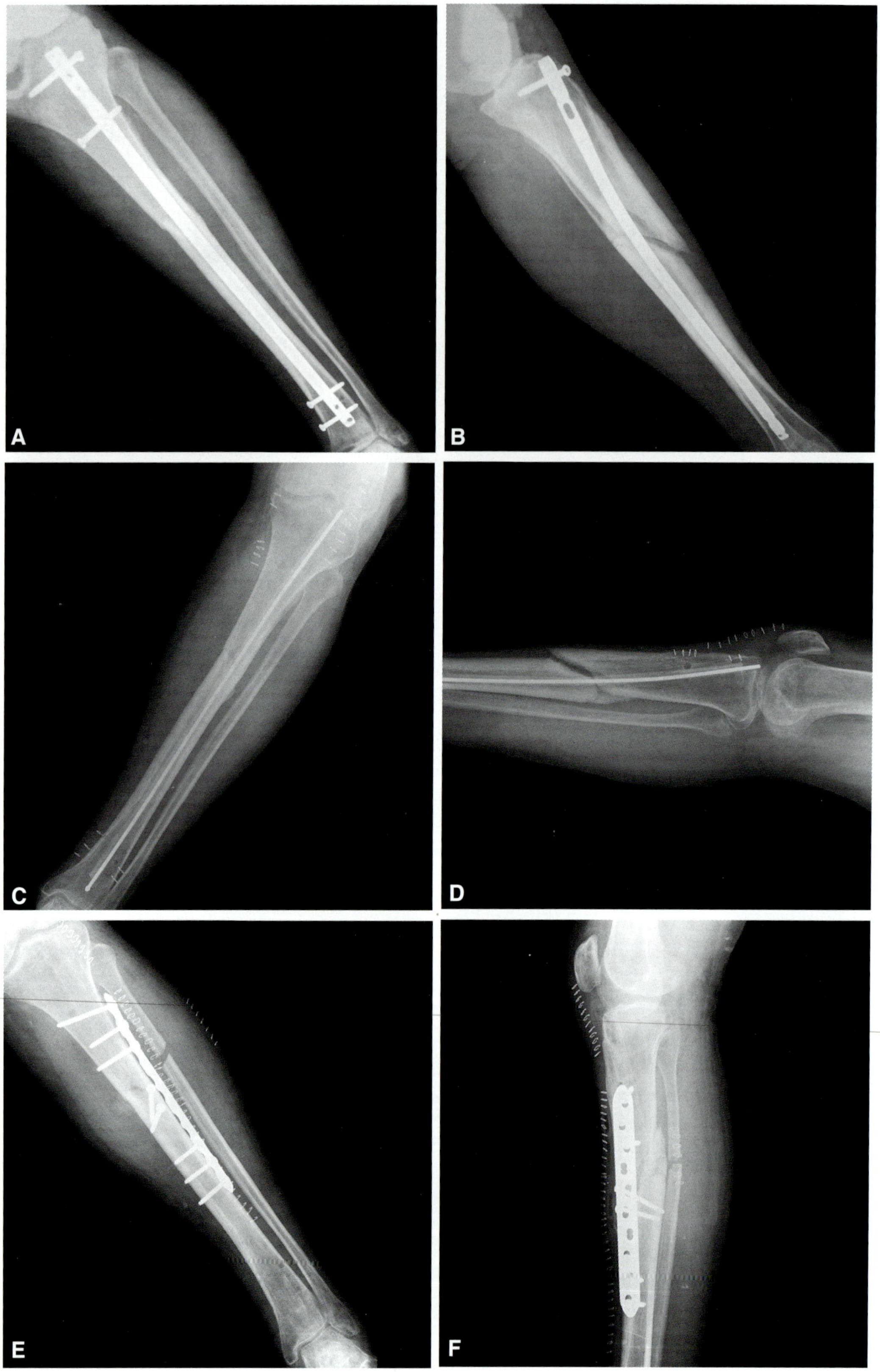

Figures 26.15A to F

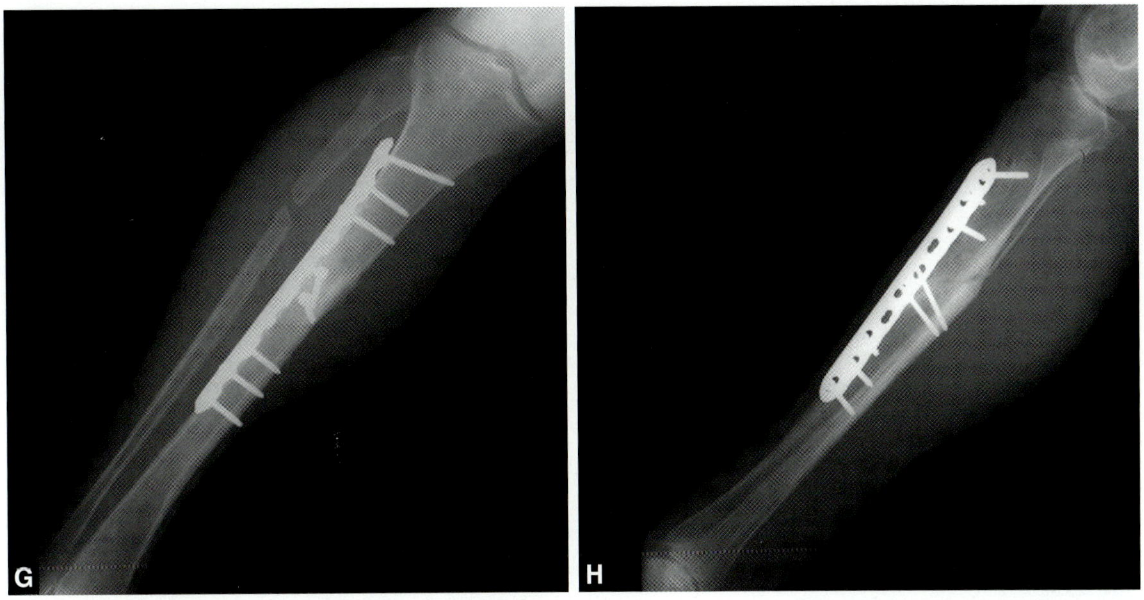

Figures 26.15A to H: Treatment of an aseptic, atrophic nonunion of the tibia: removal of nail and compression plating with autogenous bone graft. (A) Anteroposterior (AP) and (B) lateral images of atrophic nonunion of the tibia; (C) Due to an elevated C-reactive protein and some suspicion for possible infection, implants were removed, cultures were taken, and an antibiotic spacer nail was placed as shown in AP and (D) lateral images; (E) Cultures were negative for infection and the spacer nail was removed and compression plating with autogenous iliac crest bone graft was placed as shown on AP and (F) lateral images; (G) AP and (H) lateral images demonstrating union of the fracture.

of the hypertrophic nonunion. If the authors make this diagnosis radiographically, his treatment plan depends mainly on the time since the injury. For the tibial shaft, he generally will not perform revision surgery for this until at least 6 months which has been supported by the SPRINT study.[17] If a patient is having pain at the fracture site and an obvious hypertrophic appearance of callus is seen without fracture healing, the authors usually initiate activity modification. This often just means telling the patient to "take it easy" and try to limit the amount of ambulation they are doing or using a cane to limit weight bearing on the affected limb. If it is beyond 6 months and simple rest is not sufficient to allow the fracture to heal, he considers nonunion repair. As opposed to atrophic nonunions, bone grafting of the nonunion site is generally not required and treatment is based on providing improved stability of the fracture. If there is a nail in place, this can be exchanged for a larger reamed nail. If the fracture was treated nonoperatively, surgical stabilization with compression plating, nailing or external fixation can be performed.

This particular case is that of a 65-year-old gentleman whose occupation involves light labor and he suffered from a proximal third tibial nonunion (Figs 26.16A to C). He had been initially treated nonoperatively but continued to have pain and difficulties ambulating. On examination, there were no open wounds or mechanical instability, although there was some tenderness at the fracture site. Radiographs demonstrated a hypertrophic nonunion with a classic elephant foot appearance. This had been troubling him for nearly 1 year and he had already been treated with conservative management consisting of immobilization and rest which had failed. Therefore, he was indicated for nonunion repair with compression lateral plating. Since the fracture was relatively proximal, an anterolateral approach was utilized and the anterior compartment muscles were carefully elevated off of the proximal tibia. The fracture site itself was not disturbed or mobilized, but a small fibular segment resection was performed in order to allow compression of the tibia. The locking periarticular plate was then applied laterally and locked screws were placed proximally. The AO articulating tensioning device (push-pull device) was then applied to the distal end of the plate and compression was performed. Cortical screws were then applied distally and one lag screw was placed across the fracture for

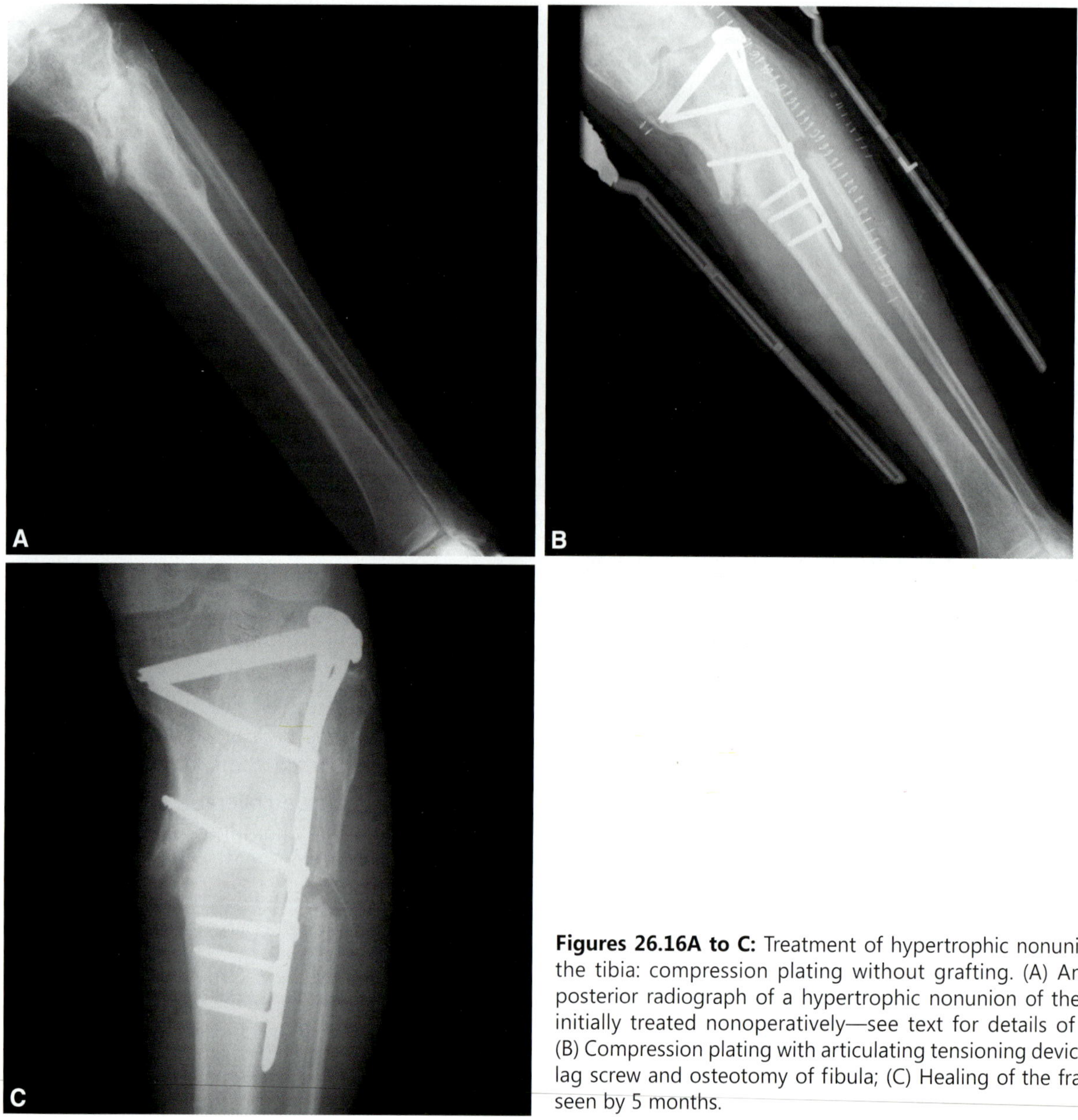

Figures 26.16A to C: Treatment of hypertrophic nonunion of the tibia: compression plating without grafting. (A) Anteroposterior radiograph of a hypertrophic nonunion of the tibia initially treated nonoperatively—see text for details of case; (B) Compression plating with articulating tensioning device and lag screw and osteotomy of fibula; (C) Healing of the fracture seen by 5 months.

additional compression. This patient went on to heal and returned to his usual occupation without further complication.

The important principles of this case are as follows:

- Hypertrophic nonunions are simply treated by increasing the stability and/or reducing the stresses across the fracture site. This can be accomplished by rest, immobilization, providing fixation or increasing the strength of the fixation if it had already been done.
- The fracture site is typically left undisturbed in hypertrophic nonunion surgery.
- If treated properly, hypertrophic nonunions can be expected to heal more reliably than atrophic nonunions.

Case 5: Treatment of Acute Tibial Bone Loss with Massive Autogenous Bone Grafting

Bone loss is usually the result of severe open fractures of the tibia and subsequent debridement and not necessarily is considered a complication. Bone loss can also be the result of debridements of the tibia due to infection. It is often accompanied by soft tissue loss and therefore skeletal reconstruction is performed either in conjunction with a plastic surgeon or by an orthopedic surgeon alone who is skilled in plastic surgical reconstructive methods in the lower extremity. Soft tissue reconstructive methods can include simple measures such as local tissue transfer or stretching or more complex techniques such as free tissue transfer. One must be careful not to move too slowly up the "reconstructive ladder" and risk infection due to a failed local rotational flap when a free flap was really necessary.

This case involves a 40-year-old male who was struck by a car sustaining a grade 3B open tibia fracture which was treated with irrigation and debridement and external fixation (Figs 26.17A to O). He returned to the OR for serial debridements, antibiotic bead placement and exchanges, and negative pressure wound therapy. Aggressive bony debridement of devitalized bone fragment was performed in order to minimize the chances of infection. At this point his tibial bone defect measured 4.5 cm. On hospital day 11, he underwent removal of the external fixator, IM nailing of the tibia and syndesmotic repair, and placement of an antibiotic spacer block consisting of PMMA with tobramycin and vancomycin as described in Case 1 into the defect. Instead of making beads, a shaped block is placed into the defect to provide antibiotic treatment, fill dead space, prevent ingrowth of fibrous tissue and create a membrane which can host mesenchymal stem cells as described by Masquelet.[10] After fixation and spacer block placement was done, a latissimus dorsi free flap was performed by our plastic surgical consultant.

Six weeks after free flap coverage, the patient was brought back to the OR for elevation of the flap, removal of the antibiotic spacer and autogenous bone grafting with medullary bone harvested from the ipsilateral femur. The membrane surrounding the spacer block was left in place. An alternative to iliac crest bone grafting, the femoral canal is a site for harvest of autologous graft which can often be obtained in abundance and was appropriate for this patient's 4.5 cm defect. The Reamer Irrigator Aspirator (RIA–Synthes, Paoli, PA) is a useful device for obtaining graft in this manner. The patient was placed in the supine position with a rolled blanket under the ipsilateral buttock and the piriformis starting point was utilized as in femoral nailing (trochanteric entry portal can also be used). The initial guidewire and opening reamer was utilized first to open the canal. This was followed by placement of the ball-tipped guidewire and insertion of the oversized, extremely sharp reamer which was attached to a suction device. As reaming was performed, IM bone was harvested and suctioned into a canister with a filter. The guidewire can be directed into the medial or lateral condyle of the distal femur in order to obtain additional bone graft. After the graft was harvested, it was packed into the bone defect in the center of which was the IM nail. The flap was inset back in place and the wound was closed. The bone graft went on to consolidate and the fracture healed 6 months later and the free flap eventually assumed a more cosmetically aesthetic appearance.

The important principles of this case are as follows:

- Aggressive bone debridement in grade 3 open tibia fractures is required to prevent deep infection.
- External fixation can be performed on initial presentation, but conversion to IM nailing should be performed within 2 weeks if possible in order to prevent canal colonization and infection from the Shanz pins.
- Definitive soft tissue coverage should also be performed within 1–2 weeks in order to prevent colonization and infection.
- Antibiotic cement PMMA beads can be successfully used initially, but an antibiotic spacer block is better after flap coverage is performed as an interim step before bone grafting.
- If sufficient autologous bone graft cannot be obtained, Ilizarov methods as described in Figure 26.14 above can be utilized to reconstruct the bone defect via distraction osteogenesis.

Case 6: Treatment of Compartment Syndrome of the Leg

Compartment syndrome of the leg is now a well recognized condition which when diagnosed is treated with immediate fasciotomy of the compartments. Increased intracompartmental pressure can be due to fractures, ischemia, crush injury and reperfusion injury. A compartment syndrome occurs when the pressure increases to the point of causing tissue ischemia, which

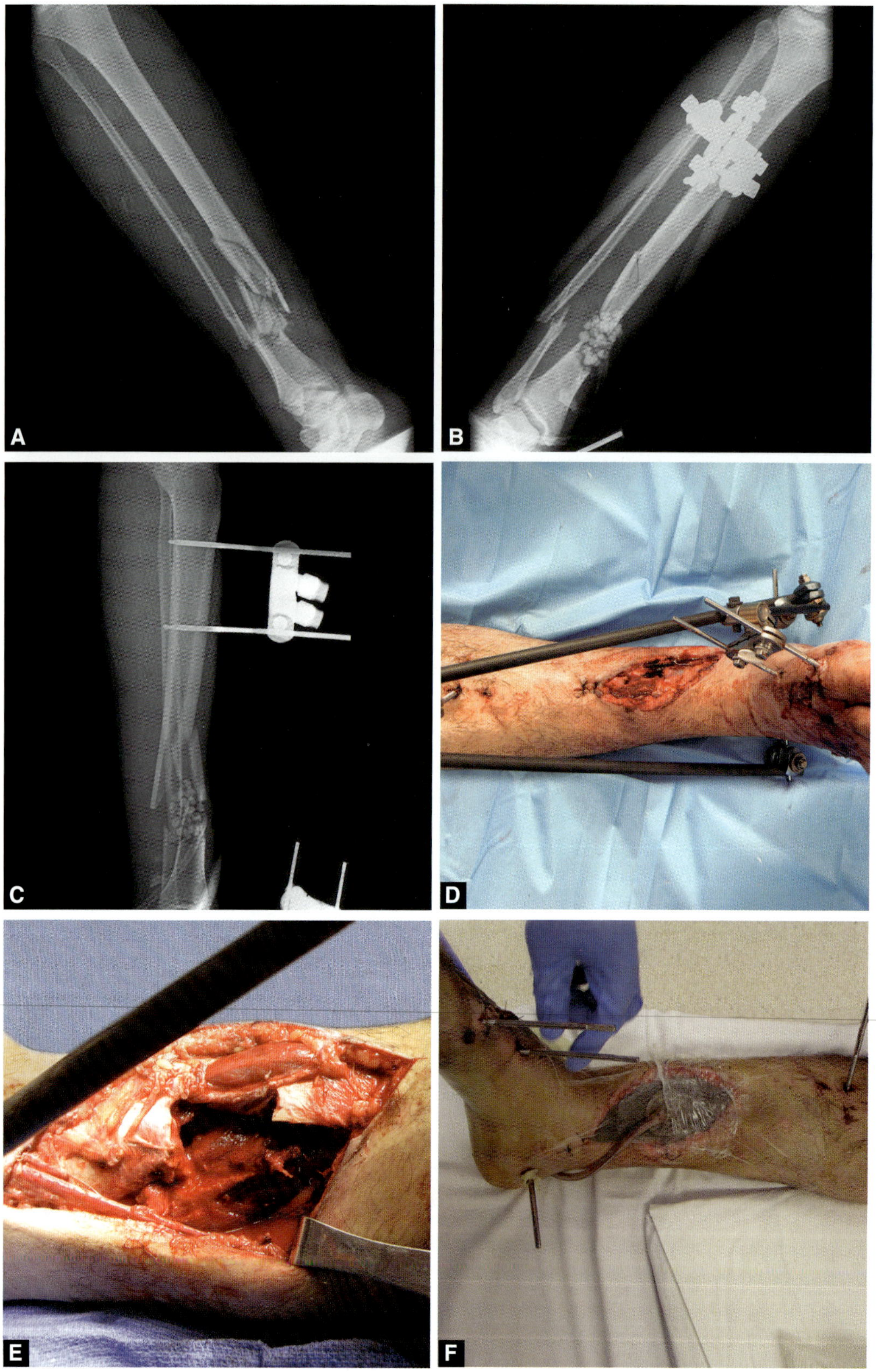

Figures 26.17A to F

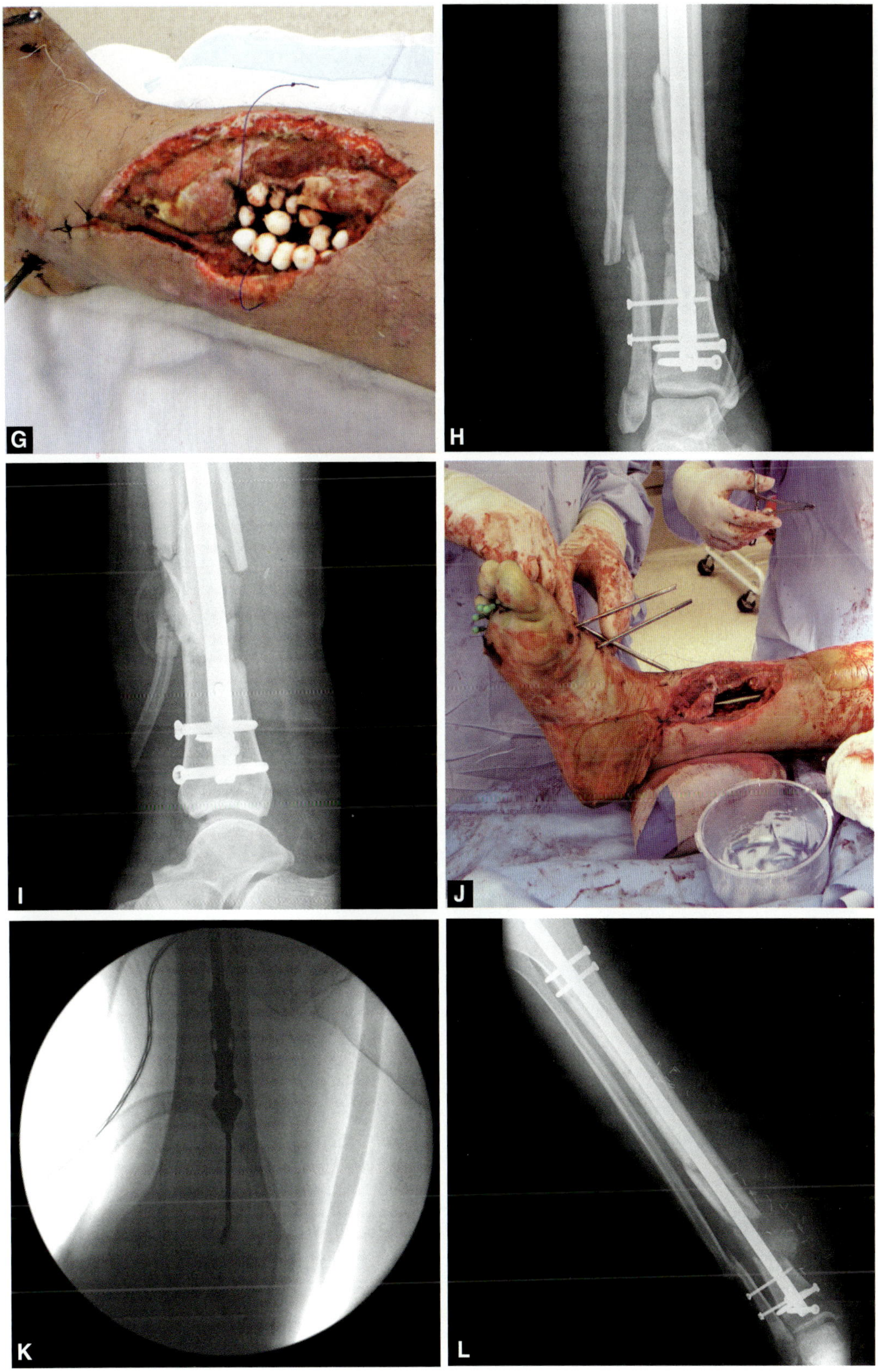

Figures 26.17G to L

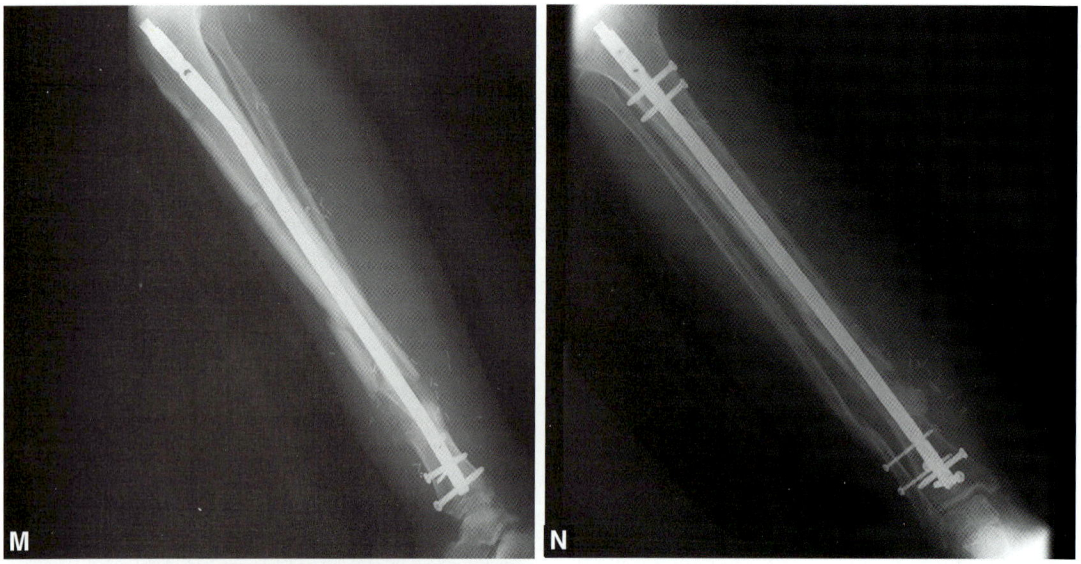

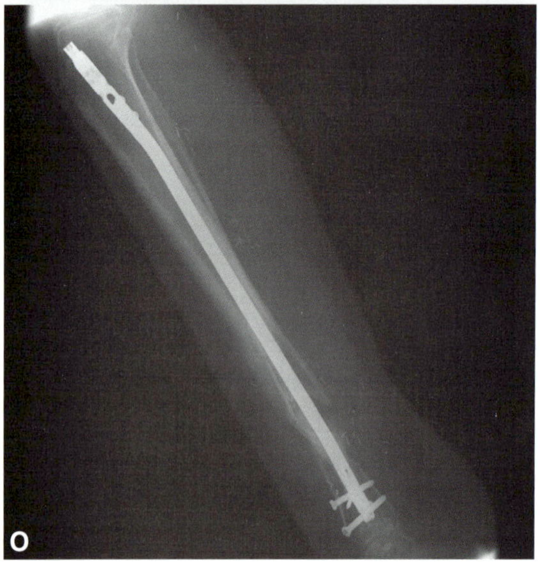

Figures 26.17A to O: Treatment of acute tibial bone loss from trauma: massive autogenous bone grafting after spacer block placement. (A) Radiograph of grade 3B open tibia fracture on initial presentation; (B to D) Debridement, external fixation, and antibiotic bead placement is performed. Multiple open metatarsal fractures were also treated; (E) Additional aggressive debridement of all devitalized bone fragments have resulted in a 4.5 cm tibial bone defect; (F) Negative pressure wound therapy and; (G) antibiotic polymethylmethacrylate (PMMA) bead therapy with external fixation is continued; (H to J) Removal of the external fixator, intramedullary nailing, syndesmotic repair, antibiotic cement spacer block placement and free latissimus muscle flap was done at hospital day 11; (K) Six weeks later, the flap was elevated and the spacer was removed. Autogenous ipsilateral femoral medullary bone graft is harvested with a Reamer Irrigator Aspirator (see text for details). Graft is packed into the defect as shown on; (L) anteroposterior (AP) and (M) lateral postoperative radiographs; (N) The fracture is healed at 6 months post bone grafting as shown on AP and (O) lateral radiographs.

can lead to a vicious cycle of increased swelling leading to decreased perfusion of the muscles and soft tissues. Ultimately, tissue death can occur which is irreversible and can lead to permanent disability. Diagnosis is usually made with clinical signs of not only a swollen leg, but pain out of proportion to the condition (particularly pain with passive stretch of the muscles in the involved compartment), paresthesias, pallor and pulselessness. As the condition progresses, symptoms typically appear in that order and it is important to make the diagnosis before pallor and pulseless occur. If the diagnosis is uncertain or difficult to make due to the mental status of the patient (or if the patient is intubated), intracompartmental pressure measurements should be taken. The authors usually use a handheld intracompartmental pressure monitor (Stryker, Mahwah, NJ). Recent data suggests that diastolic pressure–intracompartmental pressure (delta P) less than 30 mm Hg is a better indicator of the need for fasciotomy rather than an absolute pressure of 30 mm Hg.[19]

Once a diagnosis of acute compartment syndrome is made, the patient should be taken immediately to surgery for fasciotomy. Either a two incision (medial and anterolateral) or one incision (lateral) can be done to perform fasciotomies of all four compartments (Figs 26.18A to H). In the two incision fasciotomy technique, the medial incision is used to access and decompress the superficial and deep posterior compartments. The anterolateral incision is used to access and decompress the anterior and lateral compartments. Care should be taken to avoid undermining the anterior flap in order to avoid devascularization of the anterior skin flap which is often traumatized by the initial injury. The single incision lateral fasciotomy technique avoids this potential problem by virtue of only utilizing one incision. The incision is placed directly laterally and all four compartments are accessed and decompressed through this.

After fasciotomy is completed, loosely applied but abundant dressings are placed. The authors do not change these dressings outside of the OR particularly if a fracture is involved for fear of nosocomial colonization of these large open wounds. He brings the patient back to the OR every 3 days until the wound is either closed or covered with a skin graft. In the OR, the wound is gently irrigated, swelling of the limb is assessed regarding safety of wound closure and tissue is assessed for viability and debrided if necessary. On the second or third trip to the OR, the surgeon will use a shoelace or "Roman sandal" technique in order to provide tension across the wound in order to facilitate wound closure. The authors have found that negative pressure wound therapy alone is not as effective with regard to facilitating wound closure, even if the sponge is undersized in an attempt to pull the wound edges together. Negative pressure wound therapy is, however helpful in keeping the drainage in a closed system to prevent soaked dressings and wound infection. These benefits can be realized along with the benefits of progressive wound approximation by combining the negative pressure wound therapy with the shoelace approximation method. As is the case with open fractures, the authors try to achieve fasciotomy wound coverage or closure within 1–2 weeks. Wound closure is preferable to skin grafting but closure is not always possible unfortunately due to persistent swelling.

The important principles about compartment syndrome management are:

- Do not miss a compartment syndrome! Have a high index of suspicion with tibia fractures. This should be the surgeon's primary concern when managing any patient with a tibial shaft fracture. Obtunded or intubated patients might require intracompartmental pressure monitoring due to the difficulties with physical examination. Pressure monitors are also indicated in equivocal cases in which the diagnosis is uncertain.
- Once a diagnosis is made, immediate fasciotomy surgery is performed. This is an orthopedic emergency and timing of treatment is more critical than it is for open fractures, for example. Fasciotomy should be performed within 6–8 hours once a diagnosis is made in order to have the best chance of muscle tissue survival.
- Either a one- or two-incision decompressive fasciotomy procedure can be performed.

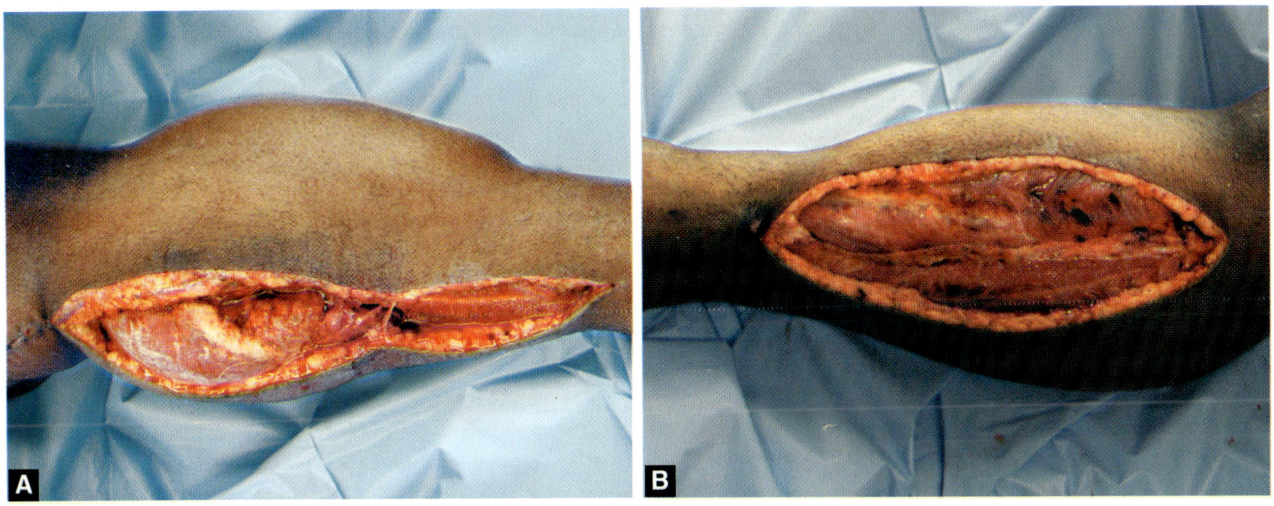

Figures 26.18A and B

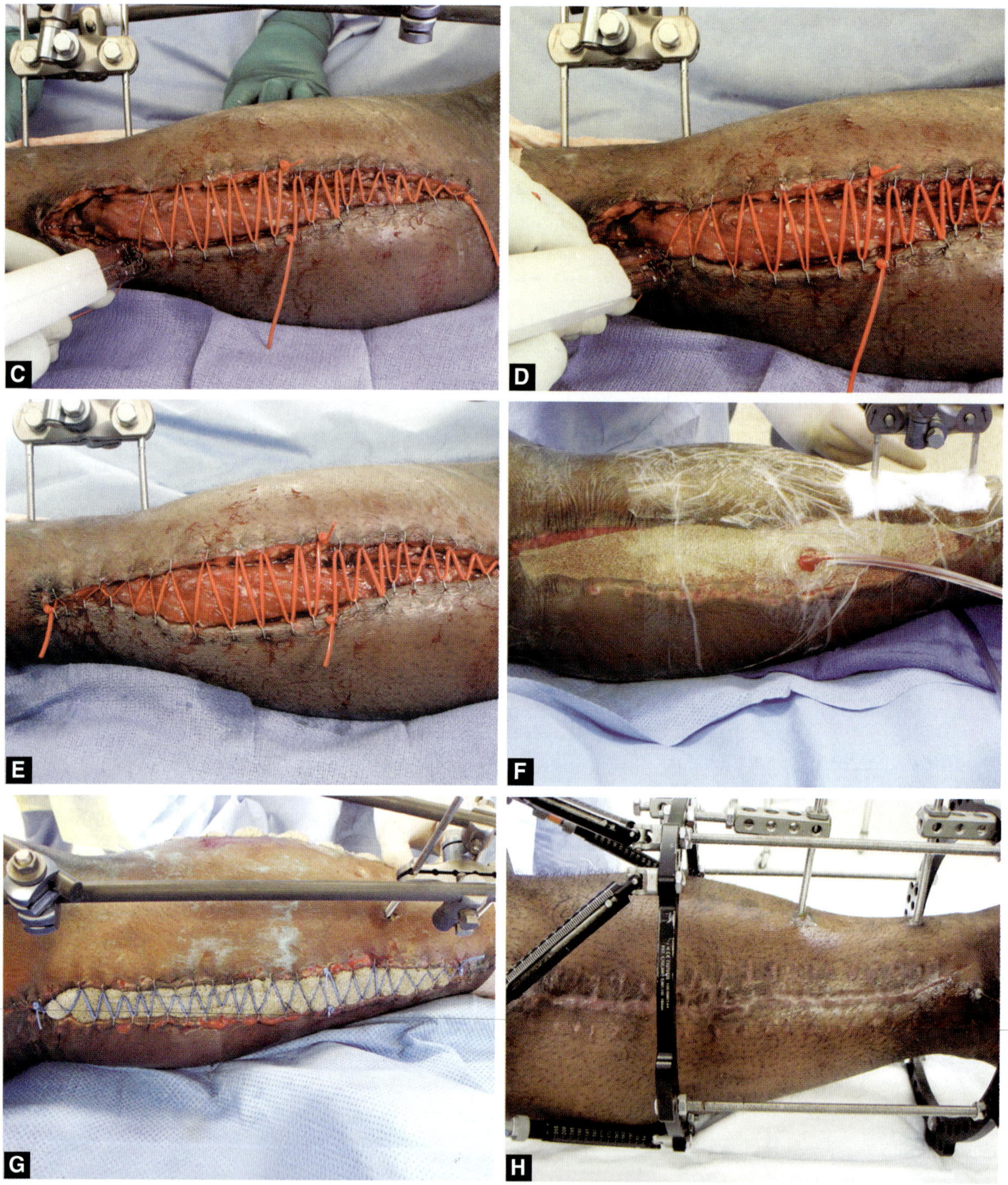

Figures 26.18A to H: Treatment of compartment syndrome of the leg: fasciotomy wound management. (A) The two-incision fasciotomy of the leg utilizes the medial incision for access and decompression of the superficial and deep posterior compartments; (B) The anterolateral incision accesses and decompresses the anterior and lateral compartments; (C to E) The shoelace or "Roman sandal" method utilizes a skin stapler and vessel loops to gently tension the skin edges when it is safe to do so; (F) Negative pressure wound therapy can also be used both as a closed drain system as well as a method to try and close the wound. This is generally not as effective as the shoelace method; (G) The same wound shown with both a negative pressure wound therapy for drainage control and the shoelace tension method to better approximate the skin; (H) This wound was closed by 10 days after fasciotomy.

- Do not allow wounds to become contaminated particularly if fractures are involved and either close or skin graft these incisions within 1–2 weeks in order to reduce the chance of colonization and infection.

Summary

Tibial shaft fracture management can be challenging and potentially fraught with complications. Nonunion and infection is more common than in other fractures and the surgeon must proceed cautiously but deliberately in order to achieve good results. Intramedullary nailing is the mainstay of treatment of most tibial diaphyseal fractures, although not as universal as in the femoral shaft. The surgeon should always consider the development of compartment syndrome in any patient with tibial shaft fractures but should be even more alert in obtunded patients and in high energy injuries. Proper preoperative planning and efficient but careful execution of OR protocols and surgical techniques should avoid most surgical complications. However, if these are to occur, there are well described methods of treating these complications, many of which are outlined above in the case examples.

References

1. Bucholz RW, Heckman JD, Court-Brown CM. Rockwood and Green's Fractures in Adults, 6th Edition; 2006. pp. 2080-143.
2. Court-Brown CM, McBirnie J. The epidemiology of tibial fractures. J Bone Joint Surg. 1995;77B:417-21.
3. Küntscher G. The Küntscher method of intramedullary fixation. J Bone Joint Surg. 1958;40A:17-26.
4. Templeman DC, Marder RA. Injuries of the knee associated with fracture of the tibial shaft. J Bone Joint Surg. 1989;71A:1392-5.
5. Keating JF, Kuo RS, Court-Brown CM. Bifocal fractures of the tibia and fibula. J Bone Joint Surg. 1994:76B:395-400.
6. Müller ME, Nazarian S, Koch P, et al. The comprehensive classification of fractures of long bones. Berlin: Springer-Verlag. 1990.
7. Nelson G, Kelly P, Peterson L, et al. Blood supply of the human tibia. J Bone Joint Surg Am. 1960;42-A:625-36.
8. Tornetta PT III, Riina J, Geller J, et al. Intraarticular anatomic risks of tibial nailing. J Orthop Trauma. 1999;13:247-51.
9. McConnell T, Tornetta P III, Tilzey J, et al. Tibial portal placement: the radiographic correlate of the anatomic safe zone. J Orthop Trauma. 2001;15:207-9.
10. Keating JF, Orfaly R, O'Brian PJ. Knee pain after tibial nailing. J Orthop Trauma. 1997;11:10-3.
11. Jarmo AK, Toivanen JA, Vaisto O, et al. Anterior knee pain after intramedullary nailing of fractures of the tibial shaft: an eight-year follow-up of a prospective, randomized study comparing two different nail-insertion techniques. J Bone Joint Surg Amer. 2002;84:580-5.
12. Roberts CS, Pape HC, Jones AL, et al. Evolving concepts in the treatment of patients who have sustained orthopaedic trauma. J Bone Joint Surg. 2005,87A:434-49.
13. Tornetta P, Collins E. Semiextended position for intramedullary nailing of the proximal tibia. Clin Orthop. 1996;328:185-9.
14. Court-Brown CM, Gustilo T, Shaw AD. Knee pain after intramedullary nailing: its incidence, etiology, and outcome. J Orthop Trauma. 1997;11:103-5.
15. Court-Brown CM, Christie J, McQueen MM. Closed intramedullary tibial nailing. Its use in closed and type I open fractures. J Bone Joint Surg. 1990;72B:605-11.
16. Brinker MR, O'Connor D, Monla Y, et al. Metabolic and endocrine abnormalities in patients with nonunions. Current Orthop Practice. 2008;19:430-42.
17. SPRINT Investigators, M. Bhandari, G. Guyatt et al. Randomized trial of reamed and unreamed intramedullary nailing of tibial shaft fractures. J Bone Joint Surg Am. 90(12). 2006; 2567 78.
18. Pelissier PH, Masquelet AC, Bareille R, et al. Induced membranes secrete growth factors including vascular and osteoinductive factors and could stimulate bone regeneration. J Orthop Res 2004;22:73-9.
19. McQueen MM, Court-Brown CM. Compartment monitoring in tibial fractures—the pressure threshold for decompression. J Bone Joint Surg. 1996;78-B:99-104.

Chapter 27

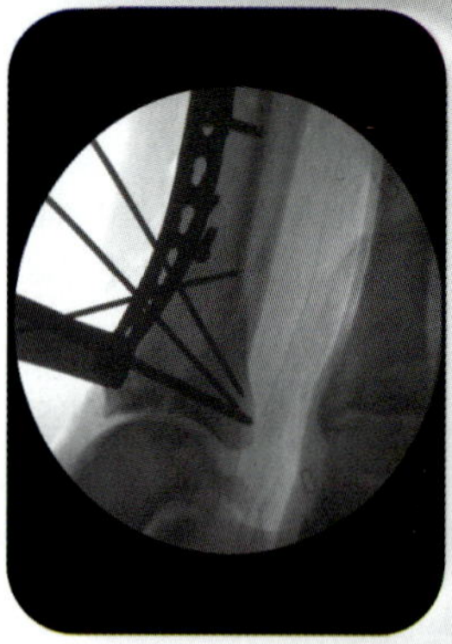

Distal Tibia Fractures

Michael Suk, Megan Manthe, Saqib Rehman

Chapter Outline

Introduction
Diagnosis
Classification
Surgical Indications
- Nonoperative Management
- Surgical Evolution

Surgical Anatomy, Positioning, Approaches and Techniques
- Applied Surgical Anatomy
- Staged Approach
- Postoperative Care
- Special Considerations

Outcomes
Complications
Authors' Preferred Management of Select Complications
- Case 1: Treatment of Recalcitrant Nonunion of the Distal Tibial Shaft and Pilon Fracture with Nonunion Repair and Fusion of the Ankle and Subtalar Joints with Retrograde Fusion Nail
- Case 2: Treatment of Nonunion Repair of Distal Tibia Fracture with Revision Open Reduction and Internal Fixation and Autologous Bone Grafting
- Case 3: Treatment of Infected Nonunion of the Distal Tibia with Radical Resection and Bone Transport Distraction Osteogenesis
- Case 4: Treatment of an Aseptic Malunion/Nonunion of the Distal Tibia with Osteotomy and Open Reduction and Internal Fixation

Summary

Introduction

Distal tibia fractures that involve the tibiotalar articulation (pilon) have long been both challenging to manage as well as difficult to predict outcomes, especially in the most severe forms, particularly with increasing degrees of severity. The treatment of pilon fractures has evolved from one of early primary fixation to a staged management with fewer complications and improved outcomes. Fractures occurring at the distal articular surface of tibia account only for roughly 3–10% of all tibia fractures, equal to less than 1% of fractures of the lower extremity.[1-3] The incidence is higher in men than women, most often occurring in the third and fourth decades of life.

Pilon fractures often result from high-energy accidents such as motor vehicle collisions and falls from substantial height, where there is an axial load component causing the talus to compress proximally onto distal tibial articular surface. This loading mechanism sets pilon fractures apart from more predictable common ankle fractures described by Lauge-Hansen[4] that result from primarily indirect and torsional forces and are of much lower energy. The rapid axial loading component of pilon fractures has a propensity to cause significant comminution at the distal tibial articular surface, lending to their uncertain outcomes even after fixation. With high-energy failure (fracture) of the distal tibia, the energy released is subsequently imparted to the soft tissues, often causing rapid and significant swelling, fracture blisters, open wounds, local skin necrosis and impaired perfusion among other soft tissue complications related to the soft tissue envelope. The shift of attention to protection and limited stripping and handling of soft tissues is a major factor associated with improved outcomes.

Potential complications include malunion, delayed or nonunion, deep infection, osteomyelitis, stiffness and ankle arthrosis. In order to lessen the threat of potential complications and optimize outcomes, appropriate management of pilon fractures requires a solid understanding of the injury mechanism, appropriate evaluation of fracture pattern, knowledge of surgical anatomy and proficiency in many surgical options.

Diagnosis

As many pilon fractures are the results of high-energy accidents, every evaluation should begin with standard advanced trauma life-support protocol. From here, typical physical examination findings associated with pilon fractures include pain and swelling at the distal tibia. Often times, there is an obvious deformity (Figs 27.1A to D).

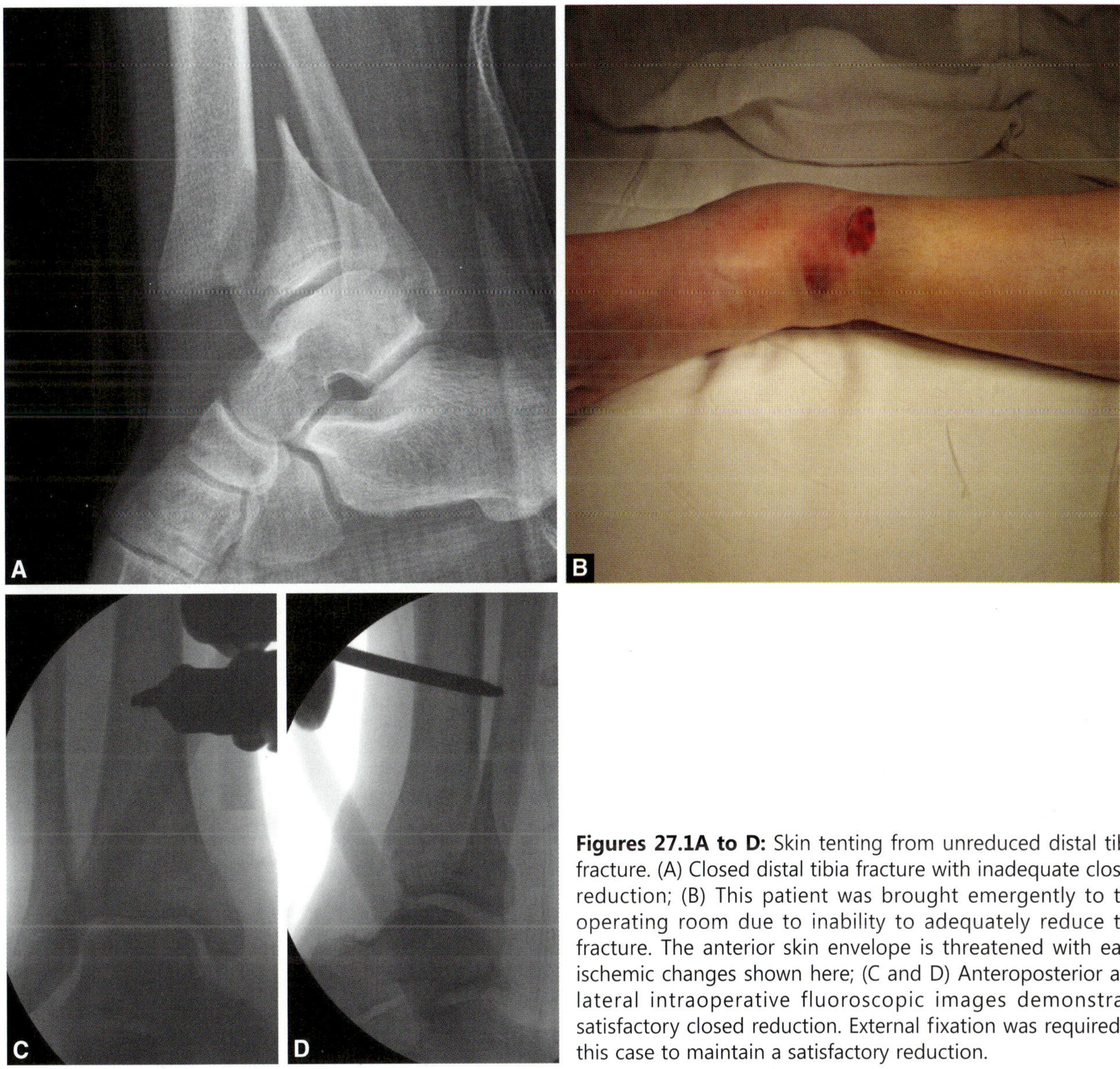

Figures 27.1A to D: Skin tenting from unreduced distal tibia fracture. (A) Closed distal tibia fracture with inadequate closed reduction; (B) This patient was brought emergently to the operating room due to inability to adequately reduce the fracture. The anterior skin envelope is threatened with early ischemic changes shown here; (C and D) Anteroposterior and lateral intraoperative fluoroscopic images demonstrate satisfactory closed reduction. External fixation was required in this case to maintain a satisfactory reduction.

Open wounds need to be addressed with administration of appropriate antibiotics, determination of amount of gross contamination, and often prompt bedside irrigation prior to initial splinting to grossly realign the limb, while reducing any displacement of talus (Fig. 27.2). Assessment of perfusion and neurological function is performed during the initial physical examination. Temporary splinting can minimize gross motion at the fracture site, thereby relieving pain, skin pressure and protecting further soft tissue damage. The resultant swelling is often abrupt, yet will certainly increase as the inflammatory process ensues; therefore, extremity elevation may also be helpful. Fracture blisters may form as early as 6–8 hours after injury, and the differentiation between clear and hemorrhagic contents is important in surgical timing. It has been shown that hemorrhagic blisters result from complete separation of the epidermis from the dermis and significant wound complications occur, if incisions are made through these tissues prior to re-epithelialization (Figs 27.3A and B).[5,6]

The degree of soft tissue injury in tibial pilon fractures may be described using the Tscherne classification scheme (Fig. 27.4).[7] Although compartment syndrome is rare with pilon fractures, it has occurred in those fractures having diaphyseal extension. Therefore, one should beware of early signs and symptoms including severe and increasing pain, pain with passive stretch of extensor hallucis longus (EHL), weakness of EHL, sensory changes in deep peroneal distribution and tense compartments. Open fractures are commonly described using the Gustilo and Anderson

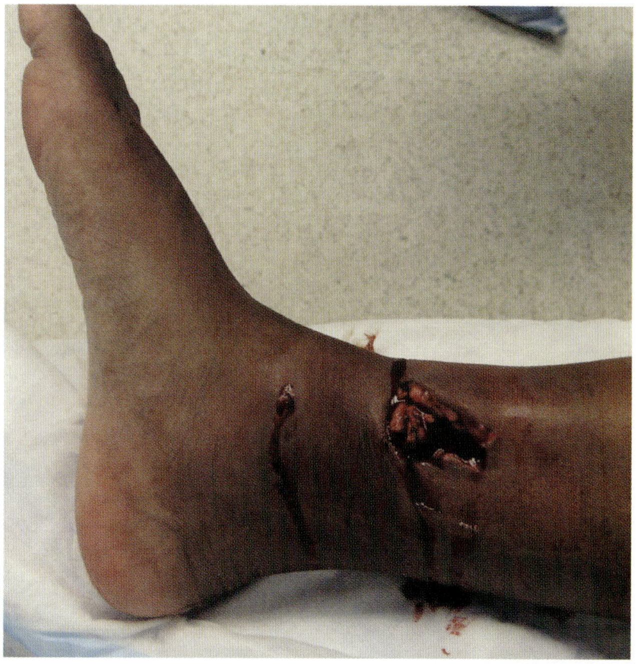

Figure 27.2: Open tibial fracture with medial wounds. Emergent irrigation and debridement is required in these injuries.

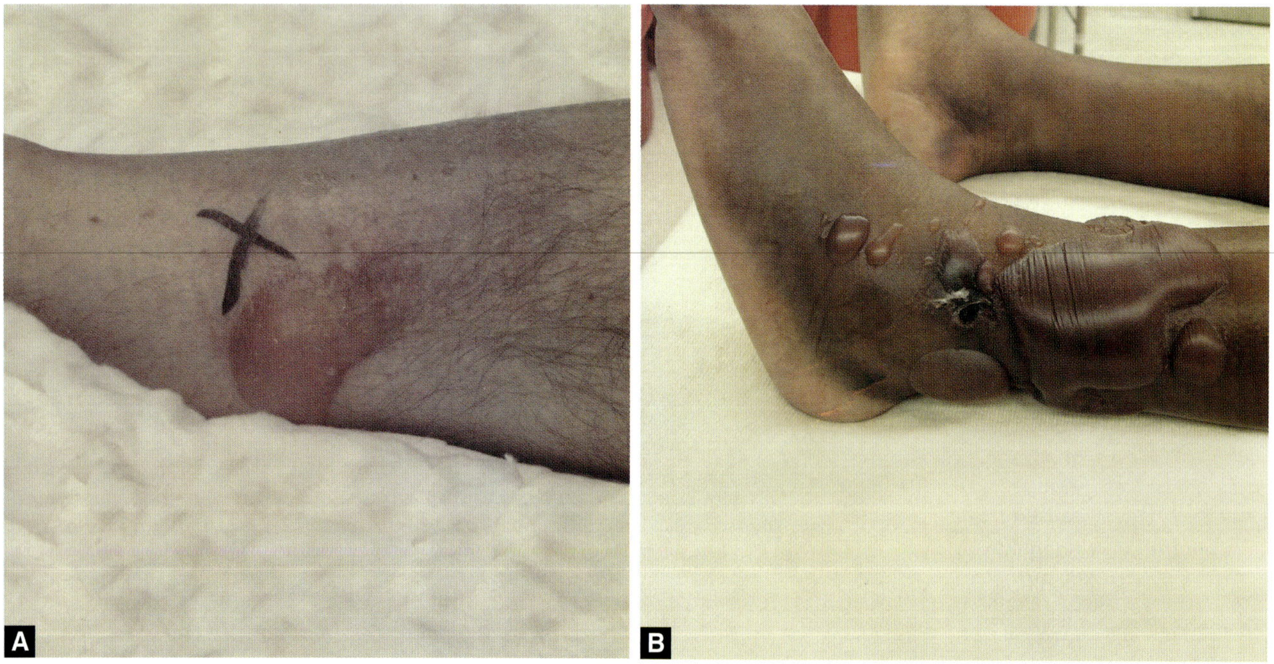

Figures 27.3A and B: Fracture blisters associated with distal tibial fractures. (A) Serous fracture blister; (B) Multiple hemorrhagic blisters (dark colored). A few smaller serous blisters are also seen anteriorly at the ankle.

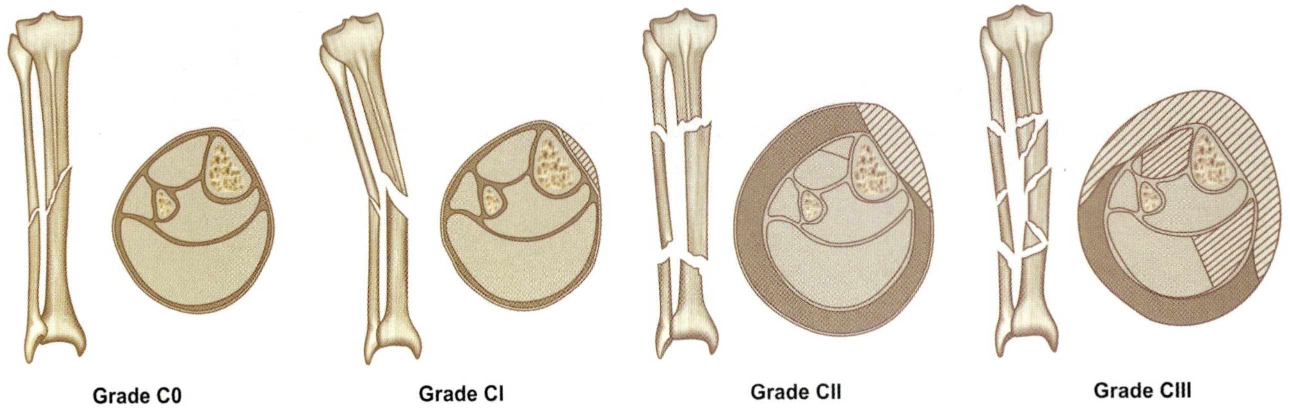

Figure 27.4: Tscherne classification of soft tissue injury associated with closed fractures. Grade C0: Minimal soft tissue damage. Indirect violence. Simple fracture patterns; Grade CI: Superficial abrasion or contusion caused by pressure from within. Mild to moderately severe fracture configuration; Grade CII: Deep, contaminated abrasion associated with localized skin or muscle contusion. Impending compartment syndrome. Severe fracture configuration; Grade CIII: Extensive skin contusion or crush. Underlying muscle damage may be severe. Subcutaneous avulsion. Decompensated compartment syndrome.

classification, which not only describes the soft tissue wound and underlying fracture pattern, but also guides antibiotic coverage (Table 27.1).[2,8] Since the soft tissue envelope is potentially severely disrupted in pilon fractures, dependence versus elevation of the extremity can not only affect the surgical timing, but overall soft tissue integrity, which is directly related to outcomes.

Radiographs for suspected tibial pilon fractures begin with anteroposterior (AP), mortise and lateral views and are essential for proper preoperative planning. Fracture characteristics easily depicted in plain radiographs include proximal extensions, multiple fragments, impacted segments, bone loss and osteopenia, all of which can further complicate surgical management. Disruption of the ankle mortise is important to recognize, reduce and immobilize during initial management not only to protect the soft tissue envelope, but also to relieve abnormal contact pressures on the articular cartilage that could lead to further chondrocyte death. With standard radiographs, one can often see how foot position at the time of injury dictates fracture pattern.[4,9,10] A plantar-flexed foot creates a large posterior tibial fragment, whereas a dorsiflexed foot creates a compressive fracture of the anterior tibia (Figs 27.5A and B). Similarly, with the foot in a neutral position, there are purely vertical forces that create a Y-shaped fracture with both anterior and posterior components. The gross degree of comminution both articular and metaphyseal is also often easily depicted from standard ankle radiographs.

Table 27.1: Open fractures—Gustilo classification

Type I	Open fracture with a skin wound <1 cm in length and clean
Type II	Open fracture with a laceration >1 cm in length without extensive soft tissue damage, flaps, or avulsions
Type III	Open segmental fracture with >10 cm wound with extensive soft tissue injury or a traumatic amputation (special categories in Type III include gunshot fractures and open fractures caused by farm injuries)
III_A	Adequate soft tissue coverage
III_B	Significant soft tissue loss with exposed bone that requires soft tissue transfer to achieve coverage
III_C	Associated vascular injury that requires repair for limb preservation

The presence or absence of an associated fibula fracture is important for preoperative planning. An associated fibula fracture occurs in approximately 70–85% of pilon fractures.[11] Associated fibula fractures are characterized as tension failure or compression failure. Tension failure of fibula will present as a varus deformity and requires a medial buttress to prevent varus malunion. Compression failure of fibula will present as a valgus deformity and requires a lateral buttress plate to prevent valgus malunion. An intact fibula often depicts a varus compressive force resulting in impaction on the medial articular surface. A computerized tomography (CT) scan of the pilon fracture is often required for preoperative

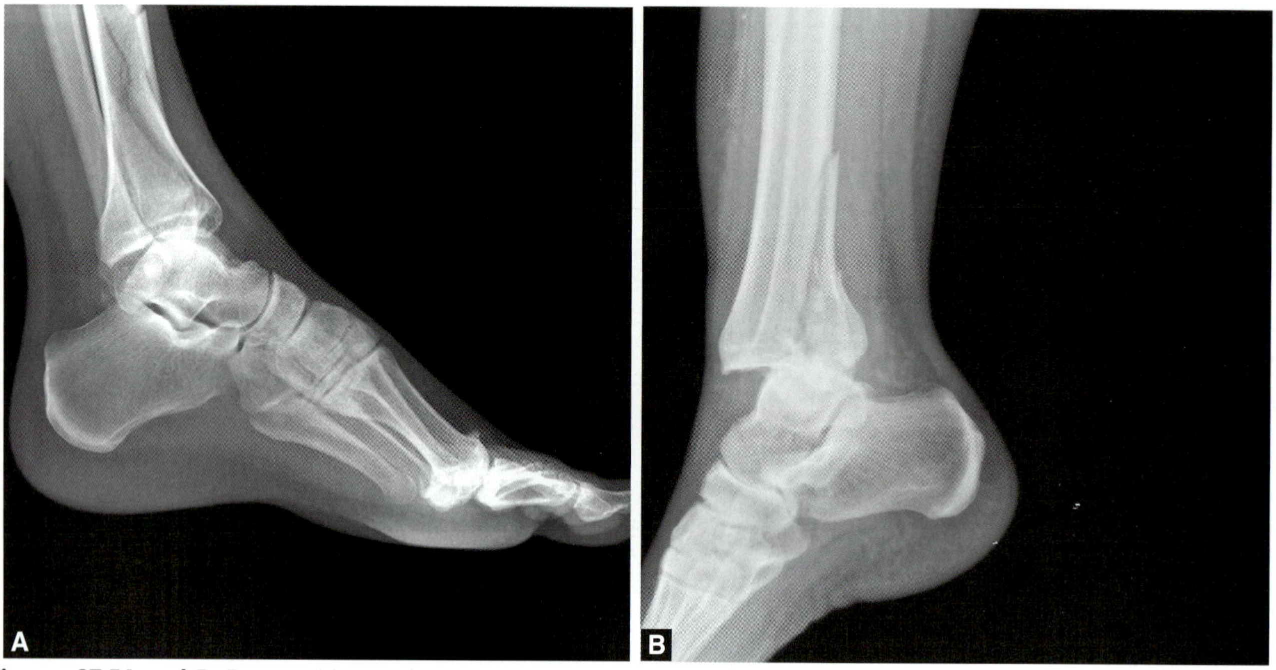

Figures 27.5A and B: Foot position at the time of impact can determine the site of plafond fracture. (A) Axial loading with dorsiflexion typically results in an anterior plafond fracture; (B) Axial loading with plantar flexion typically results in a posterior plafond fracture.

planning to further delineate fracture comminution and impaction. This is often most useful after limb length has been restored, especially when there are many small and potentially rotated fragments. Evaluation and understanding of axial CT images allows for more rapid and accurate surgical treatment, while limiting soft tissue disruption and stripping.

DISTAL TIBIA FRACTURES DIAGNOSIS: Pearls and Pitfalls

- Due to the thin soft tissue envelope of the lower leg and ankle, skin tenting and open wounds are common and must be ruled out with careful physical examination
- Fracture blisters can also compromise surgical approaches and must be carefully managed
- Fracture pattern can suggest the likely mechanism involved

Classification

There are a number of different classification systems available to describe pilon fractures. Some are more descriptive than others; however, the goals with any classification system are that it is reproducible and reliable and in some way, directs treatment. Certainly, with pilon fractures, the aim is to match the treatment technique with fracture type and soft tissue injury. The Ruedi and Allgower classification scheme is based upon increasing degrees of comminution;[10] whereas, the AO/OTA classification system is the most descriptive (Figs 27.6 and 27.7).[12,13] Each classification system has limitations in reliability, yet both provide framework in decision making.

Surgical Indications

Nonoperative Management

Operative treatment of pilon fractures is almost always the standard of care. There are however, few instances, where nonoperative management is acceptable. Truly nondisplaced fracture patterns or those patients with absolute contraindications to surgery, such as paraplegics or those with significant unstable medical comorbidities, can be treated with closed reduction and plaster immobilization, although displacement is common.[14] In those treated nonoperatively, progressive weight bearing is dictated as healing is demonstrated on subsequent radiographs. Closed reduction and cast immobilization is ineffective at reducing displaced fragments or correcting articular impaction, solidifying the notion that only few

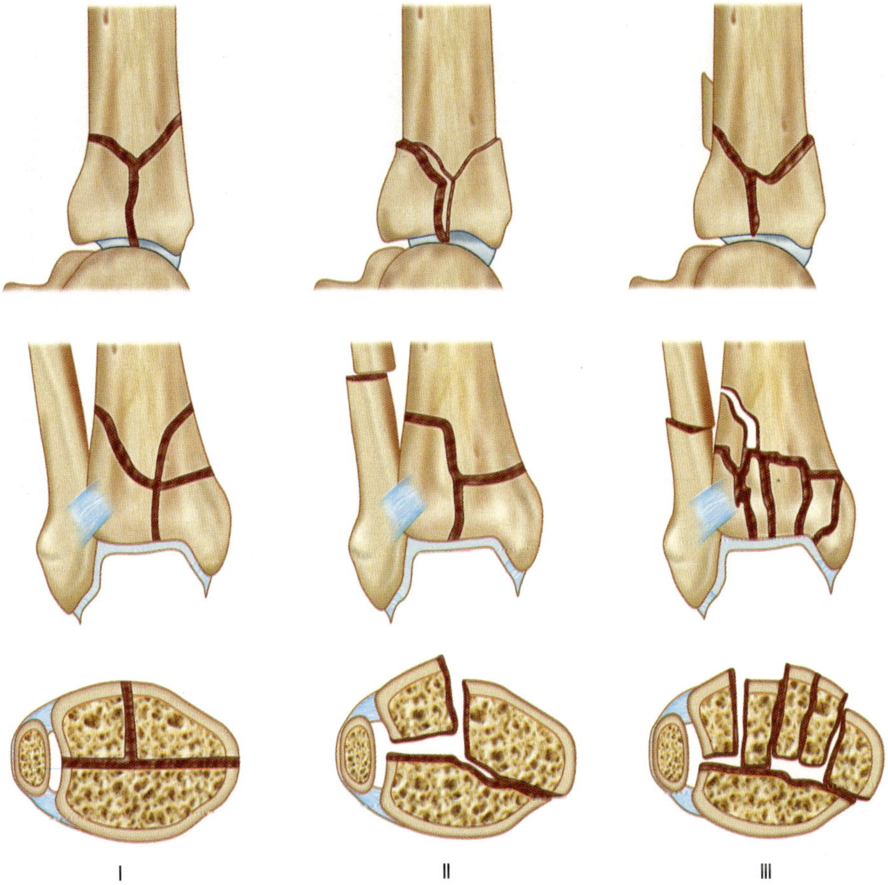

Figure 27.6: Ruedi and Allgower classification of distal tibia fractures. Type I: Minimally displaced intra-articular fracture; Type II: Displaced intra-articular fracture; Type III: Comminuted and displaced intra-articular fracture.

pilon fractures are amenable to closed methods of treatments. Furthermore, as cast immobilization is often maintained until the appearance of radiographic bony healing, significant joint stiffness is a problem commonly encountered (Fig. 27.8).

Surgical Evolution

The only true absolute operative indications are open fractures and those associated with vascular injuries, yet relative indications such as 2 mm articular incongruity and 10° of angular malalignments in any plane also exist.[11,15] The long-term and even short-term complications of post-traumatic noncongruent articular surfaces are reasons for these relative surgical indications. The goals of surgical treatment are to obtain stable anatomical reduction and fixation, while allowing early range of motion. Prior to 1963, outcomes of surgical management of severe pilon fractures were dismal. Complications such as skin sloughing, repeated surgeries, osteomyelitis and amputations were frequent. In 1963, the AO introduced principles of open reduction and internal fixation (ORIF), wherein the framework of modern-day fracture care began.[12] Guidelines included meticulous soft tissue dissection, limited stripping of fracture fragments, indirect reduction, anatomical reduction and stable fixation. Yet still, relative success after surgical treatment of pilon fractures prior to 2000 was low, with good results ranging from 30–60%, many having high rates of deep infection and repeated surgery, some complications as high as 70%[16-18] (note that many studies reporting higher success rates after pilon fixation were of lower energy mechanisms, not higher grade 43C1–3 type fractures).

Poor outcomes after ORIF prompted the evolution of staged protocols typically initially stabilized with a spanning external fixation, the extremity brought out to length, and time was allowed for the soft tissue envelope to heal, an average 12–24 days. After soft tissue

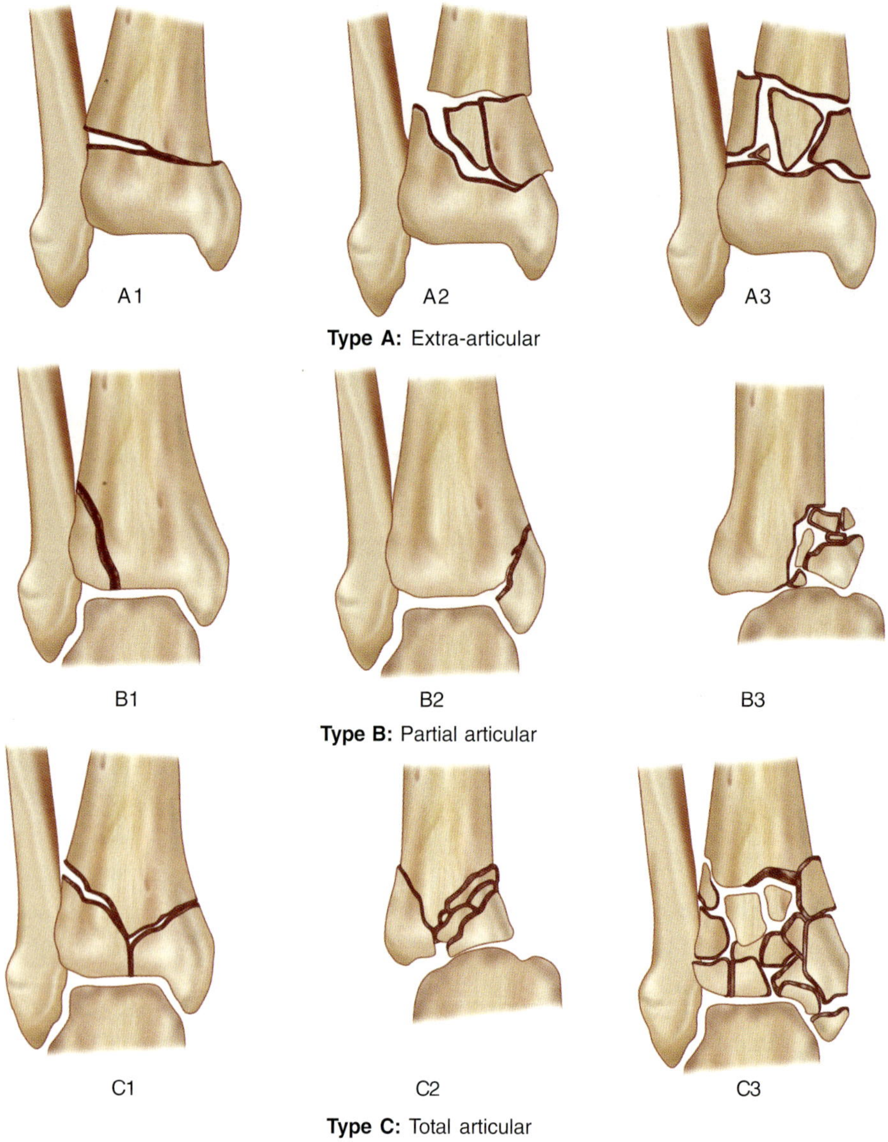

Figure 27.7: AO/OTA classification of distal tibia fractures. Type A: Extra-articular fracture; Type B: Partial articular fracture; Type C: Complete articular fracture; The three types and nine groups of the AO/OTA classification of distal tibia fractures are illustrated. The three types of fractures are extra-articular, partial articular and total articular, and they are divided into nine groups based on the amount of comminution.

compromise had resolved, formal ORIF was performed. Patterson and Sirkin each published literature in 1999 demonstrating the benefits of staged protocols. Sirkin treated 56 tibial pilon fractures with immediate fibular ORIF and ankle spanning external fixation. After an average delay of 12.7–14 days, formal ORIF was performed on the distal tibia with only 1.8% wound dehiscence and 3.6% infection rate. Patterson similarly treated 21 consecutive C3 tibial pilon fractures with fibular ORIF and spanning external fixation initially. After an average delay of 24 days, formal ORIF was performed resulting in no infection, no soft tissue complications and 77% good results.[19,20] Watson and colleagues in 2000 also adopted a staged protocol, where the extremity was first placed into calcaneal traction. To allow for soft tissue improvement, definitive ORIF was completed after an average delay of 5 days. At follow-up of 4.9 years, good or excellent results were seen in 60–93% of cases, stratified according to AO fracture classification.[21] Blauth in 2001 found that patients treated in a staged manner had less pain, a higher proportion

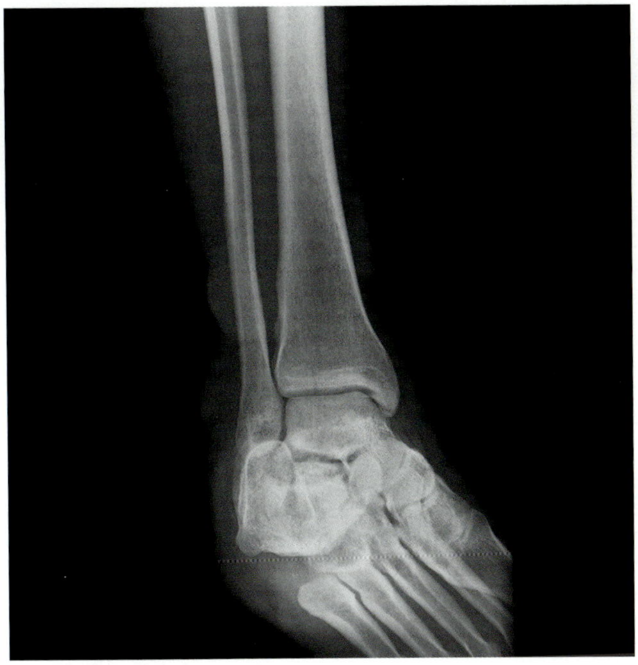

Figure 27.8: A nondisplaced tibial pilon fracture. This can be successfully treated nonoperatively.

returned to previous occupation and fewer limitations of leisure activity, when compared to those treated with other methods.[21] Today, many options are available for the treatment of pilon fractures. These include hybrid external fixation, small wire external fixation, ORIF, ankle spanning external fixation, articulated ankle spanning external fixation and limited internal fixation and external fixation (Figs 27.9A to C). Surgical decision-making directs the strategy of fixation chosen; however, a combination of different techniques is frequently adopted.

Surgical Anatomy, Positioning, Approaches and Techniques

Applied Surgical Anatomy

The surgical anatomy of the pilon region demands knowledge of not only the osseous components, but the ligamentous, muscular and neurovasculature architecture as well (Fig. 27.10). The osseous anatomy includes the tibia and fibula, as well as their articulations with the talus. The articular surface of the distal tibia is concave to accept the talar dome, while having anterior and posterior extensions. The fibula extends distally relative to the tibia, and is firmly attached by anterior and posterior tibiofibular ligaments. The integrity of these ligaments becomes relevant, when reducing the tibial articular surface, as these intact ligaments often aid in reduction. It is the maintenance of these ligaments that help create commonly observed fracture patterns: Volkmann's fragment attached to posterior talofibular ligament (PTFL), Chaput fragment attached to anterior talofibular ligament (ATFL) and the medial fragment attached to deltoid ligament. Similarly, changes in the length or rotation of the distal fibula (a potential complication when fixing highly comminuted fibula fractures during Stage 1 of pilon fractures) can inhibit anatomical fixation of anterolateral and posterolateral segments of the tibia.

Staged Approach

The most common surgical approaches to the distal tibia are anterolateral, anteromedial and posterolateral; the chosen surgical approach is dictated by mechanically appropriate location of fixation. Regardless of approach chosen, be mindful to avoid incisions through bad skin as well as avoidance of tight closures.

The anterolateral approach is the most useful for majority of complete articular fractures of the distal tibia, as well as some partial articular and extra-articular variants (Figs 27.11A to K). It provides excellent visualization of the entire articular surface. The skin incision is parallel to the fourth metatarsal distally and may extend to the talonavicular joint. It is centered at the ankle joint and runs parallel to and in between the tibia and fibula proximally. Beware of the superficial peroneal nerve, which crosses the incision proximal to the ankle joint. Throughout the dissection, maintain full-thickness skin flaps to assure late skin viability after closure. With deep dissection, remain posterolateral to the anterior tibial vessels and deep peroneal nerve. Finally, arthrotomy is performed close to the fracture line defining the anterolateral fragment, while protecting the ATFL. Proximally, this can be made extensile between anterior compartment of the leg and lateral surface of the tibial shaft. If direct medial or posteromedial fixation is required, this is done through a separate incision.

The anteromedial approach is also extensile and provides excellent visualization of the entire articular surface (Figs 27.12A to H). The skin incision is curvilinear over the anterior compartment, lateral to the tibial crest

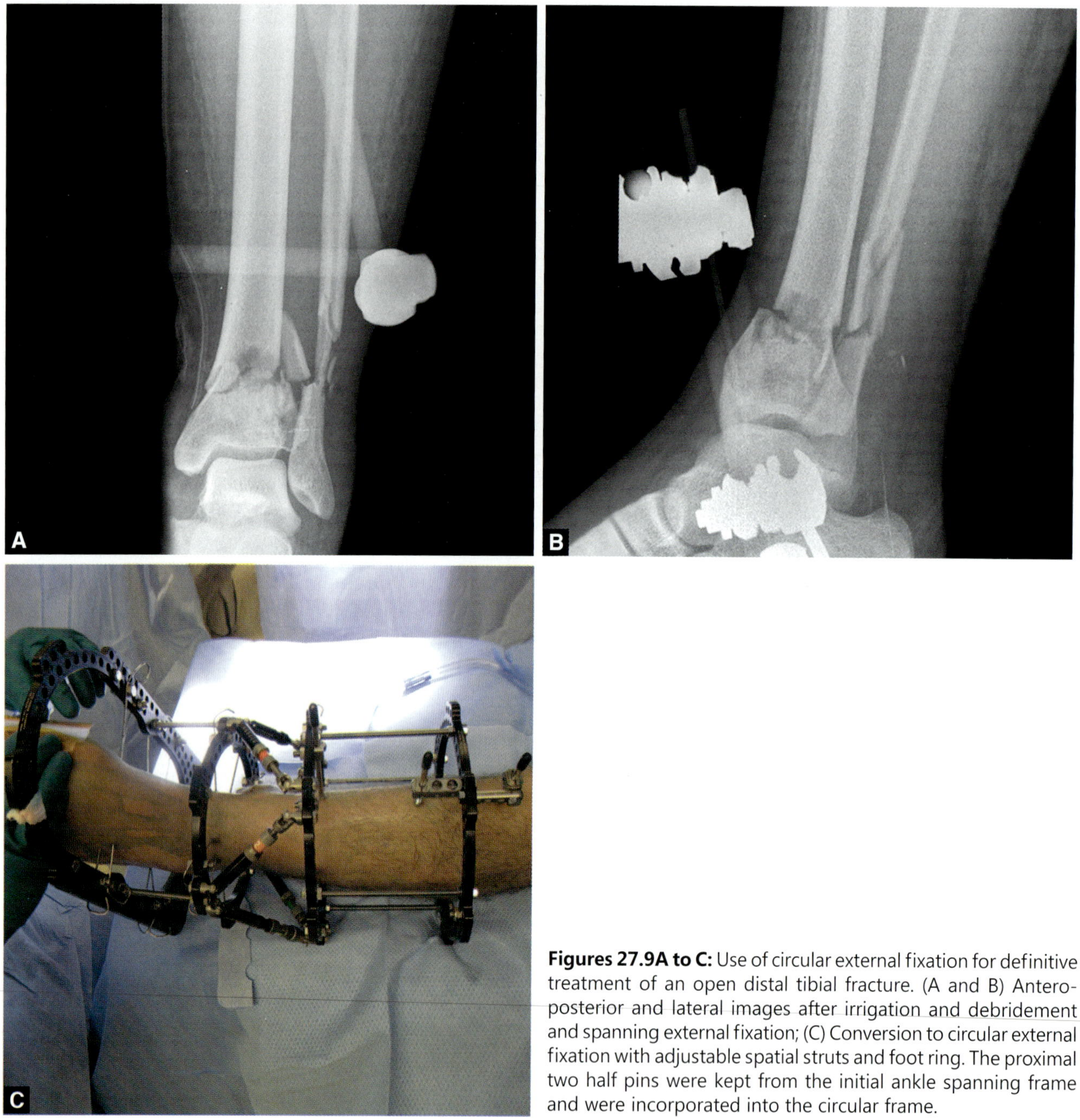

Figures 27.9A to C: Use of circular external fixation for definitive treatment of an open distal tibial fracture. (A and B) Antero-posterior and lateral images after irrigation and debridement and spanning external fixation; (C) Conversion to circular external fixation with adjustable spatial struts and foot ring. The proximal two half pins were kept from the initial ankle spanning frame and were incorporated into the circular frame.

and is directed toward the navicular tubercle. The saphenous vein is identified and exposure is limited distally. Important to keep in mind is the unforgiving nature of medial soft tissue envelope, as one should assure healthy tissue prior to create the full-thickness anteromedial skin flap. With deep dissection, remain medial to the tibialis anterior tendon, avoiding injury to the paratenon. The extensor retinaculum is incised and an anteromedial capsulotomy is performed at the joint level, again protecting the integrity of the deltoid and ATFL.

The use of posterolateral approach is limited to fibular fixation and cortical reductions of the posterolateral fragments to the tibial metaphysis (Figs 27.13A to E and 27.14). Articular visualization is virtually impossible due to distal extension of the posterior malleolus. A straight posterolateral skin incision is placed anterior to peroneal

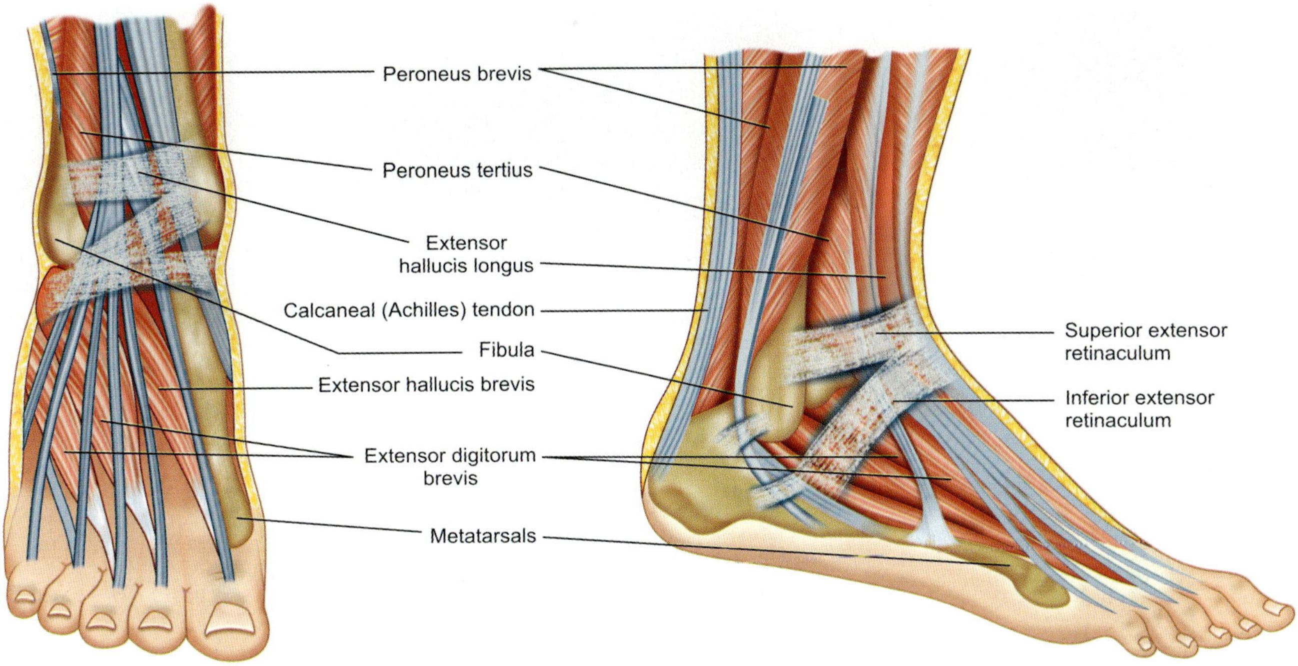

Figure 27.10: Anatomy of the ankle joint.

tendons. Both the sural nerve distally and superficial peroneal nerve proximally are protected. Deep dissection develops the posterolateral border of peroneal tendons and the tibia is exposed from lateral to medial. The PTFL and posterior joint capsule are respected at all times, as are periosteal attachments, especially if an additional anterior approach is anticipated.

A novel lateral approach to definitively treat tibial pilon fractures was recently described in 2007 by Grose and colleagues.[22] The development of lateral approach was based on the ability to create thick skin flaps, while allowing excellent visualization for articular reduction, thereby reducing potential soft tissue complications, while achieving anatomical reconstruction. There are two specific exclusions from the use of lateral approach: (1) the fracture cannot have impacted articular fragments, where the fracture line exits very medially at the anterior aspect of the tibia, and (2) there cannot be soft tissue compromise along the anterior border of the fibula. The lateral approach begins with a skin incision along the anterior fibula border from the most proximal fracture line and extends up to 3–4 cm distal to the ankle joint. Care should be taken to protect the superficial peroneal nerve. Blunt dissection posteriorly allows for fibula reduction, recreating a stable lateral column. Blunt dissection anteriorly is performed to the level of interosseous membrane. A large elevator is used to develop a plane between the interosseous membrane and contents of the anterior compartment, exposing the entire lateral tibial surface. This lateral approach has been found to result in 93% anatomical reduction with a low infection rate and wound dehiscence rate of 4.5% each.[22]

Stage 1

As previously mentioned, the first stage of pilon fracture surgical management is external fixation to stabilize the fracture, maintain reduction at length, while allowing the soft tissue envelope to heal. An additional benefit of using external fixation initially is that it provides a portable traction device before definitive treatment, allowing the patient to mobilize and to be discharged home in the interim. If needed, the fixator can be prepped into the surgical field and used as a distraction device during the definitive fixation procedure (Figs 27.15A to E). Many configurations of external fixation are available including tibial-talar, tibial-calcaneal, bridged, articulated, unilateral, triangular, circular and semicircular. We prefer one of the simplest forms in most cases with two pins on anteromedial face of the tibial shaft and one transfixion

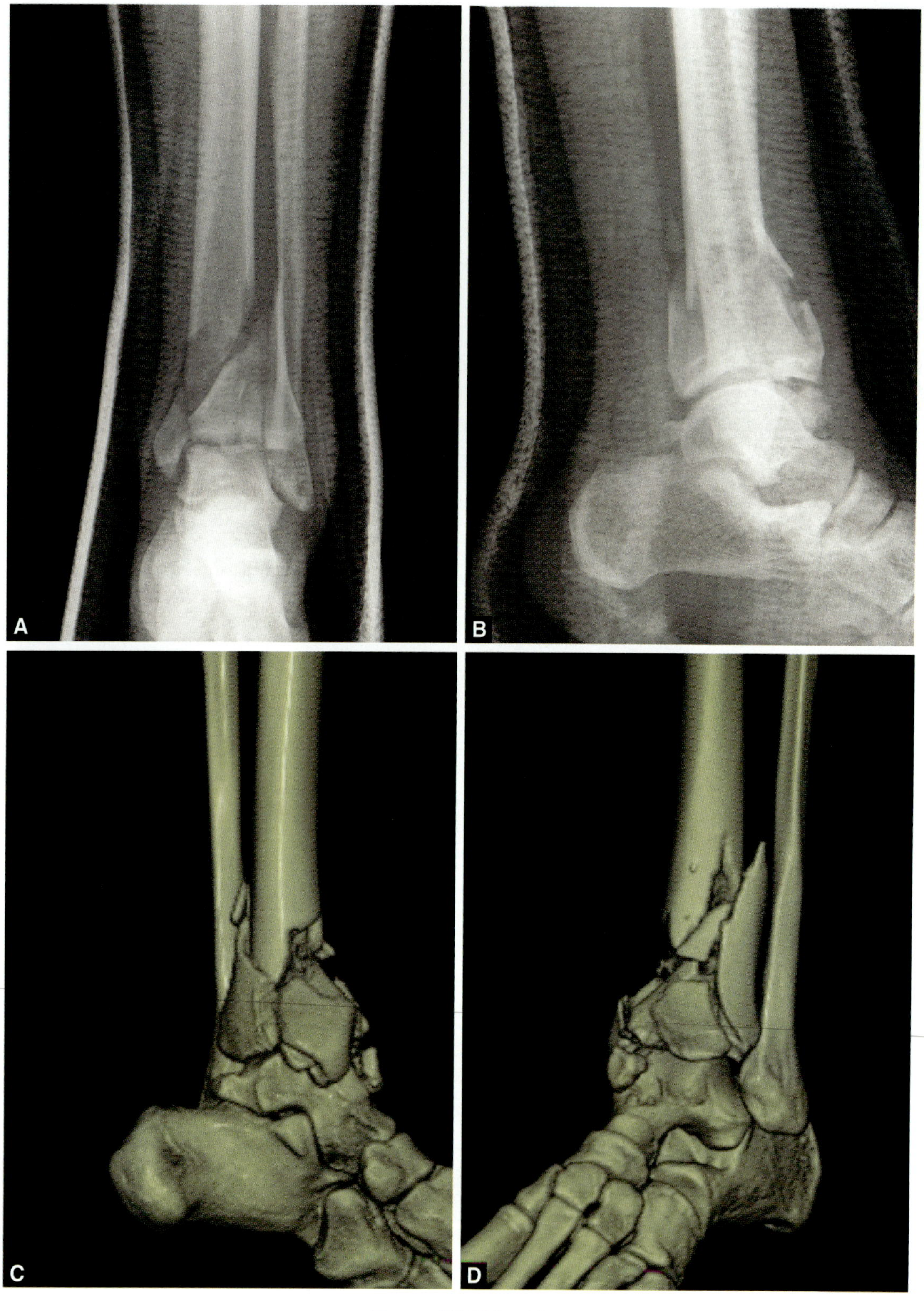

Figures 27.11A to D

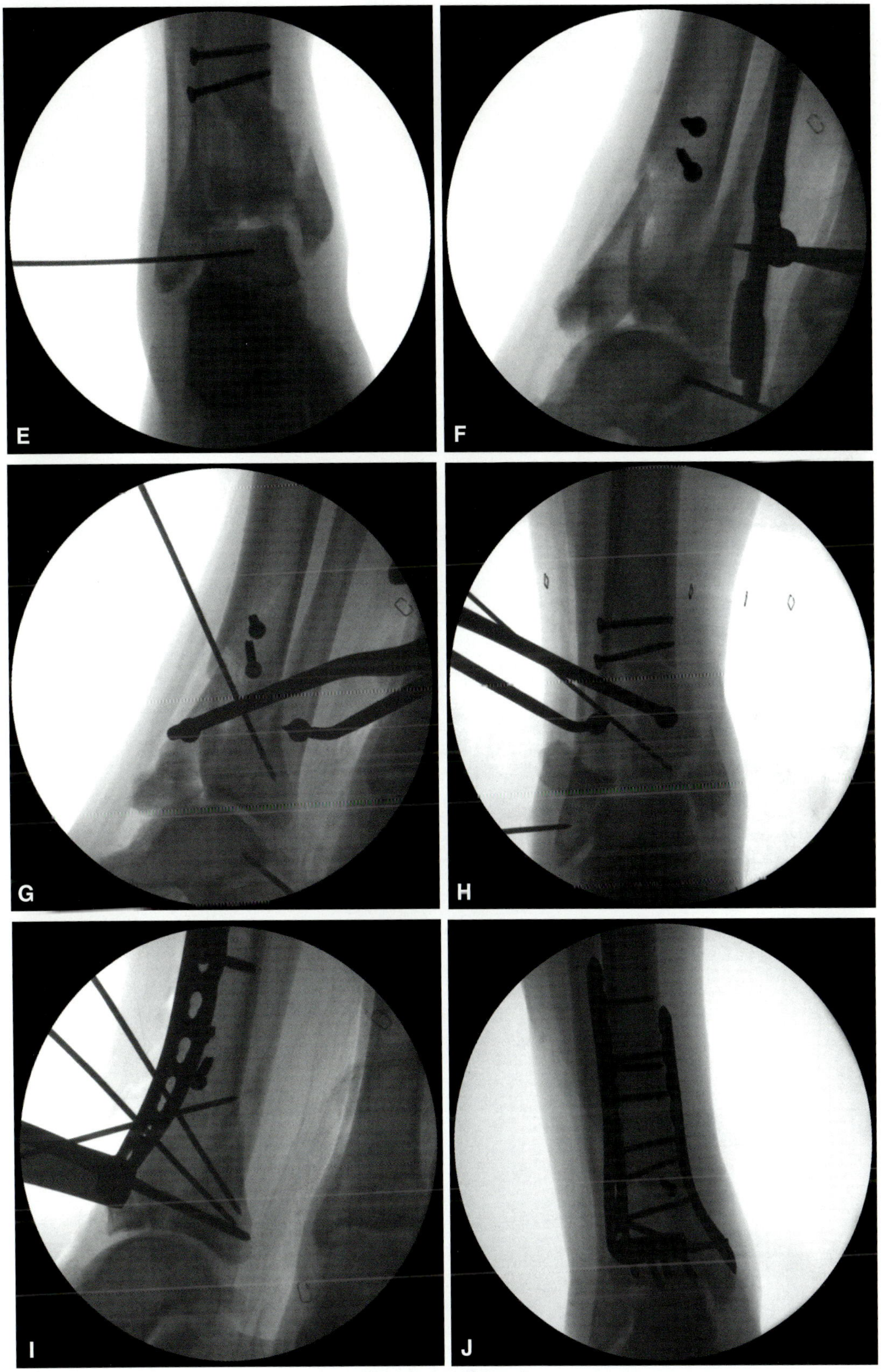

Figures 27.11E to J

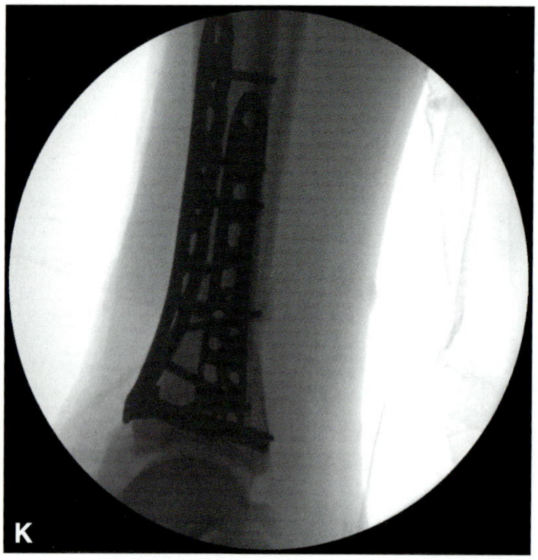

Figures 27.11A to K: Anterolateral approach for open reduction and internal fixation of a tibial pilon fracture. (A and B) Antero-posterior and lateral radiographs; (C and D) Three-dimensional CT images of a comminuted tibial pilon fracture; (E) Instead of using a large distractor, the intact fibula allows manual distraction of the ankle and placement of a Steinman pin from fibula to talus, maintaining slight distraction; (F to H) After initial lag screw fixation of metadiaphyseal fragments, the posterior articular fragment is reduced with the use of a pelvic reduction forcep; (I to K) Multiple intraoperative images demonstrate anterolateral and percutaneous medial locked plating of the distal tibia fracture.

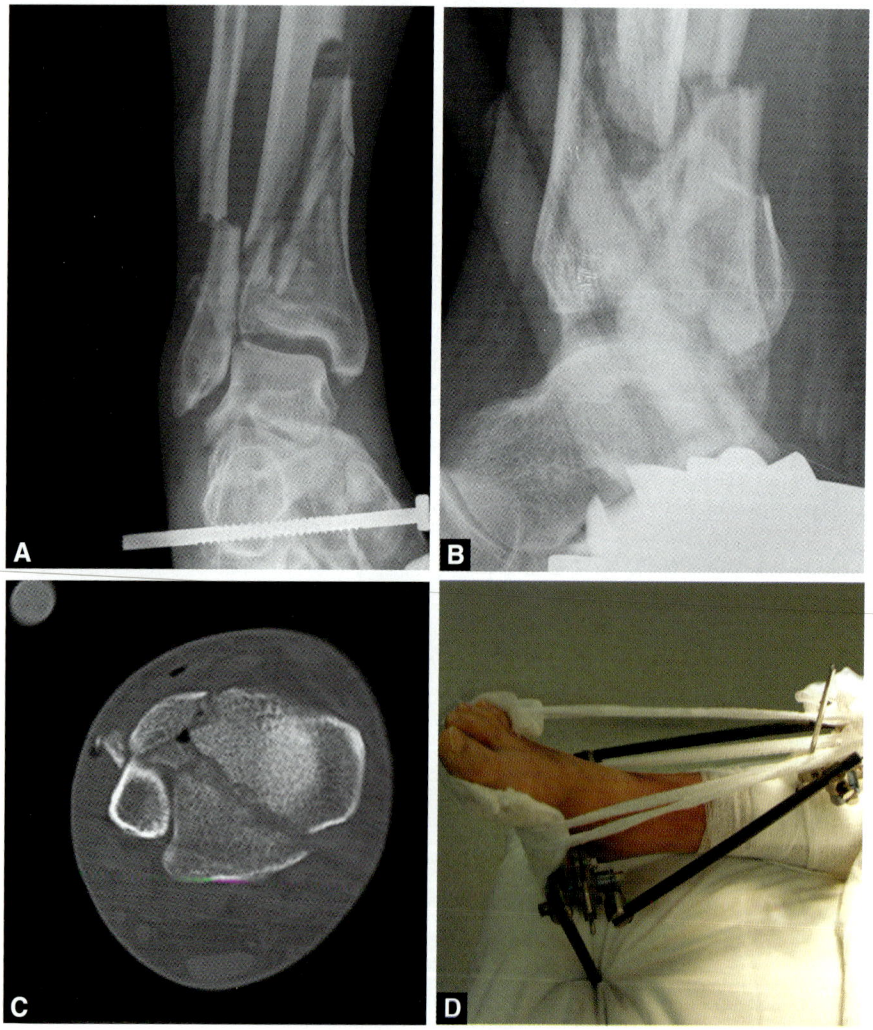

Figures 27.12A to D

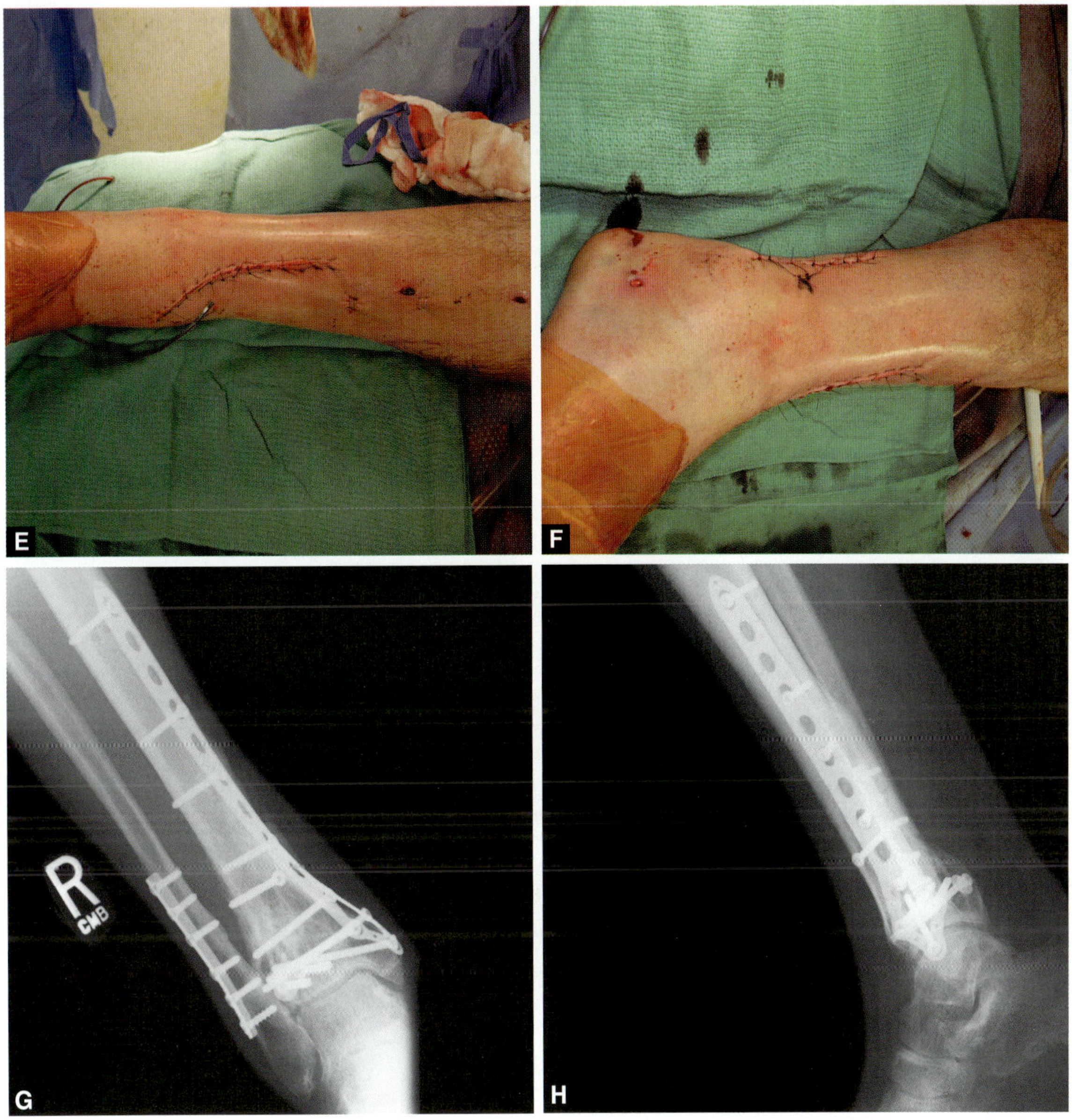

Figures 27.12A to H: Anteromedial approach for open reduction and internal fixation (ORIF) of a tibial pilon fracture. (A to C) Anteroposterior and lateral radiographs and axial CT scan of an open distal tibial fracture treated with irrigation, debridement and spanning external fixation; (D) Spanning external fixation with "hammock" to prevent equinus contracture. Alternatively, metatarsal pins can be placed and fixed to the frame; (E and F) Anteromedial and lateral approaches were done for ORIF of both distal tibia and fibula fractures. A small lateral open fracture wound is also seen; (G and H) Anteroposterior and lateral images after removal of external fixation and ORIF at follow-up demonstrating fractures healed. In this case, although anteromedial fixation was performed due to the metadiaphyseal fracture pattern, anterolateral fixation is also an option.

pin through the calcaneus. An extra fixation pin into midfoot cuneiforms or metatarsals may be necessary in order to keep the foot in neutral position and the talus well reduced beneath the tibia, certainly in fracture patterns with a large posterior fragment. This bridging configuration is quick and easy to apply, as well as safe, since the fixation elements are not placed directly in the distal tibia. The fixator should keep the extremity at length, but not distracted, which could result in a number of iatrogenic complications including neurovascular compromise and compartment syndrome. Pin placement in subcutaneous locations will minimize local irritation. The pins should never be placed

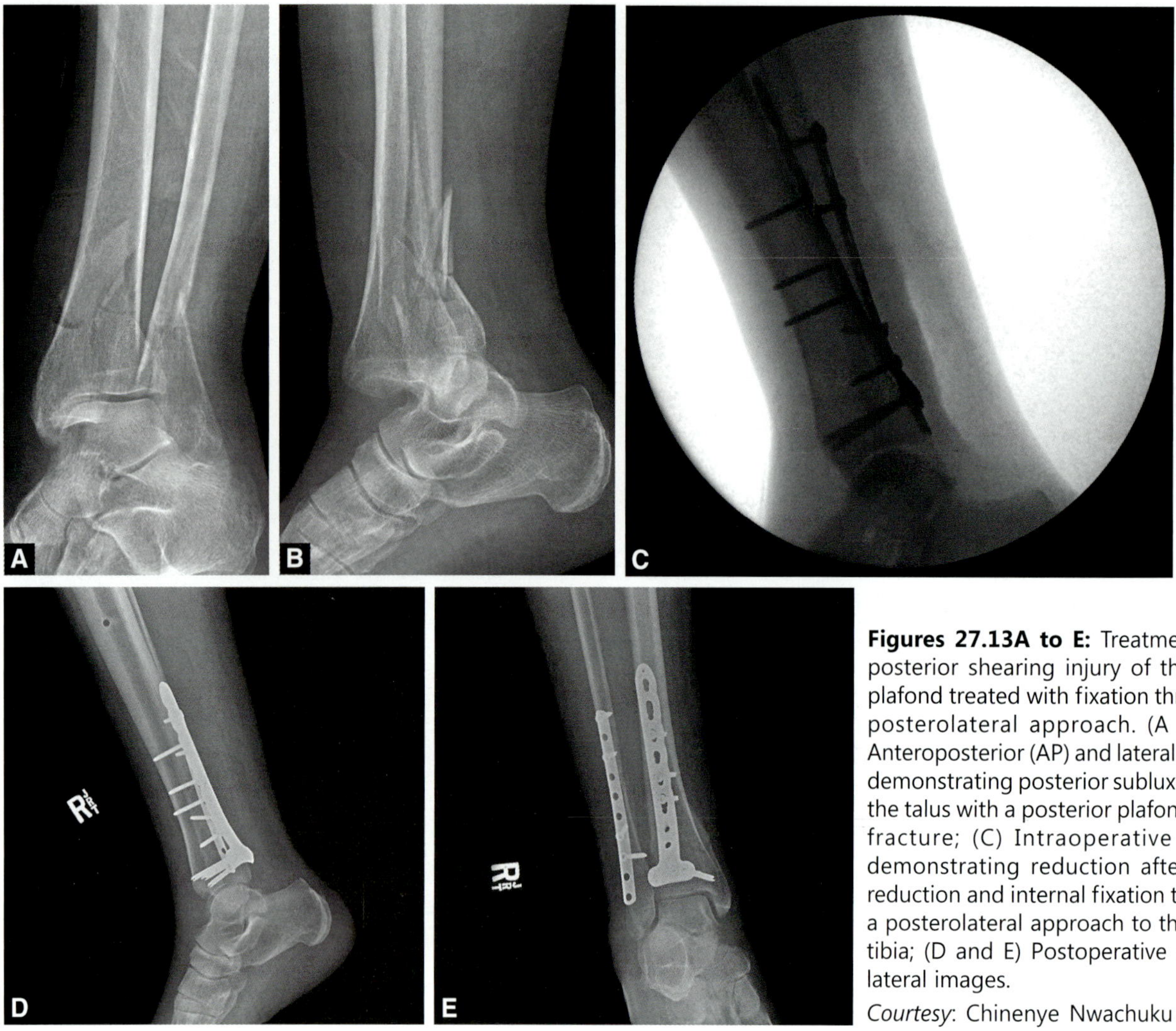

Figures 27.13A to E: Treatment of a posterior shearing injury of the tibial plafond treated with fixation through a posterolateral approach. (A and B) Anteroposterior (AP) and lateral images demonstrating posterior subluxation of the talus with a posterior plafond shear fracture; (C) Intraoperative image demonstrating reduction after open reduction and internal fixation through a posterolateral approach to the distal tibia; (D and E) Postoperative AP and lateral images.

Courtesy: Chinenye Nwachuku

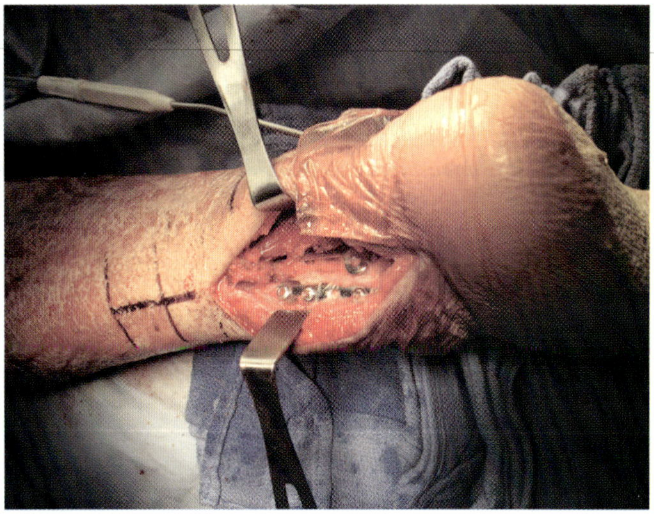

Figure 27.14: Intraoperative image of the posterolateral approach to the distal tibial plafond and distal fibula. This is performed between the peroneal musculature and flexor hallucis longus. The patient is prone and the fibula is towards bottom of the image.

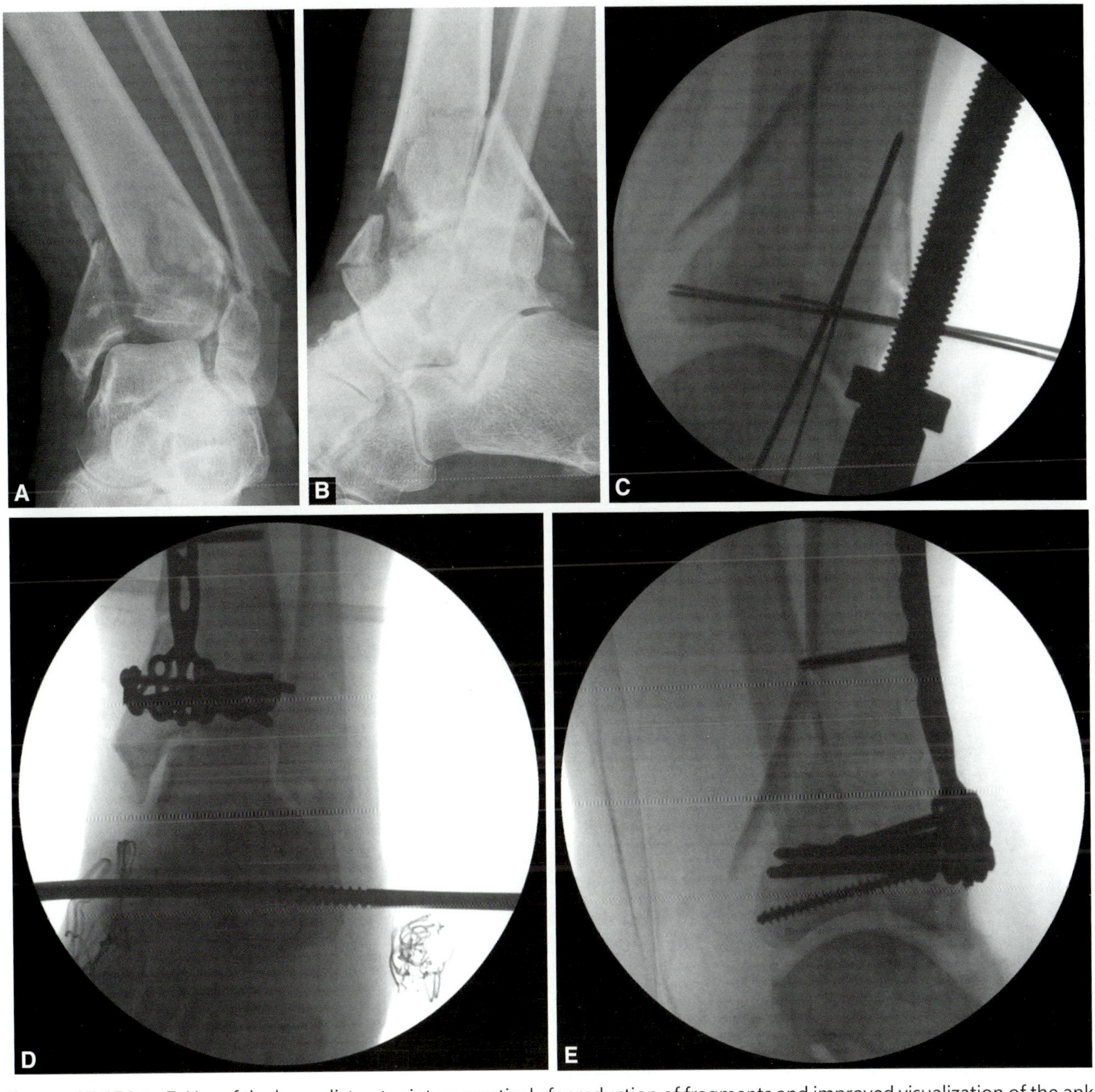

Figures 27.15A to E: Use of the large distractor intraoperatively for reduction of fragments and improved visualization of the ankle joint. (A and B) Anteroposterior and lateral radiographs of a comminuted tibial pilon and fibula fracture; (C to E) The patient had been initially treated with spanning external fixation. At the time of definitive fixation, the frame was removed and pins were kept in place for the procedure. The large distractor was placed utilizing the previous pins as shown. After provisional reduction and fixation with pins, an anteromedial malleable locked plate was placed for fixation. The distractor was then removed.

near anticipated surgical incisions. Increasing stiffness of the external fixator construct can be accomplished by adding sidebars, decreasing the distance of sidebar from center of the bone, increasing the separation of pins across the fracture fragment and increasing the number or diameter of pins (Figs 27.16A to G). Anatomical fibular fixation can frequently indirectly reduce the tibia due to its strong ligamentous attachments, as well as create a stable lateral column (see Figs 27.12A to H). It is often treated with direct open reduction through a posterolateral incision, which provides adequate skin bridge (minimum 7 cm), if an anterolateral approach is chosen for the distal tibia

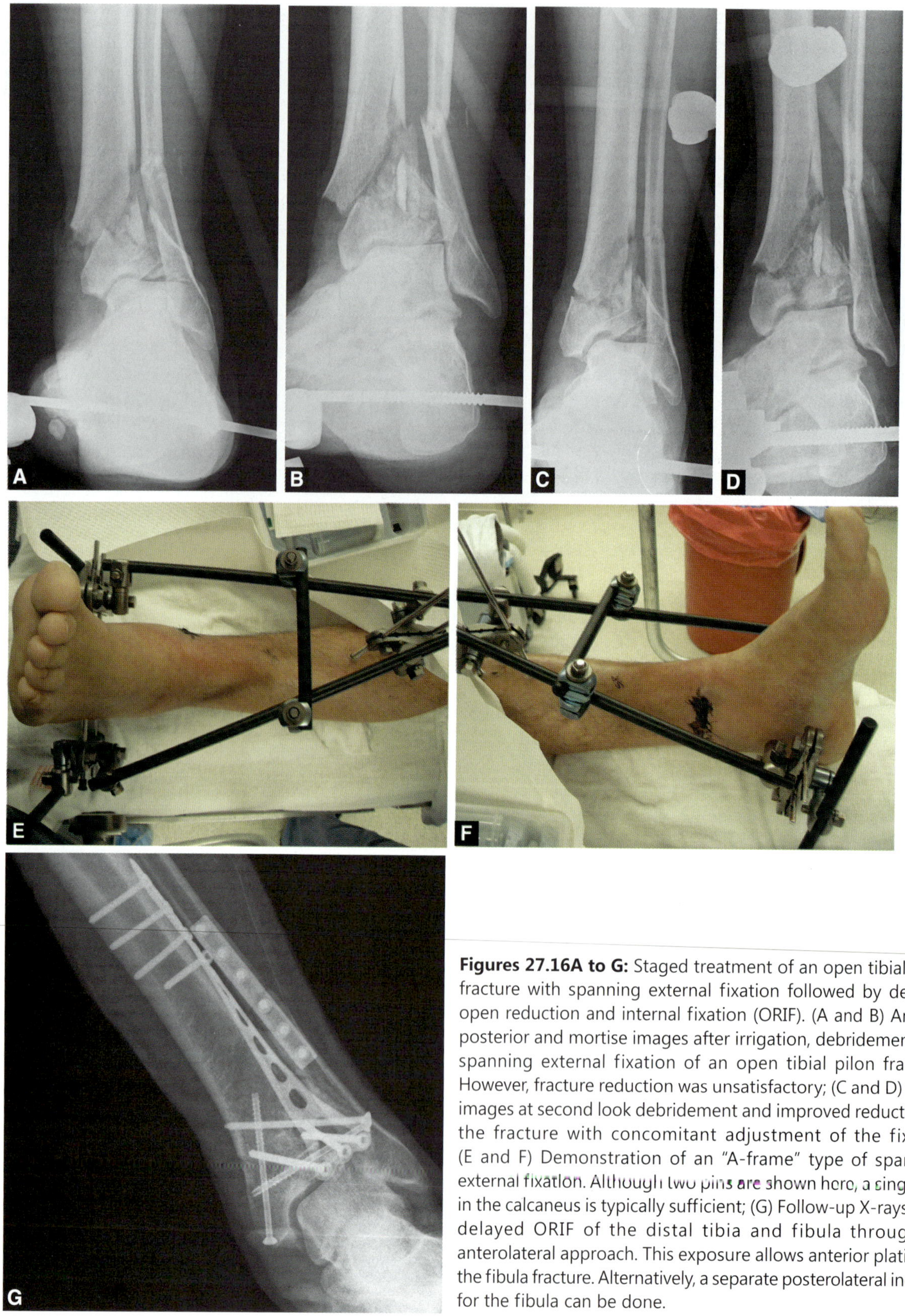

Figures 27.16A to G: Staged treatment of an open tibial pilon fracture with spanning external fixation followed by delayed open reduction and internal fixation (ORIF). (A and B) Anteroposterior and mortise images after irrigation, debridement and spanning external fixation of an open tibial pilon fracture. However, fracture reduction was unsatisfactory; (C and D) Same images at second look debridement and improved reduction of the fracture with concomitant adjustment of the fixator; (E and F) Demonstration of an "A-frame" type of spanning external fixation. Although two pins are shown here, a single pin in the calcaneus is typically sufficient; (G) Follow-up X-rays after delayed ORIF of the distal tibia and fibula through an anterolateral approach. This exposure allows anterior plating of the fibula fracture. Alternatively, a separate posterolateral incision for the fibula can be done.

reduction.[23-25] In our opinion, fibula fixation during Stage 1 should only be performed for simple oblique or transverse fracture patterns of the fibula, if there is confidence in obtaining anatomical reduction and that further surgical approaches will not be compromised. Furthermore, a malreduced distal fibula could inhibit the accuracy of distal tibial reduction, leading to impingement and malunion.

Timing: Timing for definitive treatment in pilon fractures is critical. Poor surgical timing virtually guarantees a poor outcome. The abrupt swelling that occurs with pilon fractures is initially the result of fracture hematoma. By 8–12 hours post injury, interstitial edema develops, further potentiating soft tissue compromise. The delay in definitive treatment may be days to weeks, and is dependent upon the severity of soft tissue injury, the speed of improvement, as well as the surgical treatment plan. Surgeons must wait for the subsidence of swelling, which typically takes 7–14 days.[11,19–21,23,26] It should be noted that a delay of greater than 3 weeks may create additional problems at the time of surgery. Beyond the average time frame, accumulation of granulation tissue at the site of injury occurs, signs of disuse osteoporosis arise, and bone resorption at the fracture site make ORIF technically more demanding and the likelihood of a achieving an anatomical articular reduction decreases. Vigilance toward the soft tissue envelope is imperative for appropriate surgical timing. Adequate evaluation of soft tissues includes assessment of swelling, visualize nature and extent of fracture blisters, allow hemorrhagic blisters to re-epithelialize prior to create a traversing incision,[5,6] recognition of the return of skin wrinkles, and a complete understanding of anticipated invasiveness of the planned surgical approach.

Definitive Treatment Planning: Characterizing the fracture fragments from CT and injury radiographs guides the request for appropriate surgical instruments, determination of the final fixation construct and allows for more rapid surgical treatment with less dissection of soft tissues. Axial cuts from the CT scan obtained after external fixation provide the most specific and helpful information in surgical planning. When evaluating the injury radiographs, consideration must be made toward the primary failure mode. For instance, varus angulation of the distal tibia as commonly occurs with tension failure of the fibula will require a medial buttressing implant to prevent varus malunion. Similarly, valgus angulation of the distal tibia that commonly occurs with a compressive failure of the fibula will require an anterolateral buttress plate at the distal tibia. In some cases, both anterior and medial fixation is required (Figs 27.17A to D). Common instruments typically required for definitive treatment include pointed reduction clamps, dental picks, Kirschner (K-wires), small- and mini-fragment screws, multiple-sized plates (locking plates for patients with osteopenia or those with metaphyseal bone loss), bone tamps and distracters. Patients are most often positioned supine on a radiolucent table and a pneumatic tourniquet is used for better visualization of the surgical field intraoperatively.

Stage 2

The general approach for reconstruction of the distal tibial articular surface was outlined by Ruedi and Allgower in 1969.[11] The steps in sequential order are: correction of fibular length, anatomical reconstruction of tibial articular surface, bone grafting of metaphyseal defects and stable fixation by reattachment of metaphysis to diaphysis. Waddell proposed a further detailed description of pilon fixation: (1) restoration of fibular length, (2) anterior ankle arthrotomy, (3) external fixator for ankle distraction, (4) restoration of articular fragments in stepwise fashion—lateral fragments, central, bone graft and medial fragments, (5) anterolateral versus medial buttress plating.[27]

Fibula fixation is often the first step, as it often creates the foundation for a stable lateral column, if length and rotation are accurately reproduced. Anatomical reduction of the fibula may also reduce anterolateral and posterolateral fragments of the tibia due to maintained integrity of the ATFL and PTFL. It is the surgeon's preference in determining whether the fibula is fixed in stage one or two, as well as in plate choices, where one-third tubular, 3.5 mm dynamic compression plates and antiglide plates are often available. In instances of severe fibular comminution potentially leading to nonanatomical reduction, the fibula may best be fixed after distal tibial reconstruction, so as to avoid impingement that could prevent anatomical reduction of the tibiotalar articulation and excess loads on the lateral articular surface.[12,23,28]

Reconstruction of articular fragments often begins with the lateral column. Hematoma, debris and early callus are removed from the fracture fragments prior to temporarily stabilization with K-wires. Typically, the sequence of reduction begins with posterolateral fragment, then posteromedial, central, anterior and anterolateral, sequentially. The anterolateral and medial fragments can be rotated around their ligamentous attachments to better visualize the

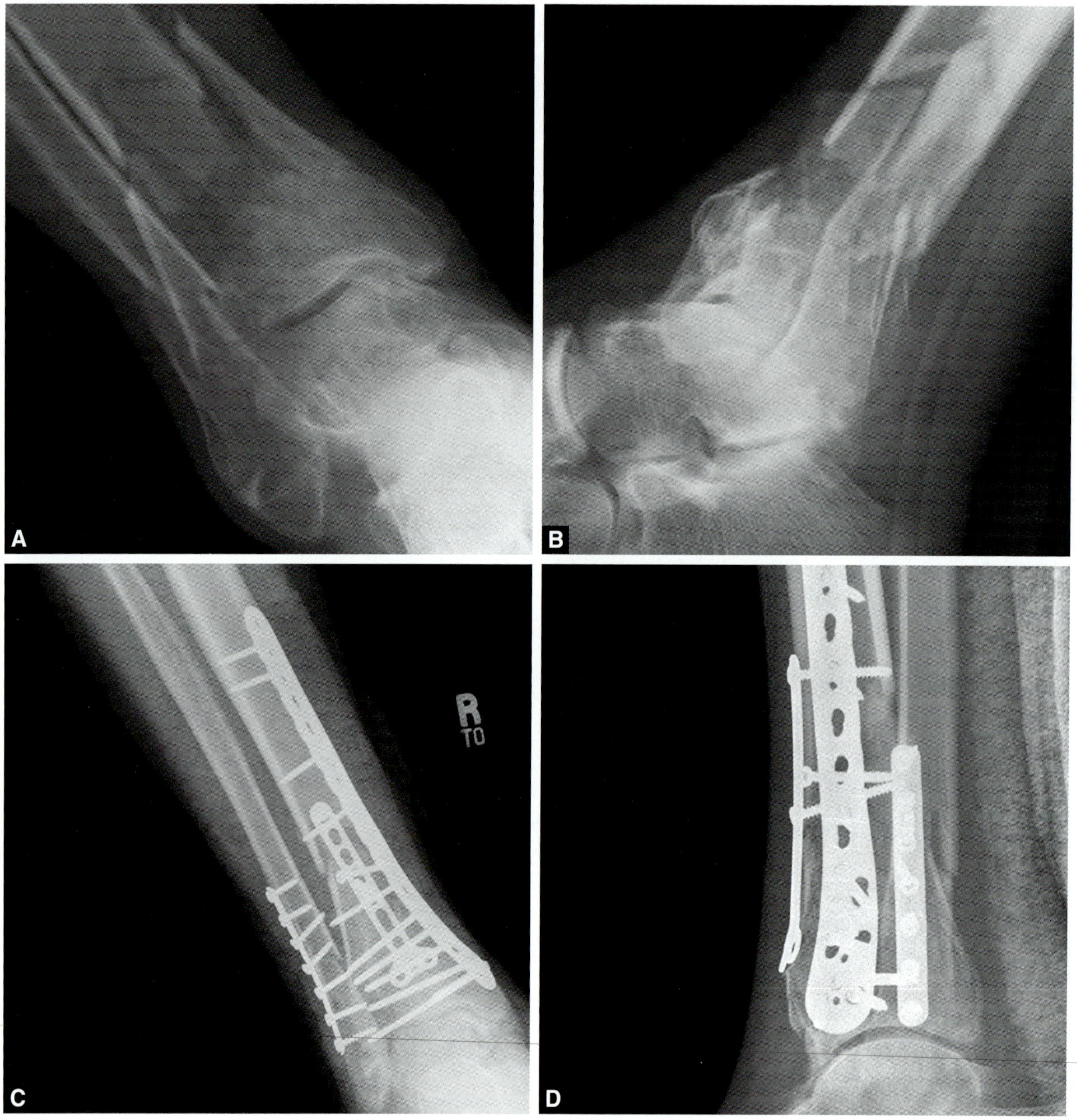

Figures 27.17A to D: Use of both anterior and medial fixation for a comminuted distal tibia fracture. (A and B) Preoperative and (C and D) postoperative radiographs of a comminuted tibial pilon fracture, which was treated with anterior and medial plate fixation through an anteromedial exposure. In this case, the anterior plate acts as a spring plate for supporting comminuted fragments.

posterior aspect of the tibial plafond and any central impaction. The articular surface of talus serves as a template for adequate reduction of the tibial plafond. Once anatomical reduction is verified both visually and fluoroscopically, K-wires are replaced with small-fragment screws with the goal of achieving interfragmentary compression.

Impaction often leaves defects between the joint and shaft after the articular surface is elevated and reduced. Bone graft is placed in these defects prior to plate fixation.

Although the "gold standard" is autologous iliac crest bone graft, cancellous allograft chips and bone substitutes are available without any morbidity associated with the harvest of autologous bone graft.

Once the articular surface has been reduced and bone graft has been utilized to fill remaining bone defects, the overall fracture configuration is fixed with buttress plating. The location of plating is dependent upon the initial injury radiographs, which depict the mode of failure. Most pilon fractures fail in varus and therefore, are ultimately stabilized with a medial buttress plate. An anterolateral L-shaped plate is used for those fractures that initially failed in valgus. For improved fit about the distal tibia, the plates need to be contoured prior to use. Also available are small clover-leaf plates, T-shaped plates and percutaneous anatomical specific plates that are precontoured for anteromedial and anterolateral tibia.

Partial articular (AO/OTA type B) distal tibia fractures are treated with direct articular visualization and reduction with surgical approach chosen based on the best access to the fragment involved. Fixation in these cases is by interfragmentary compression and buttress plate fixation in most cases (Figs 27.18A to D).

Postoperative Care

Elevation is critical for first few days after ORIF is performed on pilon fractures. Surgery in itself is a sort of second-hit phenomenon after the initial injury that will again initiate an inflammatory response. Therefore, strict elevation will help protect the skin closure from any wound dehiscence resulting from excessive swelling. A drain is often placed at the time of definitive surgery to decrease the amount of retained fluid within the wound. The drain is typically removed after 48 hours, or when the output drops to below 15 ml/8 hours. Prophylactic antibiotic coverage is continued for 24 hours. Once the surgical wounds have sealed after typically 48 hours, gentle ankle and subtalar range of motion exercises are initiated. A dorsiflexion splint is also used until the patient begins weight bearing in order to prevent an equinus contracture. Patients are kept non-weight bearing for 8–12 weeks, and then undergo progressive weight bearing to full weight bearing over the course of 4 weeks.[23,29] Union typically is achieved by 10–16 weeks.[15,19,20,23]

Special Considerations

Open fractures complicate the already arduous task of fixing pilon fractures. Patients should receive appropriate intravenous (IV) antibiotics at first notice of the open fracture. These are typically continued prophylactically for 72 hours after injury, or modified and continued based on specificity of a positive culture. Debridement and irrigation are meticulously accomplished in the operating room. Most wounds tend to be medial sided, owing to their thin subcutaneous nature (See Fig. 27.2). One should always plan for subsequent procedures and avoid extending wound edges in such a way that may create a nonviable flap when combined with subsequent planned surgical approach for fixation. Retain all articular fragments, while at times diaphyseal devitalized cortical fragments may be removed. Keep in mind that defects noted in this first debridement stage may be filled with antibiotic beads until definitive fixation, which also helps maintain length and prevent soft tissue interposition. After thorough debridement and irrigation are completed, the extremity is placed into external fixation to re-establish extremity length and assist in resolution of swelling. Certain grossly contaminated wounds are often taken back to the operating room for multiple washouts until infection can be definitively ruled out. In rare instances, with a low energy, simple articular fracture pattern, primary ORIF can be accomplished with minimally invasive techniques through the open wound. Confidence in timeliness and completeness of the debridement are absolute prerequisites for this rare primary fixation.

A solid understanding of a number of different surgical considerations, including choice of implant, will help minimize operative risk. First and foremost, delay until definitive surgical treatment, while stabilized in external fixation certainly decreases soft tissue complications. However, excessive delays are not without risk. Delays longer than 3–4 weeks have increased risk of pin-tract infections, increased difficulty in surgical reduction, as well as patient dissatisfaction and intolerance to the frame.[30,31] Therefore, it is imperative that the soft tissue envelope should be checked weekly for resolution of inflammation and return of skin wrinkles so that surgery can be scheduled in an appropriate time frame. Surgical considerations such as using tissue sparing indirect techniques as well as

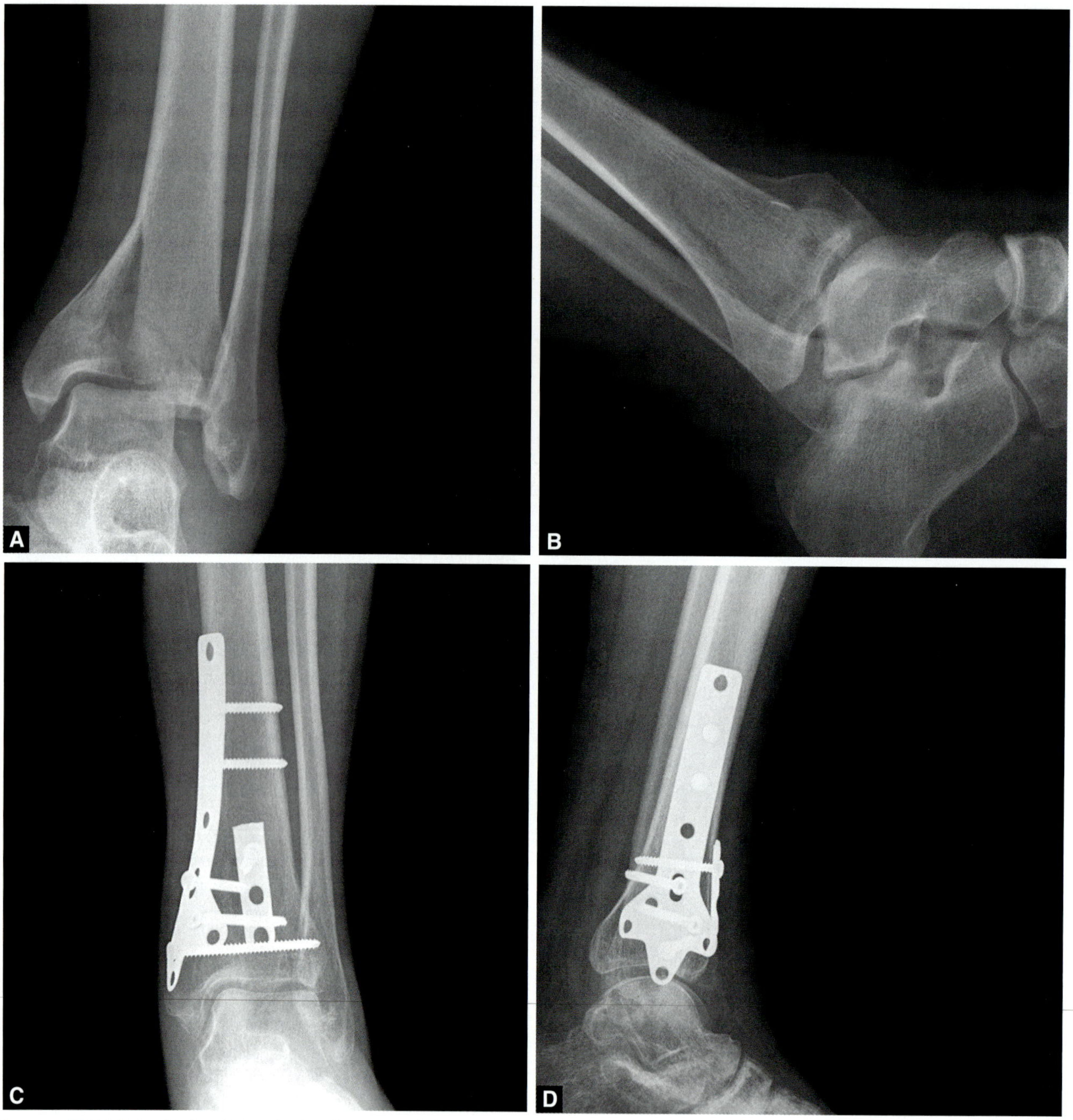

Figures 27.18A to D: Partial articular fracture of the medial plafond treated with open reduction and internal fixation and traditional nonlocked buttress plate fixation. (A and B) Anteroposterior (AP) and lateral preoperative radiographs demonstrating the fracture. Note that the posterior cortex and posterior articular surface are intact. An anteromedial approach was utilized and ORIF was performed; (C and D) Standard cloverleaf plate buttress fixation was performed with an accessory anterior spring plate as shown on postoperative AP and lateral radiographs.

avoiding anteromedial incisions when possible (higher risk of wound complications due to its thin subcutaneous nature) will also decrease operative risk. Finally, the evolution of small, lower profile implants has not only improved patient satisfaction of outcomes, but again, has decreased the risk of wound complications.

Extra-articular distal tibial fractures require special consideration. Many are still of high energy and therefore, require delayed fixation as the soft tissue envelope remains at risk. Already described are anteromedial and anterolateral approaches, which can be extended to allow fixation of extra-articular distal tibial fractures. They may be fixed with anteromedial or lateral plating techniques. Extra-articular spiral fractures of lower energy may be fixed with lag screw fixation followed by a neutralization plate using the anteromedial approach. The option of intramedullary nail fixation for extra-articular distal tibial fractures also becomes available with inclusion of locking screws near the distal tip of the nail. Typically, the malleolar fractures are stabilized first. The nail itself will not assist in reducing the fracture due to the large volume of cancellous bone at the metaphysis; therefore, maintenance of tibial alignment and reduction during all stages of fixation is imperative (reaming, nail delivery, distal interlock screw placement). This can be achieved by temporary unicortical plating, percutaneous clamps, ensuring the guidewire is center-center, fibular plating to establish a stable lateral column, and screws that are 90° to one another to assist in control of the distal most segment.[1,2]

STAGED TREATMENT OF PILON FRACTURES: Pearls and Pitfalls

- Pilon fractures requiring reconstruction are best treated by a staged approach at most institutions and in most surgeon's hands. This involves initial spanning external fixation followed by delayed ORIF and reconstruction of articular fragments. Partial articular fractures and centers with round-the-clock availability of surgeons with experience in treating pilon fractures are possible exceptions
- Fibular fixation at the time of spanning external fixation should only be done in cases with simple fibular fracture patterns that can be confidently fixed anatomically. Ideally, there should also be a clear understanding of where the incisions for definitive treatment will be placed. When in doubt (which is frequently the case), it is better to leave the fibula and let the fixator keep fractures out to length
- Fixator pins should be placed proximal enough in the tibial shaft, so that they are out of the zone of future tibial plate fixation. Whereas these distant pins make the frame less rigid, they still provide traction across the fracture and are not meant to be definitive treatment devices in most cases
- If possible, attempts should be made to keep the foot relatively plantigrade with adjunctive straps, slings, foot plates or fixator pins in the foot, if necessary
- Computerized tomography scanning is best done after spanning external fixation for proper reconstructive preoperative planning

ANTEROMEDIAL APPROACH AND OPEN REDUCTION AND INTERNAL FIXATION: Pearls and Pitfalls

- Consider this approach for medial partial articular fractures and those with clear need for medial-sided support
- Extremely thin patients and patients with skin compromise on the medial distal leg can preclude the safe placement of fixation medially
- During dissection, try not to disrupt the paratenon over the tibialis anterior tendon. If wound healing becomes a problem, an exposed tendon without paratenon coverage will be more difficult to treat

ANTEROLATERAL APPROACH AND OPEN REDUCTION AND INTERNAL FIXATION: Pearls and Pitfalls

- Consider this approach for fractures involving better access to the anterolateral plafond fragments and any case with skin compromise over the medial distal leg and ankle
- The superficial peroneal nerve will be directly in the field throughout the case. Take care not to excessively retract or injure this, and warn the patient of potential dorsal foot sensory disturbances postoperatively
- Whereas, distal lateral malleolus fractures requiring fixation will require a separate posterolateral incision, many distal fibula shaft fractures can be fixed anteriorly through the same anterolateral pilon exposure

POSTEROLATERAL APPROACH AND OPEN REDUCTION AND INTERNAL FIXATION: Pearls and Pitfalls

- Consider this approach for fractures that have primarily a posterior shearing component, particularly with posterior subluxation or dislocation of the talus. Direct buttressing of the posterior plafond fragments is best achieved with this approach
- It is also an alternative approach to the plafond for cases in which the anteromedial or anterolateral soft tissues and skin are not amenable to surgical incisions
- Do not expect to have good visualization of the tibiotalar joint. The joint is difficult or impossible to properly view from the posterolateral approach. If both direct posterior buttressing as well as reduction of centrally-impacted fragments are required, then sequential surgical approaches might be necessary
- The fibula can be reduced and fixed through the same surgical approach for the majority of fracture patterns

Outcomes

If severe complications are avoided, most pilon fractures heal after initial treatment. Yet, even after near-anatomic union, many follow-up studies continue to show suboptimal results with significant pain and arthrosis. There are many nonsurgical factors, both patient related and resultant from the initial injury that are directly related to outcomes after surgical treatment of pilon fractures. All axial loading injuries damage the articular cartilage and cause some, almost instantaneous, chondrocyte death. It is the severity of the initial injury that has a significant impact on the prognosis of joint function. Even after stable anatomical reduction and fixation is achieved, there is a high prevalence of post-traumatic osteoarthritis, certainly in the AO type 43-C3 fracture patterns. Anatomical articular reduction and stable fixation will absolutely optimize eventual ankle function; however, many studies have shown that the initial articular injury may have the largest impact on overall postoperative function.[15,29,32] Another study by DeCoster and associates found that patients' subjective assessment of their outcome was not related to the quality of reduction or the severity of articular injury, concluding that soft tissue injury and complications have a high impact on patient's perception of successful treatment.[33] Furthermore, patient factors such as diabetes, immunosuppression, smoking history, alcoholism and peripheral vascular disease further complicate the already delicate condition of soft tissue injuries associated with pilon fractures, thus affecting potential outcomes. What has been shown through multiple reports is a decrease in the complication rate and improvement in near anatomical union in those pilon fractures treated with a staged protocol.[6,10,13]

Complications

Complications are encountered that result from both the injury and treatment. Stiffness, soft tissue compromise, pin-tract infection, deep infection, osteomyelitis, malunion, nonunion and arthritis continue to arise as complications; although, the incidence of each has decreased since more attention has been placed on the protection of soft tissues. Stiffness is common and appears to be the same regardless of which treatment technique is chosen. Most patients will lose about 10° of dorsiflexion and plantarflexion,[19] yet will still have a functional extremity and joint. Soft tissue compromise is often correlated with injury severity although it has certainly decreased in incidence since the evolution of staged protocols and delayed primary fixation.[19–21,29] It is likely attributed to poor vascularity, especially over the anteromedial surface of the tibia; and can lead to wound dehiscence, skin sloughing, stasis ulceration and infection.[34] Most pin-tract infections are successfully treated with oral antibiotics and adequate pin-site care. Pin-site infections not cured with antibiotics may need aggressive debridement and irrigation as well as IV antibiotics. Most infections originate in the soft tissues and spread deep to the bone. Similar to wound complications, higher rates of infection appear related to perform ORIF during the acute period.[15] Chronic osteomyelitis is one of the most devastating complications. It was more common previously when incisions were made through compromised tissues and often led to arthrodesis and even amputation.[34] Malunion and nonunion are more common after higher-energy, more severe pilon fractures, likely due to more soft tissue stripping. The treatment of malunion and nonunion is difficult and often requires a combination of correction of the deformity, bone grafting and repeated stabilization. Arthrosis will likely always be a potential complication after an articular fracture, resulting from the initial irreversible cartilage damage. It will occur in essentially 100% of those patients with poor reduction, yet often times, the report of pain or lack thereof does not correspond with the radiographical images after a traumatic event. The initial treatment for arthrosis after pilon fractures remains activity modification, nonsteroidal anti-inflammatory drugs and rocker-bottom shoes to reduce pain. If these conservative measures fail, tibiotalar arthrodesis and total ankle arthroplasty are potential surgical options and must be tailored to each specific patient's condition and needs.

Authors' Preferred Management of Select Complications

Case 1: Treatment of Recalcitrant Nonunion of the Distal Tibial Shaft and Pilon Fracture with Nonunion Repair and Fusion of the Ankle and Subtalar Joints with Retrograde Fusion Nail

This case involves a 52-year-old female nurse, who was involved in a motor vehicle crash sustaining an open distal tibia and fibula fracture with extension into the distal tibial shaft. She was initially treated with irrigation and debridement and spanning external fixation. Subsequently, she underwent delayed surgical reconstruction of the distal tibia and fibula, which unfortunately resulted in a nonunion. Nonunion repair was attempted three times with bone grafting and revision fixation (first time with autografting, second time with bone morphogenetic protein-7 (BMP-7) and allograft, and third time with concentrated iliac crest stem cells and allograft), unfortunately without success (Figs 27.19A and B). At this point, it had been 4 years since her original injury, and she had not been able to ambulate comfortably with fracture bracing and was unable to work due to persistent pain and instability. An infection workup including serological testing, nuclear scanning and bone biopsies and cultures did not reveal any obvious sign of infection. On physical examination, there was apparent motion at the fracture site, but no obvious motion at the ankle or subtalar joints.

At this point, the surgeon discussed her options with her and a decision was made to either consider a below-knee amputation and prosthetic fitting, or one more attempt at reconstruction to try and get her fractures heal. She did not wish to proceed with an amputation, as her foot was still sensate and toes were mobile. However, her ankle was painful and stiff, and radiographic review demonstrated degenerative changes of the ankle joint. Reconstructive options included another attempt at nonunion repair with or without fusion of the ankle joint. With her multiple surgical incisions, previous failures with plate fixation and the need for a stable limb to walk on, we decided to perform nonunion repair with fusion of the ankle joint and retrograde nail fixation. The subtalar joint did not absolutely require fusion, but was already completely stiff as a result of her exceedingly prolonged immobilization. Retrograde nail fixation would require subtalar joint fusion as well as ankle joint fusion.

Medial and lateral surgical approaches were performed to remove the broken implants and debride the nonunion site of fibrous tissues, until there was bony bleeding. Both approaches were used to prepare the ankle joint surfaces for fusion. The lateral approach was extended to the subtalar joint and joint surfaces were prepared for fusion. Retrograde fusion nail fixation was performed as shown in Figures 27.19C to E. Autograft bone was performed at the ankle and subtalar joints as well as the metadiaphyseal tibial nonunion. She was subsequently immobilized in a fracture brace and was allowed to bear weight at 3 months postoperatively. Although, she did go on to heal, a stress fracture occurred at the tip of the nail, which fortunately did not displace, but was temporarily painful, preventing ambulation for several weeks. Ultimately, her fractures healed and joints fused successfully and she was able to return to work as a nurse (Figs 27.19F and G).

The key points of this case are as follows:

- The retrograde fusion nail is considered a salvage treatment and not the first line for the management of distal tibial nonunions. It requires fusion of both the ankle and subtalar joints, which is not frequently indicated. However, in this case, she had already failed other multiple attempts and her ankle joint was painful and arthritic.
- If there was any sign of infection or history of infection during the course of treatment of this patient, the

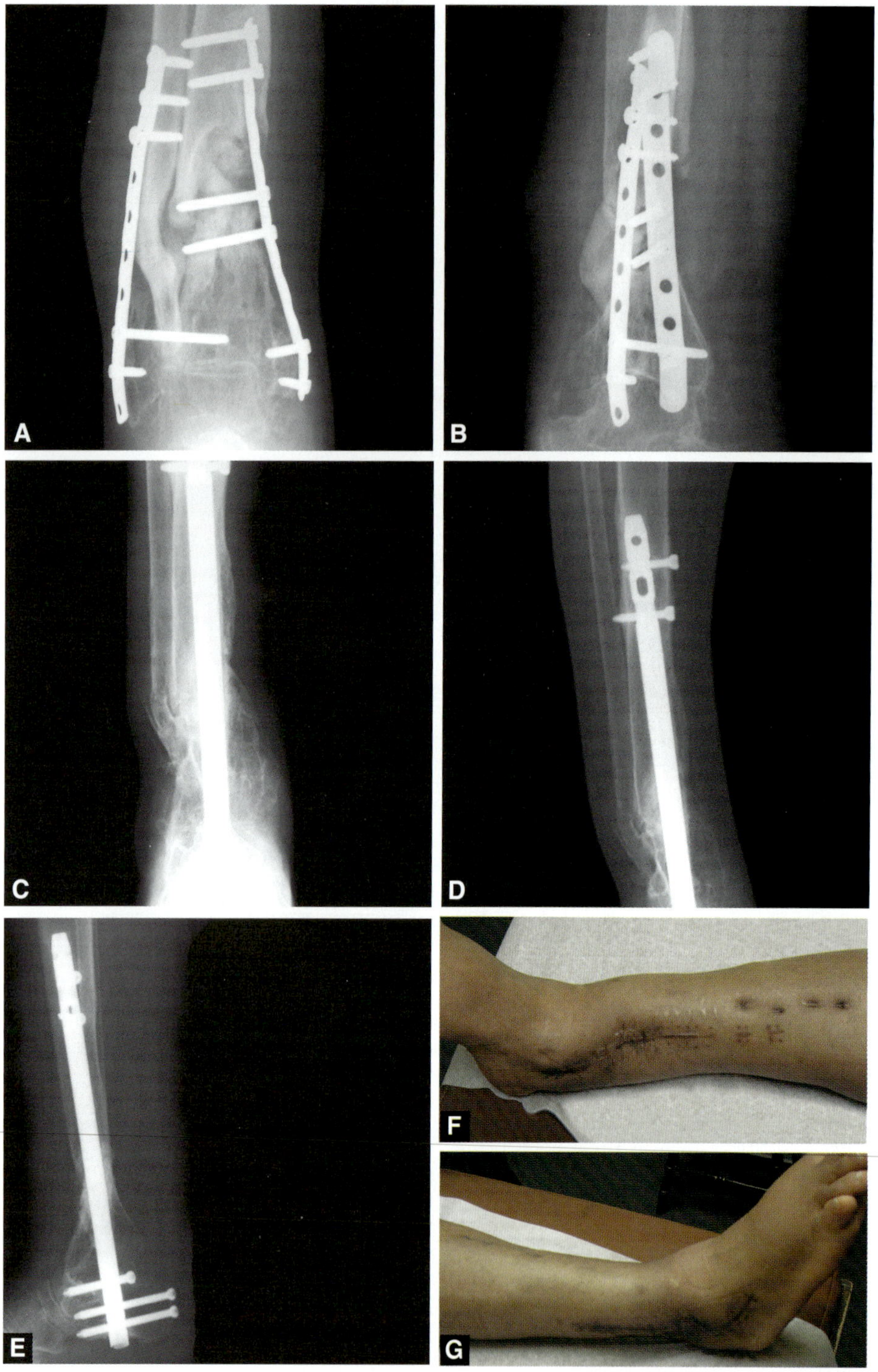

Figures 27.19A to G: Management of nonunion of the distal tibia with post-traumatic arthritis of the ankle joint with retrograde fusion nail. (A and B) Anteroposterior and lateral views of the ankle after multiple surgeries for an open distal tibial fracture including attempted nonunion repair. Post-traumatic arthritis of the tibiotalar joint and persistent metadiaphyseal nonunion are apparent; (C to E) Multiple follow-up radiographs after nonunion repair with bone grafting and fusion of ankle and subtalar joints. Both the nonunion site and visions are healed. The deformity created a stress riser at the proximal tip of the nail. This developed a stress fracture, which is healed in these radiographs; (F and G) Clinical images at 1 year post fusion and nonunion repair at which point, the patient had returned to work.

surgeon would be more hesitant to use the retrograde nail and instead, would consider circular external fixation methods. However, the nail does not require pin care and the inconveniences of fixator management. Although weight bearing may be technically possible with the frame, most patients with foot rings will not bear weight, thereby delaying return to function. The nail also gives the surgeon more confidence in allowing earlier weight bearing than with plate and screw fixation.
- Stress fractures and intraoperative fractures at the proximal tip of the nail can occur particularly in a case in which some deformity exists (like this particular case).

Case 2: Treatment of Nonunion Repair of Distal Tibia Fracture with Revision Open Reduction and Internal Fixation and Autologous Bone Grafting

This case involves a 30-year-old male, who sustained a closed intra-articular distal tibia and fibula fractures as a result of an assault. This was initially treated with spanning external fixation and percutaneous wire fixation of articular fragments (Figs 27.20A to D). At this point, he was referred to the surgeon for further management. After 2 weeks, he underwent what was hoped to be definitive reconstruction of his distal tibia and fibula fractures through anteromedial and lateral approaches. After surgical repair, he started range of motion exercises at 2 weeks and was allowed weight bearing at 3 months. At 5 months, he still had significant pain with and without weight bearing, and had been unable to return to work. Radiographs and CT scan demonstrated that the fracture was incompletely healed (Figs 27.20E to G). A workup for infection including blood tests—Erythrocyte sedimentation rate (ESR) and C-reactive protein (CRP) and nuclear scanning were negative. In the absence of any positive or equivocal testing, bone biopsy specimens were not obtained and he was indicated for nonunion repair of the distal tibia rather than continuing to wait. The medial plate had also become somewhat prominent in this patient, even after removal of one symptomatic distal screw. The stable-appearing fixation did not require revision otherwise, but in this case, a decision was made to revise to prevent further prominence and irritation. Although the plate was quite thin, the contouring and positioning was not perfect, subsequently resulting in prominence distally.

Nonunion repair was performed with revision internal fixation with a locked medial plate, excision of all intervening fibrous tissue and autologous iliac crest bone grafting. The fibula was left alone. The fracture went on to heal and the patient was able to return to work without further complications (Figs 27.20H to K).

The key points of this case are as follows:
- In contradistinction to the preceding case, there was no indication for fusion of the ankle. Bone grafting with osteoinductive material was indicated for an atrophic nonunion, which was derived from the iliac crest in this case.
- In this case, the plate required revision due to imperfect contouring and resultant skin irritation distally. However, the alignment and fixation was otherwise satisfactory. If the plate had not been irritating him, I would have considered leaving the fixation and performed bone grafting alone. In general, if the fixation is adequate in the setting of an atrophic nonunion, bone grafting can be done, while leaving the fixation in place.

Case 3: Treatment of Infected Nonunion of the Distal Tibia with Radical Resection and Bone Transport Distraction Osteogenesis

This case involves a 54-year-old man who sustained a grade 2 open distal tibia and fibula fractures with significant metadiaphyseal involvement. This was initially treated with multiple debridements and spanning external fixation with percutaneous reduction and screw fixation of the distal tibial articular fragments. Unfortunately, a deep infection occurred before definitive reduction and internal fixation could be performed. After multiple debridements and antibiotic bead treatment, an infected nonunion persisted (Fig. 27.21A). This was treated by multiple bony debridements and attempts at bone grafting with both autogenous and off the shelf BMPs. Intermittent drainage also persisted indicating failure of eradication of chronic osteomyelitis. Two years after his initial injury, the surgeon made a decision to proceed with radical resection, application of a bone transport frame and placement of an antibiotic spacer block at the distal metadiaphyseal tibia.

A proximal corticotomy was performed and standard methods of distraction osteogenesis were performed (Fig. 27.21B). His infection was successfully eradicated and his bone transport was successful. Bone grafting was repeated at the docking site distally at 4 months and this

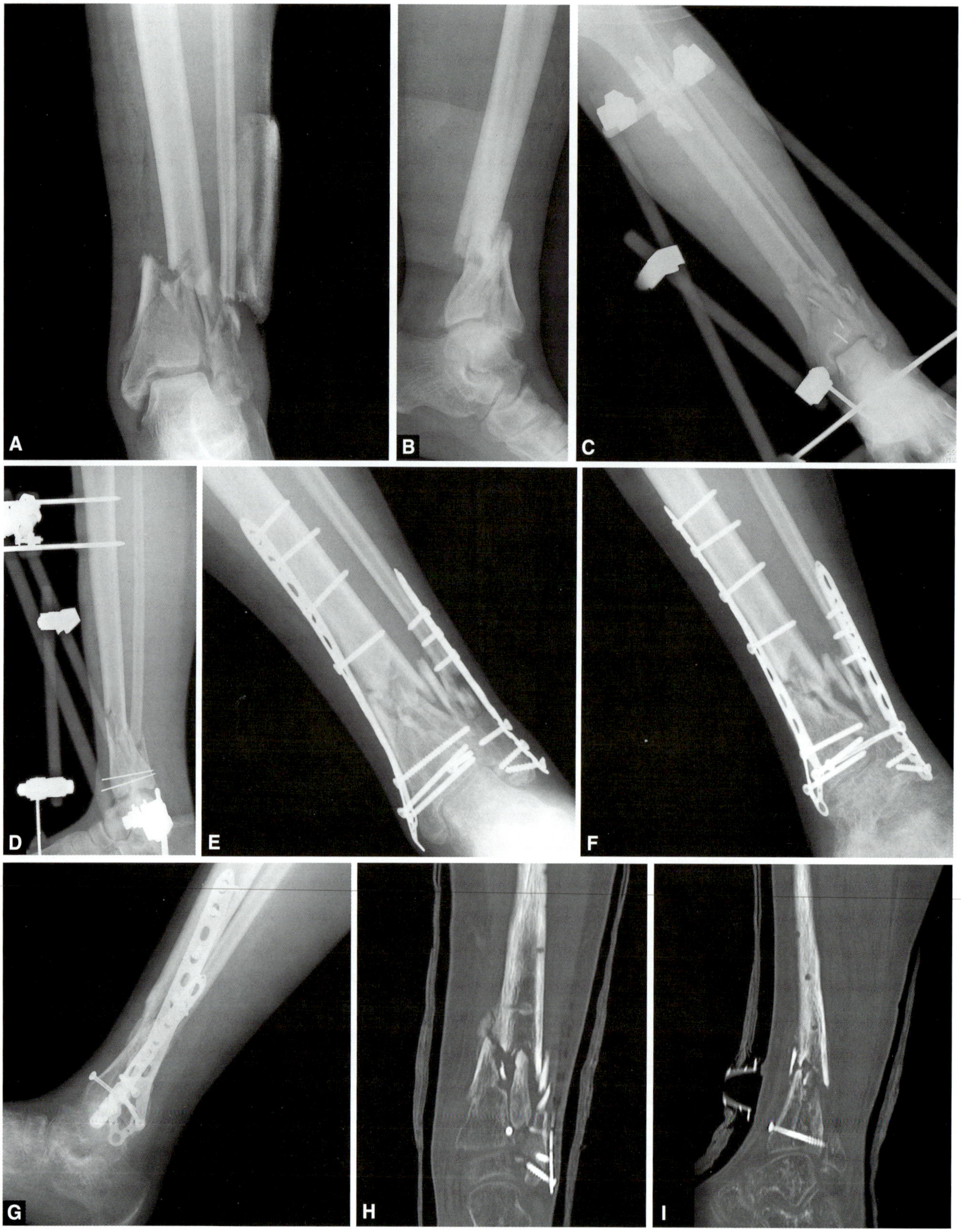

Figures 27.20A to I

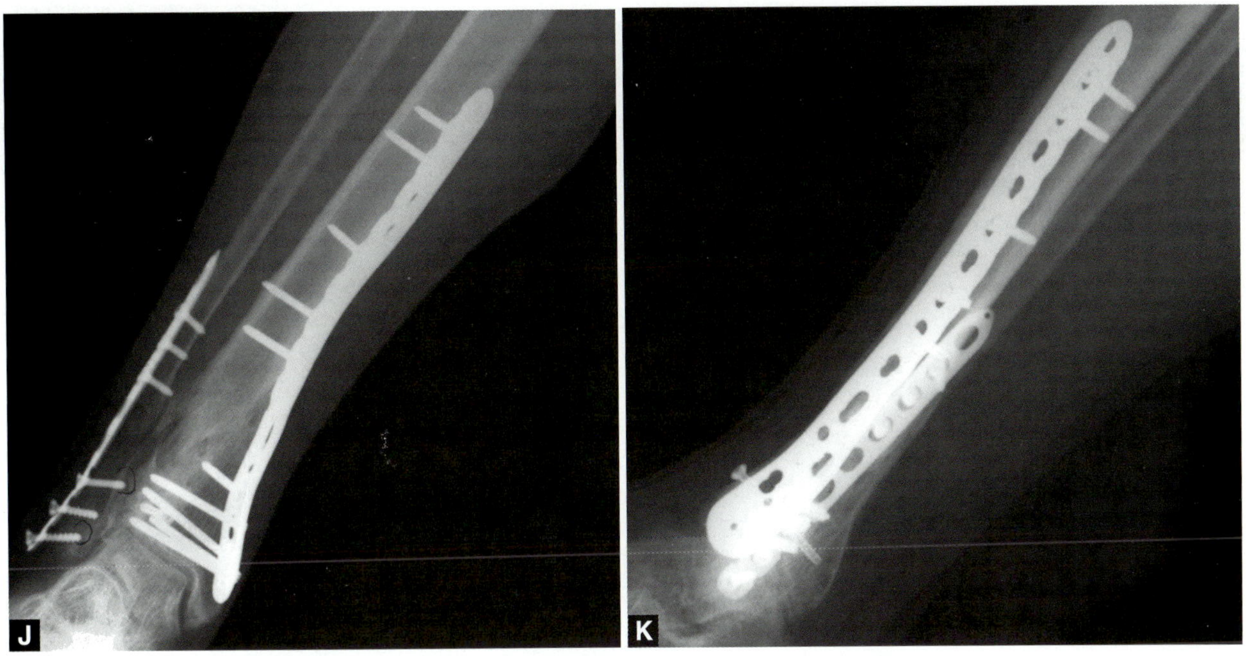

Figures 27.20A to K: Management of nonunion of the distal tibia with revision open reduction and internal fixation (ORIF) and autografting. (A and B) Anteroposterior and lateral radiographs demonstrating a displaced tibial pilon fracture; (C and D) This was treated with spanning external fixation and pinning of the articular fragments; (E to G) Anteroposterior mortise and lateral views of the ankle 5 months after ORIF of the distal tibia and fibula; (H and I) CT scan images demonstrated nonunion of the distal tibia; (J and K) Nonunion repair was performed with revision of fixation to a locked distal tibial plate and autografting. Anteroposterior and lateral images here show the fracture healed at final follow-up.

went on to heal. He was allowed to ambulate in the fixator; although, it remained for 13 months from the time of application, until it was removed. He was ambulatory with minimal overall pain, but was unable to return to his usual work of driving a truck. The ankle went on to autofuse, the nonunion site healed and the site of distraction osteogenesis proximally remodeled very well. There was no sign of recurrence of osteomyelitis (Figs 27.21C and D).

The key points of this case are as follows:

- For recalcitrant osteomyelitis, a decision must be made in accordance to the classical principles as outlined by Dr George Cierny. This patient had persistent infection with drainage, was an otherwise good physiological host with no systemic or other local disease to challenge fracture healing, and was very compliant with good understanding of the Ilizarov fixator. He had tolerated his previous fixator treatments well. He was therefore, a good candidate for this procedure, which was successful in eradicating his infection. The converse would be true as well, i.e. the surgeon would not perform this procedure, if he did not meet all these conditions.
- Bone transport in this case was extra-articular, simplifying the treatment. If an intra-articular infected nonunion needs similar treatment, the debridement of the plafond and talar dome needs to be done and the docking will essentially be an attempt at ankle fusion. In this patient's case, a painless autofusion of the ankle had already occurred.

Case 4: Treatment of an Aseptic Malunion/Nonunion of the Distal Tibia with Osteotomy and Open Reduction and Internal Fixation

In this case, a 28-year-old female sustained a comminuted, Reudi-Allgower type III tibial pilon fracture, which was initially treated with external fixation. It was definitively treated with screw fixation and external fixation. Unfortunately, she went on to develop an apex-anterior deformity with pain and inability to place the foot plantigrade on the ground (Figs 27.22A and B). This persisted for 2 years and she was referred to the surgeon for definitive management. An infection workup including blood tests (ESR and CRP) and nuclear medicine scanning was negative for any obvious infection. Her main complaint was the pain and inability to place the foot flat. Radiographs and CT scanning demonstrated incomplete healing and angulation of the fracture, but satisfactory alignment of the articular surface (Figs 27.22A to D).

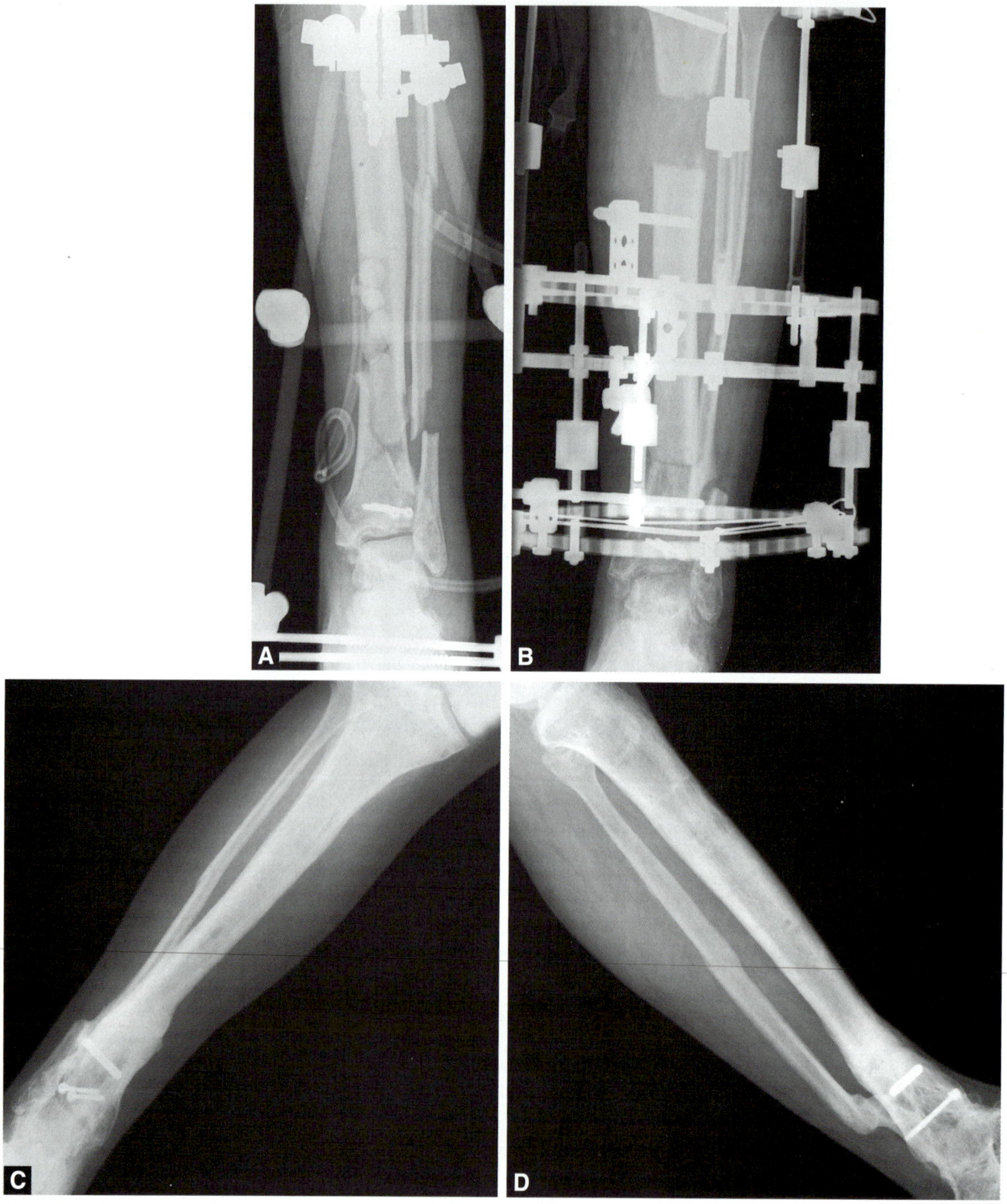

Figures 27.21A to D: Management of a recalcitrant infected extra-articular distal tibial nonunion with resection and bone transport distraction osteogenesis. (A) Initial treatment was with serial irrigation and debridement and spanning external fixation. Infection was treated with serial debridement and antibiotic bead exchange; (B) After failures with local bony debridements and subsequent bone grafting, his persistent infected nonunion was treated with resection and bone transport. Shown here is a radiograph after frame placement, corticotomy, removal of the antibiotic spacer block, transport of the segment and docking; (C and D) Anteroposterior and lateral radiographs at latest follow-up, nearly 2 years after the application of bone transport frame, demonstrating healing of the docking site after bone grafting and good consolidation of the proximal site of distraction osteogenesis.

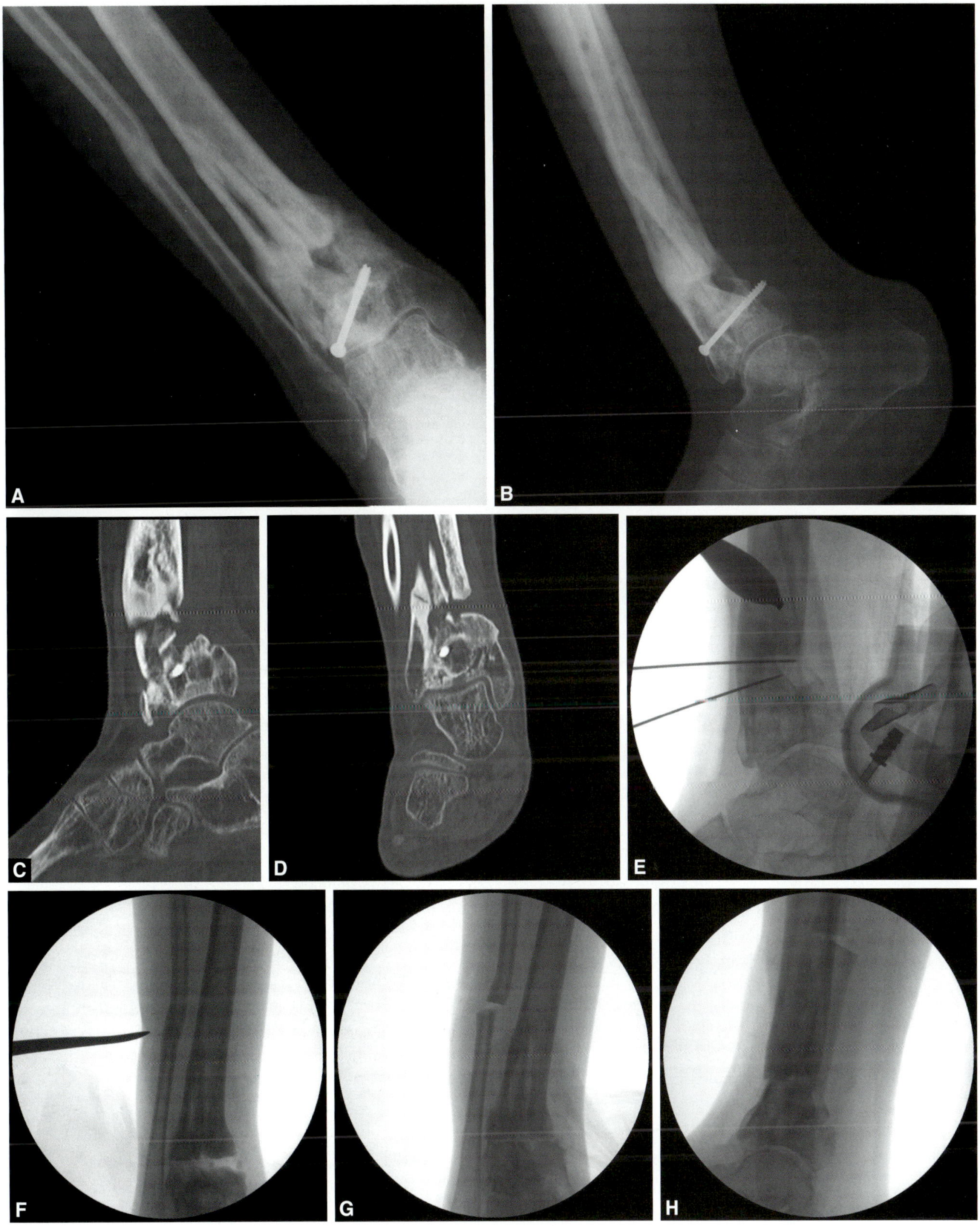

Figures 27.22A to H

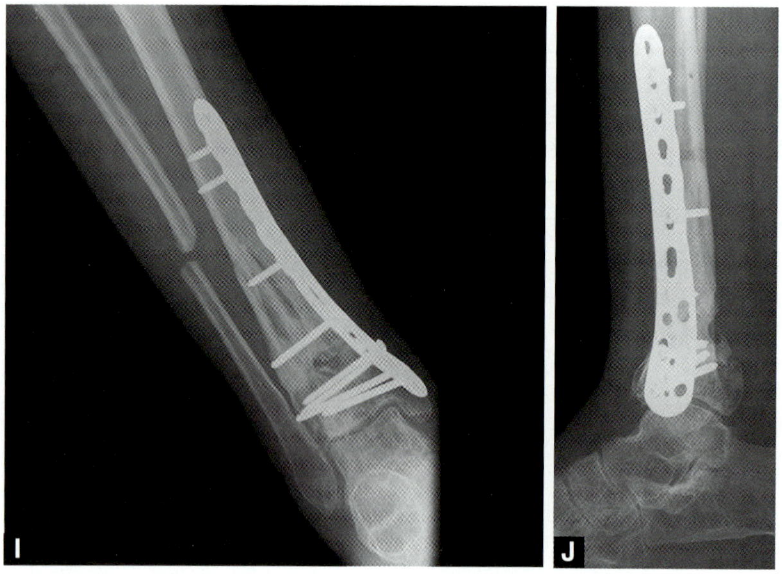

Figures 27.22A to J: Management of malunion/nonunion of a distal tibial fracture. (A to D) Radiographs and CT images demonstrating partial bony union with apex anterior angulation 2 years after treatment of a tibial pilon fracture; (E to H) Treatment with osteotomy and anteromedial plate fixation is shown. After tibial osteotomy, fibular osteotomy is performed. The osteotomy is compressed and fixed with a periarticular medial distal tibia locked plate; (I and J) Anteroposterior and lateral images at final follow-up demonstrating a healed osteotomy with satisfactory overall alignment. Slight overcorrection was done due to posterior ankle contracture.

She was indicated for osteotomy, deformity correction ORIF with compression fixation without bone grafting 2 years after her initial injury. This was performed with an anteromedial surgical approach, osteotomy of the tibia and fibula, and fixation (Figs 27.22E to H). Fixation could also have been performed with an anterolateral plate. A slight overcorrection was performed due to persistent posterior capsular and achilles contracture. She went on to heal without complications and her pain improved to the point that she could return to work (Figs 27.22I and J).

Summary

Pilon fracture management is challenging and has historically been burdened with devastating complications. With advances and evolution in the treatment strategy, the complication rate has certainly decreased, yet the long-term outcome remains suboptimal. A staged protocol, with protection and awareness of the fragility of the soft tissue envelope along with anatomical articular reduction currently gives the patient the best available outcome. Further long-term outcome studies with regard to staged protocol may help moderate pilon fracture management in the future.

References

1. Browner ED, Levine AM, Jupiter JB, et al. Skeletal Trauma: Expert Consult, 4th edition. Philadelphia: Saunders-Elsevier; 2006.
2. Bucholz RW, Heckman JD, Court-Brown C, et al. Rockwood and Green's Fractures in Adults, 6th edn. Philadelphia: Lippincott Williams & Wilkins; 2006.
3. Court-Brown CM, McBirnie J. The epidemiology of tibial fractures. J Bone Joint Surg Br. 1995;77(3):417-21.
4. Lauge-Hansen N. Fractures of the ankle. V. Pronation-dorsiflexion fracture. AMA Arch Surg. 1953;67(6):813-20.
5. Giordano CP, Koval KJ. Treatment of fracture blisters: a prospective study of 53 cases. J Orthop Trauma. 1995;9(2):171-6.
6. Varela CD, Vaughan TK, Carr JB, et al. Fracture blisters: clinical and pathological aspects. J Orthop Trauma. 1993;7(5):417-27.
7. Tscherne H, Gotzen L. Fractures with Soft-Tissue Injuries. Berlin: Springer-Verlag; 1984. pp. 1-58.
8. Gustilo RB, Anderson JT. Prevention of infection in the treatment of one thousand and twenty-five open fractures of the long bones: retrospective and prospective analysis. J Bone Joint Surg Am. 1976;58(4):453-8.
9. Ruedi T. Fractures of the lower end of the tibia into the ankle joint: results nine years after open reduction and internal fixation. Injury. 1973;5(2):130-4.

10. Ruedi TP, Allgower M. The operative treatment of intra-articular fractures of the lower end of the tibia. Clin Orthop Relat Res. 1979;(138):105-10.
11. Ruedi T, Allgower M. Fractures of the lower end of the tibia into the ankle joint. Injury. 1969;1:92-9.
12. Muller ME, Allgower M, Schneider R, et al. In: Tscherne H, Schatzker kJ (Eds). Manual of Internal Fixation Techniques Recommended by the AO Group. New York: Springer-Verlag; 1979. pp. 146, 147, 208-10, 214-5, 586-612.
13. Muller MEN, Nazarian S, Koch P, et al. The Comprehensive Classification of Fractures of Long Bones. New York: Springer-Verlag; 1987. pp. 170-9.
14. Brumback RJ, McGarvey WC. Fractures of the tibial plafond. Evolving treatment concepts for the pilon fracture. Orthop Clin North Am. 1995;26(2):273-85.
15. Wyrsch B, McFerran MA, McAndrew M, et al. Operative treatment of fractures of the tibial plafond. A randomized prospective study. J Bone Joint Surg Am. 1996;78(11): 1646-57.
16. McNamara MG, Heckman JD, Corley FG. Severe open fractures of the lower extremity: a retrospective evaluation of the mangled extremity severity score (MESS). J Orthop Trauma. 1994;8(2):81-7.
17. Ovadia DN, Beals RK. Fractures of the tibial plafond. J Bone Joint Surg Am. 1986;68(4):543-51.
18. Teeny SM, Wiss DA. Open reduction and internal fixation of tibial plafond fractures. Variables contributing to poor results and complications. Clin Orthop Relat Res. 1993;(292):108-17.
19. Patterson MJ, Cole JD. Two-staged delayed open reduction and internal fixation of severe pilon fractures. J Orthop Trauma. 1999;13(2):85-91.
20. Sirkin M, Sanders R, DiPasquale T, et al. A staged protocol for soft tissue management in the treatment of complex pilon fractures. J Orthop Trauma. 1999;13(2):78-84.
21. Blauth M, Bastian L, Krettek C, et al. Surgical options for the treatment of severe tibial pilon fractures: a study of three techniques. J Orthop Trauma. 2001;15(3):153-60.
22. Grose A, Gardner MJ, Hettrich C. Open reduction and internal fixation of tibial pilon fractures using a lateral approach. J Orthop Trauma. 2007;21(8):530-7.
23. Borrelli J Jr, Catalano L. Open reduction and internal fixation of pilon fractures. J Orthop Trauma. 1999;13(8):573-82.
24. Leone VJ, Ruland R, Meinhard B. The management of the soft tissues in pilon fractures. Clin Orthop Relat Res. 1993;(292):315-20.
25. Mast JW, Spiegal PG, Pappas JN. Fractures of the tibial pilon. Clin Orthop Relat Res. 1988;(230):68-82.
26. Helfet DL, Koval K, Pappas J, et al. Intra-articular "pilon" fracture of the tibia. Clin Orthop Relat Res. 1994;(298): 221-8.
27. Waddell JP. Tibial plafond fractures. In: Tscherne H, Schatzker J (Eds). Major Fractures of the Pilon, the Talus and the Calcaneus. Heidelberg, New York: Springer-Verlag; 1993. pp. 43-8.
28. Williams TM, Marsh JL, Nepola JV, et al. External fixation of tibial plafond fractures: is routine plating of the fibula necessary? J Orthop Trauma. 1998;12(1):16-20.
29. Watson JT, Moed BR, Karges DE, et al. Pilon fractures. Treatment protocol based on severity of soft tissue injury. Clin Orthop. 2000;(375):78-90.
30. Fogel GR, Morrey BF. Delayed open reduction and fixation of ankle fractures. Clin Orthop Relat Res. 1987;(215): 187-95.
31. Mast JW, Teipner WA. A reproducible approach to the internal fixation of adult ankle fractures: rationale, technique, and early results. Orthop Clin North Am. 1980; 11(3):661-79.
32. Crutchfield EH, Seligson D, Henry SL, et al. Tibial pilon fractures: A comparative clinical study of management techniques and results. Orthopedics. 1995;18(7):613-7.
33. DeCoster TA, Willis, MC, Marsh JL, et al. Rank order analysis of tibial plafond fractures: does injury or reduction predict outcome? Foot Ankle Int. 1999;20(1):44-9.
34. McFarran MA, Smith SW, Boulas HJ, et al. Complications encountered in the treatment of pilon fractures. J Orthop Trauma. 1992;6(2):195-200.

Chapter 28

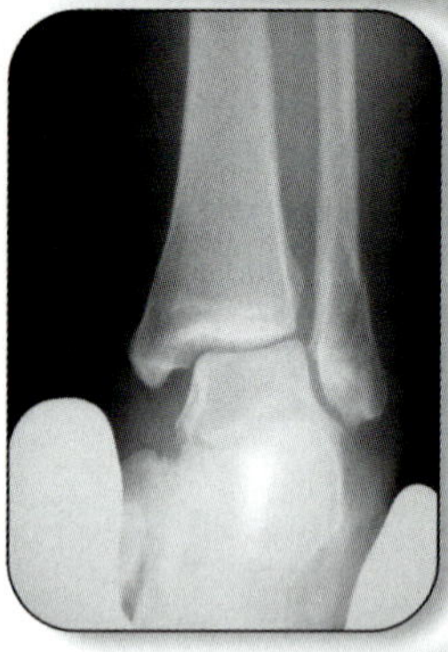

Ankle Fractures and Syndesmotic Injuries

Nirmal Tejwani, Sanjit Konda, Steven Gross

Chapter Outline

Introduction
Diagnosis
Classification
Surgical Indications
- Lateral Malleolar Fractures
- Bimalleolar Fractures
- Posterior Malleolar Fractures
- Syndesmotic Injuries
- Open Ankle Fractures
- Role of External Fixation

Surgical Anatomy, Positioning and Approaches
- Applied Anatomy
- Positioning
- Surgical Approach

Surgical Techniques
- Technique 1: Open Reduction and Internal Fixation (ORIF) of Distal Fibula and Diaphyseal Fibula Fractures
- Technique 2: Operative Fixation of Medial Malleolus Fractures
- Technique 3: ORIF of Posterior Malleolar Fractures
- Technique 4: ORIF of Syndesmotic Injuries of the Ankle

Outcomes
Complications
- Infection and Wound Breakdown
- Early Loss of Hardware Fixation
- Malunion
- Nonunion
- Late Syndesmotic Widening and Neglected Syndesmotic Instability
- Peroneal Tendonitis

Authors' Preferred Management of Select Complications
- Case 1: Treatment of Early Infection and Wound Breakdown
- Case 2: Treatment of Painful Nonunion of a Medial Malleolus Fracture
- Case 3: Loss of Reduction with Early Post-traumatic Arthrosis Treated with Arthrodesis

Summary

Introduction

Ankle fractures are frequently encountered by the orthopedic surgeon. The incidence of these injuries appears to be increasing. Kannus et al. found a three-fold increase in the number of ankle fractures in elderly Finnish patients from 1970 to 2000.[1] However, these injuries may be sustained by an individual in any age group. The incidence of ankle fractures follows a bimodal distribution with the highest rate occurring in young males and elderly females.[2]

The normal anatomic movement of the ankle joint is created by the motion of the talus within the ankle mortise. The ankle is primarily responsible for allowing plantar flexion and dorsiflexion; minimal rotation is tolerated due to the congruity of the tibiotalar joint in the coronal plane. It is not surprising, therefore, that ankle fractures are typically caused by a rotational mechanism. These injuries frequently result from low-energy insults, such as simple falls. Given the low-energy rotational mechanisms that result in ankle fractures, most injuries are closed fractures and open ankle fractures are estimated to account for only 2% of the total number.[2] Successful treatment is based on ensuring a stable reduction of the talus within the mortise by restoring the anatomic relationships of the joint.

Diagnosis

A focused musculoskeletal assessment of the affected lower extremity must be performed. Examination of the ankle should be accompanied by evaluation of the remainder of the limb, as well as the other extremities, for associated injuries. Typically the injured ankle is swollen and ecchymotic. Any gross deformity about the ankle should alert the clinician to the possibility of a fracture-dislocation, which should be reduced as soon as possible to relieve abnormal tension on soft tissue and neurovascular structures, as well as to reduce pressure necrosis of the articular surface of the tibial plafond and talar dome.

The condition of the soft tissues should be evaluated as well. Surgical intervention is often best delayed in the presence of excessive swelling and/or fracture blisters (Fig. 28.1). Though open ankle fractures are uncommon, the limb should be circumferentially inspected for any open wounds. A casual inspection may miss this important finding, so a thorough evaluation should be performed.

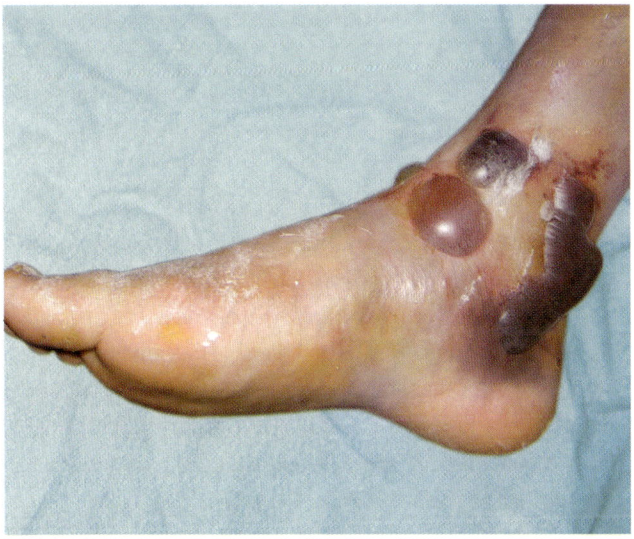

Figure 28.1: Fracture blisters about the ankle. Hemorrhagic blisters as shown here are considered to be a higher risk for infection than serous blisters.

It is important to assess the ankle for tenderness and to note the location of the tenderness. The presence of anteromedial soft tissue tenderness often indicates injury to the deltoid ligament, which can have important ramifications for treatment. The entire length of the tibia and fibula should be palpated as this can demonstrate evidence of associated injuries. Tenderness and crepitus at the proximal fibula indicates a proximal fibular fracture which in the setting of a medial malleolus fracture or a deltoid rupture indicates a longitudinal rupture of the syndesmosis and interosseus membrane between the tibia and fibula (Maisonneuve variant). A positive "squeeze test" defined as pain at the level of the ankle joint with compression of the fibula against the tibia at the level of the midcalf suggests an injury to the distal tibiofibular syndesmosis.

Range of motion of the ankle is typically very painful for patients who have sustained an ankle fracture and many patients will refuse to actively range the joint. This is particularly true if the tibiotalar joint is subluxed or dislocated. Nonetheless, a careful neurovascular exam must be performed upon initial evaluation as well as after any attempts at manipulation or reduction.

Associated injuries in the setting of an acute ankle fracture are difficult to diagnose given the associated soft-tissue swelling and diffuse ankle pain. Fractures of the metatarsals, talus and calcaneus can be present. Tendon ruptures, including the Achilles tendon, can occur as well. Appropriate imaging studies should be ordered if clinical suspicion is high for these associated injuries.

The standard radiographic ankle series includes anteroposterior (AP), lateral and oblique (mortise) views. The mortise view is obtained by internally rotating the ankle approximately 15° from the AP view. Full-length views of the tibia and fibula are indicated if there is tenderness proximally along the fibular shaft. The radiographs of the ankle should be scrutinized not only for evidence of a fracture but also for abnormalities in the normal contour of the ankle mortise and the normal relationship of distal tibiofibular joint. On the AP view, an increased tibiofibular clear space (normal < 5 mm) or decreased tibiofibular overlap (normal > 10 mm) suggests injury to the syndesmosis. On the mortise view, widened tibiotalar medial clear space (normal < 5 mm) indicates disruption of the deltoid ligament. The lateral view should be inspected for congruency of the talar dome with the tibial plafond, with the dome centered under the tibia.

In the event that there is a lateral malleolus fracture in the absence of any medial malleolus fracture, it is extremely important to assess the integrity of the deltoid ligament. If the deep deltoid ligament is disrupted, the talus is rendered unstable beneath the plafond. A "stress view" should be obtained in this circumstance if the medial clear space appears normal on the nonstressed mortise radiograph, particularly if there is tenderness over the deltoid ligament. This view is obtained by positioning the ankle for a standard mortise view, then applying an external rotation force to the dorsiflexed foot while stabilizing the tibia. An increase in the medial clear space greater than 5 mm indicates incompetence of the deltoid ligament (Figs 28.2A and B).[3]

Computed tomography (CT) is usually not required in the evaluation of ankle fractures, as plain radiographs typically provide enough information to properly evaluate and treat the injury. CT is most helpful when there is suspicion of plafond impaction or posterior malleolus fracture that is incompletely visualized on radiographs. If suspicion for associated bony injuries in the hindfoot is high, CT can help evaluate these as well.

Magnetic resonance imaging (MRI) of the ankle provides information primarily about the soft tissues. This imaging modality can provide additional information on damage to tendinous or ligamentous structures. Syndesmosis injuries not readily apparent on plain radiographs can be identified on MRI. In cases of borderline stress radiographs of the ankle where there may not be complete rupture of the deep deltoid ligament, MRI can be an important adjunctive test (Fig. 28.2C). However, physical examination and plain radiographs are almost always sufficient to diagnose ankle fractures, syndesmotic injuries and associated ankle instability in the acute setting.

ANKLE FRACTURES AND SYNDESMOTIC INJURIES DIAGNOSIS: Pearls and Pitfalls

- Physical examination should focus on locating specific areas of tenderness, inspecting for open wounds and evaluating neurovascular integrity
- Plain radiographs with ankle stress views are typically insufficient for diagnosis of ankle fractures, syndesmotic injuries and associated ankle instability
- Stress radiographs should be obtained in all cases of lateral malleolar fracture without medial malleolar injury to evaluate the integrity of the deltoid ligament
- Advanced imaging modalities are usually unnecessary but can be used to diagnose associated injuries, if clinical suspicion is high

Classification

There are several ways to classify ankle fractures. The descriptive classification system is a straightforward method of communicating the extent of bony injury. A fracture of a single malleolus is a unimalleolar injury and described as either an isolated medial, lateral, or posterior malleolus fracture. Fractures of both the lateral and medial malleoli are termed bimalleolar fractures. When the posterior malleolus is also involved, it is described as a trimalleolar fracture.

Ankle fractures can also be described as stable or unstable. Stable injuries refer to those injuries in which the talus is stable beneath the tibial plafond. This implies integrity of the medial stabilizing structures, most notably the medial malleolus and the deep deltoid ligament. By contrast, unstable fractures are those in which either of these structures are disrupted and the talus is subsequently prone to subluxation and/or dislocation. Generally speaking, this classification scheme remains the most clinically relevant as it alludes to the need for surgical intervention in unstable injuries.

The Lauge-Hansen classification system is predicated upon a rotational mechanism of injury.[4] The various fracture types are named by the position of the foot at the time of injury combined with the direction of the force applied to the ankle. The four major patterns are: (1) supination-external rotation (SER), (2) supination-adduction (SA), (3) pronation-external rotation (PER), and (4) pronation-abduction (PA). Various subtypes are described and depend on the severity of injury (Figs 28.3A to D).

By contrast, the Danis-Weber classification is based on the location of the fibula fracture relative to the syndesmosis.[5,6] A Weber type A fibula fracture is below the level

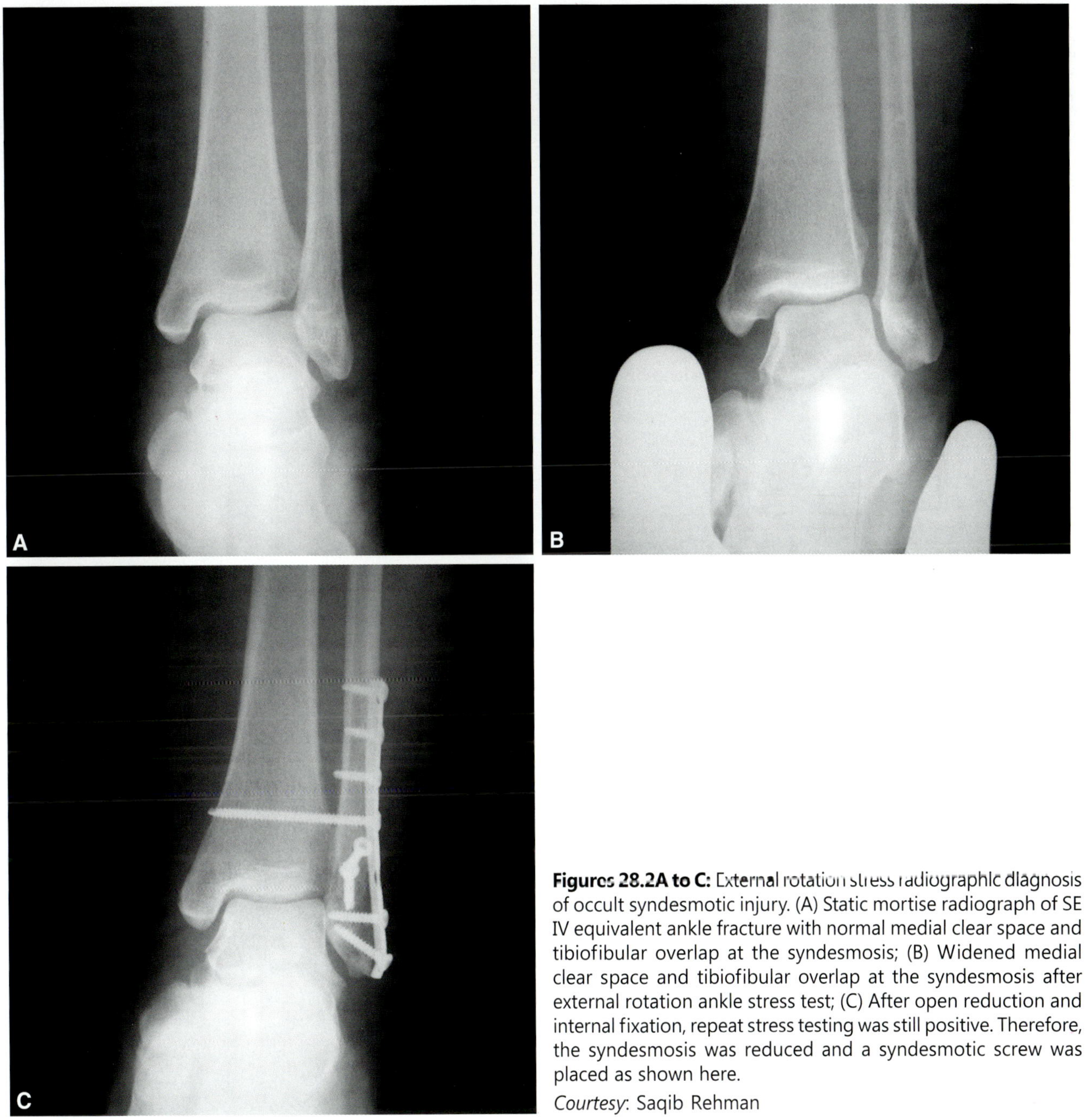

Figures 28.2A to C: External rotation stress radiographic diagnosis of occult syndesmotic injury. (A) Static mortise radiograph of SE IV equivalent ankle fracture with normal medial clear space and tibiofibular overlap at the syndesmosis; (B) Widened medial clear space and tibiofibular overlap at the syndesmosis after external rotation ankle stress test; (C) After open reduction and internal fixation, repeat stress testing was still positive. Therefore, the syndesmosis was reduced and a syndesmotic screw was placed as shown here.

Courtesy: Saqib Rehman

of the syndesmosis. Type B fractures are at the level of the syndesmosis. Type C fractures are above the syndesmosis. Despite this classification scheme's close association with the syndesmosis, it does not consistently predict the presence or degree of syndesmotic injury (Fig. 28.4).

AO/OTA classification system incorporates the Weber classification scheme but expands upon it.[7] The numeric designation for ankle fractures is 44. The basic fracture types in this system (A, B, C) correspond to the Weber types. Further subtypes are used to describe associated injuries about the ankle mortise, including the medial malleolus and syndesmosis. The AO system is the most comprehensive of the numerous classification schemes in use today.

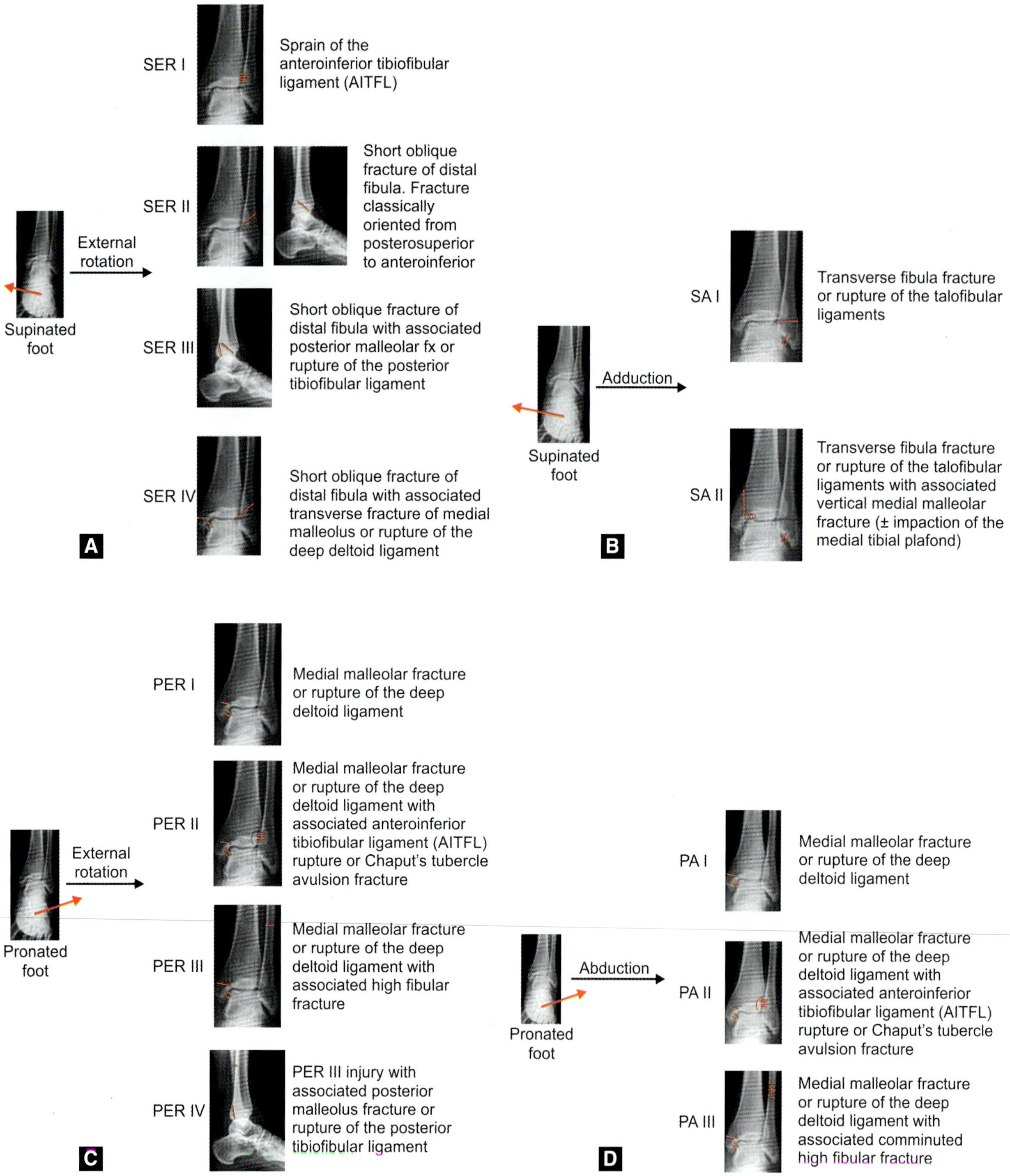

Figures 28.3A to D: Lauge-Hansen classification system of malleolar ankle fractures.

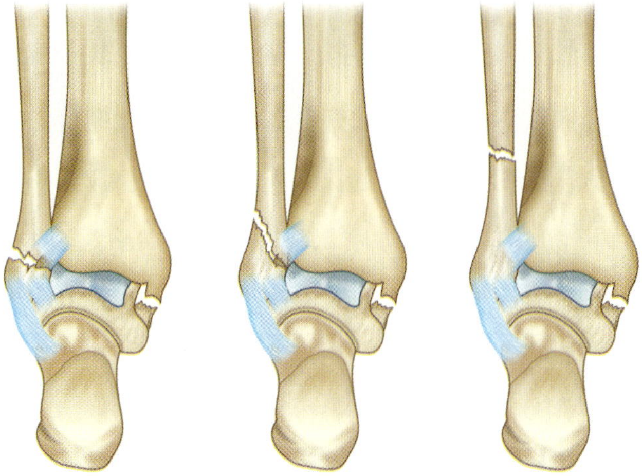

Figure 28.4: Radiograph of ankle demonstrating the Danis-Weber classification system. Type A denotes fractures distal to the ankle syndesmosis. Type B denotes fractures at the level of the syndesmosis. Type C denotes fractures above the level of the syndesmosis.

Surgical Indications

The decision to operate on an ankle fracture is based on the instability of the fracture pattern and the inability of nonoperative treatment to maintain a congruent ankle mortise and a reduced syndesmosis. Even 1 mm of talar displacement decreases the joint contact surface by 42%[8] so anatomic reduction of the talus within the ankle mortise is essential to prevent early arthritic changes of the ankle joint.

Lateral Malleolar Fractures

For isolated fractures of the lateral malleolus, fixation is necessary only if there is associated compromise to the deep deltoid ligament. This is evidenced by lateral talar displacement and an increase in the medial clear space greater than 5 mm on AP, mortise and ankle stress view radiographs. In equivocal cases, MRI can be a useful confirmatory study, as recent literature has demonstrated that the deep deltoid ligament may still be intact even when the stress test is positive.[9] When surgery is indicated, direct repair of the deltoid ligament is unnecessary. The surgeon will only need to approach the medial aspect of the joint in the case of an incarcerated portion of the ligament hindering congruent reduction of the talus. A plate and screw construct is the standard method of internal fixation of the lateral malleolus.

Bimalleolar Fractures

In the setting of a bimalleolar ankle fractures, both the lateral and medial malleolus must be fixed. The indications for fixation of an isolated medial malleolus fracture are not as clearly defined. We advocate fixation of this particular fracture when any significant displacement exists, in order to maintain articular congruity and reduce the chances of nonunion. Depending on the size of the fragment and the quality of bone, a number of different constructs may be employed. Options include lag screws, a tension band construct, or medial plating.

Posterior Malleolar Fractures

Fixation of a posterior malleolar fracture is necessary, if there is greater than 25% involvement of the articular surface. This has classically been advocated for the purposes of restoring articular congruity and ankle stability. However, recent literature has also demonstrated that fixation of the posterior malleolus contributes to stability of the syndesmosis.[10] For fractures of the posterior malleolus, lag screws or a posterior plate offer satisfactory fixation. Trimalleolar ankle fractures only require fixation of the posterior malleolus if the above criteria are met. Otherwise, addressing the medial and lateral malleolus alone is sufficient treatment to restore ankle stability.

Syndesmotic Injuries

Rupture of the syndesmosis can lead to instability of the mortise even in the absence of any malleolar fractures. Typically, though, syndesmotic disruption occurs in the setting of bony injury about the ankle. Syndesmotic disruption is commonly seen in Weber C or Lauge-Hansen PER type IV ankle fracture patterns where the rotational mechanism of injury results in diaphyseal fibular fractures. However, even Weber B or Lauge-Hansen SER type II and PA type III ankle fracture patterns can result in syndesmotic injury. The most reliable way to assess the integrity of the syndesmosis complex is through the intraoperative "cotton test," which is performed after fixation of all malleolar fractures is complete (Fig. 28.5). Alternatively, an external rotation stress test can

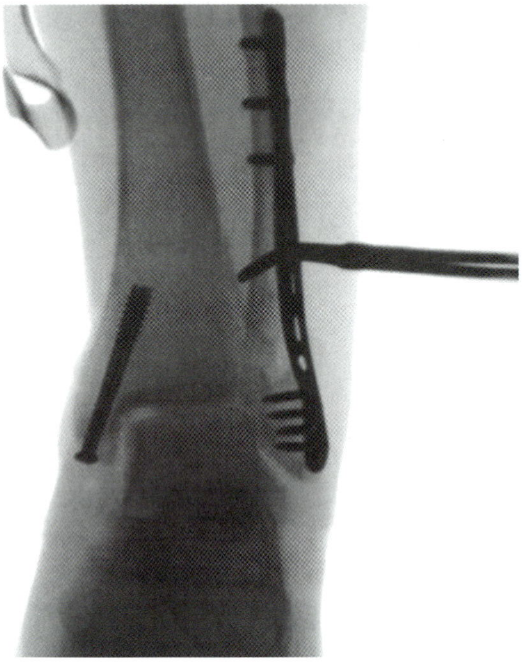

Figure 28.5: Example of the "cotton test" to evaluate the integrity of the ankle syndesmosis after fixation of this supination-external rotation type IV equivalent ankle fracture.

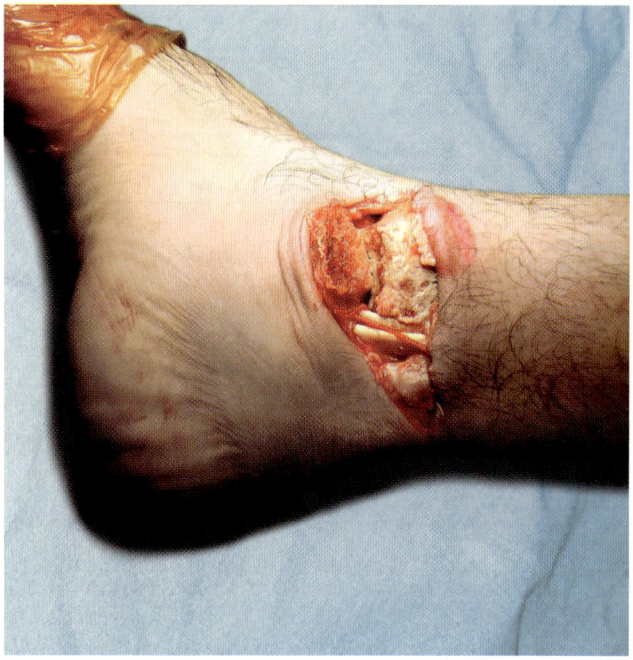

Figure 28.6: Open ankle fracture with a medial open wound (classically transverse) secondary to tension failure with medial displacement of medial malleolus through the wound.

be performed. If either test demonstrates syndesmotic instability, internal fixation with one or two screws is indicated.

Open Ankle Fractures

Open ankle fractures are usually associated with a medial open wound (classically transverse) secondary to tension failure and resulting in medial displacement of the distal tibia through the wound (Fig. 28.6). Management of open fractures requires urgent irrigation and debridement (I and D) along with fracture stabilization with either external fixation, (if there is associated contamination or significant fracture comminution or soft tissue damage) or internal fixation if feasible. Wounds can be closed primarily over a drain, however, if significant swelling is present and the wound edges cannot be approximated without tension then a negative pressure wound therapy device, such as the vacuum assisted closure (V.A.C, Kinetic Concepts, Inc., San Antonio, TX) can be applied to decrease swelling, to promote granulation tissue formation in the wound bed and to act as a sterile dressing. Antibiotics should be continued until the wound is closed.

Role of External Fixation

External fixation of an ankle fracture is typically reserved for those patients whose medical comorbidities or condition of the soft tissues preclude an open procedure at the fracture site. External fixation can also be helpful as adjunctive neutralization when splinting or bracing may not be suitable due to body habitus limitations (i.e. extreme morbid obesity), particularly in open fractures requiring wound management (Figs 28.7A to E). Different frame arrangements exist. External fixation can be used as a definitive procedure when needed (Fig. 28.7F). It is also useful for maintaining an anatomic reduction while awaiting improvement in the soft tissue envelope with an ultimate plan to perform definitive internal fixation.

Surgical Anatomy, Positioning and Approaches

Applied Anatomy

Effective treatment of ankle fractures requires a sound understanding of the anatomy surrounding the entire ankle

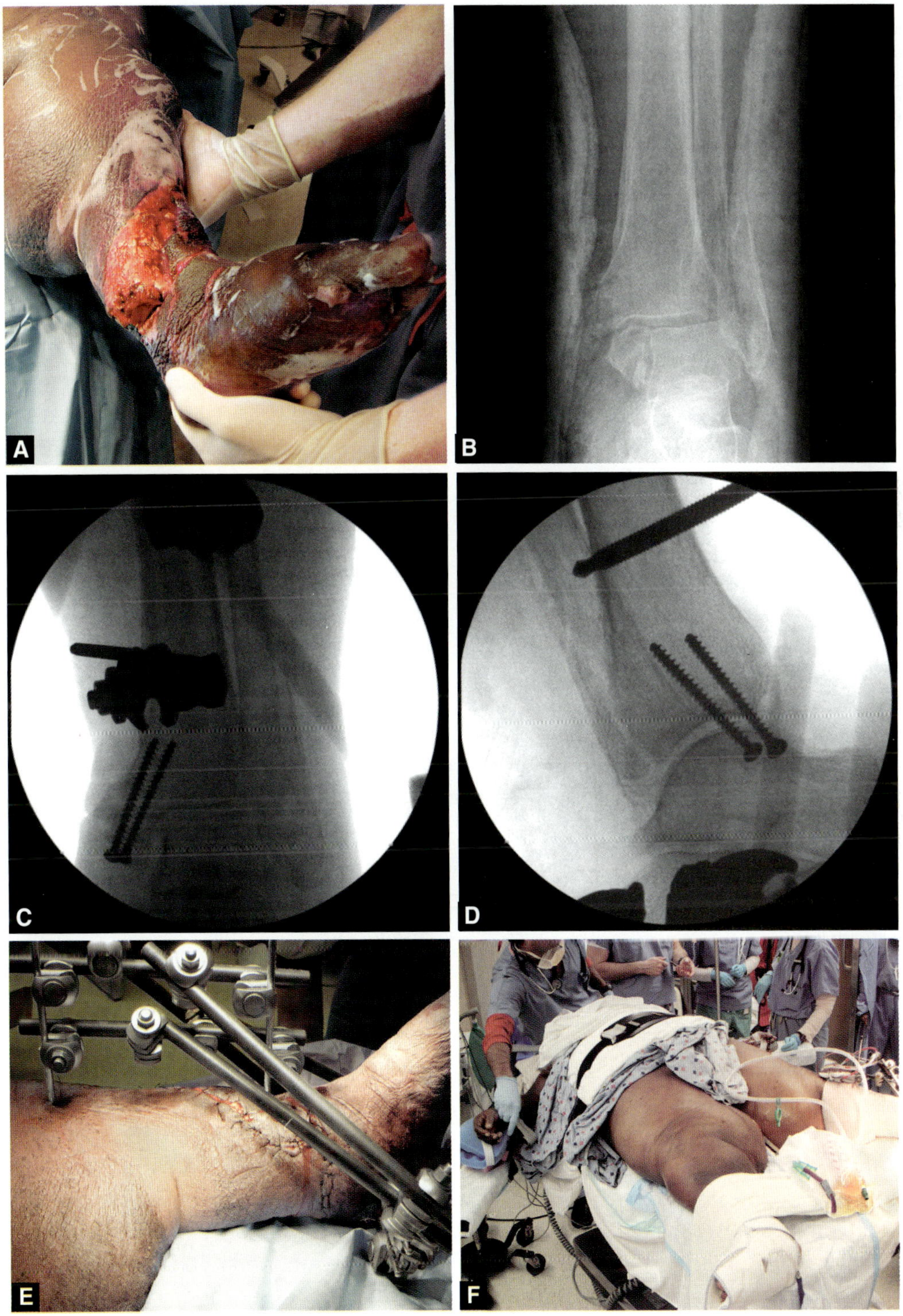

Figures 28.7A to F: Open ankle fracture dislocation with morbid obesity treated with limited ORIF and spanning external fixation. (A) Open ankle fracture dislocation in an 83-year-old female with entire tibial plafond exposed and dislocated medially; (B) Anteroposterior (AP) radiograph demonstrating medial and lateral malleolar fractures; (C and D) AP and lateral intraoperative fluoroscopic images after screw fixation of the medial malleolus and spanning external fixation. A posterior malleolar fracture is also seen here; (E and F) Wound debridement was completed, skin approximated over suction drain and spanning external fixation is demonstrated. Due to her body habitus and need for wound checks, it was felt that external fixation was preferable to splinting or casting.

Courtesy: Saqib Rehman

joint. Various sensory nerve branches and neurovascular bundles cross the ankle joint and can be damaged during the surgical approach to the lateral malleolus, medial malleolus and posterior malleolus.

The ankle joint consists of the tibiotalar articulation. The medial malleolus, lateral malleolus and posterior malleolus provide medial, lateral and posterior support to the ankle joint, respectively. The ankle mortise refers to the tibiotalar articulation in the coronal plane and is externally rotated 15° relative to the coronal plane of the tibia. The talar dome is wider anteriorly and narrower posteriorly, therefore, when assessing congruency of the ankle mortise the ankle must be dorsiflexed to neutral otherwise radiographs will demonstrate a falsely widened medial clear space.

The distal 2–3 cm of the fibula is devoid of muscular attachments and is directly subcutaneous. The peroneus brevis and longus tendons run directly posterior to the distal fibula in the peroneal groove. At the level of the distal fibula, the peroneus brevis lies anterior to peroneus longus directly against the fibula and its muscle belly extends to the level of the ankle joint. The peroneal tendons are maintained in the peroneal groove by the superior peroneal retinaculum which runs from the calcaneus to the posterior distal tip of the fibula. The peroneal longus and brevis muscle bellies are innervated by the superficial peroneal nerve (SPN) and serve to evert the foot. The SPN, a branch of the common peroneal nerve, emerges from the lateral compartment fascia approximately 7–10 cm proximal to the distal tip of the fibula and crosses to the anterolateral aspect of the distal tibia running subcutaneously. Care must be taken during surgical approaches to the fibula proximal to the subcutaneous portion to avoid cutting the SPN which can lead to a painful neuroma as well loss of sensation over the dorsum of the foot. Anterior to the lateral border of the fibula is the peroneus tertius which originates from the distal fibula and interosseus membrane and is innervated by the deep peroneal nerve. The terminal branch of the peroneal artery runs just medial to the distal tip of the fibula and can be injured if dissection in this area does not remain sub-periosteal. The sural nerve runs posterior to the distal fibula with the short saphenous vein and it is at risk for injury during the posterior approach to the distal tibia. The sural nerve supplies sensation to the lateral aspect of the foot. It is not usually encountered during the lateral approach to the distal fibula.

The medial malleolus is a directly subcutaneous structure and similar to the distal fibula, is also devoid of muscular attachments. It is comprised of an anterior colliculus and a posterior colliculus where the superficial and deep deltoid ligaments attach, respectively. The saphenous nerve is the terminal branch of the femoral nerve and divides into two branches that run along either side of the saphenous vein. The saphenous nerve supplies innervation to the medial aspect of the foot. Both the saphenous nerve and vein run along the anterior aspect of the medial malleolus and must be protected and mobilized during the surgical approach to this structure. Lying directly posterior to the medial malleolus are the posterior tibialis tendon, flexor digitorum longus tendon, posterior tibial artery, tibial nerve and flexor hallucis longus (FHL) tendon. Proximal to the ankle joint, only the posterior tibial tendon and FHL tendon are enveloped by the flexor retinaculum. Distal to the ankle joint, the flexor retinaculum extends from the posterior aspect of the medial malleolus to the calcaneus and overlies all the aforementioned structures. These three muscles running directly posterior to the medial malleolus are innervated by the tibial nerve. The tibial nerve also supplies sensation to the plantar surface of the foot. Dissection along the posterior aspect of the medial malleolus should be performed carefully to avoid injury to these tendinous and neurovascular structures.

The posterior malleolus is the posterior distal aspect of the tibia and provides posterior stability to the ankle. This structure is connected to the posterior distal fibula via the posterior inferior tibiofibular ligament and the inferior transverse ligament. The inferior transverse ligament provides the primary ligamentous support to posterior ankle stability. Lying posterior to the posterior malleolus is the muscle belly of the FHL. Of the posterior deep posterior compartment muscles, the FHL muscle belly extends the most distally and is the only muscle belly visible at the level of the ankle joint.

The ankle syndesmosis is the ligamentous complex that maintains congruity between the distal tibiofibular joint. It is comprised of four ligaments: the anterior inferior tibiofibular ligament, the interosseus ligament, the posterior inferior tibiofibular ligament and the inferior transverse ligament. The distal fibula lies in the incisura which is a groove in the posterolateral aspect of the distal tibia.

Positioning

The supine position is the most commonly utilized position for treatment of lateral malleolus fractures, diaphyseal fibula fractures, medial malleolus fractures and some posterior malleolus fractures (via anterior to posterior percutaneous screw fixation). A radiolucent flat table [e.g. Jackson flat table® or a table with a radiolucent extension (e.g. AMSCO table®)] should be utilized. A bump is placed under the ipsilateral hip to maintain neutral rotation of the ankle. Neutral rotation is achieved when the patella points directly towards the ceiling. Without a bump, the ankle tends to lie in an externally rotated position due to the naturally occurring 15° of hip anteversion. This makes it more difficult to access the lateral malleolus and more difficult to obtain adequate intraoperative AP, mortise and lateral radiographs of the ankle joint. A ramp made of bedsheets or a commercially available foam support (e.g. Bone Foam, Excel Medical Solutions, Plymouth, MN) is placed under the ipsilateral leg to lift it above the contralateral leg to make obtaining intraoperative lateral radiographs easier.

The prone position can be utilized to access large posterior malleolus fractures, as well as lateral malleolus fractures and diaphyseal fibula fractures. A radiolucent flat table or a table with a radiolucent extension should be utilized. Two bumps are placed on either side of the patient's chest wall and abdomen to elevate these structures from the bed to allow for adequate chest wall and abdominal excursion during respiration. A small foam pad is placed under each knee and the contralateral foot and ankle to prevent pressure necrosis. A sterile bump placed under the dorsum of the ankle is used intraoperatively to elevate the affected ankle from the table to make obtaining intraoperative lateral radiographs easier. It is more difficult to fix medial malleolar fractures via this prone position; however, it can be accomplished via judicious use of intraoperative fluoroscopy.

Surgical Approach

The lateral approach to the distal fibula is straightforward as the distal fibula is subcutaneous and without muscular attachments. A straight lateral incision will expose the lateral surface of the distal fibula. This same approach can be utilized to fix an injured syndesmosis. If the incision is extended proximally to access diaphyseal fibular fractures, the internervous plane utilized is between the peroneus brevis muscle (innervated by the SPN) and the peroneus tertius muscle (innervated by the deep peroneal nerve). The peroneus brevis muscle is retracted posteriorly and the peroneus tertius muscle is retracted anteriorly. The SPN is identified (most commonly in the anterior skin flap) and protected as it pierces the lateral compartment fascia and travels anteriorly in the subcutaneous tissues.

The posterolateral approach to the posterior malleolus and the distal fibula utilizes the internervous plane between the peroneus brevis muscle (innervated by the SPN) and the FHL muscle (innervated by the tibial nerve). Initiate the approach by incising the deep fascia of the leg in-line with the longitudinal skin incision halfway between the Achilles tendon and posterior aspect of the distal fibula to expose the underlying peroneal brevis and FHL muscles. Next, incise the peroneal retinaculum located at the level of the ankle joint and retract the peroneal brevis muscle and peroneus longus tendon laterally to expose the FHL muscle origin along the posterior border of the fibula. Incise the deep posterior compartment fascia overlying the FHL muscle in-line with the skin incision and sharply reflect its origin from the posterior fibula to expose the posterior border of the fibula and retract it medially. To expose the posterior malleolus, continue reflecting the FHL sharply off the interosseus membrane and retract it medially until the posterior malleolus is visualized. The sural nerve runs with the short saphenous vein in the subcutaneous tissues posterior to the lateral malleolus. Therefore, this nerve should be identified and protected in the superficial portion of the dissection.

The anteromedial approach to the medial malleolus is straightforward as the medial malleolus is subcutaneous and without muscular attachments. A longitudinal incision centered over the medial malleolus and curved slightly anteriorly over the distal aspect of the malleolus gives exposure of the both the lateral and anterior aspect of the malleolus. This allows for direct visualization of anatomic reduction in both the coronal and sagittal planes. The saphenous vein and two branches of the saphenous nerve run together along the medial malleolus in the subcutaneous tissue. This nerve should be identified and protected during the approach. The posterior tibial tendon lies directly posterior to the medial malleolus and care should be taken when dissecting in this area.

Surgical Techniques

Technique 1: Open Reduction and Internal Fixation (ORIF) of Distal Fibula and Diaphyseal Fibula Fractures

Preoperative Planning

Instrumentation necessary to have during the case includes small fragment instrumentation and fluoroscopy. Additional instrumentation that will be helpful to have available include Kirchner (K) wires and fracture reduction tools. We routinely use a thigh tourniquet inflated to 100 mm Hg above systolic blood pressure prior to making incision. The most common implant to use for fibular fracture fixation is a one-third tubular plate. Supination-external rotation type ankle fractures have a unique distal fibular fracture pattern extending from anteroinferior to posterosuperior that is amenable to both lateral plating or posterior or posterolateral plating. If lateral plating is performed, the fracture fragments can be lagged together with an anterior to posterior or posterior to anterior 3.5 mm cortical lag screw placed via standard AO lag technique. The lateral plate serves as a neutralization plate with this method of fixation (Fig. 28.8). If posterior or posterolateral plating is performed, the plate serves an antiglide function by preventing superior migration of the distal fibular fracture fragment (Figs 28.9A and B). A 3.5 mm cortical lag screw can be placed through the plate if the fracture pattern allows. Diaphyseal fibular fractures are routinely fixed with a laterally placed plate. In osteoporotic bone, several techniques can be utilized to enhance fixation. Refer to the complications section (early loss of hardware fixation) for a list of techniques that can be considered to enhance fixation.

Technique

Make a 5 cm longitudinal incision centered over fibular shaft and extended 1 cm distal to the tip of the fibula for distal fibular fractures or, in the case of fibular diaphyseal fractures, the incision is centered at the fracture site. Incise through skin and subcutaneous fat. Continue with sharp dissection directly to the distal fibula creating a thick flap for later repair over the implanted hardware. In the proximal portion of the incision use long curved Mayo scissors to spread the soft tissues and identify the SPN.

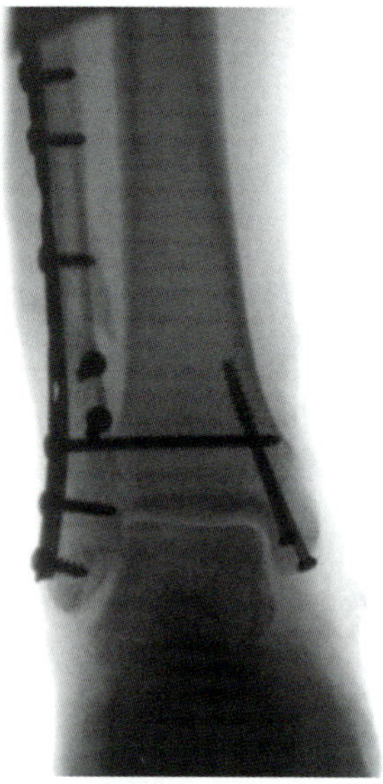

Figure 28.8: Anteroposterior radiograph of an ankle demonstrating lag screw fixation of a fibular fracture with a neutralizing one-third tubular plate, one 4.0 mm quadricortical syndesmotic screw placed through the one-third tubular plate and two parallel partially threaded screws to fix a medial malleolus fracture.

Once down to bone, sharply excise a 2 mm cuff of periosteum proximal and distal to the fracture to more clearly identify the fractured cortices of the fibula. Curette and irrigate the fracture site to clear out hematoma and soft tissue entrapped in the fracture site and to more clearly visualize the fracture edges.

Place a one-third tubular plate flush to bone and hold it in place with serrated bone holding forceps (or plate-holding forceps) on the proximal fragment. This recreates a lateral (or posterior) cortical strut to which the distal fragment can be reduced. Make sure to hold the plate with the forceps between holes to create the maximum amount of compression of the plate to bone. Reduce the fracture and hold the reduction in place using another pair of serrated bone holding forceps holding the plate against the distal fibular fragment. In cases of significant comminution, it may be difficult to assess by direct visualization if anatomic fibular length has been restored.

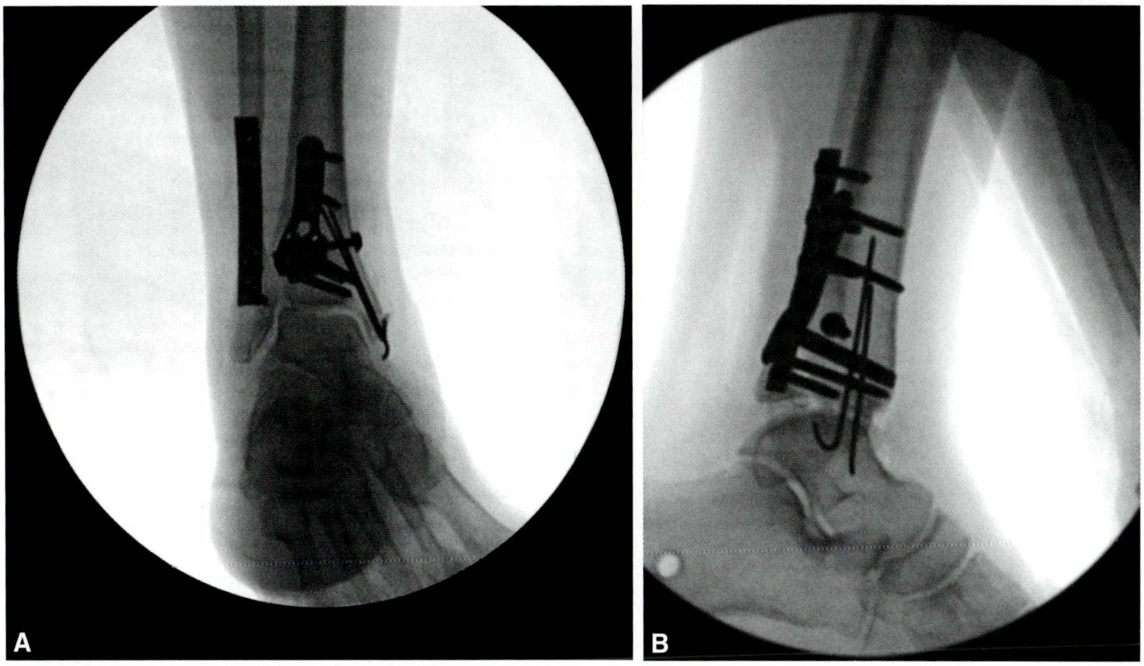

Figures 28.9A and B: Anteroposterior and lateral radiograph of an ankle demonstrating posterior plating of distal fibular fracture using the antiglide mode of one-third tubular plate, posterior plating of posterior malleolus fracture with a distal tibia plate (a one-third tubular plate can also be used), and tension-band technique to repair a medial malleolus fracture.

Anteroposterior fluoroscopic images should be taken in this scenario to confirm restoration of the normal congruent relationship between the tip of the distal fibula and the lateral process of the talus known as the "dime sign" (Fig. 28.10). Another method to assess restoration of fibular length is to take a fluoroscopic AP image of the unaffected ankle and measure the talocrural angle, the angle subtended by a line parallel and tangential to the joint line and a line tangential to the intermalleolar axis (normal is 8–12°) (Fig. 28.11). This measured talocrural angle should be restored on the injured extremity.

Once the fracture is reduced, a cortical screw should be placed in the plate to compress the plate to bone. If the plate is placed posteriorly in an antiglide fashion, then the first screw placed should be in the screw hole just proximal to the superior extent of the fracture line. This creates an antiglide effect that prevents further superior displacement of the distal fragment. Next, an assessment should be made if a lag screw can be placed across the fracture site and if feasible this can be performed at this stage either through the plate or directly on bone. Finally, screw holes are filled as necessary to achieve secure fixation of the fractured fibula. Final AP, mortise and lateral

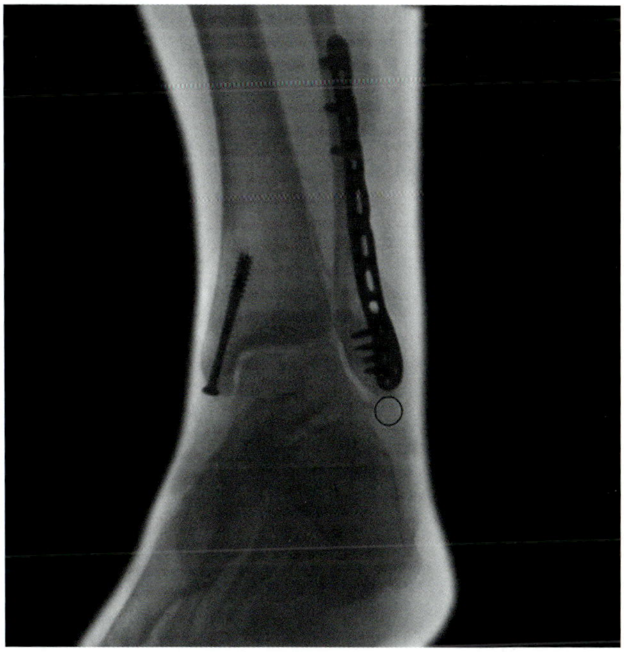

Figure 28.10: Radiograph of ankle fracture after open reduction and internal fixation demonstrating appropriate restoration of fibular length as evidenced by the presence of the "dime sign" (circle).

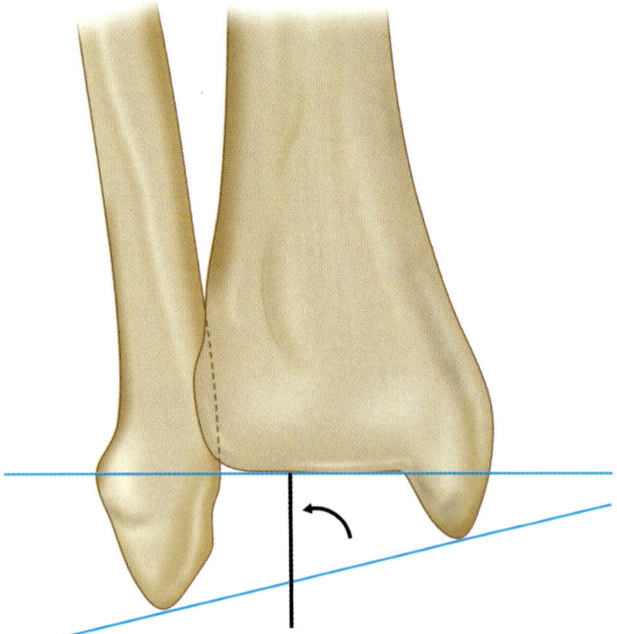

Figure 28.11: Measurement of the talocrural angle to determine accurate restoration of fibular length.

fluoroscopic images are obtained to confirm anatomic reduction of the fibula and restoration of the ankle mortise.

Next, an assessment of the integrity of the distal tibia-fibula syndesmosis is made. The "cotton test" is performed by placing a clamp around the fibula and applying a lateral stress under an AP or mortise fluoroscopic view. Decreased tibiofibular overlap (normal $\geq$ 10 mm overlap on AP, and mortise views) is indicative of a syndesmotic injury that necessitates fixation. See Section on Surgical Technique: Technique 4—syndesmosis repair—for an in-depth description of the repair technique.

At the level of the distal fibula, the lack of soft tissue coverage makes it difficult to place soft tissue over the plate for closure. We attempt to close any available soft tissue over the plate with 2-0 vicryl suture as a layer of cushion between the plate. Subcutaneous buried sutures placed in this area tend to cause skin irritation and have a tendency to form suture abscesses, therefore, we prefer to close skin directly with a 3-0 nylon suture in a vertical mattress fashion. Xeroform gauze dressing and sterile 4x4 gauze dressing are placed over the wound. The leg is wrapped in sterile cotton roll dressings and a standard short leg plaster splint is applied for immediate post-operative comfort. The patient is made non-weight-bearing for six weeks postoperatively at which time weight-bearing is progressively advanced. The patient is allowed to actively plantarflex and dorsiflex the ankle to prevent ankle stiffness once the surgical wounds are healed and sutures removed at approximately 7–10 days postoperatively.

ORIF OF DISTAL FIBULAR AND DIAPHYSEAL FIBULA FRACTURES: Pearls and Pitfalls

- In osteoporotic bone, it is advisable to have a locking plate available to enhance fracture fixation
- Shortening of comminuted fibular fractures will lead to malreduction of the ankle mortise
- This can be avoided by recreating the normal relationship between the tip of the distal fibula and the lateral processes of the talus the "dime sign"
- Test the integrity of the syndesmosis after fixing the fibula in isolated fibular fractures (and medial malleolus in the case of bimalleolar fractures) (and medial malleolus and posterior malleolus in the case of trimalleolar fractures)

Technique 2: Operative Fixation of Medial Malleolus Fractures

Preoperative Planning

Instrumentation necessary to have during the case includes small fragment instrumentation and fluoroscopy. Additional instrumentation that will be helpful to have available include K-wires, fracture reduction tools and heavy non-absorbable suture. We routinely use a thigh tourniquet inflated to 100 mm Hg above systolic blood pressure prior to making incision. The most common fracture pattern is a transverse medial malleolar fracture (as seen in supination-external rotation, PER and PA ankle fractures), and this is the best fixed with two parallel 4.0 mm x 40 mm partially threaded lag screws placed in parallel fashion perpendicular to the fracture line (Fig. 28.8). Supination-adduction ankle fractures produce a vertical fracture line. These fractures can be fixed with either two 4.0 mm partially threaded screws placed parallel to the joint line or a one-third tubular plate placed in buttress fashion (Fig. 28.12). Extremely, comminuted medial malleolus fractures can also be fixed with a one-third tubular plate used as a bridging construct. Small transverse medial malleolar fractures such as anterior or posterior collicular fractures or very distal medial malleolar fractures will be unable to accept two 4.0 mm screws, therefore, these fracture patterns can be adequately secured using a tension band construct (Figs 28.9A and B).

Technique

Make a 4 cm gently curved incision over the anteromedial aspect of the ankle overlying the medial malleolus. Identify and mobilize the saphenous vein and two branches of the saphenous nerve that run together and cross the surgical field. Expose the lateral and anterior aspect of the fractured medial malleolus as this will allow for easier reduction.

Excise a 2 mm cuff of periosteum proximal and distal the fracture site to more easily identify the fractured cortices of the medial malleolus. Curette and irrigate the fracture site to clear out hematoma and soft tissue entrapped in the fracture site and to more clearly visualize the fracture edges. A dental pick can be used to evert the distal fracture fragment and expose the tibiotalar joint. The talar dome should be inspected for osteochondral lesions and/or articular surface damage that may have occurred at the time of the injury. Thoroughly, irrigate the joint to remove soft tissue and bone fragments that may have displaced into the joint.

Once the joint has been irrigated and the fracture cortices exposed, the fracture is reduced. To reduce transverse medial malleolus fractures, we prefer to use one of two techniques. In the first technique, a dental pick can be used to manipulate the distal fragment until reduction is achieved and a 1.6 mm K-wire is then placed across the fracture perpendicular to the fracture in the center of the fragment to hold this reduction. By placing the K-wire in the center of the distal fracture fragment, room is left anterior and posterior to this wire to achieve good spread between the two parallel lag screws that will be placed perpendicular to the fracture. In the second technique to achieve reduction, a pointed reduction clamp is used to achieve reduction. A pilot hole is drilled proximal to the fracture site using a 2.5 mm drill to secure the proximal tine of the reduction clamp and the distal tine of the reduction clamp secures the distal fragment. Again, the distal tine should be placed in the middle of the distal fragment to allow for one lag screw each to be placed anterior and posterior to the distal tine.

Reduction should be checked using fluoroscopy to ensure restoration of the ankle mortise prior to placement of lag screws. Once anatomic reduction is confirmed, two 4.0 mm x 40 mm partially threaded cannulated lag screws are placed across the fracture site perpendicular to the orientation of the fracture to achieve compression at the fracture site. The starting point of the screws is the distal tip of the medial malleolus. One screw should be placed anterior and the other screw posterior to the reduction clamp or K-wire to achieve good spread of the lag screws. These screws should be placed under AP fluoroscopy to ensure that they do not penetrate into the ankle joint. Placing the lag screws too close to each other negates the anti-rotatory effect of using two screws by effectively creating one large screw about which the distal fragment can rotate.

In the case of comminuted medial malleolus fractures where cortical apposition of the fractured fragments is difficult to achieve, a one-third tubular plate using 3.5 mm cortical screws spanning the fracture site is used in bridging mode (Figs 28.12A and B). Appropriate length, rotation and restoration of the ankle mortise is confirmed under fluoroscopy.

In the case of vertical shear fractures of the medial malleolus, as is common in SA type ankle fractures, it is difficult to place lag screws perpendicular to the fracture site from the common location of the distal tip of the medial malleolus. In this case, if there is sufficient bone in the distal fragment that is proximal to the ankle joint, two 4.0 mm partially threaded lag screws can be placed across the fracture site above the ankle joint and parallel to the joint line. If there is insufficient bone in the distal fragment to achieve adequate fixation, a one-third tubular plate using 3.5 mm cortical screws can be used in antiglide mode to achieve fixation.

In the case of small medial malleolar fractures that are too small for lag screw fixation as is the case in isolated anterior or posterior collicular fractures, a tension band construct can be used. In this technique, two K-wires are placed into the distal fracture fragment perpendicular to the fracture line securing the fragment in the anatomically reduced position. A bicortical screw and washer is placed

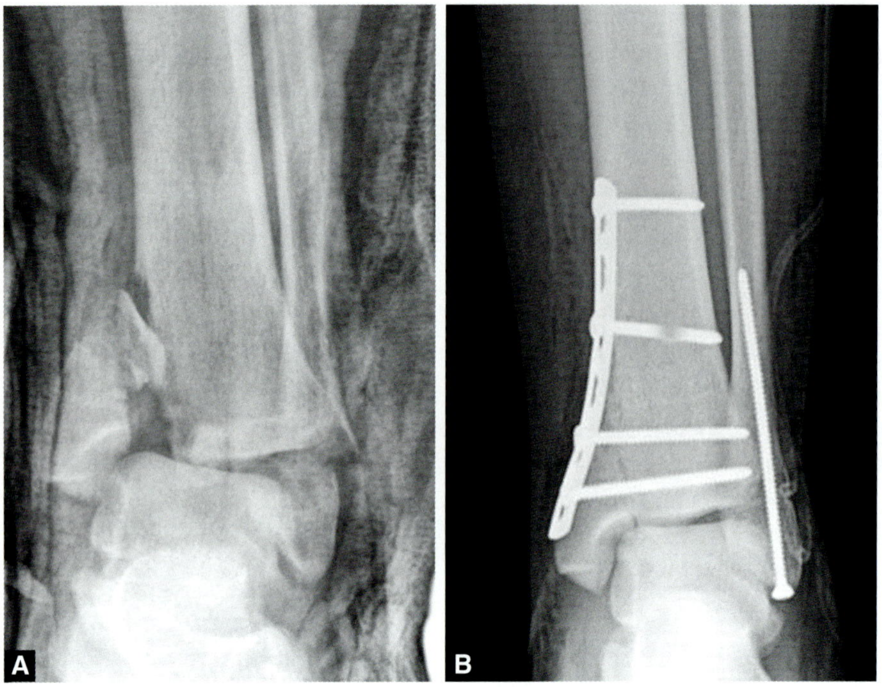

Figures 28.12A and B: Anteroposterior radiograph of ankle demonstrating supination-adduction vertical shear type medial malleolus fracture before and after open reduction and internal fixation with the use of a one-third tubular plate used with antiglide technique.

approximately 2 cm proximal to the fracture line above and parallel to the ankle joint. Prior to securing the screw or washer to bone, a heavy nonabsorbable suture (#5 ethibond or #2 fiberwire) is secured around the proximal screw or washer and the 2 distal K-wires in a figure-of-eight fashion. The screw is then firmly secured around the suture and the K-wires are bent, cut and then tamped into the distal fragment until they are no longer prominent.

Note that if a medial malleolus fracture is fixed in conjunction with a fibular fracture, the ankle syndesmosis must be stressed after fixation of both these fractures to evaluate its integrity. The "cotton test" is performed by placing a towel clip around the fibula and applying a lateral stress under AP or mortise view fluoroscopy. Decreased tibiofibular overlap (normal ≥ 10 mm overlap on AP and mortise views) is indicative of a syndesmotic injury that necessitates fixation. See Section on Surgical Technique: Technique 4—syndesmosis repair—for an in-depth description of the repair technique.

At the level of the medial malleolus, the lack of soft tissue coverage over the medial malleolus causes subcutaneous buried sutures, placed in this area, to cause skin irritation and have a tendency to form stitch abscesses. Therefore, we prefer to close skin directly with a 3-0 nylon suture in a vertical mattress fashion. Xeroform gauze dressing and sterile 4x4 gauze dressing are placed over the wound. The leg is wrapped in sterile webril and a standard short leg plaster splint is applied for immediate postoperative comfort. The patient is made non-weight-bearing for 6 weeks postoperatively at which time weight-bearing is progressively advanced. The patient is allowed to actively plantarflex and dorsiflex the ankle to prevent ankle stiffness once the surgical wounds are healed and sutures removed at approximately 7–10 days postoperatively.

OPERATIVE FIXATION OF MEDIAL MALLEOLUS FRACTURES: Pearls and Pitfalls

- In transverse medial malleolar fractures, expose the lateral and anterior aspect of the fracture to allow for anatomic reduction in both sagittal and coronal planes. This will reduce fluoroscopy time as reduction of the lateral and anterior aspect of the fracture indicates that the distal fragment is not malrotated. This should be confirmed under fluoroscopy

- Pointed reduction forceps or a 1.6 mm K-wire are used to reduce transverse medial malleolar fractures and should be placed in the middle of the distal fragment. This allows for adequate spread between two lag screws. If the two lag screws are placed too close together, they will act as a single screw thereby losing their anti-rotation function
- Place lag screws under fluoroscopy to ensure that they are perpendicular to the fracture line and that they do not penetrate the ankle joint
- Consider use of a small plate to bridge the fracture site in significantly comminuted medial malleolus fractures
- Consider use of a tension band technique to achieve secure fixation in the case of isolated anterior or posterior collicular fractures of the medial malleolus

Technique 3: ORIF of Posterior Malleolar Fractures

Preoperative Planning

Instrumentation necessary to have during the case includes small fragment instrumentation and fluoroscopy. Additional instrumentation that will be helpful to have available include K-wires and fracture reduction tools. We routinely use a thigh tourniquet inflated to 100 mm Hg above systolic blood pressure prior to making incision. Posterior malleolar fractures typically result from an axial load vector to a plantarflexed foot resulting in a characteristic vertical shear fracture pattern of the posterior distal tibia in the coronal plate. If an adequate closed reduction is obtained, these fracture fragments can be fixed with two percutaneous anterior to posterior 4.0 mm partially threaded cannulated lag screws (Fig. 28.13). If an open reduction is required to obtain an anatomic reduction (via the posterolateral approach to the ankle joint), then either two posterior to anterior directed 4.0 mm partially threaded lag screws or a one-third tubular plate placed in antiglide fashion along the distal tibia can be performed (Figs 28.9A and B). In the case of a posterior malleolar fracture with an associated distal fibular fracture, consideration should be given to accessing both fracture fragments via the posterolateral approach to the ankle joint (see Section on Surgical Approach).

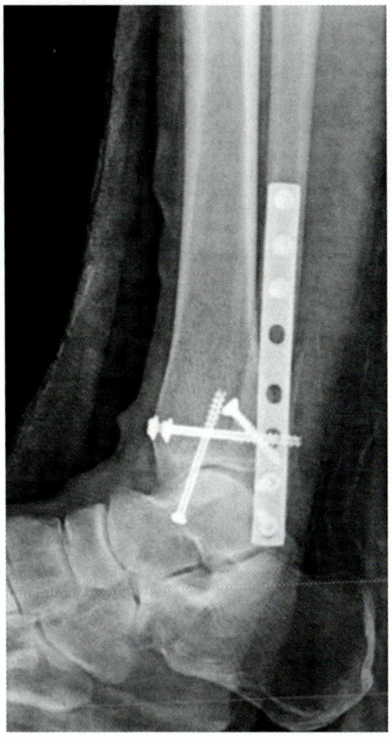

Figure 28.13: Lateral radiograph of ankle demonstrating closed reduction of posterior malleolus fracture and percutaneous fixation with two anterior to posterior 4.0 mm partially threaded cannulated lag screws.

Technique

To attempt closed reduction of a posterior malleolus fracture, in the supine position place the posterior tine of a large pointed reduction clamp percutaneously just lateral to the Achilles tendon and secure it against the posterior malleolus. Next, make a stab incision just through skin anteriorly at the level of the distal tibia just between the extensor digitorum longus and peroneus tertius tendons and place the anterior tine of the large pointed reduction clamp against the anterior cortex of the distal tibia. Visualize the reduction using lateral fluoroscopic images.

Once anatomic reduction is achieved, place two percutaneous 1.6 K-wires from anterior to posterior. It is advisable to make two 1 cm longitudinal skin incisions approximately 1–2 cm apart for each K-wire and subsequent screw. A blunt hemostat should be used to separate the soft tissues to ensure the anterior neurovascular bundle (tibialis anterior artery and deep peroneal nerve) is mobilized out the way of the projected K-wire and screw path. A soft tissue protector is placed directly on the anterior cortex of the tibia and the K-wires are then placed without fear of penetrating or wrapping the neurovascular bundle. Alternatively, advance the K-wires by oscillating to prevent wrapping up the neurovascular bundle. Next, the hemostat is placed back through the incision to keep the soft tissue separated around the K-wire and the 4.0 mm partially threaded cannulated screws are placed sequentially. Reduction is confirmed via lateral fluoroscopic images.

Open reduction of small posterior malleolar fractures is best achieved through a posterolateral approach to the ankle joint. Identify and protect the sural nerve which runs with the short saphenous vein in the layer superficial to the deep fascia surrounding the Achilles and peroneal tendons. Once the posterior malleolus is identified, obtain reduction with either a large pointed reduction clamp or K-wires. Reduction is confirmed on lateral fluoroscopic images. Fixation is achieved with two 4.0 mm partially threaded lag screws. Ensure that the lag screws are not placed too close together otherwise they will act as a single screw about which the posterior malleolus will be able to rotate.

Larger posterior malleolus fractures may achieve more stable fixation with a one-third tubular plate placed in antiglide fashion along the posterior aspect of the distal tibia. Again, the posterolateral approach to the ankle joint is used to visualize the fractured posterior malleolus.

Once the fracture is identified and cleared of interposed periosteum in usual fashion, reduction is achieved using either large pointed reduction clamps or K-wires. Once anatomic reduction is confirmed on lateral fluoroscopic images, the one-third tubular plate is contoured to the posterior aspect of the distal tibia. The screw hole just proximal to the fracture site is filled first to create an axilla at the apex of the fracture that prevents further proximal displacement of the fracture. Screw holes proximal and distal to the fracture are then filled with bicortical screws until secure fixation is achieved. Anatomic reduction of the fracture and ankle joint is confirmed on lateral fluoroscopic images.

Incisions for percutaneously placed anterior to posterior lag screws are closed with 3-0 nylon. If a posterolateral approach to the ankle joint is used, the subcutaneous layer is closed with buried 2-0 vicryl suture and the skin is closed with 3-0 nylon in vertical mattress fashion. Xeroform gauze dressing and sterile 4x4 gauze dressing are placed over the wound. The leg is wrapped in sterile webril and a standard AO short leg plaster splint is applied for immediate postoperative comfort. The patient is made non-weight-bearing for six weeks postoperatively at which time weight-bearing is progressively advanced. The patient is allowed to actively plantarflex and dorsiflex the ankle to prevent ankle stiffness once the surgical wounds are healed and sutures removed at approximately 7–10 days postoperatively.

ORIF OF POSTERIOR MALLEOLAR FRACTURES: Pearls and Pitfalls

- Closed reduction and percutaneous anterior to posterior lag screw fixation of posterior malleolus fractures is most easily performed in the supine position with the image intensifier set-up to take lateral fluoroscopic images
- Use a soft tissue protector or oscillating drill technique is used when placing percutaneous K-wires for the anterior to posterior 4.0 mm partially threaded cannulated lag screws. This ensures that the anterior neurovascular bundle (tibialis anterior artery and deep peroneal nerve) will not become wrapped up during insertion
- The prone position facilitates exposure during the posterolateral approach to the ankle. Additionally, both lateral malleolar and posterior malleolar fractures can be accessed through this approach. However, it is more difficult to fix medial malleolar fractures in this position

Technique 4: ORIF of Syndesmotic Injuries of the Ankle

Preoperative Planning

Instrumentation necessary to have during the case includes small fragment instrumentation, a large pointed reduction clamp and fluoroscopy. Controversy exists regarding the optimum screw configuration for syndesmotic fixation. Traditionally, either one 4.0 mm quadricortical screw (screw achieving distal cortical fixation in the lateral tibia) or two 3.5 mm tricortical screws (screw achieving distal cortical fixation in the medial tibia) are used to obtain secure syndesmotic fixation. In ankle injuries involving the syndesmosis that do not require full exposure of the fibula

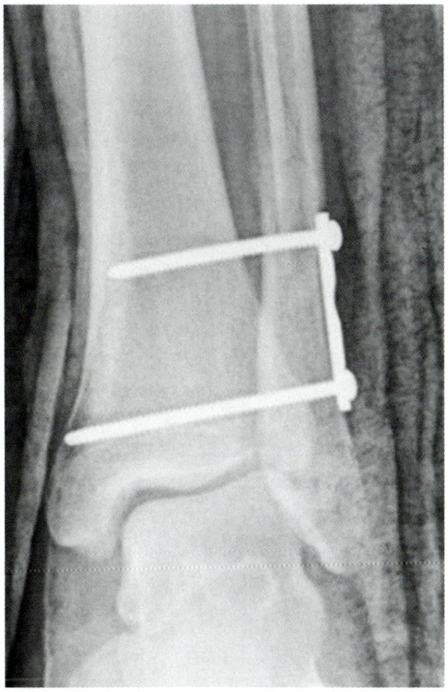

Figure 28.14: Anteroposterior radiograph of the ankle demonstrating repair of the ankle syndesmosis using two tricortical 3.5 mm cortical screws using a 3-hole one-third tubular plate as a washer.

for separate fixation, the syndesmosis can be repaired open or percutaneously using either one cannulated 4.0 mm quadricortical screw or two cannulated 3.5 mm tricortical screws (Fig. 28.14). In ankle fractures that require fixation of the fibula, the syndesmosis can be repaired with one 4.0 mm quadricortical screw or two 3.5 mm tricortical screws placed through a laterally placed one-third tubular plate (Fig. 28.8). If a posterior or posterolateral one-third tubular plate is used in antiglide fashion to fix the fibular fracture, then the syndesmosis screws are placed directly through the lateral fibula.

Technique

In the case of bimalleolar fractures, bimalleolar fracture equivalents (SER type ankle fractures with a medial deltoid rupture) and trimalleolar fractures, the ankle syndesmosis must be tested to determine if it is stable or unstable after fixation of all fracture fragments. The "cotton test" tests for syndesmosis instability and is performed by placing a towel clip around the fibula and applying a lateral stress under AP or mortise view fluoroscopy. Decreased tibiofibular overlap (normal $\geq$ 10 mm overlap on AP and mortise views) is indicative of a syndesmotic injury that necessitates fixation.

A bump is placed under the distal tibia to elevate the calcaneus off the bed. This prevents anterior displacement of the distal fibula relative to the distal tibia which can lead to malreduction of distal fibula in the incisura. A large pointed reduction clamp is placed along the intermalleolar axis on the apex of lateral malleolus and the medial malleolus. Because the intermalleolar axis is externally rotated approximately 30° from the coronal plane of the distal tibia, if the ankle joint is facing directly anterior (confirm by ensuring the patella is pointing toward the ceiling), then the reduction clamp should also be externally rotated relative to the distal tibia. Reduce the distal fibula into the incisura and confirm under AP and mortise fluoroscopic views that the tibiofibular overlap is normalized. Confirm under lateral fluoroscopic views that the distal tip of the fibula is sitting in posterior third of the distal tibia (the location of the incisura). If there is concern about the adequacy of the reduction, the syndesmosis should be visualized through the lateral approach to the fibula by sharply dissecting supraperiostially over the anterior aspect of the fibula 1–2 cm above the level of the ankle joint. The distal fibula should be observed to lie concentrically reduced within the incisura.

Either one quadricortical 4.0 mm screw or two 3.5 mm tricortical screws are placed from lateral to medial and oriented 30° externally rotated relative to the coronal plane of the distal tibia. Reduction is again confirmed using AP, mortise and lateral fluoroscopic imaging. Direct visualization of the syndesmosis is performed if there is concern regarding the adequacy of the reduction.

Incisions for percutaneously placed syndesmotic screws are closed with 3-0 nylon in vertical mattress fashion. If a lateral approach to the fibula is used to either fix an associated fibular fracture of directly visualize the syndesmosis, we prefer not to place subcutaneous buried sutures in this area because they have a tendency to cause skin irritation and form stitch abscesses. Therefore, we prefer to close skin directly with a 3-0 nylon suture in a vertical mattress fashion. Xeroform gauze dressing and sterile 4 x 4 gauze dressing are placed over the wound. The leg is wrapped in sterile webril and a standard short leg plaster splint is applied for immediate postoperative comfort. The patient is made non-weight-bearing for 6 weeks postoperatively at which time weight-bearing is progressively advanced. The patient is allowed to actively plantarflex and dorsiflex the ankle to prevent ankle stiffness once the surgical wounds are healed and sutures removed at approximately 7–10 days postoperatively. It is common for syndesmotic screws to break once full weight-bearing is allowed given the relative motion at ankle syndesmosis. We routinely do not remove these broken screws as they typically go unnoticed and do not cause further discomfort for the patient.

ORIF OF SYNDESMOTIC INJURIES OF THE ANKLE: Pearls and Pitfalls

- Place a bump under the distal tibia to prevent anterior translation of the distal fibula relative to the incisura. An anteriorly directed force on the calcaneus will cause anterior displacement of the distal fibula through ligamentotaxis via talocalcaneal interosseus ligaments and talofibular ligaments
- Radiographically, the syndesmosis is reduced if on AP and mortise fluoroscopic views of the ankle the tibiofibular overlap is ≥ 10 mm and on a lateral view the distal tip fibula lies along the posterior one-third of the tibia
- If there is concern regarding adequate reduction of the syndesmosis, the distal fibula articulation with the tibial incisura should be visualized through the lateral approach to the fibula
- Either one 4.0 mm quadricortical screw or two 3.5 mm tricortical screws can be used to achieve secure fixation of the syndesmosis

Outcomes

The literature has demonstrated that patients can expect reasonable improvement in their ankle symptoms over time following surgical fixation. Egol et al. reported on the functional outcomes of patients following surgery.[11] At one year, 88% of patients had either no or mild ankle pain and 90% had either no limitations or limitations only in recreational activities. Patients experienced significant improvement in their function between the 6 month and one year time points. Predictors of better outcome included age less than 40 years, male sex, absence of diabetes and lower ASA class. In another study, these same factors were shown to be predictive of return to sporting activities.[12]

In a different series, Lash et al. found similar outcomes evaluating patients two years after ankle fracture.[13] Overall, 77% of patients achieved a good or excellent outcome. Nonetheless, this study also reported residual functional difficulties in many patients, especially those who sustained unstable ankle fractures and were treated surgically. Philips et al. in a randomized prospective trial of 71 patients, found that outcomes for patients with unstable fracture patterns were better in those who underwent surgery, though the difference was not statistically significant.[14]

For unstable ankle fractures, patient outcome appears to worsen when the medial and/or posterior malleoli are fractured in addition to the lateral malleolus. Tejwani et al. reported on patients with SER-IV ankle fractures with 1 year follow-up.[15] They found that Short Musculoskeletal Functional Assessment (SMFA) scores were significantly lower in patients who sustained a medial malleolus fracture than in those who had deltoid ligament rupture without medial bony injury. Bhandari et al. also found that a medial malleolus fracture was predictive of a worse outcome.[16] The presence of a posterior malleolar component to an unstable ankle fracture has likewise been reported as an independent predictor of a worse outcome at 1 year.[17] The above findings suggest that, in rotational ankle fractures, bony injuries imply a more severe insult to the ankle than ligamentous ones.

For patients who sustain disruption of the syndesmosis, adequate fixation is crucial to achieving an optimal outcome. Pettrone et al. in a series of 146 ankle fractures found that radiographic evidence of preoperative syndesmotic disruption was not associated with a worse outcome.[18] However, the presence of postoperative syndesmotic instability did adversely affect the final outcome. Another series similarly identified adequate syndesmotic reduction as the primary factor affecting functional outcomes in patients who required trans-syndesmotic fixation.[19] Egol et al. found that the need for syndesmotic fixation predisposed patients to a worse outcome than the need for malleolar fixation alone.[20] Though the literature contains conflicting reports of the prognostic effect of syndesmotic injury, attaining anatomic fixation of this lesion gives patients the best chance for a favorable result.

The presence of preexisting comorbidities can also affect patient outcomes. A large review of diabetic ankle fracture patients found that this population had a higher in-hospital mortality rate and postoperative complication rate, as well as a longer length of stay than non-diabetic patients.[21] Similarly, peripheral vascular disease has been shown to adversely affect postoperative outcomes.[22] The effect of obesity on long-term outcomes following ankle fractures is less clear, with conflicting reports on whether it serves as an independent risk factor for a worse result.[23,24] Nonetheless, we believe that patients with significant comorbidities, including obesity, should be counseled preoperatively that their postoperative course and overall outcome may be unfavorably affected by their conditions.

Complications

Complications are common in the management of operative fixation of ankle fractures and include; (1) infection and wound breakdown; (2) early loss of hardware fixation; (3) malunion; (4) nonunion; (5) late syndesmotic widening or neglected syndesmotic instability; and (6) peroneal tendonitis.

Infection and Wound Breakdown

The rates for all ankle fractures treated operatively range from 0.93–8.6%.[14,25,26] The wide range of reported rates in the literature is due to lack of separation of superficial and deep infection rates. In a large review of the California discharge database of 57,183 patients who underwent open ORIF of ankle fractures, SooHoo et al. reported a wound infection rate of 1.4% based on the need for readmission to the hospital for treatment within 90 days of discharge.[22] Diabetic patients, in particular, have a much higher rate of wound breakdown and early infection due to decreased perfusion of soft tissues resulting from chronic microvascular changes. Smaller studies reporting solely on operatively treated ankle fractures in diabetic patients have reported infection rates ranging from 12% to 46%.[27-29]

Superficial infections after operatively treated ankle fractures presents as cellulitis and can be managed with antibiotics. Marginal wound necrosis usually results from wound closure under high tension and can lead to a superficial infection. This type of skin breakdown can be managed with local wound care with the addition of antibiotics if a superficial infection develops. Deep infections commonly present with frank wound dehiscence and should be managed with I and D of the wound. A sequelae of a deep wound infection is a septic ankle and the ankle joint should also be irrigated thoroughly if there is concern for this complication. Intravenous antibiotic therapy should be initiated and hardware should be retained if fixation is secure. If fixation is unstable, then hardware should be removed and either external fixation or casting should be performed to provide some stability of the ankle to allow healing of the fracture.

The most important factor to reduce the incidence of infection after operatively treated ankle fractures is to delay surgery until there is reduced swelling of the soft tissue envelope of the ankle. Surgery should be delayed until the normal wrinkles of the skin around the ankle return indicating sufficiently reduced swelling of the ankle, i.e. the "wrinkle test". Blisters can be unroofed and silver sulfadiazine cream can be applied to promote re-epi-thelialization of the blister bed prior to surgery.[30] Surgical incisions should avoid blisters if possible, atraumatic surgical technique should be utilized and tourniquet use should be minimized to reduce the incidence of infection and wound breakdown.

Early Loss of Hardware Fixation

This most commonly occurs in osteoporotic bone. This can lead to malunion and nonunion of ankle fractures. To prevent this complication several strategies exist. Locking one-third tubular plates can be utilized to allow for decreased chance of screw pullout from the osteoporotic bone. Posterior fibular plating of distal fibular fractures allows for increased fixation strength compared to lateral plating. Screws placed distal the ankle joint can achieve bicortical purchase with posterior plating because the screws are extra-articular compared to screws placed with a lateral plate which must remain unicortical to prevent penetration into the ankle joint. With lateral plating, tricortical screw fixation can be used with screw purchase in the tibia used to enhance fixation stability. K-wires inserted from the tip of the distal fibula proximally across the fracture site prior to screw placement allow for interference fit of screws providing increased stability of the construct. Bone cement inserted into predrilled screw holes is another technique for enhancing screw fixation in osteoporotic bone.

Malunion

Malunion is an uncommon complication of operatively treated ankle fractures and more commonly results from nonoperatively treated unstable ankle fractures. Malunion of the fibula results from either shortening or external rotation of the distal fibula. This leads to lateral talar shift and altered contact forces of the tibiotalar joint.[31] Malunion of fibula fractures is more common in the case of comminuted fractures where cortical keys for bony apposition are absent. To prevent malunion in this scenario, intraoperative fluoroscopy is imperative. The "dime sign" and the talocrural angle of the unaffected ankle can be used as intraoperative markers to establish the appropriate fibular length (see Section on Surgical Technique: Technique 1). Malunion of medial malleolar fractures is due to rotatory malalignment during operative reduction and can be prevented by adequately exposing both the lateral and anterior aspect of the fracture. This allows for anatomic bony apposition in both the sagittal and coronal plane making malreduction less likely. Malunions that result in an incongruent mortise require revision surgery to restore a congruent mortise to achieve the best functional outcome.

Nonunion

Nonunion is another uncommon complication of operatively treated ankle fractures and is more commonly seen in conservatively managed unstable ankle fractures. Nonunion of medial malleolar fractures are more common than nonunion of lateral malleolar fractures.[32] Nonunion of operatively treated ankle fractures are usually secondary to interposed soft tissue at the fracture site that was never removed at the time of surgery. To prevent nonunion of operatively treated ankle fractures, we recommend thorough debridement of interposed soft tissue at the fracture site and minimal periosteal stripping around the fracture site. Symptomatic nonunion of the medial malleolus, lateral malleolus, or posterior malleolus warrant revision of the nonunion to achieve stable fixation.

Late Syndesmotic Widening and Neglected Syndesmotic Instability

This negatively affects patient functional outcome.[18,33,34] Intraoperative stress radiographs obtained after fixation of all bony injuries are essential to diagnose this injury. We routinely use the "cotton test" in which we place a clamp around the fibula and apply a lateral stress to the fibula and observe under AP fluoroscopic imaging if there is increase in tibiofibular overlap greater than 10 mm (normal $\leq$ 10 mm). Weening and Bhandari reviewed the functional outcome of 39 patients, who underwent syndesmotic screw fixation and showed that the only significant predictor of functional outcome was anatomic reduction of the syndesmosis.[19] If there is any concern regarding the adequacy of the syndesmotic reduction, then direct visualization of the syndesmosis should be performed to ensure that the distal fibula is resting congruently within the tibial incisura.

Peroneal Tendonitis

This is most commonly associated with posterior plating of distal fibular fractures. Treadwell and Fallet reported a 2.8% rate of peroneal tendonitis in 71 patients treated with antiglide plating of Weber B distal fibular fractures.[35] To reduce the incidence of this complication, we recommend contouring the distal tip of the one-third tubular plate to fit snuggly against the convex surface of the distal fibula. Peroneal tendonitis generally resolves after hardware removal.

Authors' Preferred Management of Select Complications

Case 1: Treatment of Early Infection and Wound Breakdown

A 48-year-old female sustained a twisting injury to her right ankle while walking in high heels in a busy subway station. Physical examination in the emergency room revealed a grossly swollen ankle without open wounds. Radiographic evaluation revealed a SER rotation type IV ankle fracture-dislocation. The patient underwent closed reduction in the emergency room and was sent home in a plaster splint with instructions for strict elevation. She was re-evaulated in the office setting five days after her injury where physical examination revealed significantly decreased ankle swelling. She had a positive "wrinkle test". The patient underwent operative fixation of the ankle fracture 10 days after the injury where she received

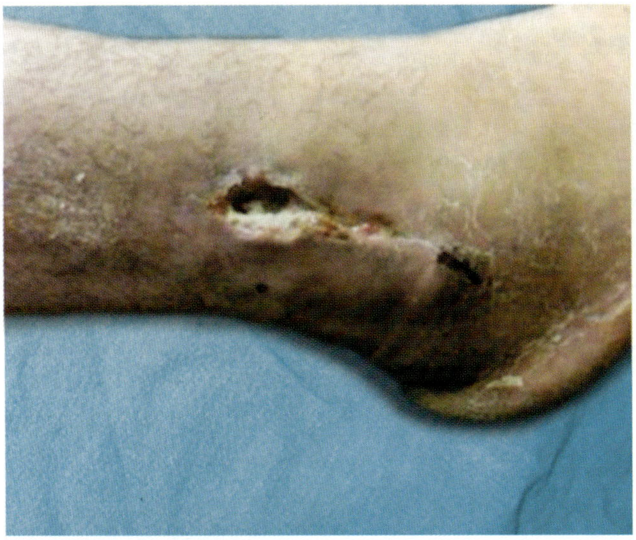

Figure 28.15: Lateral ankle incision dehiscence and breakdown, 10 days after open reduction and internal fixation (ORIF) of an ankle fracture.

a one-third tubular plate placed in antiglide fashion along the posterior fibula and two 4.0 mm partially threaded cannulated lag screws into the medial malleolus. The patient was discharged on postoperative day 0. The patient returned to the office on postoperative day 10 for removal of sutures where her lateral wound was noted to have serous drainage from the distal one-third of the wound with associated dehiscence of the distal incision (Fig. 28.15). Given the concern for deep infection, the patient was admitted to the hospital for I and D of the lateral wound in the operating room for the initiation of broad-spectrum antibiotic therapy.

In cases of suspected acute deep infection of operatively treated ankle fracture, we hold antibiotic therapy until intraoperative deep cultures are obtained in order to increase the positive bacterial yield of these cultures. If the fixation construct is stable, which is most commonly the case, we retain the hardware to allow for fracture healing. We use pulse-lavage irrigation and mechanical scrubbing of the metal hardware to decrease the bacterial load and associated biofilm layer on the metal implants. After intraoperative cultures are obtained, we start empiric intravenous antibiotic therapy to cover both Gram-positive and Gram-negative bacterial organisms. At our institution, we routinely use 1 gram IV vancomycin dosed every 12 hours to cover methicillin-resistant *Staphylococcus aureus* and 3.375 grams of piperacillin or tazobactam every 6 hours to cover Gram-positive and Gram-negative organisms as well as anaerobic organisms. Patients with deep infections require chronic antibiotic therapy to ensure eradication of the infection; therefore, we place a peripherally inserted central catheter to administer 4–6 weeks of intravenous antibiotic therapy. In conjunction with an infectious disease consulting physician, we follow weekly infectious laboratory values including white blood cell count, erythrocyte sedimentation rate and C-reactive protein (CRP) to determine when the infection has cleared and antibiotics can be stopped. Once the fracture has healed, we will remove hardware if the infection has not been eradicated as determined by the previously mentioned infection laboratory values or a persistently draining wound. If the infection has been eradicated, then we opt to leave the hardware in place.

Case 2: Treatment of Painful Nonunion of a Medial Malleolus Fracture

A 55-year-old obese male smoker with a past medical history significant for diabetes sustained a supination-eversion type IV ankle fracture to his left ankle. Injury radiographs revealed a reduced ankle joint and a minimally displaced medial malleolus fracture. After risks, benefits and alternatives of operative and nonoperative treatment of this fracture pattern were explained to the patient, the patient opted for nonoperative treatment in a cast despite our recommendation for operative fixation. The patient was placed into a short-leg cast for 12 weeks and made non-weight-bearing. At the time of cast removal, the patient remained tender to palpation over the medial malleolus and radiographs of the ankle demonstrated a frank radiolucency at the site of the fracture without evidence of bridging callus (Fig. 28.16A).

In cases of medial malleolar nonunion with either associated pain and/or joint incongruity, it is necessary to obtain fracture healing to both decrease pain and restore the ankle mortise. This patient was taken to the operating room and an anteromedial approach to the medial malleolus was used to expose the nonunion site. The nonunion site was cleared of fibrous tissue and atrophic callus. Autogenous iliac crest cancellous bone graft was obtained from the ipsilateral iliac crest and placed into the nonunion site to promote bone healing.

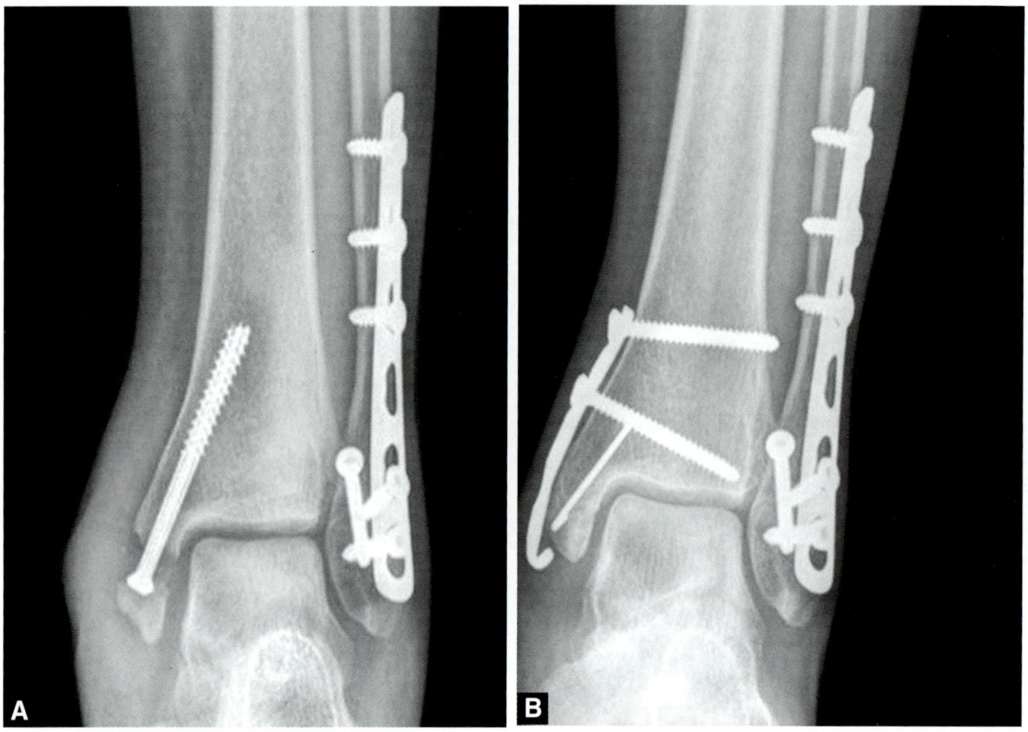

Figures 28.16A and B: Anteroposterior radiograph of (A) medial malleolus nonunion after operative fixation and (B) after revision of fixation with plate and K-wire.

Two 4.0 mm 40 mm partially threaded lag screws were placed perpendicular to the fracture site in parallel fashion to obtain secure fixation of the medial malleolus. Postoperatively, given the patient's multiple risk factors to retard fracture healing, the patient was given an external bone stimulator and made non-weight-bearing for an additional 12 weeks. Serial radiographs obtained in the interim revealed progressive healing of the medial malleolus. At 3 months follow-up, the patient was non-tender to palpation at the fracture site and radiographs of the ankle demonstrated effacement of the radiolucency that defined the fracture site indicating that the medial malleolus had healed (Fig. 28.16B).

Case 3: Loss of Reduction with Early Post-traumatic Arthrosis Treated with Arthrodesis

(Courtesy of Saqib Rehman)

A 70-year-old female sustained a low energy fall with a resulting bimalleolar ankle fracture. This was determined to be an unstable injury and was subsequently treated with open reduction and internal fixation. Her concurrent medical conditions include hypertension, congestive heart failure, diabetes mellitus, hypothyroidism, sarcoidosis and major depressive disorder. Her initial postoperative course was reportedly uneventful with good fracture alignment. However, she was then temporarily lost for follow-up for 2 months. Although it was recommended that she be non-weight-bearing, she was noted to be weight-bearing at her follow-up with pain, complete loss of alignment, broken and loose implants and obvious signs of post-traumatic arthrosis of the tibiotalar joint (Figs 28.17A and B). At this point, she was referred to the author for further care.

On examination, valgus instability as suggested on the radiograph was demonstrated clinically. There were no open wounds or obvious concerns for infection other than the fact that the fracture did not heal. The valgus could be corrected to neutral with manipulation, but bracing was required to at least partially maintain this. Given her pain, instability, poor alignment and nonunion, she was indicated for operative reconstruction. Radiographs appeared to demonstrate post-traumatic arthrosis of the tibiotalar joint. Therefore, arthrodesis was chosen as her definitive treatment. It was felt that even if revision ORIF were successful in maintaining alignment, painful post-traumatic arthritis may result in an unsatisfactory result. Furthermore, it did not appear that revision ORIF would work given that her previous attempt at ORIF failed and her diabetes comorbidity. Also, repeated ankle surgeries on a diabetic patient increase the risk for infection, so one definitive procedure would be the preferred treatment.

In order to rule out the possibility of infection as an etiology for the nonunion, a workup was performed in order to rule this out. Unfortunately, there are no tests which are highly sensitive and specific for occult osteomyelitis. Even deep bone biopsies can often yield negative cultures when there is obvious infection. Nevertheless, the surgeon generally performs a workup in suspicious cases in which the definitive treatment might be affected by the discovery of a deep occult infection. In her case, blood tests including a CRP and a sedimentation rate were ordered as well as a tagged white blood cell nuclear scan. These tests all yielded normal results as did a bone biopsy and culture (Figs 28.17C and D). At this point, she was indicated to proceed to removal of the implants and arthrodesis of the tibiotalar joint. The patient was informed that bone morphogenetic protein 2 (BMP-2) would likely be used in an off-label manner (i.e. not used according to Federal Drug Administration-approved indications).

Given her difficulties with maintaining non-weight-bearing restrictions, her diabetes and possibly poor bone quality, compression with locked plate fixation was chosen as her treatment rather than screws alone. External fixation was also an option, but not particularly attractive (due to difficulties for the patient) and was unnecessary given the lack of obvious infection. Previous surgical incisions were utilized (medially and laterally). The broken implants were removed, the distal fibula was resected and the remaining articular cartilage of the tibiotalar joint surfaces was debrided with curettes. An attempt was made to create congruent bone surfaces and compression was performed. Local autogenous graft supplemented with cancellous autograft was utilized in addition to BMP-2 (infuse). Fixation was performed with a stainless steel proximal humeral locked plate which was properly contoured for use in this manner (also used off-label) as shown in Figures 28.17E and F. Neutral plantigrade position was maintained with 5° of external rotation and valgus was neutral (5° of valgus would have been more preferable). Splinting and bracing was utilized until union was achieved at 9 months (Figs 28.17G and H). She was ambulatory at this time with satisfactory function although screw loosening and slight ankle dorsiflexion developed before union (Fig. 28.17H).

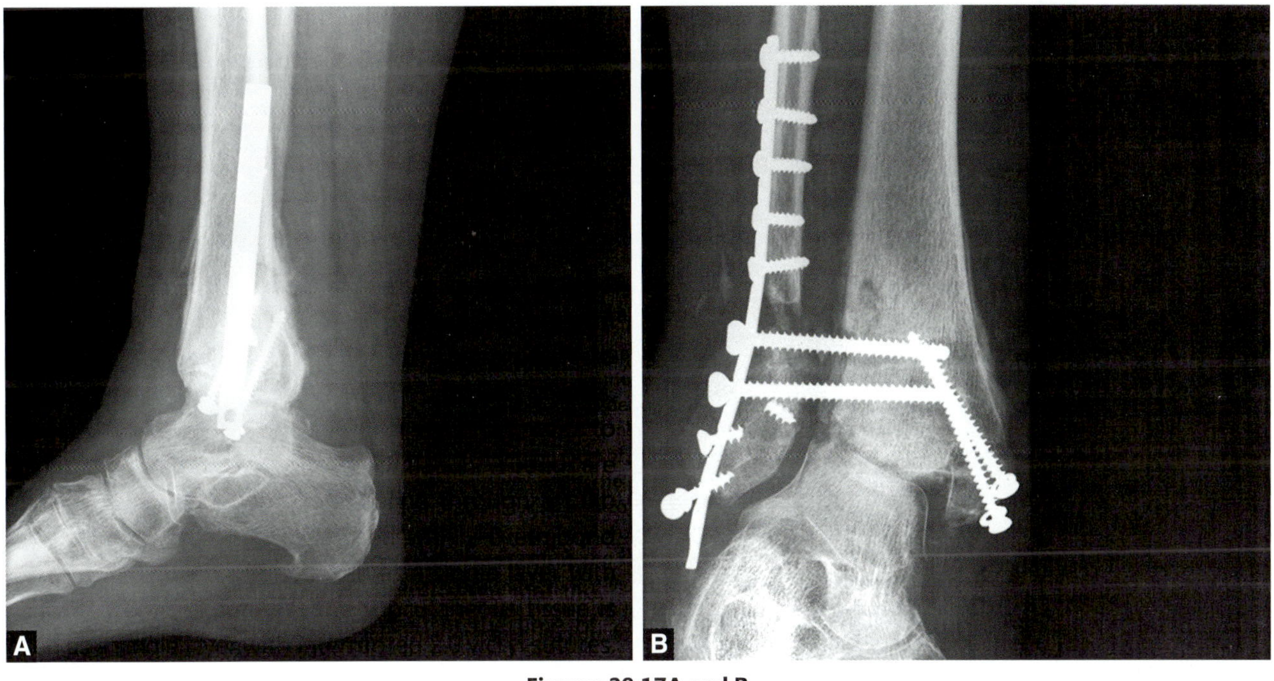

Figures 28.17A and B

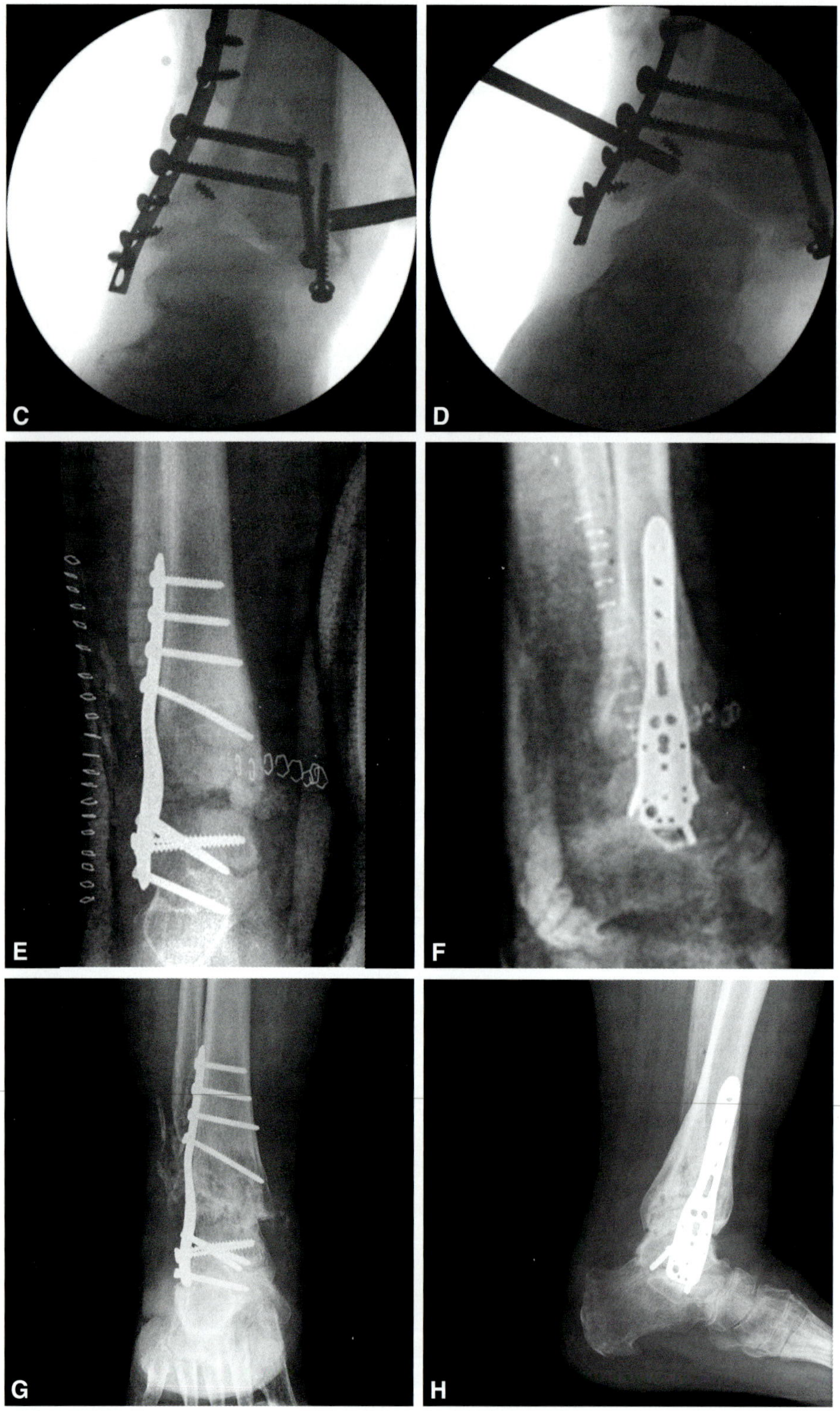

Figures 28.17A to H: Loss of reduction and post-traumatic arthrosis treated with arthrodesis. (A and B) Anteroposterior (AP) and lateral radiographic images of the ankle after previous open reduction and internal fixation and syndesmotic repair of an unstable bimalleolar ankle fracture; (C and D) A workup for occult deep infection included operative biopsies and cultures of both the medial and lateral malleoli; (E and F) AP and lateral radiographs after removal of implants and ankle arthrodesis with bone graft and locked compression plating; (G and H) AP and lateral radiographs after successful radiographic ankle fusion.

The key points of this case are as follows:

- Diabetes is a significant risk for nonunion and loss of fixation. Immobilization and delay of weight-bearing is required to prevent such complications
- Infection needs to be ruled out in cases of nonunion such as this
- Arthrodesis is generally a successful salvage procedure for cases in which post-traumatic arthrosis of the ankle has occurred. Total ankle arthroplasty is also an option, but still has not produced superior results in post-traumatic ankle arthrosis
- In diabetic patients, stronger fixation is generally wise. Therefore, although plate fixation is not typically done for ankle fusions, it was chosen in this case for this reason.

Summary

Ankle fractures are one of the most common fractures orthopedics surgeons face and their incidence is increasing. Operative fixation of unstable ankle fractures and syndesmotic injuries have shown to result in good to excellent patient outcomes. Fibular fractures are adequately fixed with a one-third tubular plate and screw construct placed in either a lateral or posterior or posterolateral position depending on the location and orientation of the fracture pattern. Transverse medial malleolar fractures are routinely fixed with two parallel lag screws, however, one-third tubular plates can be used in either bridging or antiglide mode if the fracture is significantly comminuted or has a vertical shear pattern, respectively. Posterior malleolar fractures can be fixed with either two lag screws or a one-third tubular plate used in antiglide mode. Syndesmotic injures not associated with common injury patterns can be easily missed if not stressed intraoperatively but are easily reduced and fixed with screws placed across the syndesmosis.

Potentially the most devastating complication following operative treatment of ankle fractures is the development of wound breakdown and deep infection. Ankle fractures should only undergo operative fixation when swelling has subsided to allow a tension-free closure. Additionally, atraumatic surgical technique and placing incisions to avoid areas of fracture blistering can lead to a decreased incidence of these complications. Other complications the surgeon may encounter include malunion and nonunion of the fracture, missed syndesmotic instability and early loss of hardware fixation. Being prepared to handle these complications will allow the surgeon to optimize the care for his or her patient.

References

1. Kannus P, Palvanen M, Niemi S, et al. Increasing number and incidence of low-trauma ankle fractures in elderly people: Finnish statistics during 1970-2000 and projections for the future. Bone. 2002;31:430-3.
2. Court-Brown CM, McBirnie J, Wilson G. Adult ankle fractures—an increasing problem? Acta Orthop Scand. 1998;69:43-7.
3. Park SS, Kubiak EN, Egol KA, et al. Stress radiographs after ankle fracture: the effect of ankle position and deltoid ligament status on medial clear space measurements. J Orthop Trauma. 2006;20:11-8.
4. Lauge-Hansen N. Fractures of the ankle. II. Combined experimental-surgical and experimental-roentgenologic investigations. Arch Surg. 1950;60:957-85.
5. Danis R. Les fractures malleolaires. In: Danis R (Ed). Theorie et Pratique de l'Osteosynthese. Paris: Masson et Cie; 1949. pp. 133-65.
6. Weber B. Die Verletzungen des oberen Sprungelenkes, 2nd edition. Bern: Hans Huber; 1972.
7. Fracture and dislocation compendium. Orthopaedic Trauma Association Committee for Coding and Classification. J Orthop Trauma. 1996;10 Suppl 1:v-ix, 1-154.
8. Ramsey PL, Hamilton W. Changes in tibiotalar area of contact caused by lateral talar shift. J Bone Joint Surg Am. 1976;58:356-7.
9. Koval KJ, Egol KA, Cheung Y, et al. Does a positive ankle stress test indicate the need for operative treatment after lateral malleolus fracture? A preliminary report. J Orthop Trauma. 2007;21:449-55.
10. Gardner MJ, Brodsky A, Briggs SM, et al. Fixation of posterior malleolar fractures provides greater syndesmotic stability. Clin Orthop Relat Res. 2006;447:165-71.
11. Egol KA, Tejwani NC, Walsh MG, et al. Predictors of short-term functional outcome following ankle fracture surgery. J Bone Joint Surg Am. 2006;88:974-9.
12. Colvin AC, Walsh M, Koval KJ, et al. Return to sports following operatively treated ankle fractures. Foot Ankle Int. 2009;30:292-6.
13. Lash N, Horne G, Fielden J, et al. Ankle fractures: functional and lifestyle outcomes at two years. ANZ J Surg. 2002; 72:724-30.

14. Phillips WA, Schwartz HS, Keller CS, et al. A prospective, randomized study of the management of severe ankle fractures. J Bone Joint Surg Am. 1985;67:67-78.
15. Tejwani NC, McLaurin TM, Walsh M, et al. Are outcomes of bimalleolar fractures poorer than those of lateral malleolar fractures with medial ligamentous injury? J Bone Joint Surg Am. 2007;89:1438-41.
16. Bhandari M, Sprague S, Hanson B, et al. Health-related quality of life following operative treatment of unstable ankle fractures: a prospective observational study. J Orthop Trauma. 2004;18:338-45.
17. Tejwani NC, Pahk B, Egol KA. Effect of posterior malleolus fracture on outcome after unstable ankle fracture. J Trauma. 2010;69:666-9.
18. Pettrone FA, Gail M, Pee D, et al. Quantitative criteria for prediction of the results after displaced fracture of the ankle. J Bone Joint Surg Am. 1983;65:667-77.
19. Weening B, Bhandari M. Predictors of functional outcome following trans-syndesmotic screw fixation of ankle fractures. J Orthop Trauma. 2005;19:102-8.
20. Egol KA, Pahk B, Walsh M, et al. Outcome after unstable ankle fracture: effect of syndesmotic stabilization. J Orthop Trauma. 2010;24:7-11.
21. Ganesh SP, Pietrobon R, Cecilio WA, et al. The impact of diabetes on patient outcomes after ankle fracture. J Bone Joint Surg Am. 2005;87:1712-8.
22. SooHoo NF, Krenek L, Eagan MJ, et al. Complication rates following open reduction and internal fixation of ankle fractures. J Bone Joint Surg Am. 2009;91:1042-9.
23. Bostman OM. Body-weight related to loss of reduction of fractures of the distal tibia and ankle. J Bone Joint Surg Br. 1995;77:101-3.
24. Strauss EJ, Frank JB, Walsh M, et al. Does obesity influence the outcome after the operative treatment of ankle fractures? J Bone Joint Surg Br. 2007;89:794-8.
25. Lindsjo U. Operative treatment of ankle fracture-dislocations. A follow-up study of 306/321 consecutive cases. Clin Orthop Relat Res. 1985:28-38.
26. Mak KH, Chan KM, Leung PC. Ankle fracture treated with the AO principle—an experience with 116 cases. Injury. 1985;16:265-72.
27. Jones KB, Maiers-Yelden KA, Marsh JL, et al. Ankle fractures in patients with diabetes mellitus. J Bone Joint Surg Br. 2005;87:489-95.
28. Blotter RH, Connolly E, Wasan A, et al. Acute complications in the operative treatment of isolated ankle fractures in patients with diabetes mellitus. Foot Ankle Int. 1999;20: 687-94.
29. Low CK, Tan SK. Infection in diabetic patients with ankle fractures. Ann Acad Med Singapore. 1995;24:353-5.
30. Strauss EJ, Petrucelli G, Bong M, et al. Blisters associated with lower-extremity fracture: results of a prospective treatment protocol. J Orthop Trauma. 2006;20:618-22.
31. Thordarson DB, Motamed S, Hedman T, et al. The effect of fibular malreduction on contact pressures in an ankle fracture malunion model. J Bone Joint Surg Am. 1997;79: 1809-15.
32. Mendelsohn HA. Nonunion of malleolar fractures of the ankle. Clin Orthop Relat Res. 1965;42:103-18.
33. Leeds HC, Ehrlich MG. Instability of the distal tibiofibular syndesmosis after bimalleolar and trimalleolar ankle fractures. J Bone Joint Surg Am. 1984;66:490-503.
34. Chissell HR, Jones J. The influence of a diastasis screw on the outcome of Weber type-C ankle fractures. J Bone Joint Surg Br. 1995;77:435-8.
35. Treadwell JR, Fallat LM. The antiglide plate for the Danis-Weber type-B fibular fracture: a review of 71 cases. J Foot Ankle Surg. 1993;32:573-9.

Chapter **29**

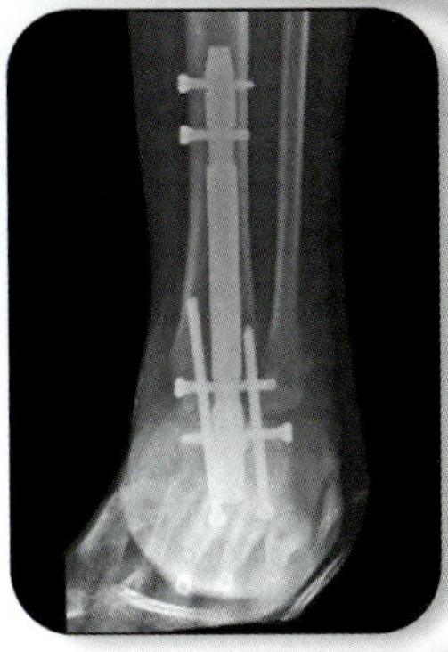

Hindfoot Fractures

Frank Liporace, Matthew Frank

Chapter Outline

Introduction
FRACTURES OF THE CALCANEUS
Diagnosis
Physical Examination
Classification
Surgical Indications
Surgical Procedure
Surgical Anatomy, Positioning and Approaches
Surgical Techniques
Technique 1: Essex-Lopresti Technique
Technique 2: Lateral Extensile Approach to the Calcaneus
Technique 3: Medial Approach to the Calcaneus
Outcomes
Complications
Tibiotalocalcaneal Fusion with an Intramedullary Nail
FRACTURES OF THE TALUS
Diagnosis
Classification
Surgical Indications
Surgical Anatomy, Positioning and Approaches
Surgical Techniques
Anteromedial Approach to the Talar Neck
Anterolateral Approach to the Talar Neck
Complications
Avascular Necrosis
Malunion
Arthritis
Authors' Preferred Management of Select Complications
Case: Chronic Infection after ORIF of an Extruded Talus
Summary

Introduction

Though they account for less than 4% of all fractures, fractures of the talus and calcaneus portend a high incidence of morbidity. For a greater part of 20th century many of these fractures were treated conservatively but in the last 20 years operative fixation has become a viable and in many instances, a superior treatment strategy owing to technological innovations in orthopedic hardware and the evolution of surgical technique. Irrespective of these advances, many fractures of both the calcaneus and talus continue to be vexing injuries rife with wound complications and lacking a true consensus of management. The authors' review will summarize the recent literature on surgical approaches to calcaneal and talar fractures with a brief discussion of contemporary treatment options and surgical techniques. Lastly, the authors will discuss the various complications and their associated treatments.

FRACTURES OF THE CALCANEUS

Diagnosis

A history of a fall from height, a motor vehicle accident or a similar mechanism should suggest a possible injury to the hindfoot. Intra-articular injuries are more common in young males who tend to sustain higher energy mechanisms of injury. A thorough history should be obtained ensuring to rule out other areas of injury or pain. The pain associated with a fracture of the calcaneus is often so severe that other significant injuries are ignored. Compression fractures of the spine are common (seen in 10–15% of the cases), as are compression type injuries to other areas of the bony skeleton, such as the proximal femur.

Documenting chronic medical conditions, such as diabetes, peripheral vascular disease or malignancy must be recognized as they may affect the prognosis. The clinician must be vigilant about prior injuries or surgeries in the affected area. It is equally important to document current and recent medication use and inquire about social habits, such as alcohol and tobacco consumption, which can have profound effects on surgical outcome.

Physical Examination

Patients with a fracture of the calcaneus may present with the following: pain, edema, ecchymosis, deformity of the heel or plantar arch, and an inability to bear weight on the injured foot. Observe all areas for evidence of open injury, particularly areas with overlying lacerations.

The hindfoot should be palpated, the clinician should hold the heel of the patient's foot in the palm of the hand and gently squeeze. Elicited pain suggests calcaneal fracture. One should not ignore close examination of the ankle (malleoli), base of the 5th metatarsal, talus, navicular and lisfranc joint. A hematoma or pattern of ecchymosis extending distally to the sole of the foot is specific for calcaneal fractures and is known as the Mondor's sign. Deformity of the heel or plantar arch (widening or broadening of the arch) is seen secondary to the displacement of the lateral calcaneal border outward along with accompanying edema. This leads to inability or difficulty with weight bearing on the affected side and limited or absent inversion/eversion of the foot.

Check for posterior tibial and dorsalis pedis pulses, and compare these to the uninjured side. Ensure that distal capillary refill is 2 seconds or less. This is of vital importance particularly in patients with preexisting peripheral vascular disease. If pulses cannot be palpated, a Doppler ultrasound should be used to document the presence/absence of distal pulses. A vascular consult is obtained in the face of vascular insufficiency regardless of its acute or chronic nature.

Pay particular attention to the presence of any paresthesia, edema, pallor, diminished pulses or severe pain with passive flexion of the toes that might suggest compartment syndrome of the foot. Examine the knee, ankle and midfoot for tenderness, ecchymosis or swelling. Radiographs of the knee, ankle and foot may be indicated if positive findings are noted.

As many as 7% of the patients with a calcaneus fracture may have fracture of the contralateral heel. Given the appropriate mechanism of injury (i.e. a fall from height), care must be taken to examine both lower extremities thoroughly to exclude the presence of bilateral injuries.

FRACTURES OF THE CALCANEUS: Pearls and Pitfalls

- Perform thorough neurovascular exam
- Obtain computed tomography (CT)
- Respect soft tissue
- Look for concomitant injuries

Classification

The X-rays or radiographs: Axial—determines primary fracture line and displays the body, tuberosity, middle and posterior facets. Lateral—determines Bohler's angle. Oblique/Brodén's view displays the degree of displacement of the primary fracture line.

Computed tomographic scan (both axial and coronal views) to classify the degree of injury to the posterior facet and lateral calcaneal wall

The Sanders classification is based on the coronal CT reconstructions. The coronal CT image that shows the posterior facet in widest profile is chosen; next mark 2 vertical lines to divide the posterior facet into 3 equal sections; (hence: A-lateral, B-central, C-medial); the final line marks the vertical border of the sustentaculum; fractures which lie in the medial zones will be more difficult to visualize and hence, will be more difficult to fix. The classification is broken down as follows:

- Type II fractures: Two part
- Type III fractures: Three part fracture with depression of posterior facet
- Type IV: Severely comminuted (consider primary fusion)

Surgical Indications

Significant debate remains as to what is the best course of treatment following a calcaneal fracture, particularly following operative management of displaced or intra-articular fractures. Nonoperative management is preferable when there is no impingement of the peroneal tendons and the fracture segments are not displaced (or are displaced less than 2 mm). Nonoperative care is also recommended when despite the presence of a fracture, proper weight-bearing alignment has been adequately maintained and articulating surfaces are not disturbed. Extra-articular fractures are generally treated conservatively. Patients who are over the age of 50 years or who have pre-existing health conditions, such as diabetes or peripheral vascular disease, are also commonly treated using nonoperative techniques. Patients receiving non-operative management are 5.5 times more likely to require primary subtalar arthrodesis at some point in the future. Surgical repair is recommended in calcaneal fractures which present with displaced fracture segments, impinged peroneal tendons or entrapped medial compartments. Buckley et al. 2002 study postulated that anatomic restoration of the articular surface did not necessarily translate into better clinical outcomes. In a prospective, randomized trial of 424 patients with intraarticular calcaneal fractures, the study reported equivocal outcomes when comparing operative and nonoperative cohorts. The study concluded that women and non-workers' compensation patients under the age of 29 with a moderately low Bohler's angle and intra-articular step off of less than or equal to 2 mm had favorable outcomes with operative management.[1,2] A 10–16% incidence of wound complication is associated with operative management.[3] Using the classifications of Sanders, nonoperative and operative treatment courses are preferred for the following grades of calcaneal fracture:

- Type I: Nonoperative management of immobilization or early mobilization
- Type II/III (Sanders): Operative management commonly including open reduction and internal fixation (ORIF)
- Type IV (Sanders): Nonoperative management for non-salvageable comminuted fractures or operative management consisting of ORIF with primary arthrodesis

Surgical Procedure

The goals of operative management of a calcaneal fracture include: (1) restoration of normal heel height and length; (2) realignment of the posterior facet of the subtalar joint, (3) restoration of the mechanical axis of the hindfoot. Surgical repair is often delayed 3–14 days after the fracture, especially in the presence of significant edema or fracture blister formation to allow for some reduction of swelling.

Surgical Anatomy, Positioning and Approaches

The calcaneus transmits body weight to the ground and creates a robust lever for the muscles of the calf. Consequently, anatomical restoration is requisite for the preservation of subtalar joint function. The superior calcaneal surface is comprised of three articular facets; the posterior facet, the largest of the three, along with the less stout middle and anterior facets comprise the inferior aspect of the subtalar joint.[4] The posterior facet is convex assuming a saddle shape, sloping posteromedially in its support of the talar body. Conversely, the anterior and middle facets are flatter and support the talar neck and head, respectively. Paradoxically though smaller, the anterior and middle facets support more weight per unit area than the posterior facet.[2] A small oblique nonarticular groove marks the region between the posterior facet and the anterior and middle facets. This houses the insertion point of the interosseous ligament, the inferior extensor retinaculum and the joint capsule of the posterior facet.[5]

Two crucial angles are seen on the lateral radiograph of the calcaneus. Bohler's angle, usually between 20° and 40°, is formed by 2 lines; the first line is drawn from the highest point of the anterior process of the calcaneus to the highest point of the posterior facet. The second line runs tangential to the superior edge of the tuberosity.

A decrease in this angle may indicate collapse of the weight-bearing surface—posterior facet. The collapse results in the transfer of load to the anterior facet of the calcaneus. The second angle, the crucial angle of Gissane, is seen directly inferior to the lateral process of the talus and is represented by 2 strong cortical struts that extend laterally and form an obtuse angle.[5-7]

The first strut extends along the lateral border of the posterior facet and the second extends anteriorly to the beak of the calcaneus. Medially, the sustentaculum tali supports the middle facet and acts as a fulcrum for the traversing flexor hallucis longus (FHL). The dense bone of the sustentaculum tali serves as a welcome medium for screw purchase. Immediately dorsal to the sustentaculum tali lies the neurovascular bundle and the remnants of the deep posterior compartment. Classically, calcaneal reconstruction was predicated on the restoration of the articular surface with particular attention to the posterior facet however, it is now understood that appropriate reconstruction of the three-dimensional spatial relationships between the 3 articular facets is of paramount importance.[8]

Displaced intra-articular fractures of the calcaneus are usually the result of high-energy trauma most often secondary to a fall from height or a motor vehicle accident. Initial assessment should include plain radiographs including Brodén views to adequately assess the posterior facet. Recently, treatment has focused on the restoration of the articular surface of the posterior facet. Sanders has demonstrated through CT analysis that articular restoration is feasible, if comminution of the posterior facet is limited to 3 or fewer fracture fragments. Although there are numerous variations in fracture patterns that have been described with intra-articular calcaneal fractures, two major fracture fragments, the anteromedial and posterolateral have been accepted. Carr et al. found that two primary fracture lines were consistently derived from the fracture model. The first line originated at the angle of Gissane and propagated to the medial calcaneal cortex. The second line extends from the anterior process of the tuberosity creating medial and lateral pieces and exiting either through the anterior facet or the calcaneal cuboid joint.[7] A sustenacular "constant" fragment frequently maintains its spatial relationship with the talus because of its firm attachment to the interosseous and medial ligament. However, if the energy and direction of force is severe enough even this relationship can be disturbed. Essex-Lopresti's earlier work described both a tongue-type and a joint depressed fracture pattern. These fracture lines represent secondary fractures that either exit behind or below the posterior facet. Additionally, the posterior facet may be comminuted or rotated plantarly about an intact calcaneal tuber.[2]

Currently, the goals of ORIF are similar to those originally outlined by Bohler in 1931, namely accurate anatomic reduction of the subtalar joint, restoration of calcaneal anatomy, stable fixation and early range of motion.[9] Timing of surgery has been long debated. The soft tissue envelope should be able to accommodate the physiological stresses of surgical dissection. Waiting up to 2–3 weeks for "adequate wrinkling" is advocated by most when performing formal open approaches. Premature open treatment may induce a cascade of untoward sequelae, such as necrosis, infection ultimately leading to increased morbidity at times as severe as amputation.[10]

Although the lateral right-angled approach is often used for the surgical treatment of calcaneal fractures, it has been shown to carry a high rate of wound complications that in some cases lead to amputation.[11-13] The precarious nature of the soft tissue about the lateral calcaneus is derived from the scarcity of the soft tissue envelope coupled with its tenuous vascularity. The vascularity of the region is derived from a vascular arcade consisting of an anastomisis of three arteries: the lateral calcaneal artery (a branch of the peroneal artery)—rami calcaneareas laterales, venterolateral tarsal artery (a branch of the dorsalis pedis) and the lateral malleolar artery (branching off from the anterior tibialalis artery).[14]

A recent cadaveric study showed that the arcade's arch was reliably located at the border of the lateral extensile incision. Incorrect execution of the lateral extensile incision potentially places the lateral soft tissue at grave risk for serious ischemic injury. The rate of these complications varies greatly in the literature where the incidence of minor wound dehiscence exceeds 25% in some studies. In Bezes et al's study of 257 fractures the reported incidence of skin necrosis was 10%.[3] The rate of complications after ORIF of calcaneal fractures is directly correlated with respect to body mass index, smoking, single-layered closure and extended time between injury and surgery. Furthermore, the lateral right-angled approach offers limited access to the medial aspect of the calcaneus which includes the sustentacular fragment.

Surgical Techniques

Technique 1: Essex-Lopresti Technique

For stabilization of isolated tongue-type fragments or those attached to a simple articular injury, the Essex-Lopresti technique is often instituted. A Shantz pin is placed through a stab incision into the posterior tuberosity from a posterior-to-anterior direction, in-line with the superior border of the posterior tuberosity and ending just short of the posterior facet (Figs 29.1A and B). The Schanz pin is then manipulated to reduce the general alignment of the posterior tuberosity and calcaneus as per the Essex-Lopresti maneuver.[15] Finally, multiple 2.7 mm, 3.5 mm or cannulated 4.0 mm and 4.5 mm screws are positioned through stab incisions to cross and stabilize the fracture lines as preoperatively planned based on radiographs and CT.

Technique 2: Lateral Extensile Approach to the Calcaneus

When dealing with more complex intra-articular injuries and associated comminution, the "standard L-shaped approach" is often utilized. The L-shaped extensile lateral approach was developed by Letournel as a modification of Palmer's and Kocher's lateral approach[16] and involves the elevation of full thickness flaps that incorporate the peroneal tendons; it is the workhorse incision of modern day calcaneal ORIF. It provides access for the direct reduction of the posterior facet, the posterolateral fragment and any anterolateral fragments. The incision begins just anterior to the Achilles tendon slightly above the superior aspect of the calcaneus. The incision is carried distally below the peroneal tendon and sural nerve in a curved fashion along the plantar lateral border of the calcaneus terminating at the calcaneal cuboid joint. A curved incision is recommended to lower the potential risk of devascularization vis-a-vis a centrally sharp or 90° edge.[17] A full thickness flap is created to include the periosteum, subcutaneous tissue, peroneal tendons and sural nerve. The flap is reflected superiorly to expose the entire lateral wall, superior calcaneus, subtalar and calcaneal-cuboid joints. The lateral approach necessitates the indirect fracture reduction of the aforementioned fragments in the restoration of their anatomic relationship to the anteromedial or "constant" fragment.

After conducting the dissection, the lateral wall is removed and placed on the back table (Fig. 29.2A). Next, the areas of impacted posterior facet articular surface are disimpacted, removed if necessary for realignment

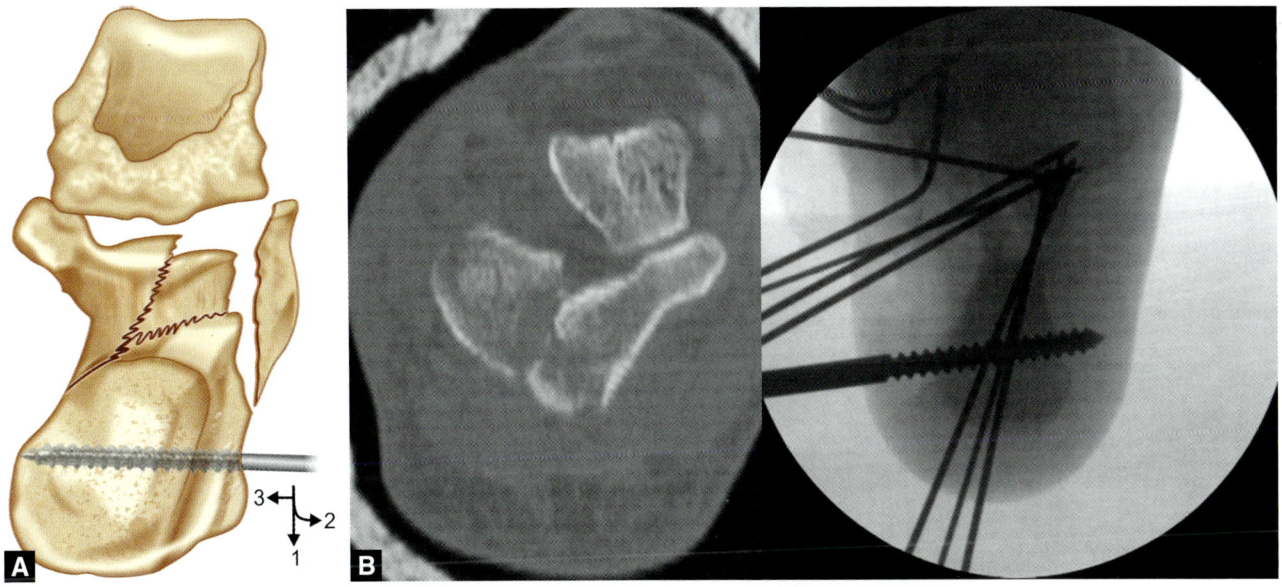

Figures 29.1A and B: The Essex-Lopresti technique. (A) Pictorial demonstration of correct Schanz pin placement prior to distraction and correction of shortening; (B) Preoperative computed tomography and intraoperative fluoroscopic image after Schanz pin placement, reduction of shortening and varus and temporary wire fixation.

and back table provisional stabilization. Then the application of a 5.0 mm Schanz pin is applied in a lateral-to-medial direction in the posterior tuberosity. An elevator is placed in the fracture line between the sustentacular fragment and the posterior tuberosity fragment to allow for disimpaction. Finally, manual manipulation of the posterior tuberosity to attain overall calcaneal length and height is conducted (Fig. 29.2B). As well, the heel is "brought out of varus" with the aid of this Schanz pin to correct width. Finally, the posterior tuberosity is provisionally stabilized to the sustenacular fragment with the aid of multiple Kirschner wires (K-wires). At that juncture, the posterior facet articular fragments that had been previously disimpacted are reapproximated in their native location with application of independent lag screw fixation into the sustenacular fragment. Often these articular fragments have the dense cortical apex of the angle of Gissane attached. Finally, anterior comminution and displacement is addressed and provisionally reduced and pinned. Ultimately, the lateral wall is replaced and a laterally based perimeter plate is applied with additional lag screw fixation through the plate for the posterior facet.

Technique 3: Medial Approach to the Calcaneus

The medial approach allows direct reduction of the posterolateral and anteromedial fragments parallel with the principle fracture line. The medial neurovascular structures must be identified and protected. In contrast to the lateral approach, the medial approach allows the direct reduction with visualization of the subtalar facets, posterolateral fracture fragments and the freeing of the FHL tendon. The medial approach is based on its ability to facilitate the anatomic restoration of the tuberosity and the superomedial fragment. Ultimately, the restoration of these elements is necessary for proper anatomic restoration of the posterior facet.

Liporace et al. presented data on more than 20% incidence of sustenacular displacement with intra-articular, displaced calcaneal fractures involving the posterior facet, making the "constant fragment" not so constant. In an effort to deal with the issues of morbidity, complications and problems associated with extensile incisions in the "watershed" zone the authors used a modified lateral approach that may be combined with a medial approach in instances of sustenacular displacement. As well, this protocol allows earlier treatment of these fractures.[18]

A medial approach aids in reducing this angulation and with fixation of the sustentaculum to the posterior tuberosity. A lateral approach is still necessary for anatomic reduction of the posterior facet and calcaneocuboid joint. Laterally, a curvilinear incision over the sinus tarsi that extends toward the anterior process allows excellent

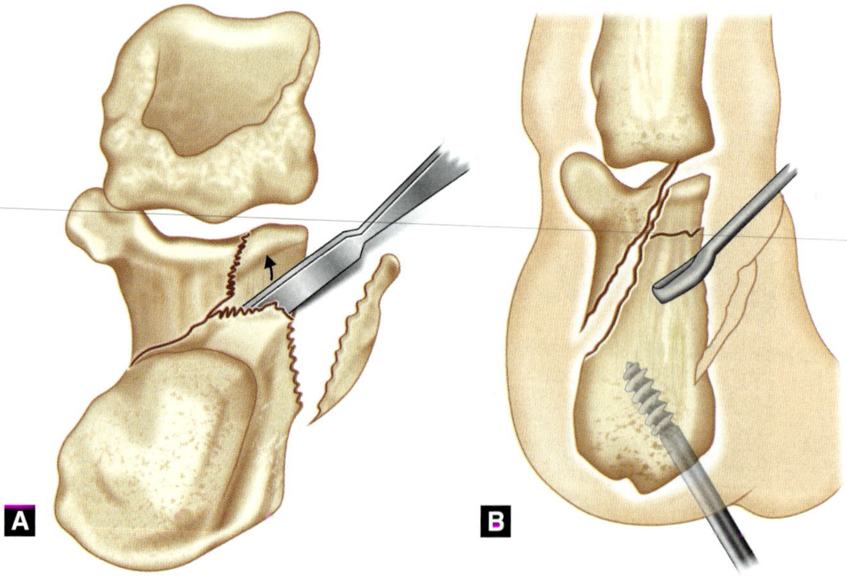

Figures 29.2A and B: Lateral extensile approach to the calcaneus. (A) Removal of the lateral wall gives access to the primary fracture line and the articular fragments; (B) A Schanz pin in the tuberosity helps to reduce shortening and varus to the "constant" sustentacular fragment.

visualization of the posterior facet and calcaneocuboid joint while mitigating concerns about wound healing associated with a right-angled incision. A small limb of the modified Ollier approach that was ultimately used in definitive care, was made to aid in tuberosity reduction. This approximated a 3–4 cm incision, approximately 2 cm distal to the fibula, going between tangential lines drawn along the most posterior and anterior aspects of the fibula. This incision is then carried another 3–4 cm distally toward the calcaneal-cuboid joint. The extensor digitorum brevis (EDB) is elevated dorsally and the sinus tarsi fat is debrided. The peroneal tendons are maintained within their sheath and mobilized as needed. Disimpaction of the articular fragments may be done and percutaneously a Schanz pin may be applied into the posterior tuberosity to allow manipulation as needed. As well, this approach allows direct visualization superiorly of the posterior facet when a varus stress is applied to the subtalar joint. Visualization from lateral to medial at the level of the angle of Gissane is also quite feasible. If there is a concomitant impaction injury of the distal fibula, the posterior aspect of the incision may be curved proximally to allow reduction and fixation of the fibula as needed, while avoiding the "watershed" zone (Figs 29.3A and B).

With sustenacular displacement or in an effort to provide assistance with posterior tuberosity reduction and fixation, a medial approach may be concurrently performed. This will allow reduction plus screw or mini-fragment buttress plate fixation to recreate the "constant" fragment and maintain posterior tuberosity reduction. A 6–8 cm incision is made at a 45° angle from proximal posterior to distal anterior plantar. This incision is centered over a point halfway between the posterior distal aspect of the medial malleolus and the most posterior plantar aspect of the foot. Dissection is carried full-thickness to posterior tuberosity. Then a full-thickness flap may be elevated distally to the sustentaculum, protecting important structures within the flap. Based on preoperative CT planning, the incision may be made slightly flatter relative to the plantar aspect of the foot but deep dissection will require care in the area of the neurovascular structures (Figs 29.4A and B). Definitive fixation may be accomplished

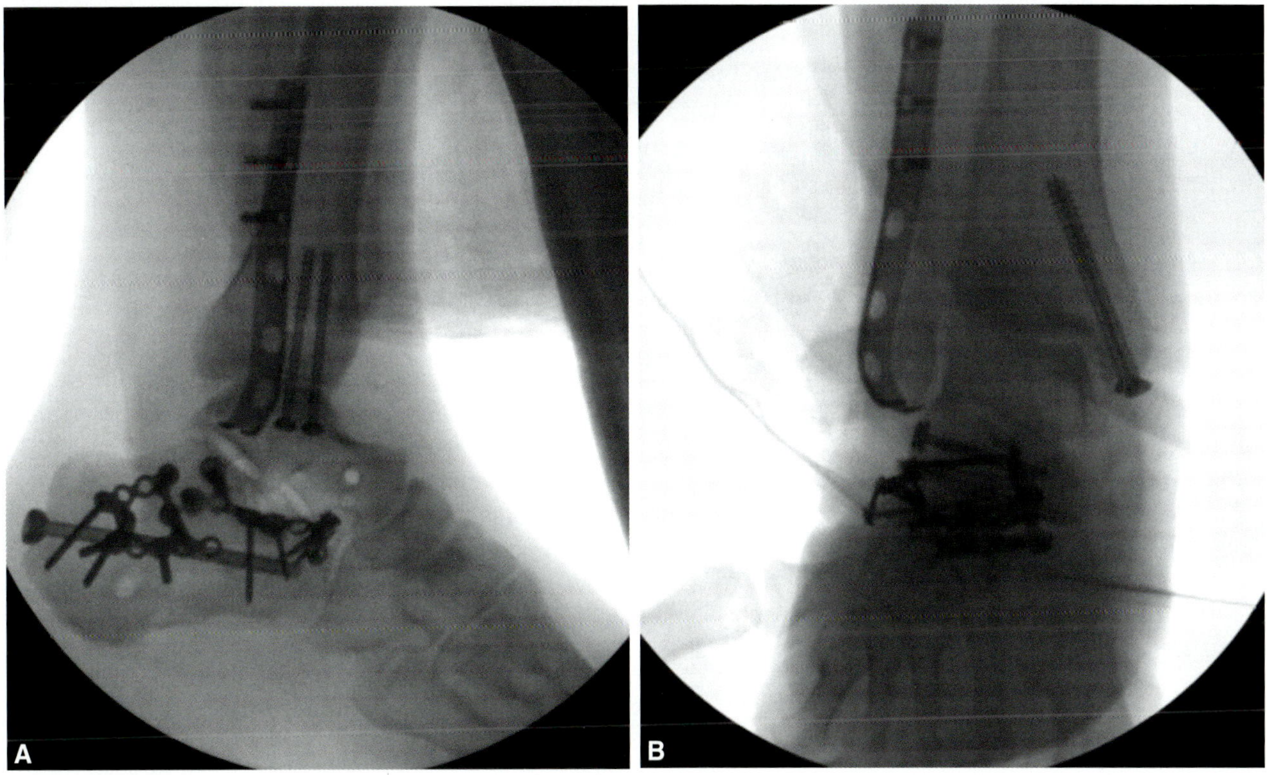

Figures 29.3A and B: Lateral extensile approach to the calcaneus with concomitant ankle fractures. (A and B) Anteroposterior and lateral images of a case exemplify how the proximal aspect of the lateral incision can be gently curved into a lateral approach to the ankle to allow for fixation of the lateral malleolus in combination injuries.

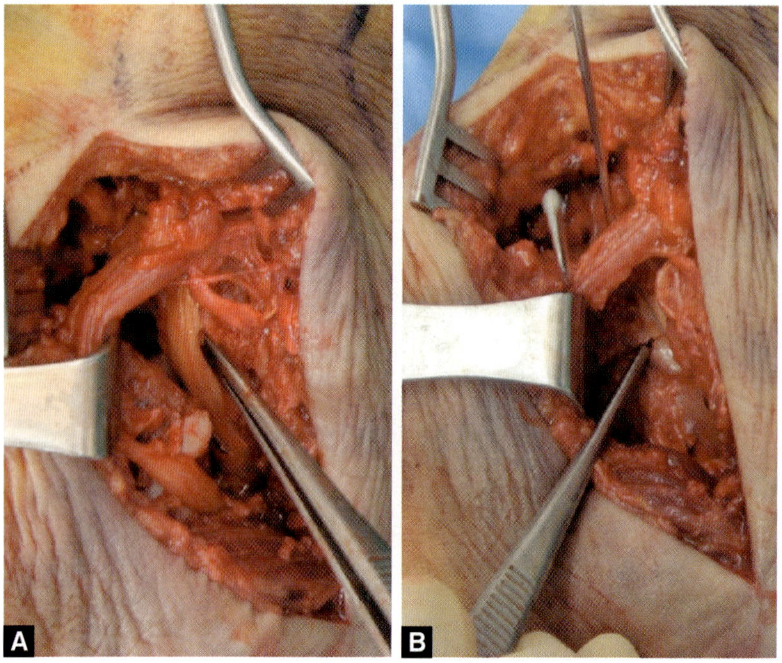

Figures 29.4A and B: Medial approach to calcaneal fractures. (A) Note the neurovascular bundle; (B) Note the medial aspect of calcaneal posterior facet and talar articular cartilage.

through both the approaches with modular foot (2.0 mm and 2.4 mm plates and screws), as well as cannulated screws. Fixation of the sustenacular fragment to both the posterior tuberosity and the posterior facet may be accomplished in all cases. Lateral column fixation is also conducted with either modular foot plates or multiple long cannulated screws (Figs 29.5A to E).

The medial approach for ORIF of calcaneal fractures can also be utilized with open fractures which frequently have a medial open wound requiring debridement (Figs 29.6A to I). If the wound can be adequately debrided and the patient is relatively at a lower risk for infection (e.g. nonsmoker, not diabetic), reduction and fixation and bone grafting, if necessary, can be performed.

FRACTURE OF THE CALCANEUS: Pearls and Pitfalls

- Develop full thickness flaps do not undercut soft tissue
- Respect soft tissue. Do not perform definitive open procedure on swollen or edematous tissue
- Be wary of the sustentacular "constant" fragment, as this piece is not always constant
- Do not neglect proximal peroneal examination to rule out peroneal subluxation

Outcomes

Surgical wound management involves layered closure with deep hemovac drain placement and overlying vacuum-assisted closure (VAC) dressing application for 48 hours to promote neoangiogenesis, increased local blood flow, decreased edema and decreased subcutaneous hematoma. Stannard et al. has shown a positive benefit with VAC application over surgical incisions in tenuous wounds.[19] Theoretically, angiogenesis, increased blood flow and decreased interstitial fluid can contribute to successful wound healing. Sutures are removed at 3 weeks and patients are begun in physical therapy. Patients remain non-weight bearing for a total of 12 weeks. The authors have applied this protocol to a total of 38 fractures. To date, postoperative CT scans obtained on all fractures show anatomic or near-anatomic reduction (<2 mm displacement) at the posterior facet, restoration of Bohler's and Gissane's angles and reconstitution of heel height, width and length. The wound complication rate with the use of this protocol is 2.6% (1 in 38 fractures that required operative debridement and antibiotics).

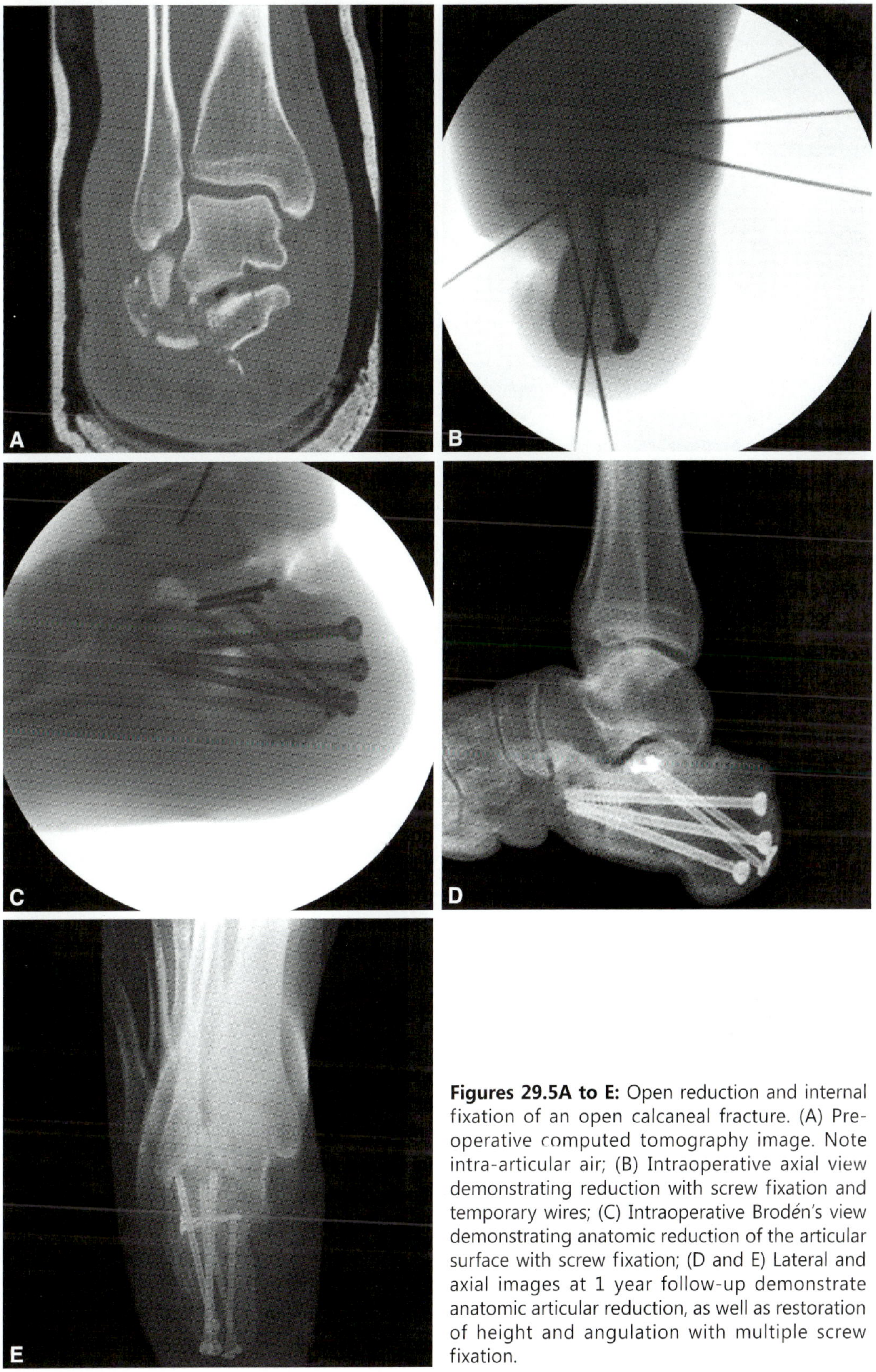

Figures 29.5A to E: Open reduction and internal fixation of an open calcaneal fracture. (A) Preoperative computed tomography image. Note intra-articular air; (B) Intraoperative axial view demonstrating reduction with screw fixation and temporary wires; (C) Intraoperative Brodén's view demonstrating anatomic reduction of the articular surface with screw fixation; (D and E) Lateral and axial images at 1 year follow-up demonstrate anatomic articular reduction, as well as restoration of height and angulation with multiple screw fixation.

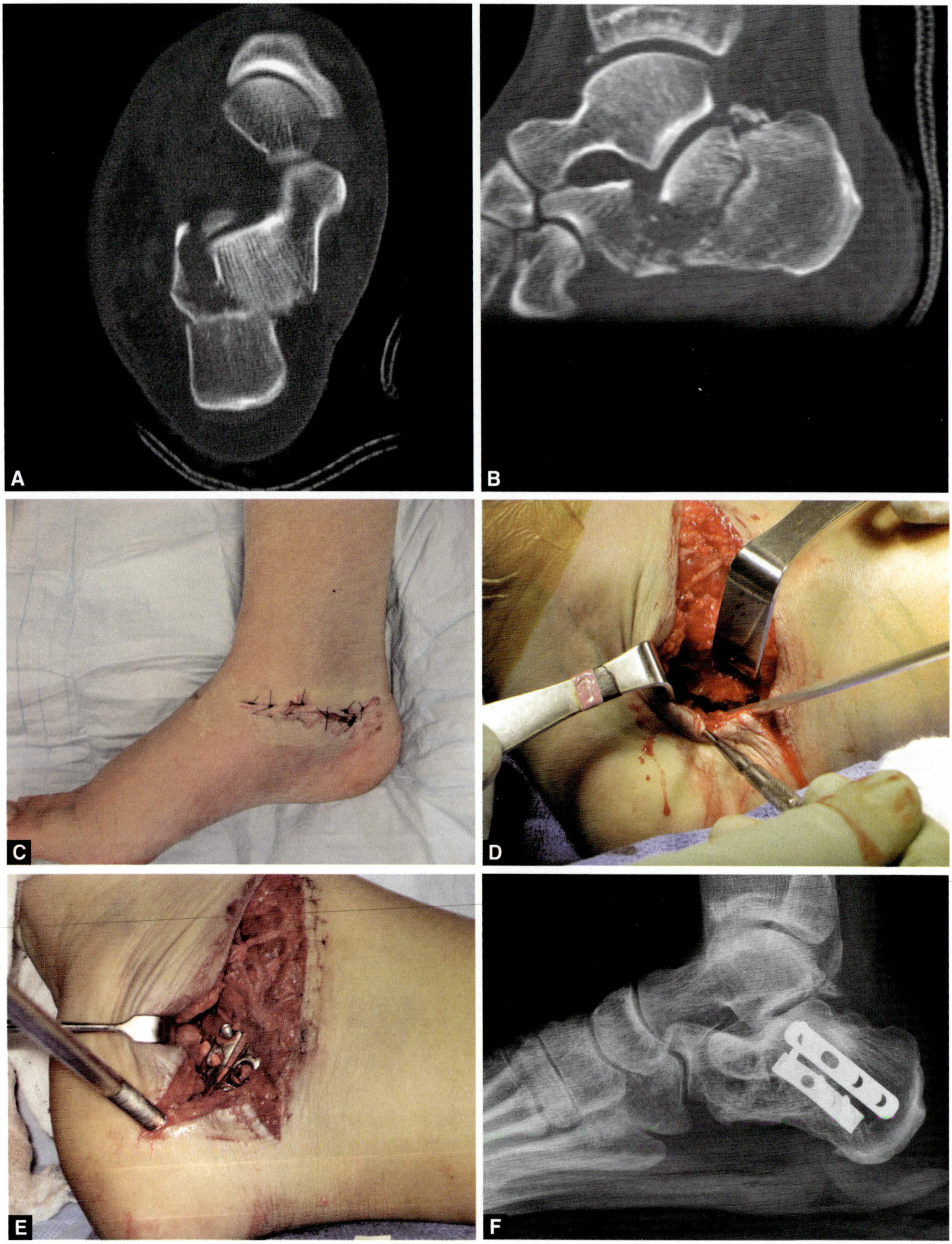

Figures 29.6A to F

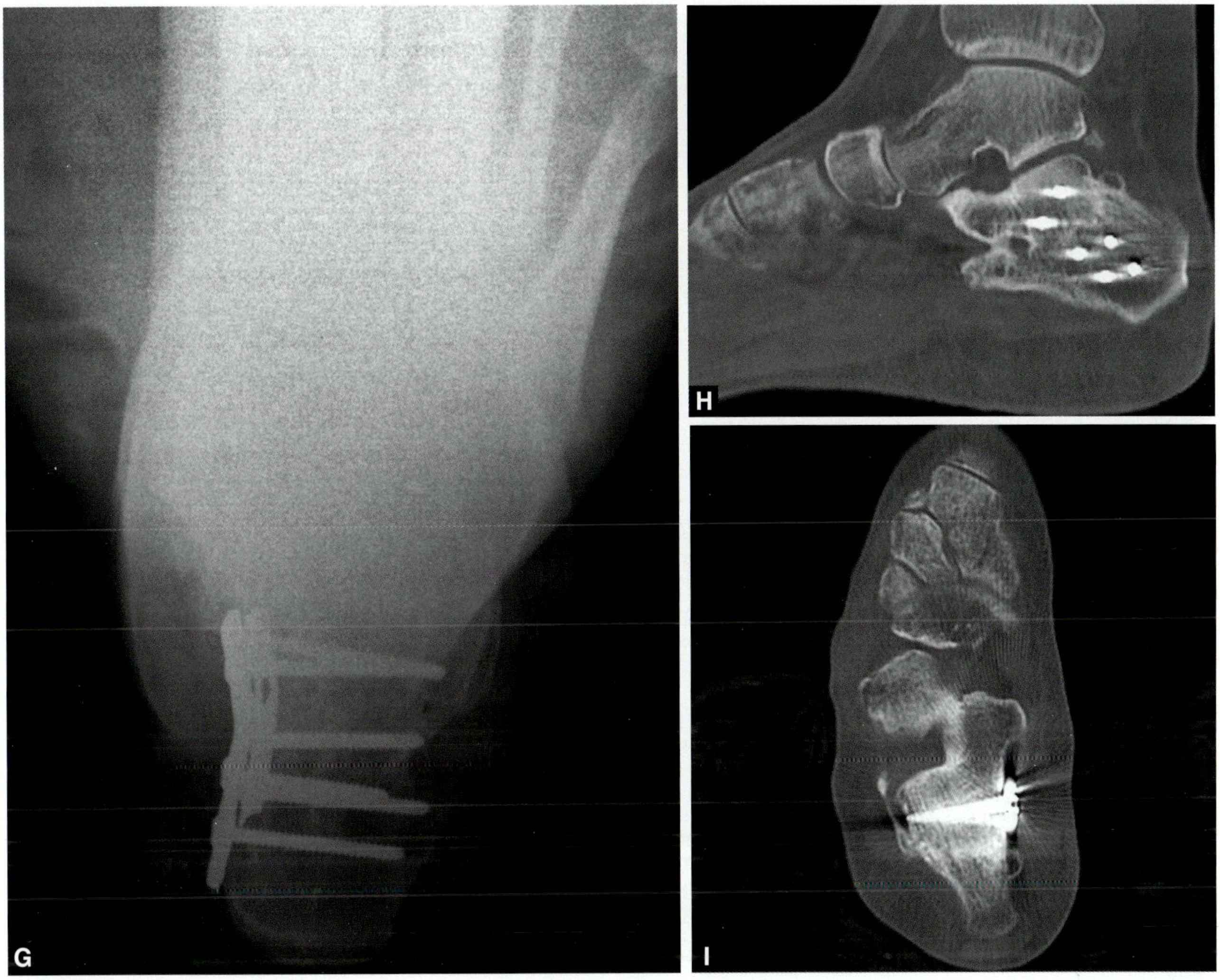

Figures 29.6A to I: Open reduction and internal fixation (ORIF) of an open calcaneal fracture from a medial exposure. (A and B) Computed tomography images demonstrate minimal intra-articular involvement but significant displacement with some bone loss; (C) Wound appearance after initial irrigation, debridement and wound closure; (D and E) Intraoperative images during ORIF demonstrate fracture displacement initially, then plate fixation and bone grafting with two one-third tubular plates and calcium triphosphate graft substitute; (F and G) Lateral and axial radiographs, as well as (H and I) computed tomography images demonstrate healed fracture with good overall alignment.

Complications

The importance of striving for anatomic reduction cannot be overemphasized. The aim of surgical treatment should be the re-establishment of calcaneal architecture. In the post-traumatic setting, failure to restore calcaneal width and calcaneal height can cause insidious pain and disability for the patient. Displacement of the lateral wall causes heel widening which itself can lead to lateral impingement of the peroneal tendons and the sural nerve. Loss of height (Figs 27.7A to K) which is easily discerned by a diminished Bohler's angle, adversely affects the talocural joint and alters gait mechanics.[20] Inability to control the calcaneal tuberosity may lead to persistent hindfoot varus, which has far reaching implications. A varus hindfoot means the transverse tarsal joint remains locked altering gait mechanics and over time leading to post-traumatic arthritis in adjacent joints by means of eccentric loading.[20]

Classifying the malunion via the Stephens and Sanders classification is a good first step but one must elicit a good history and physical exam as well. Radnay and colleagues reported on over 60 patients who have suffered a displaced intra-articular calcaneus fracture. There were 2 cohorts, the first of which were managed initially with ORIF and subsequently underwent *in situ* subtalar fusion. The second group was managed initially nonoperatively later developed a symptomatic painful malunion. The patients in this group subsequently underwent a subtalar

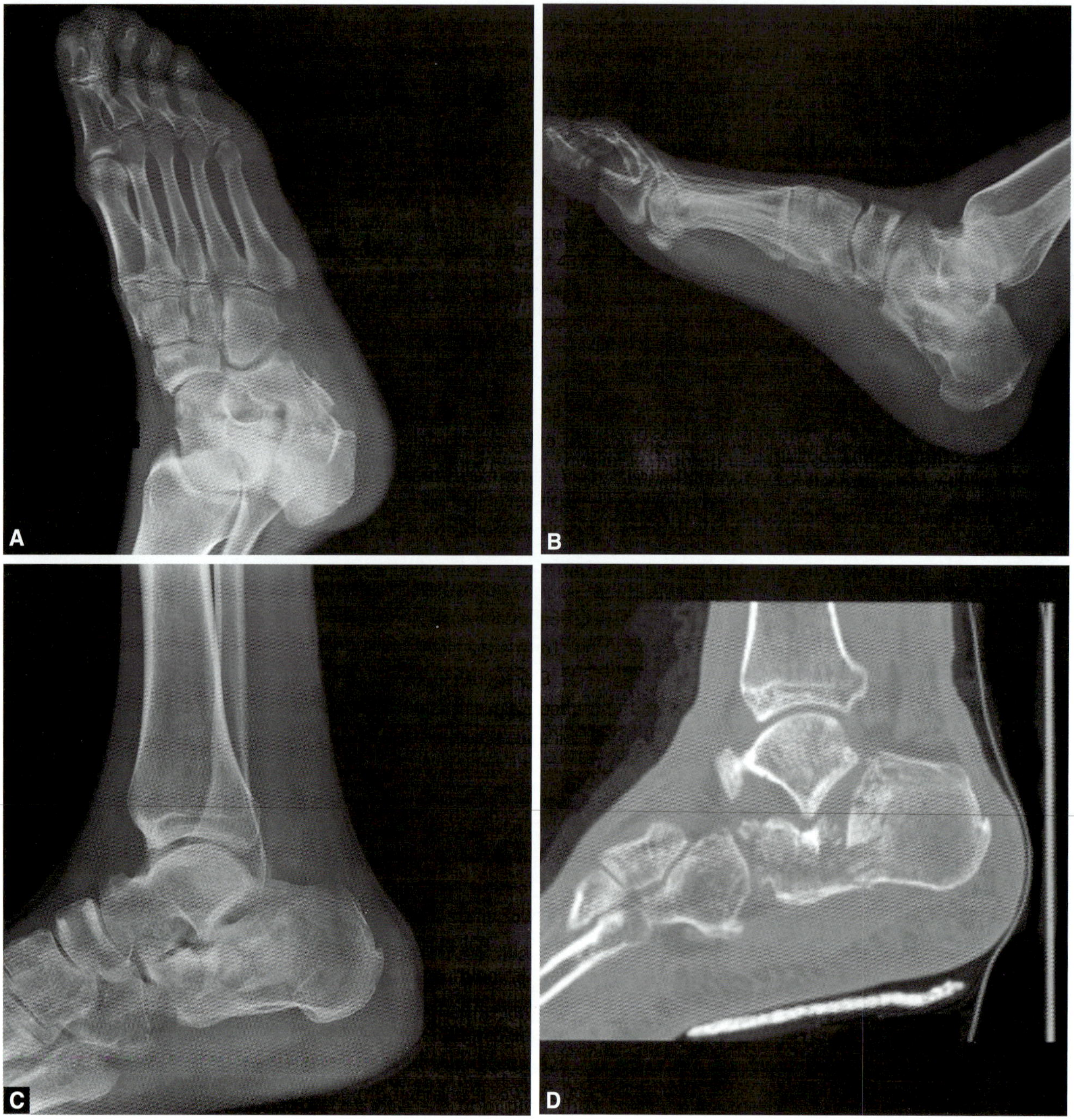

Figures 29.7A to D

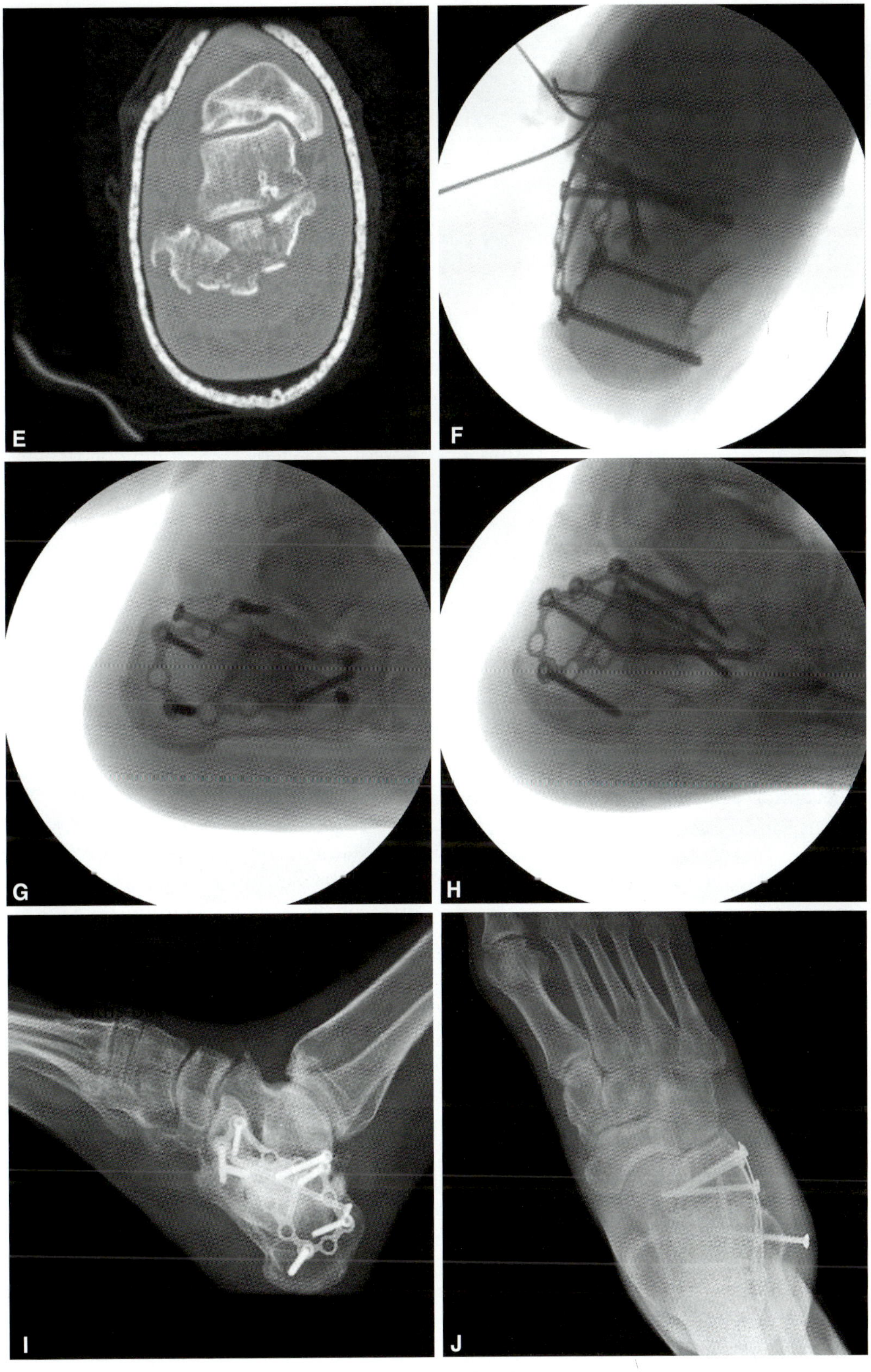

Figures 29.7E to J

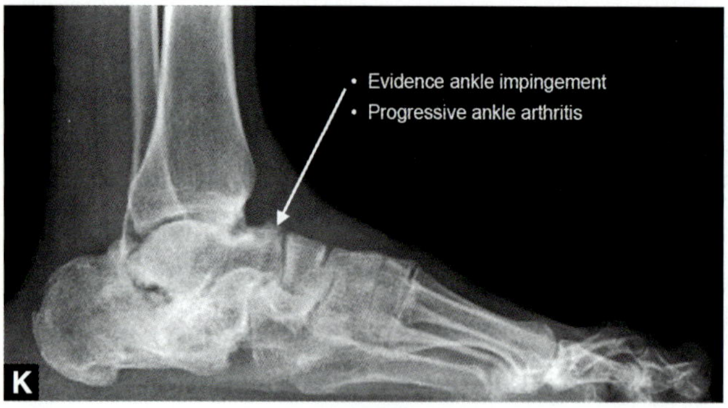

Figures 29.7A to K: Infection and loss of reduction after open reduction and internal fixation of calcaneal fracture. (A to C) Radiographs of an intra-articular calcaneal fracture; (D and E) Sagittal and coronal computed tomography images taken preoperatively; (F to H) Intraoperative lateral, axial and Brodén's views demonstrating restoration of height, articular congruity and Bohler's angle; (I and J) Lateral and anteroposterior views demonstrating loss of reduction with implant loosening at 3 months with the patient presenting with deep infection; (K) Follow-up radiograph after implant removal demonstrating loss of height, a horizontal talus, progressive ankle and subtalar arthritis and anterior ankle impingement.

distraction arthrodesis. The authors found the ORIF group had more favorable outcomes after fusion because ORIF restores "calcaneal shape, alignment and height, which facilitates the fusion procedure and establishes an opportunity to create a better long-term functional result".[21]

Calcaneal fractures often are accompanied by soft tissue complications. These complications can occur both before and after surgical intervention. If the soft tissues are not amenable to fixation, i.e. there is no wrinkling of the glabellar skin then surgery should be delayed, in the setting of an unstable fracture an external fixator should be applied. When wound breakdown occurs after fixation, a plastic surgery consult should be sought and a decision made regarding the application of a negative pressure dressing and eventual skin grafting with or without musculocutaneous flap application.

Tibiotalocalcaneal Fusion with an Intramedullary Nail

In situations where degenerative changes with or without rigid deformity have occurred in both the ankle and subtalar joints, a tibiotalocalcaneal (TTC) fusion is a very viable option. Laterally based approach for the subtalar joint can be extended proximally along the fibula and a subsequent distal fibula resection to gain access to the ankle joint. At times, access to the medial shoulder of the ankle joint will require a small, anteromedial ankle approach concomitantly. The resected distal fibula can be morselized and used to fill any defect. The distal tibia articular surface and the talar dome articular surface should be prepared as described for preparation of the talar and calcaneal surfaces for fusion.

Alternatively, the ankle joint can be reached via a direct anterior approach. This is centered-based on the mortise, extending 5 cm proximal and 3 cm distal to the ankle joint. Care is taken to avoid the superficial peroneal nerve and its branches. Deep dissection can be done on either side of the extensor digitorum longus while taking care of the deep peroneal neurovascular bundle. A recent retrospective review of 49 pilon fractures noted low complication rate and minimal soft tissue disturbance after direct anterior approach.[22]

FRACTURES OF THE TALUS

Diagnosis

For the purposes of this chapter the authors will limit their discussion of talus fractures to those of the talar neck and body. Talar neck fractures account for approximately half of all talus fractures owing to its stout shape and relatively weak cortex. Fractures of the talus are either intra-articular or result in joint incongruity by extra-articular axial displacement.[23] Historically, talus fractures carried with them high mortality reported upwards of 80% in the mid 19th century.[24] Treatment has evolved from astragalectomy to contemporary ORIF leading to marked improvement in functional outcome.[25-27]

Roughly half of the talus fractures result from a fall from height and the other half as a result of motor vehicle accidents with indirect force accounting for less than 10% of all fractures.[23] Clinical assessment often reveals significant swelling and hematoma about the ankle. Patients are unable to bear weight and have drastically reduced range of motion at the ankle, subtalar and midtarsal joints. In patients who have experienced a fracture-dislocation examination will reveal bony prominence with skin at risk signs of pallor, blistering and eventually skin necrosis. It is

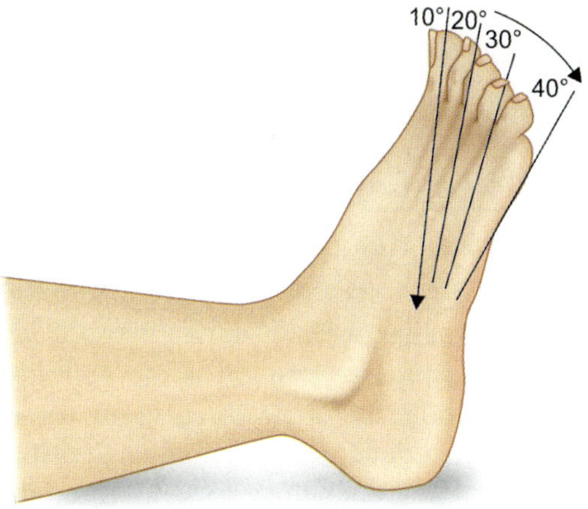

Figure 29.8: Brodén's views of the subtalar joint. Multiple images are taken as shown. This is a useful intraoperative image when assessing posterior facet articular reduction.

important not to overlook the hindfoot in polytrauma patients. A thorough neurovascular exam is warranted in these injuries. If pulses are not readily palpable then the dorsalis pedis and posterior tibial pulses should be detected with Doppler ultrasound. Compartment syndrome should be ruled out, this may mean performing compartment measurements in the unconscious or obtunded patient.

Standard radiographs are obtained including a Broden view (Fig. 29.8) to adequately assess the subtalar joint and a Canale view (Figs 29.9A and B) to assess the talar neck. Computed tomography scans are performed with axial images through the tibiotalar and subtalar joints with subsequent coronal and sagittal reconstructions to further elucidate the extent of injury including the precise fracture pattern, the degree of comminution, the assessment of surrounding structures/articulations and moreover, to plan operative intervention.

FRACTURES OF THE TALUS
DIAGNOSIS (TALUS): Pearls and Pitfalls

- Perform thorough neurovascular exam
- Obtain computed tomography
- Respect soft tissue
- Obtain reduction in fracture-dislocation to avoid skin necrosis

Classification

The Hawkins classification modified by Canale and Kelly has proven in many studies to be prognostic of overall outcome and the incidence of avascular necrosis

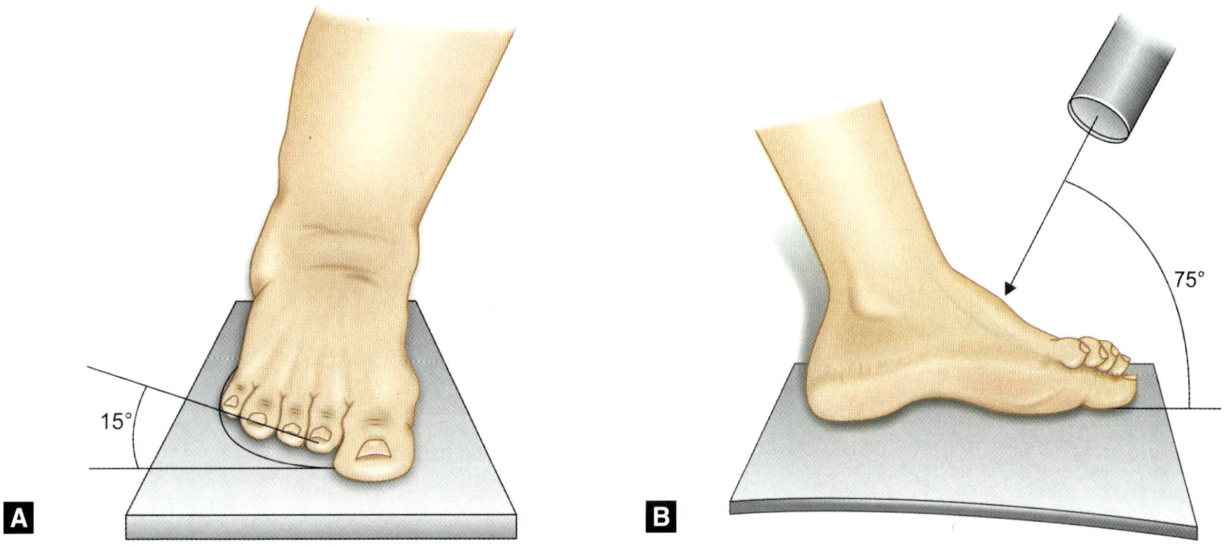

Figures 29.9A and B: Canale view of the talar neck and head.

(AVN).[3,25,26,28] Type I Hawkins fracture is a nondisplaced fracture. Type II fractures involve an associated subtalar subluxation/dislocation. Type III fractures have both an associated subtalar and ankle dislocation. Type IV (Canale and Kelley) is a Type III fracture with an associated talonavicular subluxation or dislocation (Fig. 29.10).

Because fractures of the talar body involve both the ankle joint and the posterior facet of the subtalar joint, accurate reconstruction of a congruent articular surface is required. As with talar neck fractures, talar body fractures with associated dislocation have a higher incidence of osteonecrosis. In the simplest sense, talar body fractures can be divided into three groups: group I is proper or cleavage fractures (horizontal, sagittal, shear or coronal); group II (talar process or tubercle fractures); and group III (compression or impaction fractures).[29]

Surgical Indications

The decision to operate on these fractures should be based upon the presence of an open fracture, fracture-displacement and the condition of the soft tissue envelope. In the face of a fracture-dislocation or a severely displaced talar neck or body fracture with contraindications for immediate open reduction, a closed reduction should be attempted with the patient under conscious sedation. For displaced talar neck fractures the forefoot is initially

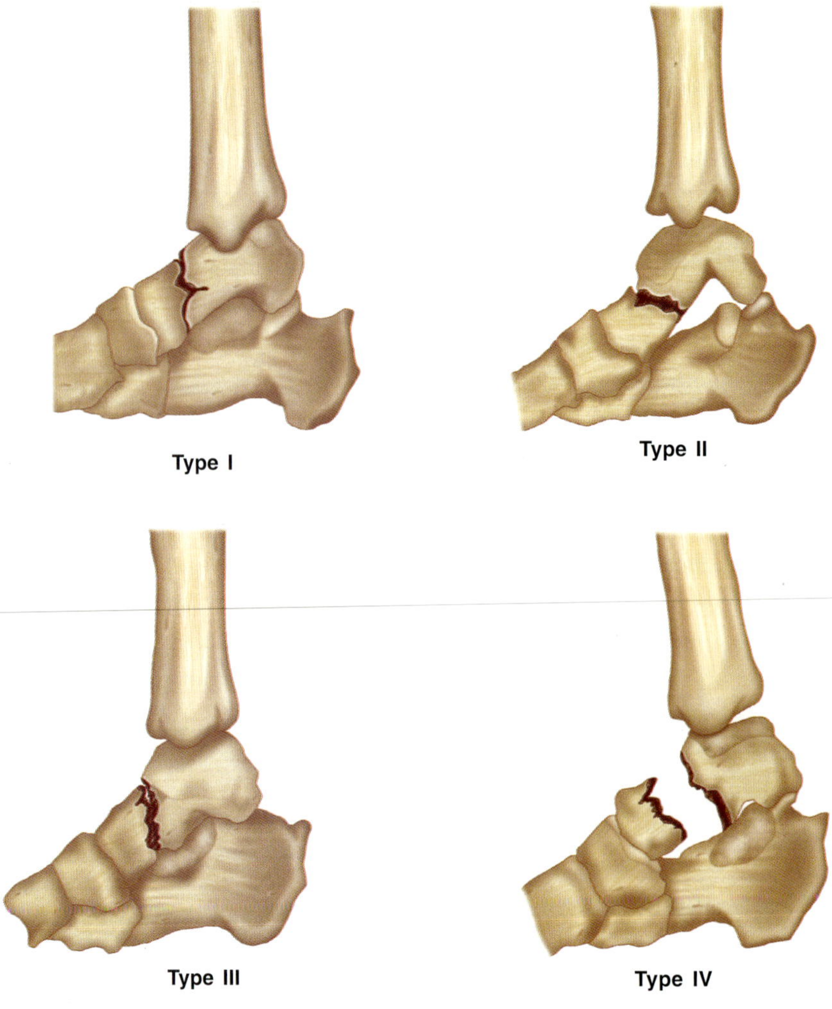

Figure 29.10: Hawkins classification of talar neck fractures.

hyperdorsiflexed followed by forceful plantar flexion while maintaining downward/axial pull on the heel. Displaced talar body fractures can be reduced with direct manipulation of the fracture fragment again with axial traction on the hindfoot.

The goal of treatment of talar neck fractures is anatomic reduction, which requires attention to rotation, length and alignment of the neck. Biomechanical studies on cadavers have shown why precisely reducing talar neck fractures leads to better outcome. As demonstrated in a cadaveric study, displacements of as little as 2 mm were found to significantly alter the contact characteristics of the subtalar joint with dorsal and medial or varus displacement causing the greatest change. The weight-bearing load characteristics changed, and contact stress was actually less in the anterior and middle facets but was more localized in the posterior facet.[30] In another study, where varus alignment was created via a medially based osteotomy of the talar neck, the hindfoot was severely affected; the altered foot position included internal rotation of the calcaneus, heel varus, and forefoot adduction.[31] The altered hindfoot mechanics with a talar neck fracture are a major contributor to development of subtalar post-traumatic arthrosis.

Timing of surgery remains controversial, however recent literature has moved away from the previous convention that a closed talar neck fracture was a true orthopedic emergency. Kellam et al.[32] concluded that the severity of injury and the quality and maintenance of reduction have much greater bearing on long-term outcome as opposed to timing of surgery. Lindvall et al.[25] compared patient outcomes in surgical patients treated within 6 hours to delayed surgery. They found no appreciable difference in outcome. However they comment that overall the open fractures in their series fared much worse than did the closed fractures, with a much lower union rate, a higher osteonecrosis rate and substantially higher reoperation and infection rate. Displaced talar body fractures often result in significant morbidity'.[25] Vallier et al. reporting on radiographic findings of 26 talar body fractures with a minimum follow-up of 1 year, noted a 38% incidence of AVN, 65% incidence of post-traumatic tibiotalar arthritis and 34% incidence of post-traumatic subtalar arthritis. Like talar neck fractures, worse outcomes were noted in association with comminuted fractures, associated talar neck fractures and open fractures.[27] Sneppen et al. (1977) reviewed 51 patients with talar body fractures. The patients with significant talar compression had a greater than 50% incidence of ankle arthritis; if the talus exhibited a shearing pattern of injury, the incidence of post-traumatic arthritis in both the ankle and subtalar joints was 41%, with a further nearly, a quarter of patients exhibiting osteoarthritis in either ankle or subtalar joints. They concluded that results in talar body fractures are directly related to the severity of the initial injury and warned of poor long-term prognosis in patients that had suffered subluxation and articular damage to the subtalar and talotibial joints at the time of the initial injury.[33]

Surgical Anatomy, Positioning and Approaches

The talus has unique morphology and function: it has no muscular attachments, two third of its surface is comprised of cartilage and it has a tenuous blood supply. The talus is an integral part of three essential joints of the foot. The convex talar head articulates with the concavity of the navicular to form the talonavicular joint. Inferiorly, the talus articulates with the calcaneus to form the subtalar joint, and superiorly it articulates with the tibia to form the ankle joint. The sulcus tali is a deep grove formed by the plantar borders of the anterior/medial facet and the posterior facet. It is oriented about 40° posterolateral to antero-medial; its broad lateral extent forms the sinus tarsi while the medial side forms the tarsal canal in concert with its paired calcaneal sulcus. The sinus tarsi and tarsal canal house, both the interosseous ligament complex—a strong broad attachment between the talus and calcaneus—and the anastomosis between the arteries of the tarsal canal and sinus that provide the blood supply to about two-thirds of the talar body.

In a recent article by Helfet and Lorich examining the arterial supply of the talus, they found that the posterior tibial artery provided a total of four branches to the talus. There was significant variability as to where each of these branches arose but all specimens had a robust anastomotic network between the posterior tibial and peroneal arteries around the posterior tubercle of the talus. The artery of the tarsal canal anastomosed with the artery of the tarsal sinus—itself a branch of the peroneal artery, not only within the tarsal canal but within the "osseous architecture of the talus itself." They also noted the presence of an anastomotic network between the posterior and anterior tibial arteries around the medial and superior surfaces of the talar neck. The authors conclude, "We therefore recommend using extreme caution during surgical dissection to prevent unnecessary additional injury to the vasculature. Specifically, great care must be taken to avoid dissection dorsally and plantarly during both approaches to avoid injury to branches from the dorsalis pedis artery and the anastomotic network in the tarsal canal respectively"[34] (Figs 29.11 and 27.12).

The evolution of surgical reduction techniques is a result of the attainment of greater understanding of the variability of the fracture patterns. This variability dictates the development of myriad surgical reduction and provisional fixation techniques. Patients may be placed in the lateral or prone position for most of the techniques based on surgical preference. The prone position is often preferred with bilateral injuries to allow fixation bilaterally under a prep and drape.

Surgical Techniques

Anteromedial Approach to the Talar Neck

The anteromedial approach remains the workhorse incision for displaced talar neck fractures. In addressing talar body fractures the incision may be extended proximally and a medial malleolar osteotomy can be performed to gain improved exposure. To approach the medial aspect, an incision starting at the level of the tibiotalar joint, posterior to the medial malleolus is extended along the course of the posterior tibial tendon towards the talonavicular joint. Dissection is carried down and the interval between the tibialis anterior and posterior tendons is developed. If the talonavicular capsule is opened, this must be securely closed upon conclusion of the procedure. If a medial malleolar osteotomy is required, then an osteotomy at the level of the shoulder of the tibiotalar joint, extending proximally at a 45–60° angle can be made. This osteotomy may be transverse or chevron type. Some recommend predrilling for two screws for ultimate fixation.

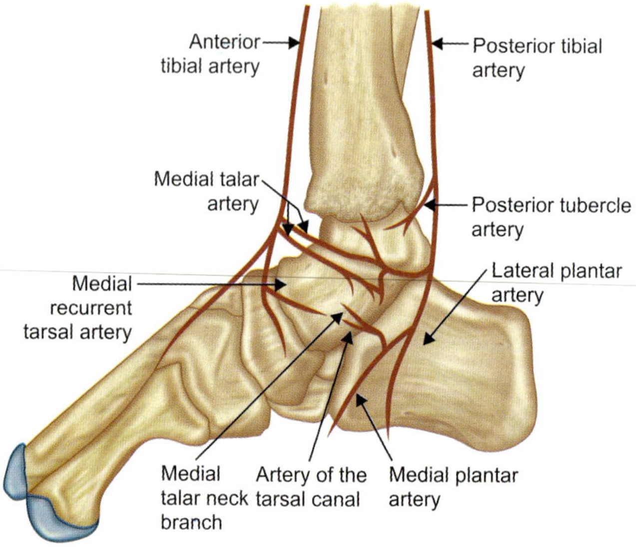

Figure 29.11: Medial vascular structures pertinent to talar neck fractures.

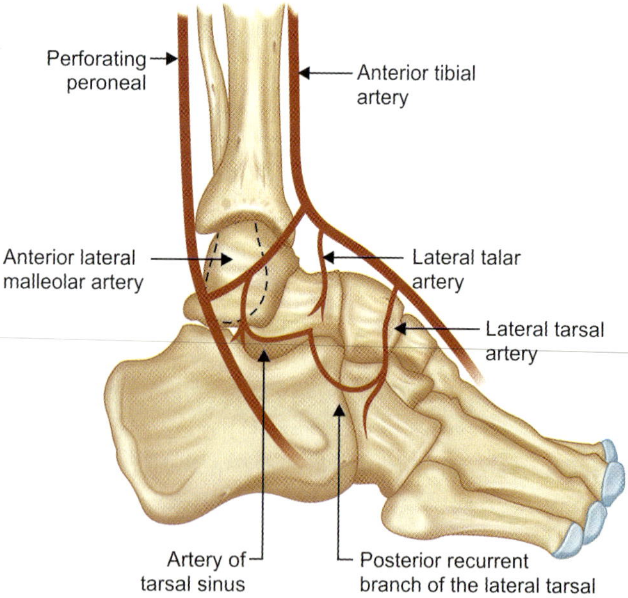

Figure 29.12: Lateral vascular structures pertinent to talar neck fractures.

The osteotomy can be started with a saw but completed with an osteotome to avoid removing the curve of the saw blade from the articular surface so as not to change the curvature of the shoulder of the ankle joint.

Anterolateral Approach to the Talar Neck

To approach the lateral aspect of the talus, either an incision from the lateral distal tip of the fibula toward the base of the fourth metatarsal can be made, or a Bohler's incision (Fig. 29.13). The topographic anatomic landmarks used are Chaput's tubercle and the area between the shafts of the third and fourth metatarsals. Begin the incision about 5 cm proximal to the ankle joint and slightly medial to Chaput's tubercle and extend it distally in a straight line toward the base of the third and fourth metatarsals (Figs 29.14A and B). It is imperative to avoid the creation of partial thickness skin flaps during the dissection. As the superficial peroneal nerve is identified and protected, the dissection continues through the subcutaneous tissue to expose the superior and inferior extensor retinaculum, and the tendons of the extensor digitorum longus, peroneus tertius, hallucis brevis, and the extensor hallucis longus (Figs 29.14A and B). Both the superior and inferior extensor retinacula are divided. Next, the tendons of the extensor digitorum longus and peroneus tertius, the deep peroneal nerve and the dorsalis pedis artery are mobilized medially. In the distal aspect of the incision, the muscle belly of the EDB is visualized and, if greater exposure is required, they can be either retracted laterally or detached from its origin and reflected distally. The lateral branch of the deep peroneal nerve and the lateral tarsal artery that arise at this level, care should be taken to preserve these structures. The incision is then carried down to the level of periosteum of the tibia proximally, the capsule of the ankle and the calcaneocuboid joint distally.[35]

At this juncture, the perforating branch of the peroneal artery is encountered in the interval between the tibia and fibula at the proximal edge of the incision and it should be either ligated or cauterized. The periosteum and capsule are divided and the sinus tarsi fat and the capsule of Chopart's joint are then incised. The dissection continues toward the articulation of the cuboid and the fourth metatarsal. Once finished, the exposure allows access to the calcaneocuboid joint, the talonavicular joint and a majority of the talar neck, the posterior facet of the subtalar joint, the anterior aspect of the ankle joint and the anterior face of the distal tibia (Figs 29.15A to K). Once the surgical procedure is completed, the tendons and neurovascular structures are released. The closure begins with the repair

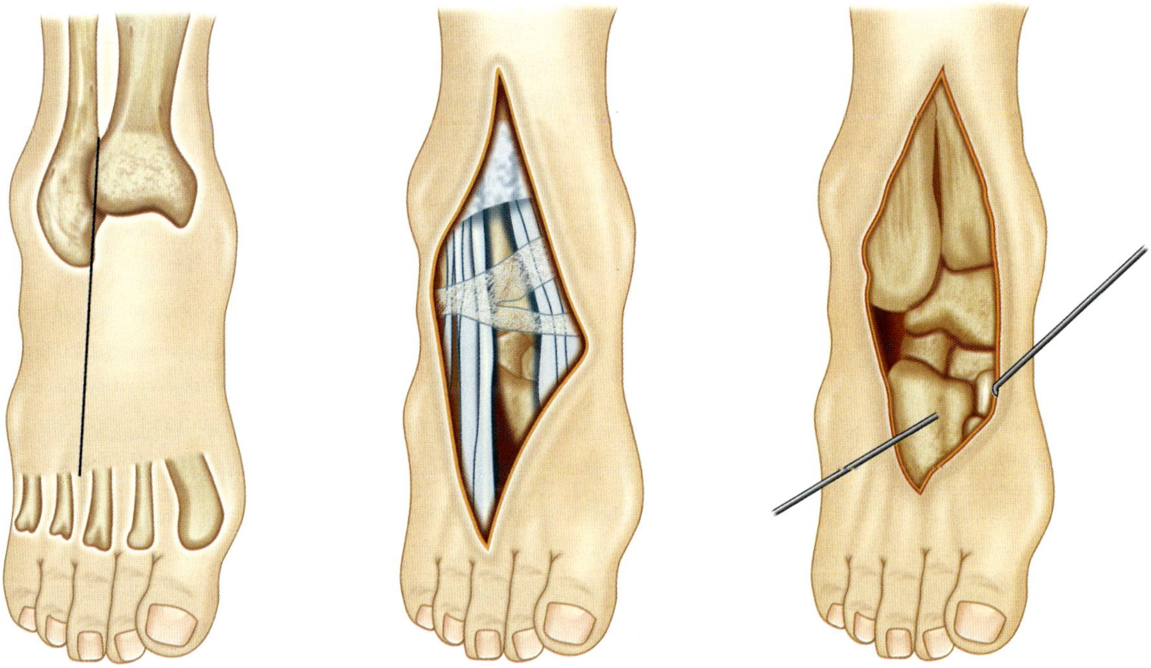

Figure 29.13: Bohler's incision for anterolateral exposure of the talar neck.

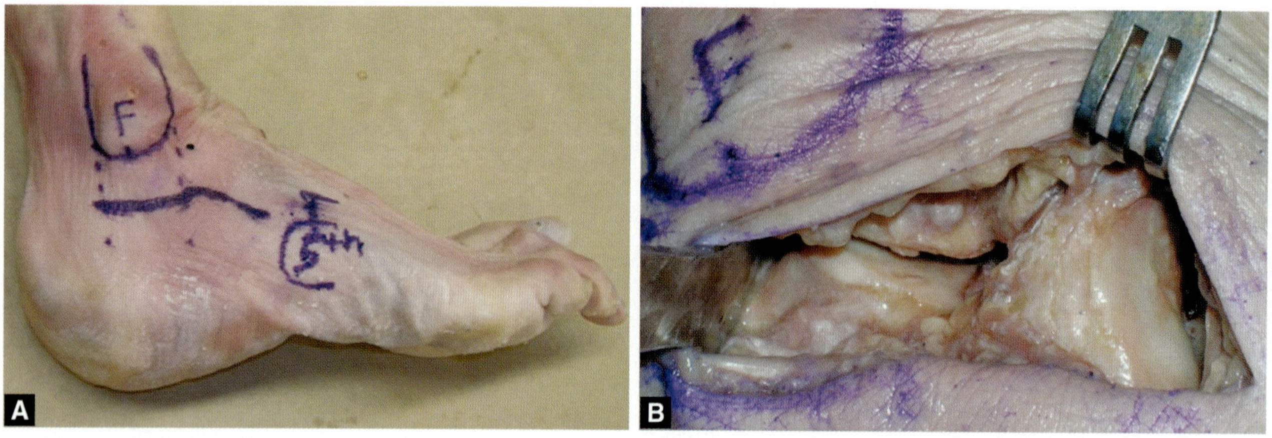

Figures 29.14A and B: Exposure of the subtalar joint from a lateral approach. (F: Fibula; 5th: Base of fifth metatarsal).

of the superior and inferior extensor retinaculum followed by the subcutaneous layer. The skin can be approximated with either interrupted nylon sutures or a subcuticular closure, and a drain may be left in the sinus tarsi if there is concern regarding the formation of a hematoma.[35] Whichever incision is used, cutaneous branches of the superficial peroneal nerve should be preserved, and the EDB elevated from plantar to dorsal.

Of note, in comminuted fractures of the talar neck, the risk of flexion and varus can occur if solely medial bony landmarks are reconstituted. Frequently, there is less comminution along the lateral neck at the juncture with the lateral process. This can provide a good key to the appropriate length and alignment of the talus. To allow for fragment specific fixation, use of small and mini-fragment screws and plates can be helpful.

ANTEROMEDIAL AND ANTEROLATERAL APPROACH TO THE TALAR NECK:
Pearls and Pitfalls

- Do not neglect plantar-medial comminution
- Do not neglect extension proximal to the lateral process of the talus which would involve the talar body
- With higher energy injuries, utilize two approaches with care to have apposition be based on the least comminuted side (most often this is the lateral side) to avoid coronal and sagittal deformity (most frequently varus and flexion)
- Avoid iatrogenic disruption of the deep deltoid arterial branches

Complications

Numerous complications have been described, including osteonecrosis, delayed union, infection, malunion, nonunion and post-traumatic arthritis. In the literature, the rate of talar neck malunion approaches 30%.[3,36] The degree of fracture comminution can make achieving an anatomic reduction more difficult, and the rate of malunion can be expected to be higher in comminuted fractures as compared with noncomminuted fractures.[37] The consequences of malunion are numerous and include varus malalignment resulting in decreased subtalar range of motion, subtalar arthritis and lateral column overload. Talar neck and body fractures are associated with several commonly observed late complications, which may be related to the severity of injury, the surgery itself or a combination of the two. Early complications include wound issues that, at times, can be avoided with careful attention to the placement of surgical incisions and the timing of surgical treatment as the authors have outlined above. In cases of talar body dislocation, early surgical management is necessary to avoid skin necrosis secondary to pressure from the displaced segment. The use of two approaches has not been associated with wound complications.[25-27] Nonunion is uncommon but late complications include AVN, post-traumatic arthritis of the ankle and subtalar joints and malunion.

Avascular Necrosis

Avascular necrosis frequently occurs after fractures of the talar neck and has been reported in 10–50% of cases. There

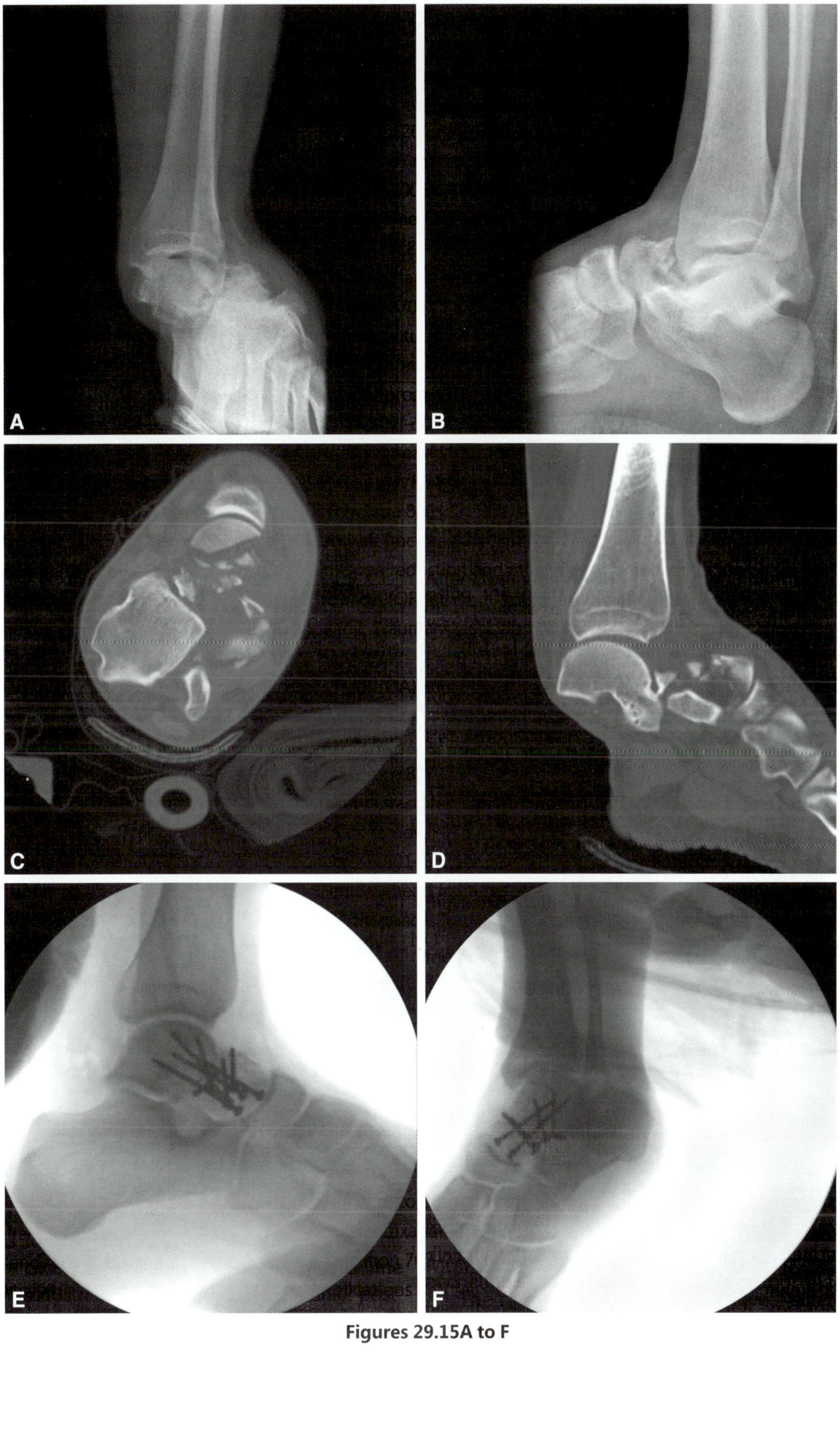

Figures 29.15A to F

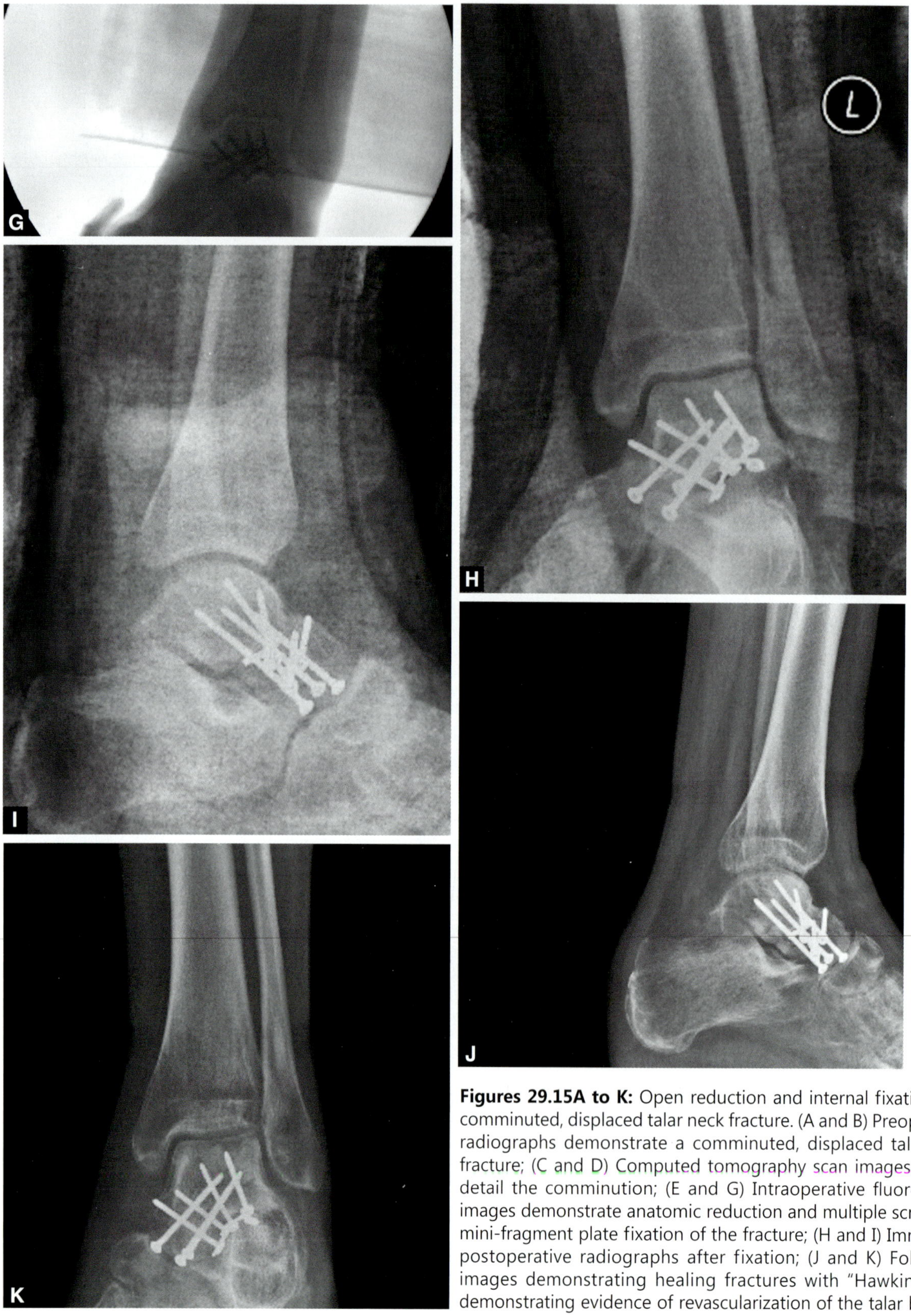

Figures 29.15A to K: Open reduction and internal fixation of a comminuted, displaced talar neck fracture. (A and B) Preoperative radiographs demonstrate a comminuted, displaced talar neck fracture; (C and D) Computed tomography scan images further detail the comminution; (E and G) Intraoperative fluoroscopic images demonstrate anatomic reduction and multiple screw and mini-fragment plate fixation of the fracture; (H and I) Immediate postoperative radiographs after fixation; (J and K) Follow-up images demonstrating healing fractures with "Hawkins sign" demonstrating evidence of revascularization of the talar body.

is an increased incidence of AVN with increasing fracture displacement as predicted by the Hawkins classification. Most patients will have some evidence of increased density on X-ray evaluations following a neck fracture; this finding does not necessarily portend talar collapse or a poor clinical outcome. A significant percentage of these cases will undergo revascularization with resolution of the sclerosis, while others will have persistence of sclerosis without collapse. Avascular necrosis with talar body collapse is a very ominous complication that results in pain with associated ankle and subtalar joint arthritis. Complex secondary reconstructive procedures are needed. Open wounds are associated with an increased rate of AVN in both talar body and talar neck injuries with reported incidences ranging from 69–86%.[25,27]

Malunion

Malunion of the talar neck is due to either surgical malreduction or loss of reduction prior to healing of a previously reduced fracture. The common deformity patterns include: shortening, varus and dorsiflexion. These late deformities pantomime injury displacement patterns found in the acute setting of injuries with advanced comminution. Varus talar neck malunion is directly associated with both a loss of subtalar motion and a loss of foot eversion.[31] This complication is best avoided by accurately reducing the fracture on the tension side (typically plantar and lateral), combined with stable fixation spanning the comminuted zones (typically dorsal and medial). Plate fixation placed on the side with the most comminution may assist in minimizing late deformity.[30] Acute bone grafting at the time of fixation is often necessary if a void exists dorsally and medially after the proper length of the talar neck has been re-established.

Arthritis

Peritalar stiffness and arthritis commonly occur after both talar neck and talar body fractures. Subtalar joint arthritis occurs more frequently after talar neck fractures, with an incidence of 60–100%. The incidence is directly correlated with the Hawkins classification type.[26] Talar body fractures have increased rate of arthritis at the ankle joint. Despite X-ray evidence of joint space narrowing in many patients, there is usually little need for secondary reconstructive procedures.[25,39]

To date, salvage procedures after talar malunions with joint involvement have consisted primarily of arthrodesis of the affected joints. Numerous studies have described ankle, subtalar, talonavicular, tibiotalocalcaneal or triple arthodesis for post-traumatic arthritis, malunion, nonunion or AVN.[3,36,40-44] As total ankle arthroplasty has become more accepted, some have espoused its use as an alternative to ankle arthrodesis in cases with isolated ankle arthritis.[45] However, the use of total ankle replacement may not be optimal in the setting of post-traumatic AVN or in the presence of poor bone quality that exists after the removal of pseudarthroses of the talus. This is of particular importance as some authors have reported that the talar component is more prone to failure than the tibial component.[46-48] Furthermore, at present, no reliable arthroplasty option exists for the subtalar and talonavicular joints. Although arthrodeses reportedly provide substantial pain relief, functional impairment prevails and the long-term outcome is limited due to the development of degenerative changes in adjacent joints.[49,50] The results of triple arthrodesis for the treatment of varus malalignment of the talar neck have been reported to be unsatisfactory.[3] Anatomical reconstruction of malunited talar fractures with preservation of the essential joints is of the utmost importance.

Subtalar Fusion

The decision to perform a subtalar fusion is based primarily on the patient's symptoms in concert with radiographic evidence of degenerative changes and/or progressive deformity (i.e. coronal hindfoot deformity, flattened talus, etc.). If nonoperative measures, such as anti-inflammatory medications, injections or bracing fail to provide adequate relief then a fusion is considered. Incision is based on prior incisions and soft tissue quality.

The following is a description of subtalar fusion technique providing there is no evidence of significant deformity. If a previously done "L-shaped" incision exists from prior calcaneal ORIF, then this can be used in a similar manner as for the initial surgery but may require proximal extension to allow better access to the subtalar joint. The original plate and screws may be removed and the articular cartilage and subchondral bone denuded from the posterior facets of the calcaneus and talus, respectively. If there is evidence of a modified sinus tarsi incision, then this can be used. Subsequent "shingling" of the bony articular surfaces with an osteotome or subchondral drilling with a 2.0 mm drill bit should be done to promote vascularization of the surfaces. Next, the surfaces should be approximated and the hindfoot maintained in 5° of valgus. Next, two guidewires for 7.3 mm cannulated screws should be inserted percutaneously from the plantar/posterior aspect of the posterior tuberosity of the calcaneus across the joint and into the talar body. Measurement should be made after countersinking is performed and based on bone quality. Partially threaded screws are chosen with screw threads that will only reside in the talus and not cross the joint. Wires are removed and closure proceeds.

Subtalar Fusion with Bone Block Arthrodesis

If significant horizontal displacement of the talus has progressed over time with or without depression of the posterior facet of the calcaneus with varus, then consideration for a bone block arthrodesis of the subtalar joint should be done. If possible, especially in a situation that had previous nonsurgical management, a vertical incision approximately 8–10 cm long, in line with the posterior aspect of the fibula and centered over the subtalar joint should be considered. This vertical incision will present less of an issue during closure after deformity correction, especially when there is a horizontal talus and a shortened calcaneus, in comparison to a horizontal incision. Full thickness flaps and care to avoid sural nerve and peroneal tendon injury is paramount. The exostectomy of a protuberant lateral wall of the calcaneus can be done if necessary. Once the approach is complete, similar debridement and preparation of the articular aspects of the talus and calcaneus should be done.

Then a percutaneous medial-to-lateral 5.0 mm Schanz pin should be applied in the plantar-posterior aspect of the talus. A second Schanz pin should be placed percutaneously medial-to-lateral in the distal third of the tibial shaft. A femoral distractor can be applied to both of these to promote lengthening of the hindfoot, realignment and correction of varus deformity.

Tricortical iliac crest can be harvested, preferably from the patient or bone bank. If autograft is chosen, the ipsilateral iliac region must be prepped as well. An incision is made from the anterior superior iliac spine (ASIS) proximally along the iliac crest for approximately 10–12 cm. Care must be taken not to violate the lateral femoral cutaneous nerve. The avascular line between the abductors of the hip and the external oblique musculature is developed to the ilium along the outer table, to the iliac crest and then subperiosteal deep to the iliacus on the inner table. The appropriate sized segment of bone is chosen based on the gap after deformity correction. Preferably this is harvested from the area of the gluteal ridge with the strongest bone approximated 4–6 cm proximal to the ASIS. Tight, layered closure should then be done.

Once the graft is harvested and shaped, it should be tightly impacted in the gap created by deformity correction with the femoral distractor. Provisionally fix the graft with K-wires. Then place two guidewires for 7.3 mm cannulated screws similarly to those done in a fusion without deformity but utilize 2 fully threaded screws to maintain the correction of deformity. Pack morselized allograft with or without autograft (calcaneal lateral wall exostectomized bone) around the area to be fused.

Tibiotalocalcaneal Fusion with an Intramedullary Nail

In situations where degenerative changes with or without rigid deformity have occurred in both the ankle and subtalar joints, a TTC fusion is a very viable option. Laterally based approach for the subtalar joint can be extended proximally along the fibula and a subsequent distal fibula resection to gain access to the ankle joint. At times, access to the medial shoulder of the ankle joint will require a small, anteromedial ankle approach concomitantly. The resected distal fibula can be morselized and used to fill any defects. The distal tibia articular surface and the talar dome articular surface should be prepared as described for preparation of the talar and calcaneal surfaces for fusion.

Alternatively, the ankle joint can be reached via a direct anterior approach. This is centered on the mortise, extending 5 cm proximal and 3 cm distal to the ankle joint. Care is taken to avoid the superficial peroneal nerve and its branches. Deep dissection can be done on either side of the extensor digitorum longus while taking care of the deep peroneal neurovascular bundle. A recent retrospective review of 49 pilon fractures noted low complication rates and minimal soft tissue disturbance after direct anterior approach.[22]

Once the articular surfaces have been prepared the aligned tibia, talus and calcaneus can be pinned provisionally. A 2–3 cm plantar incision can be made to allow introduction of the guidewire for the opening reamer for the TCC-type nail chosen. Standard nailing steps as per the nail's manufacturer's specifications can be done. Most nails allow for compression, which is preferable.

Authors' Preferred Management of Select Complications

Case: Chronic Infection after ORIF of an Extruded Talus

The following case is illustrative of many of the operative principles, perils and salvage techniques that the authors have discussed. This case involves a 69-year-old male who sustained, among other orthopedic injuries, an extruded left talus—open fracture-dislocation of his talus, with concomitant ipsilateral calcaneal fracture, bimalleolar-equivalent ankle fracture, partial tear of the peroneus brevis tendon and dysvascular limb (Figs 29.16A and B). The patient had a roughly 16 cm long open wound that began on the lateral aspect of the ankle about 8 cm proximal to the distal extent of the fibula. The wound extended distally and medially towards the midline and then curved around posteriorly in the direction of the calcaneal tuberosity posterior to the fibula. On day 1, he underwent ORIF of his calcaneal, ankle and talus fractures. The talar extrusion was completed and reconstruction was performed on the back table after the talus underwent 3 successive 10-minute soaks in a saline solution augmented with polymixin and bacitracin. Additionally, his peroneal brevis tendon was repaired and an external fixator applied (Figs 29.16C and D). The vascular team performed a femoral to below the knee synthetic bypass graft after angiography revealed a complete occlusion of the superficial femoral artery. The wounds were closed with 3-0 vicryl subcutaneously and 3-0 nylons on skin. Twenty days later the patient returned to the operating room with plastic surgery for debridement of necrotic tissue that had developed in the area about his open wound. The wound was debrided and cultured. A negative pressure dressing was applied. Infectious disease service was consulted and the patient was started on empiric therapy and transitioned to targeted antibiotic therapy after the cultures revealed infection with Methicillin-resistant Staphylococcus aureu and pseudomonas aeruginosa. Within 4–5 months of the initial injury, it was evident that the talus had progressed to an infected nonunion. In anticipation of a tibiocalcaneal fusion the patient underwent an irrigation and debridement, talectomy, and placement of tobramycin and vancomycin impregnated bone cement (Figs 29.16E and F). The wound closure was done in concert with the plastic surgery team who placed a split-thickness skin graft.

Two months subsequent to the talectomy the patient underwent definitive fusion of his tibiocalcaneal joint with a retrograde fusion nail, as well as fusion of his calcaneal cuboid and talonavicular joints with adjunctive osteo-inductive bone graft materials (demineralized bone matrix and bone morphogenetic protein). His wound was reapproximated with in a layered fashion and a wound VAC was placed on the closed incision to facilitate a complex wound healing in a known vasculopathic patient (Figs 29.16G to I). A bone stimulator was also applied in an attempt to improve bony fusion. Unfortunately, the split thickness skin graft failed and required further debridement. After numerous attempts at salvage the patient ultimately agreed to and underwent below-the-knee amputation approximately 9 months after his initial injury due to chronic infected nonunion (Figs 29.16J and K).

An alternative to retrograde fusion nail for a similar situation is ring external fixation as shown in Figures 29.17A to D for a different patient with osteomyelitis after ORIF of an extruded talus.

Summary

Hindfoot fractures continue to be vexing injuries rife with wound complications and lacking a true consensus of management. Currently, the extensile lateral approach for the calcaneus and the anteromedial approach for the talus are the workhorse incisions. However, owing to the precarious vasculature to both the osseous and soft tissue milieu of the hindfoot, there is an impetus to develop hybrid techniques and limited exposures to optimize reduction and limit complications. Regardless of the prevailing treatment, close attention must be paid to soft tissue management and timing of intervention. Despite assiduous adherence to modern treatment principles,

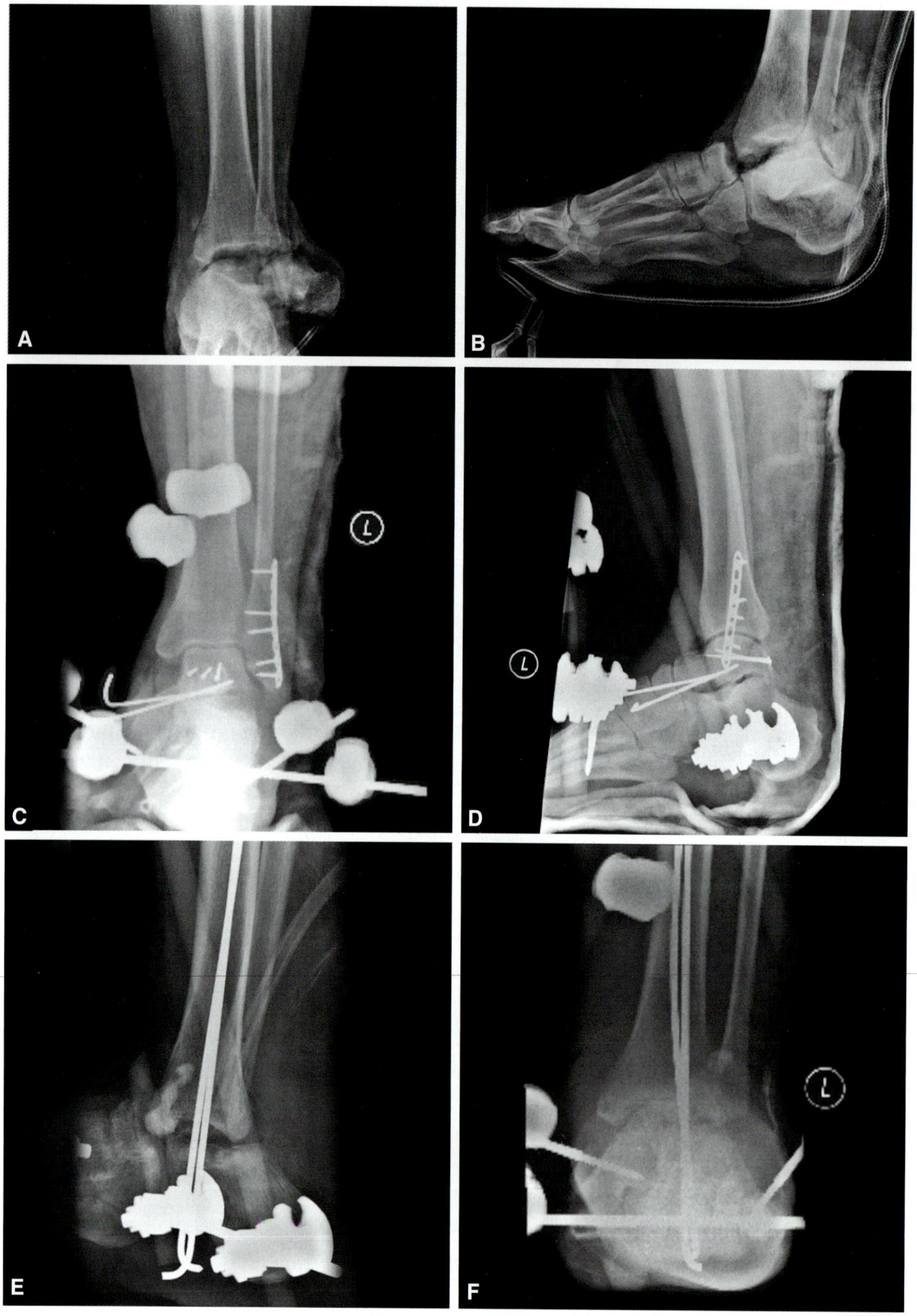

Figures 29.16A to F

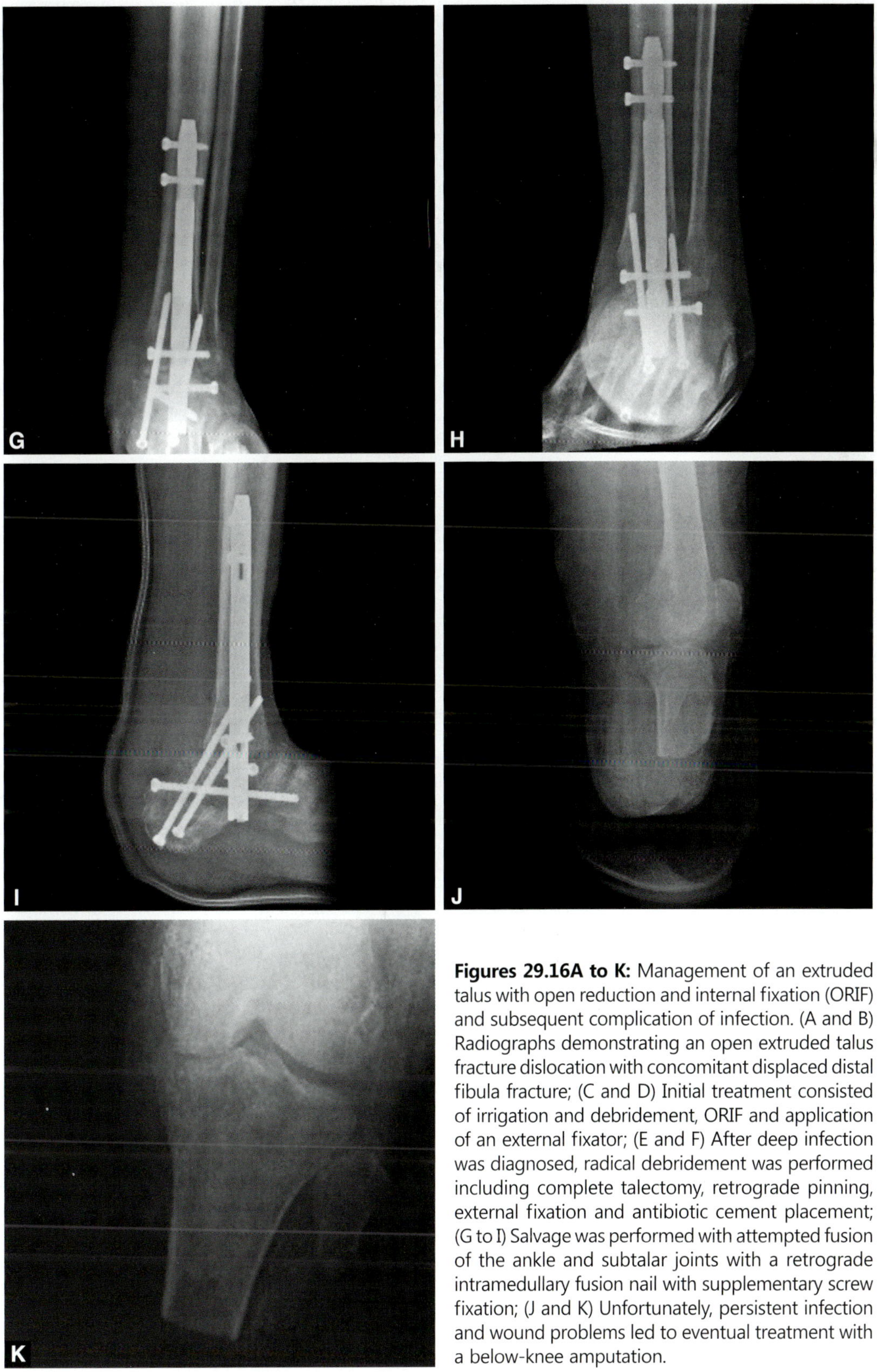

Figures 29.16A to K: Management of an extruded talus with open reduction and internal fixation (ORIF) and subsequent complication of infection. (A and B) Radiographs demonstrating an open extruded talus fracture dislocation with concomitant displaced distal fibula fracture; (C and D) Initial treatment consisted of irrigation and debridement, ORIF and application of an external fixator; (E and F) After deep infection was diagnosed, radical debridement was performed including complete talectomy, retrograde pinning, external fixation and antibiotic cement placement; (G to I) Salvage was performed with attempted fusion of the ankle and subtalar joints with a retrograde intramedullary fusion nail with supplementary screw fixation; (J and K) Unfortunately, persistent infection and wound problems led to eventual treatment with a below-knee amputation.

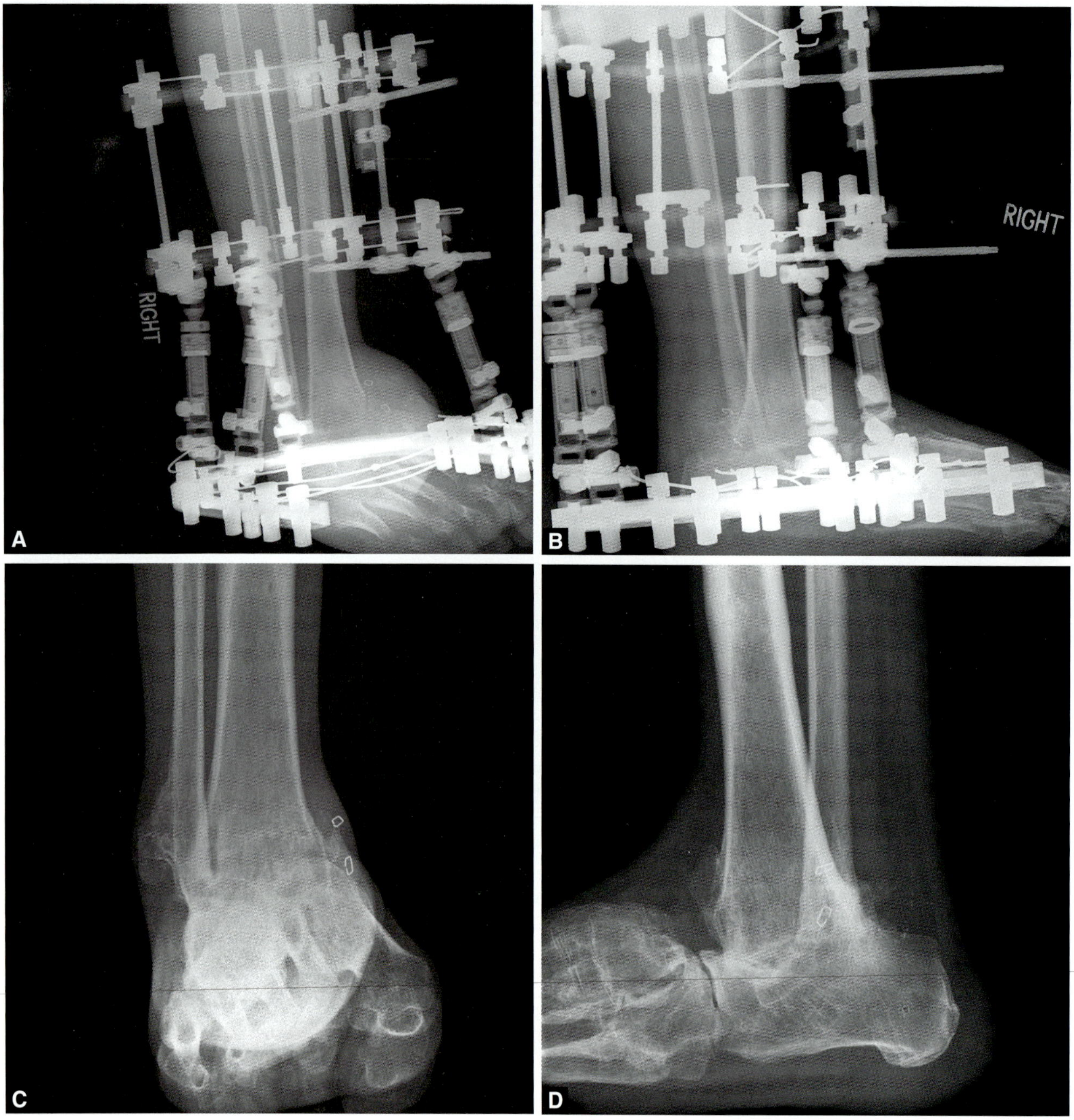

Figures 29.17A to D: Alternative management of an extruded talus with open reduction and internal fixation (ORIF) and subsequent complication of infection. (A and B) Radiographs demonstrating ankle after radical debridement of chronic osteomyelitis of the talus after initial attempts at ORIF. Fusion was performed with a ring fixator, compression and vancomycin-impregnated calcium sulfate pellets; (C and D) Successful fusion was achieved without evidence of residual infection. Although the patient has extreme shortening as a result of the talectomy, he is ambulatory with a shoe lift.

Courtesy: Saqib Rehman

complications are unavoidable and frequent. The authors hope that they have outlined a rational approach to diagnostic strategies, treatment modalities and salvage procedures for fractures of the calcaneus, talar neck and talar body.

References

1. Heier KA, Infante AF, Walling AK, et al. Open fractures of the calcaneus: soft-tissue injury determines outcome. J Bone Joint Surg. 2003;85-A(12):2276-82.
2. Harty M. Anatomic considerations in injuries of the calcaneus. Orthop Clin North Am. 1973;4(1):179-83.
3. Bezes H, Massart P, Delvaux D, et al. The operative treatment of intra-articular calcaneal fractures. Indications, technique, and results in 257 cases. Clin Orthop Relat Res. 1993;(290):55-9.
4. Soeur R, Remy R. Fractures of the calcaneus with displacement of the thalamic portion. J Bone Joint Surg Br. 1975;57(4):413-21.
5. Browner BD, Jupiter JJ, Levine AM, et al. Skeletal Trauma, 4th edition. Volume 2. Philadelphia, PA: WB Saunder; 2009. pp. 2585-748.
6. Koski A, Kuokkanen H, Tukiainen E. Postoperative wound complications after internal fixation of closed calcaneal fractures: a retrospective analysis of 126 consecutive patients with 148 fractures. SJS. 2005;94(3):243-5.
7. Bezes H, et al. The operative treatment of intra-articular calcaneal fractures. Indications, technique, and results in 257 cases. Clin Orthop Relat Res. 1993;(290):55-9.
8. Gilmer PW, Herzenberg J, Frank JL, et al. Computerized tomographic analysis of acute calcaneal fractures. Foot Ankle. 1986;6(4):184-93.
9. McLaughlin HL. Treatment of late complications after os calcis fractures. Clin Orthop Relat Res. 1963;30:111-5.
10. Watson TS. Soft tissue complications following calcaneal fractures. Foot Ankle Clin. 2007;12(1):107-23.
11. Essex-Lopresti P. The mechanism, reduction technique, and results in fractures of the os calcis. Br J Surg. 1952; 39(157): 395-419.
12. Watson TS. Soft tissue complications following calcaneal fractures. Foot Ankle Clin. 2007;12(1):107-23.
13. Al-Mudhaffar M, Prasad CV, Mofidi A. Wound complications following operative fixation of calcaneal fractures. Injury. 2000;31(6):461-4.
14. Borrelli J, Jr, Lashgari C. Vascularity of the lateral calcaneal flap: a cadaveric injection study. J Orthop Trauma. 1999; 13(2):73-7.
15. Howard JL, Buckley R, McCormack R, et al. Complications following management of displaced intra-articular calcaneal fractures: a prospective randomized trial comparing open reduction internal fixation with nonoperative management. J Orthop Trauma. 2003;17(4):241-9.
16. Palmer I. The mechanism and treatment of fractures of the calcaneus; open reduction with the use of cancellous grafts. J Bone Joint Surg Am. 1948;30A(1) 2-8.
17. Harvey EJ, Grujic L, Early JS, et al. Morbidity associated with ORIF of intra-articular calcaneus fractures using a lateral approach. Foot Ankle. 2001;22(11):868-73.
18. Liporace F, Berberian WS, Najarian RG, Lin SS. Displacement of the sustentacular fragment in intra-articular calcaneus fractures. Paper #62, Annual Meeting of the Orthopaedic Trauma Association, Denver, CO, October 2008.
19. Stannard JP, Robinson JT, Anderson ER, et al. Negative pressure wound therapy to treat hematomas and surgical incisions following high-energy trauma. J Trauma. 2006; 60(6):1301-6.
20. Banerjee R, Saltzman C, Anderson RB, et al. Management of calcaneal malunion. J Am Acad Orthop Surg. 2011; 19(1):27-36.
21. Radnay CS, Clare MP, Sanders RW. Subtalar fusion after displaced intra-articular calcaneal fractures: does initial operative treatment matter? Surgical technique. J Bone Joint Surg Am. 2010,92 Suppl 1 Pt 1:32-43.
22. McCann PA, Jackson M, Mitchell ST, et al. Complications of definitive open reduction and internal fixation of pilon fractures of the distal tibia. Int Orthop. 35(3):413-8.
23. Rammelt S, Zwipp H. Talar neck and body fractures. Injury. 2009;40(2):120-35.
24. Syme J. Contribution to the pathology and practice of surgery 1848. Edinburgh: Sutherland and Knox.
25. Lindvall E, Haidukewych G, DiPasquale T, et al. Open reduction and stable fixation of isolated, displaced talar neck and body fractures. J Bone Joint Surg Am. 2004;86-A(10):2229-34.
26. Vallier HA, Nork SE, Barei DP, et al. Talar neck fractures: results and outcomes. J Bone Joint Surg Am. 2004;86-A(8):1616-24.
27. Vallier HA, Nork SE, Benirschke SK, et al. Surgical treatment of talar body fractures. J Bone Joint Surg Am. 2004;86-A Suppl 1(Pt 2):180-92.
28. Hawkins LG. Fractures of the neck of the talus. J Bone Joint Surg Am. 1970;52(5):991-1002.
29. Fortin PT, Balazsy JE. Talus fractures: evaluation and treatment. J Am Acad of Orthop Surg. 2001;9(2):114-27.
30. Sangeorzan BJ, Wagner UA, Harrington RM, et al. Contact characteristics of the subtalar joint: the effect of talar neck misalignment. J Orthop Res. 1992;10(4):544-51.

31. Daniels TR, Smith JW, Ross TI. Varus malalignment of the talar neck. Its effect on the position of the foot and on subtalar motion. J Bone Joint Surg Am. 1996;78(10): 1559-67.

32. Kellam J, Bosse M, Obremskey W. Timing of surgical fixation of talar neck fractures. Paper 2745. Presented at: Orthopaedic Trauma Association General Meeting. Salt Lake City, Utah. 2003.

33. Sneppen O, Christensen SB, Krogsoe O, et al. Fracture of the body of the talus. Acta orthop Scand. 1977;48(3): 317-24.

34. Prasarn ML, Miller AN, Dyke JP, et al. Arterial anatomy of the talus: a cadaver and gadolinium-enhanced MRI study. Foot Ankle Int. 2010;31(11):987-93.

35. Herscovici D, et al. Bohler incision: an extensile anterolateral approach to the foot and ankle. J Orthop Trauma. 2000; 14(6):429-32.

36. Frawley PA, Hart JA, Young DA. Treatment outcome of major fractures of the talus. Foot Ankle Int. 1995;16(6): 339-45.

37. Charlson MD, Parks BG, Weber TG, et al. Comparison of plate and screw fixation and screw fixation alone in a comminuted talar neck fracture model. Foot Ankle Int. 2006;27(5):340-3.

38. Fleuriau Chateau PB, Brokaw DS, Jelen BA, et al. Plate fixation of talar neck fractures: preliminary review of a new technique in twenty-three patients. J Orthopc Trauma. 2002; 16(4):213-9.

39. Elgafy H, Ebraheim NA, Tile M, et al. Fractures of the talus: experience of two level 1 trauma centers. Foot Ankle Int. 2000;21(12):1023-9.

40. Gagneux E, Gerard F, Garbuio P, et al. [Treatment of complex fractures of the ankle and their sequellae using trans-plantar intramedullary nailing]. Acta Orthop Belg. 1997; 63(4):294-304.

41. Kitaoka HB, Patzer GL. Arthrodesis for the treatment of arthrosis of the ankle and osteonecrosis of the talus. J Bone Joint Surg Am. 1998;80(3):370-9.

42. Rockett AK, Mangum G, Mendicino SS. Bilateral intra-osseous cystic formation in the talus: a complication of subtalar arthroeresis. J Foot Ankle Surg: official publication of the American College of Foot and Ankle Surgeons. 1998; 37(5):421-5.

43. Chou LB, Mann RA, Yaszay B, et al. Tibiotalocalcaneal arthrodesis. Foot Ankle Int. 2000;21(10):804-8.

44. Easley ME, Trnka HJ, Schon LC, et al. Isolated subtalar arthrodesis. J Bone Joint Surg Am. 2000;82(5):613-24.

45. Hintermann B, Valderrabano V. Total ankle replacement. Foot Ankle Clin. 2003;8(2):375-405.

46. Buechel FF, Buechel FF, Pappas MJ. Ten-year evaluation of cementless Buechel-Pappas meniscal bearing total ankle replacement. Foot Ankle Int Am. 2003;24(6):462-72.

47. Knecht SI, Estin M, Callaghan JJ, et al. The Agility total ankle arthroplasty. Seven to sixteen-year follow-up. J Bone Joint Surg Am. 2004;86-A(6):1161-71.

48. Spirt AA, Assal M, Hansen ST. Complications and failure after total ankle arthroplasty. J Bone Joint Surg Am. 2004;86-A(6):1172-8.

49. Coester LM, Saltzman CL, Leupold J, et al. Long-term results following ankle arthrodesis for post-traumatic arthritis. J Bone Joint Surg Am. 2001;83-A(2):219-28.

50. Fuchs S, Sandmann C, Skwara A, et al. Quality of life 20 years after arthrodesis of the ankle. A study of adjacent joints. J Bone Joint Surg Br. 2003;85(7):994-8.

Chapter 30

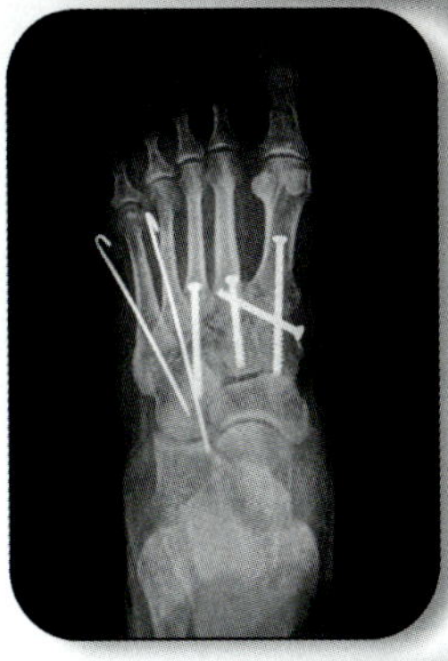

Midfoot and Forefoot Fractures

Jamal Ahmad

Chapter Outline

Introduction
Diagnosis
Classification
Surgical Indications
- Open Reduction and Internal Fixation
- Closed Reduction and Percutaneous Pinning
- Midfoot Fusion or Arthrodesis

Surgical Anatomy, Positioning and Approaches
- Applied Anatomy
- Positioning
- Approaches

SURGICAL TECHNIQUES
Technique 1: Open Reduction and Internal Fixation of Lisfranc Fracture-dislocations
Technique 2: Midfoot Arthrodesis for Lisfranc Fracture-dislocations with Irreparable Joint Damage
Technique 3: Open Reduction and Internal Fixation of Extra-articular First-fourth Metatarsal Fractures
Technique 4: Open Reduction and Internal Fixation of Proximal Fifth Metatarsal Fractures
Technique 5: Open Reduction and Internal Fixation of Hallucal Fracture-dislocations
Technique 6: Open Reduction and Internal Fixation of Hallucal Sesamoid Fractures
Outcomes
Complications
- Postoperative Infection
- Wound Complications
- Post-traumatic Arthritis
- Nonunion
- Compartment Syndrome

Author's Preferred Management of Select Complications
- Case 1: Treatment of Post-traumatic Midfoot Arthritis after ORIF of a Lisfranc Injury
- Case 2: Nonunion vs Refracture of a Proximal Zone Two Fifth Metatarsal Fracture
- Case 3: Treatment of Compartment Syndrome of the Foot

Summary

Introduction

There is a wide variety of midfoot and forefoot fractures and dislocations. A proper understanding of these injuries begins with an appreciation for the complex anatomy of the midfoot and forefoot.

The midfoot consists of the three cuneiforms, cuboid and the first-fifth proximal metatarsals. The joints of the midfoot are known as the tarsometatarsal (TMT) or Lisfranc joint complex, the latter being named after Dr Jacques Lisfranc de Saint-Martin (1787–1847), who described amputations through these joints while working as an army field surgeon.[1] These involve the naviculo-cuneiform, cuboid-cuneiform, inter-cuneiform and first-fifth TMT joints, which are specifically the first metatarsal-medial cuneiform, second metatarsal-intermediate cuneiform, third metatarsal-lateral cuneiform, fourth metatarsal-cuboid and fifth metatarsal-cuboid joints. Midfoot stability is based on its unique joint anatomy and ligamentous restraints. The first-fifth TMT joints are arranged in a Roman arch pattern, with the second TMT joint being recessed as the keystone of the complex between the medial and lateral cuneiforms. The first-third TMT joints are relatively rigid, while the fourth-fifth are more mobile. The first-third TMT joints provide arch support and act as a lever arm for foot propulsion. The fourth-fifth TMT joints allow the foot to accommodate to uneven ground. Multiple dorsal, interosseous and plantar ligaments, with the latter being the strongest of the three, support the TMT joints. While there is no first-second proximal inter-metatarsal ligament, the medial cuneiform is stabilized to the second metatarsal by the Lisfranc ligament, which is the largest at the midfoot.

The forefoot consists of the first-fifth distal metatarsals, hallucal medial and lateral sesamoids, first-fifth proximal phalanges, second-fifth middle phalanges and first-fifth distal phalanges. The joints of the forefoot include the metatarsophalangeal (MTP), the first toe or hallucal interphalangeal (IP), the second-fifth proximal inter-phalangeal (PIP) and the second-fifth distal interphalangeal (DIP) joints. The distal intermetatarsal ligaments, the plantar plates at the MTP joints, the phalangeal collateral ligaments and balance between the flexor and extensor tendons provide forefoot stability (Fig. 30.1).

As over 20 bones and joints comprise the midfoot and forefoot, there are many different types of fractures and/or dislocations that can be seen. Since this is a surgical text, those injuries that are unstable and warrant operative treatment shall be emphasized. Such conditions include: (1) Lisfranc injuries; (2) extra-articular first-fourth metatarsal fractures; (3) proximal fifth metatarsal fractures; (4) hallucal fractures and/or dislocations and; (5) hallucal

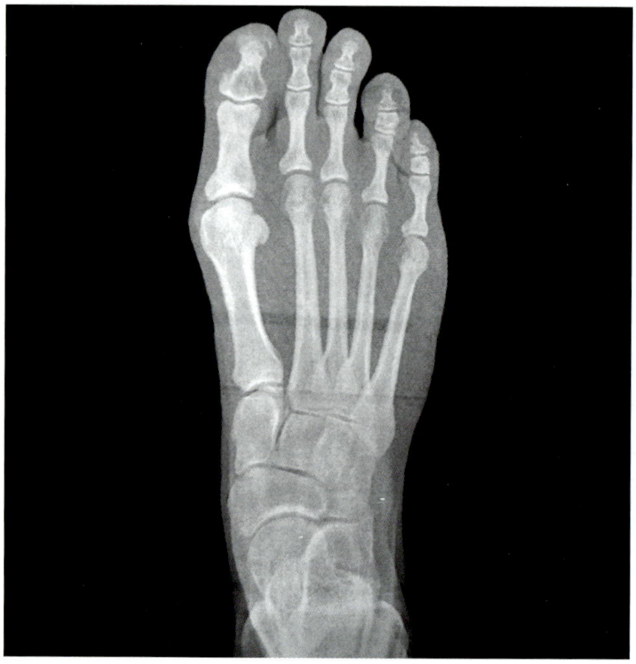

Figure 30.1: Midfoot and forefoot radiographic anatomy. Note that the base of the second metatarsal is recessed at the intermediate cuneiform; the parabolic appearance of the first-fifth metatarsal heads.

sesamoid fractures. Additional forefoot injuries include lesser phalangeal fractures and lesser MTP, PIP and DIP dislocations, which are often successfully treated with nonsurgical management.

Lisfranc fracture-dislocations account for 0.2% of all fractures. Causes range from those due to direct high-energy versus indirect lower-energy trauma. Direct injuries involve forces applied from dorsal to plantar at the TMT joints. Indirect injuries typically involve an axial load applied to the TMT joints while the forefoot is twisted and the entire foot is plantarflexed. Lisfranc fracture-dislocations can vary widely based on the amount of bony and/or ligamentous injury. It is important to note that some injuries can result in purely ligamentous Lisfranc dislocations, which can be missed or neglected on initial evaluation. The severity of such dislocations does not become apparent until the subacute or chronic phase, when irreversible midfoot instability develops.[2] As the midfoot loses its inherent stability, post-traumatic arthritis occurs and the foot develops a rigid planovalgus deformity.

Extra-articular first-fifth metatarsal fractures account for 2% of all fractures. There are three types based on location: (1) base; (2) shaft; and (3) head and/or neck. Such injuries may present with single or multiple metatarsal involvement. Many of these fractures are due to high-energy trauma, such as motor vehicle accidents, falls from a height, or crush injuries. As the first metatarsal is critical in gait and bearing weight, much less displacement is tolerated than in the central metatarsals.

Proximal fifth metatarsal fractures are further classified into three types: (1) tuberosity or styloid fractures; (2) Jones fractures at the metaphyseal-diaphyseal junction and; (3) diaphyseal stress fractures. Initially, tuberosity fractures were thought to be due to action of the peroneus brevis while the hindfoot is inverted. Recent studies suggest that acute contracture of the lateral band of the plantar aponeurosis is the true mechanism of injury[3] Jones fractures are named after Sir Robert Jones, who first described this injury in 1902.[4] The injuries are infamous as they are located in an area of the bone that is less vascular than the tuberosity and diaphysis.[5] These injuries are thought to be due to forefoot adduction as the foot is plantarflexed. Diaphyseal stress fractures are pathologic in which the bone is subject to repetitive distraction forces.

Injuries to the hallux include both fractures and dislocations. Most hallucal fractures are due to direct injuries in which a heavy object falls on the toe. Such injuries are common among manual laborers. Most first MTP dislocations are dorsal where an axial load is applied to the joint while it is hyperdorsiflexed. This causes the plantar plate to rupture from its origin at the plantar first metatarsal neck. With further dorsiflexion, the plantar plate and sesamoids follow the proximal phalanx as it dislocates over the metatarsal head. Such injuries are most often seen following motor vehicle accidents or contact sports. Akin to the first MTP joint, the majority of first IP joint dislocations are also dorsal as an axial load is applied to the joint while it is hyperdorsiflexed.

The hallucal medial and lateral sesamoids are vulnerable to injury due to their unique location and function. Both sesamoids are invested by the flexor hallucis brevis (FHB) and articulate with the plantar first metatarsal head to allow for smooth, painless weight-bearing at the first metatarsal. Specifically, the sesamoids elevate the first metatarsal head while increasing the mechanical advantage of FHB function. Most sesamoid fractures are caused by a hyperdorsiflexion of the first MTP joint, as seen in football and soccer players.

Many factors are important in successful treatment of midfoot and forefoot fractures and dislocations. These include restoration of articular congruity, stable bony fixation, achievement of bony healing and avoidance of complications such as post-traumatic arthritis and nonunion.

Diagnosis

The physical examination of the injured foot begins with a thorough evaluation of its neurovascular status. The sural, tibial and superficial peroneal nerves (SPN) provide sensation to the skin of the lateral, plantar and combined dorsal and medial aspects of the foot, respectively. The deep peroneal nerve innervates the skin of the foot's first web space. In addition, the tibial and deep peroneal nerves innervate the flexor and extensor muscles of the foot, respectively. Peripheral pulses and capillary refill should be checked and compared with the contralateral foot to assess perfusion. The proximity of the dorsalis pedis artery to the central midfoot places it at risk with Lisfranc injuries and their treatment. When the dorsalis pedis pulse is not palpable, additional testing such as an arterial duplex ultrasound or angiography may be necessary to complete an adequate vascular assessment. Neurovascular examination should be repeated after any closed reduction maneuvers and the foot should be exposed enough for additional repeat examinations without compromising overall joint stability.

It is critical to examine the foot's soft tissue at the time of initial injury and regularly thereafter. High-energy injuries can often cause open wounds, closed blisters and severe soft tissue swelling. Open fracture wounds typically occur at the dorsum of the foot. It is especially important to avoid overlooking small wounds. All open wounds should be assessed for size and then treated with emergent irrigation and debridement (I and D). Fracture blisters contain either serum or blood, the latter being indicative of greater soft tissue trauma. While there is no universal consensus for treatment of acute fracture blisters, author's personal preference is to drain these with a needle, leave the skin intact and cover them with a non-adherent dressing such as xeroform or adaptic gauze. When acutely swollen, the foot must be assessed for compartment syndrome. Early signs of compartment syndrome are pain out of proportion to the injury or with passive toe motion. Later signs include pallor, paralysis, diminished pulses and paresthesias. Objective compartment measurements that indicate compartment syndrome are when any of the foot's nine compartments (medial, lateral, superficial, adductor, calcaneal and four interossei) have a pressure greater than 30 mm Hg or within 30 mm Hg of the patient's diastolic pressure.[6,7] This situation requires emergent compartment release or fasciotomy as treatment. When the foot does not have compartment syndrome, it is still important to note how swollen it may be. Performing open surgical treatment on the foot before its soft tissue has a chance to improve carries a higher risk of surgical wound complications such as dehiscence. In certain situations, it is not abnormal to delay definitive surgical treatment for up to 2–3 weeks if it takes that long for the soft tissue to improve. Ultimately, the timing of surgical treatment depends upon an optimal condition of the foot's soft tissue.

Diagnostic imaging of the midfoot and forefoot starts with a full series of radiographs. This involves antero-posterior (AP), lateral and an oblique 30° views. Tangential sesamoid films should be included if a patient has a suspected first ray or sesamoid injury (Fig. 30.2).

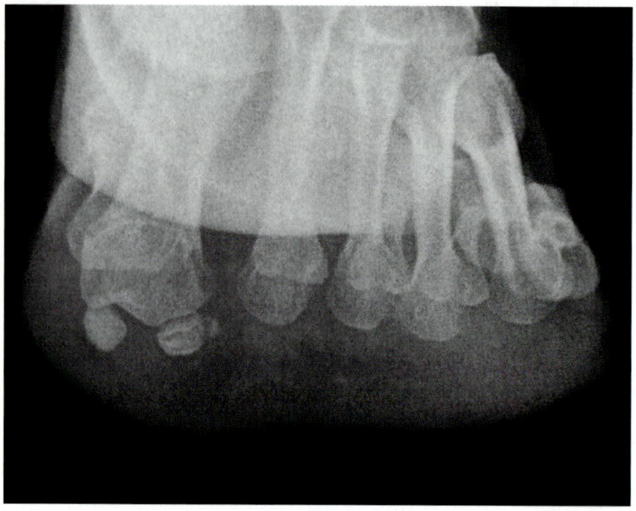

Figure 30.2: A tangential sesamoid radiograph. This particular patient has a fibular sesamoid fracture.

Radiographs of the contralateral, uninjured foot can also be obtained for comparative purposes. Non-weight-bearing films are sufficient to guide treatment if fracture and/or joint instability are clear. However, if such radiographs show neither, then weight-bearing films are critical in assessing the patient's injury severity. While this may be painful for patients to perform soon after their injuries, these can be important in determining possible fracture and/or joint instability. If patients are unable to bear weight on their foot for radiographs initially, another attempt at weight-bearing films should be done within 7–10 days. By this time, most patients are able to provide weight-bearing foot radiographs. It is rare that a radiographic exam under anesthesia is required to assess the complete nature of the patient's injury. Radiographic signs of Lisfranc injuries include TMT joint disturbances, widening of the space between the second metatarsal base and the medial cuneiform where the Lisfranc ligament courses and "fleck signs" which are avulsion fractures at the TMT joint (Fig. 30.3).[8]

Computed tomography (CT) may be a necessary adjuvant for imaging of certain midfoot and forefoot injuries. In general, CT scans are invaluable and recommended for assessing most intra-articular fractures. This becomes particularly important in managing Lisfranc fracture-dislocations as CT scans are highly accurate in measuring extent of bony injury, fracture comminution and intra-articular extension and amount of joint incongruity. The surgeon routinely obtains CT scans on all patients with Lisfranc injuries regardless of radiographic appearance so as to not miss any subtle bony or joint injuries. CT scans can also be useful for better definition of intra-articular hallux or lesser MTP injuries.

Magnetic resonance imaging (MRI) has limited uses for managing acute midfoot and forefoot injuries. However, it has been recently used to diagnose purely ligamentous Lisfranc injuries in which patients have significant midfoot pain but no radiographic signs of acute ligamentous

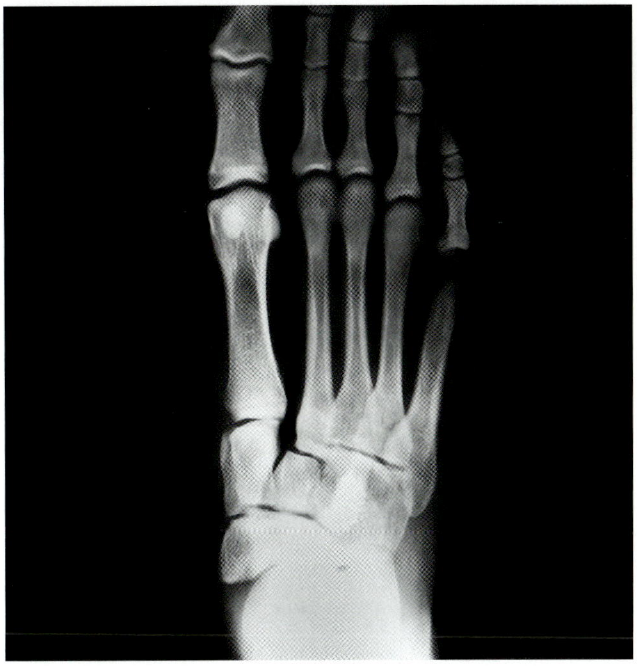

Figure 30.3: An example of a Lisfranc injury limited to the Lisfranc ligament. Note the significant widening between the base of the second metatarsal and the medial cuneiform.

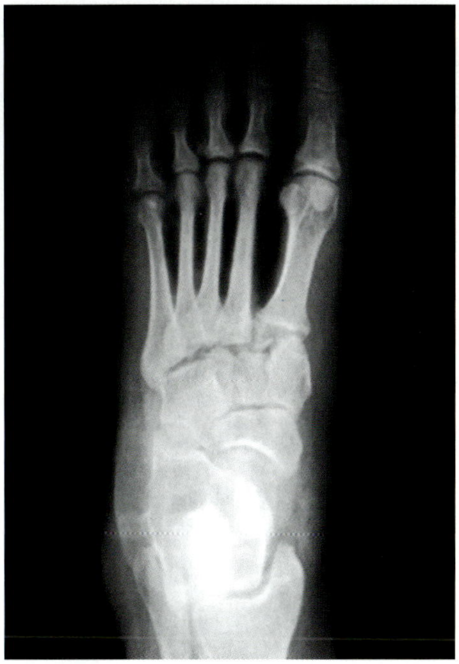

Figure 30.4: Type A, complete homolateral Lisfranc fracture-dislocation. Note the lateral displacement of the first-fifth proximal metatarsals.

instability.[9] Detection of such subtle injuries is critical as missing or neglecting them can lead to early post-traumatic midfoot instability and/or arthritis. While MRI can be an important imaging tool, it is important to realize that findings of Lisfranc ligament injury can be highly dependent on both the quality of the images and the physician interpreting them.

MIDFOOT AND FOREFOOT FRACTURES DIAGNOSIS: Pearls and Pitfalls

- Open wounds, neurovascular status and soft tissue compartments should be assessed with vigilance
- Fracture blisters should be drained and dressed, leaving the roof of skin intact
- Non-weight-bearing radiographs are sufficient when there is overt bony and/or ligamentous instability. Weight-bearing films can be useful in determining unstable fractures and/or dislocations
- CT scans are invaluable for characterizing and preoperative planning of intra-articular fracture-dislocations. MRIs are useful when evaluating a patient that may have a ligamentous Lisfranc injury despite normal radiographs. Surgical treatment is best performed when the foot's soft tissue is optimal. It is not unreasonable to delay surgery as long 10–14 days under such circumstances

Classification

Several classification systems for Lisfranc fracture-dislocations have been proposed. Historical descriptions include Quenu and Kuss' original classification and Hardcastle's modification of this.[10,11] The author recommends using Myerson's categorization of these injuries, which are divided into three primary types.[8] Type A injuries are known as complete homolateral injuries with total first-fifth TMT joint incongruity. All five metatarsals dislocate as a single unit in a single direction, which can be dorsal, plantar or lateral (Fig. 30.4).

Type B injuries are called incomplete homolateral injuries with partial TMT joint incongruity. These are further classified into medial B1 and lateral B2 patterns of injury. Type B1 injuries only involve the first TMT joint while B2 injuries include one or more of the second-fifth TMT joints (Fig. 30.5).

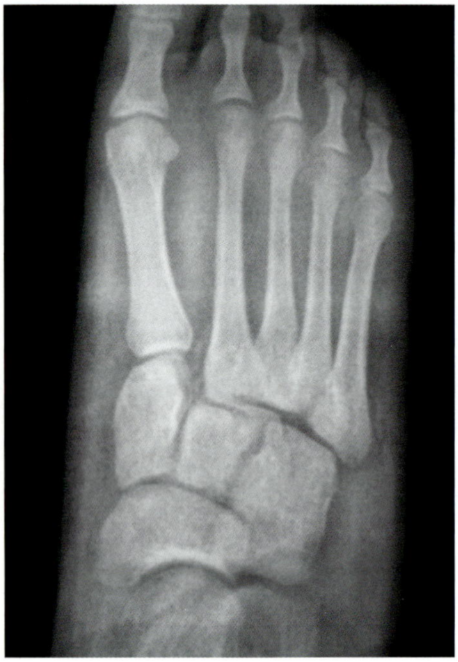

Figure 30.5: Type B2, incomplete homolateral Lisfranc fracture-dislocation. Note the lateral displacement of the second-fourth proximal metatarsals while the first tarsometatarsal (TMT) joint is stable.

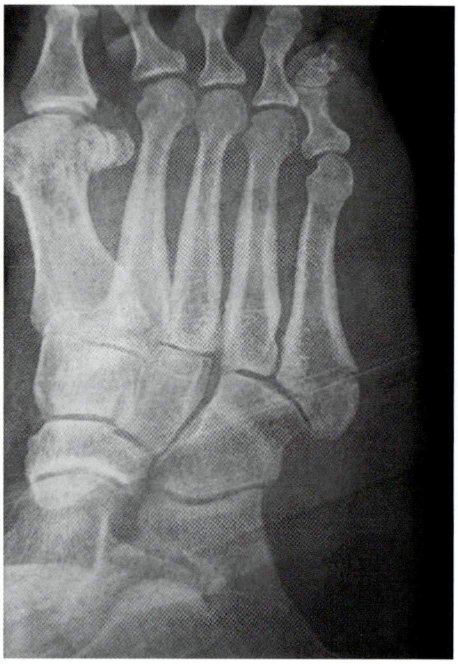

Figure 30.6: Zone 1 fifth metatarsal fracture.

Finally, type C injuries are known as divergent injuries in which the first TMT joint is dislocated medially and any of the second-fifth TMT joints are dislocated laterally. These are further divided into partial C1 and total C2 injuries in which some and then all of the second-fifth TMT joints are involved respectively.

Extra-articular first-fifth metatarsal fractures are of three types based on location: (1) base; (2) shaft and; (3) head and/or neck. Proximal fifth metatarsal fractures are further classified based on their location or zone. Zone 1 fractures occur at the tuberosity or styloid. Zone 2 or Jones fractures occur at the metaphyseal-diaphyseal junction. Zone 3 fractures occur at the diaphysis, but are typically stress fractures rather than acute injuries (Figs 30.6 and 30.7).

Hallucal joint injuries include fractures at the MTP or IP joints. First proximal phalangeal (PP) fractures are either intra-articular or extra-articular. Intra-articular fractures at the MTP joint are regarded as basal while those at the IP joint are considered condylar. Extra-articular PP fractures are regarded as shaft fractures. Most first distal phalangeal (DP) are known as tuft fractures (Figs 30.8A and B).

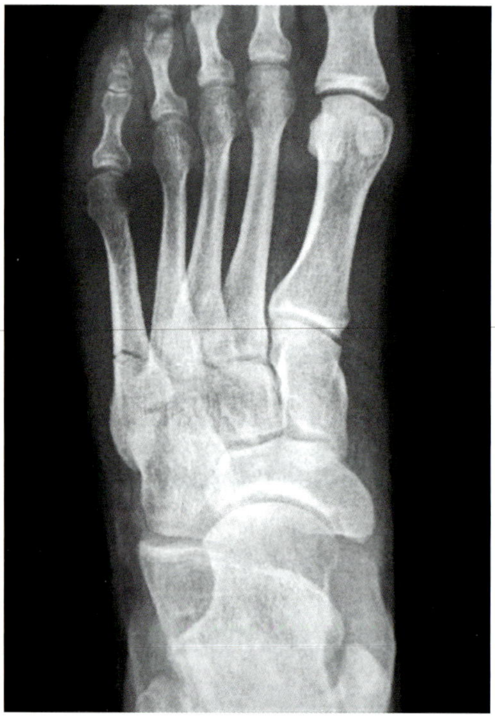

Figure 30.7: Nondisplaced zone 2 fifth metatarsal "Jones" fracture.

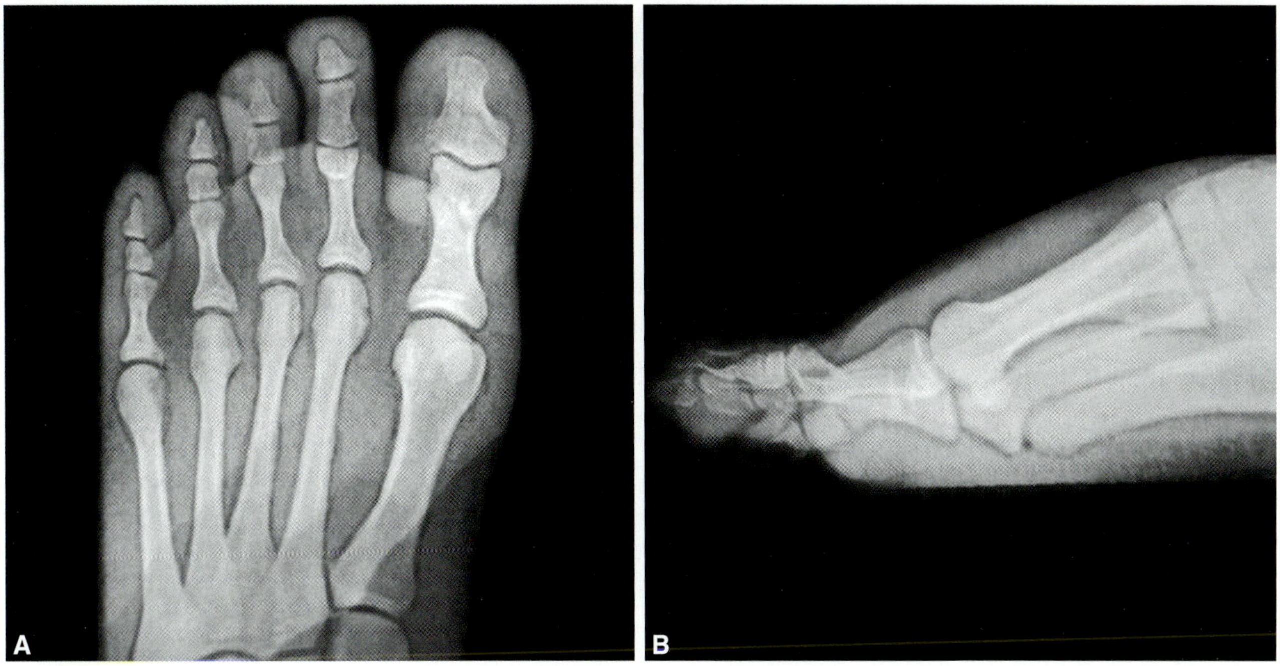

Figures 30.8A and B: An example of a displaced, angulated first proximal phalangeal (P1) fracture that accompanies a nondisplaced second proximal phalangeal fracture. Note the dorsal angulation of the hallux on the lateral radiograph.

Hallucal joint injuries also encompass first MTP and IP joint dislocations, the majority of which are dorsal. Jahss classifies dorsal first MTP joint dislocations based on the stability of the plantar plate-sesamoid complex.[12,13] In type I dislocations, the plantar plate and sesamoids remain intact. However, this results in plantar incarceration of the first metatarsal head. Attempts at closed reduction only further tighten the intact ligaments around the metatarsal head. Ultimately, these dislocations often require open reduction with an arthrotomy. In contrast, Type II and III dislocations present with injury to either the plantar plate or sesamoids. Type IIA and IIIA dislocations are those in which the plantar plate is partially and completely ruptured respectively. Most of these injuries are treated successfully with closed reduction. Type IIB dislocations are those in which one or both of the sesamoids are fractured and the plantar plate is partially torn. Type IIIB dislocations are those in which one or both of the sesamoids are fractured and the plantar plate is completely torn. If the distal pole of the sesamoid is incarcerated in the MTP joint, closed reduction is often unsuccessful. Ultimately, these types IIB and IIIB dislocations may require open reduction with an arthrotomy. Miki classifies dorsal first IP joint dislocations into two types based on the ability to realign the joint.[14] For the first IP joint to dislocate, the plantar plate must be completely ruptured in all cases. The difference between types I and II injuries is that the plantar plate is incarcerated in the joint in the former, but not in the latter. As a result, the IP joint can often be reduced closed in type II injuries, but not in type I dislocations.

Hallucal sesamoid fractures involve either the medial tibial or lateral fibular sesamoid. Acute injuries to both sesamoids are very rare. While no specific classification system exists for these fractures, author describes them based on location. Fractures occur in three types: (1) the proximal one-third or pole; (2) the middle third or waist and; (3) the distal one-third or pole.

Surgical Indications

While Lisfranc fracture-dislocations encompass a wide spectrum of presentations, most are routinely treated operatively. These injuries are often unstable with ligamentous injury and/or intra-articular fracture displacement and comminution. Since osteochondral fragments and soft tissue often become interposed at the TMT joints, closed treatment with casting is not sufficient to provide articular congruity. The only injury in which nonsurgical management is sufficient would be an isolated partial disruption or sprain of the Lisfranc ligament with neither arch collapse nor greater than 2 mm of diastasis between the medial cuneiform and the second metatarsal.

Surgical indications for extra-articular first-fifth metatarsal fractures are based on which and how many metatarsals are involved. As the first metatarsal is critical for gait, balance and weight-bearing, bony displacement is poorly tolerated. First metatarsal fractures that display any angulation, rotation, shortening, comminution, or greater than 2 mm of displacement are best treated with surgery. In contrast, a greater degree of malalignment can be tolerated in the lesser metatarsals. Lesser metatarsal fractures with more than 10° of angulation and rotation and 1 cm of shortening and displacement are appropriate for operative treatment. Patients with multiple metatarsal fractures should be given greater consideration for surgical management, as these tend to be high-energy injuries. Certain patients with nondisplaced zone 2 fifth metatarsal fractures could also be treated surgically.[15] These patients would be ones that engage in prolonged high-demand activities to their feet, such as athletes or manual laborers. The justification for this aggressive approach is that these proximal fifth metatarsal fractures are at higher risk for nonunion due to their location in a watershed area of bony blood supply.

Surgical indications for hallucal and sesamoid fractures and dislocations vary based on articular involvement. As the first MTP joint is critical for gait, balance and weight-bearing, displacement of the joint or the first PP is poorly tolerated. Intra-articular hallucal fractures with 2 mm or more of displacement are appropriate for surgical treatment. Extra-articular first PP fractures that display any angulation, rotation, shortening, comminution or greater than 5 mm of displacement are also best treated with surgery. Most first DP fractures involve the tuft and do well with nonsurgical treatment. Certainly, any hallucal dislocation that cannot be reduced closed warrants an open reduction. This is typically the case for all Type I dislocations of the MTP or IP joints. Acute sesamoid fractures that are appropriate for surgery are those that are displaced by 1 cm or more.

In general, midfoot and forefoot fractures and/or dislocations are indicated for operative management in the presence of bony displacement and/or joint incongruity that cannot be restored through closed means. It is important to understand that up to 1 cm of displacement can be endured at most extra-articular lesser metatarsal and toe injuries, but more than 2 mm of displacement is poorly tolerated at joints and at the first metatarsal. Other situations that warrant surgical treatment include open fractures, vascular injury and polytrauma patients. Surgical management techniques may be divided into three main categories: open reduction and internal fixation (ORIF), closed reduction and percutaneous pinning (CRPP) and joint fusion or arthrodesis.

Open Reduction and Internal Fixation

This method is employed most frequently in the surgical management of midfoot and forefoot fractures and/or dislocations. ORIF restores stability and anatomical relationships through rigid fixation. The inter-cuneiform and first-third TMT joints require partially threaded cancellous screws to restore stability, while the more mobile fourth-fifth TMT joints do well with Kirschner wire (K-wire) fixation. Single screw or wire fixation may be difficult in those Lisfranc injuries with severe bone loss or comminution. Such situations necessitate plate and screw fixation to restore foot length and alignment. Historically, extra-articular first-fourth metatarsal fractures were treated with single wires or screws due to their smaller size. Over the past 10 years, fracture fixation technology has improved to the point where there are mini-fragment plates and screws to provide an internal buttress and optimal stability to these injuries. The proximal fifth metatarsal is traditionally fixed with a partially threaded intramedullary cancellous screw. As an alternative, some surgeons use a tension-band wire construct with or without screws as treatment. Hallucal and sesamoid fractures are managed with mini-fragment screws. Newer technologies, such as smaller implants, have arguably improved fixation in cases where rigid fixation had been previously difficult to obtain.

Closed Reduction and Percutaneous Pinning

Closed reduction and percutaneous pinning (CRPP) is indicated as a temporary treatment in situations where definitive ORIF cannot be performed due to the condition of the soft-tissue, but acute skeletal stability is required.

An example would be a complete Lisfranc fracture-dislocation due to a crush injury. Patients with severe soft tissue injuries can benefit from temporary CRPP. This can restore skeletal length, allow access to the skin and soft tissues and prevent further injury from instability. Patients that require vascular repair and/or compartment release are also indications for temporary CRPP in order to protect the vascular repair and allow access for wound care.

Midfoot Fusion or Arthrodesis

It is important to recognize that certain Lisfranc injuries are better suited with a fusion or arthrodesis of the involved TMT joints rather than ORIF. Some fracture-dislocations may present with such severe bone loss and cartilage injury that the TMT joints cannot be restored to normalcy. Missed or neglected subacute and chronic Lisfranc injuries are another situation that can cause permanent TMT joint damage simply due to the time elapsed between injury and its recognition. Trevino et al. found that success rates of ORIF decrease when performed on injuries that were older than 6 weeks due to articular cartilage damage and ligament attenuation seen at the time of surgery.[16] Following their randomized and prospective study, Ly and Coetzee have recently argued that all acute ligamentous Type A (complete homolateral) and C2 (complete divergent) Lisfranc dislocations are best treated with a primary fusion rather than an attempt at ORIF.[17] However, this matter remains open to debate. The surgeon reserves midfoot fusion as primary treatment for Lisfranc injuries that present with severe joint injuries in which the cartilage cannot be restored and/or are over 6 weeks old. Akin to ORIF, the arthrodesis is limited to affected joints. The inter-cuneiform and first-third TMT joints can be fused with single screws or plate and screw constructs. Historically, the fourth-fifth TMT joints have also been fused if they are involved in these specific Lisfranc injuries. Over the past 15 years, concerns arose regarding potential detrimental effects on gait if the more mobile fourth-fifth TMT joints are fused. This led to the practice of an interposition arthroplasty, rather than an arthrodesis, of these joints with either local tendons or ceramic spacers.[18] If the surgeon needs to address the fourth-fifth TMT joints, they do so with a resection arthroplasty and interpose the extensor digitorum brevis (EDB) to maintain space.

Surgical Anatomy, Positioning and Approaches

Applied Anatomy

Understanding the anatomy of the midfoot and forefoot is critical to effective surgical treatment of its fractures and dislocations. The midfoot is organized in three columns: the first TMT joint is medial; the second and third TMT joints are central; and the fourth and fifth TMT joints are lateral. The medial and central columns act as a rigid lever that connects the hindfoot to the forefoot and provide shock absorption. In contrast, the lateral column exhibits more motion than the medial and central columns. The primary function of the lateral column is to provide accommodation to uneven ground. This has surgical implications as patients may tolerate decreased motion at the lateral column poorly. It is critical to realize that midfoot stability is provided by the unique joint anatomy and ligamentous restraints at the TMT joints. The first-fifth TMT joints are arranged in a Roman arch pattern, with the second TMT joint being recessed as the keystone of the complex. Dorsal, interosseous and plantar ligaments further support the joints. The forefoot is divided into five rays where each ray consists of the distal metatarsal and corresponding phalanx. As mentioned earlier, the distal inter-metatarsal ligaments, plantar plates, phalangeal collateral ligaments and flexor and extensor tendons provide stability at the forefoot.

There are important principles for surgical approaches to the midfoot and forefoot. Most fractures and/or dislocations are approached through the dorsum of the foot. The skin on the dorsum is thin and loose which facilitates retraction. In general, longitudinal skin incisions with full thickness flaps should be utilized for maximal exposure with minimal chances of skin necrosis. Prior to deep dissection, subcutaneous branches of the SPN must be identified and protected. Superficial veins are arranged in a dorsal arch and can be ligated as needed for bone and joint exposure. The extensor digitorum longus (EDL), EDB, extensor hallucis longus (EHL) and extensor hallucis brevis tendons rest just deeper to the nerves and veins. The only structure that remains at the dorsum of the foot between the extensor tendons and bones is the dorsalis pedis artery at the first proximal inter-metatarsal web space. Certainly, there are risks to the above neurovascular structures and tendons in dorsal surgical approaches to the foot. However, the main advantage in dorsal foot incisions is that there is less chance of injury to the majority of the foot's nerves, veins, arteries and tendons, which are at the plantar portion of the foot.

Certain midfoot and forefoot injuries are best exposed through surgical approaches on other areas of the foot. Isolated injuries to the first metatarsal and hallucal tibial sesamoid can be treated through a medial skin incision. Cutaneous branches of the SPN are at risk with this approach. Most fractures to the fifth metatarsal are exposed through a lateral skin incision. Cutaneous branches of the sural nerve are at risk with this approach. A plantar surgical incision is reserved for managing hallucal fibular sesamoid fractures. In addition to the risk of injuring branches of the interdigital nerve, care must be taken to avoid creating a painful scar at the weight-bearing area of the first ray.

Positioning

For most midfoot and forefoot injuries, supine positioning on a radiolucent table with a bump underneath the ipsilateral hip is recommended. This overcomes the limb's external rotation at rest and allows for simultaneous access to all midfoot columns and forefoot rays. The foot is placed at the edge of the bed such that unobstructed fluoroscopic images can be obtained easily. A pneumatic tourniquet inflated to 250 mm Hg is routinely used. In cases of isolated proximal fifth metatarsal fractures, lateral positioning with a beanbag is preferable.

Approaches

The surgical approach for ORIF of Lisfranc fracture-dislocations depends on the extent of the injury. The Lisfranc ligament, inter-cuneiform joints, and first-second TMT joints are exposed through a single longitudinal incision centered over the proximal first inter-metatarsal web space on the dorsum of the foot. The deep peroneal nerve and dorsalis pedis artery are at risk for injury with this incision. In fact, the dorsalis pedis artery travels from the dorsal to plantar foot in this area. The third-fifth TMT joints are exposed with another longitudinal incision centered over the dorsal fourth TMT joint. Single tendons from the EDL and branches of the SPN are at risk with both of these incisions. The length of these incisions should be generous and are at a minimum length of 7 cm to achieve adequate midfoot exposure. One should be aware of how proximal the midfoot is to the anterior skin crease of the ankle such that incisions are not started too distal. The strength of this approach is that it provides such a wide exposure of the Lisfranc ligament and all five TMT joints. However, the problem with these multiple incisions is a risk of poor wound healing, if the bridge of skin separating them is less than 7 cm (Fig. 30.9).

This surgical approach can change for those Lisfranc injuries that have irreparable cartilage damage that require arthrodesis as treatment. Such situations include acute high-energy injuries or when treatment is delayed longer than 6 weeks. If patients have chronic Lisfranc ligament instability or first-second TMT arthritis, the same longitudinal incision centered over the proximal first intermetatarsal web space can still be used. If patients have first-fifth TMT arthritis, the fusion is performed through three incisions. The first TMT joint is exposed through a longitudinal medial incision centered at the joint. Care is taken to avoid injuring the tibialis anterior and peroneus longus tendons at the dorsal and plantar joint,

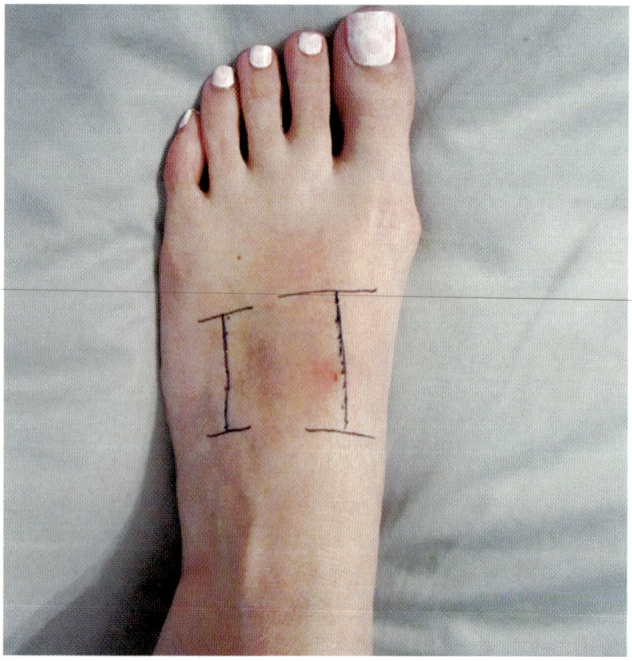

Figure 30.9: Standard dual-incision approach marked out for open reduction and internal fixation of Lisfranc injuries.

respectively. The second-third TMT joints are exposed through a longitudinal incision centered at the proximal second intermetatarsal web space. The fourth-fifth TMT joints are exposed through a longitudinal incision centered at the proximal fourth intermetatarsal web space. Since both the peroneus tertius and EDB tendons lie just superficial to the TMT joints, either one can be used to provide substance for an interpositional arthroplasty. The benefit of this approach is that it provides such a wide exposure of the five TMT joints. However, the problem with these multiple incisions is a risk of injury to tendons from the EDL and branches of the SPN. There is also a risk of poor wound healing if the bridge of skin separating them is less than 7 cm.

The surgical treatment of extra-articular metatarsal fractures also depends on the extent of the injury. The first metatarsal is exposed through a longitudinal medial incision just distal to the first TMT joint (Fig. 30.10).

The second-fourth metatarsals are visualized through a dorsal longitudinal incision distal to the TMT joints. The specific location of the incision depends on which of these are fractured. Single fractures require an incision centered directly over it. Two fractures would necessitate the incision to be at the involved inter-metatarsal web space. If the second-fourth metatarsals are all fractured, the incision should be over the third metatarsal shaft to allow wide access to all three bones. Both the proximal aspect and shaft of the fifth metatarsal can be exposed through a longitudinal incision at the lateral aspect of the bone. Branches of the sural nerve lie within the skin in this area. It is important to recognize that the peroneus brevis inserts at the base. Pros of this approach are that it provides a wide exposure of all five metatarsals with a sufficient skin bridge between incisions. However, the con with these incisions is a risk of injury to tendons from the EDL and branches of the sural nerve and SPN (Fig. 30.11).

The surgical approach to hallucal MTP and IP injuries is through dorsal incisions. The MTP joint is exposed through a longitudinal incision centered at the joint and medial to the EHL. The IP joint is approached through a "stair-case" shaped incision. The horizontal limb of the incision is centered at the IP joint. The medial and lateral ends of this incision are then extended distally proximally respectively with a longitudinal incision. Joint capsulotomies are performed through longitudinal incisions. The strengths of these incisions are that they minimize neurovascular injury and are most suited for treating dorsal dislocations of both joints. The main faults of these incisions are injury to the nail bed, EHL and branches of the SPN if carried too distal and with minimal care (Fig. 30.12).

The surgical approach to treating hallucal sesamoid fractures are through two separate incisions. The medial or tibial sesamoid is exposed with a longitudinal medial incision centered at the first metatarsal head, but placed at its inferior

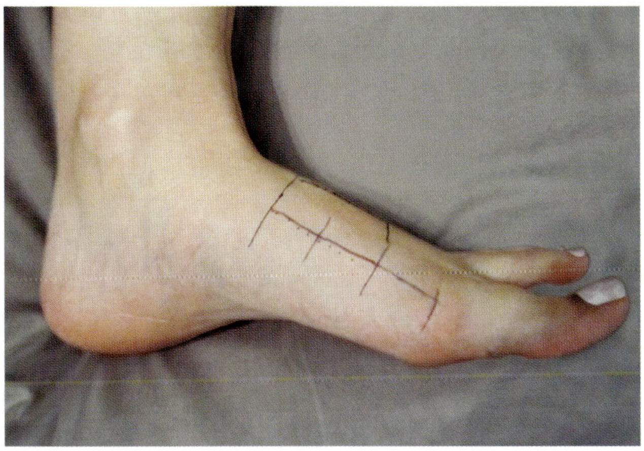

Figure 30.10: Standard incision marked out for open reduction and internal fixation of the first metatarsal.

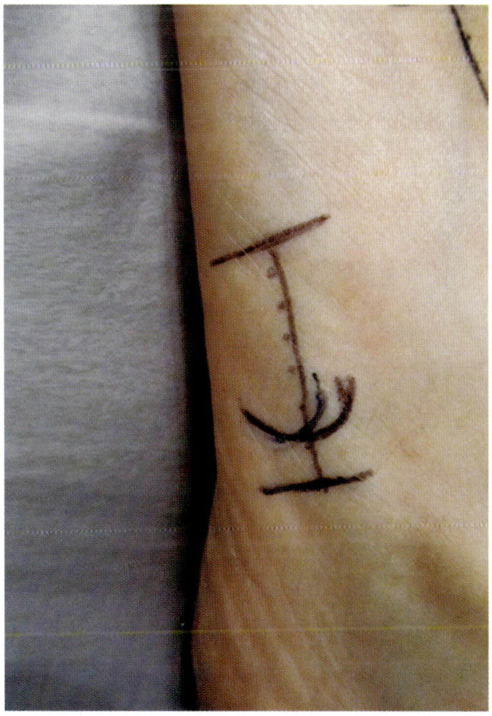

Figure 30.11: Standard incision marked out for open reduction and internal fixation of the proximal fifth metatarsal.

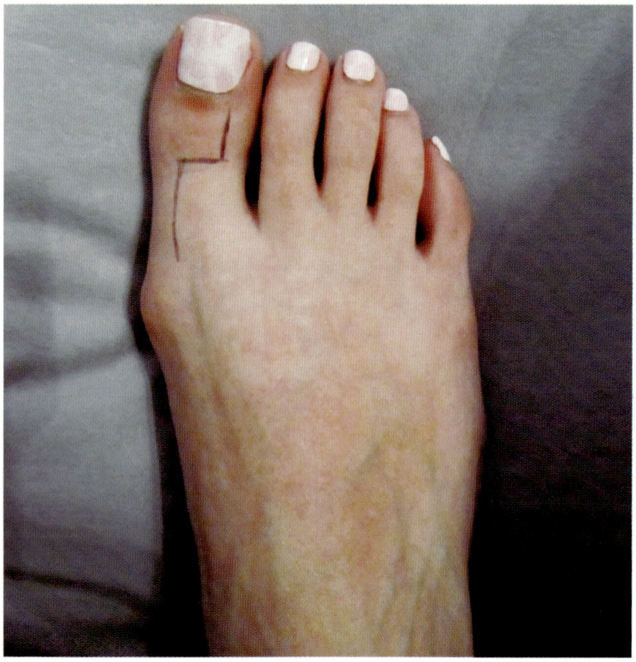

Figure 30.12: Standard incision marked out for open reduction and internal fixation of the first joint.

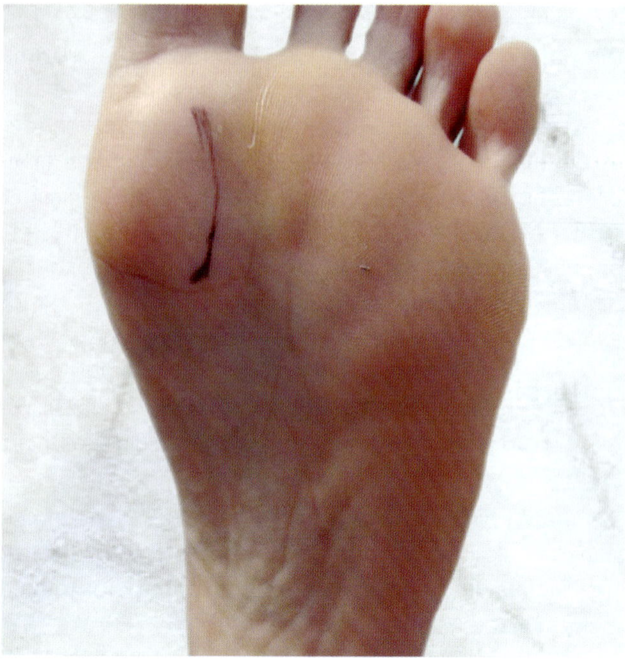

Figure 30.13: Standard incision marked out for open reduction and internal fixation of the fibular sesamoid.

aspect. The lateral or fibular sesamoid is visualized through a longitudinal curvilinear incision at the distal first intermetatarsal web space. While a dorsal incision may be adequate to expose this fibular sesamoid, a plantar incision is more useful for both visualization and treatment of fractures. Once the sesamoid is exposed, the inter-digital nerve should be exposed and retracted from the field. It is important to avoid placing the incision directly over the sesamoid and creating a scar that would be painful to walk on. The strength of these approaches is that they provide ideal exposure. However, the weakness of these incisions is the risk of digital nerve injury (Fig. 30.13).

SURGICAL TECHNIQUES

Technique 1: Open Reduction and Internal Fixation of Lisfranc Fracture-dislocations

Preoperative Planning

Anatomical Considerations

The naviculo-cuneiform, cuboid-cuneiform, inter-cuneiform and first-fifth TMT joints are arranged in a Roman arch pattern with a dorsal apex. Dorsal surgical approaches to the midfoot are ideal as they provide a wide exposure of bony and joint anatomy. Dorsal incisions involve minimal risk of injury to tendons and neurovascular structures as the plantar foot contains much more of these. However, it is important to realize that since the dorsal foot has less soft tissue coverage, implants placed through this area should not be left prominent. Palpable foot hardware may certainly cause discomfort after the injury has healed. Preoperative planning should include knowledge of the extent of the injury with radiographs and CT scans. In some instances, contralateral and comparative foot radiographs can be useful to visualize patients' normal foot anatomy.

Instrumentation and Implant Considerations

Once preoperative planning is complete, the surgeon should be sure that all appropriate instrumentation and implants are readily available. Instrumentation required for ORIF includes fracture reduction tools like medium-sized pointed tenaculums and a pneumatic or battery-powered driver and drill. A radiolucent table and fluoroscopic C-arm is needed for intraoperative imaging. If a large, rather than a portable mini, fluoroscope is used, then the surgeon may consider using a sterile "triangle" knee positioner to assist with foot placement. Using such a device would allow for the foot to rest flat on the operative table and obtain ideal AP images. Common implants used for ORIF include 0.062-inch K-wires for the fourth-fifth TMT joints and 4.0 mm partially threaded cannulated cancellous screws for the inter-cuneiform and first-third TMT joints. The advantage of using these types of screws is that they are placed over guide wires. Using such thin wires allows for provisional midfoot fixation without causing too much bony injury if initial wire placement is not ideal. When certain fracture-dislocations are difficult to realign, 2.5 mm Schanz half pins may be needed to assist in reduction maneuvers. Such pins can be drilled into the metatarsal shafts and used as "joysticks" to manipulate the proximal metatarsals into acceptable alignment.

In the event of injuries with severe bone and joint comminution, screw and/or wire fixation may be inadequate for treatment. Such situations may require plate and screw fixation to restore foot length and alignment. Medial small-fragment T-plates can be used to bridge the naviculo-medial cuneiform and first TMT joints with 3.5 mm screw fixation in the navicular and first metatarsal shaft. Dorsal 2.0 or 2.4 mm mini-fragment plates can be utilized to span the remaining naviculo-cuneiform and second-third TMT joints. These implants can also be used at the fourth-fifth TMT joints. Within the past 2 years, particular locking plates designed for specific use in the midfoot have been made available. Such implants include the Modular Foot Set (Synthes, Paoli, PA, USA) and the ALPS (Depuy, Warsaw, IN, USA). These plates come in a wide variety of widths, lengths and shapes. These implants provide a theoretical advantage of contoured designs and locking plate technology which itself can improve fixation in comminuted bone. While these materials hold promise, their use requires further study and supporting literature.

Patient Considerations

Finally, systemic and local patient factors should be assessed before performing ORIF. Patients that are not medically optimized may do poorly with the additional stress of anesthesia and midfoot surgery. Such conditions include those with hemodynamic instability, uncontrolled sepsis and multisystem organ failure. The condition of the foot's soft tissue should also be considered before performing ORIF. Local infection and skin blisters are a contraindication to ORIF. Rather, these conditions should be resolved by the time of surgery. Foot swelling should be optimized before surgery as incisions through a swollen foot have a higher risk of surgical wound complications such as compartment syndrome, dehiscence and infection. Therefore, it may be necessary to delay ORIF for 14 days or longer if takes that long for the foot's soft tissue to improve. In the presence of gross midfoot instability and severe swelling, patients are best treated in a staged manner. CRPP under anesthesia should be undertaken acutely to restore overt dislocations. Once the patient's soft tissue is optimized, the second stage of surgery would be the ORIF for definitive treatment.

Technique

The patient is placed supine on the radiolucent operating table. The patient is given a general or spinal anesthetic. The use of an indwelling epidural catheter for postoperative pain management is not recommended as this may impair a reliable postoperative neurologic and compartment examination. Intravenous antibiotics for skin flora bacterial prophylaxis should be given within one hour of skin incision. A tourniquet is placed at the calf and inflated to 250 mmHg. A rolled sheet, blanket, or bump is placed under the ipsilateral buttock to overcome the external rotation of the hip. As the foot is scrubbed and draped in sterile fashion, anti-thrombotic stockings and venodyne boots are placed on the contralateral leg.

While there are a wide variety of Lisfranc injuries, all surgical treatment starts with an incision over the proximal first inter-metatarsal web space to expose the Lisfranc ligament, inter-cuneiform joints and first-second TMT joints. During the superficial dissection, branches of the SPN are identified and protected. As the exposure deepens, the EDL is retracted laterally and the dorsalis pedis artery is protected medially. Once the inter-cuneiform and first-second TMT joints are exposed, they should be debrided free of hematoma, fibrous tissue and bony fragments. At this point, the Lisfranc ligament should be in clear view. A rongeur or curette is then used to debride or freshen both ends of the ligament. All fracture fragments are examined and debrided, leaving their soft tissue attachments intact when possible. This is particularly important if the Lisfranc ligament is injured as a bony avulsion from the base of the second metatarsal rather than as a mid-substance ligament injury. Upon identification of all fractures and dislocations that are visible through this incision, realignment can be performed in different orders depending upon the extent of injury. The surgeon starts by addressing any medial or intermediate cuneiform fractures. Most of these are horizontal, intra-articular and dorsally displaced. A tenaculum is used to compress these fractures, as a single 4.0 mm cannulated screw is placed from dorsal to plantar for each bone. The surgeon continues by compressing the base of the second metatarsal to the medial cuneiform with a tenaculum. Once this space is decreased, a guidepin is drilled retrograde from the lateral base of the second metatarsal to the medial cuneiform. The pin is advanced until it no longer protrudes laterally from the second metatarsal. AP and lateral fluoroscopic images are carefully inspected to ensure that this wire is neither too plantar nor too dorsal. Once proper wire placement is confirmed, a 4.0 mm screw is inserted over the guide wire antegrade from the medial cuneiform to the proximal second metatarsal. The surgeon proceeds by assessing the inter-cuneiform joints for persistent instability. If there is residual widening, a tenaculum is used to compress these joints and fixation is provided with a single percutaneous 4.0 mm screw from medial to lateral. The next joints that are assessed through this incision are the first and second TMT joints. If there is residual instability at either, the joint(s) are compressed with tenaculums and held reduced with guidepins drilled retrograde. These pins are angled as horizontal and parallel as possible to the metatarsal so as to increase screw length, leverage and strength. Lateral and AP fluoroscopic images are carefully inspected to ensure that the wires are not too plantar, dorsal or long. Additional images can be taken with the foot dorsiflexed to 30° for a true AP of the midfoot. Once proper wire placement is confirmed, the base of the metatarsal at the wire is notched with a countersink to ensure screw heads are not palpable. The 4.0 mm screws are then inserted retrograde over the guide wires to cross the first and/or second TMT joint(s). Once the more medial TMT joints are addressed in the above manner, the third-fifth TMT joints can be inspected fluoroscopically. If any of these joints are involved and reduce spontaneously, they can be treated percutaneously. The third TMT joint is held reduced with a retrograde guidepin, followed by a 4.0 mm screw. The fourth-fifth TMT joints are stabilized with a retrograde 0.062-inch K-wire each.

If the third-fifth TMT joints are injured and do not reduce spontaneously, they require an additional dorsal incision for proper treatment. This second incision is centered over the fourth TMT joint. During the superficial dissection, branches of the SPN are identified and protected. As the exposure deepens, the EDL is retracted medially. Once the third-fifth TMT joints are exposed, they should be debrided free of hematoma, fibrous tissue and bony fragments. All fracture fragments are examined and debrided, leaving their soft tissue attachments intact when possible. The surgeon begins treatment of the more lateral part of the midfoot with the third TMT joint. This joint is compressed with a tenaculum and held reduced with a retrograde guidepin that is angled as horizontal and parallel as possible to the third metatarsal. Once fluoroscopic images confirm proper wire placement, the base of the metatarsal at the wire is notched with a countersink to ensure the screw head is not palpable. A single 4.0 mm screw is then inserted retrograde over the guide wire to cross the third TMT joint. Finally, the fourth-fifth TMT joints are reduced and stabilized to the cuboid with a retrograde 0.062-inch K-wire each.

After fixation is provided, fluoroscopic images are performed in multiple planes to assess for acceptable bone and joint reduction and hardware placement. Midfoot stability should be confirmed clinically and radiographically. Screws and wires should be checked to make sure that they are not too dorsal, plantar or lengthy (Figs 30.14A to C and 30.15A to D).

Closure

Once normal bone and joint alignment has been restored with proper hardware placement, wound closure can begin. The tourniquet is deflated at this point to revascularize the foot and assess for bleeding vessels. Hemostasis is achieved through an electrocautery to minimize postoperative hematoma formation. Wounds are irrigated copiously with normal saline through a bulb syringe. The subcutaneous tissue is closed as a single layer with interrupted 2-0 vicryl sutures. The skin is closed as a single layer with interrupted 2-0 nylon sutures. The wounds are injected with an appropriate amount of 0.5% bupivacaine without epinephrine to provide adjuvant local

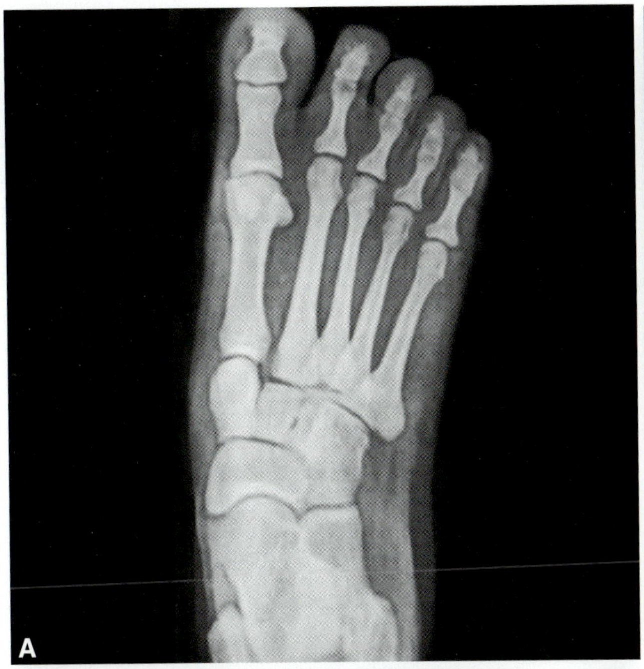

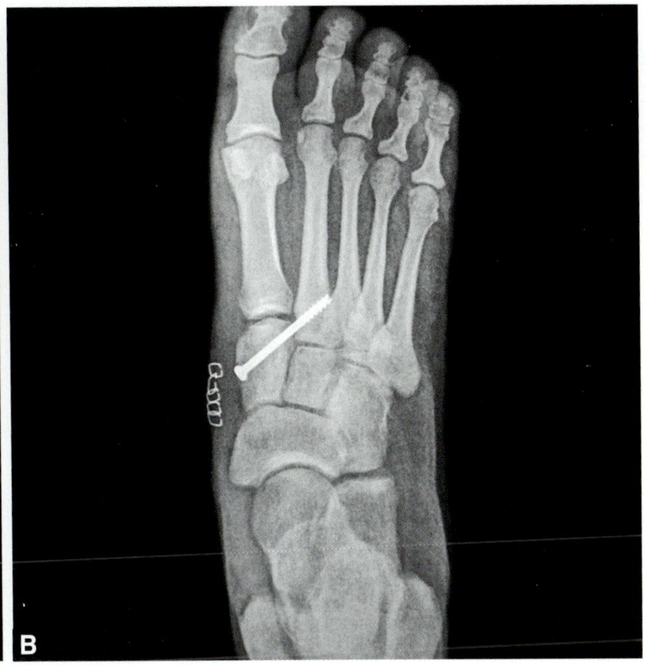

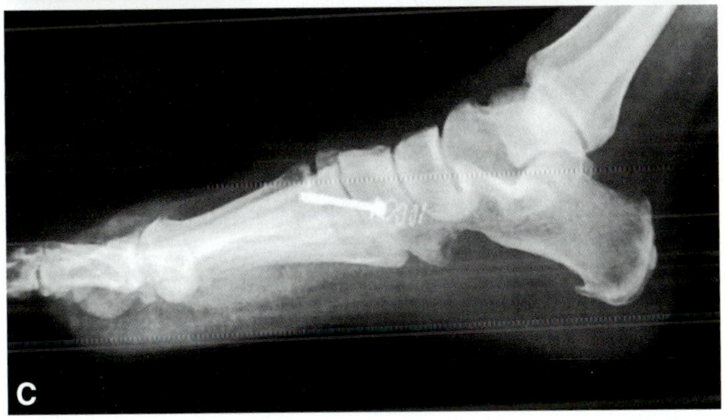

Figures 30.14A to C: Preoperative and postoperative radiographs of open reduction and internal fixation of a Lisfranc injury that only involved the Lisfranc ligament. Note the lateral radiograph confirms the screw is neither too plantar nor too dorsal.

anesthesia. Distal pulses are checked before applying the postoperative dressings. The wounds are dressed with a sterile layer of non-adherent xeroform dressing, gauze and webril cast padding. The foot is then placed in a well-padded short-leg non-weight-bearing splint. For the more severe injuries, patients are kept overnight to monitor for pain and symptoms of compartment syndrome.

Rehabilitation

Patients are followed monthly until full recovery is achieved. Immediately following surgery, they are rendered non-weight-bearing following surgery in their postoperative splint. Hip and knee range of motion (ROM) exercises are encouraged. At 2 weeks from surgery, the splint is removed and patients are fitted for a controlled ankle motion (CAM) fracture boot. The boot can be removed only for showering and sleeping. Sutures are removed at 2–4 weeks from surgery depending on how swollen the foot is. Patients are kept non-weight-bearing in the boot until six weeks from surgery once radiographs maintain normal joint alignment and show initial fracture healing. If patients have percutaneous K-wires through the fourth and/or fifth TMT joints, these wires are removed at 6 weeks from surgery, if the joints remain stable. Progressive to full weight-bearing in the boot is then allowed after 6 weeks from surgery. At this point, the boot can also be removed for regular ankle ROM exercises. The boot is used until full bony and ligamentous healing is reached, which is typically at 3–4 months from surgery. Upon full healing, patients

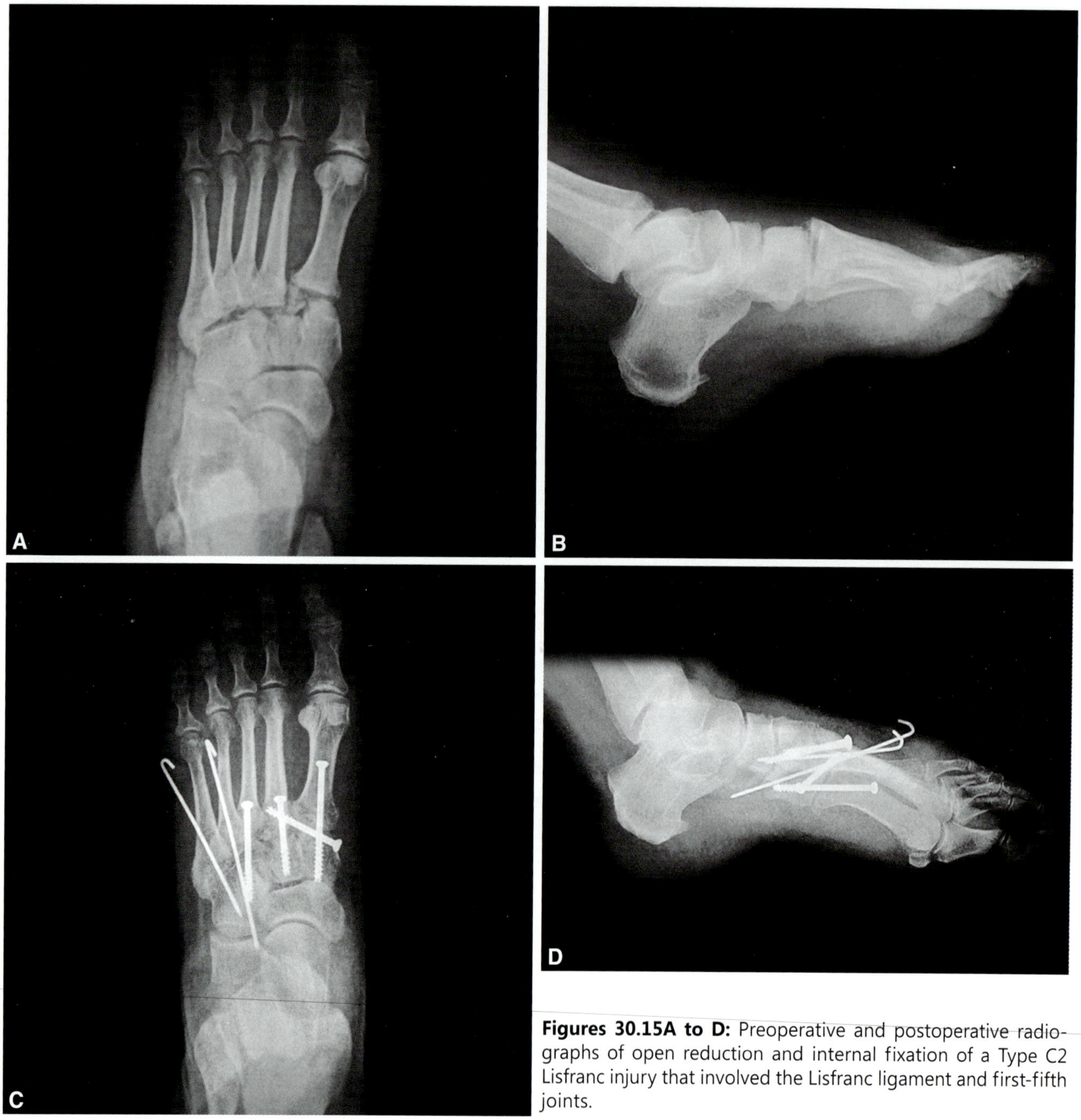

Figures 30.15A to D: Preoperative and postoperative radiographs of open reduction and internal fixation of a Type C2 Lisfranc injury that involved the Lisfranc ligament and first-fifth joints.

are allowed to start wearing normal shoes and a return to most activities of daily life. Patients are routinely fitted for custom molded orthotics to maintain midfoot stability and provide additional arch support. Physical therapy is prescribed on an individual basis if patients exhibit any residual stiffness, weakness, or gait dysfunction. A return to high-impact activities is postponed until 6–9 months from surgery when midfoot screw removal can be considered. The surgeon routinely removes screws at this point to avoid breakage and potential cartilage injury with prolonged intra-articular hardware placement.

ORIF OF LISFRANC FRACTURE-DISLOCATIONS:
Pearls and Pitfalls

- Be generous with the length of incisions. The incisions may have to be at a minimal length of 7 cm to adequately expose the TMT joints
- While there are a wide variety of Lisfranc injuries, all of their components should be addressed in sequence
- Order of fixation from first to last should be the cuneiform fractures, Lisfranc ligament, inter-cuneiform joints, second TMT joint, first TMT joint, third TMT joint, fourth TMT joint and the fifth TMT joint
- Ensure that joints are properly reduced at the time of guide wire placement. Wires crossing the TMT joints should be as horizontal and parallel as possible. Be generous with fluoroscopic images once guide wires are in place. Care should be taken to ensure that the wires are not too dorsal, plantar, or long before screws are placed over them

Technique 2: Midfoot Arthrodesis for Lisfranc Fracture-dislocations with Irreparable Joint Damage

Preoperative Planning

Patient Considerations

It is important to recognize that certain Lisfranc injuries are better suited with a fusion or arthrodesis of the involved TMT joints, rather than ORIF, as primary treatment. Some fracture-dislocations may present with such severe bone loss and cartilage injury that the TMT joints cannot be restored to normalcy. Missed or neglected Lisfranc injuries that are older than 6 weeks are another situation that can cause permanent TMT joint damage simply due to the time elapsed between injury and its recognition. Akin to ORIF, the arthrodesis is limited to affected joints. The inter-cuneiform and first-third TMT joints can be fused with single screws. In the presence of bone loss or osteopenia, these joints can be fused with plate and screw constructs as an alternative. In order to preserve some motion at the midfoot, the fourth-fifth TMT joints are addressed with a resection arthroplasty and interposition of the EDB to maintain space.

Akin to ORIF, systemic and local patient factors should be assessed before performing ORIF. Patients that are not medically optimized may do poorly with the additional stress of anesthesia and a midfoot fusion. The condition of the foot's soft tissue should also be considered before performing an arthrodesis. Local infection and skin blisters are a contraindication to surgery. Foot swelling should be optimized before surgery to minimize the risk of surgical complications such as compartment syndrome, wound dehiscence and wound infection. In the presence of acute irreparable cartilage damage, gross midfoot instability and severe swelling, patients are best treated in a staged manner. CRPP under anesthesia should be undertaken acutely to restore overt dislocations. Once the patient's soft tissue is optimized, the second stage of surgery would be the arthrodesis for definitive treatment.

Anatomical Considerations

Dorsal surgical approaches to the midfoot can still be used to perform a fusion as they provide a wide exposure of bony and joint anatomy. An alternative exposure to the first TMT joint is a medial approach to the joint. Care should be taken to avoid injury to the tibialis anterior and peroneus longus tendons as they insert at the proximal first metatarsal. Preoperative planning should include knowledge of the extent of the joint damage and deformity with radiographs, CT scans and possibly MRI imaging. In some instances, contralateral and comparative foot radiographs can be useful to visualize patients' normal foot anatomy.

Instrumentation and Implant Considerations

Once preoperative planning is complete, the surgeon should be sure that all appropriate instrumentation and implants are readily available. Instrumentation required for arthrodesis includes a micro oscillating sagittal saw, osteotomes, mallets, rongeurs, curettes, fracture reduction tools like medium-sized pointed tenaculums and a pneumatic or battery-powered driver and drill. A radiolucent table and fluoroscopic C-arm is needed for intraoperative imaging. Common implants used for arthrodesis of the inter-cuneiform and first-third TMT joints include 4.0 mm partially threaded cannulated cancellous screws. However, screw fixation may be inadequate for situations where osteopenia, bone loss and/or severe (planovalgus) deformity are present. Such conditions may require plate and screw fixation to restore foot length, alignment and stability. Small-fragment T-plates placed medially can be used to fuse the naviculocuneiform and first TMT joints. Dorsal 2.0 mm or 2.4 mm mini-fragment plates can be utilized to fuse the remaining naviculocuneiform and second-third TMT joints. Implants used to perform a resection arthroplasty of the fourth-fifth TMT joints are 0.062-inch K-wires. Over the past 2–3 years, pre-contoured locking plates and spacers specifically designed for use at the first-third and fourth-fifth TMT joints respectively have become commercially available. However, their use requires further study.

Technique

The patient is placed supine on the radiolucent operating table. The patient is given a general or spinal anesthetic. Intravenous antibiotics for skin flora bacterial prophylaxis should be given within one hour of skin incision. A tourniquet is placed at the calf and inflated to 250 mm Hg. A bump is placed under the ipsilateral buttock to overcome the external rotation of the hip. As the foot is scrubbed and draped in sterile fashion, anti-thrombotic stockings and venodyne boots are placed on the contralateral leg.

Lisfranc injuries with irreparable joint damage can present with much variety. One of the more common conditions is a missed or neglected injury to the Lisfranc ligament. This commonly presents with damage and/or instability to the inter-cuneiform and second TMT joints with widening of the space between the base of the second metatarsal and medial cuneiform. Akin to ORIF, the required surgical incision is still over the proximal first inter-metatarsal web space. Branches of the SPN are identified during the superficial dissection. As the exposure deepens, the EDL is retracted laterally and the dorsalis pedis artery is protected medially. Once the inter-cuneiform and second TMT joints are exposed, they should be debrided free of fibrous tissue and bony fragments. The Lisfranc ligament may not be visualized due to chronic attenuation. A micro-oscillating sagittal saw is used to remove the diseased cartilage at these joints and expose subchondral bone. Typically, the layer of bone removed is 2–4 mm thick. Care is taken to remove more bone from the plantar than the dorsal base of the second metatarsal, which allows for preservation of the foot's arch shape. A rongeur or curette is then used to further debride or freshen both ends of exposed cancellous bone. Restoration of midfoot stability can be performed in different orders, but author starts by compressing the base of the second metatarsal to the medial cuneiform with a tenaculum. Once this space is decreased, a guide pin is placed across it. So long as radiographs confirm appropriate wire placement that is neither too dorsal nor plantar, a 4.0 mm screw is placed over the wire. The next step is to compress the medial to intermediate cuneiform with a tenaculum to provide further stability. Fixation is then provided with a single percutaneous 4.0 mm screw from medial to lateral. Finally, the second TMT joint is compressed manually and held reduced with a retrograde guide pin. As with ORIF, the pin is placed as horizontal and parallel as possible to the metatarsal. Once proper wire placement is confirmed under fluoroscopy, the base of the metatarsal at the wire is notched with a countersink and a 4.0 mm screws is inserted over the wire to cross the second TMT joint (Figs 30.16A and B).

A two-incision approach is utilized if irreparable cartilage damage involves the first-third TMT joints. The first TMT joint is exposed through a medial incision centered at the joint. Branches of the SPN are identified and retracted from the field. The tibialis anterior and peroneus longus tendons are protected dorsally and plantarly respectively. Once the first TMT joint is exposed, it should be debrided free of fibrous tissue and bony fragments. A sagittal saw is used to remove the diseased cartilage at these joints and expose subchondral bone. Care is taken to remove a thicker layer of cartilage from the lateral medial cuneiform and plantar first metatarsal. This allows for deformity correction of the first ray if necessary. Once flat surfaces for bony apposition are prepared, the joint is held fixed with two crossing guide pins. While both are placed from dorsal to plantar, one is placed from distal to proximal and the other is placed from proximal to distal. If wire placement is acceptable, two 4.0 mm screws are placed over these wires and countersunk. The second-third TMT joints are exposed through a dorsal incision at the second proximal intermetatarsal web space. The EDL and branches of the SPN are identified and protected. Akin to the first TMT joint, fibrous tissue and bony fragments should be removed from the second-third TMT joints upon exposure. Layers of articular cartilage are then removed, with more bone removed from the plantar than the dorsal bases of the second-third metatarsals. This allows for preservation

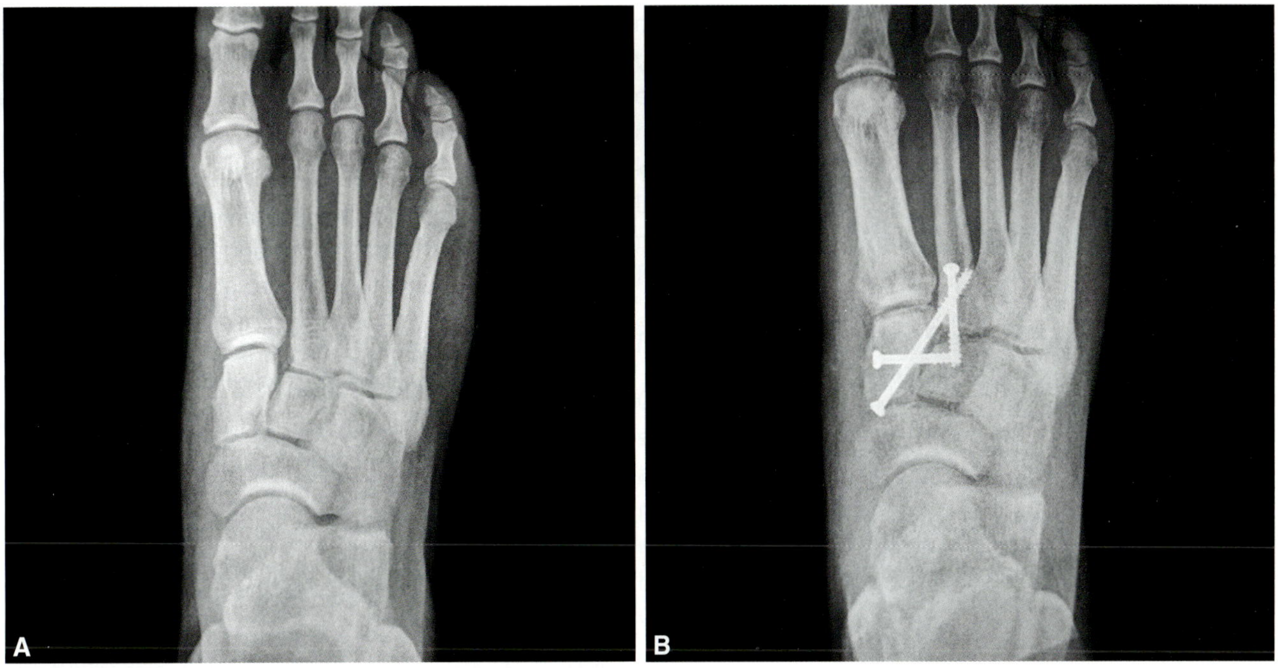

Figures 30.16A and B: (A) Neglected injury to the Lisfranc ligament. This particular patient's injury was three months old at the time of presentation. Patient was not a candidate for open reduction and internal fixation due to the time elapsed; (B) Arthrodesis involved fusion of the space between the second metatarsal and medial cuneiform, and the inter-cuneiform and second tarsometatarsal joints.

of the foot's arch shape. A rongeur or curette is then used to further debride or freshen both ends of exposed cancellous bone. Once the second-third TMT joints can be manually compressed, guide pins are placed across them. So long as radiographs confirm appropriate wire placement, a 4.0 mm screw is placed over each wire and countersunk to achieve fusion of both joints (Fig. 30.17).

If the fourth-fifth TMT joints have irreparable cartilage, they should be addressed after first-third TMT fusion. These lateral joints are exposed through an additional incision centered over the fourth proximal inter-metatarsal web space. During the superficial dissection, branches of the SPN are identified and protected. As the exposure deepens, the EDL is retracted medially. Once the fourth-fifth TMT joints are exposed, they should be debrided free of fibrous tissue and bony fragments. Layers of articular cartilage are resected with a sagittal saw. The EDB is identified, ligated proximally and placed into both joints. With the EDB acting as an interpositional material, the fourth-fifth TMT joints are reduced and stabilized to the cuboid with a retrograde 0.062-inch K-wire each (Fig. 30.18).

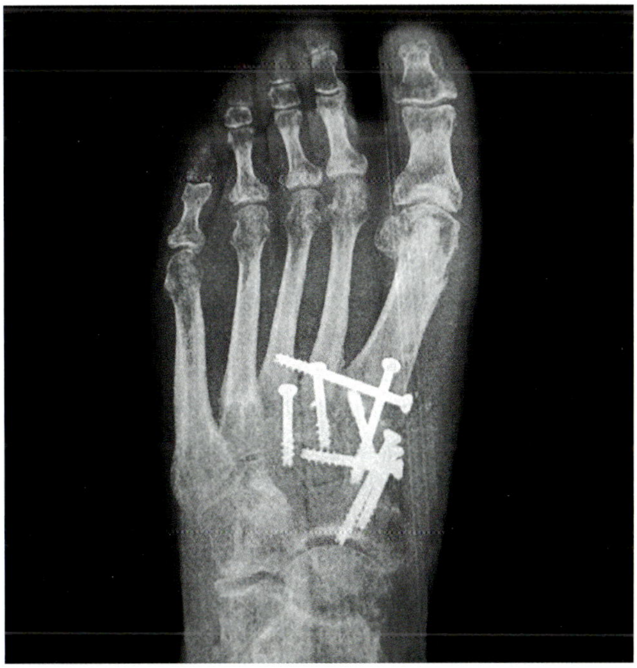

Figure 30.17: An example of a first-third tarsometatarsal and naviculocuneiform fusion.

such as compartment syndrome, dehiscence and infection. Therefore, it may be necessary to delay ORIF for 14 days or longer if takes that long for the foot's soft tissue to improve.

Technique

The patient is placed supine on the radiolucent operating table. The patient is given a general or spinal anesthetic. The use of an indwelling epidural catheter for post-operative pain management is not recommended as this may impair a reliable postoperative neurologic and compartment examination. Intravenous antibiotics for skin flora bacterial prophylaxis should be given within one hour of skin incision. A tourniquet is placed at the calf and inflated to 250 mm Hg. A rolled sheet or bump is placed under the ipsilateral buttock to overcome the external rotation of the hip. As the foot is scrubbed and draped in sterile fashion, anti-thrombotic stockings and venodyne boots are placed on the contralateral leg.

When there are multiple metatarsal fractures, the first metatarsal is treated first. The first metatarsal is exposed through a medial incision centered along the palpable bone. Branches of the SPN are identified and retracted from the field. The tibialis anterior and peroneus longus tendons are protected dorsally and plantarly respectively. Once the fracture is exposed, it should be debrided free of hematoma, fibrous tissue and bony fragments. A rongeur or curette is then used to debride or freshen both ends of the fracture. All fracture fragments are examined and debrided, leaving their soft tissue attachments intact when possible. Once the fracture is prepared and properly realigned, the plate is applied to the medial bone. The plate is placed in such a way to allow for at least two screws proximal and two screws distal to the fracture site. Anteroposterior and lateral fluoroscopic images are carefully inspected to ensure proper bone alignment and hardware placement.

Once the first metatarsal is stabilized in the above manner, the second-fourth metatarsals can be addressed through a separate dorsal incision. Specific wound placement depends on how many of these bones are fractured. A single metatarsal fracture requires the incision to be placed over it. When two of the bones are fractured, the incision should be at the corresponding inter-metatarsal web space. If all the second-fourth metatarsals are injured, the incision should be placed over the third metatarsal shaft to allow for a wide exposure. During the superficial dissection, branches of the SPN are identified and protected. As the exposure deepens, the EDL is retracted medially. Once the metatarsals are exposed, they should be debrided free of hematoma, fibrous tissue and bony fragments. All fracture fragments are examined and debrided, leaving their soft tissue attachments intact when possible. Once the fractures are prepared and properly aligned, the plates are applied to the dorsal bones. Longitudinal plates are used for mid-shaft injuries, while T-plates are used for base or neck fractures. The plate is placed in such a way to allow for at least two screws proximal and two screws distal to the fracture site. Anteroposterior and lateral fluoroscopic images are carefully inspected to ensure proper bone alignment and hardware placement (Figs 30.19 and 30.20).

After fixation is provided, fluoroscopic images are performed in multiple planes to assess for acceptable bone reduction and hardware placement. Bony stability should be confirmed clinically and radiographically. Screws and plates should be checked to make sure that they are

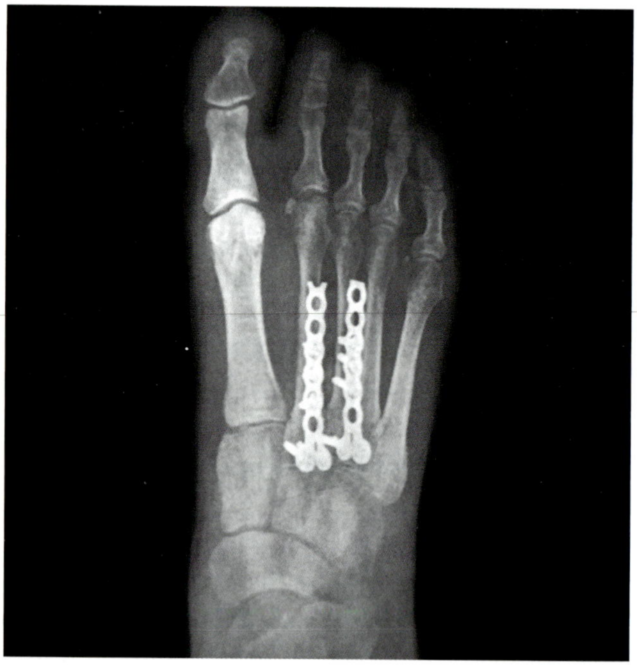

Figure 30.19: Anteroposterior radiograph demonstrating open reduction and internal fixation (ORIF) of an extra-articular metatarsal base fractures with dorsal plating.

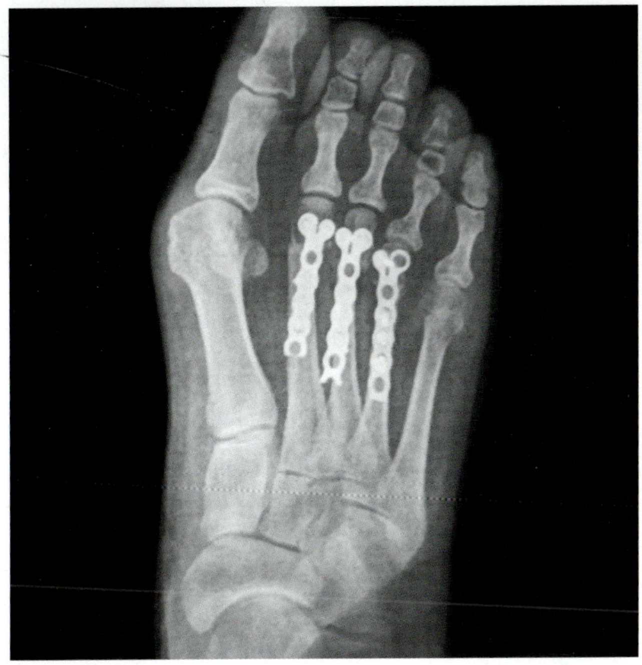

Figure 30.20: Anteroposterior radiograph demonstrating open reduction and internal fixation of an extra-articular metatarsal neck fractures with dorsal plating.

not too long. In particular, plates should not cross the TMT or MTP joints. Foci of bone loss at the fracture sites can receive bone grafting at the surgeon's discretion. When the surgeon encounters some degree of bone loss following fracture debridement, they fill these areas with Vitoss (Orthovita, Malvern, PA, USA), which is a synthetic, osteoconductive bone allograft.

Closure

Once normal bone and joint alignment has been restored with proper hardware placement, wound closure can begin. The tourniquet is deflated at this point to revascularize the foot and assess for bleeding vessels. Hemostasis is achieved through an electrocautery to minimize postoperative hematoma formation. Wounds are irrigated copiously with normal saline through a bulb syringe. The subcutaneous tissue is closed as a single layer with interrupted 2–0 vicryl sutures. The skin is closed as a single layer with interrupted 2–0 nylon sutures. Alternatively, medial skin incisions can be closed with a skin stapler. The wounds are injected with an appropriate amount of 0.5% bupivacaine without epinephrine to provide local anesthesia. Distal pulses are checked before applying the postoperative dressings. The wounds are dressed with a sterile layer of non-adherent xeroform dressing, gauze and webril cast padding. The foot is then placed in a well-padded short-leg non-weight-bearing splint. Patients that receive surgery upon all first-fourth metatarsals are kept overnight to monitor for pain and symptoms of compartment syndrome. Patients with limited metatarsal fractures can be discharged home on the day of surgery so long as they have minimal pain.

Rehabilitation

Patients are followed monthly until full recovery is achieved. Immediately following surgery, they are rendered non-weight-bearing following surgery in their postoperative splint. Hip and knee ROM exercises are encouraged. At 2 weeks from surgery, the splint is removed and patients are fitted for a CAM boot. The boot can be removed only for showering and sleeping. Sutures are removed at 2–4 weeks from surgery depending on how swollen the foot is. Patients are kept non-weight-bearing in the boot until 6 weeks from surgery once radiographs show initial fracture healing. Progressive to full weight-bearing in the boot is then allowed after 6 weeks from surgery. At this point, the boot can also be removed for regular ankle ROM exercises. The boot is used until full bony healing is reached, which is typically at 3–4 months from surgery. Upon full healing, patients are allowed to start wearing normal shoes and a return to most activities of daily life. Physical therapy is prescribed on an individual basis if patients exhibit any residual stiffness, weakness, or gait dysfunction. A return to high-impact activities is postponed until one full month from achieving full healing.

ORIF OF EXTRA-ARTICULAR FIRST-FOURTH METATARSAL FRACTURES: Pearls and Pitfalls

- Plate and screw constructs provide rigid fixation to metatarsal fractures
- The surgeon should strive to place at least three screws proximal and three screws distal to the fracture. If this is not possible due to proximity of the fracture to articular surfaces, then two proximal screws and/or two distal screws are sufficient

- T-plates work well when fractures involve the proximal base or distal neck
- Be careful with plate placement so they do not cross any joints

Technique 4: Open Reduction and Internal Fixation of Proximal Fifth Metatarsal Fractures

Preoperative Planning

Anatomical Considerations

Among all metatarsals, the fifth metatarsal is most lateral and plantar. A lateral surgical approach is used for the fifth metatarsal, which involves minimal risk of injury to tendons and neurovascular structures. However, it is important to realize that the lateral foot has scant soft tissue coverage. Implants placed through these areas should not be left prominent. Preoperative planning should include knowledge of the extent of the injury with radiographs. Most proximal fifth metatarsal fractures are transverse. In some instances, contralateral and comparative foot radiographs can be useful to visualize patients' normal foot anatomy.

Instrumentation and Implant Considerations

Once preoperative planning is complete, the surgeon should be sure that all appropriate instrumentation and implants are readily available. Instrumentation required for ORIF includes fracture reduction tools like medium-sized pointed tenaculums and a pneumatic or battery-powered drill. A radiolucent table and fluoroscopic C-arm is needed for intraoperative imaging. Common implants used for ORIF of the fifth metatarsal include a range of partially threaded cannulated cancellous screws between 4.5 mm and 6.5 mm to be placed with the intramedullary canal. Many surgeons, including author, routinely use 4.5 mm screws. In recent years, some have advocated using larger implants for larger sized bone to achieve the tightest fit possible.[19] Some thought may be given to using 0.062-inch K-wires in the presence of fracture comminution. Additional consideration may be given to supplementing intramedullary screw fixation with a tension-band wire construct, but author finds this to be unnecessary.

Patient Considerations

Finally, systemic and local patient factors should be assessed before performing ORIF. Patients that are not medically optimized may do poorly with the additional stress of anesthesia and ORIF. The condition of the foot's soft tissue should be considered before performing surgery. Local infection and skin blisters are a contra-indication to ORIF. Rather, these conditions should be resolved by the time of surgery. Foot swelling should be optimized before surgery as incisions through a swollen foot have a higher risk of surgical wound complications such as compartment syndrome, dehiscence and infection. Therefore, it may be necessary to delay ORIF for 14 days or longer if takes that long for the foot's soft tissue to improve.

Technique

The patient is given a general or spinal anesthetic. The patient is placed lateral on the radiolucent operating table with the use of a beanbag. A pillow is placed between both legs to prevent pressure sores on the contralateral leg. The use of an indwelling epidural catheter for post-operative pain management is not recommended as this may impair a reliable postoperative neurologic and compartment examination. Intravenous antibiotics for skin flora bacterial prophylaxis should be given within one hour of skin incision. A tourniquet is placed at the calf and inflated to 250 mm Hg. As the foot is scrubbed and draped in sterile fashion, anti-thrombotic stockings and venodyne boots are placed on the contralateral leg.

The fifth metatarsal is exposed through a lateral incision centered along the palpable bone. Branches of the sural nerve are identified and retracted from the field. The peroneus brevis tendon is identified and protected. Once the fracture is exposed, it should be debrided free of hematoma, fibrous tissue and bony fragments. A rongeur or curette is then used to debride or freshen both ends of the fracture. All fracture fragments are examined and debrided, leaving their soft tissue attachments intact when possible. Once the fracture is prepared and properly realigned, a guide pin is drilled into the tuberosity to access

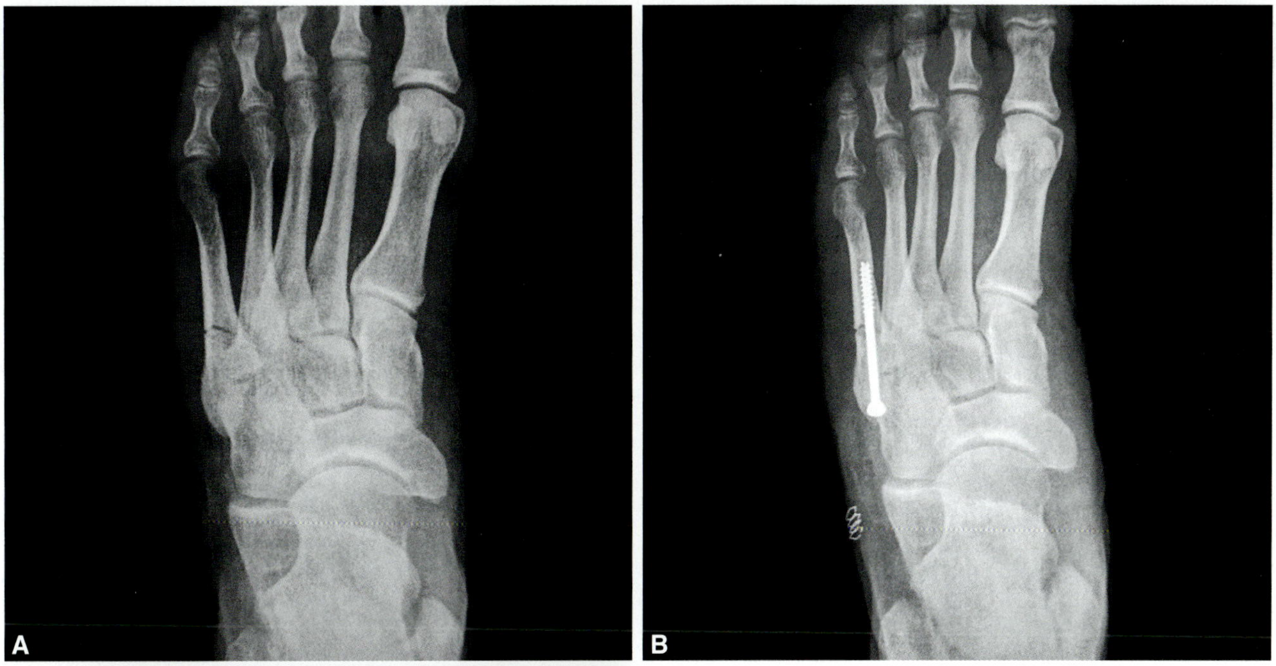

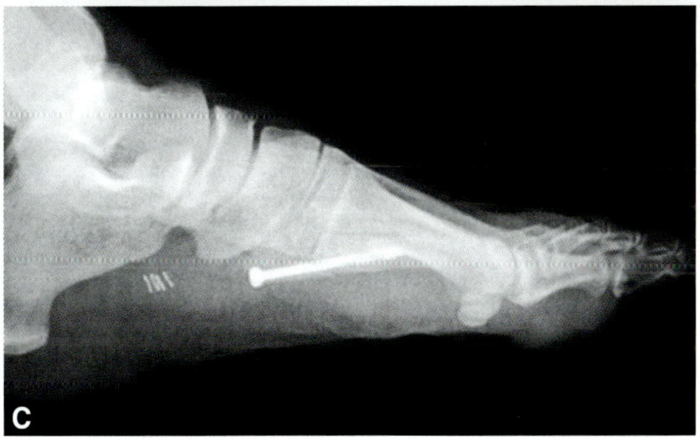

Figures 30.21A to C: Preoperative and postoperative radiographs of open reduction and internal fixation of an acute zone 2 fifth metatarsal fracture in a manual laborer.

the intramedullary canal. The guidepin is advanced past the fracture site, but no further than the metatarsal neck. Anteroposterior and lateral fluoroscopic images are carefully inspected to ensure proper bone alignment and hardware placement. Once this is confirmed, a 4.5 mm screw is placed over the wire and no further than the metatarsal neck. The screw should be long enough so its threads fully cross the fracture site and provide maximal fracture compression. However, it should not be too long that it creates a stress riser at the metatarsal neck. After screw fixation is provided, fluoroscopic images are performed in multiple planes to assess for acceptable bone reduction and hardware placement. Bony stability should be confirmed clinically and radiographically. Foci of bone loss at the fracture sites can receive bone grafting at the surgeon's discretion. When author encounters some degree of bone loss following fracture debridement, he fills these areas with Vitoss (Orthovita, Malvern, PA, USA), which is a synthetic, osteoconductive bone allograft (Figs 30.21A to C).

Closure and Rehabilitation

Treatment protocol is identical to that described in the above technique #3.

ORIF OF PROXIMAL FIFTH METATARSAL FRACTURES: Pearls and Pitfalls

- Placing patients in the lateral position for surgery facilitates fracture exposure and screw placement through the tuberosity
- Take thorough intraoperative fluoroscopic images. The guide wire and screw must be completely intramedullary
- Make certain that the screw is neither too short nor too long

Technique 5: Open Reduction and Internal Fixation of Hallucal Fracture-dislocations

Preoperative Planning

Anatomical Considerations

The hallux is critical in providing stable weight-bearing and gait patterns. The MTP joint is a complex ball-and-socket joint that provides plantarflexion and dorsiflexion with sliding and rolling. The IP joint is a hinge joint that provides additional plantarflexion and dorsiflexion. Either a dorsal or medial surgical approach can be used to expose the MTP joint. A dorsal incision is used to expose the IP joint. While these wounds involve minimal risk of injury to tendons and neurovascular structures, it is important to realize that there is scant soft tissue coverage at the first ray. Implants placed through this area should not be left prominent. Preoperative planning should include knowledge of the extent of the injury with radiographs and possibly CT scans. In some instances, contralateral and comparative foot radiographs can be useful to visualize patients' normal foot anatomy.

Instrumentation and Implant Considerations

Once preoperative planning is complete, the surgeon should be sure that all appropriate instrumentation and implants are readily available. Instrumentation required for ORIF includes a pneumatic or battery-powered drill and fracture reduction tools like 0.045-inch and 0.062 K-wires. A radiolucent table and fluoroscopic C-arm is needed for intraoperative imaging. If a large, rather than a portable mini, fluoroscope is used then the surgeon may consider using a sterile "triangle" knee positioner to assist with foot placement and obtaining ideal AP images. Common implants used for ORIF of the hallux include mini-fragment 2.0 mm cortical screws for large fracture fragments and 1.3–1.7 mm bioabsorbable pins (Orthosorb, Depuy, Warsaw, In, USA) for large osteochondral fractures. Alternatively, percutaneously placed K-wires can be used for fracture fixation.

Patient Considerations

Finally, systemic and local patient factors should be assessed before performing ORIF. Patients that are not medically optimized may do poorly with the additional stress of anesthesia and ORIF. The condition of the foot's soft tissue should be considered before performing surgery. Local infection and skin blisters are a contra-indication to ORIF. Rather, these conditions should be resolved by the time of surgery. Foot swelling should be optimized before surgery as incisions through a swollen foot have a higher risk of surgical wound complications such as compartment syndrome, dehiscence and infection. It may be necessary to delay ORIF for 14 days or longer, if takes that long for the foot's soft tissue to improve. However, joint dislocations that cannot be reduced with closed maneuvers should be treated promptly with ORIF to minimize joint injury.

Technique

The patient is placed supine on the radiolucent operating table. The patient is given a general or spinal anesthetic. The use of an indwelling epidural catheter for post-operative pain management is not recommended as this may impair a reliable postoperative neurologic examination. Intravenous antibiotics for skin flora bacterial prophylaxis should be given within one hour of skin incision. A tourniquet is placed at the calf and inflated to 250 mm Hg. A rolled sheet or "bump" is placed under the ipsilateral buttock to overcome the external rotation of the hip. As the foot is scrubbed and draped in sterile fashion, anti-thrombotic stockings and venodyne boots are placed on the contralateral leg.

The primary surgical approach to the first MTP and IP joints are through a dorsal incision over the joints. While some may expose the first MTP joint with a medial incision, author prefers a longitudinal dorsal approach for wide exposure of the joint. In contrast, the IP incision is always dorsal and shaped like a "staircase" with the horizontal limb over the IP joint and longitudinal distal and plantar extensions. Cutaneous branches of the SPN are identified and retracted medially. The EHL is identified and retracted laterally. A dorsal capsulotomy is performed to expose the MTP and IP joint fractures and/or dislocations. Once the plantar plate is identified, a 3–4 mm longitudinal incision is created in it. Longitudinal traction is applied to reduce the MTP and IP joints. If this maneuver is unsuccessful, a probe or elevator is used to displace the plantar plate and then reduce the joints with longitudinal traction. Once the fracture is exposed, it should be debrided free of hematoma, fibrous tissue and bony fragments. A rongeur or curette is then used to debride or freshen both ends of the fracture. All fracture fragments are examined and debrided, leaving their soft tissue attachments intact when possible. Once the fracture is prepared and properly realigned, the first step is to realign the joint surface. Large fracture fragments are fixed with 2.0 mm screws while osteochondral fractures are fixed with bioabsorbable pins through the joint. Fluoroscopic images are performed in multiple planes to assess for acceptable bone and joint reduction and hardware placement. Bony and joint stability should be confirmed clinically and radiographically. Screws should be checked to make sure that they are not too long. If there is any doubt regarding construct stability, supplemental K-wires can be used with percutaneous placement.

Closure

Once normal bone and joint alignment has been restored with proper hardware placement, wound closure can begin. The tourniquet is deflated at this point to revascularize the toe and assess for bleeding vessels. Hemostasis is achieved through an electrocautery to minimize postoperative hematoma formation. Wounds are irrigated copiously with normal saline through a bulb syringe. The plantar plate is closed with 2-0 ethibond suture. The joint capsule is closed as a single layer with interrupted 0 vicryl sutures. The subcutaneous tissue is closed as a single layer with interrupted 2.0 vicryl sutures. The skin is closed as a single layer with interrupted 2-0 nylon sutures. Alternatively, medial skin incisions can be closed with a skin stapler. The wounds are injected with an appropriate amount of 0.5% bupivacaine without epinephrine to provide local anesthesia. Distal pulses are checked before applying the postoperative dressings. The wounds are dressed with a sterile layer of non-adherent xeroform dressing, gauze and webril cast padding. The foot is then placed in a surgical hard-soled shoe. Patients can be discharged home on the day of surgery, so long as they have minimal pain.

Rehabilitation

Patients are followed monthly, until full recovery is achieved. Immediately, following surgery, they are rendered non weight-bearing following surgery in their postoperative surgical shoe. Knee and ankle ROM exercises are encouraged. At 2 weeks from surgery, patients are allowed to bear weight on their heel. Sutures are removed at 2–4 weeks from surgery depending on how swollen the toe is. Patients are kept in heel weight-bearing shoes until 6 weeks from surgery once radiographs show maintained joint alignment and initial fracture healing. Progressive to full weight-bearing in the shoe is then allowed after 6 weeks from surgery. At this point, the shoe can also be removed for regular first toe ROM exercises. The shoe is used until full bony healing is reached, which is typically at three months from surgery. Upon full healing, patients are allowed to start wearing normal shoes and a return to most activities of daily life. Physical therapy is prescribed on an individual basis, if patients exhibit any residual stiffness, weakness or gait dysfunction. A return to high-impact activities is postponed until one full month from achieving full healing.

ORIF OF HALLUCAL FRACTURE-DISLOCATIONS: Pearls and Pitfalls

- Dorsal incisions provide a wide surgical exposure to the hallux
- Incisions through the plantar plate may be necessary to reduce dislocations
- Mini-fragment and bioabsorbable screws provide rigid internal fixation
- K-wires can provide supplemental fixation

Technique 6: Open Reduction and Internal Fixation of Hallucal Sesamoid Fractures

Preoperative Planning

Anatomical Considerations

The tibial and fibular sesamoids are critical to normal function and stability of the hallux. They lie within the FHB tendon, but are separated from each other by the flexor hallucis longus (FHL). As they articulate with the plantar first metatarsal head, they elevate the metatarsal and provide a gliding surface for weight-bearing. A medial surgical approach is used to expose the tibial sesamoid, while a plantar incision is used to expose the fibular sesamoid. While a medial wound has minimal risk, a plantar incision has a significant risk of injury to the flexor tendons and digital nerve. Implants placed through the sesamoids should not be left prominent as they are weight-bearing bones. Preoperative planning should include knowledge of the extent of the injury with radiographs and possibly CT scans. In some instances, contralateral and comparative foot radiographs can be useful to visualize patients' normal foot anatomy.

Instrumentation and Implant Considerations

Once preoperative planning is complete, the surgeon should be sure that all appropriate instrumentation and implants are readily available. Instrumentation required for ORIF includes a pneumatic or battery-powered drill and fracture reduction tools like 0.045-inch K-wires and small tenaculums. A radiolucent table and fluoroscopic C-arm is needed for intraoperative imaging. If a large, rather than a portable mini, fluoroscope is used then the surgeon may consider using a sterile "triangle" knee positioner to assist with foot placement and obtaining ideal AP images. Common implants used for ORIF of the sesamoids include mini-fragment 1.5 mm cortical screws.

Patient Considerations

Finally, systemic and local patient factors should be assessed before performing ORIF. Patients that are not medically optimized may do poorly with the additional stress of anesthesia and ORIF. The condition of the foot's soft tissue should be considered before performing surgery. Local infection and skin blisters are a contra-indication to ORIF. Rather, these conditions should be resolved by the time of surgery. Foot swelling should be optimized before surgery as incisions through a swollen foot have a higher risk of surgical wound complications such as compartment syndrome, dehiscence and infection. It may be necessary to delay ORIF for 14 days or longer, if takes that long for the foot's soft tissue to improve.

Technique

The patient is placed supine on the radiolucent operating table. The bed should be placed in approximately 15° of reverse Trendelenburg to assist with creating a plantar incision at the hallux. The patient is given a general or spinal anesthetic. Intravenous antibiotics for skin flora bacterial prophylaxis should be given within one hour of skin incision. A tourniquet is placed at the calf and inflated to 250 mm Hg. A rolled sheet or bump is placed under the ipsilateral buttock to overcome the external rotation of the hip. As the foot is scrubbed and draped in sterile fashion, anti-thrombotic stockings and venodyne boots are placed on the contralateral leg.

The primary surgical approach to the tibial sesamoid is a medial longitudinal incision over the plantar aspect of the first MTP joint. Cutaneous branches of the SPN are identified and retracted dorsally. A medial L-shaped capsulotomy is performed at the MTP joint to expose the metatarsal head. The tibial sesamoid is then exposed at the plantar metatarsal head.

The primary surgical approach to the fibular sesamoid is a plantar, curvilinear incision over the plantar, distal first inter-metatarsal web space. The FHL is identified and retracted medially. The inter-digital nerve is visualized and retracted laterally. The FHB is identified and incised longitudinally. This serves to expose the fibular sesamoid.

Once the fractures are exposed, it should be debrided free of hematoma, fibrous tissue and bony fragments. A rongeur or curette is then used to debride or freshen both ends of the fracture. All fracture fragments are examined and debrided, leaving their soft tissue attachments intact when possible. Once the fracture is prepared and properly realigned, it is fixed with 1–2 mini-fragment screws. Plantarflexion of the first MTP joint can help with reduction of displaced fractures. Fluoroscopic images are performed in multiple planes to assess for acceptable bone and joint reduction and hardware placement. Bony and joint stability should be confirmed clinically and radiographically. Screws should be checked to make sure that they are not too dorsal, plantar, or long.

Closure

Once normal bone and joint alignment has been restored with proper hardware placement, wound closure can begin. The tourniquet is deflated at this point to revascularize the toe and assess for bleeding vessels. Hemostasis is achieved through an electrocautery to minimize postoperative hematoma formation. Wounds are irrigated copiously with normal saline through a bulb syringe. Deep structures such as the medial first MTP joint capsule and FHB are closed as a single layer with interrupted 0 vicryl sutures. The subcutaneous tissue is closed as a single layer with interrupted 2–0 vicryl sutures. The medial and plantar skin is closed as a single layer with interrupted 2–0 nylon sutures. Sutures on the plantar skin are placed in a vertical-mattress technique to avoid creating a painful plantar scar. The wounds are injected with an appropriate amount of 0.5% bupivacaine without epinephrine to provide local anesthesia. Distal pulses are checked before applying the postoperative dressings. The wounds are dressed with a sterile layer of non-adherent xeroform dressing, gauze and webril cast padding. The foot is then placed in a surgical hard-soled shoe. Patients can be discharged home on the day of surgery, so long as they have minimal pain.

Rehabilitation

Patients are followed monthly until full recovery is achieved. Immediately, following surgery, they are rendered non-weight-bearing following surgery in their postoperative surgical shoe. Knee and ankle ROM exercises are encouraged. At 2 weeks from surgery, patients are allowed to bear weight on their heel. Sutures are removed at 2–4 weeks from surgery depending on how swollen the toe is. Patients are kept in heel weight-bearing shoes until 6 weeks from surgery once radiographs show maintained joint alignment and initial fracture healing. Progressive to full weight-bearing in the shoe is then allowed after 6 weeks from surgery. At this point, the shoe can also be removed for regular first toe ROM exercises. The shoe is used until full bony healing is reached, which is typically at three months from surgery. Upon full healing, patients are allowed to start wearing normal shoes and a return to most activities of daily life. Patients are fitted with a dancer's pad to use in their shoes as needed to unload the sesamoids. Physical therapy is prescribed on an individual basis, if patients exhibit any residual stiffness, weakness, or gait dysfunction. A return to high-impact activities is postponed until 1–2 full months from achieving full healing.

ORIF OF HALLUCAL SESAMOID FRACTURES: Pearls and Pitfalls

- A medial incision exposes the tibial sesamoid. A plantar incision exposes the fibular sesamoid
- This plantar incision and its closure must be meticulous to avoid creating potential painful plantar scar
- Mini-fragment provide rigid internal fixation

Outcomes

Obtaining ideal outcomes after surgical management of both acute and chronic, neglected Lisfranc fracture-dislocations is highly dependent upon achieving anatomic bone and joint alignment. Over the past 20 years, studies with long-term follow-up of ORIF of acute injuries and midfoot fusion for chronic conditions present good functional outcomes in 65–90% of patients.[20,21] It is important to note that 40–90% of patients that had ORIF for their acute injuries progressed to develop varying degrees of post-traumatic midfoot arthritis from mild to severe. The more severe cases of joint degeneration that correlated to poorer outcomes occurred in those that had purely ligamentous Lisfranc injuries despite ORIF. This high rate of post-traumatic arthritis seen despite ORIF has led some authorities to propose primary midfoot fusion for certain acute ligamentous Lisfranc injuries.[16] To date, this matter is a source of much debate. The authors personal preference remains performing ORIF for most acute injuries and reserving arthrodesis for injuries that have irreparable joint damage like chronic or missed injuries.

There is a varying amount of literature regarding outcomes following ORIF of extra-articular metatarsal fractures. Few studies exist regarding outcomes following

ORIF of first-fourth metatarsal fractures. Most reports regarding these injuries detail how poorly patients do, if they receive nonsurgical treatment for unstable injuries.[22] In contrast, there is much more literature regarding outcomes following ORIF of fifth metatarsal fractures. Most studies report union rates as high as 100% with return to pre-injury levels of activity within 4–5 months.[23]

Scant literature exists regarding outcomes following ORIF of hallucal fracture-dislocations and sesamoid fractures. Most studies regarding surgical treatment of these injuries are limited to case series.[13] These reports reveal high rates of healing and pain relief. The most common complaint among patients following open treatment of hallucal dislocations was residual joint stiffness at a rate of 25–50%.

Complications

Surgical management of midfoot and forefoot fractures and dislocations has its fair share of complications. While there are methods to treat postoperative complications, the surgeon should be proactive and work towards minimizing risks.

Postoperative Infection

It can occur at any point following surgical treatment of foot injuries. Presentations can range from superficial cellulitis to deeper abscesses. Open fractures are at higher risk for developing infection than closed injuries. Prevention is the first step in avoiding infection. Antibiotics should be given within 1 hour of skin incision and continued for 24 hours after surgery. Skin preparation with betadine or chlorhexidine should be done with strict adherence to sterile protocol in the operating room. In addition, implants and instruments should be covered with a sterile towel until they are ready to be used.

Wound Complications

They are not uncommon following operative treatment of foot injuries. This is because the foot is prone to significant swelling following trauma and surgery. As the foot is often in a dependent position and farthest from the heart anatomically, it is also challenging for foot swelling to resolve in a timely manner. Patients are encouraged to ice and elevate their foot as much as possible before surgery to optimize the soft tissue before surgical injury. During surgery, full-thickness skin flaps are developed and carefully handled. Wounds are retracted under tension as little as possible so as to minimize injury to the skin's angiosomes. Following surgery, patients are still asked to continue to ice and elevate their foot as much as possible to minimize postoperative swelling. Sutures may be left in as long as 4 weeks to further minimize wound problems like dehiscence.

Post-traumatic Arthritis

It can occur following intra-articular fractures despite treatment and Lisfranc injuries are no exception. A high rate of Lisfranc injuries present with degenerative changes despite surgical treatment. Fortunately, this encompasses a wide range of disease from mild to severe as not all patients with arthritis have pain. While it is not possible to undo cartilaginous injury at the midfoot, certain intra-operative measures can be taken to minimize the risk of post-traumatic arthritis. Joints should be debrided thoroughly and free of bone and/or cartilage fragments. Large osteochondral fractures should be fixed with mini-fragment screws. Joints should be reduced anatomically and rigidly fixed.

Nonunion

Nonunion is a potential complication following operative treatment. In the context of managing midfoot and forefoot injuries, nonunion can apply to ORIF and midfoot fusions. Atrophic nonunions occur due to poor blood supply at the bone. Patient factors that can cause this include nicotine, steroids, diabetes, inflammatory conditions and vascular disease. Bony factors that can predispose to atrophic nonunion are periosteal injuries that can occur with stripping. Hypertrophic nonunions are due to excessive motion at the fracture or fusion site which in turn is due to poor implant stability. Other nonunions are due to infections. With all of these factors in mind, certain measures can be taken in mind to minimize the risk of nonunion. Patients are advised to stop using nicotine and steroids. With the assistance of the appropriate medical specialist, patients' medical comorbidities are optimized. Periosteal stripping is minimized during surgery. Implant strength and fracture stability is confirmed intraoperatively. Some consideration may be given to using a plate and screw construct instead of just screws for midfoot fusions in certain patients that may be at risk for poor bone healing. Patients are not advanced in weight-bearing until appropriate bony callus is seen radiographically for risk of premature hardware failure. As mentioned earlier, steps are taken to minimize the risk of infection.

Compartment Syndrome

Compartment syndrome of the foot is a serious problem, if it develops after surgical treatment of fractures. However, it can be highly distressing if it is missed as it can lead to irreversible muscle death and dysfunction. In the context of midfoot and forefoot injuries, high-energy Lisfranc injuries are at the highest risk for developing compartment syndrome postoperatively. It can be difficult to prevent compartment syndrome as this can occur following the injury itself. Epidural catheters should be avoided as they may interfere with postsurgical pain assessment. Care is taken to ensure splints are not too tight after surgery. This includes both the plaster splint as well as the layer of webril underneath the plaster. Patients with high-energy injuries that may be at risk for postoperative compartment syndrome are kept overnight for observation.

Author's Preferred Management of Select Complications

Case 1: Treatment of Post-traumatic Midfoot Arthritis after ORIF of a Lisfranc Injury

A high rate of Lisfranc injuries is present with arthritic changes despite surgical treatment, ranging from 40% to 100% among various studies. While some patients may have only mild arthritis and minimal symptoms, others may have more severe degenerative changes and debilitating pain. Nonsurgical measures, such as anti-inflammatory medication and rigid orthoses, can be attempted as the first line of treatment. Should this fail, a midfoot fusion would be the next step in treatment.

In this particular case, a 65-year-old woman sustained a closed, complete homolateral, ligamentous Lisfranc injury in a motor vehicle accident (MVA) 5 years before presenting to author. ORIF was performed within a week from her injury by another surgeon at an outside institution (Fig. 30.22). The surgery utilized a single incision through the proximal first inter-metatarsal web space and without immediate complications. Within one year from the ORIF, the same surgeon removed her hardware as she was thought to have painful hardware. When the surgeon saw her, she had developed severe post-traumatic midfoot arthritis at her first-fifth TMT joints that had failed years of non-surgical treatment. Following a discussion of nonsurgical and surgical treatment options, she agreed to undergo a midfoot fusion.

The patient received a midfoot fusion through a two-incision approach. The first incision was through her previously healed scar over the proximal first inter-metatarsal web space to expose the first-second TMT joints. Once these joints were exposed, they were debrided free of fibrous tissue and diseased articular cartilage. Care was taken to remove more bone from the plantar than the dorsal base of the first-second metatarsals, to restore an arch shape to her foot. The second incision was placed over her fourth metatarsal to expose the third-fifth TMT joints. Once these joints were exposed, they were also debrided free of fibrous tissue and diseased cartilage. Care was taken to remove more bone from the plantar than the dorsal base of the third metatarsal, to maintain the arch shape to her foot. A rongeur and curette were then used to further debride or freshen both ends of exposed cancellous bone at all five TMT joints. A third incision was created at the lateral calcaneus to harvest autogenous calcaneal bone graft. This bone graft was placed in the first-third TMT joints. The first-third TMT joints are aligned correctly with two guide pins crossing the first and first crossing the second and third each. So long as radiographs confirm appropriate wire placement, 4.0 mm screw are placed over each wire and countersunk. Once the first-third TMT joints are fused, the EDB is identified at the second incision and placed into the fourth-fifth TMT joints. With the EDB acting as an interpositional material, the fourth-fifth TMT joints are reduced and stabilized to the cuboid with a retrograde 0.062-inch K-wire each. Fluoroscopic images confirmed appropriate joint and hardware placement. Within four months, the patient healed fully and without event. To date, she has no recurrence of pain or deformity (Figs 30.22A to D).

The important principles of this case are as follows:

- Prior midfoot incisions are incorporated into revision surgical treatment approaches
- Simultaneous joint fusion and deformity correction is performed to achieve a stable, functional, plantigrade foot

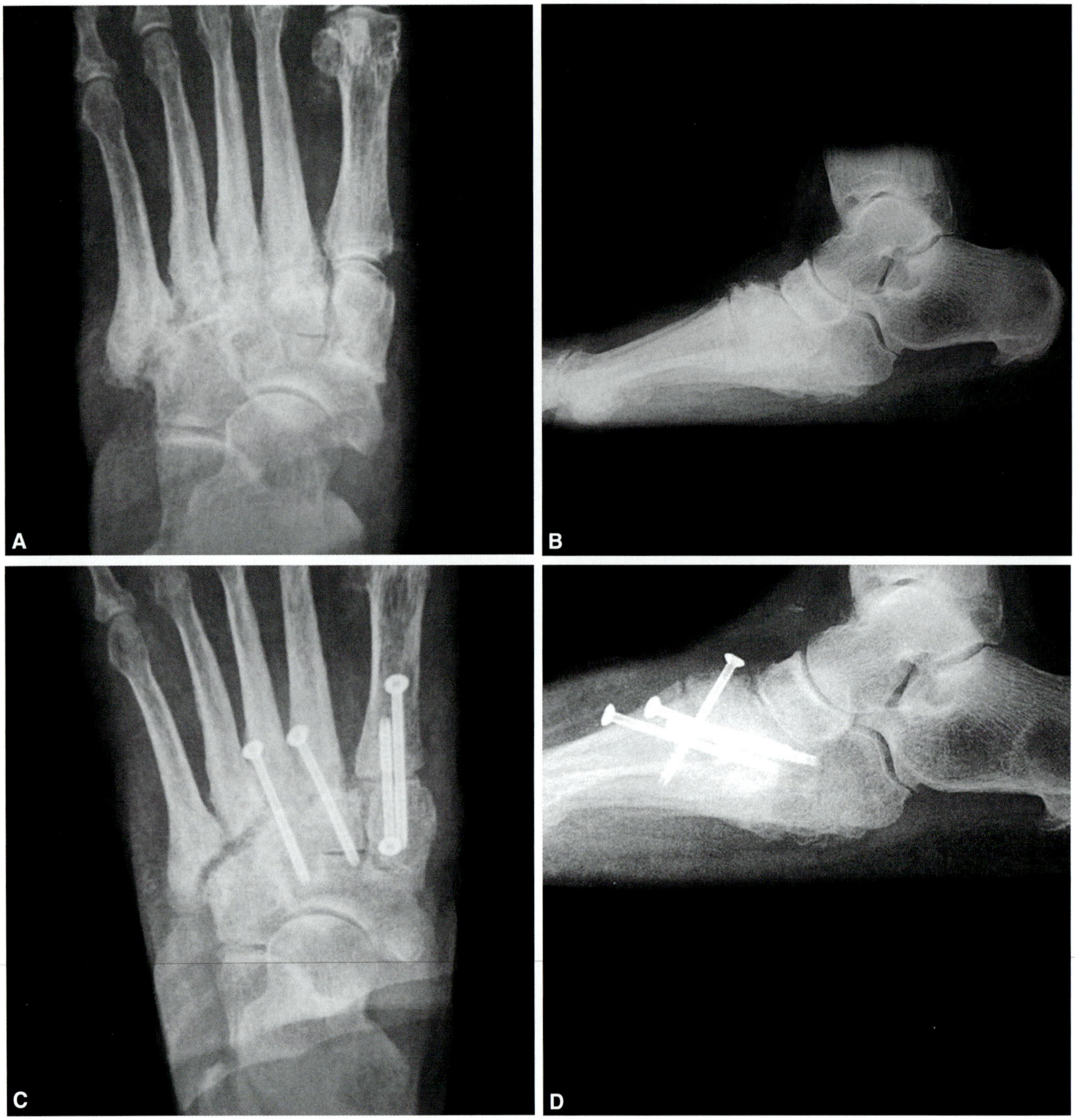

Figures 30.22A to D: Preoperative and postoperative radiographs for Case 1, a patient who developed post-traumatic midfoot arthritis following a Lisfranc injury and despite open reduction and internal fixation. The implants were subsequently removed due to presumed painful hardware. Due to painful midfoot arthritis which had failed other treatment methods, she underwent a midfoot fusion salvage procedure as shown in Figures C and D.

Case 2: Nonunion vs Refracture of a Proximal Zone Two Fifth Metatarsal Fracture

While most literature report a high union rate of ORIF of Zone two fifth metatarsal fractures, some studies reveal a significant incidence of refracture and/or nonunion among competitive athletes. Larson et al. showed four refractures and two nonunions among 15 patients that receive ORIF.[24] The authors determined the refractures to have actually healed at some point after surgery, but became reinjured. In the athletic population, the possible causes for refracture and nonunion include poor bony blood supply, poor implant strength and anatomical features that cause excessive lateral column loading like a varus hindfoot. Nonsurgical measures, such as bone stimulators and rigid orthoses, can be attempted as the first line of treatment. Should this fail, an open repair of the fifth metatarsal with autogenous bone graft may be indicated.

In this particular case, an 18-year-old woman sustained a closed, Zone two fifth metatarsal fracture while playing competitive soccer in high school 2 years before presenting to the author. ORIF was performed within a week from her injury by another surgeon at an outside institution. The surgery utilized an incision at the lateral fifth metatarsal and K-wires for fixation. While her surgery was without immediate complications, she complained of recurrent pain within 6 months. Within 1 year from the ORIF, the same surgeon removed her hardware as she was thought to have painful hardware (Figure 30.23). Upon seeing the author, she had returned to playing competitive soccer despite months of recurrent fifth metatarsal pain. Initial radiographs with author revealed a chronic fifth metatarsal fracture nonunion with minimal fracture callus. Under authors take-over care, she had failed weeks of non-surgical treatment. Following a discussion of nonsurgical and surgical treatment options, she agreed to undergo an ORIF of the fifth metatarsal with autogenous bone graft.

The patient received an ORIF of the fifth metatarsal through a two-incision approach. The first incision was through her previously healed scar over the lateral fifth metatarsal. Once the fracture nonunion was exposed, it was debrided free of fibrous tissue and bony callus under fluoroscopic guidance. The nonunion was debrided to expose bleeding subchondral bone. The intramedullary canal was broached through the tuberosity with a guide pin and reamed with as large drill bits as possible. A second incision was created at the lateral calcaneus to harvest autogenous calcaneal bone graft. This bone graft was placed in the fifth metatarsal fracture site. The largest screw that could fit in the patient's fifth metatarsal was a 5.5 mm cannulated partially threaded cancellous screw. Care was taken to ensure the screw used was neither too long nor short. Fluoroscopic images confirmed appropriate joint and hardware placement. Within three months, the patient healed fully and without event. She was fitted for a custom-molded orthotic with a lateral flare to unload the lateral column. To date, she has no recurrence of pain and has returned to playing soccer at her pre-injury level (Figs 30.23A to D).

The important principles of this case are as follows:

- Refractures and/or nonunions of the proximal fifth metatarsal should be treated aggressively in athletes
- Autogenous bone graft should be used liberally
- Successful treatment of the nonunion requires a thorough and aggressive debridement of the fracture
- A partially threaded screw that is as large as possible should be utilized

Case 3: Treatment of Compartment Syndrome of the Foot

In the context of midfoot and forefoot injuries, high-energy Lisfranc injuries are at the highest risk for developing compartment syndrome postoperatively. This can occur in any of the foot's nine compartments when the pressure within increases beyond intra-arterial pressures. Ultimately, this leads to decreased muscle and soft tissue perfusion which progresses to irreversible tissue death when left untreated. Treatment is emergent and requires decompressive fasciotomies of all nine compartments (medial, lateral, superficial, adductor, calcaneal and four interossei). A full recovery is dependent upon providing rapid treatment.

In this situation, a 16-year-old woman presented with a seven-day-old closed B2 (incomplete homolateral, lateral) Lisfranc fracture-dislocation following an MVA. She displayed instability of the Lisfranc ligament and second-fourth TMT joints. As her foot was only moderately swollen, she received ORIF that week. The procedure was performed through one incision. The primary incision was placed over the proximal first inter-metatarsal web space

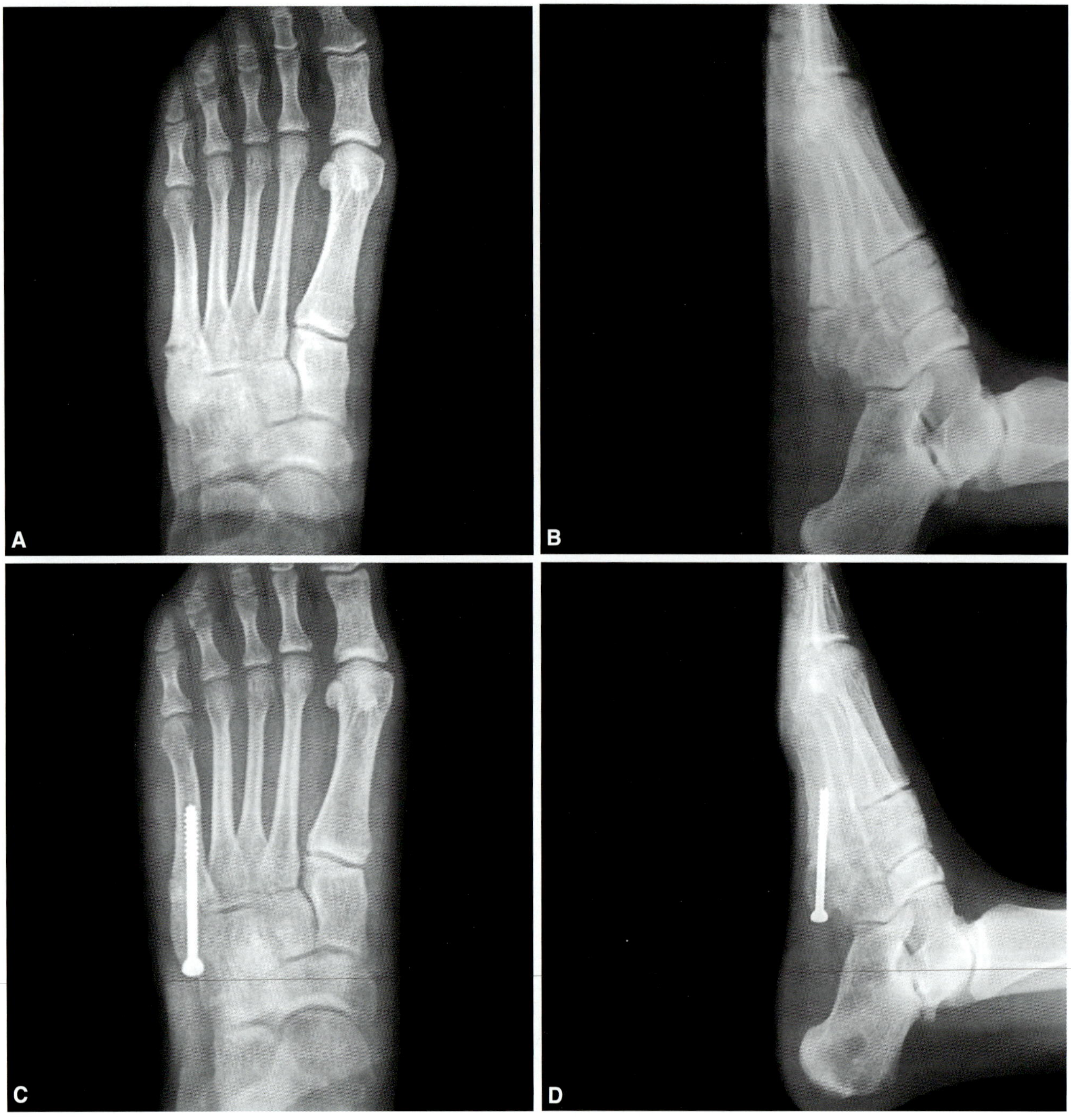

Figures 30.23A to D: Preoperative and postoperative radiographs for Case 2, a patient who developed a re-injury or nonunion of a fifth metatarsal despite open reduction and internal fixation. Patient received revision treatment with autogenous calcaneal bone graft.

to expose the Lisfranc ligament and second TMT joints. The second TMT joint was exposed and debrided free of hematoma, fibrous tissue and bony fragments. The Lisfranc ligament was visualized and also debrided. The base of the second metatarsal was compressed to the medial cuneiform with a single screw. The second TMT joint was then compressed with a single screw. This resulted in spontaneous third-fourth TMT joint reduction. As a result,

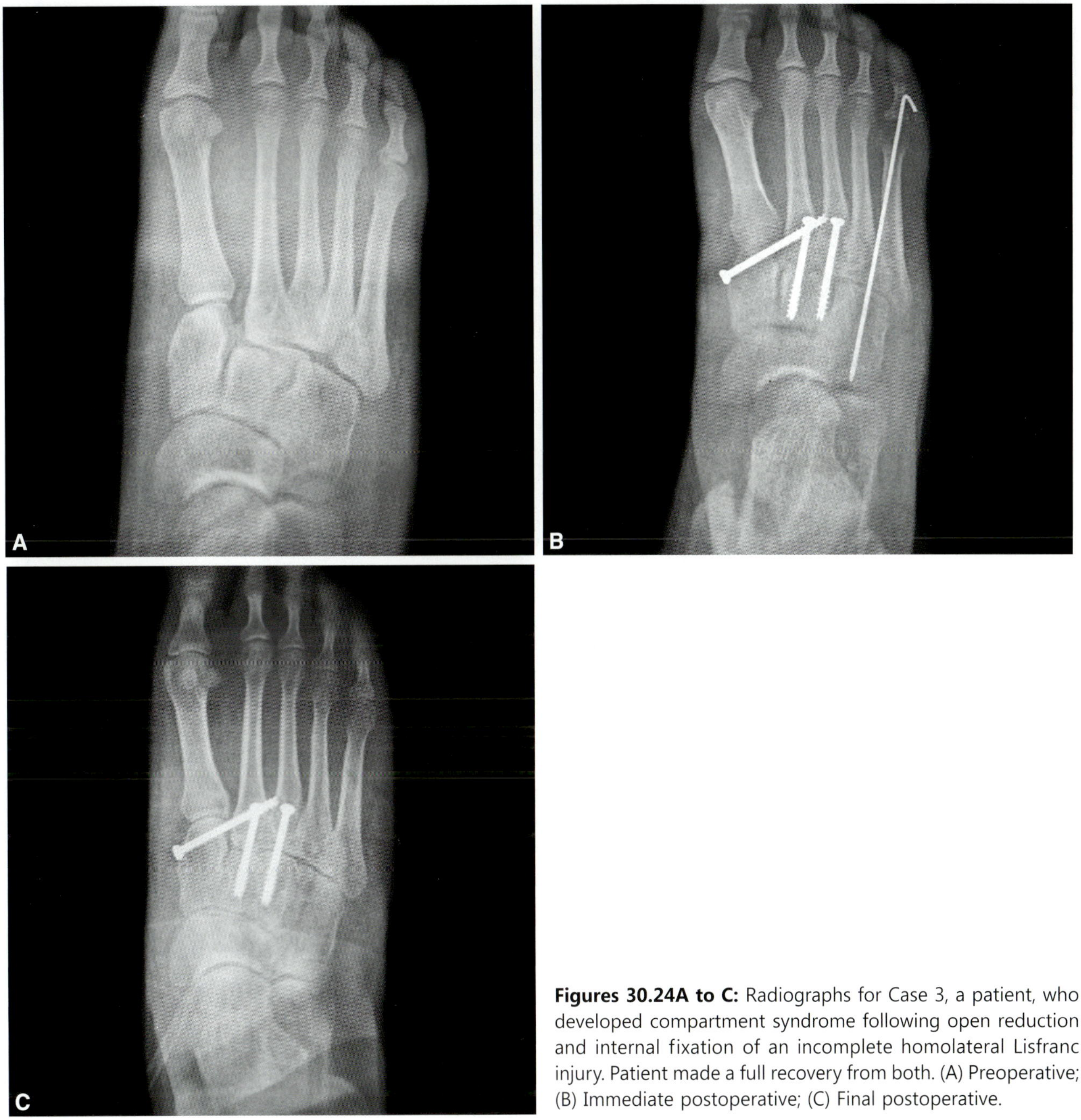

Figures 30.24A to C: Radiographs for Case 3, a patient, who developed compartment syndrome following open reduction and internal fixation of an incomplete homolateral Lisfranc injury. Patient made a full recovery from both. (A) Preoperative; (B) Immediate postoperative; (C) Final postoperative.

third TMT screw and fourth TMT wire fixation was performed percutaneously. Fluoroscopic images confirmed acceptable bone and joint reduction and hardware placement. The wounds were closed using standard technique and she was placed in a short-leg splint to stay overnight in the hospital (Figs 30.24A to C).

At 12 hours from surgery, the patient complained of increasing pain that was poorly managed with her postoperative medication. Her splint was promptly removed for a proper exam of her foot. While her foot had palpable pulses and normal sensation, she had severe swelling at her foot and pain on minimal palpation. With

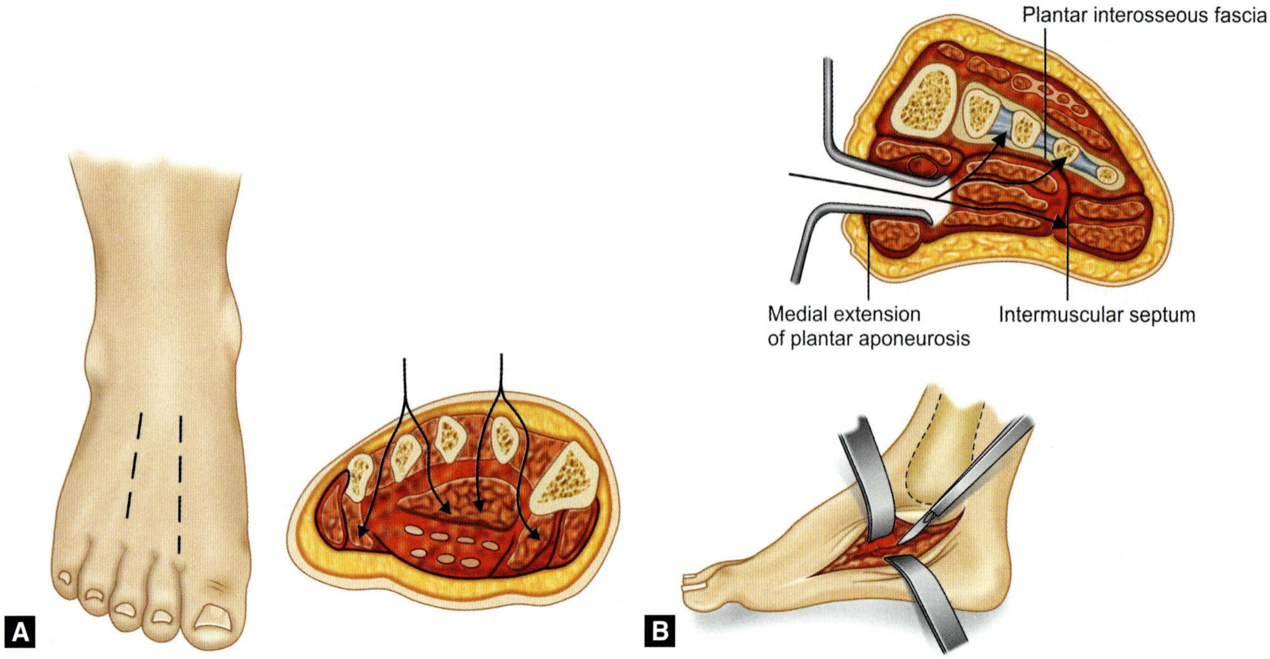

Figures 30.25A and B: Placement of incisions for foot fasciotomies. (A) Dorsal incisions shown on the skin as well as cross-sectional depiction of intended releases; (B) Medial incision with cross-sectional depiction of intended releases.

a high clinical suspicion for postoperative compartment syndrome, she was emergently taken back to receive fasciotomies of her foot. Compartment release was performed through three incisions, which is the standard of care (Figures 30.25A and B). Her dorsal foot incision was reopened to decompress the medial interossei compartments. She received a second incision on her dorsal foot over the fourth metatarsal to decompress the lateral interossei compartments. She received a third incision at her medial arch to decompress the remaining five compartments. While hematoma was evacuated from the dorsal foot, all three wounds were irrigated copiously with normal saline. After the fasciotomies were done, the author used a shoelace technique with staples and a rubber catheter to provide some tension across the wound and facilitate delayed closure. The author also began negative pressure wound therapy (NPWT) at her incisions. The author left these dressings intact and did not change them outside of the operating room for fear of infection.

The patient felt immediate pain relief following fasciotomies. She was brought back to the operating room two days later for further I and D with an assessment of the wound. By this time, her swelling had resolved and the author was able to close all three fasciotomy wounds. She was placed back in a splint and soon discharged from the hospital. Within 3½ months, the patient healed fully and without event. To date, she has neither post-traumatic midfoot arthritis nor any sequelae of compartment syndrome.

The important principles of this case are as follows:

- Have a high index of suspicion for compartment syndrome when treating high-energy injuries of the midfoot
- Treatment of foot compartment syndrome is urgent and requires three incisions to decompress all nine compartments. A full recovery is dependent upon rapid diagnosis and treatment
- NPWT with wound approximation can help to achieve delayed wound closure
- Subsequent fasciotomy wound infection after compartment syndrome can be devastating. If wounds cannot be closed within 1–2 weeks, patients will benefit from skin grafting.

Summary

Surgical management of unstable midfoot and forefoot fractures and dislocations can be challenging. ORIF with modern instrumentation is the standard treatment for most of these injuries. The only exceptions to this are Lisfranc injuries that present with irreparable cartilage damage, which are better suited for arthrodesis. Both ORIF and arthrodesis result in generally satisfactory results. Ideal outcomes are dependent on appropriate timing of surgery, preoperative planning and achieving anatomic bone and joint realignment. However, it is important to realize that complications can occur despite meticulous surgical technique. The surgeon should always be alert for the development of compartment syndrome in any patient with high-energy midfoot and forefoot injuries. Other post-surgical difficulties that can occur include post-traumatic arthritis and fracture nonunion. The surgeon should be prepared to manage both these injuries and their potential complications as they arise.

References

1. Lisfranc J. Nouvelle methode operatoire pour l'amputation partielle du pied par son articulation tarso-metatarsienne. Paris, Gibbon, 1815.
2. Aronow MS. Treatment of the missed Lisfranc injury. Foot Ankle Clin. 2006;11(1):127-42.
3. Richli WR, Rosenthal DI. Avulsion fracture of the Fifth metatarsal: experimental study of pathomechanics. AJR Am Roentgenol. 1984;143(4):889-91.
4. Jones R. Fracture of the base of the Fifth metatarsal bone by indirect violence. Ann Surg. 1902;35(6):697-700.
5. Smith JW, Arnoczky SP, Hersh, A. The intraosseous blood supply of the fifth metatarsal: implications for proximal fracture healing. Foot Ankle. 1992;13(3):143-52.
6. Perry MD, Manoli A. Foot compartment syndrome. Orthop Clin North Am. 2001;32(1):103-11.
7. Olson SA, Glasgow RR. Acute compartment syndrome in lower extremity musculoskeletal trauma. J Am Acad Orthop Surg. 2005;13(7):436-44.
8. Myerson MS, Fisher RT, Burgess, AR, et al. Fracture dislocations of the tarsometatarsal joints, end results correlated with pathology and treatment. Foot Ankle. 1986; 6(5):225-42.
9. Raikin S, Elias I, Dheer S, et al. Prediction of midfoot instability in the subtle Lisfranc injury. Comparison of magnetic resonance imaging with intraoperative findings. J Bone Joint Surg Am. 2009;91(4): 892-9.
10. Quenu E, Kuss G. Etude sur les luxations du metatarse. Review de Chirgurie Paris.1909;39.
11. Hardcastle PH, Reschauser R, Kutscha-Lissberg E, et al. Injuries to the tarsometatarsal joint: incidence, classification, and treatment. J Bone Joint Surg Br. 1982;64(3): 349-56.
12. Jahss MH. Traumatic dislocations of the first metatarsophalangeal joint. Foot Ankle. 1980;1(1):15-21.
13. Maskill JD, Bohay DR, Anderson JG. First ray injuries. Foot Ankle Clin. 2006;11(1):143-63.
14. Miki T, Yamamuro T, Kitai T. An irreducible dislocation of the great toe. Report of two cases and review of the literature. Clin Orthop Relat Res. 1988;230:200-6.
15. Rosenberg, GA, Sferra JJ. Treatment strategies for acute fractures and nonunions of the proximal fifth metatarsal. J Am Academy of Orthop Surg. 2000;8(5):332-38.
16. Trevino SG, Kodros, S. Controversies in tarsometatarsal joints. Orthop Clin North Am. 1995;26(2):229-38.
17. Ly TV, Coetzee JC. Treatment of primarily ligamentous Lisfranc joint injuries: primary arthrodesis compared with open reduction and internal fixation. A prospective, randomized study. J Bone Joint Surg Am. 2006;88(3):514-20.
18. Berlet GC, Hodges Davis W, Anderson RB. Tendon arthroplasty for basal fourth and fifth metatarsal arthritis. Foot and Ankle Int. 2002;23(5):440-6.
19. Sides SD, Fetter NL, Glisson R, et al. Bending stiffness and pull-out strength of tapered, variable pitch screws, and 6.5 mm cancellous screws in acute Jones fractures. Foot Ankle Int. 2006;27(10):821-25.
20. Richter M, Wipperman B, Krettek C, et al. Fractures and fracture dislocations of the midfoot: occurrence, causes and long-term results. Foot Ankle Int. 2001;22(5):392-98.
21. Komenda GA, Myerson MS, Biddinger KR. Results of arthrodesis of the tarsometatarsal joints after traumatic injury. J Bone Joint Surg Am. 1996;78(11):1665-76.
22. Sánchez Alepuz E, Vicent Carsi V, Alcántara P, et al. Fractures of the central metatarsal. Foot Ankle Int. 1996;17(4):200-3.
23. Porter DA, Duncan M, Meyer SJ. Fifth metatarsal Jones fracture fixation with a 4.5-mm cannulated stainless steel screw in the competitive and recreational athlete: a clinical and radiographic evaluation. Am J Sports Med. 2005; 33(5):726-33.
24. Larson CM, Almekinders LC, Taft TN, et al. Intramedullary screw fixation of Jones fractures. Analysis of failure. Am J Sports Med. 2002;30(1):55-60.

Index

Page number followed by *f* and *t* indicates figure and table respectively.

A

Acetabulum fracture 552–553
anterior column 566
anterior wall 565–566
case study
heterotopic ossification of hip 575, 577, 577*f*–578*f*, 579
infection, management of 575, 576*f*
classification 555–556, 556*t*
complications 553
DVT 573
heterotopic ossification 572–573
late instability after ORIF 575
late stage arthritis 574–575
malunion 574
nerve palsy 573
nonunions 574
pulmonary embolism 573
CT scan 556–557
epidemiology 553
hemitransverse 569–571
heterotopic ossification 572–573
obese patients and 553
percutaneous fixation 571–572
antegrade anterior column screw 571, 571*f*
ischial posterior column screw 572
LC-II screw 571
posterior column screw 572
retrograde anterior column screw 571–572
posterior column fractures 565
posterior wall fractures 564–565, 565*f*
radiographic evaluation 554
anteroposterior view 554, 554*f*
iliac oblique view 555, 555*f*
obturator-oblique view 554, 555*f*
roof-arc measurements 557, 557*f*
surgical management
anterior approach 560–563
extensile approaches 563–564, 564*f*
iliofemoral approach 561
ilioinguinal approach 561–562, 561*f*, 562*f*
indications for 557–558, 557*f*
Kocher-Langenbeck approach 558–560, 559*f*
modified Stoppa approach 562–563, 563*f*
posterior approach 558–560
trochanteric osteotomy 560, 560*f*
transverse fractures 566–567, 566*f*
T-type fractures 568–569, 569*f*–570*f*
ACL *see* Anterior cruciate ligament (ACL)
Acromioclavicular (AC) joint 360, 360*f*
Acromion process fractures 339, 340*f*
outcomes 354
surgical indications 340
Advanced trauma life support (ATLS) 335, 381, 581, 582
cervical spine injury 379
ALL *see* Anterior longitudinal ligament (ALL)
Alonso-Llames approach, distal humerus 256, 256*f*
American College of Radiology (ACR) 95
American Spinal Injury Association (ASIA)
impairment scale 386
spinal cord injury assessment form 382, 382*f*
spinal cord injury grading 384–386, 385*f*, 385*t*
Anatomy
ankle joint 903*f*
cervical spine 416–418, 416*f*, 417*f*
clavicle 365–366, 365*f*
distal femur fractures 741–742, 741*f*
distal humerus 253–255, 254*f*
elbow 229–230, 229*f*
femoral neck fractures 618–624
femoral shaft fractures 713
hand and wrist 69–72, 70*f*
humeral shaft fractures 282–283
intertrochanteric femur fractures 656–657
metacarpals 36–37, 36*f*
patellar fractures 770–771
phalangeal fractures 6–7, 6*f*
proximal humerus 309–311, 310*f*, 311*f*
proximal tibia fractures 794–795
scaphoid 99–100, 99*f*, 100*f*
scapula 340–341, 341*f*
subtrochanteric femur fractures 677, 678*f*
thoracic and lumbar spine 447–448
Ankle-brachial index 738
Ankle fractures
anteromedial approach 935–936
bimalleolar 931
classification system 928–931
AO/OTA 929
Danis-Weber 928–929, 931*f*
Lauge-Hansen 928, 930*f*

concomitant 959*f*
diagnosis 927–928
CT scan 928
MRI 928
physical examination 927
radiography 927–928
squeeze test 927
dime sign 937*f*
external fixation role 932
fracture blisters 927*f*
hardware fixation loss 945
infection 945
treatment 946–947
lateral approach 935
malunion 946
nonunion 946
open 932
ORIF 931, 936–944
fibular length restoration 937*f*, 938*f*
lateral ankle incision dehiscence 947*f*
overview 926–927
peroneal tendonitis 946
posterior malleolar fractures 931
posterolateral approach 935
surgery 931–944
applied anatomy 932–935
approaches 935–936
complications 945–951
indications 931–932
outcomes 944–945
positioning 935
techniques 936–944
syndesmotic injuries 931–932, 946
unstable 944
wound breakdown 945
Ankle syndesmosis *see* Syndesmotic injury, ankle
Antegrade femoral nailing
femoral shaft fractures 713–720, 714*f*–718*f*
Anterior cord syndrome 387*t*, 388, 388*f*
Anterior cruciate ligament (ACL) 789
Anterior ligamentous complex injury, pelvis 498, 499*f*
Anterior longitudinal ligament (ALL) 449, 451
Anterior sacroiliac (SI) ligaments 496, 498
Anterior superior iliac spine (ASIS) 561, 563, 564, 621
Anterolateral approach
distal tibia fractures 901, 904*f*–906*f*, 915
humeral shaft fractures 283–284, 285*f*, 286*f*
proximal humerus fractures 314*f*, 315
talar neck fractures 971–972
Anteromedial approach
ankle fractures 935–936
distal tibia fractures 901–902, 906*f*–907*f*, 915
talar neck fractures 970–971
Antibiotic cement-coated nails
femoral shaft fractures 724
AO/OTA classification system
acetabular fractures 556*t*
ankle fractures 929
distal femur fractures 739, 740*f*
distal tibia fractures 900*f*
femoral neck fractures 616*f*
femoral shaft fractures 710, 711*f*, 712*f*
intertrochanteric femur/hip fractures 655, 656*f*
proximal humerus fractures 303, 308*f*
proximal tibia fractures 791–792, 791*f*
scapular fractures 336*t*
subtrochanteric femur fractures 675, 676*f*
tibial shaft fractures 846–847, 847*f*
Arthritis
acetabulum fracture 574–575
femoral head fractures 601
hip dislocations 601
patellar fractures 778
proximal tibia fractures 836, 839–840
scaphoid fractures 111, 113, 113*f*, 113*t see also* Scaphoid fractures
talus fractures 975–977
Arthrodesis 948–951, 950*f*, 991, 1001*f*
Arthroplasty 618
elbow 253, 254*f*, 264–265, 264*f*, 268
phalangeal fractures 19, 19*f*, 20*f*
radial head 228–229
Articular fragments, reconstruction 611–613
ASIA *see* American Spinal Injury Association (ASIA)
ASIF *see* Swiss Association for the Study of Internal Fixation (ASIF)
ASIS *see* Anterior superior iliac spine (ASIS)
Atlas-dens interval (ADI) 389*t*
Atlas fractures 396 *see also* Cervical spine injuries
classification of 397–398, 397*f*
clinical symptoms 397
injury mechanism 396
management 401
Gardner-Well tongs 403, 403*f*
Halo ring and vest orthotics 401–403, 402*f*
skeletal traction 403
ATLS *see* Advanced trauma life support (ATLS)
Autologous bone graft 188
Avascular necrosis (AVN) 309, 612
femoral neck fractures 640 *see also* femoral neck fractures
proximal humerus fractures 327, 330, 330*f*
scaphoid fractures 111, 112*f*
talus fractures 972–975
Axial dislocations 61, 61*f*, 68

B

Bag of bones method 253
BAI *see* Basion-axial interval (BAI)
Bare area 200
Basicervical femoral neck fractures 618
Basion-axial interval (BAI) 391–392, 393*f*
Basion-dental interval (BDI) 393*f*
Beach-chair position 311, 311*f*, 351, 352, 366, 366*f*
Bennett's fractures 34, 34*f see also* Metacarpal fractures
Bicondylar fractures 791 *see also* Proximal tibia fractures
dual plating 812, 813*f*–815*f*

hybrid circular external fixation 815–822, 818*f*–820*f*
locked plating 812–815, 816*f*–817*f*
Bimalleolar ankle fractures 931
Biplanar fluoroscopy 717
Blade plate management, subtrochanteric femur fractures 691–694, 692*f*, 693*f*
Blocking screws 748
subtrochanteric femur fractures 680, 682*f*
Blunt dissection 621
BMP *see* Bone morphogenic proteins (BMP)
Bone block arthrodesis, talus fractures 966–981
Bone morphogenic proteins (BMP) 759, 825
Bone scan, subtrochanteric femur fractures 673
Both bone fractures 169*f*, 171 *see also* Forearm fractures
intramedullary fixation 183, 184*f*–185*f*
surgical fixation 181–183, 182*f*
surgical indications 172
Brachial artery 172, 173
Brachial plexopathy 621
Brachial plexus 359
neurapraxia 374
Brachium, anatomy of 282–283
Bridge plating 45, 46
comminuted fractures 865
midshaft clavicle fixation 363
proximal metaphyseal tibial fracture 869*f*–870*f*
Brodén's views, subtalar joint 967*f*
Brooke and Jenkin's technique, C1–C2 fusion 426, 426*f*
Brown-Sequard syndrome 386–388, 387*t*, 388*f*
Bryan and Morrey approach, distal humerus 256
Burst fractures 448*f*, 449, 457–458, 458*f* *see also* Thoracic and lumbar spine fractures
stable 450, 454*f*
surgical management 462–463
unstable 450–451, 453, 454*f*
Buttress pin plate 162, 164*f*, 165*f*

C

Calcaneus fractures 954–966 *see also* Talus fractures
classification 954–955
concomitant ankle fractures 959*f*
diagnosis 954
displaced intra-articular fractures 956
Essex-Lopresti technique 957
grades 955
intramedullary nail 966
lateral extensile approach 957–958, 958*f*, 959*f*
medial approach 958–960, 960, 960*f*
ORIF 961*f*
infection and loss of reduction 964*f*–966*f*
medial exposure 962*f*–963*f*
physical examination 954
soft tissue complications 966
surgery
anatomy 955–956
techniques 957–960
sustenacular displacement 959–960
tibiotalocalcaneal fusion 966
Calcar of proximal humerus 310, 310*f*
CAM fracture boot *see* Controlled ankle motion (CAM) fracture boot
Campbell approach, distal humerus 255
Canadian C-spine rules 394*f*
Canadian Orthopaedic Trauma Society 359, 821
Cannulated screw fixation
anatomic considerations 625, 625*f*, 627*f*
instrumentation, patient positioning 625–626
pearls and pitfalls 629
technique 626–627, 628*f*, 629*f*, 631*f*
Capitate fractures 60 *see also* Carpal fractures and perilunate dislocations
Capitellum fractures 256, 265–266, 265*f*, 266*f*
Capsular reinforcements, types 618, 620
Capsulotomy 621
role of 640
C-arm fluoroscopy 625
Carpal dislocations 67
Carpal fractures 53–54
capitate 60
carpal dislocations 61–63
classification 55–63
complications 81–85
management of, case studies on 85–92
diagnosis 54
CT scans 55
history examination 54–55
MRI 56, 58*f*
physical examination 55
radiographic 54*f*, 55, 56*f*, 57*f*
hamate fractures 60
incidence 54
injury mechanism 54
lunate fractures 59–60, 60*f*
open reduction and internal fixation
of other carpal bone fractures 77
of perilunate dislocations 77–80
of scaphoid fractures 74–76, 75*f*, 76*f*
scaphoid fractures 58–59, 58*f*, 59*f*
see also Scaphoid fractures
surgical management
anatomy relevant to 69–72
dorsal midline approach 72–73, 73*f*
modified distal Henry approach 72
outcomes 80–81, 81*f*
patient positioning 72
techniques 74–80
trapezial fractures 59
triquetral fractures 59, 59*f*, 60*f*
Carpal instability 85
Carpometacarpal (CMC) joint, fracture-dislocations at 30–31, 34–35
see also Metacarpal fractures
CAS *see* Computer assisted surgery (CAS)
Cast immobilization, scaphoid fractures 94–95, 98

Causalgia 159
CBC *see* Complete blood count (CBC)
Central cord syndrome 386, 387*t*, 388*f*
Cephalomedullary nailing, subtrochanteric femur fractures 684–689, 685*f*–688*f*
Cerclage wire 771
Cervical spine injuries 379
  anatomy related to 416, 416*f*, 417*f*
    lower cervical spine 417–418
    upper cervical spine 416–417, 416*f*
  atlas fractures 397–398, 397*f*, 401–403, 402*f*, 403*f*
  case study
    lateral mass screws 444–445, 444*f*
    neglected C2–C3 fracture 442–443, 443*f*
    nonunion 441–442, 442*f*
  classification and scoring of 384–386
  cleared spine 394–395
  clinical evaluation 381
    local examination 381
    neurologic examination 381–384
  complications
    anterior fixation related 440–441, 440*t*
    due to lateral mass fixation 439
    injury-related 439
  CT scan 389, 391, 392*f*
  Hangman's fracture 398, 400–401, 400*f*, 400*t*, 401*f*, 404–405, 405*f*
  history/physical examination 379, 381
  incomplete 386–389
  injury mechanism 379
  lower 379
  motor examination 383–384
  MRI 380*f*, 389, 391, 392*f*
  occipital condyle fractures 395–396, 396*f*
  occipitocervical dislocation 396, 397*f*
  odontoid fractures 398, 399*f*, 399*t*, 404, 404*f*, 405*f*
  radiographic evaluation 379*t*, 380*f*, 389, 389*t*, 390*f*–391*f*, 393*f*
  rectal examination 384
  sensory examination 383
  subaxial cervical fractures 401, 405–416
  surgical management
    anterior approach 418–419
    anterior corpectomy and fusion 431–433, 433*f*, 434*f*, 435*f*
    C1–C2 fusion 421–426
    C2 odontoid fixation 426–427, 428*f*, 429*f*–430*f*, 431*f*
    C2 pars fixation 427, 429–430, 431*f*, 432*f*
    C1 posterior fixation 420–421, 420*f*, 421*f*
    lateral mass screw fixation 433, 435, 436*f*, 437*f*, 438*f*
    outcomes 438–439
    posterior approach 419
  upper 379
Chance fractures 451
Clavicle fractures 358–359
  anatomy related to 365–366, 365*f*
  case study
    nonunion repair 374–375, 375*f*
    nonunion repair with secondary brachial plexopathy 376, 376*f*
  classification
    Allman system 361, 361*f*
    Neer system 361, 362*f*
  complications 373
    brachial plexopathy 374
    hardware complications 374
    malunion 374
    nonunions 373–374
    thoracic outlet syndrome 374
    wound breakdown 374
  diagnosis 359–361
    CT scans 360
    MRI 360
    neurological evaluation 359
    physical examination 359
    radiographic evaluation 360, 360*f*
  distal third 361–362
  lateral 359, 369, 371, 371*f*, 372*f*, 373
  midshaft 359, 361, 361*f*, 362*f*, 367–369, 371–373
  nonoperative treatment 358–359
  surgical management
    approaches 366
    coracoclavicular screw fixation 371, 372*f*
    distal clavicle fixation 363–365, 364*f*
    indications for 361–365
    midshaft clavicle fixation 362–363, 364*f*, 367–368, 368*f*
    outcomes 371–373
    patient positioning 366, 366*f*
    plate fixation 362–363, 364*f*, 367–368, 368*f*
    Rockwood pin fixation 364*f*, 369, 370*f*
    transarticular and hook plate fixation 369, 371*f*
  treatment 358–359
Closed reduction and percutaneous pinning (CRPP)
  midfoot and forefoot fractures 990–991
  phalangeal fractures 4, 5*f*, 8, 10*f*, 13*f*
Cobb elevator 621
Cobra retractors 559
Colles fracture 128 *see also* Distal radius fractures
Comminuted fractures, bridge plating 865
Compartment syndrome
  bicondylar fractures 812
  foot 1013
    ORIF 1017
    treatment 1015–1018
  forearm 168
  leg, 887
    fasciotomy 890–891, 891*f*–892*f*
    management principles 891–893
    tibial shaft fractures and 846, 872
    treatment of 887–893, 891*f*–892*f*
  periscapular musculature 354
  proximal tibia fractures 786
  tibial plateau fractures 797–798
Complete blood count (CBC) 728
Complex elbow dislocations 224, 224*f*, 227*f*

Complex regional pain syndrome (CRPS) 159
Compression plate fixation 44–45, 46, 47*f*
Computed tomography (CT)
 acetabulum fracture 556–557
 ankle fractures 928
 carpal fractures and perilunate dislocations 55
 clavicle fractures 360
 distal femur fractures 739, 739*f*
 distal humerus fractures 250–251, 252*f*
 femoral head fractures and hip dislocations 582–583, 585*f*
 femoral neck fractures 612, 614*f*
 femoral shaft fractures 710
 forearm fractures 170
 metacarpal fractures 32, 33*f*
 midfoot and forefoot fractures 986
 Olecranon fractures 193, 195, 195*f*
 pelvic ring and sacral injuries 496
 proximal humerus fractures 303, 305*f*, 306*f*
 proximal tibia fractures 786
 scaphoid fractures 97
 subtrochanteric femur fractures 673, 683, 683*f*
 thoracic and lumbar spine fractures 455, 455*f*, 458*f*, 459, 461*f*
Computer assisted surgery (CAS) 683
 subtrochanteric femur fractures 683
Concomitant ankle fractures 959*f*
Condylar fractures, of phalanx 15, 15*f*
Constant shoulder scores (CSS) 359
Continuous passive motion (CPM) 777
Controlled ankle motion (CAM) fracture boot 997
Coracoclavicular (CC) ligaments 361, 362*f*
Coracoclavicular screw fixation, clavicle fractures 364*f*, 371, 372*f*
Coracoid process fractures 338–339, 339*f*
 operative technique 353
 outcomes 354
 surgical indications 340
Corona mortis 510, 510*f*, 562, 562*f*
Coronoid fracture 232, 239, 240*f*
Cortical ring sign 55, 57*f*
Cortical screw fixation 871
CPM *see* Continuous passive motion (CPM)
Craniocervical ligaments 417, 417*f*
C-reactive protein (CRP) 831
CRPP *see* Closed reduction and percutaneous pinning (CRPP)
Cruciate paralysis 386
Crush injury 846
CT *see* Computed tomography (CT)

D

Damage control orthopedics 726–727, 726*f*
 see also Femoral shaft fractures
Deep vein thrombosis (DVT) 694
 acetabulum fracture 573
 subtrochanteric femur fractures 695
Deltopectoral approach, proximal humerus fractures 312, 313*f*
Diaphyseal fibula fractures, ORIF 936–938
Dime sign 937*f*
Direct ulnar approach, forearm fractures 173, 174*f*
Disabilities of the arm, shoulder and hand (DASH) scores 359
Displaced femoral neck fractures
 instrumentation, implant and patient positioning 629, 632, 634*f*, 636*f*
 preoperative planning and anatomic consideration 629
 technique 632
Displaced intra-articular fractures, calcaneus 956
Dissolving pedicle sign 461
Distal femur fractures 737–738
 case study
  atrophic nonunion with stable implant 759, 761*f*, 762*f*
  chronic deep infection 759–764, 762*f*, 763*f*
  nonunion with implant failure 758–759, 760*f*
 classification 739
  AO/OTA Müeller's classification 739, 740*f*
 complications
  knee stiffness 756–757
  malunion 758
  nonunion 757–758
 diagnosis 738*f*
  CT scan 739, 739*f*
  MRI 739
  pearls and pitfalls 739
  X-rays 738, 739*f*
 outcomes 756
 surgical management
 acute knee arthroplasty 741
 anatomy 741–742, 741*f*
 external fixation 741
 intramedullary fixation 741
 lateral approach 742, 743*f*
 medial subvastus 743–745
 minimally invasive plate osteosynthesis plating 745, 746*f*
 positioning 742, 743*f*
 retrograde intramedullary nail 747–749, 747*f*
 type B fracture 751–753, 752*f*, 754*f*
 type C fracture 749–751, 750*f*, 751*f*
Distal fibular fractures
 ORIF 936–938
 posterior plating 937*f*
Distal humerus fractures 249
 anatomy related to 253–255, 254*f*
 case study
  elbow stiffness 268–270
  ulnar neuropathy 270–272
 classification 251–252
 complications 267
  elbow stiffness 267
  heterotopic ossification 267–268
  nonunion 268
  ulnar neuropathy 268
 diagnosis 250–251
  CT scan 250–251, 252*f*
  physical examination 250
  radiographic evaluation 250, 250*f*, 251*f*

incidence 249
nonoperative treatment 253
surgical management
approaches 255–257, 256*f*, 257*f*
elbow arthroplasty 253, 254*f*, 264–265, 264*f*
external fixation 253
indications for 252–253
open reduction and internal fixation 253, 257–263
outcomes 267
patient positioning 255, 255*f*
Distal interphalangeal (DIP) joint 7, 21
Distal radioulnar joint (DRUJ) 131*f*, 143, 143*f*, 154, 157, 161*f*, 162, 167, 168, 170–172, 178, 181, 224
Distal radius fractures 128–130
anatomy related to 143–144, 143*f*–145*f*
case study
intra-articular screw placement 159–162, 160*f*, 161*f*
loss of reduction 162, 163*f*–165*f*
classification 136–137, 136*f*
AO classification 136, 136*f*
Fernandez's 137, 138*f*, 139*f*
Frykman's 136
three-column theory 137, 140*f*
diagnosis 130–136
history examination 130
MRI scan 133
neurovascular functions assessment 130
physical examination 130
radiographic evaluation 129*f*, 130–131, 131*f*–133*f*
injury mechanism 128, 129*f*
intra-articular 160*f*
and perilunate dislocations 134, 135*f*
and radiocarpal dislocations 133–134, 134*f*, 135*f*
surgical management 137
closed reduction and external fixation 140, 141*f*
closed reduction and internal fixation 141*f*, 142
and complications 158–159
dorsal approach 145, 145*f*, 146*f*
extensile flexor carpi radialis approach 148
extensile volar-ulnar approach 148
modified Henry approach 148
open reduction and internal fixation 141*f*, 142, 142*f*
outcomes 158
patient positioning 145
radial approach 145
techniques 137, 140, 140*f*, 141*f*, 148–157
trans-FCR approach 145–148, 146*f*
volar approach 145–148
surgical techniques 148–157
dorsal plating 157
external fixation 150–151, 150*f*, 151*f*
intramedullary nailing 151–154, 152*f*–153*f*
Kirschner wire fixation 148–150, 149*f*
volar plating 154–157, 155*f*, 156*f*
treatment 130
unstable and displaced 130, 163*f*–164*f*
Distal tibia fractures 894–924
anterior and medial fixation 912*f*
anterolateral approach 901, 904*f*–906*f*, 915
anteromedial approach 901–902, 906*f*–907*f*, 915
aseptic malunion/nonunion, treatment 921–924
circular external fixation 902*f*
classification systems 898
AO/OTA classification 900*f*
Ruedi and Allgower 899*f*
closed 895*f*
complications 916–924
arthrosis 917
chronic osteomyelitis 916
malunion and nonunion 916–917, 923*f*–924*f*
management 917–924
soft tissue compromise 916
diagnosis 895–898
extra-articular 914–915
fibula fixation 911
fracture blisters 896*f*
infected nonunion, management 919–921
lateral approach 903
nonoperative management 888–889
nonunion repair, treatment 919
ORIF 899–901, 904*f*–907*f*, 915, 916
partial articular fracture 914*f*
overview 894–895
partial articular 913, 914*f*
posterolateral approach 902–903, 916
intraoperative image 908*f*
posterior shearing injury treatment 908*f*
postoperative care 913
recalcitrant nonunion, management 915–919, 922*f*
skin tenting 895*f*
soft tissue injury 896–897, 897*f*
special consideration 913–915
staged treatment 901–913, 915
first stage 903–911
second stage 911–913
spanning external fixation 910*f*
timing 911
surgical anatomy 901
surgical evolution 899–901
treatment outcomes 916
Dorsal extension block pinning, phalangeal fractures 15, 16*f*
Dorsal intercarpal (DIC) ligament 100, 100*f*
Dorsal plate fixation, distal radius fractures 142, 157, 159
Double-arc sign 250, 251*f*
Drill holes 324, 325*f*
DRUJ *see* Distal radioulnar joint (DRUJ)
DVT *see* Deep vein thrombosis (DVT)

Dynamic compression plate 182*f*, 183
  humeral shaft fractures 287
  olecranon fractures 198, 198*f*, 208
Dynamic external fixation, phalangeal fractures 15–16, 17*f*

E

East Baltimore lift 587 *see also* Femoral head fractures and hip dislocations
EDB *see* Extensor digitorum brevis (EDB)
Elbow 229–230, 229*f*
  instability 243, 246*f*, 247
  ligamentous stabilizers of 230, 230*f*
  stiffness 242
Empty vertebral body sign 461
Erythrocyte sedimentation rate (ESR) 831
Essex-Lopresti injury 243
Exchange nailing, tibia infection treatment 876, 877*f*–879*f*
Extensile volar-ulnar approach 148
Extensor digitorum brevis (EDB) 991
Extensor pollicis longus (EPL) tendon 105, 106*f*, 143
Extensor tendon adhesions 51
External fixation
  ankle fractures 932
  distal radius fractures 140, 141*f*, 150–151, 151*f*, 159
  phalangeal fractures 6
Extra-articular first-fifth metatarsal fractures 988
  with dorsal plating 1004*f*
  ORIF 1003–1006
    preoperative planning 1003–1004
    rehabilitation 1005
    technique 1004–1005
    wound closure 1005
  surgical indications 990
  surgical treatment of 993
Extra-articular metatarsal neck fractures, ORIF 1005*f*

F

Farabeuf/pelvic reduction clamp and screws, anterior pelvic fixation 511, 513*f*
Fasciotomy, leg compartment syndrome 890–891, 891*f*–892*f*
Fat pad sign 225
FCR *see* Flexor carpi radialis (FCR)
FDA *see* Food and Drug Administration (FDA)
Femoral circumflex artery
  lateral 618
  medial 618
Femoral head fractures and hip dislocations 581–582
  Allis maneuver 587
  case study
    nonunion and osteonecrosis management 606–609, 607*f*, 608*f*
    osteonecrosis management 605–606, 605*f*, 606*f*
  classification 585, 585*f*–587*f*
    Levin 585
    Pipkin 585, 587*f*, 587*t*
    Thomas and Epstein 585, 587*t*
  complications
    heterotopic ossification 602–603, 602*f*, 604*f*
    osteonecrosis 601–602
    post-traumatic arthritis 601
    residual instability 603–604
    retained loose bodies 603
    sciatic nerve injury 603
  diagnosis 582–583, 583*f*
    CT scan 582–583, 585*f*
    MRI 583
    pearls and pitfalls 583, 585
    radiographic evaluation 584*f*
    X-rays 582
  East Baltimore lift 587
  incidence 581
  Kocher-Langenbeck approach 592, 593
  osteosynthesis 590
  rehabilitation 600
  Smith-Peterson incision 593
  Stimson gravity technique 587
  surgical management
    anatomy 590–592
    anterolateral approaches 593
    arthroscopic excision 594–595
    indications 585–590, 588*t*, 589*f*, 591*f*, 592*f*
    Kocher-Langenbeck posterior approach 597–598, 597*f*, 598*f*
    patient positioning 592
    posterior approaches 593
    Smith-Peterson approach 595–597, 595*f*, 596*f*
    transtrochanteric approaches 593–594, 594*f*
    trochanteric flip osteotomy 598–600
  Watson-Jones incision 593
Femoral neck fractures 611–612
  basicervical 618
  case study
    angled blade plate fixation 642–645, 646*f*–650*f*
    loss of fixation 650–651
    subtrochanteric femur fracture 645–650
    total hip arthroplasty 640–642, 644*f*
  classification 613–617, 616*f*
    Garden 614, 617*f*
    Pauwels 617, 617*f*
  complications 641*f*
    avascular necrosis 640
    nonunion 639–640
  diagnosis 612
    CT scan 612, 614*f*
    MRI 612, 615*f*
    pearls and pitfalls 613
    physical examination 612
    radiographic evaluation 612, 613*f*
  health care expenditures 611
  outcomes 639
  radiographs 613*f*
  screw placement 629*f*
  surgical management
    anatomy and positioning 618–624
    closed reduction/cannulated screw fixation 625–629
    hemiarthroplasty 632–639

indications 618
ORIF of displaced 629–632
Femoral nerve palsy 573
Femoral shaft fractures 708–709
associated femoral neck fractures 727, 728*f*
case study
femur fracture infection 731–732, 731*f*, 732*f*
femur nonunion 730–731, 730*f*, 731*f*
classification 710
AO/OTA 710, 711*f*, 712*f*
Winquist-Hansen 710, 711*f*
complications
heterotopic ossification 730
infection 729
leg length discrepancy 729
malunion 728–729
nonunion 728
pudendal nerve palsy 730
damage control orthopedics 726–727, 726*f*
diagnosis
CT scan 710
history/physical examination 710
imaging 710
pearls and pitfalls 710
floating knee 727
gunshot wounds 725–726, 726*f*
open fractures 725
outcomes 725
surgical management
anatomy and positioning 713
antegrade femoral nailing 713–720, 714*f*–718*f*
antibiotic cement-coated nails 724
intramedullary nailing 712
plate fixation 712, 713*f*
retrograde intramedullary nailing 720–723, 720*f*, 721*f*
traction pin placement 723
vascular injuries 727
FHL tendon *see* Flexor hallucis longus (FHL) tendon
FiberWire 804
Fibula fixation, distal tibia fractures 911
Fibular length, restoration 937*f*, 938*f*
Fibular sesamoid fracture 986*f*
tangential sesamoid radiograph 986*f*
Finger alignment, metacarpal fractures and 31
Fixation failure, olecranon fractures 214, 217–219, 218*f*
Flexion distraction injuries, spine 451
Flexor digitorum profundis (FDP) 143
Flexor hallucis longus (FHL) tendon 934
Flexor pollicis longus (FPL) 143
Floating knee 727 *see also* Femoral shaft fractures
Food and Drug Administration (FDA) 825
Forearm fractures 167–168, 169*f*
anatomy related to 167–168, 168*f*, 172–173
both bones fractures 171, 172
case study
nonunions 186–188, 188*f*
synostosis 188–190, 189*f*, 190*f*
classification 170–171
complications 184
infection 185, 186*f*
malunion 186
nonunions 186
synostosis 186, 187*f*
diagnosis 168
CT scan 170
MRI 170
neurovascular examination 168
radiographic evaluation 168–170, 169*f*
Galeazzi fractures 170–172
incidence 168
injury mechanism 168
Monteggia fracture 170, 171–172, 171*f*
radial shaft fractures 170, 172
surgical management
direct ulnar approach 173
Henry approach 173, 174*f*
indications 171–172
outcomes 183–184
patient positioning 173
techniques 173–183
Thompson approach 173
ulnar shaft fracture 170, 171
Fracture blisters
ankle fractures 927*f*
associated with distal tibia fractures 896*f*
Frankel scale, spinal cord injury 384

G

Galeazzi fractures 169f, 170–171 *see also* Forearm fractures
surgical approach 178, 180*f*, 181, 181*f*
surgical indications 172
Gallie technique, C1–C2 fusion 425–426, 426*f*
Garden classification, femoral neck fractures 614, 617*f*
Gardner-Well tongs 403, 403*f*
Gerdy's tubercle 795
Gilula's lines 55, 56*f*
Glenohumeral joint 342*f*
Glenoid fractures 337–338, 338*f*
exposure of 342*f*
operative technique 348–349, 351–352, 351*f*
outcomes 354
surgical indications 340
Glenopolar angle 337, 337*f*
Goel-Harm's technique, C1–C2 fusion 424–425, 424*f*, 425*f*
Greater sigmoid notch 200
Guidewire placement, tibial shaft fracture 854, 855*f*
Gunshot wounds 725–726, 726*f* *see also* Femoral shaft fractures

H

Hallucal fracture-dislocations
ORIF 1008–1009
rehabilitation 1009
technique 1008–1009
wound closure 1009
preoperative planning 1008

Hallucal joint injuries 988–989
  surgical approach 993
Hallucal sesamoid fractures 989
  ORIF 1010–1011
    preoperative planning 1010
    rehabilitation 1011
    technique 1010–1011
    wound closure 1011
  surgical approach 993–994
  surgical indications 990
Halo ring 401–403, 402*f*
Halo vest 396, 401
Hamate fractures 60, 67
Hangman's fracture 398, 400–401, 400*f*, 400*t*, 401*f*, 404–405, 405*f*
Hardware complications, olecranon fractures 213–214
Hardware fixation, ankle fractures 945
Harris Hip Scores 639
Hemiarthroplasty
  femoral neck fractures
    instrumentation, implant and patient positioning 636
    pearls and pitfalls 639
    preoperative planning 632, 635–636
    technique 636–637, 638*f*
  proximal humerus fractures 324–326, 325*f*, 328
Hemi-hamate reconstruction, phalangeal fractures 18–19, 18*f*
Hemorrhagic blisters, ankle fractures 927*f*
Henry approach, forearm fractures 173, 174*f*
Henry approach, modified, volar distal radius 148
Herbert's classification system, scaphoid fractures 97, 98*t*
Heterotopic ossification (HO) 582, 602–603, 602*f*, 604*f*, 730
    see also Femoral shaft fractures
  acetabulum fracture 572–573
  distal humerus fractures 267–270, 271*f*
  elbow dislocations 241–242
  olecranon fractures 215, 216*f*
Hindfoot fractures
  calcaneus fractures 954–966
  overview 953
  talus fractures 966–981
Hip joint, ligaments 618, 620*f*
HO *see* Heterotopic ossification (HO)
Hoffa fracture 739, 739*f*, 753–756, 755*f*
    see also Distal femur fractures
Hohmann retractor 749
Hook plate fixation
  clavicle fractures 364, 364*f*
  olecranon fractures 198, 198*f*, 206, 208, 208*f*
Horner's syndrome 359
Hospital for special surgery (HSS) 821
HSS *see* Hospital for special surgery (HSS)
Humeral shaft fractures 276–277, 277*f*
  anatomy related to 282–283
  case management
    nonunion 296–300, 297*f*–299*f*
    radial nerve injury 295–296, 295*f*
  classification 279–281, 280*f*
  complications
    iatrogenic fracture extension 294–295
    insertion site morbidity 294
    nonunion 294
    radial nerve palsy 294
  diagnosis 277–279, 278*f*, 279*f*
    neurovascular examination 277–278, 278*f*
    physical examination 277
    radiographic evaluation 278–279, 279*f*
  nonoperative management 281
  open fractures 279, 281
  pathologic 276, 277*f*
  surgical management
    anterolateral approach 283–284, 285*f*, 286*f*
    indications for 281, 281*t*
    intramedullary nailing 281–282, 282*f*, 288–293, 291*f*–292*f*
    medial approach 286–287
    open reduction internal fixation 281, 282*f*, 287–288, 288*f*, 289*f*
    outcomes 293–294
    patient positioning 283, 284*f*
    posterior approach 284, 286*f*
    triceps-sparing approach 285
    triceps-splitting approach 285
Humpback deformity 100, 101*f*, 111
Hypertrophic nonunion, tibia 883–886, 886*f*
Hypovolemic shock 381

I

Iliac crest pin 501, 502*f* *see also* Pelvic ring and sacral injuries
Iliofemoral ligament 620
Iliosacral screw insertion, retropelvic fixation 517–537, 518*f*–539*f*
  prone technique 524–537, 527*f*–537*f*
    imaging 524–527
    insertion technique 527–529
    sacral dysmorphism 531–533
    sacral fracture style screws 530–531
    sacroiliac style screws 530
    sacroiliac *vs.* sacral style screws 529–530
    S2 screws 533–535
    transiliac-transsacral screws 535–536, 536*f*–538*f*
  supine technique 517–524, 518*f*–524*f*
Iliotibial (IT) band 795
Ilizarov method 876
  chronic osteomyelitis 880
Incisions
  metacarpal fractures 37, 37*f*
  olecranon 202, 202*f*
  phalangeal fractures 7, 7*f*
Infections
  forearm fractures 185, 186*f*
  olecranon fractures 217
  proximal humerus fractures 327
Interosseous ligaments 498
Interphalangeal (IP) joint 2, 7
Intertrochanteric femur/hip fractures
  case study
    lag screw cut-out 667, 668*f*
    nonunion 667, 669f, 670*f*
  classification 655
    AO/OTA 655, 656*f*
  complications 666–667

diagnosis 654–655
MRI 655
pearls and pitfalls 655
radiographic evaluation 655
incidence 654
outcomes 663–666
surgical management
anatomy and positioning 656–658, 657*f*, 658*f*
fracture reduction 658–659, 659*f*, 660*f*
indications 655
intramedullary nailing 661–663
ORIF 659–661
types of 655
Intramedullary devices, for midshaft clavicle fixation 363 *see also* Clavicle fractures
Intramedullary (IM) nailing
calcaneus fractures 966
distal radius fractures 141*f*, 142, 151–154, 152*f*–153*f*, 159
distal tibial metadiaphyseal fracture 863–871
humeral shaft fractures 281–282, 282*f*, 288–293, 291*f*–292*f*, 293
of intertrochanteric femur/hip fractures
pearls and pitfalls 663
preoperative planning 661–662
technique 662–663, 662*f*, 664*f*–665*f*
olecranon fractures 199–200, 199*f*, 209, 210*f*
proximal humerus fractures 321–324, 322*f*, 323*f*
subtrochanteric femur fractures 679
talus fractures 976–977
tibia 857*f*
tibial shaft fractures 849–871
acute infection treatment 873*f*–875*f*
patient assessment 850
portal preparation 852*f*
preoperative planning 849–850
proximal 858–863
reamed, locked 849–858
technique 850–858
Ischiofemoral ligament 620
IT band *see* Iliotibial (IT) band

J

Jersey finger fractures 20–21
Joint stiffness, after finger fracture fixation 27
Judet approach, scapula 343, 344*f*
Judet quadricepsplasty 757

K

Kaplan approach, radial head fractures 231, 232*f*
Kirschner (K) wires 4
distal femur fractures 745, 746*f*
distal radius fractures 141*f*, 142, 148–150, 149*f*, 158
femoral neck fractures 632
lateral clavicle fractures 369
olecranon fractures 202–206, 203*f*–204*f*
patellar fractures 771
proximal humerus fractures 316
proximal tibia fractures 801
scaphoid fractures 99, 101, 104*f*, 105
subtrochanteric femur fractures 691
Knee Society Pain Score 757
Knee Society Rating Scale (KSRS) 836
Kocher approach, radial head fractures 231, 232*f*
Kocher-Langenbeck approach 592, 593 *see also* Femoral head fractures
Koch's biomechanical study, subtrochanteric femur fractures 677
KSRS *see* Knee Society Rating Scale (KSRS)
Kyphoplasty 468, 469*f*, 470*f*

L

Lag screw fixation 44, 45–46, 46*f*
Lateral collateral ligament (LCL) 230, 230*f*, 231, 237*f*–238*f*, 239, 239*f*, 247, 789
Lateral malleolar fractures 931
Lateral mass screw fixation, cervical spine injuries 433, 435, 436*f*, 437*f*, 438*f*, 439
Lateral ulnar collateral ligament (LUCL) complex 224, 229, 229*f*
Lauge-Hansen classification system, ankle fractures 928, 930*f*
LCL *see* Lateral collateral ligament (LCL)
Leg length discrepancy 729 *see also* Femoral shaft fractures
Less invasive stabilization system (LISS) 756
Levin classification, femoral head fractures 585
Lisfranc fracture-dislocation 987*f*
classification systems 987–989
homolateral
complete 987*f*
incomplete 988*f*
midfoot arthrodesis 999–1003
preoperative planning 999–1000
rehabilitation 1002–1003
technique 1000–1002
wound closure 1002
ORIF 994–999
anatomical factors 994
instrumentation and implant 994–995
patient factors 995
preoperative planning 994–995
rehabilitation 997–999
technique 995–996
wound closure 996–997
ROM exercises 997
two-incision approach 1001–1002
Lisfranc injury 987*f*
diagnosis 986–987
ORIF radiographs 997*f*, 998*f*
Lisfranc ligament, neglected injury 1001*f*
LISS *see* Less invasive stabilization system (LISS)
Lister's tubercle 105, 106*f*, 143, 143*f*
LMWH *see* Low molecular weight heparin (LMWH)
Locked plates 307, 326
Log-roll maneuver 381
Long oblique fracture, reduction 851*f*

Long radiolunate (LRL) ligament 70, 70*f*
Low molecular weight heparin (LMWH) 827
Lunate dislocations 61
Lunate fractures 59–60, 60*f*, 143, 144*f*, 165*f*
see also Carpal fractures and perilunate dislocations
Lysholm scores 725

M

Magerl's technique, C1–C2 fusion 421–424, 422*f*, 423*f*
Magnetic resonance imaging (MRI)
ankle fractures 928
carpal fractures 56
clavicle fractures 360
distal femur fractures 739
distal radius fractures 133
femoral head fractures and hip dislocations 583
femoral neck fractures 612, 615*f*
forearm fractures 170
intertrochanteric femur fractures 655
midfoot and forefoot fractures 986–987
proximal tibia fractures 786
scaphoid fractures 96–97, 97*f*
subtrochanteric femur fractures 673
thoracic and lumbar spine fractures 455, 456*f*, 459–460
Malleolar ankle fractures 930*f*
lateral 931
posterior 931
Mallet fractures 21–22, 22*f*
Malunion
acetabulum fracture 574
ankle fractures 946
clavicle fractures 374
forearm fractures 186
metacarpal fractures 51
olecranon fractures 214
phalangeal fractures 23–26, 25*f*
proximal humerus fractures 327
radial head fractures 242
scapular fractures 354
talus fractures 975
Mayo scissors 621
Mayo stand cover 621
Medial collateral ligament (MCL) 229, 229*f*, 230, 789
Medial coronoid approach, radial head fractures 231–232, 233*f*
Medial femoral circumflex artery (MFCA) 583
Medial malleolus fractures 948*f*
nonunion, treatment 947–948
operative fixation 938–941
supination-adduction vertical shear type 940*f*
transverse 940
Medial open wound, open ankle fractures 932*f*
Medial wounds, open tibial fracture 896*f*
Median nerve 71, 172
compression of 130
Metacarpal fractures 30–31
anatomy related to 36–37, 36*f*
case study
finger stiffness 51, 51*f*
tendon rupture 51–52, 52*f*
classification 33–35, 33*t*, 34*f*
closed reduction, pinning 40–44, 41*f*–43*f*
Bennett fractures 47–48, 48*f*, 49*f*
Bouqet pinning 41*f*
cross pinning 40, 41*f*
crucifix pinning 40, 41*f*, 42*f*, 43
intramedullary pinning 41*f*, 43, 43*f*
transarticular pinning 41*f*, 44
transverse pinning 41*f*
complications 50
malunion 51
nonunion 51
stiffness 50–51
diagnosis 31–33
CT scan 32, 33*f*
physical examination 31, 31*f*
radiographic evaluation 31–32,32*f*
etiologies 30
fifth metacarpal neck fracture 30,31*f*
incidence 30
surgical management
approaches for 37–38, 37*f*, 38*f*, 39*f*
basal thumb metacarpal fractures 35–36
indications for 35–36
metacarpal shaft fractures 35
outcomes 50
patient positioning 37
pinning technique 40–44, 41*f*–43*f*, 47–48, 48*f*, 49*f*
plate and screw fixation 38–39, 49*f*, 44–47, 45*f*–47*f*, 48, 50*f*
Wagner approach 38, 39*f*
thumb 30, 32–33
Metacarpophalangeal (MP) joints 2, 6, 31
open wounds 31
stiffness 51
Metatarsophalangeal (MTP) joints 984
Methicillin-resistant *Staphylococcus aureus* (MRSA) 872
MFCA *see* Medial femoral circumflex artery (MFCA)
Midaxial approach, radial head fractures 231, 232*f*
Midfoot and forefoot fractures 983–1019
anatomy related to 984, 984*f*
classification systems 987–989
compartment syndrome 1013
treatment 1015–1018
diagnosis 985–987
computed tomography 986
imaging 986
MRI 986–987
physical examination 985
radiographs 986
soft tissue examination 985–986
hallucal joint injuries 988–989
management 1013–1018
midfoot fusion 991
nonunion 1012–1013
vs refracture 1015
ORIF 990, 994–999, 1003–1011
overview 983–985
postoperative infection 1012
post-traumatic arthritis 1012
treatment 1013
proximal fifth metatarsal fractures 985

proximal phalangeal fractures 988, 989*f*
standard dual-incision 992*f*
standard incision 993*f*–994*f*
surgery
anatomy 991–992
approaches 992–994
complications 1012–1018
indications 989–991
outcomes 1011–1012
positioning 992
techniques 994–1012
wounds 1012
Midfoot fusion 991
Minimally invasive plate osteosynthesis (MIPO) 745
proximal metaphyseal tibial fracture 869*f*–870*f*
Monteggia fractures 169*f*, 170 *see also* Forearm fractures
Bado classification 170, 171*f*
surgical approach 178, 179*f*
surgical indications 171–172
Moore classification, proximal tibia fractures 792, 792*f*, 793*f*
Morel-Lavallee lesion 496, 497*f*
Motor index scoring 384
MRI *see* Magnetic resonance imaging (MRI)
MRSA *see* Methicillin-resistant *Staphylococcus aureus* (MRSA)
MTP joints *see* Metatarsophalangeal (MTP) joints
Müeller's classification, distal femur fractures 739

N

Naviculocuneiform fusion 1001*f*
Nerve palsy, acetabulum fracture 573
Neurogenic shock 381
vs. hypovolemic shock 381
Neurovascular examination
forearm fractures 168
humeral shaft fractures 277–278, 278*f*
Nightstick fractures 170 *See also* Ulnar shaft fractures
Nonsteroidal anti-inflammatory drugs (NSAIDs) 835
Nonunion
acetabulum fracture 574
ankle fractures 946
clavicle fractures 359, 373–374
distal humerus fractures 268, 272–273, 273*f*, 274*f*
distal tibia
post-traumatic arthritis 918*f*
revision ORIF 921*f*
femoral neck fractures 639–640
femoral shaft fractures 728
forearm fractures 186–188, 188*f*
humeral shaft 294, 296–300, 297*f*–299*f*
intertrochanteric femur/hip fractures 667, 669*f*, 670*f*
medial malleolus fracture 947–948
midfoot and forefoot fractures 1012–1013
olecranon fractures 214–215, 214*f*
patellar fractures 777, 780*f*, 781*f*
proximal tibia fractures 831–836
radial head fractures 242–243
scaphoid fractures 95, 110–111, 111*f*
subtrochanteric femur fractures 696–697
NSAID *see* Nonsteroidal anti-inflammatory drugs (NSAIDs)

O

OA *see* Osteoarthritis (OA)
Obturator artery 618
Occipital condyle fractures 395–396, 396*f* *see also* Cervical spine injuries
Occipitocervical dislocations 316, 317*f* *see also* Cervical spine injuries
Odontoid fractures 398, 398*f*
classification of 399*f*, 399*t*
management 404, 404*f*, 405*f*
Type III 399*f*
Olecranon fractures 192, 192*f*
anatomy related to 200–201, 200*f*
case study
fixation failures 217–219, 218*f*
classification 195
Colton 195
Mayo 195, 196*f*
Schatzker 195
and complex elbow fractures 193, 194*f*
complications 213
fixation failure 214
hardware complications 213–214
heterotopic ossification 215, 216*f*
infection 217
malunions 214
nonunions 214–215, 214*f*
proximal radioulnar joint injury 215, 217, 217*f*, 219, 220*f*
stiffness 215
ulnar neuropathy 217
diagnosis
CT scans 193, 195, 195*f*
physical examination 193
radiographic evaluation 193
injury mechanisms 192
surgical management
excision with triceps advancement 200, 200*f*, 211–212, 211*f*
indications for 195–200
intramedullary nailing 198–200, 199*f*, 209, 210*f*
outcomes 212–213
patient positioning 201–202, 201*f*
plate fixation 198, 198*f*, 206–209, 207*f*, 208*f*
posterior approach 202, 202*f*
tension band fixation 197–198, 197*f*, 202–206, 203*f*–204*f*
Olecranon osteotomy 256, 257*f*
Open ankle fractures 932
dislocation with morbid obesity 933*f*
with medial open wound 932*f*
Open fractures 725 *see also* Femoral shaft fractures
Open reduction and internal fixation (ORIF) 16–17, 17*f*

ankle fractures 931
calcaneus fractures 961*f*
capitellum fracture 265–266, 265*f*, 266*f*
carpal bones and fragments 77, 77*f*
compartment syndrome, foot 1017
diaphyseal fibula fractures 936–938
of displaced femoral neck fractures
  instrumentation, implant and patient positioning 629, 632, 634*f*, 636*f*
  preoperative planning and anatomic consideration 629
  technique 632
distal femur fractures 740–741
  type B3/Hoffa 753–756, 755*f*
  type B/unicondylar 751–753, 752*f*, 754*f*
  type C 749–751, 750*f*, 751*f*
distal fibular fractures 936–938
distal humerus fractures 253, 257–263
  extra-articular 258, 259*f*–261*f*
  intra-articular 258, 262*f*
distal radius fractures 141*f*, 142, 142*f*, 158
distal tibia fractures 899–901
extra-articular first-fifth metatarsal fractures 1003–1006
extruded talus 977, 978*f*–979*f*, 980*f*
  of fibula 857*f*
hallucal fracture-dislocations 1008–1009
hallucal sesamoid fractures 1010–1011
humeral shaft fractures 281, 282*f*, 287–288, 288*f*, 289*f*, 293
of intertrochanteric femur/hip fractures
  pearls and pitfalls 661
  preoperative planning 659
  technique 659–660, 661*f*
Lisfranc fracture-dislocation 994–999
midfoot and forefoot fractures 990, 994–999, 1003–1011
open calcaneus fractures 961*f*–963*f*
partial articular fracture 914*f*
perilunate dislocations 77–80, 78*f*–79*f*
phalangeal fractures 5, 5*f*, 8, 14*f*, 15, 17, 26, 26*f*
proximal fifth metatarsal fractures 1006–1008
proximal humerus fractures 315–321, 317*f*, 318*f*–319*f*, 320*f*–321*f*
proximal metaphyseal tibial fracture 869*f*–870*f*
scaphoid fractures 74–76, 98
  dorsal approach 105, 106*f*, 107*f*
  volar approach 101–104, 102*f*–104*f*
tibial diaphyseal fracture 864–870
  indications 864–865
  technique 865
tibial shaft fracture 866*f*–868*f*
ORIF *see* Open reduction and internal fixation (ORIF)
Orthopaedic Trauma Association (OTA) 613, 767
Osteoarthritis (OA) 590
Osteomyelitis
  1Λ 872
  chronic, cure 877
  distal tibia fractures 916
  implants removal 876
Osteonecrosis 601–602 *see also* Femoral head fractures
OTA *see* Orthopaedic Trauma Association (OTA)

P

Palmaris longus (PL) 69
Paraplegia 386
Patellar fractures
  case study 778–784
    knee stiffness 778, 783–784
    partial or total patellectomy 778
    revision fixation 778
  classification 767–770
  complications
    arthritis 778
    hardware irritation 777
    infection 777, 779*f*, 780*f*
    knee stiffness 777–778, 782*f*, 783*f*
    loss of reduction 777
    nonunion 777, 780*f*, 781*f*
  diagnosis 766–767, 768*f*, 769*f*
    pearls and pitfalls 767
    physical examination 766–767
    radiographic evaluation 767
    saline load test 767
  management
    anatomy and positioning 770–771
    indications 770
    partial patellectomy 770
  outcomes 777
  surgical management
    partial patellectomy 773–776
    tension band technique 771–773
Patient positioning *see* Positioning, patient
Pauwels angle 629, 632
Pauwels classification, femoral neck fractures 617, 617*f*
PCL *see* Posterior cruciate ligament (PCL)
Pedicle fracture 484
Pelvic C-clamp 520–521
Pelvic instability 497 *see also* Pelvic ring and sacral injuries
Pelvic ring and sacral injuries 495–496
  anterior ligamentous complex injury 498, 499*f*
  classification 496–499, 499*f*
  complications, management of
    errant placement of anterior external fixation pins 541, 543, 543*f*
    nonunion of pelvis after anterior external fixation 544, 548–550, 548*f*–550*f*
    percutaneous treatment of pelvic fracture nonunion 543–544, 547*f*–549*f*
    unstable injury with malreduction of posterior ring 538–539, 540*f*–542*f*, 541

diagnosis 496
clinical evaluation 496, 497*f*
CT scan 496
radiographic evaluation 496, 498*f*
sacral fracture classification 499, 499*f*
surgical management 499–501, 500*f*, 501*f*
anterior iliac crest pin insertion 501–502, 502*f*–505*f*
anterior pelvic fixation 505, 507–517
external fixation of pelvis 501–505
iliosacral screw insertion 517–537, 518*f*–539*f*
medullary ramus screws 513–516, 516*f*
supra-acetabular pins insertion 502, 502*f*, 505, 506*f*–508*f*
symphyseal plate fixation 507–513, 510*f*–515*f*
unstable 500*f*, 501*f*
Perched facets 409
Percutaneous fixation
distal radius fractures 142
scaphoid fractures 98, 110
dorsal approach 107–110, 109*f*
volar approach 105, 107, 108*f*
Periarticular locking plates 258, 258*f*
olecranon fractures 198, 198*f*
Perilunate dislocations 54, 55, 57*f*, 61, 62*f*, 63*f*, 81 *see also* Carpal fractures
greater arc 134, 135*f*
Peroneal nerve palsy 621
Peroneal tendonitis, ankle fractures 946
Pfannenstiel approach, anterior pelvic fixation 508–511, 510*f*
Phalangeal fractures 1–2
anatomy related to 6–7, 6*f*
classification 2, 4
comminuted 2, 4
complications 23
malunion 23–26, 25*f*
stiffness 24, 26–27, 26*f*
condylar fracture 15, 15*f*
diagnosis 2
pearls and pitfalls 2
physical examination 2, 3*f*
radiograph evaluation 2, 4*f*
ultrasound 2
diaphyseal 11–12, 13*f*, 14*f*
distal 4, 20–21, 22*f*
extra-articular 4, 8, 10*f*
incidence 1
injury mechanisms 1
intra-articular 4, 12*f*, 15
Jersey finger fractures 20–21
mallet fracture 21–22, 22*f*
middle 4, 15–19, 16*f*–20*f*
nondisplaced 4
proximal 4, 8, 8*f*, 10–11, 10*f*, 11*f*, 12*f*
spiral 4
surgical management 7–8
CRPP 4, 5*f*
dorsal approach 8, 8*f*
external fixation 6
incisions placement 7, 7*f*
indications 4–6
midaxial approach 8, 9*f*
ORIF 5, 5*f*
positioning 7
techniques 8–21
volar approach 8, 9*f*
transverse 2
treatment 1–2
Physical examination
carpal fractures and perilunate dislocations 55
clavicle fractures 359
distal humerus fractures 250
distal radius fractures 130
femoral neck fractures 612
femoral shaft fractures 710
humeral shaft fractures 277
metacarpal fractures 31, 31*f*
olecranon fractures 193
patellar fractures 766–767
phalangeal fractures 2, 3*f*
proximal humerus fracture 303
proximal tibia fractures 786
scaphoid fractures 95, 95*f*
subtrochanteric femur fractures 673
Pilon fractures *see* Distal tibia fractures
PIN *see* Posterior interosseous nerve (PIN)
Pin tract infection 159
Pipkin classification, 585, 587*f*, 587*t*
Piriformis tendon 622
Plafond fracture, foot position and 898*f*
Plate and screw fixation
Bennett fractures 48, 50*f*
metacarpal neck fractures 44, 45*f*
metacarpal shaft fractures 44–47, 46f, 47*f*
midshaft clavicle fixation 362–363, 364*f*, 367–368, 368*f*
olecranon fractures 198, 198*f*, 206–209, 207*f*, 208*f*
PMMA *see* Polymethylmethacrylate (PMMA)
Pneumatic tourniquet 749
Poller screws 748
Polymethylmethacrylate (PMMA) 466, 468, 822, 875, 875*f*
Popliteal artery 738
Positioning, patient
ankle fractures 935
calcaneus fractures 955–956
distal femur fractures 742, 743*f*
femoral head fractures and hip dislocations 592
femoral neck fractures 618–622
femoral shaft fractures 713
forearm fractures 173
humeral shaft fractures 283, 284*f*
intertrochanteric femur fractures 657, 657*f*, 658*f*
metacarpal fractures 37
patellar fractures 770–771
phalangeal fractures 7
proximal humerus fractures 311–312, 311*f*, 312*f*
proximal tibia fractures 794–795
subtrochanteric femur fractures 677–678
talus fractures 970
tibial shaft fractures 848

Posterior cord syndrome 387*t*, 388–389, 388*f*
Posterior cruciate ligament (PCL) 789
Posterior interosseous nerve (PIN) 71, 172, 230
Posterior longitudinal ligament (PLL) 449
Posterior malleolar fractures 931
  anatomic reduction 941–942
  closed reduction 941*f*
  open reduction 942
  ORIF 941–942
Posterior malleolus 934
Posterior sacroiliac (SI) ligaments 498
Posterior superior iliac spine (PSIS) 564
Posterior vertebral angle 454–455
Posterior vertebral height 454–455
Posterolateral approach
  ankle fractures 935
  distal tibia fractures 902–903, 916
Post-traumatic arthritis 1012
  Lisfranc injury 1013, 1014*f*
  treatment 1013
Post-traumatic arthrosis
  loss of reduction 948–951, 949*f*–950*f*
Powers ratio 389*t*, 393*f*, 396
Pronator quadratus (PQ) muscle 143
Proximal femoral locking plate
  subtrochanteric femur fractures 679, 689–691, 690*f*
Proximal femur, anatomy 619*f*
Proximal fifth metatarsal fractures 985
  ORIF 1006–1008
  preoperative planning 1006
  rehabilitation 1005
  technique 1006–1007
  wound closure 1005
Proximal humerus fractures 302
  anatomy related to 309–311, 310*f*, 311*f*
  bone graft substitutes 317–318, 318*f*–319*f*
  case study
    failure of fixation followed by hemiarthroplasty 328, 330, 330*f*
    failure of fixation followed by revision of fixation 328, 329*f*
    ORIF followed by infected nonunion 330–332, 331*f*
  classification 303, 307*f*, 308*f*
    AO/OTA classification system 303, 308*f*
    Neer classification 303, 307*f*
  complications 327–328
    avascular necrosis 327
    hemiarthroplasty-related 328
    infection 327
    varus malunion 327
  cortical thickness measurement 306, 309*f*
  diagnosis 302–303
    CT scan 303, 305*f*, 306*f*
    history examination 302–303
    physical examination 303
    radiographic imaging 303, 304*f*
  in elderly 309
  head-split 318, 320–321, 320*f*–321*f*
  incidence 302
  surgical management
    anterolateral acromial approach 314*f*, 315, 316
    deltopectoral approach 312, 313*f*
    hemiarthroplasty 324–326, 325*f*
    indications for 304, 306–309
    intramedullary nailing 321–324, 322*f*, 323*f*
    open reduction internal fixation 315–321, 317*f*–321*f*
    outcomes 326–327
    patient positioning 311–312, 311*f*, 312*f*
  treatment 302
Proximal interlocking, tibial shaft fractures 854
Proximal interphalangeal (PIP) joint 6, 15, 18–19, 20*f*, 21
Proximal phalangeal fractures 988, 989*f*
Proximal radioulnar joint (PRUJ) injury, olecranon fractures 215, 217, 217*f*, 219, 220*f*
Proximal tibia fractures 785
  case study
    infection 830–831, 831*f*–833*f*
    loss of fixation 827–830, 828*f*–830*f*
    malunion and nonunion 831–836, 834*f*–835*f*, 837*f*–839*f*
    post-traumatic arthritis 836–840
  classification
    AO/OTA 791–792, 791*f*
    Moore 792, 792*f*, 793*f*
    Schatzker 790–791, 790*f*
  diagnosis
    associated injuries 789–790
    CT scan 786
    imaging 786–787, 787*f*, 788*f*
    mechanism of injury 787–789
    MRI 786
    pearls and pitfalls 790
    physical examination 786
  surgical management
    anatomy and positioning 794–796, 795*f*, 796*f*
    bicondylar fractures 812–822
    emergent treatment 796–799, 798*f*–800*f*
    indications 792
    lateral fracture dislocations 804, 804*f*
    medial plateau fracture 805, 806*f*, 807*f*
    posterolateral fracture 801–805
    posteromedial fracture 805–811, 808*f*–811*f*
    postoperative care 826–827
    pure depression fracture 801, 803*f*
    repair 794
    split depression fracture 801, 802*f*
    split fracture 799–801
    tibial plateau fracture 822–826, 823*f*, 824*f*, 826*f*
Pseudorotator cuff rupture 335
Ptotic eyelid 359–360
Pubofemoral ligament 620
Pudendal nerve palsy 730
Pulmonary embolism, acetabulum fracture 573

Q

Quadricepsplasty 757
  Judet 757
  Thompson 757

R

Radial head fractures 223
  anatomy related to 229–230, 229*f*, 230*f*
  case study
    elbow instability 246*f*, 247
    longitudinal forearm instability 243–247
  classification 226, 228*f*
    Broberg and Morrey 226, 228*f*
    Hotchkiss 226
    Mason 226
  complications
    elbow instability 243
    elbow stiffness 242
    Essex-Lopresti injury 243
    heterotopic ossification 241–242
    longitudinal instability of forearm 243
    malunions 242
    nonunion 242–243
  diagnosis 224–226
    CT scan 226
    physical examination 224
    radiographic evaluation 225–226, 225*f*
  with elbow dislocations 223–224, 224*f* (*see also* Complex elbow dislocations)
  injury mechanism 223
  isolated 223, 224*f*
  nonoperative treatment 228
  surgical management 226, 228–229
    indications for 226, 228–229
    Kaplan approach 231, 232*f*
    Kocher approach 231, 232*f*
    medial coronoid approach 231–232, 233*f*
    midaxial approach 231, 232*f*, 233
    outcomes 240–241
    patient positioning 230, 231*f*
    radial head arthroplasty 235, 236*f*
    radial head fixation 233–235, 234*f*
    terrible triad repair 235–240, 237*f*–240*f*
  and terrible triad injuries 224
Radial sensory nerve 71, 172
Radial shaft fractures 169*f*, 170 *See also* Forearm fractures
  fixation 175–176
    dorsal fixation 177–178
    Henry's volar approach 176–177, 177*f*
  surgical indications 172
Radiocarpal dislocations 61, 61*f*, 67, 133, 134*f*, 135*f*
Radiographs
  acetabulum fracture 554–555, 554*f*, 555*f*
  clavicle fractures 360, 360*f*
  distal humerus fractures 250, 250*f*, 251*f*
  distal radius fractures 129*f*, 130–131, 131*f*–133*f*
  femoral neck fractures 612, 613*f*
  forearm fractures 168–170, 169*f*
  humeral shaft fractures 278–279, 279*f*
  intertrochanteric femur/hip fractures 655
  metacarpal fractures 31–32, 32*f*
  olecranon fractures 193
  patellar fractures 767
  pelvic radiographic triad 496, 498*f*
  phalangeal fractures 2, 4*f*
  proximal humerus fractures 303, 304*f*, 305*f*
  scaphoid fractures 95, 96*f*
  thoracic and lumbar spine fractures 454–455, 454*f*, 454*t*, 457*f*, 458*f*, 460*f*
Radioscaphocapitate ligament (RSCL) 95, 100, 100*f*
Radioscapholunate (ligament of Testut) ligament 70, 70*f*
Radius 168, 168*f*
Rami fractures, pubic 507
Range of motion (ROM) 785
  elbow 224
  hip and knee 997
Reamer irrigator aspirator (RIA) 706, 722
Reaming, tibial shaft fracture 854, 855*f*, 866*f*
Reconstruction nails, subtrochanteric femur fractures 679
Rectus femoris, heads 621
Reflex sympathetic dystrophy 159
Rehabilitation
  extra-articular first-fifth metatarsal fractures 1005
  hallucal fracture-dislocations 1009
  Lisfranc fracture-dislocation 997–999, 1002–1003
  proximal fifth metatarsal fractures 1005
Retrograde intramedullary nail
  distal femur fractures 747–749, 747*f*
  femoral shaft fractures 720–723, 720f, 721*f*
  pearls and pitfalls 722, 749
RIA *see* Reamer irrigator aspirator (RIA)
Rockwood pin fixation, clavicle fractures 364*f*, 369, 370*f*
Rolando's fractures 34, 34*f* *see also* Metacarpal fractures
ROM *see* Range of motion (ROM)
Roof-arc measurements 557, 557*f*
RSCL *see* Radioscaphocapitate ligament (RSCL)
Russell-Taylor classification, of subtrochanteric femur fractures 674–675, 675*f*

S

SA *see* Shear angle (SA)
Sacral sparing 382
Sacrum, fractures of 499, 499*f* *see also* Pelvic ring and sacral injuries
Saline load test, patellar fractures 767
Sandwich sign 461
Scaphocapitate ligament (SCL) 100, 100*f*
Scaphoid fractures 54, 54*f*, 94–95
  anatomy related to 99–100, 99*f*, 100*f*

case study
nonunions without AVN 118–123, 121*f*–122*f*
proximal pole nonunions with AVN 113–114, 116–118, 117*f*–120*f*
stage III SNAC wrist 123–126, 124*f*–125*f*
classification 97–98, 98*t*
complications 95, 110
arthritis 111, 113, 113*f*, 113*t*
avascular necrosis 111, 112*f*
delayed union 81
malunion 83
nonunion of scaphoid 81–83, 82*f*
nonunions 110–111, 111*f*
osteoarthritis 83, 83*f*, 84*f*
criteria for displacement and instability 98*t*
diagnosis 95
bone scan 97
CT scan 97
MRI 96–97, 97*f*
pearls and pitfalls 97
physical examination 95, 95*f*
radiographic evaluation 95, 96*f*
displaced 65–67
distal pole 98
Herbert's classification 58–59, 58*f*
incidence 94
management 94–95, 98
headless compression screws 98–99
nonoperative treatment 98
ORIF 98
percutaneous fixation 98
nondisplaced 63–65, 64*f*, 65*f*, 66*f*
ORIF of 74
mini-open dorsal approach 76, 76*f*
open volar approach 74, 76
percutaneous volar technique 74, 75*f*
postoperative management 76
outcomes 80–81, 81*f*
proximal pole 101, 105
Russe's classification 59, 59*f*
surgical indications 63–67
surgical management
approaches to 101
dorsal ORIF 105, 106*f*, 107*f*
dorsal percutaneous fixation 107–110, 109*f*
outcomes 110
positioning 100–101
volar ORIF 101–104, 102*f*–104*f*
volar percutaneous fixation 105, 107, 108*f*
unstable 98, 101
Scaphoid nonunion advanced collapse (SNAC) 83, 83*f*, 84*f*, 111, 113, 113*f*
stages 113, 113*t*, 114*f*
surgical management 113, 115*f*–116*f*
Scapholunate interosseous ligament (SLIL) 99
Scapholunate ligament (SLL) 85, 133
Scapula and glenoid fractures 334–335
anatomy related to 340–341, 341*f*
case study
glenoid fossa malunion 355
scapular neck malunion 355–356
classification 335–339
complications 354
compartment syndrome 354
iatrogenic nerve injury 354
intrathoracic scapular impaction 355
malunion 354
and concomitant injuries 335
diagnosis 335
surgical management
anterior approach 341–343
indications for 339–340
outcomes 353–354
posterior approach 343–344
techniques for 345–353
Scapular body fractures 337
operative technique 345, 346*f*–347*f*
surgical indications 339
Scapular neck fractures 337
operative technique 345–346, 348, 349*f*–350*f*
surgical indications 340
Schanz screws 511
Schatzker classification, proximal tibia fractures 790–791, 790*f*
Sciatic nerve injury 603 *see also* Femoral head fractures and hip dislocations
Sciatic nerve palsy 573
SCL *see* Scaphocapitate ligament (SCL)
Screw fixation 265, 266*f*
metacarpal head fractures 38–39, 40*f*
olecranon fractures 199, 199*f*
scaphoid fractures 98–99
Seinsheimer's classification, of subtrochanteric femur fractures 673–674, 674*f*
Sensory index scoring 383
Serous fracture blister 896*f*
Shear angle (SA) 812
Short Musculoskeletal Functional Assessment (SMFA) scores 944
Short radiolunate (SRL) ligament 70, 70*f*
SIGN nail *see* Surgical Implant Generation Network (SIGN) nail
Skin tenting, distal tibia fractures 895*f*
SLL *see* Scapholunate ligament (SLL)
Sloppy lateral position 311, 312*f*, 316
SMFA scores *see* Short Musculoskeletal Functional Assessment (SMFA) scores
Smith-Peterson incision 593 *see also* Femoral head fractures and hip dislocations
SNAC *see* Scaphoid nonunion advanced collapse (SNAC)
Space available for cord (SAC) 389*t*
Space of Poirier 70
Spinal fractures *see* Cervical spine injuries
Spinal shock 382
Spine evaluation, in trauma patients 394
Canadian C-spine rules 394*f*
clinical clearance 394
conscious, symptomatic patients 394–395

SPN *see* Superficial peroneal nerve (SPN)
Steinmann pin 658
Sternoclavicular (SC) joint 360, 360*f*
Stiffness
  elbow 242, 267
  metacarpal fractures 50–51
  olecranon fractures 215
  phalangeal fractures 24, 26–27, 26*f*
Stimson gravity technique 587 *see also* Femoral head fractures and hip dislocations
Subaxial cervical fractures 401, 405–406 *see also* Cervical spine injuries
  compressive extension injuries 411–413, 413*f*
  compressive flexion injuries 407–408, 408*f*
  distractive extension injuries 414–415, 414*f*, 415*f*
  distractive flexion injury 408–411, 409*f*–412*f*
  lateral extension injuries 415–416, 416*f*
  vertical compression injuries 406–407, 406*f*, 407*f*
Subscapularis split technique 342–343
Subscapularis tenotomy technique 343
Subtalar fusion, talus fractures 975–976
Subtalar joint, Brodén's views 967*f*
Subtrochanteric femur fractures 672–673
  case study
    intertrochanteric femur fracture 698–701, 699*f*, 700*f*
    pertrochanteric femur fracture 701, 702*f*, 703*f*
    proximal femur locking plate 703–706, 704*f*, 705*f*
  classification
    AO/OTA 675, 676*f*
    Russell-Taylor 674–675, 675*f*
    Seinsheimer's 673–674, 674*f*
  complications and management
    DVT 695
    loss of fixation and malunion 695–696, 696*f*
    malrotation 697–698
    nonunion 696–697
  diagnosis
    bone scan 673
    CT scan 673
    diagnostic imaging 673
    MRI 673
    pearls and pitfalls 673
    physical examination 673
  occurrence 673
  outcomes 694–695
  surgical management 678–679
    anatomy 677, 678*f*
    95° angled plates 679
    blade plate 691–694, 692*f*, 693*f*
    CAS 683
    cephalomedullary nailing 684–689, 685*f*–688*f*
    clinical assessment 683
    CT scan 683, 683*f*
    definitive fixation 677
    fluoroscopic measurement 680
    intramedullary nails 679
    intraoperative assessment 683–684
    lesser trochanteric profile 680–681
    positioning 677–678
    postoperative protocol 694
    preoperative planning 679–680
    proximal femoral locking plate 679, 689–691, 690*f*
    reconstruction nails 679
    reduction technique 680, 681*f*, 682*f*
    temporizing measures 675–677
    trochanteric nails 679
Superficial peroneal nerve (SPN) 934
Supra-acetabular pin 501, 502*f*, 506*f*, 507*f* *see also* Pelvic ring and sacral injuries
Supraclavicular nerves 365, 365*f*
Supracondylar femur fractures 737
Suprascapular nerve, injury to 354
Surgical Implant Generation Network (SIGN) nail 850
Suture placement, proximal humerus fractures 324, 325*f*
Swimmer's view 389, 391*f*, 393*f*
Syndesmotic injury, ankle
  anatomy 934–935
  cotton test 932*f*, 938, 940
  late 946
  occult, diagnosis 929*f*
  open reduction and internal fixation 942–944
    preoperative planning 942–943
    technique 943–944
  repair 943*f*
Synostosis, forearm fractures 186, 187*f*, 188–190, 189*f*, 190*f*

T

TAD *see* Tip-apex distance (TAD)
Talar neck fractures *see also* Talus fractures
  anterolateral approach 971–972
  anteromedial approach 970–971
  Bohler's incision 971*f*
  Hawkins classification 967–968, 968*f*
  medial vascular structures 970*f*
  ORIF comminuted, displaced 973*f*–974*f*
  treatment 969
Talus fractures 966–981 *see also* Calcaneus fractures
  arthritis 975–977
  avascular necrosis 972–975
  chronic infection management 977
  classification 967–968
  malunion 975
  subtalar fusion 975–976
  surgery
    anatomy 969–970
    positioning 970
  tibiotalocalcaneal fusion 976–977
Tarsometatarsal (TMT) joints 983–984
  first-third 1001*f*, 1002*f*
  incongruity 987–988

irreparable cartilage 1001
midfoot fusion 991
Taylor Spatial Frame 758
Tension band technique, in patellar fractures *see also* Patellar fractures
closure 773
fracture reduction techniques 771–773, 772*f*–775*f*
instrumentation and implant consideration 771
pearls and pitfalls 773
rehabilitation 773
surgical approach 771
Terrible triad injuries 224, 226*f*, 227 *see also* Radial head fractures
Terry Thomas sign 55, 57*f*
Tetraplegia 386
TFCC *see* Triangular fibrocartilage complex (TFCC)
Thomas and Epstein classification 585, 587*t* *see also* Femoral head fractures and hip dislocations
Thompson approach, forearm fractures 173, 174*f*
Thompson quadricepsplasty 757
Thoracic and lumbar spine fractures 447–448
burst fracture 448*f*
burst fractures 457–459, 458*f*, 459*f*
case study
failure to recognize fracture patterns 488–489
implant failure 488
missed systemic injury 489, 490*f*
post-traumatic kyphosis 485–487, 486*f*, 487*f*
Chance fracture. 461*f*
classification 448
Allen-Ferguson 450
AO 451–452, 451*f*
Boehler's 448
column concept 449
Denis 449–450, 449*f*
load sharing 452
McAfee's 450–451, 450*f*
TLICS 452, 452*f*, 453*f*
complications
anterior approach 484–485
chronic 485
posterior approach 483–484
compression fractures 455–457, 457*f*
diagnosis 453
CT scans 455, 455*f*, 458*f*, 459, 461*f*
MRI 455, 456*f*, 459–460
radiographic evaluation 454–455, 454*f*, 454*t*, 457*f*, 458*f*, 460*f*
flexion distraction injury 448*f*, 459–461, 459*t*, 460*f*, 463–464
fracture dislocation 448*f*, 462, 464*f*
surgical management
anterior decompression and fixation 471–476, 474*f*, 475*f*
indications for 462–465
kyphoplasty 468, 469*f*, 470*f*
outcomes 481–483
percutaneous pedicle screw fixation 468–471, 470*f*, 471
percutaneous stabilization 466–471
percutaneous vertebroplasty (VP) 465–468, 465*f*, 466*f*, 467*f*
posterior decompression and fixation 476–481, 477*f*–480*f*
unstable thoracolumbar injuries 459–462, 460*f*, 461*f*
wedge compression fractures 448*f*
Thoracic outlet syndrome 360, 374
Thoracolumbar fractures 448 *see also* Thoracic and lumbar spine fractures
concept of instability 442–453
Thoracolumbar injury classification system (TLICS) 449, 452, 452*f*, 453*f*
Thoracolumbar junction 448
Thoracolumbar sacral orthosis (TLSO) 462
Thumb epibasal fractures 34, 34*f* *see also* Metacarpal fractures
Tibia 845
anteromedial aspect 848
nonunion of 871
aseptic, atrophic, treatment 882–883, 884*f*–85*f*
established infected, treatment 876–880, 887*f*–879*f*
hypertrophic, treatment 883–886, 886*f*
Tibial bone loss, acute
massive autogenous bone grafting 886–887, 888*f*–890*f*
Tibial shaft fractures 845–893
classification 846–848
AO-OTA 846–847
Gustilo and Anderson 847
Tscherne 847–848
compartment syndrome 846, 872
treatment of 887–893, 891*f*–892*f*
complications 871–872
infection 871
malalignment and malunion 871–872
management 872–893
nonunion of tibia 871
crush injury 846
diagnostic imaging techniques 846
guidewire placement 854, 855*f*
instrumentation and implant 849–850
intramedullary nailing 849–871
acute infection treatment 873*f*–875*f*
patient assessment 850
portal preparation 852*f*
preoperative planning 849–850
reamed, locked 849–858
technique 850–858
ORIF 868*f*
outcomes, treatment 871
overview 845–846
physical examination 846
positioning 848
proximal 858–863
proximal interlocking 854
surgery 848–871
anatomy 848–849
techniques 849–871
traction 848–849

Tibiotalocalcaneal (TTC) fusion
calcaneus fractures 966
talus fractures 976–977
Tip-apex distance (TAD) 659
TMT arthritis, surgical approach 992–993
TMT joints *see* Tarsometatarsal (TMT) joints
Total hip arthroplasty 642
Traction pin placement
femoral shaft fractures 723
pearls and pitfalls 723
Traction, tibial shaft fractures 848–849
Transarticular plate fixation
lateral clavicle 364*f*, 369, 371*f*
Trans-flexor carpi radialis (trans-FCR) approach, volar distal radius 146–148, 147*f*
Transiliac-transsacral screws 535–536, 536*f*–538*f*
Translational injuries, spine 451
Transolecranon fracture-dislocations 193
Transverse dislocations 61, 68–69, 68*f*
Trapezial fractures 59 *see also* Carpal fractures and perilunate dislocations
Traumatic spondylolisthesis of C2 *see* Hangman's fracture
Triangular fibrocartilage complex (TFCC) 133, 181
Triceps-sparing approach, distal humerus 256, 256*f*
Tricortical iliac crest 976
Triquetral fractures 59, 59*f*, 60*f*, 67 *see also* Carpal fractures and perilunate dislocations
Trochanteric flip osteotomy 598–600, 599*f*
Trochanteric nails 662
subtrochanteric femur fractures 679
Tscherne classification
soft tissue injury, closed fractures 897*f*
tibial shaft fractures 847–848
TTC fusion *see* Tibiotalocalcaneal (TTC) fusion

U

Ulna 168, 168*f*
Ulnar nerve 71, 172, 173, 201, 232
Ulnar neuropathy
distal humerus fractures 268
olecranon fractures 217
Ulnar shaft fractures 169*f*, 170 *see also* Forearm fractures
fixation 173–175, 173*f*, 175*f*, 176*f*
isolated 170
surgical indications 171
Ulnocarpal ligaments 70, 70*f*
Ulnohumeral joint 229
Ultrasound, phalangeal fractures 2
Unicondylar fractures 751–753 *see also* Distal femur fractures
pearls and pitfalls 753

V

Varencline 835
Vascularized bone graft (VBG) 101, 111, 113–114, 118, 118*f*
Vertebroplasty 465–468, 465*f*, 466*f*, 467*f*
Volar intercalated segment instability (VISI) 85
Volar locking plates 142, 142*f*, 161
Volar plate arthroplasty 19, 19*f*
Volar plate fixation
distal radius fractures 141*f*, 142, 142*f*, 145*f*, 154–157, 155*f*, 156*f*, 159
and malpositioning of screws 159–162, 160*f*, 161*f*

W

Wackenheim line 389*t*, 393*f*
Watson-Jones anterolateral approach 642
Watson-Jones incision 593 *see also* Femoral head fractures and hip dislocations
WBC *see* White blood cell (WBC)
Weber clamp application, anterior pelvic fixation 511, 512*f*
Wedge compression fractures 407–408, 448*f*, 450, 455–457, 457*f* *see also* Thoracic and lumbar spine fractures
diagnosis 455, 457, 457*f*
surgical management 462
Well-leg compartment syndrome 625
White blood cell (WBC) 831
Winquist-Hansen classification, femoral shaft fractures 710, 711*f*
Wounds
breakdown, ankle fractures 945
midfoot and forefoot fractures 1012

X

X-rays *see also* Radiographs
distal femur fractures 738, 739*f*
femoral head fractures and hip dislocations 582